D1377247

To view the website, please go to: http://www.compgyn.com

Please enter the following passcode when prompted:

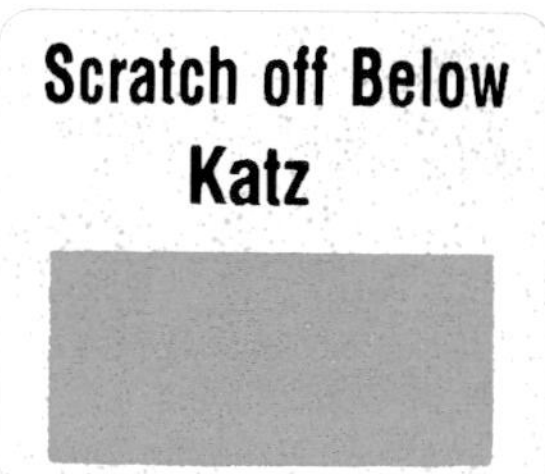

THIS PASSCODE WILL BE USED TO CREATE A USERNAME THE FIRST TIME YOU ENTER THE WEBSITE

Technical Support

For technical problems with the use of this site, please contact our specialist support operators at:

- Tel: 800-401-9962 (inside the United States)
- +1-314-995-3200 (outside the United States)
- Monday – Friday, 7:30 AM - 7:00 PM CT
- Fax: +1-314-997-5080

Comprehensive Gynecology

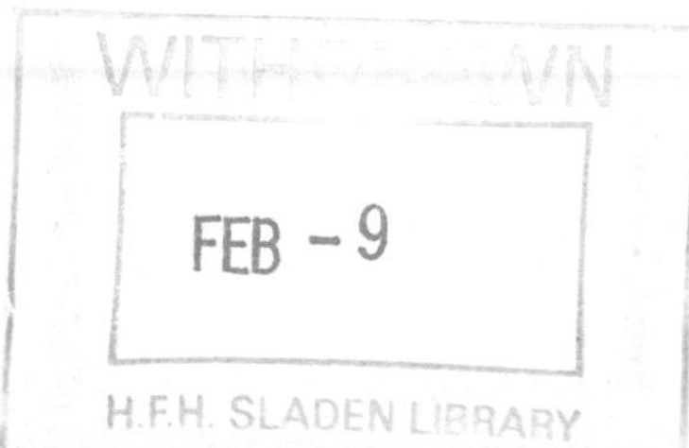

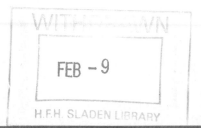

5th Edition

Comprehensive Gynecology

Vern L. Katz, MD
Clinical Professor
Department of Obstetrics and Gynecology
Oregon Health Sciences University
Portland, Oregon
Adjunct Professor
Department of Human Physiology
University of Oregon
Director of Perinatal Services
Sacred Heart Medical Center
Eugene, Oregon

Gretchen M. Lentz, MD
Associate Professor and Director, Women's Health
Adjunct Associate Professor of Urology
University of Washington
Seattle, Washington

Rogerio A. Lobo, MD
Professor and Chair of Obstetrics and Gynecology
Columbia University School of Medicine
New York, New York

David M. Gershenson, MD
Professor and Chairman, Gynecologic Oncology
The University of Texas M.D. Anderson Cancer Center
Houston, Texas

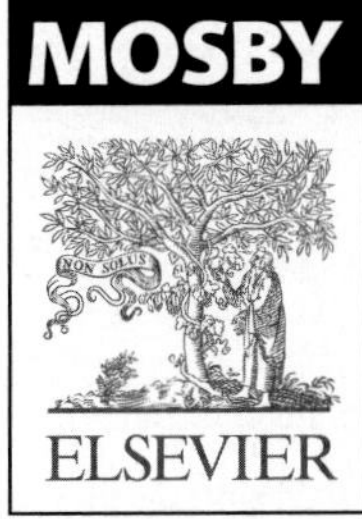

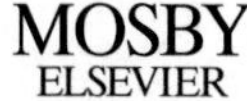

MOSBY
ELSEVIER

1600 John F. Kennedy Boulevard
Suite 1800
Philadelphia, PA 19103-2899

COMPREHENSIVE GYNECOLOGY FIFTH EDITION ISBN 978-0-323-02951-3

Notice

Knowledge and best practice in this field are constantly changing. As new research and experience broaden our knowledge, changes in practice, treatment and drug therapy may become necessary or appropriate. Readers are advised to check the most current information provided (i) on procedures featured or (ii) by the manufacturer of each product to be administered, to verify the recommended dose or formula, the method and duration of administration, and contraindications. It is the responsibility of the practitioner, relying on their own experience and knowledge of the patient, to make diagnoses, to determine dosages and the best treatment for each individual patient, and to take all appropriate safety precautions. To the fullest extent of the law, neither the Publisher nor the Editors assume any liability for any injury and/or damage to persons or property arising out or related to any use of the material contained in this book.

Previous editions copyrighted 2001, 1997, 1992, 1987.

Library of Congress Cataloging-in-Publication Data
Comprehensive gynecology/Vern L. Katz... [et al.]–5th ed.
p.; cm.
Includes bibliographical references and index.
ISBN 978-0-323-02951-3
1. Gynecology. I. Katz, Vern L.
[DNLM: 1. Genital Diseases, Female. 2. Genital Neoplasms, Female. WP 140 C737 2007]
RG101.C726 2007
618.1–dc22

2006050720

Acquisitions Editor: Rebecca Schmidt Gaertner
Developmental Editor: Deidre Simpson
Project Manager: David Saltzberg
Design Direction: Lou Forgione

Printed in China

Last digit is the print number: 9 8 7 6 5 4 3 2 1

Contributors

Diane C. Bodurka, MD
Associate Professor
Department of Gynecologic Oncology
The University of Texas M.D. Anderson Cancer Center
Houston, Texas

Fillmore Buckner, MD, JD
Clinical Professor Emeritus of Obstetrics and Gynecology
University of Washington School of Medicine
Seattle, Washington
Past President
American College of Legal Medicine
Schaumberg, Illinois

Edith Cheng, MD, MS
Associate Professor
Director, Prenatal Diagnosis
Department of Obstetrics and Gynecology
Adjunct Associate Professor, Medical Genetics
Department of Internal Medicine
University of Washington
Seattle, Washington

Robert L. Coleman, MD
Professor and Director of Clinical Research
Department of Gynecologic Oncology
The University of Texas M.D. Anderson Cancer Center
Houston, Texas

Ann Jeannette Davis, MD
Professor
Department of Obstetrics and Gynecology
Dartmouth University School of Medicine
Hanover, New Hampshire

Deborah Jean Dotters, MD
Director, Gynecologic Oncology
Northwest Gynecologic Oncology
Eugene, Oregon

Linda O. Eckert, MD
Associate Professor of Obstetrics and Gynecology
University of Washington
Seattle, Washington

Michael Frumovitz, MD, MPH
Department of Gynecologic Oncology
The University of Texas M.D. Anderson Cancer Center
Houston, Texas

David M. Gershenson, MD
Professor and Chairman, Gynecologic Oncology
The University of Texas M.D. Anderson Cancer Center
Houston, Texas

Anuja Jhingran, MD
Associate Professor
Radiation Oncology
The University of Texas M.D. Anderson Cancer Center
Houston, Texas

Vern L. Katz, MD
Clinical Professor
Department of Obstetrics and Gynecology
Oregon Health Sciences University
Portland, Oregon
Adjunct Professor
Department of Human Physiology
University of Oregon
Director of Perinatal Services
Sacred Heart Medical Center
Eugene, Oregon

John J. Kavanagh, MD
Department of Gynecologic Oncology
The University of Texas M.D. Anderson Cancer Center
Houston, Texas

Charles Kunos, MD, PhD
Assistant Professor
Department of Radiation Oncology
University Hospitals Case Medical Center
Case Comprehensive Cancer Center
Cleveland, Ohio

Gretchen M. Lentz, MD
Associate Professor and Director, Women's Health
Adjunct Associate Professor of Urology
University of Washington
Seattle, Washington

Charles Levenback, MD
Professor and Deputy Chairman
Department of Gynecologic Oncology
The University of Texas M.D. Anderson Cancer Center
Houston, Texas

Rogerio A. Lobo, MD
Professor and Chair of Obstetrics and Gynecology
Columbia University School of Medicine
New York, New York

Karen Lu, MD
Associate Professor
Department of Gynecologic Oncology
The University of Texas M.D. Anderson Cancer Center
Houston, Texas

Daniel R. Mishell, Jr., MD
The Lyle G. McNeile Professor and Chairman
Department of Obstetrics and Gynecology
Keck School of Medicine
University of Southern California
Los Angeles, California

Kenneth L. Noller, MD, MS
Louis E. Phaneuf Professor and Chair
Department of Obstetrics and Gynecology
Tufts University School of Medicine
Boston, Massachusetts

Brian M. Slomovitz, MD
Assistant Professor
Department of Obstetrics and Gynecology
Weill Medical College of Cornell University
Assistant Professor
Department of Obstetrics and Gynecology
New York Presbyterian Hospital
New York, New York

Fidel A.Valea, MD
Professor
Department of Gynecologic Oncology
Duke University School of Medicine
Durham, North Carolina

Steven E. Waggoner, MD
Professor, Obstetrics and Gynecology
University Hospitals of Cleveland
MacDonald Women's Hospital
Cleveland, Ohio

S. Diane Yamada, MD
Associate Professor
Chief, Section of Gynecologic Oncology
Department of Obstetrics and Gynecology
University of Chicago Medical Center
Chicago, Illinois

Preface

"Medicine is not only a science; it is an art. It does not consist of compounding pills and plasters; it deals with the very processes of life, which must be understood before they may be guided."

Paracelsus

The improvement of women's health is our privilege and responsibility as gynecologists. More than 20 years ago, the original four editors created *Comprehensive Gynecology* as part of that goal. In this fifth edition, the creators have passed this task on. All generations in medicine see their mentors and teachers as giants. Drs. Droegemueller, Herbst, Mishell, and Stenchever are giants. Their efforts, dedication, and achievements for women's health, for education, and for the advancement of knowledge are overwhelming and will last for decades. They have affected tens of thousands of physicians worldwide. We cannot thank them enough.

In this fifth edition, we have updated the principles and theories of gynecologic physiology and disease. New management options are discussed, and outdated treatment protocols are revised. Recent research necessitated major changes in the menopause and genetics chapters, and the DES chapter was folded into the chapters on miscarriage and vaginal neoplasia. New topics, such as legal considerations, in our field have necessitated new chapters. The sections on adenomyosis have been updated and included in the chapter on benign disease. New treatments for ectopic pregnancy, miscarriage, malignancy, and urologic problems have been emphasized. Importantly, we continue to emphasize evidence-based medicine in reviewing literature.

Because we learn from the past, many aspects of older hypotheses and treatment strategies are noted for newer physicians and students to appreciate. For these younger physicians and for more seasoned clinicians we have recommendations for using this text. Always remember that our understanding of medicine changes rapidly, particularly with the expanding knowledge of genetics, molecular biology, and imaging. The accepted dogmas of today will be but historical footnotes next year. Thus, we all must continue to learn and revise our knowledge and understanding of our art.

Vern L. Katz
Gretchen M. Lentz
Rogerio A. Lobo
David M. Gershenson

Acknowledgments

The editors of this edition wish to acknowledge a few of the many scientists, clinicians, and mentors who have contributed to past editions on which we have built and also to this edition. Drs. William Droegemueller, Arthur L. Herbst, Daniel R. Mishell, Jr., and Morton A. Stenchever top the list. In addition, thanks to Marta Abrams, Jan Hammanishi, Phillip Patton, and Carolyn Westoff.

We also wish to express our deepest thanks and love to our families, who have lent incredible support and encouragement during the long hours of work on this edition.

Contents

PART I
BASIC SCIENCE

PART II
COMPREHENSIVE EVALUATION OF THE FEMALE

PART III
GENERAL GYNECOLOGY

PART I

BASIC SCIENCE

Fertilization and Embryogenesis 1

Meiosis, Fertilization, Implantation, Embryonic Development, Sexual Differentiation

Edith Cheng and Vern L. Katz

KEY TERMS AND DEFINITIONS

Acrosome Reaction. The process by which the cap over the head of the sperm, the acrosome, is removed to expose the portion of the sperm head containing the hydrolytic enzymes, which makes it possible for the sperm to penetrate the cells and structures investing the egg. This process is involved in capacitation but is not necessarily the same response as capacitation.

Anlage. The cell mass that gives rise to a specific organ or structure. Also called the primordium.

Bivalent. Paired homologous chromosomes seen at metaphase of the first meiotic division.

Blastocyst. The stage of the conceptus that follows the morula stage. It consists of a fluid-filled cavity surrounded by trophoblasts with embryonic cells at one pole.

Blastula. The stage of embryonic development that follows the morula stage. At this stage a cyst (blastocyst) forms within the cell mass, and early differentiation begins.

Capacitation. The morphologic, physiologic, and biochemical changes that a sperm goes through to be capable of penetrating the cumulus oophorus, corona radiata, and zona pellucida of the egg. It involves the sequentially timed release of a series of hydrolytic enzymes, which allows the sperm to digest a passage through the aforementioned structures.

Chemotaxis. The attraction of the sperm to the ova.

Chemokinesis. The stimulation of sperm motility.

Chiasmata. Points of attachment of homologous chromosomes during meiosis, where the exchange of genetic material occurs.

Cleavage. The first cell division of the fertilized ovum (zygote).

Conceptional Age. The age of the conceptus from the time of fertilization.

Conceptus. The fertilized oocyte and its derivatives at all stages of development from fertilization until birth and including all extraembryonic membranes.

Cumulus Oophorus. The cell mass that invests the egg. It is a remnant of the primitive sex cords of the embryonic ovary.

Embryo. The developmental stage of the conceptus after the development of the primitive streak and until all major organs are developed. In the human, it begins at about conceptional day 14 and ends when organ development is complete. The definition of the end of the embryonic period is not entirely agreed upon by authorities but is probably between postconceptional days 36 and 49.

Fertilization. The point at which one spermatozoon penetrates the oocyte. This is the stage before the pronuclei are formed.

Gartner Duct. Remnants of the mesonephric (wolffian) duct system often found in the broad ligament and beside the uterus, cervix, and vagina of the adult woman.

Gestational Age. The stage of the embryo counting from the first day of the last menstrual period. On average, it is about 2 weeks longer than conceptional age, assuming a 28-day menstrual cycle.

Implantation. The process by which the early embryo burrows within the endometrial lining of the uterus.

Mesonephros. The mesodermal anlage of the male sexual duct system.

Metanephros. The anlage of the adult kidney.

Morula. A ball of cells composing the early embryo that produces both the embryo and the placenta and membranes. Each cell is totipotential.

Oogenesis. The development of the oocyte from an oogonium by meiosis.

Paramesonephric (Müllerian) Duct. The anlage of the female sex duct system that gives rise to the fallopian tube, uterus, and cervix in the adult woman.

Polar Body. The daughter cell produced during oogenesis at first and second meiotic division (first and second polar body); it contains a nucleus and minimal cytoplasm. For each polar body the nuclear material is similar to the nucleus of the ovum at the same stage.

Primordium. An early embryonic structure that further differentiates into an adult structure.

Sister Chromatid Exchange. The exchange of chromosomal material between

KEY TERMS AND DEFINITIONS *Continued*

the identical arms of a chromosome; the arms are separated except at the centromere and at the sites of exchanges.

Spermatogenesis. The development of mature sperm from spermatogonia by meiosis.

Synapsis. The pairing process that brings together homologous chromosomes of maternal and paternal origin during meiosis.

Syngamy. The active union of the sperm and the egg to form a zygote.

Teratogen. An endogenous or exogenous substance that causes the formation of an anomaly.

Teratogenesis. The process of developing an anomaly of an organ or organs.

Zona Pellucida. The translucent belt consisting of a noncellular layer of mucopolysaccharide that is deposited at the periphery of the ovum while it is in the ovary and continues to surround the egg, the conceptus, and the morula until the stage of implantation.

Zygote. The one-cell stage of the fertilized ovum after pronuclear membrane breakdown but before first cleavage occurs.

Several areas of medical investigation have brought increased attention to the processes of fertilization and embryonic development, including teratology, stem cell research, immunogenetics, and assisted reproductive technology. The preimplantation, implantation, and embryonic stages of development in the human can now be studied because of the development of newer techniques and areas of research. This chapter considers the processes of oocyte meiosis, fertilization and early cleavage, implantation, development of the genitourinary system, and sex differentiation. Chapter 2 (Reproductive Genetics) continues with a discussion of closely related issues of genetics.

THE OOCYTE AND MEIOSIS

The oocyte is a unique and extremely specialized cell. Initially, during the process of oocyte meiosis, the genetic variability of the species is ensured. Later, the oocyte develops the ability to facilitate fertilization and to provide the energy system to support early embryonic development.

The primordial germ cells in both males and females are large eosinophilic cells derived from endoderm in the wall of the yolk sac. These cells migrate to the germinal ridge by way of the dorsal mesentery of the hindgut by ameboid action by 6 weeks. In the human female, oogenesis begins with the multiplication of the diploid oogonia through multiple rounds of mitosis to produce primary oocytes, reaching a peak number of 6 to 7 million during the first 10 to 12 weeks of gestation. The numbers then rapidly decline to 2 to 4 million by birth, and at menarche, only about 400,000 remain in the ovary.

The meiotic process begins as mitosis is ending in the fetal ovary. Oocytes in the early stage (prophase) of meiosis may be seen at 10 to 12 weeks' gestation. Meiosis is the mechanism by which diploid organisms reduce their gametes to a haploid state so that they can recombine again during fertilization to become diploid organisms. In humans, this process reduces 46 chromosomes (or 23 pairs) to 23 chromosome structures in the gamete. The haploid gamete contains only one chromosome for each homologous pair of chromosomes, so that it has either the maternal or paternal chromosome for each pair, but not both. Meiosis is also the mechanism by which genetic exchange is completed through chiasma formation and crossing over between homologous chromosome pairs. In humans, all of this is completed during fetal life of the yet to be born female.

Two meiotic cell divisions are required to produce haploid gametes. The first, known as the reduction division, division I, or meiosis I, is complicated, and in the human female occurs over a time span from fetal life to menarche. Of the five stages, prophase I lasts the longest, occurs exclusively during fetal life, and sets the stage for genetic exchange that ensures genetic variation in our species.

The oocytes complete prophase before entering a quiescent period. Reentry into meiosis is signaled by the endocrine changes of puberty. In the mature cycle, usually one oocyte each month will complete meiosis I as a function of ovulation and meiosis II if fertilization occurs. Thus it is in fetal life that the ovary makes all of the oocytes that the adult women will have for reproduction.

In the human female, oogonia enter meiosis in "waves" (Fig. 1-1), that is, not all oogonia enter meiosis at the same time. The initiating signal or signals are unknown, but cytologic evidence suggests that oocytes represent the first substage of prophase, leptotene, in the human fetal ovary as early as 10 weeks' gestation. With increasing gestational age, greater proportions of oocytes in later stages of meiosis may be observed, and by the end of the second trimester of pregnancy, the majority of oocytes in the fetal ovary have cytologic characteristics that are consistent with the diplotene/dictyotene substages of prophase I of meiosis I (the stage at which the oocytes are arrested until ovulation) (Fig. 1-2).

The structural characteristics of the chromosomes in prophase of meiosis I in human oogenesis are seen in Figure 1-3. Interphase I has not yet been observed in the fetal ovary cytologically. It is a time when DNA replication takes place, thus transforming the diploid oogonia with a DNA content of $2N$ to an oocyte with a DNA content of $4N$. Each chromosome is duplicated, and the identical copies, called sister chromatids, of each chromosome are tightly held together along their length. Leptotene is proportionately the most abundant of all the prophase I substages in the early gestations. Cells in this meiotic phase are characterized by a large nucleus with fine, diffuse, stringlike chromatin evenly distributed within the nucleus. Chromatin of homologous pairs occupies "domains" and does not occur as distinct linear strands of chromosomes. By this stage each chromosome has replicated, and the DNA content is now $4N$. The zygotene substage (Fig. 1-3A) is defined by the initiation of pairing, which is characterized by the striking appearance of the synaptonemal complex formation in some of the chromosomes (Fig. 1-3B).

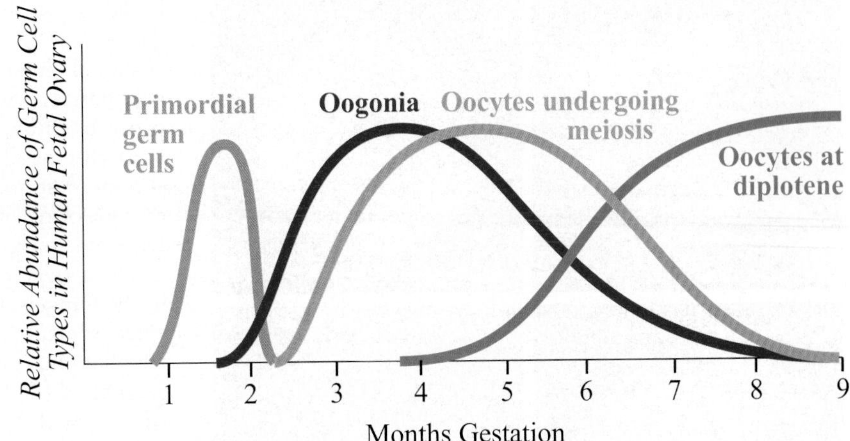

Figure 1-1. Diagrammatic representation of the different meiotic cell types and their proportions in the ovary during fetal life. (Courtesy of Edith Cheng, MD.)

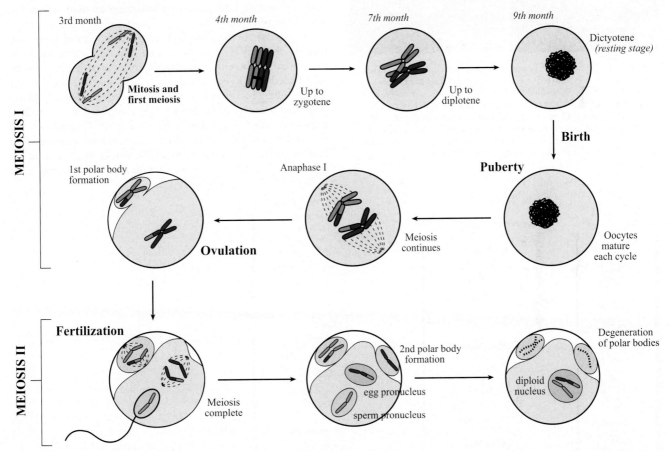

Figure 1-2. Diagram of oocyte meiosis. For simplicity, only one pair of chromosomes is depicted. Prophase stages of the first meiotic division occur in the female during fetal life. The meiotic process is arrested at the diplotene stage ("first meiotic arrest"), and the oocyte enters the dictyotene stages. Meiosis I resumes at puberty and is completed at the time of ovulation. The second meiotic division take place over several hours in the oviduct only after sperm penetration. (Courtesy of Edith Cheng, MD.)

There is cytologic evidence of chromosome condensation and linearization, and the chromatin is seen as a fine, stringlike structure. The pachytene substage is the most easily recognizable period of the prophase and is characterized by clearly defined chromosomes that appear as continuous ribbons of thick beadlike chromatin. By definition, this is the substage in which all homologs have paired. In this substage, the paired homologs are structurally composed of four closely opposed chromatids and is known as a tetrad. The frequency of oocytes in pachytene increases with gestational age and peaks in the mid second trimester of pregnancy (about 20–25 weeks' gestation). The diplotene substage is a stage of desynapsis that occurs as the synpatonemal complex dissolves and the two homologous chromosomes pull away from each other. However, these

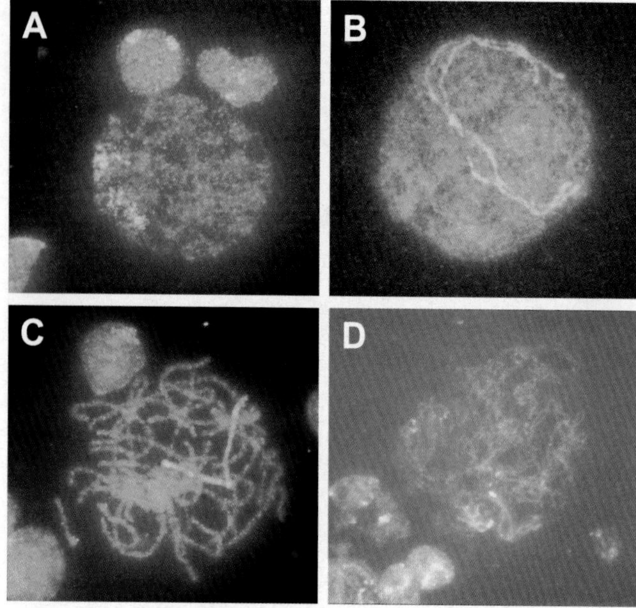

Figure 1-3. Fetal ovary with fluorescent in-situ hybridization. The first three images are meiotic cells from a 21-week fetal ovary. **A,** Fluorescent in situ hybridization (FISH) with a whole chromosome probe for chromosome X was completed to visualize the pairing characteristics of the X chromosome during leptotene. **B,** Zygotene. **C,** Pachytene. **D,** Image of a meiotic cell from a 34-week fetal ovary that underwent dual FISH with probes for chromosomes 13 (*green signal*) and 21 (*red signal*) to illustrate the pairing characteristics of this substage of prophase in meiosis I. (Courtesy of Edith Cheng, MD.)

bivalents, which are composed of a maternally and a paternally derived chromosome, are held together at the centromere and at sites of chiasma formation that represent sites where crossing over has occurred. In general, chiasma formation occurs only between chromatids of homologous pairs and not between sister chromatids. Usually, one to three chiasma occur for each chromosome arm. Oocytes at this stage of prophase I constitute the majority of third-trimester fetal and newborn ovaries. Diplotene merges with diakinesis, the last substage of meiosis I, and is a stage of transition to metaphase, lasting many years in the humans. Oocytes are arrested at this stage until puberty, when sometime before ovulation, metaphase, anaphase, and telophase are completed. The result is two daughter cells, which are diploid (2*N*) in DNA content, but contain 23 chromosome structures, each containing two closely held sister chromatids. One daughter cell, the oocyte, receives the majority of the cytoplasm, and the other becomes the first polar body when ovulation occurs. Both the oocyte and the polar body are present within the zona pellucida.

In contrast to the long and complex process of meiosis I, meiosis II is rapid, and the oocyte advances immediately to metaphase II where the sister chromatids for each chromosome are aligned at the equatorial plate, held together and on the spindle fibers by the centromere of the chromosome. If sperm penetration occurs, then meiosis II is completed in the oviduct with union of the sperm and oocyte nucleus, and extrusion of the first and second polar bodies. In the male, meiosis generates four haploid gametes of equal reproductive potential, whereas in the female, only one oocyte is generated for reproduction (Fig. 1-4).

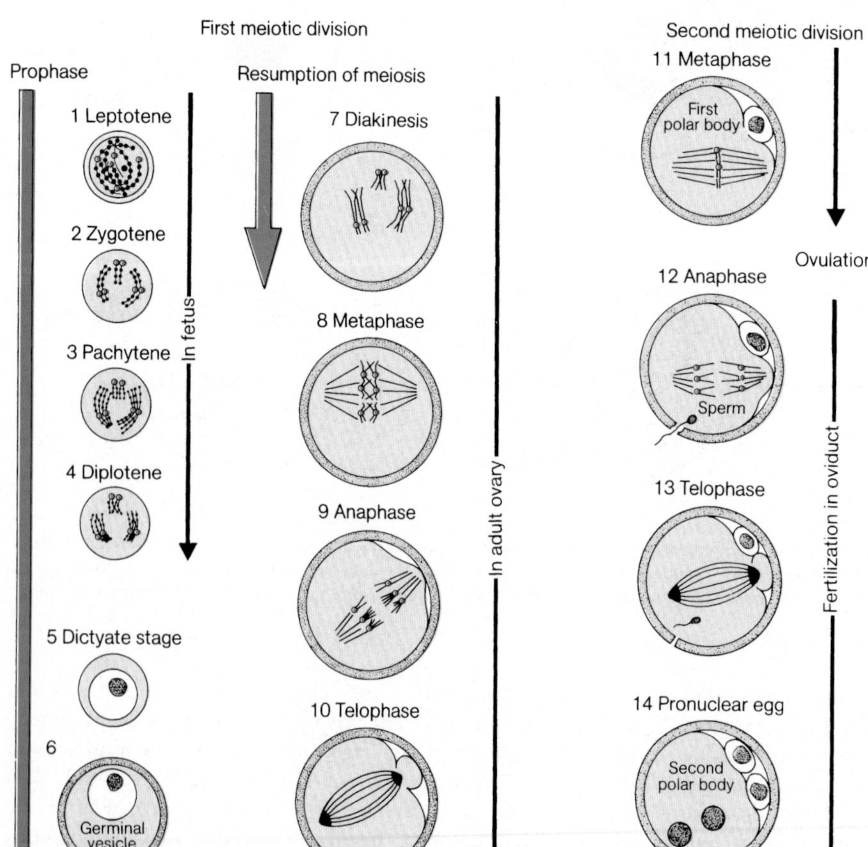

Figure 1-4. Diagram of oocyte meiosis. For simplicity, only three pairs of chromosomes are depicted (1–4). Prophase stages of the first meiotic division, which occurs in most mammals during fetal life. The meiotic process is arrested at the diplotene stage ("first meiotic arrest"), and the oocyte enters the dictyate stages (5–6). When meiosis is resumed, the first maturation division is completed (7–11). Ovulation occurs usually at the metaphase II stage (11), and the second meiotic division (12–14) takes place in the oviduct only after sperm penetration. (From Tsafriri A: Oocyte maturation in mammals. In Jones RE (ed): The Vertebrate Ovary. New York, Plenum, 1978. With kind permission of Springer Science and Business Media.)

FERTILIZATION AND EARLY CLEAVAGE

In most mammals, including humans, the egg is released from the ovary in the metaphase II stage (Fig. 1-5). When the egg enters the fallopian tube, it is surrounded by a cumulus of granulosa cells (cumulus oophorus) and intimately surrounded by a clear zona pellucida. Within the zona pellucida are both the egg and the first polar body. Meanwhile, spermatozoa are transported through the cervical mucus and the uterus and into the fallopian tubes. During this transport period the sperm undergo two changes: capacitation and acrosome reaction. These changes activate enzyme systems within the sperm head and make it possible for the sperm to transgress the cumulus oophorus and the zona pellucida (Fig. 1-6).

The sperm are attracted to an egg through the process known as chemotaxis, which is related to capacitation of the sperm. The process is aided by the binding of progesterone to a surface receptor on the sperm. This allows an increase in intracellular calcium ion concentration, which increases sperm motility (chemokinesis). Once the sperm has passed the barrier of the zona pellucida, it attaches to the cell membrane of the egg and enters the cytoplasm. When the sperm enters the cytoplasm, intracytoplasmic structures, the coronal granules, arrange themselves in an orderly fashion around the outermost portion of the cytoplasm just beneath the cytoplasmic membrane, and the sperm head swells and gives rise to the male pronucleus. The egg completes its second meiotic division, casting off the second polar body to a position also beneath the zona pellucida. The

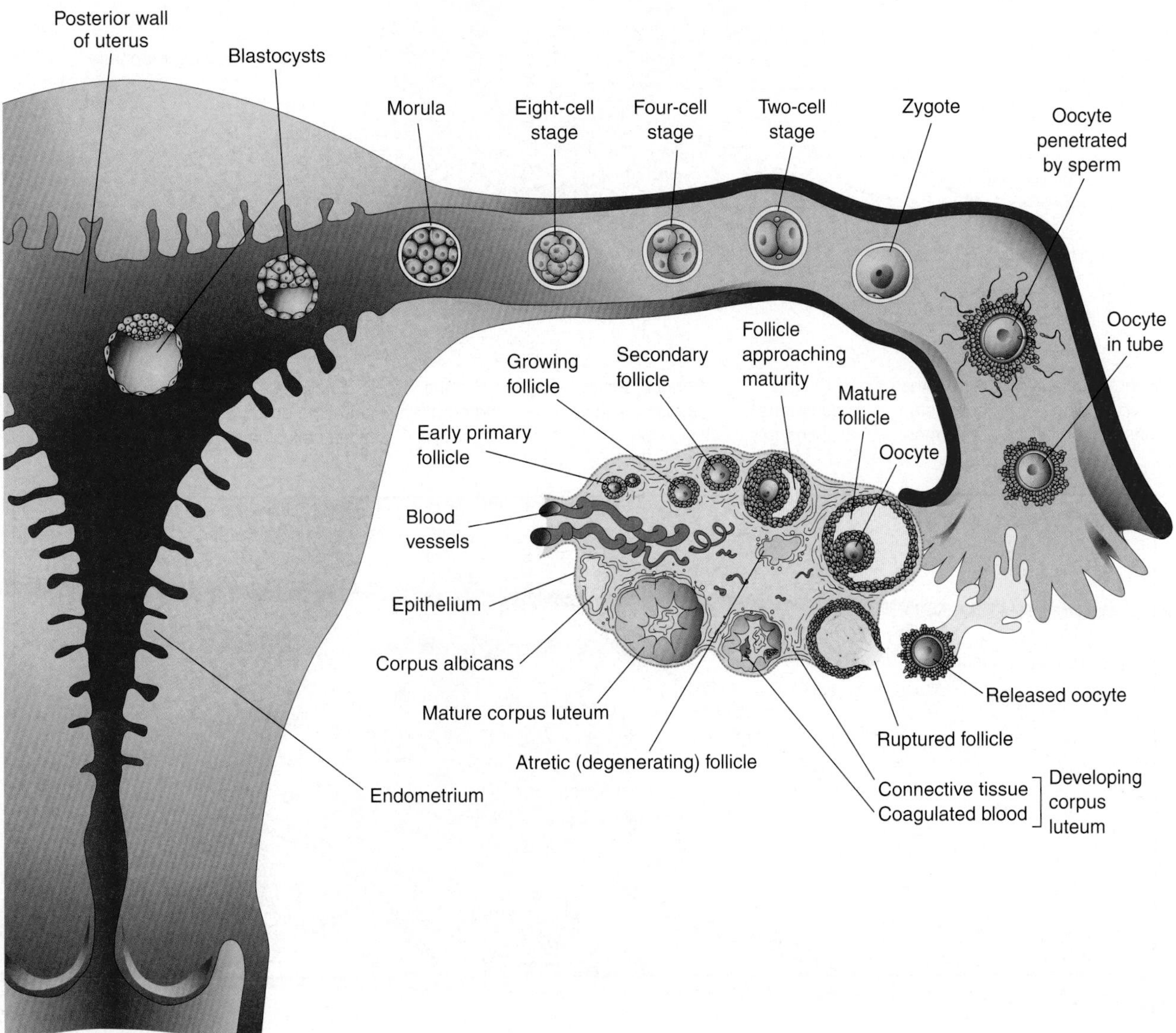

Figure 1-5. Summary of the ovarian cycle, fertilization, and human development during the first week. Stage 1 of development begins with fertilization in the uterine tube and ends when the zygote forms. Stage 2 (days 2–3) comprises the early stages of cleavage (from 2 to about 32 cells, the morula). Stage 3 (days 4–5) consists of the free (unattached) blastocyst. Stage 4 (days 5–6) is represented by the blastocyst attaching to the posterior wall of the uterus, the usual site of implantation. The blastocysts have been sectioned to show their internal structure. (From Moore KL, Persaud TVN: The Developing Human: Clinically Oriented Embryology, 7th ed. Philadelphia, WB Saunders, 2003.)

female pronucleus swells as well. In most mammals the male pronucleus can be recognized as the larger of the two. The pronuclei, which contain the haploid sets of chromosomes of maternal and paternal origin, do not fuse in mammals. However, the nuclear membranes surrounding them disappear, and the chromosomes contained within each membrane arrange themselves on the developing spindle of the first mitotic division. In this way the diploid complement of chromosomes is reestablished, completing the process of fertilization.

Cell division (cleavage) then occurs, giving rise to the two-cell embryo (Fig. 1-7). The first division takes about 20 hours to complete, and the actual phase of fertilization generally occurs in the ampulla of the fallopian tube. A significant number of fertilized ova do not complete cleavage for a number of reasons, including failure of appropriate chromosome arrangement on the spindle, specific gene defects that prevent the formation of the spindle, and environmental factors. Importantly, teratogens acting at this point are usually either completely destructive

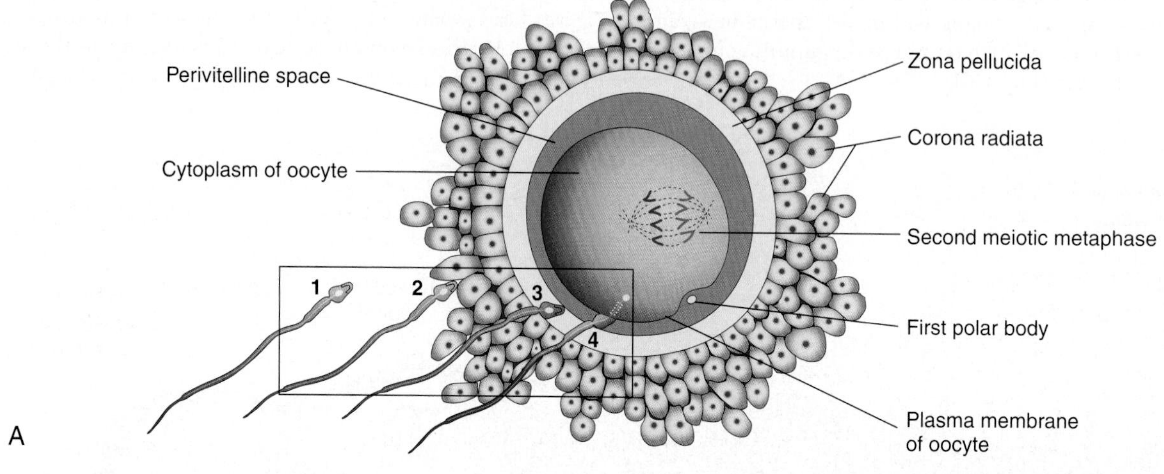

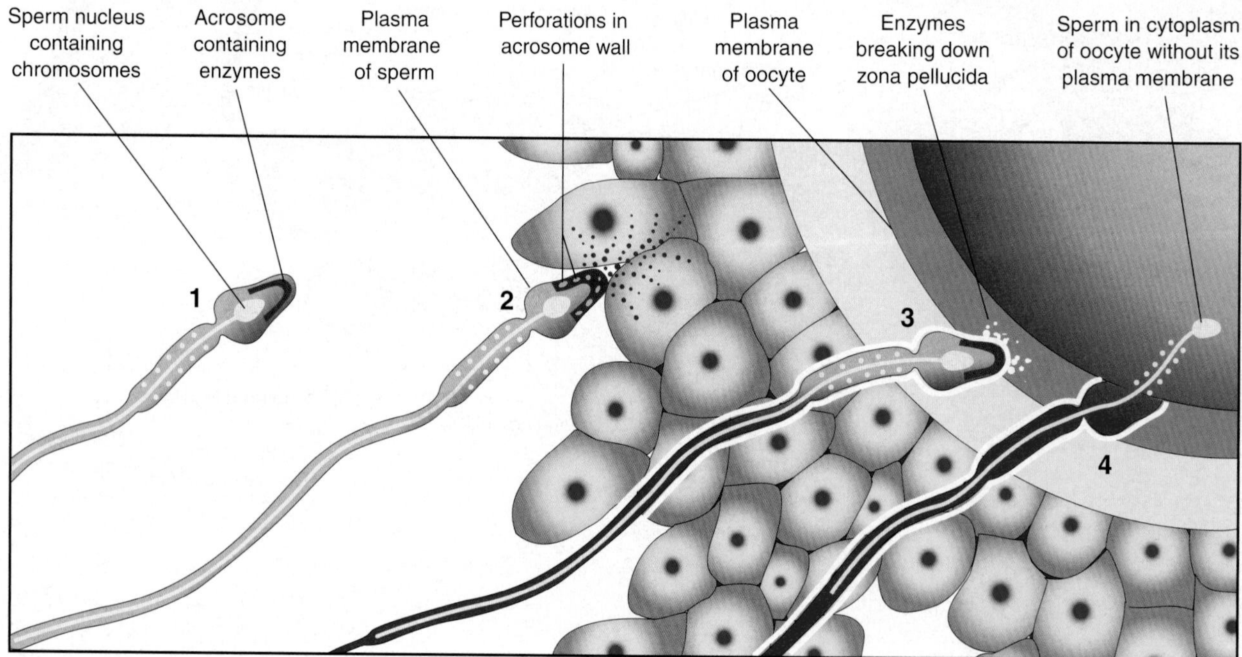

Figure 1-6. Acrosome reaction and a sperm penetrating an oocyte. The detail of the area outlined in **A** is given in **B**. Sperm during capacitation, a period of conditioning that occurs in the female reproductive tract. 2, Sperm undergoing the acrosome reaction, during which perforations form in the acrosome. 3, Sperm digesting a path through the zona pellucida by the action of enzymes released from the acrosome. 4, Sperm after entering the cytoplasm of the oocyte. Note that the plasma membranes of the sperm and oocyte have fused and that the head and tail of the sperm enter the oocyte, leaving the sperm's plasma membrane attached to the oocyte's plasma membrane. (From Moore KL, Persaud TVN: The Developing Human: Clinically Oriented Embryology, 7th ed. Philadelphia, WB Saunders, 2003.)

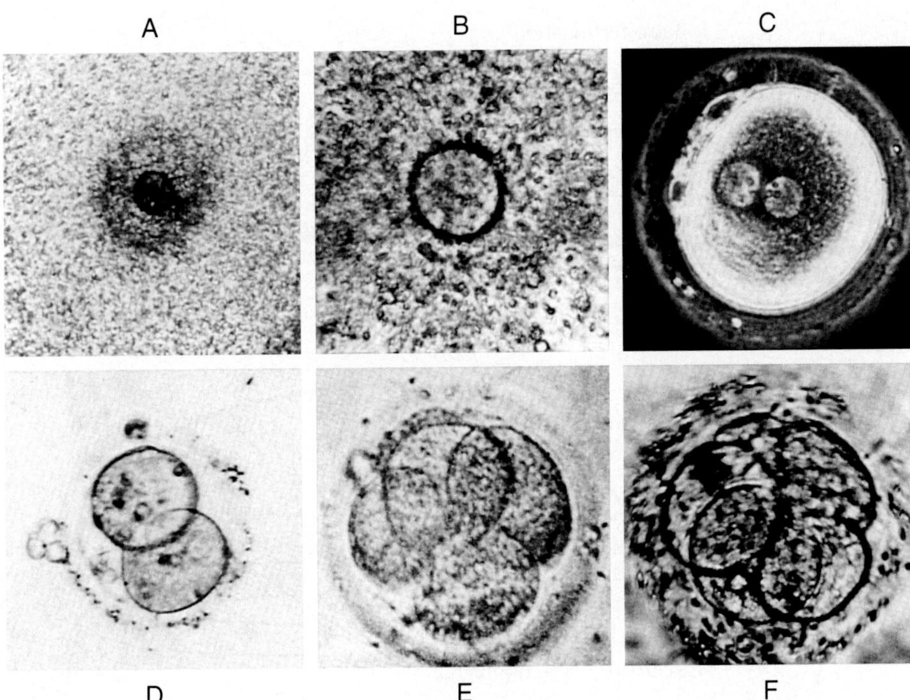

Figure 1-7. Six photomicrographs of fresh, unmounted human eggs and embryos. **A,** Early maturing oocyte. **B,** Mature oocyte surrounded by granulosa cells, zona pellucida visible. **C,** Fertilized oocyte demonstrating male and female pronuclei and both polar bodies. **D,** Two-cell zygote. **E,** Four-cell embryo. **F,** Eight-cell embryo. (Courtesy of Edith Cheng, MD.)

or cause little or no effect. Twinning may occur by the separation of the two cells produced by cleavage, each of which has the potential to develop into a separate embryo. Twinning may occur at any stage until the formation of the blastula, since each cell is totipotential. Both genetic and environmental factors are probably involved in the causation of twinning.

Morula and Blastula Stage: Early Differentiation

After the first mitotic division the cells continue to divide as the embryo passes along the fallopian tube and enters the uterus. This process takes 3 to 4 days after fertilization in the human, and the embryo may arrive at the uterus in any form, from 32 cells to the early blastula stage. In the human, implantation generally takes place 3 days after the embryo enters the uterus.

Implantation depends on the development of early trophoblastic cells during the blastula stage. These cells digest away the zona pellucida and allow the embryo to fix to the wall of the uterus and subsequently to burrow within the endometrium. The development of the blastula and the separation of the embryonic disk cells from the developing trophoblastic cells together make up the first stage of differentiation in the embryo. Again, at this stage of development, teratogens are generally either completely destructive or have little or no effect, since each of the cells of the early embryonic disk is pluripotent. Differentiation within the embryonic disk, however, proceeds fairly rapidly, and if separation of cells and twinning occur at this point, the twins are frequently conjoined in some fashion.

Advances in assisted reproductive technology and genetics now provide practitioners assess to the early embryo for preimplantation genetic diagnosis (PGD) of single-gene or chromosome disorders (Fig. 1-8). This technique, initiated in the United Kingdom in the late 1980s, involves the removal of one or two cells at the cleavage stage (six to eight cells) at day 2 to 4 after fertilization using highly sophisticated micromanipulation techniques. For PGD of single-gene disorders, DNA is extracted from the cell(s), amplified by PCR (polymerase chain reaction), and tested for the gene mutation in question. Embryos containing the mutation are discarded (not transferred), and embryos in which the mutation in question in not detected are saved. Some of these may be transferred into the primed uterine cavity as in any in vitro fertilization (IVF) cycle. For PGD of chromosomal defects such as aneuploidy or structural rearrangements, fluorescent in situ hybridization (FISH) is completed on the one or two cells removed from each embryo for only the chromosomal abnormality in question. PGD must be completed within 12 to 24 hours of embryo biopsy in order to transfer appropriate embryos into the uterus.

IMPLANTATION

Implantation has been noted to occur in the human embryo as early as day 6 after ovulation (Table 1-1). For implantation to take place, the zona pellucida must be removed from the developing blastocyst, which occurs because of enzyme action produced either by cells of the blastocyst or by some endometrial enzymes. Endometrial capillaries in contact with the invading syncytiotrophoblast are engulfed to form venous sinuses at or about $7^1/_2$ days after conception and are seen abundantly by day 9. Endometrial spiral arteries are not invaded at this point. The endoplasmic reticulum of the syncytiotrophoblast is probably responsible for the synthesis of human chorionic gonadotropin (HCG), which is well developed by 11 days after ovulation. Transfer is most likely through the venous sinuses before intact circulation to the developing embryo has been established. HCG be transmitted to maternal circulation since

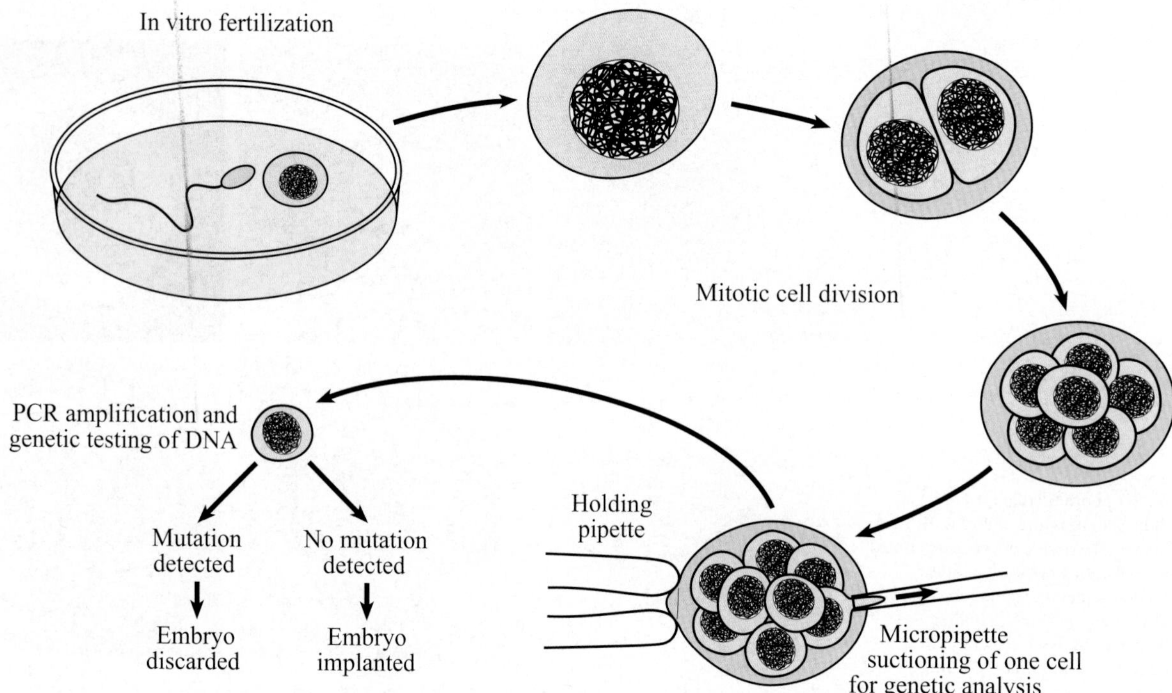

Figure 1-8. Schematic illustration of preimplantation diagnosis. PGD requires in vitro fertilization technology to achieve pregnancy. After fertilization, one or two blastomeres are removed at the six- to eight-cell stage from each embryo. For gene mutational analysis, the DNA is extracted and amplified several hundred-fold. Embryos without the mutation are kept and transferred. (Courtesy of Edith Cheng, MD.)

Table 1-1 Events of Implantation

Event	Days after Ovulation
Zona pellucida disappears	4–5
Blastocyst attaches to epithelial surface of endometrium	6
Trophoblast erodes into endometrial stroma	7
Trophoblast differentiates into cytotrophoblastic and syncytial trophoblastic layers	7–8
Lacunae appear around trophoblast	8–9
Blastocyst burrows beneath endometrial surface	9–10
Lacunar network forms	10–11
Trophoblast invades endometrial sinusoids, establishing a uteroplacental circulation	11–12
Endometrial epithelium completely covers blastocyst	12–13
Strong decidual reaction occurs in stroma	13–14

it is responsible for maintaining the corpus luteum. HCG has been detected in the peripheral blood of the mother as early as 6 days after ovulation, but is always seen by the twelfth day. The concentration doubles every 1.2 to 2 days, reaching its highest point at 7 to 9 weeks of pregnancy.

Early Organogenesis in the Embryonic Period

During the third week after fertilization, the primitive streak forms in the caudal portion of the embryonic disk, and the embryonic disk begins to grow and change from a circular to a pear-shaped configuration. At that point the epithelium facing superiorly is considered ectoderm and will eventually give rise to the developing central nervous system, and the epithelium facing downward toward the yolk sac is endoderm. During this week the neuroplate develops with its associated notochordal process. By the sixteenth day after conception the third primitive germ layer, the intraembryonic mesoderm, begins to form between the ectoderm and endoderm. Early mesoderm migrates cranially, passing on either side of the notochordal process to meet in front in the formation of the cardiogenic area. The heart soon develops from this area. Later in the third week extraembryonic mesoderm joins with the yolk sac and the developing amnion to contribute to the developing membranes. An intraembryonic mesoderm develops on each side of the notochord and neural tube to form longitudinal columns, the paraxial mesoderm. Each paraxial column thins laterally into the lateral plate mesoderm, which is continuous with the extraembryonic mesoderm of the yolk sac and the amnion. The lateral plate mesoderm is separated from the paraxial mesoderm by a continuous tract of mesoderm called the intermediate mesoderm. By the twentieth day, paraxial mesoderm begins to divide into paired linear bodies known as somites. About 38 pairs of somites form during the next 10 days. Eventually a total of 42 to 44 pairs will develop, and these will give rise to body musculature.

Angiogenesis, or blood vessel formation, can be seen in the extraembryonic mesoderm of the yolk sac by day 15 or 16. Embryonic vessels can be seen about 2 days later and develop when mesenchymal cells known as angioblasts aggregate to form masses and cords called blood islands. Spaces then appear within these islands, and the angioblasts arrange themselves around these spaces to form primitive endothelium. Isolated vessels form channels and then grow into adjacent areas by endothelial budding. Primitive blood cells develop from endothelial cells as the vessels develop on the yolk sac and allantois. However, blood formation does not begin within the embryo until the second month of gestation, occurring first in the developing liver and later in the spleen, bone marrow, and lymph nodes. Separate mesenchymal cells surrounding the primitive endothelial vessels differentiate into muscular and connective tissue elements. The primitive heart forms in a similar manner from mesenchymal cells in the cardiogenic area. Paired endothelial channels, called heart tubes, develop by the end of the third week and fuse to form the primitive heart. By the twenty-first day, this primitive heart has linked up with blood vessels of the embryo, forming a primitive cardiovascular system. Blood circulation starts about this time, and the cardiovascular system becomes the first functioning organ system within the embryo. All the organ systems form between the fourth week and seventh week of gestation.

A teratogenic event that takes place during the embryonic period gives rise to a constellation of malformations related to the organ systems that are actively developing at that particular time. Thus cardiovascular malformations tend to occur because of teratogenic events early in the embryonic period, whereas genitourinary abnormalities tend to result from later events. Teratogenic effects before implantation often cause death but not malformations.

The effects of a particular teratogen depend on the individual's genetic makeup, other environmental factors in play at the time, the embryonic developmental stage during which the teratogenic exposure occurred, and in some cases the dose of the teratogen and the duration of exposure. Some teratogens in and of themselves are harmless, but their metabolites cause the damage. Teratogens may be chemical substances and their by-products, or they may be physical phenomena, such as temperature elevation and irradiation. Teratogen exposure after the forty-ninth day of gestation may injure or kill the embryo or cause developmental and growth retardation but usually will not be responsible for specific malformations. The period of embryonic development is said to be complete when the embryo attains a crown–rump length of 30 mm, corresponding in most cases to day 49 after conception.

DEVELOPMENT OF THE GENITOURINARY SYSTEM

The development of the genital organs is intimately involved with the development of the renal system.

Renal Development

Nephrogenic cords develop from the intermediate mesoderm as early as the 2-mm embryo stage, beginning in the more cephalad portions of the embryo. Three sets of excretory ducts and tubules develop bilaterally. The first, the pronephros, with its pronephric ducts, forms in the most cranial portion of the embryo at about the beginning of the fourth week after conception. The tubules associated with the duct probably have no excretory function in the human. Late in the fourth week a second set of tubules, the mesonephric tubules, and their accompanying mesonephric ducts begin to develop. These are associated with tufts of capillaries, or glomeruli, and tubules for excretory purposes. Thus the mesonephros functions as a fetal kidney, producing urine for about 2 or 3 weeks. As new tubules develop, those derived from the more cephalad tubules degenerate. Usually about 40 mesonephric tubules function on either side of the embryo at any given time.

The metanephros, or permanent kidney, begins its development early in the fifth week of gestation and starts to function late in the seventh or early in the eighth week. The metanephros develops both from the metanephrogenic mass of mesoderm, which is the most caudal portion of the nephrogenic cord, and from its duct system, which is derived from the metanephric diverticulum (ureteric bud). It is a cranially growing outpouching of the mesonephric duct close to where it enters the cloaca. The metanephric duct system gives rise to the ureter, the renal pelvis, the calyces, and the collecting tubules of the adult kidney. A critical process in the development of the kidney requires that the cranially growing metanephric diverticulum meets and fuses with the metanephrogenic mass of mesoderm so that formation of the kidney can take place. Originally the metanephric kidney is a pelvic organ, but by differential growth it becomes located in the lumbar region.

The fetus produces urine throughout all the periods of gestation, but the placenta handles the excretory functions of the fetus. The urine produced by the fetus contributes to the amniotic fluid. The fetus may swallow the amniotic fluid and recirculate it through the digestive system. This seems to be an important factor in regulating the amount of amniotic fluid present in the fetus. Congenital abnormalities that impair normal development or function of the fetal kidneys generally result in little or no amniotic fluid (oligohydramnios or anhydramnios), whereas structural abnormalities of the gastrointestinal tract or neuromuscular conditions that prevent the fetus from swallowing can lead to excess amniotic fluid (polyhydramnios).

Bladder and Urethra

The embryonic cloaca is divided by the urorectal septum into a dorsal rectum and a ventral urogenital sinus. The urogenital sinus, in turn, is divided into three parts: the cranial portion—the vesicourethral canal, which is continuous with the allantois; a middle pelvic portion; and a caudal urogenital sinus portion, which is covered externally by the urogenital membrane. The epithelium of the developing bladder is derived from the endoderm of the vesicourethral canal. The muscular layers and serosa of the bladder develop from adjacent splanchnic mesenchyme. As the bladder develops, the caudal portion of the mesonephric ducts is incorporated into its dorsal wall. The portion of the mesonephric duct distal to the points where the metanephric duct is taken up into the bladder becomes the trigone of the bladder. Although this portion is mesoderm in origin, it is probably epithelialized eventually by endodermal epithelium from the urogenital sinus. In this way the ureters, derived from the metanephric duct, come to open directly into the bladder.

In the male the mesonephric ducts open into the urethra as the ejaculatory ducts. Also in the male, mesenchymal tissue surrounding the developing urethra where it exits the bladder develops into the prostate gland, through which the ejaculatory ducts traverse. Figure 1-9 demonstrates graphically the development of the male and female urinary systems.

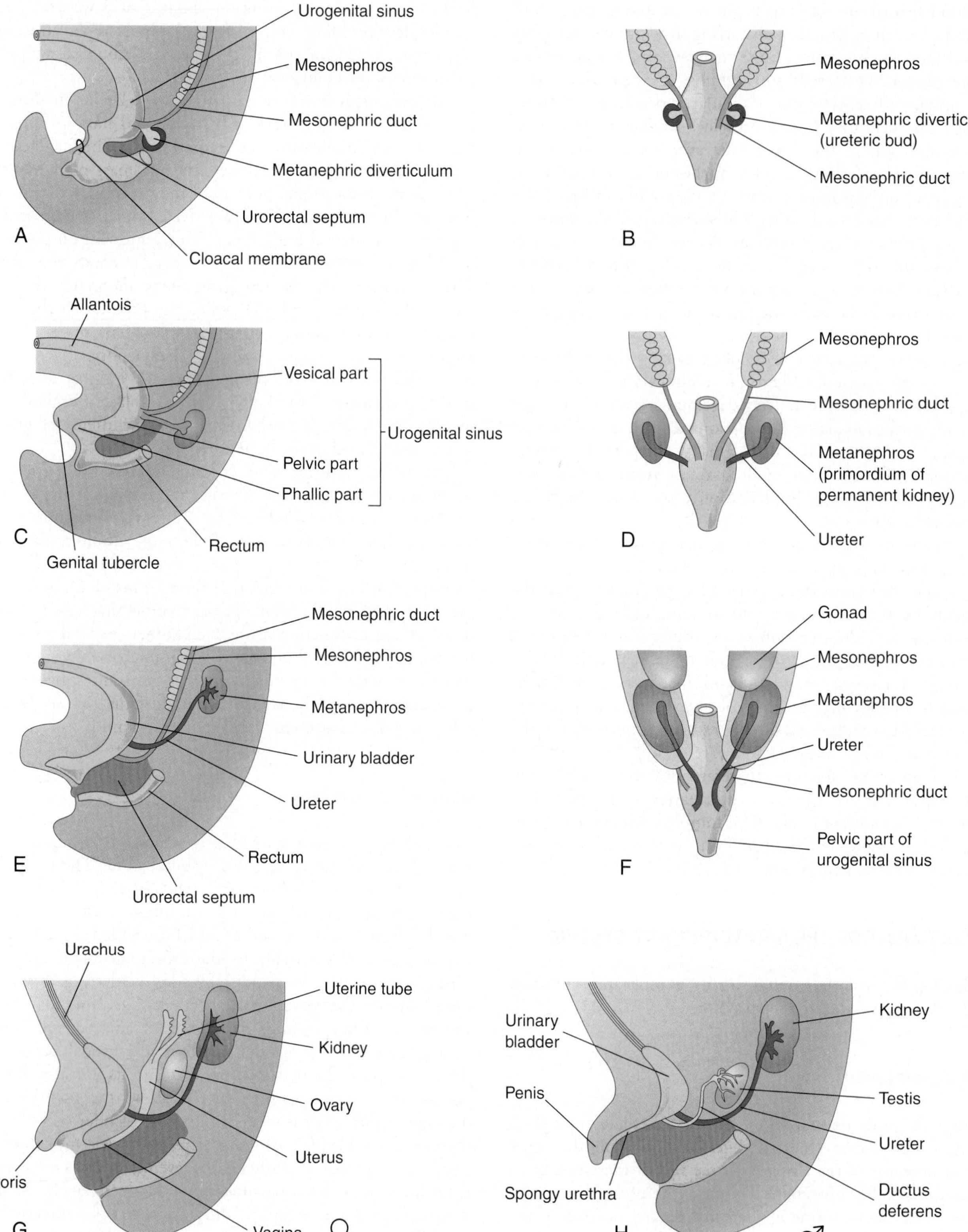

Figure 1-9. Diagrams showing division of the cloaca into the urogenital sinus and rectum; absorption of the mesonephric ducts; development of the urinary bladder, urethra, and urachus, and changes in the location of the ureters. **A,** Lateral view of the caudal half of a 5-week embryo. **B, D,** and **F,** Dorsal views. **C, E, G,** and **H,** Lateral views. The stages shown in **G** and **H** are reached by the twelfth week. (From Moore KL, Persaud TVN: The Developing Human: Clinically Oriented Embryology, 7th ed. Philadelphia, WB Saunders, 2003.)

The epithelium of the female urethra is derived from endoderm of the vesicourethral canal. The urethral sphincter develops from a mesenchymal condensation around the urethra after the division of the cloaca in the 12- to 15-mm embryo. Following the opening of the anal membrane at the 20- to 30-mm stage, the puborectalis muscle appears. At 15 weeks' gestation, striated muscle can be seen, and a smooth muscle layer thickens at the level of the developing bladder neck, forming the inner part of the urethral musculature. Thus the urethral sphincter is composed of both central smooth muscle and peripheral striated muscle. The sphincter develops primarily in the anterior wall of the urethra in a horseshoe or omega shape.

SEX DIFFERENTIATION

Genetic sex is determined at the time of conception. A Y chromosome is necessary for the development of the testes, and the testes are responsible for the organization of the sexual duct system into a male configuration and for the suppression of the paramesonephric (müllerian) system. In the absence of a Y chromosome or in the absence of a gonad, development will be female in nature. General phenotypic development of the female seems to be a neutral event, only slightly related to maternal estrogen activity.

Sex differentiation occurs from genes that are coded on the Y chromosome. The primary determinant is the *SRY* gene, sometimes called the testis-determining factor. The *SRY* gene is found on the short arm of the Y chromosome. The *SRY* gene influences Sertoli cell differentiation, development of cells in the mesonephric ridge, and male architectural development of the gonad, including blood vessels and other structures of the testes. Several other genes, including those that express steroidogenic factor-1, WT1, DAX1, on other chromosomes are also necessary for normal testicular development. Male gonadal development precedes female development (Fig. 1-10). The secretion of testosterone and antimüllerian hormone (AMH) from the testes steers the further development of the rest of the genital tracts.

An interesting bit of evidence for the importance of the *SRY* gene in the development of male sexual differentiation is seen in the 45,X/47,XYY mosaics. Hsu reviewed the phenotypes of 15 postnatally diagnosed cases and found that 8 were female, 3 male, and 4 intersex. She postulated that the sex reversal occurred because of deletion or mutation of the *SRY* gene. To date, multiple mutations of the *SRY* gene have been reported, and all are associated with sex reversals (female phenotype). In very rare male individuals, a Y chromosome may be absent, but the *SRY* gene may be located on another chromosome, most commonly the X chromosome. Other rare genetic causes of gonadal dysgenesis may occur from mutations or deletions in a number of other genes that influence hormonal and cellular differentiation.

During the fifth week after conception, coelomic epithelium, later known as germinal epithelium, thickens in the area of the medial aspect of the mesonephros. As germinal epithelial cells proliferate, they invade the underlying mesenchyme, producing a prominence known as the gonadal ridge. In the sixth week the primordial germ cells, which have formed at about week 4 in the wall of the yolk sac, migrate up the dorsal mesentery of the hindgut and enter the undifferentiated gonad. These cells may differentiate into the testes or ovaries. For the formation of a testis, the H-Y antigen must be activated. The somatic cells of the primitive gonadal ridge then differentiate into interstitial cells (Leydig cells) and Sertoli cells. As they do so, the primordial

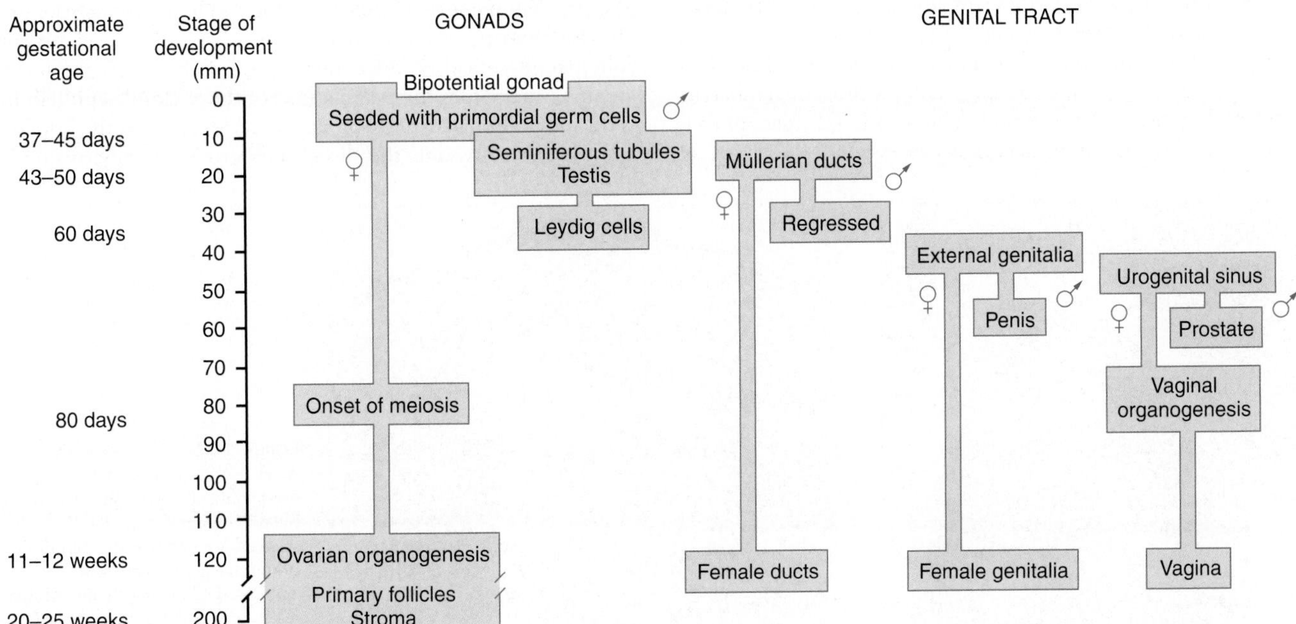

Figure 1-10. Development of sexual differentiation in the human. Note the lag from male to female development. (Modified from Grumbach MM, Hughes IA, Conte FA: Disorders of Sex Differentiation. In Larsen PR, Kronenberg HM, Melmed S, Polonsky KS (eds): Williams Textbook of Endocrinology, 10th ed. Philadelphia, WB Saunders, 2003, p 870.)

germ cells and Sertoli cells become enclosed within seminiferous tubules, and the interstitial cells remain outside these tubules. The H-Y antigen can be demonstrated in Sertoli cells at this stage but not in the developing germ cells. Sertoli cells are encased in the seminiferous tubules in the seventh and eighth weeks. In the eighth week Leydig cells differentiate and begin to produce testosterone. At this point the mesonephric (wolffian) duct differentiates into the vas deferens, epididymis, and seminal vesicles, while the paramesonephric duct is suppressed because of the secretion and action of AMH.

Primary sex cords, meanwhile, have condensed and extended to the medullary portion of the developing testes. They branch and join to form the rete testis. The testis therefore is primarily a medullary organ, and eventually the rete testis connects with the tubules of the mesonephric system and joins the developing epididymal duct.

In specific androgen target areas, testosterone is converted to 5-α-dihydrotestosterone by the microsomal enzyme Δ-4-5-α-reductase. Data suggest that two androgens—testosterone and its metabolite, dihydrotestosterone—are involved in sexual differentiation in the male fetus, with selective roles for each hormone during embryogenesis; that is, dihydrotestosterone stimulates the testes and scrotum, and testosterone stimulates the prostate gland.

Androgen action must be initiated at the target areas. Testosterone enters the cell and either is bound to a cytoplasmic receptor or, in certain target tissue, is converted to dihydrotestosterone. Dihydrotestosterone in such cells would then bind to a cytoplasmic receptor. Afterward, the androgen-receptor complex gains access to the nucleus, where it binds to chromatin and initiates the transcription of messenger ribonucleic acid. This leads to the metabolic process of androgen action.

For normal male development in utero, the testes must differentiate and function normally. At a critical point, AMH, produced by Sertoli cells, and testosterone, secreted by Leydig cells, must be produced in sufficient amounts. AMH acts locally in suppressing the müllerian duct system, and testosterone acts systemically, causing differentiation of the mesonephric duct system and affecting male development of the urogenital tubercle, urogenital sinus, and urogenital folds. Thus the masculinization of the fetus is a multifactorial process under a variety of genetic controls. Genes on the Y chromosome are responsible for testicular differentiation. Enzymes involved in testosterone biosynthesis and conversion to dihydrotestosterone are regulated by genes located on autosomes. The ability to secrete AMH is a recessive trait coded on either an autosome or the X chromosome, and genes for development of cytoplasmic receptors of androgens seem to be coded on the X chromosome.

Development of the ovary occurs at about the eleventh or twelfth week, though the primordial germ cells have migrated several weeks earlier to the germinal ridge (Fig. 1-11). Two functional X chromosomes seem necessary for optimal development of the ovary. The effect of an X chromosome deficiency is most severe in species in which there is a long period between the formation and use of oocytes (i.e., the human). Thus in 45,X and 46,XY females, the ovaries are almost invariably devoid of oocytes. On the other hand, germ cells in the testes do best when only one X chromosome is present; rarely do they survive in the XX or XXY condition.

When non-Y-bearing oocytes enter the differentiating gonad, the primary sex cords do not become prominent but, instead, break up and encircle the oocytes in the cortex of the gonad (in contrast to the structure of the XY gonad). This occurs at about 16 weeks' gestation, and the isolated cell clusters derived from the cortical cords that surround the oocytes are called primordial follicles. No new oogonia form after birth, and many of the oogonia degenerate before birth. Those that remain grow and become primary follicles to be stimulated after puberty. The processes of gonadal development are schematically summarized in Figure 1-12.

Genital Duct System

Early in embryonic life, two sets of paired genital ducts develop in each sex: the mesonephric (Wolffian) ducts and the paramesonephric (Müllerian) ducts. The mesonephric duct development precedes the paramesonephric duct development. The paramesonephric ducts develop on each side of the mesonephric ducts from the evaginations of the coelomic epithelium. The more cephalad ends of the ducts open directly into the peritoneal cavity, and the distal ends grow caudally, fusing in

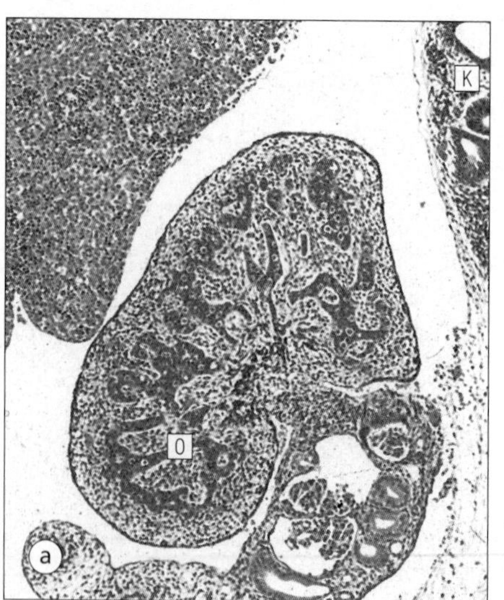

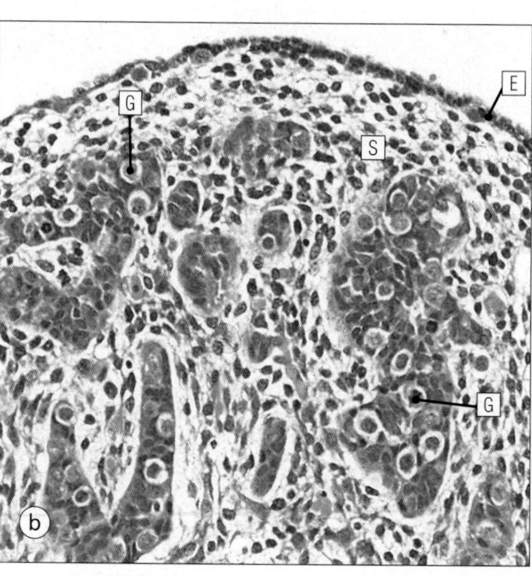

Figure 1-11. Ovary in embryo. **A,** The developing ovary (O) in a 9-week-old embryo is shown close to the developing kidney (K). **B,** At this stage of development the columns of primordial germ cells (G) are embedded in a mesenchymal stroma (S) covered by a layer of cuboidal surface cells (E). (From Stevens A, Lowe J: Human Histology, 3rd ed. Philadelphia, Elsevier Mosby, 2005, p 357.)

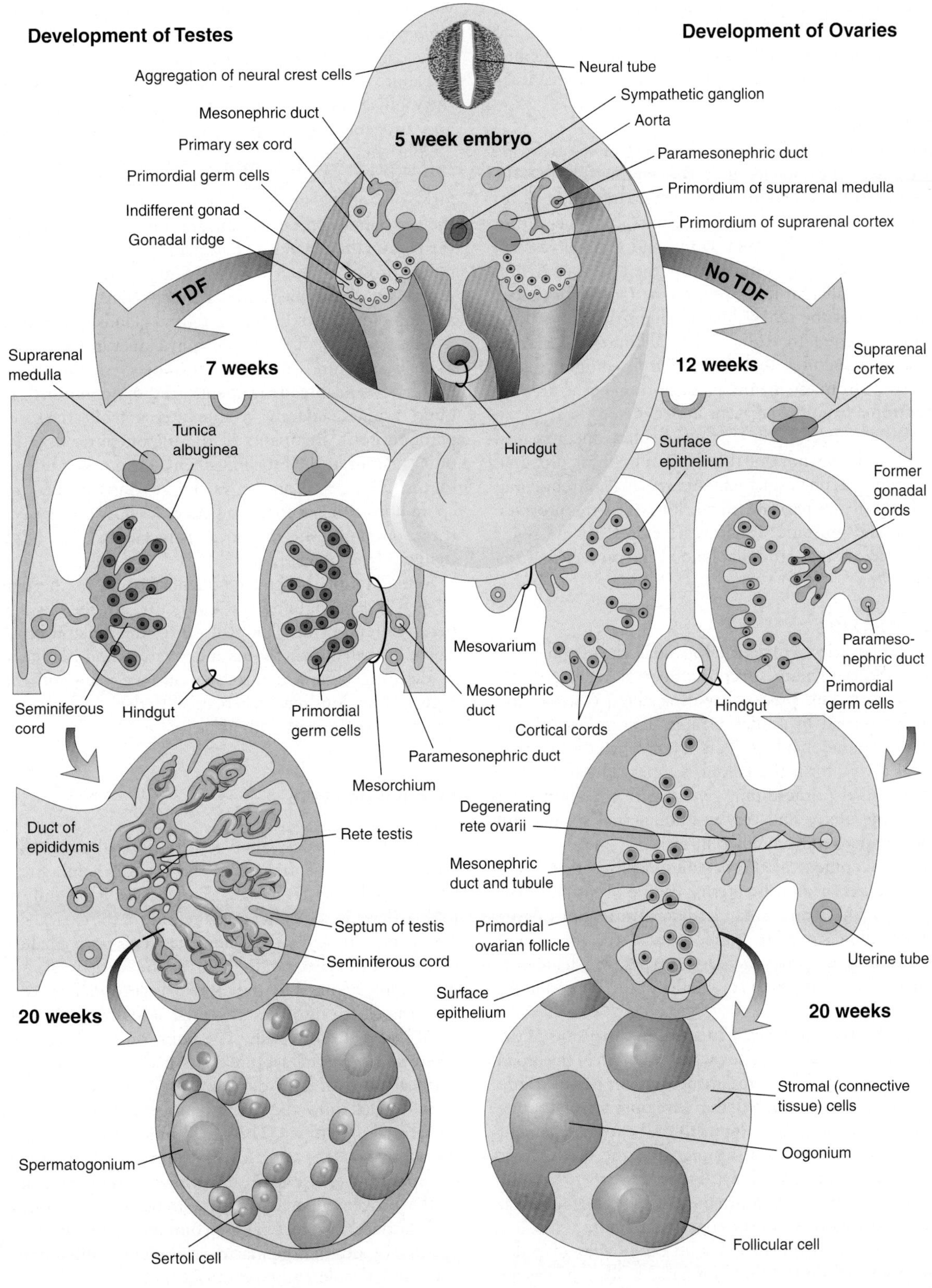

Figure 1-12. Schematic illustration showing differentiation of the indifferent gonads of a 5-week embryo (top) into ovaries or testes. Left side shows the development of testes resulting from the effects of the testis-determining factor (TDF), also called the SRY gene, located on the Y chromosome. Note that the gonadal cords become seminiferous cords, the primordium of the seminiferous tubules. The parts of the gonadal cords that enter the medulla of the testis form the rete testis. In the section of the testis at the bottom left, observe that there are two kinds of cells: spermatogonia derived from the primordial germ cells and sustentacular (Sertoli) cells derived from mesenchyme. Right side shows the development of ovaries in the absence of TDF. Cortical cords have extended from the surface epithelium of the gonad, and primordial cells have entered them. They are the primordia of the oogonia. Follicular cells are derived from the surface epithelium of the ovary. (From Moore KL, Persaud TVN: The Developing Human: Clinically Oriented Embryology, 7th ed. Philadelphia, WB Saunders, 2003.)

the lower midline to form the uterovaginal primordium. This tubular structure joins the dorsal wall of the urogenital sinus and produces an elevation, the müllerian tubercle. The mesonephric ducts enter the urogenital sinus on either side of the tubercle.

Male Genital Ducts

Some seminiferous tubules are produced in the fetal testes during the seventh and eighth weeks after conception. During the eighth week interstitial (Leydig) cells differentiate and begin to produce testosterone. At this point the mesonephric duct differentiates into the vas deferens, epididymis, and seminal vesicles, and the müllerian anlage is suppressed by the action of AMH, previously called müllerian-inhibiting factor (MIF), produced by the Sertoli cells of the testes. The development of the prostate gland was referred to earlier. The bulbourethral glands, which are small structures that develop from outgrowths of endodermal tissue from the membranous portion of the urethra, incorporate stroma from the adjacent mesenchyme.

The most distal portion of the paramesonephric duct remains, in the male, as the appendix of the testes. The most proximal end of the paramesonephric duct remains as a small outpouching within the body of the prostate gland, known as the prostatic utricle. Rarely, the prostatic utricle is developed to the point where it will excrete a small amount of blood and cause hematuria in adult life.

Female Genital Ducts

In the presence of ovaries or of gonadal agenesis, the mesonephric ducts regress, and the paramesonephric ducts develop into the female genital tract. This process begins at about 6 weeks and proceeds in a cephalad to caudal fashion. The more cephalad portions of the paramesonephric ducts, which open directly into the peritoneal cavity, form the fallopian tubes. The fused portion, or uterovaginal primordium, gives rise to the epithelium and glands of the uterus and cervix. Endometrial stroma and myometrium are derived from adjacent mesenchyme.

Failure of development of the paramesonephric ducts leads to agenesis of the cervix and the uterus. Failure of fusion of the caudal portion of these ducts may lead to a variety of uterine anomalies, including complete duplication of the uterus and cervix or partial duplication of a variety of types, which are outlined in Chapter 12 (Congenital Anomalies of the Reproductive Tract).

Peritoneal reflections in the area adjacent to the fusion of the two paramesonephric ducts give rise to the formation of the broad ligaments. Mesenchymal tissue here develops into the parametrium.

Pietryga and Wózniak studied the development of uterine ligaments, documenting the development of the round ligament at the eighth week, the cardinal ligaments at the tenth week, and the broad ligament at week 19. From weeks 8 to 17, the round ligament is connected to the uterine tube. Beginning at week 18, it comes to arise from the edge of the uterus.

The vagina develops from paired solid outgrowths of endoderm of the urogenital sinus—the sinovaginal bulbs. These grow caudally as a solid core toward the end of the uterovaginal primordium. This core constitutes the fibromuscular portion of the vagina. The sinovaginal bulbs then canalize to form the vagina. Abnormalities in this process may lead to either transverse or horizontal vaginal septa. The junction of the sinovaginal bulbs with the urogenital sinus remains as the vaginal plate, which forms the hymen. This remains imperforate until late in embryonic life, although occasionally, perforation does not take place completely (imperforate hymen).

Failure of the sinovaginal bulbs to form leads to agenesis of the vagina. The precise boundary between the paramesonephric and urogenital sinus portions of the vagina has not been established.

Auxiliary genital glands in the female form from buds that grow out of the urethra. The buds derive contributions from the surrounding mesenchyme and form the urethral glands and the paraurethral glands (Skene glands). These glands correspond to the prostate gland in males. Similar outgrowths of the urogenital sinus form the vestibular glands (Bartholin glands), which are homologous to the bulbourethral glands in the male.

The remnants of the mesonephric duct in the female include a small structure called the appendix vesiculosa, a few blind tubules in the broad ligaments (the epoophoron), and a few blind tubules adjacent to the uterus (collectively called the paroophoron). Remnants of the mesonephric duct system are often present in the broad ligaments or may be present adjacent to the uterus and/or the vagina as Gartner duct cysts. The epoophoron or paroophoron may develop into cysts. Cysts of the epoophoron are known as paraovarian cysts (Chapter 18, Benign Gynecologic Lesions).

Remnants of the paramesonephric duct in the female may be seen as a small, blind cystic structure attached by a pedicle to the distal end of the fallopian tube—the hydatid of Morgagni. Table 1-2 categorizes the adult derivatives and residual remnants of the urogenital structures in both the male and the female. Figure 1-13 outlines schematically the development of the internal sexual organs in both sexes.

External Genitalia

In the fourth week after fertilization, the genital tubercle develops at the ventral tip of the cloacal membrane. Two sets of lateral bodies—the labioscrotal swellings and urogenital folds—develop soon after on either side of the cloacal membrane. The genital tubercle then elongates to form a phallus in both males and females. By the end of the sixth week, the cloacal membrane is joined by the urorectal septum. The septum separates the cloaca into the urogenital sinus ventrally and the anal canal and rectum dorsally. The point on the cloacal membrane where the urorectal septum fuses becomes the location of the perineal body in later development. The cloacal membrane is then divided into the ventral urogenital membrane and the dorsal anal membrane. These membranes then rupture, opening the vulva and the anal canal. Failure of the anal membrane to rupture gives rise to an imperforate anus. With the opening of the urogenital membrane, a urethral groove forms on the undersurface of the phallus, completing the undifferentiated portion of external genital development. Differences between male and female embryos can be noted as early as the ninth week, but the distinct final forms are not noted until 12 weeks' gestation (Fig. 1-14).

Androgens (testosterone and dihydrotestosterone), produced by the testes and by peripheral conversion of testosterone in target cells, respectively, are responsible for the masculinization of the undifferentiated external genitalia in males. The phallus

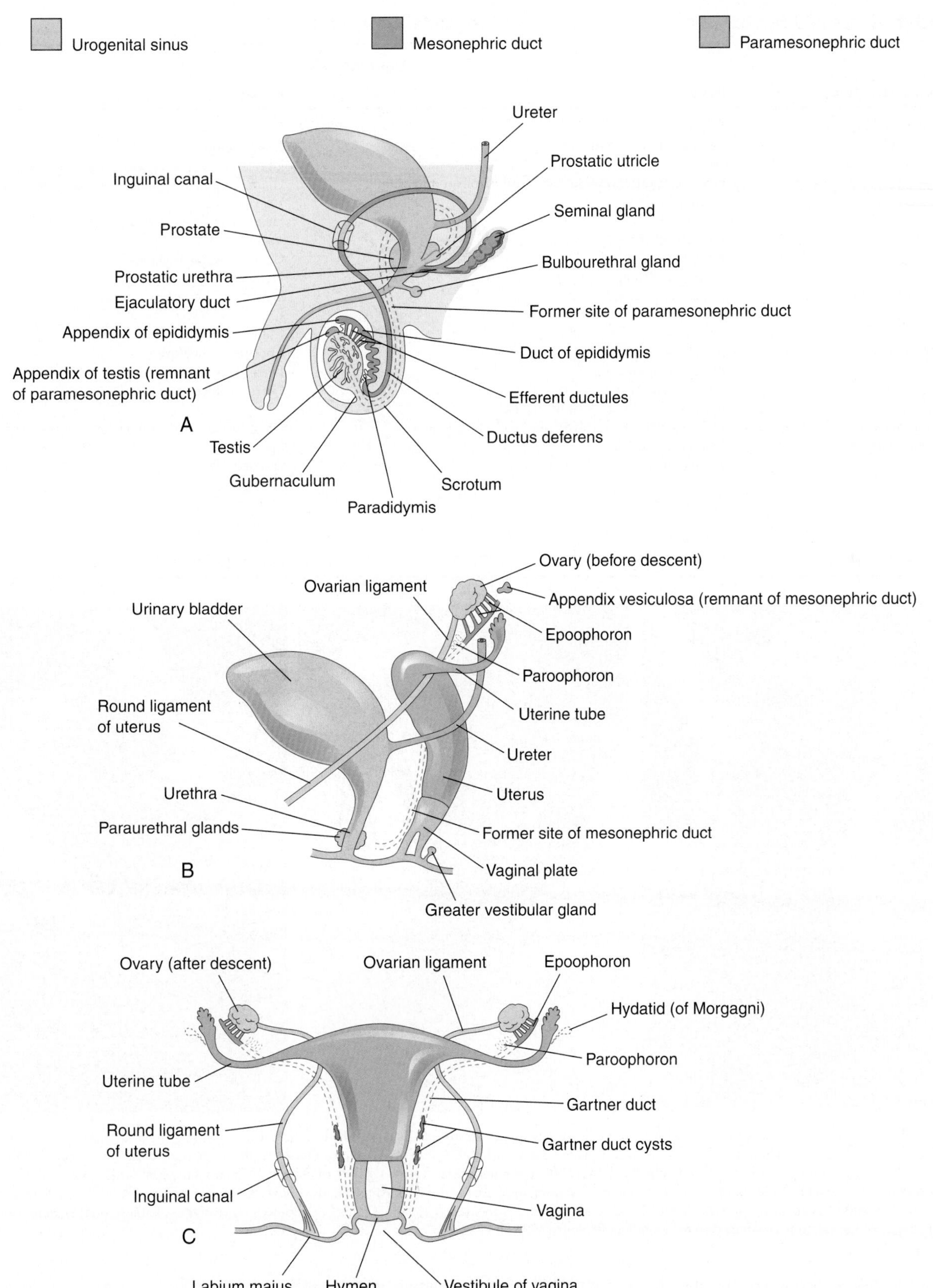

Figure 1-13. Schematic drawings illustrating development of the male and female reproductive systems from the genital ducts and urogenital sinus. Vestigial structures are also shown. **A,** Reproductive system in a newborn male. **B,** Female reproductive system in a 12-week fetus. **C,** Reproductive system in a newborn female (From Moore KL, Persaud TVN: The Developing Human: Clinically Oriented Embryology, 7th ed. Philadelphia, WB Saunders, 2003.)

Table 1-2 Male and Female Derivatives of Embryonic Urogenital Structures

	DERIVATIVES	
Embryonic Structure	**Male**	**Female**
Labioscrotal swellings	Scrotum	Labia majora
Urogenital folds	Ventral portion of penis	Labia minora
Phallus	Penis	Clitoris
	Glans, corpora cavernosa penis, and corpus spongiosum	Glans, corpora cavernosa, bulb of the vestibule
Urogenital sinus	Urinary bladder	Urinary bladder
	Prostate gland	Urethral and paraurethral glands
	Prostatic utricle	Vagina
	Bulbourethral glands	Greater vestibular glands
	Seminal colliculus	Hymen
Paramesonephric duct	Appendix of testes	Hydatid of Morgagni
		Uterus and cervix
		Fallopian tubes
Mesonephric duct	Appendix of epididymis	Appendix vesiculosis
	Ductus of epididymis	Duct of epoophoron
	Ductus deferens	Gartner's duct
	Ejaculatory duct and seminal vesicle	—
Metanephric duct	Ureters, renal pelvis, calyces, and collecting system	Ureter, renal pelvis, calyces, and collecting system
Mesonephric tubules	Ductuli efferentes	Epoophoron
	Paradidymis	Paroophoron
Undifferentiated gonad	Testis	Ovary
Cortex	Seminiferous tubules	Ovarian follicles
Medulla	—	Medulla
	Rete testis	Rete ovarii
Gubernaculum	Gubernaculum testis	Round ligament of uterus

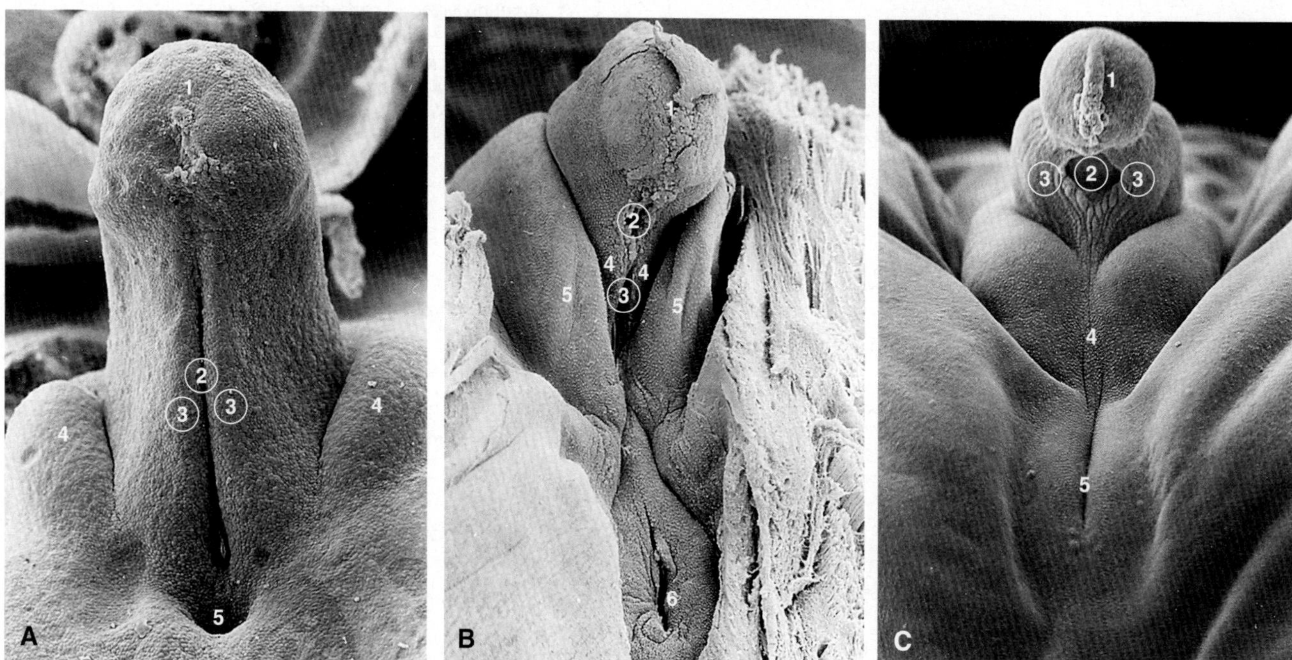

Figure 1-14. Scanning electron micrographs (SEMs) of the developing male external genitalia. **A,** SEM of the perineum during the indifferent state of a 17-mm, 7-week embryo (×100). 1, Developing glans of penis with the ectodermal cord. 2, Urethral groove continuous with the urogenital sinus. 3, Urogenital folds. 4, Labioscrotal swellings. 5, Anus. **B,** External genitalia of a 7.2-cm, 10-week female fetus (×45). 1, Glans of clitoris. 2, External urethral orifice. 3, Opening into urogenital sinus. 4, Urogenital folds (labia minora). 5, Labioscrotal swelling (labia majora). 6, Anus. **C,** SEM of the external genitalia of a 5.5-cm, 10-week male fetus (×40). 1, Glans of penis with ectodermal cord. 2, Remains of urethral groove. 3, Urogenital folds in the process of closing. 4, Labioscrotal swelling fusing to form the raphe of the scrotum. 5, Anus. (From Moore KL, Persaud TVN: The Developing Human: Clinically Oriented Embryology, 7th ed. Philadelphia, WB Saunders, 2003.)

grows in length to form a penis, and the urogenital folds are pulled forward to form the lateral walls of the urethral groove on the undersurface of the penis. These folds then fuse to form the penile urethra. Defects in fusion of various amounts give rise to various degrees of hypospadias. The skin at the distal margin of the penis grows over the glans to form the prepuce (foreskin). The vascular portion of the penis (corpora cavernosa penis and corpus cavernosum urethrae) arises from the mesenchymal tissue of the phallus. Finally, the labioscrotal swellings grow toward each other and fuse in the midline to form the

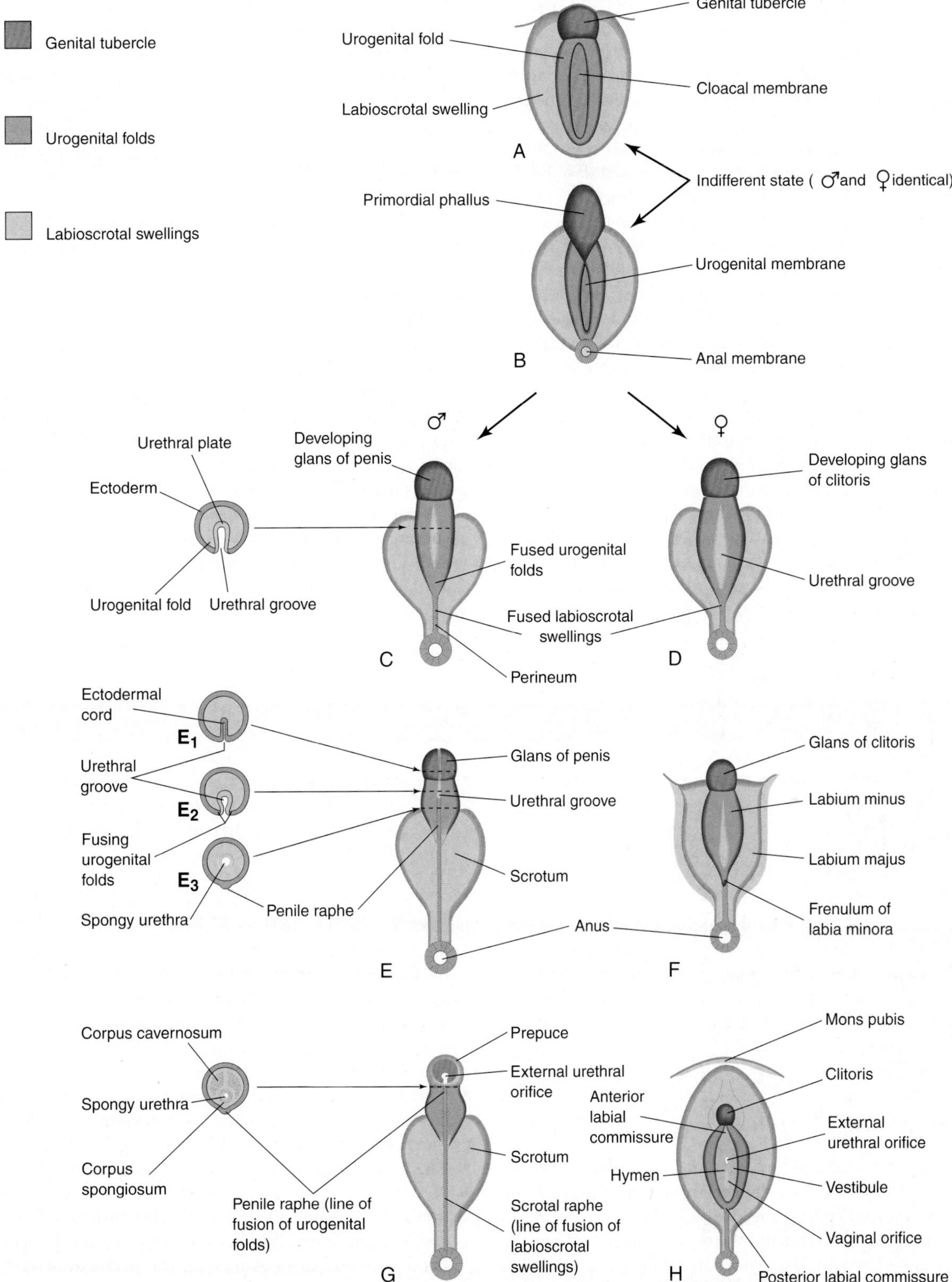

Figure 1-15. Development of the external genitalia. **A** and **B,** Diagrams illustrating the appearance of the genitalia during the indifferent state (fourth to seventh weeks). **C, E,** and **G,** Stages in the development of male external genitalia at 9, 11, and 12 weeks, respectively. To the left are schematic transverse sections of the developing penis, illustrating formation of the spongy urethra. **D, F,** and **H,** Stages in the development of female genitalia at 9, 11, and 12 weeks, respectively. (From Moore KL, Persaud TVN: The Developing Human: Clinically Oriented Embryology, 7th ed. Philadelphia, WB Saunders, 2003.)

scrotum. Later in embryonic life, usually at about the twenty-eighth week, the testes descend through the inguinal canal guided by the gubernaculum.

Androgen receptors have been found in the fetus in the corpus cavernosum and the stroma of the inner prepuce, scrotum, and periphery of the glans penis. The periurethral mesenchyme, the early progenitor of the corpus spongiosum is also very rich in androgen receptors. The epithelium of the preputial skin, penile shaft skin, and scrotal skin are initially androgen-receptor-negative. No estrogen receptors have been noted in these regions, suggesting that maternal estrogen has no direct influence on male genital development. Female external genital structures also contain androgen receptors, and the distribution of androgen receptors resembles that of the male. This would explain why female genitalia can be masculinized if exposed to high androgen levels early in gestation. Diseases of incomplete or absent masculinazation of a male (XY karyotype) fetus may occur for three reasons: (1) inadequate or deficient secretion of androgens or peripheral conversion of testosterone to dihydrotestosterone, (2) absence or deficient receptors, or (3) deficient or absent AMH.

Feminization of the undifferentiated external genitalia occurs in the absence of androgen stimulation. The embryonic phallus does not demonstrate rapid growth and becomes the clitoris. Urogenital folds do not fuse except in front of the anus. The unfused urogenital folds form the labia minora. The labioscrotal folds fuse posteriorly in the area of the perineal body but laterally remain as the labia majora. Beyond 12 weeks' gestation, the labioscrotal folds will not fuse if the fetus is exposed to androgens, though masculinization may occur in other organs of the external genitalia. The labioscrotal folds fuse anteriorly to form the mons pubis. A portion of the urogenital sinus between the level of the hymen and the labia develops into the vestibule of the vagina, into which the urethra, the vagina, and the ducts of Bartholin glands enter. The work of Kalloo and coworkers demonstrated that female external genitalia are intensely estrogen-receptor-positive compared with the genitalia of the male. These receptors may be seen primarily in the stroma of the labia minora and in the periphery of the glans and interprepuce. The presence of such receptors suggests that there may be a direct role of maternal estrogens in the development of female external genitalia. This is in contrast to the long-held belief that female genital development was passive and occurred in the absence of androgens. Virilization, masculinazation, of a female (karyotype XX) fetus may occur from exposure to androgens, either from the mother or through fetal androgens due to genetic deficiencies in the steroid biosynthetic pathway such as occurs in congenital adrenal hyperplasia.

The ovaries do not descend into the labioscrotal folds. A structure similar to the gubernaculum develops in the inguinal canal, giving rise to the round ligaments, which suspend the uterus in the adult. Figure 1-15 summarizes the development of the external genitalia in each sex.

KEY POINTS

- Oocyte meiosis is arrested at prophase I from the fetal period until the time of ovulation.
- Fertilization occurs in the ampulla of the fallopian tube before the second polar body is cast off.
- After fertilization, first cell division leading to the two-cell embryo takes 20 hr.
- The human embryo enters the uterus somewhere between 3 and 4 days after conception. Preimplantation genetic diagnosis in conjunction with IVF techniques could be accomplished at this time. By the time the embryo enters the uterus, it will be between the 32-cell and blastocyst stages of development.
- Implantation occurs when trophoblastic cells contact endometrium and burrow beneath the surface by enzymatic action. This generally takes place 3 days after the embryo enters the uterus.
- Twinning may occur at any time until the formation of the blastula, after which time each cell is no longer pluripotent.
- The earliest fetal epithelium to develop is the ectoderm; the second is the endoderm; and the third is the mesoderm.
- HCG is secreted by the syncytiotrophoblast at about the time of implantation. It doubles in quantity every 1.2–2 days until 7–9 weeks' gestation.
- Angiogenesis is seen by day 15 or 16. Embryonic heart function begins in the third week of gestation.
- Organogenesis is complete by postconception day 49.
- The mesonephric duct system gives rise in the male to the epididymis, vas deferens, and seminal vesicles. Remnants of the mesonephric duct system in the female remain as parovarian cysts and the Gartner duct.
- The paramesonephric duct system develops in the female to give rise to the fallopian tube, uterus, and cervix. Remnants give rise to the hydatid of Morgagni at the end of the fallopian tubes. Remnants in the male remain as the appendix of the testes and prostatic utricle. This duct system is suppressed in the male by the action of AMH.
- The vagina develops from the sinovaginal bulbs, which are outgrowths of the urogenital sinus. Failure of these bulbs to form leads to agenesis of the vagina.
- The adult kidney develops from the metanephros, and its collecting system (ureter and calyceal system) develops from the metanephric (ureteric) bud from the mesonephric duct.
- The urinary bladder develops from the urogenital sinus.
- A Y chromosome is responsible for the development of testes. Without the presence of a Y chromosome, the gonadal development is usually that of an ovary or is undifferentiated. If no testicular tissue is present, the paramesonephric duct system develops into a phenotypic female configuration, and the mesonephric duct system is suppressed.
- The genital tubercle elongates to form the penis in the male and the clitoris in the female.
- Two functional X chromosomes are necessary for optimal development of the ovary.

BIBLIOGRAPHY

Recommended Reading

Delhanty JD, Harper JC: Pre-implantation genetic diagnosis. Ballieres Best Pract Res Clin Obstet Gynaecol 14(4):691, 2000.

Feckner P: The role of Sry in mammalian sex determination. Acta Paediatr Jpn 38:380, 1996.

Moore KL, Persaud TVN: The Developing Human: Clinically Oriented Embryology, 7th ed., Philadelphia, 2003, WB Saunders.

General References

Amice B, Bercovic JP, Nahoul K, et al: Increase in H-Y antigen-positive lymphocytes in hirsute women: Effects of cyproterone acetate and estradiol treatment. J Clin Endocrinol Metab 68:58, 1989.

Blackmore P, Beebe S, Danforth D, Alexander N: Progesterone and 19-alpha-hydroxyprogesterone level stimulators of calcium influx in human sperm. J Biol Chem 265:1376, 1990.

Bourdelat D, Barbet JP, Butler-Browne GS: Fetal development of the urethral sphincter, Eur J Pediatr Surg 2:35, 1992.

Cohen-Dayag A, Ralt D, Tur-Kaspa I, et al: Sequential acquisition of chemotactic responsiveness by human spermatozoa. Biol Reprod 50:786, 1994.

Cheng EY, Gartler SM: A fluorescent in situ hybridization analysis of X chromosome pairing in early human meiosis. Hum Genet 94:389, 1994.

Coutelle C, Williams C, Handyside A, et al: Genetic analysis of DNA from single human oocytes: A model for preimplantation diagnosis of cystic fibrosis. BMJ 229(6690):22, 1989.

GeneTests: Medical Genetics Information Resource (database online). Educational Materials: Preimplantation diagnosis. University of Washington, Seattle. 1993–2005. Available at http://www.genetests.org. Accessed 2/2005.

Handyside AH, Pattinson JK, Penketh RJ, et al: Biopsy of human preimplantation embryos and sexing by DNA amplification. Lancet 1(8634):347, 1989.

Hartman CG: Science and the Safe Period: A Compendium of Human Reproduction, Huntington, NY, RE Krieger, 1972.

Harvey VR, Jackson DI, Hextal PJ, et al: DNA binding activity of recombinant SRY from normal males and XY females. Science 225:453, 1992.

Heap RV, Flint AP, Gadsby JE: Role of embryonic signals in the establishment of pregnancy. BMJ 35:129, 1979.

Hsu L: Phenotype/karyotype correlations of Y chromosome aneuploidy with emphasis on structural aberrations in postnatally diagnosed cases. Am J Med Genet 53:108, 1994.

Kalloo NB, Gearhart JP, Barrack ER: Sexually dimorphic expression of estrogen receptors, but not of androgen receptors in human fetal external genitalia. J Clin Endocrinol Metab 77:692, 1993.

Kokoua A, Homsy Y, Lavigne JF, et al: Maturation of the external urinary sphincter: A comparative histotopographic study in humans. J Urol 150:617, 1993.

Koopman P, Gubbay J, Vivian N, et al: Male development of chromosomally female mice transgenic for Sry. Nature 351:117, 1991.

Lovell-Badge R: Sex determining gene expression during embryogenesis. Philos Trans R Soc Lond B Biol Sci 27:339, 1993.

Mohr LR, Trounson AO, Leeton JF, Wood C: Evaluation of normal and abnormal human embryo development during procedures in vitro. In Beier HM, Lindner HR (eds): Fertilization of Human Egg in Vitro, Berlin, Springer-Verlag, 1983.

Moor RM, Warnes RM: Meiosis in mammalian oocytes. Br Med Bull 35:97, 1979.

Oeheninger S, Blackmore P, Morshedi M, et al: Defective calcium influx and acrosome reaction (spontaneous and progesterone-induced) in spermatozoa of infertile men with severe teratozoospermia. Fertil Steril 61:349, 1994.

Parhar RS, Yagel S, Lala PK: PGE-2-mediated immunosuppressive by first trimester: Human decidual cells block activation of maternal leukocytes in the decidua with potential antitrophoblast activity. Cell Immunol 120:61, 1989.

Patton HD, Fuchs AF, Hill EB, et al: Textbook of Physiology, vol 2, Philadelphia, WB Saunders, 1989.

Pietryga E, Wózniak W: The development of the uterine ligaments in human fetuses. Folia Morphol 51:181, 1992.

Ralt D, Goldenberg M, Fetterolf P, et al: Sperm attraction of follicular factor(s) correlated with human egg fertilizability. Proc Natl Acad Sci USA 88:2840, 1991.

Ralt D, Manor M, Cohen-Dayag A, et al: Chemotaxis and chemokinesis of human spermatozoa to follicular factor. Biol Reprod 50:774, 1994.

Sinclair AH, Berta P, Palmer MS, et al: A gene from the human sex-determining region encodes a protein with homology to a conserved DNA-binding motif. Nature 346:240, 1990.

Thomas P, Meiezel S: Phosphatidylinositol 4,5-bisphosphate hydrolysis in human sperm stimulated with follicular fluid on progesterone is dependent on Ca^{++} influx. Biochem J 264:539, 1989.

Tsafriri A: Oocyte maturation in mammals. In Jones RE (ed): The Vertebrate Ovary. New York, Plenum, 1978.

Tsafriri A, Bar-Ami S, Lindner HR: Control of the development of meiotic competence in an oocyte maturation in mammals. In Beier HM, Lindner HR (eds): Fertilization of the Human Egg in Vitro, Berlin, Springer-Verlag, 1983.

Villanueva-Diaz C, Arias-Martinez J, Bernejo-Martinez L, Vadillo-Ortega F: Progesterone indices human sperm chemotaxis. Fertil Steril 64:1183, 1995.

Whittingham DG: In-vitro fertilization, embryo transfer and storage. Br Med Bull 35:105, 1979.

Yang J, Seres C, Philibet D, et al: Progesterone and RU 486: Opposing effects on human sperm. Proc Natl Acad Sci USA 91:529, 1994.

Reproductive Genetics

2

Gene Structure, Mutation, Molecular Tools, Types of Inheritance, Counseling Issues, Oncogenes

Edith Cheng and Vern L. Katz

KEY TERMS AND DEFINITIONS

Allele. One of the alternative versions of a gene that occupy a given locus (the physical location of a gene).

Centromere. A region of a chromosome, forming a point at which the chromatids are held together during meiosis and mitosis. A primary constriction, the centromere, divides the chromosome into two "arms" designated p and q.

Chimerism. The presence of two different cell populations derived from two separate conceptuses within the same individual. Acquired chimerism is a result of transplantation.

Chromatid. A constituent strand of a chromosome seen in prophase, after division of the chromosomes.

Chromatid Break. Separation in chromatin material in only one chromatid arm.

Chromosome. Threadlike structures of chromatin containing genetic information (DNA) located in the cell nucleus.

Codon. A sequence of 3 bases in a DNA molecule specifying the code for a specific amino acid.

Deletion. The loss of a sequence of DNA of varying amounts from a chromosome.

Exon. The coding region of a gene.

Expressivity. The degree to which the features of a genetic defect is expressed.

Fragment. A small piece of chromosome separated from its centromere.

Gene. A unit of genetic information, a sequence of nucleotides that forms the code for the production of a functional product.

Genome. A complete complement of genes in a gamete, an individual, a population, or a species.

Genotype. The genetic make-up of an individual, the alleles at one locus.

Insertion. A condition in which a segment of DNA from one chromosome is inserted into another chromosome.

Intron. Noncoding region of a gene. A gene will have many introns intervening between the coding regions (exons).

Inversion. A condition occurring when a chromosome suffers two breaks with a 180° rotation of the fragments. If the centromere is involved in the inversion, the condition is called a pericentric inversion. If the centromere is not included, it is called a paracentric inversion.

Isochromosome. An abnormal chromosome that is produced by a transverse split instead of the usual longitudinal split of the centromere. The daughter chromosome formed will have either of the two identical arms while the other arm is missing.

Karyotype. An arrangement of all the chromosomes of a cell at metaphase in descending order of size.

Locus. The physical location of a gene on a chromosome. There may be alternative forms of the gene (alleles).

Mosaicism. The presence of two or more genetically different cell types derived from a single zygote within the same individual. This is not to be confused with chimera, in which the different cell types in one individual are derived from two different zygotes.

Mutation. A permanent and heritable alteration in DNA sequence.

Nondisjunction. The failure of a pair of chromosomes to separate during meiosis or mitosis. In meiosis, if one daughter cell receives both members of the chromosome pair, after fertilization a triple number of the chromosome, or a trisomic state, exists in each cell.

Oncogene. A gene that acts in a dominant fashion to unregulate cell growth and proliferation, resulting in tumor development.

Penetrance. The fraction of individuals with a mutation that actually demonstrates any clinical features of the mutation. Generally refers to autosomal dominant conditions.

Phenotype. The observed characteristics of a gene. This can be biochemical, physical, or physiological.

Pleiotropic. Description of genes that have multiple diverse clinical effects on the affected individual.

Polymerase Chain Reaction (PCR). The process by which a small segment of DNA may be amplified to produce larger amounts of materials for analysis.

Polymorphism. Natural variations of a gene, DNA sequence, or chromosome that does not have adverse clinical consequence. Generally, the frequency of a polymorphism in the general population is at least 0.01 (1%) or greater than that which would occur by recurrent mutation alone.

Restriction Endonucleases. Bacterial enzymes that recognize and cut specific nucleotide sequences in the double-stranded DNA molecule at specific sites.

Restriction Fragment Length Polymorphism (RFLP). The study of DNA fragments produced by restriction endonucleases has demonstrated that normal individuals may have variations in the DNA

Continued

KEY TERMS AND DEFINITIONS *Continued*

sequences without the presence of an abnormality. RFLPs are generated using restriction endonucleases and can indirectly identify mutations in a gene that is near a polymorphic site.

Ribonucleic Acid (RNA). A single-helix nuclear protein that serves several purposes in the cell. It is composed of a sugar (ribose), a phosphate, and a purine or pyrimidine base.

Translocation. The transfer of a segment of chromosome material from one chromosome to another.

A number of illnesses and conditions have a genetic basis. In some cases the problem arises from a single-point mutation within a gene, whereas others may involve changes in multiple genes or in an interreaction of genes and environmental factors. Finally, some conditions are the result of chromosome abnormalities of a variety of types. Although this chapter cannot provide a complete course in genetics, it attempts to offer an understanding of the genetic basis of conditions of particular interest to the gynecologist.

GENE STRUCTURE, EXPRESSION, AND MUTATION

Genetic information is stored in the form of deoxyribonucleic acid (DNA) molecules, which are made up of a linear sequence of nucleotides intertwined together as a double helix. The backbone of the linear DNA molecule is composed of a phosphate and a pentose sugar (deoxyribose) to which is attached a nitrogen base. Four such bases are found in a DNA molecule: two purines [adenine (A) and guanine (G)] and two pyrimidines [thymine (T) and cytosine (C)]. Purine and pyrimidine occur in equal amounts; A is always paired with T in the two strands of the double helix, and G is always paired with C. These associations allow for accuracy both in the replication of the DNA molecule and in the translation of a genetic message from the DNA molecule to a single-strand ribonucleic acid (RNA) molecule known as *messenger RNA* (mRNA). The message is transmitted in such a fashion that a configuration with three bases in sequence (codon) represents a code, known as the *genetic code,* for an amino acid. With the message of the gene encoded on the mRNA, the latter leaves the nucleus of the cell, attaches to a cytoplasmic structure (the ribosome), and then attracts amino acids by means of smaller RNA molecules known as *transfer RNA (tRNA).* Transfer RNA molecules each carry a specific amino acid and have three bases, which match the code of the mRNA, following the A-to-T and G-to-C pairings. In the RNA molecule, uracil (U) is substituted for thymine. When all segments of the message are covered, the amino acids are spliced together and the protein determined by the message is complete and free for use in the cell and for transport from the cell. Figure 2-1 schematically demonstrates this process.

In its simplest form, a gene is a sequence of codons that, when transcribed and translated, will become a functional product. However, with the exception of a few organisms, the sequences of base pairs that actually form a gene in eukaryotes are very complex and provide many opportunities for different types of mutations to occur. Figure 2-2 illustrates the structure of a typical human gene. Most genes have a promoter region and transcriptional start point, both of which are necessary to begin transcription. Within the gene itself, regions of coding sequences (exons) are interspaced with noncoding regions (introns). At the end of the gene, there is a termination site and other regulatory elements that end the transcriptional process for that gene.

Transcription occurs through both intron and exon portions of the gene and beyond the position on the chromosome that corresponds to the most distal part of the gene. The resulting primary RNA transcript then undergoes many post-transcriptional modifications, including splicing out the introns and splicing together the exons, placing a "chemical cap" on the 5′ end and a "tail" of adenosine nucleotides (poly A) at the 3′ end. The poly A tail appears to stabilize the mature mRNA, which is now ready for transport into the cytoplasm for translation. In the cytoplasm, after translation, the resultant protein often undergoes further post-translational modifications.

A gene mutation occurs when there has been a change in the genetic code; these changes are the source of genetic variation. The mutation may involve changing a single base, known as a point mutation, or a larger segment, in which bases are removed, duplicated, or inserted. Mutations occur as a result of environmental damage to DNA, through errors during DNA replication or repair, and through uneven crossing over and genetic exchange during meiosis. The loss or gain of bases may disrupt the reading frame of the triplet codons. The consequences depend on the location of the mutation: In a promoter region, it may enhance or prevent transcription; in splice site junctions between introns and exons, there may be duplications or deletions of those sequences such that the resulting mRNA cannot be translated into a functional product; or mutations could affect the poly A tail and thus the stability of the mRNA. The position of the mutation in the gene is also important; a mutation at the beginning of the gene can be so disruptive that transcription ceases at the site of the mutation. No mRNA is generated and therefore, no gene product. Conversely, a mutation at the end of the gene may result in a truncated but still translatable mRNA, leading to a partially functional gene product. Point mutations within the gene could result in an amino acid substitution, leading to different products with altered functions. Figure 2-3 demonstrates such an occurrence for sickle cell anemia caused by the substitution of a single base at a single point. The cystic fibrosis transmembrane conductance regulator (CFTR) gene is an example of a gene for which over 1000 mutations or alleles have been described to date. Some genes also have regions that are more prone (hot spots) to mutational events.

In spite of the potential clinical importance of mutations, only a small fraction of the genome, about 2% to 5% actually encodes protein or has regulatory significance. In addition, most base pair changes in coding sequences do not lead to a change in amino acid substitution. These mutations are known as silent

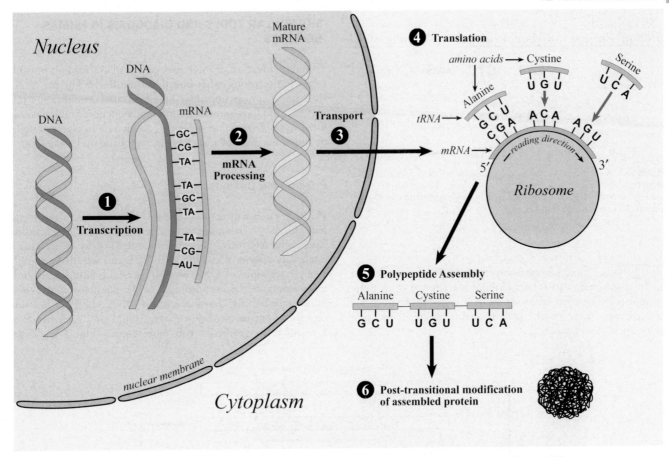

Figure 2-1. Schematic representation of polypeptide production from genetic message to final product. (Courtesy of Edith Cheng, MD.)

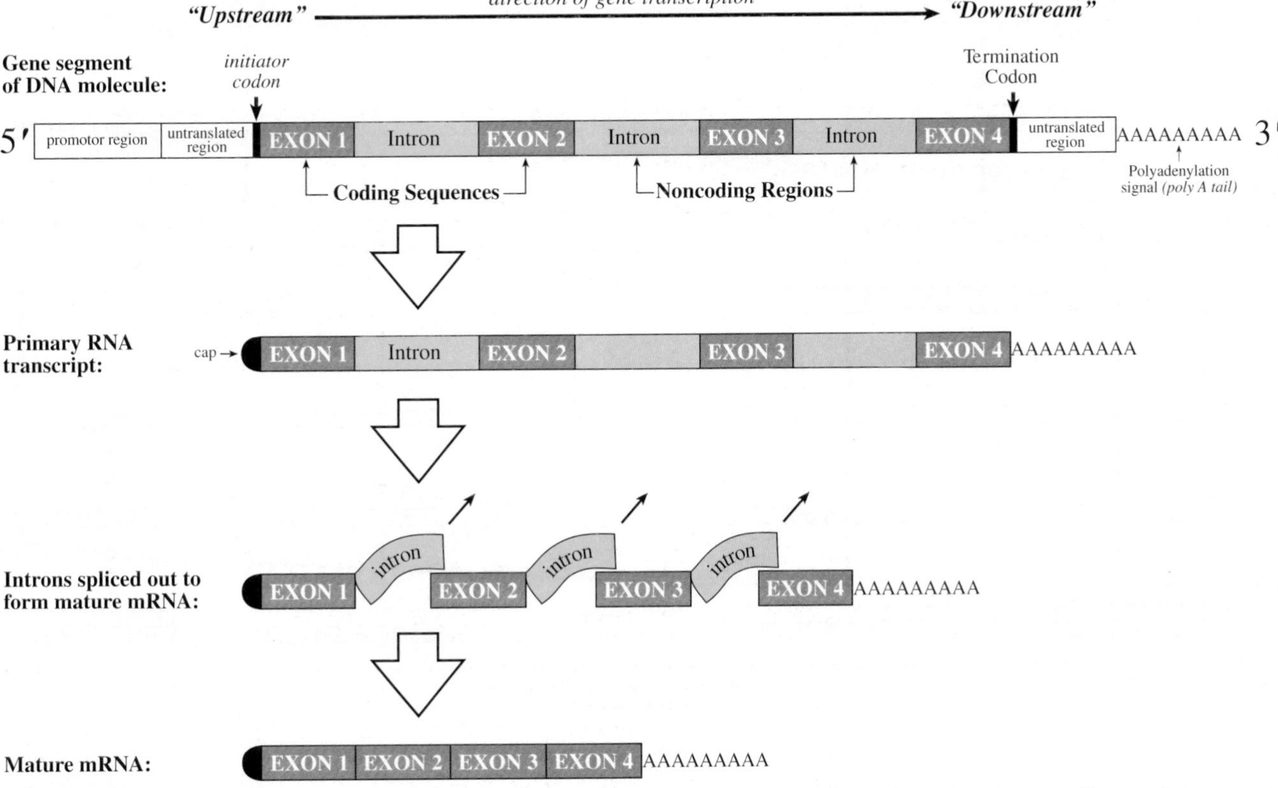

Figure 2-2. Structure of typical human gene and its processing to become a mature mRNA transcript for translation. Mutations can affect any of these steps. (Courtesy of Edith Cheng, MD.)

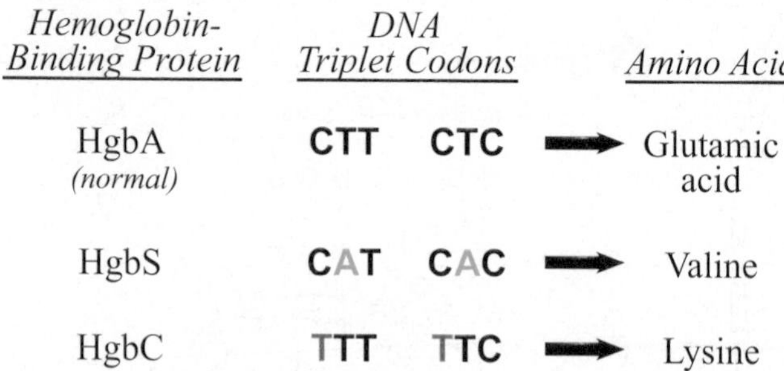

Hemoglobin-Binding Protein
DNA Triplet Codons
Amino Acid
HgbA (normal)
CTT CTC
Glutamic acid
HgbS
CAT CAC
Valine
HgbC
TTT TTC
Lysine

Figure 2-3. A single base pair substitution in the same DNA triplet codon for glutamic acid at amino acid position 6 for normal hemoglobin results in hemoglobin S (valine in sickle cell disease), or hemoglobin C (lysine in Hgb C disease). (Courtesy of Edith Cheng, MD.)

substitutions. These benign substitutions are generally passed on from generation to generation and are referred to as polymorphisms. The term *mutation* then, is generally reserved for new changes in the genetic code that lead to altered function and clinical consequences.

MOLECULAR TOOLS AND DIAGNOSIS IN HUMAN GENETICS

Technical advances in molecular genetics have made it possible to study mutations either directly or indirectly. The use of polymerase chain reaction (PCR) permits rapid amplification of a sequence of DNA or multiple different sequences simultaneously for analysis. This section will cover common molecular techniques of which the gynecologist should have a basic understanding.

Polymerase Chain Reaction

PCR has essentially revolutionized DNA diagnostics and medicine. Our daily laboratory assessment of the subject's medical issues now rely heavily on material amplified by PCR. This is essentially a form of cloning since PCR can selectively amplify a single sequence of DNA or RNA several billion-fold in only a few hours. By taking advantage of the double-stranded complimentary pairing characteristics of DNA, the PCR reaction separates (denatures) the two strands and uses each strand as a template to synthesize two more copies (Fig. 2-4). Target

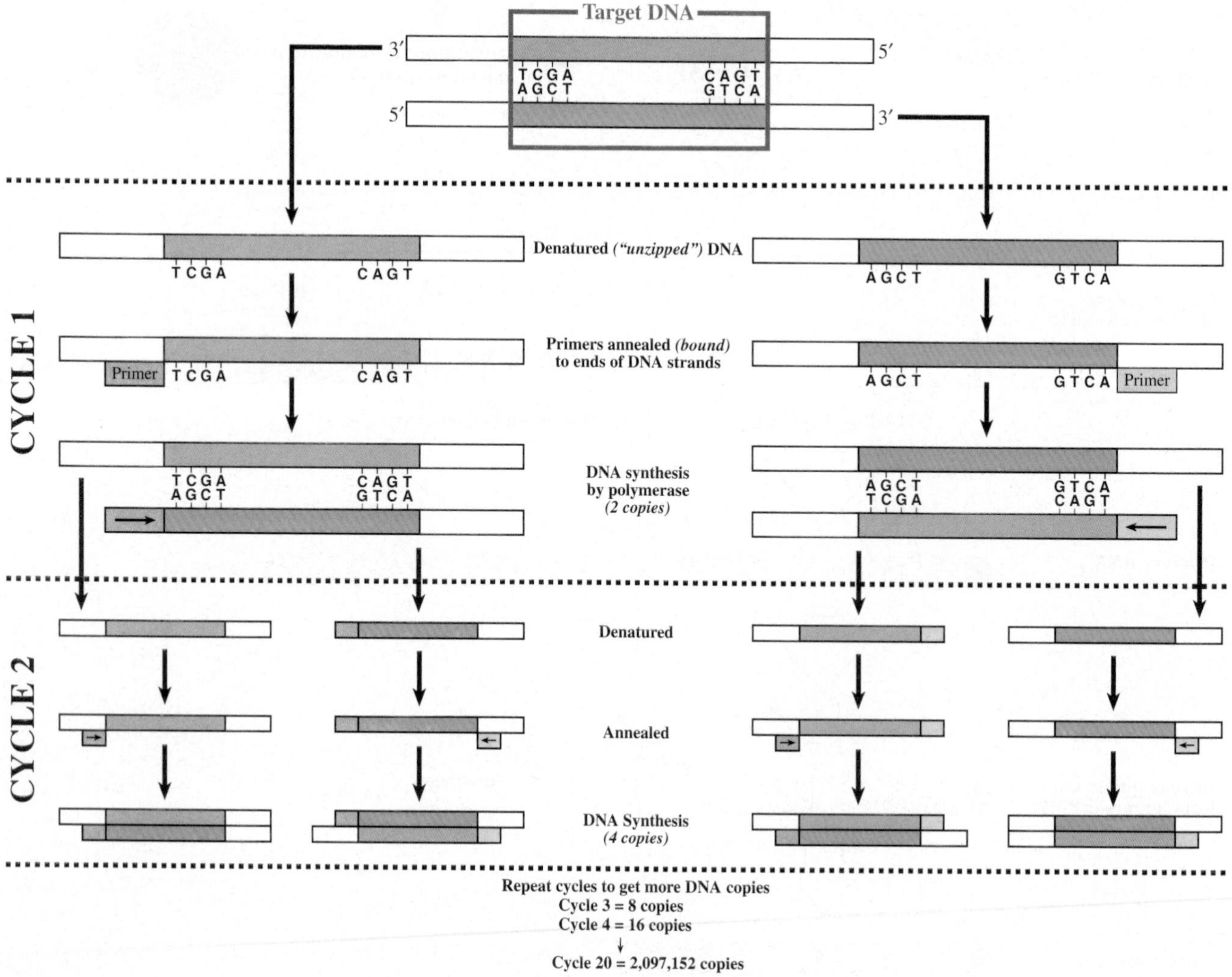

Figure 2-4. Schematic representation of the polymerase chain reaction (PCR). (Courtesy of Edith Cheng, MD.)

sequences of DNA flanked by primers undergo repeated cycles of heat penetration, hybridization with primers, and DNA synthesis, resulting in an exponential amplification of the target DNA sequence.

Restriction Endonucleases and Restriction Fragment Length Polymorphisms

The key to the analysis of DNA sequences has been the discovery of a group of more than 1000 bacterial enzymes, called restriction endonucleases, that recognize and cut specific nucleotide sequences in the double-stranded DNA molecule. The sites of their action are known as restriction sites. Each enzyme recognizes a unique sequence of nucleotides, usually a palindrome of 4 to 8 base pairs (bp) in length, and will cut the double-stranded DNA molecule wherever the specific site is recognized. For example, *Hin*dIII cuts the palindromic site 5′-AAGCTT-3′ at A and T. Table 2-1 lists some of the more commonly used restriction endonucleases and there cut sites. Restriction endonucleases are used to digest a sample of DNA (e.g., extracted from a subject for carrier testing) into a collection of DNA fragments in varying sizes. These fragments are then separated by gel electrophoresis according to size and denatured into single strands, which are then transferred (blotted) onto a nitrocellulose or nylon filter. The single-stranded DNA sequences of interest are then hybridized with the known sequence, which has been radioactively labeled (probe). The hybridized sequences are then detected. This method, known as Southern blotting, permits identification of specific DNA fragments of interest and in some cases, the number of copies of the fragment. Figure 2-5 is an example of how Southern blotting is used to detect the sickle cell gene. Some cut sites of restriction endonucleases result in "sticky ends," such as those generated by *Eco*RI. This property of *Eco*RI is used to create recombinant DNA. Benign base pair changes at cut sites that alter the recognition site of a restriction endonuclease will result in a change in the fragment size

Table 2-1 Examples of Common Restriction Endonucleases, Their Source and Their Recognition Sequence

Restriction Enzymes	Source	Recognition Sequence
*Bam*HI	*Bacillus amyloliquefaciens* H	5′-G^GATC C-3′ 3′-C CTAG^G-5′
*Eco*RI	*Escherichia coli* RY 13	G^AATT C C TTAA^G
*Hae*III	*Haemophilus aegyptius*	GG^CC CC^GG
*Hin*dIII	*Haemophilus influenzae* R_d	A^AGCT T T TCGA^A
*Not*I	*Nocardia otitidis-cavarium*	GC^GGCC GC CG CCGG^CG
*Sau*3A	*Staphylococcus aureus* 3A	^GATC CTAG^
*Ser*II	*Streptomyces stanford*	CC GC^GG GG^CG CC

^ = cleavage sites.
From Thompson MW, Thompson HFV: Genetics in Medicine, 6th ed. Philadelphia, WB Saunders, 1991.

generated. Mutations within a gene or near a gene can also alter the recognition sites of restriction endonucleases, which will generate an altered length of DNA fragment containing the gene of interest. These restriction fragment length polymorphisms (RFLPs) can be used to follow the transmission of a gene in a family.

Microarray DNA Analysis

Microarray technology, first introduced in 1995, permits the expression and analysis of thousands of genes simultaneously. Initially it was used to understand the molecular basis of cancer and the biological behavior of tumors (Fig. 2-6). This powerful tool can provide a "molecular fingerprint" of an individual's disease and is referred to as gene expression profiling (GEP). Molecular differences revealed by gene expression patterns of individuals with the same condition, such as, type II diabetes, may give insights into the mechanisms contributing to the disease, to its prognosis, and to more specific treatments, such as individualized drug therapy. The use of microarrays have expanded into areas of genetic diagnosis, in which, simultaneous screening for many different genetic conditions in an individual is now possible. In the near future, it will be possible to routinely perform prenatal diagnosis on a sample of amniotic fluid for many conditions on a single microarray chip.

Genetic Testing: Direct and Indirect Methods

For many genetic conditions, the gene and its mutations (e.g., cystic fibrosis) responsible for the condition have been molecularly characterized. In these conditions, direct testing for the actual mutation in an affected individual to confirm the clinical diagnosis, or to provide presymptomatic diagnosis or prenatal diagnosis would be possible by obtaining DNA from the subject. Direct testing or typing of the disease causing the mutation can be accomplished by sequencing the gene itself or through analysis of RFLPS. As in the case with sickle cell anemia, the mutation within the gene itself leads to an alteration that removes a cut site, resulting in a larger fragment that is associated with the mutation. This example also illustrates that the entire hemoglobin gene does not have to be analyzed to identify the mutation responsible for sickle cell anemia.

When "direct testing" is not possible, as in the case when the disease-causing gene has not be isolated, when the gene is too large to sequence, or when a mutation cannot be directly found, indirect testing using linkage analysis is the alternative strategy. This approach does not involve direct examination of the disease-causing mutation. The simplest explanation for this concept is that DNA markers located (or tightly linked) to the presumptive disease-causing gene/mutation are used as road maps to identify the travel or passage of the gene from an affected parent to an at-risk offspring. This strategy requires that the affected individual has markers that are informative, in other words, unique or distinctive from markers of the nonaffected individual. Multiple family members, both affected and unaffected must have DNA available for analysis in order for this approach to be informative. The "markers" are often RFLPs. Figure 2-7 uses autosomal dominant breast cancer as an example

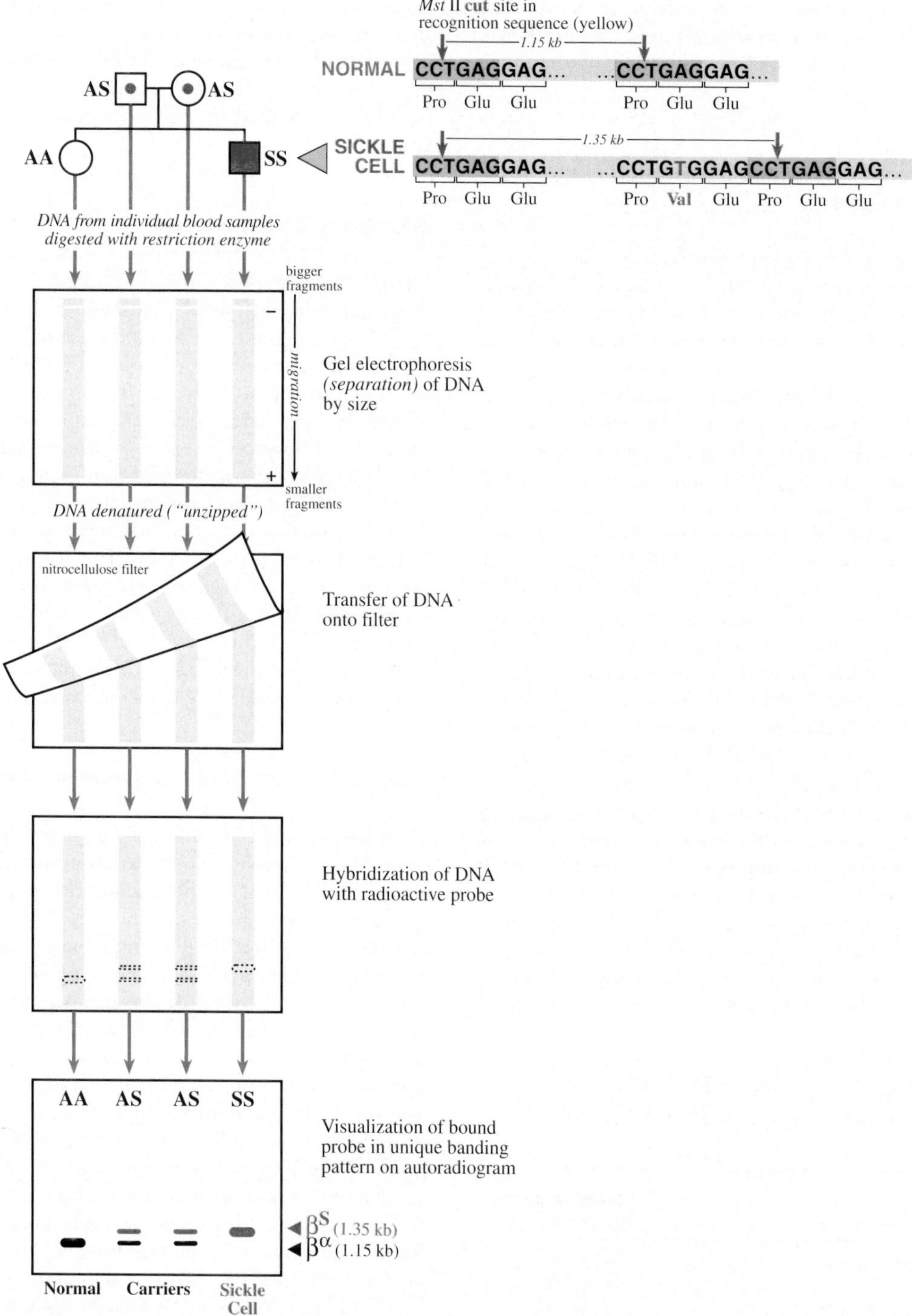

Figure 2-5. Schematic representation of the Southern blot procedure—in the case, for diagnosis of sickle cell disease. Genomic DNA from the carrier parents, an unaffected daughter, and the affected son are extracted from a sample of peripheral blood. The DNA samples are digested with restriction enzymes and fragmented into smaller pieces. In this case, the restriction enzyme *Mst*II is used specifically because it recognizes the normal sequences that encompass the codons for glutamic acid at position 6 of the hemoglobin A polypeptide. The DNA fragments are separated based on size by gel electrophoresis, then transferred (blotted) onto a nitrocellulose filter. The DNA of the filter paper is then hybridized with a specifically labeled DNA probe containing the sequences of interest. The fluorescent or radioactive probe is visualized as bands at sites where the genomic DNA has hybridized with the labeled DNA. (Courtesy of Edith Cheng, MD.)

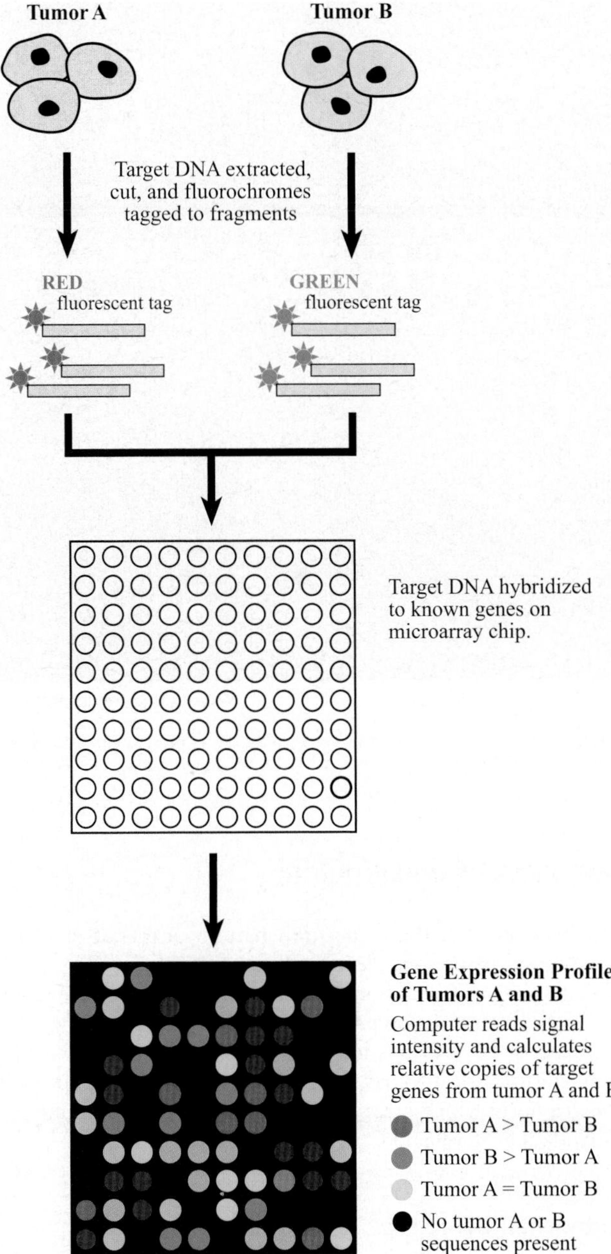

Figure 2-6. Schematic example of how microarray technology can be used to study or compare gene expression patterns from different sources. Here, it is used to compare the gene expression profiles of two different tumors. However, one can easily substitute DNA from two individuals with diabetes. (Courtesy of Edith Cheng, MD.)

of how linkage studies are used to predict the inheritance of a gene for which direct mutational analysis is not possible.

Molecular Cytogenetics

Molecular cytogenetic technology is a powerful tool to analyze chromosome abnormalities (deletions, additions, rearrangements) that are not visible using traditional karyotyping and microscopy. The most widely used procedure is fluorescent in

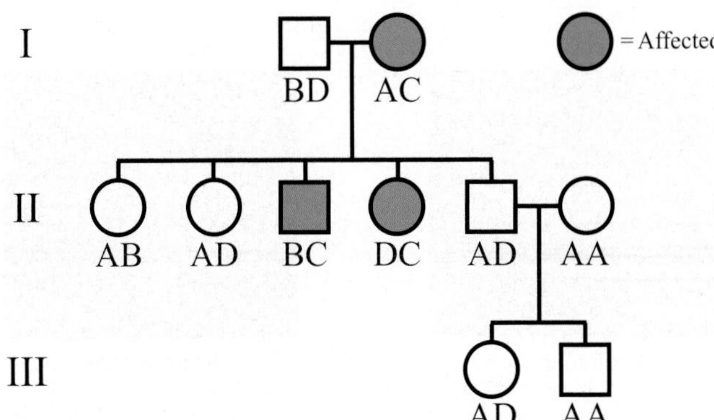

Figure 2-7. Hypothetical autosomal dominant condition illustrating the principle of indirect mutational analysis. Genetic markers A, B, C, D are used. In this pedigree, it appears that the condition segregates (travels) with marker C. Therefore, the male and female in generation III, who did not inherit marker C are not expected to manifest the condition. (Courtesy of Edith Cheng, MD.)

situ hybridization (FISH). Like PCR and Southern blotting, FISH takes advantage of the complimentary nature of DNA. In this approach, denatured DNA sequences labeled with a fluorescent dye are hybridized onto denatured chromosomes that have been immobilized onto a slide. The chromosomes are then viewed with a wavelength of light that excites the fluorescent dye (Fig. 2-8). FISH is used commonly to screen for chromosome aneuploidy in amniotic fluid cells in prenatal diagnosis (Fig. 2-9). FISH is also a powerful tool to confirm or diagnose syndromes that are due to microdeletions of segments of chromosome material (Fig. 2-10). FISH is also used to identify the actual physical location of a gene or to order a series of DNA sequences or genes on a chromosome.

Two other powerful diagnostic and investigational tools for human chromosome analysis directly expanded from FISH technology are comparative genome hybridization (CGH) and

WCP: Chromosomes 1 and 4

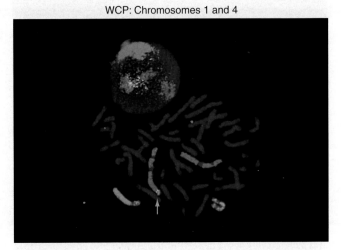

Figure 2-8. Example of FISH (fluorescent in situ hybridization) with whole-chromosome DNA (whole-chromosome paint—WCP) from chromosomes 1 (*red signal*) and 4 (*green signal*) hybridized onto a metaphase nucleus containing all 46 chromosomes. This FISH study revealed a translocation of a piece of material from chromosome 4 onto chromosome 1. (Courtesy of Lisa Shaffer, PhD, Washington State University).

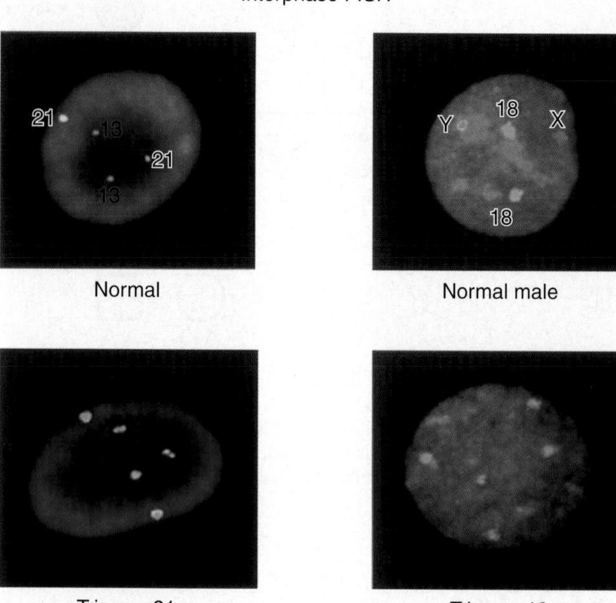

Figure 2-9. Interphase FISH on amniotic fluid cells to screen for aneuploidy. (Courtesy of Edith Cheng, MD.)

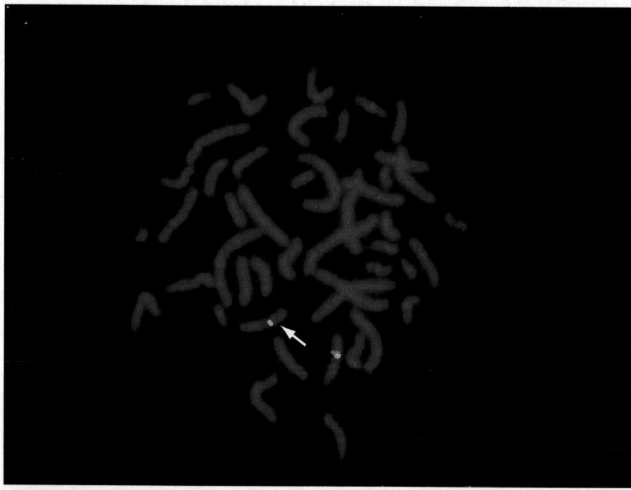

Figure 2-10. Example of FISH technology in the diagnosis of microdeletion syndromes. Here, standard karyotyping appears to be normal. However, using FISH microdeletion probes, this child was discovered to have a submicroscopic deletion (*arrow*) of the terminal section of the long arm of chromosome 1. The other chromosome containing the red signal is the normal chromosome (Courtesy of Lisa Shaffer, PhD, Washington State University).

spectral karyotyping (SKY). CGH is used to measure differences in copy number or dosage of a particular chromosome segment. Its widest application is in the study of gene dosage in normal and cancer cell lines. The second technique, SKY, uses the FISH principle to visualize all 24 chromosomes by "painting" with chromosome-specific probes in different colors simultaneously. Because each chromosome probe emits its own unique wavelength of fluorescence, and therefore color, structural rearrangements and chromosome fragments can be identified (Fig. 2-11).

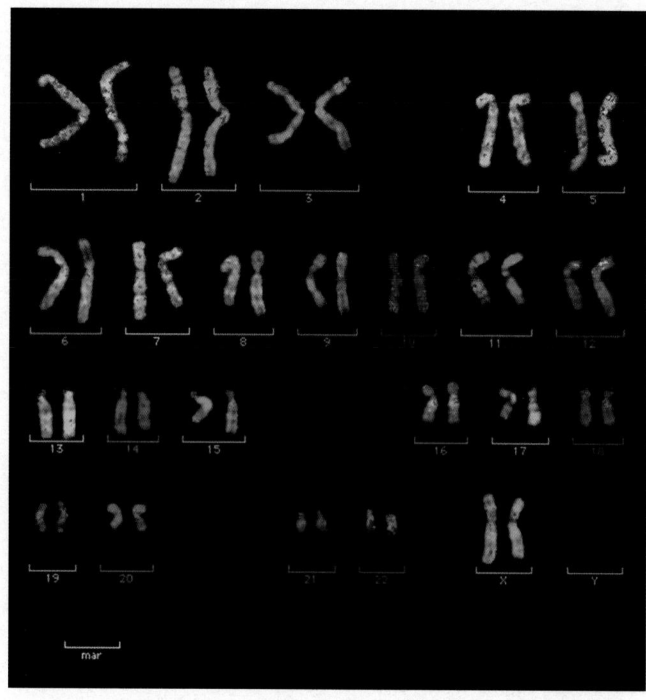

Figure 2-11. Example of spectral karyotyping (SKY) on standard metaphase chromosomes (Courtesy of Lisa Shaffer PhD, Washington State University).

PATTERNS OF INHERITANCE

Any evaluation of the segregation pattern of a trait or disease in a family requires the development of a pedigree (Fig. 2-12). This graphic representation of family history data assists in determining the transmission pattern of the gene. In some conditions, the pattern of transmission and the constellation of clinical characteristics of affected individuals in the pedigree provides the diagnosis, which otherwise would not be evident if only one individual was evaluated.

Autosomal Dominant

In an autosomal dominant mode of inheritance, only one copy of the mutated gene is required for expression of the trait, and the individual is said to be heterozygous for the trait. There are over 4000 known autosomal dominant conditions, and most occur in the heterozygous form in affected individuals. With a few exceptions, autosomal dominant conditions occurring in the homozygous form (two copies of the affected gene) are rare, the phenotype is more severe, and are often lethal.

The general characteristics of autosomal dominant inheritance are illustrated in Figure 2-13 and summarized as follows:

1. Every affected individual has an affected parent (unless this is a new mutation—to be discussed later). The inheritance pattern is vertical.
2. If reproductively fit, the affected person has a 50% risk of transmitting the gene with each pregnancy.
3. The sexes are affected equally.

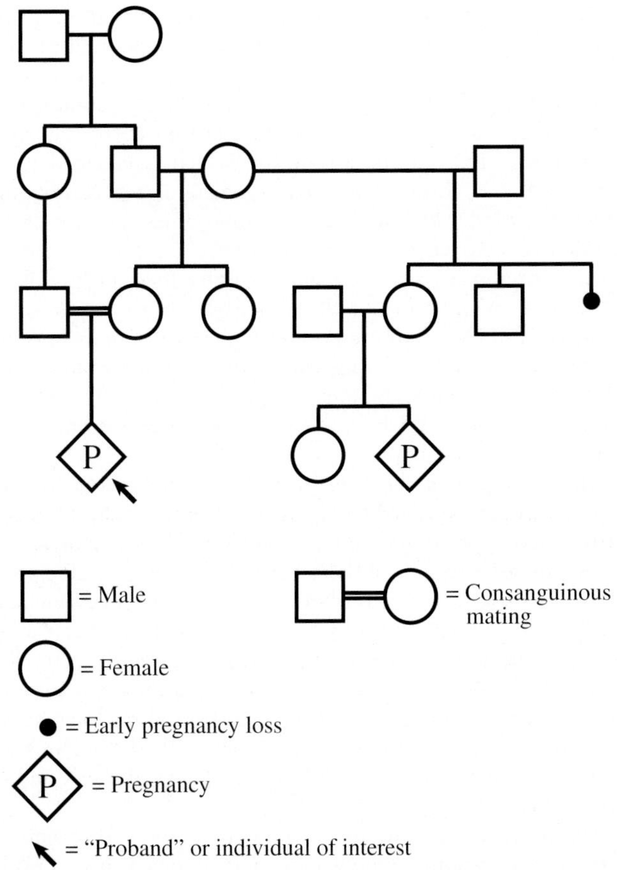

Figure 2-12. Standard figures and nomenclature for a pedigree. (Courtesy of Edith Cheng, MD.)

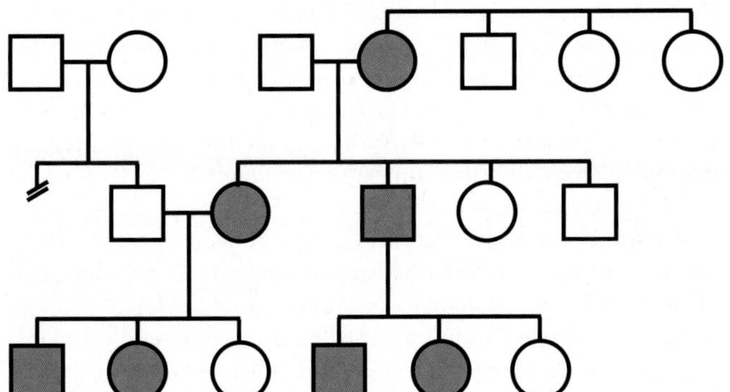

Figure 2-13. Example of autosomal dominant inheritance. (Courtesy of Edith Cheng, MD.)

4. There is father-to-son transmission.
5. An individual who does not carry the mutation will have no risk of transmission to his or her offspring.

Three additional properties associated with, but not exclusive to, autosomal dominant traits are variable expressivity, penetrance, and new mutations. Variable expressivity describes the severity of the phenotype in individuals who have the mutation. Some autosomal dominant conditions have a clear clinical demarcation between affected and unaffected individuals. However, some conditions express the clinical consequences of the mutation in varying degrees among members of the same family and between different families. These differences in expression are modified by age, sex of the affected individual, the individual's genetic background, and by the environment. Variable expression of a condition can lead to difficulties in diagnosis and interpretation of inheritance pattern. Penetrance refers to the probability that a gene will have any clinical manifestation at all in a person known to have the mutation. A condition is 100% penetrant if all individuals with the mutation have any clinical feature of the disease (no matter how minor). A number of autosomal dominant conditions are the result of new mutations. For example, about 70% of achondroplasia occur as new mutations. Because this condition has 100% penetrance, the recurrence risk in subsequent pregnancies in the normal parents of an affected child is not 50%, but the risk to the offspring of the affected is 50%. If an autosomal dominant condition is associated with poor reproductive fitness, then the likelihood that the cases occurred due to new mutation is greater.

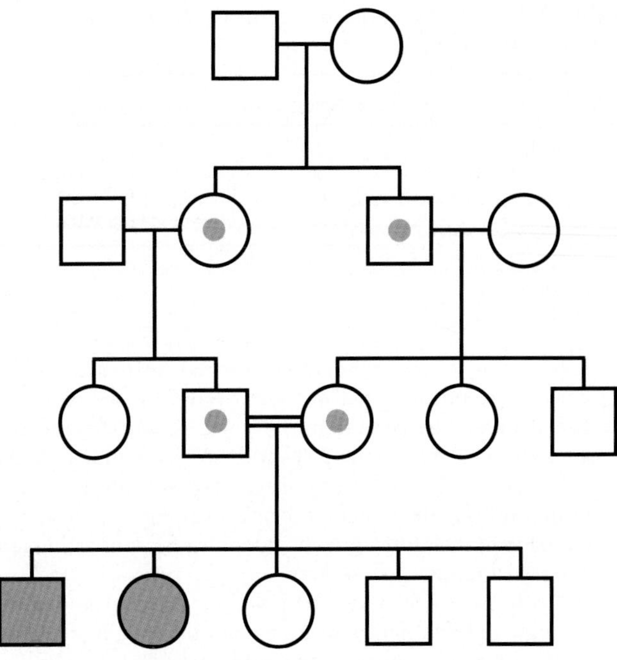

Figure 2-14. Pedigree illustrating autosomal recessive inheritance. Here, the parents of the affected children are first cousins as denoted by the double line connecting them. (Courtesy of Edith Cheng, MD.)

Autosomal Recessive

Autosomal recessive conditions are rare and require the affected individual to have two copies of the mutant allele (homozygous) in order to manifest the condition. In the heterozygote carrier, the product of the normal allele is able to compensate for the mutant allele and prevent occurrence of the disease. Figure 2-14 is a typical pedigree illustrating autosomal recessive inheritance. The following general statements can be made about an autosomal recessive trait:

1. The characteristic will occur equally in both sexes.
2. For an offspring to be at risk, both parents must be have at least one copy of the mutation.

Table 2-2 Carrier Frequencies for Cystic Fibrosis in Different Populations

Ethnicity	Chance of Being Carrier	Chance Both Carriers*
European descent	1 in 29	1 in 841
Hispanic American	1 in 46	1 in 2,116
African American	1 in 65	1 in 4,225
Asian American	1 in 90	1 in 8,100

*The chance for an affected child being born to these couples is the chance that both are carriers times 1/4.

3. If both parents are heterozygous (carrier) for the condition, 25% of the offspring will be homozygous for the mutation and manifest the condition, 50% will be carriers and unaffected. The remaining 25% will not have inherited the mutation at all, will be unaffected, and will not be at risk of transmitting the mutation to any offspring.
4. Consanguinity is often present in families demonstrating rare autosomal recessive conditions.
5. If the disease is relatively rare, it will be clustered among the siblings, and will not be seen among other family members such as ancestors, cousins, aunts and uncles.

Because autosomal recessive conditions require two copies of the mutant allele, and because most matings are not consanguineous, counseling couples about the risk for an autosomal recessive condition requires knowledge of the carrier frequency of the condition in the general population. Cystic fibrosis is an example of the importance of knowing the population in which screening/counseling is being provided (Table 2-2). Depending on the ethnic group of the mother and father, the risk for a child having cystic fibrosis could be as high as 1 in 1936 ($1/22 \times 1/22 \times 1/4$) if they are of Caucasian (European) descent, or negligible if they are of Asian descent.

X-Linked Trait

The human X chromosome is quite large, containing about 160 million base pairs, or about 5% of the nuclear DNA. Of the 500 genes that have been mapped to the X chromosome, 70% are known to be associated with disease phenotypes. Diseases caused by genes on the X chromosome are said to be X-linked and most are recessive. In contrast, the Y chromosome is quite small, about 70 million base pairs, and contains only a few genes.

The expression of genes located on the X chromosome demonstrate a unique characteristic known as dosage compensation, which was put forth by Mary Lyon in the 1960s to explain the equalization of X-linked gene products in males and females. Achievement of dosage compensation is through the principles of X inactivation, also known as the Lyon hypothesis. The tenets of the Lyon hypothesis are:

1. One X chromosome in each cell is randomly inactivated in the early female embryo (soon after fertilization).
2. The inactivation process is random: either the paternally or maternally derived X chromosome is chosen. The female is thus a mosaic for genes located on the X chromosome.
3. All descendants of the cell will have the same inactive X chromosome.

The Lyon hypothesis is supported by clinical evidence derived from animal and human observations of traits located on the X chromosome, such as the calico cat pattern of red and black patches of fur on female cats, but not on male cats. In humans, male and females have equal quantities of the enzyme glucose-6-phosphate dehydrogenase (G6PD), which is encoded by a gene on the X chromosome. Barr bodies, or sex chromatin, which are condensed, inactive X chromosomes found only in females, are cytogenetic evidence that only one X chromosome is transcriptionally active in females. The mechanism for X inactivation is unknown at this time, but clearly requires the presence of the X inactivation center, which has been mapped to the proximal end of the long arm of the X chromosome (Xq). This center contains an unusual gene call XIST (X-inactive specific transcript), which seems to control X inactivation, which cannot occur in its absence.

The principles of the Lyon hypothesis remain true for the majority of genes located on the X chromosome. The silencing of these genes appears to occur as a function of DNA methylation at the promoter regions of these genes. However, several regions remain genetically active on both chromosomes. They include the pseudoautosomal regions located at the tips of the long and short arms, which are the regions that contain the genes for steroid sulfatase, the Xg blood group, and Kallman syndrome (hypogonadism and anosmia). The pseudoautosomal region on the short arm shares extensive homology with the Y chromosome and is the region involved in the pairing of the X and Y chromosome at meiosis.

Another exception to the Lyon hypothesis is that one X chromosome is nonrandomly, preferentially inactivated. This is observed for most cases of translocations between an X chromosome and an autosome. If the translocation is balanced, the structurally normal X chromosome is preferentially inactivated. If the translocation is unbalanced, then the structurally normal X chromosome is always active. These nonrandom patterns of inactivation are an attempt to minimize the clinical consequences of the chromosomal rearrangement. Studies can be done to look at patterns of inactivation, as in the case of prenatal diagnosis, to predict the clinical consequences of a de novo X/autosome translocation in the fetus.

Random inactivation confers a mosaic state for the carrier female. The normal allele is able to compensate for the abnormal allele (as in autosomal recessive traits), and carrier females of X-linked recessive conditions usually do not have clinical manifestations of the disease. Occasionally however, there is skewed or less than 50-50 chance of inactivation such that the X chromosome carrying the normal allele is inactivated more frequently. In such cases, carrier females display some features of the condition and are referred to as manifesting heterozygotes. Manifesting heterozygotes have been described for hemophilia A, Duchenne muscular dystrophy, and X-linked color blindness.

Genetic counseling of recurrent risks for X-linked recessive condition depends on the sex of the affected parent and of the offspring. Figure 2-15 is a pedigree illustrating X-linked recessive inheritance, the characteristics of which are:

1. Affected individuals are usually males unless X chromosome activation is skewed in the carrier female or the female is homozygous for the trait.

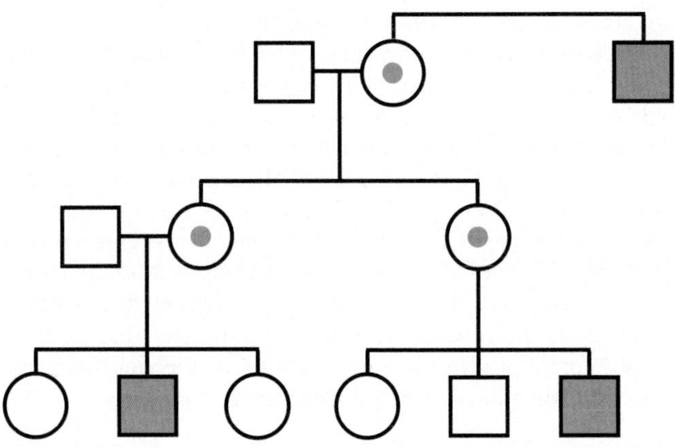

Figure 2-15. Pedigree illustrating X-linked recessive condition. (Courtesy of Edith Cheng, MD.)

2. The affected males in a kindred are related through females.
3. The gene is not transmitted from father to son.
4. All daughters of affected males will be carriers.
5. Daughters of carrier females have a 50% chance of being carriers; sons of carrier females have a 50% chance of being affected.

X-linked Dominant Inheritance

The major feature of X-linked dominant inheritance is that all heterozygotes, both male and female, manifest the condition. Although the pedigree may resemble autosomal dominant inheritance, the distinguishing feature is that affected males never have affected sons, and all daughters of affected males are affected. There are usually more affected females than males, and the majority of the females are heterozygotes.

Atypical Patterns of Inheritance

Trinucleotide-Repeat Disorders: Unstable Mutations

In the early 1990s a new class of genetic conditions was recognized as being due to unstable dynamic mutations in a gene. In the previous section, the diseases and their inheritance patterns were due to mutations that were passed on from generation to generation in a stable form. That is, all affected members in a family had the identical inherited mutation. In 1991, however, a number of reports began to describe a new class of genetic conditions in which the gene mutation was dynamic and would change with different affected individuals within a family. The most common group of disorders is known as triplet, or trinucleotide-repeat, disorders. More than a dozen diseases are now known to be associated with unstable trinucleotide repeats (Table 2-3).

These conditions are characterized by an expansion of variable size, within the affected gene, of a segment of DNA that contains a repeat of three nucleotides such as CAGCAGCAG (CAG)*n*, or CCGCCG(CCG)*n*. These triplet repeats are unstable in that they tend to expand as the gene is passed on from generation to generation. The molecular mechanism is most likely misalignment at the time of meiosis. The result of increasing triplet expansion is progressively earlier onset or more severe manifestation of disease with each successive generation. This phenomenon is known as anticipation and is generally characteristic of genetic conditions caused by unstable repeats.

The commonality of this group of genetic condition stops at the shared molecular mechanism. Each disease, otherwise, has its own features. Some, such as myotonic dystrophy, are inherited in an autosomal dominant pattern, but others, such as Friedrich's ataxia, are autosomal recessive conditions. The susceptibility of the triplet repeat to expand also depends on the parent of origin, paternal in Huntington's disease, and exclusively maternal in fragile X syndrome.

Fragile X Syndrome

Fragile X syndrome, although a disease within the unstable triplet group, is discussed in this section because of its unique molecular and clinical characteristics. This is the most common heritable form of moderate mental retardation and is second to Down syndrome among the causes of mental retardation in males. The gene is located on the X chromosome at Xq27.3 and causes a pattern of abnormalities, including mental retardation and characteristic facial features in at least 1 in 4000 male births. The condition is due to an expansion of the triplet repeat CGG located in the untranslated region of the first exon of the gene called *FMR1* (fragile X mental retardation 1). The triplet expansion blocks normal function of the *FMR1* gene, thus causing the syndrome.

Normal individuals have about 8 to 50 copies of the CGG triplet, whereas affected individuals have from 200 to over 1000 copies. Individuals with an intermediate number of copies (52–200) are known as premutation carriers; this level of "expansion" renders the triplet-repeat segment unstable. These carriers are generally unaffected but are at risk for having affected children or descendants if the premutation expands in

Table 2-3 Some Commonly Known Disorders Associated with Unstable Triplet Repeats

				REPEAT NUMBER		
Disease	**Inheritance Pattern**	**Triplet Repeat**	**Location of Expansion**	**Normal**	**Unstable**	**Affected**
Huntington's disease	Autosomal dominant	CAG	Exon coding region	<36	29–35	>35
Fragile X	X-linked	CGG	5′ untranslated region	<55	56–200	>200
Myotonic dystrophy	Autosomal dominant	GTG	3′ untranslated region	<35	50–100	>100
Spinal cerebellar ataxias*	Autosomal dominant	CAG	Exon	<40	Different for each subtype	>40
Friedrich's ataxia	Autosomal recessive	GAA	Intron of gene	<33	34–65	>65

*Spinal cerebellar ataxias are a heterogeneous group of conditions, all of which appear to be associated with a CAG repeat. Each subtype has its own specific range of normal, unstable, and affected repeat sizes

successive generations. The premutation, however, can be passed on without expanding.

Long-term follow-up of premutation carriers has revealed that these individuals are not necessarily "unaffected." Premature ovarian failure has been associated with female premutation carriers, and in men, a new syndrome of atypical adult-onset ataxia has now been described.

Although the unstable triplet is transmitted in an X-linked pattern, the probabilities of the different phenotypes are far from traditional X-linked inheritance. Understanding of this feature of the fragile X syndrome is crucial to genetic counseling and assessing recurrence risks. The possible outcomes of the offspring of a premutation carrier female are:

1. Male offspring: Three possibilities
   a. Unaffected by not having inherited the X chromosome with the premutation.
   b. Unaffected by inheriting the X chromosome with the premutation, which did *not* expand (about 20% of the time); this male however, is at risk for passing the premutation to his daughters, who in turn will be at risk for having affected children. Therefore, for this male, his grandchildren will be at risk for the fragile X syndrome.
   c. Affected by having inherited the abnormal X chromosome, in which the premutation also expanded to a full mutation.
2. Female offspring: Four possibilities
   a. Unaffected by not having inherited the X chromosome with the premutation.
   b. Unaffected by inheriting the X chromosome with the premutation that did *not* expand.
   c. Unaffected, but inherited the X chromosome *with* an expansion—about 50% of females with the expansion appear to be clinically unaffected.
   d. Affected by inheriting the X chromosome with an expansion.

Genomic Imprinting and Uniparental Disomy

Genomic imprinting and uniparental disomy refers to the differential activation or expression of genes depending on the parent of origin. In contrast to Mendel's hypothesis that the phenotype of a gene is no different if inherited from the mother or the father, there is now a group of diseases in which the parent of origin of a gene or chromosome plays a role in the phenotype of the affected individual. The best studied examples of this mechanism are molar pregnancies and Prader–Willi syndrome (PWS) and Angelman syndrome (AS). PWS is characterized by obesity, hyperphagia, small hands and feet, hypogonadism, and mental retardation. In about 70% of cases, cytogenetic deletion of the proximal arm of the paternally inherited chromosome 15 is observable at 15q11-q13. In contrast, the same deletion of the maternally inherited chromosome 15 results in a different phenotype (AS) of severe mental retardation, short stature, spasticity, and seizures. More interestingly, 30% of subjects with PWS do not have a cytogenetic deletion, but rather, inherit two intact chromosomes 15 from the mother. No genetic information on chromosome 15 is inherited from the father. This is referred to as maternal uniparental disomy. As expected, individuals with Angelman syndrome without a cytogenetic deletion have two copies of the paternally derived chromosome 15 and no chromosome 15 from the mother—a condition termed paternal uniparental disomy. These findings indicate that at least for the region of 15q11-q13, the expression of the PWS phenotype is brought on by the absence of a paternal contribution of the genes in this region. Likewise, the expression of Angelman syndrome is due to the absence of the maternal contribution of genes located at 15q11-q13. The genes in this region are said to be "imprinted" because their parent of origin has been "marked."

Many regions of the human genome have now demonstrated evidence of imprinting. Knowledge of diseases that occur as a result of imprinting has implications in prenatal diagnosis, especially when mosaicism is encountered.

Germline Mosaicism

Mosaicism is defined as the presence of two or more genetically different cell lines in the same individual or tissue derived from a single zygote. Females, because of X inactivation, are mosaics for genes on the X chromosome. Mosaicism, however, is not necessarily evenly or randomly distributed throughout the body. In other words, using the entire body as the whole organism, an individual is mosaic either because different organs or tissues have genetically different cells, but each organ or tissue has the same cell line, or because the genetically different cell lines are dispersed throughout many tissues in the body. The distinction between these two types of mosaicism is particularly important in making a prenatal diagnosis in cases in which mosaicism is identified in amniotic fluid cells. One cannot be confident that a trisomy 21 phenotype, such as mental retardation, would be less severe because of mosaicism. The brain cells could be all trisomy 21, but the cells of the skin could all be normal diploid.

In germline mosaicism, the implication is that the mutation is present in only one parent and arose during embryogenesis in all or some of the germ cells but few or none of the somatic cells of the embryo. This concept was developed to explain recurrence of a genetic condition in a sibship (usually autosomal dominant) in which incorrect diagnosis, autosomal recessive inheritance, reduced penetrance, or variable expression could not be the reason for the recurrence. The best example of germline mosaicism is osteogenesis imperfecta type II (lethal form). At the molecular level, the mutation causing the condition is dominant, that is, only one copy of the abnormal gene is necessary to cause this perinatal lethal condition. Yet, there are families in which multiple affected pregnancies are seen in the same couple, or, one parent has recurrences with different partners. If the spontaneous mutation rate for an autosomal dominant mutation is 1 chance in 10^5, then the probability of two independent spontaneous mutations for the same lethal autosomal dominant condition is $(1/10^5)^2$, a highly unlikely event. Germline mosaicism is now well documented for about 6% of cases of osteogenesis imperfecta type II. Unfortunately, the exact recurrence risk is difficult to assess because the proportion of gametes containing the mutation is unknowable.

Mitochondrial Inheritance—Maternal Inheritance

The majority of inherited conditions occur as a result of mutations in the DNA of the nucleus (nuclear genome). However, a growing number of conditions due to abnormalities of the mitochondria have now been identified. Because the mitochondrial apparatus and its function are under the control of both nuclear and mitochondrial genes, diseases affecting the mitochondria do not follow the typical mendelian pattern of inheritance.

Each human cell contains a population of several hundred or more mitochondria in its cytoplasm. Most of the subunits that make up the mitochondrial apparatus are encoded by the nuclear genome. However, mitochondria have their own DNA molecules, which contain a small fraction of genes whose product are vital to the function of the cell. Mitochondrial DNA (mtDNA), which was completely sequenced in 1981, is small, about 16.5 kilobase pairs (kbp) in size, and is packaged as a circular chromosome located in the mitochondria. The replication process is self-sufficient, with the molecule coding for 37 genes. These genes code for two types of rRNA, 22 tRNAs, and 13 of 87 polypeptides that are subunits of the oxidative phosphorylation pathway (OXPHOS). The other 74 polypeptides are encoded by nuclear DNA. Therefore, mitochondrial diseases can be caused by mutations in the mtDNA or in the nuclear genes that code for components of the OXPHOS system.

Since the primary function of the OXPHOS complex is to provide energy (ATP) for the cell, mutations that affect the OXPHOS complex will likely result in cell dysfunction and death. The organs most affected would be those that depend heavily on mitochondria. The diseases that result are generally neuromuscular in nature, such as encephalopathies, myopathies, ataxias, and retinal degeneration, but the mutations have pleiotropic effects.

The first pathogenic mutations in mtDNA were identified in the early 1990s. They include mutations in the coding regions of genes that alter the activity of an OXPHOS protein, mutations in tRNA or rRNA genes that impair mitochondrial protein synthesis, or rearrangements that result in deletions or duplications of the mtDNA molecule. The lack of mtDNA repair mechanisms and constant exposure to oxygen free radicals may explain the high mutation rate of mtDNA (10 times that of nuclear DNA, which has a spontaneous mutation rate of 1 in 10^5).

The most significant characteristic of mitochondrial diseases caused by mutations in mtDNA is that they are all maternally inherited. Leber's hereditary optic neuropathy (LHON) is a well known mitochondrial disease in which rapid, bilateral loss of central vision occurs. Males and females are affected equally, and all affected individuals are related through maternal lineage. This is because the cytoplasm of the ovum is abundant with mitochondria, but the sperm contain very few mitochondria. Therefore, an individual's mitochondria (and its DNA) is essentially all inherited from the mother. If the mother has an mtDNA mutation, then all of her children will inherit that mutation. When a mutation arises in the DNA of a mitochondrion in the cytoplasm of the ovum, it is at first one mutation in one mitochondrion. However, as replication and division of this mutated mitochondrion occurs, they become randomly distributed among the normal mitochondria and between the daughter cells. One daughter cell by chance may contain a large population of mitochondria with the mutation, but the other has none or very little. Fertilization of the egg with a large proportion of mitochondria containing the mutation would result in an offspring that is at risk for manifesting a mitochondrial disease.

A second feature is that of variable expression. Within each cell and tissue, there is a threshold for energy production below which the cells will degenerate and die. Organ systems with large energy requirements will be most susceptible to mitochondrial abnormalities. Thus, if there is an mtDNA mutation, the severity of the mitochondrial disease will depend on the proportion of mitochondria with the mutation that the individual inherited from his or her mother, and the susceptibility of different tissues to altered ATP metabolism.

Abnormalities of mitochondrial function caused by mutations in the nuclear genome will, however, exhibit traditional mendelian inheritance patterns with autosomal dominant and recessive, as well as X-linked conditions now being observed. A few conditions occur as sporadic, somatic mutations and have little or no recurrence risk. Table 2-4 lists some of the currently known mitochondrial diseases and their inheritance patterns. However, mitochondrial dysfunction has now been found to be associated with many conditions, including diabetes, Alzheimer's disease, Parkinson's disease, and human oocyte aging.

Table 2-4 Some Mitochondrial Disorders and Their Features

	Disease	Features	Inheritance Pattern
Mitochondrial DNA Mutations	**Leber's hereditary optic neuropathy (LHON)**	Blindness, rapid optic nerve death in young adulthood	Maternal
	Leigh disease (NARP)	**N**europathy, **a**taxia, **r**etinitis **p**igmentosa, mental retardation, lactic acidosis	Maternal
	MERRF	**M**yotonic **e**pilepsy, **r**agged **r**ed **f**ibers in muscle, ataxia, sensorineurodeafness	Maternal
	MELAS	**M**itochondrial **e**ncephalopathy, **l**actic **a**cidosis, **s**trokelike episodes, sensorineurodeafness	Maternal
Nuclear DNA Mutations	**Friedreich's ataxia**	Limb movement abnormalities, dysarthria, absent tendon reflexes, triplet repeat affecting gene that codes for mitochondrial protein (Frataxin)	Autosomal recessive
	Barth syndrome	Dilated cardiomyopathy, cyclic neutropenia, skeletal myopathy, growth deficiency, abnormal mitochondria	X-linked
	Wilson disease	Copper accumulation in brain and liver leading to cirrhosis, parkinsonism, and dystonia	Autosomal recessive

Multifactorial Inheritance

Multifactorial inheritance is defined as traits or characteristics produced by the action of several genes, with or without the interplay of environmental factors. A number of structural abnormalities occurring as isolated defects and not part of a syndrome, such as cleft lip with or without cleft palate , open neural tube defect (including anencephaly and spina bifida), and cardiac defects are examples of such conditions. When both parents are normal and an affected child is produced, the chance of recurrence is generally between 2% and 5% for any given pregnancy. Because the underlying mechanisms by which the genes and the environment interact to cause these conditions are unknown, genetic counseling of recurrent risks must measure the observed recurrence risks in collections of families to generate a population-based empiric risk. These risk rates, however, are modified by ethnicity, the sex of the carrier parent, the sex of the affected parent and at-risk offspring, the presence of the defect in one or both parents, the number of affected family members, and by consanguineous parentage.

Chromosome Abnormalities

A variety of chromosome abnormalities may occur during meiosis or mitosis (see Chapter 1, Fertilization and Embryogenesis). They fall into several general categories, and many clinical conditions are associated with each type. Although it is impossible within the scope of this chapter to discuss every clinical condition associated with a known chromosome abnormality, an attempt is made to categorize the specific types of anomalies and the more common problems seen by obstetricians and gynecologists that relate to these anomalies. Several conditions are dealt with in more detail in other chapters of this book.

Numerical Chromosomal Abnormalities

Two terms are used in the description of numerical chromosomal abnormalities: aneuploidy refers to an extra or missing chromosome, such as in trisomy 21 (Down syndrome) or monosomy X (Turner syndrome), respectively; polyploidy refers to numerical chromosome abnormalities in which there is an addition of an entire complement of haploid chromosomes, such as in triploidy, in which three haploid sets occur (69, XXX or XXY or XYY).

Numerical or aneuploid chromosome abnormalities involve either autosomes or sex chromosomes. Most occur as the result of nondisjunction during meiosis or mitosis in which homologous chromosome pairs fail to disjoin. The result in meiosis is that one daughter cell receives two copies of the homologs and the other receives none. Fertilization with a gamete containing a normal chromosome complement will result in a zygote that is either trisomic or monosomic (Fig. 2-16). Molecular studies for the parent of origin have identified that the majority of autosomal aneuploidies result from nondisjunctional errors in maternal meiosis I.

The majority of trisomic conceptions are nonviable, and autosomal trisomies have been seen in abortus material in all but chromosomes 1 and 17. However, trisomies 21, 18, 13, and 22 result in live births and are associated with advanced maternal age (Fig. 2-17). Trisomy 13 (Patau syndrome) occurs in approximately 1/10,000 live births. The syndrome is characterized by gross multiple structural defects involving the midline (holoprocencephaly, cleft lip/palate, cardiac defects), and postaxial

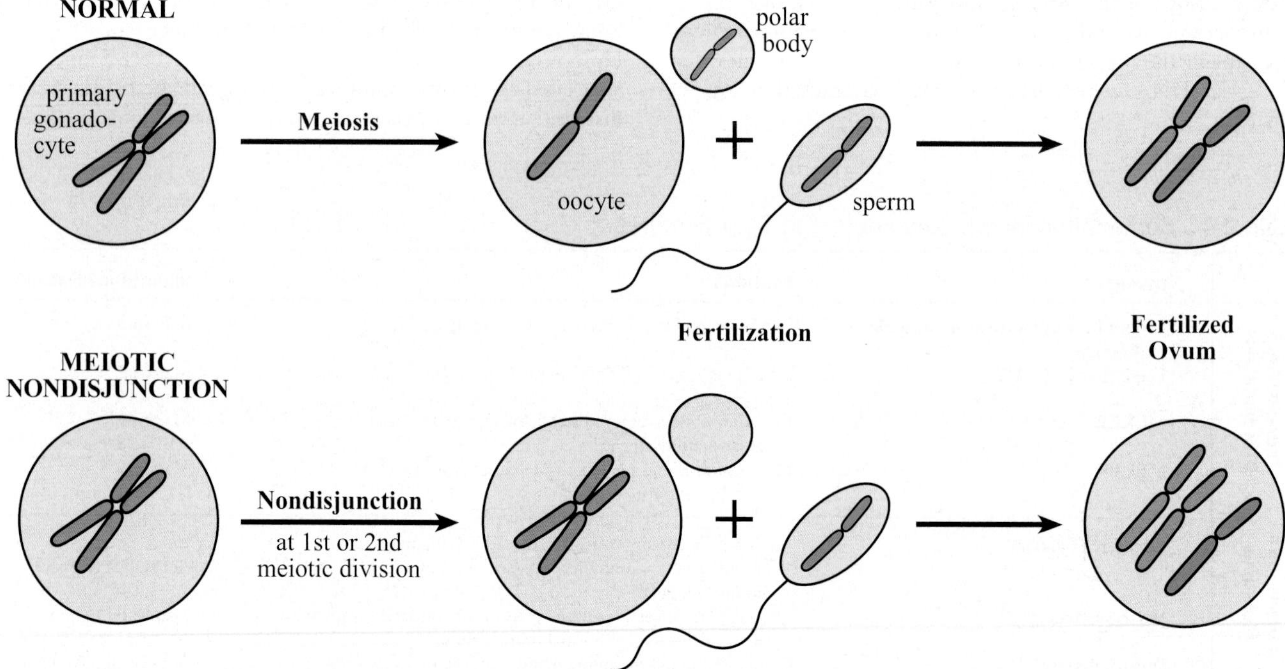

Figure 2-16. Graphic representation of meiotic nondisjunction. (Courtesy of Edith Cheng, MD.)

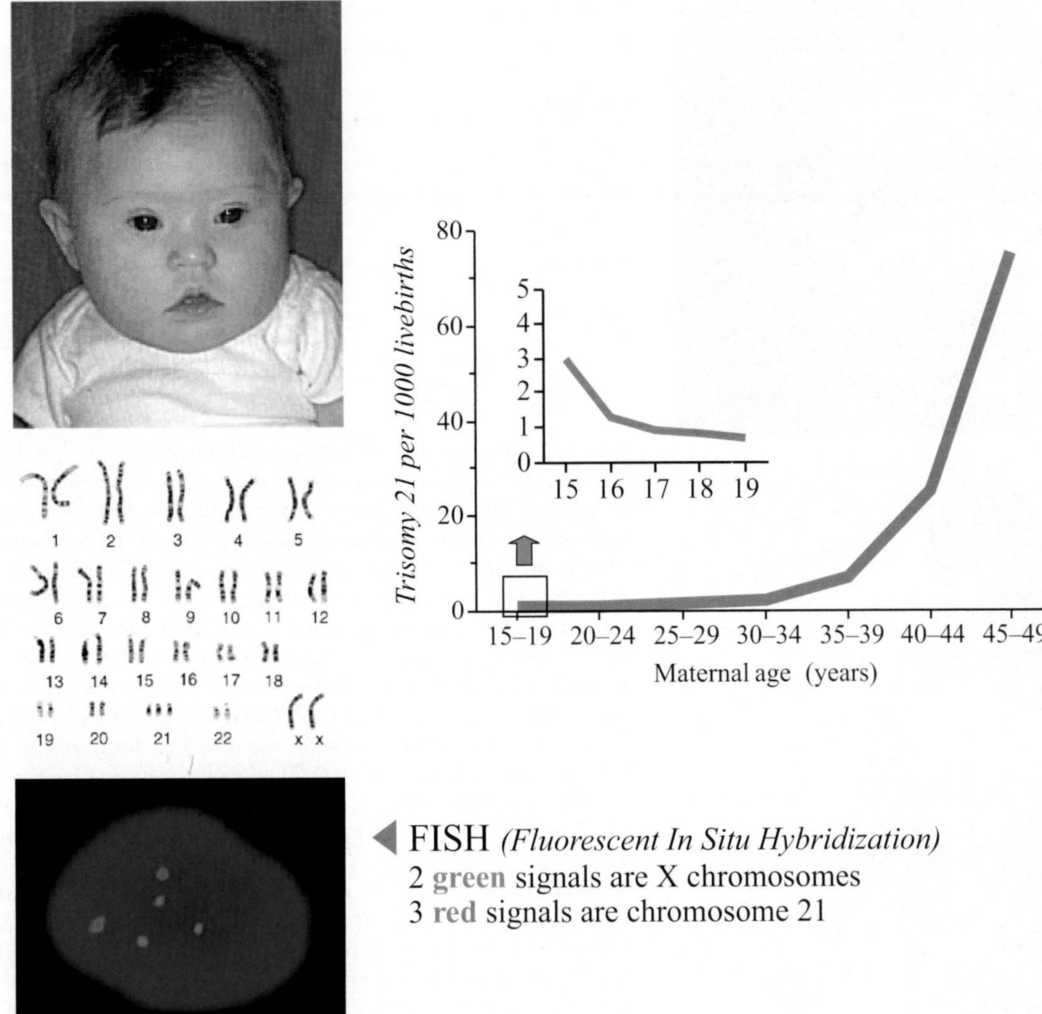

Figure 2-17. Trisomy 21 infant with karyotype demonstrating three separate chromosomes 21. Interphase FISH illustration of screening for trisomy 21. Graph illustrating the maternal age association and increasing risk for aneuploidy. Note that there is an increased risk at the peripubertal ages as well. (Courtesy of Edith Cheng, MD.)

polydactyly. Trisomy 18 (Edwards syndrome) is found in 1/6,000 live births and is associated with prenatal growth restriction, rocker bottom feet, and cardiac and renal defects. Trisomy 21 is the most common viable autosomal trisomy and has an incidence of 1/800 live births. The majority (95%) of individuals with Down syndrome have trisomy 21, that is, three separate copies of chromosome 21 because of maternal nondisjunction. However, about 2% to 3% of individuals with clinical Down syndrome have a structural rearrangement (robertsonian translocation—to be discussed in the next section) and another 1% to 3% are mosaic for trisomy 21. Trisomy 22 has been seen in a few live-born individuals and is associated with severe neurologic impairment. Monosomic states involving autosomes are extremely rare and generally lethal.

Sex chromosome aneuploidy usually occurs in the trisomic state. Monosomy Y is lethal and has never been seen in a clinical situation or even in an abortus. Monosomy of the X chromosome (45,X), however, is the typical finding in the condition known as Turner syndrome. However, because most 45,X conceptions are lethal, the actual incidence of live female births is about 1/5000. At birth, Turner syndrome is characterized by lymphedema, hypotonia, and webbed neck. Girls with Turner syndrome have short stature, a broad chest with wide spaced nipples, cubitus valgus (widened carrying angle of the arms), and gonadal dysgenesis resulting in lack of secondary sex characteristics, amenorrhea, and infertility (Fig. 2-18). Other features include congenital heart disease (coarctation of the aorta is the most common), kidney disease, and hypertension in later life. Intelligence is normal although spatial perception abnormalities are common. Hormonal supplementation during puberty allows girls with Turner syndrome to develop secondary sex characteristics.

Unlike autosomal trisomies in which the majority are maternally derived, the 45,X karyotype occurs through paternal nondisjunction and is not associated with advanced maternal or paternal age. There is no increased recurrence for 45,X, which accounts for 50% of women with Turner syndrome. Another 30% to 40% of individuals are mosaic for the 45,X cell line

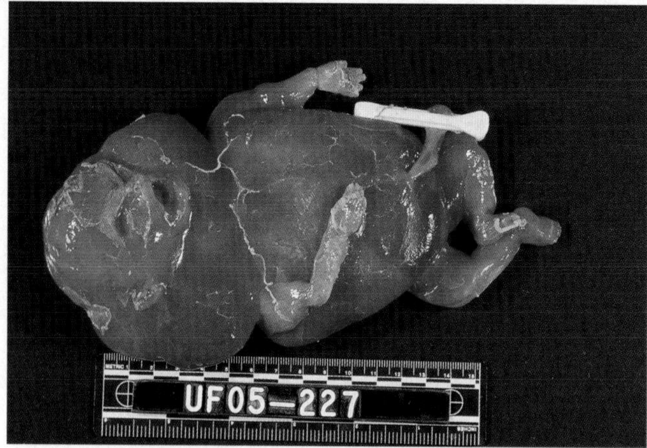

A

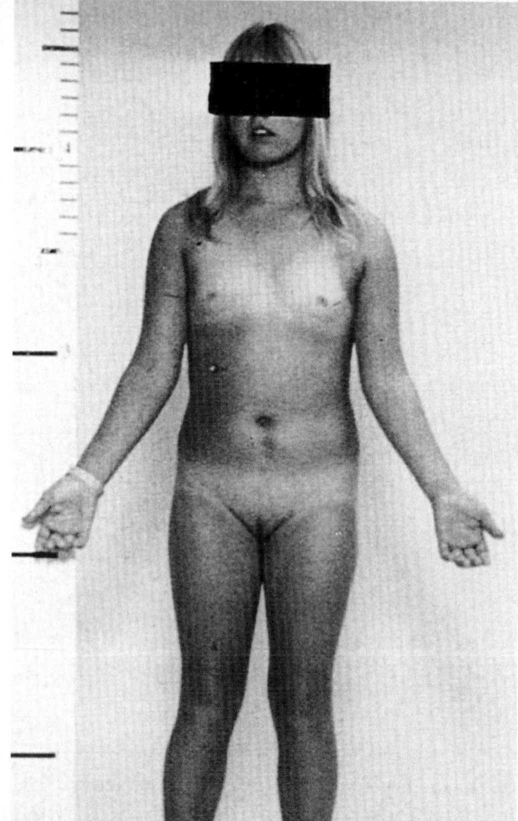

B

Figure 2-18. **A,** Photo of a 20-week fetus with Turner syndrome, 45,X. This fetus was diagnosed during a routine 20-week ultrasound for anatomy and growth and was found to have a large cystic hygroma and hydrops. The autopsy revealed a complex cardiac defect, abnormal kidneys, streaked ovaries, and malrotation of the gut with the appendix in the left lower quadrant (Courtesy of Drs. W. Tony Parks and Corrine Fligner, Department of Pathology, University of Washington). **B,** A 17-year-old woman with Turner syndrome. Note the short stature, poor sexual development, and increased carrying angles at elbows. Subject also has webbing of the neck.

and another cell line (usually 46,XX) because of postzygotic nondisjunction during mitosis. The clinical features of these women will vary depending on the proportion of normal 46,XX cell lines present. However, females who are mosaic with a 45,X/46,XY karyotype are at an increased risk for gonadoblastoma. Therefore, women suspected of having Turner syndrome should have a chromosomal analysis, not only for diagnosis, but for exclusion of mosaicism for a 46,XY cell line. The remaining 10% to 20% of individuals with Turner syndrome have a structural abnormality of the X chromosome (Table 2-5). Occasional correlation between phenotype and the type of structural abnormality has lead investigators to examine the genes responsible for ovarian development and function and other features associated with Turner syndrome. For example, women with 46,X,i(Xq) are indistinguishable from women with 45,X, whereas women with a deletion of the long arm of X (Xq) often only have gonadal dysfunction, and women with deletions of the short arm of X (Xp) have short stature and congenital malformations.

Table 2-5 Karyotypes discovered in Subjects with Phenotypic Characteristics of Turner Syndrome

Karyotype	Error
45,X	Deletion X
45,Xi(Xq)	Deletion Xp, Isochromosome Xq
45,X,Xq	Deletion Xp
45,X/46,XX	Mosaicism
45,X/46,XX/47,XXX	Mosaicism
45,X/46,XY	Mosaicism
45,X/46,XY/47,XYY	Mosaicism
45,XringX	Ring chromosome
46,XX	Phenotype with normal karyotype

Other trisomies involving the sex chromosomes are seen in 47,XXX, 47,XXY (Klinefelter syndrome), and 47,XYY karyotypes. The incidence of 47,XXX is approximately 1/1000 live female births and is due to maternal nondisjunction associated with increasing maternal age. Most women are phenotypically normal with exception of possible mild developmental delay; fertility is normal and there may be a slightly increased risk for offspring with aneuploidy involving the sex chromosomes and autosomes. Klinefelter syndrome, 47,XXY, is a common sex chromosome abnormality associated with maternal age and occurs in 1/1000 live male births. Clinical features include tall gynecoid stature, gynecomastia (with an increased risk for breast cancer), and testicular atrophy. Mental retardation is not a typical feature, but affected individuals may have IQ scores that are lower than those of their siblings. Nondisjunction during spermatogenesis involving the Y chromosome leads to 47,XYY. These males may be taller than average, but are otherwise phenotypically normal. Contrary to previous and outdated observational studies, this sex chromosome aneuploidy is not associated with violent crime. However, behavioral problems such as attention deficit disorder may be observed.

Nondisjunctional events during mitosis in the early embryo (after fertilization) will produce individuals with cell populations containing different chromosome numbers. This condition, known as *mosaicism,* may involve the autosomes or the sex chromosomes. The actual phenotype depends on the proportion of aneuploid and euploid cells in the embryo and in the specific organs or tissues involved.

Structural Chromosome Abnormalities

Chromosome breaks and rearrangements may lead to no obvious phenotypic consequences (genetically balanced), loss or gain of chromosomal material (genetically imbalanced) that produce abnormalities, or abnormalities due to interruption of a critical gene at the breakpoint site on the chromosome. Types of structural rearrangements include translocations (reciprocal and robertsonian), insertions, inversions, isochromosomes, duplications, and deletions. The rate of formation of balanced rearrangements is generally very low, 1.6×10^{-4}, although some chromosomal segments are more prone to breakage (hotspots) than others. This section will discuss the clinical and reproductive implications of some of these structural rearrangements.

Balanced Reciprocal Translocations. Translocations occur as a result of a mutual and physical exchange of chromosome (genetic) material between nonhomologous chromosomes. Balanced reciprocal translocations are found in about 1/11,000 newborns. Figure 2-19 is an example of a hypothetical balanced translocation between the short arms (p arm) of two chromosomes. The carrier of a reciprocal balanced translocation is usually phenotypically normal. However, the carrier is at an increased risk for producing offspring who are chromosomally abnormal. In meiosis, the two pairs of nonhomologous chromosomes involved in the translocation resolve their pairing difficulties by forming a quadriradial. Three segregation possibilities are illustrated in Figure 2-19, but only one segregation (alternative) pattern will result in genetically balanced gametes. Of the six possible gametes, four are partially monosomic and trisomic, one has a normal complement of chromosomes, and the other contains a pair of reciprocally balanced translocation chromosomes (like its parent). The viability of the genetically unbalanced gametes depends on the chromosomes involved in the reciprocal translocation, the size of the translocated chromosome material, and the sex of the carrier. In addition, most reciprocal translocations are unique to a family, and, consequently, the reproductive fitness of the carrier depends on the carrier's sex and nature of the translocation. In general, however, the recurrence for an unbalanced conception is 3% to 5% for male carriers, and 10% to 15% for female carriers of reciprocal balanced translocations.

A second and important type of translocation is the robertsonian translocation. This is a structural rearrangement between the acrocentric chromosomes: chromosome pairs 13, 14, 15, 21, and 22. In this structural rearrangement, the short arms (p arms) of two nonhomologous chromosomes are lost, and the long arms fuse at the centromere, forming a single chromosome structure. Figure 2-20 is an example of a robertsonian translocation involving chromosomes 14 and 21. The phenotypically normal carrier of a robertsonian translocation has 45 chromosomes in each cell because the two acrocentric chromosomes involved in the translocation have formed into one chromosome structure. This person is genetically balanced, that is, he or she has two copies of each chromosome. However, the gametes are at risk to be unbalanced. As in reciprocal translocations, the chromosomes involved in the rearrangement resolve the pairing of homologous segments at meiosis by forming a triad as seen in Figure 2-21. The chromosomes can segregate into gametes in one of three patterns. Only one segregation pattern (alternate) results in normal offspring, one gamete will have a normal chromosome complement, and the other will be a balanced carrier with 45 chromosome structure, like its parent. The other two segregation patterns result in

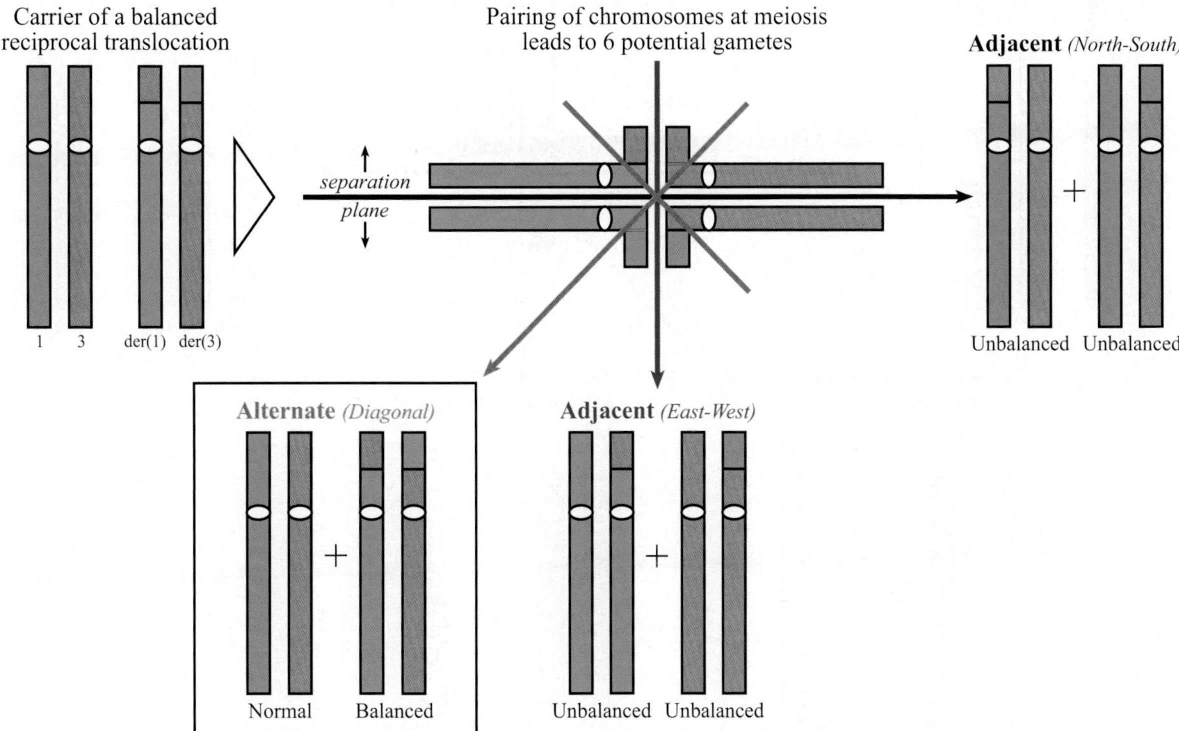

Figure 2-19. Schematic representation of segregation patterns of a diploid gamete with a reciprocal balanced translocation. Here, exchanges have occurred between the short arms of chromosomes 1 and 3. The two pairs of chromosomes pair in a quadriradial fashion. There are three potential axes in which the cell can divide. Only two of the six potential gametes will be genetically balanced. (Courtesy of Edith Cheng, MD.)

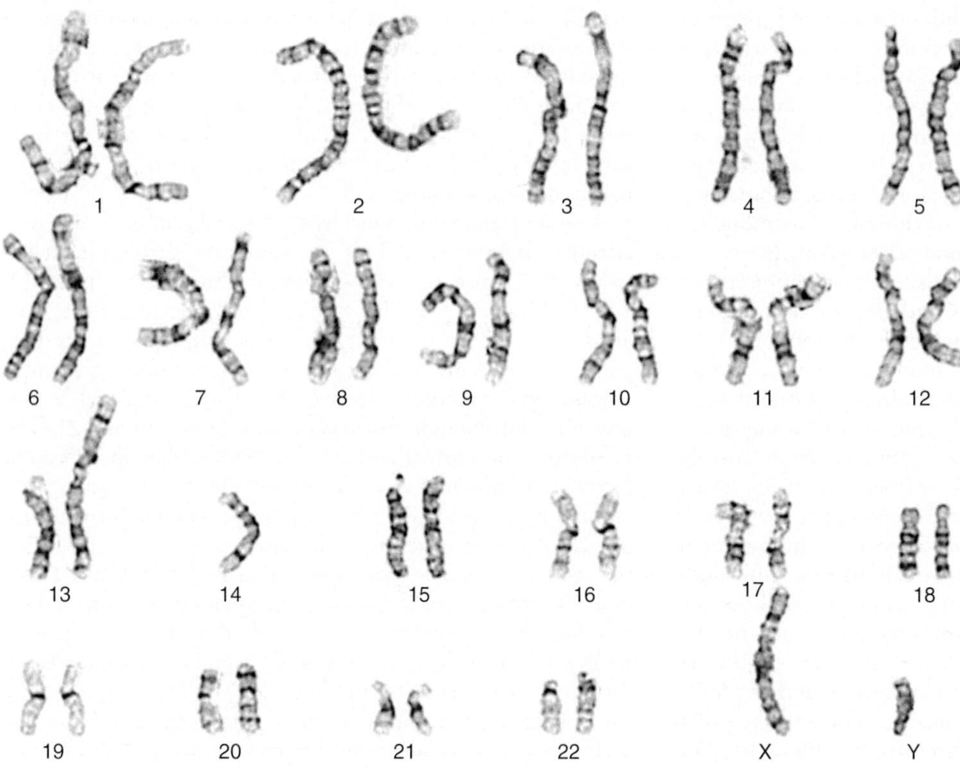

Figure 2-20. Karyotype demonstrating a robertsonian translocation between chromosomes 13 and 14. Notice that there are only 45 chromosome structures, but this male is genetically diploid. (Courtesy of Edith Cheng, MD.)

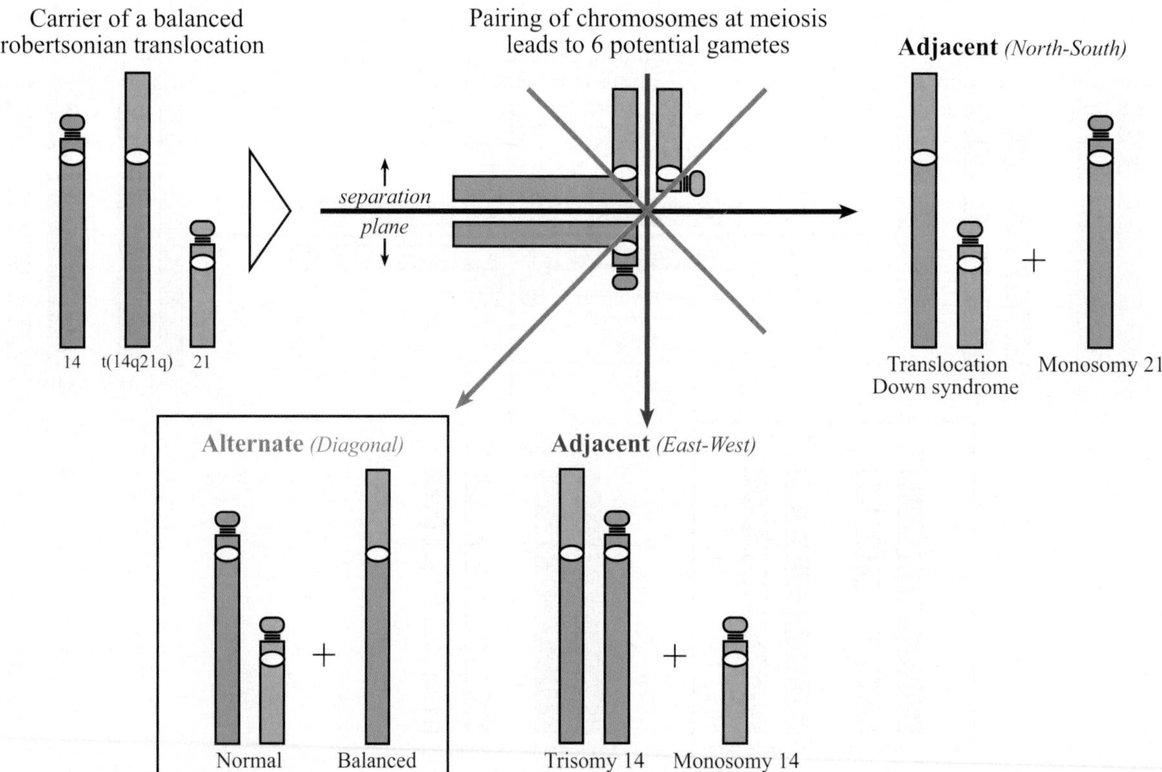

Figure 2-21. Schematic representation of the segregation patterns of a diploid gamete with a robertsonian translocation. Six potential gametes are formed, but only two are genetically balanced. One of the six gametes containing the 14/21 translocation and the free chromosome 21 will result in a conception with Down syndrome. (Courtesy of Edith Cheng, MD.)

chromosomally unbalanced gametes that are monosomic for chromosome 21 or 14 (both lethal), or trisomic for chromosome 14 (lethal). In addition, one of the gametes will have the robertsonian (14q;21) translocation, and, if fertilized, the resultant offspring will have Down syndrome. The risk for recurrence of translocation Down syndrome depends on parent of origin (10% to 15% for maternal carriers, and 1% to2% for paternal carriers).

One very important exception in translocation Down syndrome is that associated with a 21q21q translocation. Here, the chromosome structure is composed of two chromosomes 21. Although this chromosome rearrangement is extremely rare, this translocation confers a 100% risk that the carrier will have abnormal gametes and 100% of viable gametes will result in a conception with Down syndrome.

Chromosome inversions occur when two breaks occur on a chromosome followed by a 180° turn of the segment and reinsertion at its original breakpoints. Thus, if a sequence of markers on a chromosome is ABCDEFGHIJ, but an inversion occurs between markers D and H, the sequence of markers becomes ABCHGFEDIJ. If the centromere is included in the inverted segment, it is called a *pericentric inversion*. If the centromere is not involved, then the inversion is called a *paracentric inversion*. Chromosome inversions are generally considered balanced and usually do not confer an abnormal phenotype unless one of the breakpoints disrupts a critical gene. Inversions, however, do interfere with pairing at meiosis and can result in gametes with chromosome abnormalities.

Isochromosomes occur as a result of the chromosome dividing along the horizontal axis rather than the longitudinal axis at the centromere. The result is a chromosome that has two copies of one arm and no copies of the other. Isochromosomes involving autosomes are generally lethal because the resultant conception will be both trisomic and monosomic for genetic information. However, isochromosome involving the long are of the X chromosome (iso Xq) is compatible with life.

Finally, deletions and duplications of chromosome segments arise from unequal crossing over at meiosis, or from crossing over during pairing of inversions or reciprocal translocations. Breaks resulting in loss of chromosome material at the tip are called *terminal deletions,* and loss of chromosome material beween two breaks within a chromosome is called an *interstitial deletion*. There are several well documented terminal deletion syndromes, including cri-du-chat (5p-) syndrome, characterized by microcephaly, profound mental retardation, growth retardation, a unique facial appearance, and a distinctive "cat-like" cry. Most cases occur as a de novo chromosome deletion of the tip of the short arm (p arm) of chromosome 5, but approximately 10% to 15% arise as a consequence of a parental reciprocal translocation involving chromosome 5 and another chromosome.

Microdeletion/Duplication or Contiguous Gene Syndromes. The discussion in the previous section described only phenotypes that were associated with chromosome abnormalities visible with traditional cytogenetic techniques and light microscopy that imply involvement of large segments of chromosomes containing a large number (hundreds) of genes. In the last decade, high-resolution chromosome banding and advances in molecular cytogenetics technology have revealed a new class of chromosome syndromes known as microdeletion,

Table 2-6 Common Microdeletion/Contiguous Gene Syndromes

		CHROMOSOME		
Syndrome	**Incidence**	**Location**	**Abnormality**	**Size (Mb)**
Sotos	Rare	5q35	Deletion	2.2
Smith–Magenis	1/25,000	17p11.2	Deletion and duplication	4
Williams	1/20,000–1/50,000	7q11.23	Deletion	1.6
Charcot–Marie–Tooth (*CMTIA/HNLPP*)	1/10,000	17p12	Duplication and deletion	1.5
DiGeorge/ Velocardiofacial	1/4,000		Deletion	1.5
Cat's eye	Rare	22q11	Duplication	3
der(22)	Rare			3
Neurofibromatosis I	1/40,000–1/80,000	17q11.2	Deletion	1.5

or contiguous gene, syndromes in which the involved chromosome region(s) are submicroscopic and so small that molecular cytogenetic techniques such as fluorescent in situ hybridization (FISH) is necessary to localize the affected region. Table 2-6 lists some of the more commonly recognized syndromes, most of which are due to deletions although some duplication syndromes have now been identified. The phenotypes of these conditions are due to the absence (or duplication) of multiple contiguous genes within the involved region. These regions are small, usually about 1.5 to 3 Mb (compared with traditional chromosome banding and microscopy, which has a resolution requirement of at least 5 Mb). Fine mapping of the breakpoints in some of these conditions has implicated unequal or abnormal recombination between low-copy repetitive DNA sequences in the area of the deleted or duplicated regions. The discovery of microdeletion/duplication or contiguous gene syndromes has been important in clinical genetics and genetic counseling in that it finally provides a diagnosis, recurrence risk, and prenatal diagnosis for a large group of syndromes that previously had no cytogenetic confirmation. Moreover, these "naturally occurring" sequestered small regions of contiguous genes have provided a powerful tool for developmental geneticists to decipher the critical genes for normal human development. For example, the 22q11 region appears to be rich in genes responsible for specific congenital heart defects and craniofacial anomalies.

Chromosome Abnormalities and Pregnancy Outcome

The incidence and types of chromosome abnormalities differ between spontaneous abortions, stillbirths, and live births. Experience from pregnancies achieved by assisted reproductive technology indicates that 15% of fertilized ova fail to divide. Another 15% fail to implant, and 25% to 30% are aborted spontaneously at previllous stages. Of the roughly 40% of fertilized ova that survive the first missed menstrual period, as many as one fourth are aborted spontaneously, so that only about 30% to 35% of fertilized ova actually result in live-born infants. Chromosome and lethal genetic abnormalities play a major role in early losses. Thirty to 60% of first-trimester abortuses are found to have a chromosome abnormality of which approximately 50% are due to autosomal trisomies. Certain chromosomes

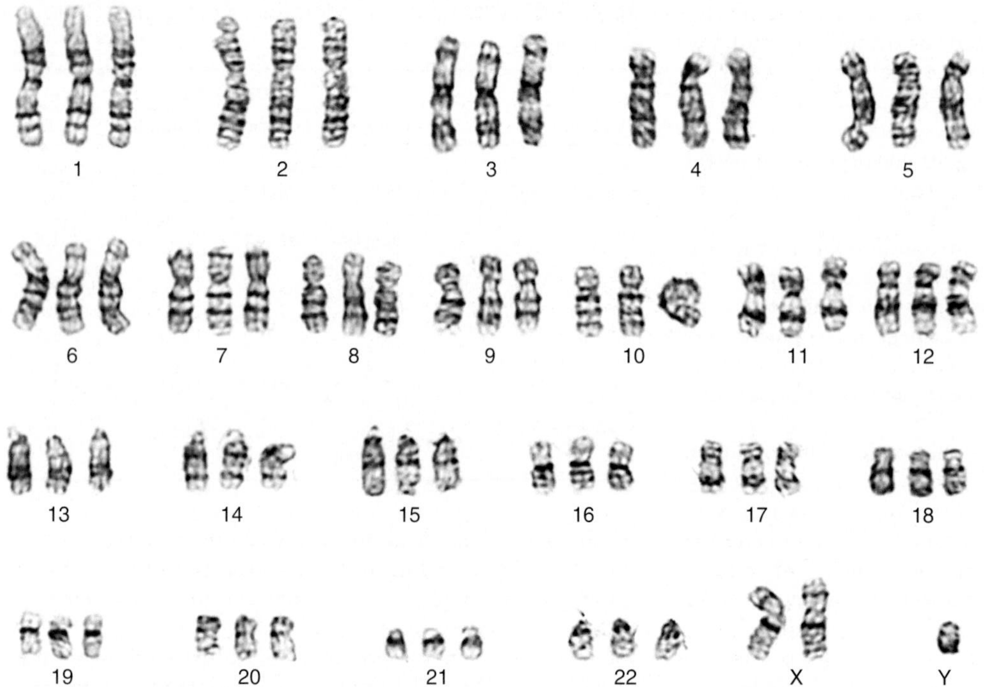

Figure 2-22. Karyotype of a partial mole containing 69 chromosomes (triploid). The nomenclature is 69, XXY. (Courtesy of Edith Cheng, MD.)

are more commonly involved than others; for example, trisomy 16 accounts for one third of trisomic abortuses. Autosomal monosomies are extremely rare, accounting for less than 1% of chromosomally abnormal abortuses. This may reflect selection at the gametic level in that the gamete with monosomy is not viable. Triploidy accounts for 16% of spontaneous abortions. Turner syndrome due to 45,X is by far the most common chromosome abnormality, accounting for 20% of spontaneous abortions that are chromosomally abnormal. This topic is discussed further in Chapter 16, Spontaneous and Recurrent Abortion.

Molar Gestations

Molar gestations comprise two clinical entities: the syndrome of associated triploidy, also known as partial moles and the hydatidiform, or complete, mole. Each has a distinctive chromosome abnormality and different clinical consequences. Triploidy (three chromosome complements) is found in 16% of abortuses with chromosome abnormalities (Fig. 2-22). They occur as a consequence of errors in meiosis or from double fertilization of a single ovum. The clinical features of a triploid pregnancy depend on the parent of origin of the extra set of chromosomes. In two thirds of cases, there is one maternal set and two paternal sets of chromosomes, resulting in poor embryonic development but a large hydropic placenta, the partial mole. Conversely, if there is an extra maternal set, an anomalous and growth-restricted fetus and a small fibrotic placenta are seen. Thus, triploidy is an example of imprinting in which the parent of origin of genetic information is marked and important for development.

In contrast to the triploid, partial mole, the complete mole is diploid with a 46,XX karyotype. The chromosomes are all paternally derived. When genetic markers are used to characterize the two sets of paternal chromosome, all of the markers are homozygous. Complete moles arise through the fertilization of an anucleated oocyte and subsequent duplication of the haploid chromosome complement (23,X) of the sperm. The absence of maternal contribution results in the development of abundant, hydropic trophoblastic tissue, and no recognizable embryonic tissue.

The clinical features of molar gestations indicate that normal pregnancies require both maternal and paternal genetic contributions, with the paternal genome being important for extraembryonic development and the maternal genome necessary for fetal development. Molar gestations and trophoblastic disease are discussed further in Chapter 35 (Gestational Trophoblastic Disease).

KEY POINTS

- Base pairing in DNA molecules is always A–T and G–C, and in RNA molecules is always A–U and G–C.
- Endonuclease enzymes cleave specific nucleotide pairs, making DNA fragment evaluation and gene cloning possible. More than 200 different endonucleases exist.
- Through a process known as polymerase chain reaction (PCR), small fragments of DNA may be cloned to produce larger amounts of the same material suitable for analysis.
- When a heterozygous individual who has an autosomal dominant trait mates with a normal individual, 50% of their offspring will have the trait.

KEY POINTS *Continued*

- When two individuals who carry an autosomal recessive trait mate, 25% of their offspring will demonstrate the trait and 50% will be carriers.
- X-linked recessive characteristics are transmitted from maternal carriers to male offspring and will affect 50% of such male offspring.
- In general, if a couple produces an offspring with a multifactorial defect and the problem has never occurred in the family, it can be expected to be repeated in 2% to 5% of subsequent pregnancies.
- The findings always present in 45,X Turner syndrome are shortness of stature and sexual infantilism.
- A variety of different karyotypes have been discovered in individuals with the phenotype of Turner syndrome.
- Nondisjunctional events have been described in every autosome except chromosomes 1 and 17. The risk of producing a second conceptus with a nondisjunctional event is approximately 1%.
- Conditions always seen in individuals with Klinefelter syndrome (47,XXY) are tallness of stature and azoospermia. One third of these individuals have gynecomastia.
- Of ova penetrated by sperm, 15% fail to implant, and 25% to 30% are aborted spontaneously at a previllous stage. Of the 40% that survive the first missed menstrual period, as many as one fourth abort spontaneously. From 30% to 35% of ova penetrated by sperm end in live-born individuals.
- Between 30% and 60% of known aborted conceptuses have chromosome abnormalities. Half of these have autosomal trisomies; 20% 45,X; 14% to 19% triploidy; 3% to 6% tetraploidy; and 3% to 4% chromosome rearrangements.
- Of live-born infants with chromosome abnormalities, about 0.8% to 1% have 45,X; 36.8% have other sex chromosome abnormalities; 21% have autosomal trisomies; and balanced chromosome translocations occur in 32.4%. About 3.2% have unbalanced translocation abnormalities.
- One in 200 women has recurrent (three or more) abortions, with chromosome abnormalities occurring in about 4.8% of the mothers and 2.4% of the fathers.
- When chromosome 21 is present as part of a robertsonian translocation with a D group chromosome, the chance of transmission of an unbalanced karyotype (leading to an offspring with Down syndrome) is 10% to 15% if the mother is the carrier and 1% to 2% if the father is the carrier.
- Hydatidiform moles are either diploid (46,XX or 46,XY) or triploid. The chromosomes of the diploid type, usually seen in true moles, are completely derived from paternal chromosomes. Triploid moles have at least two haploid sets derived from paternal origin.

BIBLIOGRAPHY

American College of Obstetrics and Gynecology: Update on carrier screening of cystic fibrosis. Committee Opinion Number 325, December 2005.

Benn PA, Hsu L: Prenatal diagnosis of chromosomal abnormalities through amniocentesis. In Milunsky A (ed): Genetic Disorders and the Fetus, 5th ed. Baltimore and London, The Johns Hopkins University Press, 2004.

Berchuck A, Kohler MF, Marks JR, et al: The p53 tumor suppressor gene frequently is altered in gynecologic cancers. Am J Obstet Gynecol 170:246, 1994.

Boue J, Boue A, Lazar P: Retrospective and prospective epidemiological studies of 1500 karyotyped spontaneous human abortions. Teratology 12:11, 1975.

Boue A, Gallano P: A collaborative study of segregation of inherited chromosome structural rearrangements in 1356 prenatal diagnoses. Prenat Diagn 4:45, 1984.

Bretherick KL, Kluker MR, Robinson WP: High normal FMR1 repeat sizes are associated with premature ovarian failure. Hum Genet 117:376, 2005.

Creasy MR, Crolla JA, Alberman ED: A cytogenetic study of human spontaneous abortion using banding techniques. Hum Genet 31:177, 1976.

Cummings FC, Zoghbi HY: Fourteen and counting: unraveling trinucleotide repeat diseases. Hum Mol Genet 9:909, 2000.

Deveriendt K, Vermeesch JR: Chromosomal phenotypes and submicroscopic abnormalities. Hum Genom 1:126, 2004.

Dewhurst J: Fertility in 47,XXX and 45,X patients. J Med Genet 15:132, 1978.

Erlich A, Gelfand DH, Saiki RK: Specific DNA amplification. Nature 331:46, 1988.

Evans HJ, Prosser J: Tumor-suppressor genes: cardinal factors in inherited predisposition to human cancers. Environ Health Perspect 98:25, 1992.

Ford EHR: Human chromosomes. New York, Academic Press, 1973.

Fortuny A, Carrio A, Soler A, et al: Detection of balanced chromosome rearrangements in 445 couples with repeated abortion and cytogenetic prenatal testing in carriers. Fertil Steril 49:774, 1988.

Hagerman PJ, Hagerman RJ: The fragile-X premutation: a maturing perspective. Am J Hum Genet 74:805, 2004.

Hamerton JL, Canning N, Ray M, Smith S: A cytogenetic survey of 14,069 newborn infants. I. Incidence of chromosome abnormalities. Clin Genet 8:223, 1975.

Harnden DG, Klinger HP (eds): An International System for Human Cytogenetic Nomenclature. Published in collaboration with Cytogenet Cell Genet, Basel, Switzerland, S Karger, 1985.

Johns DR: Mitochondrial DNA and disease. N Engl J Med 333:639, 1995.

Jones KL: Smith's Recognizable Patterns of Human Malformation, 6th ed. Philadelphia, Elsevier Saunders, 2006.

Jorde LB, Carey JC, Bamshad MJ, White RL: Medical Genetics, 2nd ed. St. Louis, Mosby, 1999.

Kajii T, Nikawa N: Origin of triploidy and tetraploidy in man: Cases with chromosome markers. Cytogenet Cell Genet 18:109, 1977.

Kajii T, Ohama K: Androgenetic origin of hydatidiform mole. Nature 268:633, 1977.

Kerem B-S, Rommens JM, Buchanan JA, et al: Identification of the cystic fibrosis gene: Genetic analysis. Science 245:1073, 1989.

Kotzot D: Complex and segmental uniparental disomy (UPD): Review and lessons from rare chromosomal complements. J Med Genet 38:497, 2001.

Ledbetter DH, Engel E: Uniparental disomy in humans; development of an imprinting map and its implications for prenatal diagnosis. Hum Mol Genet 4:1757, 1995.

Lubinsky MS: Female pseudohermaphroditism and associated anomalies. Am J Med Genet 6:123, 1980.

Malkin D, Li FP, Strong LC, et al: Germ line p53 mutations in a familial syndrome of breast cancer, sarcomas, and other neoplasms. Science 250:1233, 1990.

McKinlay Gardner RJ, Sutherland GR: Chromosome abnormalities and genetic counseling, 3rd ed. New York, Oxford University Press, 2004.

McKusick VA: Mendelian inheritance in man. Baltimore, The Johns Hopkins Press, 1978.

Miki Y, Swensen J, Shattuck-Eidens P, et al: A strong candidate for the breast and ovarian cancer susceptibility gene BRCA1. Science 266:66, 1994.

Morison IM, Reeve IM: A catalogue of imprinted genes and parent-of-origin effects in humans and animals. Hum Mol Genet 7:1599, 1998.

Nussbaum RL, McInnes RR, Willard HF: Thompson and Thompson Genetics in Medicine, 6th ed. Philadelphia, WB Saunders, 2001.

Roman E: Fetal loss rates and their relation to pregnancy order. J Epidemiol Community Health 38:29, 1984.

Schmike RN: Genetics and Cancer in Man. Edinburgh, Churchill Livingstone, 1980.

Shepard TH, Fantel AG: Embryonic and early fetal loss. Clin Perinatol 6:219, 1979.

Shoffner JM: Maternal inheritance and the evaluation of oxidative phosphorylation diseases. Lancet 348:1283, 1996.

Stene J, Stene E, Mikkelsen M: Risk for chromosome abnormality at amniocentesis following a child with a non-inherited chromosome aberration. Prenat Diagn 4:81, 1984.

Stephenson MD: Frequency of factors associated with habitual abortion in 197 couples. Fertil Steril 66:24, 1996.

Uehara S, Nata M, Nagae M, et al: Molecular biologic analyses of tetragemetic chimerism in a true hermaphrodite with 46,XX/46,XY. Fertil Steril 63:189, 1995.

Watkins PC: Restriction fragment length polymorphism (RFLP): Applications in human chromosome mapping and genetic disease research. BioTechniques 6:310, 1988.

Watson JD, Hopkins NH, Roberts WJ, et al: Molecular biology of the gene, 4th ed. Menlo Park, CA, Benjamin-Cummings, 1987.

Women's Health Care Physicians: Genetics in Obstetrics and Gynecology American College of Obstetricians and Gynecologists. June 30, 2002.

Reproductive Anatomy 3

Gross and Microscopic, Clinical Correlations

Vern L. Katz

KEY TERMS AND DEFINITIONS

Auerbach's Plexus. A network of twin vessels within the tunica muscularis of the ureters.

Apocrine Gland. A gland that produces secretions formed partially from the secreting cells of the gland itself.

Bladder Neck. That part of the bladder that is continuous with the urethra.

Canal of Nuck. A tubular process of peritoneum that accompanies the round ligament into the inguinal canal. It is generally obliterated in the adult but sometimes remains patent.

Carunculae Myrtiformes. Small nodules of fibrous tissue at the vaginal orifice that are remnants of the hymen.

Cornua. The superolateral aspects of the uterine cavity; the anatomic areas where the oviducts enter the uterine cavity.

Cul-de-sac of Douglas. A deep pouch formed by the most caudal extent of the parietal peritoneum. It is anterior to the rectum, separating the uterus from the large intestine.

Eccrine Gland. A simple sweat-producing gland in which the secreting cells are maintained intact during production of secretions.

Fimbria Ovarica. One of the largest finger-like projections of the distal end of the oviducts. The fimbria ovarica usually attaches the oviducts to the ovary.

Frankenhäuser's Plexus. An extensive concentration of both myelinated and nonmyelinated nerve fibers located in the uterosacral ligaments and supplying primarily the uterus and the cervix.

Fundus. The dome-shaped top of the uterus.

Genitocrural Fold. The skin line dividing the external female genitalia and the medial aspects of the thigh.

Isthmus. The short area of constriction in the lower uterine segment.

Parametria. The extraperitoneal fatty and fibrous connective tissue immediately adjacent to the uterus. The parametria lie between the leaves of the broad ligament and in the contiguous area anteriorly between the cervix and the bladder.

Pelvic Diaphragm. A thin, muscular layer of tissue that forms the inferior border of the abdominal pelvic cavity. The primary muscles of the pelvic diaphragm are the levator ani and coccygeus muscles.

Perineum. The region between the thighs bounded anteriorly by the vulva and posteriorly by the anus.

Plexus. A mixture of preganglionic and postganglionic fibers; small, inconsistently placed nerve ganglia; and afferent sensory fibers. In the female pelvis a plexus also may be termed a nerve.

Plicae Palmatae. Longitudinal folds in the mucous membrane of the endocervical canal. The secondary branching folds are called arbor vitae.

Posterior Fourchette. The fold of skin that joins the labia minora at their inferior margins.

Presacral Nerves. A midline plexus of nerves that contains the most important components of the pelvic autonomic nerves. The presacral nerves are located in the retroperitoneal connective tissue from the fourth lumbar vertebra to the hollow over the sacrum. (Also termed the superior hypogastric plexus.)

Rugae. Numerous transverse folds of the vagina in women of reproductive age.

Space of Retzius. The area lying between the bladder and symphysis pubis, bounded laterally by the obliterated hypogastric arteries.

Urachus. The adult remnant of the embryonic allantois.

Urogenital Diaphragm. A strong, muscular membrane that occupies the area between the symphysis pubis and the ischial tuberosities. Posteriorly, the urogenital diaphragm inserts into the central point of the perineum.

Vestibular Bulbs. Two elongated masses of erectile tissue situated on either side of the vaginal orifice. They are homologous to the bulb of the penis in the male.

The organs of the female reproductive tract are classically divided into the external and the internal genitalia. The external genital organs are present in the perineal area and include the mons pubis, clitoris, urinary meatus, labia majora, labia minora, vestibule, Bartholin's glands, and periurethral glands. The internal genital organs are located in the true pelvis and include the vagina, uterus, cervix, oviducts, ovaries, and surrounding supporting structures. This chapter integrates the basic anatomy of the female pelvis with clinical situations.

Embryologically the urinary, reproductive, and gastrointestinal tracts develop in close proximity. This relationship continues throughout a woman's life span. In the adult the reproductive organs are in intimate contact with the lower urinary tract and large intestines. Because of the anatomic proximity of the genital and urinary systems, altered pathophysiology in one organ often produces symptoms in an adjacent organ. The gynecologic surgeon should master the intricacy of these anatomic relationships to avoid major surgical complications.

This chapter does not duplicate the completeness of anatomic texts or surgical atlases; it concentrates on the norms of human anatomy. The reader must appreciate that wide individual differences in anatomic detail exist among patients. Understanding these variations is one of the greatest challenges of clinical medicine.

EXTERNAL GENITALIA

Vulva

The vulva, or pudendum, is a collective term for the external genital organs that are visible in the perineal area. The vulva consists of the following: the mons pubis, labia majora, labia minora, hymen, clitoris, vestibule, urethra, Skene's glands, Bartholin's glands, and vestibular bulbs (Fig. 3-1).

The boundaries of the vulva extend from the mons pubis anteriorly to the rectum posteriorly and from one lateral genitocrural fold to the other. The entire vulvar area is covered by keratinized, stratified squamous epithelium. The skin becomes thicker, more pigmented, and more keratinized as the distance from the vagina increases.

Mons Pubis

The mons pubis is a rounded eminence that becomes hairy after puberty. It is directly anterior and superior to the symphysis pubis. The hair pattern, or escutcheon, of most women is triangular. Genetic and racial differences produce a variety of normal hair patterns, with approximately one in four women having a modified escutcheon that has a diamond (malelike) pattern.

Labia Majora

The labia majora are two large, longitudinal, cutaneous folds of adipose and fibrous tissue. Each labium majus is approximately 7 to 8 cm in length and 2 to 3 cm in width. The labia extend from the mons pubis anteriorly to become lost in the skin between the vagina and the anus in the area of the posterior fourchette. The skin of the outer convex surface of the labia majora is pigmented and covered with hair follicles. The thin skin of the inner surface does not have hair follicles but has many sebaceous glands. Histologically the labia majora have both sweat and sebaceous glands (Fig. 3-2). The apocrine glands are similar to those of the breast and axillary areas. The size of the labia is related to fat content. Usually the labia atrophy after menopause. The labia majora are homologous to the scrotum in the male.

Labia Minora

The labia minora, or nymphae, are two small, red cutaneous folds that are situated between the labia majora and the vaginal orifice. They are more delicate, shorter, and thinner than the labia majora. Anteriorly, they divide at the clitoris to form superiorly the prepuce and inferiorly the frenulum of the clitoris. Histologically they are composed of dense connective tissue with erectile tissue and elastic fibers, rather than adipose tissue. The skin of the labia minora is less cornified and has many sebaceous glands but no hair follicles or sweat glands. The labia minora and the breasts are the only areas of the body rich in sebaceous glands without hair follicles. Among women of reproductive age, there is considerable variation in the size of the labia minora. They are relatively more prominent in children and postmenopausal women. The labia minora are homologous to the penile urethra and part of the skin of the penis in males.

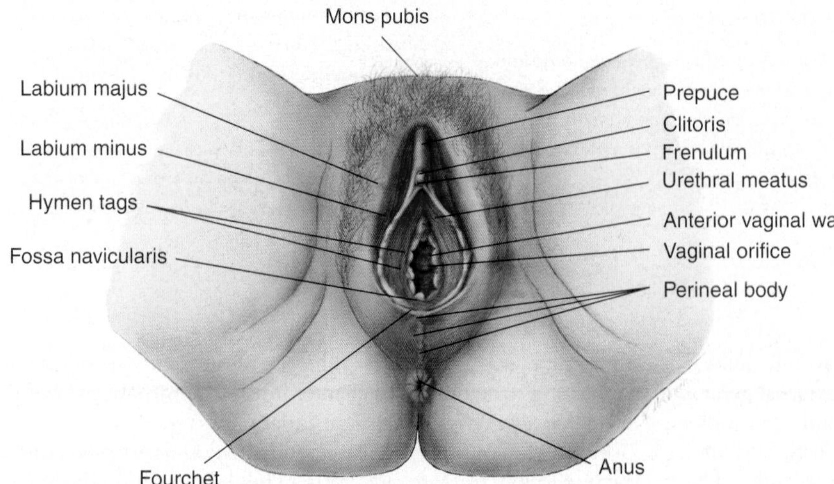

Figure 3-1. The structures of the external genitalia that are collectively called the vulva. (Redrawn from Pritchard JA, MacDonald PC, Gant NF: Williams' Obstetrics, 17th ed. New York, Appleton-Century-Crofts, 1985, p 8.)

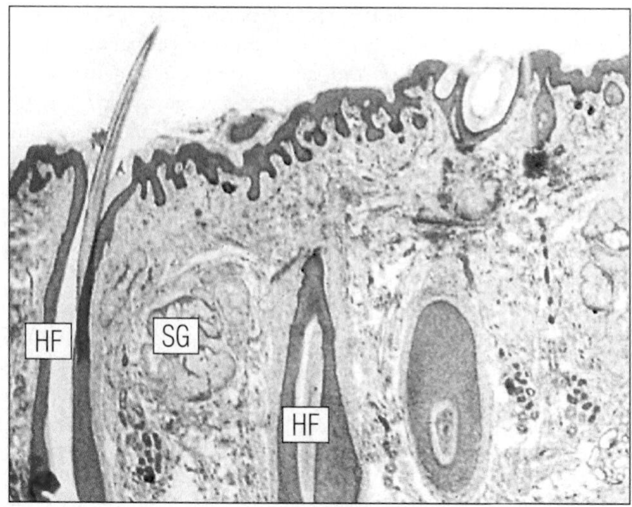

Figure 3-2. Histologic section from the labia majora. HF, hair follicles; SG, sebaceous glands. Note the eccrine glands and ducts. (From Stevens A, Lowe J: Human Histology, 3rd ed., Philadelphia, Elsevier, 2002, p 346.)

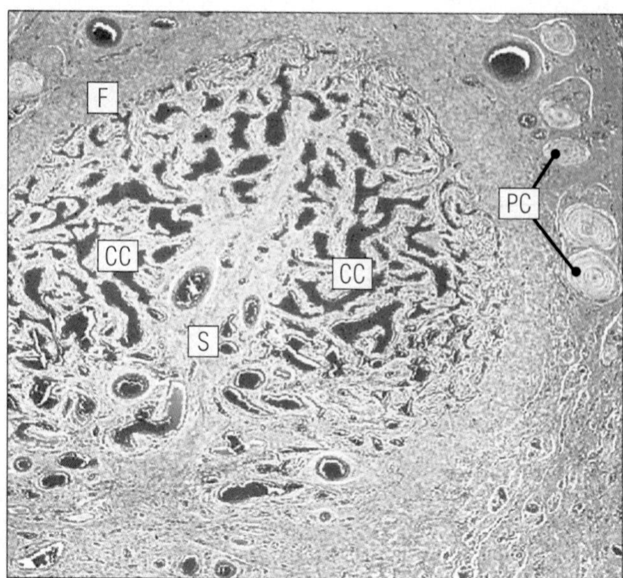

Figure 3-3. A histologic section of the clitoris. Note the two corpus cavernosa (CC), the septum (S), and the fibrous-collagenous sheath (F). Multiple nerve endings may be seen surrounding the clitoris. PC, pacinian touch corpuscles. (From Stevens A, Lowe J: Human Histology, 3rd ed. Philadelphia, Elsevier, 2002, p 346.)

Hymen

The hymen is a thin, usually perforated membrane at the entrance of the vagina. There are many variations in the structure and shape of the hymen. The hymen histologically is covered by stratified squamous epithelium on both sides and consists of fibrous tissue with a few small blood vessels. Small tags, or nodules, of firm fibrous material, termed *carunculae myrtiformes,* are the remnants of the hymen identified in adult females.

Clitoris

The clitoris is a short, cylindrical, erectile organ at the superior portion of the vestibule. The normal adult glans clitoris has a width less than 1 cm, with an average length of 1.5 to 2 cm. Previous childbearing may influence the size of the clitoris, but age, weight, and oral contraceptive use do not change the anatomic dimensions. Usually, only the glans is visible, with the body of the clitoris positioned beneath the skin surface. The clitoris consists of a base of two crura, which attach to the periosteum of the symphysis pubis. The body has two cylindrical corpora cavernosa composed of thin-walled, vascular channels that function as erectile tissue (Fig. 3-3). The distal one third of the clitoris is the glans, which has many nerve endings. The clitoris is the female homologue of the penis in the male.

Vestibule

The vestibule is the lowest portion of the embryonic urogenital sinus. It is the cleft between the labia minora that is visualized when the labia are held apart. The vestibule extends from the clitoris to the posterior fourchette. The orifices of the urethra and vagina and the ducts from Bartholin's glands open into the vestibule. Within the area of the vestibule are the remnants of the hymen and numerous small mucinous glands.

Urethra

The urethra is a membranous conduit for urine from the urinary bladder to the vestibule. The female urethra measures 3.5 to 5 cm in length. The mucosa of the proximal two thirds of the urethra is composed of stratified transitional epithelium, whereas the distal one third is stratified squamous epithelium. The distal orifice is 4 to 6 mm in diameter, and the mucosal edges grossly appear everted.

Skene's Glands

Skene's glands, or paraurethral glands, are branched, tubular glands that are adjacent to the distal urethra. Usually Skene's ducts run parallel to the long axis of the urethra for approximately 1 cm before opening into the distal urethra. Sometimes the ducts open into the area just outside the urethral orifice. Skene's glands are the largest of the paraurethral glands; however, many smaller glands empty into the urethra. Skene's glands are homologous to the prostate in the male.

Bartholin's Glands

Bartholin's glands are vulvovaginal glands that are located beneath the fascia at about 4 and 8 o'clock, respectively, on the posterolateral aspect of the vaginal orifice. Each lobulated, racemose gland is about the size of a pea. Histologically the gland is composed of cuboidal epithelium (Fig. 3-4). The duct from each gland is lined by transitional epithelium and is approximately 2 cm in length. Bartholin's ducts open into a groove

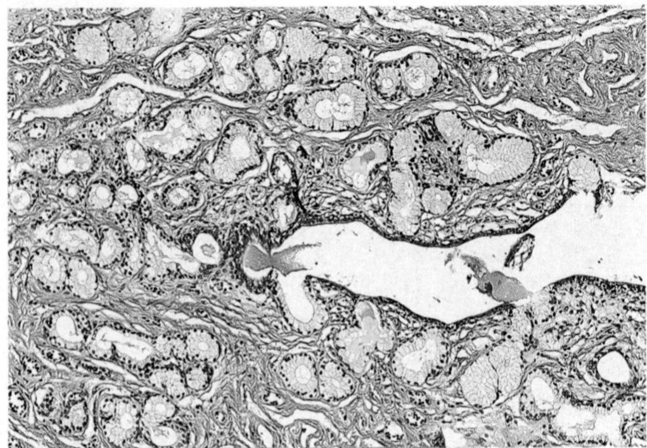

Figure 3-4. A histologic section of a Bartholin's gland. Note the multiple alveoli draining into a central duct. (From Shea CR, Stevens A, Dalziel KL, Robboy SJ: Vulva. In Robboy SJ, Anderson MC, Russell P [eds]: Pathology of the Female Reproductive Tract. Edinburgh, Churchill Livingstone, 2002, p 36.)

between the hymen and the labia minora. Bartholin's glands are homologous to Cowper's glands in the male.

Vestibular Bulbs

The vestibular bulbs are two elongated masses of erectile tissue situated on either side of the vaginal orifice. Each bulb is immediately below the bulbocavernosus muscle. The distal ends of the vestibular bulbs are adjacent to Bartholin's glands. They are homologous to the bulb of the penis in the male.

CLINICAL CORRELATIONS

The skin of the vulvar region is subject to both local and general dermatologic conditions. The intertriginous areas of the vulva remain moist, and obese women are particularly susceptible to chronic infection. The vulvar skin of a postmenopausal woman is sensitive to topical cortisone and testosterone but insensitive to topical estrogen. The most common large cystic structure of the vulva is a Bartholin's duct cyst. This condition may become painful if the cyst develops into an acute abscess. Chronic infections of the periurethral glands may result in one or more urethral diverticula. The most common symptoms of a urethral diverticulum are similar to the symptoms of a lower urinary tract infection: urinary frequency, urgency, and dysuria.

Vulvar trauma such as straddle injuries frequently results in large hematoms or profuse external hemorrhage. The richness of the vascular supply and the absence of valves in vulvar veins contribute to this complication. The abundant vascularity of the region promotes rapid healing, with an associated low incidence of wound infection in episiotomies or obstetric tears of the vulva.

The subcutaneous fatty tissue of the labia majora and mons pubis are in continuity with the fatty tissue of the anterior abdominal wall. Infections in this space such as cellulites and necrotizing fasciitis are poorly contained, and may extend cephaladly in rapid fashion.

INTERNAL GENITALIA

Vagina

The vagina, is a thin-walled, distensible, fibromuscular tube that extends from the vestibule of the vulva to the uterus. The potential space of the vagina is larger in the middle and upper thirds. The walls of the vagina are normally in apposition and flattened in the anteroposterior diameter. Thus the vagina has the appearance of the letter H in cross section (Fig. 3-5).

The axis of the upper portion of the vagina lies fairly close to the horizontal plane when a woman is standing, with the upper portion of the vagina curving toward the hollow of the sacrum. In most women an angle of at least 90° is formed between the

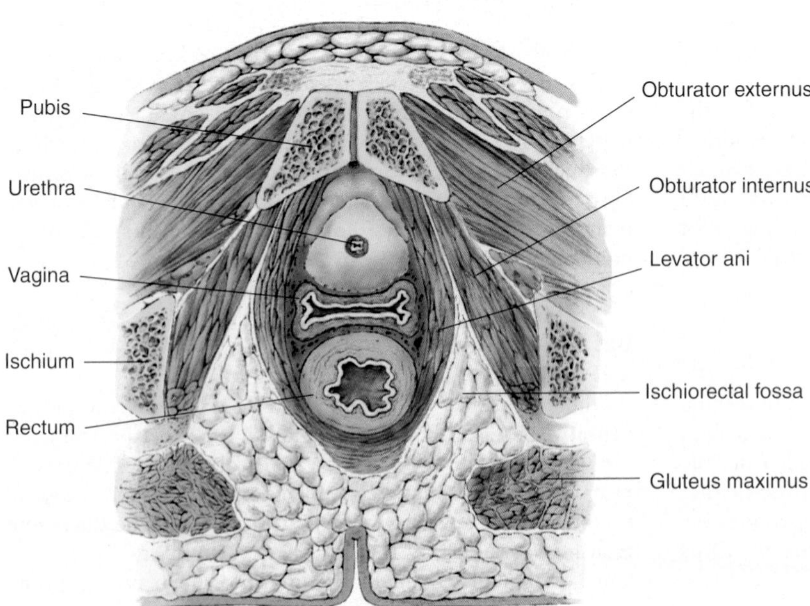

Figure 3-5. A schematic drawing of a cross section of the female pelvis, demonstrating the H shape of the vagina. Note the surrounding levator ani muscle. (Redrawn from Pritchard JA, MacDonald PC, Gant NF: Williams' Obstetrics, 17th ed. New York, Appleton-Century-Crofts, 1985, p 12.)

axis of the vagina and the axis of the uterus (Fig. 3-6). The vagina is held in position by the surrounding endopelvic fascia and ligaments.

The lower third of the vagina is in close relationship with the urogenital and pelvic diaphragms. The middle third of the vagina is supported by the levator ani muscles and the lower portion of the cardinal ligaments. The upper third is supported by the upper portions of the cardinal ligaments and the parametria.

The vagina of reproductive-age women has numerous transverse folds, termed *rugae.* They help provide accordion-like distensibility and are more prominent in the lower third of the vagina. The cervix extends into the upper part of the vagina. The spaces between the cervix and attachment of the vagina are called *fornices.* The posterior fornix is considerably larger than the anterior fornix; thus the anterior vaginal length is approximately 6 to 9 cm in comparison with a posterior vaginal length of 8 to 12 cm.

Histologically the vagina is composed of four distinct layers. The mucosa consists of a stratified, nonkeratinized squamous epithelium (Fig. 3-7). If the environment of the vaginal mucosa is modified, as in uterine prolapse, then the epithelium may become keratinized. The squamous epithelium is similar microscopically to the exocervix, although the vagina has larger and more frequent papillae that extend into the connective tissue. The normal vagina does not have glands. The next layer is the lamina propria, or tunica. It is composed of fibrous connective tissue. Throughout this layer of collagen and elastic tissue is a rich supply of vascular and lymphatic channels. The density of the connective tissue in the endopelvic fascia varies throughout the longitudinal axis of the vagina. The muscular layer has many interlacing fibers. However, an inner circular layer and an outer longitudinal layer can be identified. The fourth layer consists of cellular areolar connective tissue containing a large plexus of blood vessels.

The vascular system of the vagina is generously supplied with an extensive anastomotic network throughout its length. The vaginal artery originates either directly from the uterine artery or as a branch of the internal iliac artery arising posterior to the origin of the uterine and inferior vesical arteries. The vaginal arteries may be multiple arteries on each side of the pelvis. There is an anastomosis with the cervical branch of the uterine artery to form the azygos arteries. Branches of the internal pudendal, inferior vesical, and middle hemorrhoidal arteries also contribute to the interconnecting network and the longitudinal azygos arteries.

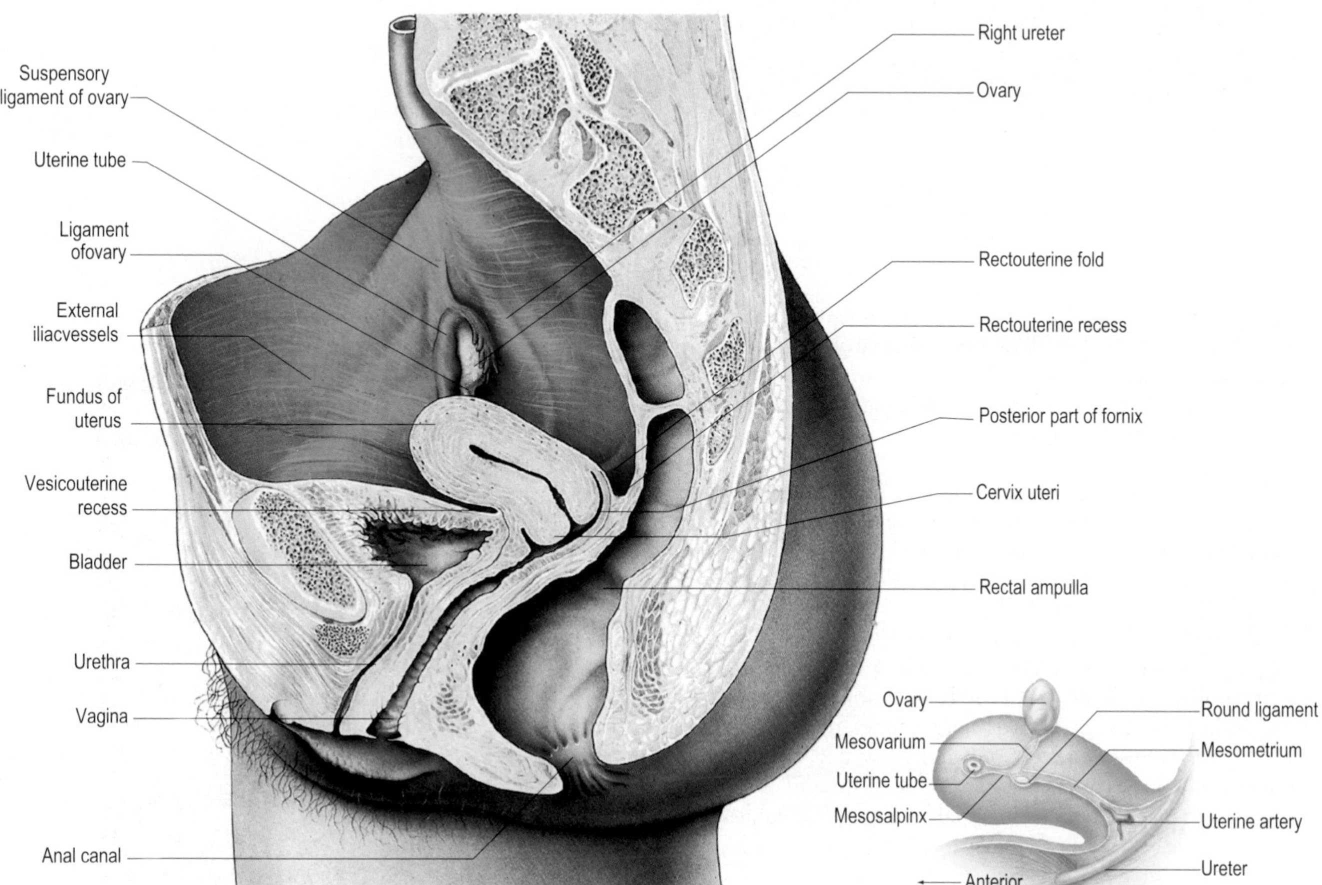

Figure 3-6. A median sagittal section through the pelvis. The peritoneum is shaded blue. Note the proximal vagina at a close to horizontal axis and in a near 90° juxtaposition to the uterus. In this woman, the uterus is anteflexed. (From Standring S [ed]: Gray's Anatomy, 39th ed. Edinburgh, Elsevier Churchill Livingstone, 2005, p 1321.)

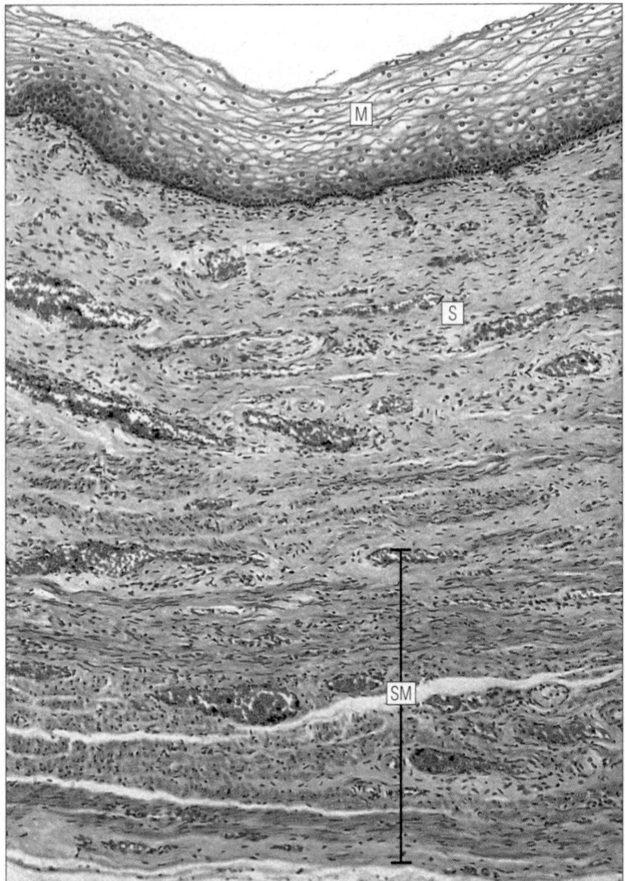

Figure 3-7. Histologic section of the vaginal squamous epithelium (M). Submucosa (S) is well vascularized. (Lamina propria). SM, smooth muscle. (From Stevens A, Lowe J: Human Histology, 3rd ed. Philadelphia, Elsevier, 2002, p 347.)

The venous drainage is complex and accompanies the arterial system. Below the pelvic floor the principal venous drainage occurs via the pudendal veins. The vaginal, uterine, and vesical veins, as well as those around the rectosigmoid, all provide venous drainage of the venous plexuses surrounding the middle and upper vagina.

The nerve supply of the vagina comes from the autonomic nervous system's vaginal plexus, and sensory fibers come from the pudendal nerve. Pain fibers enter the spinal cord in sacral segments two to four. There is a paucity of free nerve endings in the upper two thirds of the vagina.

The lymphatic drainage is characterized by its wide distribution and frequent crossovers between the right and left sides of the pelvis. In general the primary lymphatic drainage of the upper third of the vagina is to the external iliac nodes, the middle third of the vagina drains to the common and internal iliac nodes, and the lower third has a complex and variable distribution, including the common iliac, superficial inguinal, and perirectal nodes.

CLINICAL CORRELATIONS

In clinical practice anatomic descriptions of pelvic organs are derived from Latin roots, such as the word *vagina* comes from the Latin word for sheath. In contrast, the names for surgical procedures of pelvic organs are derived from Greek roots. *Colpectomy, colporrhaphy,* and *colposcopy* are derived from *kolpos* (fold), the Greek word for the vagina, or salpingectomy from the Greek word for tube.

Clinicians should consider the H shape of the vagina when they insert a speculum and inspect the walls of the vagina. The posterior fornix is an important surgical landmark, since it provides direct access to the cul-de-sac of Douglas. The distal course of the ureter is an important consideration in vaginal surgery. Ureteral injury has occurred as a result of vaginally placed sutures to obtain hemostasis with vaginal lacerations. The anatomic proximity and interrelationships of the vascular and lymphatic networks of the bladder and vagina are such that inflammation of one organ can produce symptoms in the other. For example, vaginitis sometimes produces urinary tract symptoms, such as frequency and dysuria.

Gartner's duct cyst, a cystic dilation of the embryonic mesonephros (Fig. 3-8), is usually present on the lateral wall of the vagina. However, in the lower third of the vagina these cysts are present anteriorly and may be difficult to distinguish from a large urethral diverticulum.

An interesting phenomenon is the source of vaginal lubrication during intercourse. For years there was speculation on how an organ without glands is able to "secrete" fluid. Vaginal lubrication occurs from a transudate produced by engorgement of the vascular plexuses that encircle the vagina. This richness of vascualrization allows many drugs to readily enter the systemic circulation when placed in the vagina.

The anatomic relationship between the long axis of the vagina and other pelvic organs may be altered by pelvic relaxation

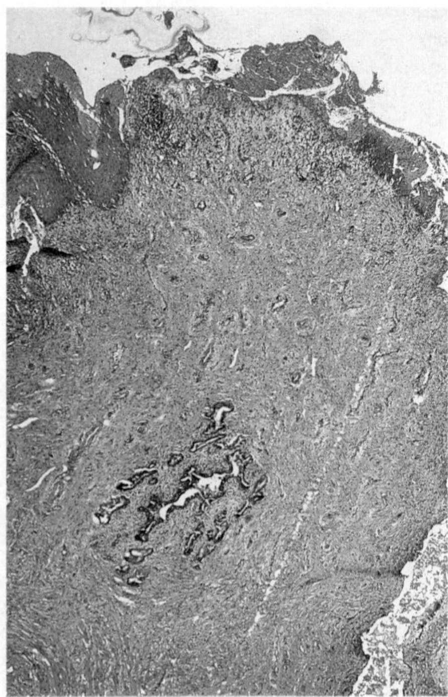

Figure 3-8. Mesonephric duct remnant in the vaginal wall. (From Robboy SJ, Anderson MC, Russell P [eds]: Pathology of the Female Reproductive Tract. Edinburgh, Churchill Livingstone, 2002, p 77.)

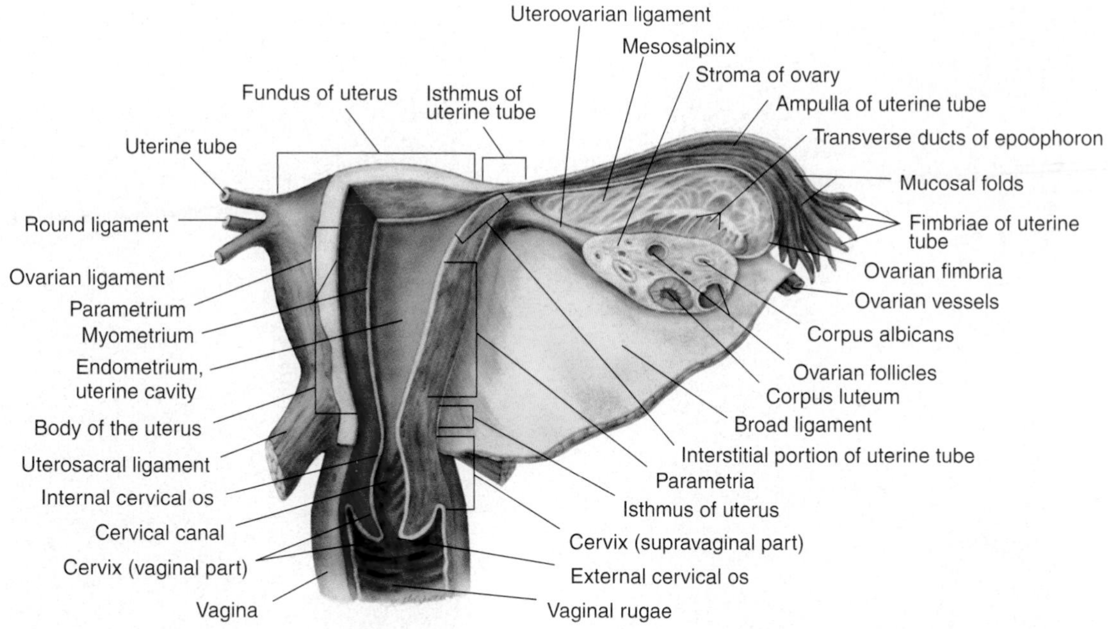

Figure 3-9. A schematic drawing of a posterior view of the cervix, uterus, fallopian tube, and ovary. Note that the cervix is divided by the vaginal attachment into an external portio segment and a supravaginal segment. Note that the uterus is composed of the dome-shaped fundus, the muscular body, and the narrow isthmus. Note the fimbria ovarica, or ovarian fimbria, attaching the oviduct to the ovary. (Redrawn from Clemente CD: Anatomy: A Regional Atlas of the Human Body, 3rd ed. Baltimore-Munich, Urban & Schwarzenberg, 1987.)

resulting primarily from the trauma of childbirth. Atrophy or weakness of the endopelvic fascia and muscles surrounding the vagina may result in the development of a cystocele, rectocele, or enterocele. One of the popular operations for vaginal vault prolapse is fixation of the apex to the vagina to the sacrospinous ligament. A rare complication of this operation is massive hemorrhage. The arterial bleeding is usually from the inferior gluteal or pudendal arteries.

Cervix

The lower, narrow portion of the uterus is the cervix. The word *cervix* originates from the Latin word for neck. The Greek word for neck is *trachelos,* and when the cervix is removed, the surgical procedure is termed *trachelectomy.* The cervix may vary in shape from cylindrical to conical. It consists of predominantly fibrous tissue in contrast to the primarily muscular corpus of the uterus.

The vagina is attached obliquely around the middle of the cervix; this attachment divides the cervix into an upper, supravaginal portion and a lower segment in the vagina called the *portio vaginalis* (Fig. 3-9). The supravaginal segment is covered by peritoneum posteriorly and is surrounded by loose, fatty connective tissue—the parametrium—anteriorly and laterally.

The canal of the cervix is fusiform, with the widest diameter in the middle. The length and width of the endocervical canal varies; it is usually 2.5 to 3 cm in length and 7 to 8 mm at its widest point. The width of the canal varies with the parity of the woman and changing hormonal levels. The cervical canal opens into the vagina at the external os of the cervix. In the majority of women the external os is in contact with the posterior vaginal wall. The external os is small and round in nulliparous women. The os is wider and gaping following vaginal delivery. Often lateral or stellate scars are residual marks of previous cervical lacerations.

The mucous membrane of the endocervical canal of nulliparous women is arranged in longitudinal folds, called plicae palmatae, with secondary branching folds, the arbor vitae (Fig. 3-10). These folds, which form a herringbone pattern, disappear following vaginal delivery.

A single layer of columnar epithelium lines the endocervical canal and the underlying glandular structures. This specialized

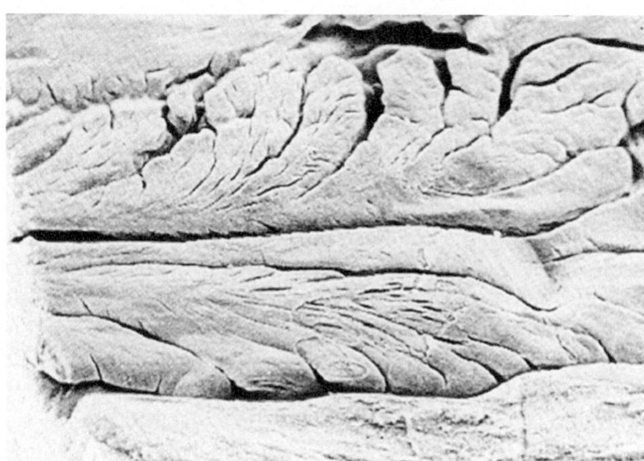

Figure 3-10. An electron micrograph of the endocervical canal, demonstrating the arbor vitae. These folds and crypts provide a reservoir for sperm. (From Singer A, Jordan JA: The anatomy of the cervix. In Jordan JA, Singer A [eds]: The Cervix. Philadelphia, WB Saunders, 1976, p 18.)

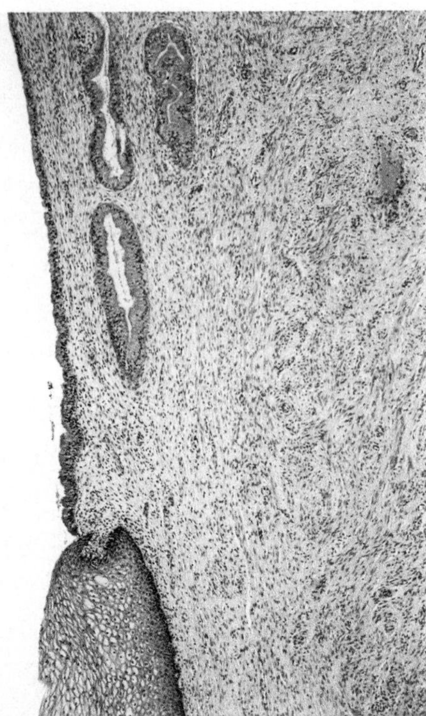

Figure 3-11. A histologic section through the squamocolumnar junction of the cervix. Note the abrupt transformation from squamous to columnar epithelium. (From Standring S [ed]: Gray's Anatomy, 39th ed. Edinburgh, Elsevier Churchill Livingstone, 2005, p 1335.)

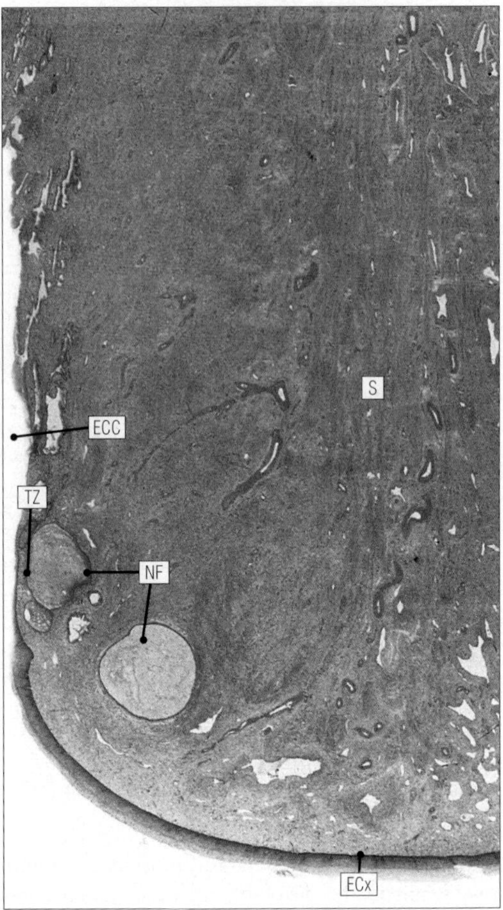

Figure 3-12. A low-power histologic section of the cervix. The stroma (S), has a small amount of smooth muscle. The ectocervix (Ecx) is covered in stratified squamous epithelium. The endocervix (ECC) is lined by tall columnar cells. NF-nabothian follicles, a normal finding, and TZ-transformation zone. (From Stevens A, Lowe J: Human Histology, 3rd ed. Philadelphia, Elsevier, 2002, p 349.)

epithelium secretes mucus, which facilitates sperm transport. An abrupt transformation usually is seen at the junction of the columnar epithelium of the endocervix and the nonkeratinized stratified squamous epithelium of the portio vaginalis (Fig. 3-11). The stratified squamous epithelium of the exocervix is identical to the lining of the vagina.

The dense, fibromuscular cervical stroma is composed primarily of collagenous connective tissue and mucopolysaccharide ground substance. The connective tissue contains approximately 15% smooth muscle cells and a small amount of elastic tissue (Fig. 3-12). However, there are few muscle fibers in the distal portions of the cervix.

It is not surprising that the cervical and uterine vascular supplies are interrelated. The arterial supply of the cervix arises from the descending branch of the uterine artery. The cervical arteries run on the lateral side of the cervix and form the coronary artery, which encircles the cervix. The azygos arteries run longitudinally in the middle of the anterior and posterior aspects of the cervix and the vagina. There are numerous anastomoses between these vessels and the vaginal and middle hemorrhoidal arteries. The venous drainage accompanies these arteries. The lymphatic drainage of the cervix is complex, involving multiple chains of nodes. The principal regional lymph nodes are the obturator, common iliac, internal iliac, external iliac, and visceral nodes of the parametria. Other possible lymphatic drainage includes the following chains of nodes: superior and inferior gluteal, sacral, rectal, lumbar, aortic, and visceral nodes over the posterior surface of the urinary bladder. The stroma of the endocervix is rich in free nerve endings. Pain fibers accompany the parasympathetic fibers to the second, third, and fourth sacral segments.

CLINICAL CORRELATIONS

The major arterial supply to the cervix is located on the lateral cervical walls at the 3 and 9 o'clock positions, respectively. Therefore a deep figure-of-eight suture through the vaginal mucosa and cervical stroma at 3 and 9 o'clock helps to reduce blood loss during procedures such as cone biopsy. If the gynecologist is overzealous in placing such a hemostatic suture high in the vaginal fornix, it is possible to compromise the course of the distal ureter.

The transformation zone of the cervix is an important anatomic landmark for clinicians. This area encompasses the transition from stratified squamous epithelium to columnar epithelium. Dysplasia of the cervix develops within this transformation zone. The position of a woman's transformation zone, in relation to the long axis of the cervix, depends on her age and hormonal status.

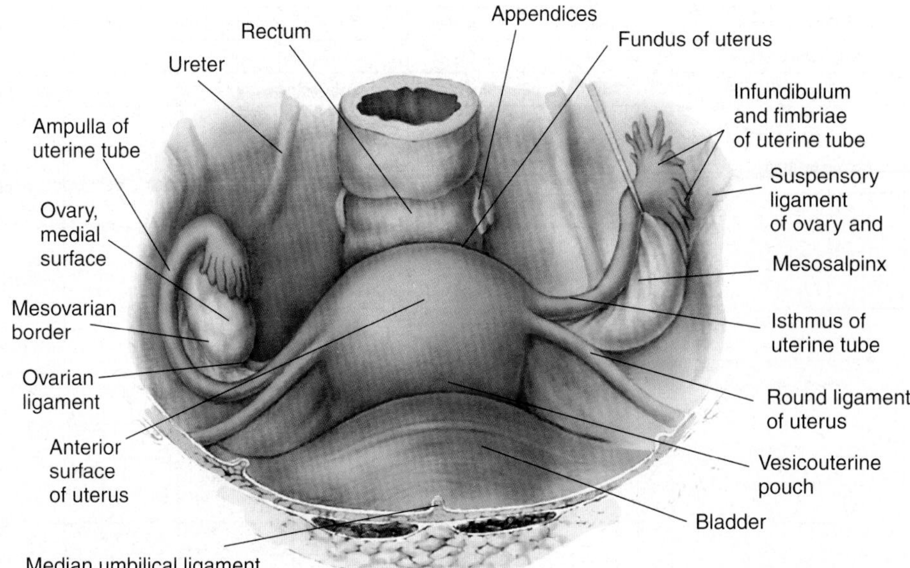

Figure 3-13. The organs of the female pelvis. The uterus is surrounded by the bladder anteriorly, the rectum posteriorly, and the folds of the broad ligaments laterally. (Redrawn from Clemente CD: Anatomy: A Regional Atlas of the Human Body, 3rd ed. Baltimore-Munich, Urban & Schwarzenberg, 1987.)

The endocervix is rich in free nerve endings. Occasionally, women experience a vasovagal response during transcervical instrumentation of the uterine cavity. Serial cardiac monitoring during insertion of intrauterine devices demonstrates a reflex bradycardia in some women. The sensory innervation of the exocervix is not as concentrated or sophisticated as that of the endocervix or external skin. Therefore, usually the exocervix may be cauterized by either cold or heat without major discomfort to the patient.

Uterus

The uterus is a thick-walled, hollow, muscular organ located centrally in the female pelvis. Adjacent to the uterus are the urinary bladder anteriorly, the rectum posteriorly, and the broad ligaments laterally (Figs. 3-6 and 3-13). The uterus is globular and slightly flattened anteriorly; it has the general configuration of an inverted pear. The short area of constriction in the lower uterine segment is termed the *isthmus* (Fig. 3-14). The dome-shaped top of the uterus is termed the *fundus.* The lower edge of the fundus is described by an imaginary line drawn between the site of entrance of each oviduct. The size and weight of the normal uterus depend on previous pregnancies and the hormonal status of the individual. The uterus of a nulliparous woman is approximately 8 cm long, 5 cm wide and 2.5 cm thick and weighs 40 to 50 g. In contrast, in a multiparous woman, each measurement is approximately 1.2 cm larger, and normal uterine weight is 20 to 30 g heavier. The upper limit for weight of a normal uterus is 110 g. The capacity of the uterus to enlarge during pregnancy results in a 10- to 20-fold increase in weight at term. After menopause the uterus atrophies in both size and weight.

The cavity of the uterus is flattened and triangular. The oviducts enter the uterine cavity at the superolateral aspects of the cavity in the areas designated the cornua. In the majority of women, the long axis of the uterus is both anteverted in respect to the long axis of the vagina and anteflexed in relation

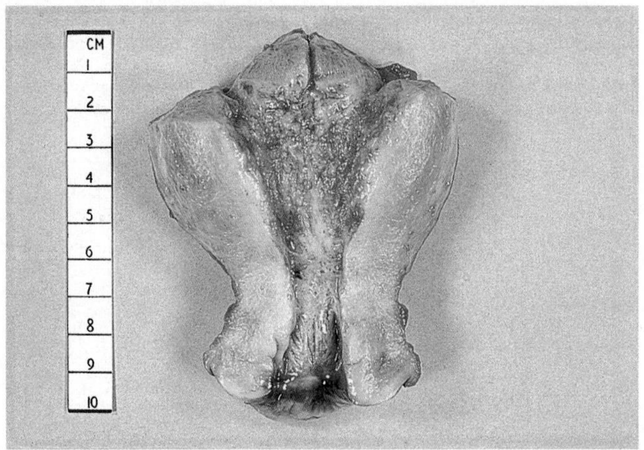

Figure 3-14. A surgical specimen of a uterus that has been opened. (From Robboy SJ, Anderson MC, Russell P [eds]: Pathology of the Female Reproductive Tract. Edinburgh, Churchill Livingstone, 2002, p 241.)

to the long axis of the cervix. However, a retroflexed uterus is a normal variant found in approximately 25% of women.

The uterus has three layers, similar to other hollow abdominal and pelvic organs. The thin, external serosal layer comprises the visceral peritoneum. The peritoneum is firmly attached to the uterus in all areas except anteriorly at the level of the internal os of the cervix. The wide middle muscular layer is composed of three indistinct layers of smooth muscle. The outer longitudinal layer is contiguous with the muscle layers of the oviduct and vagina. The middle layer has interlacing oblique, spiral bundles of smooth muscle and large venous plexuses. The inner muscular layer is also longitudinal. The endometrium is a reddish mucous membrane that varies from 1 to 6 mm in thickness, depending on hormonal stimulation (Fig. 3-15). The uterine glands are tubular and composed of tall columnar epithelium. The cells of the endometrial stroma resemble embryonic connective tissue with scant cytoplasm and large nuclei (Fig. 3-16). The endometrium may be divided into an inner stratum basale and an

Day of Cycle		Before 14	15-16	17	18	19-22	23	24-25	26-27	28+
Post-ovulatory day		-	1-2	3	4	5-8	9	10-11	12-13	14+
Cycle phases		Proliferative	'Interval'	Early secretory		Mid-secretory			Late secretory	Menstrual
Key feature		Mitoses	Mitoses and subnuclear vacuoles	Maximum subnuclear vacuoles	Subnuclear vacuoles present	Stromal edema	Focal decidua around spiral arteries	Patchy decidua	Extensive decidua	Stromal crumbling
Microscopic features of functional zone	**Stroma**	Loose stroma. Mitoses	Same as proliferative	Loose stroma, scanty mitoses	Loose stroma	Stromal edema	Focal decidua around spiral arteries. Edema prominent	Decidua throughout stroma. Some edema	Extensive decidua. Prominent granulated lymphocytes	Stromal crumbling. Hemorrhage
	Glands	Straight to tightly coiled tubules. Mitoses	Some subnuclear vacuoles, otherwise as prolifertaive	Extensive subnuclear vacuoles	Dilated glands. Some subnuclear vacuoles	Dilated glands with irregular outline. Luminal secretion		'Saw tooth' glands	Prominent 'saw tooth' glands	Disrupted glands. Secretory exhaustion. Regeneraing epithelium
Appearances		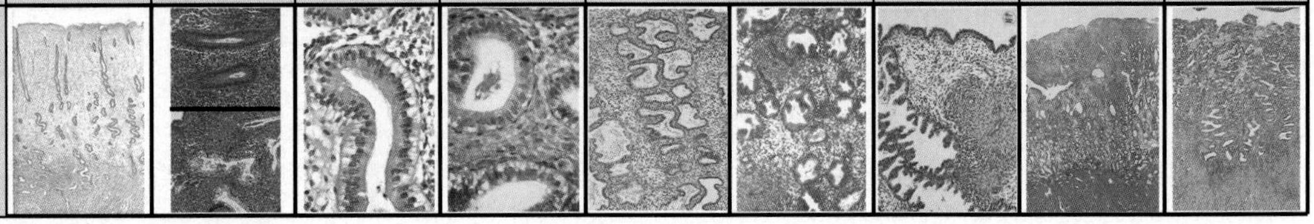								

Figure 3-15. The endometrium is responsive to the hormonal changes of the menstrual cycle. Glands and stroma change activity and thus histologic appearance throughout the cycle. (From Robboy SJ, Anderson MC, Russell P [eds]: Pathology of the Female Reproductive Tract. Edinburgh, Churchill Livingstone, 2002, p 248.)

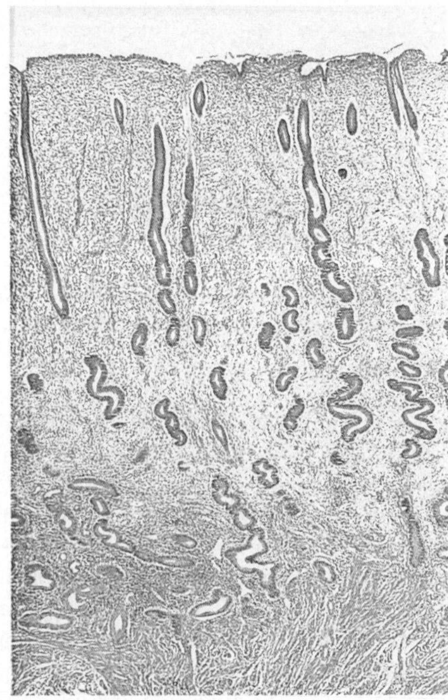

Figure 3-16. Low-power histologic section of proliferative endometrium. (From Robboy SJ, Anderson MC, Russell P [eds]: Pathology of the Female Reproductive Tract. Edinburgh, Churchill Livingstone, 2002, p 248.)

outer stratum functionale. The stratum functionale may be further subdivided into an inner compact stratum and a more superficial spongy stratum. Only the stratum functionale responds to fluctuating hormonal levels.

The arterial blood supply of the uterus is provided by the uterine and ovarian arteries. The uterine arteries are large branches of the hypogastric arteries, whereas the ovarian arteries originate directly from the aorta. The veins of the pelvic organs accompany the arteries. Therefore venous drainage from the fundus goes to the ovarian veins and blood from the corpus exits via the uterine veins into the iliac veins. The lymphatic drainage of the uterus is complex. The majority of lymphatics from the fundus and the body of the uterus go to the aortic, lumbar, and pelvic nodes surrounding the iliac vessels, especially the internal iliac nodes. However, it is possible for metastatic disease from the uterus to be found in the superior inguinal nodes transported via lymphatics in the round ligament.

In contrast to other pelvic organs, the afferent sensory nerve fibers from the uterus are in close proximity to the sympathetic nerves. Afferent nerve fibers from the uterus enter the spinal cord at the eleventh and twelfth thoracic segments. The sympathetic nerve supply to the uterus comes from the hypogastric and ovarian plexus. The parasympathetic fibers are largely derived from the pelvic nerve and from the second, third, and fourth sacral segments.

CLINICAL CORRELATIONS

Removal of the uterus is termed *hysterectomy,* which is derived from the Greek word *hystera,* meaning womb. The symptoms of primary dysmenorrhea are treated successfully in most women by prostaglandin synthetase inhibition. Rarely is a woman's pain not controlled by oral medication. However, it is possible to alleviate uterine pain by cutting the sensory nerves that accompany the sympathetic nerves. This operation is termed a *presacral neurectomy.* During the operation the gynecologist must be careful to avoid injuring the ureters and also careful to control hemorrhage from vessels in the retroperitoneal space.

The position of the fundus of the uterus in relation to the long axis of the vagina is quite variable. Not only are there differences between individual women but also in the same woman secondary to normal activity. In some women the uterus is anteflexed or anteverted, whereas in others the normal position is retroflexed or retroverted. In the 1930s and 1940s a retroflexed uterus was believed to be one of the primary causes of pelvic pain. To alleviate this condition many women underwent an anterior uterine suspension. Modern gynecologists have abandoned the suspension operation as a treatment for pelvic pain.

The arterial blood supply enters the uterus on its lateral margins. This relationship allows morcellation of an enlarged uterus to facilitate removal of multiple myomas without appreciably increasing blood loss during vaginal hysterectomy.

Methods of transcervical female sterilization designed to occlude the tubal ostia at the uterine cornua have been attempted for many years. Procedures that blindly inject caustic solutions into the uterine cornua have a high percentage of failure. Individual differences in size and shape of the uterine cavity and muscular spasm of this region are the primary reasons that sufficient amounts of the caustic chemicals do not reach the fallopian tubes in up to 20% of patients.

Oviducts

The paired uterine tubes, more commonly referred to as the *fallopian tubes* or *oviducts,* extend outward from the superolateral portion of the uterus and end by curling around the ovary (Fig. 3-17). The oviducts are also referred to using the prefix "salpingo," from the Greek *salpinx,* meaning a tube. The tubes

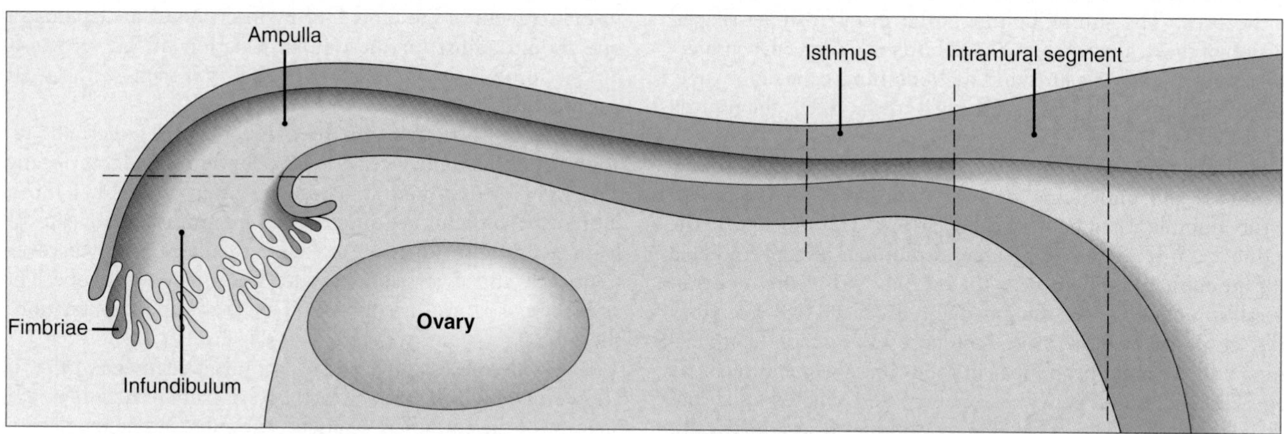

A

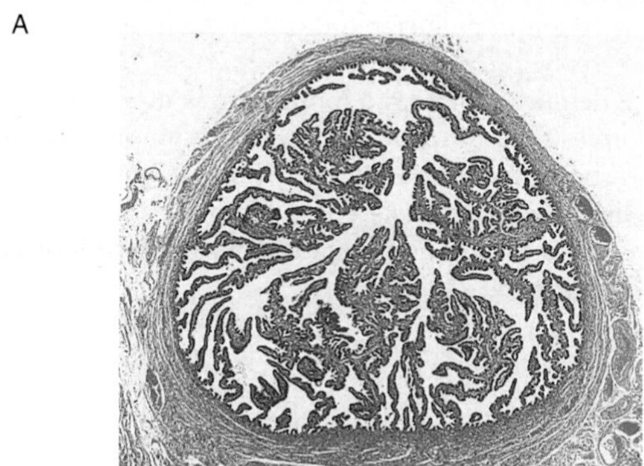

B

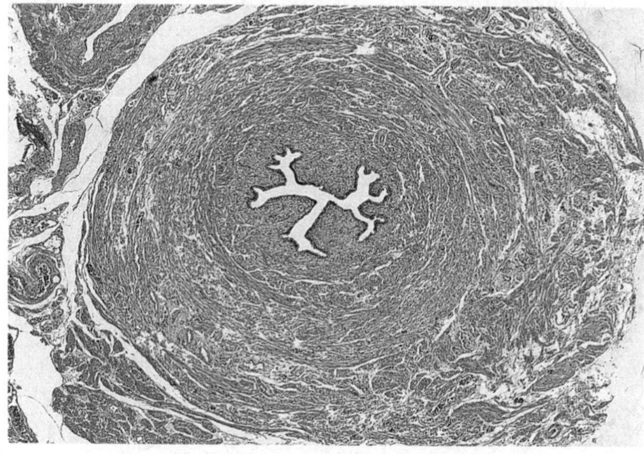

C

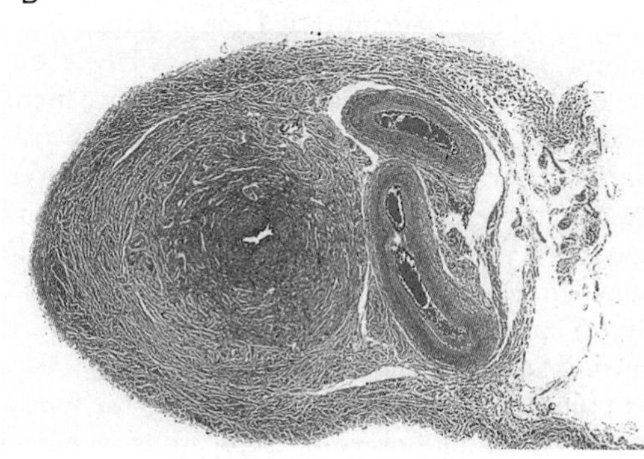

D

Figure 3-17. The fallopian tube. **A.** Schematic representation. Note that the intramural segment is within the uterine body. **B,** Low-power histologic section from the ampulla. **C,** Section from the isthmus of the tube. **D,** Section from the isthmus. Note the thick muscular wall. (**A, B,** and **D,** from Stevens A, Lowe J: Human Histology, 3rd ed. Philadelphia, Elsevier, 2002, p 354; **C,** from Robboy SJ, Anderson MC, Russell P [eds]: Pathology of the Female Reproductive Tract. Edinburgh, Churchill Livingstone, 2002, p 416.)

are contained in a free edge of the superior portion of the broad ligament. The mesentery of the tubes, the mesosalpinx, contains the blood supply and nerves. The uterine tubes connect the cornua of the uterine cavity and the peritoneal cavity. The ostia into the endometrial cavity are 1.5 mm in diameter, whereas the ostia into the abdominal cavity are approximately 3 mm in diameter.

The oviducts are between 10 and 14 cm in length and slightly less than 1 cm in external diameter. Each tube is divided into four anatomic sections. The uterine intramural, or interstitial, segment is 1 to 2 cm in length and is surrounded by myometrium. The isthmic segment begins as the tube exits the uterus and is approximately 4 cm in length. This segment is narrow, 1 to 2 mm in inside diameter, and straight. The isthmic segment has the most highly developed musculature. The ampullary segment is 4 to 6 cm in length and approximately 6 mm in inside diameter. It is wider and more tortuous in its course than other segments. Fertilization normally occurs in the ampullary portion of the tube. The infundibulum is the distal trumpet-shaped portion of the oviduct. From 20 to 25 irregular finger-like projections, termed *fimbriae,* surround the abdominal ostia of the tube. One of the largest fimbriae is attached to the ovary, the fimbria ovarica.

The tube contains numerous longitudinal folds, called plicae, of mucosa and underlying stroma. Plicae are most prominent in the ampullary segment (see Fig. 3-17). The mucosa of the oviduct has three different cell types. Columnar ciliated epithelial cells are most prominent near the ovarian end of the tube and overall compose 25% of the mucosal cells (Fig. 3-18). Secretory cells, also columnar in shape, compose 60% of the epithelial lining and are more prominent in the isthmic segment. Narrow peg cells are found between secretory and ciliated cells and are believed to be a morphologic variant of secretory cells. The stroma of the mucosa is sparse. However, there is a thick lamina propria with vascular channels between the epithelium and muscular layers. The smooth muscle of the tube is arranged into inner circular and outer longitudinal layers. Between the peritoneal surface of the tube and the muscular layer is an adventitial layer that contains blood vessels and nerves.

The arterial blood supply to the oviducts is derived from terminal branches of the uterine and ovarian arteries. The arteries anastomose in the mesosalpinx. Blood from the uterine artery supplies the medial two thirds of each tube. The venous drainage runs parallel to the arterial supply. The lymphatic system is separate and distinct from the lymphatic drainage of the uterus. Lymphatic drainage includes the internal iliac nodes and the aortic nodes surrounding the aorta and the inferior vena cava at the level of the renal vessels.

The tubes are innervated by both sympathetic and parasympathetic nerves from the uterine and ovarian plexuses. Sensory nerves are related to spinal cord segments T11, T12, and L1.

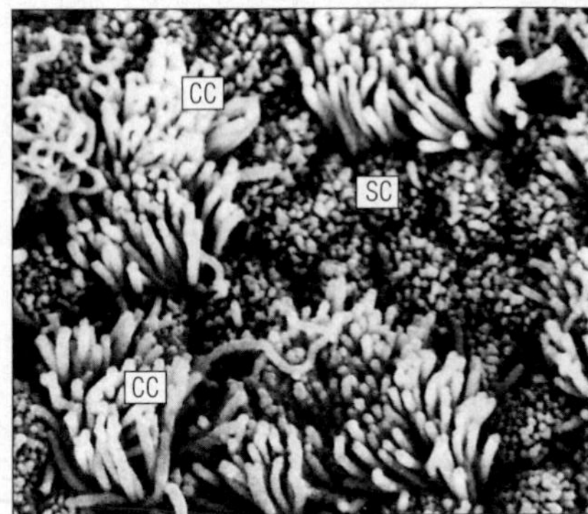

Figure 3-18. Electron micrograph of the tubal mucosa from the ampulla. CC, ciliated cells; SC, secretory cells. (From Stevens A, Lowe J: Human Histology, 3rd ed. Philadelphia, Elsevier, 2002, p 354.)

CLINICAL CORRELATIONS

The vast majority of ectopic pregnancies occur in the oviduct. The acute abdominal and pelvic pain that women with an ectopic pregnancy experience is believed to be caused by hemorrhage. The most catastrophic bleeding associated with ectopic pregnancy occurs when the implantation site is in the intramural segment of the tube. During insertion of the laparoscope, one should adjust for the caudal deviation in the vertical axis of the umbilicus in extremely obese women with a large panniculus.

The isthmic segment of the oviduct is the preferred site to apply an occlusive device, such as a clip, for female sterilization. The right oviduct and appendix are often adjacent. Clinically it may be difficult to differentiate inflammation of the tube from acute appendicitis. Accessory tubal ostia are discovered frequently and always connect with the lumen of the tube. These accessory ostia are usually found in the ampullary portion of the tube.

The wide mesosalpinx of the ampullary segment of the tube allows torsion of the tube, which occasionally results in ischemic atrophy of the ampullary segment. Paratubal or paraovarian cysts can reach 5 to 10 cm in diameter and occasionally are confused with ovarian cysts before surgery.

Although a definitive anatomic sphincter has not been identified at the uterotubal junction, a temporary physiologic obstruction has been identified during hysterosalpingography. Sometimes clinicians may alleviate this temporary obstruction by giving the patient intravenous sedation, a paracervical block, or intravenous glucagon.

Ovaries

The paired ovaries are light gray, and each one is approximately the size and configuration of a large almond. The surface of the ovary of adult women is pitted and indented from previous ovulations. The ovaries contain approximately 1 to 2 million oocytes at birth. During a woman's reproductive lifetime, about 8000 follicles begin development. The growth of many follicles is blunted in various stages of development; however, approximately 300 ova eventually are released. The size and position of the ovary depend on the woman's age and parity. During the reproductive years, ovaries weigh 3 to 6 g and measure approximately 1.5 cm × 2.5 cm × 4 cm. As the woman ages, the ovaries become smaller and firmer in consistency.

In a nulliparous woman who is standing, the long axis of the ovary is vertical. The ovary in nulliparous women rests in a depression of peritoneum named the ovarian fossa. Immediately adjacent to the ovarian fossa are the external iliac vessels, the ureter, and the obturator vessels and nerves.

Three prominent ligaments determine the anatomic mobility of the ovary (Fig. 3-19). The posterior portion of the broad ligament forms the mesovarium, which attaches to the anterior border of the ovary. The mesovarium contains the arterial anastomotic branches of the ovarian and uterine arteries, a plexus of veins, and the lateral end of the ovarian ligament. The ovarian ligament is a narrow, short, fibrous band that extends from the lower pole of the ovary to the uterus. The infundibular pelvic ligament, or suspensory ligament of the ovary, forms the superior and lateral aspect of the broad ligament. This ligament contains the ovarian artery, ovarian veins, and accompanying nerves. It attaches the upper pole of the ovary to the lateral pelvic wall.

The ovary is subdivided histologically into an outer cortex and an inner medulla (Fig. 3-20). The ovarian surface is covered by a single layer of cuboidal epithelium, termed the *germinal epithelium.* This term is a misnomer because the cells are similar to those of the coelomic mesothelium, which forms the peritoneum, and because the germinal epithelium is not related to the histogenesis of graafian follicles. If the ovary is transected, numerous transparent, fluid-filled cysts are noted throughout the cortex. Microscopically these are graafian follicles in various stages of development, active or regressing corpus luteum, and atretic follicles. The stroma of the cortex is composed primarily of closely packed cells around the follicles. These specialized connective tissue cells form the theca. The medulla contains the ovarian vascular supply and a loose stroma. The specialized polyhedral hilar cells are similar to the interstitial cells of the testis.

Each of the ovarian arteries arises directly from the aorta just below the renal arteries. They descend in the retroperitoneal space, cross anterior to the psoas muscles and internal iliac vessels, and enter the infundibulopelvic ligaments, reaching the mesovarium in the broad ligament. The ovarian blood supply enters through the hilum of the ovary. The venous drainage of the ovary collects in the pampiniform plexus and consolidates into several large veins as it leaves the hilum of the ovary. The ovarian veins accompany the ovarian arteries, with the left ovarian vein draining into the left renal vein, whereas the right ovarian vein connects directly with the inferior vena cava.

The lymphatic drainage of the ovaries is primarily to the aortic nodes adjacent to the great vessels at the level of the renal veins. Metastatic disease from the ovary occasionally takes a shorter course to the iliac nodes. The autonomic and sensory nerve fibers accompany the ovarian vasculature in the infundibulopelvic ligament. They connect with the ovarian, hypogastric, and aortic plexuses.

CLINICAL CORRELATIONS

The size of the "normal" ovary during the reproductive years and the postmenopausal period is important in clinical practice. Before menopause a normal ovary may be up to 5 cm in length. Thus a small physiologic cyst may cause an ovary to be 6 to 7 cm in diameter. In contrast, the normal atrophic postmenopausal ovary usually cannot be palpated during pelvic examination.

It is important to emphasize that the ovaries and surrounding peritoneum are not devoid of pain and pressure receptors. Therefore it is not unusual for a woman during a routine pelvic examination to experience discomfort when normal ovaries are palpated bimanually.

Attempts have been made to alleviate chronic pelvic pain by performing an ovarian denervation operation by cutting and ligating the infundibulopelvic ligaments. This operation has been abandoned because of the high incidence of cystic degeneration of the ovaries, which resulted from the interruption of their primary blood supply that was associated with the neurectomy procedure.

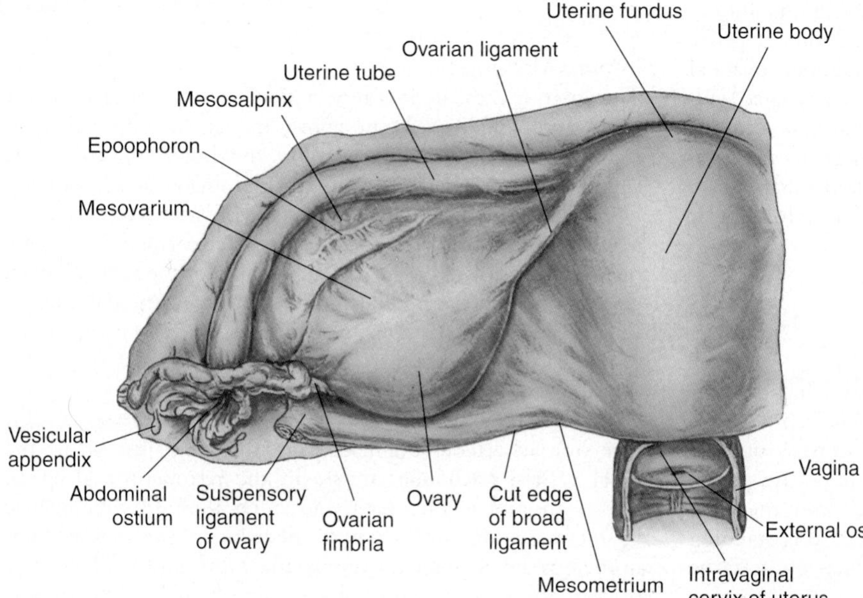

Figure 3-19. The posterior aspect of the broad ligament-spread out to demonstrate the ovary. (From Standring S [ed]: Gray's Anatomy, 39th ed. Edinburgh, Elsevier Churchill Livingstone, 2005, p 1322.)

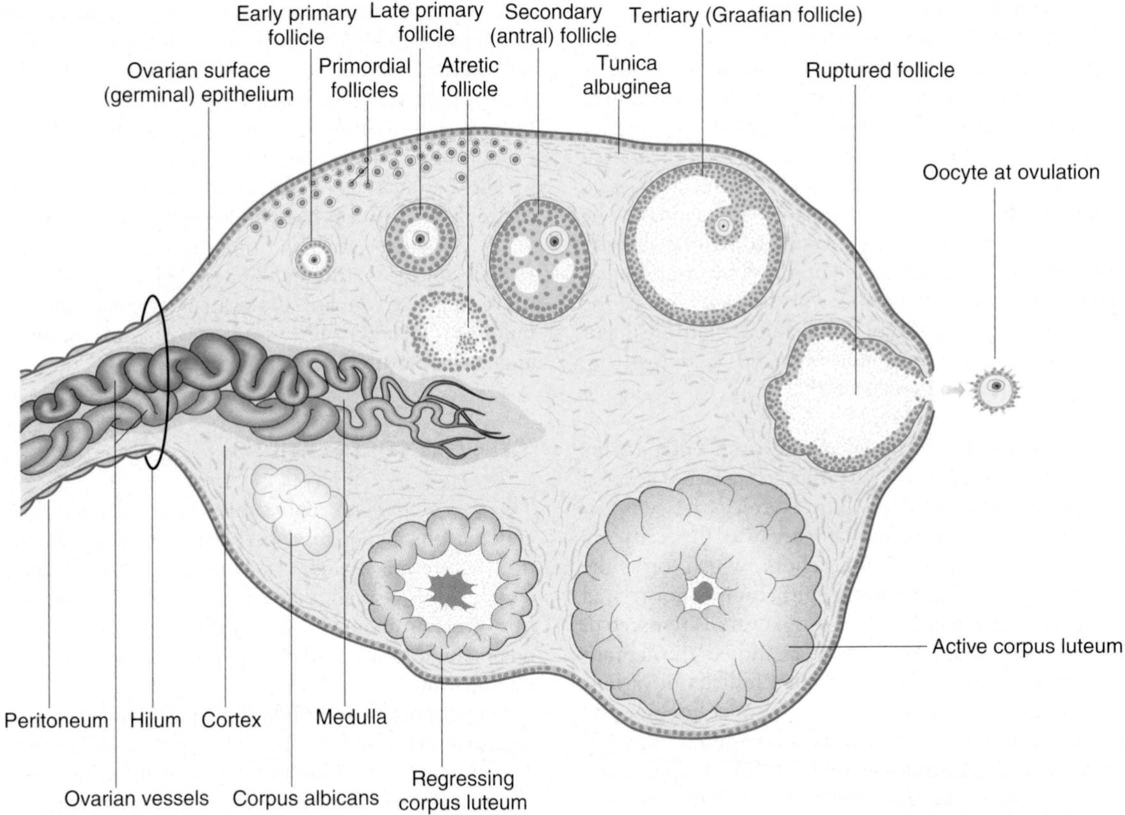

Figure 3-20. A schematic drawing of the ovary. Note the single layer of cuboidal epithelium called the *germinal epithelium.* Note the graafian follicles in different stages of development. (From Standring S [ed]: Gray's Anatomy, 39th ed. Edinburgh, Elsevier Churchill Livingstone, 2005, p 1324.)

The close anatomic proximity of the ovary, ovarian fossa, and ureter is emphasized in surgery to treat severe endometriosis or pelvic inflammatory disease. It is important to identify the course of the ureter in order to facilitate removal of all of the ovarian capsule that is adherent to the peritoneum and surrounding structures so as to avoid immediate ureteral injury and residual retroperitoneal ovarian remnants in the future. Prophylactic oophorectomy is performed at the time of pelvic operations in postmenopausal women. Sometimes bilateral oophorectomy is technically more difficult when associated with a vaginal procedure in contrast to an abdominal hysterectomy. Vaginal removal of the ovaries may be facilitated by identifying the anatomic landmarks similar to the abdominal approach and separately clamping the round ligaments and infundibular pelvic ligaments.

VASCULAR SYSTEM OF THE PELVIS

Several generalizations should be made in describing the network of arteries that bring blood to the female reproductive organs. The arteries are paired, are bilateral, and have multiple collaterals (Fig. 3-21). The arteries enter their respective organs laterally and then unite with anastomotic vessels from the other side of the pelvis near the midline. There is a long-standing teaching generalization that the pelvic reproductive viscera lie within a loosely woven basket of large veins with numerous interconnecting venous plexuses. The arteries thread their way through this interwoven mesh of veins to reach the pelvic reproductive organs, giving off numerous branching arcades to provide a rich blood supply.

Arteries

Inferior Mesenteric Artery

The inferior mesenteric artery, a single artery, arises from the aorta approximately 3 cm above the aortic bifurcation. It supplies part of the transverse colon, the descending colon, the sigmoid colon, and the rectum and terminates as the superior hemorrhoidal artery. The inferior mesenteric artery is occasionally torn during node dissections performed in staging operations for gynecologic cancer. Because of the rich collateral circulation from the middle and inferior hemorrhoidal arteries, the inferior mesenteric artery can be ligated without compromise of the distal portion of the colon.

Ovarian Artery

The ovarian arteries originate from the aorta just below the renal vessels. Each one courses in the retroperitoneal space, crosses anterior to the ureter, and enters the infundibulopelvic ligament. As the artery travels medially in the mesovarium, numerous small branches supply the ovary and oviduct. The ovarian artery unites with the ascending branch of the uterine

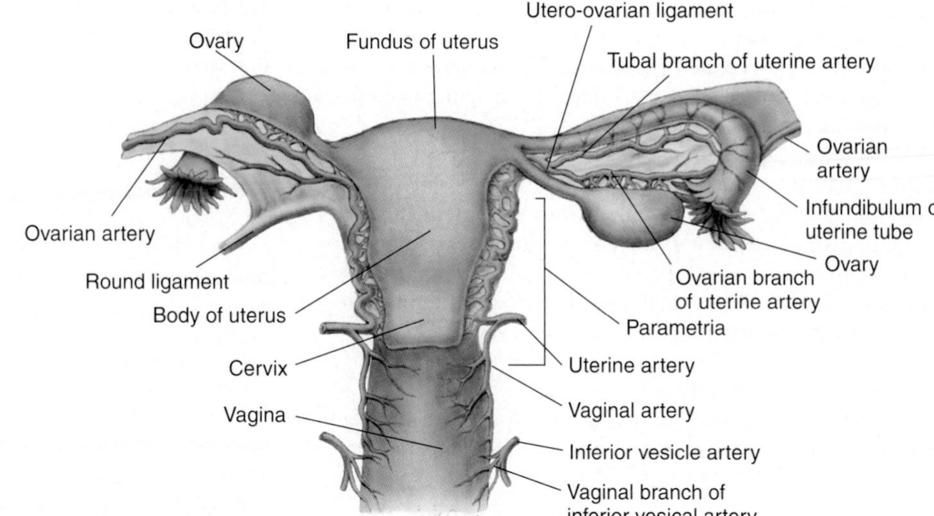

Figure 3-21. The arteries of the reproductive organs. Note the paired arteries entering laterally and freely anastomosing with each other. (Redrawn from Clemente CD: Anatomy: A Regional Atlas of the Human Body, 3rd ed. Baltimore-Munich, Urban & Schwarzenberg, 1987.)

artery in the mesovarium just under the suspensory ligament of the ovary.

Common Iliac Artery

The bifurcation of the aorta occurs at the level of the fourth lumbar vertebra, forming the two common iliac arteries. Each common iliac artery is approximately 5 cm in length before the vessel divides into the external iliac and hypogastric arteries.

Hypogastric Artery (Internal Iliac Artery)

The hypogastric arteries are short vessels, each approximately 3 to 4 cm in length. Throughout their course they are in close proximity to the ureters, which are anterior, and to the hypogastric veins, which are posterior. Each hypogastric artery branches into an anterior and a posterior division (or trunk). The posterior trunk gives off three parietal branches: the iliolumbar, lateral sacral, and superior gluteal arteries. The anterior trunk has nine branches. The three parietal branches are the obturator, internal pudendal, and inferior gluteal arteries. The six visceral branches include the umbilical, middle vesical, inferior vesical, middle hemorrhoidal, uterine, and vaginal arteries. The superior vesical artery usually arises from the umbilical artery. The individual branches of the hypogastric artery may vary from one woman to another.

Uterine Artery

The uterine artery arises from the anterior division of the hypogastric artery and courses medially toward the isthmus of the uterus. Approximately 2 cm lateral to the endocervix, it crosses over the ureter and reaches the lateral side of the uterus. The ascending branch of the uterine artery courses in the broad ligament, running a tortuous route to finally anastomose with the ovarian artery in the mesovarium (Fig. 3-22). Through its circuitous route in the parametrium, the uterine artery gives off numerous branches that unite with arcuate arteries from the other side. This series of arcuate arteries develops radial branches that supply the myometrium and the basalis layer of the endometrium. The arcuate arteries also form the spiral

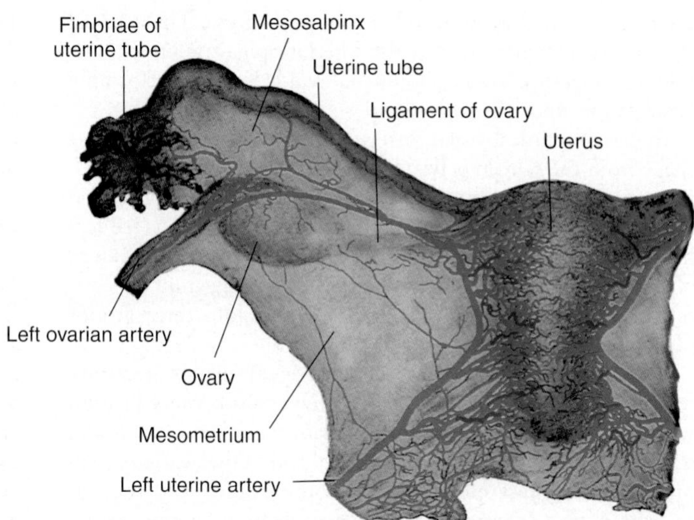

Figure 3-22. A photograph of an injected specimen demonstrating the rich anastomoses of the uterine and ovarian arteries. (From Warwick R, Williams PL: Gray's Anatomy, 35th ed. Edinburgh, Churchill Livingstone, 1973, p 1361.)

arteries of the functional layer of the endometrium. The descending branch of the uterine artery produces branches that supply both the cervix and the vagina. In each case the vessels enter the organ laterally and anastomose freely with vessels from the other side.

Vaginal Artery

The vaginal artery may arise either from the anterior trunk of the hypogastric artery or from the uterine artery. It supplies blood to the vagina, bladder, and rectum. There are extensive anastomoses with the vaginal branches of the uterine artery to form the azygos arteries of the cervix and vagina.

Internal Pudendal Artery

This artery is the terminal branch of the hypogastric artery and supplies branches to the rectum, labia, clitoris, and perineum.

Veins

The venous drainage of the pelvis begins in small sinusoids that drain to numerous venous plexuses contained within or immediately adjacent to the pelvic organs. Invariably there are numerous anastomoses between the parietal and visceral branches of the venous system. In general the veins of the female pelvis and perineum are thin-walled and have few valves.

The veins that drain the pelvic plexuses follow the course of the arterial supply. Their names are similar to those of the accompanying arteries. Often multiple veins run alongside a single artery. One special exception is the venous drainage of the ovaries. The left ovarian vein empties into the left renal vein, whereas the right ovarian vein connects directly with the inferior vena cava.

CLINICAL CORRELATIONS

Although the external iliac artery and its branches do not supply blood directly to the pelvic viscera, they are important landmarks in surgical anatomy. The fact that the external iliac artery gives rise to the obturator artery in 15% to 20% of women must be considered in radical cancer operations with associated node dissections of the obturator fossa. The external iliac artery also gives rise to the inferior epigastric artery. The inferior epigastric artery should be avoided when performing laparoscopic operative procedures.

In certain clinical situations associated with profuse hemorrhage from the female pelvis, hypogastric ligation is performed. Because of the extensive collateral circulation, this operation does not produce hypoxia of the pelvic viscera but reduces hemorrhage by decreasing the arterial pulse pressure. The extent of collateral circulation after hypogastric artery ligation depends on the site of ligation and may be divided into three groups (Table 3-1).

In cases of intractable pelvic hemorrhage, it may be necessary to supplement the effects of bilateral hypogastric artery ligation with ligation of the anastomotic sites between the ovarian and uterine vessels. Ligation of the terminal end of the ovarian artery preserves the direct blood supply to the ovaries, and there is no fear of the subsequent cystic degeneration of the ovaries that may occur after ligation of the vessels in the infundibulopelvic ligaments. Arterial embolization provides an alternative approach to ligation. A catheter is advanced under fluoroscopic visualization, and small particulate material is injected to produce hemostasis in the bleeding vessels. This less invasive technique, when appropriate, may preserve fertility. A rare condition that presents an interesting challenge to the clinician is a congenital arteriovenous (A-V) malformation in the female pelvis. Most of these A-V fistulas are treated with preoperative embolization and subsequent operative ligation.

One of the treatments for repetitive embolization arising from a thrombosis in the female pelvis is the placement of a vascular umbrella into the inferior vena cava. Collateral circulation exists between the portal venous system of the gastrointestinal tract and the systemic venous circulation through anastomosis in the pelvis, especially in the hemorrhoidal plexus. The pelvic veins also anastomose with the presacral and lumbar veins. Thus, though rare, patients may develop trophoblastic emboli to the brain without the trophoblast being filtered by the capillary system in the lungs.

Table 3-1 Collateral Arterial Circulation of the Pelvis

Branches from Aorta

Ovarian artery—anastomoses freely with uterine artery
Inferior mesenteric artery—continues as superior hemorrhoidal artery to anastomose with middle and inferior hemorrhoidal arteries from hypogastric and internal pudendal
Lumbar and vertebral arteries—anastomose with iliolumbar artery of hypogastric
Middle sacral artery—anastomoses with lateral sacral artery of hypogastric

Branches from External Iliac Artery

Deep iliac circumflex artery—anastomoses with iliolumbar and superior gluteal of hypogastric
Inferior epigastric artery—gives origin to obturator artery in 25% of cases, providing additional anastomoses of external iliac with medial femoral circumflex and communicating pelvic branches

Branches from Femoral Artery

Medial femoral circumflex artery—anastomoses with obturator and inferior gluteal arteries from hypogastric
Lateral femoral circumflex artery—anastomoses with superior gluteal and iliolumbar arteries from hypogastric

Reprinted with permission from Mattingly RF, Thompson JD: Te Linde's Operative Gynecology, 6th ed. Philadelphia, JB Lippincott, 1985.

LYMPHATIC SYSTEM

External Iliac Nodes

The external iliac nodes are immediately adjacent to the external iliac artery and vein (Figs. 3-23 and 3-24). There are two distinct groups: one situated lateral to the vessels and the other posterior to the psoas muscle. The distal portion of the posterior group is enclosed in the femoral sheath. The majority of lymphatic channels to this group of nodes originates from the vulva, but there are also channels from the cervix and lower portion of the uterus. The external iliac nodes receive secondary drainage from the femoral and internal iliac nodes.

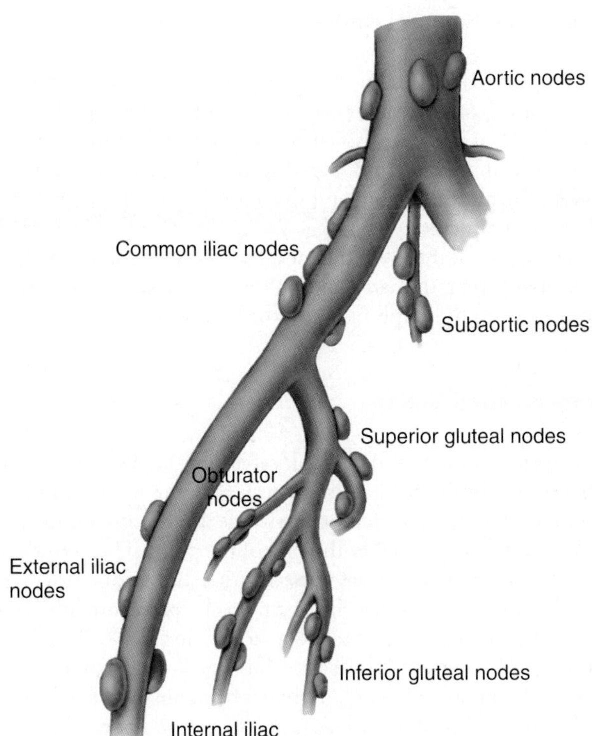

Figure 3-23. Schematic view of the pelvic lymph nodes. (From Plentl AA, Friedman EA: Lymphatic System of the Female Genitalia. Philadelphia, WB Saunders, 1971, p 13.)

Internal Iliac Nodes

The internal iliac nodes are found in an anatomic triangle whose sides are composed of the external iliac artery, the hypogastric artery, and the pelvic sidewall. Included in this clinically important area are nodes with special designation, including the nodes of the femoral ring, the obturator nodes, and the nodes adjacent to the external iliac vessels. This rich collection of nodes receives channels from every internal pelvic organ and the vulva, including the clitoris and urethra.

Common Iliac Nodes

The common iliac nodes are a group of nodes located adjacent to the vessels that bear their name and are between the external iliac and aortic chains. Most of these nodes are found lateral to the vessels. To remove this chain, it is necessary to dissect the common iliac vessels away from their attachments to the psoas muscle. This group receives lymphatics from the cervix and the upper portion of the vagina. Secondary lymphatic drainage from the internal iliac, external iliac, superior gluteal, and inferior gluteal nodes flows to the common iliac nodes.

Inferior Gluteal Nodes

A small group of lymph nodes, the inferior gluteal nodes, are located in anatomic proximity to the ischial spines and are adjacent to the sacral plexus of nodes. It is difficult to remove these nodes surgically. The nodes receive lymphatics from the cervix, the lower portion of the vagina, and Bartholin's glands. This group of nodes secondarily drains to the internal iliac, common iliac, superior gluteal, and subaortic nodes.

Superior Gluteal Nodes

The superior gluteal nodes are a group of nodes found near the origin of the superior gluteal artery and adjacent to the medial and posterior aspects of the hypogastric vessels. The superior gluteal nodes receive primary lymphatic drainage from the

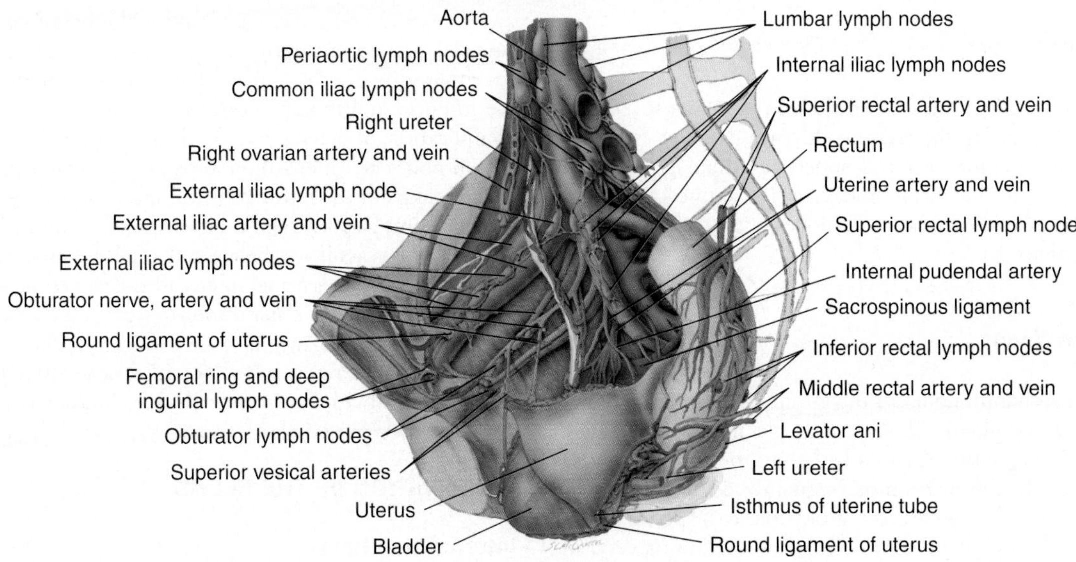

Figure 3-24. A lateral view of the female pelvis demonstrating the extensive lymphatic network. Note that most of the lymphatic channels follow the courses of the major vessels. (Redrawn from Clemente CD: Anatomy: A Regional Atlas of the Human Body, 3rd ed. Baltimore-Munich, Urban & Schwarzenberg, 1987.)

cervix and the vagina. Efferent lymphatics from this chain drain to the common iliac, sacral, or subaortic nodes.

Sacral Nodes

The sacral nodes are found over the middle of the sacrum in a space bounded laterally by the sacral foramina. These nodes receive lymphatic drainage from both the cervix and the vagina. Secondary drainage from these nodes runs in a cephalad direction to the subaortic nodes.

Subaortic Nodes

The subaortic nodes are arranged in a chain and are located below the bifurcation of the aorta, immediately anterior to the most caudal portion of the inferior vena cava and over the fifth lumbar vertebra. The primary drainage to this chain of nodes is from the cervix, with a few lymphatics from the vagina. This group is the first secondary chain to receive the efferent lymphatics as lymph flow progresses in a cephalad direction from the majority of other pelvic nodes.

Aortic Nodes

The many aortic nodes are immediately adjacent to the aorta on both its anterior and lateral aspects, predominantly in the furrow between the aorta and inferior vena cava. Primary lymphatics drain from all the major pelvic organs, including the cervix, uterus, oviducts, and especially the ovaries. The aortic chain receives secondary drainage from the pelvic nodes. In general, primary afferent lymphatics drain into the nodes over the anterior aspects of the aorta, whereas secondary efferent drainage from other pelvic nodes is found in those nodes situated lateral and posterior to the aorta.

Rectal Nodes

The rectal nodes are found subfascially and in the loose connective tissue surrounding the rectum. Primary drainage from the cervix flows to the superior rectal nodes, and drainage from the vagina appears in the rectal nodes in the anorectal region. Secondary drainage from the rectal nodes goes to the subaortic and aortic groups.

Parauterine Nodes

The number of lymph nodes in the group of parauterine nodes is small; most frequently there is a single node immediately lateral to each side of the cervix and adjacent to the pelvic course of the ureter. Though anatomists frequently do not comment about the parauterine nodes, the group receives special attention in radical surgical operations to treat uterine or cervical malignancy. Primary drainage to this node originates in the vagina, cervix, and uterus. Secondary drainage from this node is to the internal iliac nodes on the same side of the pelvis.

Superficial Femoral Nodes

The superficial femoral nodes are a group of nodes found in the loose, fatty connective tissue of the femoral triangle between the superficial and deep fascial layers. These lymph nodes receive lymphatic drainage from the external genitalia of the vulvar region, the gluteal region, and the entire leg, including the foot. Efferent lymphatics from this group of nodes penetrate the fascia lata to enter the deep femoral nodes. Plentl and Friedman have stated that this area undoubtedly represents the greatest concentration of lymph nodes in the female (Fig. 3-25).

Deep Femoral Nodes

The deep femoral nodes are located in the femoral sheath, adjacent to both the femoral artery and the vein within the femoral triangle. The femoral triangle is the anatomic space lying immediately distal to the fold of the groin. The boundaries of the femoral triangle are the sartorius and adductor longus muscles and the inguinal ligament. Each space contains, from medial to lateral, the femoral vein, artery, and nerve. This chain receives the primary lymphatics for the lower extremity and receives secondary efferent lymphatics from the superficial lymph nodes and thus the vulva. This group of lymph nodes is in direct continuity with the iliac and internal iliac chains.

CLINICAL CORRELATIONS

A precise knowledge of pelvic lymphatics is important for the gynecologic oncologist who is surgically determining the extent of spread of a pelvic malignancy. Aortic and pelvic lymphadenectomy operations require precise knowledge of normal anatomy and possible anomalies in both the urinary and vascular systems. The fact that most lymphatic metastatic spread from ovarian carcinoma occurs in a cephalad direction should be emphasized. This explains the importance of sampling aortic and subaortic nodes during second-look operations for ovarian cancer. In carcinoma of the vulva, lymphatic drainage may occur to either side of the pelvis. Thus bilateral node dissections are important. Pelvic hemorrhage is the most common acute complication of a lymph node dissection because most pelvic lymph nodes are in anatomic proximity to major pelvic vessels. Lymphocysts in the retroperitoneal space are the most common chronic complication associated with radical node dissections.

For many years it was believed that all the superficial femoral nodes drained to a sentinel node called *Cloquet's node.* Cloquet's node, by the present classification system, would be one of the most proximal and medial of the nodes in the external iliac chain. Cloquet's node is only of historical interest, since the assumption is neither anatomically nor clinically correct.

INNERVATION OF THE PELVIS

Internal Genitalia

The innervation of the internal genital organs is supplied primarily by the autonomic nervous system. The sympathetic

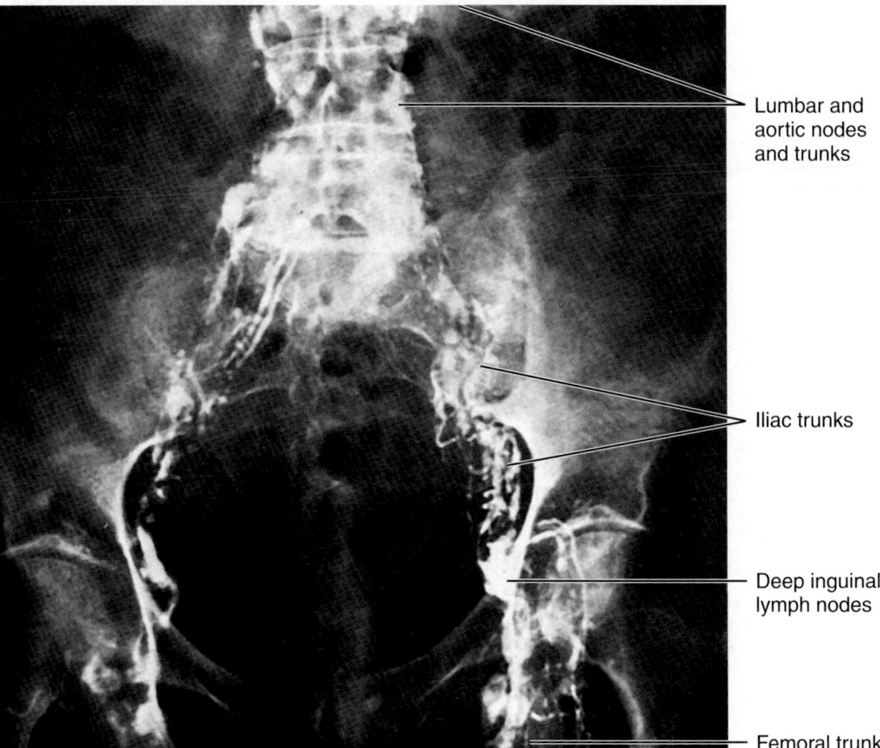

Figure 3-25. A lymphangiogram of the pelvis and lumbar areas. This X-ray film shows the course of the lymphatics from the deep femoral nodes into the iliac nodes. Note the extensive network of nodes in the inguinal region. (From Clemente CD: A Regional Atlas of the Human Body, 3rd ed. Baltimore-Munich, Urban & Schwarzenberg, 1987.)

portion of the autonomic nervous system originates in the thoracic and lumbar portions of the spinal cord, and sympathetic ganglia are located adjacent to the central nervous system. In contrast, the parasympathetic portion originates in cranial nerves and the middle three sacral segments of the cord, and the ganglia are located near the visceral organs. Although the fibers of both subdivisions of the autonomic nervous system frequently are intermingled in the same peripheral nerves, their physiologic actions are usually directly antagonistic. As a broad generalization, sympathetic fibers in the female pelvis produce muscular contractions and vasoconstriction, whereas parasympathetic fibers cause the opposite effect on muscles and vasodilation.

The semantics of pelvic innervation are confusing and imprecise. A *plexus* is a mixture of preganglionic and postganglionic fibers; small, inconsistently placed ganglia; and afferent (sensory) fibers. Throughout both the anatomic and surgical literature, a plexus may also be termed a *nerve.* For example, the superior hypogastric plexus is also called the *presacral nerve.*

Although autonomic nerve fibers enter the pelvis by several routes, the majority are contained in the superior hypogastric plexus, which is a caudal extension of the aortic and inferior mesenteric plexuses. The superior hypogastric plexus is found in the retroperitoneal connective tissue. It extends from the fourth lumbar vertebra to the hollow over the sacrum. In its lower portion the plexus divides to form the two hypogastric nerves, which run laterally and inferiorly. These nerves fan out to form the inferior hypogastric plexus in the area just below the bifurcation of the common iliac arteries. The nerve trunks descend farther into the base of the broad ligament, where they join with parasympathetic fibers to form the pelvic plexus. Both motor fibers and accompanying sensory fibers reach the pelvic plexus from S2, S3, and S4 via the pelvic nerves, or nervi erigentes. From the pelvic plexus secondary plexuses are adjacent to all pelvic viscera, namely, the rectum, anus, urinary bladder, vagina, and Frankenhäuser's plexus in the uterosacral ligaments. Frankenhäuser's plexus is extensive and contains both myelinated and nonmyelinated fibers passing primarily to the uterus and cervix, with a few fibers passing to the urinary bladder and vagina. The ovarian plexus, like the blood supply to the ovaries, is not part of the hypogastric system. The ovarian plexus is a downward extension of the aortic and renal plexuses.

It is impossible to separate afferent, sensory fibers from pelvic organs into morphologically independent tracts. The majority of fibers accompany the vascular system from the organ and then enter plexuses of the autonomic nervous system before eventually entering white rami communicates to the cell bodies in dorsal root ganglia of the spinal column. The major sensory fibers from the uterus accompany the sympathetic nerves, which enter the nerve roots of the spinal cord in segments T11 and T12. Thus, referred uterine pain is often located in the lower abdomen. In contrast, afferents from the cervix enter the spinal cord in nerve roots of S2, S3, and S4. Referred pain from cervical inflammation is characterized as low back pain in the lumbosacral region.

External Genitalia

The pudendal nerve and its branches supply the majority of both motor and sensory fibers to the muscles and skin of the vulvar region. The pudendal nerve arises from the second, third, and fourth sacral roots. It has an interesting course in which it initially leaves the pelvis via the greater sciatic foramen. Next,

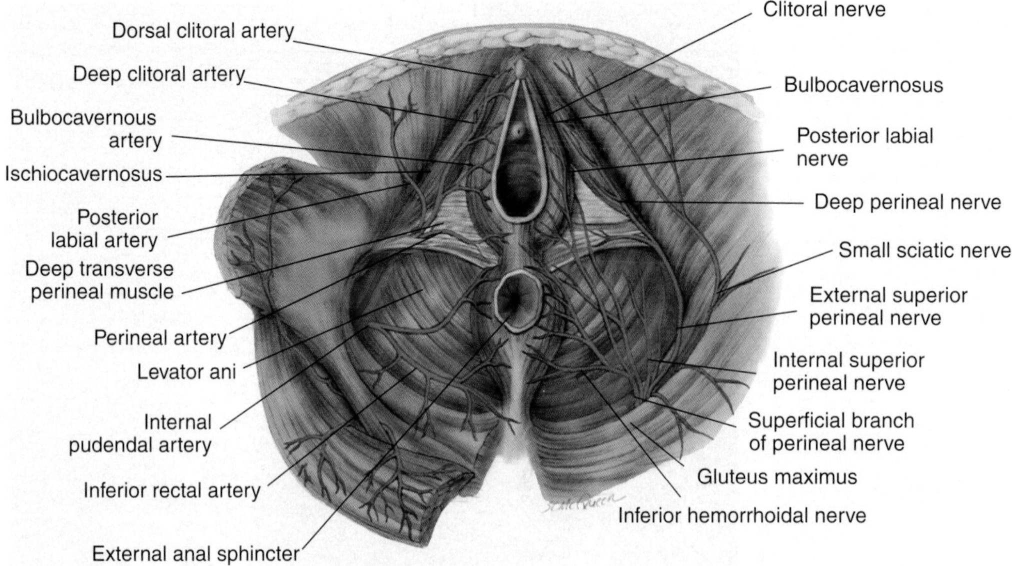

Figure 3-26. A posterior view of the female perineum demonstrating the pudendal nerve emerging externally. The nerve divides into three segments as it passes out of the pelvis: the inferior hemorrhoidal nerve and the deep and superficial perineal nerves. The clitoral nerve is the terminal branch of the deep perineal nerve. (Redrawn from Mattingly RF, Thompson JD: Te Linde's Operative Gynecology, 6th ed. Philadelphia, JB Lippincott, 1985, p 49.)

it crosses beneath the ischial spine, running on the medial side of the internal pudendal artery. The pudendal nerve then reenters the pelvic cavity and travels in Alcock's canal, which runs along the lateral aspects of the ischial rectal fossa. As the nerve reaches the urogenital diaphragm, it divides into three branches: the inferior hemorrhoidal, the deep perineal, and the superficial perineal (Fig. 3-26). The dorsal nerve of the clitoris is a terminal branch of the deep perineal nerve.

The skin of the anus, clitoris, and medial and inferior aspects of the vulva is supplied primarily by distal branches of the pudendal nerve. The vulvar region receives additional sensory fibers from three nerves. The anterior branch of the ilioinguinal nerve sends fibers to the mons pubis and the upper part of the labia majora. The genital femoral nerve supplies fibers to the labia majora, and the posterior femoral cutaneous nerve supplies fibers to the inferoposterior aspects of the vulva.

CLINICAL CORRELATIONS

An unusual but troublesome postoperative complication of gynecologic surgery is injury to the femoral nerve. During abdominal hysterectomy the femoral nerve may be compromised by pressure from the lateral blade of a self-retaining retractor in the area adjacent to where the femoral nerve penetrates the psoas muscle. During vaginal hysterectomy the femoral nerve may be injured from exaggerated hyperflexion of the legs in the lithotomy position, since hyperflexion produces stretching and compression of the femoral nerve as it courses under the inguinal ligament.

Because of the low density of nerve endings in the upper two thirds of the vagina, women are sometimes unable to determine the presence of a foreign body in this area. This explains how a "forgotten tampon" may remain unnoticed for several days in the upper part of the vagina until its presence results in a symptomatic discharge, abnormal bleeding, or odor. Infrequent but serious complications of pudendal nerve block are hematomas from trauma to the pudendal vessels and intravascular injection of anesthetic agents. The vessels or nerves are in close anatomic proximity to the ischial spine.

The fallopian tube is one of the most sensitive of the pelvic organs when crushed, cut, or distended, a fact that is appreciated in performing tubal ligations with the patient under local anesthesia. Damage to the obturator nerve during radical pelvic operations does not affect the pelvis directly. Although the nerve has an extensive pelvic course, its motor fibers supply the adductors of the thigh and its sensory fibers innervate skin over the medial aspects of the thigh.

DIAPHRAGMS AND LIGAMENTS

Pelvic Diaphragm

The pelvic diaphragm is a wide but thin muscular layer of tissue that forms the inferior border of the abdominopelvic cavity. Composed of a broad, funnel-shaped sling of fascia and muscle, it extends from the symphysis pubis to the coccyx and from one lateral sidewall to the other. The primary muscles of the pelvic diaphragm are the levator ani and the coccygeus (Fig. 3-27). This structure is the evolutionary remnant of the tail-wagging muscles in lower animals.

The muscles of the pelvic diaphragm are interwoven for strength, and a continuous muscle layer encircles the terminal portions of the urethra, vagina, and rectum. The levator ani muscles constitute the greatest bulk of the pelvic diaphragm

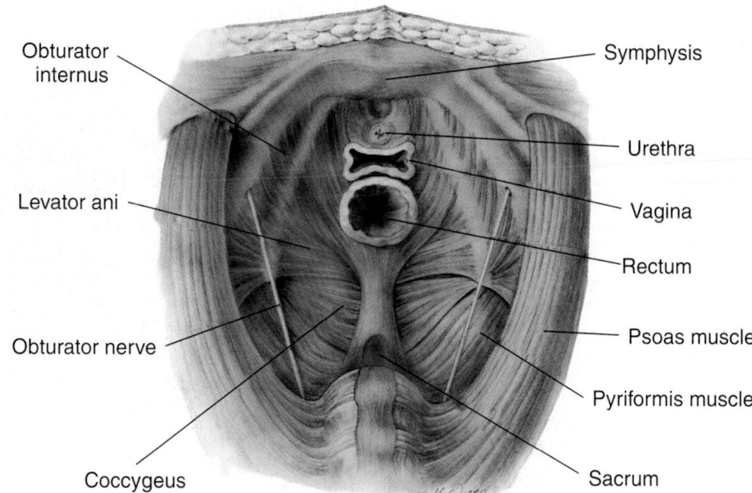

Figure 3-27. A superior view of the pelvic diaphragm and the pelvic floor. The primary muscles that compose this funnel-shaped sling are the coccygeus and the levator ani. (Redrawn from Mattingly RF, Thompson JD: Te Linde's Operative Gynecology, 6th ed. Philadelphia, Lippincott, 1985, p 41.)

and are divided into three components, which are named after their origin and insertion: pubococcygeus, puborectalis, and iliococcygeus. Some refer to the pubococcygeus muscles by a more descriptive name—the *pubovisceral muscle.* The coccygeus is a triangular muscle that occupies the area between the ischial spine and the coccyx.

The paired levator ani muscles act as a single muscle and functionally are important in the control of urination, in parturition, and in maintaining fecal continence. Zacharin (1980) proposed that these muscles function as a "pelvic trampoline." The pelvic diaphragm is important in supporting both abdominal and pelvic viscera and facilitates equal distribution of intraabdominal pressure during activities such as coughing.

Urogenital Diaphragm

The urogenital diaphragm, also called the *triangular ligament,* is a strong, muscular membrane that occupies the area between the symphysis pubis and ischial tuberosities (Fig. 3-28) and stretches across the triangular anterior portion of the pelvic outlet. The urogenital diaphragm is external and inferior to the pelvic diaphragm. Anteriorly, the urethra is suspended from the pubic bone by continuations of the fascial layers of the urogenital diaphragm. The free edge of the diaphragm is strengthened by the superficial transverse perineal muscle. Posteriorly, the urogenital diaphragm inserts into the central point of the perineum. Situated farther posteriorly is the ischiorectal fossa. Located more superficially are the bulbocavernosus and ischiocavernosus muscles.

The urogenital diaphragm has two layers that enfold and cover the striated, deep transverse perineal muscle. This muscle surrounds both the vagina and the urethra, which pierce the diaphragm. The pudendal vessels and nerves, the external sphincter of the membranous urethra, and the dorsal nerve to the clitoris are also found within the urogenital diaphragm. The deep transverse perineal muscle is innervated by branches of the pudendal nerve. The major function of the urogenital diaphragm is support of the urethra and maintenance of the urethrovesical junction.

Ligaments

The pelvic ligaments are not classic ligaments but are thickenings of retroperitoneal fascia and consist primarily of blood and lymphatic vessels, nerves, and fatty connective tissue. Anatomists call the retroperitoneal fascia *subserous fascia,* whereas surgeons refer to this fascial layer as *endopelvic fascia.* The connective tissue is denser immediately adjacent to the lateral walls of the cervix and the vagina.

Broad Ligaments

The broad ligaments are a thin, mesenteric-like double reflection of peritoneum stretching from the lateral pelvic sidewalls to the uterus (Fig. 3-29). They become contiguous with the uterine serosa, and thus the uterus is contained within two folds of peritoneum. These peritoneal folds enclose the loose, fatty connective tissue termed the *parametrium.* The broad ligaments afford minor support to the uterus but are conduits for important anatomic structures. Within the broad ligaments are found the following structures: oviducts; ovarian and round ligaments; ureters; ovarian and uterine arteries and veins; parametrial tissue; embryonic remnants of the mesonephric duct, and wolffian body, and secondary two ligaments; the mesovarium; and the mesosalpinx. The round ligament is composed of fibrous tissue and muscle fibers. It attaches to the superoanterior aspect of the uterus, anterior and caudal to the oviduct, and runs via the broad ligament to the lateral pelvic wall. It, too, offers little support to the uterus. The round ligament crosses the external iliac vessels and enters the inguinal canal, ending by inserting into the labia majora in a fanlike fashion. In the fetus a small, finger-like projection of the peritoneum, known as *Nuck's canal,* accompanies the round ligament into the inguinal canal. Generally, the canal is obliterated in the adult woman.

Cardinal Ligaments

The cardinal, or Mackenrodt's, ligaments extend from the lateral aspects of the upper part of the cervix and the vagina to the pelvic wall. They are a thickened condensation of the subserosal fascia and parametria between the interior portion of the two folds of peritoneum. The cardinal ligaments form the

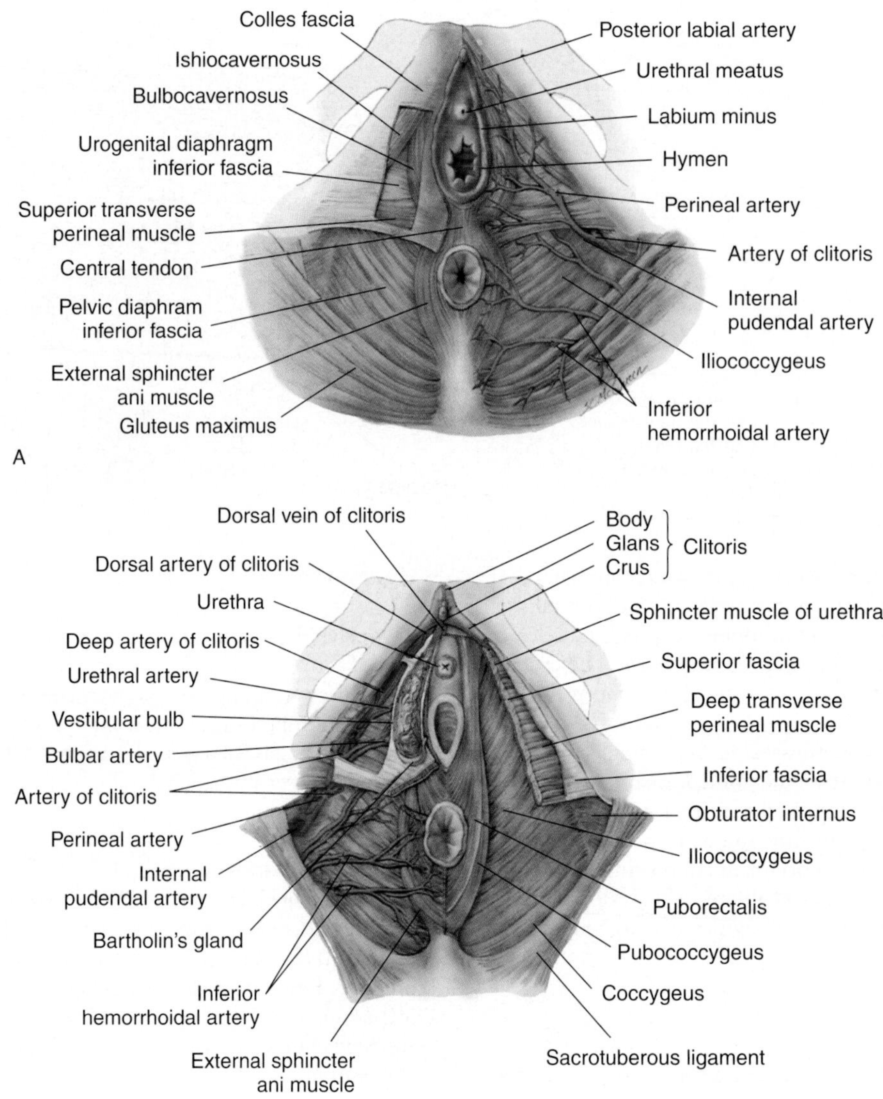

Figure 3-28. **A,** Schematic views of the perineum demonstrating superficial structures. Note the two layers of the urogenital diaphragm enfolding the deep transverse perineal muscle. **B,** Schematic views of the perineum demonstrating superficial structures and deeper structures. (Redrawn from Pritchard JA, MacDonald PC, Gant NF: Williams' Obstetrics, 17th ed. New York, Appleton-Century-Crofts, 1985, p 14.)

base of the broad ligaments, laterally attaching to the fascia over the pelvic diaphragm and medially merging with fibers of the endopelvic fascia. Within these ligaments are found blood vessels and smooth muscle. The cardinal ligaments help to maintain the anatomic position of the cervix and the upper part of the vagina and provide the major support of the uterus and cervix.

Uterosacral Ligaments

The uterosacral ligaments extend from the upper portion of the cervix posteriorly to the third sacral vertebra. They are thickened near the cervix and then run a curved course around each side of the rectum and subsequently thin out posteriorly. The external surface of the uterosacral ligaments is formed by an inferoposterior fold of peritoneum at the base of the broad ligaments. The middle of the uterosacral ligaments is composed primarily of nerve bundles. The uterosacral ligaments serve a minor role in the anatomic support of the cervix.

CLINICAL CORRELATIONS

The posterior fibers of the levator ani muscles encircle the rectum at its junction with the anal canal, thereby producing an abrupt angle that reinforces fecal continence. Surgical repair of a displacement or tear of the rectovaginal fascia and levator ani muscles resulting from childbirth is important during posterior colporrhaphy. Normal position of the female pelvic organs in the pelvis depends on mechanical support from both fascia and muscles. Vaginal delivery sometimes results dysfunction of the anal sphincter. Etiology of this problem may be direct

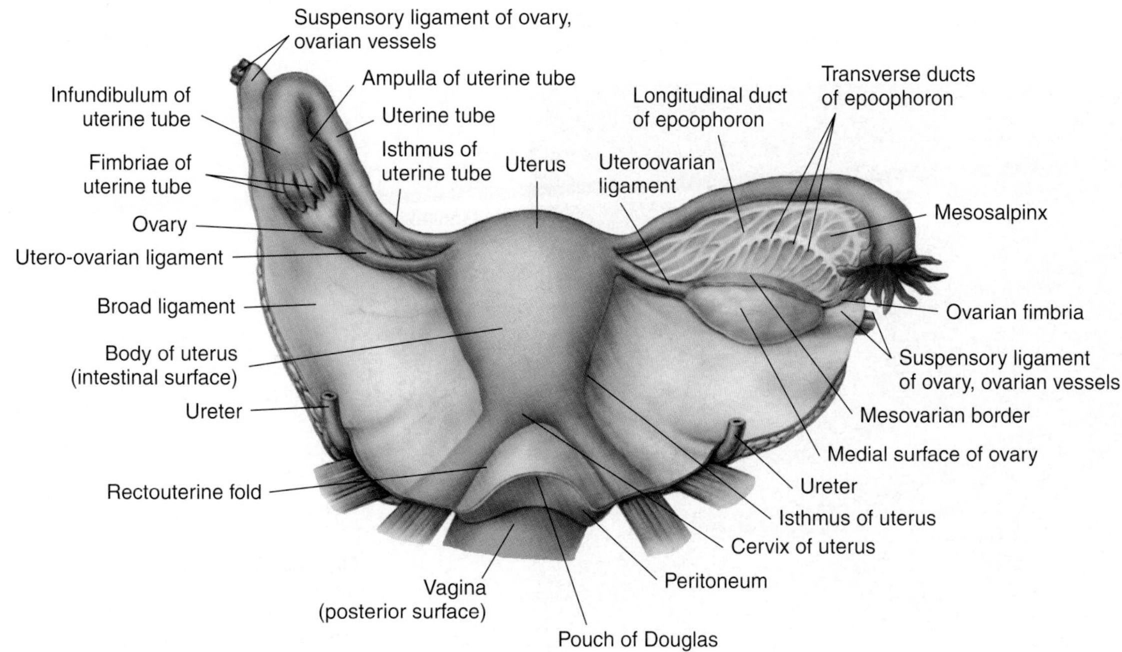

Figure 3-29. A schematic drawing of the broad ligament, posterior view. Note the many structures contained within the broad ligament. Note the posterior aspect of the rectouterine fold, called the cul-de-sac, or pouch, of Douglas. (Redrawn from Clemente CD: Anatomy: A Regional Atlas of the Human Body, 3rd ed. Baltimore-Munich, Urban & Schwarzenberg, 1987.)

injury to the striated muscles of the pelvic floor or damage to the pudendal and presacral nerves during labor and delivery.

The round ligament is an important surgical landmark in making the initial incision into the parietal peritoneum to gain access to the retroperitoneal space. Direct visualization of the retroperitoneal course of the ureter is an important step in many pelvic operations, including dissections in women with endometriosis, pelvic inflammatory disease, large adnexal masses, broad ligament masses, and pelvic malignancies. A cyst of Nuck's canal may be confused with an indirect inguinal hernia. When a large amount of fluid is placed in the abdominal cavity, postoperative bilateral labial edema may develop in some women because of patency of the canal of Nuck.

During pelvic surgery, traction on the uterus makes the uterosacral and cardinal ligaments more prominent. There is a free space approximately 2 to 4 cm below the superior edge of the broad ligament. In this free space there are no blood vessels, and the two sides of the broad ligament are in close proximity. Often gynecologic surgeons utilize this area to facilitate clamping of the anastomosis between the uterine and ovarian arteries.

NONGENITAL PELVIC ORGANS

Ureters

The ureters are whitish, muscular tubes, 28 to 34 cm in length, extending from the renal pelves to the urinary bladder. The ureter is divided into abdominal and pelvic segments. The diameters vary. The abdominal segment is approximately 8 to 10 mm in diameter. The pelvic segment is approximately 4 to 6 mm. A congenital anomaly of a double, or bifid, ureter occurs in 1% to 4% of females. Ectopic ureteral orifices may occur in either the urethra or the vagina.

The abdominal portion of the right ureter is lateral to the inferior vena cava. Four arteries and accompanying veins cross anterior to the right ureter. They are the right colic artery, the ovarian vessels, the ileocolic artery, and the superior mesenteric artery. The course of the left ureter is similar to its counterpart on the right side in that it runs downward and medially along the anterior surface of the psoas major muscle.

The iliopectineal line serves as the marker for the pelvic portion of the ureter. The ureters run along the common iliac artery and then cross over the iliac vessels as they enter the pelvis (Fig. 3-30). There is a slight variation between the two sides of the female pelvis. The right ureter tends to cross at the bifurcation of the common iliac artery, whereas usually the left ureter crosses 1 to 2 cm above the bifurcation.

The ureters follow the descending, convex curvature of the posterolateral pelvic wall toward the perineum. Throughout its course the ureter is retroperitoneal in location. The ureter can be found on the medial leaf of the parietal peritoneum and in close proximity to the ovarian, uterine, obturator, and superior vesical arteries (Fig. 3-31). The uterine artery lies on the anterolateral surface of the ureter for 2.5 to 3 cm. At approximately the level of the ischial spine, the ureter changes its course and runs forward and medially from the uterosacral ligaments to the base of the broad ligament. There the ureter enters into the cardinal ligaments. In this location the ureter is approximately 1 to 2 cm lateral to the uterine cervix and is surrounded by a plexus of veins. A cross-sectional study, by Hurd and colleagues, using compute tomography of women with normal anatomy, evaluated the distance from the ureter to the lateral aspect of

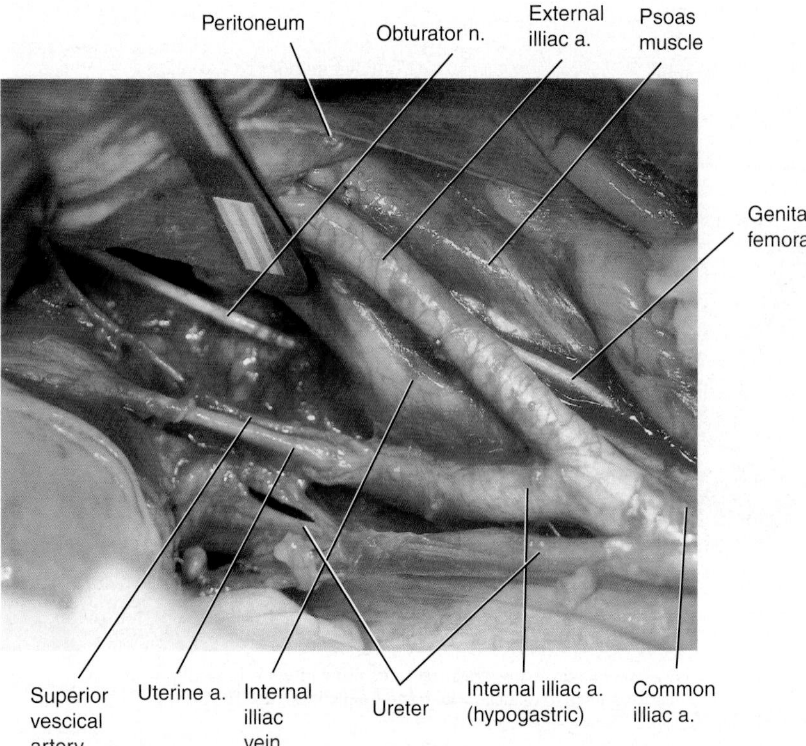

Figure 3-30. Photograph taken during a dissection of the lateral pelvic wall at the time of a radical hysterectomy. Note the ureter coursing over the common iliac artery in close proximity to the bifurcation. The ureter then drops under and very close to the uterine artery. The retractor is lifting the internal iliac vein. (Courtesy Deborah Jean Dotters, MD, Eugene, OR.)

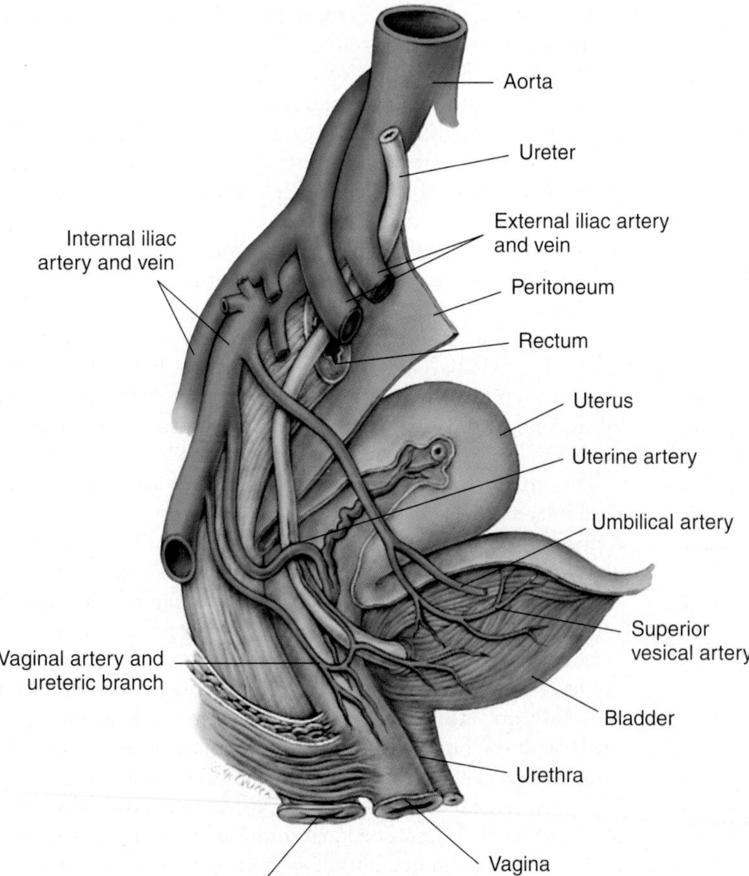

Figure 3-31. A schematic drawing of the female pelvis, lateral view, demonstrating the ureter's relation to the major arteries. Note the uterine artery crossing over the ureter. (From Buchsbaum HJ, Schmidt JD: Gynecologic and Obstetric Urology. Philadelphia, WB Saunders, 1978, p 24.)

the cervix. The measurement of the closest distance in any individual women was (median of all subjects) 2.3 cm ± .8 cm. However, the authors noted that in 12% of women, the ureter was less than 0.5 cm from the cervix (Fig. 3-32). This finding emphasizes the caution needed in surgery to prevent ureteral injury. This close proximity also underscores the fact that ureteral injury may be unavoidable in some women. The ureter then runs upward (ventral) and medially in the vesical uterine ligaments to obliquely pierce the bladder wall. Just before entering the base of the bladder, the ureter is in close contact with the anterior vaginal wall.

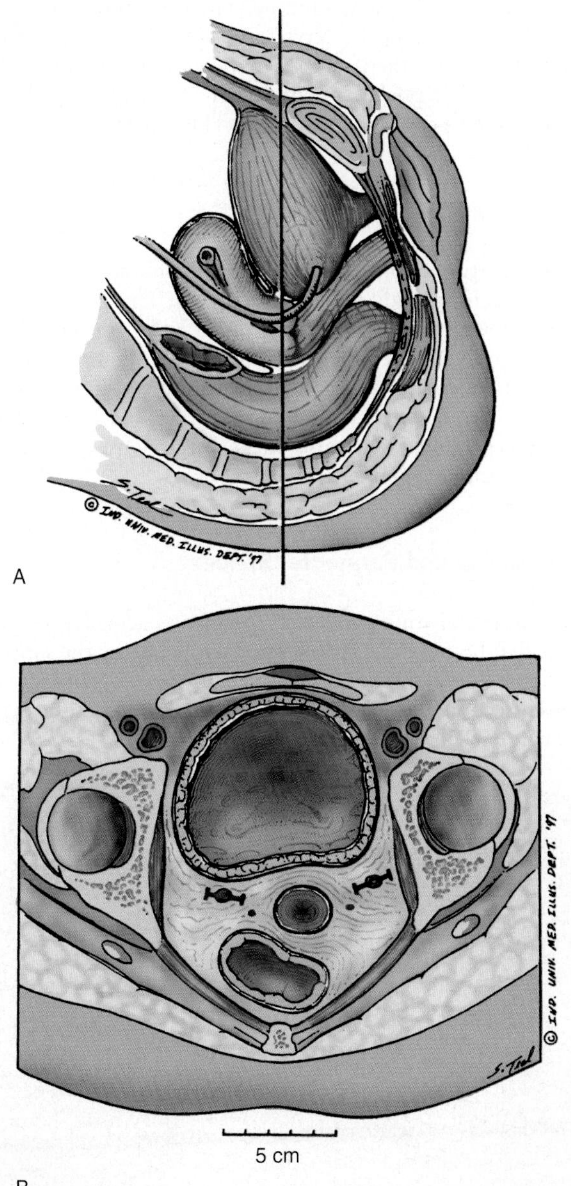

Figure 3-32. Average location of the ureters in relation to the cervix. **A,** Sagittal view representing the plane from the CT cut noted in **B.** The most proximal point from the ureter to the cervix. Bars represent standard deviation. (From Hurd WW, Chee SS, Gallagher KL, et al: Location of the ureters in relation to the uterine cervix by computed tomography. Am J Obstet Gynecol 184:338, 2001.)

The ureter has a rich arterial supply with numerous anastomoses from many small vessels that form a longitudinal plexus in the adventitia of the ureter. Parent vessels that send branches to this arterial plexus surrounding the ureter include the renal, ovarian, common iliac, hypogastric, uterine, vaginal, vesical, middle hemorrhoidal, and superior gluteal arteries. The ureter is resistant to injury resulting from devascularization unless the surgeon strips the adventitia from the muscular conduit.

Urinary Bladder

The urinary bladder is a hollow muscular organ that lies between the symphysis pubis and the uterus. The size and shape of the bladder vary with the volume of urine it contains. Similarly, the anatomic proximity to other pelvic organs depends on whether the bladder is full or empty. The superior surface of the bladder is the only surface covered by peritoneum. The inferior portion is immediately adjacent to the uterus. The urachus is a fibrous cord extending from the apex of the bladder to the umbilicus. The urachus, which is the adult remnant of the embryonic allantois, is occasionally patent for part of its length. The base of the bladder lies directly adjacent to the endopelvic fascia over the anterior vaginal wall. The bladder neck and connecting urethra are attached to the symphysis pubis by fibrous ligaments. The prevesical or retropubic space of Retzius is the area lying between the bladder and symphysis pubis and is bounded laterally by the obliterated hypogastric arteries. This space extends from the fascia covering the pelvic diaphragm to the umbilicus between the peritoneum and transversalis fascia.

The mucosa of the anterior surface of the bladder is light red and has numerous folds. The inferoposterior surface delineated by the two ureteral orifices and the urethral orifice is the trigone. The trigone is a darker red than the rest of the bladder mucosa and is free of folds. When the bladder is empty, the ureteral orifices are approximately 2.5 cm apart. This distance increases to 5 cm when the bladder is distended. The muscular wall of the bladder, the detrusor muscles, is arranged in three layers. The arterial supply of the bladder originates from branches of the hypogastric artery: the superior vesical, inferior vesical, and middle hemorrhoidal arteries. The nerve supply to the bladder includes sympathetic and parasympathetic fibers, with the external sphincter supplied by the pudendal nerve.

Rectum

The rectum is the terminal 12 to 14 cm of the large intestine. The rectum begins over the second or third sacral vertebra, where the sigmoid colon no longer has a mesentery. After the large intestine loses its mesentery, its anatomic posterior wall is in close proximity to the curvature of the sacrum. Anteriorly, peritoneum covers the upper and middle thirds of the rectum. The lowest one third is below the peritoneal reflection and is in close proximity to the posterior wall of the vagina.

The rectum empties into the anal canal, which is 2 to 4 cm in length. The anal canal is fixed by the surrounding levator ani musculature of the pelvic diaphragm (see Fig. 3-5). The external sphincter of the anal canal is a circular band of striated muscle. Recent studies of the cross-sectional anatomy of the external anal sphincter by both ultrasound and magnetic resonance imaging have identified two distinct layers of the external anal sphincter. With MRI with 3-D reconstruction, Hsu and colleagues noted three separate components to the external sphincter: a main muscle body, a separate encircling subcutaneous band of muscles, and bilateral wing-shaped muscle bands that attach near the ischiopubis. They are a subcutaneous and a deep layer. The rectum, unlike other areas of the large intestine, does not have teniae coli or appendices epiploicae. The arterial supply of the rectum is rich, originating from five arteries: the superior hemorrhoidal artery, which is a continuation of the inferior mesenteric; the two middle hemorrhoidal arteries; and the two inferior hemorrhoidal arteries. Approximately 10% of carcinomas of the large bowel occur within the rectum. Therefore during rectal examination special emphasis to palpate the entire circumference of the rectum, not just the area of the rectovaginal septum, is an important part of screening for colon cancer.

CLINICAL CORRELATIONS

The anatomic proximity of the ureters, urinary bladder, and rectum to the female reproductive organs is a major consideration in most gynecologic operations. Surgical compromise of the ureter may occur during clamping or ligating of the infundibulopelvic vessels, clamping or ligating of the cardinal ligaments, or wide suturing in the endopelvic fascia during an anterior repair, even with apparent normal anatomy and utmost surgical care. Operative injuries to the bladder or ureter occur in approximately 1 out of 100 major gynecologic operations. Bladder injuries are approximately five times more common than ureteral injuries. Two of the classic ways to differentiate a ureter from a pelvic vessel are (1) visualization of peristalsis after stimulation by a surgical instrument and (2) visualization of Auerbach's plexuses, which are numerous, wavy, small vessels that anastomose over the surface of the ureter. Injury to the ureter or bladder during urethropexy operations for genuine stress incontinence are common. Therefore, most urogynecologists routinely inject indigo carmine and either open the bladder or perform cystoscopy near the end of the operative procedure.

For years, gynecologic teachers have referred to the area in the base of the broad ligament near the cervix where the uterine artery crosses the ureter as the area where "water flows under the bridge."

The urinary bladder, if properly drained, will heal rapidly after a surgical insult if the blood supply to the bladder wall is not compromised. This capacity allows the gynecologist to use a suprapubic cystostomy tube without fear of fistula formation.

One of the surgical approaches for urinary stress incontinence is to suspend the periurethral tissue to either the symphysis pubis or Cooper's ligaments. Occasionally, this surgical approach is complicated by a significant amount of postoperative venous bleeding. A subfascial hematoma may extend as high as the umbilicus in the space of Retzius. One of the most common causes of female urinary incontinence is defective connective tissue, especially in the periurethral connective tissue, the pubourethral ligaments, and pubococcygeus muscles.

Rectal injury may occur during vaginal hysterectomy with associated posterior colporrhaphy. In the middle third of the vagina the distance between vaginal and rectal mucosa is only a few millimeters, and usually the connective tissue is densely adherent and should be separated by sharp dissection. The rectum bulges anteriorly into the vagina in this area, producing a further challenge during the operative procedure.

OTHER STRUCTURES

Cul-de-sac of Douglas

The cul-de-sac of Douglas is a deep pouch formed by the most caudal extent of the parietal peritoneum. The cul-de-sac is a potential space and is also called the *rectouterine pouch* or *fold* (Figs. 3-29 and 3-33). It is anterior to the rectum, separating the uterus from the large intestine. The parietal peritoneum of the cul-de-sac covers the cervix and upper part of the posterior vaginal wall, then reflects to cover the anterior wall of the rectum. The pouch is bounded on the lateral sides by the peritoneal folds covering the uterosacral ligaments.

Parametria

The parametria are the coats of extraperitoneal fatty and fibrous connective tissues adjacent to the uterus. The parametria lie between the leaves of the broad ligament and in the contiguous area anteriorly between the cervix and bladder. This connective tissue is thicker and denser adjacent to the cervix and vagina, where it becomes part of the connective tissue of the pelvic floor. The parametria may also thicken in response to radiation, pelvic cancer, infection, or endometriosis.

Paravescical and Pararectal Spaces

The paravesical and pararectal spaces are actually potential spaces that become true spaces when developed by the surgeon. Development of these spaces is very useful in pelvic lymph node dissection and in radical pelvic surgery because it makes the anatomic landmarks so clear.

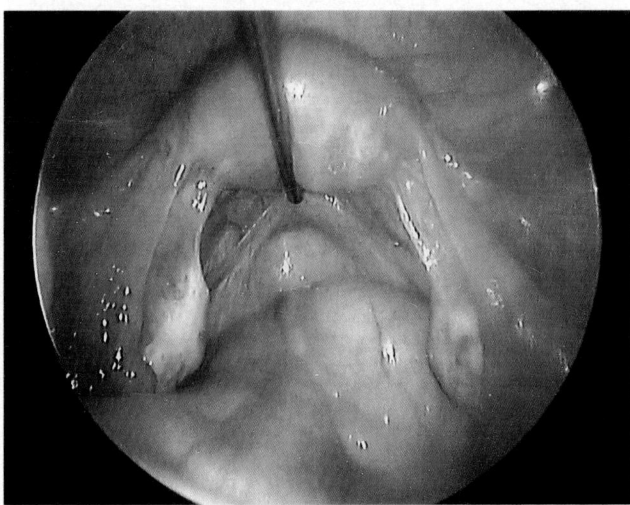

Figure 3-33. Laparoscopic visualization of a normal pelvis. The probe is elevating the uterus to expose the cul-de-sac of Douglas. (Courtesy of Burke Beller.)

The paravesical space is bordered medially by the bladder and upper vagina and is contiguous with, but lateral to, the space of Retzius. Laterally, it is bordered by the obturator fossa and the external iliac vessels. Inferiorly, it is bordered by the pubic ramus, and superiorly by the cardinal ligament.

The pararectal space is developed by dissecting the adventitial tissue within the broad ligament, between the ureter (medially), and the internal iliac vessels (laterally). More deeply, the medial border is the rectum. Superiorly, the pararectal space is limited by the sacral hollow. Inferiorly, it is limited by the cardinal ligament, containing the uterine artery. The paravesical and pararectal spaces are actually potential spaces that become true spaces when developed by the surgeon. Development of these spaces is very useful in pelvic lymph node dissection and in radical pelvic surgery because the anatomic landmarks become so clear.

CLINICAL CORRELATIONS

The parametria and cul-de-sac of Douglas are important anatomic landmarks in advanced pelvic infection and neoplasia. Intrauterine infection, cervical carcinoma, and endometrial carcinoma may penetrate the endocervical stroma or the myometrium and secondarily may invade the loose connective tissue of the parametria.

The pouch of Douglas is easily accessible in performing transvaginal surgical procedures. Vaginal tubal ligation may be the procedure of choice in massively obese women. Posterior colpotomy is frequently chosen for drainage of a pelvic abscess occurring in the cul-de-sac of Douglas.

When the paravescial and pararectal spaces have been developed and the uterus is held on traction medially, the pelvic anatomy; including the ureter, internal and external iliac vessels, obturator fossa, and the cardinal ligament, with the uterine artery crossing the ureter, can be clearly and readily identified.

Many women with uterine prolapse have an associated enterocele, which is a hernia that protrudes between the uterosacral ligaments. Occasionally the cul-de-sac of Douglas is obliterated by the inflammatory process associated with either endometriosis or advanced malignancy.

KEY POINTS

- The labia majora are homologous to the scrotum in the male. The labia minora are homologous to the penile urethra and a portion of the skin of the penis in males.
- The clitoris is the female homologue of the penis in the male. Skene's glands are homologous to the prostate gland in the male.
- The average length of the clitoris is 1.5 to 2 cm. Clinically, in determining clitoromegaly width is more important and should be less than 1 cm, for it is difficult to actually measure the length of the clitoris.
- The female urethra measures 3.5 to 5 cm in length. The mucosa of the proximal two thirds of the urethra is composed of stratified transitional epithelium, and the distal one third is stratified squamous epithelium.
- When a woman is standing, the axis of the upper portion of the vagina lies close to the horizontal plane, with the upper portion of the vagina curving toward the hollow of the sacrum.
- The lower third of the vagina is in close anatomic relationship to the urogenital and pelvic diaphragms.
- The middle third of the vagina is supported by the levator ani muscles and the lower portion of the cardinal ligaments.
- The primary lymphatic drainage of the upper third of the vagina is to the external iliac nodes, the middle third of the vagina drains to the common and internal iliac nodes, and the lower third has a wide lymphatic distribution, including the common iliac, superficial inguinal, and perirectal nodes.
- Descriptive terms for pelvic organs are derived from the Latin root, whereas terms relating to surgical procedures are derived from the Greek root.
- The length and width of the endocervical canal vary. The width of the canal varies with the parity of the woman and changing hormonal levels. It is usually 2.5 to 3 cm in length and 7 to 8 mm at its widest point.
- The fibromuscular cervical stroma is composed primarily of collagenous connective tissue and ground substance. The connective tissue contains approximately 15% smooth muscle cells and a small amount of elastic tissue.
- The major arterial supply to the cervix is located in the lateral cervical walls at the 3 and 9 o'clock positions.
- The pain fibers from the cervix accompany the parasympathetic fibers to the second, third, and fourth sacral segments.
- The transformation zone of the cervix encompasses the border of the squamous epithelium and columnar epithelium. The location of the transformation zone changes on the cervix depending on a woman's hormonal status.
- The uterus of a nulliparous woman is approximately 8 cm long, 5 cm wide, and 2.5 cm thick and weighs 40 to 50 g. In contrast, in a multiparous woman each measurement is approximately 1.2 cm larger and normal uterine weight is 20 to 30 g heavier. The maximal weight of a normal uterus is 110 g.
- In the majority of women, the long axis of the uterus is both anteverted in respect to the long axis of the vagina and anteflexed in relation to the long axis of the cervix. However, a retroflexed uterus is a normal variant found in approximately 25% of women.
- The arterial blood supply of the uterus is provided by the uterine and ovarian arteries. The uterine arteries are large branches of the anterior division of the hypogastric arteries, whereas the ovarian arteries originate directly from the aorta.
- Afferent nerve fibers from the uterus enter the spinal cord at the eleventh and twelfth thoracic segments.
- The oviducts are 10 to 14 cm in length and are composed of four anatomic sections. Closest to the uterine cavity is the interstitial segment, followed by the narrow isthmic

Continued

KEY POINTS *Continued*

segment, then the wider ampullary segment, and distally the trumpet-shaped infundibular segment.

- The right oviduct and appendix are often anatomically adjacent. Clinically it may be difficult to differentiate inflammation of the upper portion of the genital tract and acute appendicitis.
- During the reproductive years the ovaries measure approximately 1.5 cm × 2.5 cm × 4 cm.
- The ovary in nulliparous women rests in a depression of peritoneum named the *fossa ovarica.* Immediately adjacent to the ovarian fossa are the external iliac vessels, the ureter, and the obturator vessels and nerves.
- Three prominent ligaments determine the anatomic mobility of the ovary: the mesovarian, the ovarian ligament, and the infundibulopelvic ligament.
- The arterial supply of the pelvis is paired, bilateral, and has multiple collaterals and numerous anastomoses.
- The extent of collateral circulation after hypogastric artery ligation depends on the site of ligation and may be divided into three groups: branches from the aorta, branches from the external iliac arteries, and branches from the femoral arteries.
- The internal iliac nodes are found in an anatomic triangle whose sides are composed of the external iliac artery, the hypogastric artery, and the pelvic sidewall. This rich collection of nodes receives channels from every internal pelvic organ and the vulva, including the clitoris and urethra.
- The femoral triangle is the anatomic space lying immediately distal to the fold of the groin. The boundaries of the femoral triangle are the sartorius and adductor longus muscles and the inguinal ligament.
- The pudendal nerve and its branches supply the majority of both motor and sensory fibers to the muscles and skin of the vulvar region.
- The femoral nerve may be compromised by pressure on the psoas muscle during abdominal surgery and by hyperflexion of the leg during vaginal surgery.
- The pelvic diaphragm is important in supporting both abdominal and pelvic viscera and facilitates equal distribution of intraabdominal pressure during activities such as coughing. The levator ani muscles constitute the greatest bulk of the pelvic diaphragm.
- The major function of the urogenital diaphragm is support of the urethra and maintenance of the urethrovesical junction.
- Contained within the broad ligaments are the following structures: oviducts; ovarian and round ligaments; ureters; ovarian and uterine arteries and veins; parametrial tissue; embryonic remnants of the mesonephric duct and wolffian body, and two secondary ligaments.
- The cardinal ligaments provide the major support to the uterus.
- A congenital anomaly of a double, or bifid, ureter occurs in 1% to 4% of females.
- When the urinary bladder is empty, the ureteral orifices are approximately 2.5 cm apart. This distance increases to 5 cm when the bladder is distended.
- The distal ureter enters into the cardinal ligament. In this location the ureter is approximately 1 to 2 cm lateral to the uterine cervix and is surrounded by a plexus of veins. In approximately 12% of women the cervix will be less than 0.5 cm from the cervix.
- Two ways of distinguishing the ureter from pelvic vessels are (1) identification of peristalsis after stimulation with a surgical instrument and (2) identification of Auerbach's plexuses.
- Surgical compromise of the ureters may occur during clamping or ligating of the infundibulopelvic vessels, clamping or ligating of the cardinal ligaments, or wide suturing in the endopelvic fascia during an anterior repair.
- The following three important axioms should be in the forefront of decision making during difficult gynecologic surgery: (1) do not assume that the anatomy of the left and right side of the pelvis are invariably identical mirror images; (2) during difficult operations with multiple adhesions operate from known anatomic areas into the unknown; and (3) from the sage advice of a distinguished Canadian gynecologist, Dr. Henry McDuff:

> If the disease be rampant and the anatomy obscure,
> And the plans of dissection not pristine and pure,
> Do not be afraid, nor faint of heart,
> Try the retroperitoneum, it's a great place to start.

REFERENCES

Aronson MP, Bates SM, Jacoby AF, et al: Periurethral and paravaginal anatomy: An endovaginal magnetic resonance imaging study. Am J Obstet Gynecol 173:1702, 1995.

Beckmann CRB, Lipscomb GH, Murrell L, et al: Instruction in surgical anatomy for gynecology residents using prosected human cadavers. Am J Obstet Gynecol 170:148, 1994.

Benedetti-Panici P, Maneschi F, Scambia G, et al: Anatomic abnormalities of the retroperitoneum encountered during aortic and pelvic lymphadenectomy. Am J Obstet Gynecol 170:111, 1994.

Benedetti-Panici P, Scambia G, Baiocchi G, et al: Anatomical study of para-aortic and pelvic lymph nodes in gynecologic malignancies. Obstet Gynecol 79:498, 1992.

Cruikshank SH, Stoelk EM: Surgical control of pelvic hemorrhage: Method of bilateral ovarian artery ligation. Am J Obstet Gynecol 147:724, 1983.

DeLancey JOL: Anatomy and biomechanics of genital prolapse. Clin Obstet Gynecol 36:897, 1993.

DeLancey JOL: Structural anatomy of the posterior pelvic compartment as it relates to rectocele. Am J Obstet Gynecol 180:815, 1999.

Fenner DE, Kriegshauser JS, Lee HH, et al: Anatomic and physiologic measurements of the internal and external anal sphincters in normal females. Obstet Gynecol 91:369, 1998.

Grant JCB: An Atlas of Anatomy, 9th ed. Baltimore, Williams & Wilkins, 1991.

Hahn L: Clinical findings and results of operative treatment in ilioinguinal nerve entrapment syndrome. Br J Obstet Gynaecol 96:1080, 1989.

Hoffman MS, Lynch C, Lockhart J, Knapp R: Injury of the rectum during vaginal surgery. Am J Obstet Gynecol 181:274, 1999.

Hsu Y, Fenner DE, Weadock WJ, DeLancy JO: Magnetic resonance imaging and 3-dimensional analysis of external anal sphincter anatomy. Obstet Gynecol 106:1259, 2005.

Hurd WW, Chee SS, Gallagher KI, et al: Location of the ureters in relation to the uterine cervix by computed tomography. Am J Obstet Gynecol 184:336, 2001.

Jelen I, Bachmann G: An anatomical approach to oophorectomy during vaginal hysterectomy. Obstet Gynecol 87:137, 1996.

Koelbl H, Strassegger H, Riss PA, Gruber H: Morphologic and functional aspects of pelvic floor muscles in patients with pelvic relaxation and genuine stress incontinence. Obstet Gynecol 74:789, 1989.

Kurman RJ: Blaustein's Pathology of the Female Genital Tract, 4th ed. New York, Springer-Verlag, 1994.

Krantz KE: The anatomy of the urethra and anterior vaginal wall. Am J Obstet Gynecol 62:374, 1951.

Krantz KE: Innervation of the human vulva and vagina. Obstet Gynecol 12:382, 1958.

Netter FH: Reproductive system, vol 2. The CIBA Collection of Medical Illustrations. Summit, NJ, CIBA Pharmaceutical Products, 1983.

Nichols DH, Randall CL: Vaginal Surgery, 4th ed. Baltimore, Williams & Wilkins, 1996.

Novak ER, Woodruff JD: Gynecologic and Obstetric Pathology, 8th ed. Philadelphia, WB Saunders, 1979.

Pelosi MA III, Pelosi MA: Alignment of the umbilical axis: an effective maneuver for laparoscopic entry in the obese patient. Obstet Gynecol 92:869, 1998.

Peschers UM, DeLancey JOL, Fritsch H, et al: Cross-sectional imaging anatomy of the anal sphincters. Obstet Gynecol 90:839, 1997.

Plentl AA, Friedman EA: Lymphatic System of the Female Genitalia: The Morphologic Basis of Oncologic Diagnosis and Therapy. Philadelphia, WB Saunders, 1971.

Richardson AC: The rectovaginal septum revisited: Its relationship to rectocele and its importance in rectocele repair. Clin Obstet Gynecol 36:976, 1993.

Robboy SJ, Anderson MC, Russell P (eds): Pathology of the Female Reproductive Tract. Edinburgh, Churchill Livingstone, 2002.

Shull B: Using videography to teach retropubic space anatomy and surgical technique. Obstet Gynecol 77:640, 1991.

Standring S: Gray's Anatomy, 39th ed. Philadelphia, Elsevier, 2005.

Stevens A, Lowe J: Human Histology, 3rd ed. Philadelphia, Elsevier Mosby, 2005.

Thakar R, Clarkson P: Bladder, bowel and sexual function after hysterectomy for benign conditions. Br J Obstet Gynaecol 104:983, 1997.

Thompson JR, Gibb JS, Genadry R, et al: Anatomy of pelvic arteries adjacent to the sacrospinous ligament: Importance of the coccygeal branch of the inferior gluteal artery. Obstet Gynecol 94:973, 1999.

Ulmsten U, Falconer C: Connective tissue in female urinary incontinence. Curr Opin Obstet Gynecol 11:509, 1999.

Vedantham S, Goodwin SC, McLucas B, Mohr G: Uterine artery embolization: An underused method of controlling pelvic hemorrhage. Am J Obstet Gynecol 176:938, 1997.

Verkauf BS, Von Thron J, O'Brien WF: Clitorial size in normal women. Obstet Gynecol 80:41, 1992.

Wall LL: The muscles of the pelvic floor. Clin Obstet Gynecol 36:910, 1993.

Wynn RM, Jollie WP: Biology of the Uterus, 2nd ed. New York, Plenum Publishing, 1989.

Zacharin RF: The suspensory mechanism of the female urethra. J Anat 97:423, 1963.

Zacharin RF: Pulsion enterocele: Review of functional anatomy of the pelvic floor. Obstet Gynecol 55:135, 1980.

Reproductive Endocrinology 4

Neuroendocrinology, Gonadotropins, Sex Steroids, Prostaglandins, Ovulation, Menstruation, Hormone Assay

Rogerio A. Lobo

KEY TERMS AND DEFINITIONS

Activin. Peptide with a similar structure to inhibin but an opposite action. Activins stimulate pituitary follicle-stimulating hormone (FSH) release and ovarian estradiol production.

Affinity (*K*). Degree to which a hormone binds to its receptor. Affinity is determined by the degree to which the hormone structurally fits, or interlocks, with the receptor.

Arcuate Nucleus. A group of nerve cells lying in the medial portion of the hypothalamus just above the median eminence. Nerve cells in the arcuate nucleus are the major source of gonadotropin-releasing hormone (GnRH) secretion.

Aromatization. Synthesis of a phenolic, or aromatic, benzene ring, as occurs during conversion of testosterone to estradiol.

Atresia. Process of regression of preantral follicles.

Autocrine. Producing hormonal effects by intracellular communication.

Bioassay. Measurement of the amount of hormone present in a substance by determining its effect on a target organ in an animal and comparing it with the effect produced by a known (standard) amount of hormone.

Catechol Estrogens. Steroids that structurally resemble both estrogens and catecholamines and have only a weak estrogenic action.

Coefficient of Variation (CV). Mathematical technique for measuring precision of assay after results of measurement of same substance are calculated several times in one assay (intra-assay *CV*) or in several assays (interassay *CV*).

Cortical Granules. Particles in ooplasm that are released into the surface membrane after one sperm penetrates the ovum. They may act to block further sperm penetration.

Cross-reaction. Interference in immunoassay by a substance that is not being measured but reacts with the antibody to a lesser degree than the hormone being measured. It thus alters the results of the assay.

Desensitization (Down-Regulation). The condition wherein a hormone is secreted or administered for a prolonged period and produces an inhibitory instead of a stimulatory response because of saturation of its receptor.

Dominant Follicle. Follicle that enlarges to about 2 cm in diameter and eventually ovulates.

Eicosanoids. Class of fatty acid derivatives that includes prostaglandins, thromboxanes, and leukotrienes. Eicosanoids are derived from the unsaturated fatty acid form of eicosanoic acid and have a high degree of biologic activity. The most important precursor of the eicosanoids is arachidonic acid.

β-Endorphin. A potent opioid peptide (more potent than morphine) that is concentrated in the hypothalamus and pituitary. It inhibits luteinizing hormone (LH) secretion.

Extraglandular Conversion. Process whereby one steroid is converted to another steroid in tissue other than endocrine organs.

Follicle-Stimulating Hormone (FSH). A glycoprotein with a molecular weight of 33,000 daltons that is composed of a nonspecific α subunit and a specific β subunit. The primary action of FSH in the female is to stimulate granulosa cell synthesis.

Germinal Vesicle. Nuclear material that is surrounded by a membrane, visible histologically, and that is present in the primary oocyte.

Gonadotropin-Releasing Hormone (GnRH). A decapeptide synthesized in and secreted by the hypothalamus at periodic intervals to stimulate gonadotropin release from the pituitary gland.

Gonadotropin-Releasing Hormone Analogue (GnRH Analogue). GnRH analogues are proteins that have various amino acid substitutions of the 10 amino acids found in the parent molecule that increase potency and half-life.

Growth Factors. Small peptides or polypeptides that interact with cell membrane receptors and usually promote cell proliferation and/or differentiation.

Hormone Receptors. Proteins on the cell membrane or within the cell of the target tissue that bind to a specific molecule of a hormone (ligand) for the purpose of eliciting a biologic response. Hormone receptors bind only to ligands of a specific hormone and thus are hormone specific.

Hypothalamus. Portion of the base of the brain that is located just below the optic chiasm and that has a major role in regulating the hormones involved in reproductive endocrinology.

Inhibin. A polypeptide dimer composed of an α and a β subunit joined by disulfide bonds. This hormone is produced by ovarian granulosa cells and inhibits FSH secretion.

Continued

KEY TERMS AND DEFINITIONS *Continued*

Leptin. A peptide secreted by adipose tissue. It is believed to be a peripheral signal of amount of fat stores.

Leukotrienes. Derivatives of unsaturated eicosanoic acid, particularly arachidonic acid, which do not have a closed ring structure but have a similar system of assignment of letters and numeric subscripts. Their biologic effects are not completely understood but appear to stimulate smooth muscle.

Luteinizing Hormone (LH). A glycoprotein with a molecular weight of 28,000 daltons that is composed of a nonspecific α subunit and a specific β subunit. The primary action of LH in the female is to stimulate ovarian steroid synthesis.

Median Eminence (Infundibulum). The portion of the neurohypophysis lying in the midline at the base of the hypothalamus. It is connected to the infundibular stalk and the posterior (neural) lobe of the pituitary gland.

Metabolic Clearance Rate (MCR). Volume of plasma, serum, or blood that is cleared of the steroid per unit of time (e.g., measured in liters per day).

Monoclonal Antibody. Single type of antibody produced by the spleen cell of a mouse that was injected with antigen. The spleen cell is subsequently fused with a myeloma cell to form a hybridoma cell in order to produce large quantities of the antibody.

Neurohypophysis. The portion of the hypothalamus consisting of the median eminence, infundibular stalk, and posterior lobe of the pituitary.

Neuromodulator. A substance that affects the action of a neurotransmitter.

Neurotransmitter. Biogenic amines secreted by a nerve cell that produce an action on another cell.

Nonradioactive Immunoassays. Assays that do not use a radioactive marker but act by the same principle. These include the chemiluminescent immunoassay, fluoroimmunoassay, and enzyme immunoassay, which uses excess antigen, and enzyme-linked immunosorbent assay (ELISA), which uses excess antibody.

Oogonia. Primordial female germ cells with a full chromosomal complement that are present in the fetal ovary.

Paracrine. Producing hormonal effects by diffusion to contiguous cells.

Primary Follicle (Preantral Follicle). Immature oocyte covered by multiple layers of granulosa cells but without an antrum.

Primary Oocyte. Female germ cell in the diplotene stage of first meiotic division.

Primordial Follicle. Immature oocyte covered by a single layer of granulosa cells.

Production Rate. Amount of steroid that enters the circulation per unit of time (usually measured in milligrams or micrograms per day).

Prostaglandins. Prostanoids with a cyclopentane ring and two side chains. The different letters assigned to the various prostaglandins refer to different substitutions in the cyclopentane ring, and the numbers in the subscript of the letter indicate the number of double bonds in the side chain.

Prostanoids. Family of closely related lipids that include prostaglandins and thromboxanes. They have the basic structure of prostanoic acid, which consists of 20 carbon atoms arranged in a ring structure with two side chains.

Radioimmunoassay (RIA). Technique of measurement of hormone using a specific antibody raised against the hormone (antigen). The antigen competes for binding to the antibody with a radioactively labeled form of the same antigen.

Second Messenger. A substance, usually a cyclic nucleotide, that is activated when a protein hormone attaches to its receptor to induce changes within the cell.

Sex Hormone-Binding Globulin (SHBG). A serum globulin that has a high affinity for dihydrotestosterone, testosterone, and estradiol estrogens and androgens (also called testosterone–estrogen-binding globulin [TeBG]).

Standard Curve. Curved line that results from connecting the endpoints derived from assay of different amounts of known (standard) hormone plotted graphically against the amount of hormone present.

Stratum Basale. Thin, lowermost portion of endometrium that overlies the muscularis and consists of primordial glands and densely cellular stroma.

Stratum Functionale. Thick, uppermost portion of endometrium that grows under the influence of estrogen. It is composed of a thin superficial stratum compactum and an underlying broader stratum spongiosum.

Thromboxanes. Prostanoids with an oxane ring instead of a cyclopentane ring. Letters and numeric subscripts are assigned similar to those used with prostaglandins.

Transcription. Generation of messenger RNA from a segment of DNA produced by the hormone-receptor complex in the nucleus.

Transformation. The change in receptor configuration produced by a steroid that allows the receptor-hormone complex to undergo translocation.

Zona Pellucida. Mucopolysaccharide coat surrounding the oocyte that allows only sperm of the same species to penetrate the ovum.

The endocrinologic regulation of the reproductive system is extremely complex. Much information has been accumulated in the past three decades, and new information is constantly becoming available. Entire books have been written about each aspect of reproductive endocrinology. In this chapter, only the basic information required for understanding this complex process will be presented. Specifically the physiology of gonadotropin-releasing hormone (GnRH) secretion will be emphasized.

No single organ that secretes hormones involved in the reproductive process acts independently. Nevertheless, for ease of understanding, each organ and its principal hormones will be discussed as a unit. Information in this chapter will include the central nervous system control of GnRH secretion, GnRH action on gonadotropin secretion, gonadotropin effects on the ovary, and ovarian steroid effects on the uterus. The positive and negative feedback control of the various organs involved in human reproduction will be presented. The regulation of prolactin secretion is discussed in Chapter 39 (Hyperprolactinemia, Galactorrhea, and Pituitary Adenomas). Because of space limitations, even though the adrenal and thyroid hormones have a profound influence on the reproductive system, a discussion of adrenal and thyroid endocrinology will not be included in this text.

NEUROENDOCRINOLOGY OF GNRH SECRETION

Genes Controlling GnRH

GnRH is secreted as a 92-amino-acid precursor protein (Fig. 4-1), which is encoded on the short arm of chromosome 8 (8p 11.2-p 21). A GnRH-associated peptide (GAP), which is a 56-amino-acid part of the precursor protein, is able to inhibit prolactin and stimulate gonadotropin secretion. The GnRH receptor has been found in several organs besides the pituitary.

It is now clear that GnRH-2 also exists (p Glu-His-Trp-Ser-His-Gly-Trp-Tyr-Pro-Gly) and is encoded on the short arm of chromosome 20 (20 p13). GnRH-2 activity is predominantly outside of the CNS (eg, ovary)

GnRH-secreting cells arrive in the brain from its origins in the olfactory area. Beginning in the medial olfactory placode, from where the sense of smell originates, the cells migrate along a cranial nerve projecting from the nose to the septal-preoptic nuclei in the brain. In Kallman's syndrome, mutations arising, which prevent normal neuronal migration in this area, result in deficiency of GnRH and the lack of a sense of smell. Although X-linked transmission is most common, inheritance may also be either autosomal dominant or recessive.

The cell bodies of the hypothalamic neurons that produce GnRH are concentrated mainly in two areas: the anterior hypothalamus and the medial basal (tuberal) hypothalamus. In the latter area, the greatest number of GnRH-producing neurons are in the arcuate nucleus (Fig. 4-2). From these areas, GnRH is transported along the axons of these neurons, which terminate in the median eminence around the capillaries of the primary portal plexus. The nerve cells that transport GnRH from the arcuate nucleus to the median eminence are called the *tuberoinfundibular tract.*

The median eminence, or infundibulum, together with the infundibular stalk and posterior (neural) lobe of the pituitary, make up the neurohypophysis. The three components of the neurohypophysis share a common capillary network and have a direct arterial blood supply from the hypophyseal arteries. The capillaries of the median eminence have a fenestrated epithelium similar to that of peripheral tissue, which allows passage of large molecules. These capillaries differ from those present in the brain, and thus the median eminence is outside the blood–brain barrier.

The nerve cell terminals of the tuberoinfundibular tract secrete GnRH directly into the portal circulation, which carries the hormone to the gonadotropin-containing cells in the anterior lobe of the pituitary. The pars tuberalis of the anterior lobe of the pituitary (adenohypophysis) receives its vascular supply from pituitary portal vessels and is located adjacent to the base of the hypothalamus and the pituitary stalk (see Fig. 4-2). Unlike the neurohypophysis, the adenohypophysis has no direct arterial blood supply and receives all of its blood from the portal

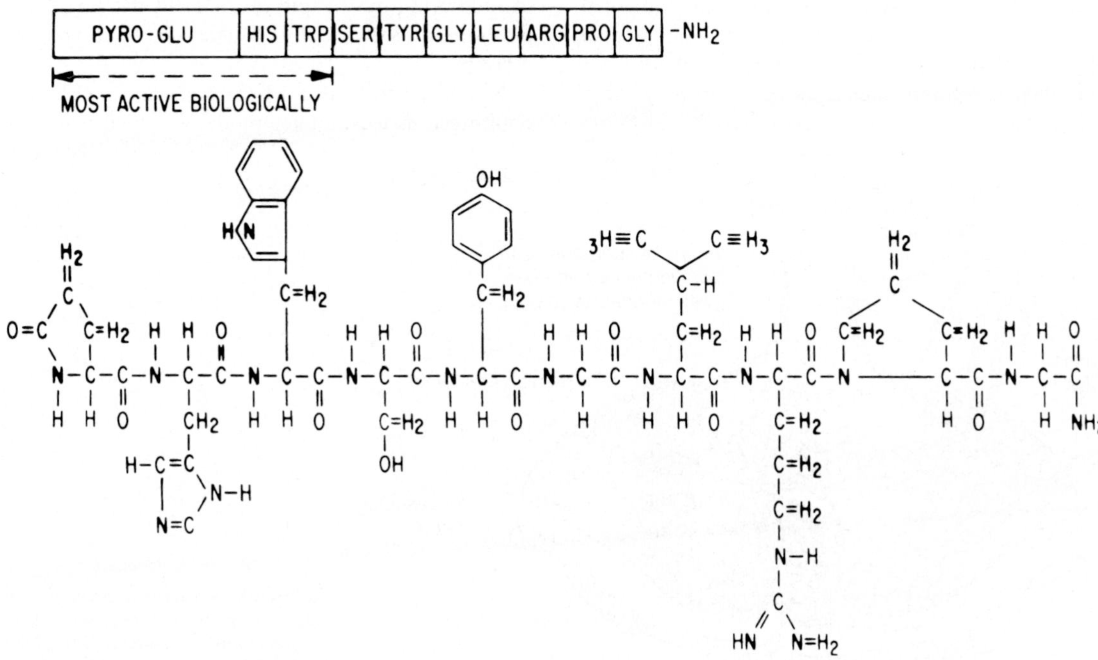

PYRO-GLU	HIS	TRP	SER	TYR	GLY	LEU	ARG	PRO	GLY	$-NH_2$

MOST ACTIVE BIOLOGICALLY

Figure 4-1. Amino acid sequence of gonadotropin-releasing hormone (GnRH). (From Kletzky OA, Lobo RA: Reproductive neuroendocrinology. In Mishell DR Jr, Davajan V, Lobo RA [eds]: Infertility, Contraception and Reproductive Endocrinology, 3rd ed. Cambridge, MA, Blackwell Scientific, 1991.)

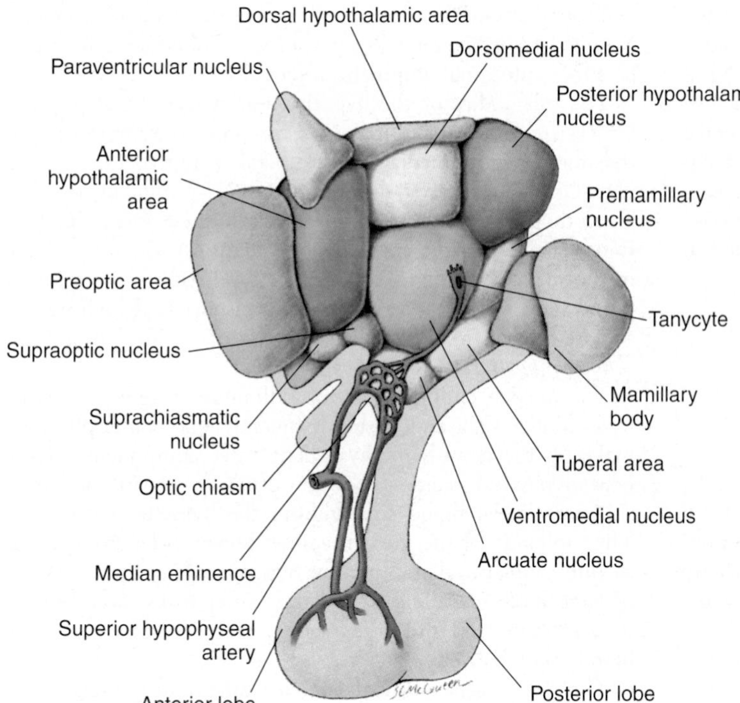

Figure 4-2. Nuclear organization of hypothalamus, shown diagrammatically in sagittal plane as it would appear from third ventricle. Rostral area is to left and caudal to right. Pituitary gland is shown ventrally. (Redrawn from Moore RY: Neuroendocrine mechanisms: Cells and systems. In Yen SSC, Jaffe R [eds]: Reproductive Endocrinology: Physiology, Pathophysiology and Clinical Management. Philadelphia, WB Saunders, 1986.)

vessels. After leaving the pituitary gland, the circulation returns to the neurohypophyseal capillary plexus, allowing pituitary hormones to help regulate the secretion of GnRH from the median eminence.

In addition to this major route of GnRH transport, an alternative route may exist. Axons of the tuberoinfundibular tract may transport GnRH directly into the third ventricle. A specialized ependymal cell, the tanycyte, extends from the lumen of the third ventricle into the outermost zone of the median eminence (Fig. 4-3). Because GnRH is transported into the portal system when it is administered into the third ventricle, it has been postulated that transport occurs via the tanycytes and their microvilli. Thus GnRH can be released both in large amounts periodically via the tuberoinfundibular tract (cyclic release) and in a low-grade continuous transependymal manner (tonic release) via the tanycytes.

In humans, GnRH is secreted in a pulsatile manner and has a half-life of only 2 to 4 minutes. The amplitude and frequency of the pulse vary throughout the menstrual cycle, with the frequency being more rapid in the follicular phase, about 1 pulse per hour, and slower in the luteal phase, about 1 pulse in 2 to 3 hours.

Knobil performed a series of elegant experiments using an oophorectomized monkey model in which endogenous GnRH

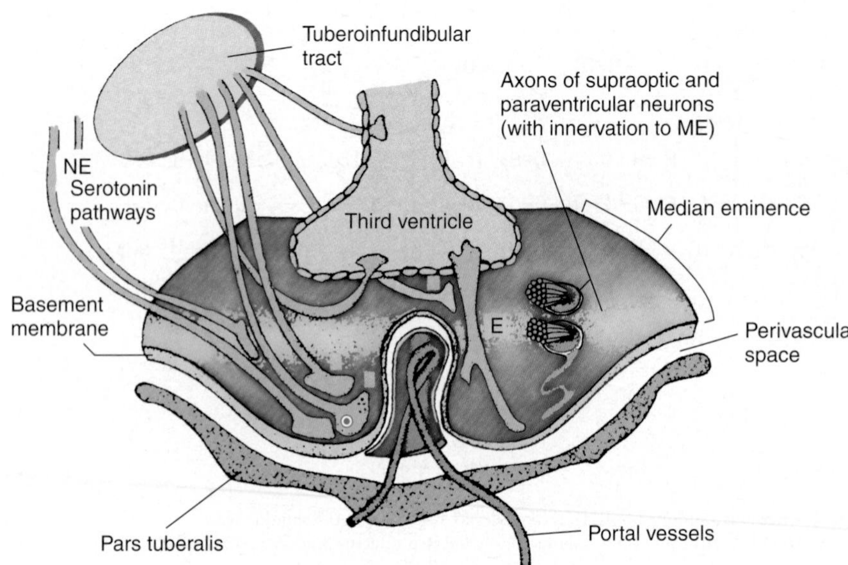

Figure 4-3. Schematic diagram showing tanycytes (E), stretching between third ventricle and outer portion of median eminence (ME). NE, norepinephrine. (From Reichlin S: Neural control of the pituitary gland: Normal physiology and pathophysiologic implications. In Current Concepts. Kalamazoo, MI, Upjohn Publications, 1978.)

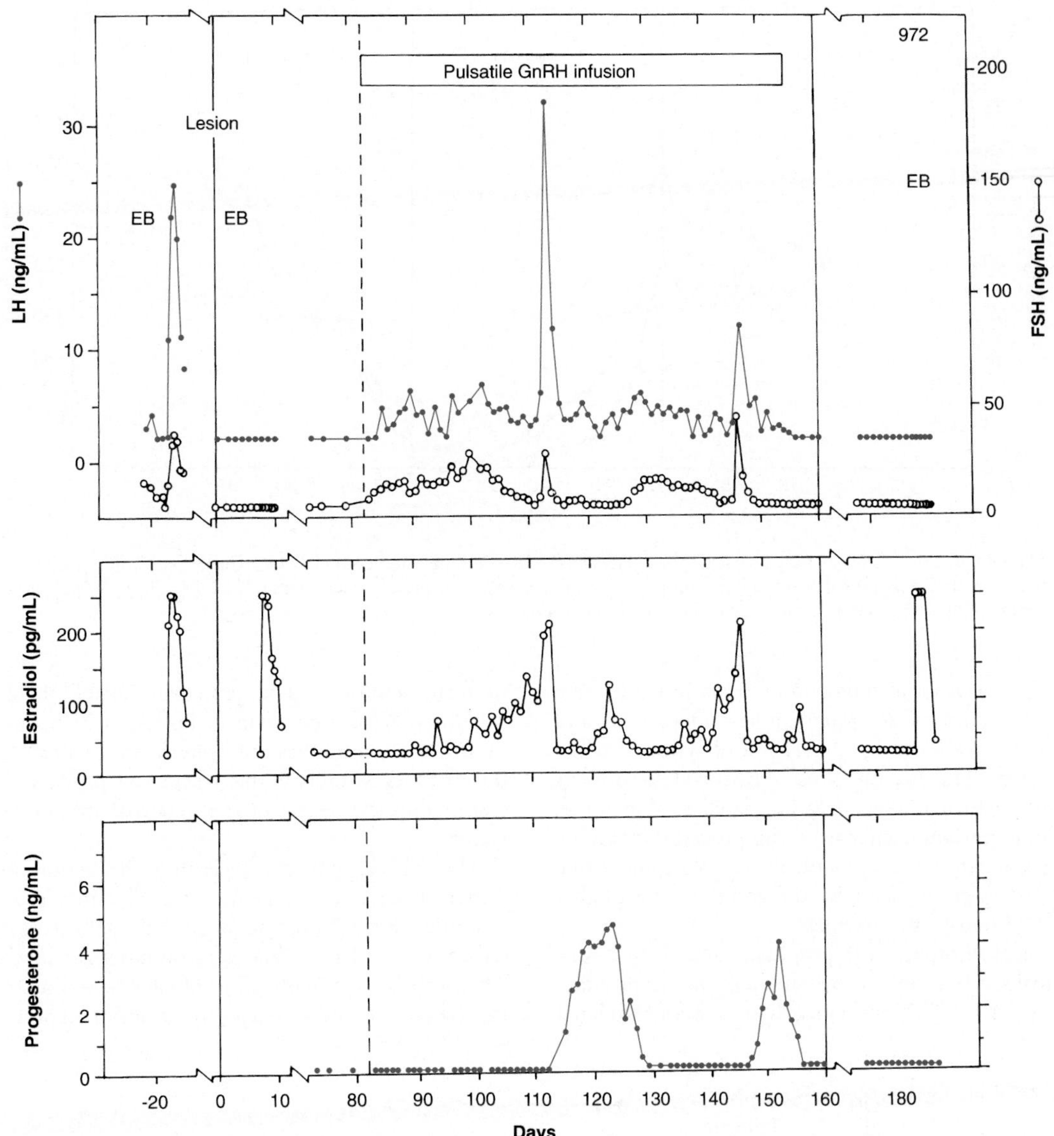

Figure 4-4. Induction of two ovulatory menstrual cycles by administration of pulsatile GnRH replacement (1 μg/min for 6 minutes, once every hour) in a rhesus monkey with hypothalamic lesion that had abolished endogenous GnRH secretion. Estradiol benzoate (EB) elicited gonadotropin response before placement of lesion but not afterward. (Redrawn from Knobil E, Plant TM, Wildt L, et al: Control of the rhesus monkey menstrual cycle: Permissive role of hypothalamic gonadotropin-releasing hormone. Redrawn with permission from Science 207:1371. Copyright 1980 AAAS.)

secretion had been abolished by a lesion in the hypothalamus. These investigators showed that altering the interval of GnRH pulses interferes with gonadotropin secretion. If exogenous GnRH pulses were administered every hour, a midcycle gonadotropin surge occurred (Fig. 4-4). However, when the pulse frequency was increased to five pulses per hour, gonadotropin secretion was inhibited (Fig. 4-5). Decreasing GnRH pulse frequency to once every 3 hours decreased the levels of luteinizing hormone (LH) and increased those of follicle-stimulating hormone (FSH); in addition, no gonadotropin surge occurred. Decreasing the amount of exogenous GnRH also inhibited gonadotropin release.

Crowley and coworkers have demonstrated that some women with anovulation (hypothalamic amenorrhea) and amenorrhea without a known cause have altered pulse frequency or amplitude of GnRH secretion or both. Thus, the control of episodic GnRH secretion is extremely important for the maintenance of normal ovulatory cyclicity. The amplitude and frequency of GnRH secretion by the hypothalamus are regulated not only by the feedback of two ovarian steroids, estradiol and progesterone, but also by gonadotropins through the humoral input pathway. Amplitude and frequency also are modulated by several neurotransmitters and neuromodulators within the brain through a neural input pathway.

Neurotransmitters

The most important neurotransmitters involved in reproductive neuroendocrinology are two catecholamines, dopamine and

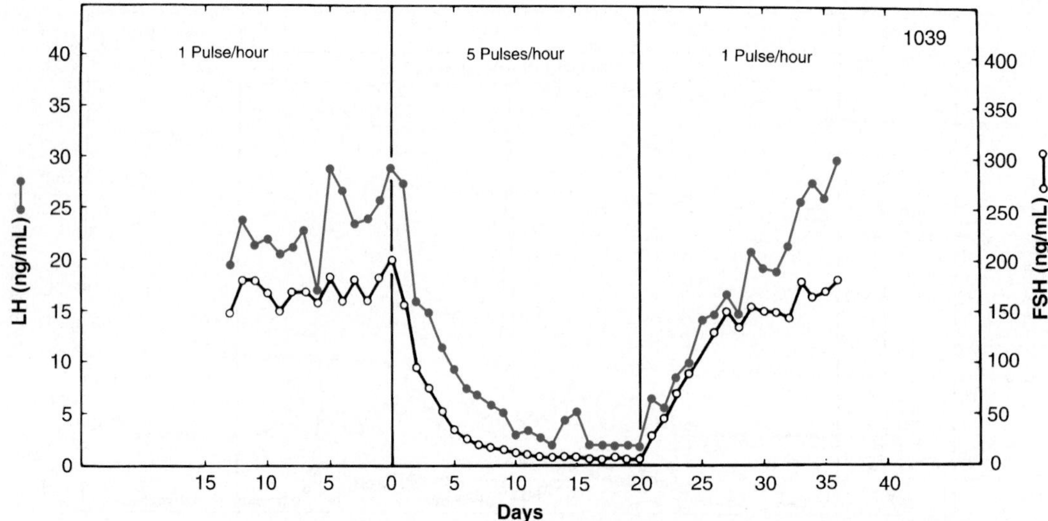

Figure 4-5. Same rhesus monkey preparation as in Figure 4-4. Gonadotropin suppression in which GnRH pulse is increased to five per hour and is restored by returning to the physiologic frequency of one pulse per hour. (From Knobil E: The neuroendocrine control of the menstrual cycle. Recent Prog Horm Res 36:53, 1980.)

norepinephrine, as well as an indolamine, serotonin. All three of these neurotransmitters are monoamines. Dopamine and norepinephrine are produced by conversion of tyrosine in the midbrain (Fig. 4-6). The enzyme tyrosine hydroxylase converts tyrosine to dopa, which is then decarboxylated to dopamine. Pyridoxine is an important coenzyme in this process. Dopamine oxidase converts dopamine to norepinephrine. Norepinephrine is then converted to epinephrine by the addition of a methyl group by a methyl transferase enzyme.

The precursor of serotonin is tryptophan, which is first converted to 5-hydroxytryptophan by the enzyme tryptophan hydroxylase (Fig. 4-7). This substance is then decarboxylated to form serotonin. The principal metabolite of serotonin is 5-hydroxyindoleacetic acid (5-HIAA), which can be measured in urine. Serotonin has not been shown to affect GnRH release, but it does stimulate the release of prolactin, probably by stimulating the release of the hypothalamic prolactin-releasing factor.

The current concept regarding the action of neurotransmitters is that the biogenic catecholamines modulate GnRH pulsatile release. Norepinephrine is thought to exert stimulatory effects on GnRH, while serotonin exerts inhibitory effects. The probable mode of action of catecholamines is to influence the frequency and perhaps the amplitude of GnRH release.

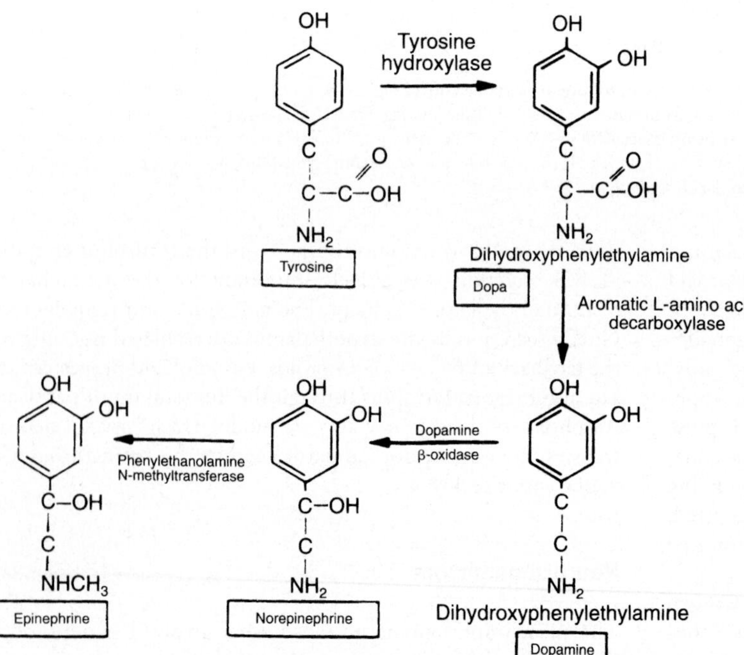

Figure 4-6. Metabolic pathways of dopamine, norepinephrine, and epinephrine synthesis. (From Kletzky OA, Lobo RA: Reproductive neuroendocrinology. In Mishell DR Jr, Davajan V, Lobo RA [eds]: Infertility, Contraception and Reproductive Endocrinology, 3rd ed. Cambridge, MA, Blackwell Scientific, 1991.)

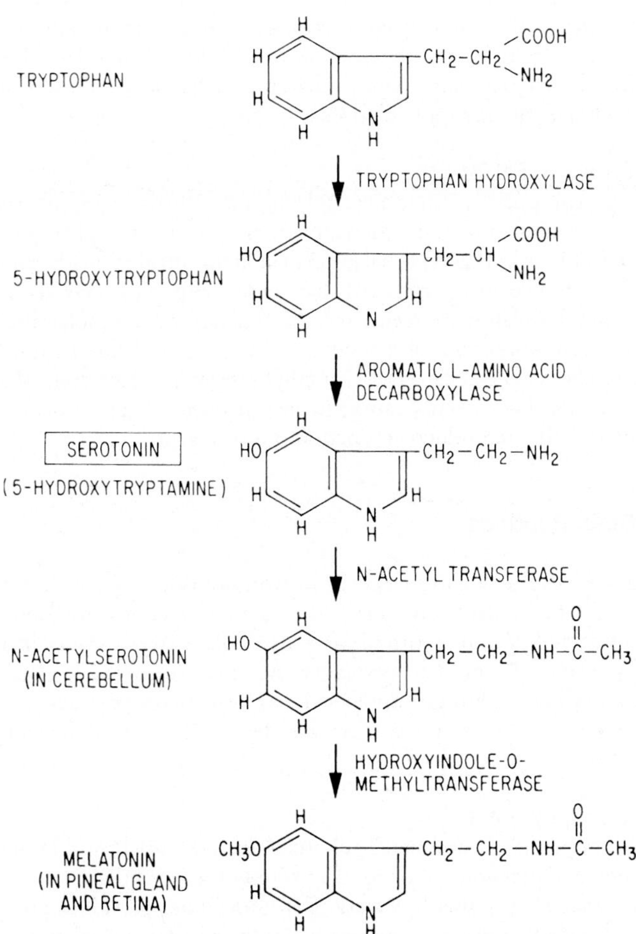

Figure 4-7. Metabolic pathway of serotonin synthesis. (From Kletzky OA, Lobo RA: Reproductive neuroendocrinology. In Mishell DR Jr, Davajan V, Lobo RA [eds]: Infertility, Contraception and Reproductive Endocrinology, 3rd ed. Cambridge, MA, Blackwell Scientific, 1991.)

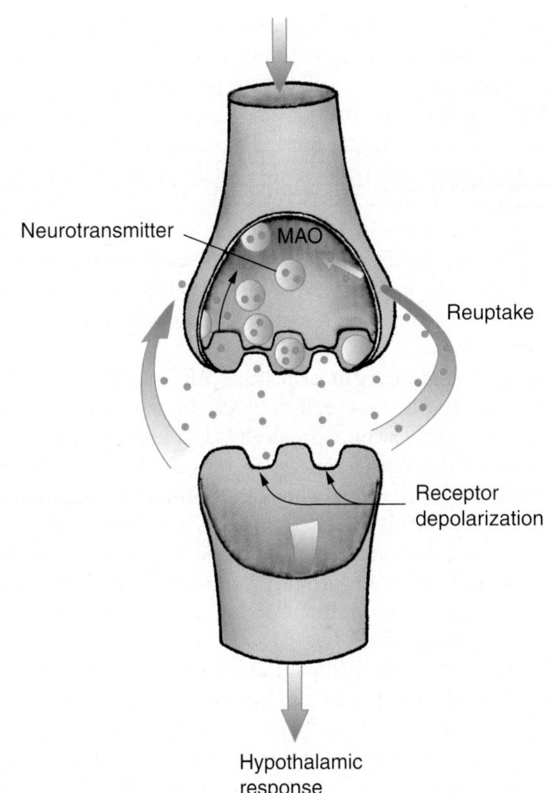

Figure 4-8. A stimulus induces release of stored neurotransmitter by exocytosis. Most of it is taken up again; the rest binds to a specific receptor, resulting in hypothalamic response. MAO, Monoamine oxidase. (From Kletzky OA, Lobo RA: Reproductive neuroendocrinology. In Mishell DR Jr, Davajan V, Lobo RA [eds]: Infertility, Contraception and Reproductive Endocrinology, 3rd ed. Cambridge, MA, Blackwell Scientific, 1991.)

Thus pharmacologic or physiologic factors that affect pituitary function probably do so by altering catecholamine synthesis or metabolism, and thus the pulsatile release of GnRH.

The intravenous administration of dopamine to both men and women is associated with a suppression of circulating prolactin and gonadotropin levels. Dopamine does not exert a direct effect on gonadotropin secretion by the anterior pituitary; instead its effect is mediated through inhibition of GnRH release in the hypothalamus. Although the exact chemical nature of the endogenous prolactin-inhibiting hormone remains unknown, overwhelming evidence indicates that dopamine is the hypothalamic inhibitor of prolactin secretion. Thus dopamine may directly suppress hypothalamic GnRH activity and pituitary prolactin secretion.

Mechanism of Action and Pharmacologic Effects

The effects of neurotransmitters on the secretion of hypothalamic hormones probably are exerted by different mechanisms. One possible mechanism is through a direct cell-to-cell connection or a multisynaptic communication whereby the neurotransmitter is released by the terminal nerve and depolarizes the receptor site on a hypothalamic cell (Fig. 4-8). Depolarization results in the release of a specific hormone from the hypothalamic cell.

These specific effects of neurotransmitters on hypothalamic cells can be altered by the systemic administration of certain drugs. For example, methyldopa and α-methyl-*p*-tyrosine can block dopamine and norepinephrine synthesis by inhibiting tyrosine hydroxylase. Reserpine and chlorpromazine interfere with norepinephrine, dopamine, and serotonin binding and storage. Finally, and clinically important, the frequently prescribed tricyclic antidepressants inhibit the reuptake of neurotransmitters, whereas other medications such as propranolol, phentolamine, haloperidol, and cyproheptadine act by blocking the receptors at the level of the hypothalamus.

As a consequence of receiving such medications, many patients develop disorders such as galactorrhea and oligoamenorrhea. These clinical entities are a result of either hyperprolactinemia or alterations in GnRH-gonadotropin secretion.

Neuromodulators

Opioids

Receptors for the opioid peptides are present in the brain. There are three subgroups of opiates: enkephalins, endorphins (α, β, γ), and dynorphins. β-Endorphin (β-EP) contains 31 amino acids, is 5 to 10 times as potent as morphine, and is concentrated mainly in the arcuate nucleus and median eminence of the hypothalamus, as well as the pituitary gland. β-EP has also been localized in the placenta, pancreas, gastrointestinal (GI) tract, and in seminal fluid. The concentrations of endorphins are about 1000 times higher in the pituitary than in the hypothalamus. Infusion of β-EP results in an increase in prolactin and a decrease in LH, the latter occurring by an inhibitory effect on GnRH neurons in the hypothalamus. It is now believed that the opiates alter GnRH release by modulating synthesis of substances in the catecholamine pathway, principally norepinephrine.

Peripheral measurement of plasma β-EP is difficult to interpret because it does not reflect levels in the central nervous system (CNS) circulation. Specifically, the pituitary or peripheral pool of β-EP (or both) appears to be separate from the pool within the hypothalamus. Therefore peripheral measurements of β-EP reflect pituitary and non-CNS secretions rather than those from the hypothalamus. Another difficulty results from the low peripheral concentration of β-EP. In addition, cross-reactivity with β-lipotropins occurs in the immunoassays currently used for β-EP.

Therefore, to study β-EP action, experiments are performed using infusions of naloxone, an opioid antagonist. Infusion of greater than 1 mg/hr blocks brain opioid activity and results in an increase of LH in the late follicular and luteal phases but not in the early follicular phase or postmenopausally. This suggests that both estrogen and progesterone increase levels of β-EP in the brain (Fig. 4-9). The increase in β-EP may account for the decreased frequency of GnRH pulses in the luteal phase.

Prostaglandins

Hypothalamic levels of prostaglandins may modulate the release of GnRH. Administration of prostaglandin E_2 significantly increases GnRH levels in the portal blood. Furthermore, a physiologic role of prostaglandins in regulating or modulating the secretion of GnRH is supported by experiments demonstrating that the midcycle surge of LH can be abolished in the rat and ewe by the administration of aspirin or indomethacin, which blocks the synthesis of prostaglandins. Clinical studies in women have also shown that prostaglandin inhibition at midcycle can disrupt ovulation.

Catechol Estrogens

The compounds 2-hydroxyestradiol and 2-hydroxyestrone, as well as their 3-methoxy derivatives, are present in higher concentrations in the hypothalamus than are prostaglandins E_1 and E_2. It has been hypothesized that these compounds may act as neuromodulators by regulating the function of catecholamines through inhibition of tyrosine hydroxylase and competition for the enzyme catechol-*O*-methyltransferase. However, the evidence that catechol estrogens have a major effect on neuromodulating reproductive function is insufficient.

Brain Peptides

Many peptides can function as neurotransmitters, but most act locally to regulate autocrine and paracrine functions. Although pituitary hormone synthesis and secretion is largely controlled by classic hormonal messenger systems, considerable local intercellular communications exist as well. Brain peptides that function as neurotransmitters are described in the following sections.

Neuropeptide Y

Neuropeptide Y stimulates pulsatile release of GnRH and in the pituitary potentiates gonadotropin response to GnRH. It thus may facilitate pulsatile secretion of GnRH and gonadotropins. In the absence of estrogen, neuropeptide Y inhibits gonadotropin secretion. Because undernutrition is associated with an increase in neuropeptide Y and increased amounts have been measured in cerebrospinal fluid of women with anorexia nervosa and bulimia nervosa, it has been proposed that neuropeptide Y is one of the factors linking altered nutrition and reproductive function.

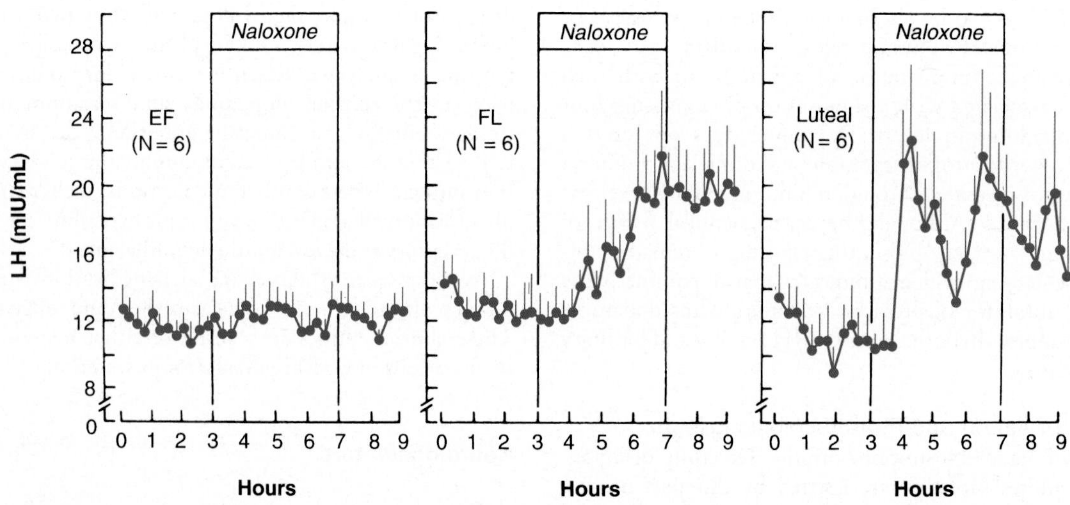

Figure 4-9. Infusion of naloxone, an opiate receptor antagonist, elicits incremental change of LH in subjects during late follicular (LF) and midluteal phases of cycle (but not in early follicular [EF] phase), indicating progressive increase in endogenous opioid inhibition of GnRH secretion, especially during luteal phase. (From Quigley ME, Yen SSC: The role of endogenous opiates in LH secretion during the menstrual cycle. J Clin Endocrinol Metab 51:179, 1980. © 1980 by The Endocrine Society.)

Angiotensin II

Several components of the renin–angiotensin system are present in the brain. Receptors for angiotensin II are found in various pituitary cell types, suggesting that angiotensin II affects the secretion of pituitary hormones by local action. In addition, angiotensin II in the hypothalamus appears to influence the effects of norepinephrine and dopamine on the releasing factors that control gonadotropin and prolactin secretion.

Somatostatin

Somatostatin is a hypothalamic peptide that inhibits the release of growth hormone, prolactin, and thyroid-stimulating hormone (TSH) from the pituitary.

Galanin

Galanin is released into the portal circulation in pulsatile fashion. It positively influences LH secretion. Galanin secretion is inhibited by dopamine and somatostatin and stimulated by thyroid-releasing hormone (TRH) and estrogen.

Activin and Inhibin

Activin and inhibin are produced by the gonads and are peptide members of the transforming growth factor-β family. These peptides have opposing effects on FSH secretion. Inhibin selectively diminishes FSH but not the release of LH, while activin stimulates FSH but not LH release.

Follistatin

Follistatin is an ovarian peptide that has also been called FSH-suppressing protein because of its main action: inhibition of FSH synthesis and secretion and the FSH response to GnRH. Follistatin also binds to activin and in this manner decreases the activity of activin.

Melatonin

Melatonin is produced by the pineal gland and is an indolamine converted from tryptophan. Secretion is influenced by darkness with increased levels occurring at night. This activity inhibits the episodic release of GnRH. Melatonin may also be important for circadian rhythms (higher at night) and is influenced by seasons with higher levels in the winter months.

Leptin

Leptin, produced by adipose cells, can act on the hypothalamus (where it enhances GnRH release). Leptin correlates with fat mass being elevated in obesity, but also exhibits a negative correlation with androgen levels, particularly dehydroeipandrosterone sulfate (DHEAS). It is likely that leptin also has a role in the pituitary, ovary, and also the endometrium, where it may have a role in implantation. Leptin may also be related to higher insulin levels, which in turn is positively correlated with enhanced GnRH release.

GNRH ACTION

When GnRH reaches the anterior lobe of the pituitary, it stimulates the synthesis and release of both LH and FSH from the same cell in the pituitary gland. Thus, whereas the hypothalamic control of prolactin is both inhibitory (dominant) and stimulatory, the hypothalamic control of gonadotropins is only stimulatory. Peptide hormones, such as GnRH, bind to specific receptors on the surface membrane of the target cell, in contrast to steroid hormones, which pass through the cell membrane to bind to intracellular receptors.

Protein hormone receptors are of high molecular weight (200,000 to 300,000 daltons), and each receptor binds a single molecule of the protein. Polypeptide hormones, including LH, FSH, and prolactin, although highly soluble in aqueous media, have low solubility in lipids and thus do not readily pass the lipid barrier of the target cell's plasma membrane. After the protein hormone binds to its transmembrane receptor, the hormone receptor complex may be brought through the cell membrane to protect it from other interactions. This process is called *internalization.* In addition to hormone-receptor complex internalization, the hormone message may be transmitted into the cell by transmembrane signaling via at least three known pathways: (1) production of an intracellular second messenger, which increases phosphorylation of regulatory proteins to produce a cellular response; (2) production of a membrane-bound second messenger; or (3) membrane-bound cystosolic phosphorylation activity triggered by hormone binding at the extracellular interface (Fig. 4-10*A* and *B*).

When a protein hormone binds to its specific receptor, it activates or inhibits the enzyme adenylate cyclase, the second messenger, which in turn changes the concentration of adenosine 3′5′-cyclic monophosphate (cyclic AMP, cAMP). The cAMP then activates protein kinase in the cytoplasm by binding its regulatory subunit, thereby dissociating this subunit from its catalytic subunit. When the regulatory subunit of the protein kinase is freed from the catalytic subunit, the latter subunit is able to transfer a phosphate from adenosine triphosphate (ATP) to the protein substrate. This action modifies the biologic function of the protein to produce a cellular response. Within a specific cell there are specific isoforms of adenylate cyclase, which explains the translation of specific cellular events. In addition, there is an intracellular amplification system of the hormonal signal (see Fig. 4-10*B*).

At the pituitary gonadotropin cell membrane, GnRH binding is facilitated by the action of calcium and prostaglandin. Intracellular calcium regenerates both cAMP and GMP. The hormone-receptor complex activates membrane-bound adenylate cyclase, which stimulates cAMP production and activates a protein kinase by dissociating its regulatory component from the catalytic subunit. The catalytic subunit then phosphorylates the membrane protein to increase calcium permeability. This change allows calcium to enter the cell. Entry of calcium into the cell mediates the response to hormones, which is itself a second-messenger system. Calcium activates the release of stored LH and FSH, producing a stimulus–secretion coupling analogous to muscle excitation–contraction coupling. Enhanced LH and FSH synthesis is also seen and may involve altering ribosomal phosphorylation to increase messenger ribonucleic acid (mRNA) translation. GnRH receptor synthesis is also stimulated by GnRH action. Differential secretion of LH and FSH is attained by feedback of steroid and peptide hormones on the gonadotrophs.

When GnRH is administered to humans in a bolus, a rapid increase occurs in circulating LH, which peaks at 30 minutes, and in FSH, which peaks at 60 minutes. Levels of both LH and

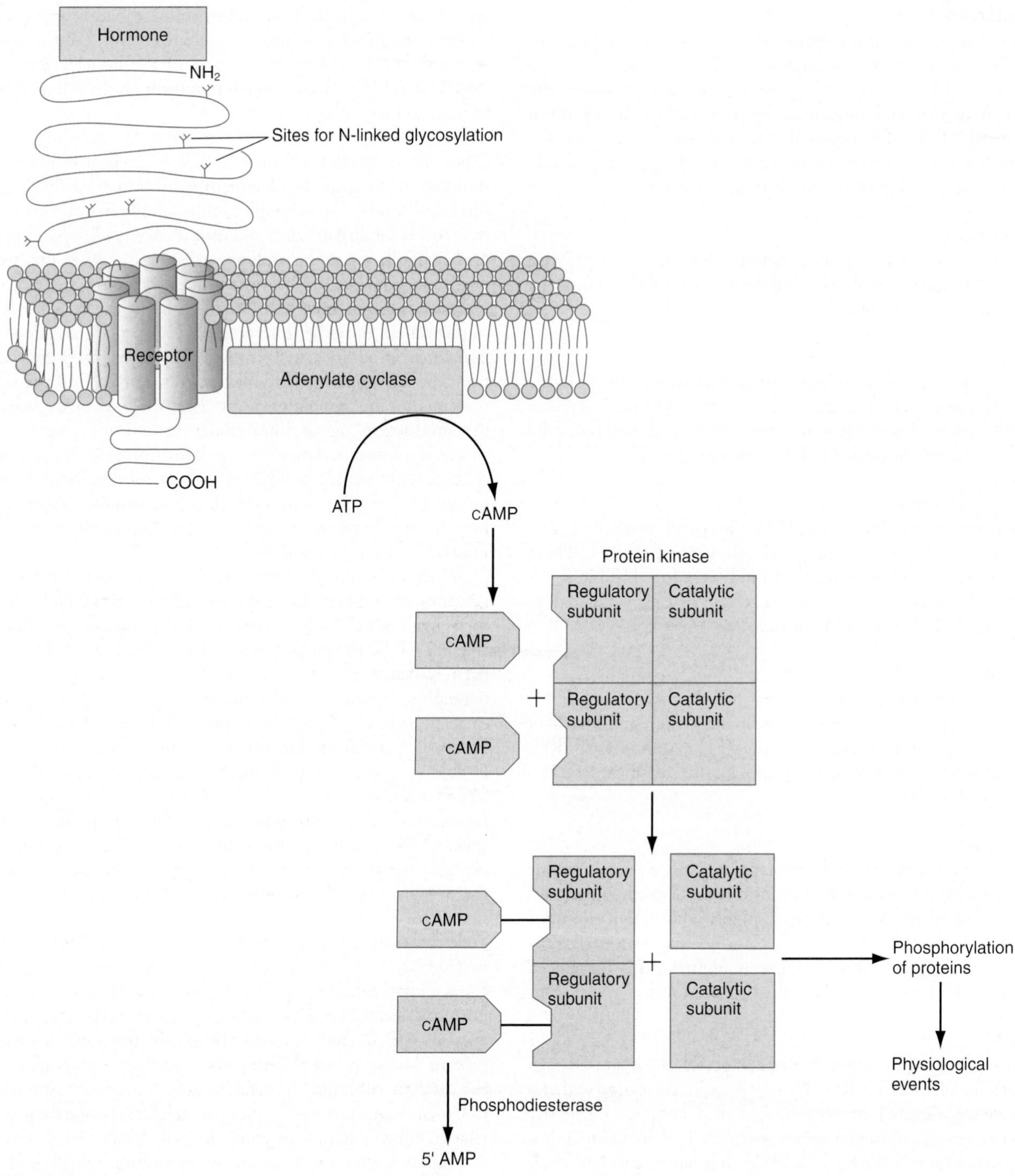

Figure 4-10. **A** and **B,** Protein hormones attach to their membrane receptor and activate an adenylate cyclase/cAMP second-messenger system. As shown in panel **B,** at various points downstream from cAMP production, amplification of the signal occurs. (Adapted from Speroff L, Fritz M (eds): Clinical Gynecologic Endocrinology and Infertility. New York, Lippincott Williams & Wilkins, 2005, pp 71–72.)

FSH return to baseline after 3 hours. With a constant infusion of GnRH, there is a biphasic release of LH but not of FSH. Yen has theorized that the initial rise represents the release of previously synthesized LH (first pool), and the second rise represents the release of newly synthesized LH (second pool) (Fig. 4-11). The combined size of both pituitary sensitivity (first pool) and reserve (second pool) has been called the functional capacity of the gonadotrophs. However, if GnRH continues to be infused, gonadotropin secretion is inhibited, probably because the receptors are saturated and are unable to continue to stimulate release of the second messenger (Fig. 4-12). Although maximal hormonal stimulation occurs when only a small percent-

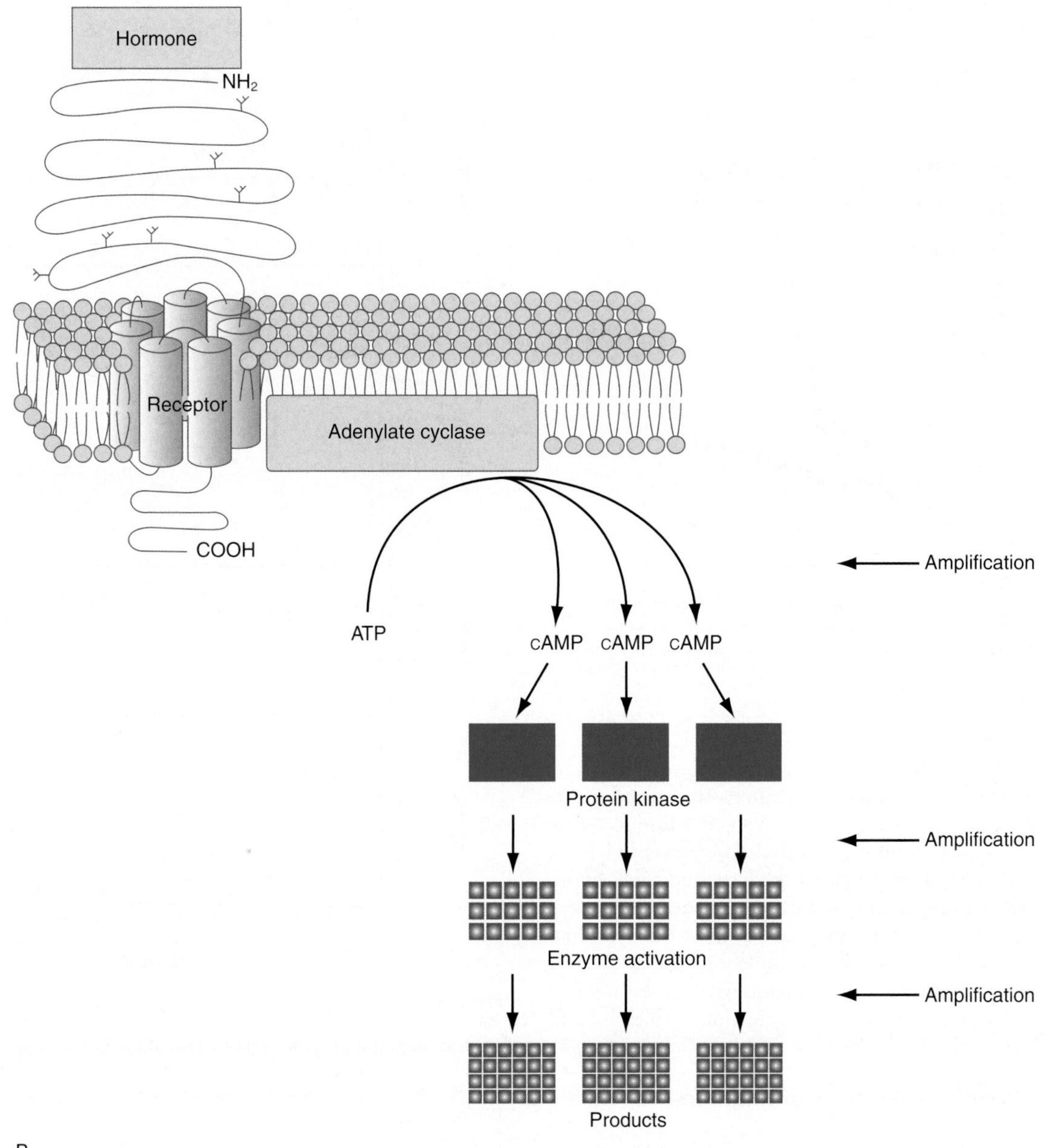

Figure 4-10. ***Cont'd,*** **B**

age of the target cell receptors are bound by hormone, when stimulation is maximal the unoccupied receptors become refractory to hormone binding for 12 to 72 hours. This phenomenon has allowed frequent administration of GnRH analogues to be used clinically.

GnRH analogues are synthesized by substitution of amino acid 6 in the parent molecule with a *d*-amino acid or replacement of amino acid 10 with an *N*-ethylamide (Na-CH_2-CH_3) or Aza-Gly (NHNHCO) moiety. The various agonists have greater potencies (15 to 200 times) and longer half-lives (1, 3, 6 hours) than GnRH. The agonists initially simulate gonadotropic release (flare). This effect lasts from 1 to 3 weeks. After this time, as the GnRH receptors become saturated with the constantly administered analogue, the stimulatory effect of the periodic release of endogenous GnRH on the pituitary gland is blocked. The process is called *desensitization,* or *down-regulation.* Therefore these analogues are used clinically to treat various steroid hormone-dependent entities.

Initial attempts to synthesize GnRH antagonists were hindered by allergic reactions induced by histamine release. In 1985 the GnRH agonist leuprolide acetate was approved for the palliative treatment of prostate cancer. Leuprolide is also available in several depot forms, which allows for the monthly or quarterly intramuscular administration for women with endometriosis and leiomyomata uteri. Although therapy has been shown to be effective, bone mineral content has decreased and hot flashes occur as a result of low estradiol levels. Adding low-dose estrogen or progestins (or both) to this therapy has proven to be successful.

A potent GnRH-antagonist, Nal-Glu, with less severe histamine reactions was the first of this class to be used clinically.

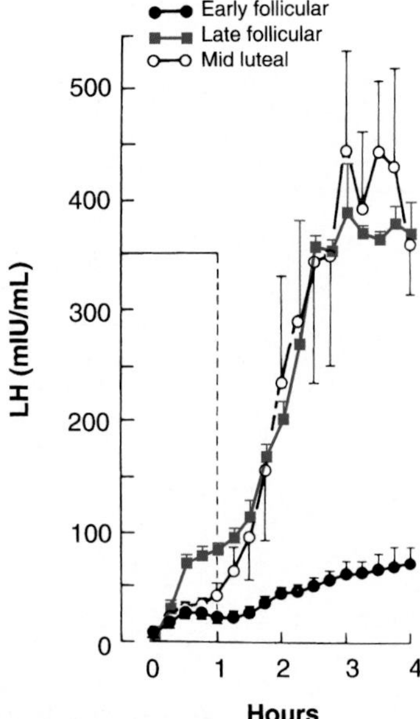

Figure 4-11. Quantitative LH release from first and second pool during GnRH infusion. Dotted line separates two pools. (From Hoff JD, Lasley BL, Wang CF, Yen SS: The two pools of pituitary gonadotropin: Regulation during the menstrual cycle. J Clin Endocrinol Metab 44:302, 1977. ©1977 by The Endocrine Society.)

Nal-Glu has been shown to decrease serum LH levels effectively when administered in a single dose (in a dose- and time-dependent manner) in both men and women without a flare effect. Nal-Glu acutely inhibits ovulation and affects LH more than FSH while decreasing estradiol levels at midcycle. Applications of GnRH antagonists have focused primarily in assisted reproductive technologies for down-regulation of the hypothalmopituitary axis during ovarian stimulation cycles. Newer applications of GnRH antagonists, including the treatment of uterine leiomyomas, are still under investigation. Tables 4-1 and 4-2 list clinical applications of GnRH agonists and available agonists and antagonists.

Table 4-1 Clinical Applications of GnRH and Its Agonists

Activation of Pituitary–Gonadal Function (GnRH)

Delayed puberty
Cryptorchidism
Functional hypothalamic amenorrhea
Hypogonadotropic hypogonadism (Kallmann's syndrome)

Pituitary–Gonadal Inhibition (Agonists)

Precocious puberty
Hormone-dependent tumors
- Endometriosis
- Uterine leiomyoma
- Breast cancer
- Prostatic cancer

Suppression of ovarian function in polycystic ovary syndrome and in vitro fertilization
Premenstrual syndrome
Dysfunctional uterine bleeding including clotting disorders

Contraception

Suppression of spermatogenesis
Ovulation inhibition

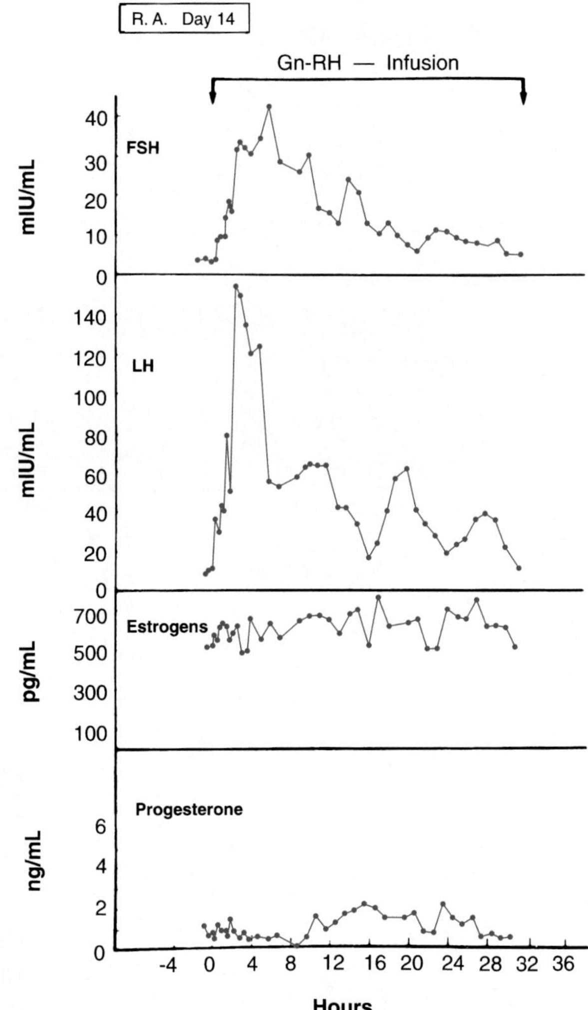

Figure 4-12. Mean serum FSH, LH, estrogen, and progesterone levels during 30-hour continuous infusions of GnRH at midcycle phase in three normal women. (From Jewelewicz R, Ferin M, Dyrenfurth I, et al: Long-term LH, RH infusions at various stages of the menstrual cycle in normal women. In Beling CG, Wenitz AC [eds]: The LH-releasing Hormone. New York, Masson Publishing, 1980.)

GONADOTROPIN STRUCTURE AND FUNCTION

LH and FSH are glycoproteins of high molecular weight, 28,000 and 37,000 daltons, respectively. They each have the same α subunit (14,000 daltons) of about 90 amino acids, which is similar in structure to the α subunit of TSH and human chorionic gonadotropin (HCG). The β subunits of all these hormones have different amino acids and carbohydrates and provide specific biologic activity. The α and β subunits are joined by disulfide bonds. The sialic acid content of each hormone increases with the duration of biologic action from one or two molecules in LH, which has a half-life of 30 minutes, to five molecules in FSH, which has a half-life of 3.9 hours. In the female, although the two gonadotropins act synergistically,

Table 4-2 GnRH Agonists and Antagonists Available for Clinical Use

	Structure	Mode of Administration
Agonists		
GnRH decapeptide	pGlu-His-Trp-Ser-Tyr-Gly-Leu-Arg-Pro-Gly-NH_2	Pulsatile pump
Leuprolide (Lupron)	pGlu-His-Trp-Ser-Tyr-DLeu-Leu-Arg-Pro-NHEt	Subcutaneous, depot implant
Buserelin (Suprefact, Suprecur, Suprefact depot)	pGlu-His-Trp-Ser-Tyr-DSer(*O*Bu)-Leu-Arg-Pro-NHEt	Subcutaneous, nasal, depot
Nafarelin (Synarel)	pGlu-His-Trp-Ser-Tyr-D2Nal-Leu-Arg-Pro-GlyNH_2	Subcutaneous, nasal
Histrelin (Supprelin)	pGlu-His-Trp-Ser-Tyr-DHis(Bzl)-Leu-Arg-Pro-AzaglyNH_2	Subcutaneous
Goserilin (Zoladex)	pGlu-His-Trp-Ser-Tyr-DSer(*O*'Bu)-Leu-Arg-Pro-AzaglyNH_2	Subcutaneous, depot
Gonadorelin pamoate (Decapeptyl)	pGlu-His-Trp-Ser-Tyr-DTrp-Leu-Arg-Pro-GlyNH_2	Subcutaneous, depot
Antagonists		
Cetrerolix	[Ac-DNal^1,DCpa^2,DPal^3,DCit^6,DAla^{10}] GnRH	Subcutaneous
Ganirelix	[Ac-D-Nal^1, DCpa^2,D-Pal^3, D-hArg$(Et)_2$ ^{6},hArg$(Et)_2$^{8},D-Ala^{10}] GnRH	Subcutaneous
Abarelix	[Ac-DNal^1,DCpa^2,Dpal^3,NMeTyr^5,DAsn^6,Lys(iPr)^8]GnRH	Subcutaneous

LH acts primarily on the theca cells to induce steroidogenesis, whereas FSH acts primarily on the granulosa cells to stimulate follicular growth. FSH release is greater than LH release until puberty, when the normal menstrual cycle is established and LH secretion overtakes that of FSH. After menopause the LH/FSH ratio is again reversed. This preferential inhibition of FSH release during the reproductive years results from increasing levels of both estradiol and inhibin.

Receptors for LH exist on the theca cells at all stages of the cycle; they are on granulosa cells after the follicle matures under the influence of FSH and estradiol, as well as on the corpus luteum. Each gonadal target tissue cell contains between 2000 and 30,000 membrane receptors. Maximal stimulation of hormonal activity occurs when less than 5% of these receptors are bound with hormone. The main action of LH is to stimulate androgen synthesis by the theca cells and progesterone synthesis by the corpus luteum through stimulation of intracellular cAMP production (Fig. 4-13). The precise action of LH on granulosa cells has not been determined, but it probably acts synergistically with FSH to help follicular maturation. LH stimulates several other metabolic events in the ovary, such as amino acid transport and RNA synthesis. LH may also induce ovulation by stimulating a plasminogen activator that decreases tensile strength of the follicle wall before follicular rupture occurs.

FSH receptors exist primarily on the granulosa cell membrane. In addition to stimulating LH receptors on this cell membrane, FSH activates the aromatase and the 3β-hydroxysteroid dehydrogenase enzymes within the cell by increasing cAMP. FSH stimulation of isolated granulosa cells in vitro produces only small amounts of estrogen; however, when androgens or theca cells are added, large amounts of estrogen are produced. These data support the two-cell hypothesis of estrogen production. This hypothesis proposes that LH acts on the theca to produce androgens (androstenedione and testosterone), which are then transported to the granulosa cells, where they are aromatized to estrogens (estrone and estradiol) by the action of FSH (see Fig. 4-13). The aromatase enzyme catalyzes this conversion.

Concomitant with increased estrogen production, mitosis is stimulated in granulosa cells, augmenting cell number. Estradiol and FSH receptor production is increased as well, maintaining intracellular cAMP levels as circulating FSH decreases. In granulosa cells primed by exposure to large amounts of estradiol and FSH, LH acts synergistically with FSH to increase LH receptors and induces luteinization of the follicle, thereby increasing progesterone production. Premature delivery of LH will disrupt the process, resulting in premature luteinization, whereas the capacity of the follicle to respond to estrogen appears to determine whether it will mature or become atretic.

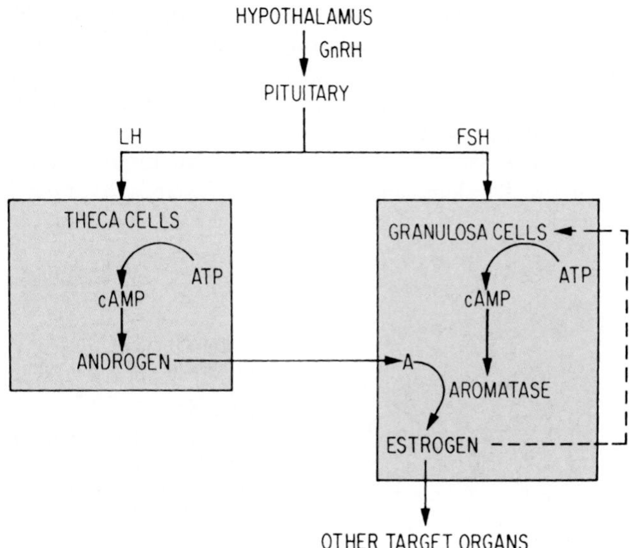

Figure 4-13. Action of gonadotropins on ovary: LH stimulates theca cell to synthesize androgen by cyclic-AMP (cAMP)-mediated action. FSH stimulates granulosa cells to activate aromatase via c-AMP-mediated action. Aromatase in granulosa cell converts androgen to estrogen, which is then utilized by target organs. Estrogen also stimulates granulosa cell proliferation. A, androgens; ATP, adenosine triphosphate; GnRH, gonadotropin-releasing hormone; LH, luteinizing hormone. (From a concept in Schulster D, Burstein S, Cooke BA: Control of gonadal steroidogenesis by FSH and LH. In Shulster D [ed]: Molecular Endocrinology of the Steroid Hormones. London, John Wiley & Sons, 1976.)

LH also stimulates prostaglandin synthesis by intracellular production of cAMP. Prostaglandin may play a role in follicle rupture, since the prostaglandin content of preovulatory follicles increases at the time of the gonadotropin surge and may stimulate smooth muscle contraction. Progesterone augments the activity of proteolytic enzymes, which act together with prostaglandins to promote follicular degradation and rupture. Plasminogen activator (PA) concentration also increases in the midcycle follicle, and its action is enhanced by LH. Follicle rupture is blocked by administration of PA inhibitors in vivo.

At the level of the ovary, follicular recruitment and initial growth take place independently of gonadotropic hormones. Animal studies have demonstrated that follicular development can proceed to the antrum stage in the absence of gonadotropic influence. Although several hundred follicles probably start to grow, the vast majority will degenerate and no more than about 30 precursor follicles are likely to become gonadotropic-dependent and be present at the beginning of the menstrual cycle. Of these only a few under physiologic conditions, with optimal FSH/LH stimulation, will be selected for further growth and development. It is believed that the rescue of follicles from degeneration by FSH is achieved by reducing androgenicity and by maintaining a predominately estrogenic environment. Initially this is accompanied by FSH indirectly by stimulating activin production and later by directly metabolizing LH-induced thecal androgens to estrogens through stimulation of the aromatizing process in granulosa cells. Lastly, the selection of the dominant follicle is marked by its increased sensitivity to FSH and its ability to produce a high concentration of estrogen, as well as its ability to modulate gonadotropin secretion (Fig. 4-14). The dominant follicle is usually established by day 7 of the cycle.

GONADAL REGULATION BY GROWTH FACTORS

Insulin-like Growth Factors (IGFs)

The growth factor family consists of two peptides, namely IGF-I and IGF-II, which have structural homology to proinsulin. The IGFs are produced at multiple sites throughout the body, and serum levels do not vary throughout the menstrual cycle, thus underscoring the importance of their autocrine/paracrine functions. They bind to type I and type II IGF receptors on target cells, with the type I receptor mediating most of their actions. Although circulating, the IGFs remain bound to a family of binding proteins (IGFBPs) that regulate IGF action in target tissues.

IGF-I stimulates basal and gonadotropin-induced steroidogenesis in both theca and granulosa cells. It enhances FSH-induced increases in cAMP, LH receptors, proteoglycan, and basal inhibin synthesis in granulosa cells. Although the granulosa cell is the primary site of IGF-I production in the ovary, the receptor is made in both granulosa and theca cells, thus suggesting a plausible regulatory mechanism for the two compartments of ovarian steroidogenesis.

IGF-II is secreted by granulosa cells and enhances steroidogenesis in both theca and granulosa cells. Receptors have been found in the granulosa cell. Although insulin is not produced

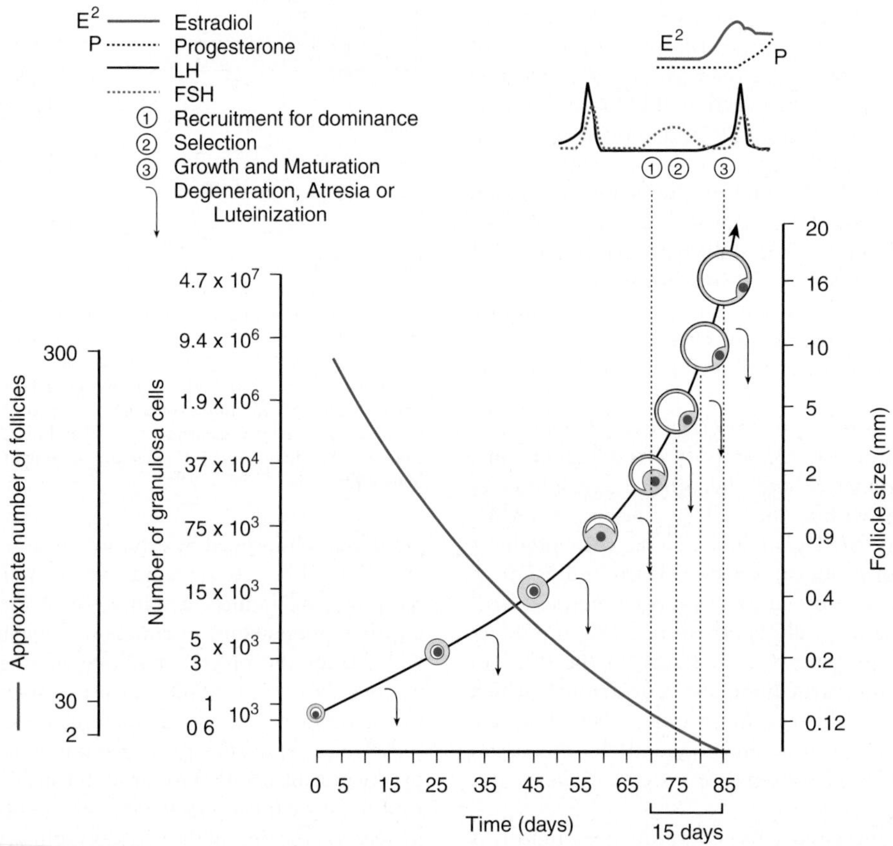

Figure 4-14. Time required for oocyte development capable of gonadotropic responsiveness. FSH, follicle-stimulating hormone; LH, luteinizing hormone. (From Lunenfeld B: The ovary—control from above and within. Aust N Z J Obstet Gynaecol 34:265, 1994.)

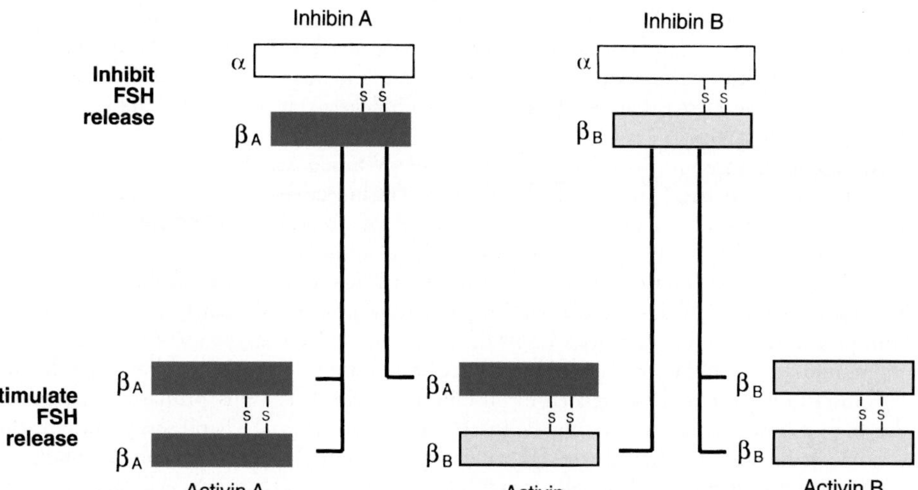

Figure 4-15. Chemical relationships of inhibins and activins. S, disulfide bond. (From Hylka VW, di Zerega GS: Reproductive hormones and their mechanisms of action. In Mishell DR Jr, Davajan V, Lobo RA [eds]: Infertility, Contraception and Reproductive Endocrinology, 3rd ed. Cambridge, MA, Blackwell Scientific, 1991.)

by the ovary, it may affect ovarian steroidogenesis by several mechanisms. Insulin is known to interact with granulosa cell receptors and may bind to IGF-I receptors at high concentration. Furthermore, insulin is partially responsible for regulating circulating levels of IGFBPs, which are decreased in women with polycystic ovarian syndrome, insulin resistance, and hyperinsulinemia. It is thus plausible that the androgenic characteristics of these syndromes are secondary to insulin acting via the type 1 receptor in ovarian stroma.

Inhibin, Activin, and Follistatin

Substantial evidence exists to suggest that inhibin, activin, and follistatin play critical roles in ovarian steroidogenesis. Inhibin and activin are glycoproteins consisting of two subunits that are connected by disulfide bonds. The subunits are highly conserved evolutionarily, which understates the importance of their roles in ovarian steroidogenesis. Inhibin consists of one type of alpha (alpha) and one of two beta (A-beta and B-beta) subunits, whereas activin consists of two of the same beta units from inhibin (A-beta/A-beta, A-beta/B-beta, B-beta/ B-beta) (Fig. 4-15).

The two bioactive inhibins, inhibin A and inhibin B, each have molecular weights of 32,000 daltons and are believed to possess identical biologic functions. The predominant sites of production include granulosa cells, testicular Sertoli cells, the corpus luteum, and the placenta. Inhibin production is primarily regulated in a positive fashion by FSH levels, although evidence is emerging that various autocrine and paracrine factors may alter its release. Inhibin is characterized by its ability to preferentially inhibit FSH release over LH release (Fig. 4-16). Its local actions within the ovary appear to be confined to stimulation of thecal androgen production and inhibitory effects on oocyte maturation. The menstrual cycle is characterized by low inhibin levels during the early and midfollicular phases, with

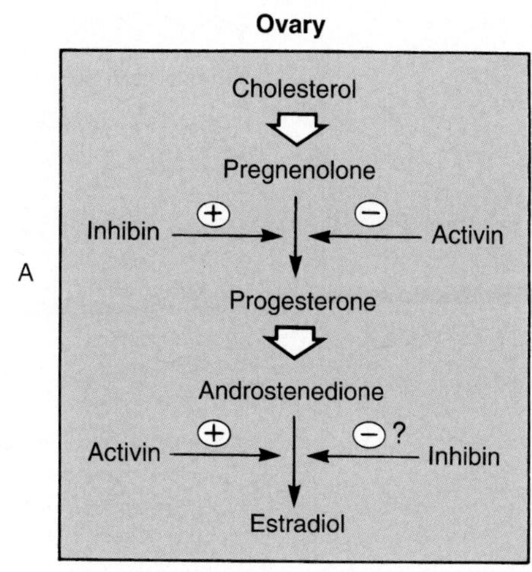

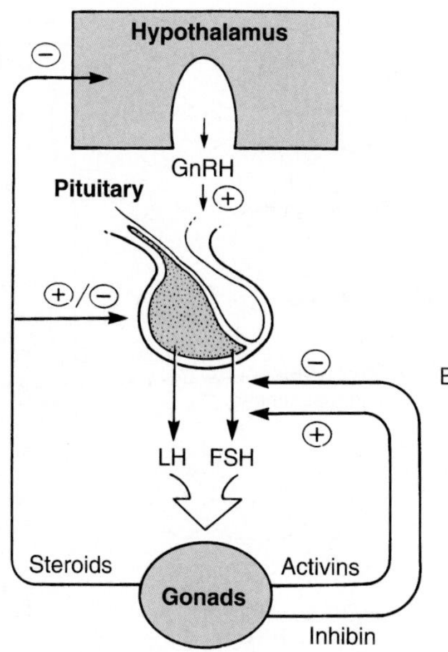

Figure 4-16. A, Generalized schemata showing involvement of activins and inhibins A, in hypothalamic-hypophyseal-gonadal axis. **B,** Regulation of steroidogenesis intragonadally by activins and inhibins. FSH, follicle-stimulating hormone; GnRH, gonadotropin-releasing hormone; LH, luteinizing hormone. (From Hylka VW, di Zerega GS: Reproductive hormones and their mechanisms of action. In Mishell DR Jr, Davajan V, Lobo RA [eds]: Infertility, Contraception and Reproductive Endocrinology, 3rd ed. Cambridge, MA, Blackwell Scientific, 1991.)

a rise a few days after the midcycle LH surge, and subsequent peak in the mid to late luteal phase. Their levels decrease dramatically in the perimenopause and menopause and may be the permissive factor that results in elevated FSH levels at this stage of life.

Although all three forms of activin are found in humans, activin A (A-beta/A-beta) predominates in women. The bioactive forms of these molecules have a molecular weight of 28,000 daltons. At the levels of the pituitary, the activins stimulate FSH release in opposition to inhibin. Their paracrine/autocrine functions include aromatase activity and progesterone production, promotion of folliculogenesis via its differentiating effects on granulosa cells, and prevention of premature luteinization.

Follistatin is structurally unrelated to inhibin or activin. It is also highly conserved evolutionarily. Follistatin is derived from a single gene and is cleaved and glycosylated, resulting in several bioactive forms. Functionally, it inhibits FSH release by binding activin, thus preventing activin's bioactivity. Furthermore, follistatin inhibits many of activin's paracrine/autocrine functions, but it may also directly affect granulosa cells, that is, acceleration of the rate of oocyte maturation.

Transforming Growth Factor α/β and Epidermal Growth Factor

Transforming growth factors α (TGF-α) and β (TGF-β) share significant homology with the β subunit of the inhibin and activin molecules. Within the ovary, they both bind with equal affinity to a common receptor. TGF-α and epidermal growth factor (EGF) are potent regulators of granulosa cell proliferation and differentiation. They have been demonstrated to inhibit both gonadotropin-supported granulosa cell differentiation and follicular cell steroidogenesis. TGF-β promotes growth and cAMP accumulation in granulosa cells and enhances FSH-induced increases in aromatase and LH receptors. TGF-β also inhibits follicular cell growth and thus facilitates follicle cell growth.

Interleukin-1

Interleukin-1 (IL-1) is a polypeptide cytokine that is predominately produced and secreted by macrophages, but within the ovary, it is also produced by theca-interstitial cells and granulosa cells following follicular rupture. Regulation within the ovary is primarily determined by local progesterone concentrations. It possesses antigonadotropic activity as it suppresses the functional and morphologic luteinization of granulosa cells. In addition, evidence exists to support that it may play a central role in the preovulation cascade of follicular rupture.

PROSTAGLANDINS AND RELATED COMPOUNDS

Arachidonic acid, the most abundant and important precursor for the biosynthesis of eicosanoids in humans, is formed from linoleic acid and is supplied in the diet. Arachidonic acid is released from membrane phospholipids by lipases, which are activated by various stimuli.

The biosynthesis of prostanoids takes place through the cyclic endoperoxides prostaglandin G (PGG) and prostaglandin H (PGH) (Fig. 4-17). PGG, through which all prostanoids are formed, is itself formed from one of the three precursor fatty acids by the microsomal enzyme prostaglandin synthetase. The formation of endoperoxides and their subsequent conversion

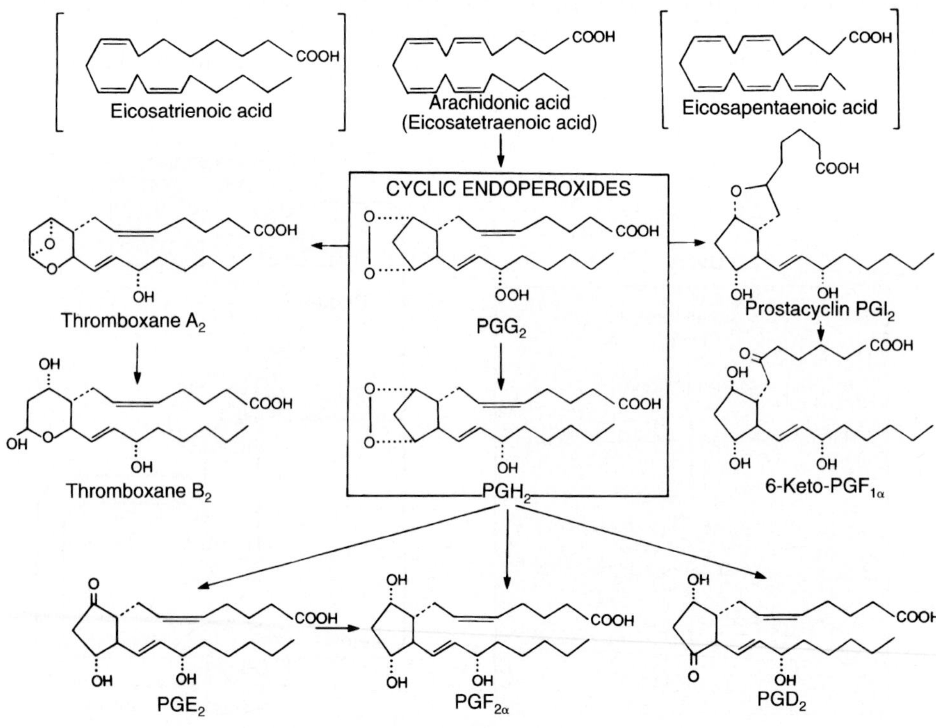

Figure 4-17. Biosynthesis of prostanoids. PG, prostaglandin. (From Stanczyk FZ: Prostaglandins and related compounds. In Mishell DR Jr, Davajan V, Lobo RA [eds]: Infertility, Contraception and Reproductive Endocrinology, 3rd ed. Cambridge, MA, Blackwell Scientific, 1991.)

to prostanoids is very rapid. Since prostanoids are then released immediately from the cell, measurement of tissue or serum levels of prostanoids does not accurately reflect in vivo levels before biopsy or blood collection.

The biosynthesis of prostanoids can be inhibited by several groups of compounds, including the nonsteroidal antiinflammatory drugs (NSAIDs) type 1 (aspirin and indomethacin, which inhibit endoperoxide formation) and type 2 (phenylbutazone), which inhibit action of endoperoxide isomerase and reductase. Corticosteroids can also inhibit prostanoid formation by decreasing precursor phospholipid hydrolysis and release (Fig. 4-18).

In contrast to steroid hormones, which are stored and act at target organs distant from their source, prostanoids are produced intracellularly shortly before they are released and generally act locally. Specific prostanoids can have variable effects on different tissues, as well as variable effects on the same organ, even when released in the same concentration (Table 4-3). One important effect is their ability to modulate the responses of endogenous stimulators and inhibitors, such as ovarian stimulation by LH, which is modulated by $PGF_2\alpha$, which in turn regulates ovarian receptor availability.

Eicosanoids have a wide variety of biologic effects throughout the body and an important role in reproductive system function. Prostaglandins have an important role in ovarian physiology. They help control early follicular growth by increasing blood supply to certain follicles and inducing FSH receptors on granulosa cells of preovulatory follicles. Both PGE_2 and $PGF_2\alpha$ are concentrated in the follicular fluid of preovulatory follicles and may assist the process of follicular rupture by facilitating proteolytic enzyme activity in the follicular walls. Prostaglandins may help regulate the life span of the corpus luteum. PGE_2 is probably luteotropic, and $PGF_2\alpha$ results in luteolysis.

Prostaglandins also have potent effects on oviductal motility, mediating the stimulatory estrogen effect and the inhibitory progesterone effect on oviductal muscular contractility. They also act to delay passage of the fertilized ovum into the uterus by influencing uterotubal junction activity. In the cervix, PGE_2 relaxes the smooth muscle, whereas $PGF_2\alpha$ causes the muscle to contract.

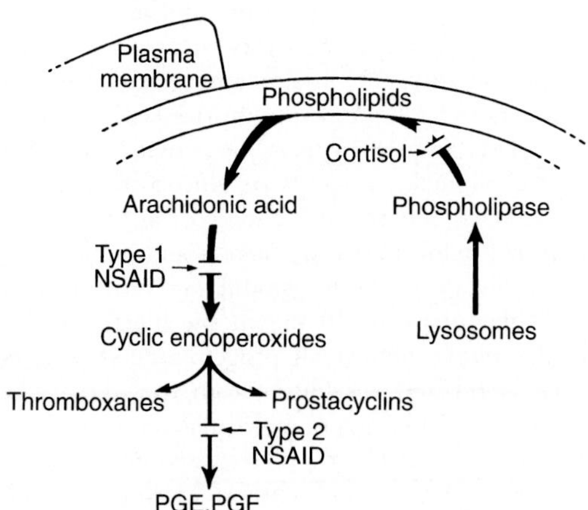

Figure 4-18. Inhibition of enzymes involved in biosynthesis of prostanoids. NSAID, nonsteroidal antiinflammatory drug; PG, prostaglandin. (From Stanczyk FZ: Prostaglandins and related compounds. In Mishell DR Jr, Davajan V, Lobo RA [eds]: Infertility, Contraception and Reproductive Endocrinology, 3rd ed. Cambridge, MA, Blackwell Scientific, 1991.)

Table 4-3 Effects of Eicosanoids

Prostaglandins	Effects
PGI_2, PGE_2, PGD_2	Vasodilation Cytoprotection Platelet aggregation Leukocyte aggregation Cyclic-AMP formation IL-1 and IL-2 formation
$PGF_{2\alpha}$	Vasoconstriction Bronchoconstriction Smooth muscle contraction
TXA_2	Vasoconstriction Platelet aggregation Lymphocyte proliferation Bronchoconstriction
LTB_1	Vascular permeability Leukocyte aggregation IL-1 formation IL-2 formation Natural killer cell cytotoxicity Chemoattractant
LTC_4, LTD_4	Bronchoconstriction Vascular permeability

IL, interleukin; LT, leukotriene; PG, prostaglandin; PGI_2, prostacyclin; TX, thromboxane.

Many prostanoids are produced by the endometrium. These include PGE_2, $PGF_2\alpha$, PGI_2, and thromboxane A_2 (TXA_2). Concentrations of PGE_2 and $PGF_2\alpha$ increase progressively from the proliferative to the secretory phase. The highest levels are found during menstruation. These prostaglandins help regulate myometrial contractility and appear to be important in regulating the process of menstruation.

OVARIAN STEROIDS

Chemistry

Steroids are lipids that have a basic chemical structure or nucleus. The nucleus consists of three six-carbon rings (A, B, and C) joined to a five-carbon atom (D) ring that is called cyclopentanoperhydrophenanthrene, or gonane (Fig. 4-19). The molecular weight of most steroid hormones is in the range of 250 to 550 daltons. Steroids such as progesterone and estradiol are insoluble in water but dissolve readily in organic solvents such as diethyl ether and chloroform. In contrast, steroids that have a sulfate or glucuronide group attached (conjugated steroids), such as DHEAS and pregnanediol glucuronide, are water-soluble.

Steroids are named according to a generally accepted convention that is used to determine their systemic (scientific) names. Most steroid hormones also have common (trivial) names, such as progesterone and estradiol, which are generally used instead of the scientific names. The carbon atoms of steroids are numbered as shown in Figure 4-20. Functional groups above the plane of the molecule are preceded by the β symbol and shown in the structural formula by a solid line, whereas those below the plane are indicated by an α symbol and a dotted line.

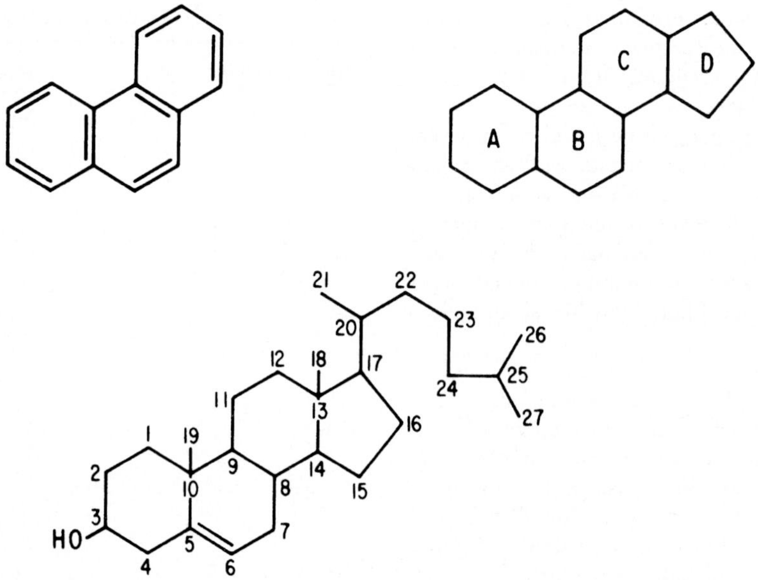

Figure 4-19. Phenanthrene *(top left)*. Cyclopentanoperhydrophenanthrene nucleus *(top right)*, in which the three 6-carbon rings *(A, B, and C)* resemble the phenanthrene ring system and the five-carbon ring *(D)* resembles cyclopentane. Cholesterol *(bottom)* is the common biosynthetic precursor of steroid hormones. Numbers *1* to *27* indicate the conventional numbering system of carbon atoms in steroids. (From Stanczyk FZ: Steroid hormones. In Lobo RA, Mishell DR Jr, Paulson RJ, Shoupe D [eds]: Mishell's Textbook of Infertility, Contraception and Reproductive Endocrinology, 4th ed. Malden, MA, Blackwell Science, 1997.)

The symbol Δ indicates a double bond, and those steroids with a double bond between carbon atoms 5 and 6 (cholesterol, pregnenolone, 17-hydroxypregnenolone, and dehydroepiandrosterone) are called Δ^5 steroids, whereas those with a double bond between carbon atoms 4 and 5 (progesterone, 17-hydroxyprogesterone, androstenedione, testosterone as well as all mineralocorticoids and glucocorticoids) are Δ^4 steroids.

Biosynthesis

All steroids in the body are formed from acetate, a two-carbon compound. The first step in its conversion to a variety of steroids is the formation of cholesterol, a 27-carbon steroid, via a complex series of reactions (11 steps). All sex steroids and corticosteroids are derived by stepwise degradation of cholesterol. The steroidogenic acute regular l(StAR) protein is thought to be the regulator of acute cholesterol transfer into the mitochondria for adrenal and ovarian steroidogenesis. Corticosteroids, pregnenolone, 17-hydroxypregnenolone, progesterone, and 17-hydroxyprogesterone have 21 carbon atoms. Androgens, DHEA, DHEAS, androstenedione and testosterone have 19 carbon atoms. Estrogens (estrone and estradiol) have 18 carbon atoms and a phenolic or aromatic ring A.

The first step in ovarian steroid biosynthesis is transformation of cholesterol to pregnenolone by hydroxylation of carbon-20 and carbon-22 and cleavage between these atoms. This process reduces the carbon-27 compound cholesterol to the carbon-21 compound pregnenolone. From pregnenolone, ovarian steroid biosynthesis proceeds along two major pathways under the influence of specific enzymes: (1) the Δ^5 pathway through 17-hydroxypregnenolone and DHEA to Δ^5 androstenediol and (2) the Δ^4 pathway through progesterone and 17-hydroxyprogesterone to androstenedione and testosterone (see Fig. 4-20). LH stimulates this synthesis. Androstenedione and testosterone are interconverted, and the former can be converted to estrone and the latter to estradiol, respectively, by the aromatase enzyme. This enzymatic process aromatization results in loss of the carbon-19 methyl group and formation of the aromatic ring in the carbon-18 steroid.

The ovary secretes three primary steroids: estradiol, progesterone, and androstenedione. These hormones are the chief secretory products of the maturing follicle, corpus luteum, and stroma, respectively. The ovary also secretes, in varying amounts, pregnenolone, 17-hydroxyprogesterone, testosterone, DHEA, and estrone. Because the ovaries lack 21-hydroxylase, 11β-hydroxylase, and 18-hydroxylase activity, they are unable to synthesize mineralocorticoids or glucocorticoids. Each day the ovary secretes between 0.1 and 0.5 mg of estradiol, with the amount being lowest during menses and highest just before ovulation. Daily progesterone production varies from 0.5 mg in the follicular phase to 20 mg in the luteal phase. During the follicular phase, almost all progesterone is secreted from the adrenal gland and very little from the ovary. The ovary secretes between 1 and 2 mg of androstenedione, less than 1 mg of DHEA, and about 0.1 mg of testosterone daily. Androgen metabolism and corticosteroid synthesis are discussed in Chapter 40 (Hyperandrogenism).

In addition to gonadal steroid biosynthesis, steroid metabolism occurs in extraglandular tissues. Interconversion of androstenedione and testosterone, as well as estrone and estradiol, takes place outside the ovaries, mainly by oxidation of the latter

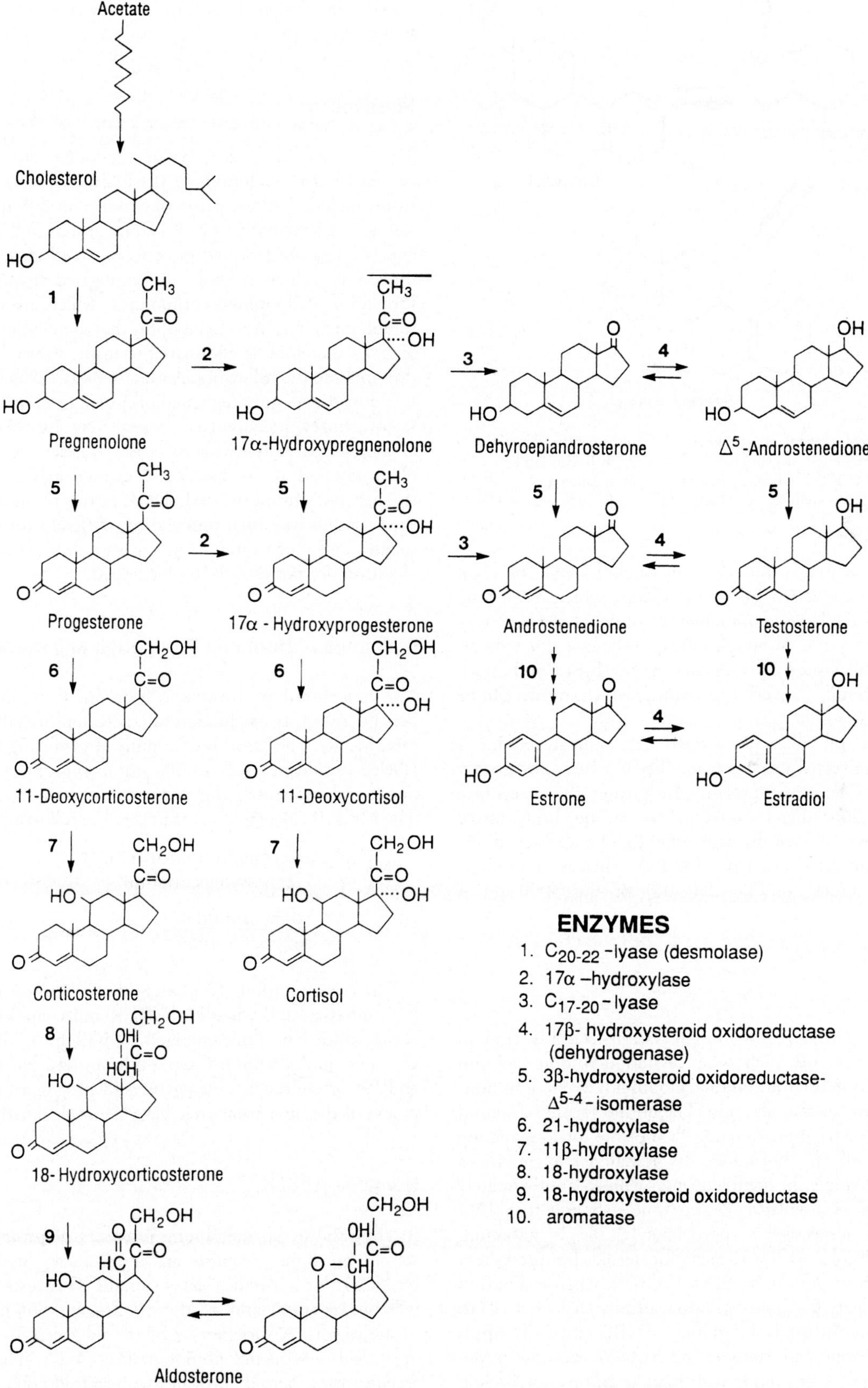

Figure 4-20. Biosynthesis of androgens, estrogens, and corticosteroids. (From Stanczyk FZ: Steroid hormones. In Lobo RA, Mishell DR Jr, Paulson RJ, Shoupe D [eds]: Mishell's Textbook of Infertility, Contraception and Reproductive Endocrinology, 4th ed. Malden, MA, Blackwell Science, 1997.)

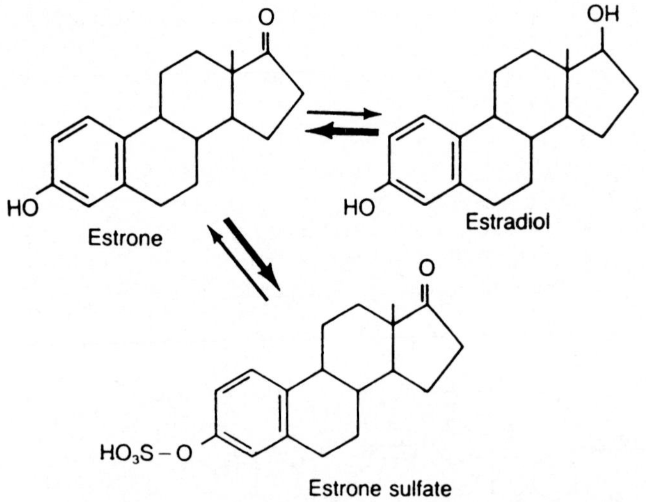

Figure 4-21. Interconversion of three principal circulating estrogens. (From Stanczyk FZ: Steroid hormones. In Lobo RA, Mishell DR Jr, Paulson RJ, Shoupe D [eds]: Mishell's Textbook of Infertility, Contraception and Reproductive Endocrinology, 4th ed. Malden, MA, Blackwell Science, 1997.)

steroids to the former, thus reducing their biologic potency. Estrone is also converted to estrone sulfate, which has a long half-life and is the largest component of the pool of circulating estrogens (Fig. 4-21). Although estrone sulfate is not biologically active, sulfatases in tissues such as the breast and endometrium can readily convert it to estrone, which in turn can be converted to estradiol.

MacDonald and colleagues showed that androstenedione is peripherally converted to estrone in adipose tissue. The greater the amount of fat tissue present, the greater the percentage of androstenedione that is converted to estrone. In a normal individual about 1.3% of the daily 3000 μg of androstenedione produced is converted to estrone (40 μg), whereas in an obese individual as much as 7% (200 μg) of the 3000 μg is converted.

Transport

After they are secreted into the circulation, steroids bind to either specific proteins, such as sex hormone-binding globulin (SHBG) and corticosteroid-binding globulin (CBG), or to nonspecific proteins, such as albumin. The bound form of a steroid hormone represents approximately 95% of the total circulating concentration of the hormone; the remainder is unbound ("free"). For example, in premenopausal women approximately 65% and 30% of circulating testosterone is bound to SHBG and albumin, respectively; approximately 2% is unbound. SHBG and CBG have a low capacity for steroids but bind them with high affinity ($K_a = 1 \times 10^8$ to 1×10^9), whereas albumin has a high capacity but binds with low affinity ($K_a = 1 \times 10^4$ to 1×10^6). Albumin binds all steroids. SHBG primarily binds dihydrotestosterone, testosterone, and estradiol (in order of decreasing affinity). CBG binds with highest affinity to cortisol, corticosterone, and 11-deoxycortisol, and, to a lesser extent, to progesterone. Circulating levels of each of the globulins are increased by estrogen; SHBG levels are also increased by obesity and hyperthyroidism and lowered by androgens and hypothyroidism.

Metabolism

The liver and, to a small extent, the kidney are the major sites of metabolism of steroids in the body. Transformation mechanisms include hydroxylation of carbons on different sites of the steroid nucleus, reduction of ketone groups and double bonds, and conjugation (formation of sulfates and glucuronides). The process by which steroids are conjugated involves the transformation of lipophilic compounds, which are only sparingly soluble in water, into metabolites that are readily water-soluble and can therefore be eliminated in urine. Examples of conjugation include the following: About 10% to 15% of progesterone is transformed to pregnanediol-3-glucuronide, which is the major urinary metabolite of progesterone. Estradiol and estrone are converted in the liver to estriol. These three estrogens are often referred to as the *classic* estrogens because they were the first ones to be isolated. These estrogens are conjugated by the liver and intestinal mucosa into different forms of estrogen sulfates and glucuronides, such as estrone sulfate, estradiol-17-glucuronide, and estriol-16-glucuronide.

Dynamics of Hormone Production and Metabolism

The concentration of a steroid hormone in serum or plasma is dependent on its production rate (PR) and metabolic clearance rate (MCR). The MCR is determined by infusing a radioactively labeled steroid in tracer amounts at a constant rate over several hours and measuring the tracer concentration at steady state. The MCR is calculated according to the following formula:

$$\text{MCR} = \frac{\text{tracer administered/time}}{\text{tracer concentration}}$$

$$= \frac{\text{counts/min/day}}{\text{counts/min/liter}} = \text{Liters/day}$$

The concentration (C) of steroid can be measured by radioimmunoassay, and when both MCR and C are known, the PR is determined by multiplying the MCR by C: PR = MCR × C = liters/day × amount/liter = amount/day. Normal C, MCR, and PR of androgens, estrogens, and progesterone at different phases of the menstrual cycle have been calculated (Table 4-4).

Hormone Action

In contrast to the membrane receptors of protein hormones, steroid hormone receptors are intracellular. Steroid hormone receptors bind a specific class of steroids. Thus, estrogen receptors will bind natural and synthetic estrogens but not progestins or androgens. A superfamily of steroid receptors exists with a great deal of sequence homology (Fig. 4-22). The affinity of a receptor for a steroid correlates with steroid potency. For example, the estrogen receptor has a greater affinity for estradiol than for estrone or estriol. After the steroid hormone (S) is bound to its receptor (R), a hormone-receptor (SR) complex forms.

Table 4-4 Plasma Concentrations (C), Metabolic Clearance Rates (MCR), and Production Rates (PR) of Androgens, Estrogens, and Progesterone During Menstrual Cycle

		PLASMA CONCENTRATION*				PRODUCTION RATE (MG/DAY) (PR = C × MCR)	
Steroid Hormone	**Phase of Cycle**	**Mean**	**Range**	**Units**	**Metabolic Clearance Rate Plasma* (L/day)**	**Mean**	**Range**
Androstenedione	†	1.4	0.7–3.1	ng/mL	2000	2.8	1.4–6.2
Testosterone	†	0.35	0.15–0.55	ng/mL	700	0.25	0.1–0.4
Dehydroepiandrosterone	†	4.2	2.5–7.8	ng/mL	1600	6.7	4.8–12.5
Dehydroepiandrosterone sulfate	†	1.6	0.8–3.4	μg/mL	7	11.2	5.6–23.8
Estradiol	Follicular	44	20–120	pg/mL	1350	0.059	0.027–0.162
	Preovulatory	250	150–600	pg/mL	1350	0.338	0.203–0.810
	Luteal	110	40–300	pg/mL	1350	0.149	0.054–0.405
Estrone	Follicular	40		pg/mL	2200	0.088	
	Preovulatory	170		pg/mL	2200	0.374	
	Luteal	92		pg/mL	2200	0.202	
Estrone sulfate	Follicular	470		pg/mL	146	0.069	
	Luteal	890		pg/mL	146	0.130	
Progesterone	Follicular	0.2	0.06–0.37	ng/mL	2300	0.46	0.14–0.85
	Luteal	8.9	4.3–19.4	ng/mL	2300	20.5	9.9–45.0

*These values may vary somewhat depending on investigator and method.
†Unspecified. No major changes during menstrual cycle.
From Stanczyk FZ: Steroid hormones. In Mishell DR Jr, Davajan V, Lobo RA (eds): Infertility, Contraception and Reproductive Endocrinology, 3rd ed. Cambridge, MA, Blackwell Scientific, 1991.

Steroid hormone receptors are located in either the cytoplasm or nucleus. They are maintained in an inactive state by association with heat shock proteins. Hormone binding leads to disassociation of the heat shock proteins and conformational changes (transformation) that allow it to bind to the hormone-responsive element (HRE) of nuclear DNA. Thereafter, mRNA is generated from a segment of DNA (transcription). The mRNA migrates into the cytoplasm, where it attaches to ribosomes and translates information so that they synthesize new protein (Fig. 4-23).

The magnitude of the signal to the cell depends on the concentration of both hormones (S) and receptors (R), as well as on the affinity (*K*) of the receptor for hormone. Thus the hormone effect may be altered by receptor concentration and affinity, as well as by concentration of the hormone in the circulation. Affinity is quantitatively characterized by a constant derived from the law of mass action.

$$S + R \underset{K_d}{\overset{K_a}{\rightleftharpoons}} SR$$

The association constant, K_a, is determined by dividing the rate constant for association, k_a, by the rate constant for dissociation, k_d. The dissociation constant, K_d, is the inverse of K_a; therefore, $K_d = 1/K_a$. K_d is equal to the concentration of the hormone when half the receptor sites are occupied. Steroid hormones are present in concentrations of 10^{-10} to 10^{-8} M, and most steroid receptors have a K_d of 10^{-9}. It should be emphasized that these processes are greatly modulated by numerous other coactivator and corepressor factors (see Fig. 4-23). The different tissue response to estrogen and estrogen-like compounds depends on the sum of these various interactions, particularly the expression pattern of various coactivators and corepressors in the particular tissue.

In addition, steroids can activate signals independent of nuclear interactions (nongenomic). These very rapid effects are mediated from the membrane through a series of kinases and second messengers including cAMP.

Estrogen stimulates the synthesis of both estrogen and progesterone receptors in target tissues such as the endometrium. Progestins inhibit the synthesis of both estrogen and progesterone receptors. Thus, the estrogen/progesterone receptor content in the endometrium peaks about midcycle and then decreases (Fig. 4-24). Mitotic activity and endometrial growth rates, therefore, peak at midcycle. Progestins also increase the intracellular synthesis of estradiol dehydrogenase, which converts the more potent estradiol to the less potent estrone, further decreasing estrogenic activity in the target cell.

Antiestrogens, such as clomiphene or tamoxifen, bind to the estrogen receptor but initiate little transcription. Thus, estrogen receptors are depleted without new receptor synthesis or estrogenic action.

EFFECTS OF HORMONES ON SPECIFIC REPRODUCTIVE FACTORS

Ovarian Gametogenesis (Oogenesis)

Oogenesis begins in fetal life when the primordial germ cells migrate to the genital ridge. These germ cells, oogonia, increase in number by mitotic division from about 600,000 in the second month to 7 million in the seventh month of fetal life. The oogonia then begin meiotic division and are called primary oocytes. Just prior to birth the primary oocytes, which now number 2 to 4 million, undergo meiosis until they reach the diplotene stage of the prophase, which is also called the germinal vesicle stage (for further details refer to Chapter 1, Fertilization and Embryogenesis). The oocytes stay quiescent or undergo atresia until puberty, at which time some of the oocytes mature and resume their meiotic division under the stimulatory influence of FSH.

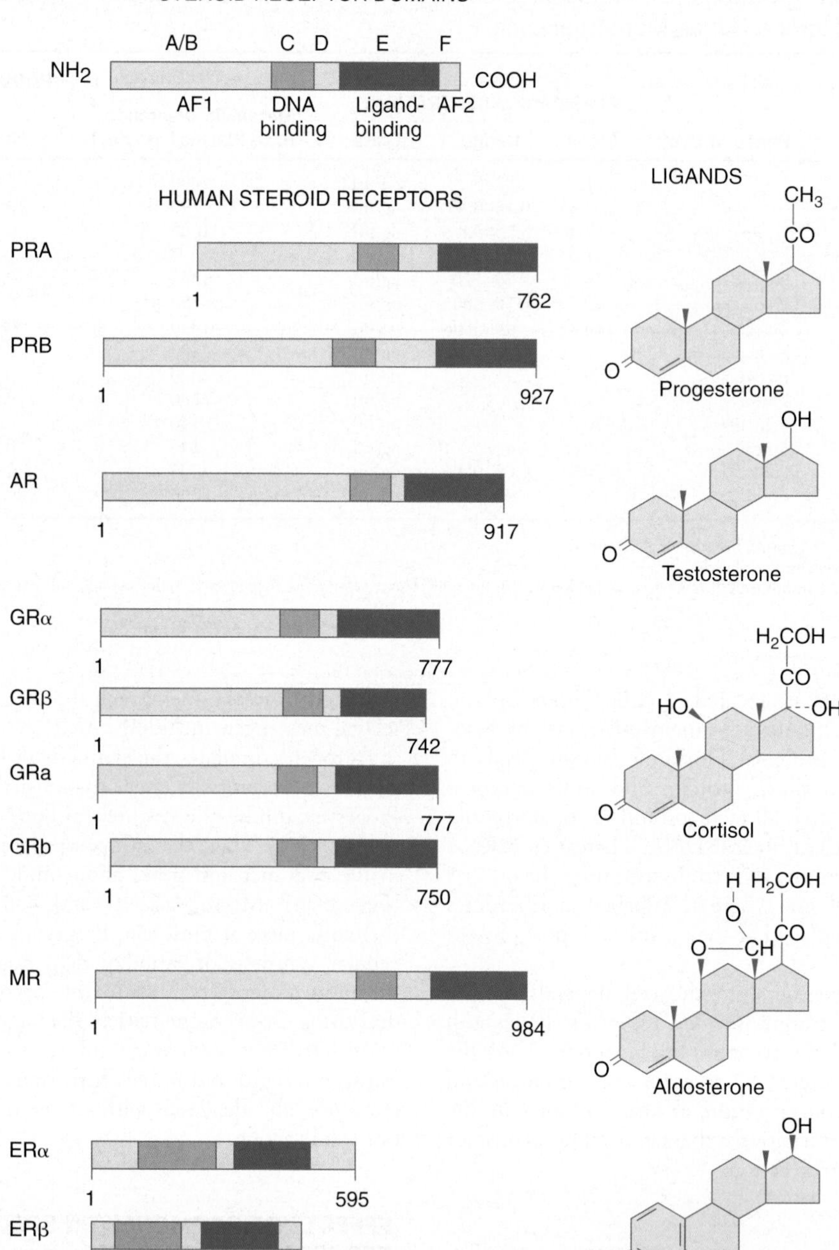

Figure 4-22. Schematic diagram of the primary structure or a generic steroid receptor and its functional domains; the primary structure of human steroid receptors, their isoforms, and their physiologic ligands. Numbers indicate amino acid residues. Note that there is a fair amount of sequence homology among this family of receptors. (Modified from Strauss J, Barbieri R: Yen and Jaffe's Reproductive Endocrinology, 5th ed. Philadelphia, Elsevier, 2004.)

Leptin, a peptide secreted by adipose tissue, is thought to be a peripheral signal of fat stores. Rodent models deficient for leptin or leptin receptor activity demonstrate hyperphagia and obesity. A role for leptin in reproduction is supported by the observation that mice lacking leptin fail to undergo puberty, the presence of leptin in the human ovarian follicle, and a possible role in the endometrium and in implantation. Frisch proposed that a critical weight must be reached in order to elicit menarche and maintain menstruation. Leptin may therefore act as a peripheral messenger to the central nervous system in order to elicit the pattern of GnRH secretion necessary for puberty.

The primary oocyte that is still in the diplotene stage of its first meiotic division is covered by a single layer of granulosa cells and constitutes the primordial follicle. Even without gonadotropin stimulation, some primordial follicles develop into

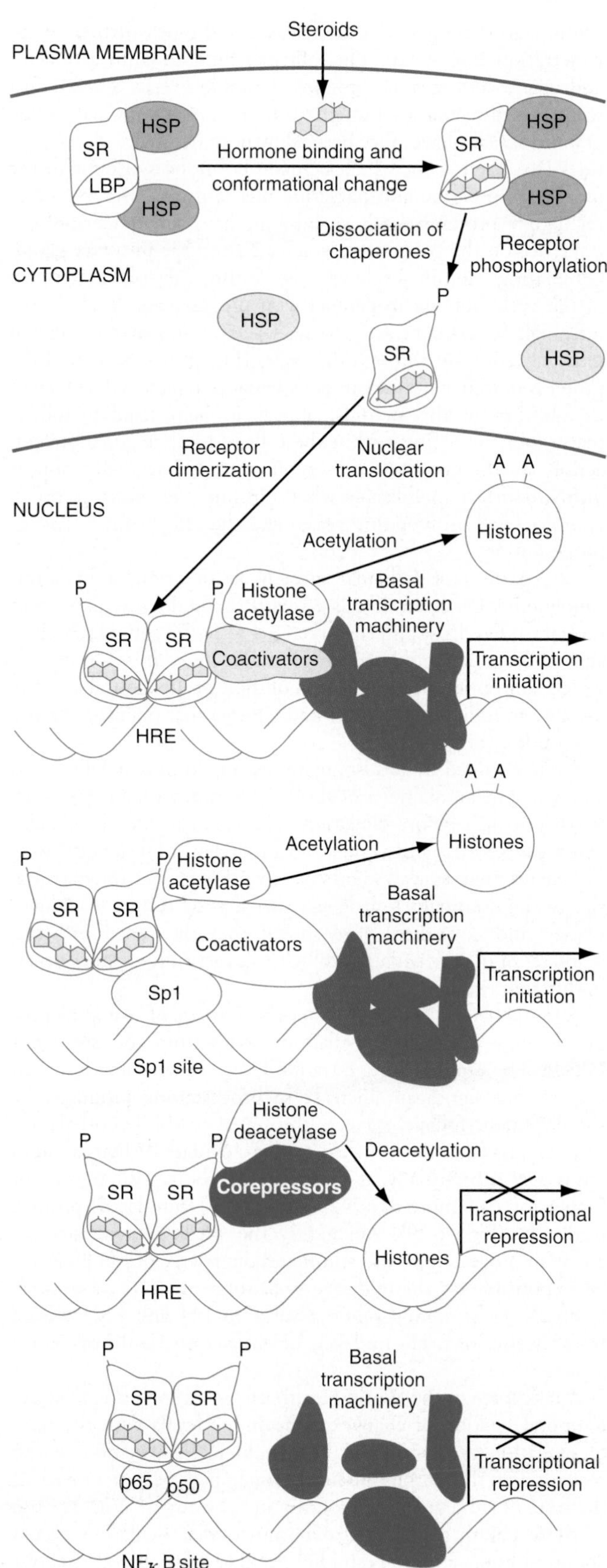

Figure 4-23. General mechanism of action for cytoplasmic steroid receptors as described in the text. A, acetyl group; HSP, heat shock protein; HRE, hormone response element; LBP, ligand-binding pocket; P, phosphate group, SR, steroid receptor. The steroid receptor is chaperoned to the nucleus by coactivators where binding occurs. Additional binding of the ligand/receptor complex in the nucleus by a variety of possible (tissue specific) coactivators and corepressors influence specific transcriptional events. (Modified from Strauss J, Barbieri R: Yen and Jaffe's Reproductive Endocrinology, 5th ed. Philadelphia, Elsevier, 2004.)

primary (preantral) follicles, which are oocytes covered by multiple layers of granulosa cells (Fig. 4-25). This FSH-independent process occurs in all premenopausal women during the nonovulatory states of childhood, pregnancy, and oral contraceptive use, as well as during ovulatory cycles. However, only in the presence of FSH in ovulatory cycles do some of those primary follicles develop to the antrum stage. Without the FSH stimulation, all follicles become atretic.

Under the influence of FSH the number of granulosa cells in the primordial follicle increases dramatically, and the follicle matures into a primary (preantral) follicle. As the number of granulosa cells increases under the influence of LH and FSH, there is a concomitant parallel increase in estradiol production and secretion as FSH stimulates aromatase synthesis. Estradiol stimulates preantral follicle growth, prevents follicle atresia, and

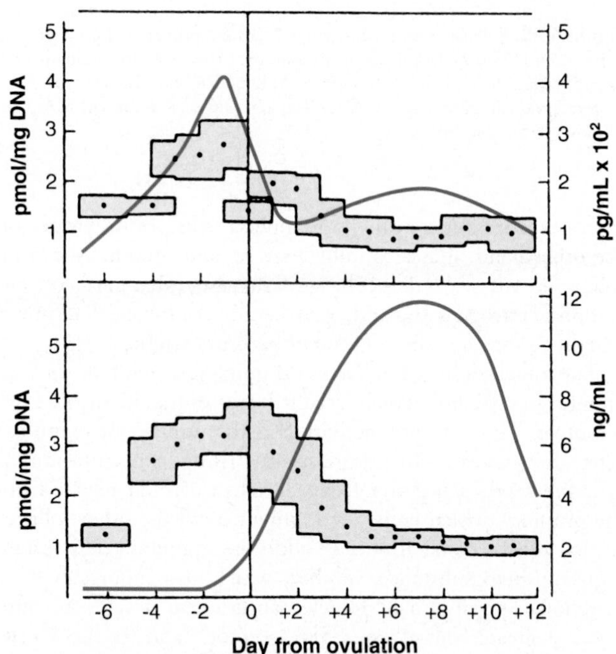

Figure 4-24. Estradiol and progesterone receptors in endometrial cells during normal menstrual cycle. Concentrations of estradiol receptor *(upper panel)* and of total progesterone receptor *(lower panel)* for each day of cycle were pooled with those of adjacent days. Each point represents the mean of pooled values. It is surrounded by a rectangle, with its abscissa extending from preceding to following day to account for imprecision of dating and with its ordinate equal to twice the standard error of the mean. Curves represent mean values of plasma estradiol *(upper panel)* and progesterone *(lower panel)*. (From Levy C, Robel P, Gautray JP, et al: Estradiol and progesterone receptors in human endometrium: Normal and abnormal menstrual cycles and early pregnancy. Am J Obstet Gynecol 136:646, 1980.)

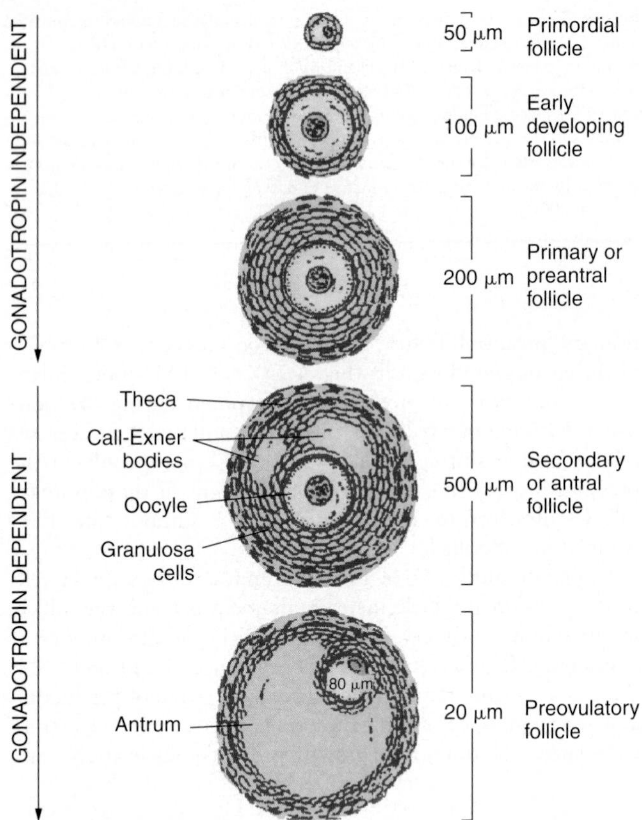

Figure 4-25. Follicle development. Progress beyond primary follicle stage depends on FSH stimulation. (From Paulson RJ: Oocytes: from development to fertilization. In Mishell DR Jr, Davajan V, Lobo RA [eds]: Infertility, Contraception and Reproductive Endocrinology, 3rd ed. Cambridge, MA, Blackwell Scientific, 1991.)

increases FSH action on the granulosa cells. Testosterone, on the other hand, increases follicle atresia and prevents preantral follicle growth. Ross and colleagues suggested that local concentration of estrogens and androgens within the follicle determines whether a specific follicle grows or becomes atretic.

The follicle destined to become dominant secretes the greatest amount of estradiol, which in turn increases the density of FSH receptors. Thus, mitotic activity and the number of granulosa cells also increase. In addition, the rising concentration of estradiol exerts a negative feedback effect of FSH release from the pituitary, which halts development of all the other follicles so that they become atretic. In addition, granulosa cells secrete a glycoprotein substance, inhibin, which also suppresses FSH secretion. The dominant follicle continues to develop because it has a greater density of FSH receptors, and its theca cells become more vascularized than the other follicles, allowing more FSH to reach its receptors.

As the oocyte develops, it becomes surrounded by the zona pellucida, and fluid accumulates in the follicle. The zona pellucida is a mucopolysaccaride coat containing specific protein sites that allow only spermatozoa of the same species to penetrate and fertilize the ovum. Underneath the zona pellucida is the vitelline membrane, which surrounds the ooplasm. Cortical granules form just below this membrane as the oocyte matures. Once the zona pellucida has been penetrated by a single sperm cell, these granules are released and block further sperm penetration (Fig. 4-26). The follicular fluid contains estrogens, androgens, and various proteins. Granulosa cells are not just recipients of regulatory protein hormones. As mentioned earlier, granulosa cells have also been shown to secrete various peptides (see Table 4-3), which regulate hormone synthesis in the ovary via autocrine and paracrine mechanisms. Some of those regulatory proteins, such as inhibin, have an endocrinologic influence on the gonadotropin release from the pituitary gland. Circulating inhibin levels are low during the follicular phase of the cycle but rise in parallel with progesterone levels in the luteal phase. In contrast, plasma levels of free activin remain relatively constant through the cycles (Fig. 4-27). Several of the proteins in follicular fluid are now being characterized, and they, in addition to the steroids, appear to help regulate follicle maturation by acting within the follicle to alter gonadotropin action. As the granulosa cells proliferate, LH receptors appear on their surface membrane; when LH binds to these receptors, granulosa cell proliferation ceases and the cells begin to secrete progesterone.

The pattern of follicular growth, as determined by ultrasonography, has been correlated with the endocrine pattern in several studies. Eissa and coworkers, as well as Zegers-Hochschild and colleagues, correlated these parameters in 43 cycles in which conception occurred. Both of these groups found a steady increase in follicular diameter and volume that parallels the rise in estradiol (Fig. 4-28).

As determined by ultrasonography, the dominant follicle has a maximal mean diameter of about 19.5 mm, with a range of 18 to 25 mm just before ovulation. The mean maximal follicular volume is 3.8 mL, with a range of 3.1 to 8.2 mL. The investigators just mentioned, as well as others, have shown that the maximal size of the dominant follicle can vary among different women. Lemay and coworkers have shown that the mean maximal diameter of the preovulatory follicle can vary in the same woman in different cycles.

About 80% of the approximately 500 µg of estradiol produced daily just before ovulation comes from the dominant follicle. The rapidly rising estradiol levels, in combination with a small but significant increase in progesterone produced by the dominant follicle, serve as the signal to the hypothalamo-pituitary axis that the follicle is ready to ovulate. When estradiol levels rise substantially at midcycle, to about 200 pg/mL or higher for 2 or more days, LH secretion is stimulated (positive feedback) (Fig. 4-29). Apparently the small preovulatory increase in progesterone also stimulates the release of LH and may be responsible for the midcycle FSH surge. Thus, by a positive feedback, these steroids elicit a surge in LH and FSH release from the pituitary. The midcycle LH surge initiates the ovulatory process.

A task force of the World Health Organization correlated the temporal relation of changes in hormone levels with the time of ovulation as determined by histologic examination of the maturity of the corpus luteum, which had been removed at the time of subsequent laparotomy in 78 women. With the use of those parameters, it was determined that ovulation occurs about 24 hours after the estradiol peak. Ovulation occurs about 32 hours after the initial rise in LH levels and about 12 to 16 hours after the peak of LH levels in serum (Table 4-5). Using ultrasonography to detect the time of ovulation, Lemay

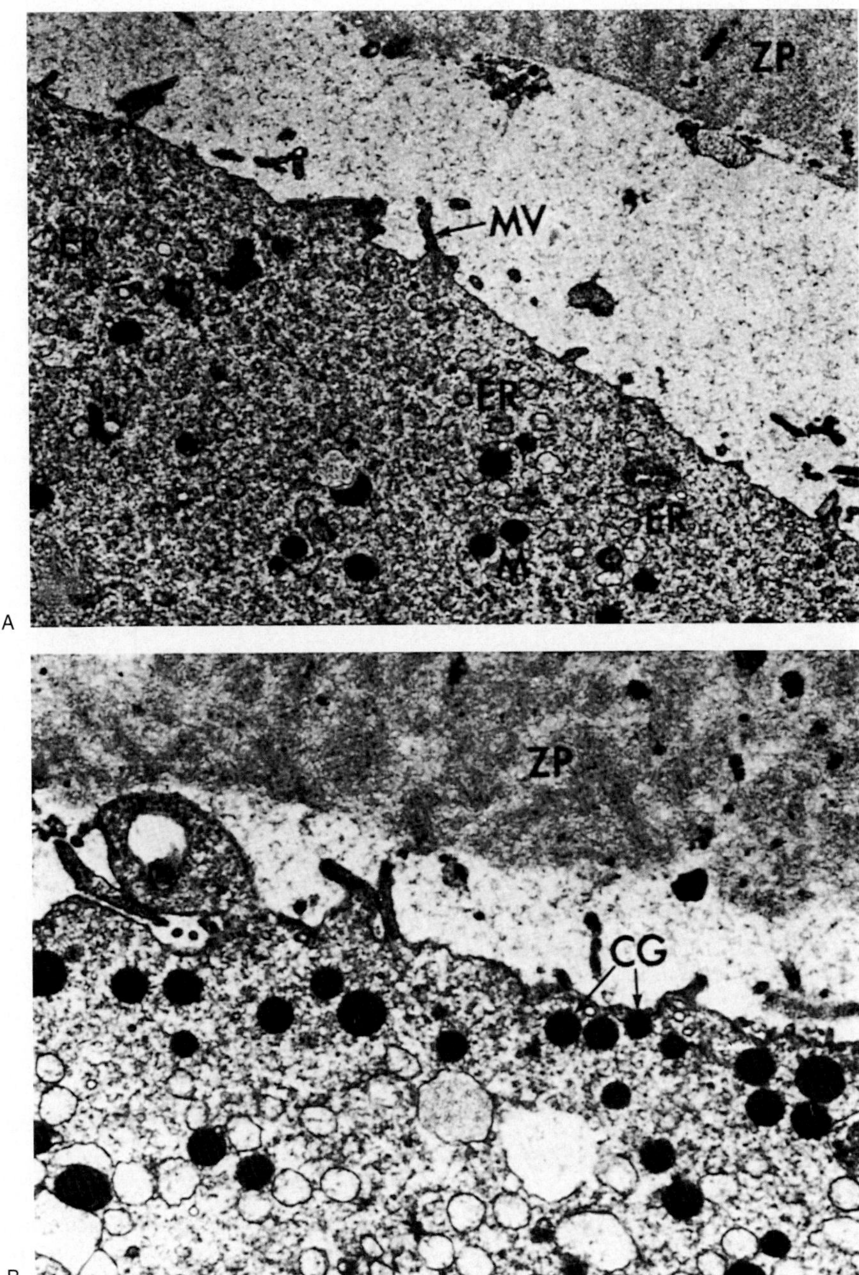

Figure 4-26. A, Surface of fertilized ovum, showing absence of cortical granules. A few microvilli (MV) are projecting into perivitelline space, which has been widened by retraction of ooplasm from zona pellucida (ZP). Dense mitochondria (M) and large vesicular components of endoplasmic reticulum (ER) are visible in ooplasm. The egg was fixed 3 hours after insemination in vitro. (×15,400.) **B,** Surface of unfertilized ovum that had been inseminated for 3 hours. Numerous extremely electron-dense cortical granules (CG) are present beneath vitelline membrane. ZP has a fine fibrillar appearance. (×19,600.) (Reprinted from Fertility and Sterility, 33, Lopata A, Sathananthan AM, McBain JC, et al, The ultrastructure of the preovulatory human egg fertilized in vitro, 12. Copyright 1980, with permission from The American Society for Reproductive Medicine.)

and coworkers reported that ovulation occurs between 18 and 48 hours after the initial rise in LH levels. With serial ultrasound definition and LH measurements, Eissa and coworkers and Zegers-Hochschild and colleagues reported that in conception cycles, ovulation usually occurs within 24 hours and always within 48 hours after the LH peak.

The midcycle LH surge initiates germinal vesicle disruption, and metaphase I is completed. As the oocyte enters metaphase II, the first polar body appears. Completion of meiosis and extrusion of the second polar body occur only when a spermatozoon penetrates the ovum. In preparation for follicular rupture, LH stimulates synthesis of both $PGF_2\alpha$ and PGE_2 and

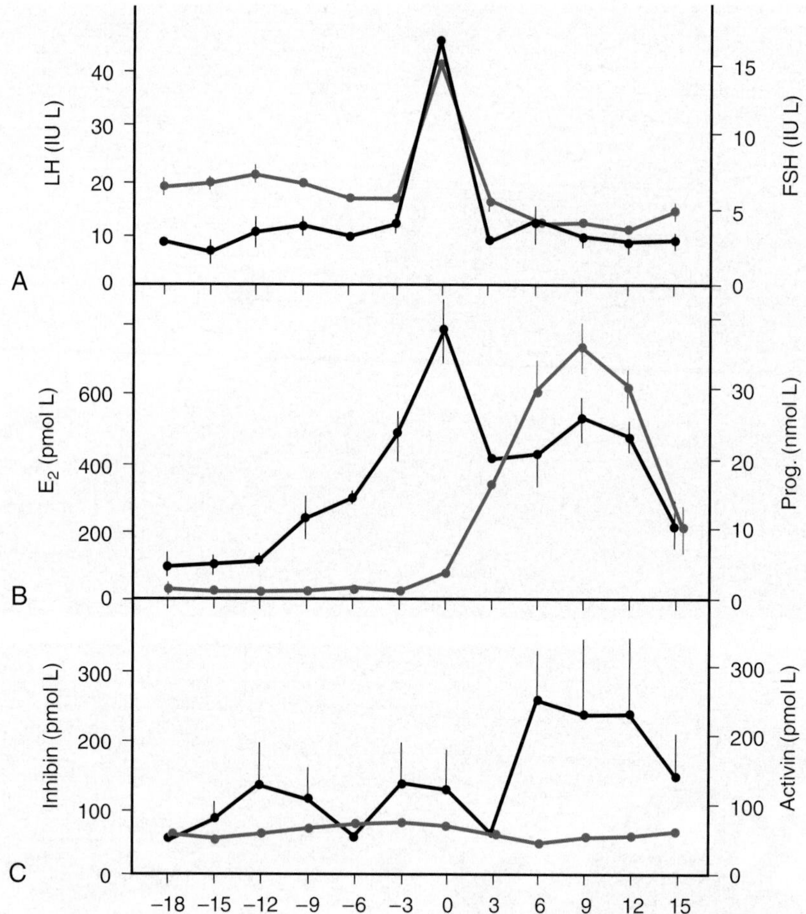

Figure 4-27. Hormonal profiles of four normal subjects during menstrual cycle. Day 0 was defined as the day corresponding to a surge of LH and FSH. **A,** Plasma levels of LH (*blue circles*) and FSH (*black circles*). **B,** Levels of E_2 (*blue circles*) and progesterone (*black circles*). **C,** Plasma levels of inhibin (*blue circles*) and activin (*black circles*). Each *point* represents the mean of four subjects, and *vertical bars* represent the standard error of the mean. (Courtesy of Demura R, Suzuki T, Tajima S, et al: Human plasma free activin and inhibin levels during the menstrual cycle. J Clin Endocrinol Metab 76:1080, 1993.)

Table 4-5 Range of Observed Times from Defined Hormonal Events and Time of Ovulation

	TIME OF OVULATION (HR) FROM RISE TO PEAK			
	FIRST SIGNIFICANT RISE		PEAK	
Hormone	**Median**	**Range**	**Median**	**Range**
17β-Estradiol	82.5	48–168	24.0	0–48
LH	32.0	24–56	16.5	8–40
FSH	21.1	8–24	15.3	8–40
Progesterone	7.8	0–32	—	—

From World Health Organization: Temporal relationships between ovulation and defined changes in the concentration of plasma estradiol-17 beta, luteinizing hormone, follicle-stimulating hormone, and progesterone. I. Probit analysis. World Health Organization, Task Force of Methods for the Determination of the Fertile Period, Special Programme of Research, Development and Research Training in Human Reproduction. Am J Obstet Gynecol 138:383–390, 1980.

proteolytic enzymes (collagenase). The rise in FSH levels stimulates production of a plasminogen activator, which converts plasminogen to the proteolytic enzyme plasmin. Plasmin helps to detach the cumulus from the parietal granulosa cells and thus aids in the process of extrusion of the egg and cumulus at the time of follicle rupture.

After the oocyte is extruded, the amount of follicular fluid is markedly reduced, the follicular wall becomes convoluted, and the follicular diameter and volume greatly decrease. These changes are detectable by ultrasonography (Fig. 4-30). As the granulosa and theca cells become luteinized, they take up lipids and lutein pigment, giving them a yellow coloration. The granulosa cell layer becomes vascularized only after ovulation. Under the influence of LH, the corpus luteum produces progesterone in amounts of about 20 μg/24 hr and also secretes estradiol. High LH levels are necessary for the support of corpus luteum secretory function. In case of conception, the production of progesterone in the corpus luteum continues under the stimulatory action of human chorionic gonadotropin secreted by the syncytiotrophoblast.

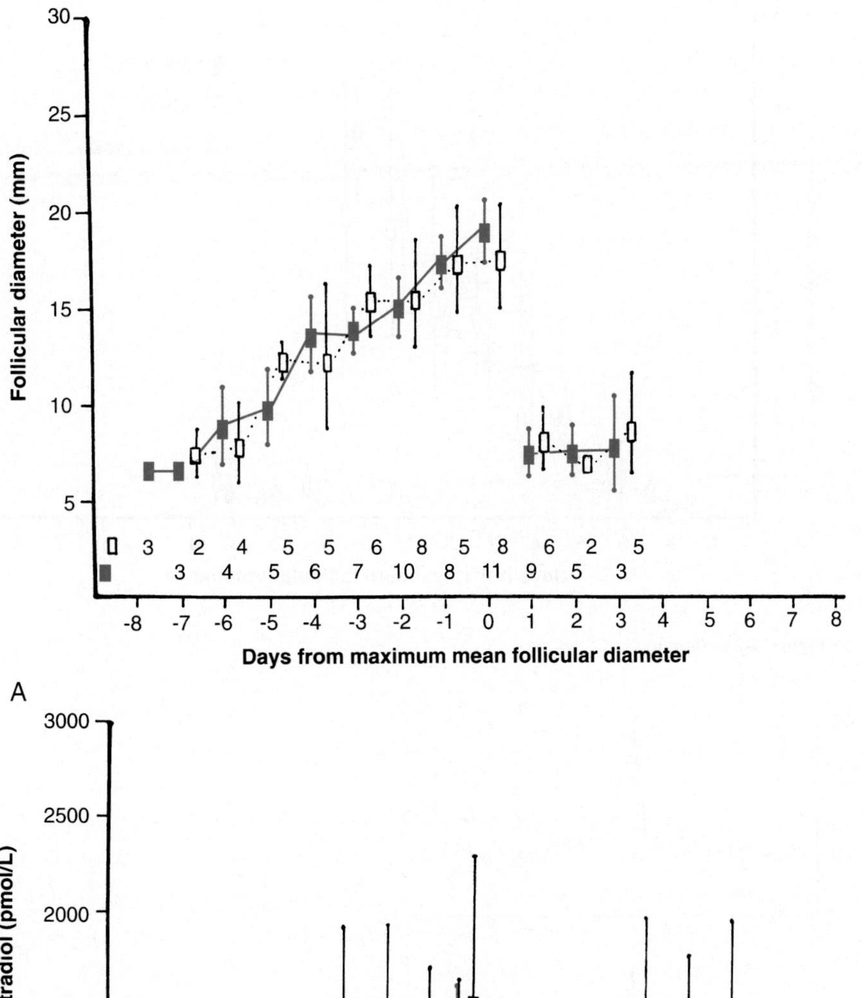

Figure 4-28. Correlation of follicular diameter with follicular growth and follicular volume with estradiol in 11 spontaneous and 8 induced conception cycles. **A**, Follicular diameter. **B**, Serum estradiol concentrations. **C**, Follicular volume. The shaded bars show spontaneous cycles and the open bars represent induced or stimulated cycles. (Adapted from Fertility and Sterility, 45, Eissa MK, Obhrai MS, Docker MF, et al, Follicular growth and endocrine profiles in spontaneous and induced conception cycles, 191. Copyright 1986, with permission from The American Society for Reproductive Medicine.)

Continued

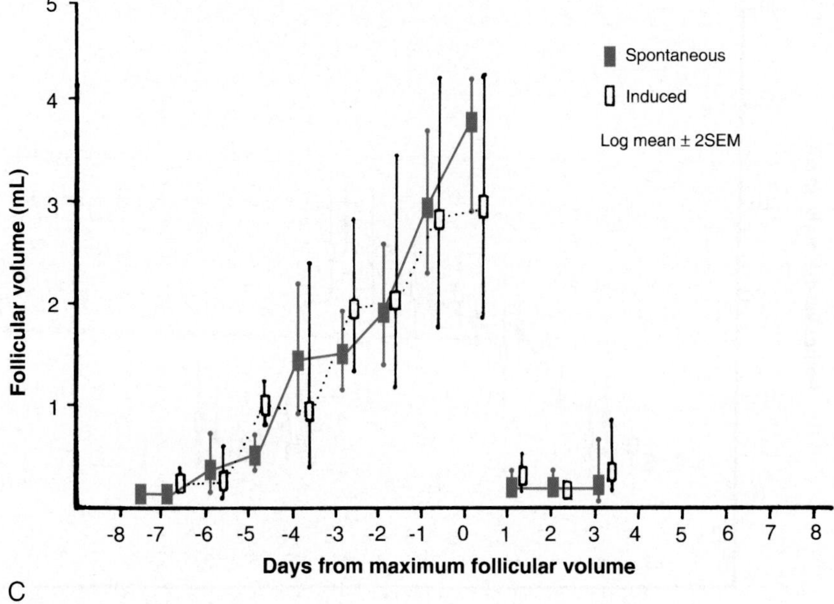

Figure 4-28. ***Cont'd,*** C.

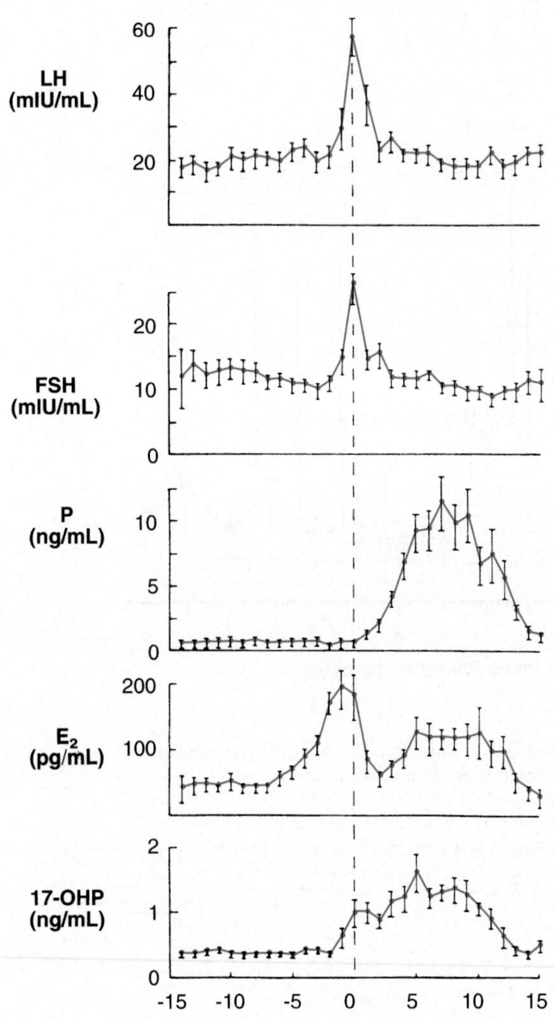

Figure 4-29. Means and standard errors of serum luteinizing hormone (LH), follicle-stimulating hormone (FSH), progesterone (P), estradiol (E_2), and 17-hydroxyprogesterone (17-OHP) levels measured in nine women daily during entire ovulatory menstrual cycle. Individual daily results were grouped according to day of midcycle LH peak and averaged. (From Thorneycroft IH, Mishell DR Jr, Stone SC, et al: The relation of serum 17-hydroxyprogesterone and estradiol-17-beta levels during the human menstrual cycle. Am J Obstet Gynecol 111:947, 1971.)

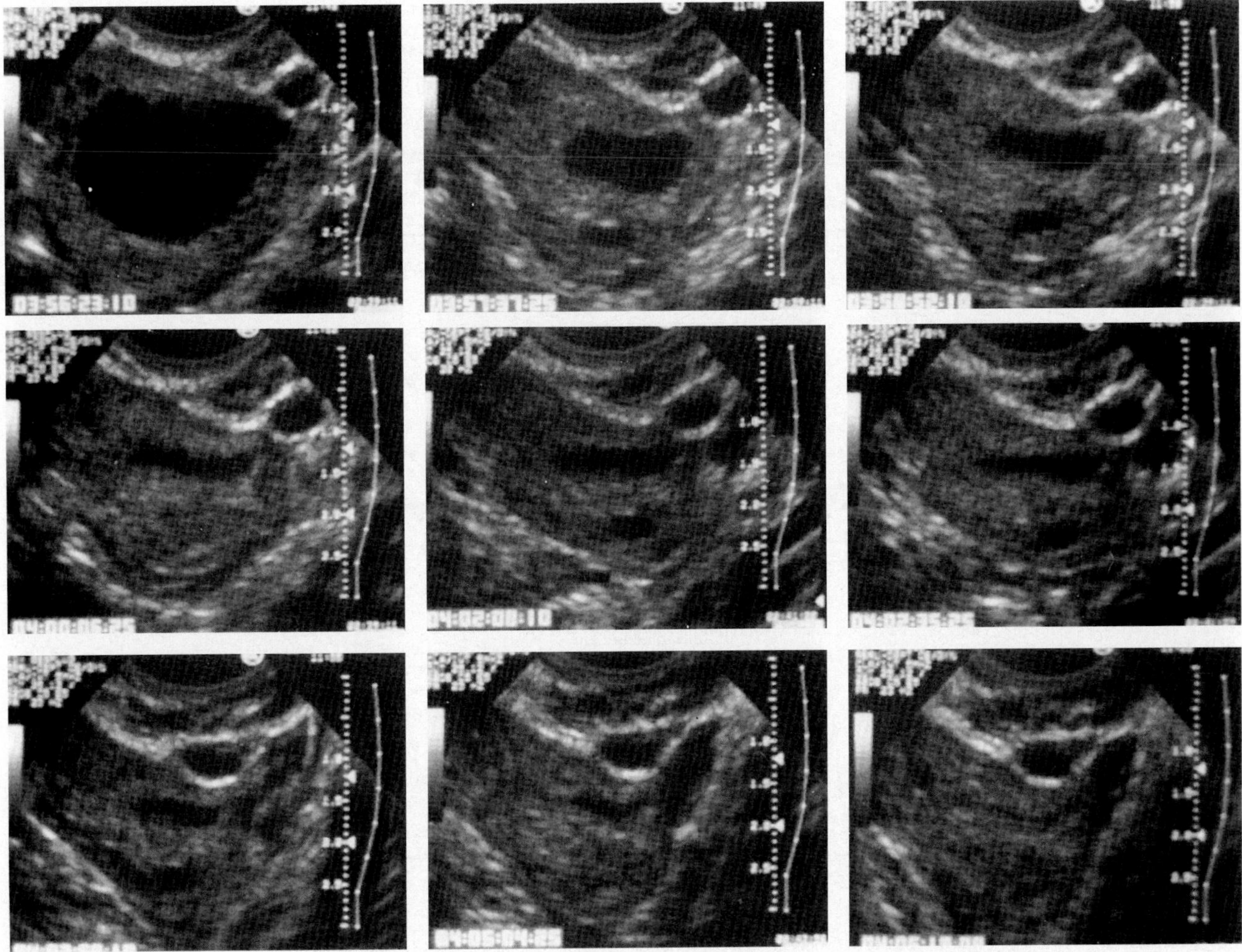

Figure 4-30. Sequence of images recorded during an ovulation research study. This ovulation took 10 minutes an 56 seconds from onset to complete follicular evacuation. Images are shown at intervals of 1 minute and 14.5 seconds. The first half of the follicular fluid was evacuated in 20 seconds; the remainder was evacuated over the next 10 minutes and 36 seconds. Time code values representing hours, minutes, seconds, and video frame are seen in the lower right corner of each image. (Adapted from Hanna MD, Chizen DR, Pierson RA: Characteristics of follicular evacuation during human ovulation. J Ultrasound Obstet Gynecol 4:488, 1994.)

Levels of progesterone steadily increase in the serum after ovulation and plateau about 1 week later, after which they decline unless pregnancy occurs. The increasing levels of progesterone and estradiol exert a negative feedback on FSH and LH secretion. Estradiol inhibits mainly FSH (negative feedback), whereas progesterone inhibits mainly LH. There is also evidence that luteal estradiol production exerts a local luteolytic action. It is postulated that increased intraovarian progesterone concentration prevents follicle maturation in that ovary in the subsequent cycle.

As luteolysis occurs and estradiol and progesterone levels decline, there is less negative feedback. Therefore, FSH and LH levels begin to rise before the onset of menstruation to stimulate follicular growth for the next cycle.

Estradiol and progesterone exert both a direct inhibitory effect on pituitary gonadotropin synthesis and secretion, and an effect on GnRH release, altering the frequency as well as the amplitude of GnRH pulses. The steroid feedback on GnRH release occurs by a direct effect on the neurotransmitters (dopamine and norepinephrine) and the neuromodulators (β-endorphin) in the arcuate nucleus.

Three studies by Reame and colleagues, Crowley and co-workers, and Filicori and associates have shown that the frequency of LH peaks, and presumably of GnRH pulses, changes throughout the menstrual cycle when blood sampling was performed every 10 minutes. In sleep, there is a close relationship between the frequency of GnRH pulses in portal blood and the frequency of LH pulses in the peripheral circulation. In the early follicular phase, LH pulses occur about once every 90 minutes, with an absence of pulsation during sleep (Fig. 4-31). The frequency of LH pulses significantly increases in the middle and late follicular phases to about one pulse per hour throughout the day and night. The amplitude of LH pulses is low and decreases somewhat between the early and middle follicular phases; however, during the late follicular (preovulatory) phase, LH amplitude significantly increases (Fig. 4-32). LH pulse frequency progressively slows in the luteal phase from about one pulse every 90 minutes in the early luteal phase to about

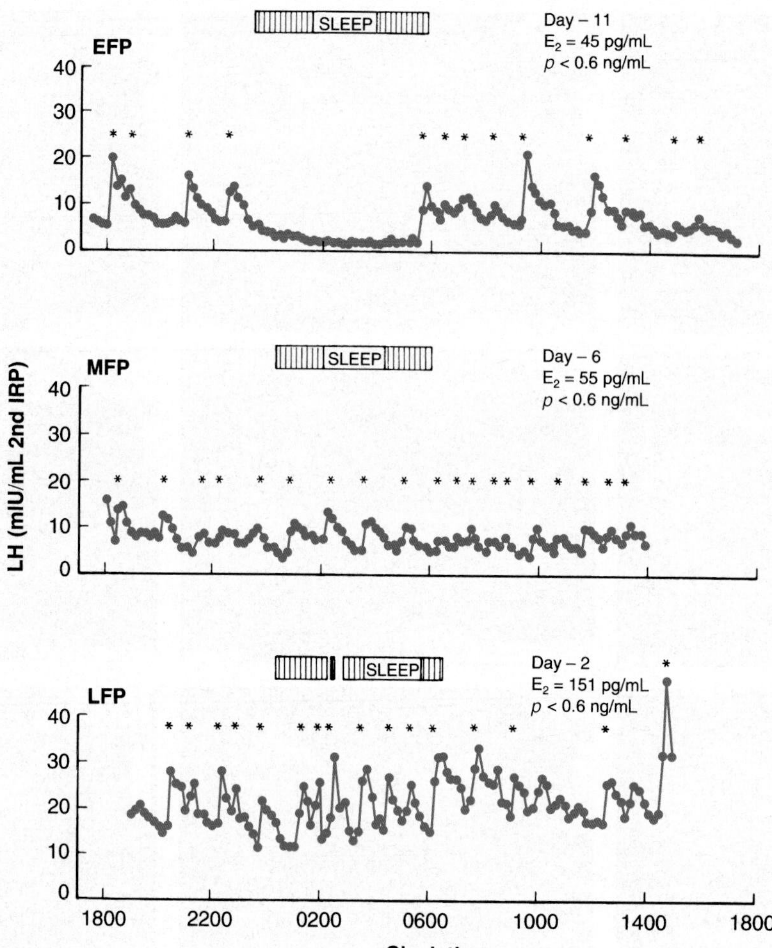

Figure 4-31. Patterns of episodic LH secretion throughout follicular phase of menstrual cycle. Representative examples of early follicular phase (EFP), midfollicular phase (MFP), and late follicular phase (LFP) series are shown. Stage of follicular phase is indicated from Day 0. LH pulsations are indicated by asterisks. Levels of prostaglandin E_2 and progesterone represent mean of samples obtained at 6-hour intervals. Sleep is indicated by hatched bars. P, progesterone. (From Filicori M, Santoro N, Merriam GR, et al: Characterization of the physiological pattern of episodic gonadotropin secretion throughout the human menstrual cycle. J Clin Endocrinol Metab 62:1136, 1986.)

one every 3 hours in the late luteal phase (Fig. 4-33). The amplitude of LH pulses varies after ovulation, with a bimodal distribution of small and large pulses. Overall mean LH levels are higher in the luteal phase than in the follicular phase (Fig. 4-34). Similar changes in FSH pulsation in peripheral blood do not occur, probably because of its longer half-life.

The increase in frequency of LH pulses during the late follicular phase is probably important in stimulating follicular secretion of estradiol, since 80% of LH pulses are followed by a rise in circulating estradiol levels. An increased amplitude of LH pulses is observed during the midcycle LH surge, probably because of either an increased frequency of GnRH pulsations or the positive feedback effect of increasing levels of estradiol and progesterone on increasing gonadotropin responsiveness to GnRH. Middle to late luteal LH pulses stimulate progesterone production. Bächström and colleagues and Filicori and coworkers have shown that beginning in the midluteal phase, progesterone is secreted in a pulsatile manner, with increases occurring immediately following an LH pulse (see Fig. 4-33). The variations in LH pulse amplitude and the slower frequency in the midluteal phase are probably caused by the negative feedback effects of progesterone and estradiol. Filicori and coworkers have postulated that the decrease in LH frequency is due to an action of progesterone on hypothalamic release of GnRH, possibly being mediated through increased levels of β-endorphin, whereas the decrease in amplitude of LH pulses is due to a negative feedback effect of progesterone on the pituitary.

The patterns of FSH and LH levels obtained by radioimmunoassay (RIA) measurements in serum are similar to the patterns observed by bioassay of urinary extracts, except that the midcycle FSH peak occurs 2 days later and is more pronounced, probably because of the longer half-life of FSH in serum (Fig. 4-35). The amounts of urinary FSH and LH excretion are about 1 to 10 IU/24 hr, whereas serum levels fluctuate between 1 to 100 mIU/mL.

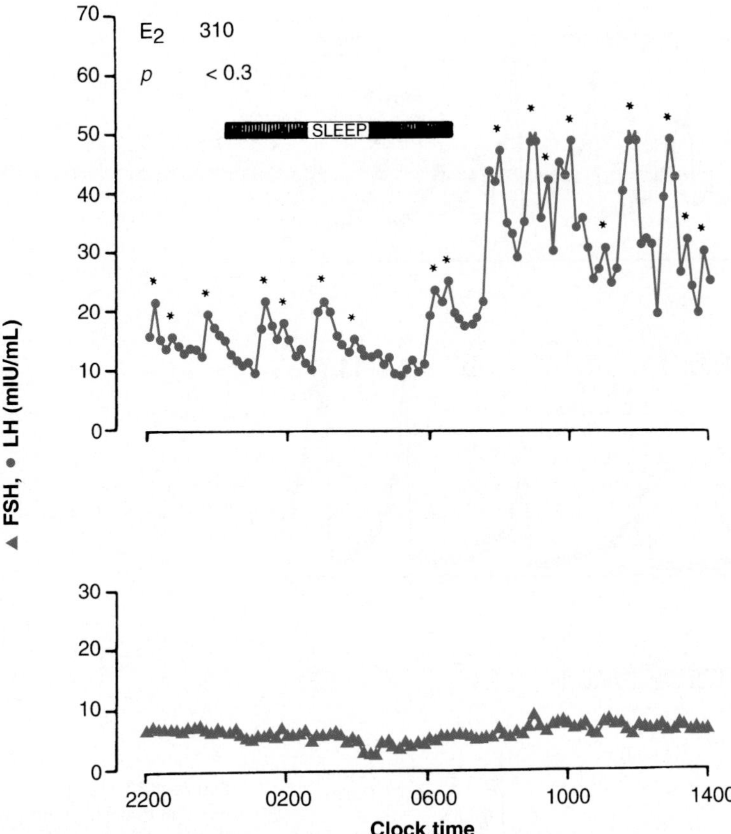

Figure 4-32. Luteinizing hormone (LH) secretory response in normal woman studied on day of LH surge. Note increase in amplitude and frequency of GnRH secretion, absence of any day–night variation, and discernible FSH pulsations. E_2, prostaglandin E_2; FSH, follicle-stimulating hormone. (From Crowley WF, Filicori M, Spratt DI, et al: The physiology of gonadotropin-releasing hormone (GnRH) secretion in men and women. Recent Prog Horm Res 41:473, 1985.)

Excretion of the three classic estrogens—estrone, estradiol, and estriol—is lowest during the early follicular phase, peaks just before LH peaks, decreases shortly thereafter, and rises in the luteal phase, after which it falls again. The luteal-phase rise of these estrogens is of smaller amplitude but longer duration than the preovulatory peak (Fig. 4-36). Midcycle peak urinary excretion of all three estrogens is about 50 to 75 μg/24 hr. Serum levels of estradiol follow a similar pattern throughout the cycle, rising from less than 50 pg/mL in the early follicular phase to 200 to 500 pg/mL at midcycle and having a broad luteal-phase peak level of about 100 to 150 pg/ mL (see Fig. 4-29).

The major metabolite of progesterone excreted in the urine is pregnanediol. Levels of pregnanediol are less than 0.9 μg/24 hr before ovulation (mean, 0.4 μg/24 hr) and consistently greater than 1 μg/24 hr (mean, 3 to 4 μg/24 hr) after ovulation (Fig. 4-37). Progesterone levels in serum are less than 1 ng/mL before ovulation and reach midluteal levels of 10 to 20 ng/mL. In cycles followed by conception, several investigators have reported that progesterone levels are always greater than 9 ng/mL. However, as progesterone is secreted in a pulsatile manner with wide fluctuations in its serum levels, a single low serum value may not be indicative of a lack of corpus luteum formation or of an inadequate corpus luteum.

Levels of the steroid metabolite 17-hydroxyprogesterone increase concomitantly with the increase of the LH surge, indicating a shift of steroidogenesis from the Δ^5 to the Δ^4 pathway (see Figure 4-29). Levels of 17-hydroxyprogesterone then fall and rise again in the midluteal phase as progesterone and estradiol levels increase. About 4 to 6 days before the onset of menses, levels of estradiol, progesterone, and 17-hydroxyprogesterone all begin to decline.

During midcycle the first event is a rise in estradiol. When estradiol reaches peak levels, there is an abrupt increase (surge) in LH and FSH (Fig. 4-38). The increase in LH reaches a peak in about 18 hours, and peak levels plateau for about 14 hours, after which there is a decline. The mean duration of the LH surge is about 24 hours. Beginning about 12 hours before the onset of the LH surge, there is an increase of both progesterone and 17-hydroxyprogesterone. With the occurrence of the LH peak there is a decline in estradiol and a further increase in progesterone. This shift in steroidogenesis in favor of progesterone instead of estradiol production is brought about by the luteinization of the granulosa cells produced by LH.

Levels of numerous other hormones have been measured in serum throughout the cycle and summarized in the excellent review by Diczfalusy and Landgren. Serum levels of

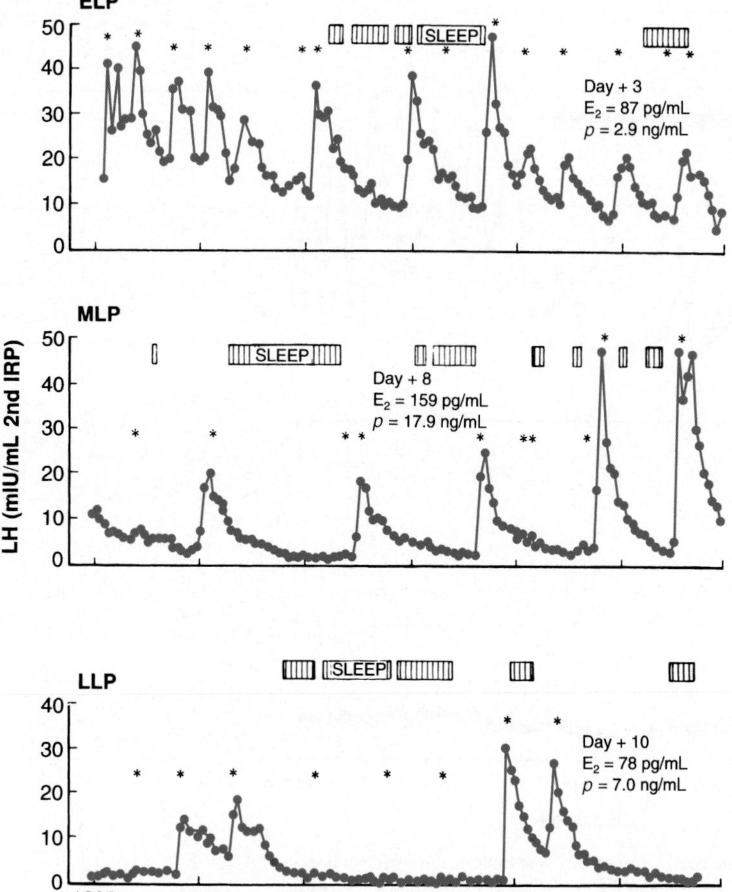

Figure 4-33. Patterns of episodic luteinizing hormone (LH) secretion throughout luteal phase of menstrual cycle. Representative examples of early (ELP), middle (MLP), and late (LLP) series are shown. Stage of luteal phase is indicated as post-day 0. P, progesterone. (From Filicori M, Santoro N, Merriam GR, et al: Characterization of the physiological pattern of episodic gonadotropin secretion throughout the human menstrual cycle. J Clin Endocrinol Metab 62:1136, 1986.)

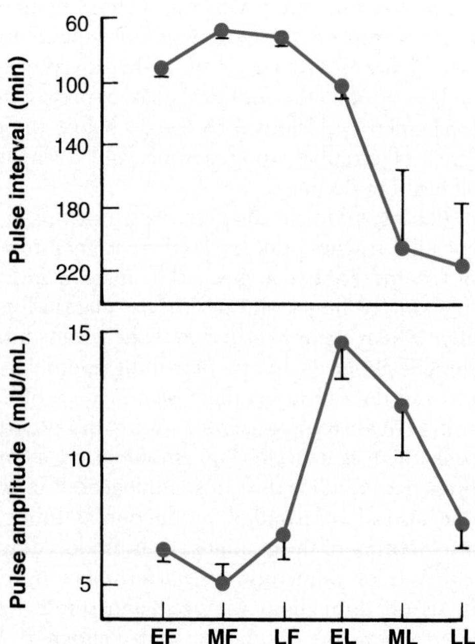

Figure 4-34. LH interpulse interval and amplitude during different stages of menstrual cycle. Data shown were obtained by pulse analysis and are expressed as means (*circles*) and standard errors (*vertical bars*). EF, early follicular phase; EL, early luteal phase; LF, late follicular phase; LL, late luteal phase; MF, midfollicular phase; ML, midluteal phase. (From Filicori M, Santoro N, Merriam GR, et al: Characterization of the physiological pattern of episodic gonadotropin secretion throughout the human menstrual cycle. J Clin Endocrinol Metab 62:1136, 1986.)

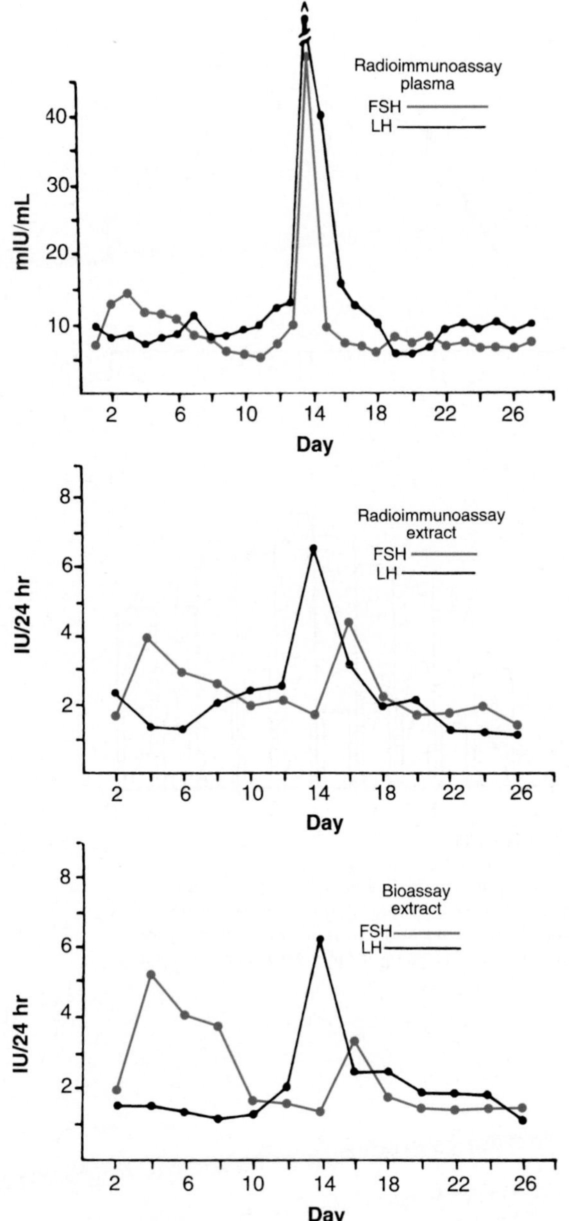

Figure 4-35. Serum follicle-stimulating hormone (FSH) and luteinizing hormone (LH) measured by radioimmunoassay (RIA) and urinary FSH and LH measured by both RIA and bioassay through an entire ovulatory menstrual cycle. (From Stevens VC: Comparison of FSH and LH patterns in plasma, urine and urinary extracts during the menstrual cycle. J Clin Endocrinol Metab 29:904, 1969. © 1969 by The Endocrine Society.)

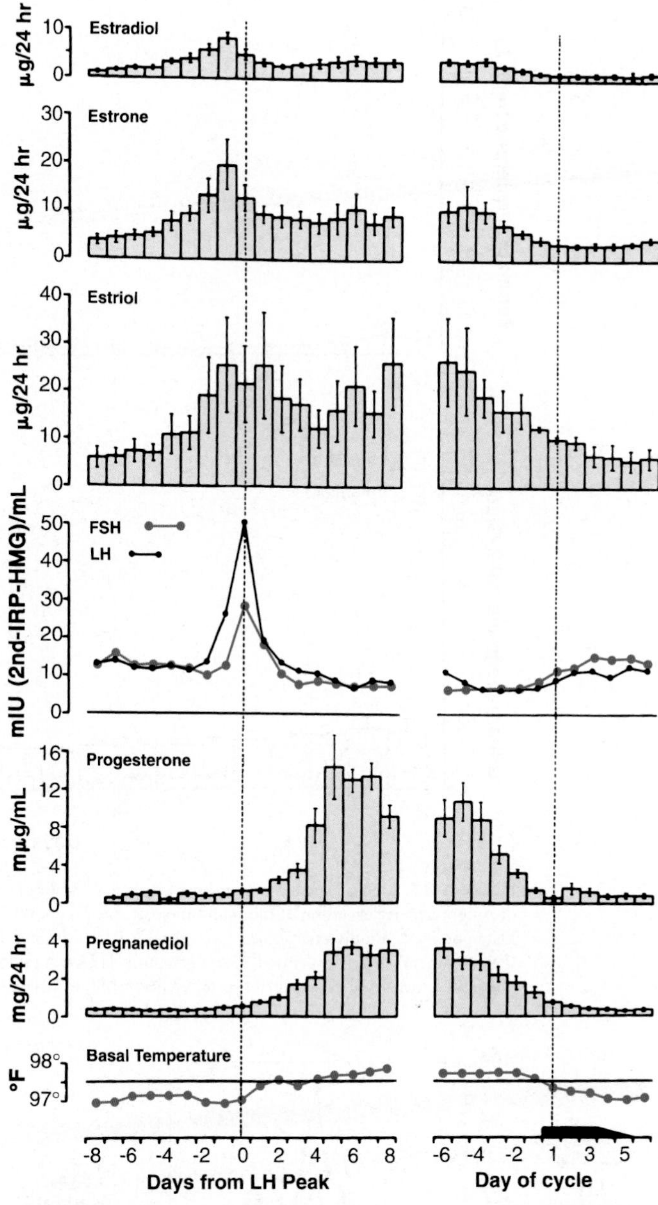

Figure 4-36. Mean serum follicle-stimulating hormone (FSH) and luteinizing hormone (LH) levels, urinary estrogen levels, pregnanediol excretion, and basal body temperatures measured daily in five women during ovulatory menstrual cycle. Bars depict standard errors. Individual results were grouped according to day of midcycle LH surge (*left*) or first day of menstruation (*right*) and averaged. 2nd IRP-HMG, Second International Reference Preparation of human menopausal gonadotropin. (From Goebelsmann UT, Midgley AR Jr, Jaffe RB: Regulation of human gonadotropins: VII. Daily individual urinary estrogens, pregnanediol and serum luteinizing and follicle stimulating hormones during the menstrual cycle. J Clin Endocrinol Metab 29:1222, 1969. © 1969 by The Endocrine Society.)

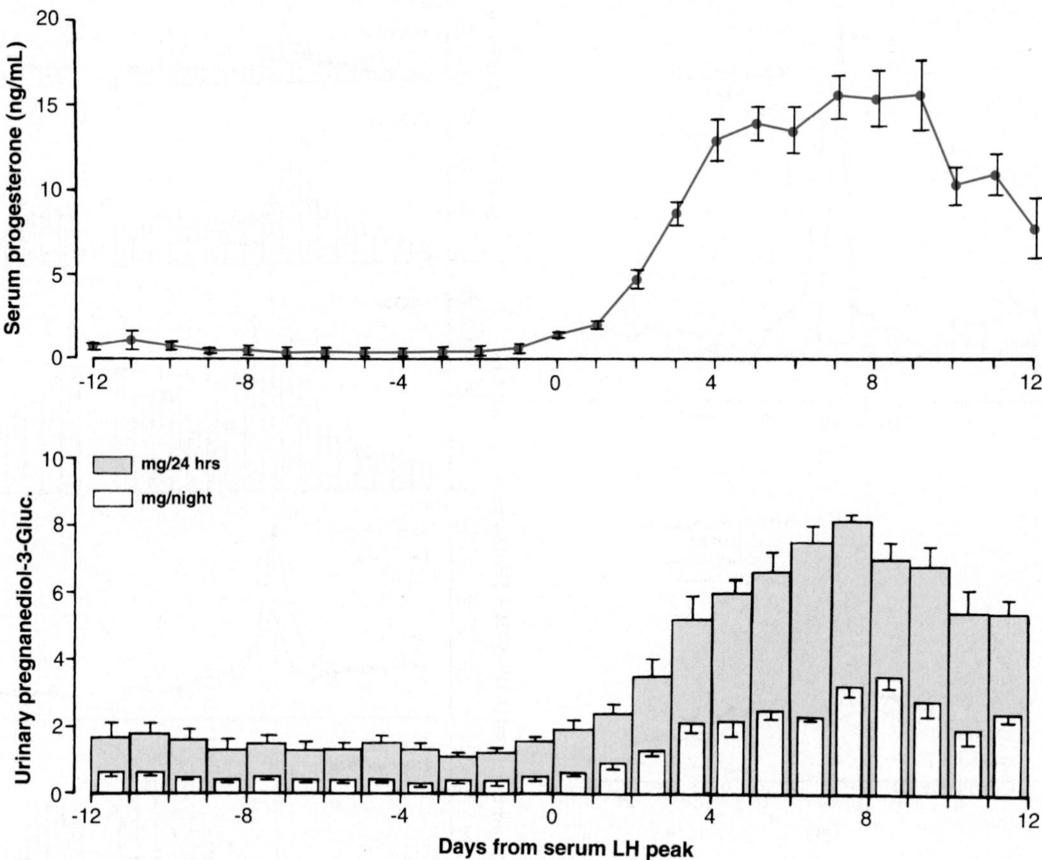

Figure 4-37. Means and standard errors of daily 8 AM serum progesterone concentrations and 24-hour (8 AM to 8 AM) and overnight urinary excretion of radioimmunoassayable pregnanediol-3-glucuronide in seven women during entire menstrual cycle. Data obtained in individual subjects were grouped according to day of midcycle luteinizing hormone (LH) peak and averaged. (From Stanczyk FZ, Miyakama I, Goebelsmann UT: Direct radioimmunoassay of urinary estrogen and pregnanediol glucuronides during the menstrual cycle. Am J Obstet Gynecol 137:443, 1980.)

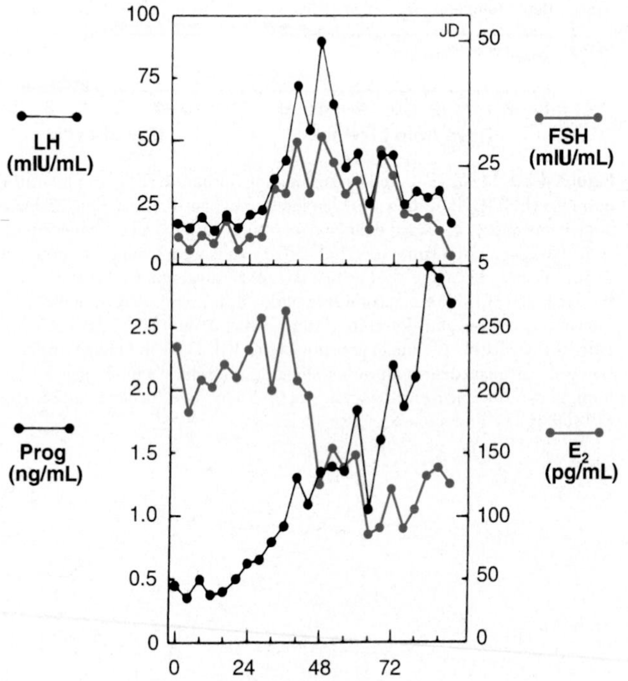

Figure 4-38. Serum follicle-stimulating hormone (FSH), luteinizing hormone (LH), estradiol (E_2), and progesterone (Prog) levels around midcycle. (From Thorneycroft IH, Sribyatta B, Tom WK, et al: Measurement of serum LH, FSH, progesterone, 17-hydroxy-progesterone and estradiol-17beta levels at 4-hour intervals during the periovulatory phase of the menstrual cycle. J Clin Endocrinol Metab 39:754, 1974. © 1974 by The Endocrine Society.)

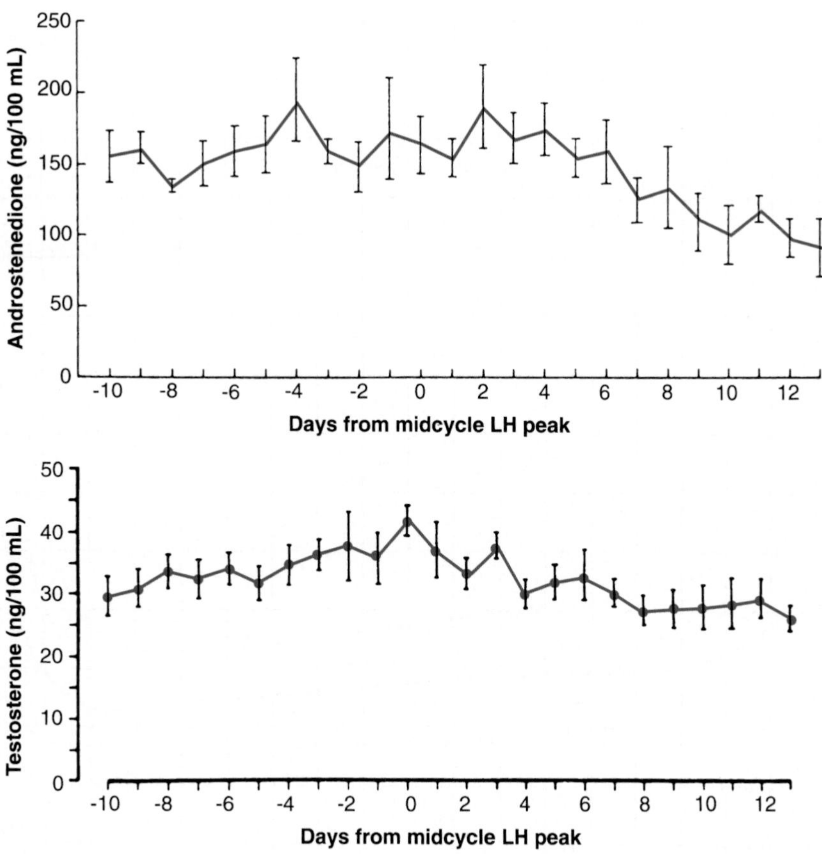

Figure 4-39. *Upper panel:* Means (*points*) and standard errors (*vertical bars*) of serum androstenedione concentrations measured in six women daily during entire ovulatory menstrual cycle. Individual daily results were grouped according to day of preovulatory serum estradiol peak and averaged. *Lower panel:* Means and standard errors of serum testosterone concentrations measured daily in eight women during entire ovulatory menstrual cycle. Individual daily results were grouped according to day of midcycle LH peak and averaged. (From Ribeiro WO, Mishell DR Jr, Thorneycroft IH: Comparison of the patterns of androstenedione, progesterone, and estradiol during the human menstrual cycle. Am J Obstet Gynecol 119:1026, 1974; and Goebelsmann UT, Arce JJ, Thorneycroft IH, et al: Serum testosterone concentrations in women throughout the menstrual cycle and following HCG administration. Am J Obstet Gynecol 119:445, 1974.)

androstenedione and testosterone change little during the cycle, but levels tend to peak at midcycle (Fig. 4-39). Serum TSH levels also remain relatively constant, while adrenocorticotropic hormone (ACTH) and growth hormone (GH) have a preovulatory peak. Prolactin levels appear to be slightly higher in the luteal phase.

Menstrual Cycle Length

The mean age of menarche is about 13 years, and the mean age of menopause is about 51 years. Therefore women have menses for a duration of about 38 years. Menstrual cycle length varies among different women and for an individual woman at different times of her life. The most information regarding menstrual cycles comes from the classic study of Treloar and colleagues, who analyzed 275,947 menstrual intervals recorded by more than 2700 women over prolonged periods. Analysis of these data revealed that menstrual cycle length is most irregular in the 2 years after menarche and the 3 years before menopause, times of life during which anovulatory cycles are most frequent (Table 4-6). During these times of life, both shortened and prolonged cycle lengths are common, with the latter being more frequent (Fig. 4-40).

Menstrual cycle length is least variable between the ages of 20 and 40 years. During this time there is a gradual decrease

Table 4-6 Means and Standard Deviations in Days for Menstrual Intervals at Selected Ages

Age	Mean (Days)	Standard Deviation (Days)
2 yr after menarche	32.20	8.38
20 yr	30.09	3.94
25 yr	29.84	3.45
30 yr	29.30	3.16
35 yr	28.22	2.67
40 yr	27.26	2.83
3 yr before menopause	33.20	14.24

Data from Treloar AE, Boynton RE, Behn BG, Brown BW: Variation of the human menstrual cycle through reproductive life. Int J Fertil 12:77–126, 1967.

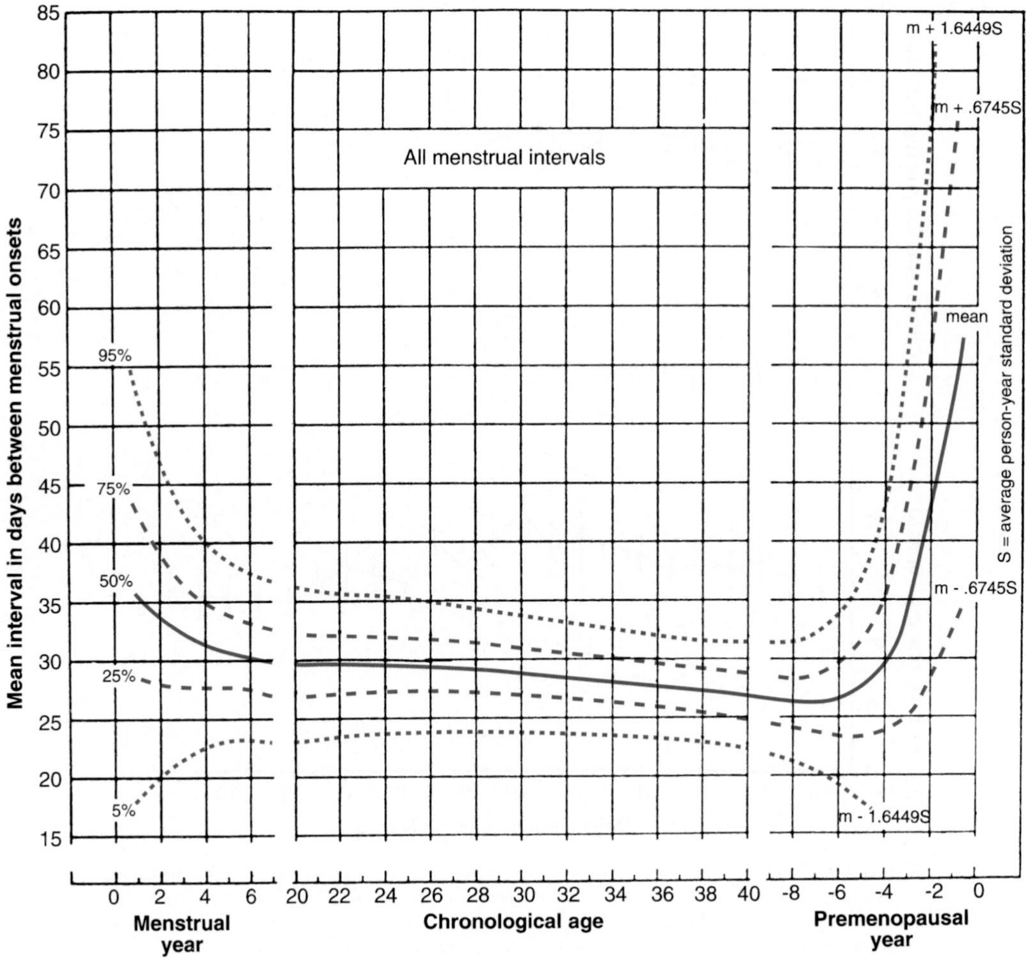

Figure 4-40. Normal curve contours for distribution of menstrual intervals in three zones of menstrual life. (From Treloar AE, Boynton RE, Behn BG, Brown BW: Variation of the human menstrual cycle through reproductive life. Int J Fertil 12:77, 1967.)

of mean cycle length. The follicular phase length defined as the interval from the onset of menstruation up to, but not including, the day of the LH peak decreases with age from 14.2 to 10.4 for women age 18 to 24 and 40 to 44 years, respectively. However, between these ages, menstrual cycle length still varies in an individual woman, as recorded by the women, with the most regular duration of menstrual cycles among the several thousand studied by Vollman for many years (Fig. 4-41). It is generally accepted that the mean duration of menstrual cycle length is 28 ± 7 days, with the occurrence of shorter cycles (<21 days) being called polymenorrhea and that of longer cycles (>35 days) being called oligomenorrhea. The mean duration of menstrual flow is 4 ± 2 days.

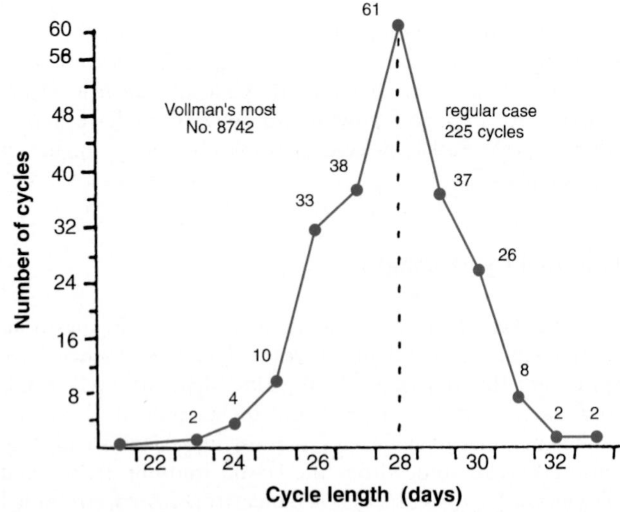

Figure 4-41. Frequency distribution of cycle lengths of Vollman's "most regular" subject. (From Hartman CG: The Irregularity of the Menstrual Cycle. In Science and the Safe Period. Huntington, NY, RE Krieger, 1972.)

Endometrial Histology

Human endometrium is made up of two basic layers: the stratum basale, which lies above the myometrium, and the stratum functionale, lying between the stratum basale and the uterine lumen. The stratum basale consists of primordial glands and densely cellular stroma, which changes little throughout the menstrual cycle and does not desquamate at the time of menstruation. The stratum functionale is divided into two layers. The superficial, narrow stratum compactum consists of the necks of the glands and densely populated stromal cells. The underlying, broader stratum spongiosum consists primarily of glands with less densely populated stroma and large amounts of interstitial tissue. The stratum functionale grows during the cycle, and a portion of it desquamates at the time of menses.

After menstruation, the endometrium is only 1 to 2 mm thick and consists mainly of the stratum basale and a portion of the spongiosum. Under the influence of estrogen, the stratum functionale proliferates greatly by multiplication of both glandular and stromal cells. Mitotic figures are abundant. In the late follicular phase, the glands become more tortuous in appearance. As estrogen levels peak immediately before ovulation, the cells lining the glandular lumina undergo pseudostratification (Fig. 4-42).

Just after ovulation, glycogen-rich subnuclear vacuoles appear in the base of the cells lining the glands (Fig. 4-43). This subnuclear vacuolization is the first histologic indication of the effect of progesterone but is not evidence that ovulation has occurred. As progesterone levels increase in the early luteal phase, the glycogen-containing vacuoles ascend toward the gland lumina. Soon thereafter, the contents of the glands are released into the endometrial cavity. The glycogen provides energy to the free-floating blastocyst, which reaches the endometrial cavity about 3½ days after fertilization. Implantation occurs 1 week after fertilization.

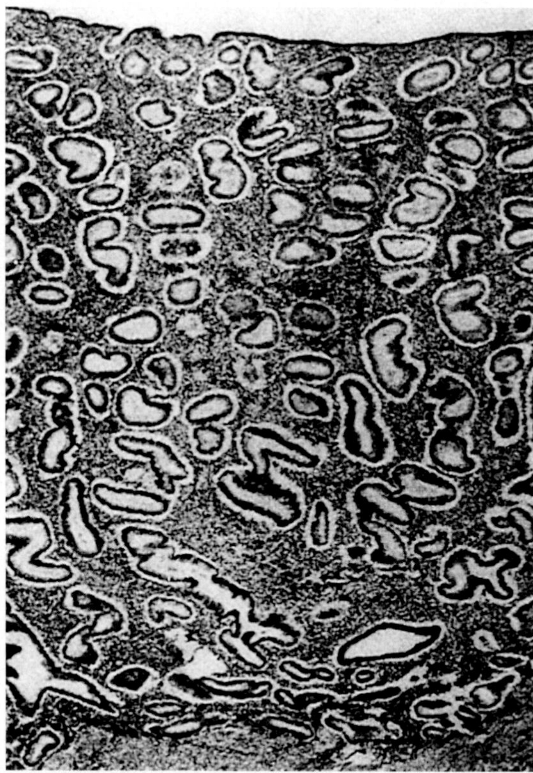

Figure 4-42. Early-interval endometrium. (From Novak E, Novak ER [eds]: Textbook of Gynecology, 4th ed. Baltimore, Williams & Wilkins, 1952.)

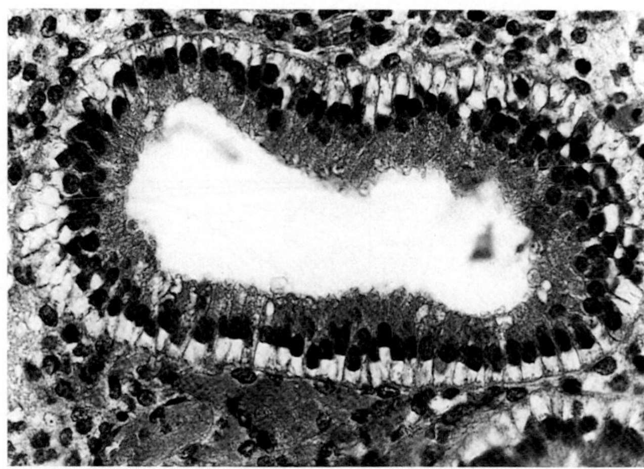

Figure 4-43. Subnuclear vacuoles lining base of endometrial gland 2 to 3 days after ovulation. (×500; reduced by 22%.) (From March CM: The endometrium in the menstrual cycle. In Mishell DR Jr, Davajan V, Lobo RA [eds]: Infertility, Contraception and Reproductive Endocrinology, 3rd ed. Cambridge, MA, Blackwell Scientific, 1991.)

In the midluteal phase the glands become increasingly tortuous and the stroma becomes more edematous and vascular (Fig. 4-44). During the secretory phase, several specific proteins are produced by the endometrium. The two major proteins are placental proteins 14 and 12 (PP14 and PP12). The former is also called pregnancy-associated endometrial protein (PEP), and α_2-pregnancy-associated endometrial globulin, as well as glycodelin. PP12 is also called α-uterine protein and chorionic α_2-globulin. PP14 is not actually a placental protein, but rather a major secretory product of glandular epithelium during the secretory phase. Circulating levels of PP14 correlate with serum progesterone levels, but the exact purpose of PP14 has not been determined. In addition, other peptide hormones, growth factors, and prostaglandins are produced by the endometrium

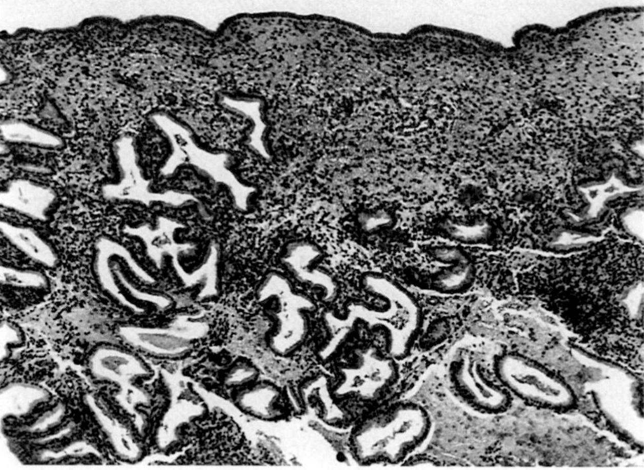

Figure 4-44. Maximal secretory activity characteristic of 7 to 8 days after ovulation. (×90; reduced by 22%.) (From March CM: The endometrium in the menstrual cycle. In Mishell DR Jr, Davajan V, Lobo RA [eds]: Infertility, Contraception and Reproductive Endocrinology, 3rd ed. Cambridge, MA, Blackwell Scientific, 1991.)

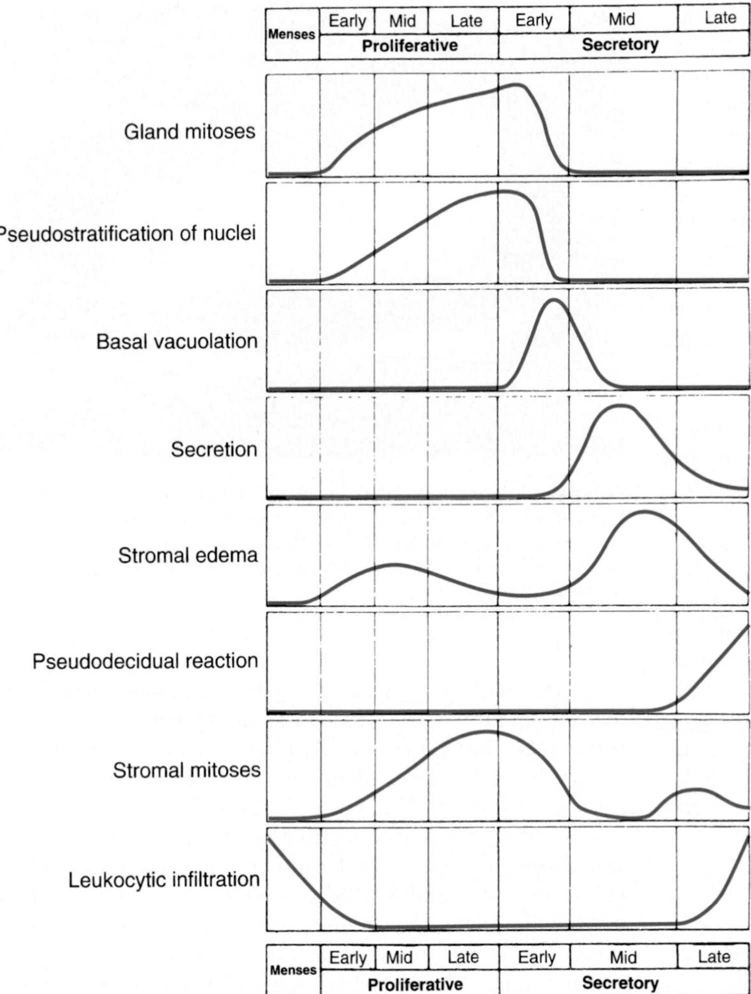

Figure 4-45. Patterns of histologic changes throughout menstrual cycle. (Modified from Fertility and Sterility, 1, Noyes RW, Hertig AT, Rock J, Dating the endometrial biopsy, 3. Copyright 1950, with permission from The American Society for Reproductive Medicine.)

and may have roles in the development of the decidualized endometrium. If implantation of the blastocyst does not occur in the late luteal phase and HCG is not produced to maintain the corpus luteum, the glands begin to collapse and fragment. Subsequently, polymorphonuclear leukocytes and monocytes infiltrate the glands and stroma, autolysis of the functional zone of the endometrium occurs, and desquamation begins. Other proteins involved in endometrial cyclicing include matrix metallaproteinases (MMPs), which are regulated by sex steroids and are important for tissue breakdown (Fig. 4-45). Other proteins such as leukocyte inhibitory factor (LIF) and tumor necrosis factor (TNF) are particularly important around the time of implantation.

The histologic pattern of the endometrium has been correlated with the phase of the menstrual cycle in the classic study of Noyes and coworkers (Fig. 4-46). This subjective method of correlating the degree of maturation of the endometrium is relatively imprecise. Several blind studies have demonstrated wide variability of both interobserver interpretation and intraobserver interpretation at different intervals. Recently, hormonal levels have been correlated with endometrial indices based on quantitative morphometric analysis. Li and colleagues noted that this methodology could produce a significant correlation with chronologic dating of the length of the luteal phase when only 5 of 17 morphometric measurements were used. These five measurements were (1) the frequency of mitosis per 1000 gland cells, (2) the amount of secretion in gland lumen, (3) the amount of gland cell pseudostratification, (4) the proportion of glands infused by gland cells, and (5) the amount of predecidual reaction. These authors concluded that use of these objective morphometric criteria resulted in better correlation with the actual length of the luteal phase than did histologic dating by the method of Noyes and coworkers. Numerous authors have now confirmed the day of LH surge is a more appropriate dating correlate than the onset of the next menstrual cycle (Fig. 4-47).

With the use of serial vaginal sonography of normal ovulatory women, Bakos and associates reported that the endometrial thickness, including both the anterior and posterior layers, steadily increased from a mean of about 4 mm in the early follicular phase to about 12 mm at the time of ovulation (Fig. 4-48). The mean endometrial thickness remained at 12 mm during the luteal phase. Endometrial volume showed a similar pattern.

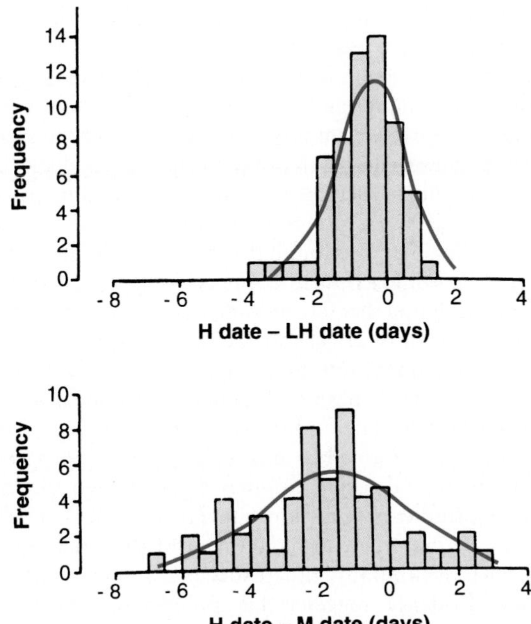

Figure 4-46. Frequency distribution of difference between histologic dating (*top*) and chronologic dating (*bottom*) by each method. H date, mean value of histologic dating by two observers; LH date, chronologic dating derived from luteinizing hormone (LH) surge; M date, chronologic dating derived from onset of next menstrual period. Normal curve has been fitted to frequency distribution according to bar chart. (Reprinted from Fertility and Sterility, 48, Li TC, Rogers AW, Lenton EA, et al, A comparison between two methods of chronological dating of human endometrial biopsies during the luteal phase, and their correlation with histologic dating, 928. Copyright 1987, with permission from The American Society for Reproductive Medicine.)

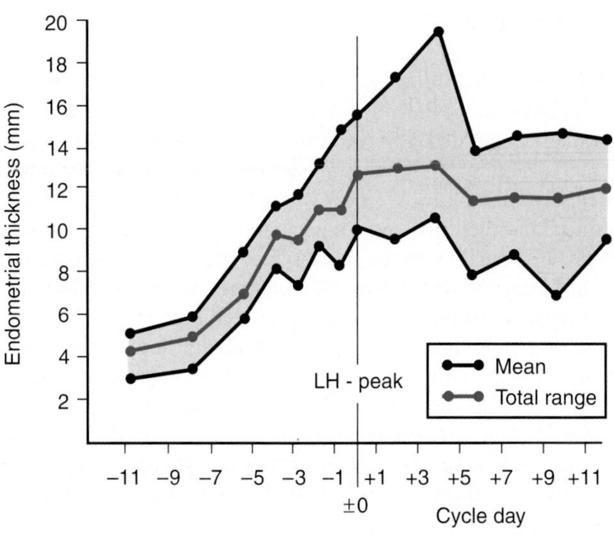

Figure 4-47. The endometrial thickness (in millimeters) measured by transvaginal ultrasound, presented as the mean and the total range, in 16 women during an ovulatory cycle. Each point on the curve represents a minimum of six observations. LH, luteinizing hormone.

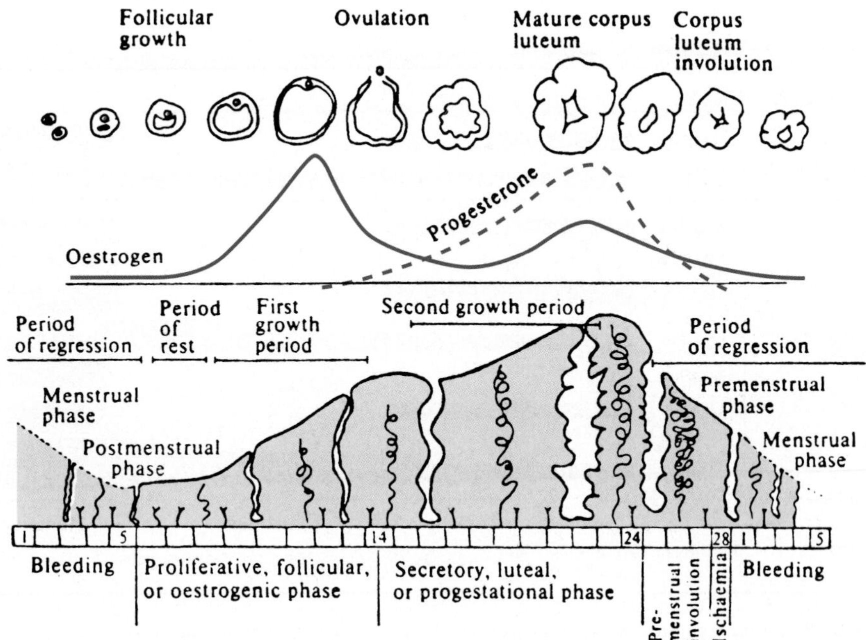

Figure 4-48. Diagram of changes in normal human ovarian and endometrial cycles. (From Shaw ST Jr, Roche PC: Menstruation. In Finn CA [ed]: Oxford Reviews of Reproduction and Endocrinology, Vol 2. London, Oxford University Press, 1980.)

Menstruation

Older classical studies by Markee and Bartelmez who observed menstrual changes in the anterior chamber of the eye of rhesus monkeys suggested a hypoxic theory for the initiation of menstrual bleeding; an ischemic necrosis was thought to initiate menstrual shedding. We now know based on human perfusion studies that their data are not accurate. Indeed a nuclear protein, hypoxia-inducible factor, is not increased at menstruation as would be expected if hypoxia occurred. Rather the initiation of menstrual sloughing occurs as a result of enzymatic digestion of tissue. This in turn is hormonally dependent in that progesterone withdrawal induces the expression of MMPs (Fig. 4-49). At the end of this process, coagulation takes over, a platelet plug first occurs with the more organized coagulation cascade following; then vasoconstriction of vessels occurs and re-epithelialization of endometrial tissues occur as estrogen levels rise.

Nogales-Ortiz and colleagues also found extreme variability in the extent of endometrial exfoliation. They found that usually only the entire compactum and some parts of the spongiosum were shed, but in some areas nearly the entire endometrium was desquamated. Desquamation of the endometrium occurs mainly in the fundus, not in the isthmus or cornual areas. As early as 36 hours after the onset of menses, regeneration of surface epithelium from the glandular stumps begins even as endometrial shedding continues.

Ferenczy, using scanning as well as transmission electron microscopy, reported that the endometrium remained intact in the cervical and isthmic areas. His studies revealed that re-epithelialization of the desquamated endometrium began 2 to 3 days after menses began and was completed in 48 hours. Ferenczy and coworkers performed historadioautography studies and concluded that repair of the desquamated endometrium occurred by both epithelial outgrowth from the mouths of the basal glands and by ingrowth from the endometrium in the cervical and isthmic areas that had not been desquamated. They believe that regeneration of the endometrial surface occurs as a local reaction to injury and is not mediated by ovarian steroid hormones, whose levels are very low at this time of the cycle.

In 1978, Flowers and Wilborn performed a histologic, histochemical, and ultrastructural study of endometrial biopsy specimens obtained from a group of menstruating women. In these detailed studies, they also found that the only cells desquamated are from the compactum and upper spongiosum layers. In addition, they found that few endometrial cells undergo necrosis. Instead, the majority of cells in the endometrium survive and undergo regression in size by autophagocytosis, heterophagocytosis, and release of enzymes. Endometrial autophagocytosis is carried out by lysosomes, which digest the cytoplasm; heterophagocytosis is performed by macrophages, which phagocytose debris from stromal tissue; enzymes digest the reticular fibers. More recent studies have demonstrated that interleukin-8 (IL-8) levels may be important in recruitment of these macrophages. IL-8 attracts neutrophils into tissues and causes them to degranulate. Evidence suggests that progesterone may inhibit endometrial production of IL-8. Thus, decreasing progesterone levels in the late luteal phase may allow increased production of IL-8 in the endometrial cells, leading to leukocyte immigration and degranulation. Progesterone maintains the stability of the lysosomes, which contain enzymes that degrade the substances providing support for the growing endometrium such as mucopolysaccharides, collagen, and reticulum. The MMPs degrade structural elements of the extracellular matrix and basement membrane. Enzymes in the lysosomes degrade the substances that make up the supporting growth substance of the endometrium: the mucopolysaccharides, collagen, and reticulum.

Other changes within the endometrial cells may also contribute to disorganization of the endometrium during menstruation. Recent studies have determined that expression of proteins,

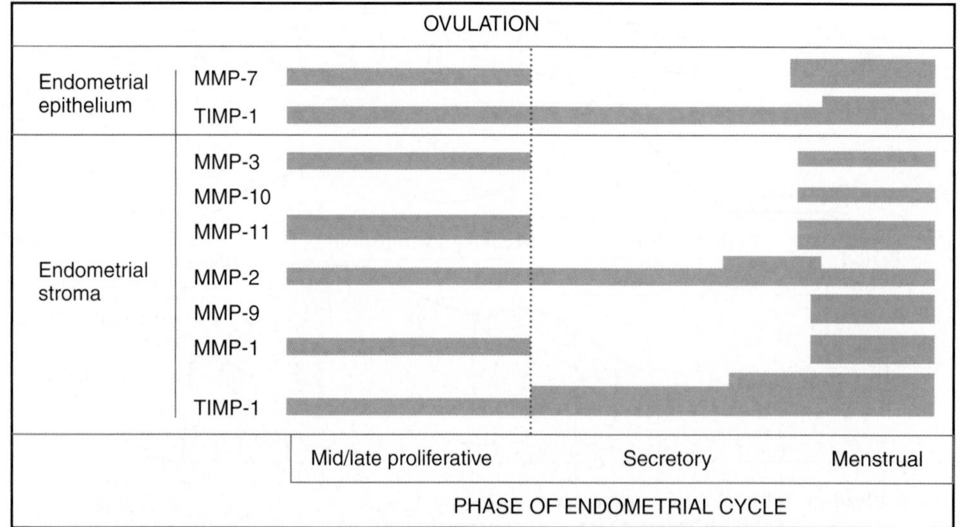

Figure 4-49. Schematic of matrix metalloproteinase (MMP) expression in the human endometrium during the menstrual cycle. The pattern of expression varies during the menstrual cycle and is influenced by estrogen and progesterone. TIMP-1, tissue metalloproteinase-1. (Modified from Rodgers WH, Matrisan LM, Giudice LC, et al: Patterns of matrix metalloproteinase expression in cycling endometrium imply differential functions and regulation by steroid hormones. J Clin Invest 94:946–953,1994.)

important in epithelial cell–cell-binding in human endometrium, changes throughout the menstrual cycle. These proteins include E-cadherin, α- or β-catenin, β-actin, and desmoplalkin I/II. Menstrual shedding is associated with disorganization of the site-specific distribution of these proteins. Therefore, menstruation may also be the result of withdrawal of steroid hormones, leading to the dissolution of integrity of the tight, gap, intermediate and desmosomal junctions that bind the epithelial, stromal, and glandular cells. These changes have not been observed in the basalis layer, which is not shed during the menstrual phase.

After this sequence of events, the cells are reorganized in structure and participate in the new proliferative process as described earlier, and the same cells that previously formed the secretory endometrium also form the new proliferative endometrium. Thus menstruation in humans is probably a combination of superficial tissue shedding brought about by ischemia, increases in IL-8, lysis from hydrolytic enzymes from macrophages, and loss of cell–cell-binding proteins followed by reorganization and regeneration of endometrial cells.

When implantation occurs, in the absence of menstruation, a complex interaction of the substances comes into play (Fig. 4-50).

TECHNIQUE OF HORMONE ASSAY

Bioassay

Measurement (assay) of reproductive hormones was initially done by bioassay techniques. Hormones such as the gonadotropins were measured in urine. Bioassays measure the biologic response (growth) of target organs of certain animals (usually rats, rabbits, or mice), which is produced by administering different concentrations of the substances to be assayed, such as in urinary extracts. First, various dilutions of a known (standard) preparation of hormone are administered. The varying increases in weight of the target organ in the animal are then used to develop a dose-response curve against which the response of the substance being assayed is determined.

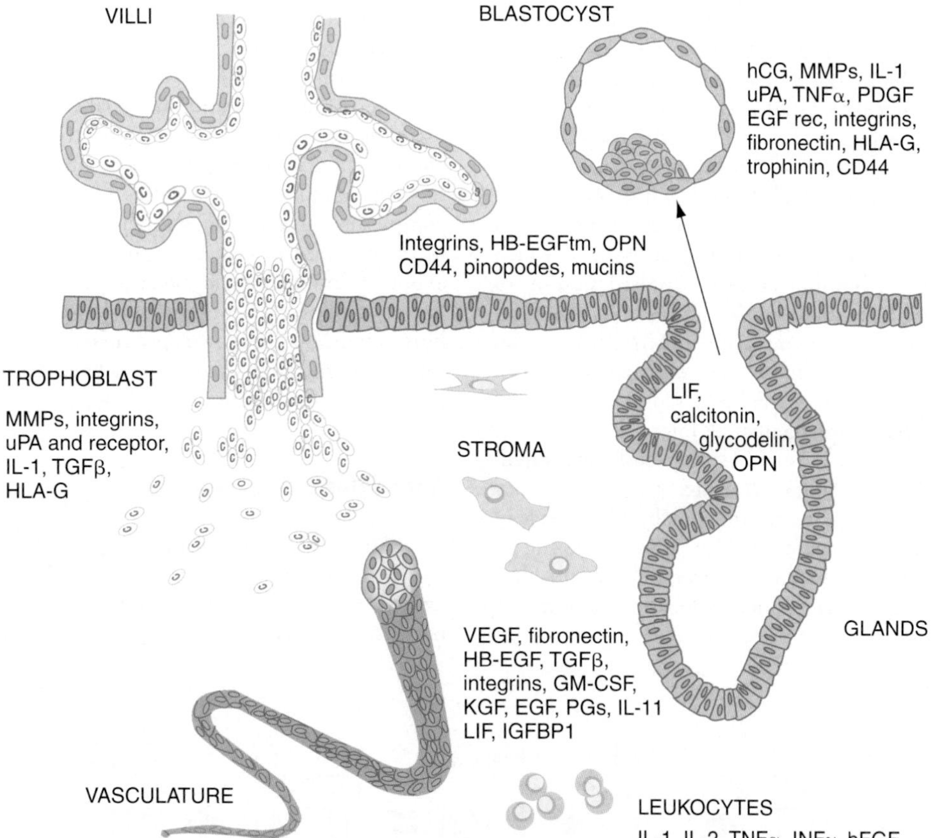

Figure 4-50. Implantation is a complex process involving the elaboration of adhesion molecules, cytokines and growth factors, each secreted by the blastocyst, the trophoblast as well as by endometrial glands, stroma, blood vessels and resident leukocytes. bFGF, basic fibroblast growth factor; GM-CSF, granulocyte-macrophage colony-stimulating factor; HB-EGF, heparin-binding epidermal growth factor; HLA-G, human leukocyte antigen-G; IGFBP, insulin-like growth factor-binding protein; IL, interleukin; INF-γ, interferon gamma; KGF, keratin growth factor; LIF, leukocyte inhibitory factor; MMPs, metalloproteinases; OPN, osteopontin; PDGF, platelet-derived growth factor; PGs, prostaglandins; TGF, transforming growth factor; TNFα, tumor necrosis factor α; uPA, urokinase-type plasminogen activator; VEGF, vascular endothelial growth factor. (Modified from Strauss J, Barbieri R: Yen and Jaffe's Reproductive Endocrinology, 5th ed. Philadelphia, Elsevier, 2004.)

Chemical Methods

Chemical assay methods were developed to measure urinary sex steroid levels in women. These assays lack the sensitivity to quantify steroid levels in blood (serum or plasma). Three basic procedural steps are performed in chemical assays of steroids. First, the steroids undergo hydrolysis to remove the conjugate (sulfate or glucuronide group). This is necessary because steroids in urine are present almost entirely in a conjugated form. Second, the steroids are extracted by organic solvents from the urinary hydrolysate. The final basic step is purification of the steroid by column chromatography. The amount of steroid is then quantified by measurement of the color reaction, using either colorimetry or the more sensitive fluorometry. A more sensitive chemical method of measurement of steroids is gas chromatography, an extremely tedious procedure.

Radioimmunoassay

In 1959, Yalow and Berson developed the technique of RIA, which provided the method of measuring extremely small amounts of hormone in serum or plasma. Use of this technique has greatly increased the knowledge of reproductive endocrinology. RIA allows a much greater number of assays to be performed than does bioassay or chemical assay, in addition to having much greater sensitivity and needing less than 1 mL of serum or plasma for testing. However, this technique measures only the immunologic property of a hormone, not its biologic effects. The two effects frequently differ in magnitude.

The basic principle of RIA involves competition between a radioactively labeled and an unlabeled antigen, both of which are present in excess, for binding sites on a limited amount of antibody. To produce a standard curve that permits measurement of a hormone in the serum or plasma, the investigator uses a standard preparation of the hormone to be measured (antigen). Varying known amounts of the unlabeled (cold) antigen and the labeled (hot) antigen are incubated for a time with an antibody raised specifically against the antigen to be measured, and an antigen–antibody complex is formed (Fig. 4-51). Since there is always an excess of labeled and unlabeled antigen in the reaction, some of each type of antigen is always bound to the antibody and some always remains free in solution after the incubation. After a predetermined incubation period, the bound complex is separated from the excess free antigen in solution, usually by the addition of an antibody (second antibody) raised against the first antibody, the amount of tracer present in either the bound or free component (usually the bound complex) is measured by a radioactive analyzer (counter). A standard curve is then constructed by plotting the counts per minute measured in the bound components obtained from assaying the various dilutions of the standard preparation, against the mass of antigen used. The type of curve varies with the scale of the abscissa (Fig. 4-52).

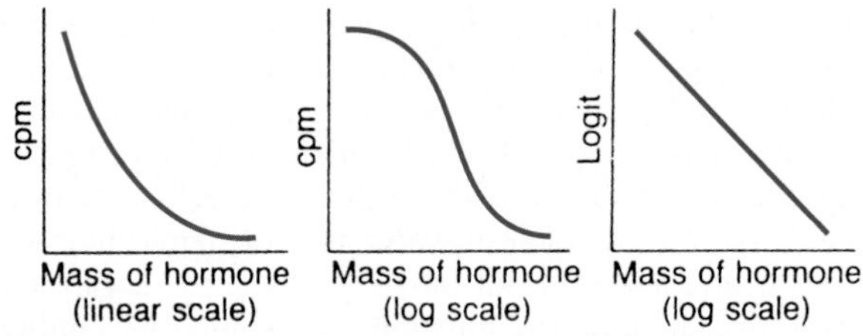

Figure 4-52. Standard curve using linear scale (*left*) or log scale (*center and right*) for the abscissa and linear (*left and center*) or logit (*right*) for the ordinate. cpm, counts per minute. (From Nakamura RM, Stanczyk FZ: Immunoassays. In Lobo RA, Mishell DR Jr, Paulson RJ, Shoupe D [eds]: Mishell's Textbook of Infertility, Contraception and Reproductive Endocrinology, 4th ed. Malden, MA, Blackwell Science, 1997.)

For measurement of the amount of hormone in the unknown specimen, the same amount of labeled antigen and antibody used for the standard curve preparation are also added to an aliquot of the unknown specimen. After incubation and separation, the amount of tracer that is bound in the antigen–antibody complex is counted. The number of counts per minute measured in the complex is located on the ordinate, and from this point a line is intersected on the standard curve. A perpendicular line is dropped to the abscissa to determine the amount of hormone in the unknown specimen. Rapid calculations of hormone concentrations can be performed by use of a programmed calculator or by a computer.

Antibodies

In contrast to steroid hormones, protein hormones themselves are antigenic and can produce antibody formation. Since steroids are haptens and are not antigenic by themselves, they need to be attached to a carrier protein (usually bovine serum

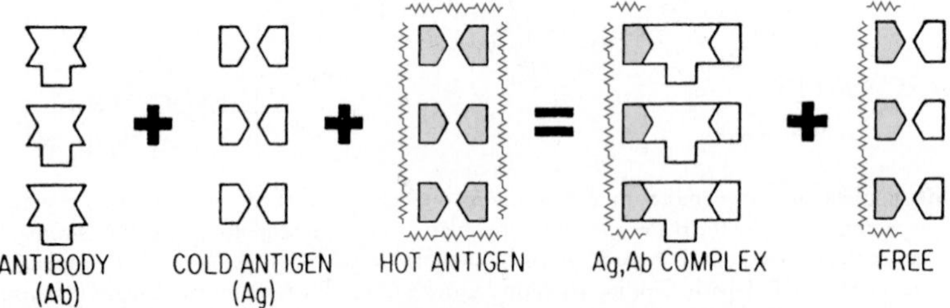

Figure 4-51. Schematic representation of monoclonal antibody production. (From Nakamura RM, Stanczyk FZ: Immunoassays. In Lobo RA, Mishell DR Jr, Paulson RJ, Shoupe D [eds]: Mishell's Textbook of Infertility, Contraception and Reproductive Endocrinology, 4th ed. Malden, MA, Blackwell Science, 1997.)

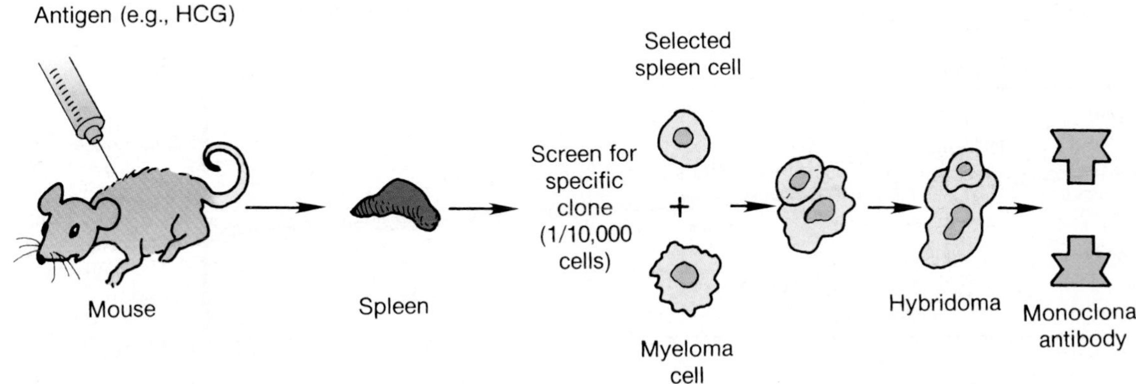

Figure 4-53. Schematic representation of monoclonal antibody production. (From Nakamura RM, Stanczyk FZ: Immunoassays. In Lobo RA, Mishell DR Jr, Paulson RJ, Shoupe D [eds]: Mishell's Textbook of Infertility, Contraception and Reproductive Endocrinology, 4th ed. Malden, MA, Blackwell Science, 1997.)

albumin) to induce antibody formation. Even with the injection of purified antigens, there is a degree of cross-reaction of most hormone antibodies (polyclonal) with other hormones. To increase assay specificity, antibodies are now being produced to eliminate the variability and heterogeneity of antibodies produced by several injections of antigen. Monoclonal antibodies are produced by first injecting the antigen into a mouse to induce an immunologic reaction in its spleen (Fig. 4-53). The spleen cells are screened to find those particular ones (clones) capable of secreting a single antibody type. These cells are then fused with a myeloma cell from the same species to form a hybrid or hybridoma cell. Because of the immortality of the myeloma cell in culture, the hybridoma continually secretes antibodies characteristic of the selected spleen cell. This clone line is maintained in culture to provide homogenous monoclonal antibody molecules, which are used for sensitive and specific immunoassays of protein hormones.

Antigens

To produce standard curves, varying amounts of known pure preparations of hormone need to be utilized. Since steroid hormones are available as chemically pure preparations, the amount added to form the standard curve and determine the amount in the unknown can be expressed in terms of absolute mass or weight, such as nanograms (10^{-9}) or picograms (10^{-12}). Thus, the results obtained from different laboratories should be constant. However, most European laboratories express the results in terms of nanomoles instead of nanograms. For most steroids, about 3 nmol/L is equivalent to 1 ng/mL.

Protein hormones, however, being of high molecular weight, are not available in pure form. Therefore, the results of measuring unknown samples need to be expressed in terms of the amount of a standard reference preparation by use of standard extracts of the hormone obtained from collections of urine, serum, or pituitary glands. Thus, the levels of hormone measured by laboratories using different standards do not always agree, and clinicians should be aware of the normal levels used by these laboratories. The protein standard is frequently an international reference preparation, and the results are usually expressed in international units.

Assay Markers

As described earlier, quantitation in an RIA is carried out by measuring the radioactive antigen (assay marker). The use of radioisotopes for RIA has become a negative factor in recent years because of the problems associated with radioactive waste disposal. During the past few years, major advances have occurred in both the development of new instruments and the identification of new nonradioactive markers. When coupled to assay antigens, these result in assays whose markers are almost as sensitive as RIA and sometimes are as sensitive as the most sensitive RIA. Use of these markers has rejuvenated the field of immunoassays by allowing individuals without training in the use of radioisotopes to perform these assays. One can easily extend this use to the home, and "home kits" are becoming readily available. Examples of nonradioactive markers are given in the next section.

Types of Immunoassays

Because of advances made in the development of nonradioactive markers to replace the radioactive markers used in RIAs, many new types of assays, some related and others not related, to RIAs, have been established. All these assays, however, use the antigen–antibody interaction and thus are now usually referred to as immunoassays. Immunoassays can be categorized not only on the basis of whether they use excess antigen or excess antibody, but also according to whether they use a radioactive tracer. A categorization of some of the most frequently used types of immunoassays in reproductive endocrinology laboratories is shown in Table 4-7.

The basic principle of the nonradioactive immunoassays that use antigen excess is the same as that of RIA (Fig. 4-54). The nonradioactive immunoassay uses a nonradioactive tag, such as fluorescein in the fluorometric immunoassay (FIA), luminol in the chemiluminescent immunoassay (CIA), and an alkaline phosphatase conjugate in the enzyme immunoassay (EIA). Quantification of these tags is achieved by use of a fluorometer in the FIA and a luminometer in the CIA. In the EIA, quantification is carried out by addition of a specific substrate. For example, *p*-nitrophenylphosphate is used with

Table 4-7 Types of Immunoassays

Assay Type	Examples
Excess Antigen	
Radioactive	Radioimmunoassay (RIA)
Nonradioactive	Chemiluminescent immunoassay (CIA)
	Fluoroimmunoassay (FIA)
	Enzyme immunoassay (EIA)
Excess Antibody	
Radioactive	Immunoradiometric assay (IRMA)
Nonradioactive	Enzyme-linked immunosorbent assay (ELISA)

alkaline phosphatase, and the product formed, *p*-nitrophenol, can be measured spectrophotometrically.

Two of the most widely used excess-antibody assays in clinical reproductive endocrinology laboratories are the immunoradiometric assay (IRMA) and the enzyme-linked immunosorbent assay (ELISA). In the IRMA the principle involves the use of excess radiolabeled antibody that binds to the antigen, followed by removal of excess antibody. At present the two-site IRMA (Fig. 4-55) is often employed. It requires the addition of a second antibody attached to a solid phase, such as a bead.

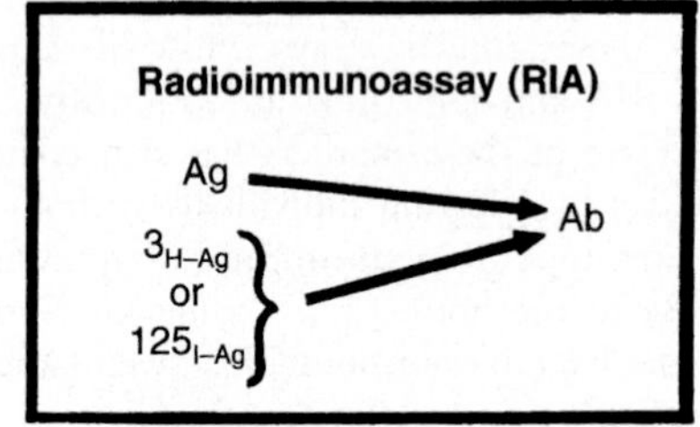

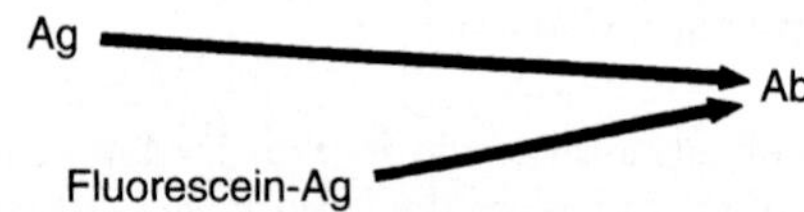

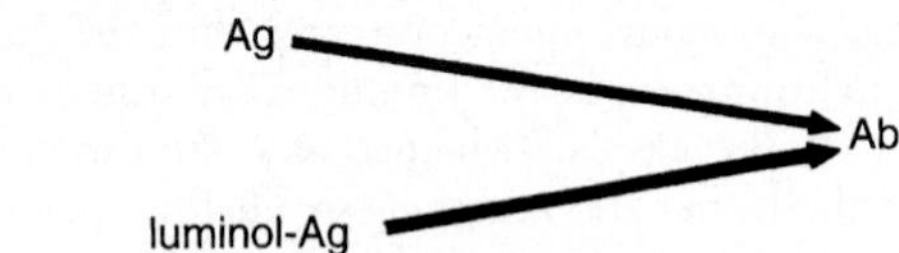

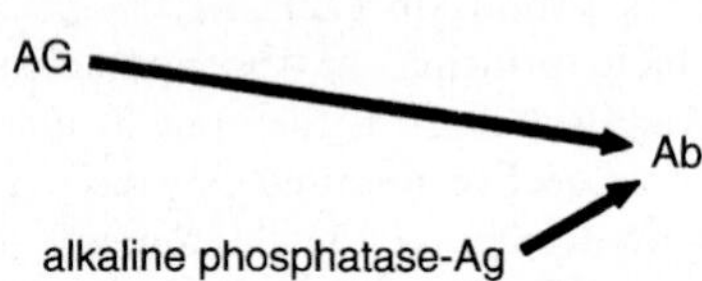

Figure 4-54. Competition between excess antigen (Ag) (analyte or standard) and excess radioactive or nonradioactive antigen (marker) for a limited amount of antibody (Ab). (From Stanczyk FZ: Immunoassays. In Lobo RA, Mishell DR Jr, Paulson RJ, Shoupe D [eds]: Mishell's Textbook of Infertility, Contraception and Reproductive Endocrinology, 4th ed. Malden, MA, Blackwell Science, 1997.)

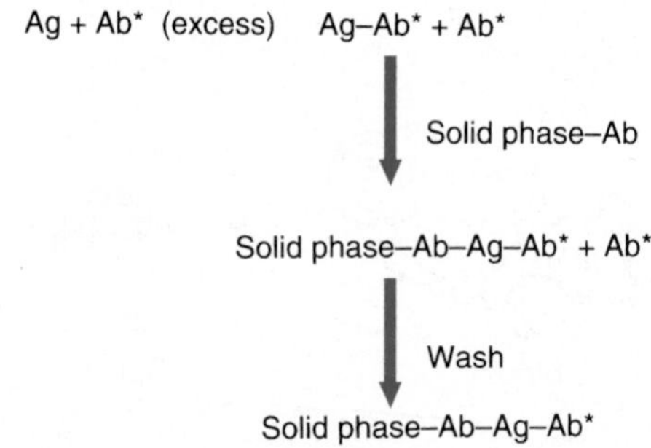

Figure 4-55. Principle of the immunoradiometric assay. Ag, antigen; Ab, antibody. (From Stanczyk FZ: Immunoassays. In Lobo RA, Mishell DR Jr, Paulson RJ, Shoupe D [eds]: Mishell's Textbook of Infertility, Contraception and Reproductive Endocrinology, 4th ed. Malden, MA, Blackwell Science, 1997.)

The second antibody differs from the first one in that the second is not radioactive and recognizes a different site on the antigen. Since the complex formed is attached to a solid phase, it can be readily separated from the excess radioactive antibody by centrifugation. The amount of radioactivity measured in the final complex is directly proportional to the concentration of standard used to prepare the standard curve and the concentration of analyte in the specimen. This is in contrast to the inverse relationship between the "bound" radioactivity and standard concentrations observed in a radioimmunoassay.

In the ELISA, antigen is bound to an excess of antibody, which is attached to a solid phase, such as a plastic tube or plate (Fig. 4-56). Once the antigen–antibody complex is formed, an antibody–enzyme conjugate is added. The antibody in this conjugate is directed against an antigenic site different from that recognized by the first antibody. The result is a "sandwich" type of complex, thus the term *sandwich ELISA.* Following the addition of the appropriate substrate for the enzyme, the resulting product is measured spectrophotometrically. The relationship between the product concentration and concentration of standard or analyte is similar to that obtained by IRMA.

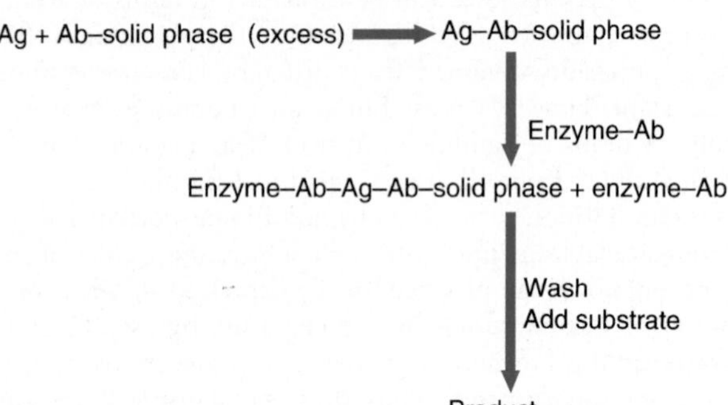

Figure 4-56. Principle of the enzyme-linked immunosorbent assay. Ag, antigen; Ab, antibody. (From Stanczyk FZ: Immunoassays. In Lobo RA, Mishell DR Jr, Paulson RJ, Shoupe D [eds]: Mishell's Textbook of Infertility, Contraception and Reproductive Endocrinology, 4th ed. Malden, MA, Blackwell Science, 1997.)

Table 4-8 95% Confidence Limits of Hormones Used in Reproduction

	PHASE OF MENSTRUAL CYCLE			
Hormone	**Follicular**	**Midcycle**	**Luteal**	**Menopause**
LH (mIU/mL)	4.0–20.0	43–145	3–18	>40
FSH (mIU/mL)	3.2–9.0	10–18	3–9	>30
Prolactin (ng/mL)	8.0–20.0	0–22	10–30	8–25
Estradiol (pg/mL)	30–140	150–480	50–250	10–30
Progesterone (ng/mL)	0.5–1.0	0.8–2.0	3.0–31	0.5–1.0
Testosterone (ng/dL)	20–85	20–85	20–85	8–30*
Free testosterone (ng/dL)	1.2–9.9	1.2–9.9	1.2–9.9	3–13†
DHEAS (μg/mL)	0.5–2.8	0.5–2.8	0.5–2.8	0.2–1.5

*In oophorectomized women the range is 1–18 ng/dL.
†In oophorectomized women the range is 1–10 ng/dL.
DHEAS, dehydroepiandrosterone sulfate; FSH, follicle-stimulating hormone; LH, leuteinizing hormone.
From Nakamura RM, Stanczyk FZ: Immunoassays. In Mishell DR Jr, Davajan V, Lobo RA (eds): Infertility, Contraception and Reproductive Endocrinology, 3rd ed. Cambridge, MA, Blackwell Scientific, 1991.

Four characteristics of assays apply to each of these techniques: sensitivity, specificity, accuracy, and precision. Sensitivity is the least amount of substance that can be measured in the assay. Specificity is the ability of the assay to measure only one substance and not allow the measurement to be altered by the presence of other substances (cross-reaction). Accuracy is the ability to measure the exact amount of substance in the sample; thus specimens (quality controls) containing known low and high values of the substance to be measured are always included in each assay. Precision is the ability of the assay to consistently reproduce the same results. Precision is determined by measuring the within-assay, or intra-assay, coefficient of variation (CV) and the between-assay, or interassay, CV. The intra-assay CV is calculated by determining the amounts of a known sample measured in about 10 replicates in the same assay.

$$CV = \frac{\text{standard deviation}}{N\ \text{mean}} \times 100$$

The interassay CV is determined by measuring the same unknown sample on different days. The intra-assay CV should be less than 10%, and the interassay CV should be less than 15% for satisfactory precision of the assay.

The normal range of values of hormones in normal women is frequently expressed in terms of the mean level plus the mathematically calculated 95% confidence limits (±2 SD). However, the distributions of hormone levels in the menstrual cycles of a group of women with normal ovulation have been shown to follow a log-normal distribution instead of a gaussian (normal) distribution. Although results of normal values usually vary from laboratory to laboratory, the 95% confidence limits of measurement of reproductive hormones among women in our laboratory are listed in Table 4-8 as a guide of normality.

KEY POINTS

- The hypothalamic hormone that controls gonadotropin release, namely gonadotropin-releasing hormone (GnRH), is a decapeptide.
- The cell bodies of the hypothalamic neurons that produce GnRH are concentrated mainly in two areas: the anterior hypothalamus and the medial basal (tuberal) hypothalamus.
- GnRH can be released both in large amounts periodically via the tuberoinfundibular tract (cyclic release) and in a low-grade continuous transependymal fashion (tonic release) via the tanycytes.
- GnRH is secreted in a pulsatile manner. The amplitude and frequency of the pulses vary throughout the menstrual cycle. The frequency is rapid in the follicular phase, about one pulse per hour, and slower in the luteal phase, about one pulse every 2 or 3 hours.
- The most important neurotransmitters involved in reproductive neuroendocrinology are two catecholamines, dopamine and norepinephrine, as well as an indolamine, serotonin.
- Infusion of β-endorphin results in an increase in prolactin and a decrease in luteinizing hormone (LH), the latter occurring by an inhibitory effect on GnRH neurons in the hypothalamus.
- Peripheral measurement of plasma β-endorphin levels does not reflect levels in the central nervous system circulation.
- The peptide hormones, such as GnRH, bind to specific receptors on the surface membrane of the target cell, in contrast to steroid hormones, which pass through the cell membrane to bind to intracellular receptors.
- When a protein hormone binds to its specific receptor, it activates or inhibits the enzyme adenyl cyclase, the second messenger, which in turn changes the concentration of adenosine 3′,5′-cyclic monophosphate (cyclic-AMP, cAMP).
- The various growth factors provide hormonal effects within the ovary by both autocrine and paracrine mechanisms.
- Inhibin inhibits pituitary follicle-stimulating hormone (FSH) release, whereas in the ovarian follicle inhibin stimulates

Continued

KEY POINTS *Continued*

progesterone and inhibits estradiol production. Activins have an opposite action to inhibins by stimulating pituitary FSH release and opposing ovarian action by inhibiting progesterone and stimulating estradiol.

- Biosynthesis of prostanoids from arachidonic acid and other precursors takes place via the cyclic endoperoxides, prostaglandins G and H (PGG and PGH). Prostanoids are produced intracellularly shortly before they are released and generally act locally, in contrast to steroids.
- Following a single intravenous bolus of GnRH, the LH levels peak in 30 minutes and FSH in 60 minutes.
- With a constant infusion of GnRH there is a biphasic release of LH but not of FSH. The initial increase of LH occurs 30 minutes, and the second, 90 minutes after the start of the infusion.
- When stimulation by hormone is maximal, the unoccupied receptors become refractory to hormone binding for 12 to 72 hours. This phenomenon has allowed frequent administration of GnRH analogues to be used clinically to inhibit FSH and LH levels, and thus decrease steroidogenesis.
- GnRH analogues are synthesized by substitution of amino acids in the parent molecule at the 6 and 10 positions. The various agonists have greater potencies and longer half-lives than the parent GnRH.
- LH and FSH have the same α subunit, which is similar in structure to the α subunit of thyroid-stimulating hormone (TSH) and human chorionic gonadotropin (HCG). The β subunits of all these hormones have different amino acids and carbohydrates, which provide specific biologic activity.
- The half-life of LH is more rapid (30 minutes) than that of FSH (3.9 hours).
- LH acts primarily on the theca cells to induce steroidogenesis, whereas FSH acts primarily on the granulosa cells to stimulate follicular growth.
- LH acts on the theca cells to produce androgens, which are then transported to the granulosa cells, where they are aromatized to estrogens.
- After sufficient LH receptors have been produced by the action of FSH and estradiol, LH acts directly on the granulosa cells to cause luteinization and production of progesterone.
- The ovary secretes three principal steroid hormones: estradiol from the follicle, progesterone from the corpus luteum, and androstenedione from the stroma.
- Pregnenolone, 17-hydroxypregnenolone, progesterone, 17-hydroxyprogesterone, and corticosteroids have 21 carbon atoms; androgens (testosterone and androstenedione) have 19 carbon atoms; estrogens have 18 carbon atoms and a phenolic ring A.
- Because the ovaries lack 21-hydroxylase, 11-β-hydroxylase, and 18-hydroxylase reductase activity, they are unable to synthesize mineralocorticoids or glucocorticoids.
- Estradiol and estrone are interconverted outside the ovary. Estrone is then converted to estrone sulfate, which has a long half-life and is the largest component of the pool of circulating estrogens.
- The greater the amount of fat tissue present, the greater is the percentage of androstenedione that is converted to estrone. In a normal individual, about 1.3% of the daily 3000 μg of androstenedione produced is converted to estrone (40 μg), whereas in an obese individual as much as 7% of the 3000 μg is converted (200 μg).
- The process by which steroids are conjugated involves the transformation of lipophilic compounds, which are only sparingly soluble in water, into metabolites (sulfates and glucuronides) that are readily water-soluble and can therefore be eliminated in urine. Progesterone first undergoes extensive reduction of its double bond and ketone group(s) before it is conjugated. Its major urinary metabolite is pregnanediol glucuronide. The major urinary metabolites of estradiol and estrone are glucuronides and sulfates of estrone, estradiol, and estriol.
- Sex hormone-binding globulin (SHBG) primarily binds dihydrotestosterone, testosterone, and estradiol. About 65% of circulating testosterone is bound to SHBG and 30% to albumin. Approximately 2% remains unbound or free.
- Corticosteroid-binding globulin (CBG) binds with highest affinity to cortisol, corticosterone, and 11-deoxycortisol, and to a lesser extent to progesterone.
- Estrogen stimulates the synthesis of both estrogen and progesterone receptors in target tissues, and progestins inhibit the synthesis of both estrogen and progesterone receptors.
- Just before birth the primary oocytes, which at that time number 2 to 4 million, reach the diplotene stage, also called the germinal vesicle stage of development.
- Estradiol stimulates preantral follicle growth, reduces follicular atresia, and increases FSH action on the granulosa cells. Testosterone increases follicular atresia and prevents preantral follicle growth.
- The follicle destined to become dominant secretes the greatest amount of estradiol, which in turn increases the density of FSH receptors.
- With ultrasound it has been found that there is a steady increase in follicular diameter and volume that parallels the rise in estradiol. The dominant follicle has a maximal mean diameter of about 19.5 mm, with a range of 18 to 25 mm just before ovulation. The mean maximal follicular volume is 3.8 mL, with a range of 3.1 to 8.2 mL.
- Ovulation occurs about 24 hours after the estradiol peak, as well as 32 hours after the initial rise in LH, and about 12 to 16 hours after the peak of LH levels in serum.
- The midcycle LH surge initiates germinal vesicle disruption, and metaphase I is completed. As the oocyte enters metaphase II, the first polar body appears. Completion of meiosis and extrusion of the second polar body occur only when a sperm penetrates the ovum.
- By serial ultrasound observation and LH measurements, ovulation usually occurs within 24 hours and always within 48 hours after the peak in LH.
- Beginning in the midluteal phase, progesterone is secreted in a pulsatile manner, occurring immediately following an LH pulse.
- Serum levels of estradiol rise from less than 50 pg/mL in the early follicular phase to 200 to 500 pg/mL at midcycle and have a broad luteal-phase peak level of about 100 to 300 pg/mL.

KEY POINTS *Continued*

- Progesterone levels in serum are less than 1 ng/mL before ovulation and reach midluteal levels of 10 to 20 ng/mL.
- During a normal ovulatory cycle at midcycle, the first event is a rise in estradiol. When estradiol reaches peak levels, there is an abrupt increase (surge) in LH and FSH. The increase in LH reaches a peak in about 18 hours, and peak levels plateau for about 14 hours, after which there is a decline. The mean duration of the LH surge is about 24 hours. Beginning about 12 hours before the onset of the LH surge, there is an increase of both progesterone and 17-hydroxyprogesterone.
- With the occurrence of the LH peak, there is a decline in estradiol and a further increase in progesterone. This shift in steroidogenesis in favor of progesterone instead of estradiol production is brought about by the luteinization of the granulosa cells produced by LH.
- Menstrual cycle length is most irregular in the 2 years after menarche and the 3 years before menopause, times of life during which anovulatory cycles are most frequent.
- The mean duration of menstrual cycle length is 28 ± 7 days, with menstruation in which cycles occur at more frequent intervals (<21 days) being called polymenorrhea, and that in which cycles are less frequent (>35 days) being called oligomenorrhea. The mean duration of menstrual flow is 4 ± 2 days.
- Only the spiral arteries that supply the upper two thirds of the endometrium become coiled and constrict.
- After menstruation, regeneration of the endometrium comes from cells in the spongiosum that were previously a portion of the secretory endometrium and not from the stratum basale, as previously believed.
- The endometrium produces growth factors, prostaglandins, and peptide hormones, including a specific peptide called pregnancy-associated endometrial protein.
- The subjective method of correlating the degree of maturation in the endometrium by histologic visualization is relatively imprecise, and more precise indices based on quantitative morphometric analysis have been developed. To date the endometrium most accurately, the maturation should be correlated with the days after LH peak, not the number of days before the onset of the next menstrual period.
- There are extreme variations in the amounts of endometrial shedding in different areas of the same uterus, as well as variations among different uteri removed by hysterectomy.
- Menstruation in humans is probably a combination of some superficial tissue shedding, brought about by ischemia and the presence of hydrolytic enzymes and possibly relaxin, as well as mainly by tissue regression and reorganization of the endometrial cells.
- Just after ovulation, glycogen-rich subnuclear vacuoles appear in the base of the cells lining the glands. This subnuclear vacuolization is the first histologic indication of the effect of progesterone, but is not evidence that ovulation has occurred.
- Enzyme-linked immunosorbent assay (ELISA), or "sandwich," techniques have been developed to measure protein hormones (e.g., LH, FSH, HCG), with the use of monoclonal antibodies against the α and β subunits. The endpoint is a color reaction and can be read in a spectrophotometer.
- There are four characteristics of hormone assays that establish their reliability: sensitivity, specificity, accuracy, and precision.

BIBLIOGRAPHY

Bächström CT, McNeilly AS, Leask RM, et al: Pulsatile secretion of LH, FSH, prolactin, oestradiol and progesterone during the human menstrual cycle. Clin Endocrinol 17:29, 1982.

Bakos O, Lundkvist O, Wide L, Bergh T: Ultrasonographical and hormonal description of the normal ovulatory menstrual cycle. Acta Obstet Gynecol Scand 73:790, 1994.

Brzech PR, Jakimiuk J, Agarwal SK, et al: Serum immunoreactive leptin concentrations in women with polycystic ovary syndrome. J Clin Endocrinol Metab 81:4166, 1966.

Chehab FF, Mounzih K, Lu R, Lim ME: Early onset of reproductive function in normal female mice treated with leptin. Science 275:88, 1997.

Chikasawa K, Araki S, Tameda T: Morphological and endocrinological studies on follicular development during the human menstrual cycle. J Clin Endocrinol Metab 62:305, 1986.

Clark JR, Dierschke DJ, Wolf RC: Hormonal regulation of ovarian folliculogenesis in rhesus monkeys. III. Atresia of the preovulatory follicle induced by exogenous steroids and subsequent follicular development. Biol Reprod 25:3320, 1981.

Crowley WF Jr, Filicori M, Spratt DI, et al: The physiology of gonadotropin-releasing hormone (GnRH) secretion in men and women. Recent Prog Horm Res 41:501, 1985.

Diczfalusy E, Landgren BM: Hormonal changes in the menstrual cycle. In Diczfalusy E, Diczfalusy A (eds): Regulation of Human Fertility. Copenhagen, Scriptor, 1977.

di Zerega GS, Hodgen GD: The interovarian progesterone gradient: A trial and temporal regulator of folliculogenesis in the primate ovarian cycle. J Clin Endocrinol Metab 54:495; 1982.

Eissa MK, Obhrai MS, Docker MF, et al: Follicular growth and endocrine profiles in spontaneous and induced conception cycles. Fertil Steril 45:191, 1986.

Felberbaum RE, Germe U, Ludwig M, et al: Treatment of uterine fibroids with a slow-release formulation of the gonadotropin releasing hormone antagonist Cetrorlix. Human Reprod 13(6):1660, 1998.

Ferenczy A: Studies on the cytodynamics of human endometrial regeneration. Am J Obstet Gynecol 124:64, 1976.

Filicori M, Santoro N, Merriam GR, et al: Characterization of the physiological pattern of episodic gonadotropin secretion throughout the human menstrual cycle. J Clin Endocrinol Metab 62(6):1136, 1986.

Flowers CE, Wilborn WH: New observations on the physiology of menstruation. Obstet Gynecol 51:16, 1978.

Frisch RE: Body fat, menarche, and reproductive ability. Semin Reprod Endocrinol 3:45, 1985.

Knobil E: The neuroendocrine control of the menstrual cycle. Recent Prog Horm Res 36:53, 1980.

Laughlin GA, Yen SSC: Serum leptin levels in women with polycystic ovarian syndrome: The role of insulin resistance/ hyperinsulinemia. J Clin Endocrinol Metab 82:1692, 1997.

Lemay A, Maheux R, Faure N, et al: Reversible hypogonadism induced by a LH-RH agonist (Buserelin) as a new therapeutic approach for endometriosis. Fertil Steril 41:863, 1984.

Li TC, Dockery P, Rogers AW, et al: How precise is histologic dating of endometrium using the standard dating criteria? Fertil Steril 51:759, 1989.

Li TC, Rogers AW, Lenton EA, et al: A comparison between two methods of chronological dating of human endometrial biopsies during the luteal phase, and their correlation with histologic dating. Fertil Steril 48:928, 1987.

Li TC, Rogers AW, Dockery P, et al: A new method of histologic dating of human endometrium in the luteal phase. Fertil Steril 50:52, 1988.

Lin D, Sugawara T, Strauss JF, III, et al: Role of steroidogenic acute regulatory protein in adrenal and gonadal steroidogenesis. Science 267;1828, 1995.

MacDonald PC, Rombant RP, Siitari PK: Plasma precursion of estrogen. I. Extent of conversion of plasma Δ4 in adrenalectamized females. J Clin Endocrinol 27:1103, 1967.

McLennan CE, Rydell AH: Extent of endometrial shedding during normal menstruation. Obstet Gynecol 26:605, 1965.

Nogales-Ortiz F, Puerta J, Nogales FF Jr: The normal menstrual cycle, J Obstet Gynecol 51:259, 1978.

Nolan JJ, Olefsky JM, Nyce MR, et al: Effect of troglitazone on leptin production: studies in vitro and in human subjects. Diabetes 45:1276, 1996.

Reame N, Sauder SE, Kelch RP, et al: Pulsatile gonadotropin secretion during the human menstrual cycle: Evidence for altered frequency of gonadotropin-releasing hormone secretion. J Clin Endocrinol Metab 59:328, 1984.

Reissman T, Felberbaum R, Diedrich K, et al: Development and applications of luteinizing hormone-releasing hormone antagonists in the treatment of infertility: An overview. Hum Reprod 10(8):1974-81, 1995.

Ross GT, Cagrille CM, Lipsett MB, et al: Pituitary and gonadal hormones in women during spontaneous and induced ovulatory cycles. Recent Prog Horm Res 26:1, 1970.

Treloar AE, Boynton RE, Borghild BG, et al: Variation of the human menstrual cycle through reproductive life. Int J Fertil 12:77, 1967.

Yalow RS, Berson SA: Assay of plasma insulin in human subjects by immunological methods. Nature 184:1648, 1959.

Zegers-Hochschild F, Lira CG, Parada M, et al: A comparative study of the follicular growth profile in conception and nonconception cycles. Fertil Steril 41:244, 1984.

Evidence-Based Medicine and Clinical Epidemiology 5

Vern L. Katz

KEY TERMS AND DEFINITIONS

Attributable Risk. The excess cases or the fraction of a disease in the population that is due to a particular factor or exposures. Also the population excess rate or the rate difference.

Bias. Any effect, at any stage of investigation or inference, tending to produce results that departs systematically from the true values (to be distinguished from random error). The term *bias* does not necessarily carry an imputation of prejudice or other subjective factor, such as the experimenter's desire for a particular outcome. This differs from conventional usage in which bias refers to a partisan point of view.

Case-Control Study. A study that starts with the identification of persons with the disease (or other outcome variable) of interest and a suitable control (comparison, reference) group of persons without the disease. The relationship of an attribute to the disease is examined by comparing the diseased and nondiseased with regard to how frequently the attribute is present or, if quantitative, the levels of the attribute in each of the groups.

Clinical Practice Guideline. A systematically developed statement designed to assist clinician and patient decisions about appropriate health care for specific clinical circumstances.

Cohort. 1. The component of the population born during a particular period and identified by period of birth so that its characteristics (e.g., causes of death and numbers still living) can be ascertained as it enters successive time and age periods. 2. The term *cohort* has broadened to describe any designated group of persons who are followed or traced over a period of time, as in cohort study (prospective study).

Cohort Study. Involves identification of two groups (cohorts) of patients one that received the exposure of interest and one that did not, and following these cohorts forward for the outcome of interest.

Confidence Interval, Confidence Limits. A range of values determined by the degree of presumed random variability in the data, within which the point estimate is thought to lie, with the specified level of confidence. The boundaries of a confidence interval are the confidence limits. The confidence interval is symmetric around the point estimate. If the confidence interval overlaps 1.0, the change in risk is statistically insignificant.

Confounding. A situation in which the effects of two processes are not separated. The distortion of the apparent effect of an exposure brought about by the association with other factors that can influence an outcome.

Epidemiology. The study of the distribution and determinants of health-related states and events in a population, and the application of this study to control of health problems.

Evidence-Based Medicine. The conscientious, explicit, and judicious use of current best evidence in making decisions about the care of individual patients. The practice of evidence-based medicine means integrating individual clinical expertise with the best available external clinical evidence from systematic research.

Incidence. The proportion of new cases of the target disorder in the population at risk during a specified time interval.

Meta-Analysis. A systematic review that uses quantitative methods to summarize the results. Meta-analysis is a collection of techniques to produce a pooled effect estimate from several studies.

Observational Study (nonexperimental study, survey). Epidemiologic study in situations where nature is allowed to take its course; changes or differences in one characteristic are studied in relation to changes or differences in other(s), without the intervention of the investigator.

Odds Ratio (cross-product ratio, relative odds). The ratio of two odds. Consider the following notation for the distribution of a binary exposure and a disease in a population or a sample:

	Exposed	Unexposed
Disease	*a*	*b*
No disease	*c*	*d*

The odds ratio (cross-product ratio) is *ad/bc*. The exposure-odds ratio for a set of case-control data is the ratio of the odds in favor of exposure among the cases *(a/b)* to the odds in favor of exposure among noncases *(c/d)*. This reduces to *ad/bc*. With incident cases, unbiased subject selection, and a rare disease (say, less than 2% cumulative incidence rate over the study period), *ad/bc* is an approximate estimate of the risk ratio.

Outcomes. All possible results that may stem from exposure to a causal factor or from preventive or therapeutic interventions; all identified changes in health status arising as a consequence of the handling of a health problem.

Positive Predictive Value. Proportion of people with a positive test who have the target disorder.

Power. Relative frequency with which a true difference (of specified size) between populations would be detected by the experiment or test. It is equal to 1 minus the probability of type II error.

KEY TERMS AND DEFINITIONS *Continued*

Precision. The quality of being sharply defined or stated. One measure of precision is the number of distinguishable alternatives from which a measurement was selected, sometimes indicated by the number of significant digits in the measurement. Another measure of precision is the standard error of measurement, the standard deviation of a series of replicate determinations of the same quantity. In statistics, precision is defined as the inverse of the variance of a measurement or estimate.

Random Error (sampling error). Error due to chance, when the result obtained in the sample differs from the result that would be obtained if the entire population ("universe") were studied. Two varieties of sampling error are type I, or alpha error, and type II, or beta error. In an experiment, if the experimental procedures do not in reality have any effect, an apparent difference between experimental and control groups may nevertheless be observed by chance, a phenomenon known as type I error. Another possibility is that the treatment is effective but by chance the difference is not detected on statistical analysis-type II error. In the theory of testing hypothesis, rejecting a null hypothesis when it is incorrect is called "type I error." Accepting a null hypothesis when it is incorrect is called "type II error."

Randomized Control Clinical Trial (RCT). A group of subjects is randomized into an experimental group and a control group. These groups are followed up for the variables/outcomes of interest.

Relative Risk. The ratio of the risk of disease or death among those exposed to the risk divided by those unexposed; this usage is synonymous with risk ratio. Alternatively, the ratio of the cumulative incidence rate in those exposed relative to the cumulative incidence rate in those unexposed (i.e., the cumulative incidence ratio). The term *relative risk* has also been used synonymously with odds ratio and, in some biostatistical articles, has been used for the ratio of the forces of morbidity. The use of the term *relative risk* for several different quantities arises from the fact that for rare diseases (e.g., most cancers) all the quantities approximate one another. For common occurrences (e.g., neonatal mortality in infants under 1500 g birth weight), the approximations do not hold.

Risk Ratio (RR). The ratio of risk measured in the treated group (ERR) to risk measured in the control group. Used in randomized trials and cohort studies: RR = ERR/CER.

Sensitivity. The proportion of persons in the screened population who truly have the disease and are identified as diseased by the screening test. Sensitivity is the measure of the probability of correctly diagnosing a case or the probability that any given case will be identified by the test.

Specificity. The proportion of truly nondiseased persons who are so identified by the screening test. It is a measure of the probability of correctly identifying a nondiseased person with a screening test.

Surrogate Marker. A measured observation in a study that is used to approximate a clinical endpoint.

Systematic Review. A summary of the medical literature that uses explicit methods to perform a thorough literature search and critical appraisal of individual studies and that uses appropriate statistical techniques to combine these valid studies.

Therapeutic equipoise. The situation at which the relative therapeutic values and risks of two treatments are approximately equivalent.

The ongoing explosion of knowledge in the basic and clinical sciences presents a challenge to clinicians. The fundamental task of medical science is to take the knowledge of embryology, genetics, anatomy, and endocrinology and apply this knowledge to clinical problems. The leap from bench to bedside, however, is vast and uncertain, and the results can be inadequate. Clinical epidemiology comprises a set of methods that can help us directly at the bedside as well as inform public health decisions. The results of observational epidemiologic studies, such as case reports, help by generating hypotheses about diseases that can be tested in the laboratory. Experimental studies in humans, the randomized clinical trials (RCT), serve to test hypotheses that arise in the laboratory to see if they may apply to clinical practice as predicted. The main goal of trials is to move from association to the establishment of cause and effect, and to assess efficacy of treatments.

This chapter presents the basics of epidemiologic study design and the statistical terminology commonly used to present results of clinical studies; statistical methods per se are not covered here. We also discuss approaches for interpreting study results. Finally, we consider new, explicit approaches to combining data from different studies that are used to prepare evidence reviews and clinical guidelines. This information will help the clinician read and interpret the clinical literature.

EVIDENCE-BASED MEDICINE

Evidence-based medicine relies on the assessment of our full body of knowledge, which is usually not limited to a single study. The process of evidence-based medicine starts with formulating a specific clinical question and then finding the best and most appropriate research evidence. Research evidence only rarely applies exactly to an individual, or to her particular clinical problem. Therefore, the research evidence must be evaluated for specific context, and integrated with clinical expertise as well as the preferences and values of each woman. The process is motivated by the need for up-to-date and valid information regarding diagnosis, prognosis, therapy, and preventive services. Practicing evidence-based medicine has become possible in large part because of the development of information systems that allow us to search for relevant clinical data. At best, we can look for data using the Internet right at the bedside or in the clinic to address specific questions that apply to a current individual. The bedside practice of evidence-based medicine can be efficient and practical if we learn to find and use sources that synthesize and summarize the effects of the interventions we are interested in.

To make the assessment of evidence more uniform, a grading system that rates studies according to quality is often used (Table

Table 5-1 Categorizing the Level of Evidence

Level	Evidence
I	Blinded randomized controlled trial
II-1	Controlled trials without randomization
II-2	Well-designed cohort and case-control studies
II-3	Cross-sectional studies, studies with external control groups, or ecologic studies
III	Case series evidence-derived from report of an expert committee, which itself used a scientific approach.

Modified from The periodic health examination. Canadian Task Force on the Periodic Health Examination. CMAJ 121:1193–1254, 1979.

5-1). This grading system rates blinded randomized clinical trial as the highest level of evidence. Following this are controlled trials without randomization. The next level of evidence comes from cohort studies and case-control studies. Although results taken from cross-sectional studies, studies that rely on external control groups, and ecologic studies are a lesser level of evidence, they often remain valuable specifically because of the lack of higher levels of evidence. All of these sources of evidence are more valuable than opinion, regardless of the credentials of the individual, committee, or organization that might publish an opinion. The lowest grade are case series. The basic element or unit, as described by Grimes and Schulz (2002a, pp 145–149), is the case report. This is not to say that case reports are not valuable. It was through a report of a few cases of unusual infections and disturbed immunity that AIDS was first described. Case reports, series, and cross-sectional studies are hypothesis-generating. They do not prove causality, though!

Individual studies often have imprecise results, statistical methods to combine results from several studies sometimes can be helpful. *Meta-analysis* is a collection of techniques to produce a pooled effect estimate from several studies. Meta-analysis at its best involves pooling and reanalyzing raw data from several similar randomized trials to produce a result with a tighter confidence interval. Several statistical approaches are used, but the main purpose of any meta-analysis is to improve precision. Many meta-analyses combine data from observational studies (rather than randomized trials), but these must be interpreted with extreme caution because the individual studies always vary in population, entry criteria, case definition, and exposure definitions, and these differences make combining the data problematic. This is particularly true if the analysis combines data from published tables rather than combining the raw data from the original studies. If the results from individual studies disagree in direction or report very different results, then meta-analysis is not appropriate. Often the main value of a meta-analysis proves to be the rigorous approach to collecting, evaluating, and presenting together all of the relevant data regarding a particular problem.

Because of the clinical need for good evidence, and because of the need for synthesis of evidence that goes beyond opinion, additional approaches to reviews are being developed and used. *Systematic reviews* include a comprehensive review and evaluation of the literature. Systematic reviews are reported using a standardized format that must include a detailed description of the search strategy used to identify the relevant literature and the results of the search. Systematic reviews also carry out critical appraisal of the studies they evaluate. Critical appraisal employs a rigid standardized assessment of the relevance and quality of each study. The goal of systematic reviews is to synthesize the literature regarding a specific clinical question and to use an approach that will minimize bias and random error.

Journal articles may present a summary of an evidence review, but readers generally have to go to sources on the Web to find complete documentation of these reviews. The major source of systematic reviews is the Cochrane Collaboration (www.cochrane.org). This collaboration is an international organization that aims to help people make well-informed decisions about health care by preparing, maintaining, and promoting the accessibility of systematic reviews of the effects of health care interventions. There are review groups for more than 50 areas of medicine including several that are relevant to gynecology; the groups in each area prepare and electronically publish systematic reviews. The U.S. Preventive Services Task Force also performs systematic reviews regarding clinical preventive services; these are published in book form and increasingly as electronic publications by the Agency for Healthcare Research and Quality (ARHQ). To help translate these often lengthy reviews into briefer, clinically useful documents, many professional groups have begun to issue practice guidelines to assist clinicians in making patient care decisions. An electronic collection of such guidelines is now available; to be accepted for electronic publication, the guideline must specify the search strategy that was used to obtain the evidence and must specify the methods of data synthesis (www.guidelines.gov).

Recommendations are often graded, but the systems for grading evidence and practice recommendations are continuing to evolve. In general, recommendations for or against clinical interventions need to specify whether they are based on ample or sparse evidence, and whether the evidence comes from randomized trials or from lesser studies. Even with recommendations based on ample evidence from RCTs, clinicians will always need to decide individually whether the available evidence applies to their practice setting and whether it applies directly to their specific patient's problem.

ESSENTIALS OF STUDY DESIGN

The basic purpose of an epidemiologic study is to estimate the relationship between an exposure and an outcome in order to assess causality. An exposure can be a behavior, a genetic factor, a screening program, or any aspect of a treatment. An outcome might be a symptom, a measure of functional status, the development of disease, or a change in the course of an existing disease. Some studies are primarily descriptive, providing statistics about incidence, prevalence, and mortality rates of diseases in particular populations. Descriptive studies are important to the clinician in order to provide a context—the most dramatic new research findings always must be interpreted with respect to the frequency and characteristics of the disease in one's own patient population. Descriptive studies can also help generate new hypotheses, but studies with this design do not serve to test hypotheses or answer etiologic questions. No matter the plausibility, every clinician must read descriptive studies with a cautious interpretation. The most basic element or unit of the descriptive study is the case report. Case reports are valuable initial descriptions of unusual infections and abnormal immune responses.

More valuable to evidence-based medical practice are analytic epidemiologic studies that focus on establishing an association between a particular exposure (e.g., hormone replacement therapy) and the risk of a particular disease or outcome (e.g., reduction in the incidence of osteoporotic fractures). Analytic epidemiologic studies can be classified as experimental or observational. In experimental studies, the clinical investigator controls exposure to the factor of interest—the dependent variable. Experimental studies, or randomized controlled trials, are characterized by the prospective assignment of study participants to a study group (who receive the factor of interest, typically a new treatment) or a placebo, no treatment, or standard care group. Study groups, usually two, but often many more, are then followed over time to evaluate differences in outcomes. The outcomes may include prevention or cure of a disease, reduction in severity of the condition, or differences in costs, quality of life, or side effects between the treatments. The great feature of RCTs is that, through randomizing participants, they can equalize all other factors that might influence the study outcome and leave only the effect of the study treatment itself. RCTs usually provide the best evidence for making clinical decisions. Blinded RCT are superior to nonblinded because the investigators will not interpret the results with a bias. Despite the theoretical superiority of the RCT approach, these studies provide the best evidence only if the study has been thoughtfully designed, implemented with extraordinary care, and analyzed appropriately.

Subjects recruited for a trial must receive information about the study purpose, its procedures, the likely risks and benefits, and the available alternatives. Both ethical and practical considerations may limit the use of randomized trials to answer clinical questions. It is clearly unethical to expose anyone to a potential cause of disease simply to learn about its cause; thus patients would not be randomized to smoking in order to learn about the effect of tobacco on the ovary. RCTs are rarely used to address etiologic questions. To study the effect of a treatment, making comparisons with a placebo control group is usually most efficient. However, if an effective and accepted treatment exists, it is not ethical to use a placebo control group for studies of serious conditions in which the subject may experience harm due to lack of effective treatment. If the condition is mild, the treatment period is brief, or effective treatment is not generally available, many investigators believe that a placebo control group is ethical. For a clinician to recruit or refer patients into a clinical trial, it is essential the clinician believe, based on current evidence, that the study treatments may be similar or at least balanced in benefits and harms. This belief state is called *therapeutic equipoise.* If a clinician believes that evidence already exists to indicate a treatment is superior, then it is not ethical to recruit subjects into a comparative trial. In contrast, if the superior treatment is unclear, then a randomized trial is the most ethical approach for all patients because it provides them with an equal chance to undergo the better treatment and also may provide an unbiased answer to the clinical question more quickly so all future patients can benefit. Clearly, it is critical to be honest and humble about our current state of knowledge prior to planning any randomized clinical trial.

One problem, as mentioned earlier, is that subjects and controls in RCT are often special populations that may not be generalizable. This potential weakness of randomized trials is a problem of external validity. Can the results from a specific population with a tightly controlled treatment regimen be generalized to a diverse population in clinical practice—or as is often stated, "the real world." Often, the more sophisticated and complex the protocol, the greater the difference between RCT results and general clinical outcomes. This has been referred to as the difference between efficacy—"can it work," and effectiveness—"will it work." Importantly, RCT often use surrogate markers to substitute for clinical outcomes. Surrogate markers are easier to measure in shorter periods of time than the true clinical endpoint. However, surrogate markers may not always equate with the disease process being assessed. For example, the effects of a medication on lowering cholesterol is not necessarily the same as the prevention of heart attacks. Because osteoporotic fractures are rare and occur over a long time period, interventions may be assessed by the surrogate marker of bone mineral density. Fractures and bone mineral density change are not the same. Lactation lowers bone mineral density, and breast feeding does not necessarily increase the risk of fractures. When interpreting RCT surrogate markers must be used with caution.

Practical considerations frequently determine whether a clinical question will be addressed using a randomized trial. Acute clinical problems in which every patient has a relevant outcome in a short period of time are ideal to study using clinical trials. Gynecologic examples include comparisons of short-term pain or febrile morbidity following different surgical approaches, comparisons of cure rates or side effects in the treatment of infections, or pregnancy rates following different infertility treatment regimens. For clinical problems like these, clinicians should be able to rely on RCT data. In contrast, RCTs to study long-term or rare outcomes are much more difficult to carry out. If a treatment outcome is rare or takes years to develop (cancer being an excellent example of both), one needs a very large study over years or decades to answer the clinical question. Often cohort trials will be used to evaluate rare outcomes. Even when large trials like the Women's Health Initiative are implemented, clinicians usually have to rely on other data for clinical decision making during the many years before study results are available. Finally, because of the time, effort, and expense involved in carrying out an RCT, many questions of great clinical interest have not yet been addressed in this way.

Observational studies, in which the investigator does not control the exposure, provide an alternative approach to answering clinical questions. Depending on the data collection process, observational studies are classified as cross-sectional, cohort, or case-control studies. Cross-sectional studies generate prevalence data by examining the relationship between exposure and the outcomes of interest in a defined population at a single point in time. With reference to only a designated moment in time, these studies are not able to provide as strong causal evidence. However, cross-sectional studies can highlight associations that deserve additional evaluation.

Epidemiologic studies that may be used to provide stronger evidence than a cross-sectional analysis are cohort and case-control studies (Fig. 5-1). A cohort study selects a group of individuals at risk for the outcome of interest and divides them

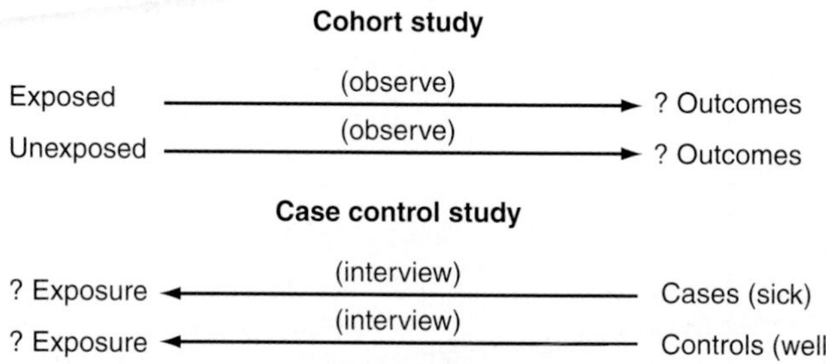

Figure 5-1. Schematic diagram of methodology used to estimate risk of exposure to outcome in cohort and case-control studies.

into subgroups based on the presence or absence of one or more exposures to be studied. Subgroups are then evaluated over time to count the outcomes as they occur. Unlike RCTs, in cohort studies, the exposure is selected by the individual subject, not by the investigator. Most studies of the long-term health effects of contraceptive methods have employed a cohort design where the subjects themselves decided which contraceptive method to use. A particular difficulty of this approach is that the subjects almost certainly differ in many characteristics beyond the main exposure of interest. When these other characteristics are related to both the exposure and the risk of experiencing an outcome, they can confound the results of the study. Age, for instance, is nearly always a confounding variable. Advancing age increases the risk of a heart attack and most other diseases and is also associated with very decreased use of oral contraceptives. If age is not accounted for in a statistical analysis, it might appear that oral contraceptives provide enormous protection against heart attacks because all of the (older) women experiencing heart attacks are not oral contraceptive users anymore. To the extent that information is collected about known or suspected confounding factors, it is possible to control their effect in the statistical analysis, and precise adjustment for age is needed in most studies. Adjustment techniques can work only for confounding variables that an investigator knows about and measures. A reason that RCTs provide stronger evidence than observational studies is that randomization balances confounding variables across the study groups, even confounders that are not recognized to be important at the time the study is performed.

A strength of cohort studies is the possibility of assessing many different outcomes over time, but a weakness is often the need to wait many years until enough outcomes occur to allow an analysis. Thanks to computerized databases of medical information, cohort studies can now sometimes be done historically; that is, the research question is formulated and the analyses are done years after the data have been collected and recorded for routine uses. This approach can be quick and very cost-effective, but the value of such studies is completely dependent on the quality of the original data. Information from large databases is dependent on exclusions, data entry, and limited input to name only a few factors.

Case-control studies are always retrospective. Study participants are selected on the basis of already having the outcome of interest (the case group) or of not having that outcome (the control group). Case status needs to be carefully defined and should include all cases of new-onset disease drawn from an identifiable population. Controls should be sampled from the same population; the purpose of the control group is to estimate the frequency in the population of the exposures being studied if there were no relationship with the disease being studied. In the past, investigators often found it convenient to select controls from among other patients found in the same hospital as the cases, but choosing controls from the general population is highly preferable. Similar to all studies (no matter the type) the ability to generalize from the study population to all populations determines the external validity of the study; its generalizability is a key feature. All clinicians evaluating a study should assess the study's "external validity." After identifying the cases and controls, data are then gathered, usually by interview, concerning past exposures. The exposure information from cases and controls is then compared quantitatively to obtain an estimate of risk. Case-control studies are quite useful for evaluating rare occurrences. As with cohort studies, statistical adjustment techniques are needed to account for confounding variables. The quality of the results from these studies is dependent on uniform, meticulous interview techniques when collecting data from cases and controls. Recall bias is a particular problem.

The case-control study is often the best approach to study rare diseases. A case-control study including only 8 cases and 31 controls was able to identify the strong association between vaginal adenocarcinoma and in utero exposure to diethylstilbestrol (DES). Although a randomized trial of DES had been performed to evaluate its now-recognized ineffectiveness in preventing spontaneous abortion, that study was not large enough or long enough to identify a rare cancer that was identified in daughters 20 years later.

The best experiment, to test causality, is the randomized, controlled trial. The investigator may control for differences between two groups except the treatment or exposure. This kind of evidence provides the strongest support for causal relationships. If a relative risk is strong, at least greater than 2.0 or less than 0.5, causality is a more likely explanation. Weaker associations can often be explained instead by confounding variables, and weak associations are frequently overinterpreted by enthusiastic investigators, worried patients, or sensationalistic media. Statistical testing is used to detect whether a study's findings are due to a chance occurrence—the traditional p value is the indication that of the finding likelihood that the results were "accidental" small sample size and low study power increases the likelihood of a chance result.

PRESENTATION OF STUDY RESULTS

Epidemiologic studies use a quantitative approach to describing both exposures and outcomes. Whether RCT, cohort study, or case-control study, all of these studies attempt to present their results as a single number, usually referred to as the point estimate, that quantifies the relationship between the exposure and the outcome. This number is an estimate of the truth rather than the truth itself because each study, however large, includes only a sample of all the people who are affected by the exposure–outcome relationship. The point estimate expresses the strength of the association between the exposure and outcome. In an RCT or a cohort study, the point estimate is

Table 5-2 Interpretation of Relative Risk (RR) and Odds Ratio (OR) Values

RR and ORs < 1.0 indicate protection from outcome.
RRs and ORs > 1.0 indicate risk of outcome.
RRs and ORs = 1.0 indicate no association to outcome.
For both RR and OR, the further away the value is from 1.0 the stronger the relationship.

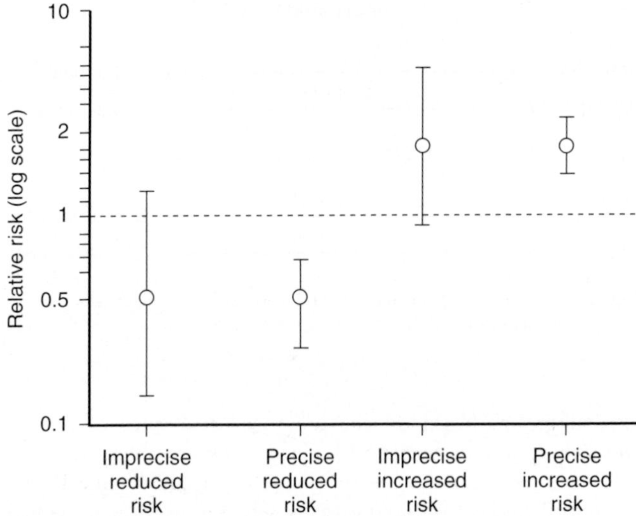

Figure 5-2. Examples of point estimates (*open circles*) and confidence intervals (*between the cross bars*) of two studies with reduced risk and two studies with increased risk. If confidence interval overlaps 1.0, the change in risk is statistically insignificant.

the relative risk (RR). Risk in the study subjects is the number of cases or outcomes that occur over time. The RR is simply the risk of disease (or other outcome) among the exposed or treated subjects divided by the risk in the unexposed subjects. A case-control study does not measure risk directly, but calculates its results as an odds ratio (OR), which is generally equivalent to a RR from a cohort study (Table 5-2).

If there is no association at all between the exposure and outcome, then the RR or OR would be 1.0. RRs and ORs greater than 1.0 indicate an increased risk of the outcome. RRs and ORs less than 1.0 indicate a decreased risk of the outcome. For both RRs and ORs the further away the value is from 1.0, the stronger the relationship between the exposure and the outcome (Fig. 5-2). Investigators do not limit the presentation of all of their analyses to a single point estimate. Usually RRs are presented separately for different doses (e.g., estrogen levels in the oral contraceptive) or durations of exposure (e.g., pack-years of cigarette smoking) or for subgroups of subjects (e.g., those with or without a family history of the outcome).

The RR is based on results from the people in a particular study and not the entire universe, thus there is always a possibility of sampling error. The quantitative description of the study results needs to include a measure of this uncertainty. The confidence interval is widely used to express the precision of the point estimate; a wide confidence interval indicates less precision, and a narrow confidence interval indicates more. In general, the larger the study, the narrower the confidence interval. There are several cautions about interpreting confidence intervals correctly. First, the confidence interval indicates only uncertainty that is due to the play of chance; it does not inform us about uncertainty in the results due to other factors such as uncontrolled confounding or peculiarities of the population that was studied or poor study quality. Second, a wide confidence interval does not mean there is no association between the exposure and the outcome; even an imprecise point estimate remains the best answer and the best explanation of the relationship until that estimate is supplanted by results from larger or better studies. Finally, confidence intervals are often drawn as a straight line around the point estimate to show the width of their range; this might seem to suggest that the location of the true point estimate would be equally likely to fall anywhere within that interval. In fact, the confidence interval could better be shown as a bell-shaped curve centered on the point estimate, and the true point estimate thus is most likely to be close to the center of the range.

Relative risk estimates do not take into account the incidence or the importance of the problem being evaluated. A relative risk of 4 says that the outcome increases 400% in exposed individuals compared with unexposed individuals. This increase often causes great worry or excitement, but needs to be interpreted in the context of the frequency of the outcome. For instance, the incidence of venous thromboembolism (VTE) in young women without using oral contraceptives is about 1 in 10,000, and the incidence while using oral contraceptives is 4 in 10,000; thus the relative risk is 4. The absolute risk of VTE is still low in both groups of women with a difference in risk of 3 in 10,000. The risk in the exposed minus the risk in the unexposed is the risk difference. The *risk difference* describes the size of the effect in absolute terms. This is also called *attributable risk,* and it is very useful for putting large relative risks into a clinically useful perspective. This is also called the *absolute risk reduction* when a benefit is identified, and the *absolute risk increase* when a harm is identified.

For clinicians and patients, even the calculation of absolute risk differences in a population may not seem a very helpful way to assess possible risks and benefits in personal terms. An alternative calculation looks at the complementary concept: how many patients need to be treated to observe one benefit or one adverse event? The number of patients who need to be treated to achieve one additional good outcome is the reciprocal of the absolute risk reduction (the risk difference for good outcomes). The number of patients who, if they received the treatment, would lead to one additional patient being harmed, compared with patients not receiving the treatment, is the reciprocal of the absolute risk increase (the risk difference for bad outcomes). Thus, using the example of oral contraceptives, with a treatment effectiveness of about 97%, and a risk of VTE of 4 in 10,000, the number needed to treat (NNT) to avoid one pregnancy is 1.03 (the reciprocal of 0.97, which is the absolute risk reduction) and the number needed to harm (NNH), that is, to experience one extra VTE, is 3333 (the reciprocal of 3 in 10,000, which is the absolute risk increase). The effectiveness of oral contraceptives and other contraceptives is extraordinarily high, and because pregnancy is extremely common in the absence of contraception, the NNT is close to 1, that is, one treatment yields one good outcome. In contrast, for most preventive services, the outcome to prevent is less common and the treatment is less effective;

thus, in providing drug therapy to prevent osteoporotic fractures in menopausal women, the NNT is generally greater than 20. Calculations of NNT and NNH are increasingly being used to calculate the potential benefits and harms of therapies, preventive services, and screening tests. A benefit of these calculations is that they allow us to compare benefits and harms across different treatment strategies.

INTERPRETATION OF STUDY RESULTS

Most associations found in a study do not represent a cause and effect relationship. We can attempt to assess whether causation is a good explanation of an association based on the quality of the study, the design of the study, and other specific criteria. Making these assessments is a critical part of evidence-based medicine. Studies must be free of bias, or in other words, have internal validity. Grimes and Schulz (2002b) have described three main categories of bias that distort the internal validity of a study: selection, information, and confounding bias.

Selection bias is an error due to systematic differences in characteristics between those selected to participate in the study and those who are not selected. For instance, women without health insurance might never have a chance to enter a study because they cannot be seen at the center where the study is offered; women who are very busy with work and home responsibilities might not have the time to meet study requirements; study results thus may only apply to the subset of women who have an opportunity to enter a study. Biases may also be due to diagnostic testing. For instance, women who take oral contraceptives may see their physician more often than women who have undergone tubal ligation. Consequently, women using oral contraceptives may undergo more screening and diagnostic tests, and diseases may be uncovered more often in this group.

Information bias may occur when data about subjects are obtained differently in the different study groups. An example is recall bias. This occurs because recall of information is affected by illness, which can be a major problem for retrospective studies. Women (or their families) with an illness may recall in great detail all events they believe might be associated with the illness, whereas healthy controls may not remember similar exposures. Sometimes information in the study group is obtained by chart review, but in the control group, interviewers or mail surveys are used to collect data. Several other factors can bias the assessment of information. First, is the intense surveillance of patients who are placed on a new therapy compared with those taking an older, conventional therapy. This often leads to more complete identification of adverse events among those using newer therapy. Conversely, the long-term users of any treatment tend to be unusually healthy and free of side effects because all those who don't tolerate the treatment will have stopped using it. These biases tend to make new treatments appear more dangerous and old treatments safer than they really are.

Confounding biases exist when the exposure creates associated conditions that may affect outcomes. For example, women who have undergone surgery for cervical cancer will usually have general anesthesia, but women being treated with radiation don't. In theory the anesthesia may produce side effects unrelated to the specific outcomes of surgery vs. radiation. Confounding

Table 5-3 Bradford-Hill Criteria for Causation

Experiment	Investigator control or laboratory experiments
Strength	Size of RR (>2.0 or <0.5)
Consistency	Similar RR in several studies
Gradient	Dose-response relationship
Biologic plausibility	Physiologic explanation for association
Specificity	Outcome only associated with intervention
Temporality	Exposure precedes outcome
Analogy	Similar association in other related diseases or exposures
Coherence	Evidence from different sources fits together

RR, relative risk.
From Bradford-Hill A: Principles of Medical Statistics, 9th ed. New York, Oxford University Press, 1971, p 309.

biases are one of the most common problems of observational studies. Often statistical techniques, such as multivariate analysis and logistic regression, are used to help eliminate confounders.

Distinguishing whether findings in a study are associations or are causal is essential to clinical care. If an association is strong (i.e., the relative risk is far from 1.0) and precise (i.e., narrow confidence intervals), and if the risk or benefit is clinically important based on the context, then it is particularly important to assess causality. The Bradford-Hill criteria are a valuable approach to differentiate causality from association (Table 5-3). In the United States these criteria are often referred to as the surgeon general's criteria because of their initial use in interpretation of evidence regarding cigarette smoking and lung cancer. Most of the principles of causality are intuitive.

The presence of a dose-response effect or duration-response effect also supports a causal association as when a higher dose or a longer treatment is associated with a better treatment response. In contradistinction, peculiar dose-response effects indicate the need for more study to understand the effect. Biologic plausibility also needs to be considered in evaluating results, especially from observational studies; our knowledge of physiology can often support, refute, or indicate a need for more data. The notion of specificity can be more challenging to apply. One exposure to one outcome is an appealing and parsimonious approach to scientific explanation, and when a relationship is that specific, causality is likely. Conversely, when an exposure is related to a wide range of bad outcomes—or good ones—one must suspect a placebo effect is operating or an unsuspected bias. As a caution against dismissing such relationships too easily: One early argument rejecting the adverse health effects of cigarette smoking was that the very wide range of adverse effects was too nonspecific to be true! It seems obvious that an exposure causes an outcome only if it precedes the outcome. An important weakness of cross-sectional studies is that they often cannot establish the temporality of the relationship being evaluated. Even with stronger study designs, our lack of knowledge about the timing of the preclinical onset of a condition can make it difficult to obtain exposure information for the biologically important interval. Seeking analogies can help clarify a possible cause-and-effect relationship. We need to consider whether similar agents or drugs are known to have similar effects. We also need to consider whether the same exposure is known to cause similar diseases. Finally, coherence of the evidence demands that the previously listed criteria be considered in conjunction with all of our other knowledge.

KEY POINTS

- Epidemiologic studies link laboratory bench research to the bedside.
- Randomized controlled trials (RTCs) provide the strongest level of evidence to link cause and effect and are used to test hypotheses.
- Randomized trials may not be practical to study outcomes that are extremely rare or take many years to develop.
- Cohort studies are often excellent for studying a single exposure that may lead to a wide range of outcomes.
- Case-control studies are excellent for studying rare diseases and for evaluating a wide range of exposures.
- Descriptive studies, including cross-sectional and ecologic studies, help generate hypotheses and also can illuminate the size and context of a health problem.
- Evidence-based medicine helps provide firm basis for clinical decisions.

REFERENCES

Recommended Readings

Grimes DA, Schulz KF: An overview of clinical research: the lay of the land. Lancet 359:57, 2002a.

Grimes DA, Schulz KF: Bias and causal associations in observational research. Lancet 359:248, 2002b.

Summerskill W: Evidence-based practice and the individual. Lancet 365:13, 2005.

General References

Bradford-Hill A: Principles of medical statistics, 9th ed. New York, Oxford University Press, 1971.

Fletcher RH, Fletcher SE, Wagner EH: Clinical epidemiology, the essentials, 2nd ed. Baltimore, Williams & Wilkins, 1988.

Grimes DA, Schulz KF: Cohort studies: Marching towards outcomes. Lancet 359:341, 2002.

Grimes DA, Schulz KF: Descriptive studies: What they can and cannot do. Lancet 359:145, 2002.

Herbst AL, Poskanzer DC, Robboy SJ, et al: Prenatal exposure to stilbestrol. A prospective comparison of exposed female offspring with unexposed controls. N Engl J Med 13:334, 1975.

Kelsey JL, Whittemore AS, Evans AS, Thompson WD: Methods in Observational Epidemiology, 2nd ed. New York, Oxford University Press, 1996.

Last JM: A Dictionary of Epidemiology. New York, Oxford University Press, 1983.

Meinert CL, Tonascia S: Clinical Trials, Design, Conduct, and Analysis. New York, Oxford University Press, 1986.

Petitti DB: Meta-Analysis, Decision Analysis, and Cost-Effectiveness Analysis: Methods for Quantitative Synthesis in Medicine, 2nd ed. New York, Oxford University Press, 2000.

Sackett DL, Haynes RB, Guyatt GH, Tugwell P: Clinical Epidemiology: A Basic Science for Clinical Medicine, 2nd ed. Boston, Little, Brown, 1991.

Sackett DL, Straus SE, Richardson WS, et al: Evidence-Based Medicine: How to Practice and Teach EBM, 2nd ed. New York, Churchill Livingstone, 2000.

Schulz KF, Grimes DA: Case-control studies: Research in reverse. Lancet 359:431, 2002.

U.S. Preventive Services Task Force: Guide to Clinical Preventive Services, 2nd ed. Alexandria, Va, International Medical Publishing, 1996.

Medical, Legal, and Ethical Issues 6

Fillmore Buckner and Gretchen M. Lentz

KEY TERMS AND DEFINITIONS

Abandonment. Unilateral dismissal by the physician without proper notice to the patient or failure to keep an express promise when there is still a need for continuing care.

Civil Law. A codified system of written laws adopted by a jurisdiction.

Common Law. Laws made largely by judicial interpretation.

Fiduciary. Having a special relationship toward another that imposes legal duties to act responsibly and in good faith to protect that party's interests.

Informed Consent. The physician's fiduciary duty to give the patient all the information needed for the patient to make an intelligent decision about therapies offered.

Malpractice. Patient injury secondary to failure to exercise that degree of care used by reasonably careful physicians of like qualifications.

Negligence. Failure to extend the degree of diligence and care that a reasonably and ordinarily prudent person would exercise.

Tort. A civil wrong for which legal action can be taken to recover damages resulting from negligence.

A doctor who knows nothing of the law
and a lawyer who knows nothing of medicine
are deficient in essential requisites of their professions.

—David Paul Brown 1795–1872

British North America inherited its law, as it did its language, from England. Most of the European countries originally occupied by the Romans adopted a form of law based on the Roman law codes. That law is called *civil law*. England's law, on the other hand, was based mainly on Scandinavian (Danish) law with a dose of folk law of undetermined origin thrown in. It was called the *common law*. One should not be deceived by its name. It was not law designed to protect the common man. It takes its name from the fact that it was the law that was common to all of England by about the year 1240. The two forms of law differ significantly.

Civil law is a codified system of law. That is, the law is spelled out in a series of written laws adopted by the jurisdiction. Civil law, therefore, tends to be fairly static. Common law is largely law made by judges. It may incorporate some statutory elements on specific issues, but even statutes are subject to judicial interpretation. Judges in the civil law are academics specially trained for their positions and act as prosecutor, judge, and jury. Civil law is, therefore, inquisitorial in nature and heavily dependent on the written word. In contrast, common law is an adversarial system in which the oral argument between the parties plays a much larger role. Judges are chosen from the practicing bar and are not usually academics. The judge is essentially a referee and instructs the jury, who make the ultimate decision on the merits of the case. In common law, the law is made by judges who hear a disputed case on appeal. Those decisions become precedent for future cases. However, higher appellate courts or future appellate courts of the same level can overturn or overrule a prior decision if circumstances change or new information develops. Therefore, change, albeit slow and irregular, is a constant element of the common law.

Under the early common law, cases were more or less confined to one of three categories. By far the most important cases were those in the field of property law. Real property was the basis of the wealth and economy of England, and it was natural for such cases to flood the courts. The concept of enforcing promises also played heavily in the development of commerce, and contracts were second in their demand for court time. To bring any civil action a king's writ was needed, and the writ covered only recognized wrongs that might be remedied. Finally there was criminal law, the enforcement of society's code of conduct. As one can readily see, little attention was paid to compensating the individual for personal wrongs (tort law). Doctors were therefore immune to suit for what we would call malpractice today. Technically some suits might have been pursued as contract suits, but written contracts were highly unusual between a physician and his patient, and without the written document such suits became almost impossible for the plaintiff to win.

In 1346 the black (bubonic) plague arrived in Italy. It spread over Europe rapidly, but did not reach England until 1348. The major effect of the epidemic occurred between 1348 and 1351, but bubonic plague became endemic and continued more or less uninterrupted until 1381. It is estimated that between 1348 and 1351, 50% of the population died, and by 1381 two thirds of the English population was decimated by the epidemic. (Because there was no accurate census at the time, such figures are estimates based on church records, burial records, tax rolls, and contemporary accounts.)

The loss of manpower was a major blow to the English economy. Overnight, people became as important as real property (land) and personal property (including livestock) in the English economy. Therefore, a physician's mistake that deprived the economy of a worker became an important enough matter to be brought before the courts. Physicians suddenly lost their immunity for practice errors. Actually it was an even worse scenario: The physician became strictly liable for an unfavorable outcome, and because there was no tort law (law compensating the individual for personal wrongs), the physician was prosecuted under the criminal law for mayhem. By 1364, it had become obvious that this was too draconian a remedy, and two property terms that had been previously used in livestock cases were introduced to permit civil malpractice cases. "Trespass" (trespass by force and arms) was charged for direct injury and "trespass on the case" for indirect injury.

These concepts, refined over the centuries, were brought to the North American colonies and adopted almost entirely by the American court system after independence. In the early 1800s the modern concept of negligence replaced trespass and trespass on the case in English courts. In the period of rapid industrialization following the Civil War, American courts did the same. (The elements of a cause of action in negligence are undoubtedly well known to the majority of readers, but are repeated here for completeness):

1. A duty, recognized by the law requiring the individual or entity to conform to a certain standard of conduct;
2. A failure to conform to the standard required;
3. A reasonably close connection between the failure to conform with the standard required and the resultant damage (subject to tests of legality, reasonableness and public policy)—what is usually summed up as "proximate cause";
4. Actual injury, damage or loss.

Our founding fathers divided the court system into two separate systems: the federal court system and the state court system. Over the years, both systems have become remarkably similar in their rules of evidence and civil procedure, and today most state courts are trilevel, as are the federal courts. Federal courts have jurisdiction over:

Cases that arise from the constitution, federal statute, and treaties
Cases affecting ambassadors, counsels, public ministers
Admiralty and maritime cases
Cases between states
Cases between a state and a citizen of another state; between citizens of different states; and between an American citizen and foreign state or foreign citizens

Federal cases must involve a substantial financial value (an ever increasing value as determined by statute. The federal court system is definitely not interested in jurisdiction of small claims).

Under Article VI (commonly referred to as the supremacy clause) of the constitution, federal law "...shall be the supreme Law of the Land; and the Judges in every State shall be bound thereby;..."

There is at least one federal district court for each state. District court cases are heard before a single judge. The opinions are published and may be cited in future cases, but carry minimal weight as precedent. There are 13 circuit courts of appeal, which hear appeals from district courts. Cases before circuit courts of appeal are heard by three judges. Their published opinions become precedent. Finally, appeals from the circuit courts of appeal go to the United States Supreme Court. Published Supreme Court cases are the highest level of precedent.

As can be seen from the list of federal jurisdictions, most tort cases including malpractice cases will be heard in state court systems. As mentioned earlier, most are organized much as the federal system. Most frequently each county has a court. These courts are frequently named superior courts to distinguish them from lesser courts such as municipal or justice of the peace courts. The county court cases are rarely published and have no practical value as precedent. Appeals from the county courts are heard by one or more state courts of appeal. Cases from state courts of appeal cases are published and have substantial value as precedent in that state's cases and some value as precedent in other states' cases. Appeals from the state courts of appeal are heard by the state supreme court. The state supreme court's published opinions have the highest value as precedent in that state and are given careful consideration as precedent in other states.

REPRODUCTIVE MEDICINE AND THE COURTS

No area of medicine has received as much court scrutiny, legal scholar review, social comment and even presidential directives as have the fields of obstetrics and gynecology. In addition, three of the six most expensive malpractice claim categories for 2003 fall within the realm of the obstetrician/gynecologist's practice (pregnancy/birth claims, failure to diagnose breast cancer, failure to diagnose cervical cancer). Unfortunately each of the issues that has come before American courts deserves a volume of its own to discuss adequately and a chapter in a general textbook of gynecology can do little but cover the generalities and list the more important issues the courts have addressed.

Since a 1927, eugenics case validating a Virginia compulsory sterilization law (*Buck v. Bell*, 274 U.S. 200 [1927]. See also, *Skinner v. Oklahoma*, 316 U.S. 535 [1942]), the United States Supreme Court has issued a continuing series of opinions that have established our present gynecologic legal environment. In *Griswold v. Connecticut,* 381 U.S. 479 (1965) (see also *Carey v. Population Services International*, 431 U.S. 678 [1977]), the Supreme Court held that the right to privacy applies to the use of contraceptives and struck down state laws that prohibited their distribution and sale. The well known case of *Roe v. Wade* (*Roe v. Wade*. 410 U.S. 113 [1973]) applied the same principle to state laws applied to abortion. However, even these supposedly well established court cases have long histories of challenges by state courts on issues such as waiting periods, spousal and parental notice, reporting requirements, second opinions, procedure facilities and methods, public funding, harassment of facilities and clients, and have undergone modifications based on legal concepts as varied as constitutional equal protection and informed consent. Some constitutional scholars have speculated that the whole concept of reproductive privacy is in danger of being overturned by an ever more conservative Supreme Court influenced by an increasingly militant religious right (see *Thornburgh v.. ACOG*, 471 U.S. 1014 [1986], 5 to 4 decision with dissent questioning validity of *Roe v. Wade*). As a result, the prudent practicing gynecologist must research the ever-changing local, state, and federal statutes and decisions governing every aspect of his or her practice. In the next section are some general defensive strategies for the gynecologist to observe in clinical practice. These strategies are not promoted as a substitute for good communication with patients, knowledge of your jurisdiction's law, or proper, honest, fair, considerate, unbiased treatment of patients.

PHYSICIAN'S DEFENSIVE STRATEGIES

Abandonment

Unilateral dismissal of the patient by the physician without proper notice to the patient is popularly conceived of as being the entire tort of abandonment. However, failure to keep an express promise (being present for a delivery, making a house call, or treating with a particular modality are common examples), failure to give proper discharge instructions, or abrogating your authority to a less qualified individual are much more likely to result in charges of abandonment. This is particularly true in the case of the obstetrician/gynecologist, in which the courts consider the physician/patient relationship to be particularly personal and private.

Physician's Defense Strategy

Explain your coverage arrangements in a patient brochure and document that the patient has received it. Do not sign out to family practitioners or partially trained gynecologists. If house officers are going to be involved in the patient's care, explain their role and do not allow them to exceed the stated role. Do not make express promises if there is even a minimal chance a change of circumstances will prevent you from keeping your promise.

Abortion

See the preceding discussion. Two subsequent Supreme Court cases (*Webster v. Reproductive Health Services*, 109 S. Ct. 1759 [1989]; *Planned Parenthood v. Casey*, 112 S. Ct. 2791 [1992]) have greatly expanded the local control of abortion, and preabortion procedures.

Physician's Defense Strategy

Seek local legal counsel. Make sure all aspects of your abortion practice conform to local, state, and federal law. Insist on an opinion letter that covers preabortion, abortion, and post-abortion issues. Do not do the procedure without "on advice of counsel" protection. Get timely legal reviews.

Acronyms

In every teaching hospital in the country that the authors have visited or reviewed records from, resident physicians have a system of acronyms or codes that they think of as secret to communicate comments about patients. Unfortunately, those acronyms and codes rarely are original or defy interpretation. Juries view them as the work of flippant, uncaring, pompous, and condescending care givers, and use of such codes badly injures the hospital or physician's defense and is unprofessional.

Physician's Defense Strategy

Avoid bad acronyms (some of the more common to avoid: NTB, not too bright; AMF, adios my friend; MFC, measure for coffin; FLK/FLM/FLF, funny looking kid/mom/father; UKD, ugly kid disease; GORK, god only really knows) and symbols even if they truly express your frustration in caring for a patient. DIIK or a sketch of Casper the Ghost (Damned if I Know and Spooky) may truly be as close to a diagnosis as anyone will ever make prior to autopsy. But when the autopsy physician comes up with a diagnosis mentioned in a footnote in a last month's New England Journal, a foolproof case for the defense is in serious jeopardy.

Assisted Reproductive Technology

The entire area of assisted reproductive technology (ART) is plagued with unresolved issues. Not even the legal status of the embryo, preembryo, or fetus has been established with any uniformity. Furthermore, the use of fetal tissue has been the subject of state bans, federal court cases overturning the bans (see *Margret v. Edwards*, 794 F.2d 994 [5th Cir. 1986]; See also, *Lifchez v. Hartigan*, 735 F.Supp. 1361 [N.D. 1990]), presidential directives, and the dissolution of ethical advisory committees. Cases involving the marital status, economic status, parental suitability, and psychological screening of patients have all come before the courts (as a result of "do it yourself" manuals and "mail order" sperm banks, four states have specific statutes requiring artificial insemination by a physician). Cases involving the medical screening, genetic screening, psychological screening, frequency of use, and payment of sperm donors have also come before the courts. The disposal of unused fertilized eggs or preembryos has been the subject of a series of court cases since the mid 1970s (actually predating the first reported successful in vitro fertilization [IVF] pregnancy). The use of surrogate mothers, the rights of surrogates, and the payment of surrogates has been a constant subject of law review articles and has been addressed differently by several state legislatures and still other opinions by state attorneys general. Numerous governmental inquiries and several cases involving ART clinic record keeping, informed consent, reporting, and statistical methods have taken place. In addition, nowhere in medicine does basic contract law play a greater role than in ART, and many a night's sleep has been lost over a failure to consider the remotest possibility in a clinic–patient–spouse contract or spouse–spouse contract.

Physician's Defense Strategy

To the best of the author's knowledge, only eight states have adopted the Uniform Parentage Act of 1973 in regard to artificial insemination (AI), but more than 40 states have a direct or indirect individual act affecting AI. When it comes to the more technical ART techniques the variability is even greater. The prudent gynecologist will engage in ART in a center with written protocols; sufficient laboratories and personnel to guarantee proper social, genetic, psychological, and medical screening of patients and donors; sufficient numbers of patients to keep care giver's skills sharp; sufficient storage space to keep a frozen preembryo for as long as required by law or contract; readily available legal help; and a written opinion letter from the state's attorney general's office certifying that the clinic is in compliance with the state's legal requirements.

Cancellations and "No Shows"

Cancellations and "no shows" of follow-up patients appointments are often ignored in the busy clinic or office. They can be, and are, frequently responsible for subsequent malpractice suits.

Physician's Defense Strategy

Each cancellation or no show should be documented in the chart. The chart should then be reviewed by the treating physician and, where appropriate, a letter or phone call made to the patient. All efforts to communicate with the patient should be documented.

Coverage Arrangements

As mentioned earlier improper coverage arrangements may lead to charges of abandonment. Poor communication among coverage groups frequently leads to offended patients and can be the first step on the path to a malpractice suit.

Physician's Defense Strategy

The previously mentioned strategy applies here:

1. List your coverage arrangements in your new patient brochure.
2. Sign out to qualified individuals.
3. Do not make specific promises as to your presence or procedures.
4. In addition, coverage groups should meet regularly to exchange information and maintain protocols.
5. Problem patients should be known to the entire group.
6. All after-hours care should be carefully documented and entered in the medical record either contemporaneously or at the latest the next business day.
7. All medical records should be available to all members of the group.

When you have the coverage:

1. Don't put geographic barriers between you and the patient (although it is not written in stone, The Emergency Medical treatment and Active Labor Act and other federal regulations and cases based thereon would indicate that you should be able to reach your patient's bedside within **thirty** (30) minutes).
2. Do not drink alcohol or take drugs (even prescription drugs) that can affect your cognition or cause somnolence.
3. Document all phone calls. Err on the side of caution.
4. Emergency physicians are great, but emergency departments are often overworked and slow and you are inserting an intervening opinion between you and the patient. An "I will meet you at the emergency room!" has been a great relief to many a patient and many a physician.

Contraception and Sterilization

Contraceptive methods and sterilization procedures can involve the physician in multiple issues of informed consent, treatment of minors, emancipation of minors, and court-ordered procedures, wrongful pregnancy as well as wrongful life and wrongful birth suits.

Physician's Defense Strategy

There is no escaping the necessity of researching your state's requirements. However, no where in obstetrics/gynecology practice is the communication with the patient more important. A thorough, unbiased informed consent is required. In addition, be careful of your terms. A tubal transection should be truly a tubal transection and a piece of tube sent as a pathology specimen is a splendid proof that the tube was sectioned. A clamped, crushed, or cauterized tube signed out as a tubal transection is a much less satisfactory form of evidence at a subsequent trial.

Fraud and Abuse

In 1972, as part of the first amendments to the Medicaid and Medicare rules and regulations, Congress passed antifraud and abuse regulations. The first such laws were hardly more than "a slap on the wrist." However, in 1977 Congress made those laws draconian. False statements, which include:

1. Knowingly and willfully making or causing to be made any false statement or representation of a material fact in seeking to obtain any benefit or payment
2. Fraudulently concealing or failing to disclose information affecting one's rights to a payment
3. Converting any benefit or payment rightfully belonging to another, and
4. Presenting or causing to be presented a claim for a physician's service knowing that the individual who furnished the service was not licensed as a physician.

These also encompass false claims, bribes, kickbacks, rebates or "any remuneration" and are felonies with a maximum of 5 years in jail and a $25,000.00 fine possible for ***each*** such offense. (The law states that any provider who knowingly and willfully solicits, pays, offers, or receives, any remuneration, in cash or in kind, directly or indirectly, overtly or covertly, to induce or in return for arranging for or ordering items or services that will be paid for by Medicare or Medicaid will be guilty of a felony). These rules and regulations essentially made it impossible to practice without violating some aspect of the fraud and abuse laws. It was, however, 10 years before the laws were refined in the Medicaid–Medicare Patient Protection Act of 1987 which provided some "safe harbors" to free normal course of business procedures. Since 1987, the government has pursued fraud and abuse cases with ever-increasing vigor. In 2003, settlements in fraud and abuse cases netted the government close to $2 billion (*Wall Street Journal,* A1, Friday, June 11, 2004). The real danger to the physician is not the fine that may force him or her into bankruptcy or the unusual imposition of jail time (to date, the government has seemed more interested in recovering cash and calling a halt to illegal practices than it has in jailing doctors), but the felony conviction that may result in the automatic loss of the license to practice. Thus Medicare/Medicaid fraud and abuse is a far more dangerous hazard than is malpractice.

Physician's Defense Strategy

Have your patients sign in whether they have come for an office visit or just a procedure. If you are worried about privacy issues, use a privacy sign in sheet that prevents subsequent signers from seeing who has signed in before (Colwell Publishing provides several styles of such sheets and they are very likely supplied by local firms as well.)

Don't unbundle procedures that are supposed to be bundled on a physician's visit. Don't unbundle surgical procedures. Don't charge for procedures done by another licensed provider or charge for physician's services if the physician is not physically present. Send your personnel to an accredited coding course and make sure your coding is being done in an accurate manner. Do not be tempted to code up. Time studies and statistics are against you. Finally, beware of the "coding consultant" who promises to increase your accounts receivable.

Informed Consent

Physicians continually ask for a foolproof informed consent form. Informed consent has little to do with a form. Informed consent has to do with the physician's fiduciary duty to his or her patient. As the patient's fiduciary, it is the physician's duty to give the patient all the information needed for the patient to make an intelligent decision about the therapies suggested. The information given must be accurate for published studies and compared with the physician's own figures, unbiased by the physician's privileges or other agenda, and presented in language the patient in question can understand in view of her education, intelligence, experience, and social standing. The information should include the diagnosis; a description of the suggested treatment; an explanation of what the treatment is thought to accomplish; the hoped for prognosis with the treatment; the possible side effects and possible adverse happenings with treatment; the therapeutic alternatives, their benefits, and possible adverse and side effects; and the patient's prognosis with the alternative and no therapy.

Physician's Defense Strategy

Give the woman all the information called for and document it in the medical record. Ask her is she has any questions. Answer the questions, and document both the questions and the answers. Use diagrams when necessary. Add the diagrams to the medical record and ask the patient to initial the diagrams. Have the patient sign the consent form—use the statutory form if your state has one—if not, use one approved by your clinic or local medical organization and approved by your attorney. After the patient signs again ask her if she has any questions. Answer those questions, and again document both the questions and answers. Before the surgery, procedure, or therapy covered by the form, again go over the same material, answer any last-minute questions, and document the entire episode. Remember, the duty to secure informed consent is the *physician's* duty, not the nurse's duty or a hospital admission clerk's duty. It is still questionable whether the physician is legally able to delegate that duty elsewhere.

Laboratory Tests

In my experience, one of the most common reasons for malpractice suits is the unreported abnormal laboratory or X-ray finding. The usual story is that the pathologist or radiologist returns the report and the super efficient clerk, receptionist, or nurse staples it in the medical record and then files the record. The alternative story is that the report is never sent and there is no follow-up. Of course, normal clerical errors do occur in any business; nevertheless, the physician's fiduciary duty extends to communicating the results and meanings of all abnormal tests to the patient. Therefore, the failure to communicate the results of an abnormal pap smear, glucose tolerance test, or mammogram to a patient can have disastrous legal consequences.

Physician's Defense Strategy

A gynecologist must have a system to track and document all laboratory and diagnostic tests and imaging studies ordered. There is no totally satisfactory way to do this. Old-fashioned "tickler" files are the least efficient, but better than nothing. Some office-generated computer programs have been highly successful, and some of the commercially available programs even generate an automatic notification letter. In any case, the physician must track all ordered tests and make every reasonable effort to notify the patient. The notification and follow-up must be documented. Telling the patient to call for the test results does not relieve the physician of his or her duty to notify. Finally, use the information you secure. Do not order laboratory or other diagnostic tests and then ignore or belittle those results.

Medical High-Risk Patients

Elderly, frail women with or without serious concomitant conditions and women of any age with serious gynecologic or concomitant conditions are legally and medically at high risk.

Physician's Defense Strategy

Treat these women as being at high risk. Question all of your routine procedures. Check what medications (prescription, over-the-counter, and health food store) they are taking. Watch the dosages you prescribe. Make sure your staff assists them from the moment they enter the door until they are safely over the doorstep and into someone else's capable hands. To let one of these patients get on or off an examining table by herself is courting disaster. A premises liability suit can be just as expensive as a malpractice suit, and it is much easier and cheaper to bring.

Medical Records

The 1930s wag who came up with the saying, "Medical records are the malpractice witness that never dies!" offered a truism that has only increased in value over time. The world of judges and juries of 2007 expects much more than the hand-written scribbles on a 4 × 6 inch card that marked the medical record of 1930s.

Physician's Defense Strategy

If at all possible, all your records should be typed. Even the best penmanship can be misinterpreted. All records should be written or dictated contemporaneously with the event described. All records should be in English, as objective as possible, clear without confusion or ambivalence, dated, timed, signed legibly, and kept in chronological order. Chart by the subjective, objective, assessment, plan (SOAP) method whenever possible. Do not use abbreviations! (That includes abbreviations "approved" by the institution or organization. Even the most common abbreviations have multiple meanings. There will always be an expert that interprets the abbreviation in a manner contrary to your interest.) Scrivener's errors may be corrected en page. Errors of fact or substance should be corrected as a new entry placed in the chart chronologically. Do not obliterate, destroy, change, or "lose" any portion of a medical record. Such activities are termed *spoliation of evidence.* At best they may call for civil penalties at trial and at worst may constitute malpractice per se or invoke criminal penalties. In any case such spoliation of evidence makes any subsequent suit almost impossible to win. If your state or hospital or the American College of Obstetrics and Gynecology (ACOG) has a standard form that is widely used in the community, use that form or one even more extensive. Do not leave blanks on your form. If the question is worth asking it is worth recording. Although many sources advise keeping medical records for a period of 10 years after the last contact with the patient, a safer approach is to keep the record for a period that would allow a conception at the date of last visit to reach maturity and expire its statutory limitations or statute of repose in states where there is a discovery rule.

Prenatal Counseling

Prenatal counseling involves state requirements about the extent of testing, testing of ethnic groups, duties to inform parents, duties to inform third parties, the right to refuse mandatory testing, wrongful life, and wrongful birth.

Physician's Defense Strategy

There is no escaping the necessity of researching your state's requirements. Those requirements should be converted to written protocol for laboratory, clinical, communication procedures, plus a note about the right to refuse treatment. Any and all refusals should be documented and witnessed.

Prescriptions

Adverse drug events are among the most common medical errors, and although physicians are loathe to admit it, more than two thirds of all adverse drug events are caused by physician error. Transmission errors and compounding (filling the prescription) errors make up the remaining third of the errors. Proper prescribing amounts to several simple basics, the appropriate drug, the appropriate dose, the appropriate directions, the appropriate time of administration, the appropriate termination, and the appropriate refill directions. Today the appropriate drug category can preclude prescribing a drug ineffective or marginally effective for the patient's diagnosis, a drug the patient is allergic to, or a drug with adverse interactions with another drug that the woman is taking. The prescription of a drug can no longer be thought of as something a physician does "off the top of his head." He needs help from an information base that can explore the medical chart, drug interactions, recorded allergies, drug doses, and the most effective therapy, and then must transmit a legible prescription for compounding. Therefore, the best approach lies in an extensive electronic medical record and database system that is updated at least monthly and that controls prescription writing. Absent such a system we can only offer homilies.

Physician's Defense Strategy

Type or block print all orders and prescriptions.

1. Prescriptions should always be written in duplicate or triplicate (one for the patient, one for the medical record, and one as your personal permanent record.) The patient's copy should always be on safety paper.
2. Do not issue oral phone orders or call prescriptions to pharmacies; use the fax line.
3. Clear, unabbreviated syntax works best. **Never use abbreviations for drugs.**
4. Always use the leading zero; never use the trailing zero (0.4 = yes; .40 = no)
5. Spell out "units" never use the symbol "U."
6. Always specify drug strength and route of administration.
7. Avoid decimals whenever possible (1500 mg rather than 1.5 g).
8. Think carefully before you sign on the "substitution permitted" line. (Generics may have blood levels that vary as much as ±20% from the original. Therefore, if blood level is important, the potential variation of up to 40% from one refill to another should rule against a generic equivalent.)
9. Use reasonable prescription pad security. Do not leave your prescription pad exposed on your desk or in your examining rooms.
10. Be careful of multipharmacy especially in the high-risk patient, and be alert to the use of multiple psychoactive drugs including opiates.
11. Give your patients printed instructions (Several good systems are on the market, don't ignore the AMA Patient Medicinal Instructions or the USP Dispensing Information), do not depend on the nurse or pharmacist.
12. Finally, check each prescription or order you write for clarity, legibility, appropriateness of drug and dosage in relation to the information available on the drug, the patient, and the diagnosis.

Addendum: A caution about drug samples. Samples should be stored properly and with reasonable security. (Neither the patient, nor nonmedical personnel should be able to gain access to samples.) Rotate the samples appropriately, and dispose of out-of-date samples safely and legally. **Samples should be distributed by personnel with prescriptive authority only.** (Some states may permit others to do so under supervision and written protocols.) **Do not distribute samples without issuing full oral and written instructions.**

When Things Are Not Going as Expected

Physicians are used to seeing cases progress in a somewhat predictable manner. Some patients progress more rapidly than others, but, in general, the course of disease and treatment follows a course that physicians are used to. When things take an unusual turn, physicians are prone to take one or both of two destructive courses. First, they irrationally get angry at the patient, or they lose perspective on the important issues.

Physician's Defense Strategy

Hold your temper in check. A woman who is not progressing as expected is the patient you need to have the best relations with. Go out of your way to let her know that something unusual is happening and what you are doing to solve the problem. **Do not blame her!** Reevaluate your diagnostic reasoning and differential diagnosis early. Check the chart, medication orders, nurses' notes, and medications given for possible errors. Request those cultures, chemistries, and imaging studies you thought you could short cut. Do **not** reject the patient's suggestions out of hand. If it will do no harm, the expense is not overwhelming, and it is neither unethical or illegal, concede to her wishes. Do not let your ego get in your way. **Get help early!** Get a formal consultation, don't just talk to someone in the doctor's dressing room. **Get the best help available!** Don't just ask a friend because he will concur with what you are doing. Establish good relationships with quality consultants early; do not wait until you need them to help in a disaster.

KEY POINTS

- Common law is the laws passed down from England's legal system and which is interpreted by judges. It is an adversarial system.
- Most tort cases, including malpractice cases, will be heard in state court systems.
- Possibly the best advice for avoiding malpractice claims is good communication with patients and proper, appropriate, considerate, and unbiased treatment of patients.
- Informed consent has little to do with a form. Providing the patient with the information about the nature and risks of the therapies offered and documenting that discussion is the legal responsibility of the physician.
- Accurate, complete, and legible medical records that are dated and signed are critical to the physician's defense strategy.

REFERENCES

Key References

Buckner F: Spoilation (spoliation) of medical records: The destruction, alteration or loss of medical records. J Med Pract Mange 9(2):81, 1993.

Buckner F: The nature, creation, and termination of the physician-patient relationship. J Med Pract Manage 10(2):59, 1994.

Buckner F: Patient abandonment. J Med Pract Manage 10(5):239, 1995.

Buckner F: Law note on altered medical records. In Houts M: Lawyer's Guide to Medical Proof. London: Matthew Bender, 1999.

Buckner F: Generic and therapeutic substitution: The history, issues, and recommendations for practitioners. J Med Pract Manage January/February:187, 1996.

Buckner F: Physician liability to the business invitee. J Med Pract Manage Fall:146, 1991.

Buckner F: The physician/patient relationship. J Med Pract Manage 10(2):59, 1994.

Buckner F: Patient abandonment. J Med Pract Manage March 239, 1995.

Buckner F: Medical records and physician disciplinary actions. J Med Pract Manage May:2843, 1996,

Buckner F: The duty to inform, liability to third parties, and the duty to warn. J Med Pract Manage Sept:98, 1996.

Buckner F: *Cedars-Sinai Medical Center v. Superior Court* and the tort of spoliation of evidence. J Leg Med 6:1, 1999.

Woods JR, Bennett PA, Rozovsky FA: Defusing the angry patient. OBG Manage October:39, 2005.

Key Readings

Buckner F: Closing the medical office. J Med Pract Manage 4(4):2674, 1989.

Buckner F: The Uniform Health-Care Information Act: A physician's guide to record and health-care information management. J Med Pract Manage 5(3):207, 1990.

Buckner F: Cytology, pap smears, colposcopy and cervicography: An attorney's primer. Trauma 32(3):77, 1990.

Buckner F: Health care worker status: Employee vs independent contractor. J Med Pract Manage 10(1):43, 1994.

Buckner F: In vitro fertilization and the status of the pre-embryo after *Davis v. Davis*. Med Trial Tech Q 41(1):89, 1994.

Buckner F: Generic & therapeutic substitution. J Med Pract Manage 11(4):187, 1996.

Buckner F: Medical records in physician disciplinary actions. J Med Pract Manage 11(6):284, 1996.

Buckner F: *Reisner vs Regents of the University of California*: The duty to inform, liability to third parties, and the duty to warn. J Med Pract Manage 12(5):256, 1997.

Bucker F: Independent medial examiner liability. J Med Pract Manage 12(5):256, 1997.

Buckern F: The medical license as property. J Med Pract Manage 12(6):312, 1997.

Buckner F: Arbitration clauses in health care provider-patient contracts. J Med Pract Manage 14(2):98, 1998.

Buckner F: *Cedars-Sinai Medical Center vs Superior Court* and the tort for spoilation of evidence. Legal Medicine Perspectives 6(1):1, 1999.

Buckner F: The physician/patient relationship. Atlanta Med 73(4):7, 1999.

Buckner F: Mediation and medical malpractice: The physician's perspective/arbitration agreements in physician-patient contracts. Capital Univ Law Rev 28(2):307, 2000.

Buckner F: Premises liability. J Med Pract Manage 16(4):201, 2001.

Buckner F: Medical records. In Sanbar S (ed): Textbook of Legal Medicine, 5th ed. Philadelphia, Mosby, 2001.

Buckner F: Electronic mail. In Sanbar S (ed): Textbook of Legal Medicine, 5th ed. Philadelphia, Mosby, 2001.

Buckner, F: Emergency medical treatment and labor act. J Med Pract Manage 18(3):142, 2002.

Buckner F, Neiman R: Protecting the medical office from internal fraud and embezzlement. J Med Pract Manage 6(3):216, 1991.

PART II

COMPREHENSIVE EVALUATION OF THE FEMALE

History, Physical Examination, and Preventive Health Care 7

General, Gynecologic, and Psychosocial History and Examination, Health Care Maintenance, Disease Prevention

Gretchen M. Lentz

KEY TERMS AND DEFINITIONS

Anovulatory Cycle. Menstrual cycle when ovulation does not occur.

Dyspareunia. Painful intercourse.

Dysuria. Painful urination.

Ectropion. The presence of endocervical (glandular) epithelium on the portio vaginalis of the cervix. It may result from scarring of the external os, or it may be congenital.

LMP. Last menstrual period.

Menstrual Formula. Age of menarche × number of days of cycle × number of days of menstrual flow (e.g., 13 × 28 × 5).

Metaplasia. The process of covering glandular epithelium or raw areas with squamous epithelium.

Nabothian Cyst. An inclusion cyst of the cervix.

Normal Transformation Zone. Area of columnar epithelium and squamous metaplasia in the vagina or on the cervix that has normal colposcopic patterns.

PMP. Previous menstrual period.

Portio Vaginalis. The portion of the cervix exposed to the vagina.

Sexual Dysfunction. A psychologic or physiologic problem or condition that prevents the usual full participation and enjoyment of coitus.

Total Procedentia. The prolapse of the uterus and cervix through the introitus.

The first contact a physician has with a patient is critical. It allows an initial bond of trust to be developed on which the future relationship may be built. The patient will share sensitive information, feelings, and fears. The physician will gain her confidence and establish rapport by the understanding and nonjudgmental manner in which he or she collects these data.

The first contact generally involves taking a complete history, performing a complete physical examination, and ordering appropriate initial laboratory tests. In such a way the physician gains impressions of the patient's problems and needs and develops a plan for solutions. A gynecologic history includes a complete general history and adds information of gynecologic importance. In like manner the physical examination should be complete; no corners should be cut. The physician practicing obstetrics and gynecology should not assume that the patient's general medical needs are cared for by others but should assume the role of her primary physician.

This chapter focuses on the appropriate manner that a gynecologic physician should use to conduct a history and physical examination and discusses the appropriate ingredients of ongoing health maintenance. An accurate, legible, and complete medical record is an important component of the patient's care.

DIRECT OBSERVATIONS BEFORE SPEAKING TO THE PATIENT (NONVERBAL CLUES)

When meeting a patient it is important to *look* at her even before speaking. Some experienced physicians observe patients sitting in their waiting rooms before actually beginning personal contact. The general demeanor of the patient should be evaluated. Five general impressions can be transmitted both by facial expression and by posture, including happiness, apathy, fear, anger, and sadness.

A patient who is happy, self-assured, and in good personal control generally has a relaxed face with a smile and a sparkle in her eyes. She is generally sitting relaxed and will offer the physician a warm and friendly greeting. Many new patients are apprehensive about meeting a new physician, and this apprehension may modify their usual expression of good spirits. Even under these circumstances, however, their warmth shows. Happy patients returning for visits after having established a relationship with a physician are usually warm, relaxed, and responsive.

Apathetic patients generally have a blank facial expression. The eyes lack sparkle, there is little muscular movement of the face, and the mouth is generally thin and in a neutral position, neither turned up nor down. The posture may be somewhat slouched, the handshake may be weak, and answers to verbal questions are short and unemotional. Although apathetic patients may have severe emotional illness, they may also be demonstrating resignation to an imagined or serious condition or they may be responding to multiple problems, which make them feel overwhelmed.

The frightened patient frequently has a tense expression on her face; her mouth is tight and the eyes are darting and narrow. She may be perspiring but have a dry mouth. Her posture demonstrates forward leaning, and there is often endless hand activity. When she reacts, it may be grossly out of proportion to offered stimuli.

The angry patient frequently has narrowed eyes, furrowed brows, and narrow, tight lips. She may be sitting on the edge of her chair, leaning forward as if to pounce. Unlike the frightened patient, whose pose may be defensive, the angry patient radiates aggression. Her voice is usually harsh, and her overreaction to questions usually involves short, threatening phrases.

The sad patient generally sits with slouched shoulders; large, sad eyes; and a turned-down mouth. The eyes may glisten, and there may be tears. This patient is most likely depressed, and her speech reflects remorse and hopelessness.

By observing these nonverbal clues, the physician determines the appropriate style for conducting the interview. Often an opening remark appropriate to the patient's demeanor may be useful, such as, "You seem sad today, Ms. Jones," or, "I detect a note of anger in your voice, Ms. Smith. Can you tell me why that is?" By so doing, the physician projects sensitivity to the patient's feelings and genuine care with respect to her circumstances.

ESSENCE OF THE GYNECOLOGIC HISTORY

Chief Complaint

The patient should be encouraged to tell the physician why she has sought help. Questions such as, "What is the nature of the problem that brought you to me?" or, "How may I help you?" are good ways to begin. The patient should be able to present the problem as she sees it, in her own words, and should be interrupted only for specific clarification of points or to offer direction if she digresses too far. During the interview the physician should face the patient with direct eye contact and acknowledge important points of the history either by nodding or by a word or two. Such an approach allows the physician to be involved in the problem and demonstrates a degree of caring to the patient. When the patient has completed the history of her current problem, pertinent open-ended questions should be asked with respect to specific points made by the patient. This process allows the physician to develop a more detailed database. Directed questions may be asked where pertinent to clarify points. In general, however, the patient should be encouraged to tell her story as she sees it rather than to react with short answers to very specific questions. Under the latter circumstance the physician may get the answers he or she is looking for, but they may not be accurate answers.

A general outline for a gynecologic and general history is given in the following box. The outline is given in a specific order for general orientation. The information, however, may be collected through any comfortable discussion with the patient that seems appropriate in the circumstances. It is important that all aspects be covered.

History Outline

I. Observation—nonverbal clues
II. Chief complaint
III. History of gynecologic problem(s)
  A. Menstrual history—LMP, PMP
  B. Pregnancy history
  C. Vaginal and pelvic infections
  D. Gynecologic surgical procedures
  E. Urologic history
  F. Pelvic pain
  G. Vaginal bleeding
  H. Sexual status
  I. Contraceptive status
IV. Significant health problems
  A. Systemic illnesses
  B. Surgical procedures
  C. Other hospitalizations
V. Medications, habits, and allergies
  A. Medications taken
  B. Medication and other allergies
  C. Smoking history
  D. Alcohol usage
  E. Illicit drug usage
VI. Bleeding problems
VII. Family history
  A. Illnesses and causes of death of first-order relatives
  B. Congenital malformations, metal retardation, and reproductive wastage
VIII. Occupational and avocational history
IX. Social history
X. Review of systems
  A. Head
  B. Cardiovascular/respiratory
  C. Gastrointestinal
  D. Genitourinary
  E. Neuromuscular
  F. Psychiatric
  G. Depression
  H. Physical abuse
    1. Sexual abuse
      a. Incest
      b. Rape

LMP, last menstrual period; PMP, previous menstrual period.

Pertinent Gynecologic History

A pertinent gynecologic history can be divided into several parts. It begins with a menstrual history, in which the age of menarche, duration of each monthly cycle, number of days during which menses occur, and regularity of the menstrual cycles should be noted. The dates of the last menstrual period and previous menstrual period should be obtained. In addition, the characteristics of the menstrual flow, including the color, the amount of flow, and accompanying symptoms, such as cramping, sweating, headache, or diarrhea, should be noted. In general, menstruation that occurs monthly (range 21 to 40 days), lasts 4 to 7 days, is bright red, and is often accompanied by cramping on the day preceding and the first day of the period is characteristic of an ovulatory cycle. Menstruation that is irregular, often dark in color, painless, and frequently short or very long may indicate lack of ovulation. The first few cycles in teenagers or cycles in premenopausal women are frequently anovulatory and as a result may come at irregular intervals.

The second pertinent point in the gynecologic history is that of previous pregnancies. The patient should be asked specifically to list pregnancies that she has experienced, including the year of the pregnancy; the duration; the type of delivery; the size, sex, and current condition of the baby; any complications that may have occurred; and whether the infant was breast-fed and, if so, for how long. Elective terminations of pregnancy and spontaneous abortions should also be noted, including the time of gestation at termination and the circumstances under which they took place. Ectopic or molar pregnancies should also be noted, including the type of therapy that was given. When such events have occurred, obtaining old records for review is appropriate. Any pregnancy should be discussed with respect to excessive bleeding, chills, fever, known infection, or other complicating events. It is also appropriate to ask the patient about the individual who fathered each of these pregnancies so that the physician may determine the number of sexual partners the patient has had.

A history of vaginal and pelvic infections should be obtained. The patient should be asked what types of infection she has had, what treatment was received, and what complications were experienced. Risk factors for human immunodeficiency virus (HIV) infection, such as intravenous drug abuse or coitus with drug abusers or bisexual men, should be sought by direct questioning and HIV screening offered where appropriate. All hospitalizations should be reviewed as to cause and outcome.

All instances of gynecologic surgical procedures should be noted, including minor operations, such as endometrial biopsies; vulvar, vaginal, or cervical biopsies; dilation and curettage; laparoscopic examinations; and any major procedure that the patient may have undergone. When such data are elicited, dates, types of procedures, diagnoses, and significant complications should be noted. In cases where pertinent, past records, particularly operative and pathology reports, should be sought.

A careful urologic history should be taken. A history of bladder dysfunction, dysuria, loss of urine, acute or chronic bladder or kidney infections, bladder pain, urinary frequency, nocturia, or other urologic problems, such as hematuria or the passage of kidney stones, should be noted.

Symptoms of pelvic pain or discomfort should be discussed fully. Six common questions should be asked about the pain: location of the pain; timing of pain; quality of the pain such as throbbing, burning, colicky; radiation of pain to other body areas; intensity of pain on a scale of 1 to 10, with 10 being the worse pain imaginable; and duration of pain symptoms. Additional questions about what causes the pain to worsen or subside; the context of the pain symptoms; and associated triggers, signs, and symptoms may be helpful. The pain should be described, noting the presence or absence of a relationship to the menstrual cycle and its association with other events, such as coitus or bleeding.

Important Points of Sexual History

1. Sexual activity (presence of)
2. Types of relationships
3. Individual(s) involved
4. Satisfaction? Orgasmic?
5. Dyspareunia
6. Sexual dysfunction
   a. Patient
   b. Partner

Any vaginal bleeding not related to menses should be noted, as well as its relationship to the menstrual cycle and to other events, such as coitus, the use of tampons, or the use of a contraceptive device.

A complete sexual history should be obtained (see above box), and specific problems should be evaluated. The history should include whether the patient is sexually active, the types of relationships she has, whether she is orgasmic, whether she experiences pain or discomfort with coitus (dyspareunia), and whether she or her partner is experiencing problems with sexual performance (sexual dysfunction). It is important that the physician review or rehearse the types of questions that will be asked and consider the response he or she will give to less typical answers (e.g., responses concerning homosexuality or less common sexual practices). This helps prevent the physician from demonstrating surprise and thus transmitting an attitude of disapproval. Counseling women to practice safe sex to avoid contracting sexually transmitted diseases may be relevant.

Finally, the patient's contraceptive history should be investigated, including methods used, length of time they have been used, and any complications that may have arisen.

General Health History

The patient should be asked to list any significant health problems that she has had during her lifetime, including all hospitalizations and operative procedures. It is reasonable for the physician to ask about specific illnesses, such as diabetes, hepatitis, tuberculosis, or rheumatic fever, that seem likely based on what is known about the patient or about the patient's situation. Some physicians use a history checklist of the most common conditions, but a careful physician who questions appropriately can be equally effective.

Medications taken and reasons for doing so should be noted, as should allergic responses to medications. Patients should be encouraged to bring all medications, both prescription and over-the-counter drugs, including herbal preparations, to subsequent health maintenance visits.

The patient should be questioned for evidence of a bleeding or clotting problem, such as a history of hemorrhage with minor procedures, easy bruisability, or bleeding from mucous membranes.

A history of smoking should be obtained in detail, including amount and length of time she has smoked. She should be

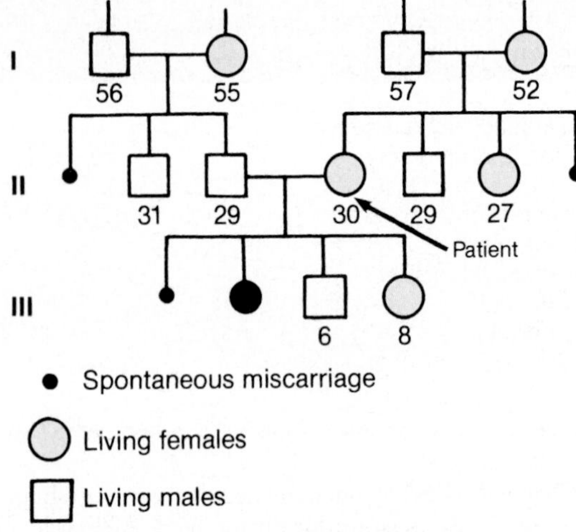

Figure 7-1. Family tree of typical gynecologic patient.

questioned about the use of illicit drugs, including marijuana, heroine, methamphetamines, and cocaine. Any affirmative answers should be followed by specific questions concerning length of use, types of drugs used, and side effects that may have been noticed. Her use of alcohol should be detailed carefully, including the number of drinks per day and any history of binge drinking or previous therapy for alcoholism.

Family History

A detailed family history of first-order relatives (mother, father, sisters, brothers, children, and grandparents) should be taken, and a family tree constructed (Fig. 7-1). Serious illnesses or causes of death for each individual should be noted. Also, an inquiry should be made about any congenital malformations, mental retardation, or pregnancy wastage in either the patient's or her husband's family. Such information may offer clues to hereditarily determined causes of reproductive problems.

Occupational and Social History

The patient should be asked to detail her and her husband's occupational histories, including jobs held and work performed. It is also useful to elicit a history of hobbies and other avocations that might affect health or reproductive capacity.

A social history should be obtained. This involves where and with whom the patient lives, other individuals in the household, areas of the world where the patient and her husband have lived or traveled, and unusual experiences that either may have had.

Safety Issues

The patient should be questioned about safety matters. She should be asked about the use of seat belts and helmets (if she rides a bicycle or motorcycle or rides a horse). She should be asked whether there are firearms in her household and, if so, whether appropriate safety precautions are taken. A question about intimate partner violence is appropriate and can be asked in a nonthreatening manner such as, "has anyone in your household threatened or physically hurt you?"

A discussion regarding whether the patient's hearing is adequate to ensure safety while she goes about her usual activities is important, especially in older women who may be suffering hearing loss, but also in younger women who may use Walkman- or iPod-type music players while they walk or jog. Appropriate footwear should be encouraged, taking into consideration the woman's usual activities, physical capabilities, and age.

Review of Systems

A complete review of systems is necessary to uncover symptoms from other areas that relate to reproduction and gynecologic problems (e.g., serious headaches, epileptic seizures, dizziness, or fainting spells). Such a history also may indicate exposure to medications that may be injurious should a pregnancy occur. The general organ systems review includes asking about constitutional systems; eyes, ears, nose and throat; skin problems; and musculoskeletal problems.

It is important to obtain a good cardiovascular/respiratory history, as well as a history of hypertension, heart disease, or chest problems, such as asthma and lack of exercise and smoking. Each of these may have an immediate effect on the patient and may also influence a future pregnancy.

Of importance to the gynecologist is a history of gastrointestinal disorders, such as functional bowel problems, diverticulitis, diverticulosis, or hepatitis. Patients should be asked about any rectal incontinence of gas or stool that they may be experiencing or have experienced in the past. Affirmative answers should be fully investigated with respect to specific illnesses and potential residuals that may affect the patient's current health or well-being.

Questions about the genitourinary system are important both from the standpoint of bladder function and as an indication of whether renal function has been or is impaired.

Neurologic or neuromuscular impairment may be important from the standpoint of the ability of the patient to carry and deliver a child without difficulty. Similarly, asking about endocrine symptoms of diabetes mellitus and thyroid disease are relevant. Menstrual abnormalities may be symptomatic of endocrine problems that affect the hypothalamic–pituitary–ovarian axis.

A history of vascular disease, including thrombophlebitis with or without pulmonary embolism, varicose veins, or other vascular problems, should be sought. If a positive history of thrombophlebitis is obtained, possible relationship to a hormonal exposure, such as pregnancy or oral contraceptive use, should be determined.

The psychiatric history should be detailed carefully for any emotional or mental disease processes. Specifically, evidence for depression and suicidal ideology should be sought. In addition, the patient should be asked specifically whether she has been sexually abused in adult life, in childhood, by a stranger, or incestuously, or raped. This topic is further discussed in Chapter

10 (Rape, Incest, and Domestic Violence). Finally, she should be questioned about the possibility of physical abuse, neglect, or intimidation, and elder abuse must not be forgotten.

ESSENCE OF COMPLETE PHYSICAL EXAMINATION

The gynecologist should perform a complete physical examination on every patient at the first visit and at each annual checkup, particularly if the gynecologist is the primary physician caring for the patient. Physical examination is a time both to gather information about the patient and to teach the patient information she should know about herself and her body.

The patient should disrobe completely and be covered by a hospital gown that ensures warmth and modesty. During each step of the examination she should be allowed to maintain personal control by being offered options whenever possible. These options begin with the presence or absence of a chaperone. The chaperone, a third party, usually a woman, serves a variety of purposes. She may offer warmth, compassion, and support to the patient during uncomfortable or potentially embarrassing portions of the examination. She may help the physician to carry out procedures, such as the Papanicolaou (Pap) smear, and in some cases she offers the physician protection from having his or her intentions misunderstood by a naive or suspicious individual. Although the presence of a chaperone is not absolutely imperative in every physician–patient relationship, the availability of one for the specific instance where it is deemed advisable should be ensured. Many clinics insist on the presence of a chaperone, and it is wise for the physician to follow local custom.

The examination should begin with a general evaluation of the patient's appearance and posture. Her weight and her blood pressure should be taken initially, and postmenopausal women should have their height measured routinely to document evidence of osteoporosis, which causes vertebral compression fractures.

The patient's eyes, ears, nose, and throat should be examined. Funduscopic examination should be performed at least annually to inspect the blood vessels of the retina and to observe the lens for evidence of early cataract formation. The patient should be inspected for evidence of upper lip or chin hair, which may indicate increased androgen activity.

The thyroid gland should be palpated for irregularities or increase in size (goiter). Discrete areas of enlargement, hardness, and tenderness should be described. The patient's neck should be palpated for evidence of adenopathy along the supraclavicular and posterior auricular chains.

The chest should be inspected for symmetry of movement of the diaphragm, percussed for areas of consolidation, and auscultated bilaterally for breath and adventitious sounds. Wheezing or rales should be noted.

The heart should be examined by palpation for points of maximum impulse, percussed for size, and auscultated for irregularities of rate and evidence of murmurs and other adventitious sounds. An older woman's neck should be auscultated for evidence of vascular bruits. The patient's heart should be auscultated in both the lying and the sitting positions.

A careful breast examination should be carried out in a systematic fashion as described in Chapter 15 (Breast Diseases).

Table 7-1 Clinical Breast Examination Elements

1. Examination of each breast with the patient sitting with arms raised, and with the patient supine
2. Attention to the entire breast mound from midsternum to the posterior axillary line and from the costal margin to the clavicle
3. Inspection and palpation to assess:
    - Skin flattening or dimpling
    - Skin erythema
    - Skin edema
    - Nipple retraction
    - Nipple eczema
    - Nipple discharge
    - Breast fixation
    - Tissue thickening
    - Palpable masses
4. Evaluation for axillary and supraclavicular lymphadenopathy

To summarize a detailed clinical breast examination, refer to Table 7-1. Research has shown the following factors are associated with a high-quality breast examination: longer duration, thorough coverage of the breast, a consistent exam pattern, use of variable pressure with the finger pads, and use of the three middle fingers. Recommending breast self-examination has been controversial as two trials do not suggest benefit from Russia and China. More research is needed on both breast self-examination and clinical breast examination. At this time the patient should be taught breast self-examination and encouraged to perform this each month.

The abdomen should be systematically examined as detailed in the following sections.

Inspection

The abdomen should be inspected for symmetry; scars, protuberance, or discoloration of the skin; and striations, which may suggest previous pregnancies or adrenal gland hyperactivity. The hair pattern should be noted. The typical female escutcheon is that of an inverted triangle over the mons pubis. A male escutcheon involves hair growth between the area of the mons pubis and the umbilicus, also known as a diamond pattern, and may indicate excessive androgen activity in the patient (Fig. 7-2).

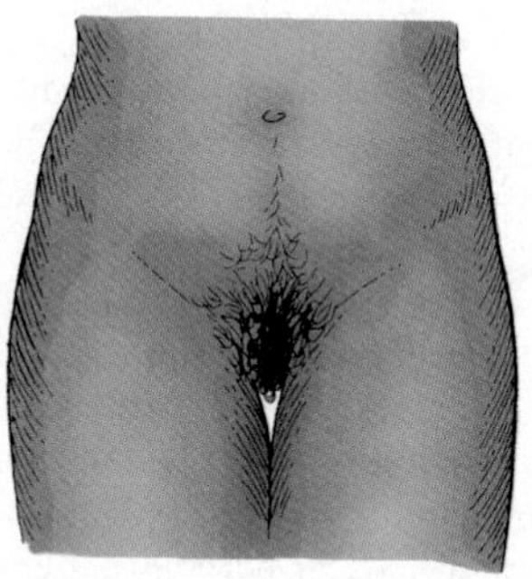
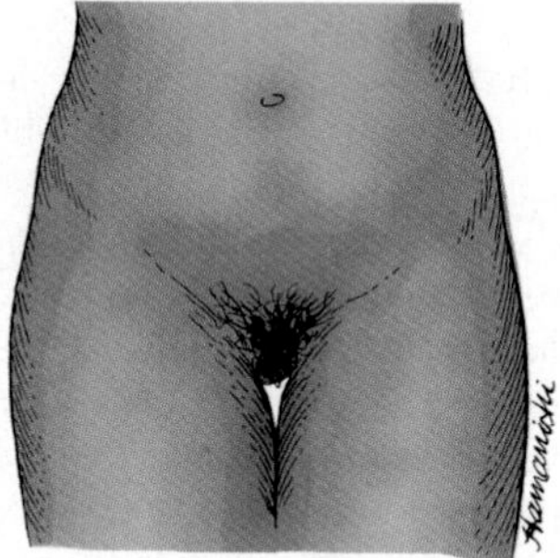

Figure 7-2. Normal female pubic hair pattern *(right)* and hair pattern of female showing male (androgenized) pattern *(left)*.

Palpation

The abdomen should be palpated for organomegaly (enlarged organs), particularly involving the liver, spleen, kidneys, and uterus; and for adnexal masses, which may be palpated abdominally, if large. Palpation also affords the possibility of noting a fluid wave, which would suggest either ascites or hemoperitoneum. Palpation also yields evidence for rigidity of the abdomen, which would imply spasm in the rectus muscles secondary to intraabdominal irritation. Where the irritation is caused by intraabdominal hemorrhage or infection, this rigidity is often evidence of an acute abdomen. During the palpation of the abdomen the physician should elicit the phenomenon of *rebound,* which also signifies intraabdominal irritation, by gently pressing the abdomen and then releasing. The release may cause pain either under the spot (direct rebound) or in a different portion of the abdomen (referred rebound). It should be noted, however, that sudden, rough pressure may cause pain even in a normal patient. Gentle pressure carried out systematically may elicit painful "trigger points."

Percussion

Percussion affords the ability to differentiate fluid waves and to outline solid organs and masses.

Auscultation

The physician should listen for bowel sounds. Hypoactive or absent bowel sounds may imply an ileus caused by peritoneal irritation of the bowel. Hyperactive bowel sounds may imply intrinsic irritation of the bowel or partial or complete bowel obstruction.

The groins should be palpated for adenopathy and inguinal hernias. The physician should also elicit the femoral pulses beneath the groin in the femoral triangles, and when these are present, the differences that may exist between the two femoral areas should be noted.

Legs should be examined for evidence of varicose veins, edema, and other lesions. In addition, it is reasonable to judge arterial circulation to the extremities by palpating pedal pulses on the dorsum of the foot.

PELVIC EXAMINATION

The pelvic examination is conducted with the patient lying supine on the examining table with her legs in stirrups. The patient may or may not desire to be draped with a sheet. Because the physician should be pointing out aspects of the patient's pelvic anatomy where possible, many patients prefer to have the head of the table elevated and to use a small hand mirror to follow the examination with the physician. In such instances, a sheet may be cumbersome. The physician should be sure the patient is as relaxed as possible and should take a few minutes to describe the procedure and allow the shy or nervous patient to prepare herself. Suggesting that the patient allow her legs to fall wide apart and concentrate on relaxing her abdominal muscles may be helpful.

Inspection

The perineum should be carefully inspected beginning with the mons pubis. The quality and pattern of the hair on the mons and the labia majora should be noted. Areas of alopecia should be noted because they may imply a skin abnormality. In general, as a woman ages, the pubic hair becomes less dense and may turn gray. During the inspection of the pubic hair the physician should look for evidence of body lice (pediculosis). Next, the skin of the perineum is inspected for redness, excoriation, discoloration, or loss of pigment and for the presence of vesicles, ulcerations, pustules, warty growths, or neoplastic growths. In addition, pigmented nevi or other pigmented lesions should be noted, as should varicose veins. Skin scars denoting previous episiotomy or other obstetric lacerations should be noted.

Next, the specific structures of the perineum should be systematically evaluated. The clitoris should be noted and its size and shape described. Normally it is 1 to 1.5 cm in length. Any irregularities or abnormalities of the labia majora or minora should be noted and carefully described. At times these areas are injured by trauma related to coitus, accidental injury, or childbearing. The patient should be questioned about evidence of trauma when appropriate.

The introitus should be observed closely. Whether the hymen is intact, imperforate, or open and whether the perineum gapes or remains closed in the usual lithotomy position should be noted.

The perineal body, the area at the posterior aspect of the labia where the muscles of the superficial perineal compartment come together, should be inspected. It represents the focal point of support for the perineum and is between the vagina and the rectum. The perianal area is then inspected for evidence of hemorrhoids, sphincter injury, warts, and other lesions (Fig. 7-3).

Palpation

The next step in the examination of the perineum involves palpation. With the second and fourth fingers of the gloved hand separating the labia minora, the urethra is inspected and the length of the urethra is palpated and "milked" with the middle finger. In this way, irregularities and inflammation of Skene's glands (periurethral glands), pus or mucus expressed, or a suburethral diverticulum can be noted. Any pus expressed from the urethra should be submitted for Gram stain and cultured, since it is frequently found to contain gonococci. The gloved hand then palpates the area of the posterior third of the labia majora, placing the index finger inside the introitus and the thumb on the outside of the labium. In this way, enlargements or cysts of Bartholin's glands are noted. This exercise should be performed on each side.

With the gloved hand holding the labia apart, the opening of the vagina should be inspected. The presence of a cystocele or a cystourethrocele should be noted. This would be seen as a bulging of vaginal mucosa downward from the anterior wall of the vagina. The presence of this abnormality may be noted

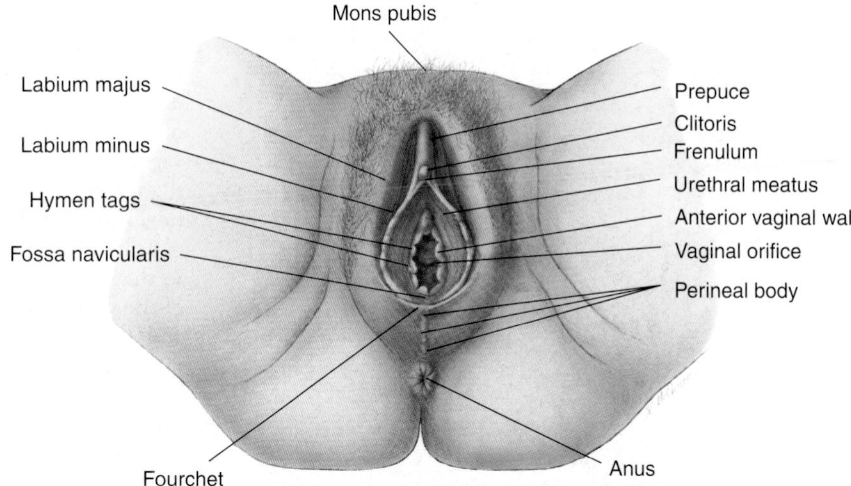

Figure 7-3. Normal female perineum. (Redrawn from Krantz KE: Anatomy of the female reproductive system. In Benson RC [ed]: Current Obstetric and Gynecologic Diagnosis and Treatment, 5th ed. Los Altos, CA, Lange Medical, 1984.)

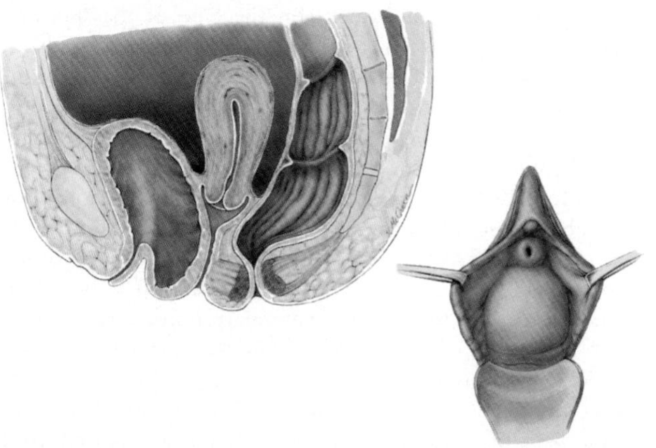

Figure 7-4. Side and direct views of cystocele. (Redrawn from Symmonds RE: Anatomy of the female reproductive system. In Benson RC [ed]: Current Obstetric and Gynecologic Diagnosis and Treatment, 5th ed. Los Altos, CA, Lange Medical, 1984.)

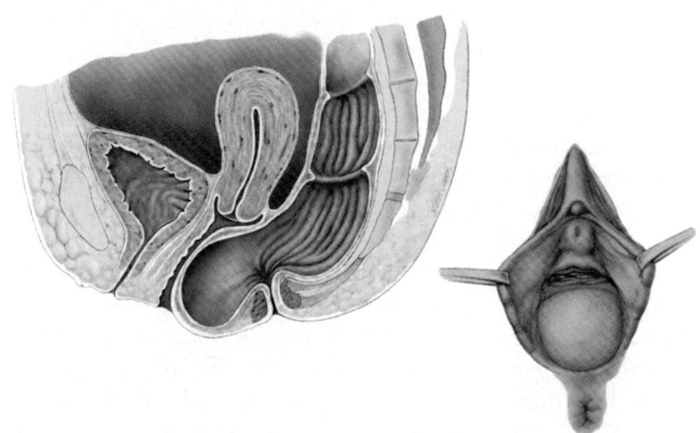

Figure 7-5. Side and direct views of rectocele. (Redrawn from Symmonds RE: Relaxations of pelvic supports. In Benson RC [ed]: Current Obstetric and Gynecologic Diagnosis and Treatment, 5th ed. Los Altos, CA, Lange Medical, 1984.)

either by simply observing or by asking the patient to bear down (Fig. 7-4). Likewise, the posterior wall should be noted for a bulging upward, which would represent a rectocele (Fig. 7-5). Also, with the patient bearing down, the cervix may become visible, indicating prolapse of the uterus. A cystic bulge in the cul-de-sac may represent an enterocele (Fig. 7-6). Each of these observations is evidence for relaxation of the pelvic supports and should be graded 1+ to 4+, with 1+ being a minimum bulge and 4+ being a bulge through the introitus. A prolapse of the cervix and uterus downward into the uterine canal can be graded in stages I, II, and III, with stage I being a minimum descent of the cervix into the vaginal canal, stage II being a descent of the cervix to the introitus, and stage III being the prolapse of the cervix or uterus through the introitus (total descensus, total procedentia) (Fig. 7-7).

The descriptions and definitions of pelvic floor relaxation problems just listed have been used in variations for many years and used by most gynecologists but not standardized until 1996. During the last decade, the International Continence

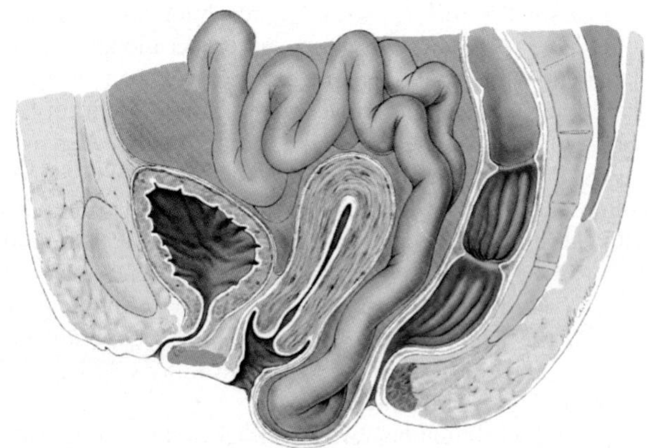

Figure 7-6. Lateral view of enterocele. (Redrawn from Symmonds RE: Relaxations of pelvic supports. In Benson RC [ed]: Current Obstetric and Gynecologic Diagnosis and Treatment, 5th ed. Los Altos, CA, Lange Medical, 1984.)

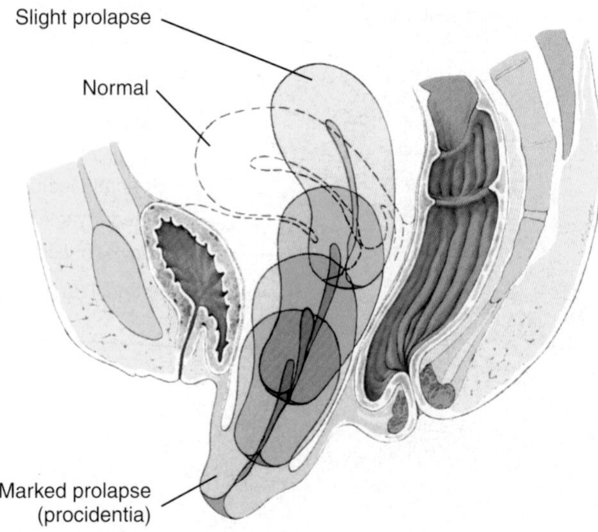

Figure 7-7. Depiction of prolapse of uterus. (Redrawn from Symmonds RE: Relaxations of pelvic supports. In Benson RC [ed]: Current Obstetric and Gynecologic Diagnosis and Treatment, 5th ed. Los Altos, CA, Lange Medical, 1984.)

Society Committee of Standardization of Terminology, Subcommittee on Pelvic Organ Prolapse and Pelvic Floor Dysfunction has been collaborating with the American Urogynecology Society and the Society of Gynecologic Surgeons to develop a standardized site-specific system for describing, quantitating, and staging pelvic support in women. Its purpose is to enhance clinical and academic communication with respect to individual patients and populations of patients. In 1996 this system was adopted by these organizations. It is discussed and defined in Chapters 20 (Anatomic Defects of the Abdominal Wall and Pelvic Floor) and 21 (Urogynecology).

Speculum Examination

After palpation the physician chooses the appropriate speculum for the patient. The typical Graves speculum generally is of three sizes: small, which is used in young children, women who have undergone tight perineal repair, or occasionally in the aged patient who has undergone severe involution; medium, used for most women; and large, which is often useful in large or obese women or those who are grand multiparas. Also available is the Pederson speculum, which is the length of the Graves speculum but narrower, for women who have not become active sexually, have never been pregnant, or have not used tampons. It is also of value for women who have undergone operations that have narrowed the vaginal diameter. For the majority of women the length of the vagina is similar, approximately 6 to 7 cm, and the Pederson or medium Graves speculum is appropriate (Fig. 7-8) for them.

The speculum should be warmed, either by a warming device or by being placed in warm water, and then touched to the patient's leg to determine that she feels the temperature is appropriate and comfortable. The speculum is then inserted by placing the transverse diameter of the blades in the anteroposterior position and guiding the blades through the introitus in a downward motion with the tips pointing toward the rectum. Because the anterior wall of the vagina is backed by the pubic symphysis, which is rigid, pressure upward causes the patient discomfort. This is avoided by following the described method of introducing the speculum. Also, in the resting state the vagina lies on the rectum and actually extends posteriorly from the introitus. The procedure may be facilitated by placing two fingers into the introitus and pressing down.

Once the blades are inserted, the speculum should be turned so that the transverse axis of the blades is in the transverse axis of the vagina. The blades should be inserted to their full length and then opened so that the physician may inspect for the position of the cervix. The cervix generally fits into the open blades with ease. If this does not occur, the physician should inspect for the position of the cervix with his or her finger and then reinsert the speculum accordingly. Once the blades are inserted and the cervix is visualized, the speculum should be opened and the introitus widened so that the cervix can be adequately inspected and a Pap smear taken. This can be done by using the screw adjustment on the base of the speculum. When inserted properly the speculum generally stays in place.

The physician then inspects the vagina and cervix. The vaginal canal is inspected during the insertion of the speculum or on its removal. The vaginal epithelium should be noted for evidence of erythema or lesions. Fluid discharge should be evaluated on slides prepared by placing one drop of vaginal secretion in one drop of sodium chloride solution, placing a cover slip over the specimen, and inspecting it for unicellular flagellated protozoa, *Trichomonas vaginalis.* The vaginal epithelial cells should also be inspected. The cells should have sharp borders and normal-appearing nuclei. Any variation from the normal appearance of cells may imply infection (see Chapter 22, Infections of the Lower Genital Tract). A drop of potassium hydroxide is placed on another slide, and a drop of vaginal secretion is placed within this. The potassium hydroxide causes lysis of the epithelial cells and trichomonads but leaves intact the mycelium of *Candida.* Thus, the presence of mycelium is helpful in diagnosing vaginal candidiasis. Vaginal lesions, such as areas of adenosis (see Chapter 12, Congenital Abnormalities of the Female Reproductive Tract), clear cystic structures (Gartner's cysts), or inclusion cysts on the lines of scars or episiotomy incisions, should be noted.

The cervix is inspected next. It should be pink, shiny, and clear. In a nulliparous individual, the external os should be round. When a woman is parous, the external os takes on a fishmouth appearance, and if there have been cervical lacerations, healed stellate lacerations may be noted (Fig. 7-9). Normally, the transformation zone (i.e., the junction of squamous and columnar epithelium) is just barely visible inside the external os. Occasionally, glandular epithelium may be present on the portio vaginalis, moving the transformation zone onto the portio. This is common in teenage girls, women who have been exposed to diethylstilbestrol in utero, some women with vaginitis, or women immediately postpartum or postabortion. Generally, this is cleared by a process of metaplasia, in which squamous epithelium covers the columnar epithelium. This process, however, may leave small areas of irregularities and inclusion cysts, called *nabothian cysts,* which may be seen in various sizes and shapes. They are of no clinical significance. Often after a woman has delivered a baby, there is lateral scarring at the 3 o'clock and 9 o'clock positions, causing an eversion of the external os so that

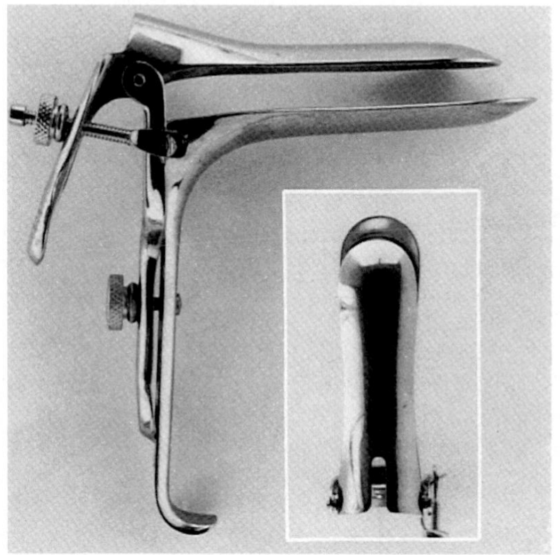

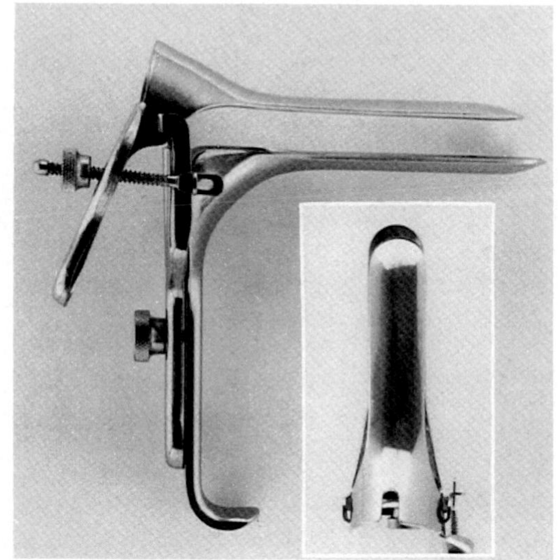

Figure 7-8. Graves *(left)* and Pederson *(right)* specula.

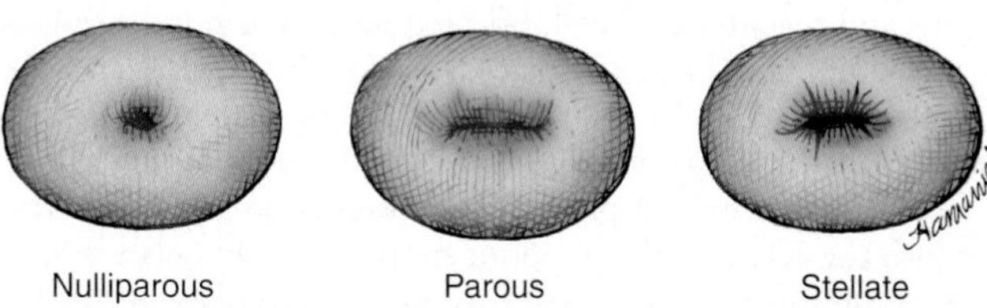

Figure 7-9. Nulliparous, parous, and stellate lacerations of cervix.

the reddened columnar epithelium is visible on the anterior and posterior lips of the cervix. If the observer looks closely, the transitional zone can be seen along the edges of this area of eversion and may be perfectly healthy. This is called an *ectropion* and is not evidence of a pathologic condition.

Any lesions of the cervix should be noted and, where appropriate, a biopsy should be performed. In a patient with acute herpes simplex, vesicles or ulcers may be noted. In a patient infected with human papillomavirus, warts (condylomata acuminata) on the cervix may also be observed.

Papanicolaou Smear

At this point in the examination a Pap smear is usually taken. In 1943 Papanicolaou and Trout published their now classic monograph demonstrating the value of vaginal and cervical cytology as a screening tool for cervical neoplasm. With the use of the Pap smear in screening programs, the incidence of invasive cervical cancer has been reduced 50%. Recently, programs focusing on cost effectiveness have suggested that the screening interval may be extended from the usual 1 year to 3 years in certain low-risk individuals after age 30. Initial screening should begin at age 21 or 3 years after the individual becomes sexually active. High-risk women, those with a history of early sexual activity and multiple partners, should be screened annually. Those patients with later exposure to coitus who have only one sexual partner and who have had three successive negative annual smears may be considered low risk and should be screened every 2 to 3 years at the discretion of the physician. A case-control study by Shy and colleagues questioned the wisdom of extending the screening interval beyond 2 years. Although no significant increase was noted in the incidence of cervical cancer in women screened every 2 years compared with those screened annually, the risk increased 3.9 times if the interval was 3 years and 12.3 times in women not screened for 10 years. The presence of risk factors did not influence these results.

A Pap smear can be performed in a number of ways. The major objective is to sample exfoliated cells from the endocervical canal and to scrape the transitional zone. It is also useful to sample the vaginal pool, although this does not usually yield as high an incidence of cervical disease as does sampling of the canal and the transitional zone. One way of performing the Pap smear is as follows:

1. After excess mucus is gently removed (routine swabbing may cause insufficient cells to be sampled), the endocervical canal is sampled with either a cotton-tipped applicator or a cytobrush, which is placed into the canal and rotated. Although both instruments generally dislodge adequate numbers of cells for study, the cytobrush appears to give more accurate results and higher yields of positive findings. The material obtained is then smeared thinly on a microscope slide by rotation of the swab or brush on the glass surface. This is labeled *endocervix* and fixed immediately either by use of a spray fixative or by immersion of the slide into a fixative solution (Fig. 7-10).
2. With an Ayres spatula or some variation thereof, the entire transformation zone is scraped and the sample smeared thinly on a second slide, which is immediately fixed. If the physician wishes a sample of the vaginal pool, this may be taken with the reverse side of the Ayres spatula and smeared on a third slide or on a second portion of the slide containing the transformation zone material (Fig. 7-11). Recent data suggest an extended-tip spatula is better for collecting endocervical cells. The best results come from using both the cytobrush and an extended-tip spatula.

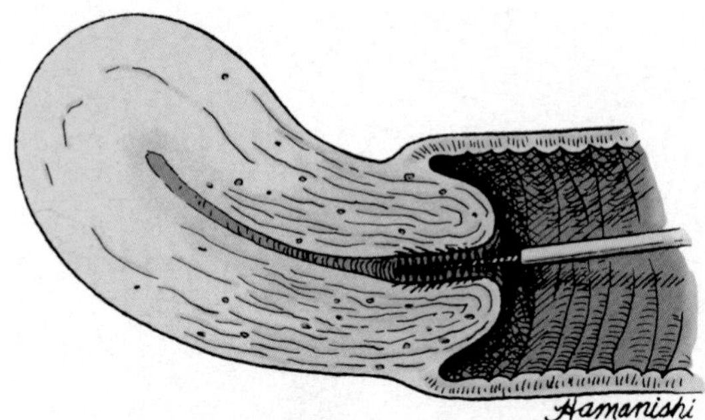

Figure 7-10. Obtaining cells from endocervix using a cytobrush.

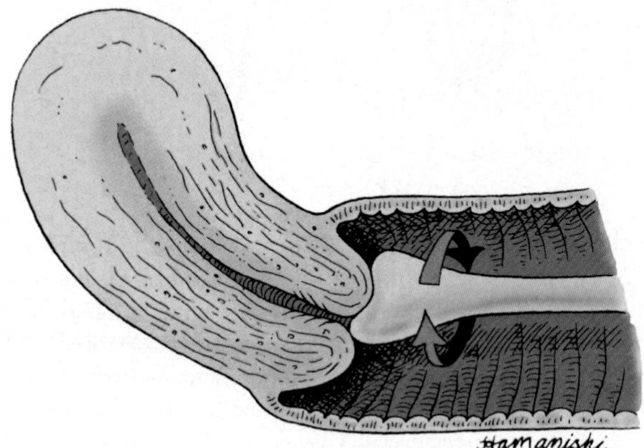

Figure 7-11. Obtaining cells from transformation zone using Ayers spatula.

A number of fixatives are available, but it is important that they be applied immediately before drying and distortion of the cells takes place. Newer liquid-based, thin-layer Pap smear preparations are available. No slides are needed. The cytobrush and spatula are used to obtain cervical cells as described earlier, and they both are placed in a liquid jar of fixative and gently rotated to dislodge cells in the liquid. Evidence-based data show both Pap slide prepared in a conventional manner and liquid-based methods for cervical cytology screening are acceptable. Pap smears may be reported using the following descriptive system (2001 Bethesda system):

Negative for Intraepithelial Lesion or Malignancy
Epithelial Cell Abnormality
Squamous cell
- Atypical squamous cells (ASC)
- Low-grade squamous intraepithelial lesions (LSIL)
- High-grade squamous intraepithelial lesions (HGSIL)
- Squamous cell carcinoma

Glandular cell
- Atypical glandular cells (AGC)
- Typical glandular cells, favor neoplastic
- Endocervical adenocarcinoma in situ (AIS)
- Adenocarcinoma

Interpretation/Result
Other nonneoplastic findings:
- Reactive
  - inflammation
  - radiation
  - intrauterine contraceptive device
- Glandular cells status posthysterectomy
- Atrophy

Organisms
- Cellular changes consistent with herpes simplex
- *Trichomonas vaginalis* infection
- Bacteria consistent with *Actinomyces* infection
- Fungal organisms
- Shift in flora suggestive of bacterial vaginosis

In most instances, particularly with new patients and women younger than 25, it is appropriate to culture for gonorrhea and *Chlamydia* using swabs that sample secretions from the endocervical canal. This step may be performed after the Pap smear.

Bimanual Examination

The bimanual examination allows the physician to palpate the uterus and the adnexa. The lubricated index and middle fingers of the dominant hand are placed within the vagina, and the thumb is folded under so as not to cause the patient distress in the area of the mons pubis, clitoris, and pubic symphysis. The fingers are inserted deeply into the vagina so that they rest beneath the cervix in the posterior fornix. The physician should be in a comfortable position at this point, generally with the leg on the side of the vaginal examining hand on a table lift and the elbow of that arm resting on the knee. The opposite hand is placed on the patient's abdomen above the pubic symphysis. The flat of the fingers are used for palpation. The physician then elevates the uterus by pressing up on the cervix and delivering the uterus to the abdominal hand so that the uterus may be placed between the two hands, thereby identifying its position, size, shape, consistency, and mobility. In the normal and non-pregnant state the uterus is approximately 6 cm by 4 cm and weighs about 70 g. It may be somewhat larger in a woman who has had children (Fig. 7-12).

Enlargement of the uterus should be described in detail. Size may be estimated in centimeters or by comparing with weeks of normal gestational age.

The uterus in two thirds of instances is anteflexed so that the abdominal hand is palpating the posterior wall of the uterus and the vaginal fingers the anterior wall. The uterus may be retroverted. If it is positioned in a straight line with the vagina, it is said to be midposition or first-degree retroverted; if it lies backward in the cul-de-sac off the direct line of the vagina, it is said to be second-degree retroverted; if it is flexed deeply into the cul-de-sac pressing toward the rectum, it is third-degree retroverted. A third-degree retroverted uterus that cannot be brought forward by manipulation is best examined by rectovaginal examination, which is described later in the chapter. The general shape of the uterus is that of a pear, with the broadest portion at the upper pole of the fundus. Generally, the uterus is mobile, and if it fails to move, it may be fixed by adhesions. The surface should be smooth; irregularities may indicate the presence of uterine leiomyomas (fibroids).

The shape of the uterus should also be described in detail. The consistency of the uterus is generally firm but not rock-hard, and

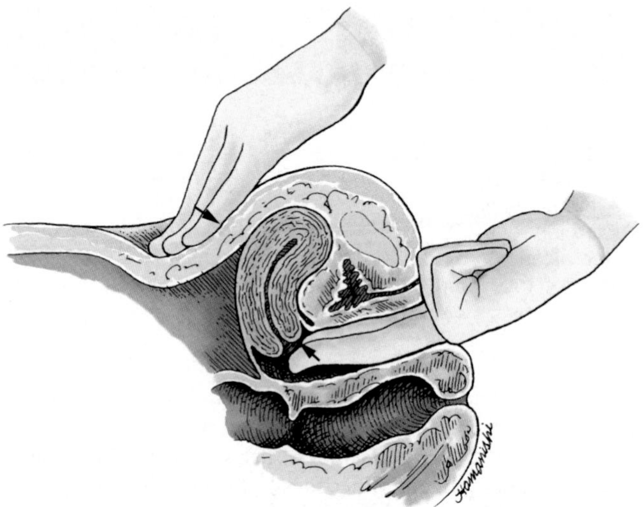

Figure 7-12. Bimanual examination of uterus.

this should be noted in the examination. Any undue tenderness caused by palpation or movement of the uterus should be noted, since it may imply an inflammatory process.

Attention is then turned to examination of the adnexa. If the right hand is the pelvic hand, the first two fingers of the right hand are then moved into the right vaginal fornix as deeply as they can be inserted. The abdominal hand is placed just medial to the anterior superior iliac spine on the right, the two hands are brought as close together as possible, and with a sliding motion from the area of the anterior superior iliac spine to the introitus, the fingers are swept downward, allowing for the adnexa to be palpated between them. A normal ovary is approximately 3 cm by 2 cm (about the size of a walnut) and will sweep between the two fingers with ease unless it is fixed in an abnormal position by adhesions. When the adnexa is palpated, its size, mobility, and consistency should be described. However, this portion of the examination should be brief, since it causes the patient a mild to moderate sickening sensation. When the right adnexa has been palpated, the left adnexa should be palpated in a similar fashion by turning the vaginal hand to the left vaginal fornix and repeating the exercise on the left side (Fig. 7-13).

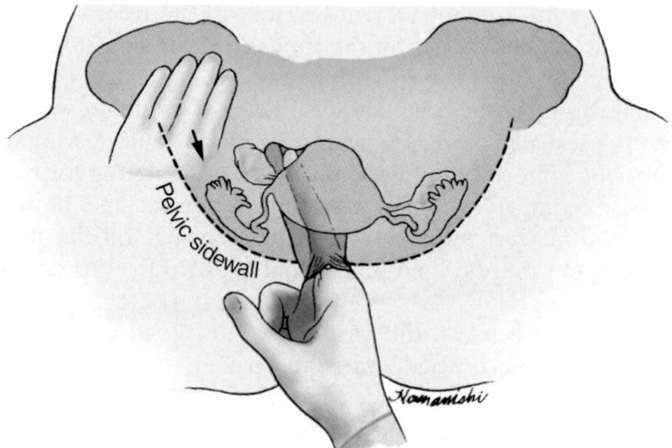

Figure 7-13. Bimanual examination of adnexa.

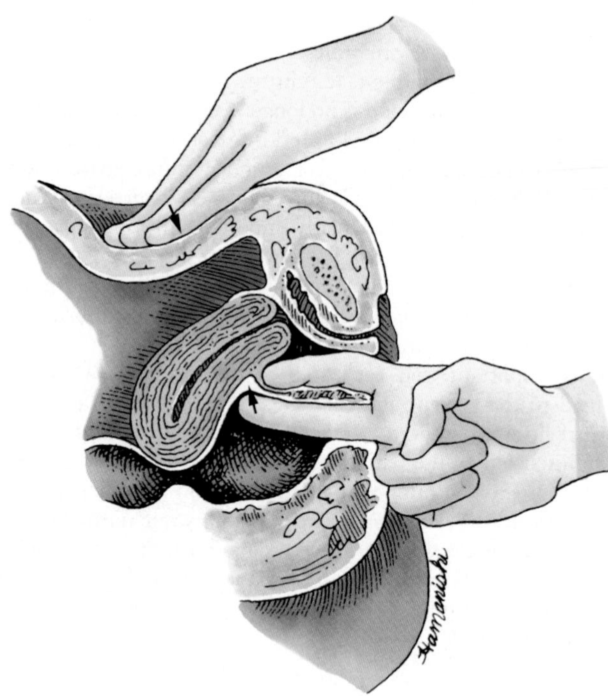

Figure 7-14. Rectovaginal examination.

Adnexa are usually not palpable in postmenopausal women because of involution and retraction of the ovary to a position higher in the pelvis. A palpable organ in such an individual may need further investigation for ovarian pathology, if enlarged.

Rectovaginal Examination

After completing the vaginal portion of the bimanual examination, the middle finger is relubricated with a water-soluble lubricant and placed into the rectum. Many physicians think the glove should be changed so as not to contaminate the rectum with vaginal organisms. The index finger is reinserted into the vagina. In this fashion the rectovaginal septum is palpated between the two fingers, and any thickness or mass is noted. The finger should also attempt to identify the uterosacral ligaments, which extend from the posterior wall of the cervix posteriorly and laterally toward the sacrum. Any thickening or beadiness of these structures may imply an inflammatory reaction or endometriosis. If the uterus is retroverted, that organ should be outlined for size, shape, and consistency at this point. It may be examined appropriately using the fingers inserted into the vagina and the rectum, as well as using the abdominal hand (Fig. 7-14).

Rectal Examination

The rectum is then palpated in all dimensions with the rectal examining finger. It should be possible to palpate as many as 70% of distal bowel lesions with the rectal finger. Because bowel cancer is common in women, particularly after the age of 35, this part of the examination should not be overlooked.

The physician should also note the tone of the anal sphincter and any other anal abnormalities, such as hemorrhoids, fissures, or masses. A stool sample taken on the rectal examining finger and tested for occult blood is no longer recommended for office screening. A recent large trial found this technique missed 95% of polyps and cancers that were found at subsequent colonoscopy. Better screening for colorectal cancer is described later in this chapter. This is particularly important in women past the age of 35 who may be at risk for bowel cancer.

At the end of the examination the physician should give the patient some facial tissue so that she may remove the lubricating jelly from her perineum before she dresses.

It is important that each step of the examination be explained to the patient and that she can be reassured about all normal findings. Wherever possible, abnormal findings should be pointed out to the patient either by allowing her to palpate the pathologic condition or by demonstrating it to her using a hand mirror. It is also appropriate to demonstrate normal structures to the patient, such as the cervix and portions of the vagina that she may be able to see with her hand mirror. The physician should use the examination as a vehicle for teaching the patient about her body.

THE ANNUAL VISIT

The annual visit is important for both health maintenance and preventive medicine reasons. Although the visit varies in emphasis depending on the patient's age, the long-term goals should be to maintain the patient in the best health and functional status possible and to promote high-quality longevity. Major preventable problems must be discussed because patient behavior can make a difference. A 1993 JAMA article estimated the root causes of American deaths and attributed 19% to tobacco, 14% to diet and activity, 5% to alcohol, 4% to microbial agents, 4% to illicit drug use, 3% to toxic agents, 2% to firearms, 1% to motor vehicles, and 1% to sexual behavior. Obviously, much of this can be altered by patients taking an active role in changing their behavior and physicians have the opportunity to advise them at the annual visit.

Although the gynecologist is generally the primary physician for women during their reproductive years, until recently this was not necessarily the case for postmenopausal women. However, it has become clear that the gynecologist with appropriate training and motivation can continue being the primary physician for older women as well.

In 1618, an English clergyman observed, "Prevention is so much better than healing because it saves the labor of being sick." In 1973 Belloc reported that in a study of women past the age of 45 the life expectancy was 7 years greater for those who routinely practiced six of seven important health habits as compared with those who practiced three or fewer (see the following box). During the annual visit physicians should therefore discuss nutrition regarding (1) proper caloric intake to maintain the patient's weight near her optimum and avoid obesity, (2) restricting saturated fat and cholesterol, and (3) understanding the need for adequate calcium in the diet and vitamin D.

At each checkup the physician should also encourage the patient to develop an exercise program appropriate for her abilities and to avoid smoking and excessive alcohol use (if she has these habits). The physician should discuss possible stressors in the patient's life, such as her relationship with her husband or partner and other family members, her satisfaction or dissatisfaction with her job, and other social problems that she may be experiencing. It is appropriate to ask questions that assess her sexual activity and gratification and questions that detect abuse or intimida-tion in her life. It is also appropriate to discuss the physical and emotional implications of loss and grief. Everyone suffers loss during his or her lifetime, and the older the patient the more likely that this is the case. Grief may be the result of a loss of a spouse or loved one, a pet, a job, a body part, or the ability to perform activities the patient has enjoyed (see Chapter 9, Emotional Aspects of Gynecology).

Good Health Habits

Eat moderately
Eat regularly
Eat breakfast
Avoid smoking
Exercise regularly
Use alcohol in moderation or not at all
Sleep 7 to 8 hours per night

The patient should be asked to bring all medications that she is taking. Prescription and over-the-counter drugs, as well as any dietary or herbal supplements, should be included. This will give the physician the opportunity to review with the patient why she is taking each one, and also to assess for possible potential adverse drug interactions. It may also be possible to tie specific drug use to an undesirable symptom the patient may be experiencing.

The annual visit is an opportunity for the physician to screen for a variety of illnesses affecting not only the reproductive organs but all of the organ systems. The visit should include an interim health history and a complete physical examination. The weight, height, and blood pressure measurements and the breast, pelvic, and rectal examinations should all be performed and recorded so that comparisons may be made from year to year. A gross assessment of the patient's hearing ability and visual acuity should be performed annually.

The American College of Obstetricians and Gynecologists Task Force on Primary Preventive Health Care recommended screening laboratory tests for the annual visit for women in different age groups (Table 7-2). It was recommended that an annual Pap smear be begun at age 21 or 3 years after a woman becomes sexually active. For women younger than 18 who are in specific high-risk groups, hemoglobin, urine testing for bacteriuria, testing for sexually transmitted diseases and human immunodeficiency virus (HIV), genetic testing, rubella titer, tuberculosis skin test, lipid profile, and hepatitis C virus testing may be appropriate.

For women between the ages of 19 and 39, an annual Pap smear should be ordered unless the patient is monogamous and after age 30 has had three consecutive normal tests and no risk factors for cervical cancer. After that and at the discretion of the physician and the patient, the testing may be done every 2 to 3 years. Human papillomavirus (HPV) typing and use

Table 7-2 Suggested Laboratory Studies for Annual Health Maintenance Visit

Age	Routine	High Risk
13–18	Pap test (annually; begin 3 years after becomes sexually active) Hepatitis B vaccine (if not immunized) Tdap booster (once between 11 and 18 years) HPV vaccine (one series between ages 9 and 26)	Hgb Urinalysis STD, HIV testing Genetic testing Rubella titer TB skin test FBS Consider additional immunizations in high-risk groups Hepatitis C virus testing
19–39	Pap test (yearly by age 21) Tdap once and Td (every 10 years) HPV vaccine (one series between ages 9 and 26)	Urinalysis Mammography (if strong family history or BRCA-1/BRCA-2 genetic mutations) FBS Cholesterol and HDL cholesterol[†] Lipid profile[‡] STD, HIV testing Genetic testing Rubella titer TB skin test Consider additional immunizations in high-risk groups TSH Hepatitis C virus testing
40–64	Pap test Mammography (annual or biannual until 50, then annual) Cholesterol (every 5 years) Colorectal screening (≥50) Tdap once and then Td (every 10 years)[‡] TSH (every 5 years beginning at 50) Fasting glucose testing (every 3 years after age 45)	Hbg Urinalysis FBS STD, HIV testing TB skin test Lipid profile[‡] Consider additional immunizations in high-risk groups Hepatitis C virus testing
65 and older	Pap test (depends on prior screening and risk factors) Mammography (continue > 70 years if no serious comorbid disease) Cholesterol (every 3–5 years) Colorectal cancer screening Bone density screening (≥every 2 years) TSH (every 5 years) FBS (every 3 years) Influenza vaccine	Hgb FBS Urinalysis STD, HIV testing Lipid profiles[‡] Hepatitis C screening

*Tdap should be given for one booster dose. Td should be used for later doses every 10 years.
[†]High risk is having diabetes, positive family history, hypertension, and/or tobacco use.
[‡]Lipid profile appropriate for family history of hyperlipidemia or premature cardiovascular disease (men < 50 years, women < 60 years), diabetes, and multiple coronary heart disease risk factors (hypertension, smoking, obesity).
FBS, fasting blood sugar; HDL, high-density lipoprotein; Hgb, hemoglobin; HIV, human immunodeficiency virus; STD, sexually transmitted disease; TB, tuberculosis; Td, tetanus–diphtheria vaccine; Tdap, tetanus toxoid, reduced diphtheria toxoid and acellular pertussis vaccine; TSH, thyroid-stimulating hormone.

for screening for cervical disease is discussed in Chapter 28 [Intraepithelial Neoplasia of the Lower Genital Tract (Cervix, Vulva)]. Women with diabetes, positive family history, hypertension, or tobacco abuse should have a fasting cholesterol and high-density lipoprotein (HDL) cholesterol test. The United States Preventive Services Task Force (USP-STF) only recommends screening for type 2 diabetes in individuals with hypertension or hyperlipidemia. For women in this age group who are at high risk, hemoglobin, urinalysis, mammography, testing for sexually transmitted diseases and HIV, rubella titer, tuberculosis skin test, TSH, and hepatitis C virus testing may be indicated.

For women between the ages of 40 and 64, annual Pap smear or as noted earlier, mammography every 1 to 2 years until age 50 and annually after that, cholesterol levels every 5 years, fasting glucose testing every 3 years after age 45 are recommended. For women in this age group who are considered high risk, hemoglobin, urinalysis, fasting glucose levels, testing for sexually transmitted diseases and HIV, tuberculosis skin test, lipid profile, TSH, colonoscopy, and hepatitis C virus testing should be considered. Women age 50 and older can be screened for colorectal cancer by several means: fecal occult blood testing (FOBT) using home testing kits every year, flexible sigmoidoscopy every 5 years, FOBT every year plus sigmoidoscopy every 5 years, double-contrast barium enema every 5 years, or colonoscopy every 10 years. Some women in high-risk groups, such as family history of colorectal cancer, should be screened earlier than age 50. Thyroid-stimulating hormone (TSH) screening is recommended every 5 years beginning at age 50.

For women who are 65 and older, Pap smears should be performed every 1 to 3 years at the discretion of the patient and physician after three consecutive normal tests. The American Cancer Society guidelines state Pap smears can be discontinued for women older than 70 years of age who have had three consecutive normal annual results or who have had no abnormal results in the past 10 years. In addition, urinalysis, mammography, cholesterol (every 3 to 5 years), colorectal cancer screening as noted earlier, and TSH every 5 years should be ordered. For women in particular high-risk groups, hemoglobin, fasting glucose, testing for sexually transmitted diseases and HIV, tuberculosis skin test, lipid profile, and hepatitis C virus testing should be considered. Bone density screening tests for osteoporosis detection can be offered at age 65 and not more frequently than every 2 years. High-risk women should be screened earlier than age 65 (steroid use chronically, family history, fracture history, physically inactive, tobacco or abuse alcohol, underweight, dementia, European or Asian ancestry, history of falls, estrogen deficiency, or poor nutrition),

Women who have undergone a hysterectomy with removal of the cervix for benign conditions can discontinue cervical cytology testing provided they have no history of cervical intraepithelial neoplasia (CIN), grade 2 or 3. There is no good evidence to date to suggest an upper age limit to stop Pap tests.

Women in the youngest age group should be given tetanus–diphtheria and acellular pertussis vaccine (Tdap) booster shots once between the ages of 11 and 18. Measles/mumps/rubella (MMR), hepatitis B vaccine, and fluoride supplementation to prevent tooth decay should be offered to those at risk. Susceptible adolescents *and* adults should be offered varicella vaccination. Meningococcal vaccine is now recommended once before entry to high school if not done at ages 11 to 12 years. For ages 19 to 39, a Tdap booster is indicated once. Then, every 10 years the regular Td (tetanus–diphtheria) booster is given.

A human papillomavirus (HPV) vaccine became available in 2006. Currently, this is recommended for females 9 to 26 years old. Ideally, the vaccine should be administered before onset of sexual activity to prevent cervical cancer and other diseases caused by certain strains of HPV.

For women between the ages of 40 and 64, the Tdap booster should be given once and then Td every 10 years. The influenza vaccine should be offered annually beginning at age 65. For women in high-risk groups, MMR, hepatitis B vaccine, influenza vaccine, and pneumococcal vaccine should be offered. Specifically, influenza vaccine should be offered to women younger than 65 with chronic medical conditions (e.g., cardiovascular or respiratory disease, diabetes, or immunosuppression). In addition, health care workers in direct patient care and caretakers of children younger than 6 months of age should be immunized.

For women who are 65 and older, the Tdap booster every 10 years should be continued, influenza vaccine should be given annually, and pneumococcal vaccine should be given once.

In addition, women in all age groups should be offered appropriate immunizations and vaccinations when they travel to other countries. Hepatitis A vaccine is available and should be offered to women of all ages.

Table 7-3 Recommended Intakes of Calcium and Vitamin D

Age (years)	Intake Calcium (mg)	Intake Vitamin D (IU)
14–18	1300	200
19–50	1000	200
51+	1200	400
71+	1200	600

Physicians should discuss risk behavior annually with their patients. In line with injury prevention, the patient should be reminded about use of seat belts and helmets and other safety concerns mentioned earlier in this chapter. Fall precautions can be discussed with elderly patients.

Exposure of the skin to ultraviolet radiation and proper precautions to avoid overexposure should be discussed. Regular dental check-ups should be encouraged. Adequate calcium and vitamin D intake for proper bone health and age appropriate intake recommendations should be reviewed at the annual visit (Table 7-3). Destructive habits such as the use of tobacco, alcohol, or drugs should be addressed, and possible remedial suggestions should be given.

Many women will ask their physician about prophylactic aspirin use. While randomized trials in men have shown that low-dose aspirin decreases the risk of a first myocardial infarction, this was not so for women in a large trial in 2005. Ridker and coworkers randomly assigned 38,876 healthy women older than 45 years of age to 100 mg of aspirin on alternate days or placebo and followed them for 10 years. Aspirin did reduce the risk of stroke by 17%, but had no significant effect on the risk of fatal or nonfatal myocardial infarction. A subgroup analysis of the 4097 women older than 65 years of age did show a significant reduction in the risk of myocardial infarction but at the cost of more gastrointestinal hemorrhages requiring transfusion. Therefore, the use of aspirin as primary prevention in women must be carefully weighed between the risks and benefits for each individual.

Promoting good health is a continuing responsibility for both the physician and the patient. It represents a challenge that includes education and observation on the physician's part and motivation on the patient's part.

KEY POINTS

- Five general impressions of patients may be gleaned nonverbally (by observation): happiness, apathy, fear, anger, and sadness.
- Menstrual history includes age of menarche, number of days of cycle, number of days of flow, presence of bleeding between menstrual periods, the date of the last menstrual period, and the date of the previous menstrual period.
- Menstrual cycles occurring just after puberty and just before menopause are frequently anovulatory and may be irregular in frequency.
- Pregnancy history should include the details of full-term and premature labors, spontaneous abortion, ectopic pregnancies, molar pregnancies, and terminations.
- A complete gynecologic evaluation should always include a sexual history, contraceptive history, and history of physical or sexual abuse.
- A detailed family history includes inquiry about congenital malformations, mental retardation, or pregnancy wastage in the families of the patient and her husband.

KEY POINTS *Continued*

- Occupational and avocational activity should be investigated for the presence of potential hazards to the patient's health.
- Annual cervical cytology screening should begin approximately 3 years after initiation of sexual intercourse, but no later than age 21.
- Pap smears should be performed every 1 to 3 years, depending on the patient's risk level, age, and Pap test history.
- Sexually active women should be evaluated at appropriate intervals for sexually transmitted diseases. Counseling women on safe sex practices to avoid contracting sexually transmitted diseases is important.
- The physician should use the occasion of the history and physical examination to teach the patient important aspects of self-evaluation.
- Goals of preventive medicine maintaining good health and function and promoting high-quality longevity.
- The physician should maintain an immunization record for each patient and offer appropriate vaccinations as recommended by public health guidelines.

BIBLIOGRAPHY

Key Readings

American College of Obstetricians and Gynecologists: Cervical cytology screening. Technical Bulletin 45. Washington, DC: American College of Obstetricians and Gynecologists, 2003.

American College of Obstetricians and Gynecologists: Primary and preventive care: Periodic assessment. Committee Opinion No. 292, Washington, DC, American College of Obstetricians and Gynecologists, 2003.

Belloc NB: Relationship of health practices and mortality. Prev Med 2:67, 1973.

U.S. Preventive Services Task Force: Screening for cervical cancer. Rockville, MD, Agency for Healthcare Research and Quality, 2003.

General References

American College of Obstetricians and Gynecologists Committee Opinion: Routine cancer screening. No. 185, Washington, DC, September 1997.

American College of Obstetricians and Gynecologists: Guidelines for Women's Health Care, Washington, DC, 1996.

American College of Obstetricians and Gynecologists: Breast cancer screening. Practice Bulletin 42. Washington, DC, American College of Obstetricians and Gynecologists, 2003.

Executive Summary of the Third Report of the National Cholesterol Education Program (NCEP): Expert panel on detection, evaluation, and treatment of high blood cholesterol in adults (Adult Treatment Panel III). JAMA 285:2486, 2001.

Hampton T: Clinical trials point to complexities of chemoprevention for cancer. JAMA 294:29, 2005.

Kosters JP, Gotzsche PC: Regular self-examination or clinical examination for early detection of breast cancer. Cochrane Database Syst Rev (2):CD003373, 2003.

Martin-Hirsch P, Jarvis G, Kitchner H, et al: Collection devices for obtaining cervical cytology samples. Cochrane Database Syst Rev (3):DC001036, 2000.

McGinnis JM, Foege WH: Actual causes of death in the United States. JAMA 270:2207, 1993.

Nichol K, Lind A, Margolis KL, et al: The effectiveness of vaccination against influenza in healthy, working adults. N Engl J Med 333:889, 1995.

Papanicolaou GN, Trout HF: Diagnosis of Uterine Cancer by Vaginal Smears. New York, The Commonwealth Fund, 1943.

Pignone M, Rich M, Teutsch SM, et al: Screening for colorectal cancer in adults at average risk: A summary of the evidence for the U.S. Preventive Services Task Force. Ann Intern Med 137(2):132, 2002.

Rex DK, Johnson DA, Lieberman DA, et al: ACG recommendations on colorectal cancer screening for average and higher risk patients in clinical practice. April 2000. [American College of Gastroenterology Web site.] Available at: *http://wwwacg.gi.org/patients/ccrk/CRC200.pdf.* Accessed October 25, 2005.

Ridker PM, Cook NR, Lee I, et al: A randomized trial of low-dose aspirin in the primary prevention of cardiovascular disease in women. New Engl J Med 352:1293, 2005.

Solomon D, Davey D, Kurman R, et al: The 2001 Bethesda System: Terminology for reporting results of cervical cytology. JAMA 287:2114, 2002.

Shy K, Chu J, Mandelson M, et al: Papanicolaou smear screening interval and risk of cervical cancer. Obstet Gynecol 74:838, 1989.

U.S Preventive Services Task Force. Screening for coronary heart disease: recommendation statement. Ann Intern Med 140(7):569, 2004.

U.S Preventive Services Task Force. Screening for high blood pressure: recommendations and rationale. Am J Prev Med 25(2):159, 2003.

U.S Preventive Services Task Force. Screening adults for lipid disorders: recommendations and rationale. Am J Prev Med 20(3 Suppl):73, 2001.

Differential Diagnosis of Major Gynecologic Problems by Age Group 8

Vaginal Bleeding, Pelvic Pain, Pelvic Mass

Gretchen M. Lentz

KEY TERMS AND DEFINITIONS

Hematocolpos. Distention of an obstructed vagina (caused by imperforate hymen or transverse septum) with blood and blood products.

Hematometria. A uterus distended with blood, secondary to partial or complete obstruction of any portion of the lower genital tract.

Levator Spasm. Spasm of the levator ani muscles frequently associated with chronic pelvic pain or vaginismus.

Menorrhagia. Heavy or prolonged menstrual flow.

Metrorrhagia. Intermenstrual bleeding.

Pain. An unpleasant sensory or emotional experience associated with actual or potential tissue damage or described in terms of such damage.

Pelvic Congestion Syndrome. Vascular engorgement of the uterus and the vessels of the broad ligament and lateral pelvic walls, which may lead to chronic pelvic pain.

Trigger Points. Painful spasm of local muscle bundles or areas of scar tissue within the abdominal wall, at times associated with chronic pelvic and lower abdominal pain.

The gynecologist will evaluate a variety of women at different periods of life for relatively few specific symptoms and signs. Perhaps the three most common of these are unusual vaginal bleeding, pelvic pain, and pelvic or abdominal mass. Although each of these complaints will be of concern to the individual patient, their diagnostic implications may vary greatly depending on the patient's age. This chapter considers unusual vaginal bleeding, pelvic pain, and pelvic or abdominal mass from the standpoint of differential diagnosis, emphasizing the differences seen at different periods of a woman's life, and includes a detailed consideration of the problem of chronic pelvic pain.

VAGINAL BLEEDING

Abnormal vaginal bleeding includes prepubertal bleeding, menorrhagia, metrorrhagia or postcoital bleeding, and postmenopausal bleeding. Although the cause of the bleeding will frequently determine the characteristics that it exhibits, the physician should develop a systematic approach to the differential diagnosis of abnormal vaginal bleeding. The following box offers an outline that can be examined when considering a patient with abnormal vaginal bleeding. In addition, Chapter 37 (Abnormal Uterine Bleeding) considers this topic in detail.

Pregnancy

The possibility of a pregnancy must be considered in any woman in her reproductive years. This possibility can be rapidly ruled out using a sensitive serum pregnancy test. If the patient is found to be pregnant and vaginal bleeding is noted, the diagnostic possibilities include implantation bleeding; threatened, inevitable, complete, or incomplete abortion; ectopic pregnancy; and molar pregnancy.

Implantation bleeding is quite common. It usually consists of minimal bleeding at about the time of the first missed menstrual period and generally lasts a very short time. Occasionally, it may be present for 1 to 2 days, with a flow similar to that of a menstrual period. Often, implantation bleeding is not perceptible to the patient but can be seen by the physician as a brownish-tinged cervical mucus if a pelvic examination is performed. Bleeding in excess of a normal menstrual flow is quite rare, and prolonged bleeding does not usually occur.

Bleeding in the first trimester of pregnancy is not uncommon. About 20% to 25% of all pregnant women spot or bleed in the first trimester. If the bleeding can be observed to be coming from the cervix and the cervix is closed, a diagnosis of threatened abortion can be made (Chapter 16, Spontaneous and Recurrent Abortion). The size of the uterus should be consistent with what is normal for the date of the pregnancy, and the uterus may or may not be contracting and tender to the touch. A threatened abortion becomes inevitable when the cervix dilates and products of conception pass through the internal os or when the bleeding is profuse.

A complete abortion is noted when the uterus has expelled its contents, the internal os is closed, the bleeding is minimal, and the uterus has returned to near normal size. It is unusual for a patient who has a complete abortion to experience significant pelvic cramping or to cramp when a uterotonic agent such as methylergonovine maleate (Methergine) is administered.

Incomplete abortion occurs when a part of the products of conception has been expelled but some remains within the uterus. The cervix is generally dilated, and there is usually

Etiology of Abnormal Vaginal Bleeding

- Pregnancy
  - Abortion
    - Threatened
    - Inevitable
    - Complete
    - Incomplete
  - Ectopic
  - Molar–trophoblastic disease
- Dysfunctional uterine bleeding
  - Postpuberty
  - During reproductive years
  - Perimenopausal
- Neoplastic
  - Vulva and vagina
  - Cervix
  - Uterine corpus
  - Fallopian tube
  - Ovary
  - Other
- Inflammatory
  - Vulvitis and vaginitis
  - Cervicitis
  - Endometritis
- Pelvic inflammatory disease
- Traumatic
- Foreign body
- Direct trauma
- Systemic diseases
  - Coagulopathies
  - Blood dyscrasias
  - Endocrinopathy
- Drug effects
- Others

bleeding, which may be profuse. The uterus is generally enlarged, and the patient may experience cramping pain. Most gestations of 6 weeks or less from the time of the last menstrual period will abort completely. Incomplete abortions become more common after 6 weeks of gestation.

A missed abortion occurs when the embryo dies but the products of conception are not expelled from the uterus. Generally, the uterus involutes so that it is smaller than expected by dates. There may be dark red or brown vaginal bleeding, often minimal in amount. Pregnancy tests may remain positive for quite some time in the face of a missed abortion.

Ectopic pregnancies are quite common and the incidence has risen since 1970 (see Chapter 17). About 20 in 1000 pregnancies end as ectopic pregnancies, but these figures vary from group to group. An ectopic pregnancy is defined as one that is implanted outside of the endometrial cavity. Thus, an ectopic pregnancy may exist in the cervix, within various portions of a fallopian tube, in the ovary, in the peritoneal cavity, and, in some rare instances, within the myometrium or a distant organ such as the spleen. A primary ectopic pregnancy in a specific organ implies that the pregnancy was implanted directly within that organ. A secondary ectopic pregnancy implies that the pregnancy ruptured from the fallopian tube and reimplanted completely or partially on another organ.

Ectopic pregnancies cause vaginal bleeding because of the separation of the decidua from the endometrium as the ectopic pregnancy dies or because of direct bleeding from the site of the ectopic pregnancy, with the blood being transported to the uterus and through the cervix. In most but not all cases the patient misses at least one menstrual period, begins to bleed from scant to significant amounts, and generally experiences pelvic pain. The pain may be limited to one side, in the case of a fallopian tube pregnancy, or may present as a more generalized pelvic pain. The pain may be similar to that experienced with pelvic inflammatory disease, but the patient with an ectopic pregnancy has a low-grade fever or is afebrile.

If the ectopic pregnancy is ruptured, intraperitoneal hemorrhage may occur and the patient may exhibit signs and symptoms of hypovolemia. Such an acute situation requires rapid intervention. It is important to remember that ectopic pregnancy is still the leading cause of pregnancy-related death during the first trimester.

Ectopic pregnancies become a diagnostic problem when they are unruptured. Vaginal bleeding occurs in about 90% of early ectopic pregnancies that are unruptured, and many patients experience pain. The uterus may be slightly enlarged or seem to be normal in size. If the ectopic pregnancy is tubal or ovarian, an adnexal mass may be noted. However, adnexal masses are not uncommon in normal pregnancies, representing the corpus luteum of pregnancy, and this may make the differential diagnosis somewhat more difficult. Adnexal tenderness may be present, but the pelvic exam can be normal with a small unruptured ectopic pregnancy.

With the availability of serum pregnancy tests, it is possible to rapidly ascertain that the patient is pregnant. When a pregnancy is diagnosed, it becomes necessary to establish whether it is intrauterine or ectopic. A vaginal ultrasound examination is indicated. If the pregnancy has progressed beyond 6 weeks' gestation, it is frequently possible to see a gestational sac within the uterine cavity. Occasionally, such a sac may be seen outside the uterine cavity in an adnexa.

Several authors have attempted to compare the levels of human chorionic gonadotropin (HCG) with the gestational age of the pregnancy and determine from this whether a normal pregnancy is developing. However, it is not yet possible to differentiate with certainty between an intrauterine and an ectopic pregnancy by relating levels of HCG to the presence or absence of a sac. In 2006, Silva and colleagues studied 200 women who were later confirmed to have an ectopic pregnancy and had at least 2 HCG values recorded. Sixty percent of subjects had a rise in HCG in 2 days and 21% of those had a rise similar to women with a viable gestation. Forty percent had an initial fall in HCG although the decline was slower than expected in 2 days compared with the decline in subjects with a completed spontaneous abortion in all but 8%. Hence, there remains too much overlap in serial HCG levels to use HCG as a sole test for evaluating women with a suspected ectopic pregnancy. This is discussed more completely in Chapter 17 (Ectopic Pregnancy).

In a patient experiencing vaginal bleeding and pelvic pain who has a positive pregnancy test and who does not exhibit a gestational sac within the uterus on ultrasound, the physician should consider the diagnosis of ectopic pregnancy. A gestational sac appearing outside the uterine cavity may be suggestive of an ectopic pregnancy, but frequent error has been noted in such diagnoses, and often the gestational sac does turn out to be intrauterine. For a stable patient, serial quantitative β-HCG levels with a follow-up transvaginal ultrasound may be necessary to differentiate an ectopic pregnancy from an intrauterine pregnancy. A study by Dart and coworkers found that women with an empty uterus at initial ultrasonography had the highest frequency of ectopic pregnancy compared with women with nonspecific fluid, echogenic material, abnormal sac, or normal sac in the uterus.

If the patient appears to have intraperitoneal bleeding, a culdocentesis may help. The presence of unclotted blood within the peritoneal cavity is evidence for intraperitoneal hemorrhage. Intraperitoneal fluid seen on ultrasound examination is also suggestive of intraperitoneal bleeding. Figure 8-1 shows an ultrasound scan of a woman with suspected ectopic pregnancy. Figure 8-2 shows an ectopic pregnancy rupturing out of the fallopian tube.

Several types of patients are at high risk for ectopic pregnancy. Prior ectopic pregnancy and prior pelvic inflammatory disease are the most important risk factors. Others include women who have undergone tubal reparative procedures, women who smoke, and those who have been exposed in utero to diethylstilbestrol (DES). Ectopic pregnancy should also be considered in users of intrauterine devices (IUDs), since IUDs only partially protect from tubular implantation. Increasing age is also a risk factor. Previous abortion has a negative association with ectopic pregnancy, but nontubal surgery and cesarean section have no association. Management of ectopic pregnancy is considered and discussed in Chapter 17 (Ectopic Pregnancy).

Another cause of abnormal vaginal bleeding associated with pregnancy is gestational trophoblastic disease (see Chapter 35). Most trophoblastic tumors are hydatidiform moles, which occur about once in every 1000 gestations in non-Asian women (rates among Southeast Asian women are 1.5 to 2.5 times higher; see Chapter 35). Although they may present in a variety of ways, the

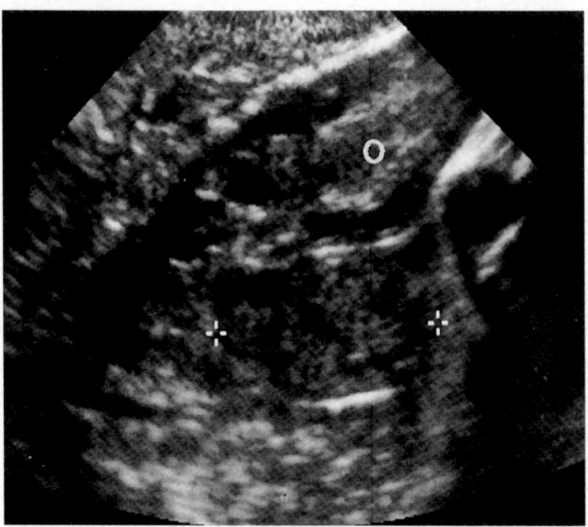

Figure 8-1. Transvaginal sonogram of a patient suspected of harboring an ectopic pregnancy. Transverse view of the left adnexa shows a hypoechoic mass (calipers) adjacent to the left ovary (O). No intrauterine pregnancy was visualized. Failure to demonstrate an intrauterine pregnancy and demonstration of a mass separate from the ovary is suggestive of ectopic pregnancy. A mass of this type generally represents a hematosalpinx. (From Callen PW: Ultrasound in Obstetrics and Gynecology, 4th ed. Philadelphia, WB Saunders, 2000, figure 33.12.)

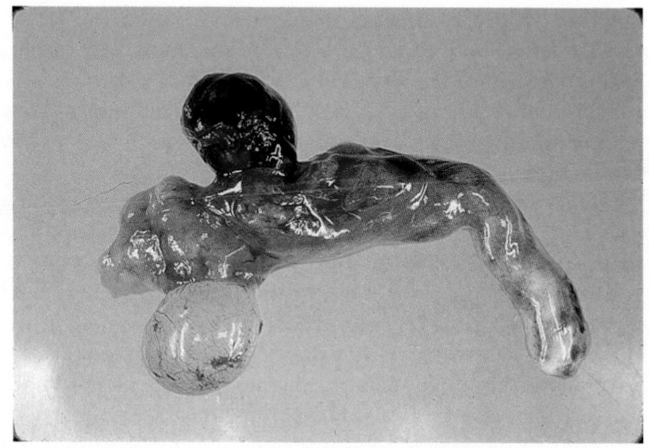

Figure 8-2. Fallopian tube with an ectopic pregnancy showing early rupture. (From Voet RL: Color Atlas of Obstetric and Gynecologic Pathology. St. Louis, Mosby, 1997, figure 5.3.)

classic molar pregnancy may include vaginal bleeding and a uterus enlarged beyond the size expected for gestational age. These findings may be associated with the passage of grapelike structures per vaginum, representing hydropic villi. At times, hypertension, edema, and proteinuria occur. Some molar pregnancies are associated with uteri that are small or normal for gestational age. In these cases the diagnosis may be suspected by an elevation of quantitative chorionic gonadotropin greater than 100,000 mIU/mL. Molar pregnancy must be differentiated from normal gestation, multiple gestation, and uterine enlargements caused by other factors, such as uterine myoma. Bleeding that occurs in the second trimester and is associated with hydatidiform mole may also be associated with a uterus that is large for gestational age; this will also need to be differentiated from hydramnios. An ultrasound examination in the late first trimester or early second trimester generally will detect hydatidiform mole and help in the differential diagnosis of other conditions, such as multiple gestation, hydramnios, and other uterine disorders.

Dysfunctional Uterine Bleeding

The endocrinology of dysfunctional uterine bleeding is discussed in Chapter 37 (Abnormal Uterine Bleeding). The frequency with which dysfunctional uterine bleeding occurs, however, is such that it is an important consideration in the differential diagnosis of abnormal vaginal bleeding. It is often a diagnosis of exclusion. The common denominator in many patients with dysfunctional uterine bleeding is anovulation or short ovulatory cycle, but this is not always the case. It is most commonly seen in the postpubertal period when normal hypothalamic function is not well established. In most instances, menstrual periods occur irregularly, often with long gaps between menses. When menses occurs, it may vary from very heavy flow to scanty flow and may continue for a number of days. The bleeding in most instances is from a nonsecretory endometrium. Occasionally, the bleeding is profuse with associated signs and symptoms of hypovolemia, requiring emergency care. Endometrial sampling will generally yield scanty nonsecretory endometrium. Rarely is any other pathologic condition noted. In a study in Montreal, Falcone and associates noted that in 61 adolescent patients,

93.4% responded to medical management, only 5 (8.2%) required dilation and curettage (D&C), and most had normal clotting factor profiles. Two had newly diagnosed hematologic problems (one had immune thrombocytopenic purpura and one had acute promyelocytic leukemia), but 29% gave a past history of some significant medical problem.

Women in the perimenopausal period who are undergoing some early evidence of ovarian failure may also experience dysfunctional uterine bleeding. Again the pattern may be one of irregularity, and the flow may vary from one that is increased in amount with clots to a scant flow with prolonged spotting. Endometrial biopsy may yield a diagnosis of nonsecretory endometrium, on histologic section, but hyperplasia of the endometrium may also be noted. In perimenopausal women it is important to differentiate dysfunctional uterine bleeding from other intrauterine disease, and endometrial sampling is indicated. An endometrial biopsy is generally sufficient to establish the appropriate diagnosis and rule out more serious conditions.

Dysfunctional uterine bleeding may also occur during the reproductive years. It may be associated with polycystic ovarian disease; thyroid or pituitary disease; or as a secondary symptom to stress, excessive weight change, or increased exercise performance. In such instances amenorrhea, oligomenorrhea, menorrhagia, or metrorrhagia may all be seen. Endometrial sampling generally produces nonsecretory endometrium; rarely is specific disease seen. In patients with polycystic ovarian disease, hyperplastic endometrium may be present. In a study of 1033 premenopausal women ages 17 to 50 who were menstruating regularly but who were complaining of abnormal menstrual bleeding, endometrial biopsy revealed normal endometrium in 93%, endometrial polyps in 2.2%, complex hyperplasia in 2.3%, atypical hyperplasia in 0.03%, and endometrial carcinoma in only 0.05%. Fifty-six percent of the patients were older than age 40, and 22.1% older than age 45. Sixteen percent were nulliparous, 7% complained of infertility, and 3.4% were diabetics. Thirty-two percent complained of menstrual bleeding lasting longer than 7 days, and 8% longer than 14 days. Irregular menstrual bleeding was experienced by one third of the patients. The diagnosis of polycystic ovarian syndrome was made in 2.3%. Risk factors for the women with hyperplasia were weight equal to or greater than 90 kg, age 45 or older, infertility, nulliparity, and a family history of colon cancer. In general, the most common cause of endometrial hyperplasia is excess estrogen, either exogenous or endogenous unopposed by progestin. So, any woman with long-term anovulatory disorders is at risk for endometrial hyperplasia and endometrial cancer and may present with abnormal vaginal bleeding. As a general guideline, an endometrial biopsy is indicated in all women older than the age of 35 with abnormal bleeding. If the woman has particular risk factors for endometrial hyperplasia or cancer, then a biopsy may be necessary in even younger women. Dysfunctional uterine bleeding is discussed more fully in Chapter 37.

Neoplastic Conditions

Although vaginal bleeding can be caused by a wide variety of neoplastic lesions, both benign and malignant, and affecting the various organs of the female reproductive tract, there are specific patterns typical of many of these (Table 8-1). In addition,

Table 8-1 Bleeding Pattern Seen in Tumors of the Reproductive Tract

Condition	Menorrhagia	Metrorrhagia	Postmenopausal Bleeding
Vulvar cancer	—	++	++
Vaginal cancer	—	++	++
Cervical cancer	—	++	++
Cervical polyp	—	++	+
Uterine myoma	++	+	—
Carcinoma of endometrium	—	—	++
Fallopian tube cancer	—	—	+
Ovarian cancer	—	±	±

++, usually occurs; +, occasionally occurs; ±, occurs rarely.

knowledge of occurrence rates of specific neoplasms in various age groups may help the physician in developing a differential diagnosis.

Cancers of the vulva and vagina may present with vaginal bleeding and usually occur in women who are in the latter reproductive years or in the postmenopausal period. Should they occur in women during the reproductive years, the bleeding is generally intermittent and therefore presents as metrorrhagia or postcoital bleeding rather than with any specific relationship to the menstrual cycle. The bleeding is generally minimal, although in advanced cases it can become profuse. An unusual vaginal tumor that may occur in teenage or young women is clear-cell cancer of the vagina, which is most often seen in women who have been exposed in utero to diethylstilbestrol (DES). Since this condition was first described by Herbst and colleagues in 1971, the actual incidence has been found to be quite low in such women. In addition, rare cases of clear-cell cancer of the vagina have been found in women who were not exposed to DES.

Tumors of the cervix are most often squamous cell carcinomas, although as many as 15% are adenocarcinomas or adenosquamous carcinomas and may be present within the endocervical canal (see Chapter 29, Malignant Diseases of the Cervix). Such lesions will generally bleed eventually, and the bleeding pattern will be one of metrorrhagia or postcoital staining. With larger lesions the bleeding may be quite profuse. Other cervical lesions, such as endocervical polyps, may also cause metrorrhagia.

The most common lesions of the uterine corpus that cause abnormal bleeding during the reproductive years are leiomyomas (fibroids). Although these are generally benign, they may become quite large and may cause menorrhagia or menometrorrhagia (see Chapter 18, Benign Gynecologic Lesions). Submucous myomas are generally associated with severe menorrhagia. Leiomyomas rarely cause vaginal bleeding in postmenopausal women. Endometrial carcinoma is the most common gynecologic malignancy. Generally, an adenocarcinoma but occasionally a sarcoma, carcinosarcoma, or some intermediate variety will cause vaginal bleeding or discharge in 90% of women (see Chapter 32, Neoplastic Diseases of the Uterus). Most of these occur in postmenopausal women and therefore would present as postmenopausal bleeding. The bleeding may be scant or profuse. Approximately 5% of endometrial adenocarcinomas occur in premenopausal women. These women most often are exposed to continuous endogenous estrogen stimulation and are often found to have polycystic ovarian disease or a functioning ovarian tumor, such as a granulosal cell tumor or a thecoma. When adenocarcinoma occurs in premenopausal women, these diagnostic possibilities should be considered.

Vaginal bleeding in association with fallopian tube cancer is quite rare and generally occurs in the postmenopausal woman. Nonetheless, scant vaginal bleeding associated frequently with a watery discharge, crampy pain, and occasionally with an adnexal mass should alert the physician to the possibility of this condition (see Chapter 34, Neoplastic Diseases of the Fallopian Tubes).

Ovarian cancers may present with vaginal bleeding, which is most often the result of intraperitoneal blood finding its way through the fallopian tube and through the uterus into the vagina. In the case of functioning ovarian tumors such as granulosal cell tumor or thecoma, the bleeding may be caused by either a hyperplastic endometrium or an endometrial cancer secondary to the estrogen stimulation.

Rarely, other intraperitoneal tumors may cause intraperitoneal bleeding with eventual vaginal bleeding from secondary passage of the blood through the reproductive tract. This is an unusual occurrence but should be considered in the differential diagnosis of unexplained vaginal bleeding.

Inflammatory Conditions

Although bleeding is not common as a symptom in inflammatory conditions, severe inflammation in tissue will often lead to capillary oozing or a small blood vessel erosion. Thus, vulvitis, vaginitis, cervicitis, and endometritis may all be associated with vaginal bleeding or spotting, generally without relationship to menses. At times, patients with acute salpingitis or tuboovarian abscess may also experience vaginal bleeding. This most likely comes from endometrial inflammation or abnormal uterine bleeding secondary to ovarian dysfunction. The symptoms and signs of inflammation, including discharge, pain, and tenderness, as well as generalized signs and symptoms of infection will help in the differential diagnosis.

Traumatic Conditions

Direct trauma to the female external genitalia and internal reproductive tract may occur secondary to accidental injury, the placement of foreign bodies within the vagina, and traumatic coitus. Direct lacerations secondary to one of these causes may lead to scant or profuse bleeding, depending on the extent of the injury. Often the bleeding is arterial and requires suture ligations. In children the insertion of foreign bodies into the vagina may lead to vaginal discharge with or without bleeding. Pencils, crayons, pieces of chalk, wads of paper, hairpins, and other items may be found. This is discussed more fully in Chapter 13 (Pediatric and Adolescent Gynecology). In adults, bleeding may be secondary to tampons or contraceptive devices. In older women bleeding may occur when a pessary is being used.

Coital lacerations may occur because of rape or as part of normal sexual function. Tears of the hymen or lacerations of the vagina when tissue is rigid may lead to severe vaginal bleeding. Occasionally, bleeding occurs from the cervix after conization or the vaginal vault after a hysterectomy. Although this often occurs shortly after the operation, there are reports of dehiscence of the upper vault years later.

Systemic Diseases

A number of systemic diseases are associated with clotting defects and therefore may present with vaginal bleeding or have vaginal bleeding associated with the natural history of the disease. These include various coagulopathies, blood dyscrasias, and endocrinopathies. In addition, patients who take medications that interfere with the normal clotting mechanism may suffer vaginal bleeding. Examples of such medications are heparin and sodium warfarin (Coumadin), which may affect the clotting mechanism directly, or agents that interfere with normal platelet function, such as salicylates and other prostaglandin synthetase inhibitors. Many such conditions can be suspected or diagnosed by history and physical examination. General laboratory studies such as complete blood count, cell smear, and assessment of the clotting mechanism will usually help discover such problems if they exist.

Postmenopausal Bleeding

Postmenopausal bleeding (PMB) accounts for 5% of all gynecologic office visits. Although PMB may be associated with a number of different conditions, it must always be investigated because many causes are premalignant or malignant. The most common premalignant and malignant causes are complex hyperplasia with atypia and carcinoma of the endometrium. These disorders are present in as many as one third of the patients evaluated for PMB in many series.

Dewhurst described the benign causes of PMB in 249 women seen at the Chelsea Hospital for Women in London (Table 8-2). A large variety of lesions were noted, and the most common

Table 8-2 Benign Conditions Causing Postmenopausal Bleeding Found in Patients Seen at the Chelsea Hospital for Women, London

Cause	Number
Atrophic vaginitis	129
Cervical polyps	65
Leiomyomata uteri	24
Endometrial hyperplasia	13
Cervical erosion	5
Trichomoniasis	3
Hematuria	2
Trauma	1
Vaginal endometriosis	1
Hemorrhoids	1
Moniliasis	1
Bartholin's gland abscess	1
Vulvar warts	1
Urethral caruncle	1
TOTAL	248

Modified from Dewhurst J: Postmenopausal bleeding from benign causes. Clin Obstet Gynecol 26:769, 1983.

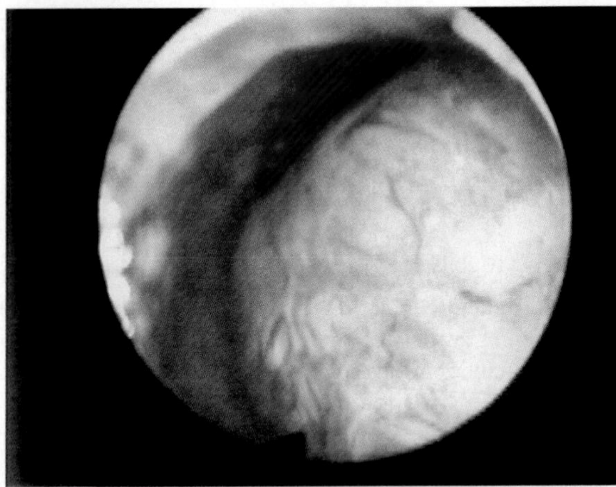

Figure 8-3. Hysteroscopy view of a large endometrial polyp in an 80-year-old woman on Tamoxifen.

single cause proved to be atrophic vaginitis. Dewhurst wisely counsels that even though an apparent benign cause of bleeding is found, women with PMB deserve a thorough evaluation to rule out a malignancy that may *also* be present. Figure 8-3 shows a large endometrial polyp found in an 80-year-old woman on Tamoxifen who presented with PMB.

Although many other lesions of the reproductive tract, both benign and malignant, may be discovered, one fourth to one third of the patients evaluated may demonstrate no obvious pathologic condition other than an atrophic endometrium.

Currently, the diagnostic procedures available for investigating PMB are endometrial biopsy, vaginal ultrasonography with endometrial thickness estimated, sonohysterography, and hysteroscopy with directed biopsy and D&C. Endometrial biopsy is comparable with D&C in detecting endometrial carcinoma with a sensitivity of between 85% and 95%, but is not accurate in diagnosing endometrial polyps or myomas. Hysteroscopy with directed biopsy can often make an accurate diagnosis but is quite costly. Endometrial biopsy coupled with sonohysterography was found to correlate well with the findings of hysteroscopy with biopsy in a study by O'Connell and colleagues. These authors found a greater than 95% correlation with a sensitivity of 94% and a specificity of 96%, suggesting that endometrial biopsy coupled with sonohysterography is a reliable office tool for identifying patients who should be considered for surgical intervention. Cost-effectiveness studies suggest that women with PMB should have an initial evaluation with an endometrial biopsy or ultrasonography. A 2002 meta-analysis by Tabor representing 3483 women with PMB found the median endometrial thickness in women with endometrial cancer was 3.7 times that of women without cancer. But, invasive testing such as endometrial biopsy was still needed as 4% of endometrial cancers would be missed even by using a relatively low endometrial thickness cutoff.

PELVIC AND ABDOMINAL PAIN

In 1994 the Taxonomy Committee of the International Association for the Study of Pain defined pain as "an unpleasant sensory and emotional experience associated with actual or potential tissue damage or described in terms of such damage." The committee further stated that pain is always subjective, with each individual learning the application of the word through experience related to injury in early life. It is always unpleasant and is, therefore, an emotional experience. They recognize that people may report pain in the absence of tissue damage or any likely pathophysiologic cause and that this may be secondary to psychological or psychosocial reasons. Blendis points out that most children and adults have experienced abdominal pain that is often short-lived and rarely associated with physical or organic cause. In many cases, both physical and psychogenic elements exist, making it impossible to tell which was the cause.

Acute Abdomen

A number of intraabdominal conditions can lead to the findings of an acute abdomen. These findings include acute pain, generally of sudden onset; tenderness to palpation; rebound tenderness; and diminished or absent bowel sounds. The pain may be caused by infection, hemorrhage, infarction of tissue, or obstruction of bowel. In the case of bowel obstruction, bowel sounds may be hyperactive. It is important to construct a differential diagnosis when signs and symptoms of acute abdomen are noted. Table 8-3 lists the more common causes of an acute abdomen and identifies the quadrant of the abdomen where findings are more likely to be positive. It should be remembered, however, that the abdominal cavity is a continuum and overlap of signs is extremely common. Disease within a tubular viscus, such as the bowel, fallopian tube, or ureter, may cause crampy pain. Frequently, patients complain of paroxysms of sharp, crampy pain interspaced with no pain at all or with periods of dull ache. Inflammatory conditions involving the ovary are frequently associated with continuous pain often described as sharp and throbbing.

Table 8-3 Conditions That May Cause Signs and Symptoms of Acute Abdomen and Abdominal Quadrants in Which They Most Often Occur

	QUADRANT			
Condition	**Right Upper**	**Right Lower**	**Left Upper**	**Left Lower**
Salpingitis	—	+	—	+
Tuboovarian abscess	±	+	±	+
Ectopic pregnancy	—	+	—	+
Adnexal torsion	—	+	—	+
Ruptured ovarian cyst	—	+	—	+
Acute appendicitis	—	+	—	—
Mesenteric lymphadenitis	—	+	—	—
Crohn's disease	—	+	—	—
Acute cholecystitis	+	±	—	—
Perforated peptic ulcer	+	±	+	±
Acute pancreatitis	+	—	+	—
Acute pyelonephritis	+	±	+	±
Renal calculus	+	+	+	+
Splenic infarct	—	—	+	—
Splenic rupture	—	—	+	—
Acute diverticulitis	—	—	—	+

+, more frequently; ±, may occur.

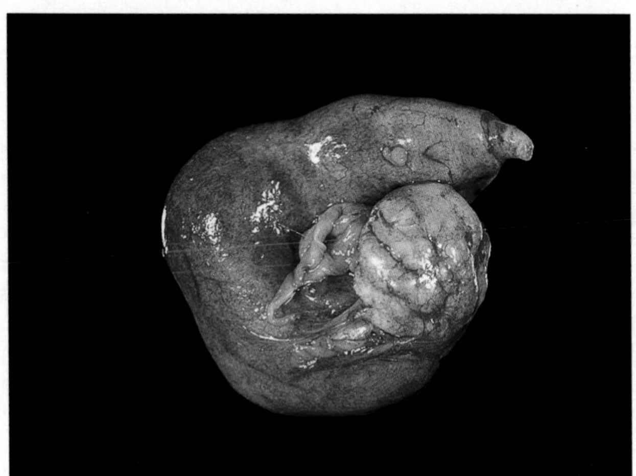

Figure 8-4. Tuboovarian abscess. (From Voet RL: Color Atlas of Obstetric and Gynecologic Pathology. St. Louis, Mosby, 1997, figure 5.11.)

Acute appendicitis, mesenteric lymphadenitis, and occasionally torsion of an adnexa may be found in preadolescent and adolescent girls. Appendicitis is, of course, a possible differential diagnosis in all age groups. It often presents initially as periumbilical pain that localizes to the right lower quadrant and is accompanied by anorexia or nausea and vomiting. Salpingitis, tuboovarian abscess, urinary tract infection, ectopic pregnancy, and ruptured ovarian cysts are common findings in those patients of reproductive age who have an acute abdomen. Patients with salpingitis tend to have a higher fever than those with appendicitis, but great variability may be observed. Although their pain may be severe, they tend to be less ill than those with appendicitis. Figure 8-4 shows a pathologic specimen of a tuboovarian abscess. However, women with these symptoms may have Crohn's disease, acute cholecystitis, perforated peptic ulcer, acute pyelonephritis, renal calculi, splenic infarct, and splenic rupture. Occasionally, they may also suffer from acute pancreatitis, which usually presents as epigastric pain often radiating to the back.

Acute abdomen in older women suggests torsion or rupture of an adnexa, acute cholecystitis, perforated ulcer, or acute diverticulitis. Pelvic inflammatory disease is less common in older women, and acute exacerbations are rare in those who have had tubal ligation.

Acute Pelvic Pain

Acute pain of gynecologic origin presents as both pelvic and lower abdominal pain. Diseases and dysfunction of the genitourinary tract, gastrointestinal tract, and musculoskeletal system may also cause pain in these regions. The following box lists a number of gynecologic and nongynecologic conditions that can cause acute onset of pelvic or lower abdominal pain.

Threatened, inevitable, or incomplete abortion generally is accompanied by midline or bilateral lower abdominal pain, usually of a crampy, intermittent nature. In such instances vaginal bleeding is generally present. When infection occurs concurrently (septic abortion), the woman generally has an elevated temperature, systemic symptoms of chills and malaise, and often an elevated white cell count and erythrocyte sedimentation rate (ESR). Rapid serum or urine pregnancy tests are generally positive.

Possible Causes of Acute Pelvic and Lower Abdominal Pain

Pregnancy-related
Abortion
Ectopic

Disorders of the Uterus and Cervix
Cervicitis
Endometritis
Degenerating myoma

Disorders of the Adnexa
Salpingitis
Tuboovarian abscess
Endometriosis (endometrioma)
Torsion of adnexa
Torsion of hydatid of Morgagni
Rupture of follicle or corpus luteum cyst
Ovarian hyperstimulation syndrome
Degenerating ovarian tumor

Nongynecologic Disorders
Appendicitis
Mesenteric lymphadenitis
Diverticulitis
Functional bowel syndrome
Cystitis
Trigonitis
Renal calculus
Musculoskeletal disorders

Ectopic pregnancy generally is associated with unilateral, continuous, crampy pain, although there may be some bilaterality to the presentation. Most ectopic pregnancies are associated with vaginal bleeding. Temperature elevation, if present, is usually minimal, and white cell count and ESR are generally normal but may be slightly elevated, particularly if there is intraperitoneal hemorrhage. Serum β-HCG is positive, and ultrasound examination may help in the diagnosis either by revealing a gestational sac in the adnexa or by ruling out the diagnosis through demonstration of a gestational sac within the uterus. Physical examination may demonstrate the presence of a mass in the adnexal region. Intraperitoneal bleeding may be suspected by seeing fluid on ultrasound examination and diagnosed by culdocentesis, with a definitive diagnosis made by laparoscopy.

Acute cervicitis, often caused by *Neisseria gonorrhoeae* or *Chlamydia trachomatis,* may frequently be associated with lower abdominal and pelvic pain. The pain is often of a dull, aching nature and may radiate to the low back or to the upper thighs. There is generally a cervical and vaginal discharge, and there may be a low-grade fever, slight leukocytosis, and slight increase in ESR. Definitive diagnosis is made by specific culture for the organism.

Endometritis may occur in *Neisseria* or *Chlamydia* infections as part of their natural history. Occasionally, douching will lead to endometritis. The pain is generally midline, pelvic, or lower

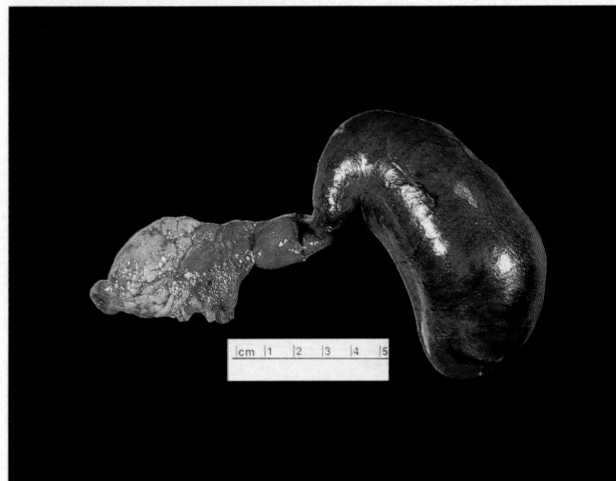

Figure 8-5. Hematosalpinx with torsion. (From Voet RL: Color Atlas of Obstetric and Gynecologic Pathology. St. Louis, Mosby, 1997, figure 5.15.)

abdominal and often aching in type (see Chapter 23, Infections of the Upper Genital Tract).

Degenerating myoma will frequently cause acute, sharp, or aching pain in the region of the myoma. Diagnosis is aided by the facts that the uterus is irregular and enlarged and that there is tenderness to palpation. There may be a mild leukocytosis, but generally laboratory parameters are normal.

Salpingitis and tuboovarian abscess have been discussed under the section on Acute Abdomen and in Chapter 23. Endometriosis is discussed in detail in Chapter 19. The pain pattern depends on the location of the endometrial implants and varies from dysmenorrhea and dyspareunia to continuous, generalized pelvic discomfort.

Torsion of the adnexa with or without an ovarian cyst or tumor may lead to acute, crampy, or continuous pain and was discussed under Acute Abdomen. It can be confused with appendicitis or pelvic inflammatory disease (PID). Occasionally, a hydatid of Morgagni will undergo torsion and give similar symptoms. Figure 8-5 demonstrates a hematosalpinx with torsion.

Rupture of an ovarian cyst may cause a sudden onset of pain. Leaking from a corpus luteum cyst generally occurs midcycle and, if it is on the right side, may be misdiagnosed as appendicitis. A hemorrhagic corpus luteum cyst may cause acute pain and is shown in Figure 8-6, and the pathologic specimen may appear like Figure 8-7. Ovarian hyperstimulation syndrome is a rare entity that may occur in women being treated with infertility medications to stimulate ovulation; it is most likely to occur if pregnancy ensues. In such instances the gestation is often found to be multiple. Ovarian hyperstimulation-like conditions may occur in women suffering from gestational trophoblastic disease and, rarely, in women with severe isoimmunization disease such as Rh isoimmunization. It is most often seen in women undergoing in vitro fertilization procedures because of the ovulation-stimulating drugs.

Degenerating adnexal tumors that have outgrown their blood supply may also cause acute-onset lower abdominal or pelvic pain.

Appendicitis, mesenteric lymphadenitis, and diverticulitis were all discussed under Acute Abdomen. Appendicitis and mesenteric lymphadenitis generally present as right lower quadrant or right pelvic pain, and diverticulitis most often presents as a left-sided pain. Young women suffering from functional bowel syndrome will often present with a crampy severe left lower quadrant pain generally made worse by emotional tension and stress. As many as 25% of young women may have this condition.

Patients suffering from cystitis may complain of lower abdominal or pelvic pain, generally midline in nature, accompanied by dysuria. Women suffering from renal calculus will generally have severe, intermittent flank pain on the side of the stone; this pain often radiates toward the lower abdomen. Interstitial cystitis is a painful bladder condition in which women present with symptoms similar to acute cystitis; however, the urine is sterile. They often have urination frequency, nocturia, and dyspareunia. The pain is typically in the suprapubic range, but can vary from the umbilicus, through the lower abdomen and pelvis, and even involve the upper thighs. Interstitial cystitis is discussed in detail in Chapter 21 (Urogynecology).

A variety of musculoskeletal disorders may also present as pelvic pain, lower abdominal pain, or backache. Slocumb has

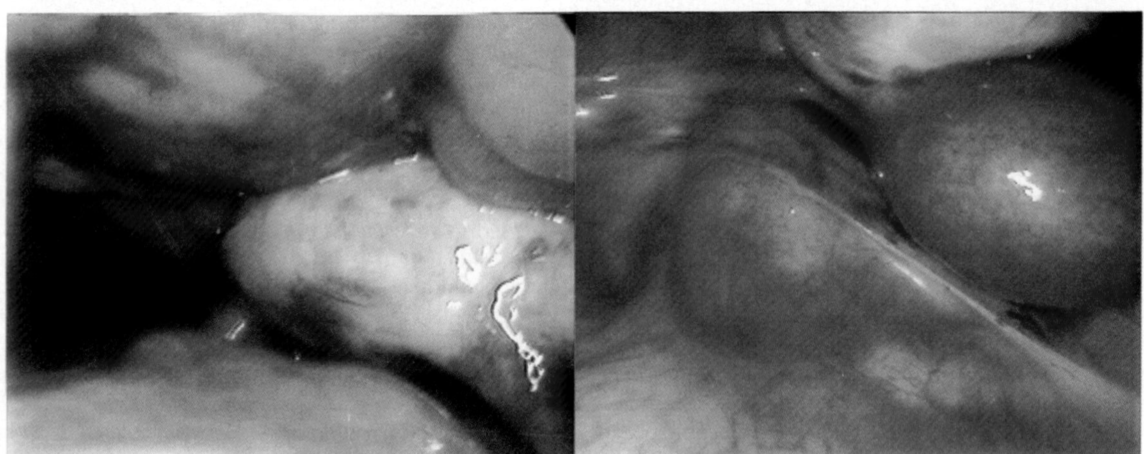

Figure 8-6. Laparoscopic view of a 33-year-old woman with a right, 7-cm hemorrhagic, ovarian cyst.

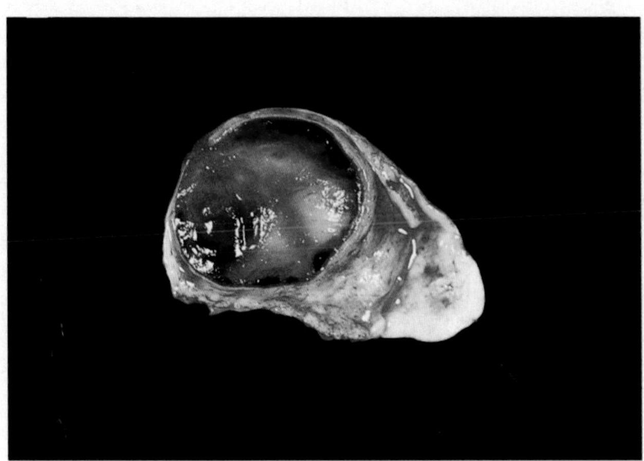

Figure 8-7. Hemorrhagic corpus luteum. (From Voet RL: Color Atlas of Obstetric and Gynecologic Pathology. St. Louis, Mosby, 1997, figure 6.5.)

called attention to the presence of "trigger points" (now called abdominal wall myofascial pain) discernible by palpation in the abdominal wall, lower back, and in the vaginal vault. Touching or stimulating these may simulate the pain about which the patient is complaining. Slocumb noted relief in several patients after the injection of these points with a local anesthetic such as 0.25% bupivacaine on one or several occasions. He notes that the pain often disappears for longer periods than the drug would be expected to cause. Because of this he speculates that in some instances chronic pelvic pain may be caused by a neurologic reflex that can be interrupted by the injection. Certainly, irritation of the musculoskeletal system by exercise or injury can produce pain that can cause the patient to believe she has internal organ disease. Perhaps the injection of "trigger points" contributes to a reassurance that this is not the case.

Pain emanating from the uterus, such as with dysmenorrhea or that associated with adenomyosis and occasionally adnexal disease, may radiate to the anterior thigh. Rarely are the inner or outer aspects of the thigh involved, and the posterior thigh is never involved with such conditions. Pain radiating to the posterior thigh generally denotes sciatic nerve involvement, and this is commonly seen with cervical cancer of an advanced nature. Occasionally, endometriosis may cause such pain by irritating the sciatic nerve.

Most pain that is limited to the lower back but not to the abdominal region is generally of musculoskeletal origin rather than from gynecologic disease.

Chronic Pelvic Pain

Chronic and recurrent pelvic pain is one of the major problems seen by the gynecologist. Dysmenorrhea (see Chapter 36, Primary and Secondary Dysmenorrhea, Premenstrual Syndrome, and Premenstrual Dysphoric Disorder) is perhaps the most common example of recurrent pelvic pain. There is no standardized definition of chronic pelvic pain, but many research papers use 6 or more months' duration of noncyclic pain as the definition. The prevalence may be as high as 15% to 20% of reproductive-age women. In addition, incompletely treated pelvic infections; recurrent pelvic infections; endometriosis; and possibly postoperative pelvic adhesions and diseases of the urinary tract, bowel, and neurologic systems may all be responsible for recurrent or persistent pelvic pain. Many who complain of chronic pelvic pain have no demonstrable pelvic disorder. Cunanan and coworkers reviewed 1194 charts of consecutive pelvic pain patients who had undergone diagnostic laparoscopy and discovered that in 355 cases a normal pelvis was found. Interestingly, of the 1194 patients, 749 had a normal pelvic examination before the diagnostic laparoscopy and, of these, 479 (63%) had abnormal findings on diagnostic laparoscopy. Of the 445 patients who had been thought to have an abnormal pelvic examination before laparoscopy, 78 (17.5%) actually had normal findings on diagnostic laparoscopy.

Kresch and associates reported the laparoscopic findings of 100 women who complained of constant pelvic pain in the same location for a minimum of 6 months. These authors compared the findings in this group with those of 50 women who were asymptomatic but who were undergoing laparoscopic tubal ligation. Overall, 83% of the group with pelvic pain had abnormal pelvic findings, whereas only 29% of the asymptomatic group demonstrated such findings. Pelvic adhesions were the most common pathologic finding, accounting for 38% of the abnormalities seen. Pelvic endometriosis accounted for 32% of the abnormal findings in the symptomatic group. These authors pointed out that when chronic pelvic pain exists in the same area for a minimum of 6 months, it is usually associated with specific pathologic conditions. However, even in this group of patients, 17% had no pelvic disorder at the time of diagnostic laparoscopy.

Between 18% and 35% of women with acute pelvic inflammatory disease have subsequent chronic pelvic pain. Why this occurs in some women and not others is unclear. Furthermore, the development of chronic pelvic pain following acute PID does not appear related to whether inpatient or ambulatory antibiotic treatment was given.

The question of whether pelvic adhesions are a frequent cause of chronic pelvic pain is as yet unanswered. Rapkin reviewed 100 consecutive laparoscopies performed because of chronic pelvic pain and compared the pelvic findings with those noted in 88 laparoscopies performed in infertility patients. A total of 26 (26%) of the pain group and 34 (39%) of the infertility group demonstrated pelvic adhesions as the only pathology seen. However, only 4 of the 34 patients in the infertility group complained of pain. Peters and colleagues performed a randomized trial of adhesiolysis in 48 patients found by laparoscopy to have American Society for Reproductive Medicine (ASRM) stage II–IV pelvic adhesions. Twenty-four underwent adhesiolysis, and 24 did not. After 9 to 12 months of follow-up, no significant differences with respect to pelvic pain were noted between the two groups. However, eight of nine women in a subgroup who had dense, vascularized (stage IV) adhesions involving the bowel showed significant improvement after adhesiolysis, whereas only one of six not given adhesiolysis reported improvement of pain. These authors concluded that pain relief might be obtained by lysing dense adhesions but probably not by lysing light or moderate adhesions.

Interstitial cystitis was mentioned in the differential diagnosis of acute pelvic pain. However, studies suggest that 38% to 85% of women coming to gynecologists for chronic pelvic pain

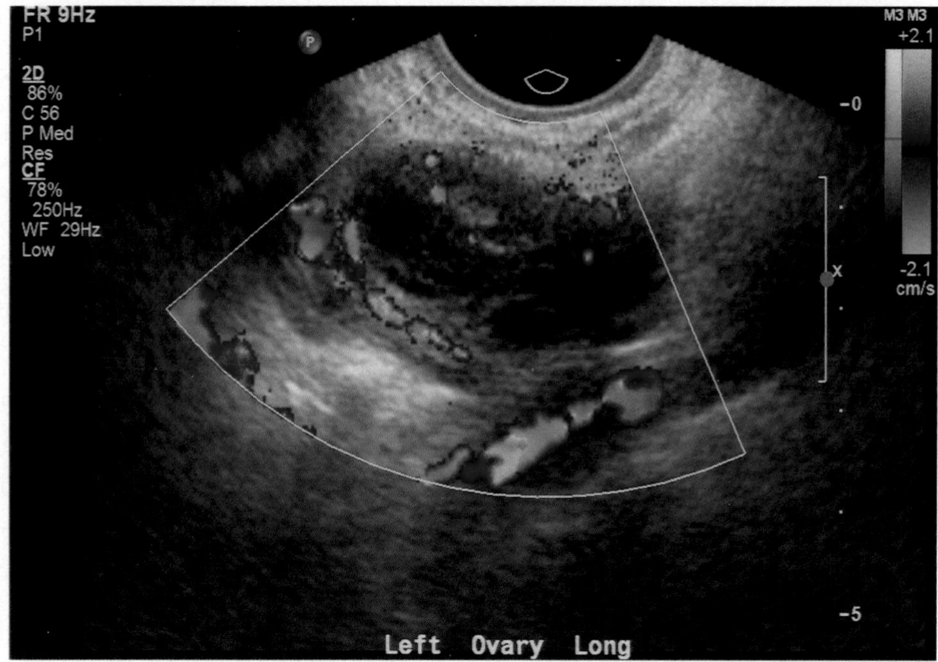

Figure 8-8. Normal left ovary in 45-year-old woman with pelvic pain.

evaluation may have interstitial cystitis. Pelvic pain may be their major complaint, and only on closer questioning can the irritative voiding symptoms be discovered.

Patients presenting with chronic pelvic pain deserve an adequate workup. In most cases this would include an ultrasound and laparoscopic examination. Often the ultrasound is normal (Fig. 8-8, left ovary) as was found in a 45-year-old woman with pelvic pain. However, laparoscopy might reveal peritoneal implants of endometriosis with normal pelvic ultrasound findings (Fig. 8-9) as in this 33-year-old woman.

The following box offers an outline of a workup for a patient with chronic pelvic pain. It is important that the physician determine not only the specific nature of the pain itself but also acquire a good understanding of the patient's basic physical, mental, and social status to determine what factors may be influencing the patient's symptom complex.

Workup of a Patient with Chronic Pelvic Pain

History
- Description and timing of pain (menstrual, intermittent, continuous, related to stress, etc.)
- Presence of pain in other parts of the body (headache, backache, etc.)
- Menstrual history and history of abnormal bleeding
- Sexual history
- Dyspareunia

Work and leisure habits
Problems involving other organ systems (urinary tract, GI tract)
Previous pelvic and abnormal infections
Previous operative procedures or diagnostic procedures
Other gynecologic disorders (e.g., endometriosis)
Social history (marital status; children; stresses in life as a child, an adolescent, and an adult; history of physical or sexual abuse or intimidation)

Physical examination
Laboratory evaluation
- CBC
- ESR
- VDRL
- Urinalysis and culture

Evaluation of GI and GU tracts (where appropriate)
Pap smear
Other studies (where appropriate)
Psychiatric evaluation
Social work evaluation
Laparoscopy
Ultrasound
CT scan, MRI
Biopsies if indicated
Cultures of cervix

CBC, complete blood count; CT, computed tomography; ESR, erythrocyte sedimentation rate; GI, gastrointestinal; GU, genitourinary; MRI, magnetic resonance imaging; VDRL, Venereal Disease Research Laboratory (syphilis test).

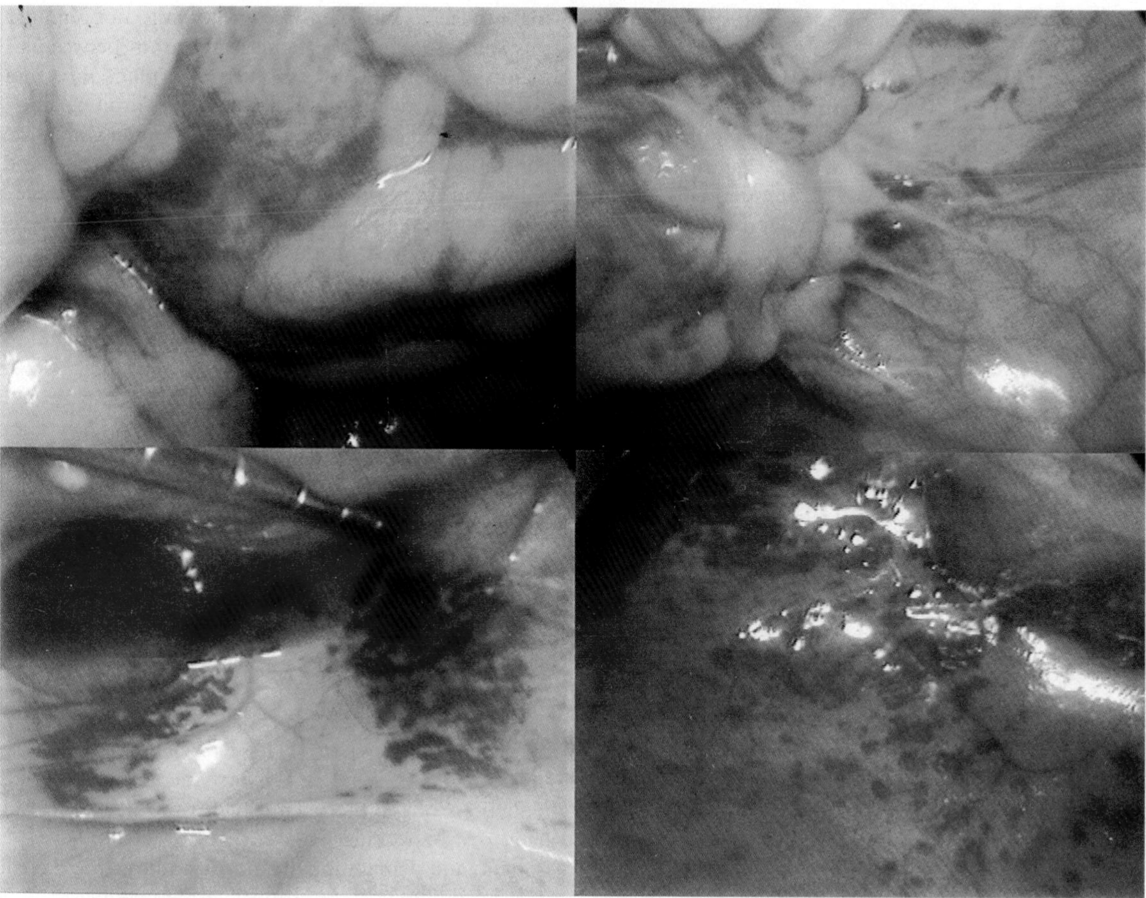

Figure 8-9. Laparoscopic view of a 33-year-old woman with chronic pelvic pain and endometriosis in the cul-de-sac.

A complete physical examination with emphasis on the effects of previous operations, infections, injuries, and, of course, a complete pelvic examination should be carried out. Appropriate diagnostic studies should be based on the history and physical exam. Cervical cultures for gonococcus and *Chlamydia,* as well as a Pap smear, are appropriate.

Laboratory data for patients with chronic pelvic pain should include a complete blood count (CBC), ESR, serologic tests for syphilis, urinalysis, and urine culture where appropriate. When indicated by history and physical findings, radiologic or ultrasound evaluation of the gastrointestinal (GI) and genitourinary (GU) tracts should be ordered.

Other studies that may be appropriate, depending on the history and physical examination, include psychiatric evaluation, social work evaluation, and biopsies if indicated. Laparoscopic examination is often indicated in such patients to discover or rule out pathologic conditions.

After completing the workup the physician may still be unable to find a cause for the chronic pelvic pain. In the past a variety of explanations were offered, including abnormal positioning of the uterus, laceration of the uterine supports, and vascular congestion of the pelvic organs. However, many of these patients have a psychosomatic disorder and benefit from counseling or treatment for depression.

Perhaps as many as 20% of all women demonstrate retroversion or retroflexion of the uterus at any given time. Rarely is the condition pathologic, and in most cases the uterus can be displaced from its posterior position in the pelvis to its normal anterior position by bimanual examination or by positioning the patient in the knee-chest position. When such anterior displacement of the uterus has been effected, the physician may place a Smith-Hodge pessary into the vagina to hold the uterus in an anterior position. If this maneuver alleviates the pain, the patient may continue to wear the pessary or may be offered a uterine suspension procedure. In most cases, however, retrodisplacement of the uterus does not appear to be a cause of pelvic pain, and replacement will make no difference in the patient's symptoms. Occasionally, the uterus is fixed in the posterior pelvis by postinflammatory or postoperative adhesions or by endometriosis. In these instances, the primary disease, not the retrodisplacement, may be responsible for the pain.

Allen and Masters defined the problem of traumatic lacerations of the uterine supports in 1955. They theorized that lacerations of the posterior leaf of the broad ligament or of the uterosacral ligament may have occurred at the time of a traumatic obstetric delivery and that with healing a greater rotation was allowed for the uterus. This condition has been called the *universal joint syndrome,* since it was theorized that the uterus could rotate freely, as with a universal joint. Many physicians have attempted to repair these so-called lacerations, and they are visible in some patients on laparoscopic examination. However, it is difficult to demonstrate a cause-and-effect relationship with pelvic pain, and a placebo effect may be responsible for occasional apparently successful outcomes.

Pelvic vascular engorgement has been observed on many occasions. Taylor defined the pelvic congestion syndrome as pain and heaviness in the pelvis that occurs after arising and becomes worse as the day progresses. On laparoscopic examination the uterus usually appears to be dusky blue and mottled, and often varicosities of the veins of the broad ligament are noted. Not all women with such findings complain of pelvic pain, and it is difficult to prove an actual cause. Beard and colleagues offered some evidence that pelvic varicosities might be a source of chronic pelvic pain. They compared 45 patients with chronic pelvic pain and no obvious pathology with 10 patients with pelvic pathology and 8 who were scheduled for tubal ligations. Each patient underwent a pelvic venogram, and the pelvic vein varicosities were graded by a radiologist blinded to the patients' complaints. A definite difference was noted in the increased diameters of the ovarian veins associated with a slower emptying time in the pelvic pain group. Beard and colleagues found very good relief of pain in 36 women with demonstrated pelvic congestion, 33 of whom had failed medical management, when total abdominal hysterectomy and bilateral salpingo-oophorectomy was performed. Hormone replacement therapy was utilized, and there was a 1-year follow-up before reevaluation.

Some patients do appear to suffer from psychosomatic disease with pelvic pain as a manifestation. Patients with chronic pelvic pain who do not seem to have obvious pathologic conditions will often reveal chaotic social histories involving both early and present life. Many of these individuals will be depressed and suffer from stress and anxiety, and some will suffer from borderline personality disorders. It is difficult to draw specific conclusions in this respect, however. Renaer demonstrated multiple symptom complaints in 12 of 24 patients with chronic pelvic pain without obvious disease. But only 1 of 22 patients suffering from chronic pelvic pain and endometriosis had such multiple symptoms. However, personality profiles developed by psychometric testing in each group failed to show differences between the two groups. A number of previous authors have pointed out that personality examinations in patients with chronic pain do not differentiate between psychogenic and organic pain.

Several investigators have noted a relationship between a history of childhood and later-life physical and sexual abuse and chronic pelvic pain. Possibly as many as 40% to 50% of women with chronic pelvic pain have a history of abuse. Harrop-Griffiths and coworkers ascertained a greater prevalence of lifetime major depression, current major depression, lifetime substance abuse history, sexual dysfunction, somatization, and an increased incidence of childhood and adult sexual abuse in a group of chronic pelvic pain patients at the time of laparoscopy compared with a group of patients without pain undergoing laparoscopy for tubal ligation or infertility.

Walling and associates studied 64 women with chronic pelvic pain, 42 women with chronic headache, and 46 pain-free women using a structured interview technique. They found that women with chronic pelvic pain had a higher lifetime prevalence of sexual abuse involving penetration or other genital or anal contact (major sexual abuse) than either of the other groups. However, with respect to physical abuse, the chronic pelvic pain group had a higher lifetime prevalence than the pain-free group but not the headache group. The difference between the headache and pain-free group was not significant—thus this study supports a specific relationship between a history of major sexual abuse and chronic pelvic pain and a more general association between physical abuse and chronic pain.

Badura and colleagues studied 46 women with chronic pelvic pain using a structured interview to assess sexual and physical abuse and somatization. The Dissociative Experience Scale was used to assess dissociation, and an abbreviated COPE scale was used to assess adaptive and maladaptive coping strategies as well as substance abuse. They found that those women in the group with self-reported sexual or physical abuse histories had significantly higher disassociation, somatization, and substance abuse scores than did the patients without such histories.

Physicians should evaluate chronic pelvic pain patients in a holistic fashion, investigating past social and emotional problems along with the physical evaluation. This makes it possible to offer specific multidiscipline therapy without suggesting to the patient that the problem is "all in her head." Placing the pain in the context of the patient's total life situation rather than as a specific isolated entity often makes a holistic approach possible.

Patients with chronic pain who do not demonstrate apparent organic causes will frequently have levator ani muscle spasm or spasm of other groups of muscle within the pelvis. Occasionally, trigger points may be defined in the anterior abdominal wall by deep digital pressure. These probably also represent spasm in local muscle bundles. These patients may also suffer from tenderness of the uterus and adnexa, which conceivably could be caused by vascular engorgement or adenomyosis. They pose difficult and demanding diagnostic and treatment challenges.

If no pathologic condition is evident but pain is persistent, physicians and patients alike have often yielded to the temptation of treating with a total hysterectomy and bilateral salpingo-oophorectomy. There is no evidence that this therapy relieves the pain in such patients and, indeed, failure to relieve the pain may lead to anger and frustration. Slocumb has shown that hysterectomy was successful in relieving pelvic pain only if dysmenorrhea was part of the symptom complex. Therefore, patients without obvious pelvic disease who have pelvic pain but not dysmenorrhea should not be offered hysterectomy. In such cases the physician should seek and treat psychosocial problems, depression, or other psychologic disease with medications, counseling, or referral to a psychiatrist or other mental health worker where appropriate. However, if reproductive tract disease exists, including endometriosis, symptomatic leiomyomata, pelvic congestion, or dysmenorrhea, it appears that 75% of these women will have improvement after hysterectomy according to observational studies.

PELVIC AND LOWER ABDOMINAL MASSES

Pelvic and lower abdominal masses may be cystic or solid and occur in any age group. They may originate from the cervix, the uterus, or the adnexa; from other organs, such as the GU tract or the bowel; or from the musculoskeletal system, vascular–lymphatic system, or nervous system. In this section the relevant incidence of pelvic and lower abdominal tumors in the various age groups will be considered and, where appropriate, means of differential diagnosis will be discussed.

Before discussing relative frequencies and types of abdominal and pelvic tumors found in different age groups, some comparisons of the more common adnexal tumors by age group are appropriate. During the reproductive years the majority of adnexal masses are follicle cysts. These tumors are functional in nature and generally disappear in 1 to 3 months. They vary in size from just a few centimeters to as large as 8 to 10 cm in diameter. They are thin-walled and frequently rupture during pelvic examination. In and of themselves they are of no clinical significance. It is likely that most women develop follicle cysts from time to time, and discovery may be related to the chance of performing a pelvic examination at the time when they exist. They rarely cause symptoms; however, when they do become large, they may cause some heaviness in the lower pelvis or in the leg. Because they are filled with follicular fluid, their rupture rarely causes any pathologic problem. A cystic adnexal mass of 5 to 8 cm that develops in a woman during the reproductive years is usually followed for at least one menstrual cycle, since functional cysts are common and the risk of malignancy is small. Transvaginal ultrasound can be very helpful in establishing a diagnosis and following the progress of a cyst. It can be reassuring to the patient and the doctor alike if a simple cyst is found. It can help differentiate between a simple and a multiloculated cyst and can rule out a solid tumor. Figure 8-10 is an example of a simple follicle cyst seen with vaginal ultrasound.

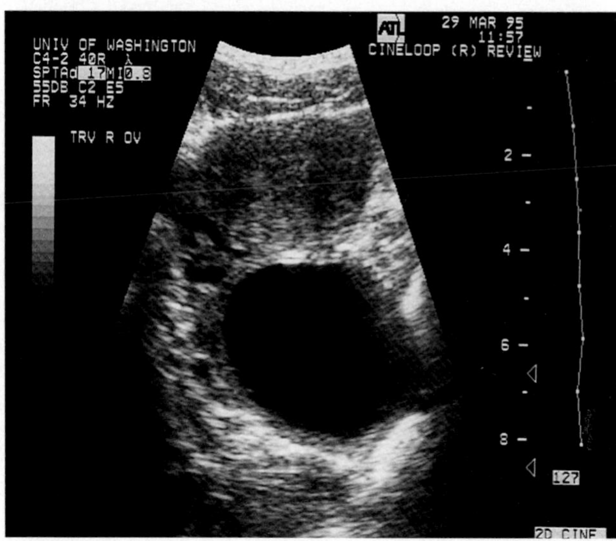

Figure 8-10. Large simple follicle cyst detected by vaginal ultrasound examination.

Also common during the reproductive years are hemorrhagic corpora lutea. These masses rarely become larger than 5 cm in diameter and frequently are somewhat tender to palpation. If they leak blood, they may mimic an ectopic pregnancy. They generally regress within a few weeks. Figure 8-11 demonstrates a 3.1-cm hemorrhagic corpus luteum on vaginal sonogram.

A number of benign and malignant neoplasms of the ovary occur quite frequently and do have special incident relationships to various age groups (see Chapters 18, Benign Gynecologic Lesions and 33, Malignant Diseases of the Ovaries). In 1968 Bennington and colleagues reviewed 443 benign and 106 malignant neoplasms of the ovary discovered in a period from 1951 to 1963 at the Oakland Kaiser Foundation Hospital. During those years, between 61,000 and 83,500 women were served annually. Because the Kaiser enrollees represented a cross section of the population in that area of California, this study made it possible to observe the relative frequency of different ovarian neoplasms within the general population. Most other studies were reported by referral institutions, and therefore the data

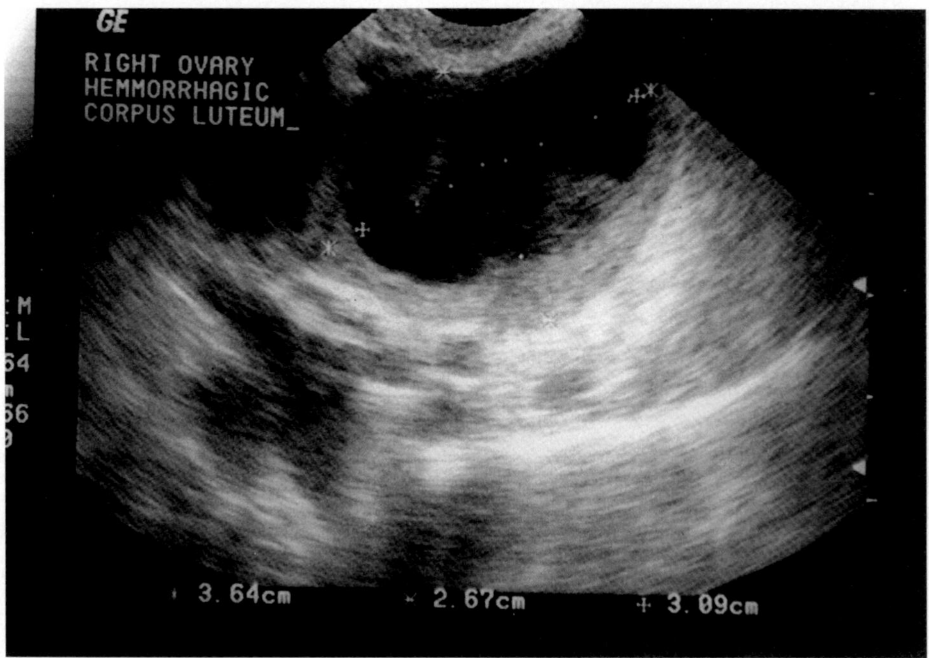

Figure 8-11. Transvaginal sonogram depicting a 3.1-cm hemorrhagic corpus luteum. (Courtesy of Steven R. Goldstein, MD, New York University School of Medicine.)

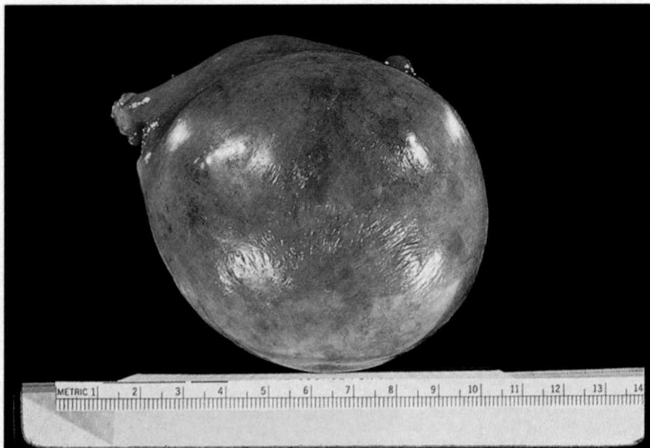

Figure 8-12. Serous cystadenoma. (From Voet RL: Color Atlas of Obstetric and Gynecologic Pathology. St. Louis, Mosby, 1997, figure 6.20.)

from the standpoint of prevalence was clouded. Thus, although this is a comparatively old study, it still represents useful data because it is an indication of incidence of various tumors in the general population. Bennington and colleagues noted that serous cystadenoma (Fig. 8-12) and benign cystic teratoma (dermoid cyst) (Fig. 8-13*A* and *B*) were the most commonly observed benign neoplasms of the adnexa. In addition, mucinous cystadenoma, Brenner tumors, thecomas, and fibromas were also seen. Table 8-4 demonstrates the age distribution and occurrence of bilaterality of 443 benign ovarian neoplasms observed by Bennington and colleagues. Although benign ovarian neoplasms were uncommon in the group up to 19 years of age, the most commonly seen benign neoplasm in this age group was the benign cystic teratoma. In the 20- to 44-year age group, serous cystadenomas were the most common benign neoplasm, with benign cystic teratomas and mucinous cystadenomas (Fig. 8-14) next in frequency. The serous cystadenomas occurred in all

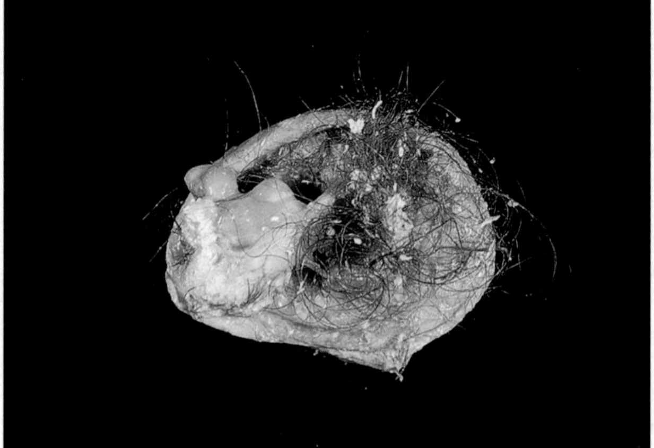

A

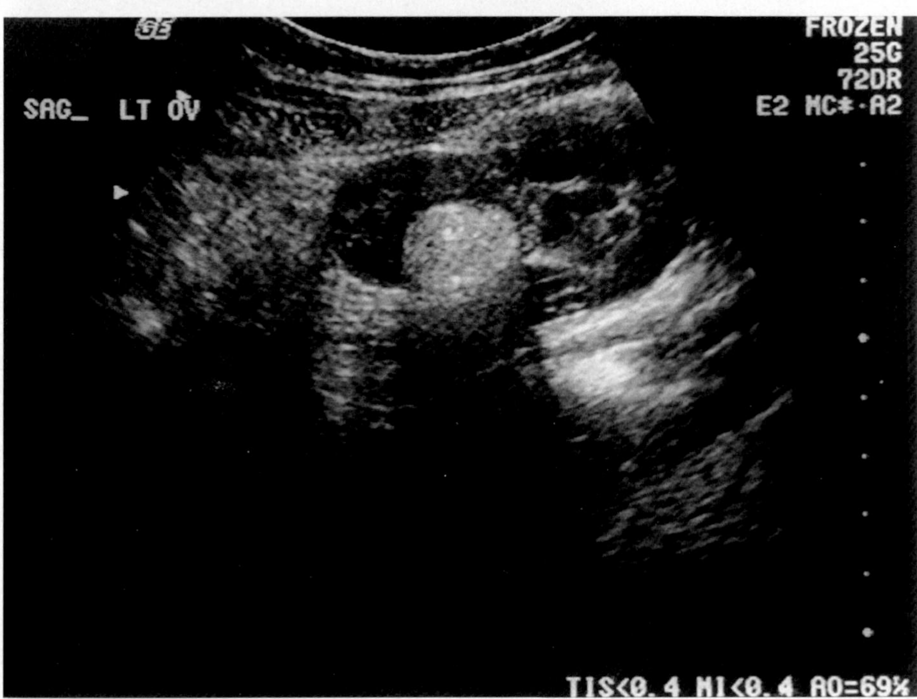

B

Figure 8-13. **A,** Dermoid. (From Voet RL: Color Atlas of Obstetric and Gynecologic Pathology. St. Louis, Mosby, 1997, figure 6.111.) **B,** Transvaginal sonogram of a dermoid cyst. (Courtesy of Steven R. Goldstein, MD, New York University School of Medicine.)

Table 8-4 Age Distribution and Laterality of 443 Benign Ovarian Neoplasms

Type	AGE						
	0–19	20–44	45–54	55–64	65–74	75+	Total
Serous Cystadenoma							
U*	4	124	35	23	10	2	198
B	1	17	3	4	2	0	27
Mucinous Cystadenoma							
U	1	42	5	5	1	0	54
B	0	1	0	0	0	0	1
Benign Teratoma							
U	8	93	12	7	2	0	122
B	0	9	1	0	0	0	10
Brenner							
U	1	4	1	0	0	0	6
B	0	0	0	0	0	0	0
Thecoma–fibroma							
U	0	11	3	8	1	1	24
B	0	0	0	1	0	0	1
Total							
U	14	274	56	43	14	3	404
B	1	27	4	5	2	0	39

*Location of neoplasm: B, bilateral; U, unilateral.
From Bennington JL, Ferguson BR, Haber SL: Incidence and relative frequency of benign and malignant ovarian neoplasms. Obstet Gynecol 32:627, 1968. Reprinted with permission from The American College of Obstetricians and Gynecologists.

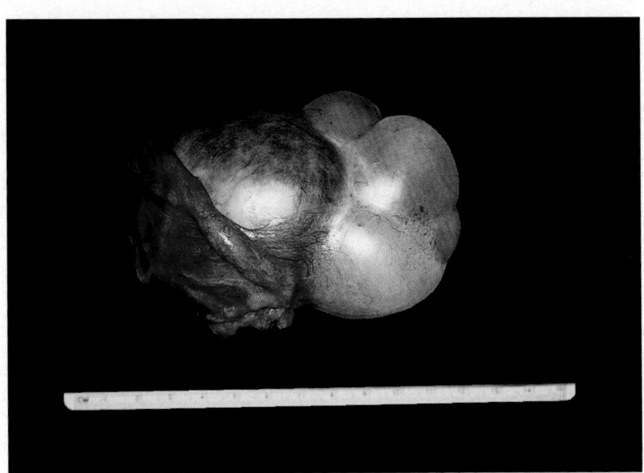

Figure 8-14. Cystadenoma mucinous. (From Voet RL: Color Atlas of Obstetric and Gynecologic Pathology. St. Louis, Mosby, 1997, figure 6.31.)

age groups but less commonly in women older than age 75. Mucinous cystadenomas occurred sporadically in all age groups, but none were seen after age 75. The majority of mucinous cystadenomas, however, occurred in women in the reproductive years. Similarly, benign cystic teratomas occurred in all age groups until age 75, but the majority occurred in the reproductive years. Brenner tumors occurred sporadically; however, none were seen after age 55. Thecomas and fibromas occurred in all age groups from 20 to beyond 75, but again the majority were in women between the ages of 20 and 64.

Malignant tumors of the ovary were not seen in the 19-year-old and younger age group of the Kaiser population except for one tumor that was metastatic to the ovary from another site. Serous cystadenocarcinoma occurred in all age groups from 20 to beyond 75 and was the most common malignant tumor seen in all age groups, but ovarian carcinomas are rare before age 40 (Fig. 8-15). Metastatic tumors to the ovary were the second most common ovarian malignant neoplasm seen in this study. Of the serous cystadenocarcinomas, 40% were bilateral, and roughly 50% of metastatic neoplasms were bilateral in all age groups. Mucinous cystadenocarcinoma was seen in all age groups from age 20 to beyond 75. In general the chance of malignancy seemed to be greater in these tumors in the older age groups. Endometrioid carcinoma occurred in a few patients in the series, as did granulosal cell carcinoma. Few other tumors were seen in this study. Table 8-5 summarizes the 106 patients with malignant ovarian neoplasm in the Bennington study by age distribution, laterality, and cell type.

Figure 8-16 plots the incidence of a number of the tumors noted in the Bennington study per 100,000 woman-years. Although their numbers of cases were relatively small, the incidence figures do demonstrate the prevalence by age of these various tumors.

Killackey and Neuwirth evaluated pelvic masses in 540 patients admitted to St. Luke's-Roosevelt Hospital in New York in 1984–1985. Of 249 patients admitted with a diagnosis of uterine myomas, 235 (94.4%) diagnoses proved to be correct, whereas benign adnexal masses were found in 7 (2.8%), cancers in 4 (1.6%), and miscellaneous findings in 3 (1.2%). Of 291 patients evaluated for "pelvic mass," benign ovarian or tubal cysts were noted in 98 (33.7%), uterine myoma in 42 (14.4%), cancers in 40 (13.7%), benign cystic teratomas in 38 (13.1%), endometriosis in 28 (9.6%), miscellaneous in 23 (7.9%), and pelvic inflammatory disease in 22 (7.6%). Table 8-6 demonstrates these diagnostic findings by patient age.

Koonings and coworkers also studied a large group of women (861) who were admitted for adnexal masses over a 10-year period. They wished to clarify the distribution of primary ovarian neoplasms by decade of life. They found that the overall risk for malignancy was 13% in premenopausal women and 45% in postmenopausal women. As seen in other studies, germ cell tumors predominated in women younger than age 40, and epithelial tumors became more frequent in the decades after age 40.

Masses in Childhood

Occasionally, babies are born with adnexal cysts that present as abdominal masses. These are generally follicular cysts secondary to maternal hormone stimulation of fetal ovaries. The cysts generally regress within the first few months of life. Thereafter, cysts and all tumors of the female pelvic organs are quite rare during childhood. Abdominal masses found in the young child are more likely to be Wilms' tumors or neuroblastomas. Tumors of the GI tract, musculoskeletal system, or lymphatic system

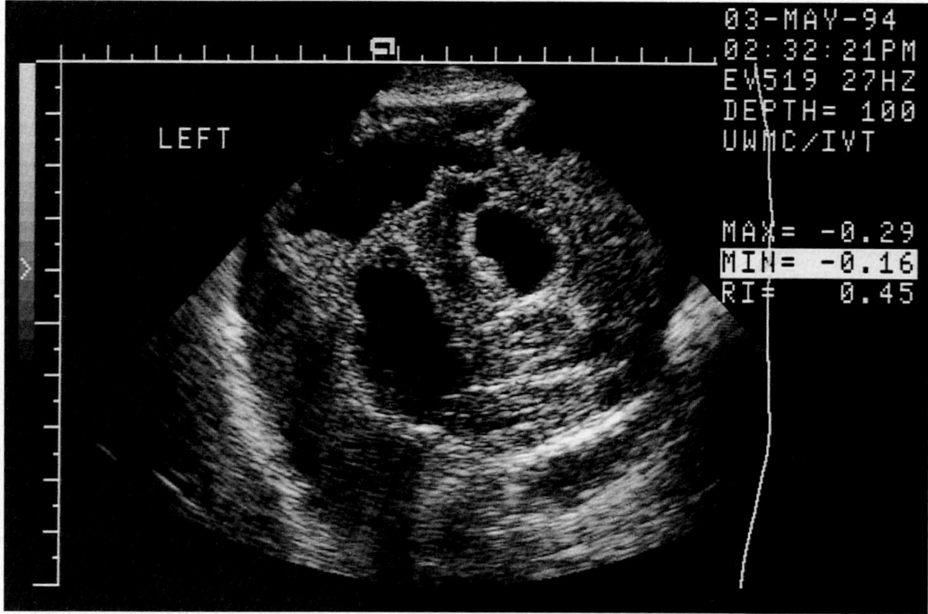

Figure 8-15. Multiloculated ovarian cyst detected by vaginal ultrasound. Pathology proved to be serous cystadenocarcinoma.

Table 8-5 Age Distribution and Laterality of 80 Primary and 26 Secondary Malignant Ovarian Neoplasms

	AGE						
Type	**0–19**	**20–44**	**45–54**	**55–64**	**65–74**	**75+**	**Total**
Serous Cystadenocarcinoma							
U*	0	8	9	10	1	2	30
B	0	7	11	3	2	1	24
Mucinous Cystadenocarcinoma							
U	0	1	0	4	1	1	7
B	0	0	0	2	1	0	3
Endometroid Carcinoma							
U	0	2	0	0	0	0	2
B	0	0	1	1	1	0	3
Granulose Carcinoma							
U	0	2	0	2	1	1	6
B	0	0	0	0	0	0	0
Other							
U	0	1†	4‡	0	0	0	5
B	0	0	0	0	0	0	0
Metastases							
U	1	3	7	1	0	0	12
B	0	7	4	3	0	0	14
Total							
U	1	17	20	17	3	4	62
B	0	14	16	9	4	1	44

*Location of neoplasm: B, bilateral; U, unilateral.
†Squamous carcinoma arising in a cystic teratoma.
‡One arrhenoblastoma, one germinoma, one malignant Brenner tumor, and one mesonephric carcinoma.
From Bennington JL, Ferguson BR, and Haber SL: Incidence and relative frequency of benign and malignant ovarian neoplasms. Obstet Gynecol 32:627, 1968. Reprinted with permission from The American College of Obstetricians and Gynecologists.

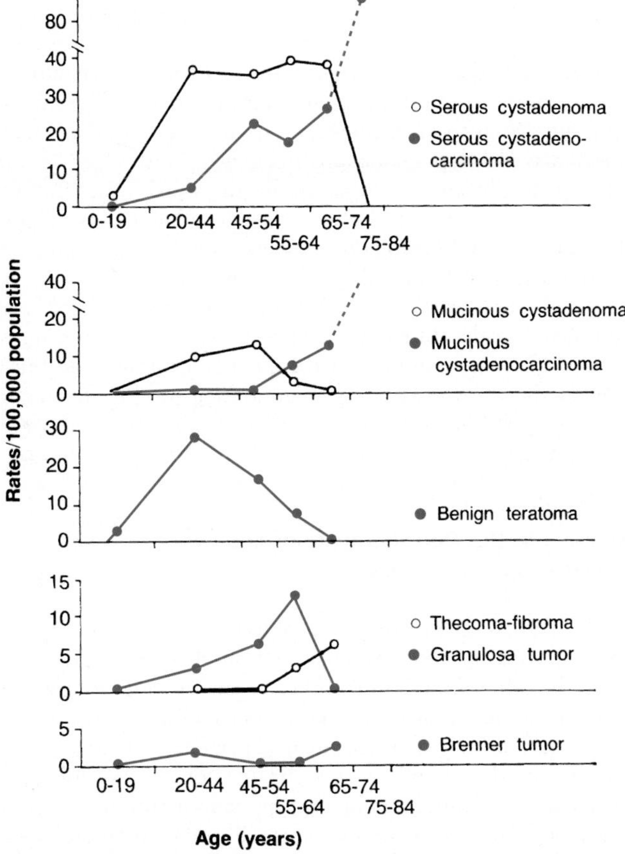

Figure 8-16. Incidence rates for ovarian tumors by age group per 100,000 women at each age interval. (From Bennington JL, Ferguson BR, Haber SL: Incidence and relative frequency of benign and malignant ovarian neoplasms. Obstet Gynecol 32:627, 1968. Reprinted with permission from The American College of Obstetricians and Gynecologists.)

may also occur occasionally. Solid or mixed solid and cystic adnexal masses are rare, but when they do occur are almost always dysgerminomas or teratomas. Mueller and associates reviewed 427 cases of dysgerminoma in 1950 and noted that 6.89% of the tumors occurred in the 1- to 10-year-old age group. Asadourian and Taylor, reviewing 105 cases of dysgerminoma in the Armed Forces Institute of Pathology experience, noted that only seven of these patients were 9 years of age or younger.

Although benign and malignant teratomas have been reported in childhood, they are quite rare before the age of 10. Caruso and colleagues reporting on 305 teratomas of the ovary, found none in children younger than age 10. However, Costin and Kennedy, reviewing 200 ovarian tumors in infants and children, found 25% to be benign cystic teratomas. Ultrasonography is useful for evaluation.

Masses in Adolescence (Menarche to 19 Years)

Once menses begins, obstruction of the lower reproductive tract, such as with imperforate hymen, agenesis of the vagina with intact cervix and uterus, or vaginal septum, may give rise to a hematocolpos or a hematometrium. Thus, abdominal or pelvic masses may occur secondary to these conditions. Other anomalies of the reproductive tract, such as obstructed uterine horns, may also give rise to a hematometrium and a pelvic mass (see Chapter 12, Congenital Abnormalities of the Female Reproductive Tract). Myomas of the uterus are rare in this age group but have been reported.

The majority of adnexal masses in this age group are functional cysts and vary in size from 3 to 10 cm. Of neoplastic ovarian tumors found, the most common is benign cystic teratoma of the ovary. In Caruso and colleagues' study of 305 teratomas of the ovary, 8.5% occurred in this age group. These tumors are generally between 5 and 10 cm in diameter, are slow-growing, and are frequently asymptomatic. Some benign cystic teratomas are larger than 10 cm. Caruso and colleagues' series of 305 teratomas found 49 measured 10 to 14 cm; 21, 15 to 19 cm; and 11, between 20 and 39 cm. They are generally found because a mass is detected on abdominal or pelvic examination. However, benign cystic teratomas may cause adnexal torsion and present as an acute abdomen. Rarely, the tumor may rupture, spilling oily, irritating contents into the peritoneal cavity and creating evidence of an acute abdomen. These tumors frequently have a thickened capsule, and rupture is unusual. Because benign cystic teratomas may contain bone or teeth, abdominal roentgenograms or ultrasound may identify these. Figure 8-13*A* and *B* demonstrates a transvaginal sonogram of a 4.0 × 3.6 cm dermoid cyst.

Solid or solid and cystic adnexal tumors, although rare in adolescence, are almost always dysgerminomas or malignant teratomas.

Table 8-6 Surgical Findings in 540 Patients Evaluated for Leiomyomata/Pelvic Masses at St. Luke's-Roosevelt Hospital 1984–1985

	NUMBER OF PATIENTS IN EACH AGE GROUP							
Surgical Diagnosis	**10–20**	**21–30**	**31–40**	**41–50**	**51–60**	**61–70**	**>70**	**Total**
Leiomyomata	0	13	99	142	19	3	0	276
Benign/functional cysts	1	24	32	23	8	9	7	104
Cancer	2	0	3	11	7	12	9	44
Benign cystic teratoma	4	17	9	3	0	3	1	37
Endometriosis	0	7	16	7	2	0	0	32
Miscellaneous	1	4	11	2	1	4	2	25
Tuboovarian abscess/ Pelvic inflammatory disease	2	7	9	4	0	0	0	22
Total	10	72	179	192	37	31	19	540

From Killackey MA, Neuwirth RS: Evaluation and management of the pelvic mass: A review of 540 cases. Obstet Gynecol 71:319, 1988.

In 137 women younger than 21 years who were found to have ovarian enlargement reported by Diamond and coworkers, 82 had ovarian neoplasms, of which 8 were borderline or malignant. All six malignant lesions were germ cell in origin. Likewise, in a study by Norris and Jensen of 353 primary ovarian neoplasms in women younger than 20 years, germ cell tumors represented 58% of cases. Of these 205 patients, 71 had benign cystic teratomas, 54 malignant teratomas, 48 dysgerminomas, and 32 embryonal carcinomas. Of the remaining cases, 67 (19%) were of epithelial origin, 62 (18%) stromal, and 19 (5%) miscellaneous.

Dysgerminomas and teratomas can vary from just a few centimeters to an extremely large size. In 117 dysgerminomas reviewed by Asadourian and Taylor, 12 were found to have other germ cell elements, including embryonal carcinoma, teratocarcinoma, and choriocarcinoma.

Cystic adnexal masses derived from mesonephric elements, such as paraovarian and paratubal cysts, are also seen in this age group. They may vary in size from 1 to 2 cm to quite large. They are thin-walled, benign entities without solid components.

Masses emanating from other organ systems in the pelvis and abdomen also occur in this age group and must be considered.

Masses during the Reproductive Years

Masses seen in women of reproductive age (20 to 44 years) may develop from the uterus and cervix, the adnexa, and other organ systems. Intrauterine pregnancy, ectopic pregnancy, and trophoblastic disease should always be considered in women of reproductive years who develop such masses. These conditions can often be ruled in or out by use of a serum pregnancy test and ultrasound. Ectopic pregnancy is generally associated with an adnexal mass, vaginal bleeding, and pelvic pain, as discussed earlier in this chapter. Trophoblastic disease may be associated with inappropriate uterine size for menstrual dates, vaginal bleeding, pelvic pain, and symptoms of toxemia of pregnancy. Adnexal enlargements caused by theca lutein cysts of the ovaries may be associated with trophoblastic disease.

Myomas of the uterus, the cervix, the round ligament, or other pelvic organs are quite common in this age group. As many as 25% to 50% of women in the reproductive years may develop myomas of the uterus and accessory organs. These tumors occur three times more frequently in blacks than in whites. The majority are benign and vary in size from very small to large enough to fill the entire abdominal cavity. These tumors are composed of smooth muscle cells in concentric whorls and are generally benign. Leiomyosarcoma occurring in such tumors is rare (0.1% to 0.5%). The tumors are usually solid but with degeneration may give the impression of a cystic consistency. Ultrasound, computed tomography (CT), or magnetic resonance imaging (MRI) scan may be helpful in making a specific diagnosis.

Rarely, myomas of the uterus occur in the cervix or lower uterine segment. They may become quite large and may put pressure on the bladder neck, causing acute urinary retention. Myomas tend to enlarge premenstrually and in pregnancy. Occasionally, cervical or lower uterine segment myomas have caused intermittent urinary retention premenstrually or during early pregnancy.

Adnexal masses in the reproductive years may involve any known ovarian tumor, as well as cysts of mesonephric origin. In this age group functional cysts of the ovary are still the most common adnexal masses found, and benign cystic teratomas are the most common neoplastic adnexal masses. During the reproductive years, endometriosis occurs, and ovarian endometriomas develop reasonably frequently in this age group. They generally are accompanied by the usual symptoms for endometriosis in association with a tender adnexal mass. Figure 8-17 depicts a bilobed endometrioma on vaginal sonogram. It measures 5.1 × 4.1 cm and 5.1 × 3.9 cm, respectively.

Tumors emanating from other organ systems should also be considered in the differential diagnosis as in other age groups. One of the more common of these is not a tumor at all but a pelvic kidney. An ultrasound or intravenous pyelogram should be useful in differentiating this entity from other pathologic conditions.

Masses in the Perimenopausal and Postmenopausal Years

In this age group (45 years and older) it is once again appropriate to consider masses originating from the uterus and cervix, from the adnexa, and from other organ systems. In general, myomas of the uterus regress postmenopausally even in the face of estrogen hormone replacement. Therefore, a uterus that is growing in size should be investigated for the possibility of malignancy. Adenocarcinoma of the endometrium, sarcomas, and mixed tumors of the uterus are all more common in the postmenopausal period, and many will be responsible for enlargement of uterine size, as well as PMB.

Adnexal masses occurring in postmenopausal women may still be benign, but the chance of malignancy increases with age. The presence of ascites and the detection of the tumor bilaterally suggest malignancy. Rulin and Preston analyzed 150 adnexal tumors in women older than 50 and noted 103 benign tumors and 47 malignant ones. Table 8-7 summarizes these tumors by size and pathologic findings. Only 1 tumor of 32 that were smaller than 5 cm proved to be malignant, whereas 6 of 55 tumors 5 to 10 cm and 40 of 63 tumors larger than

Table 8-7 Adnexal Masses in 150 Women = 50 Years

Pathology	<5 cm	5–10 cm	>10 cm
Benign Disease			
Epithelial tumors	12	26	15
Stromal and germ cell tumors	7	12	4
Nonneoplastic ovarian cysts	2	1	0
Uterine myomas	3	3	4
Nonovarian adnexal lesions	2	6	0
Absence of true mass	5	1	0
Malignant Disease			
Epithelial carcinomas	1	3	29
Borderline tumors	0	2	2
Other ovarian carcinomas	0	0	4
Nonovarian carcinoma	0	1	5
Total	32	55	63

From Rulin MC, Preston AL: Adnexal masses in postmenopausal women. Obstet Gynecol 70:578, 1987.

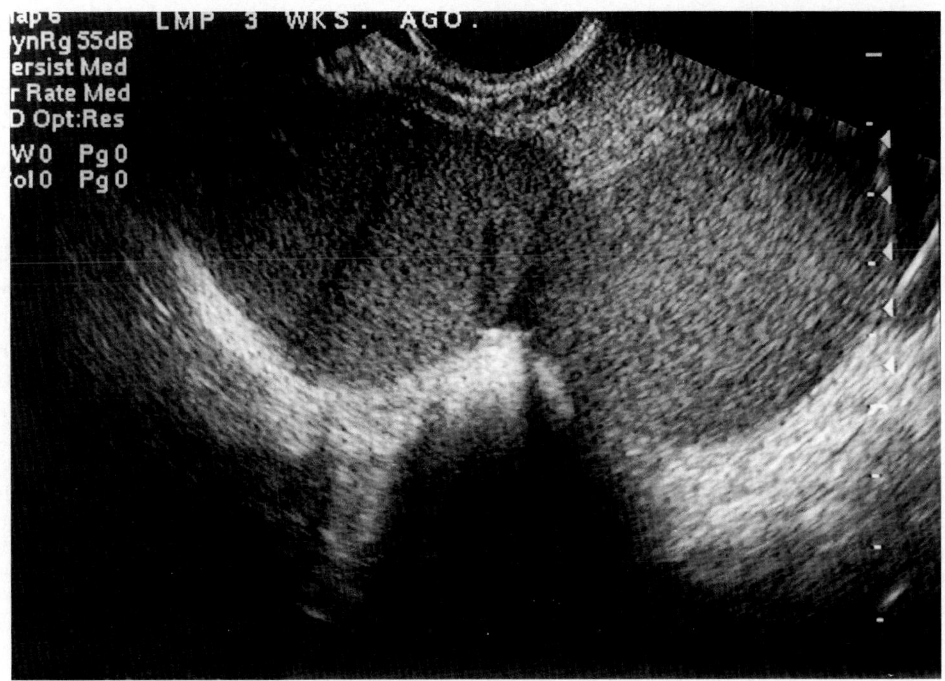

Figure 8-17. Transvaginal sonogram of a bilobed endometrioma. (Courtesy of Steven R. Goldstein, MD, New York University School of Medicine.)

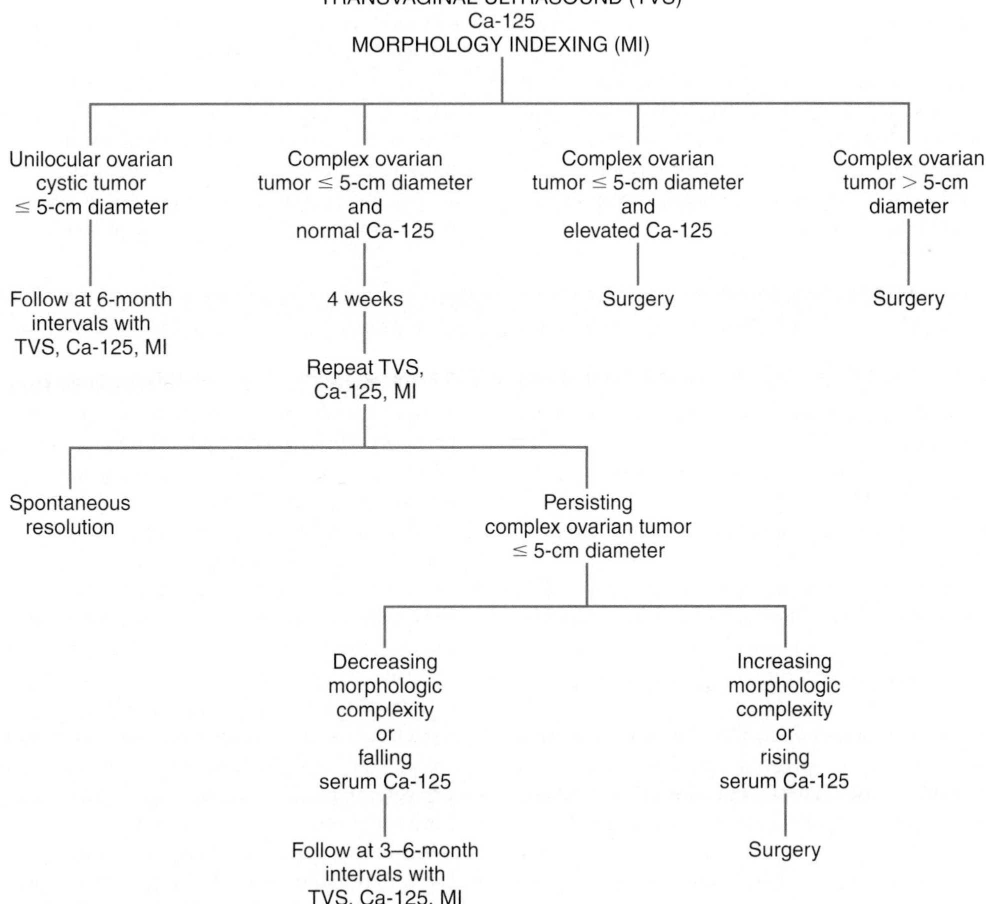

Figure 8-18. Management algorithm for postmenopausal women with an adnexal mass. Ca-125, cancer antigen-125; MI, morphologic indexing; TVS, transvaginal sonography,

10 cm were malignant. The majority of the malignant tumors were epithelial in this age group, and most were larger than 10 cm. In a similar study from Tel Aviv, Ovadia and Goldman reported that in 380 postmenopausal women operated on for adnexal masses in a 10-year period, 297 (78.2%) had benign and 83 (21.8%) had malignant tumors. They, too, showed that the chance of malignancy increased with size of tumor and with age. One third of benign adnexal masses were simple cysts. Figure 8-18 by van Nagell and DePriest suggests a management algorithm for an adnexal mass in postmenopausal women.

Endometriosis occurs primarily in women in the reproductive years; however, as many as 5% of cases do occur postmenopausally, particularly in women on hormone replacement therapy. Therefore, endometriosis of the ovaries should be part of the differential diagnosis in such women (see Chapter 19, Endometriosis).

Masses from other organ systems are quite common in this age group. Diverticulitis may be responsible for a painful left adnexal mass. Bowel tumors may present as abdominal masses, as may tumors of the kidney, the musculoskeletal system, and the lymphatic system. Blood dyscrasias and lymphomas are more common in this age group. Lymphomas may present as rapidly growing, firm masses, at times accompanied by ascites. They may develop from any abdominal or pelvic organ, including lymph nodes.

Special Considerations

A number of findings associated with abdominal mass may help direct the physician to the appropriate diagnosis. If ascites is present, as detected by physical examination or ultrasound, a malignant tumor, frequently of the ovary, is strongly suspected. Benign fibromas of the ovary may also be associated with ascites and pleural effusion (Meig's syndrome).

Defeminization or masculinization of the patient may suggest a rare masculinizing tumor of the ovary, such as a Sertoli–Leydig tumor. In the preadolescent female, precocious puberty of a heterosexual type may be the presenting symptom. In the postpubertal girl, cessation of menses and early masculinization may occur. These may also be the presenting symptoms in women in the reproductive years.

Feminizing tumors, such as granulosal cell tumors and thecomas, are more common. In the prepubertal girl they may present as precocious puberty. In the menstruating woman they may cause menometrorrhagia, and in the postmenopausal woman they may present with PMB. In a granulosal cell tumor a solid or cystic mass is readily detected. Thecomas are solid tumors and are also readily detected. Occasionally, other ovarian stromal tumors, such as a Brenner tumor, may produce sex steroids and present in a similar fashion.

Struma ovarii, a teratoma with thyroid elements, may present by developing signs of hyperthyroidism in the patient.

General Diagnostic Considerations

Specific differential diagnosis of abdominal and pelvic masses is often aided by abdominal and transvaginal ultrasound, CT, or MRI scan. In addition, special radiographic studies, such as intravenous pyelogram, barium enema, and upper GI series, may be helpful in identifying the site of the tumor. Because metastatic cancer to the ovaries is common, investigation of the patient for another primary source is often fruitful.

Tumor markers may be elevated, such as cancer antigen-125 (CA-125) in epithelial tumors, serum HCG and α-fetoprotein in germ cell tumors, and androgens or estrogens in specific hormone-producing tumors. These tests have frequent false-positive and false-negative findings and should be used only in conjunction with other diagnostic procedures.

KEY POINTS

- Bleeding in early pregnancy usually implies threatened or inevitable abortion, ectopic pregnancy, or gestational trophoblastic disease.
- Bleeding at the time of the missed menstrual period may represent implantation bleeding.
- About 90% of all ectopic pregnancies are associated with vaginal bleeding.
- Vaginal bleeding in a patient with a positive pregnancy test, lower abdominal pain, adnexal mass, and failure to demonstrate a gestational sac by ultrasound beyond 6 weeks of gestational age should suggest the possibility of an ectopic pregnancy.
- Incidence of ectopic pregnancy is increased in women who have had previous ectopic pregnancies, have undergone tubal reparative procedures, have had previous pelvic inflammatory disease, wear an IUD, or were exposed to DES in utero.
- Molar pregnancies are suggested by vaginal bleeding, uteri larger than gestational age, and serum HCG levels of 100,000 mIU/mL or greater.
- Molar pregnancy must be differentiated from normal gestation, multiple gestation, uterine enlargement because of uterine pathology and hydramnios.
- Molar pregnancies are best diagnosed with the aid of ultrasound examination.
- Dysfunctional uterine bleeding is generally associated with anovulation or short ovulatory cycle.
- Dysfunctional uterine bleeding is most commonly seen in the postpubertal period, perimenopausally, or in women during their reproductive years who have undergone excessive weight change, who are under stress, or who have embarked on a strenuous exercise program.
- Appendicitis is characterized by periumbilical pain that radiates to the right lower quadrant accompanied by loss of appetite, nausea, and vomiting. Patients with PID can have similar pain but usually have a higher fever and mild gastrointestinal symptoms and appear less ill.
- Dysfunctional uterine bleeding is often associated with polycystic ovarian syndrome and functioning ovarian tumors.

KEY POINTS—*Continued*

- Endometrial biopsy with dysfunctional uterine bleeding in younger women will generally demonstrate nonsecretory endometrium.
- Clear-cell cancer of the vagina is often associated with intrauterine DES exposure.
- Myomas of the uterus often are associated with vaginal bleeding; submucous myomas are most commonly associated with this problem.
- Of all adenocarcinomas of the endometrium, 95% occur in postmenopausal women.
- Adenocarcinoma of the endometrium found in premenopausal women is most often associated with polycystic ovarian syndrome or a functioning ovarian tumor.
- Systemic diseases that cause abnormal vaginal bleeding include coagulopathies, blood dyscrasias, and certain endocrinopathies.
- In a study of 1194 patients with chronic pelvic pain, 749 had normal pelvic examinations.
- In 749 patients with chronic pelvic pain who had normal pelvic examinations, 63% had abnormal findings at diagnostic laparoscopy.
- Of 445 patients who had abnormal pelvic examinations and a history of chronic pelvic pain, 17.5% had normal findings at the time of diagnostic laparoscopy.
- Of 100 women who reported constant pelvic pain in one place for at least 6 months, 83% had abnormal findings at diagnostic laparoscopy. Pelvic adhesions and endometriosis accounted for the majority of abnormalities seen.
- Pelvic adhesions may not be the cause of chronic pelvic pain. Whereas 26% of 100 such patients were found to have adhesions on laparoscopy, 39% of 88 patients undergoing laparoscopy for tubal ligation or infertility also had adhesions, and only 4 of these 34 patients complained of pain. Dense pelvic adhesions, especially those that are vascularized, may cause pelvic pain.
- A total of 20% of all women demonstrate retroversion or retroflexion of the uterus. This anatomic variation usually does not cause symptoms.
- Of patients with chronic pelvic pain, 50% demonstrated multiple symptom complaints.
- Personality examinations in patients with chronic pelvic pain frequently define psychosocial problems, but such testing does not determine whether the pain is psychogenic or organic in nature.
- Patients with chronic pelvic pain have been found to have a greater prevalence of lifetime major depression, current major depression, lifetime substance abuse, sexual dysfunction, somatization, and a greater incidence of childhood and adult sexual abuse.
- The majority of adnexal masses in women in the reproductive years are follicle cysts of the ovary.
- The most common benign neoplastic tumors of the ovary are serous cystadenoma and benign cystic teratoma.
- The most common benign cystic neoplasms of the ovary in the 20- to 44-year age group are benign cystic teratoma, serous cystadenoma, and mucinous cystadenoma.
- Serous cystadenocarcinoma is the most common malignant tumor in all age groups from 20 to 75 years but increases incidence with age.
- Wilms' tumor and neuroblastoma are the most common abdominal tumors in childhood.
- Dysgerminoma and teratoma are the most common solid adnexal tumors in young women.
- Most benign cystic teratomas are 10 cm or less in diameter, but about one sixth will be larger.
- Of women in the reproductive years, 25% to 50% develop myoma of the uterus.
- A total of 95% of all endometriosis occurs in women in the reproductive years.
- Of 150 adnexal tumors in women older than 50, 103 were benign. Of the malignant tumors in this age group, most were epithelial tumors. Tumors less than 5 cm were usually benign, but 40 of 63 tumors larger than 10 cm were malignant.
- Postmenopausal bleeding may be caused by a premalignant or malignant lesion of the uterus or cervix but is often associated with an atrophic endometrium.
- The most common cause of vaginal bleeding in childhood is foreign bodies in the vagina.

BIBLIOGRAPHY

Key Readings

Allen WM, Masters WH: Traumatic lacerations of uterine support. Am J Obstet Gynecol 70:500, 1955.

Asadourian LA, Taylor HB: Dysgerminoma: An analysis of 105 cases. Obstet Gynecol 33:370, 1969.

Badura AS, Reiter RC, Altmaier EM, et al: Dissociation, somatization, substance abuse, and coping in women with chronic pelvic pain. Obstet Gynecol 90:405, 1997.

Beard RW, Kennedy RG, Gangar KR, et al: Bilateral oophorectomy and hysterectomy in the treatment of intractable pelvic pain associated with pelvic congestion. Br J Obstet Gynecol 98:988, 1991.

Beard RW, Pearce S, Highman JH, Reginald RW: Diagnosis of pelvic varicosities in women with chronic pelvic pain. Lancet 2:946, 1984.

Bennington JL, Ferguson BR, Haber SL: Incidence and relative frequency of benign and malignant ovarian neoplasms. Obstet Gynecol 32:627, 1968.

Blendis LM: Abdominal pain. In Wall DP, Melzack R (eds): Textbook of Pain. New York, Churchill Livingstone, 1984.

Caruso PA, Marsh MR, Minkowitz S, Karten G: An intense clinical pathologic study of 305 teratomas of the ovary. Cancer 27:343, 1971.

Costin ME, Kennedy RLJ: Ovarian tumors in infants and children. Am J Dis Child 76:127, 1948.

Cunanan RG, Courey NG, Lippes J: Laparoscopic findings in patients with pelvic pain. Am J Obstet Gynecol 146:589, 1983.

Dewhurst J: Postmenopausal bleeding from benign causes. Clin Obstet Gynecol 26:769, 1983.

Diamond MP, Baxter JW, Pennau CG Jr, Burnett LS: The occurrence of ovarian malignancy in childhood and adolescents: A community-wide evaluation. Obstet Gynecol 71:858, 1988.

Falcone T, Desjardins C, Bourque J, et al: Dysfunctional uterine bleeding in adolescents. J Reprod Med 39:761, 1994.

Harrop-Griffiths J, Katon W, Walker E, et al: The association between chronic pelvic pain, psychiatric diagnoses, and childhood sexual abuse. Obstet Gynecol 71:589, 1988.
Herbst AL, Ulfelder H, Poskanzer DC: Adenocarcinoma of the vagina: association of maternal stilbestrol therapy with tumor appearance in young women. N Engl J Med 284:878, 1971.
Jamieson DJ, Steege JF: The association of sexual abuse with pelvic pain complaints in a primary care population. Am J Obstet Gynecol 177:1408, 1997.
Killackey MA, Neuwirth RS: Evaluation and management of the pelvic mass: A review of 540 cases, Obstet Gynecol 71:314, 1988.
Koonings PP, Campbell K, Mishell DR Jr, Grimes DA: Relative frequency of primary ovarian neoplasms: A 10-year review. Obstet Gynecol 74:921, 1989.
Kresch A, Seifer DB, Sachs LD, Barrese I: Laparoscopy in 100 women with chronic pelvic pain. Obstet Gynecol 64:672, 1984.
Mueller CW, Tompkins P, Lapp WA: Dysgerminoma of the ovary: An analysis of 427 cases. Am J Obstet Gynecol 60:153, 1950.
Peters AAW, Trimbos-Kemper GCM, Admiraal C, Trimbos JB: A randomized clinical trial on the benefit of adhesiolysis in patients with intraperitoneal adhesions and chronic pelvic pain. Br J Obstet Gynecol 99:59, 1992.
Rapkin AJ: Adhesions and pelvic pain: A retrospective study. Obstet Gynecol 68:13, 1986.
Renaer M: Gynecological pain. In Wall DP, Melzack R (eds): Textbook of Pain. New York, Churchill Livingstone, 1984.
Rulin MC, Preston AL: Adnexal masses in postmenopausal women. Obstet Gynecol 70:578, 1987.
Slocumb JC: Neurological factors in chronic pelvic pain: Trigger points and the abdominal pelvic pain syndrome. Am J Obstet Gynecol 149:536, 1984.
Slocumb JC: Chronic somatic, myofascial, and neurogenic abdominal pelvic pain. Clin Obstet Gynecol 33:145, 1990.
Tabor A, Watt HC, Wald NJ: Endometrial thickness as a test for endometrial cancer in women with postmenopausal vaginal bleeding. Obstet Gynecol 99(4):663, 2002.
Taylor HC: Vascular congestion and hyperemia. I. Physiologic basis in history of the concept. Am J Obstet Gynecol 57:211, 1949.
Taylor HC: Vascular congestion and hyperemia. II. The clinical aspects of congestion-fibrosis Syndrome. Am J Obstet Gynecol 57:637, 1949.
Walling MK, Reiter RC, O'Hara MW, et al: Abuse history and chronic pain in women: I. Prevalences of sexual abuse and physical abuse. Obstet Gynecol 84:193, 1994.

Key References

American College of Obstetricians and Gynecologyists: Clinical management guidelines for obstetrician-gynecologists. Practice Bulletin 51. Washington, DC, American College of Obstetricians and Gynecologists, 2004.
Barnhart KT, Sammel MD, Gracia CR, et al: Risk factors for ectopic pregnancy in women with symptomatic first-trimester pregnancies. Fert Steril Jul;86(1):36, 2006.
Beard RW, Kennedy RG, Gangar KF, et al: Bilateral oophorectomy and hysterectomy in the treatment of intractable pelvic pain associated with pelvic congestion. Br J Obstet Gynaecol 98:988, 1991.
Buttram VC, Reiter RC: Uterine leiomyomata: Etiology, symptomatology, and management. Fertil Steril 36:433, 1981.
Carlson KJ, Miller BA, Fowler FJ Jr: The Maine Women's Health Study: II. Outcomes of nonsurgical management of leiomyomas, abnormal bleeding, and chronic pelvic pain. Obstet Gynecol 83:566, 1994.
Carlson KJ, Miller BA, Fowler FJ Jr: The Maine Women's Health Study: I. Outcomes of hysterectomy. Obstet Gynecol 83:556, 1994.
Clark TJ, Voit D, Gupta JK, et al: Accuracy of hysteroscopy in the diagnosis of endometrial cancer and hyperplasia: A systematic quantitative review. JAMA 288(13):1610, 2002.
Clark TJ, Barton PM, Coomarasamy A, et al: Investigating postmenopausal bleeding for endometrial cancer: Cost-effectiveness of initial diagnostic strategies. Br J Obstet Gynaecol 113(5):502, 2006.
Clemons JL, Arya LA, Myers DL: Diagnosing interstitial cystitis in women with chronic pelvic pain. Obstet Gynecol 100:337, 2002.
Dart RG, Burke G, Dart L: Subclassification of indeterminate pelvic ultrasonography: Prospective evaluation of the risk of ectopic pregnancy. Ann Emerg Med 39(4):382, 2002.
Eckert LO, Hawes SE. Wolner-Hanssen PK, et al: Endometritis: The clinical-pathologic syndrome. Am J Obstet Gynecol 186(4):690, 2002.
Farquhar CM, Lethaby A, Soroter M, et al: An evaluation of risk factors for endometrial hyperplasia in premenopausal women with abnormal menstrual bleeding. Am J Obstet Gynecol 181:525, 1999.
Farquhar CM, Rogers V, Franks S, et al: A randomized controlled trial of medroxyprogesterone acetate and psychotherapy for the treatment of pelvic congestion. Br J Obstet Gynaecol 96:1153, 1989.
Green CR, Flowe-Valencia H, Rosenblum L, et al: The role of childhood and adulthood abuse among women presenting for chronic pain management. Clin J Pain 17:359, 2001.
Hillis SD, Marchbanks PA, Peterson HB: The effectiveness of hysterectomy for chronic pelvic pain. Obstet Gynecol 86:941, 1995.
Howard FM: Chronic pelvic pain. Obstet Gynecol 101:594, 2003.
Jamieson DJ, Steege JF: The prevalence of dysmenorrhea, dyspareunia, pelvic pain, and irritable bowel syndrome in primary care practices. Obset Gynecol 87:55, 1996.
Lampe A, Solder E, Ennemoser A, et al: Chronic pelvic pain and previous sexual abuse. Obstet Gynecol 96:929, 2000.
LaVecchia C, Morris HB, Draper GJ: Malignant ovarian tumours in childhood in Britain, 1962–78. Br J Cancer 48(3):363, 1983.
Lentz GM, Bavendam T, Stenchever MA, et al: Hormonal manipulation in women with chronic cyclic irritable bladder symptoms, and pelvic pain. Am J Obstet Gynecol 186:1268, 2002.
Ling FW: Randomized controlled trial of depot leuprolide in patients with chronic pelvic pain and clinically suspected endometriosis. Pelvic Pain Study Group. Obstet Gynecol 93:51, 1999.
Longstreth GF: Irritable bowel syndrome and chronic pelvic pain. Obstet Gynecol Surv 49:7, 1994.
Mathias SD, Kupperman M, Liberman RF, et al: Chronic pelvic pain: Prevalence, health-related quality of life, and economic correlates. Obstet Gynecol 87:321, 1996.
Merskey H, Bogduk N (eds): Classification of Chronic Pain. IASP Task Force on Taxonomy, 2nd ed. Seattle, WA, IASP Press, 1994, pp 209–214.
Ness RB, Soper DE, Holley RL: Effectiveness of inpatient and outpatient treatment strategies for women with pelvic inflammatory disease: Results from the Pelvic Inflammatory Disease Evaluation and Clinical Health (PEACH) Randomized Trial. Am J Obstet Gynecol 186:929, 2002.
Norris HJ, Jensen RD: Relative frequency of ovarian neoplasms in childhood and adolescence. Cancer 30:713, 1972.
O'Connell LP, Fries MH, Zerinque E, Brehrn W: Triage of abnormal postmenopausal bleeding: A comparison of endometrial biopsy and transvaginal sonohysterography versus fractional curettage with hysteroscopy. Am J Obstet Gynecol 178:956, 1998.
Ovadia J, Goldman GA: Ovarian masses in postmenopausal women. Int J Gynecol Obstet 39:35, 1992.
Paavonen J, Kiviat N, Brunham RC, et al: Prevalence and manifestations of endometritis among women with cervicitis. Am J Obstet Gynecol 152:280, 1985.
Parsons CL, Bullen M, Kahn BS, et al: Gynecologic presentation of interstitial cystitis as detected by intravesical potassium sensitivity. Obstet Gynecol 98:127, 2001.
Peterson WF, Prevost EC, Edmunds FT, et al: Benign cystic teratomas of the ovary: A clinico-statistical study of 1007 cases with review of the literature. Am J Obstet Gynecol 70:368, 1955.
Reiter RC, Gambone JC: Nongynecologic somatic pathology in women with chronic pelvic pain and negative laparoscopy. J Reprod Med 36:253, 1991.
Renaer MJ, Vertommen H, Nijs P, et al: Psychic aspects of pelvic pain in women. Am J Obstet Gynecol 134:75, 1979.
Seeber BE, Barnhart KT: Suspected ectopic pregnancy. Obstet Gynecol 107:399, 2006.
Siddall-Allum J, Rae T, Rogers V, et al: Chronic pelvic pain caused by residual ovaries and ovarian remnants. Br J Obstet Gynaecol 101:979, 1994.
Silva C, Sammel MD, Zhou L, et al: Human chorionic gonadotropin profile for women with ectopic pregnancy. Obstet Gynecol 107:605, 2006.
Simons DG, Travel JG, Simons LS. Travell & Simons' Myofascial Pain and Dysfunction: The Trigger Point Manual, vol 1: Upper Half of Body, 2nd ed. Baltimore, MD, Lippincott Williams & Wilkins, 1999.
Smith-Bindman R, Kerlikowske K, Feldstein VA, et al: Endovaginal ultrasound to exclude endometrial cancer and other endometrial abnormalities. JAMA 280(17):1510, 1998.
Soysal ME, Soysal S, Vicdan K, et al: A randomized controlled trial of goserelin and medroxyprogesterone acetate in the treatment of pelvic congestion. Hum Reprod 16:931, 2001.

Stenchever MA: Symptomatic retrodisplacement, pelvic congestion, universal joint, and peritoneal defects: Fact or fiction? Clin Obstet Gynecol 33:161, 1990.

Stovall TG, Ling FW, Crawford DA: Hysterectomy for chronic pelvic pain of presumed uterine etiology. Obstet Gynecol 75:676, 1990.

Summit RL Jr: Urogynecologic causes of chronic pelvic pain. Obstet Gynecol Clin North Am 20:685, 1993.

Swank DJ, Swank-Bordewijk SCG, Hop WCJ, et al: Laparoscopic adhesiolysis in patients with chronic abdominal pain: a blinded randomized controlled multi-centre trial. Lancet 361:1247, 2003.

Tu FF, As-Sanie AS, Steege JF: Prevalence of pelvic musculoskeletal disorders in a female chronic pain pelvic clinic. J Reprod Med 51:185, 2006.

U.S. Department of Health and Human Services: The health consequences of smoking: A report of the Surgeon General 2004. Available at *www.cdc.gov/tobaccosgr/sgr-2004/chapters.htm*. Retrieved May 31, 2006.

van Nagell JR Jr, DePriest PD: Management of adnexal masses in postmenopausal women. Am J Obstet Gynecol 193:30, 2005.

Walker EA, Sullivan ND, Stenchever MA: Use of antidepressants in the management of women with chronic pelvic pain. Obstet Gynecol Clin North Am 20:743, 1993.

Walker EA, Katon WJ, Jemelka R, et al: The prevalence of chronic pelvic pain and irritable bowel syndrome in two university clinics. J Psychosom Obstet Gynecol 12(Suppl):65, 1991.

Weiss JM: Pelvic floor myofascial trigger points: Manual therapy for interstitial cystitis and the urgency-frequency syndrome. J Urol 166:2226, 2001.

Westrom L: Effect of acute pelvic inflammatory disease on fertility. Am J Obstet Gynecol 121:707, 1975.

Zondervan KT, Yudkin PL, Vessey MP, et al: Prevalence and incidence in primary care of chronic pelvic pain in women: Evidence from a national general practice database. Br J Obstet Gynaecol 106:1149, 1999.

Zondervan KT, Yudkin PL, Vessey MP, et al: Chronic pelvic pain in the community-symptoms, investigations, and diagnoses. Am J Obstet Gynecol 184:1149, 2001.

Emotional Aspects of Gynecology 9

Sexual Dysfunction, Eating Disorders, Substance Abuse, Depression, Grief, Loss

Gretchen M. Lentz

KEY TERMS AND DEFINITIONS

Agitated Depression. A severe and rare grief reaction in which the bereaved develops tension, agitation, insomnia, feelings of worthlessness, and fantasies of the need for punishment, at times including suicide.

Anhedonia. Loss of feelings of joy and pleasure.

Anorexia Nervosa. A psychiatric disease associated with a food aversion, fear of weight gain or obesity, and a distorted body image in which the individual limits caloric intake to starvation levels. In addition to severe weight loss, there is a decreased metabolic rate and amenorrhea.

Behavior Modification. A treatment program using reward and punishment techniques to change behavior.

Binge Drinking. The consumption of five or more drinks on a specific occasion or drinking until intoxicated.

Bulimia Nervosa. A disorder that features binge eating with a sense of loss of control over eating and self-induced purging using vomiting or diarrhea (or both) as inappropriate compensatory behaviors.

Cognitive Behavior Therapy. The technique of behavior change that attempts to modify beliefs, assumptions, and thinking styles.

Delayed Grief Reaction. The postponement of the grief reaction for various reasons and for a period from days to years.

Distorted Grief Reaction. The assumption of the characteristics of the deceased by the bereaved for a prolonged period and at times in a distorted fashion, during which the bereaved often evidences no sense of loss.

Dyspareunia. Painful intercourse.

Excessive Alcohol Consumption. The consumption of greater than seven alcoholic drinks per week or three or more alcoholic drinks on a specific occasion for women is considered criteria for "at-risk" drinking.

Grief Reaction. A group of symptoms associated with loss, which generally resolves in 6 to 18 months.

Hypoactive Sexual Desire. Persistent or recurrent deficiency in sexual fantasies and desire for sexual activity.

Obesity. An eating disorder in which the individual's weight classification by body mass index (BMI) is greater than 30 kg/m^2. Severe or morbid obesity is defined as a BMI higher than 40 kg/m^2.

Orgasmic Dysfunction. Difficulty or inability in reaching orgasm.

Sexual Dysfunction. A psychological or physiologic problem or condition that prevents the usual full participation and enjoyment of coitus.

Sexual Response Curve. The graphic expression of sexual response as defined by Masters and Johnson involving four phases: excitement, plateau, orgasm, and resolution.

Vaginismus. Involuntary spasm of vaginal, introital, and levator ani muscles, causing painful sexual intercourse or preventing penetration.

During a lifetime, the individual faces several tasks and challenges. Perhaps the first is the development of an identity and the building of self-esteem. This begins in early childhood and continues through adolescence. Such development is aided by positive and nurturing forces. On the other hand, attacks against the young individual's mental or physical well-being may have a distorting influence. The quality of her self-esteem and self-perception will influence the choices she makes in life situations and will affect her personal development.

All individuals experience loss throughout their lifetime. The scope of such loss may be quite varied, including lack of accomplishment or loss of opportunity in career, the loss of a body organ or a body part, the loss of a friend or a loved one through separation or death, the loss of a relationship, or the loss of a physical or mental ability because of illness or accident. In general, loss is managed by a grieving process. The way in which the individual grieves and resolves grief often determines the degree of success in the next stage of life. The inability to handle grief appropriately may lead to lost opportunities, poor choices, and poorly developed future relationships.

The gynecologist is in an important position to help a young woman develop her self-image and to help her manage the losses that she will inevitably face. The gynecologist has the opportunity to participate with the patient in critical life events from adolescence to late in life and to provide or obtain counseling for her as she works her way through these problems.

This chapter outlines the major social problems that can arise during a woman's lifetime and will offer suggestions as to how the physician can aid the patient.

CHILDHOOD COUNSELING PROBLEMS

Self-esteem begins to develop in early childhood and is the result of positive efforts of parents and others in the child's immediate environment. Continuous reinforcement of a child's worth as an individual, by verbal and nonverbal means, should be encouraged. Touching, talking to the child in gentle ways, positively praising the child's actions, and, as the child becomes older, setting limits that are socially acceptable within the framework of the family are all reasonable steps. Punishment should be limited to reinforcing the needs for the limits set. Intimidation by verbal or physical means should be avoided. The physician may have the opportunity to suggest help for parents by offering reading material, discussing the issue directly with them, or referring them to parenting classes. In general, positive reinforcement of the child's worth as an individual mixed with appropriate warmth and love tends to build self-esteem, whereas negative statements or actions tend to tear it down. The child has little with which to compare, and if she is given negative information about herself, the tendency is to believe it.

Physical or sexual abuse in childhood can have serious consequences for the child's development. These are extreme influences and must be handled energetically when they occur or as soon afterward as they are noted. The health care professional must communicate to the child that she is a victim and in no way responsible for what has happened. Any contrary statements may have a lasting effect on the child's developing self-esteem. Issues of abuse are discussed more fully in Chapter 10 (Rape, Incest, and Domestic Violence).

Parental Loss in Childhood

A serious threat to normal emotional development in childhood is the loss of a parent by death or permanent separation. Laajus reviewed a large number of studies addressing this problem. Because the study methodology is complex, it is difficult to draw comparisons between different reports. However, a number of general observations were made. In Laajus's experience parental loss was a common finding in children referred for psychiatric treatment and was associated with a variety of pathologic and behavior disturbances. The period between the loss of a parent and the onset of the disorder is often quite long. Cognitive and emotional understanding of death and dying in children gradually evolves with age.

Tennant and colleagues, applying multiple regression analysis, believe that the earlier the separation and the longer its duration, the more maladjustment is likely to occur. The risk of developing a psychiatric disorder seems greatest if the child is younger than 5 years or an adolescent and if the child loses a parent of the same sex. Males seem more susceptible to the loss of a father than to the loss of a mother and seem to be more affected by this loss than are females. In general, their major reaction is to develop antisocial tendencies. On the other hand, loss of a father during adolescence seems to influence the emotional development of females, although the problems may not be manifested for a number of years. Loss of a mother in girls younger than 11 years seems to significantly affect development.

Some of the difficulty in clarifying the role of the loss of a mother or father in young children relates to the way parent substitutes are developed. Because maternal loss usually necessitates the finding of a care provider, often a female, the effect of maternal loss may be blunted. On the other hand, male substitution after paternal loss may not occur rapidly or at all. Tennant and colleagues showed a consistent relationship between parental loss and the development of psychiatric illness in all ages. Children between the ages of 5 and 10 years seem to be the most susceptible to behavior changes. But adolescence was also a time of important vulnerability in cases of schizophrenia, depression, and a variety of medical illnesses occurring in adolescence. The loss of a parent early in life was a frequent and significant finding in such patients, with the loss of a father being noted more frequently than the loss of a mother.

Gregory has demonstrated that parental loss is often associated with antisocial disorders, especially delinquency. The highest rates seem to occur among males who have lost their father. One study shows a 3.5-fold increase of severe crimes in a group of males who had lost one or more parents before the age of 5 years. On the other hand, the perpetration of severe crimes was less frequent among males who had experienced parental losses later in life. Anderson compared a group of delinquent and nondelinquent boys who had suffered parental loss between the ages of 4 and 7 years and demonstrated that a father substitution had occurred more frequently in the group that was not delinquent.

Counseling considerations for children and adolescents who have suffered parental loss should include attention to the child's bereavement with active help in working through the acute phase of grief followed by the incorporation of an individual into the child's life who is of the same sex as the lost parent. If the mother is deceased or absent, a loving, nurturing, and supportive female or group of females should be identified to participate in the child's care and development. This may be a grandparent, an aunt, a hired nanny, or an effective childcare program. Eventually it may be a stepmother. If the father is lost, older brothers, grandfathers, uncles, or males volunteering as "big brothers" may all be considered. In addition, surviving parents should be encouraged to protect the child as much as possible from their own grieving process and to maintain the integrity of the family unit.

Similar observations have been made with respect to the loss of a parent through separation or divorce. Hostile marital relationships seem to be more detrimental to child development than does the permanent absence of a parent by divorce or separation. Continuous discord within the family has been shown by Rutter to be associated with an increase of antisocial disorders in boys but not in girls. Tennant and colleagues investigated individuals with psychiatric disorders and looked at four causes of separation from parents during childhood. These include illness of the individual, wartime evacuation, parental illness, and marital discord. They found that parental illness and marital discord had a statistically significantly greater association with the development of psychiatric diseases than did separation because of the individual's illness or wartime evacuation.

Fergusson and coworkers performed a 15-year longitudinal study in which a sample of 935 children subjected to parental separation were evaluated at age 15 for measures of adolescent psychopathology and problem behavior. After adjusting for confounding factors, they found increased risks for problems, which included substance abuse or dependency, conduct or behavioral disorders, mood and anxiety disorders, and early-onset sexual activity, occurring at increased odds ratios of 1.07 to 3.32, with a median increase of 1.46. Males and females responded similarly.

Two review articles by Johnston and by Amato demonstrate that high-conflict divorce is associated with a two to four times increase in emotional and behavioral problems in children compared with national norms, with boys at greater risk than girls; that joint physical custody or frequent visitations lead to poorer child outcome, especially in girls; and that outcome depends on many variables, including quality time spent with the noncustodial parent, the psychological adjustment and parenting skills of the custodial parent, and the degree of economic hardship. They advise taking these factors into consideration in designing legal and therapeutic interventions.

In contrast to many reports of poorer outcomes for children of divorce, the literature is quite inconsistent. A 2005 Australian study by Ruschena actually found surprising resilience of children and adolescents. Longitudinal data from the Australian Temperament Project (ATP) studies 2443 families identified in 1983 and followed until 2000 when 1605 families remained and approximately 80% of the adolescents and parents responded to surveys. The effect of family transitions (mostly divorce or separation) on children and adolescents was no different across time with regard to behavioral and emotional adjustment, nor on academic outcomes or social competence compared with intact families. There were significant differences in conflict with parents and lower parent–child relationship quality. Also, gender differences were noted with girls having higher behavioral problems.

Methodological inconsistencies and the number of confounding issues make these studies hard to control. Gender and age of the child, financial circumstances, child temperament, interparental conflict, additional family changes like remarriage and moving probably all affect the outcome on children.

PROBLEMS IN ADOLESCENCE AND ADULTHOOD

Eating Disorders

Anorexia nervosa, bulimia nervosa, and obesity are the major eating disorders affecting adolescents and young adults. On the one hand, eating is one of the major gratifications of life and is also a readily available substitute for other forms of gratification that sometimes cannot be achieved. Today a young woman is bombarded by two very different signals stemming primarily from advertising campaigns presented on television, written media, and the Internet. The first of these involves food. Citizens of the Western world are offered foods of vast variety and unusual quantity presented in an appealing and almost demanding fashion. Stimuli to eat are seductive and almost continuous. On the other hand, the fashionable image of the American woman as depicted by the media is one of thinness. In discussing the cultural expectations of American women Garner and Garfinkel noted that a definite trend for decrease in body weight was noted between 1959 and 1978 in *Playboy* centerfold models and participants in the Miss America pageant. In both instances these women weighed significantly less than the average American woman. Furthermore, the weights of the finalists in the Miss America pageant were noted to be significantly below those of other contestants during the years 1970 through 1978. Rubenstein and Caballero recently reported a steady, statistically significant ($p < .0001$) drop in body mass index (BMI) in contestants from 1920 until 1996. In earlier years the BMI was in the range now felt to be normal (20–25 kg/m^2), but there have been an increasing number of winners in the BMI range of less than 18.5 (a level defined by the World Health Organization as undernourished), with some as low as 16.9. The image that these "ideal women" create is in severe contrast to the reality that the average weight of American women increased by several pounds during that same period. Although the ideal of thinness may have lessened during the 1980s, it seems to have been reinstated since then. A prospective 2004 study of 531 adolescent boys and girls found that the elevations in body mass, negative affect, and perceived pressure to be thin from peers predicted increases in body dissatisfaction. In contrast, a Minnesota study of 2357 adolescent students reported significantly higher body satisfaction when parental or peer attitudes encouraged healthy eating and exercising to be fit versus dieting.

Johnson and Schlundt reported that in a survey of 1200 high school girls, 48% believed that they were either overweight or very overweight, whereas only 8% considered themselves underweight. Interestingly, the mean weight of these young women was within the normal range. Because the majority believed they were overweight, 50% of those who were 14 years or older and 70% who were 18 years or older were actively dieting. Many reported the use of diuretics, diet pills, laxatives, and self-induced vomiting to lower their weight. In a similar survey in 2005, 46.8% of 1037 Italian teenage girls were dieting although less than 11% were overweight.

The effects of dieting may bring women to the attention of the gynecologist and may be responsible for symptoms that may not seem readily related to dieting. For instance, Pirke and coworkers studied 13 healthy women of normal weight who volunteered to lose 1 kg/week on an 800-calorie vegetarian diet for an average weight loss of 4.9 ± 0.7 kg. At the completion of the study, their body mass index was 99% of ideal body weight (Metropolitan Life Insurance standards). During their control cycles, each demonstrated normal gonadal function, but during the dietary cycles only two remained normal. Seven did not develop dominant follicles, and four others who did demonstrated impaired progesterone secretion by the corpus luteum. Dieting altered episodic luteinizing hormone (LH) secretion during the follicular phase, and LH concentrations and the frequency of episodic secretions were significantly reduced during the follicular phase but not during the luteal phase. Follicle-stimulating hormone (FSH) was unaltered by dieting.

Likewise, Kreipe and associates studied two groups of women who had clinical or subclinical eating disorders classified as restrictive anorexia nervosa, bulimic anorexia nervosa, normal weight bulimia nervosa, and other subclinical eating disorders and compared these with control subjects. None had weights above 110% of ideal body weight. Of 48 women with a diagnosed eating disorder, 45 (93.7%) had a menstrual abnormality consisting of amenorrhea or oligomenorrhea. Of the 22 patients with subclinical eating disorders, 21 gave a history of amenorrhea although none had this problem at present. Nine complained of oligomenorrhea. Most of these women reported weight fluctuations of 10% to 20% of ideal body weight in the past. Of the

37 controls, only 1 had a history of amenorrhea and 4 of oligomenorrhea. Thus, an eating disorder apparently can present with menstrual abnormalities even in the subclinical stages and can probably affect reproductive efficiency.

Anorexia Nervosa and Bulimia Nervosa

Although anorexia nervosa is quite uncommon in the general population (0.24–1.6 per 100,000 people), it is quite common in adolescent girls, with a lifetime risk of 0.3% to 1%, occurring in about 1 in every 100. The incidence in professional ballet dancers varies from 5% to 20%, depending on the level of competition of the ballet company, the weight standards imposed, and the number of hours of exercise required. The condition is nine times more common in women than in men. It does occur among men who must restrict their weights in training for competitive athletic events.

Sundgot-Borgen studied risk factors for eating disorders in 603 elite Norwegian female athletes ages 12 to 35. They used the Eating Disorder Inventory to classify these individuals and defined 117 at risk. Of these, 103 were given a structured clinical interview for eating disorders. A control group of 30 athletes chosen from the not-at-risk pool were also interviewed. Ninety-two of the at-risk group met the criteria for anorexia nervosa or bulimia, and the prevalence of these disorders was higher in athletes performing in sports employing leanness compared with controls. Athletes with eating disorders began sports-specific training and dieting earlier and believed that puberty had occurred too early for optimal performance. The onset of eating disorders was often associated with prolonged dieting, frequent weight fluctuation, sudden increase in training, injury, or loss of a coach.

Although various clinical signs and symptoms occur in the patient with anorexia nervosa, it basically concerns food aversion with refusal to maintain body weight at or above a minimal normal weight (<85% of ideal body weight), fear of weight gain or obesity, and a distorted body image. Three months of amenorrhea must be present to meet diagnostic criteria, which frequently disappears with weight gain. Other medical and psychiatric disorders need to be considered in the differential diagnosis of anorexia (Table 9-1). The central nervous system and endocrine considerations are discussed in Chapter 38 (Primary and Secondary Amenorrhea and Precocious Puberty).

Table 9-1 Differential Diagnosis and Physical Findings of Anorexia Nervosa

Organic Disease	Physical Findings
GI disease (i.e., inflammatory bowel disease)	Emaciation
Cancer	Dry skin
Diabetes, new onset	Excessive lanugo
Hyperthyroidism	Brittle nails
Infection (i.e., AIDs, TB)	Hair loss
Malnutrition	Bradycardia
Drug abuse	Hypotension
Adrenal Insufficiency	Little body fat
Psychiatric Disease	Peripheral edema
Affective disorder (i.e., bipolar)	
Anxiety disorder (i.e., obsessive–compulsive)	
Personality disorder	
Schizophrenia	

GI, gastrointestinal.

The American Psychiatric Association's *Diagnostic and Statistical Manual of Mental Disorders,* 4th edition (DSM-IV), lists two types of anorexia nervosa. One type involves the patient restricting food intake primarily, and the second involves regular binge eating, purging behavior, or both. Excessive, compulsive exercise may be involved. About 50% of anorectic patients use binge eating and self-induced purging.

Bulimia nervosa is defined in the DSM-IV as episodes of binge eating and a sense of loss of control over eating and inappropriate compensatory behaviors, such as self-induced vomiting or laxative abuse at least twice a week for 3 months. These women also have a preoccupation with body weight and shape and binging can lead to significant fear and anxiety. A patient with anorexia can induce vomiting and is still considered anorexic rather than bulimic if she is 15% below ideal body weight and meets the other DSM-IV criteria. Not all bulimics have low body weight. Bulimic persons may have more impulsivity and psychological problems and be more difficult to treat. In a study by Casper and colleagues 57% of bulimic patients reported vomiting after meals, in contrast to only 18% of patients with anorexia without bulimia. Bulimic persons in this series tended to be more extroverted and demonstrated symptoms of depression and anxiety, particularly with sleep disturbances. They also were more obsessional about food than were anorectics without bulimia. A third eating disorder is termed binge eating disorder and this occurs without the purging. To differentiate a binge eating disorder from obesity, the former is marked by significant distress when binge eating occurs. This binge behavior is important to recognize because the usual recommended weight loss strategies will be ineffective without attention to the biopsychosocial disease.

The cause of anorexia nervosa appears to be multifactorial, which fits with a biopsychosocial disorder. Strober and coworkers looked at the incidence of anorexia nervosa, bulimia, and subclinical anorexia nervosa in first- and second-degree relatives of anorectic patients and demonstrated that eating disorders are familial. They were, however, unable to demonstrate mechanisms responsible for these familial relationships. They suggested that genetically transmitted defects in the neurobiologic processes that control feeding behavior may be present but could not rule out specific psychologic or familial vulnerbilities, common exposure to psychologically determined environmental experiences, cotransmission, or personality traits or psychopathologic disorders that may involve eating disturbances. They also could not rule out some important combinations of all of these factors. Walters and Kendler studied a population-based sample of 2163 female twins, and noted that co-twins of twins with anorexia nervosa were at a significantly higher risk of anorexia nervosa, bulimia, major depression, and current low body mass index. Significant association was found between anorexia nervosa and major depression, bulimia, generalized anxiety disorder, alcoholism, phobia, and panic disorders. They concluded that anorexia-like syndromes are familial and share causal factors with major depression. Neurotransmitters, both norepinephrine and serotonin, may have a role in this disorder. Quite possibly, genetics, compulsive and perfectionist personality types, anxiety and depression disorders, and societal pleasures regarding appearance are all factors.

An interesting association between eating disorders and an adverse sexual experience was noted by Oppenheimer and associates. Two thirds of 78 patients with eating disorders reported such experiences and stated that thoughts of previous sexual abuse were often stressing and significant to the individuals. A total of 80% of the events occurred in childhood or adolescence, and most involved a significantly older male, usually a person known to the subject. In most cases both social taboo and personal trust were violated. The authors felt that given the nature of their study questionnaire, the incidence of such adverse sexual experience among anorectics may have been underreported. A 2001 New Zealand epidemiologic study of child sexual abuse also found higher rates of eating disorders in subjects with eating disorders compared with a group of women reporting no abuse. Furthermore, earlier menarche and paternal overcontrol independently increased the risk of developing an eating disorder.

Pope and colleagues, however, studied the incidence of childhood sexual abuse in three groups of bulimic women in three different countries (the United States, Austria, and Brazil). Although sexual abuse was reported in 24% to 36% of women in these three groups, only 15% to 32% of these women reported the abuse before the onset of bulimia and there was no increase in the incidence of childhood sexual abuse over what was reported for women in the general populations of these countries. They concluded that childhood sexual abuse is not a risk factor for bulimia. Obviously, the potential for a relationship is still not clear. However, a wide range of childhood adversities have been associated with an increased risk of eating disorders so a careful social history should be taken when an eating disorder is suspected.

Johnson and Schlundt in commenting on therapy for anorexia nervosa pointed out that the general modalities have included medication, hospitalization, nutritional support, and behavior therapy. To evaluate any therapy it is important to understand what the spontaneous remission rate might be among untreated patients. Hsu and coworkers compared three groups of patients with anorexia nervosa who were evaluated between 1968 and 1973 and were followed for 4 to 6 years. Within the group there were those treated as inpatients and as outpatients, and those not treated. Evaluation included weight gain and menstrual function. Good or fair outcomes were observed in 88% of those treated as inpatients, 77% of those treated as outpatients, and 59% of those not treated. In general, inpatient therapy consisted of hospitalization, nutritional support, various medications, and often individual or family counseling and psychotherapy. Most studies report excellent weight gain in such patients.

Few intervention strategies have been tested in controlled studies despite the significant morbidity and chronicity of anorexia. Observational studies recommend prompt refeeding and weight gain although no specific nutritional program is advised.

In severe cases, patients have been fed intravenously, given total parenteral nutrition, or given nasogastric tube feedings. Generally, these methods are used when normal feeding attempts in inpatient therapy have not been associated with weight gain. Such extreme measures are generally used in the most severe and life-threatening situations.

A number of medications have been tried with varying success. These medications have included insulin, lithium, tricyclic antidepressants, and phenothiazides, as well as high-potency vitamins. In many case-control studies these have not been found to be more effective than placebo. It is often difficult to separate the effect of a medication from the effects of counseling and psychotherapy given simultaneously. A 2006 Cochrane Database review of antidepressants found only seven randomized controlled trials. Four placebo-controlled trials did not find evidence that antidepressants hasten weight gain or improve the psychological issues. Limited studies of selective serotonin-reuptake inhibitors (SSRIs) have also not shown improved weight gain. Small uncontrolled studies do suggest nortriptyline or olanzapine may improve weight gain but well-designed trials are needed. Regarding bulimia nervosa, a 2003 Cochrane Database review of 19 trials comparing antidepressants to placebo did find a reduction in binge episodes [RR for clinical improvement 0.63 (95% CI 0.55–0.74)].

In the 1960s and 1970s therapy was often tailored to the technique of behavior modification. When controlled studies were carried out, it seemed apparent that hospitalization per se would allow for reasonable weight gain, but when behavior modification was added, the hospital course could be shortened because of accelerated weight gain. Behavior modification was based on the reward and punishment program used for a number of behavior and habituation problems. Controlled studies suggest family involvement in education and therapy improves outcomes.

More recently, however, cognitive behavior therapy has been used in the treatment of anorexia nervosa and bulimia. This therapy is aimed at bringing to the attention of the individual the fact that her beliefs, assumptions, and style of thinking have brought about a distorted body image, food aversion, phobias, and unreasonable fears of weight gain. In short, the therapy is aimed at reshaping patients' thinking processes with respect to themselves and to their body images. Cognitive behavior therapy appears to be directed toward the specific thinking disorder rather than merely to its effect. The feelings that occur related to these thoughts leads to responses that are undesirable. By correcting the negative, distorted, or inappropriate thoughts with realistic restatements, anxiety is reduced and the subsequent response may be more positive.

It is important to consider ultimate outcome in groups of patients with anorexia nervosa and bulimia. Theander, in a discussion of outcome, reviewed three long-term follow-up studies and discussed the results of his own study in Sweden. In three British studies a 5- to 6-year follow-up demonstrated good to intermediate results in 74% of patients. However, 23% of patients experienced a poor outcome, with 3% dying of the disease. In the Swedish study described by Theander with a mean observation time of 33 years, good to fair outcomes were noted in 76% of patients, poor outcomes in 6%, and death in 18%. Deaths were the result of starvation or suicide. Isager and coworkers analyzed survival data in 151 cases of anorexia nervosa, considering specifically death and relapse rates. Follow-up was from 4 to 22 years. The authors calculated the hazard of death as 0.5% per year and the hazards of relapse at 3% per year. Both hazards, however, declined steadily after therapeutic contact. Full recovery can take 5 to 7 years for treated adolescents to return to physical and psychological health. The outcomes are poorer in adults, with only 25% to 50% recovering after hospitalization.

Finally, interventions for preventing the development of eating disorders in children and adolescents are needed. Studies to date are insufficient to conclude prevention programs are beneficial, but no evidence of harm has been noted.

Obesity

The prevalence of obesity has dramatically increased in the United States. The World Health Organization (WHO) definitions for body weight are shown in Table 9-2. Weight classification by BMI is outlined in Table 9-3. Based on this definition, about one third of U.S. women are obese. WHO also describes a global epidemic of obesity, which is a major contributor to worldwide chronic disease and disability. There is a strong relationship between mortality and increased BMI above 25 kg/m^2 (and below 20 kg/m^2) (Fig. 9-1). Thirty-one percent of non-Hispanic white women were classified as obese during the period 1999–2002, with black women at a higher rate (49%), and Mexican-American women at 38%.

Severe obesity is a health hazard that carries a 12-fold increase in mortality. Often these individuals suffer complicating factors, such as hypertension, diabetes, hyperlipidemias, arthritis, increased operative morbidity and mortality, and compromised pulmonary function. Obesity has been linked to multiple obstetric and gynecologic problems, including spontaneous abortion, endometrial hyperplasia, and endometrial and breast cancer, to name a few.

Diet, exercise, and behavior modification provided by lay supervision is appropriate for those suffering from mild obesity;

Table 9-2 Body Mass Index Table

BMI	19	20	21	22	23	24	25	26	27	28	29	30	31	32	33	34	35
Height (inches)	NORMAL WEIGHT						OVERWEIGHT					OBESE					
	Body Weight (pounds)																
58	91	96	100	105	110	115	119	124	129	134	138	143	148	153	158	162	167
59	94	99	104	109	114	119	124	128	133	138	143	148	153	158	163	168	173
60	97	102	107	112	118	123	128	133	138	143	148	153	158	163	168	174	179
61	100	106	111	116	122	127	132	137	143	148	153	158	164	169	174	180	185
62	104	109	115	120	126	131	136	142	147	153	158	164	169	175	180	186	191
63	107	113	118	124	130	135	141	146	152	158	163	169	175	180	186	191	197
64	110	116	122	128	134	140	145	151	157	163	169	174	180	186	192	197	204
65	114	120	126	132	138	144	150	156	162	168	174	180	186	192	198	204	210
66	118	124	130	136	142	148	155	161	167	173	179	186	192	198	204	210	216
67	121	127	134	140	146	153	159	166	172	178	185	191	198	204	211	217	223
68	125	131	138	144	151	158	164	171	177	184	190	197	203	210	216	223	230
69	128	135	142	149	155	162	169	176	182	189	196	203	209	216	223	230	236
70	132	139	146	153	160	167	174	181	188	195	202	209	216	222	229	236	243
71	136	143	150	157	165	172	179	186	193	200	208	215	222	229	236	243	250
72	140	147	154	162	169	177	184	191	199	206	213	221	228	235	242	250	258
73	144	151	159	166	174	182	189	197	204	212	219	227	235	242	250	257	265
74	148	155	163	171	179	186	194	202	210	218	225	233	241	249	256	264	272
75	152	160	168	176	184	192	200	208	216	224	232	240	248	256	264	272	279
76	156	164	172	180	189	197	205	213	221	230	238	246	254	263	271	279	287

	OBESE				EXTREME OBESITY														
BMI	36	37	38	39	40	41	42	43	44	45	46	47	48	49	50	51	52	53	54
58	172	177	181	186	191	196	201	205	210	215	220	224	229	234	239	244	248	253	258
59	178	183	188	193	198	203	208	212	217	222	227	232	237	242	247	252	257	262	267
60	184	189	194	199	204	209	215	220	225	230	235	240	245	250	255	261	266	271	276
61	190	195	201	206	211	217	222	227	232	238	243	248	254	259	264	269	275	280	285
62	196	202	207	213	218	224	229	235	240	246	251	256	262	267	273	278	284	289	295
63	203	208	214	220	225	231	237	242	248	254	259	265	270	278	282	287	293	299	304
64	209	215	221	227	232	238	244	250	256	262	267	273	279	285	291	296	302	308	314
65	216	222	228	234	240	246	252	258	264	270	276	282	288	294	300	306	312	318	324
66	223	229	235	241	247	253	260	266	272	278	284	291	297	303	309	315	322	328	334
67	230	236	242	249	255	261	268	274	280	287	293	299	306	312	319	325	331	338	344
68	236	243	249	256	262	269	276	282	289	295	302	308	315	322	328	335	341	348	354
69	243	250	257	263	270	277	284	291	297	304	311	318	324	331	338	345	351	358	365
70	250	257	264	271	278	285	292	299	306	313	320	327	334	341	348	355	362	369	376
71	257	265	272	279	286	293	301	308	315	322	329	338	343	351	358	365	372	379	386
72	265	272	279	287	294	302	309	316	324	331	338	346	353	361	368	375	383	390	397
73	272	280	288	295	302	310	318	325	333	340	348	355	363	371	378	386	393	401	408
74	280	287	295	303	311	319	326	334	342	350	358	365	373	381	389	396	404	412	420
75	287	295	303	311	319	327	335	343	351	359	367	375	383	391	399	407	415	423	431
76	295	304	312	320	328	336	344	353	361	369	377	385	394	402	410	418	426	435	443

Evidence Report of Clinical Guidelines on the Identification, Evaluation, and Treatment of Overweight and Obesity in Adults, 1998. http://www.nhlbi.nih.gov/guidelines/obesity/bmi_tbl.pdf.

Table 9-3 Weight Classification by Body Mass Index (BMI)

Weight	BMI*
Normal Weight	18.5–24.9
Overweight	25.0–29.9
Obesity	>30
Class I	30.0–34.9
Class II	35.0–39.9
Class III	≥40

*BMI calculation = weight in kilograms/height in square meters.

diet, exercise, and behavior modification under medical supervision is appropriate for those suffering from moderate obesity; and operative intervention is appropriate for those suffering from severe obesity if conservative measures have failed. Patients suffering from severe obesity almost always have medical complications, and these often improve with weight reduction. Surgical options can provide long-term weight loss but are not without complications. A 2005 meta-analysis on surgical treatment of obesity found only a few controlled trials, but surgery was more effective for weight loss and control of some comorbid medical conditions when a patient BMI was 40 kg/m^2 or greater. Bariatric procedures used (gastric bypass, laparoscopic gastric band, vertical banded gastroplasty, and biliopancreatic diversion and switch) results in a 20% complication rate and 1% mortality. A patient with a BMI of 35 to 39 kg/m^2 appeared to do better with surgery, but more studies are needed.

When dietary and pharmacologic therapy has been used for treating severe obesity, 15% of patients suffer from severe depression and 26% from moderate depression. Depression is much less common in patients who undergo gastric reduction operations. Of these individuals, 75% report elation and a feeling of well-being. In addition, 91% of these patients state that before the operation they had required a good deal of willpower to keep from overeating, and indeed, 33% stated that they could eat another full meal after eating most of their meals. Only 14% ever felt satisfied after eating. After the operation 10% state that they require willpower to keep from eating more, and only 1% state that they could eat another full meal after eating. On the other hand, 94% feel that they could eat no more after completing the usual meal. A 2004 meta-analysis found the majority of postsurgical obesity patients have resolution or improvement in comorbid conditions such as diabetes, hypertension, hyperlipidemia, and obstructive sleep apnea.

Moderately obese patients will lose weight on diets of 1200 to 1500 Calories (Cal) and generally find this approach comfortable. However, weight loss under these circumstances takes a long time. On very low calorie diets (400 to 700 Cal), which consist mostly of protein (fish, fowl, or lean meat), dramatic change in weight can usually be accomplished in 3 months. The patient will lose 1.5 to 2.3 kg/week depending on the amount of body fat at the beginning of dieting. The major problem with such individuals is maintaining weight loss, and, in fact, most do not maintain the weight loss.

Exercise is a useful addition to diet regimens. Several studies have demonstrated that although similar weight loss can be obtained by both diet alone and diet plus exercise programs, the latter will allow for a greater loss of fat stores while maintaining muscle mass. To maintain this advantage, exercise programs must be maintained. Although exercise alone is not a good method for losing weight, studies indicate exercise is very beneficial for long-term weight management and overall health.

Craighead and associates point out that unless behavior is modified, weight loss is usually not maintained. These workers studied 145 patients who were approximately 60% overweight and divided them into three groups. Treatment continued for 6 months, and there was at least 1 year of follow-up in 99% of those who completed the therapy. Group 1 underwent behavior

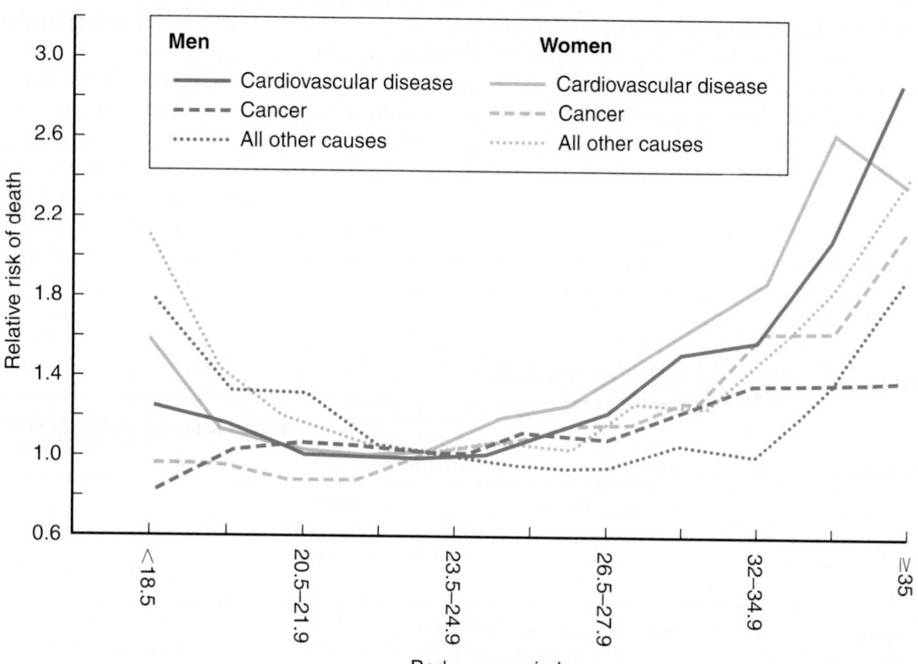

Figure 9-1. Relation between mortality and body mass index in men and women who have never smoked. (Data from Calle EE, Thun MJ, Petrelli JM, et al: Body-Mass Index and mortality in a prospective cohort of U.S. adults. N Eng J Med 341:1097, 1999.)

modification using Ferguson's *Learning to Eat* manual. They lost an average of 11.4 kg and regained only 1.8 kg during the follow-up year. Group 2 received medication therapy with an appetite suppressant, fenfluramine hydrochloride (Pondimin). They lost an average of 14.5 kg but regained 8.6 kg during the follow-up period. The third group was treated with a combination of behavior modification and medication and lost an average of 15.0 kg but regained 9.5 kg during the follow-up period. The authors concluded that behavior modification without medication was the most appropriate therapy for moderate obesity. Setting goals is important in behavior therapy, and a 5% to 10% loss of total body weight is realistic over 6 months and can decrease the severity of comorbid diseases.

Mild obesity seems to respond best to dieting, exercise, and behavior modification under lay supervision. Such individuals will generally embrace fad diets and look for magic cures. However, if placed on a nutritionally appropriate limited-caloric diet, they will generally do well if their attitudes toward eating and response to various stimuli are modified. Lay groups, such as Weight Watchers or Take Off Pounds Sensibly (TOPS), are usually quite successful for motivated individuals. Currently, there are many commercial diet centers available for referral. Most prescribe or sell low-fat foods in an attempt to achieve a diet containing about 20% fat. Because fat represents 9 Cal/g and protein and carbohydrate represent 4 Cal/g, it is possible by changing eating habits to allow a patient a considerable quantity of food without high numbers of calories. Low-carbohydrate diets have become popular, but no comparison studies have proven better long-term results with these over other diets. The use of portion-controlled servings has been demonstrated to be effective for weight loss because obese persons tend to underestimate the amount of food they consume. Educating patients to change eating habits in this fashion is the key not only to losing weight, but to maintaining the weight loss.

The FDA has approved medications for weight loss, although generally the medication must be continued for sustained benefit and there are no data past 2 years of use on outcome. Orlistat inhibits dietary fat absorption and has side effects of fecal urgency, flatulence, and oily stools. Sibutramine inhibits reuptake of neurotransmitters and affects satiation. Adverse effects include increases in heart rate and blood pressure. These drugs cause modest weight loss (2.8 to 4.8 kg) compared with placebo. A guide to selecting treatment for obesity is given in Table 9-4.

Obesity in adolescence is a variant of the problem in the general population. The percentage of young people who are overweight has more than tripled since 1980. Sixteen percent of young people (6 to 19 years old) are overweight. Being overweight in adolescence is a more powerful predictor of morbidity from cardiovascular disease than being overweight in adulthood. Because the risk for progression with increasing morbidity and mortality is great, prompt support and behavior modification are most important. School and parental involvement are important aspects of controlling the problem. Where an obese parent is also present, best results seem to be achieved when both the parent and the child undergo therapy but in separate counseling sessions. Brownell and colleagues studied 42 obese adolescents, ages 12 through 16, divided into three groups, and using 16 weeks of treatment. When the child alone attended group therapy, there was an average 3.3-kg weight loss; when the child and mother were treated together there was an average 5.3-kg weight loss; and when the child and mother were both treated but separately, there was an 8.4-kg weight loss. After 1 year of follow-up the group in which the mother and child were treated separately maintained their weight loss at a mean of 7.7 kg, whereas the other two groups had regained their previous baseline levels. Obviously, counseling and behavior modification are important in the management of obesity in both the adolescent and adult.

The Centers for Disease Control and Prevention (CDC) mentions the following promising approaches for preventing obesity: (1) breastfeeding, which is associated with a reduced risk of overweight children; (2) regular physical activity; (3) increasing physical activity in overweight people to prevent the complications associated with obesity; and (4) decreasing children's time watching television.

Sexual Function and Dysfunction

Sexual satisfaction is one of the more important human experiences, yet it has been estimated that as many as 50% of all married couples experience some sexual dissatisfaction or dysfunction. Although there is a strong physiologic basis for sexual function, it is impossible to separate sexual response from the many emotional and other contributing factors that may influence a relationship.

In 1966 Masters and Johnson published their now famous book, *Human Sexual Response,* which was a discussion of observations made on the sexual cycles of 700 subjects. It is on this important work that our current understanding of the female sexual response is based. Masters and Johnson described four phases of the sexual response: excitement, plateau, orgasm, and resolution (Fig. 9-2).

Table 9-4 Guide to Selecting Treatment

	BODY MASS INDEX CATEGORY				
Treatment	**25–26.9**	**27–29.9**	**30–34.9**	**35–39.9**	**>40**
Diet, physical activity, and behavior therapy	With comorbidities	With comorbidities	+	+	+
Pharmacotherapy		With comorbidities	+	+	+
Surgery			With comorbidities	With comorbidities	With comorbidities

The + represent the use of indicated treatment regardless of comorbidities.
The Practical Guide: Identification, Evaluation, and Treatment of Overweight and Obesity in Adults. National Heart, Lung, and Blood Institute and North American Association for the Study of Obesity. Bethesda, MD, National Institutes of Health, 2000.

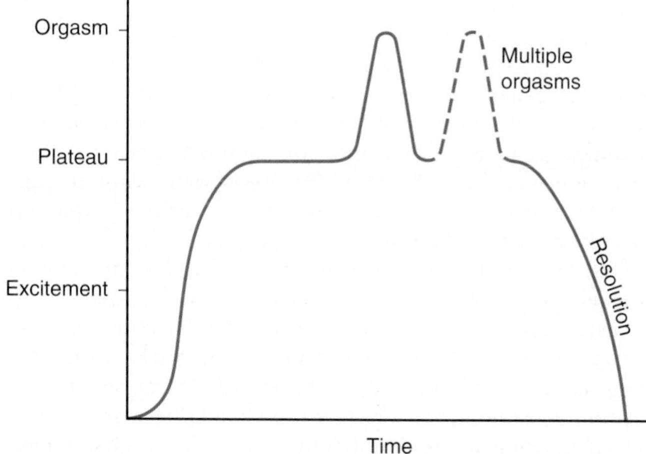

Figure 9-2. Sexual response cycle defined by Masters and Johnson. (From Masters WH, Johnson VE: Human Sexual Response. Boston, Little, Brown, 1966.)

The excitement or seduction phase may be initiated by a number of internal or external stimuli. As shown in the following box, physiologically this phase is associated with deep breathing, increase in heart rate and blood pressure, a total body feeling of warmth associated often with erotic feelings, and an increase in sexual tension. There is generalized vasocongestion, which leads to breast engorgement and the development of a maculopapular erythematous rash on the breasts, the chest, and the epigastrium, which is called the *sex flush.* There is also engorgement of the labia majora (seen particularly in multiparous women) and of the labia minora. The clitoris generally swells and becomes erect, causing it to be tightly applied to the clitoral hood. The vagina "sweats" a transudative lubricant, and the Bartholin glands may secrete small amounts of liquid. With the increasing deep breathing the uterus may tent up into the pelvis, perhaps as a result of the Valsalva maneuver. There is also a myotonic effect, which is most notable in nipple erection. Much of the response in the excitement phase is caused by stimulation of the parasympathetic fibers of the autonomic nervous system. In some cases anticholinergic drugs may interfere with a full response in this stage.

Next is the plateau stage, which is the culmination of the excitement phase and is associated with a marked degree of vasocongestion throughout the body. Breasts and their areolae are markedly engorged, as are the labia and the lower third of the vagina. The vasocongestion in the lower third of the vagina is such that it forms what has been called the *orgasmic platform,* causing a decrease in the diameter of the vagina by as much as 50% and thus allowing for greater friction against the penis. At this stage the clitoris retracts tightly against the pubic symphysis, and the vagina lengthens, with dilation of the upper two thirds. Uteri in the normal anteflex position tend to tent up more. Retroverted uteri do not.

Characteristics of Excitement Phase of Sexual Response Cycle in the Female

Deep breathing
Increased pulse
Increased blood pressure
Warmth and erotic feelings
Increased tension
Generalized vasocongestion
Skin flush
Breast engorgement
Nipple erection
Engorgement of labia and clitoris
Vaginal transudation
Uterine tenting

Characteristics of Orgasm in the Female

Release of tension
Generalized myotonic contractions
Contractions of perivaginal muscles and anal sphincter
Uterine contractions

The next stage is orgasm, in which the sexual tension that has been built up in the entire body is released. Characteristics of orgasm are listed in the above box. A myotonic response involves muscle systems of the entire body. Individuals may experience carpal spasm. Rarely, a grand–mal-type seizure may be observed. There is contraction of the muscles surrounding the vagina, as well as the anal sphincter. The uterus also contracts. Muscle contraction occurs 2 to 4 seconds after the woman begins to experience the orgasm and repeats at 0.8-second intervals. The actual number and intensity of contractions vary from woman to woman. Some women observed to have orgasmic contractions are not aware that they are having an orgasm. Masters and Johnson feel that prolonged stimulation during the excitement phase, during masturbation, or in conjunction with the use of a vibrator may lead to more pronounced orgasmic activity. Whereas the excitement phase is under the influence of the parasympathetic portion of the autonomic nervous system, orgasm seems to be related to the sympathetic portion. Medication such as antihypertensive or antidepressant drugs may affect orgasmic response.

The resolution stage is last and represents a return of the woman's physiologic state to the preexcitement level. Although a refractory period is typical of the sexual response cycle in the male, no such refractory periods have been identified in women. Therefore, new sexual excitement cycles may be stimulated at any time after orgasm. During the resolution phase the woman generally experiences a feeling of personal satisfaction and well-being.

Alternative models of the human sexual response have been proposed that differ from the linear progression of Masters and Johnson's model and also incorporate women's motivations and reasons for engaging in sex. Basson proposes that the phases overlap and may even occur in a different order. Women in established relationships may engage in sex, not because of sexual desire, but because of a desire for intimacy with their partner (Fig. 9-3).

Masters and Johnson identified the clitoris as the center of sexual satisfaction in the female. Recently, several lay publications have suggested that the cervix plays a role in sexual response, basing this theory on the fact that the cervix has a rich nerve

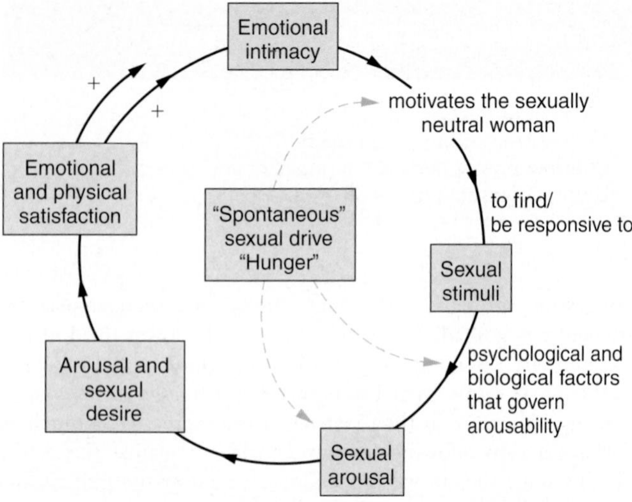

Figure 9-3. Blended intimacy-based and sexual drive–based cycles. (From Basson R: Female sexual response: The role of drugs in the management of sexual dysfunction. Obstet Gynecol 98:350, 2001.)

supply. To date, no scientific data support this theory. Sexual gratification and orgasmic behavior definitely seem to be associated with nerve endings in the clitoris, mons pubis, labia, and possible pressure receptors in the pelvis. In a study by Andersen and coworkers, 42 women ages 31 to 81 (average 50.3) who had been treated for in situ vulvar carcinoma were compared with a group of comparable women ages 30 to 61 (average 44.3) with respect to sexual function. Six of the women had undergone local therapy with laser or chemotherapy, 26 had wide excision of lesions, 9 had undergone simple vulvectomy, and 1 had undergone a radical vulvectomy. Sexual behavior patterns and desires were maintained after therapy, but a specific disruption of the phases of excitement and resolution, and to a lesser extent orgasm, were noted. The incidence of sexual dysfunction was two to three times greater in the patient group, and 30% became sexually inactive. Loss or disruption of the clitoris seemed to be the single most important factor.

Sexual Response and Menopause

Many factors contribute to sexual changes as a woman enters menopause. Aging in general is associated with the slowing of sexual response and decreases in the intensity of response. Specifically, arousal may be slower and orgasms may be less intense and less frequent. Aging may also lead to psychosocial changes affecting self-esteem in relation to desirability. Of course, hormonal changes are a factor.

The postmenopausal woman who is not on hormone replacement therapy (HRT) experiences progressive atrophy of vaginal epithelium, a change in vaginal pH, a decrease in quantity of vaginal secretions, and a decrease in the general circulation to the vagina and uterus. She may also have pelvic relaxation, including cystocele, rectocele, or prolapse of the uterus, and a general loss of vaginal tone. Women on HRT have been shown by Semmens and Semmens not to suffer the problems of vaginal atrophy and poor circulation. It is likely that HRT, therefore, prolongs the postmenopausal woman's ability to demonstrate a more normal sexual response.

A postmenopausal woman may experience other sexual probems relating to her partner, or if she is single, widowed, or divorced, to her lack of availability of male partners. In addition, her general health and the general health of her partner will play a role in her ability to respond sexually in a satisfactory manner. Couples with marital or communication problems may find that the menopause is an appropriate excuse to cease sexual activities. A concerned physician can help a couple sort out their needs and desire for sexual compatibility at this stage of life. Frequently, counseling aimed at dealing with problems of the relationship will alleviate sexual response difficulties.

Male partners of older women may suffer from medical conditions or be affected by medications they must take, with resultant decrease in arousal, difficulties in maintaining an erection, or complete impotence. The physician should ask women about sexual function and if male dysfunction is evident, should make suggestions for appropriate referral to physicians or other health care workers who may deal with the male sexual dysfunction problems. Table 9-5 lists several drugs that can affect sexual function.

Sexual Dysfunction

Sexual dysfunction is quite common. Masters and Johnson estimated that it exists in 50% of marriages. Higher percentages of dysfunction are seen in couples presenting for marital therapy. That sexual dysfunction is not necessarily incompatible with a happy marriage was noted in a study by Frank and associates, who surveyed couples felt to be well adjusted who were selected from general community groups. Of these couples, 83% rated their marriages as happy or very happy, but 63% of the women and 40% of the men gave a history of sexual dysfunction. A total of 48% of the women stated that they had difficulties becoming sexually excited, and 33% found difficulty in maintaining excitement. Of the total group, 46% of the women experienced difficulty in reaching orgasm, and 15% had never had an orgasm. Finally, 35% of the women expressed disinterest in sex. These workers' experience implies that physicians caring for women should make a special effort to uncover sexual dysfunction or poor sexual response in their patients even when the patients demonstrate general marital satisfaction. Obviously, assembling a careful history by asking general and directed questions is appropriate when dealing with a patient in a gynecologic visit. The patient should be asked if she is sexually active, if intercourse is comfortable and enjoyable (if heterosexual), and if orgasm is experienced. If she answers no to any of these questions, more specific questioning should follow with the objective of outlining the extent of the problem and the basis for it.

Sexual response problems may be the result of a previous negative sexual experience or may be secondary to emotional or physical illness. The problem may also be related to difficulties in the current relationship or to alcohol or drug abuse. Although an occasional alcohol drink may decrease inhibitions and improve sexual response, in general, alcohol is a depressant and decreases the woman's ability to become sexually aroused and to become vaginally lubricated. Drugs with antihypertensive and anticholinergic activity, as well as those active at the α- and β-receptor sites, may decrease arousal or inhibit sexual interest. Narcotics, sedatives, and antidepressive drugs such as the SSRI group may also depress sexual responsiveness. Finally, decreased arousal or ability to remain aroused may be due to distractions

Table 9-5 Drugs That May Affect Sexual Function

Drug	Adverse Effect
Acetazolamide (Diamox and others)	Loss of libido; decreased potency
Alprazolam (Xanax)	Inhibition of orgasm; delayed or no ejaculation
Amiloride (Midamor)	Impotance; decreased libido
Amiodarone (Cordarone)	Decreased libido
Amitriptyline (Elavil and others)	Loss of libido; impotence; no ejaculation
Amoxapine (Asendin)	Loss of libido; impotence; retrograde, painful, or no ejaculation
Amphetamines and related anorexic drugs	Chronic abuse; impotence; delayed or no ejaculation in men; no orgasm in women
Anticholinergics	Impotence
Atenolol (Tenormin)	Impotence
Baclofen (Lioresal)	Impotence; inability to ejaculate
Barbiturates	Decreased libido; impotence
Carbamazepine (Tegretol)	Impotence
Chlorpromazine (Thorazine and others)	Decreased libido; impotence, no ejaculation; priapism
Chlorprothixene (Taractan)	Inhibition of ejaculation; decreased intensity of orgasm
Chlorthalidone (Hygroton and others)	Decreased libido; impotence
Cimetidine (Tagamet)	Decreased libido (men and women); impotence
Clofibrate (Atromid-S)	Decreased libido; impotence
Clomipramine (Anafranil)	Decreased libido; impotence; retarded or no ejaculation (men) or orgasm (women); spontaneous orgasm associated with yawning
Clonidine (Catapres and others)	Impotence; delayed or retrograde ejaculation; inhibition of orgasm (women)
Danazol (Danocrine)	Increased or decreased libido
Desipramine (Norpramin and others)	Decreased libido; impotence; difficult ejaculation and painful orgasm
Diazepam (Valium and others)	Decreased libido; delayed ejaculation; retarded or no orgasm in women
Dichlorphenamide (Daranide and others)	Decreased libido; impotence
Digoxin	Decreased libido; impotence
Disopyramide (Norpace and others)	Impotence
Disulfiram (Antabuse and others)	Impotence
Doxepin (Adapin Sinequan)	Decreased libido; ejaculatory dysfunction
Estrogens	Decreased libido in men
Ethionamide (Trecator-SC)	Impotence
Ethosuximide (Zarontin)	Increased libido
Ethoxzolamide (Ethamide)	Decreased libido
Fenfluramine (Pondimin)	Loss of libido (frequent in women with large doses or long-term use); impotence
Fluoxetine (Prozac)	Decreased libido
Fluphenazine (Prolixin, Permitil)	Changes in libido, erection difficulties; inhibition of ejaculation
Guanabenz (Wytensin)	Impotence
Guanadrel (Hylorel)	Decreased libido; delayed or retrograde ejaculation; impotence
Guanadrel (Ismelin)	Decreased libido; impotence; delayed, retrograde, or no ejaculation
Guanfacine (Tenex)	Impotence
Haloperidol (Haldol and others)	Imptence; painful ejaculation
Hydralazine (Apresoline and others)	Impotence; priapism
Hydroxyprogesterone caproate (Delalutin and others)	Impotence
Imipramine (Tofranil and others)	Decreased libido; impotence; painful, delayed ejaculation; delayed orgasm in women
Indapamine (Lozol)	Decreased libido; impotence
Interferon (Roferon-a)	Decreased libido; impotence
Isocarboxazid (Marplan)	Impotence; delayed ejaculation; no orgasm (women)
Ketoconazole (Nizoral)	Impotence
Labetalol (Trandate, Normodyne)	Priapism; impotence; delayed or no ejaculation; decreased libido
Levodopa (Dopar and others)	Increased libido
Lithium (Eskalith and others)	Decreased libido; impotence
Maprotiline (Ludiomil)	Impotence; decreased libido
Mazindol (Sanorex, Mazanor)	Impotence; spontaneous ejaculation; painful testes
Mecamylamine (Inversine)	Impotence; decreased libido
Mepenzolate bromide (Cantil)	Impotence
Mesoridazine (Serentil)	No ejaculation; impotence; priapism
Methadone (Dolophine and others)	Decreased libido; impotence; no orgasm (men and women); retarded ejaculation
Methandrostenolone (Dianabol)	Decreased libido
Methantheline bromide (Banthine)	Impotence
Methazolamide (Neptazane)	Decreased libido (men and women); impotence; delayed or no ejaculation (men) or orgasm (women)
Methyldopa (Aldoment and others)	Decreased libido; impotence; delayed or no ejaculation (men) or orgasm (women)
Metoclopramide (Reglan and others)	Impotence; decreased libido
Metoprolol (Lopressor)	Decreased libido; impotence
Metyrosine (Demser)	Impotence; failure or ejaculation
Mexiletine (Mexitil)	Impotence; decreased libido
Molindone (Moban)	Priapism
Naltrexone (Trexan)	Delayed ejaculation; decreased potency
Naproxen (Anaprox, Naprosyn)	Impotence; no ejaculation
Norethindrone (Norlutin and others)	Decreased libido; impotence
Nortriptyline (Aventyl, Pamelor)	Impotence; decreased libido
Paragyline (Eutonyl)	No ejaculation; impotence
Paroxetine (Paxil)	Decreased libido
Perphenazine (Trilafon)	Decreased or no ejaculation
Phenelzine (Nardil)	Impotence; retarded or no ejaculation; delayed or no orgasm (men and women)
Phenytoin (Dilantin and others)	Decreased libido; impotence
Pimozide (Orap)	Impotence; no ejaculation; decreased libido
Pindolol (Visken)	Impotence
Prazosin (Minipress)	Impotence; priapism
Primidone (Mysoline and others)	Decreased libido; impotence
Progesterone	Decreased libido; impotence
Propantheline bromide (Pro-Banthine and others)	Impotence
Propanolol (Inderal and others)	Loss of libido; impotence
Protripyline (Vivactil)	Loss of libido; impotence; painful ejaculation
Rantidine (Zantac)	Loss of libido; impotence
Reserpine	Decreased libido; impotence; decreased or no ejaculation
Sertraline (Zoloft)	Decreased libido
Spironolactone (Aldactone and others)	Decreased libido; impotence
Thiazide diuretics	Impotence
Thioridazine (Mellaril and others)	Impotence; priapism; delayed, decreased, painful, retrograde, or no ejaculation
Thiothixene (Navane and others)	Spontaneous ejaculations; impotence; priapism
Timolol (Blocadren, Timolide Timoptic)	Decreased libido; impotence
Tranylcypromine (Parnate)	Impotence
Trazodone (Desyrel)	Priapism; increased libido (women); retrograde ejaculation
Trifluoperazine (Stelazine and others)	Decreased, painful, or no ejaculation; spontaneous ejaculation
Verapamil (Calan and others)	Impotence

From Med Lett Drugs Ther 29:65, 1987.

in the woman's life such as concerns for children, job, or other problems that may enter her consciousness during arousal.

Decreased sexual desire is the most common sexual dysfunction and is reported by 10% to 51% of women surveyed. Because each individual has his or her own libidinal drive, it is not surprising that couples may have some incompatibility of needs. It is important, however, that these needs and desires be discussed openly and that reasons for lack of sexual desire that may involve experiences or problems inherent in the relationship be resolved. At times the problem may be merely a failure to set aside appropriate time for intimacy. The couple should be encouraged to give sexual activity a high priority within their relationship rather than leaving it last on the list after the 11 o'clock news. Couples should be encouraged to use arousal and seduction techniques that are appropriate for their relationship. Satisfactory foreplay of a mutually enjoyable nature should be encouraged. Lack of sexual arousal is characterized by a persistent inability to attain adequate lubrication and swelling response of sexual excitement. The prevalence of this disorder is uncertain and often coexists with decreased sexual desire.

Hormonal levels are frequently obtained in evaluating desire disorders. However, there is no evidence that low testosterone levels distinguish women with sexual desire disorder from others. Davis and colleagues reported on 1021 women who had androgen levels drawn from a random recruitment in Australia. Neither total nor free testosterone or dehydroeipandrosterone sulfate (DHEAS) levels discriminated between the women with and those without low sexual function.

There are no approved medications to treat desire or arousal disorders other than estrogen for vaginal atrophy. Estrogen may improve sexual desire if hypoestrogenism is causing an overall lack of well-being from nighttime hot flashes and poor sleep or genital discomfort from atrophy. The risks of estrogen are discussed elsewhere. Androgen therapy is not at present FDA approved in women, but randomized, controlled trials have noted some benefits in postmenopausal women with hypoactive desire disorders and arousal disorders. Long-term safety and efficacy data are not available, nor are data on the use of testosterone in postmenopausal women not taking HRT. Phosphodiesterase inhibitors have not been found to be effective. Bupropion has shown some effectiveness, but further studies are needed. At present, a sound approach to female sexual dysfunction is complex and needs to assess sexual education knowledge, all forms of abuse including emotional abuse, concerns about STDs, pain, and other medical problems and everyday fatigues and stresses.

Vaginismus is a condition that is secondary to involuntary spasm of vaginal introital and levator ani muscles. Because of this spasm penetration is either painful or impossible. Lamont has attempted to classify the degrees of vaginismus, and, in a group of 80 patients, noted that 27 (34%) had first-degree vaginismus, defined as perineal and levator spasm relieved by reassurance during pelvic examination. Another 21 (26%) had second-degree vaginismus, defined as perineal spasm maintained throughout the pelvic examination. Another 18 (22.5%) demonstrated third-degree vaginismus, defined as levator spasm and elevation of the buttocks. A total of 10 (12.5%) had fourth-degree vaginismus, defined as levator and perineal spasm with withdrawal and retreat. Four of the 80 patients refused pelvic examination.

These patients frequently complain not only of pain or fear of pain with coitus or pelvic examination but also of difficulty in inserting a tampon or vaginal medication. The condition may be primary, in which case the individual has never experienced successful coitus. This problem is generally based on either early sexual abuse or aversion to sexuality in general. This leads to a form of conversion hysteria or to a lack of appropriate learning about sex secondary to cultural or familial teaching that sex is evil, painful, or undesirable. Vaginismus may also occur in patients who have been sexually active when an injury or vaginal infection has led to vaginal pain with attempted coitus. This has been seen in rape victims and in women who have had painful episiotomy repairs, severe yeast vaginitis, or vulvar vestibulitis. When the underlying cause for the vaginismus is understood, the matter may be discussed frankly with the patient and her partner to effect a relearning process that is conducive to relieving the symptoms. The actual vaginal spasm then may be relieved by teaching the patient self-dilation techniques, using fingers or dilators, in which she and her partner can participate. The period of therapy is usually short and the results good. There are little data from controlled trials, although one trial compared two desensitization techniques which were both effective.

Orgasmic dysfunction is quite common. As many as 10% to 15% of women have never experienced an orgasm through any form of sexual stimulation, and another 25% to 35% will have difficulty reaching an orgasm on any particular occasion. Many women may be orgasmic secondary to masturbation or oral sex but may not be orgasmic with penile intercourse. It is important to discern by history the extent of the patient's problem and to place it into proper perspective. If the patient is anorgasmic during intercourse but has experienced orgasms, communication with her partner may aid in bringing about an orgasm during intercourse by allowing her or her partner to stimulate her clitoral area with the intensity and timing necessary to bring about an orgasm. If the woman is anorgasmic, she may be taught masturbatory techniques to demonstrate an orgasm to her, and then these techniques may be applied to the coital situation, thereby developing the desired response during coitus. Couples should be encouraged to communicate their sexual needs so that appropriate stimulation is offered during the arousal period and during intercourse. For situation orgasmic disorder, the focus of dialogue should be the relationship. Developing this type of dialogue is often difficult but can be aided by counseling with a sensitive physician.

Dyspareunia is a sexual dysfunction where genital pain occurs before, during, or after intercourse that frequently has an organic basis. The physician should obtain a careful history of when the dyspareunia occurs (i.e., on insertion of the penis, at the midvagina during thrusting, or with deep penetration of the vault), since facts obtained by this history may point to organic causes, such as poor lubrication, a painful bladder disorder, vulvar vestibulodynia, poorly healed vaginal lacerations or episiotomy, and disease such as pelvic inflammatory disease or endometriosis. Table 9-6 lists some causes of dyspareunia. When no organic cause can be found for the dyspareunia, techniques similar to those used in evaluating and managing vaginismus are appropriate. Pelvic floor physical therapy may be beneficial for vaginismus, vulvur vestibulitis, and dyspareunia as well as sex therapy. With all the sexual pain disorders, it is not uncommon to treat the underlying organic cause with success and find

Table 9-6 Causes of Dyspareunia

Vulvodynia
Vulvar vestibulitis
Dysesthetic, generalized
Vaginitis
Yeast or other infectious agents
Desquamative inflammatory vaginitis
Skin conditions
Contact dermatitis (eczematous or contact)
Lichen sclerosis
Lichen planus
Urologic
UTI
Interstitial cystitis
Urethral diverticulum
Episiotomy
Pelvic floor myalgia (hypertonus)
Endometriosis
Leiomyomata
Pelvic inflammatory disease
Adnexal pathology
Postradiation in pelvic

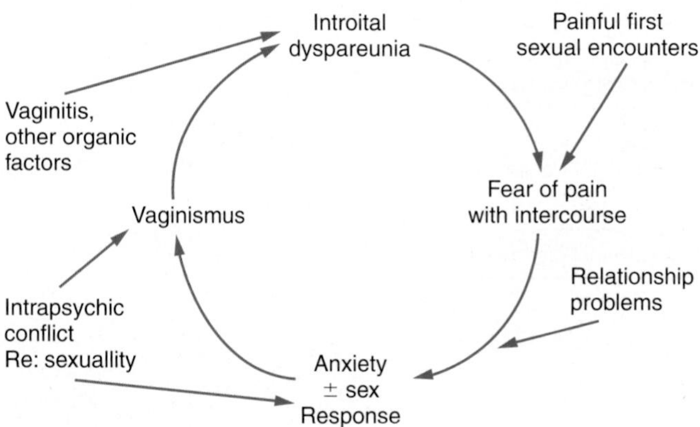

Figure 9-4. Dyspareunia and vaginismus cycle. (From Steege JF: Dyspareunia and vaginismus. Clin Obstet Gynecol 27:750, 1984.)

the pain continues. It is often muscle tension problems from the pain–tension–pain cycle that remain (Fig. 9-4). Specific pathologic conditions should, of course, be treated. At times dyspareunia can be relieved by changing coital position. Couples should be encouraged to experiment with female-dominant and side-by-side positions to see if the pain can be prevented.

An algorithm for thinking about sexual dysfunction is shown in Figure 9-5.

Female Homosexuality and Lesbian Health

Obstetricians and gynecologists are likely to care for lesbians in their practices and should be prepared to understand and have a sensitivity for their medical problems. Controversy exists around whether lesbians face unique health care problems. Certainly, emotional and social well-being are central to "health," and sexual minority women may be at risk both because of our sometimes homophobic society and because they access the health care system less frequently than their heterosexual counterparts. Little usable data are available in the literature concerning this issue, and ascertaining a patient's sexual orientation is not always easy. Bradford and colleagues completed a National Lesbian Health Care Survey with implications on mental health. Detailed questionnaires were distributed in all 50 states through a variety of lesbian organizations. The questionnaire was carefully constructed with a good deal of user input, and 1925 lesbians responded. The authors admitted that their means of ascertaining data was not and could not be a random sample of the total population of lesbians and therefore did not assume that the results of their study could be generalized. Likewise, no comparable control group of heterosexual women was obtainable given the construction of the study. Therefore, it is not possible to know whether the problems that these homosexual women suffered differed from those suffered by a comparable group of heterosexual women. Nevertheless, the survey does give some insight into the problems that these women face.

The authors discovered that 88% of the sample was open about their sexual orientation to other lesbians and gays, but only 27% was open to family members, 28% to heterosexual friends, and 17% to coworkers. Nineteen percent shared their sexual preference with no family members and 29% with no coworkers.

With respect to relationships, 60% of the group was involved in a primary relationship with another woman, 20% were single and uninvolved, and 2% were legally married to men at the time of the survey. With respect to the common concerns held by these women, 57% identified concerns over money, 31% concerns about job or school, 27% concerns about a lover, 23% responsibilities at work, and 21% family problems. Only 12% reported concerns about people knowing that they were homosexual. Many of these women felt unsafe, a third reported having suffered depression and anxiety, with 11% experiencing current depression, and 11% were currently undergoing treatment for depression. Fifty-seven percent stated that they had, at one time or another, entertained thoughts of suicide, and 18% had actually attempted suicide.

Forty-one percent of the patients gave a history of physical abuse at some time during their life, with 37% having been beaten harshly at least once. Twenty-four percent stated they had been physically abused while growing up, 16% had been abused as adults, and 6% as both adults and children.

Forty-one percent reported that they had been raped or sexually abused at least one time in their lives, with 21% reporting such attacks in childhood and 15% in adulthood. Four percent had been raped or sexually attacked both as an adult and in childhood. Nineteen percent had been victims of incest; of these, 34% were victimized by their brothers, 28% by their fathers, 27% by uncles, 18% by cousins, 9% by stepfathers, 8% by grandfathers, 3% by mothers, and 3% by sisters.

Thirty percent of the sample smoked cigarettes daily, and another 11% smoked occasionally. A third of the sample used alcohol regularly, with 6% using alcohol every day and another 25% using it at least once a week. Other surveys have found elevated rates of smoking and more alcohol consumption compared with matched controls of heterosexuals, but not all studies agree.

Forty-seven percent of the sample used marijuana at least occasionally, and 19% had tried cocaine but only 1% used it more than once a week. Eleven percent of the sample used tranquilizers, but only 1% used them daily.

Two thirds of the sample reported overeating, but only 4% indicated that they used vomiting as a means of weight control.

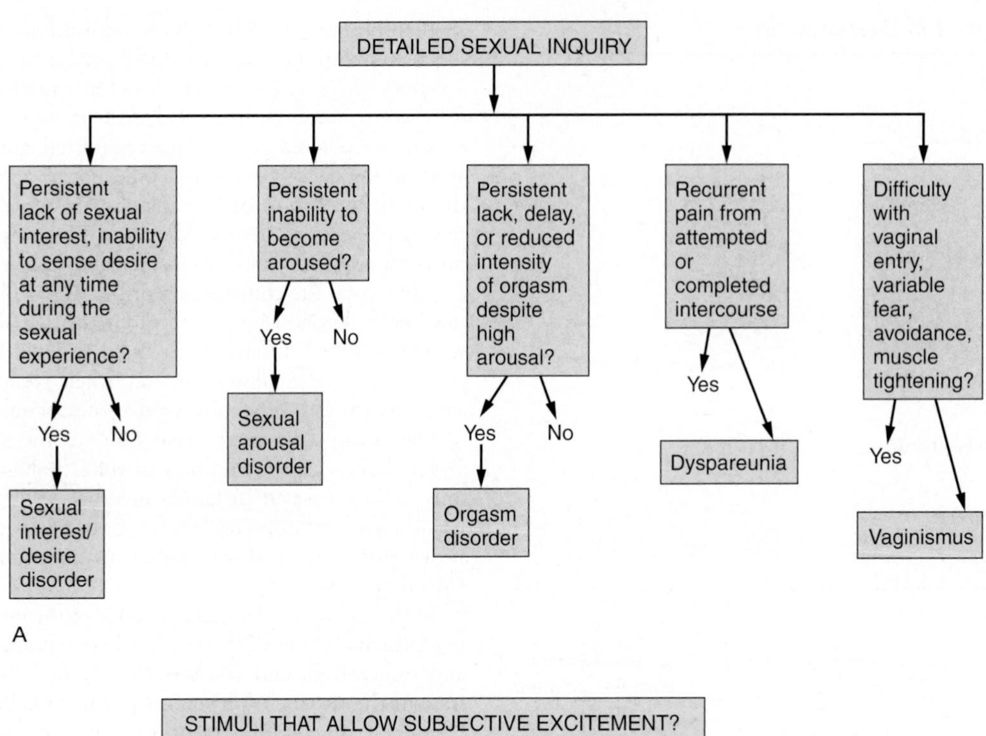

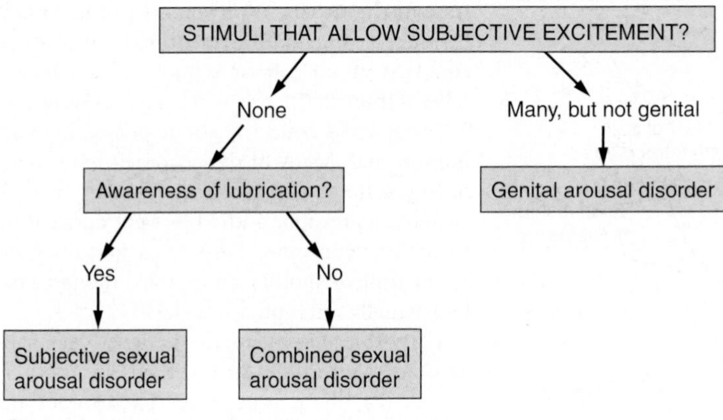

Figure 9-5. Blended sex response cycle showing many motivations to be sexual, spontaneous desire, and responsive desire accessed en route. **A,** Detailed sexual inquiry. **B,** Further assessment of arousal disorder. (From Basson R, Althof D, Davis S: Summary of the recommendations on sexual dysfunctions in women. J Sex Med 1:29, 2004.)

Seventy-three percent of the sample were in counseling or had received some counseling or mental health support from a professional at some time in the past. In general, the counseling was sought because of feeling sad or depressed (50%), feeling anxious or scared (31%), or because of loneliness (21%).

It can be seen that lesbian women have many social and emotional problems; however, whether these are in every case out of proportion with a comparable group of heterosexual women has not been demonstrated. The physician should be sensitive to these problems and attempt to offer appropriate care when such problems are discovered.

Eighty-four percent of lesbians surveyed experience a general reluctance to seek health care. Having staff, a waiting room, and health history forms with inclusive welcoming language may reinforce and support lesbian patients regarding the need for consistent health screening. Myths still exist about lesbians not needing Pap smears or sexually transmitted disease screening. Yet, approximately 80% have had sexual activity with men in the past, and 21% to 30% still may be engaging in intercourse. Provider attitudes likely influence not only the sensitivity of care but also the completeness of care.

Tobacco, Alcohol, and Drug Use

The use of tobacco, alcohol, marijuana, cocaine, and other drugs is quite common in the United States, and the abuse of these substances is not unusual. The prevalence of their use among women is variable and often age-dependent. In 1970 one third of American women of childbearing age were cigarette smokers. From 1990 to 2003, the rate of smoking by pregnant women dropped from 18.4% to 11%, with 18- and 19-year-olds having the highest rate at 18%. In 2005 the U.S. National Center for Health Statistics reported an overall smoking incidence among females of 19.4%, with rates varying by age: 21.5% in women 18 to 24, 24.2% in those in the 35 to 44 age group, and 8.3% in women older than 65 years. The overall rate came down gradually from a high of 34% in 1965 but has been fairly stable since 1990.

Alcohol use among American women is quite high, with 50.7% being current consumers in 1990, and varying by age group: 58.3% in the 18 to 44 year group, 47.6% in the 45 to 64 year group, and 31.3% in women older than 65. From 14% to 22.5% of women report drinking some alcohol while pregnant. The prevalence of alcohol dependence in primary care populations is 2% to 9%.

Sokol found in a study of pregnant women in Cleveland that only 1.2% would state that they had an alcohol problem; however, on careful questioning about alcohol consumption, 11% were noted to be heavy drinkers.

In a detailed history of marijuana use, Nahas reviewed the work of several other authors and noted that in 1970 between 7% and 20% of college students were using marijuana. In addition, he pointed out that 15% of adolescents between the ages of 12 and 17 in one series were found to be using marijuana, with an incidence of 17% among boys and 14% among girls. Recent data imply that the percentages of users are higher. In 1997, 21% of girls ages 12 to 17 were reported to have used marijuana within the past month of being surveyed, and among women ages 18 to 25, the use was 35%. The prevalence of cocaine, heroin, and other drug use is variable from group to group, but overall these uses are quite common.

It is beyond the scope of this book to discuss the health hazards of these various agents, the problems of habituation, or the social and legal considerations. It is appropriate, however, to recognize that each of these agents adversely affects the reproductive process, causes a variety of illness, and influences the health and social relationships of the users.

The obstetrician and gynecologist is in an excellent position to discourage young women from beginning to use these substances by offering educational information at the time of visits for routine checkups or during consultations for contraception. The obstetrician and gynecologist may also influence women contemplating reproduction by pointing out the potential dangers of these substances to the fetus. As the primary physician for some women, the obstetrician and gynecologist has the opportunity to periodically define activities that may be affecting the individual's health and offer education and counseling to modify these activities. Where appropriate, referrals to other health care specialists may be made.

To modify behavior in patients who abuse tobacco, alcohol, and other drugs, the physician must first identify their use. A history at the time of a routine checkup should include the following:

1. *Smoking history.* Does the patient smoke? For how long has she smoked? What substances are smoked and in what quantity? Moderate cigarette smokers (1 to 10 cigarettes per day) may be influenced to stop by simply discussing health hazards and advising that the practice be terminated. If the individual smokes fewer than 10 cigarettes a day, stopping without tapering off is appropriate, and, if motivated, the individual is usually successful. If the individual smokes more than 10 cigarettes a day, habituation may be a problem. Reducing the number of cigarettes to 10 per day may allow cessation to be successful. If not, consultation with health care professionals who may use behavioral modification therapy or medications (nicotine replacement or bupropion) is appropriate. Organized behavior modification programs to aid individuals to quit smoking are available in most communities. Many websites are available with excellent resources both for clinicians and patients. Fiore and colleagues have demonstrated, however, that 90% of successful quitters and 80% of unsuccessful quitters used individual methods similar to those described here. In their series, 47.5% of individuals who had tried to quit on their own in the previous 10 years were successful, whereas only 23.6% of those who used organized cessation methods were successful. These programs, however, were shown by the authors to aid a small group of smokers who were primarily heavy smokers. The evidence to date (2006) does not show skills training or other interventions to prevent relapse after successfully quitting smoking.
2. *Alcohol use.* Routine screening for problems with alcohol is supported by the Institute of Medicine. Many specific screening tools are available, but all get at not only the amount of alcohol consumed, but also the effect of consumption on the patient's life. This includes maladaptive patterns that cause failure to fulfill work, family, and social obligations; legal problems, other substance abuse and alcohol dependence signs like tolerance; withdrawal symptoms; desire to control use; and medical problems. One commonly used screening tool is shown in Table 9-7. To describe a particular patient's drinking habits it is necessary to take a detailed history of how many drinks per day the patient takes and the type of substance consumed (whiskey, beer, or wine). One ounce of whiskey, a wineglass (5 ounces) of wine, and 12 ounces of beer are interchangeable. Binge drinking, which is defined for women as three drinks or more per day or periodic drinking to intoxication, should be noted as should its frequency. If a patient consumes more than seven drinks per week or is a binge drinker, the physician should attempt to obtain behavior modification help for the patient. Generally, attendance at an Alcoholics Anonymous program with or without other specialized health care is indicated. If the patient does not consume large amounts of alcohol but does drink regularly, educational literature and counseling should be provided. A 2004 review by Whitlock and coworkers for the U.S. Preventive Services Task Force looked at 12 controlled trials regarding behavioral counseling interventions to reduce harmful alcohol use. Primary care providers who provided good-quality, brief, multicontact behavioral counseling reduced participants average number of drinks per week by 13% to 34% more than controls when assessed 6 to 12 months later.

Table 9-7 CAGE Questionnaire for Alcohol Screening*

C	Have you ever felt you should *"cut down"* on your drinking?
A	Have people *"annoyed"* you by criticizing your drinking?
G	Have you ever felt bad or *"guilty"* about your drinking?
E	*"Eye Opener"*: Have you ever had a drink first thing in the morning to steady your nerves or to get rid of a hangover?

*Two positive responses are considered a positive test.

3. *Marijuana use.* Marijuana is an illegal substance and has many biologic side effects. Its use should be discouraged among all patients. If marijuana is used daily, the patient's habituation must be recognized and behavior modification therapy offered. Signs of chronic marijuana use include a decrease in activities and impairment in relationships and cognitive skills. There is evidence that marijuana may increase the risk of schizophrenia and depression, although it is unclear if it triggers psychiatric illness in vulnerable people or actually causes it in nonpredisposed people.
4. *Other drug use.* Patients are frequently habituated to illegal drugs, such as cocaine and heroin, and often to prescription drugs as well (i.e., narcotics, tranquilizers, barbiturates, and amphetamines). The physician should identify the quantity and type of drug used by history and should make the appropriate referral to a health care agency. Cocaine is a major problem in the United States at present. It is addicting and gives users a sense of power and strength that they find rewarding. Because of this and the fact that users can often function reasonably well under its influence, stopping its use can be very difficult. Cocaine use and possible addiction should be inquired about by the physician in all patients and treatment vigorously suggested when its use is discovered. For instance, individuals habituated to cocaine are often treated in a fashion similar to alcoholics, using such help groups as Cocaine Anonymous. Similar advice is appropriate for methamphetamine abuse. Methamphetamine has a high potential for addiction as well as being associated with sexual risk behavior. Other amphetamine analogs are abused and are touted as sexual stimulants, such as methylenedioxymethamphetamine (MDMA, Ecstasy), methylenedioxyamphetamine (MDA, the love pill), and methylenedioxyethamphetamine (MDEA, Eve).

Of course, prevention of drug use by young people should be a primary goal. A 2006 Cochrane Database study reviewed interventions for prevention of drug abuse by people younger than age 25. The studies were too diverse to draw firm conclusions, but motivational interviews and some family interventions may have some benefit, particularly on cannabis use.

Depression

Depression is a common symptom in a variety of conditions. Patients suffering loss or grief are often depressed. Major depression in women is now estimated to be the second most frequent cause of disability in the United States. A 2005 survey of over 43,000 adults found the 12-month prevalence of major depression to be 5.3%. Female gender is a major risk factor. The lifetime risk of major depression in women is 20% to 26% compared with 8% to 12% for men, with a peak onset of depressive disorders during a woman's reproductive years (25 to 44 years of age). For women, this risk appears regardless of race or ethnicity. Research in the last 10 years has also found depression in people 65 years and older to be a major public health problem. Depression associated with psychoses such as is seen in manic–depressive (bipolar) psychosis may occur as often as 3 to 4 per 1000 people. Dorpat and Ripley noted that 9.3% of patients suffering from personality disorders, 26.9% of patients suffering from alcoholism, and 12.0% of schizophrenics had depression as a major symptom. Unfortunately, patients who suffer from depression are more prone to suicide, and psychiatric patients who commit suicide are more likely to have a depressive component to their illness.

Depression in infants and young children is frequently the result of deprivation, particularly maternal deprivation, and childhood physical or sexual trauma. It is frequently characterized by crying and behavior disorders and later by despair and withdrawal. The child may fail to eat and may eventually starve to death. If the child does not die, strong depressive symptomatology may continue into adulthood. In a 2007 prospective cohort study of 1575 subjects, Widom and colleagues reported a significantly increased risk for major depressive disorder in young adults who were subjected to child abuse and neglect.

It is useful for a gynecologist to understand how depression may present in patients. It is more than feeling sad for a short time. Depression disrupts daily life nearly all day, every day for at least 2 weeks. Early symptoms include chronic fatigue, anxiety and irritability, anhedonia (loss of feelings of joy and pleasure), decreased interest in usual pursuits including sexual activity and personal appearance, and mental changes, including poor concentration and lack of decisiveness. The individual may complain of loss of recent memory; insomnia, especially occurring shortly after falling asleep; a pessimistic outlook about the future, often associated with feelings of guilt; and a number of physical complaints including loss of appetite or a great increase in appetite; change in bowel habits, including constipation or diarrhea; headache; various aches and pains; and lack of energy. Some evidence exists that the elderly may have subsyndromal depression that doesn't meet the DSM-IV criteria for major depression. Clearly, evaluation and treatment may be warranted.

Late in the disease the patient may experience deep feelings of hopelessness, with difficulty in presenting ideas. The patient may also complain of generalized weakness, fear of impending doom from a serious illness or fear that serious problems will befall a close family member, suicidal thoughts, and, occasionally, delusions.

The physician should be alert to patients who have suffered personal loss or grief but who are still deeply depressed after 6 to 18 months of grieving. Although depression is normal in a grief situation, it should not last for a prolonged period.

The diagnosis is often suspected by simply assessing the patient's appearance and asking the usual questions concerning the patient's mood and health. Several psychological tests have been developed to assess depression and can be used in subtle cases or in the elderly. The physician should assess the degree to which the patient is depressed and whether the reason for the depression is appropriate. If the patient is grieving because of a real-life situation, the physician should demonstrate concern and offer appropriate assurance that the problem will be relieved with time.

If the degree of depression is inappropriate for the life situation, the physician should determine whether the individual has suicidal thoughts and assess whether these thoughts are likely to be put into practice. Such questions as, "Have you considered harming yourself or taking your own life?" are appropriate in this situation. If the patient states that she has had such thoughts, the degree to which she is contemplating them may be assessed

Table 9-8 Antidepressants

Functional Group	Generic name
Selective Serotonin Reuptake Inhibitors (SSRIs)	fluoxetine sertraline paroxetine citalopram escitalopram
Heterocyclic and tricyclic (TCAs)	imipramine nortriptyline amitriptyline desipramine doxepin
Monoamine Oxidase Inhibitors (MAOIs)	tranylcypromine phenelzine
Other	bupropion venlafaxine duloxetine trazadone nefazodone mirtazapine

by asking if she has considered how she would carry out the suicide or what circumstances deterred her from attempting this act. If the patient seems to be seriously considering suicide, immediate referral to a mental health worker or hospital should be made.

Patients who are depressed but give no evidence for psychosis may be helped by psychological treatment and medication. Currently, the most effective agents for this purpose are the selective SSRIs and their newer variants. Table 9-8 lists the currently available medications by functional group and by generic name. The SSRIs are effective in alleviating symptoms of depression but may have among their side effects appetite suppression, sleep disorders, and sexual dysfunction. A rare, but potentially lethal, side effect is called the serotonin syndrome. This includes change in mental status, autonomic hyperactivity, and neuromuscular problems. Patients at highest risk for serotonin syndrome often are taking additional medications like monoamine oxidase inhibitors (MAOIs) or others. A number of other newer antidepressants work on more specific neurotransmitters or receptors or work in combination as both serotonin and norepinephrine reuptake inhibitors. These newer drugs appear to have similar efficacy to the SSRIs, but less sexual dysfunction and slightly different side effect profiles.

Each of these agents causes slightly different undesirable side effects, and a specific patient's symptoms may be alleviated by switching to a different medication. Although patients may note a reduction in symptoms of depression after 1 to 2 weeks of drug use, real improvement may take as long as 1 month, and the physician may wish to continue the use of these agents for 6 months to 1 year. Many patients can use antidepressant drugs intermittently when symptomatology warrants. The dosage will need to be varied depending on the patient's response. Psychological counseling combined with antidepressant medication is associated with a higher improvement rate than drug therapy alone. Furthermore, if longer treatment is needed, the addition of psychotherapy enhances compliance with treatment. Often drug therapy is necessary to bring the patient's depression under control to an extent that allows psychotherapy or counseling to be useful. Psychotherapy alone helps about 50% of people with mild to moderate depression.

Lithium salts have been used to treat depression and are most useful in the treatment of bipolar disorder (manic–depressive psychosis). The heterocyclic and tricyclic antidepressants (TCAs) are now rarely the first choice for depression treatment because of significant anticholinergic side effects as well as sedation, weight gain, orthostatic effects, and possible cardiac arrhythmias. Concerning complementary and alternative medicines (CAMs), St. John's wort has been studied for depression. At least six randomized controlled trials have been performed plus a meta-analysis and Cochrane review showing the interest in CAMs and pointing out that better treatments are needed for depression. St. John's wort shows marked benefit for mild depression. Minimal benefits for major depression are noted in several trials, but the evidence is conflicting and some studies find benefits similar to standard antidepressants. Given the lack of quality control over supplements in the United States, quality and consistency of dosage is a concern. Also, drug interactions are an issue because St. John's wort induces the cytochrome-3A enzymes. MAOIs are also in common clinical use, but frequently have serious side effects and should be administered only by individuals well experienced in their use. MAOIs are not considered first-line treatment.

Loss and Grief

Loss is a common human experience and may affect women of all ages. The loss of a child, a spouse, or a close relative should and probably will precipitate an acute grief reaction. However, the physician must remember that a similar reaction will be precipitated by a spontaneous abortion, by the loss of a body part or organ, or by the realization that infertility and childlessness face the couple. It may also occur in women undergoing separation or divorce, losing a job, or losing a pet.

Lindemann points out that acute grief is a definite syndrome with both psychological and somatic components. In his vast experience with grieving patients he has observed that the syndrome may appear immediately after the loss or be delayed. If it is delayed, grief may appear to be absent only to occur at a future time, often in a more exaggerated fashion. At times the syndrome may occur in a distorted fashion. For successful resolution of grief, the individual must be helped to transform these distorted reactions into normal grief.

Lindemann points out that the symptomatology of normal grief is quite uniform. The individual often complains of tightness in the throat and chest, a choking sensation, a feeling of shortness of breath, and frequent sighing. An empty feeling in the abdomen, muscle weakness, and a feeling of tension and mental pain are often reported. These symptoms frequently come in waves lasting from minutes to an hour and are often dreaded by the sufferer.

Lindemann further points out that the bereaved experience disorders of the sensorium often involving a sense of unreality, a tendency to place emotional distance between themselves and other people, and a preoccupation with imagery of the deceased. At times the bereaved will assume the mannerisms of the deceased or even attempt to perform the work of the lost loved one. If the mother has died, the bereaved daughter may see the mother's face when she looks at herself in the mirror and may assume the mother's mannerisms in her speech and gestures.

There is often the perception that the deceased is nearby and can communicate.

In the immediate grief period the bereaved often feels guilt. This may directly involve the events of the death or of tasks left unfinished before the individual died. The bereaved often feels a lack of warmth and may demonstrate feelings of hostility toward others.

The burden of the grief is often so great that the individual can barely handle the maintenance activities of living, and has little energy left over for social contact or growth and development.

Most authorities feel that a normal grief reaction takes 6 to 18 months and ends when the individual has appropriately experienced the pain and suffering, placed the memory of the deceased in a proper place within the bereaved's life, and established new relationships and new life directions. In older women, however, the grieving period may be prolonged because of the limited number of diversions and opportunities available to them.

Lindemann notes, however, that abnormal grief reactions are possible and divides these into several categories. The first is the delay of reaction, which essentially is a postponement of grieving. This may be seen in an individual who is injured in an accident that kills the person to be grieved. The individual may be preoccupied with personal survival and recuperation and may not have the opportunity to grieve until this has passed. In other instances the individual may delay grieving for a long period, often years. There are often psychological reasons why this occurs, but when the grieving is finally precipitated, it may appear quite pathologic and out of context for current life situations.

A second variant is a distorted reaction. In this situation the bereaved may take on the characteristics of the deceased without evidencing a sense of loss. The bereaved may actually take on the symptoms of the lost person if that individual had experienced a prolonged illness before death.

A third abnormal reaction to grieving may be the development of a psychosomatic condition. Ulcerative colitis, rheumatoid arthritis, and asthma have all been noted to occur in approximation to bereavement. Lindemann points out that some patients suffering from these problems may improve when the grief reaction is resolved.

Other types of abnormal grief reactions include pathologic alterations in relationships with friends and relatives, inappropriate hostility toward others, behavior patterns resembling psychoses, continuing inability to make decisions or to take initiative, and performance of activities that have destructive social and economic outcomes. Finally, Lindemann notes that in the reaction of agitated depression the bereaved develops tension, agitation, insomnia, feelings of worthlessness, and fantasies of a need for punishment. In such situations suicide may be a danger. Fortunately, agitated depression is quite unusual. Lindemann feels that it may be more common in individuals who have experienced a previous depression or in those who have been intensely involved with the deceased, such as mothers who have lost young children.

Loss of a Child by Abortion, Stillbirth, or Neonatal or Infant Death

Obstetricians and gynecologists may need to counsel patients experiencing grief related to several areas of reproduction. Leppert and Pahlka counseled 22 women who had experienced spontaneous abortion. The study format was to hold a counseling session immediately after abortion and again in 4 to 6 weeks. These authors report that all women demonstrated the classic stages of grief, but that guilt was the stage that appeared the most difficult for them and their spouses to resolve. The authors thought that the unexpressed emotions relating to pregnancy loss might affect the relationship of the couple unless they are explored and defused. They suggested that the obstetrician and gynecologist make it a point to add such counseling to his or her practice routines. Bruhn and Bruhn point out that a predictable pattern of grief follows every stillbirth and perinatal death and urge physicians to work with their patients in resolving these feelings.

In addition to the physician's offering understanding and counseling, many self-help groups offer aid to parents who have lost children either in the perinatal period or in infancy. The physician should become aware of the agencies or groups that offer such help and learn the techniques used by them and to assess whether their approach fits the needs of the patient before making referrals.

The physician should also be aware of the fact that each member of the couple may grieve differently and, indeed, the style of grieving that one may exhibit may be in conflict with that of the other. Pointing out these differences and helping the couple to express their true feelings to each other may be very beneficial during this process.

An important issue in understanding the management of grief in couples who have lost infants was demonstrated in an evaluation of a group of patients by Estok and Lehman. They found that such individuals wished health care providers to acknowledge the couple's feelings of shock, guilt, and grief and to recognize the importance of their memories of the birth and of the baby. In essence, they wished the health care providers to help them sharpen the reality of the death of the child and provide support through the period after the loss rather than focus on other life events, such as the next pregnancy.

Certain aspects of bereavement should be understood by the physician in dealing with patients who are suffering grief. The loss of a child is always a serious problem. Even the loss of an adult child can have long-term sequelae. Shanfield and Swain noted that parents who have lost adult children in traffic accidents continued to grieve intensely for a prolonged period and had a higher than expected level of psychiatric symptoms and health complaints. Families that were unstable and in which problems had existed with these children suffered more guilt and more psychiatric symptoms. In addition, factors that intensified the bereavement experience were a mother losing a daughter, parents losing children who lived at home, the loss of children born early in the birth order, and the loss of multiple children in a single-car, single-driver accident. A protecting factor seemed to be a prior bereavement experience.

These observations were supported by Lundin, who used the Texas Inventory of Grief to study first-degree relatives 8 years after bereavement. He noted that relatives of persons who had died suddenly or unexpectedly suffered a more pronounced grief reaction than those who had lost someone in a death that was expected. He also noted that bereavement was greater in parents after the loss of a child than in widows or widowers who lost a spouse. The current AIDS epidemic is increasing the incidence of grief from loss of an adult child in older women.

Unplanned Pregnancy

A special counseling challenge involves the care of a woman with an unplanned pregnancy. Such individuals often suffer conflicting feelings, which may include shame and guilt for their predicament, a genuine desire to have a child, fear of social consequences, and fear for their own future and physical well-being. In addition, they may suffer from guilt about the termination of the pregnancy if abortion is considered. Although many such women have good support groups (e.g., family, significant other, friends, and religious counselors), others will rely on the physician for advice and direction. The physician should discuss all possible options with the patient, including having and raising the child, offering it for adoption, or terminating the pregnancy. Issues involving the role of the baby's father, the effect of any decision on the future life of the patient, and the risks of the procedure should be considered. The patient should be aided in reaching the most appropriate decision for her needs and then should be supported in carrying out her plan. When necessary, appropriate referrals to social agencies (e.g., adoption, abortion counseling, or welfare services) should be made.

Infertility

The inability to reproduce leads to a major life frustration and often generates a series of symptoms similar to the grief reaction. Many sequelae may occur that stress the couple's relationship. Guilt, anger, and shame may be components, depending on the social forces at play in the relationship. Sexual dysfunction may result because of the stresses imposed by the requirements of a treatment regimen or because of general dysfunction within the relationship brought about by the infertility. At times the problems associated with the infertility (e.g., endometrial implants in the cul-de-sac) may cause dyspareunia and lead to sexual dysfunction. External stresses from family and friends who continuously refer to the couple's childlessness may contribute to the tension as well.

The physician must provide the couple a complete medical evaluation, as well as being supportive of their emotional needs. The physician should discuss fully all treatment options and the chances for success. He or she should also continuously help the couple to accentuate the positives of their relationship and to consider referring them to self-help groups for infertile couples or to health care counselors who can help with the maintenance of their relationship and self-images.

Death of a Spouse

Holmes and Rahe rate the death of a spouse as one of the major life stresses among survivors, independent of age and cultural background, and state that it may contribute to a decline in physical and mental well-being of the survivor. Recent bereavement studies have confirmed that mortality rates increase in surviving spouses. Gallagher and colleagues reported the effects of acute bereavement on the indicators of mental health in widows and widowers beyond the age of 55. These workers evaluated a group from the standpoint of past grief, present grief, depression, somatic symptomatology, and self-rating of mental health status. They noted that these individuals in the early stages of their bereavement were suffering from considerable psychological distress compared with individuals of similar age who were not bereaved. They demonstrated that the degree of effect of bereavement on the patient's mental health did not vary by sex. Those conditions that were more likely to occur in one sex rather than the other occurred with incidence equal to those individuals of the same sex in the study group. Women, who tend to have a higher incidence of depression in the general population than men, demonstrated this to be the case in the same proportions among the study group.

Cross-cultural differences. Eisenbruch has pointed out that there are significant cross-cultural differences in bereavement, whereas there are great similarities in the individual grief reaction among different ethnic and cultural groups. There are differences, in general, regarding bereavement in different cultural groups, but the actual grief reaction for an individual is similar across cultural lines. Individuals from different backgrounds tend to experience difficulty with their grief when they attempt to respond in a fashion specific for the majority within the culture in which they now reside. Specific rituals, attitudes toward widowhood, mores with respect to length and type of grieving, the way in which the deceased is remembered, and the appropriate length of time for grieving and mourning may be quite different among various ethnic groups. Physicians dealing with different ethnic groups are urged to consider the points raised by Eisenbruch so as to be better able to help patients through their grieving period.

Separation and Divorce

In 2005, the number of divorces occurring annually in the United States was about 48% of the number of marriages. There are many reasons for this increase, including the emerging of women to a level of self-support, changing attitudes toward a desire to remain married, and an increased public awareness of family dysfunction, such as spouse and child abuse. Often one or both members of a divorcing couple will demonstrate evidence of grief, as well as anger, shame, and guilt. Counseling can be very useful in restoration of self-esteem and in helping the individual to emerge from the experience with the ability to survive in new relationships. Although physicians should recognize these needs in their patients who are going through separation and divorce, their primary role should be to make appropriate referrals to counselors who have the time and the skills to deal with the patient in this area.

Loss of an Organ or Body Part

Loss of a body part can be expected to bring about a grief reaction with accompanying symptoms of an emotional and somatic nature. Depression is frequently a strong component. Workers who have investigated the loss of limbs have noted this, and it is reasonable to expect that the loss of such organs as the breast or the uterus would evoke a similar reaction.

Several investigators have reported depression among posthysterectomy patients, with an incidence ranging from 4% to as high as 70%. In a review, Drummond and Field point out that the stages of the process of incorporating the loss of a uterus into the individual's self-image is similar to that of the loss of other body parts. They refer to the four stages of incorporation listed by Roberts: impact, retreat, acknowledgment, and reconstruction.

The impact stage occurs when the individual becomes aware that she has a problem with her uterus. If she is symptomatic this may be obvious. If she has been told she must lose her uterus because it is diseased, such as with cancer, she will need to make a mental adjustment to this fact. Steiner and Aleksandrowicz have pointed out that when the disease that requires operation is life-threatening or serious, the likelihood of depression is minimized. Richards has pointed out that when disease of the uterus is absent, depression is more likely to occur.

The second stage of organ loss is retreat. This is the period in which the patient accepts the need for the loss of an organ and depersonalizes it in her thinking. If denial occurs at this period, the depression that she notes later may be quite severe. The desire for a second opinion often occurs in this phase. It is a healthy response and should be encouraged.

The third stage is acknowledgment. The physician will recognize this stage because it involves the woman's repeated discussion of the procedure, the need for the procedure, and the meaning of the loss of the uterus postoperatively. It is the woman's attempt to place the procedure and the need for the procedure within the appropriate context of her life and her self-image.

The final phase is reconstruction. This involves the redefinition of her self-image without the organ. It will require acceptance by her spouse or significant other and by other members of her community of importance in this event. The physician should attempt to discuss the need for and the likely sequelae of the hysterectomy before it is performed. This discussion should include the significant other in the woman's life so that any fantasies or fears that may arise can be discussed at this point. Some men have difficulty continuing an active sexual experience with a woman who has lost her uterus. These points should be discussed ahead of time so that each realizes the implication of the operation. Conversely, some women feel that sex is for procreation only and after the removal of the uterus may respond quite differently from what the significant other has known in the past. These points, too, should be discussed before the fact.

If the individual cannot work through the four stages of loss of an organ, disruption of relationships and depression may be sequelae. In 1976, Newton and Baron noted that between 20% and 40% of couples stop having sexual intercourse after hysterectomy. They do not state whether this is a direct effect of the hysterectomy and the inability to work out feelings related to this procedure or whether other problems may have existed, allowing for the hysterectomy to be an excuse to stop experiencing intercourse. Although this is an old study, physicians should consider these points, and discuss them with the patient and her partner before embarking on an operative procedure, particularly if it is elective and the time is available for discussion.

Loss of a Pet

A final bereavement situation often overlooked by physicians but frequently important to patients is the grief associated with the death of a pet. Quackenbush reviewed the subject and concluded that animals play an important role in the human social system and may contribute greatly to the quality of life of many pet owners. In some cases where the individual lives alone and may be elderly, the animal may be the only living thing in close daily contact with the individual. It is, therefore, not unusual that when the pet dies, the owner suffers grief. Quackenbush states that understanding and sensitivity to the feelings and sense of loss that the pet owner experiences will help to facilitate the resolution of the grief.

Counseling the Dying

Dr. Elisabeth Kübler-Ross revolutionized our understanding of the death process with her classic 1969 book on the subject, *On Death and Dying*. An important paragraph taken from the first chapter describing the fear of death is quite revealing:

> When we look back in time and study old cultures and people, we are impressed that death has always been distasteful to man and will probably always be. From the psychiatrist's point of view this is very understandable and can perhaps best be explained by our basic knowledge that, in our unconscious, death is never possible in regard to ourselves. It is inconceivable for our unconscious to imagine an actual ending of our own life here on earth and if the life of ours has to end the ending is always attributed to a malicious intervention from the outside by someone else. In simple terms, in our unconscious mind we can only be killed; it is inconceivable to die of a natural cause or of old age. Therefore, death in itself is associated with a bad act, a frightening happening, something that in itself calls for retribution and punishment.

Kübler-Ross describes five stages through which an individual progresses in the acceptance of the inevitability of death: denial, anger, bargaining, depression, and acceptance. *Denial* and isolation is a temporary state brought about by the shock of learning that the individual suffers from a problem from which he or she cannot recover. The transition from denial to partial acceptance will depend on the nature of the patient's illness, how long he or she has left before death will occur, and the way in which he or she has prepared throughout life to cope with such serious situations. Kübler-Ross notes that when confronted with multiple health care providers who are likely to express the inevitable in a variety of ways, the dying person often chooses to accept the individual style of presentation that most fits her needs. During this period of adjustment, therefore, a number of different opinions may be sought and specific interpretations questioned. Inevitably, the individual may be depressed and may isolate herself from those with whom she would normally associate. Frequently, the individual may appear confused and in some cases may deny that any information about the impending death has ever been given. Most patients, according to Kübler-Ross, will go through this period long before death occurs. However, in 3 of 200 patients that she studied, acceptance of the inevitable did not occur until the very time of death.

Hospital personnel must guard against avoiding patients after having given the initial information. They must not interpret the period of the patient's denial as a distasteful circumstance with which they cannot cope. Instead they should help the patient work through this period by patiently repeating information, answering questions, and offering comfort. Terms that remove all hope, such as *terminal* or *hopeless,* should be avoided.

The second stage described by Kübler-Ross is *anger.* Staff and family members find this the most difficult one with which to cope, since the anger felt by the patient may be inappropriately displaced to everyone and everything in the environment. The physician or nurse caring for the patient falls into the unenviable position of the messenger who is hated because of the bad news he or she has brought. The health care worker who tries to make the patient comfortable may be accused of being overly solicitous, whereas the health care worker who attempts to give the patient the privacy that it is believed she seeks may be accused of being uncaring. Likewise, family members who attempt to be cheerful in visiting the patient may be accused of being glib and uncaring, whereas if they are more somber, they may be accused of being depressing. In such cases the health care worker or family member will probably experience guilt and possibly shame, and may adjust to the problem by avoiding the dying person altogether.

During the anger period the dying individual will be irritated by all stimuli. Happiness depicted on television may upset her because she feels that she is not included in it. Discussion of future plans of friends or family members will be equally depressing because the dying individual realizes that she will not be around to participate. The anger period ends when the individual can reconcile the fact that she is different from every healthy person but is still capable of being loved and accepted.

The third stage is *bargaining.* This is an attempt to postpone the inevitable by offering concessions, presumably to God. It is essentially the hope of getting more time for good behavior. In this period the individual may do charitable acts, correct past misdeeds, or reconcile damaged relationships. It is a time for relieving guilt and defusing the feeling of required punishment. It may, in many ways, be an opportunity to "put one's house in order."

The fourth stage is *depression.* Although symptoms of depression may occur in the earlier stages, depression at this stage may occur because the patient has had to cope with a number of factors associated with the illness. For instance, she may be concerned about the expenses of her care, loss of wages, and the simple fact that she feels poorly, added to the fact that she now realizes she is going to die. In addition, fears that her death will adversely affect other members of her family who depend on her may also add to her depression. Health care workers should be comfortable in allowing the patient to know that they understand the reasons for the depression. They should do everything possible to eliminate the feelings of guilt that the patient may have because of the conditions in which she finds herself. She should be made to realize that the financial burdens that may be developing or the effect that her death may have on family members and their lives are not a result of specific actions that she may have taken. In other words, she is not responsible for the condition she is in and the resulting circumstances are not legitimate reasons for her to feel guilt. Family members can be helpful by accentuating the positive aspects of the patient's life, the love they feel for her, and the happiness they have experienced with her. They should downplay the burdens that the patient's illness and death will create for them. Essentially, the patient is working through a period of grief, in this case, grief for herself.

The fifth and final stage is *acceptance.* At this point the individual has worked through the anger that she has felt for her misfortune and for those healthy individuals who do not have to die at this time and has also passed the period of depression and into a period of accepting her fate. This step will most often be achieved if there is a long enough period for the individual to work through the previous stages. Unfortunately, many die before all of these stages have been reconciled. In a very ill patient acceptance is frequently a giving in to the symptoms she has had to bear and a looking forward to relief from these symptoms that death will bring. However, Kübler-Ross points out that the acceptance stage is not necessarily this alone, because patients who are not physically suffering also will go through this stage. This is often a time when the individual takes comfort in having quality visits with family members in which positive experiences are remembered. She may also obtain comfort from interacting with representatives of her religious faith. Patients do not always follow the classic order of the stages outlined above. Many patients exhibit two or three stages simultaneously and in different order. Some patients may regress when they had reached acceptance; this may be because the family hangs on and/or unnecessary life-prolonging procedures are utilized.

A new innovation in the care of the terminally ill and their families was introduced with the hospice concept during the 1970s. There are currently many hospice organizations in the United States, offering psychosocial support to both patients and families. The service includes postdeath follow-up with the families to help them through the grieving period. Hospice organizations include free-standing institutions that offer inpatient services; community-based home programs that include both professional and volunteer services; hospital-based hospice teams, which may include physicians, nurses, social workers, chaplains, and volunteers who are in a position to minister to any patient in any bed; and hospital-based hospice units that are geographically separate from other patients and often are coordinated with a home care program.

Godkin and coworkers studied 58 bereaved spouses and their families whose loved ones had recently died of late-stage cancer after care in a hospital-based hospice service. These families in general rated hospice care significantly better than that received in prior experiences, stating that the hospice services contributed to an improved family function, greater individual well-being, and the ability of family members to cope with the situation. Over three quarters of the families reported that they were emotionally prepared and prepared in a practical sense for the death of the victim. Health problems were reported by these family members in about the same proportion as was experienced in other bereaved groups, but when these problems occurred they were dealt with within the framework of the program.

Physicians who care for chronically ill and terminal patients, particularly those suffering from cancer, should consider availing themselves of the services of such organizations within their geographic area. Hospice care developed outside the acute medical care system. The rapidly expanding field of palliative medicine incorporates hospice approaches but expands the care to patients with advanced diseases who are not immediately terminal. Interdisciplinary teams involving more traditional medical care systems guide management and decision making in advanced disease situations.

KEY POINTS

- The risk of developing a psychiatric disorder seems greatest if a child loses a parent before age 5 or in adolescence.
- The risk of developing a psychiatric disorder is greatest if a child loses a parent of the same sex.
- The highest rate of delinquency seems to occur in males who have lost their fathers unless father substitution occurs.
- Separation from parents in childhood is more likely to cause psychiatric illness when the separation is necessitated by parental illness or marital discord than when it is necessitated by the child's illness or because of wartime evacuation.
- The ideal of thinness for the American woman has increased at the same time that her actual weight has increased.
- More than half of the women between ages 24 and 54 are dieting even though they are not overweight; 75% state they do it for cosmetic reasons.
- Anorexia nervosa occurs in 1% of adolescent girls.
- Anorexia nervosa occurs in 5% to 20% of ballet dancers.
- When anorexia nervosa occurs in men, it is usually in those individuals training for competitive athletic events.
- Bulimia occurs in about 50% of anorectic patients.
- Vomiting after meals is three times as common in bulimics as it is in patients with anorexia nervosa without bulimia.
- Anorexia nervosa and bulimia occur six times more frequently in first-degree relatives than in the general population.
- Good to fair outcomes were observed in 88% of anorexia nervosa patients treated as inpatients, 77% of those treated as outpatients, and 59% of those not treated at all.
- Medications have not been useful in treating anorexia nervosa; counseling and behavior modification programs seem to be more effective.
- Long-term follow-ups of patients with anorexia nervosa calculate the hazard of death as 0.5% per year and of relapse as 3% per year. Treatment reduces these.
- Sixty-five percent of U.S. adults are either overweight or obese.
- Of patients with severe obesity who are treated with nonsurgical management, 15% suffer severe depression and 26% suffer moderate depression.
- Behavior modification without medication is the most successful therapy for moderate obesity.
- Obesity in adolescence responds best when parents and children are given behavior modification therapy in separate counseling groups.
- Half of all married couples experience some sexual dysfunction or dissatisfaction.
- The traditional sexual response cycle includes excitement, plateau, orgasm, and resolution.
- Sexual arousal is under the control of the parasympathetic portion of the autonomic nervous system.
- Orgasm is under the control of the sympathetic portion of the autonomic nervous system.
- A total of 15% of healthy women have never experienced orgasm.
- A total of 35% of healthy women in a large survey expressed disinterest in sex.
- Inhibited or hypoactive sexual desire is the most common sexual dysfunction.
- Roughly 7% to 20% of college students use marijuana.
- Smoking more than 10 cigarettes per day is evidence for habituation.
- Most smokers who successfully quit do so without behavior modification programs, but such programs seem to benefit heavy smokers.
- High-volume alcohol use for women is defined as seven alcoholic drinks per week or three drinks or more on specific occasions.
- A total of 10% of all individuals suffer depression.
- Manic–depressive (bipolar) psychoses occur in a ratio of approximately 3 to 4 per 1000 people.
- Acute grief reaction lasts 6 to 18 months but may be longer in older patients.
- Currently, the number of divorces occurring annually in the United States is about 48% of the number of marriages.
- Posthysterectomy depression occurs in 4% to 70% of women, depending on the indication for the operation and the preparation offered.
- Roberts' four stages of incorporation as an individual response to organ or body part loss are *impact, retreat, acknowledgment,* and *reconstruction.*
- Kübler-Ross defines the stages of individual progress to acceptance of the inevitability of death as *denial, anger, bargaining, depression,* and *acceptance.*
- Hospice programs are support groups for both dying patients and their families.

BIBLIOGRAPHY

Key Readings

Amato PR: Life-span adjustment of children to their parents' divorce. Future Child 4:143, 1994.

Basson R: Sexual desire and arousal disorders in women. N Engl J Med 354:1497, 2006.

Calle EE, Thun MJ, Petrelli JM, et al: Body-Mass Index and mortality in a prospective cohort of U.S. adults. N Engl J Med 341:1097, 1999.

Fergusson DM, Horwood LJ, Lynskey MT: Parental separation, adolescent psychopathology, and problem behaviors. J Am Acad Child Adolesc Psychiatry 33:1122, 1994.

Fiore MC, Novotny TE, Pierce JP, et al: Methods used to quit smoking in the United States. JAMA 263:2760, 1990.

Gallagher DE, Breckenridge JN, Thompson LW, Peterson JA: Effects of bereavement on indicators of mental health in elderly widows and widowers. J Gerontol 38:565, 1983.

Hsu LKG, Crisp AH, Harding B: Outcome of anorexia nervosa. Lancet 1:61, 1979.

Lamont J: Vaginismus. Am J Obstet Gynecol 131:632, 1978.

Lindemann E: Symptomatology and management of acute grief. Am J Psychiatry 101:141, 1944.

Maggard MA, Shugarman LR, Suttorp M, et al: Meta-analysis: Surgical treatment of obesity. Ann Intern Med 142(7):547, 2005.

Must A, Jacques PF, Dallal GE, et al: Long-term morbidity and mortality of overweight adolescents. A follow-up of the Harvard Growth Study of 1922–1935. N Engl J Med 327:1350, 1992.

Theander S: Outcome and prognosis in anorexia nervosa and bulimia: some results of previous investigations compared with those of a Swedish long-term study. J Psychiatr Res 19:493, 1985.

Wadden TA, Berkowitz RI, Womble LG: Weight loss management. N Engl J Med 353:2111, 2005.

General References

Agerbo E: Midlife suicide risk. Partner's psychiatric illness, spouse and child bereavement by suicide or other modes of death: a gender specific study. J Epidemiol Community Health 59(4):407, 2005.

Andersen BL, Turnquist D, LaPolla J, Turner D: Sexual functioning after treatment of in situ vulvar cancer: Preliminary report. Obstet Gynecol 71:15, 1988.

Anderson RE: Where's Dad? Parental deprivation in delinquency. Arch Gen Psychiatry 18:641, 1968.

Arlt W: Androgen therapy in women. Eur J Endocrinol 154:1, 2006.

Attia E, Haiman C, Walsh ET, Flater SR: Does fluoxetine augment the inpatient treatment of anorexia nervosa: Am J Psychiatry 155:548, 1998.

Bacaltchuk J, Hay P: Antidepressants versus placebo for people with bulimia. Cochrane Database Syst Rev (4):CD003391, 2003.

Bailey VJ, Farquhar C, Owen C, et al: Sexual behaviour of lesbians and bisexual women. Sex Transm Infect 79:147, 2003.

Barker MG: Psychiatric illness after hysterectomy. BMJ 2:91, 1968.

Barnes GE, Prosen H: Parental death and depression. J Abnorm Psychol 94:64, 1985.

Basson R, Althof S, Davis S: Summary of the recommendations on sexual dysfunctions in women. J Sex Med 1:24, 2004.

Basson R: Female sexual response: The role of drugs in the management of sexual dysfunction. Obstet Gynecol 98:350, 2001.

Bearer CF: Markers to detect drinking during pregnancy. Alcohol Res Health 25(3):210, 2001.

Birtchnell J: Early parent death in psychiatric diagnosis. Soc Psychiatry 7:202, 1972.

Birtchnell J: Early parent death in relation to size and constitution of sibship. Acta Psychiatr Scand 47:250, 1971.

Boggs PP, Utian WH: The North American Menopause Society develops consensus opinions (editorial). Menopause 5:67, 1998.

Bradford J, Ryan C, Rothblum ED: National Lesbian Health Care Survey: Implications for mental health care. J Consult Clin Psychol 62:228, 1994.

Bradford J: Lesbian and bisexual health: An overview for health care providers. J Watch Women Health July 10:9, 2002.

Braunstein GD, Sundwall DA, Katz M, et al: Safety and efficacy of a testosterone patch for the treatment of hypoactive sexual desire disorder in surgically menopausal women. A randomized placebo-controlled trial. Arch Intern Med 165:1582, 2005.

Brownell KD, Kelman JH, Stunkard AJ: Treatment of obese children with and without their mothers: Changes in weight and blood pressure. Pediatrics 71:515, 1983.

Bruhn DF, Bruhn P: Stillbirth: A humanistic response. Reprod Med 29:107, 1984.

Buchwald H, Avidor Y, Braunwald E, et al: Bariatric surgery: A systematic review and meta-analysis. JAMA 292:1724, 2004.

Bulik CM, Klump KL, Thornton L, et al: Alcohol use disorder comorbidity in eating disorders: A multicenter study. J Clin Psychiatry 65:1000, 2004.

Bulik CM, Sullivan PF, Fear JL, et al: Eating disorders and antecedent anxiety disorders: A controlled study. Acta Psychiatr Scand 96:101, 1997.

Bulik CM, Sullivan PF, Tozzi F: Prevalence, heritability, and prospective risk factors for anorexia nervosa. Arch Gen Psychiatry 63:305, 2006.

Casper RC, Eckert ED, Halmi KA, et al: Bulimia: Its incidence and clinical importance in patients with anorexia nervosa. Br J Psychiatry 27:1030, 1980.

Claudino AM, Hay P, Lima MS, et al: Antidepressants for anorexia nervosa. Cochrane Database Syst Rev Jan 25(1) CD004365, 2006.

Cochran SD, Mays VM Bowen D, et al: Cancer-related risk indicators and preventive screening behaviors among lesbians and bisexual women. Am J Public Health 91:591, 2001.

Craighead LW, Stunkard AJ, O'Brien R: Behavior therapy and pharmacotherapy of obesity. Arch Gen Psychiatry 38:763, 1981.

Davis SR, Davison SL, Donath S, et al: Circulating androgen levels and self-reported sexual function in women. JAMA 294:91, 2005.

DeGraaf R: New treatise concerning the generative organs of women. In Ladas AK, Whipple B, Perry JD (eds): The G-Spot and Other Recent Discoveries About Human Sexuality. New York, Holt, Rinehart & Winston, 1983.

Diagnostic and Statistical Manual of Mental Disorders, 4th ed: DSM-IV-TR, Washington, DC, American Psychiatric Association, 2000.

Diamant AL, Schuster MA, Lever J: Receipt of preventive health care services by lesbians. Am J Prev Med 19:141, 2000.

Diamant AL, Schuster MA, McGuigan K, et al: Lesbians' sexual history with men: Implications for taking a sexual history. Arch Intern Med 159:2730, 1999.

Dietrich DR: Psychological health of young adults who experienced early parent death: MMPI trends. J Clin Psychol 40:901, 1984.

Dorpat TL, Ripley HS: A study of suicide in the Seattle area. Compr Psychiatry 1:349, 1960.

Drummond J, Field PA: Emotional and sexual sequelae following hysterectomy. Health Care Women Int 5:261, 1984.

Dube SR, Anda RF, Felitti VJ, et al: Childhood abuse, household dysfunction, and the risk of attempted suicide throughout the life span. Findings from the Adverse Childhood Experiences Study. JAMA 286:3089, 2001.

Earls F: The fathers (not the mothers): Their importance and influence with infants and young children. In Chess S, Thomas A (eds): Annual Progress in Child Psychiatry and Child Development, vol 10. New York, Brunner/Mazel, 1977.

Edwards L: New concepts in vulvodynia. Am J Obstet Gynecol 189:S24, 2003.

Eisenbruch M: Cross cultural aspects of bereavement. II. Ethnic and cultural variations in the development of bereavement practices. Cult Med Psychiatry 8:315, 1984.

Eisler I, Dare C, Russell GR, et al: Family and individual therapy in anorexia nervosa: A 5-year follow-up. Arch Gen Psychiatry 54:1025, 1997.

Estok P, Lehman A: Perinatal death: Grief support for families. Birth 10:17, 1983.

Ewing JA: Detecting alcoholism: The CAGE questionnaire. JAMA 252(14):1905, 1984.

Ferguson JM: Learning to eat: Leader's manual and patient manual. Palo Alto, CA, Bull Publishing, 1975.

Field AE, Cheung L, Wolf AM, et al: Exposure to mass media and weight concerns among girls. Pediatrics 103:E36, 1999.

Fiore M, Bailey W, Cohen S, et al: Treating tobacco use and dependence. Clinical practice guideline. Rockville, MD, U.S. Department of Health and Human Services, U.S. Public Health Service, 2000.

Frank E, Anderson C, Rubinstein D: Frequency of sexual dysfunction in "normal" couples. N Engl J Med 299:111, 1978.

Garner D, Garfinkel P: Sociocultural factors in the development of anorexia nervosa. Psychol Med 10:647, 1980.

Gates S, McCambridge J, Smith LA, et al: Interventions for prevention of drug use by young people delivered in non-school settings. Cochrane Database Syst Rev Jan 25;(1):CD005030, 2006.

Godart NT, Flament MF, Curt F, et al: Anxiety disorders in subjects seeking treatment for eating disorders: A DSM-IV controlled study. Psychiatry Res 117:245, 2003.

Godkin MA, Krant MJ, Doster NJ: The impact of hospice care on families. Int J Psychiatry Med 13:153, 1983–1984.

Grafenberg E: The role of the urethra in female orgasm. Int J Sexol 3:145, 1950.

Graziottin A, Brotto LA: Vulvar vestibulitis syndrome: A clinical approach. J Sex Marital Ther 30:125, 2004.

Gregory I: Anterospective data following childhood loss of a parent. I. Pathology, performance, and potential among college students. Arch Gen Psychiatry 13:110, 1965.

Guarino R, Pellai A, Bassoli L, et al: Overweight, thinness, body self-image and eating strategies of 2,121 Italian teenagers. Sci World J 5:812, 2005.

Halmi KA, Stunkard AJ, Mason EE: Emotional responses to weight reduction by three methods: Diet, jojunoileal bypass and gastric bypass. Am J Clin Nutr 33:446, 1980.

Halmi KA, Sunday SR, Klump KL, et al: Obsessions and compulsions in anorexia nervosa subtypes. Int J Eat Disord 33:308, 2003.

Hamilton LH, Brooks-Gunn J, Warren MP: Sociocultural influences on eating disorders in professional female ballet dancers. Int J Eat Disord 4:465, 1985.

Hasin DS, Goodwin RD, Stinson FS: Epidemiology of major depressive disorder: results from the National Epidemiologic Survey on Alcoholism and Related Conditions. Arch Gen Psychiatry 62:1097, 2005.

Hay P, Bacaltchuk J, Claudino A, Ben-Tovim D, et al: Individual psychotherapy in the outpatient treatment of adults with anorexia nervosa. Cochrane Database Sys Rev 4:CD003909.
Hay PJ, Bacaltchuk J, Stefasno S: Psychotherapy for bulimia nervosa and binging. Cochrane Database Syst Rev 3:CD000562, 2004.
Hay PJ, Bacaltchuk J: Psychotherapy for bulimia nervosa and binging. Cochrane Database Syst Rev 3:CD000562, 2003.
Health, United States, 1999. US Department of Health and Human Services. Centers for Disease Control and Prevention. DHHS 99-1232, 1999.
Heiman JR, Lentz GM: Sexuality. In Seltzer VL, Pearse WH (eds): Women's Primary Health Care Office Practice and Procedures, 2nd ed. New York, McGraw-Hill, 2000, pp 453–476.
Heiman JR: Sexual dysfunction: Overview of prevalence, etiological factors, and treatments. J Sex Res 39:73, 2002.
Hoek HW, vanHoeken D: Review of the prevalence and incidence of eating disorders. Int J Eat Disord 34:383, 2003.
Holmes TH, Rahe RH: The social adjustment rating scale. J Psychosom Res 11:213, 1967.
Institute of Medicine, Solarz AL (ed): Lesbian health: Current Assessment and Directions for the Future. Washington, DC, National Academy Press, 1999, pp 48–50, 93–95.
Isager T, Brinch M, Kreiner S, Tolstrup K: Death and relapse in anorexia nervosa: Survival analysis of 151 cases. J Psychiatr Res 19:515, 1985.
Johnson WG, Schlundt DG: Eating disorders: Assessment and treatment. Clin Obstet Gynecol 28:598, 1985.
Johnston JR: High-conflict divorce. Future Child 4:165, 1994.
Kaplan HS: The New Sex Therapy. New York, Brunner/Mazel, 1974.
Kaye WH, Bulik CM, Thornton L, et al: Comorbidity of anxiety disorders with anorexia and bulimia nervosa. Am J Psychiatry 161:2215, 2004.
Kaye WH: Persistent alterations in behavior and serotonin activity after recovery from anorexia and bulimia nervosa. Ann N Y Acad Sci 817:162, 1997.
Kelly AM Wall M, Eisenberg ME, et al: Adolescent girls with high body satisfaction: Who are they and what can they teach us? J Adolesc Health 37(5):391, 2005.
Kreipe RE, Strauss J, Hodgman CH, Ryan RM: Menstrual cycle abnormalities and subclinical eating disorders: Preliminary report. Psychosom Med 51:81, 1989.
Kübler-Ross E: On Death and Dying. New York, Macmillan, 1969.
Laajus S: Parental losses. Acta Psychiatr Scand 69:1, 1984.
Lancaster T, Hajek P, Stead LF, et al: Prevention of relapse after quitting smoking: A systematic review of trials. Arch Intern Med 166:828, 2006.
Laumann EO, Paik A, Rosen RC: Sexual dysfunction in the United Sates. Prevalence and predictors. JAMA 281:537, 1999.
Lebowitz BD, Pearson JL, Schneider LS, et al: Diagnosis and treatment of depression in late life. Consensus statement update. JAMA 278:1186, 1997.
Leppert PC, Pahlka BS: Grieving characteristics after spontaneous abortion: A management approach. Obstet Gynecol 64:119, 1984.
Lew EA: Mortality and weight: Insured lives and the American Cancer Society Studies. Ann Intern Med 103:1024, 1985.
Li A, Maglione M, Tu W, et al: Meta-analysis: Pharmacologic treatment of obesity. Ann Intern Med 142:532, 2005.
Linde K, Mulrow CD, Berner M, et al: St. John's wort for depression. Cochrane Database Syst Rev (2):CD000448, 2000.
Lowe B, Spitzer RL, Grafe K, et al: Comparative validity of three screening questionnaires for DSM-IV depressive disorders and physicians' diagnoses. J Affect Disord 78:131, 2004.
Lundin T: Long-term outcome of bereavement. Br J Psychiatry 145:424, 1984.
Marazzo JM, Koutsky LA, Kiviat NB, et al: Papanicolaou test screening and prevalence of genital human papillomavirus among women who have sex with women. Am J Public Health 91:947, 2001.
Masters WH, Johnson VE: Human sexual response. Boston, Little, Brown, 1966.
Masters WH, Johnson VE: Human sexual inadequacy. Boston, Little, Brown, 1970.
McGuire H, Hawton K: Interventions for vaginismus. Cochrane Database Syst Rev (1):CD001760, 2003.
Melody GF: Depressive reactions following hysterectomy. Am J Obstet Gynecol 83:410, 1962.
Munro A, Griffiths AB: Some psychiatric nonsequelae of childhood bereavement. Br J Psychiatry 115:305, 1969.
Must A, Spadano J, Coakley EH, et al: The disease burden associated with overweight and obesity. JAMA 282:1523, 1999.
Nahas G: Marijuana: Deceptive Weed. New York, Raven, 1973.
National Center for Health Statistics: Prevalence of overweight and obesity among adults: United States, 1999–2002.
National Institutes of Health, National Heart, Lung, Blood Institute and the North American Association for the Study of Obesity in Adults. Practical guide identification, evaluation and treatment of overweight and obesity in adults, Publication No. 00-4084, Washington, DC, 2000.
National Institutes of Health, National Institute of Diabetes and Digestive and Kidney Diseases. Understanding adult obesity. Publication No. 01-3680, Washington, DC, 2001.
Nattiv A, Agostini R, Drinkwater B, Yeager KK: The female athletic triad: The interrelatedness of disordered eating, amenorrhea, and osteoporosis. Clin Sport Med 13:405, 1994.
Newton N, Baron E: Reactions to hysterectomy-fact or fiction. Prim Care 3:781, 1976.
North American Menopause Society: The role of testosterone therapy in post-menopausal women: Position statement of the North American Menopause Society. Menopause 12:497, 2005.
Oppenheimer R, Howells K, Palmer RL, Chaloner DA: Adverse sexual experience in childhood and clinical eating disorders: A preliminary description. J Psychiatr Res 19:357, 1985.
Pampallona S, Bollini P, Tibaldi G, et al: Combined pharmacotherapy and psychological treatment for depression: A systematic review. Arch Gen Psychiatry 61:714, 2004.
Parker C, Hadzi-Pavlovic D: Modification of level of depression in mother-bereaved women byparental and marital relationships. Psychol Med 14:125, 1984.
Patton GC, Coffey C, Carlin JB, et al: Cannabis use and mental health in young people: Cohort study. BMJ 325:1195, 2002.
Pirke KM, Schweiger U, Strowitzki T, et al: Dieting causes menstrual irregularities in normal weight young women through impairment of episodic luteinizing hormone secretion. Fertil Steril 51:263, 1989.
Pirke KM: Central and peripheral noradrenalin regulation in eating disorders. Psychiatry Res 62:43, 1996.
Pope HG, Jr., Mangweth B, Negrao AB, et al: Childhood sexual abuse and bulimia nervosa: A comparison of American, Austrian, and Brazilian women. Am J Psychiatry 151:731, 1994.
Practice guideline for the treatment of patients with eating disorders (revision): American Psychiatric Association/Work Group on Eating Disorders. Am J Psychiatry 157(1 Suppl):1, 2000.
Pratt BM, Woolfenden SR: Interventions for preventing eating disorders in children and adolescents. Cochrane Database Syst Rev 2:CD002891, 2002.
Presnell K, Bearman SK, Stice E: Risk factors for body dissatisfaction in adolescent boys and girls: A prospective study. Int J Eat Disord 36(4):389, 2004.
Quackenbush J: The death of a pet: How it can affect owners. Vet Clin North Am Small Anim Pract 15:395, 1985.
Racette SB, Schoeller DA, Kushner RF, Neil KM: Effects of aerobic exercise and dietary carbohydrate on energy expenditure and body composition during weight reduction in obese women. Am J Clin Nutr 61:486, 1995.
Richards DH: A posthysterectomy syndrome. Lancet 2:983, 1974.
Richards DH: Depression after hysterectomy. Lancet 2:430, 1973.
Rickert VI, Wiemann CM, Berenson AB: Ethnic differences in depressive symptomatology among young women. Obstet Gynecol 95:55, 2000.
Roberts SL: Behavioral Concepts in the Critically Ill Patient. Englewood Cliffs, NJ, Prentice-Hall, 1976.
Romans SE, Gendall KA, Martin JL, et al: Child sexual abuse and later disordered eating: A New Zealand epidemiological study. Int J Eat Disord 29:380, 2001.
Rubinstein S, Caballero B: Is Miss America an undernourished role model? JAMA 283:1549, 2000.
Ruschena E, Prior M, Sanson A, et al: A longitudinal study of adolescent adjustment following family transitions. J Child Psychol Psychiatry 46:353, 2005.
Rutter M: Parent child separation: Psychological effects on the child. J Child Psychol Psychiatry 12:233, 1971.
Sager CJ: Sexual dysfunction in marital discord. In Kaplan HS (ed): The New Sex Therapy. New York, Brunner/Mazel, 1974.
Sareen J, Fleisher W, Cox BJ, et al: Childhood adversity and perceived need for mental health care. Findings from a Canadian community sample. J Nerv Ment Dis 193:396, 2005.

Segraves RT: Croft H, Kavoussi R, et al: Bupropion sustained release (SR) for the treatment of hypoactive sexual desire disorder (HSDD) in nondepressed women. J Sex Marital Ther 27:303, 2001.

Semmens JP, Semmens EC: Sexual function in the menopause. Clin Obstet Gynecol 27:717, 1984.

Semmens JP, Wagner G: Estrogen deprivation and vaginal function in menopausal women: A study of menopausal vaginal physiology and the effect of exogenous estrogen therapy. JAMA 248:445, 1982.

Shanfield SB, Swain BJ: Death of adult children in traffic accidents. J Nerv Ment Dis 172:533, 1984.

Shifren JL, Braunstein GD, Simon JA, et al: Transdermal testosterone treatment in women with impaired sexual function after oophorectomy. N Engl J Med 343:682, 2000.

Sokol RJ: Alcohol in pregnancy: Clinical research problems. Neurobehav Toxicol Teratol 2:157, 1980.

Somboonporn W, Davis S, Seif MW, et al: Testosterone for peri- and postmenopausal women. Cochrane Database Syst Rev Oct 19;(4) CB004509, 2005

Steege JF: Dyspareunia in vaginismus. Clin Obstet Gynecol 27:750, 1984.

Steiner H, Kwan W, Shaffer TG, et al: Risk and protective factors for juvenile eating disorders. Eur Child Adolesc Psychiatry 12(Suppl 1):38, 2003.

Steiner M, Aleksandrowicz DR: Psychiatric sequelae to gynecological operations. Isr Ann Psychiatr Relat Disciplines 8:186, 1970.

Streissguth AP, Darby BL, Barr HM, et al: Comparison of drinking and smoking patterns during pregnancy over a 6-year interval. Am J Obstet Gynecol 145:716, 1983.

Strober M, Morrell W, Burroughs J, et al: A controlled family study of anorexia nervosa. J Psychiatr Res 19:239, 1985.

Stunkard AJ, Stellar E (eds): Eating and Its Disorders. New York, Raven Press, 1984.

Sundgot-Borgen J: Risk and trigger factors for the development of eating disorders in female Elite. Athletes. Med Sci Sports Exerc 26:414, 1994.

Svendsen OL, Hassager C, Christiansen C: Effect of an energy-restrictive diet, with or without exercise, on lean tissue mass, resting metabolic rate, cardiovascular risk factors, and bone in overweight postmenopausal women. Am J Med 95:131, 1993.

Svendsen OL, Hassager C, Christiansen C: Six months' follow-up on exercise added to a short-term diet in overweight postmenopausal women-effects on body composition, resting metabolic rate, cardiovascular risk factors and bone. Int J Obes Relat Metab Disord 18:692, 1994.

Szegedi A, Kohnen R, Dienel A, et al: Acute treatment of moderate to severe depression with hypericum extract WS 5570 (St. John's wort): Randomised controlled double blind non-inferiority trial versus paroxetine. BMJ 330(7490):503, 2005.

Tennant C, Smith A, Bebbington P, Hurry J: Parental loss in childhood: Relationship to adult psychiatric impairment and contact with psychiatric services. Arch Gen Psychiatry 38:309, 1981.

Urwin RE, Nunn KP: Epistatic interaction between the monoamine oxidase A and serotonin transporter genes in anorexia nervosa. Eur J Human Genet 13:370, 2005.

U.S. Department of Health and Human Services, Center for Disease Control and Prevention, National Center for Health Statistics: Prevalence of overweight and obesity among adults: United States, 1999–2002, Hyattsville, MD, 2004.

U.S. Department of Health and Human Services, Center for Disease Control and Prevention, National Center for health Statistics: Chronic disease—preventing obesity and chronic diseases through good nutrition and physical activity. Hyattsville, MD, 2005.

U.S. Department of Health and Human Services, Centers for Disease Control and Prevention, National Center for Health Statistics: Smoking. Hyattsville, MD, 2006.

U.S. Department of Health and Human Services, Public Health Service, National Institutes of Health, National Institute on Alcohol Abuse and Alcoholism: Special Report to the U.S. Congress on Alcohol and Health, 2000.

Wadden TA, Berkowitz RI, Sarwer DB, et al: Benefits of lifestyle modification in the pharmacologic treatment of obesity: a randomized trial. Arch Intern Med 161:218, 2001.

Wadden TA, Stunkard AJ, Brownell KD: Very low calorie diets: Their efficacy, safety and future. Ann Intern Med 99:675, 1983.

Waitkebica HJ: Lesbian health in primary care. Part 1: Opening your practice to the sexual minority patient. Women Health Gynecol 4(3):129, 2004.

Walters EE, Kendler KS: Anorexia nervosa and anorexic-like syndromes in a population-based female twin sample. Am J Psychiatry 152:64, 1995.

Weiner L, Rosett HL, Edelin KC, et al: Alcohol consumption by pregnant women. Obstet Gynecol 61:6, 1983.

White MA, Kohlmaier JR, Varnado-Sullivan P, Williamson DA: Racial/ethnic differences in weight concerns: Protective and risk factors for the development of eating disorders and obesity among adolescent females. Eat Weight Disord 8(1):20, 2003.

Whitlock EP, Polen MR, Green CA, et al: Behavior counseling interventions in primary care to reduce risky/harmful alcohol use by adults: A summary of the evidence for the U.S. Preventive Services Task Force. Ann Intern Med 140:557, 2004.

Whitlock EP, Williams SB, Gold R, et al: Screening and interventions for childhood overweight: A summary of evidence for the US Preventive Services Task Force. Pediatrics 116:125, 2005.

Widom CS, Dumont K, Czaja SJ: A prospective investigation of major depressive disorder and comorbidity in abused and neglected children grown up. Arch Gen Psychiatry 64:49, 2007.

Yager J, Anderson AE: Anorexia nervosa. N Engl J Med 353:1481, 2005.

Rape, Incest, and Domestic Violence 10

Discovery, Management, Counseling

Gretchen M. Lentz

KEY TERMS AND DEFINITIONS

Abuse. Aggressive behavior including acts of a sexual or physical nature, verbal belittling, or intimidation. The act may be premeditated, as when one individual wishes to gain control over another, or spontaneous, as a spontaneous response to anger or frustration.

Battered Wife Syndrome. A symptom complex occurring as a result of violence in which a woman has at any time received deliberate, severe, or repeated (more than three times) physical abuse from her husband, in which the minimal injury is bruising.

Battered Woman. Any woman over the age of 16 with evidence of physical abuse on at least one occasion at the hands of an intimate male partner.

Cycle of Battering. Three phases in the cycle of battering are noted: tension building, the act of violence, and the apology and forgiveness phase. As cycles are repeated, the second phase tends to become more violent and the third less intensive.

Domestic Violence. Violence occurring between partners in an ongoing relationship regardless of whether they are married.

Incest. Sexual intimacy with or without coitus involving a close family member. The act may include fondling, exposure, or the penetration of an orifice by the phallus or an object.

Intimate Partner Violence. Actual or threatened physical, sexual, or emotional abuse from an intimate partner (whether the same or opposite sex).

Rape. Any act of sexual intimacy performed by one person on another without mutual consent by force, by threat of force, or by the inability of the victim to give appropriate consent.

Rape-Trauma Syndrome. A set of behaviors that occur after a rape. The immediate response (acute phase) lasts hours to days and reflects a distortion or paralysis of the individual's coping mechanisms, but the outward responses vary from complete loss of emotional control to an apparently well-controlled behavior pattern. The delayed (or reorganization) phase involves flashbacks, nightmares, and a need for reorganization of thought process. It may occur months to years after the event and may involve major lifestyle adjustments.

Rape, incest, and other forms of physical and sexual abuse are very common. Physicians in general and obstetricians and gynecologists in particular are in a position to detect these problems and offer treatment and counsel when their patients are victims. In the acute state, a careful history using a compassionate and nonjudgmental approach will often allow an accurate story to be obtained. When the patient seeks medical advice at a time remote from the experience or when the experience is ongoing, the presenting chief complaint may have little to do with the actual problem. For the physician to elicit a clear picture, it is necessary to resort to open-ended questions and interviewing techniques that allow the patient to comfortably discuss truthfully the actual problem.

These patients are at risk for severe physical and emotional distress, and as victims they may suffer psychological damage to their self-image, which in turn may lead to many long-term poor choices in important life situations. Although rape, incest, and abuse will be discussed separately, there is frequently a relationship in the social pathology involved, as well as in the long-term effects that the patient must endure. In each instance appropriate physician response and physician responsibility will be discussed.

RAPE

Rape, or the sexual assault of children, women, and men, is a common act. It is defined as any sexual act performed by one person on another without that person's consent. Only recently has it become apparent how common a problem this is. From 1992 to 2000 the U.S. Department of Justice reported that for females the average annual incidence of sexual assault was 366,460, accounting for 6% of all violent crimes in 1987. All rapes, 39% of attempted rapes, and 17% of sexual assaults against females resulted in injured victims. This type of crime, however, is often underreported, and the actual incidence may be much higher. Victims are often reluctant to report sexual assault to the authorities because of embarrassment, fear of retribution, feelings of guilt, assumptions that little will be done, or simply lack of knowledge of their rights. It has been estimated that as many as 44% of women have been victims of actual or attempted sexual assault at some time in their lives and as many as 50% of these on more than one occasion. Homeless women and women with mental illness are particularly vulnerable to sexual assaults compared with the general population.

In the past, society has held many misconceptions about the rape victim, particularly female victims. These included the notion that the individual encouraged the rape by specific behavior or dress and that no person who did not wish to be raped could be raped. Furthermore, the feeling that rape was an indication of basic promiscuity was widely held. In many instances sexual assault victims were accused of lying to cause problems for otherwise innocent men. To some extent many of these societal misconceptions are held today.

Sexual assault happens to people of all ages and races in all socioeconomic groups. The very young, the mentally and physically handicapped, and the very old are particularly susceptible. Although the perpetrator may be a stranger, he or she is often an individual well known to the victim.

Some situations have been defined as variants of sexual assault. These include marital rape, which involves forced coitus or related acts without consent but within the marital relationship, and "date rape." In the latter situation the woman may voluntarily participate in sexual play, but coitus is performed, often forcibly, without her consent. Date rape is often not reported because the victim may believe she contributed by partially participating. This, however, can scar her self-esteem.

Almost all states have statutes that criminalize coitus with females under certain specified ages. Such an act is referred to as *statutory rape.* Consent is irrelevant because the female is defined by statute as being incapable of consenting.

During a rape, the victim loses control over his or her life for that period and frequently experiences anxiety and fear. When the attack is life-threatening, shock with associated physical and psychological symptoms may occur. Burgess and Holmstrom identify two phases of the rape-trauma syndrome.

The immediate, or acute, phase lasts from hours to days and may be associated with a paralysis of the individual's usual coping mechanisms. Outwardly, the victim may demonstrate manifestations ranging from complete loss of emotional control to a well-controlled behavior pattern. The actual reaction may depend on a number of factors, including the relationship of the victim to the attacker, whether force was used, and the length of time the victim was held against his or her will. Generally, the victim appears disorganized and may complain of both physical and emotional symptoms. Physical complaints include specific injuries or general complaints of soreness, eating problems, headaches, and sleep disturbances. Behavior patterns may include fear, mood swings, irritability, guilt, anger, depression, and difficulties in concentrating. Frequently, the victim will complain of flashbacks to the attack. Medical care is often sought during the acute period, and at this point it is the physician's responsibility to assess the specific medical problems and also to offer a program of emotional support and reassurance.

The second phase of the rape-trauma syndrome involves long-term adjustment and is designated the reorganization phase. During this time flashbacks and nightmares may continue, but phobias may also develop. These may be directed against members of the offending sex, the sex act itself, or nonrelated circumstances, such as a newly developed fear of crowds or heights. During this period the victim may institute a number of important lifestyle changes, including job, residence, friends, and significant others. If major complications such as the contraction of a sexually transmitted disease (STD) or a pregnancy occur, resolution may be more difficult. The reorganization period may last from months to years and generally involves an attempt on the part of the victim to regain control over his or her life. During this time medical care and counseling must be nonjudgmental, sensitive, and anticipatory. When the physician realizes that the patient is contemplating a major lifestyle change during this period, it is probably appropriate to point out to the patient why the change is being contemplated and the complicating effects it may have on the patient's overall well-being.

Physician's Responsibility in the Care of a Rape Victim

Although any individual may become a rape victim, this discussion will be limited to the care of a female, as is appropriate for a gynecology textbook. The physician's responsibility may be divided into three categories: medical, medicolegal, and supportive, as shown in the following box.

Medical

The physician's medical responsibilities are to treat injuries and to perform appropriate tests for, to prevent, and to treat infections and pregnancies. It is important to obtain informed consent before examining the patient and collecting specimens. In addition to addressing legal requirements, it helps the victim to regain control over her body and her life.

After acute injuries have been determined and stabilized, a careful history and physical examination should be performed. It is important to have a chaperone present during the taking of the history and the performance of the examination and specimen collection to reassure the victim and to provide support. The presence of such a third party probably reduces feelings of

Physician's Responsibilities in Caring for Rape–Trauma Victim

Medical
Treat injuries
Diagnose and treat STD
Prevent pregnancy

Medicolegal
Document history carefully
Examine patient thoroughly and specifically note injuries
Collect articles of clothing
Collect vaginal (rectal and pharyngeal) samples for sperm
Comb pubic hair for hair samples
Collect fingernail scrapings where appropriate
Collect saliva for secretion substance
Turn specimens over to forensic authorities and receive receipts for chart

Emotional Support
Discuss degree of injury, probability of infection, and possibility of pregnancy
Discuss general course that can be predicted
Consult with rape-trauma counselor
Arrange follow-up visit for medical and emotional evaluation in 1–4 weeks
Reassure as far as possible

vulnerability on the part of the victim. She should be asked to state in her own words what happened; if she knew the attacker, and if not, to describe the attacker; and to describe the specific act(s) performed.

A history of previous gynecologic conditions, particularly infections and pregnancy, use of contraception, and the date of last menstrual period, should be recorded. It is necessary to determine whether the patient may have a preexisting pregnancy or be at risk for pregnancy. It is also important to ascertain whether she has had a preexisting pelvic infection.

Experience derived at the Sexual Assault Center in Seattle, Washington, demonstrated that between 12% and 40% of victims who are sexually assaulted have injuries. Most of these, however, are minor and require simple reparative therapy. Only about 1% require hospitalization and major operative repair. Nonetheless, the victim will perceive the experience as having been life threatening, as in many cases it may have been. Many injuries occur when the victim is restrained or physically coerced into the sexual act. Thus, the physician should seek bruises, abrasions, or lacerations about the neck, back, buttocks, or extremities. Where a knife was used as a coercive tactic, small cuts may also be found. Erythema, lacerations, and edema of the vulva or rectum may occur because of manipulation of these areas with the hand or the penis. These are particularly common in children or virginal victims but may occur in any woman and should be looked for. Superficial or extensive lacerations of the hymen or vagina may occur in virginal victims or in the elderly. Lacerations may also be noted in the area of the urethra, the rectum, and at times through the vaginal vault into the abdominal cavity. In addition, bite marks may be noted in any of these regions. Occasionally, foreign objects are inserted into the vagina, the urethra, or the rectum and may be found in situ.

In recent years, some authorities have advised close inspection with a magnifying glass or colposcope of the vulva and vagina of infants and children suspected to be victims of rape. Muram and Elias, however, in a study of 130 prepubertal girls (mean age 5.5) identified as victims of sexual abuse, could identify evidence of trauma in 96% with unaided inspection. Four additional cases were identified by colposcopy, but the lesions were obvious on repeat unaided examination. Simple visual examination without the aid of a colposcope should be sufficient to detect signs of trauma in children.

Where oral penetration has been effected, injury of the mouth and pharynx should be looked for.

Infection. Most victims are concerned about possible infections incurred as a result of the rape, but until recently no careful follow-up studies in victims had been performed. To determine actual risk it is important to know the prevalence of existing STDs in the victim population. In 1990, Jenny and colleagues examined 204 girls and women within 72 hours of a rape and discovered that 88 (43%) were harboring at least one STD. These included *Neisseria gonorrhoeae* in 13 of 204 (6% of all tested), cytomegalovirus in 13 of 170 (8%), *Chlamydia trachomatis* in 20 of 198 (10.1%), *Trichomonas vaginalis* in 30 of 204 (14.7%), herpes simplex virus in 4 of 170 (2.4%), *Treponema pallidum* in 2 of 199 (1.0%), human immunodeficiency virus (HIV)-1 in 1 of 123 (0.8%), and bacterial vaginosis in 70 of 204 (34.3%). In 109 patients (53%) who returned for follow-up (excluding those who were found to be infected on the first visit or who were treated prophylactically), there were 3 of 71 (4%) cases of gonorrhea, 1 of 65 (0.02%) of chlamydia, 10 of 81 (12%) of trichomoniasis, and 15 of 77 (19%) of bacterial vaginosis. These authors concluded that women who were raped have a higher than average prevalence of preexisting STDs but are also at a substantial risk of acquiring such disease as a result of the assault.

Reynolds and coworkers presented a review on the risk of infection in rape victims that was the result of a MEDLINE search of the English language journals. They also noted that it was often difficult to separate new from existing infection, but placed the prevalence of STDs as follows: *N. gonorrhea* 0 to 26.3%, *C. trachomatis* 3.9% to 17%, *Treponema pallidum* 0 to 5.6%, *Trichomonas vaginalis* 0 to 19%, and HPV 0.6% to 2.3%.

Few studies are available to predict the actual risk of acquiring an STD, but *Chlamydia trachomatis* may be the most commonly acquired infection incurred under these circumstances. Most victims fear acquiring HIV as a result of a sexual attack, but current risks are probably not high depending on the population involved and the sexual acts performed. Some studies place the risk for adult rape victims of acquiring syphilis as high as 3% to 10%. These authors did not believe the risk of acquiring STDs can be quantified, but they note that the acquisition of viral STDs, including HIV, has been reported both in adults and children.

Commercial "evidence kits" are available. A speculum exam is not always necessary, but if bleeding is reported or noted on external vulvar exam, it is appropriate.

It must be remembered that infection may not be limited to the vagina but may also include the pharynx or the rectum. Specific history to raise a suspicion of this possibility should be sought. Cultures should be performed for *Neisseria gonorrhoeae* and *Chlamydia trachomatis*. Urine or nonculture nuclear amplification tests for gonorrhea and chlamydia are usually acceptable. In addition, conventional cultures of the rectum and of the oral pharynx are indicated when the history suggests that this would be productive. A wet mount for *Trichomonas vaginalis* and bacterial vaginosis and a potassium hydroxide mount for *Candida albicans* are also useful (see following box). Investigation for syphilis (RPR) is not routinely recommended at the Sexual Assault Center in Seattle, Washington, but may be done in follow-up.

Sexually Transmitted Diseases and Tests Available to Physicians Caring for a Rape-Trauma Victim

Should Perform

Gonorrhea—culture for *Neisseria gonorrhoeae*
Chlamydia trachomatis—culture
Syphilis—RPR

Could Perform

Herpes simplex—culture lesion or serology
Hepatitis B—screening serology
HIV—serology
Cytomegalovirus—serology
Condyloma virus—study lesion
Trichomonas—saline preparation
Candida—potassium hydroxide preparation

RPR, rapid plasma reagin.

Because the victim is also at risk for infection by the herpes virus, hepatitis B virus, cytomegalovirus, HIV, condyloma acuminatum, and a variety of other STDs, the physician may wish to screen for those that seem appropriate at the time the victim is seen in the acute stage. Hepatitis B vaccine is appropriate if the victim is not previously vaccinated. Tetanus prophylaxis is appropriate in some cases as well.

At follow-up visits the patient should again be investigated for signs and symptoms of the STDs, and appropriate repeat cultures and serologies should be obtained.

Prophylactic antibiotics are useful in acute rape management when the patient is concerned about contracting an STD or knows the assailant to be high risk. The patient can be given a single dose of cefpodoxime, 400 mg PO, for gonorrhea prophylaxis plus azithromycin, 1 g PO, for chlamydia prophylaxis. If the patient is pregnant, consider giving no medications and follow-up screening should be done in 2 weeks. If prophylaxis is desired, these antibiotics are class B drugs in pregnancy. This should prevent gonorrhea and *Chlamydia* infection but will have no effect on herpes, condylomata, or many of the other problems mentioned.

Pregnancy. The patient's menstrual history, birth control regimen, and pregnancy status should be assessed. If the patient is at risk for pregnancy at the time of the assault, an appropriate emergency contraception or "morning after" prophylaxis can be offered as long as the pregnancy test was negative. This is discussed more fully in Chapter 14 (Family Planning). In the experience of most sexual assault centers the chance of pregnancy occurring is quite low. It has been estimated to be approximately 2% to 4% of victims having a single, unprotected coitus. However, if the patient has been exposed at midcycle, the risk will be higher.

Holmes and associates estimated the national rape-related pregnancy rate at 5.0% and stated that among adult women 32,101 pregnancies resulted from rape each year in the United States. Many of these pregnancies occurred in women who did not receive immediate medical attention.

Medicolegal

To be meaningful, medicolegal material must be collected shortly after the assault takes place and definitely within 96 hours. Commercially manufactured "evidence kits" are available. Victims should be encouraged to come immediately to a center where they can be evaluated before bathing, urinating, defecating, washing out their mouths, changing clothes, or cleaning their fingernails. In general, evidence for coitus will be present in the vagina for as long as 48 hours after the attack, but in other orifices the evidence may last only up to 6 hours. Appropriate tests should document the patient's physical and emotional condition as judged by her history and physical examination and should include data that document the use of force, evidence for sexual contact, and materials that may help identify the offender. To document that force was used, the physician should carefully describe each injury noted and illustrate with either drawings or photographs. Detail is important, because injuries suffered by sexual assault victims have common patterns. Because *rape* and *sexual assault* are legal terms, they should not be stated as diagnoses; rather the physician should report findings as "consistent with use of force."

Documentation of sexual contact must begin with a history of when the patient had intercourse before the attack. If sperm or semen is found in the vagina or cervix of a victim, it must not be confused with such substances deposited during the victim's prior consenting sexual acts. Sexual contact will be verified by analysis of secretions from the vagina or rectum by identifying motile sperm. Nonmotile sperm may be present as well if the attack occurred 12 to 20 hours previously. In some instances, motile sperm will be noted for as long as 2 to 3 days in the endocervix. Vaginal wet mount is no longer recommended for identifying sperm as it lacks reproducibility. Manufactured "evidence kits" are available.

Table 10-1 Survival Time of Sperm

Source	Motile Sperm	Sperm	Acid Phosphatase
Vagina	Up to 8 hr	Up to 7–9 days	Variable (Up to 48 hr)
Pharynx	6 hr	Unknown	100 IU*
Rectum	Undetermined	20 to 24 hr	100 IU*
Cervix	Up to 5 days	Up to 17 days	Similar to vagina

*Minimum detectable.
From Anderson S: Sexual assault—medical-legal aspects. An unpublished training packet for pediatric house staff. Harborview Medical Center, Seattle, WA, 1980.

It is difficult to ascertain whether ejaculation occurred in the mouth, because residual seminal fluid is rapidly destroyed by bacteria and salivary enzymes, making documentation of such an event difficult after more than a few hours have passed. Seminal fluid may be found staining the skin or the clothing several hours after the attack, and this should be looked for. Because acid phosphatase is an enzyme found in high concentrations in seminal fluid, substances removed for analysis should be tested for this enzyme. Table 10-1 demonstrates the survival time of sperm in the pharynx, rectum, and cervix.

In addition to documenting that intercourse has taken place, an attempt should be made to identify the perpetrator. In this regard, all clothing intimately associated with the area of assault should be collected, labeled, and submitted to legal authorities. In addition, smears of vaginal secretions or a Pap smear should be made to permanently document the presence of sperm. Vaginal secretions needed for DNA typing should be collected by wet or dry swab and refrigerated until a pathologist can process them. In the near future tests may also be available to identify prostate specific antigen and seminal vesicle specific antigen in vaginal secretions. DNA fingerprinting is now readily available in all areas and is admissible in many jurisdictions. Pubic hair combings should be performed in an attempt to obtain pubic hair of the assailant. Saliva should be collected from the victim to ascertain whether she secretes an antigen that could differentiate her from substances obtained from the perpetrator. Finally, fingernail scrapings should be obtained for skin or blood if the victim scratched the perpetrator. Specific blood or DNA typing may be conducted to help identify the attacker. All materials collected should be labeled and turned over to the legal authority or pathologist, depending on the system used by the medical unit. A receipt should be obtained, and this should be documented in the patient's chart.

Emotional Support of the Victim

After the physical needs of the patient have been met and after the physician has carefully documented the information concerning the sexual contact, he or she should discuss with the victim the degree of injury, probability of infection or pregnancy, general course that the victim might be expected to follow with respect to these, and how follow-up to aid prevention will be carried out. The physician must allow the victim to give vent to anxieties and to correct misconceptions. The physician should reassure her, insofar as possible, that her well-being will be restored. In doing this the physician may call on other health personnel, such as individuals trained to help rape-trauma victims, to facilitate counseling and follow-up. The patient should not be released until specific follow-up plans are made and the patient understands what they are. A follow-up visit should be planned within 1 to 4 weeks to reevaluate the patient's medical, infectious disease, pregnancy, and psychological status. At this point, encouragement for continued follow-up counseling should be emphasized. It is important at each visit to emphasize to the patient *that she was a victim and holds no blame.* At each step she must be allowed to vent her feelings and to discuss her current conceptions of the problem.

It is important that the physician realize that some patients will appear to have excellent emotional control when seen immediately after a rape. This is an acute expression of the patient's defense mechanisms and should not be misinterpreted to indicate that the patient is coping with the circumstances. All the recommendations just listed should be followed *regardless* of the patient's apparent condition. Specific plans for follow-up are equally important in such an individual, because it must be anticipated that she will follow the same postrape emotional process as anyone else.

Finally, it is important to emphasize and reemphasize that at no time during the management or follow-up care of the rape victim should any comments be made by health care professionals suggesting that the patient was anything other than a victim. These women are sensitive to any accusations and insinuations and may even believe that they may have in some way been responsible for the rape. Their future well-being may be severely affected by creating such an impression.

Female genital mutilation. A form of sexual abuse only recently observed in the western world is female genital mutilation. It is a practice growing out of cultural and traditional beliefs dating back several thousand years. The World Health Organization estimates that between 85 and 200 million women undergo these procedures each year. Although they are often performed in parts of Africa, the Middle East, and Southeast Asia, they are rarely performed in the United States or the rest of the western world. About 168,000 women who have undergone such procedures currently live in the United States, and physicians may see the results of these procedures in patients who emigrate from countries where they are practiced.

The various forms of female genital mutilation include removal of the clitoral prepuce, excision of the clitoris, or removal of the clitoris and labia minora. Occasionally, the labia majora is also partially removed and the vagina partially sutured closed. The procedures are often performed between early childhood and age 14 and frequently without anesthesia under unsterile conditions by untrained practitioners. Therefore, a variety of complications often occur, including infection, tetanus, shock, hemorrhage, and death. Long-term problems include chronic infection, scar formation, local abscesses, sterility, and incontinence. In addition, depression, anxiety, sexual dysfunction, obstetric complications, and the psychosomatic conditions associated with sexual abuse may be seen. Physicians who care for women with this condition must develop an understanding of the cultural mores that lead to the performance of the procedure and the current implications on these cultural beliefs that remedial surgery may imply. Certainly the patient and her sexual partner should be involved in all decisions concerning intervention.

INCEST

Incest must be placed within the context of child sexual abuse. The actual overall incidence of such abuse is difficult to estimate, although several authorities claim that about 10% of all child abuse cases involve sexual abuse. Sarafino estimates that roughly 336,000 children are sexually abused each year in the United States. Retrospective historical data derived from adults imply that incestuous activity may be experienced by as many as 15% to 25% of all women and approximately 12% of all men. These figures seem appropriate for the population in general but vary from group to group, being higher in young prostitutes.

Sexual abuse of children may be divided into two types: the first in which the child is victimized by a stranger and the second in which a family member or friend is the perpetrator. It has been estimated that about 80% of all sexual abuse cases of children involve a family member. Rimsza and Niggemann found that only 18% of 311 children and adolescents who were evaluated for sexual abuse were assaulted by strangers.

In the case of child sexual abuse involving a stranger, the act is usually a single episode and is usually reported to the authorities. The child is capable in most instances of clearly stating what happened, and the act may involve any form of sexual activity and may have taken place because of enticement, coercion, or physical force. In such instances the child should be interviewed carefully and allowed to tell what happened. The police or protective services should be notified, and, where appropriate, the techniques used in evaluating a rape victim should be applied. Appropriate prophylaxis against infection should be employed, and counseling should be arranged with a mental health care worker, who should see the child immediately and also take the responsibility for planning long-term follow-up. The molester should be apprehended, and if it is an individual living in the home, he or she should be made to leave. Most communities have sexual abuse crisis intervention centers, and these are appropriate in such circumstances.

In each case the child should be carefully told that *he or she was a victim of a wrongful act and that in no way was he or she to blame.* Statements that imply the child might in some way have enticed the perpetrator into performing the act are inappropriate and may lead to serious compromise in the development of the child's self-esteem in the future. The welfare of siblings or other children in the household must also be considered, and an effort to discover the their status should be made.

About 80% of child sexual abuse involves a parent, guardian, other family member, mother's partner, or some other person known to the family Father–daughter incest accounts for about 75% of reported cases, with mother–son, father–son, mother–daughter, brother–sister, or incest involving another close family member constituting the remaining 25%. Brother–sister incest may be the most common form but may not be reported often.

Different states define incest in different legal terms. In some, intercourse is required; in others, it is not. Incest is noted to occur in all social groups, including cultures in which it is a stated taboo.

Families in which incestuous activity is taking place may appear normal, but family members frequently have limited contact with the outside world. Family relationships are often chaotic, including problems such as alcohol and drug abuse and severe mental illness. In father–daughter incestuous relationships the father is frequently a passive, introspective person who experiences a weak sexual relationship with the child's mother. He may therefore turn his attentions to his daughter or daughters out of loneliness, and the sexual activity may be quite affectionate. Frequently, the mother is aware of the situation, but both parents agree consciously or subconsciously that the incestuous relationship is more acceptable than an extramarital one. In such situations the daughter may assume more of the role of the wife around the house, fulfilling many homemaker duties.

Children who have been victimized by incest often feel guilty during adolescence. Many may be afraid to withdraw from the relationship out of fear that in so doing they would destroy the family and the security it provides. Such victims frequently feel humiliated and develop a weak ego and self-image. Because of this, these women may have difficulty in developing appropriate relationships with members of the opposite sex and may make poor choices in their interpersonal relationships in the future. They frequently choose chaotic family existences after they leave home. Fewer than 10% of children involved in incestuous relationships have normal psychological development at the time of evaluation. Usually, they exhibit guilt, anger, behavioral problems, unexplained physical complaints, lying, stealing, school failure, running away, and sleep disturbances.

Gynecologists may see such individuals as teenagers or young adults and may note that some or all of these complaints have been fully developed. When such a profile occurs, the gynecologist should investigate the possibility of a history of incest to fully understand the psychopathology of the patient. Appropriate questions such as, "Were you physically or sexually abused or raped as a child or adolescent?" should be asked as part of a routine history. Affirmative answers to any of these questions require specific detailed and discreet questioning of the individual involved and the circumstances of the incestuous act. The physician should assess the kinds of counseling the patient may already have experienced. Questioning should be nonjudgmental, clear, and specific. For example, the patient should be questioned about the sexual activity experienced and whether it included touching, genital manipulation, or intercourse. Often the individual is relieved to tell the health professional about her experience, because it may be something that she has never previously discussed. The knowledge that this is a common human experience and that the individual is blameless can be very helpful. The physician must then determine the necessity for an appropriate referral to a mental health worker.

Incest victims as adults frequently choose partners with inadequate personalities who may be capable of physical and sexual violence. This may be their unconscious desire to gravitate to a familiar relationship. It is equally possible that their poor social self-image may prevent them from achieving a stronger and more normal relationship.

Several studies have looked at the long-term follow-up of incest victims. Two separate studies in the 1970s, one by Lukianowicz and the other by Meiselman, found that daughters in father–daughter incestuous relationships demonstrated difficulties in sexual adjustment, including promiscuity and homosexuality. In 28 cases, 11 girls became promiscuous, as well as delinquent, and 4 of these became prostitutes. Of the 11, 5 married and had problems with sexual arousal and 4 demonstrated psychiatric symptoms of depression, anxiety, and suicidal ideology. Six, however, demonstrated no specific ill effects.

In another study by Browning and Boatman a gradual improvement in symptomatology occurred with time, regardless of whether treatment plans were followed. In specific instances of incestuous relationships with uncles, however, there was great anxiety over the possibility of repeat incest when the uncles were left at large. In this same study, violence was reported, including suicides in fathers and one murder of a mother by her son.

Earlier studies had suggested that the degree of emotional disturbance was greater the closer the relationship of the relative and that the degree was also related to whether genital contact actually took place. In a 1980 study of 796 college students Finkelhor reported that about one third of the incestuous activity occurred only once, but that in 27% the activity continued with varying frequency for more than a year. Of the involved individuals, 30% considered their experience positive, 30% negative, and the rest did not feel strongly one way or the other. In this series, women students who had sexual incestuous experiences as children were more likely to be sexually active. Experiences with siblings seemed to have a more positive effect on sexual development as long as the overall experience with the sibling was positive. Men who had sibling sexual experiences did not seem to have a higher current level of frequency of intercourse and seemed to have lower self-esteem. Thus, it is difficult to predict what overall long-term potential problems may occur in victims of incestuous experiences.

Whatever the effect childhood sexual abuse and incest may have on the development of psychological well-being and self-esteem in the victim, it is more and more clear that at least a subset of such victims develops physical complaints involving several organ systems including respiratory, gastrointestinal, musculoskeletal, and neurologic, as well as a variety of chronic pain syndromes. Forty percent to 50% of women with chronic pelvic pain report a history of abuse, either physical or sexual. Recently, chronic fatigue syndrome and bladder problems have been added to the list of problems associated with childhood sexual abuse. Therefore, physicians who have patients with such chronic problems should consider childhood sexual abuse and incest as a possible contributor and should offer counseling where appropriate as part of the treatment program.

ABUSE

Intimate Partner Violence

Domestic violence, partner abuse, intimate partner violence, the battered woman, and *spouse abuse* are terms referring to violence occurring between partners in an ongoing relationship even if they are not married. A battered woman is defined as any woman over the age of 16 with evidence of physical abuse on at least one occasion at the hands of an intimate male partner. The *battered wife syndrome* is defined as a symptom complex occurring as a result of violence in which a woman has at any time received deliberate, severe, or repeated (more than three times) physical abuse from her husband or significant male partner in which the minimal injury is bruising. *Intimate partner violence* is the CDC's currently preferred term because it allows for males or females to be the victim and intimate partners can be the same or opposite sex. Actual or threatened physical, sexual, or psychological abuse by a current or former spouse (including common-law spouses), dating partner, boyfriend or girlfriend is considered intimate partner violence. The actual physical abuse may vary from minimal activity, such as verbal abuse or threat of violence, to throwing an object, throwing an object at someone, pushing, slapping, kicking, hitting, beating, threatening with a weapon, or using a weapon. These acts may be spontaneous or intentionally planned. Most such violence is accompanied by mental abuse and intimidation. Partner abuse is often seen in conjunction with abuse of children and elderly persons in the same household.

It is difficult to ascertain the specific incidence of domestic violence, but it has been estimated that 2 million cases of domestic violence occur in the United States each year, and some authors have stated that at least 50% of family relationships are violent. In a 1984 U.S. Department of Justice study, 57% of 450,000 annual acts of family violence were committed by spouses or ex-spouses, and the wife was a victim in 93% of cases. In at least one fourth of these cases the violent acts had occurred at least three times in the previous 6 months. In 1990, FBI statistics reported similar findings. In addition, it has been estimated that between one third and one half of female homicide victims are murdered by their male partners, whereas only 12% of male homicide victims are killed by their female partners. In 1992, the AMA published guidelines for diagnosis and treatment of domestic violence. They noted that 47% of husbands who beat their wives do so three or more times per year, that 14% of ever-married women reported being raped by their current or former husbands, and that rape is a significant or major form of abuse in 54% of violent marriages. The AMA guidelines also summarized various studies noting that battered women may account for 22% to 35% of women seeking care for any reason in emergency departments (the majority of whom are seen by medical or nontrauma services) and 19% to 30% of injured women seen in emergency departments. They also noted that 14% of women seen in ambulatory care internal medicine clinics have been battered, and 28% of such women have been battered at some time. They state that 25% of women who attempt suicide, 25% who are receiving psychiatric services, and 23% of pregnant women seeking prenatal care have been victims of domestic violence. In addition, 45% to 59% of mothers of abused children have been abused and 58% of women older than 30 who have been raped have been abused. In a gynecologic clinic in England, John and colleagues surveyed a cohort of 825 women. Twenty-one percent reported physical of abuse, and of those, 48% also had forced sexual activity. Therefore, it can be seen that domestic violence and battered women are common in our society today.

The most common sites for injury are the head, neck, chest, abdomen, breast, and upper extremities. The upper extremities may be fractured as the woman attempts to defend herself. In a study from Yale, 84% of the injuries were severe enough to require medical treatment, and in 81% of the cases patients stated that the assailant had beaten them with the fists. In an English study of 100 women brought to a hostel for battered women, 44% suffered from lacerations and 59% stated that they had been kicked repeatedly. All women stated that they had been hit with a clenched fist. Fractures occurred in 32, and 9 of the women had been beaten and taken to the hostel unconscious. Other studies have demonstrated similar findings.

Murder and suicide are frequent components of the domestic violence problem. In a large study from Denver, Walker reported that three quarters of the battered patients felt that the batterer would kill them during the relationship, and almost half felt that they might kill the batterer. Of these victims, 11% stated that they had actually tried to kill the batterer, and 87% believed that they themselves would be the ones to die if someone were killed. One third of these women stated that they seriously considered committing suicide. Walker noted that victims and their attackers frequently are depressed and may move rapidly between suicidal and homicidal intent.

There is a strong relationship between spouse battering and child abuse. In Walker's study, 53% of men who abused their partners were noted also to abuse their children. Another one third had threatened to abuse their children. Interestingly, in the same relationship, 28% of the wives who themselves were abused stated that they had abused their children while living in the violent household, and an additional 6% thought that they might abuse their children at the time they were evaluated.

Physical abuse in pregnancy is quite common and may be referred to as *prenatal child abuse*. The incidence is somewhere between 1% and 20% depending on the study population. In one study, 81 of 742 (10.9%) patients visiting a prenatal clinic stated that they had been victims of abuse at some time in the past, and 29 of these women stated that the abuse had continued into the pregnancy. Violence may increase postpartum. One fifth of these noted an increase in abuse during pregnancy, and one third noted a decrease. Campbell and associates, in a study of a group of Medicaid-eligible postpartum women, noted a constellation of factors associated with violence during pregnancy. Of the patients in this study, 7% suffered battering, and significant correlates including anxiety, depression, housing problems, inadequate prenatal care, and drug and alcohol abuse were identified. The women in the study who were battered during pregnancy suffered a more severe constellation of symptoms than did those who were battered only prior to pregnancy. In the case of pregnant patients, most studies note that battering is frequently directed to the breasts and abdomen.

It is important that physicians increase their ability to recognize the signs of domestic violence and spouse abuse. A study by Hilberman and Monson demonstrated that 25% of women treated for injuries in an emergency room were victims of wife battering. The physicians who were treating these patients made the correct diagnosis originally in only 3% of cases. Viken has listed a profile of the characteristics of the abused wife. These include a history of having been beaten as a child, raised in a single-parent home, married as a teenager, and pregnant before marriage. Such women frequently visit clinics and emergency rooms with a variety of somatic complaints, including headaches, insomnia, choking sensation, hyperventilation, gastrointestinal symptoms, and chest, pelvic, and back pain. Noncompliance with the advice of physicians with respect to these complaints is frequent (see the following box).

In visits to the physician's office or emergency room the patient often appears shy, frightened, embarrassed, evasive, anxious, or passive and often cries. The batterer may accompany the patient

Somatic Complaints in Abused Women

Headaches
Insomnia
Choking sensation
Hyperventilation
Chest, back, or pelvic pain
Other signs and symptoms
- Shyness
- Fright
- Embarrassment
- Evasiveness
- Jumpiness
- Passivity
- Frequent crying
- Often accompanied by male partner
- Drug or alcohol abuse (often overdose)
- Injuries

From ACOG Technical Bulletin Number 124: The battered woman. January 1989.

on such visits and stay close at hand to monitor what is said to the physician. Thus, the woman may be hesitant to provide information about how she was injured, and the explanation given may not fit the injuries observed. Alcohol or other drug abuse is common in such individuals.

Physicians should become comfortable in asking the patient whether she has been physically abused. Every pregnant woman should be screened for intimate partner violence. Questions such as, "Has anyone hurt you or tried to injure you?" and "Have you ever been physically abused either recently or in the past?" are very appropriate introductory questions. The physician should follow up on any positive answers in a nonjudgmental manner in an attempt to learn what is happening. Physical examinations should be complete with particular attention to bruises, lacerations, burns, improbable injury, and other signs of injury. If the patient is wearing sunglasses, she should be asked to remove them so the physician can determine whether there are eye injuries. If the patient is pregnant, bruises seen on the breasts or abdomen should always be discussed. Physicians should carefully note evidence for abuse in the patient's record.

Battering acts tend to run in cycles consisting of three phases. The first phase is tension building, in which tension between the couple gradually escalates manifested by discrete acts that cause family friction. Name calling, intimidating remarks, meanness, and mild physical abuse such as pushing are common. Dissatisfaction and hostility are often expressed by the batterer in a somewhat chronic form. The victim may attempt to placate the batterer in hopes of pleasing him or calming him. She may actually believe at this point that she has the power to avoid aggravating the situation. She may not respond to his hostile actions and may even be successful from time to time in apparently reducing tensions. This, of course, will reinforce her belief that she can control the situation. As the tension phase builds, the batterer's anger is less controlled, and the victim may withdraw, fearing that she will inadvertently set off explosive behavior.

Often this withdrawal is the signal for the batterer to become more aggressive. Anything may spark the hostile act, and the acute battering then takes place. This is the cycle's second phase and is represented by an uncontrollable discharge of tension that has built up through the first phase. The attack may take the form of both verbal and physical abuse, and the victim is often left injured. In self-defense the victim may actually injure or kill the batterer. In approximately two thirds of cases reported by Walker, alcohol abuse was involved. However, the alcohol use may have been the excuse rather than the reason for the battering.

After the abuse has taken place, the third phase generally follows. In this situation, the batterer apologizes, asks forgiveness, and frequently shows kindness and remorse, showering the victim with gifts and promises. This gives the victim hope that the relationship can be saved and that the violence will not recur. Batterers are often charming and manipulative, offering the victim justification for forgiveness.

The cycles, however, do repeat themselves, with the first phase increasing in length and intensity, the battering becoming more severe, and the third phase tending to decrease in both duration and intensity. The batterer learns that he can control the victim without obtaining much forgiveness. The victim becomes more demoralized and loses her ability to leave the situation even if she has the means and opportunity to do so.

Batterers, too, tend to have a specific profile in most cases. They are men who refuse to take responsibility for their behavior, blaming their victims for their violent acts. They often have strong controlling personalities and do not tolerate autonomy in their partners. They have rigid expectations of marriage and sexual behavior and consider their wives or partners as chattel. They wish to be cared for in their most basic needs, frequently make unrealistic demands on their wives, and show low tolerance for stress. Depression and suicidal gestures are often a part of their behavior pattern, but in general they are aggressive and assaultive in most of their behavior, generally using violence to solve their problems. On the other hand, they are often charming and manipulative, especially in their relationships outside the marriage. They often exhibit low self-esteem, feelings of inadequacy, and a sense of helplessness, all of which are generally made worse by the prospects of losing their wives. It is typical behavior for male batterers to exhibit contempt for women in their usual activities. Therapy is usually ineffective and seems to work only when the man can be made to give up violence as his primary means of solving problems.

Once the physician discovers that a woman is living in an abusive relationship, it is important to acknowledge to the patient the seriousness of the situation. To do otherwise is to give the impression that the physician approves or at least accepts the violent condition. It is important to attend to the patient's injuries and to assess the patient's emotional status from the standpoint of a psychiatric condition such as a suicidal tendency, depression, anxiety reaction, or signs of abuse of drugs, alcohol, or other medications. The physician should also attempt to estimate the woman's ability to assess her own situation and her readiness to take appropriate action. If problems involving mental illness are present, a referral to an appropriate mental health worker who is sensitive to the issues of domestic violence should be made.

Physicians should determine community resources available for handling family violence. The acute situation can be helped by the police department, crisis hotline, rape relief centers, domestic violence programs, and legal aid services for abused women. Hospital emergency rooms and shelters for battered women and children are also excellent resources. Counseling and follow-up care can be offered by health care workers in these organizations or by private practitioners who specialize in the care of battered women, their spouses, and their children. Such individuals may be social workers, psychologists, psychiatrists, or other mental health workers trained specifically for this purpose. Many community hospitals, mental health departments, and community mental health services have set up counseling programs for such couples, since the problem is so common. The physician's job is to recognize the problem and either offer counseling or get counseling for the patient so that she understands her rights and alternatives and learns to protect herself and her children from future harm.

The victim of abuse very likely will not wish to leave her home because of economic concerns and a fear that the batterer may continue to pursue her. Although she may have the batterer arrested and served with restraining orders, she may be convinced that she and her children cannot be protected from the batterer. She may also believe that there is a possibility of reconciliation and of change in behavior on the part of the batterer. It is therefore reasonable to discuss an exit plan with the victim to be used should the violence recur. This exit plan should include the following:

1. Have a change of clothes packed for both her and her children including toilet articles, necessary medications, and an extra set of keys to the house and car. These can be placed in a suitcase and left with a friend or family member.
2. Keep some cash, a checkbook, and a savings account book with the friend or family member.
3. Other identification papers, such as birth certificates, social security cards, voter registration cards, utility bills, and driver's license, should be kept available, since children will need to be enrolled in school and financial assistance may have to be sought.
4. Have something special, such as a toy or book, for each child.
5. Have financial records available, such as mortgage papers, rent receipts, and an automobile title.
6. Determine a plan on exactly where to go regardless of the time of day or night. This may be to a friend or relative's house or to a shelter for battered women and children.
7. Ask neighbors to call police if violence begins.
8. Remove weapons.
9. Teach children to call 911.

Rehearsing an exit plan as one would conduct a fire drill makes it possible for the battered woman to respond even under the stress of the battering.

Long-term aid and referral of the patient, her children, and the batterer to the appropriate resources is an important aspect of the care of such patients. The American College of Obstetricians and Gynecologists has prepared a patient education brochure that physicians can keep in their offices and give to individuals who suffer from this problem. Making the brochures available in the office waiting room may encourage women with these needs to get help.

These women often suffer from severe psychiatric problems, such as anxiety, depression, post-traumatic stress disorder (PTSD) and other pathologic conditions, that may require psychotherapy. Women who are both physically and sexually assaulted have significantly higher levels of PTSD compared to women who are physically abused only. Group counseling or individual counseling may also help them to rebuild their lives as single individuals or single parents. It is frequently necessary to help them develop a skill that will enable them to be employable. Counseling programs take these things into consideration. Children of victims who may be victims as well also require counseling to avoid behavior patterns that will lead to aggressive behavior in their later lives.

Wife battering is a common problem that affects the family unit in particular and society in general. It can occur in all segments of society and reflects the violence that is a part of life today and the behavior of many. Physicians should learn to detect its presence in their patients and offer ways the victim can seek help. The help may include counseling for the victim, batterer, and children or constructing a plan for the woman to exit the relationship and rebuild her life in safety.

If the male batterer has not undergone violence elimination counseling, family counseling or intervention can be extremely dangerous as it often raises issues that exacerbate the violence and increase the risk of serious harm to the woman and her children. Therefore, this should not be advised until such time as the male batterer has addressed and eliminated his violent behavior. In general, success in such attempts with respect to the male partner is usually minimal.

Although all states have requirements for reporting child abuse, not all states require the reporting of domestic violence. However, many states have aggressive programs for intervening in domestic violence cases, and physicians should become aware of the programs in effect in their area. The patient should always be encouraged to leave a violent situation and may need community resources to help with economic and social adjustment, as well as protection for herself and her children from the violent partner.

The Elderly

The Select Committee on Aging in investigating domestic violence against the elderly held hearings before the Subcommittee of Human Services of the House of Representatives in 1980. The committee noted that approximately 500,000 to 2.5 million cases involving abuse of the elderly occur per year in the United States. The committee documented that abuse of the elderly may be as large a nationwide problem as child abuse. Usually, the abused person is a woman older than age 75, often with a physical impairment. She is generally white, widowed, and living with relatives. The abuser is generally an adult child living within the family but may also be a spouse. Counseling issues involve the entire family but particularly the individual causing the abuse. Physicians who care for geriatric patients should be alert for signs and symptoms of this type of domestic abuse; when it is found, community resources should be activated. All 50 states have passed legislation protecting the elderly from domestic violence and neglect. Forty-two states have mandatory reporting laws.

KEY POINTS

- The incidence of sexual abuse of women in the United States was estimated to be 73/100,000, accounting for 6% of all violent crimes.
- Sexual assault happens to people of all ages, races, and socioeconomic groups, but the very young, the mentally and physically handicapped, and the very old are particularly susceptible.
- Two phases of the rape-trauma syndrome occur. The first is the immediate or acute phase and lasts hours to days. The second, the reorganization stage, lasts months to years.
- In caring for rape-trauma victims, the physician's responsibilities are medical, medicolegal, and supportive.
- About 12% to 40% of victims who are sexually assaulted have injuries.
- Rape-trauma victims should always be treated as victims. At no time should guilt be implied.
- About 10% of all child abuse cases involve sexual abuse.
- As many as half a million children are sexually abused each year in the United States.
- Incestuous activity may be experienced by as many as 15% to 25% of all women and approximately 12% of all men.
- Approximately 80% of all cases of sexual abuse of children involve a family member.
- Father–daughter incest accounts for about 75% of reported cases; however, brother–sister incest may be the most common type, although it may not be reported often.
- As many as 25% of women treated for injuries in an emergency room are likely to be victims of wife battering. Diagnosis of this by a physician is rare.
- An estimated 2 million cases of domestic violence are reported in the United States each year.
- In 93% of the cases, the wife is the victim of the violence.
- More than half of the men who abuse their partners also abuse their children.
- About 10% of antepartum clinic patients may be victims of battering.
- Victims of battering demonstrate multiple somatic complaints.
- Two thirds of batterers who carry out violent acts are under the influence of alcohol, but this may be the excuse rather than the reason.
- If the male batterer has not undergone a violence elimination program, a referral of the family for family counseling should *not* be made because it may raise issues that exacerbate the violence.
- Between 500,000 and 2.5 million cases of abuse of the elderly reportedly occur in the United States each year.

BIBLIOGRAPHY

Key Readings

Browning DH, Boatman B: Incest: Children at risk. Am J Psychiatry 134:69, 1977.

Burgess AW, Holmstrom LL: Rape: Victims of crisis. Bowie, MD, RJ Brady, 1974.

Campbell JC, Poland ML, Waller JB, Ager J: Correlates of battering during pregnancy. R Nurs Health 15:219, 1992.

Finkelhor D: Sex among siblings. Arch Sex Behav 9:195, 1981.

Hilberman E, Monson K: Sixty battered women. Victimology 2:460, 1977.

Holmes MM, Resnick HS, Kilpatrick DG, Best CL: Rape-related pregnancy: Estimates and descriptive characteristics from a national sample of women. Am J Obstet Gynecol 175:320, 1996.

Jenny C, Hooton TM, Bowers A, et al: Sexually transmitted diseases in victims of rape. N Engl J Med 322:713, 1990.

Lukianowicz N: Incest. I. Paternal. II. Other types. Br J Psychiatry 120:301, 1972.

Meiselman KC: Incest: A psychological study of cases and effects with treatment recommendations. London, Jossey-Bass, 1978.

Muram D, Elias S: Child sexual abuse: Genital tract findings in prepubertal girls. II. Comparison of colposcopic and unaided examinations. Am J Obstet Gynecol 160:333, 1989.

Reynolds MW, Peipert JF, Collins B: Epidemiologic issues of sexually transmitted diseases in sexual assault victims. Obstet Gynecol Surv 55:51, 2000.

Rimsza ME, Niggemann EH: Medical evaluation of sexually abused children: A review of 311 cases. Pediatrics 69:8, 1982.

Sarafino EP: An estimate of nationwide incidence of sexual offenses against children. Child Welfare 58:127, 1979.

Viken RM: Family violence: Aids to recognition. Postgrad Med 71(5):115, 1982.

Walker LE: The battered woman syndrome. New York, Springer, 1984.

General References

American Academy of Pediatrics, Committee on Adolescence. Sexual assault and the adolescent. Peds 94:761, 1994.

American College of Obstetricians and Gynecologists: Domestic violence (Technical Bulletin Number 209). Washington, DC, ACOG, 1995.

American College of Obstetricians and Gynecologists: The Abused Woman (ACOG Patient Education Pamphlet APO83). Washington, DC, ACOG, 1989.

American College of Obstetricians and Gynecologists: Sexual Assault (Technical Bulletin Number 172). Washington, DC, ACOG, 1992.

American College of Obstetricians and Gynecologists: Female Genital Mutilation (Committee Opinion Number 151). Washington, DC, ACOG, 1995.

Bachmann GA, Moeller TP, Bennett J: Childhood sexual abuse and the consequences in adult women. Obstet Gynecol 71:631, 1988.

Barker B: Suicide by patient: Criminal charge against physician. JAMA 238(4):305, 1977.

Bowie SI, Silverman DC, Kalick SM, Edbril SD: Blitz rape and confidence rape: Implications for clinical intervention. Am J Psychother 44:180, 1990.

Campbell J, Jones AS, Dienemann J, et al: Intimate partner violence and physical health consequences. Arch Intern Med 162:1157, 2002.

Campbell JC, Soeken K: Forced sex and intimate partner violence: Effects on women's risk and women's health. Violence Against Women 51:1017, 1999.

Chang JC, Cluss PA, Ranieri LA, et al: Health care interventions for intimate partner violence: What women want. Women's Health Issues 15:21, 2005.

Chez RA: Elder abuse, the continuum of family violence. Prim Care Update OB/GYN 6:132, 1999.

Council Reports. Violence against women: Relevance for medical practitioners, Council on Scientific Affairs, American Medical Association. JAMA 267:3184, 1992.

Dienemann J, Glass N, Hyman R: Survivor preferences for response to IPV disclosure. Clin Nurs Res 14:215, 2005.

Ehrlich P, Anetzberger G: Survey of state public health departments on procedures for reporting elder abuse. Public Health Rep 106:151, 1991.

Elchalal V, Ben-Aut B, Gillis R, Brzenzinski A: Ritualistic female genital mutilation: Current status and future outlook. Obstet Gynecol Surv 92:643, 1997.

Female genital mutilation: A report of the WHO Technical Working Group, Geneva, 1995.

Flitcraft AH, Hadley SM, Hendricks-Matthews MD, et al: AMA Diagnostic and Treatment Guidelines on Domestic Violence. Chicago, AMA, 1992.
Flugel J: Psychoanalytic study of the family. London, The Hogarth Press, 1926.
Frazer M: Domestic violence: A medicolegal review. J Forensic Sci 31(4):1409, 1986.
Gazamararian JA, Lazorick S, Spitz AM, et al: Prevalence of violence against pregnant women. JAMA 275:1915, 1996.
Gelles RJ: Violence in the family: A review of research in the seventies. J Marriage Fam 42(4):873, 1980.
Gelles RJ, Cornel CP (eds): International Perspectives on Family Violence. Lexington, MA, Heath, 1983.
Gerber MR, Ganz ML, Lichter E, et al: Adverse health behaviors and the detection of partner violence by clinicians. Arch Intern Med 165:1016, 2005.
Giordano NH, Giordano JA: Elder abuse: A review of the literature. Soc Work 29:232, 1984.
Goldberg WG, Tomlanovich MC: Domestic violence, victims and emergency departments: New findings. JAMA 251(24):3259, 1984.
Hamberger LK, Ambuel B, Marbella A, et al: Physician interaction with battered women. The women's perspective. Arch Fam Med 7:575, 1998.
Hilberman E: Overview: The "wife-beater's wife" reconsidered. Am J Psychiatry 137(11):1336, 1980.
Hillard PJ: Physical abuse in pregnancy. Obstet Gynecol 66(2):185, 1985.
Holmes M, Resnick H, Kilpatrick D, et al: Rape-related pregnancy: Estimates and descriptive characteristics from a national sample of women. Am J Obstet Gynecol 175:320, 1996.
John R, Johnson JK, Kukreja S, et al: Domestic violence: Prevalence and association with gynaecological symptoms. Br J Obstet Gynecol 111:1122, 2004.
Jones JG: Sexual abuse of children. Am J Dis Child 136:142, 1982.
Kahn M, Sexton M: Sexual abuse of young children. Clin Pediatr 22:369, 1983.
Kaplan HS: The Evaluation of Sexual Disorders. New York, Brunner/Mazel, 1983.
Kempe CH: Sexual abuse: Another hidden pediatric problem. The 1977 C Anderson Aldrich Lecture. Pediatrics 62:382, 1978.
Klaus PA, Rand MR: Family Violence. Washington, DC, US Department of Justice, Bureau of Justice Statistics, 1984.
Latthe P, Migini L, Gray R, et al: Factors predisposing women to chronic pelvic pain: Systematic review. BMJ 332:749, 2006.
Lechner ME, Vogel ME, Garcia-Shelton LM, et al: Self-reported medical problems of adult female survivors of childhood sexual abuse. J Fam Pract 36:633, 1993.
Mahoney P: High rape chronicity and low rates of help-seeking among wife rape survivors in a nonclinical sample: Implications for research and practice. Violence Against Women 5:993, 1999.
Marx BP, Van Wie V, Gross AM: Date rape risk factors: A review and methodological critique of the literature. Aggression Violent Behavior 1:27, 1996.
McCauley J, Kern DE, Kolodner K, et al: Clinical characteristics of women with a history of childhood abuse. Unhealed wounds. JAMA 277:1362, 1997.
McFarlane J, Malecha A, Watson K, et al: Intimate partner sexual assault against women: Frequency, health consequences, and treatment outcomes. Obstet Gynecol 105:99, 2005.
McGrath ME, Hogan JW, Peipert JF: A prevalence survey of abuse and screening for abuse in urgent care patients. Obstet Gynecol 91:511, 1998.
Morgan SM: Conjugal terrorism: A psychological and community treatment model of wife abuse. Palo Alto, CA, R&E Research Associates, 1982.
Muram D, Hosteler BR, Jones CE, et al: Adolescent victims of sexual assault. J Adolesc Health 17:372, 1995.
Nadelson CC, Notman MT, Zackson H, et al: Follow-up study of rape victims. Am J Psychiatry 139:1267, 1982.
Pillemer K, Suitor JJ: Violence and violent feelings: What causes them among family caregivers? J Gerontol 47:S165, 1992.
Plichta SB: Intimate partner violence and physical health consequences. J Interpers Violence 19:1296, 2004.
Ramsay J, Feder G, Rivas C, et al: Advocacy interventions to reduce or eliminate violence and promote the physical and psychosocial well-being of women who experience intimate partner abuse (Protocol), The Cochrane Database Syst Rev 1:CD005043, 2005.
Rennison C, Wetchans S: Intimate partner violence. Washington, DC, U.S. Department of Justice, 2000.
Rennison DM: Rape and sexual assault: Reporting to police and medical attention, 1999–2000 (NCJ 194530). Washington, DC, U.S. Department of Justice, 2002.
Resnick HS, Holmes MM, Kilpatrick DG, et al: Predictors of post-rape medical care in a national sample of women. Am J Prev Med 19:214, 2000.
Rhynard J, Krebs M, Glover J: Sexual assault in dating relationships. J School Health 67:89, 1997.
Rodriguez MA, McLoughlin E, Nah G, et al: Mandatory reporting of domestic violence injuries to the police. What do emergency department patients think? JAMA 286:580, 2001.
Romans S, Belaise C, Martin J, et al: Childhood abuse and later medical disorders in women. An epidemiological study. Psychother Psychosom 71:141, 2002.
Sadler AG, Booth BM, Nielson D, et al: Health-related consequences of physical and sexual violence: Women in the military. Obstet Gynecol 96:473, 2000.
Sarles RM: Incest. Pediatrics 2:51, 1980.
Scarinci IC, McDonald-Haile J, Bradley LA, Richter JE: Altered pain perception and psychosocial features among women with gastrointestinal disorders and history of abuse: A preliminary model. Am J Med 97:108, 1994.
Schwarcz SK, Whittington WL: Sexual assault and sexually transmitted diseases: Detection and management in adults and children. Rev Infect Dis 12:S682, 1990.
Select Committee on Aging: Domestic violence against the elderly. Hearings before the Subcommittee of Human Services, House of Representatives, April 21, 1980, Washington, DC, 1980, US Government Printing Office.
Star B: Patterns of family violence. Soc Casework 60:339, 1980.
Steinman G: Rapid spot tests for identifying suspected semen specimens. Forensic Sci Interv 72:191, 1995.
Steward DE: Incidence of postpartum abuse in women with a history of abuse during pregnancy. CMAJ 151:1601, 1994.
Tjaden P, Thoennes N: Full report of prevalence, incidence, and consequences of violence against women survey (NCJ 183781). Washington, DC, U.S. Department of Justice, 2002.
Tjaden P, Thoennes N: Extent, nature and consequences of intimate partner violence: Findings from the national violence against women survey. Washington, DC, U.S. Department of Justice, 2000.
U.S. Department of Health and Human Services; Public Health Service; Health Resources and Services Administration: Surgeon General's Workshop on Violence and Public Health: Report. DHHS Publication No HRS-D-MC 86-1. Washington, DC, 1986, US Government Printing Office.
Walker LE: The Battered Woman, 2nd ed. New York, Springer, 2000.
Wenzl SL, Leake BD, Gelberg L: Health of homeless women with recent experience of rape. J Gen Intern Med 15:265, 2000.
Young WW, Bracken AC, Goddard MA, et al: Sexual assault: Review of a national model protocol and forensic medical evaluation. New Hampshire Sexual Assault Medical Examination Protocol Project Committee. Obstet Gynecol 80:878, 1992.
Zink T, Elder N, Jacobson J, et al: Medical management of intimate partner violence Considering the stages of change: Precontemplation and contemplation. Ann Fam Med 2:231, 2004.

Diagnostic Procedures 11

Imaging, Endometrial Sampling, Endoscopy: Indications and Contraindications, Complications

Vern L. Katz

KEY TERMS AND DEFINITIONS

Adhesiolysis. The cutting or lysis of adhesions.

Computed Tomography (CT). An imaging technique to detect soft tissue abnormalities that uses a computer to integrate differences in X-ray beam attenuation resulting from varying densities in adjacent tissue.

Endometrial Sampling. Obtaining a tissue biopsy of the endometrial lining by abrasion and by placing an instrument transcervically into the endometrial cavity.

Endometrial Stripe. A sonographic measurement of the endometrial thickness that correlates with endometrial pathology.

Falloposcopy/Salpingography. Visualization of the lumen of the fallopian tubes, usually performed transcervically with a microendoscope.

Gadolinium. A rare element used as a contrast agent for MRI scans because of its magnetically opaque nature.

Hysterosalpingography. An X-ray imaging technique whereby the uterine cavity and lumina of the fallopian tubes are visualized by injecting contrast material through the cervical canal.

Hysteroscopy. The direct visualization of the endometrial cavity using an endoscope, a light source, and a medium to distend the uterus.

Laparoscopy. Examination and inspection of the peritoneal cavity and pelvic organs by means of an endoscope and a light source.

Magnetic Resonance Imaging (MRI). An imaging technique using the resonance of hydrogen nuclei within tissue in a static magnetic field exposed to low-frequency radio waves.

Sonohysterography. A technique for ultrasonographic imaging of the uterine cavity by instilling saline transcervically through a small catheter.

Tubal Ring. A circular, clear-appearing ultrasound finding within the area of the adnexa, representing an early ectopic pregnancy.

Ultrasound. A noninvasive imaging technique using acoustic waves; modern equipment includes linear array and sector scan, endovaginal probes, and Doppler.

This chapter presents an overview of frequently used diagnostic procedures in gynecology. Indications, contraindications, and complications are included for each procedure. Detailed comparisons between modalities for specific indications are presented in the chapters pertaining to those pathologies. For those unfamiliar with the procedures, the diagnostic uses are described. Therapeutic uses are introduced, but details of these aspects of these techniques are covered elsewhere.

During the past five decades, there have been significant changes in the use of endoscopy in gynecologic practice. The fiberoptic bundle and more versatile light sources, as well as the incorporation of advances in technology, have dramatically increased the diagnostic and therapeutic capabilities of the hysteroscope and laparoscope. Colposcopy is discussed in Chapter 29 (Malignant Diseases of the Cervix). The use of computer technology has enhanced the ability of ultrasound and magnetic resonance (MR) to allow dramatic advances in imaging.

The tremendous advances in technology have led to the emergence of two directly conflicting trends in medical care. One is the increasing use of noninvasive diagnostic imaging. For example, the applications of magnetic resonance imaging (MRI) appear limitless. The conflicting trend stems from society's emphasis on cost containment, which curtails the impetus for ordering imaging procedures. As we face the future, expense is one of the foremost issues for the consumer and physician alike. The best use of limited resources should be our goal. Most diagnostic techniques have overlapping applications; thus the physician must choose the most appropriate technique for each patient. For example, it may be rare to order an MRI to stage endometrial cancer, but in a poor surgical candidate, it may be the best technique to evaluate myometrial invasion. When evaluating patients, the physician should try not to order "cafeteria style," one ultrasound, one computed tomography (CT), and then an MRI, but rather try to order the best test for the situation.

ULTRASOUND

Ultrasound, or sonography, is a noninvasive imaging technique that utilizes acoustic waves similar to sonar. Endovaginal ultrasound transducers fitted on endovaginal probes are the primary means of gynecologic imaging. The vaginal probes are placed in a sterile sheath, usually a glove or condom, prior to an examination. During the examination the woman is in a dorsal lithotomy position and has an empty bladder. Because the transducer is closer to the pelvic organs than when a transabdominal approach is employed, endovaginal resolution is usually superior.

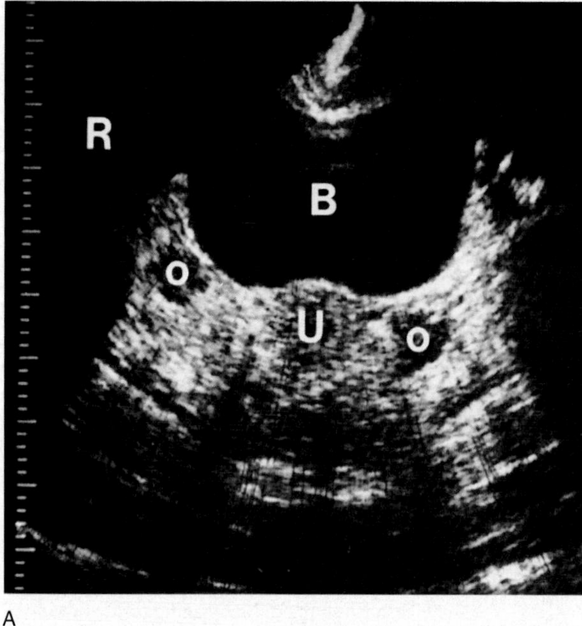

A

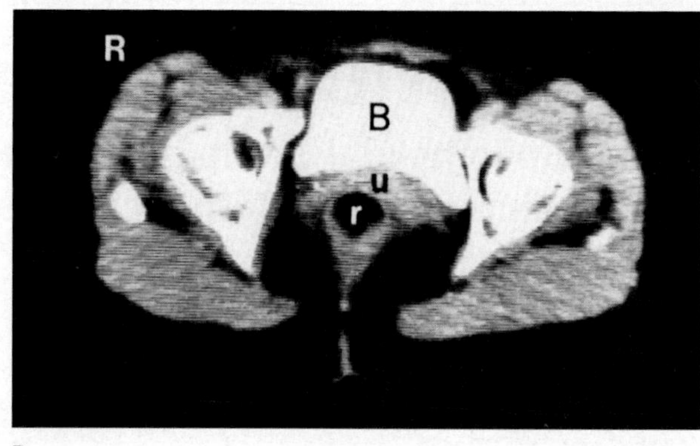

B

Figure 11-1. **A,** Transverse abdominal sonogram. **B,** CT scan of normal female pelvis. In sonogram, normal ovaries (o) and uterus (U) are seen posterior to bladder. On CT scan gas is seen in the rectum (r) posterior to the uterus; ovaries are not imaged (R, right; B, bladder). (From Sommer FG, Walsh JW, Schwartz PE, et al: Evaluation of gynecologic pelvic masses by ultrasound and computed tomography. J Reprod Med 27:47, 1982.)

However, if the pelvic structures to be studied have expanded and extend into the patient's abdomen, the organs are difficult to visualize with an endovaginal probe. Most ultrasound machines are equipped with both types of transducers.

For transabdominal gynecologic examinations, a sector scanner is preferable. It provides greater resolution of the pelvis and an easier examination than the linear array. During abdominal pelvic ultrasound examination, it is helpful for the patient to have a full bladder. This serves as an acoustic window for the high-frequency sound waves (Figs. 11-1 and 11-2). Ultrasound is more than 90% accurate in recognizing the presence of a pelvic mass, but does not establish a tissue diagnosis.

Ultrasonography employs an acoustic pulse echo technique. The transducer of the ultrasound machine is made up of piezo-electric crystals that vibrate and emit acoustic pulses. Acoustic echoes return from the tissues being scanned and cause the crystals to vibrate again and release an electric charge. The electric charges are then integrated by a computer within the ultrasound

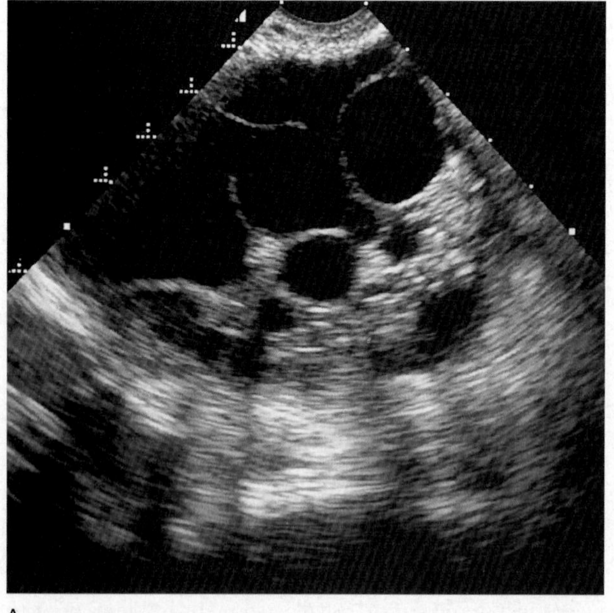

A

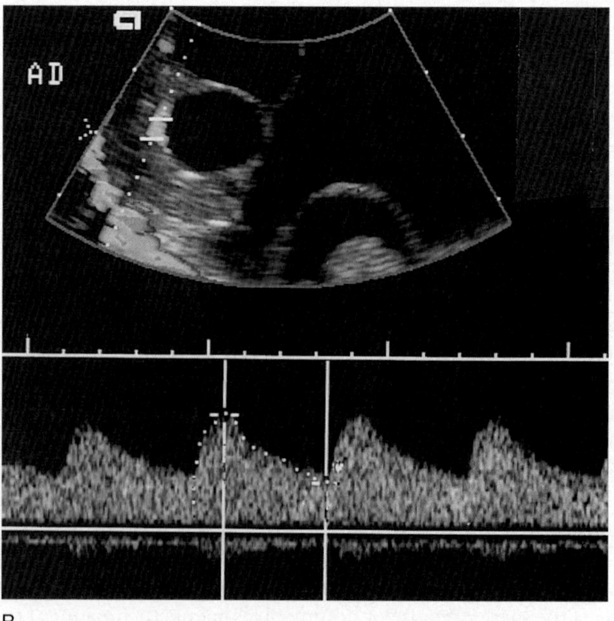

B

Figure 11-2. Ovarian cancer, contribution of Doppler in different patients. **A,** Transvaginal scan shows large multiseptated predominantly cystic mass with solid echogenic components. **B,** Same patient as part A. Spectral Doppler through area of vascularity in echogenic component (*cursors*) shows increased diastolic flow. Lowest PI obtained was 0.59 and RI 0.40. (From Salem S: The uterus and adnexa. In Rumack CM, Wilson SR, Charboneau JW (eds): Diagnostic Ultrasound, 2nd ed. St. Louis, Mosby, 1998, p 554.)

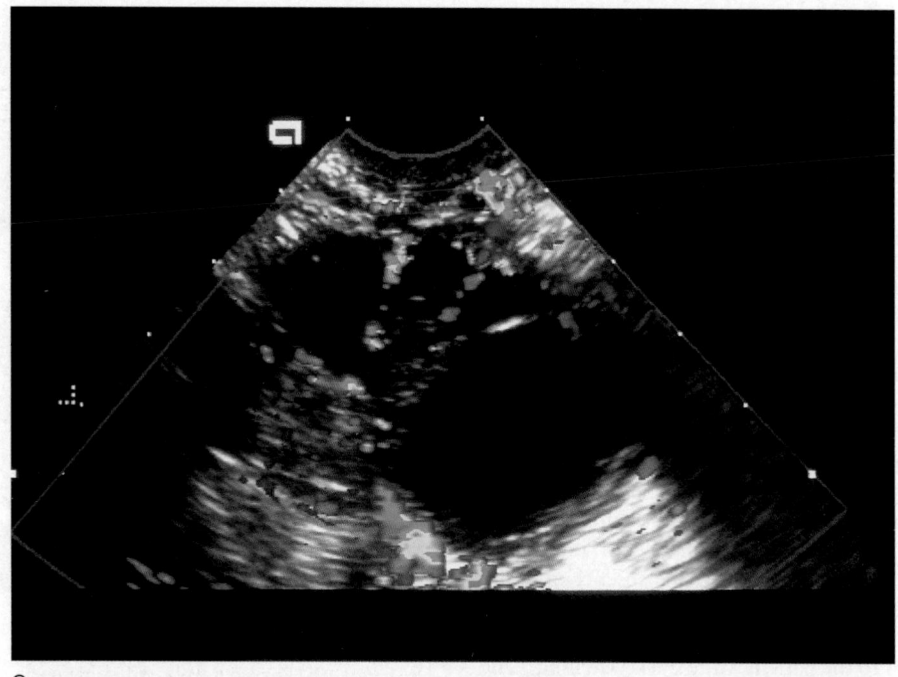

C

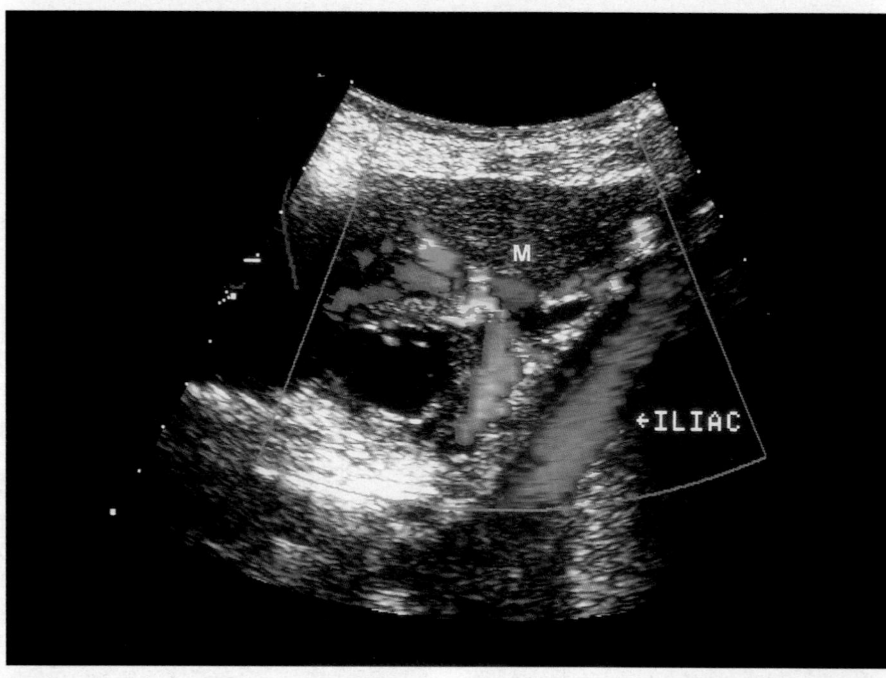

D

Figure 11-2. *cont'd,* **C,** Transvaginal color Doppler shows vascular septae in a multicystic mass. **D,** Transabdominal color Doppler shows vascularity in a predominantly solid mass (M). (From Salem S: The uterus and adnexa. In Rumack CM, Wilson SR, Charboneau JW: Diagnostic Ultrasound, 2nd ed. St. Louis, Mosby, 1998, p 554.)

machine to form the image. Present equipment provides resolution of less than 0.2 mm.

Doppler ultrasound techniques assess the frequency of returning echoes to determine the velocity of moving structures. Measurement of diastolic and systolic velocities provide indirect indices of vascular resistance. Muscular arteries have high resistance. Newly developed vessels, such as those arising in malignancies, have little vascular wall musculature and thus have low resistance. Many ultrasound signals per second may be evaluated, allowing direct measurement of blood flow. For example, this technique provides a noninvasive method of diagnosing deep vein thrombophlebitis of the legs. Color flow Doppler is a technique that usually displays shades of red and blue delineating blood flow within a neoplasm. For example, benign ovarian lesions have little color flow. When a color flow Doppler scan does demonstrate vascularity, the vascular resistance can be calculated. Low resistance is associated with malignancy, and high resistance usually is associated with normal tissue or benign disease. Color flow Doppler has been shown to be highly sensitive in evaluating ovarian malignancy.

Three-dimensional ultrasound is a computer technique in which multiple two-dimensional images are compiled to render either a surface- or volume-based image that appears to occupy space, as opposed to being flat. Three-dimensional ultrasound has of yet not been shown to have a specific diagnostic advantage in gynecology compared with other modalities.

A disadvantage of ultrasound is its poor penetration of bone and air; thus the pubic symphysis and air-filled intestines and rectum often inhibit visualization. Advantages of ultrasound include the real-time nature of the image, the absence of radiation, the ability to perform the procedure in the office before, during, or immediately after a pelvic examination, and the ability to describe the findings to the patient while she is watching. One of the most reassuring aspects of sonography is the absence of adverse clinical effects from the energy levels used in diagnostic studies.

The usefulness of ultrasound in gynecology depends largely on the pathologic conditions involved (Fig. 11-3.) Ultrasound-directed oocyte retrieval for in vitro fertilization is valuable because it allows for local anesthesia instead of retrieval by laparoscopy, which carries greater operative and anesthetic risks (Fig. 11-4). Ultrasound cannot differentiate absolutely a benign from a malignant process. However, several characteristics of ovarian masses correlate with malignancy, including septations; internal papillations—echogenic structures protruding into the mass; loculations; solid lesions, or cystic lesions with solid compo-nents; and smaller cysts adjacent to or part of the wall of the larger cyst-daughter cysts (Figs. 11-5 and 11-6).

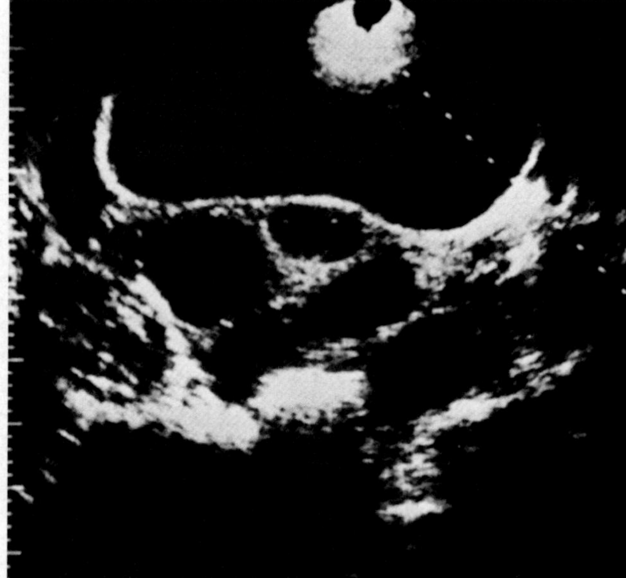

Figure 11-4. Transverse abdominal sonogram demonstrating multiple ovarian cysts in Pergonal-induced ovulation. (Reprinted from Fertility and Sterility, 37, DeCherney AH, Romero R, Polan ML, Ultrasound in reproductive endocrinology, 323. Copyright 1982, with permission from The American Society for Reproductive Medicine.)

Sonographic evaluation of endometrial pathology involves measurement of the endometrial thickness or stripe. The normal endometrial thickness is 4 mm or less in a postmenopausal woman not taking hormones. The thickness varies in premenopausal women at different times of the menstrual cycle and in women taking hormone replacement (Fig. 11-7). In this sense, a 5-mm cutoff cannot be applied to these women other than postmenopausal women. The endometrial thickness is measured in the longitudinal plane, from outer margin to outer margin, at the widest part of the endometrium. Ultrasound is not a screening tool in asymptomatic women. However, several studies

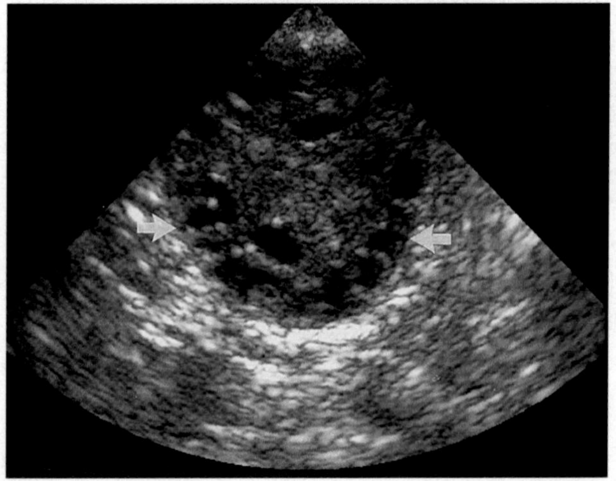

A

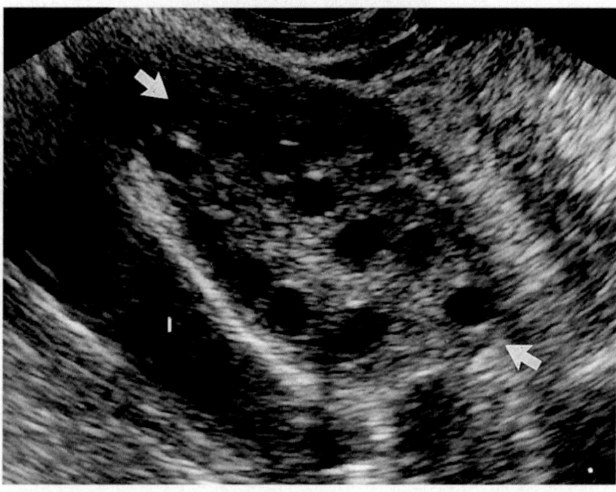

B

Figure 11-3. Polycystic ovarian disease, typical appearances. Transvaginal scans. **A,** Enlarged round ovary (*arrows*) with increased stromal echogenicity and multiple peripheral cysts; "string of pearls" sign. **B,** Enlarged ovary (*arrows*) with multiple peripheral and central cysts. I, internal iliac vein. (From Salem S: The uterus and adnexa. In Rumack CM, Wilson SR, Charboneau JW [eds]: Diagnostic Ultrasound, 2nd ed. St. Louis, Mosby, 1998, p 550.)

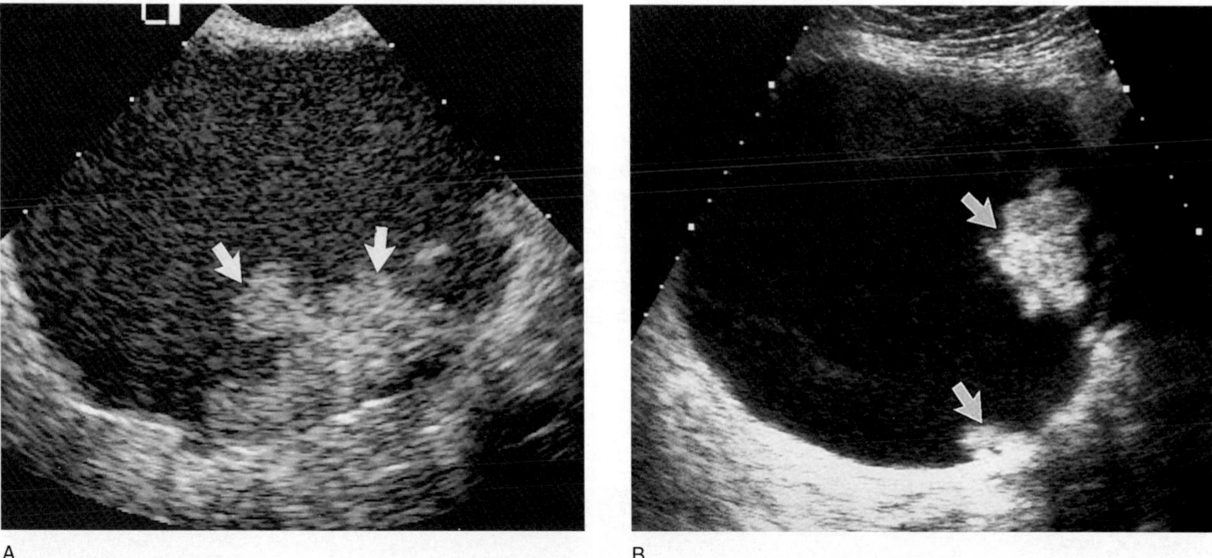

Figure 11-5. Serous cystadenocarcinoma, varying appearances. **A,** Transvaginal scan shows large cystic mass containing multiple low-level internal echoes and solid echogenic components (*arrows*). **B,** transabdominal scan shows large cystic mass with irregular solid echogenic mural nodules (*arrows*) and low-level internal echoes. (From Salem S: The uterus and adnexa. In Rumack CM, Wilson SR, Charboneau JW [eds]: Diagnostic Ultrasound, 2nd ed. St. Louis, Mosby, 1998, p 555.)

of postmenopausal women with vaginal bleeding have documented that malignancy is extremely rare in women with an endometrial thickness of 4 mm or less. Systematic reviews have noted that ultrasound may be reliably used to predict 96% to 99% of endometrial cancers in women with postmenopausal bleeding. The flip side of the coin is that 1% to 4% of malignancies will be missed using a cutoff of less than 4 mm. In addition, papillary-serous adenocarcinomas of the endometrium do not always develop endometrial stripe thickness. Two caveats for using ultrasound in screening of postmenopausal bleeding: (1) Ultrasound does not provide a diagnosis—a tissue specimen is necessary for a diagnosis. (2) All women with bleeding, no matter the endometrial thickness, need a tissue biopsy. If an endometrial biopsy obtains inadequate tissue and the endometrial thickness is 5 mm or greater, a repeat biopsy, hysteroscopically directed biopsy, or curettage should be performed.

Sonohysterography is an easily accomplished and validated technique for evaluating the endometrial cavity. The technique

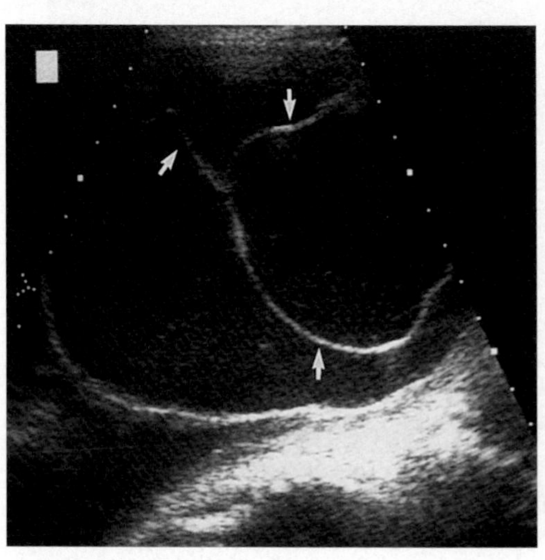

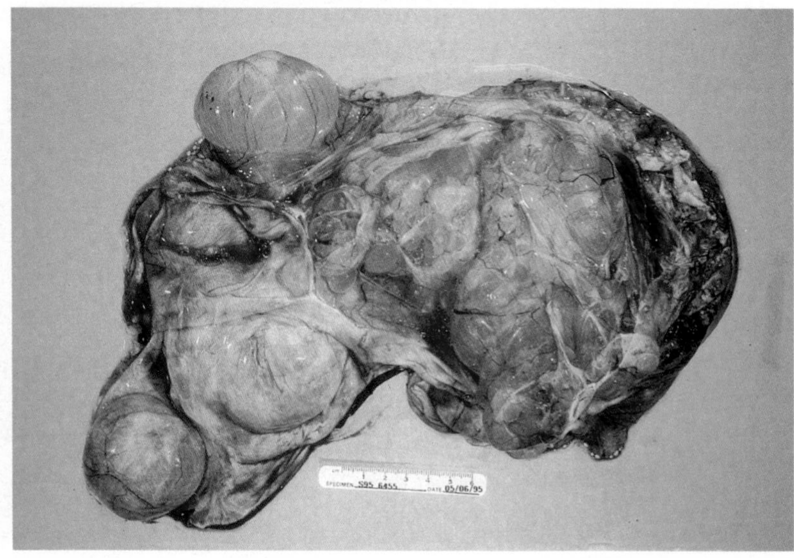

Figure 11-6. Mucinous cystadenoma. **A,** Transabdominal scan shows large cystic mass with multiple thin septations (*arrows*) and fine low-level internal echoes. **B,** Gross pathologic specimen shows multiple cystic loculations. (From Salem S: The uterus and adnexa. In Rumack CM, Wilson SR, Charboneau JW [eds]: Diagnostic Ultrasound. St. Louis, Mosby, 1998, p 556.)

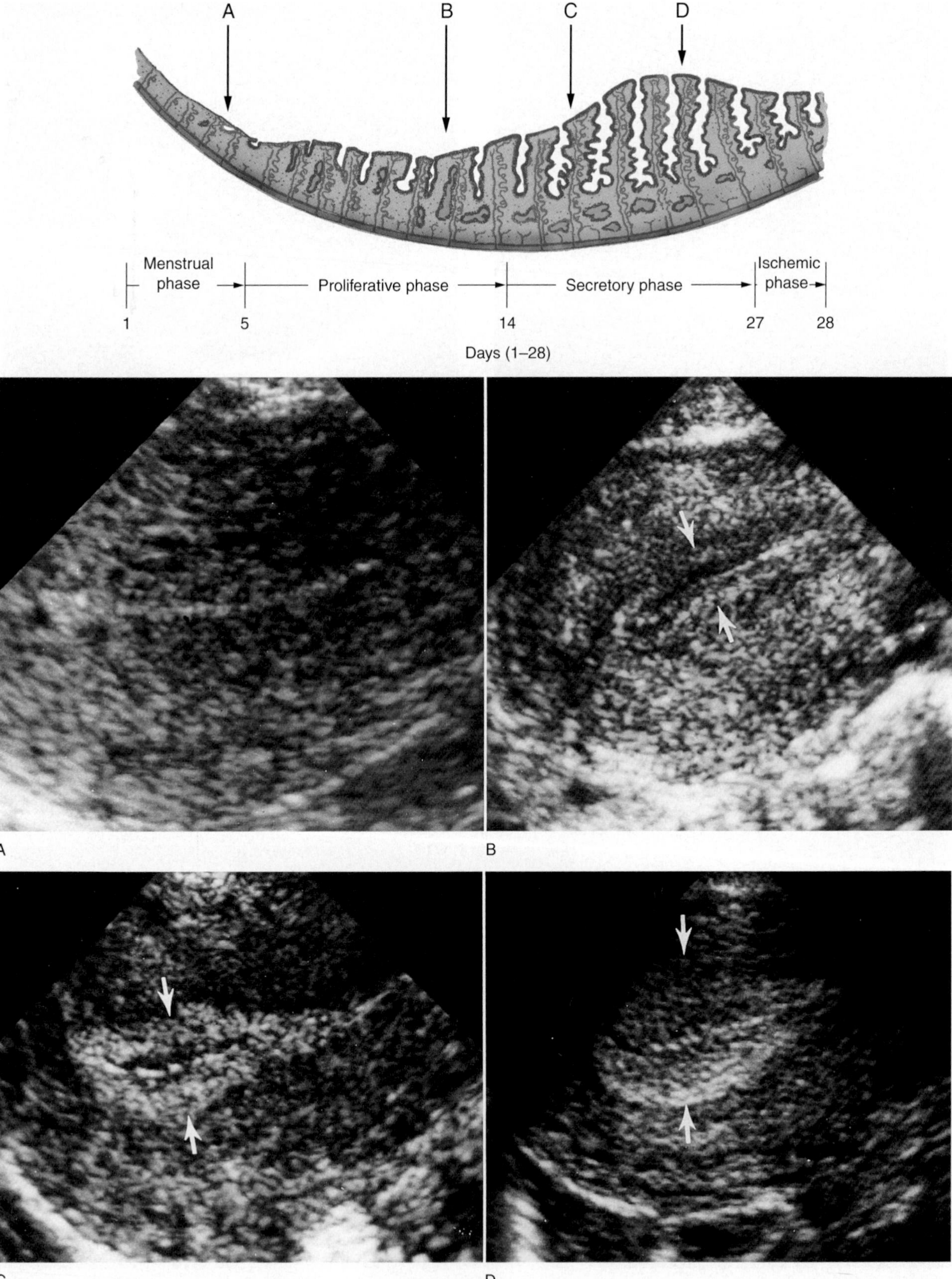

Figure 11-7. Variation in endometrium during menstrual cycle. **A,** Early proliferative phase. **B,** Late proliferative phase. **C,** Periovulatory phase. **D,** Late secretory phase. Note increase in endometrial thickness throughout the menstrual cycle. Also note multilayered appearance in the late proliferative phase. (From Fleischer AC, Kepple DM: Benign conditions of the uterus, cervix, and endometrium. In Nyberg DA, Hill LM, Bohm-Velez M, Mendelson EB [eds]: Transvaginal Ultrasound. St. Louis, Mosby–Year Book, 1992.)

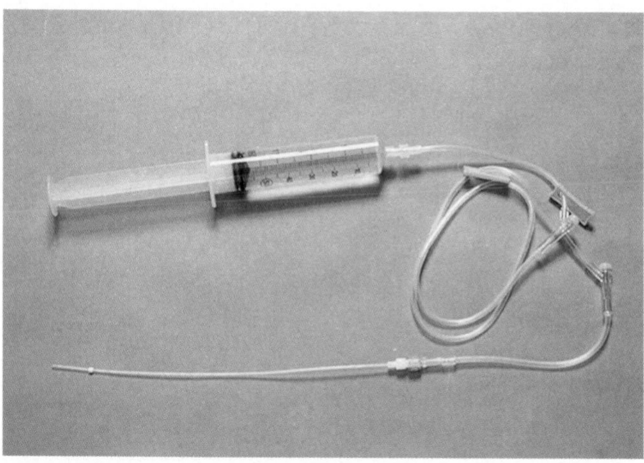

Figure 11-8. The Soules intrauterine insemination catheter for sonohysterography. (From Goldberg JM, Falcone T: Atlas of Endoscopic Techniques in Gynecology. London, WB Saunders, 2000, p 25.)

involves instilling saline into the uterine cavity. Sonohysterography is an alternative to office hysteroscopy. In this procedure, a thin balloon-tipped catheter or intrauterine insemination catheter is inserted through the cervical os and 5 to 30 mL of warmed saline is slowly injected into the uterine cavity (Fig. 11-8). Meta-analyses of sonohysterography have found the procedure to be successful in obtaining information in 95% of women, with minimal complications. Contraindications are active cervical or uterine infection. Some clinicians will have patients take a dose of ibuprofen prior to the procedure. Preferably, sonohysterography is performed in the proliferative phase of the cycle when the endometrial lining is at its lowest level. Sonohysterography has also been helpful in the evaluation of polyps, filling defects, submucous myomas, and uterine septae (Figs. 11-9 and 11-10). Importantly, sonohysterography, as with all types of ultrasound, does not make a tissue diagnosis.

Ultrasound not only provides a real-time view but also allows scanning in multiple planes and thus has some advantages over CT. Ultrasound demonstrates advanced manifestations of pelvic neoplasm such as ascites and hydronephrosis. Three-dimensional ultrasound is now in its early stages of development. Clinical applications will be evaluated over the next decade.

Ultrasound is clinically useful in the differential diagnosis of abnormalities of early pregnancy. The characteristic "snowstorm" pattern of ill-defined echogenic areas inside the uterus is pathognomonic of hydatidiform mole. Ultrasound is also of value in differentiating an intrauterine from an ectopic pregnancy. In early pregnancy the single ring inside the uterus may be either a gestational or a pseudogestational sac. The pseudogestational sac is formed by the decidual reaction that accompanies an ectopic pregnancy. Intrauterine pregnancies may be visualized as early as 4 weeks after the last menstrual period with an human chorionic gonadotropin (HCG) titer of approximately 1000 mIU/mL. A pregnancy should be routinely visualized by the fifth postmenstrual week or when the gestational sac is 4 mm or greater in diameter. Endovaginal scanning can help differentiate the tubal ring or halo (a clear, circular adnexal structure that represents an ectopic gestation) from the corpus luteum.

Sonography is the method of choice to locate a "missing" intrauterine device (IUD). It will help in diagnosing perforation of the uterus or unrecognized expulsion of the device. Endovaginal ultrasound transducers equipped with needle guides are frequently used for oocyte aspiration as part of in vitro fertilization.

The use of ultrasonography in women with pelvic infection has been disappointing. Swayne and colleagues discovered that acute pelvic inflammatory disease produced images similar to those seen in many other pelvic abnormalities. The lack of specificity in gynecology is a major limitation of ultrasonography. Gas- or fluid-filled intestines are commonly misinterpreted as gynecologic problems.

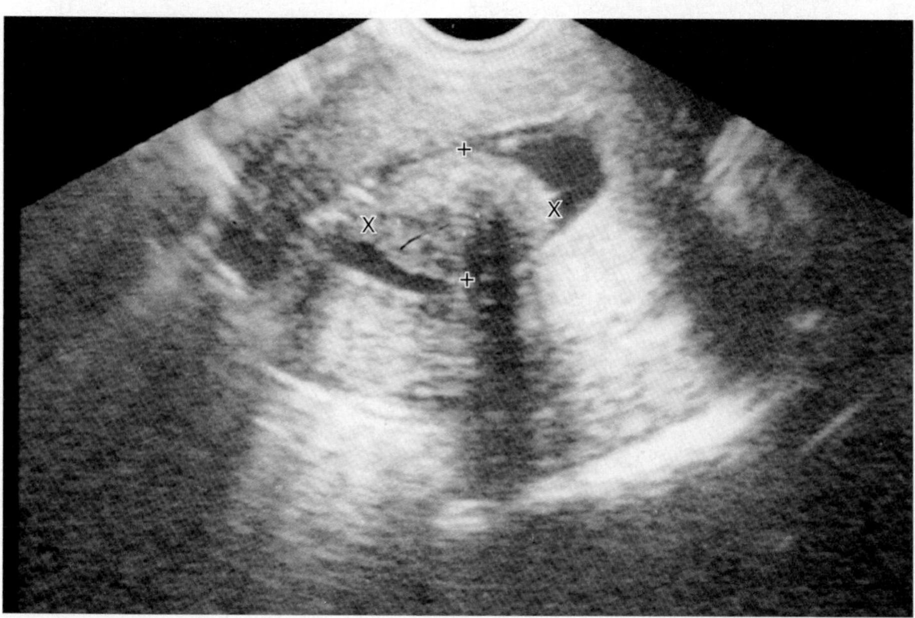

Figure 11-9. Endovaginal ultrasound using sonohysterography of an endometrial polyp in a perimenopausal woman with abnormal bleeding and secretory endometrium on endometrial biopsy. The x and + markings denote two of the dimensions of the polyp. (Courtesy of Marc A. Fritz, MD, University of North Carolina, Chapel Hill.)

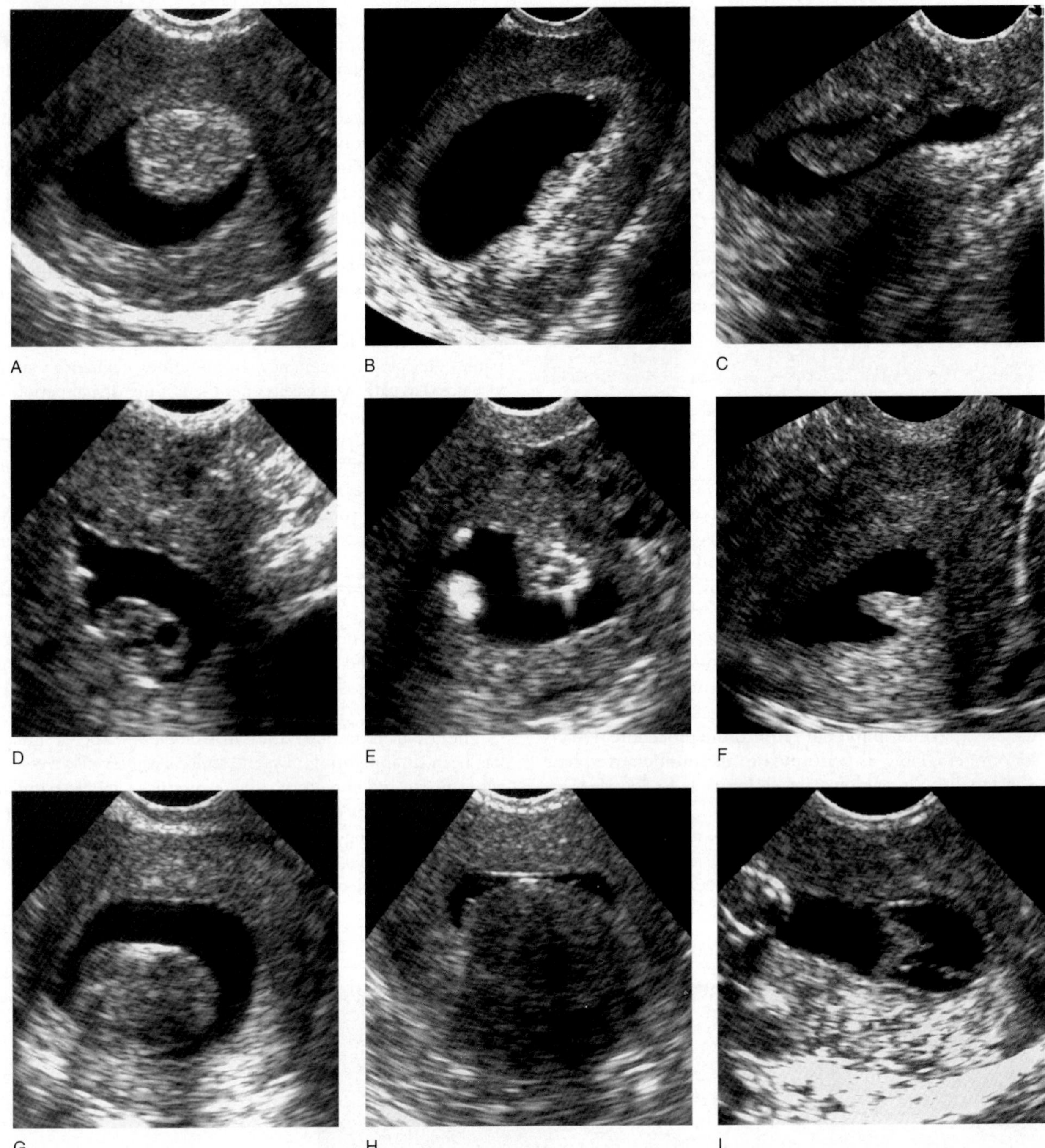

Figure 11-10. Sonohysterograms. **A,** Well-defined, round echogenic polyp. **B,** Carpet of small polyps. **C,** Polyp on a stalk. **D,** Polyp with cystic areas. **E,** Small polyp. **F,** Small polyp. **G,** Hypoechoic submucosal fibroid. **H,** Hypoechoic attenuating submucosal fibroid. **I,** Endometrial adhesions. Note bridging bands of tissue within fluid-filled endometrial canal. (From Salem S: The uterus and adnexa. In Rumack CM, Wilson SR, Charboneau JW [eds]: Diagnostic Ultrasound, 2nd ed. St. Louis, Mosby, 1998, p 538.)

Ultrasound is often used to follow growth and resolution of myomas. It has been advocated by some in the evaluation of women using tamoxifen. Ultrasound has also been suggested as an adjunctive modality for evaluation of the lower urinary tract and anatomic integrity of the rectal sphincter. Some physicians use ultrasound as a screening method to evaluate the size of the ovaries of postmenopausal women at high risk for ovarian neoplasia.

In summary, ultrasound has become an extremely valuable adjunct to the bimanual examination. In many patients, particularly obese patients, it is superior to bimanual examination alone. An endovaginal ultrasound of an early pregnancy has become a mainstay in the evaluation of the pregnant woman with first-trimester vaginal bleeding. The measurement of endometrial thickness in post- and perimenopausal vaginal bleeding is an important diagnostic test. Whether ultrasound should be used for screening for ovarian cancer is still being investigated.

COMPUTED TOMOGRAPHY

High-resolution CT is one of the leading examples of advanced technology in gynecology. CT provides detailed, two-dimensional images. Newer technologies will provide for three-dimensional images within the next decade. The ability to image anatomic areas in a cross section a few millimeters thick has varied clinical applications. CT is popular in studies of the central nervous system, and it has revolutionized the clinical practice of neurology and neurosurgery. The critics of CT cite the expense of the equipment and its adverse effect on cost containment. Proponents counter that CT scans reduce the need for other imaging techniques.

A CT scan identifies gross distortions in local anatomy by using the difference in X-ray beam attenuation that results from different densities in adjacent tissues. For example, this technique is excellent in discovering extension of pelvic cancer into the fat of the retroperitoneal space. It is also helpful in identifying peritoneal implants and abdominal fluid collections. Even so, CT definitely has its limitations. Abnormal masses are visualized, yet a definitive pathologic diagnosis cannot be established until a surgical biopsy is performed, because most masses do not have distinctive enough anatomic shapes or unique density characteristics. The CT scan may recognize a group of enlarged lymph nodes adjacent to pelvic vessels but cannot differentiate between benign hyperplasia or metastatic carcinoma. CT is often used for directed placement of needles or catheters to affect drainage from abdominal fluid collections or abscesses.

Several improvements have been made in machinery for CT since its introduction into clinical medicine. The machine rotates the X-ray beam in an arc of 180° perpendicular to the long axis of the body. A group of crystal detectors are directly opposite the narrow beam, only 2 to 10 mm wide. These crystals are capable of photon detection efficiencies of approximately 80%. The detectors measure the amount of tissue absorption, and a computer then develops two-dimensional images of the cross-sectional planes under investigation.

The best images from CT are visualized when there are significant differences in tissue densities. To enhance visualization, contrast medium may be given intravenously, orally, and/or rectally to outline the urinary and upper and lower gastrointestinal tracts. Helical CT is a modification of standard CT that uses movement of the patient combined with rotation of several X-ray registers in a spiraling fashion. Varying speeds of rotation of the X-ray beams and the addition of several X-ray registers has produced several advantages over traditional CT. A tight helix or spiral of images is obtained that may be reconstructed and manipulated by the computer to produce a more detailed image. Vascular images are of a high enough quality that in many centers, helical CT has replaced pulmonary angiography and ventilation-perfusion scans for the diagnosis of pulmonary embolism (Fig. 11-11). Helical CT provides two improvements over standard CT. The first is a much faster procedure, only a few minutes in duration. The second is many more images from differing angles. Movement artifact, such as from intestinal peristalsis, is eliminated; as a result, helical CT is the imaging modality of choice in the diagnosis of appendicitis. Using helical CT to avoid the distortion of intestinal activity, CT has been found to be up to 98% sensitive compared with up to 90% for ultrasound (Fig. 11-12). The applications for gynecology are still being evaluated.

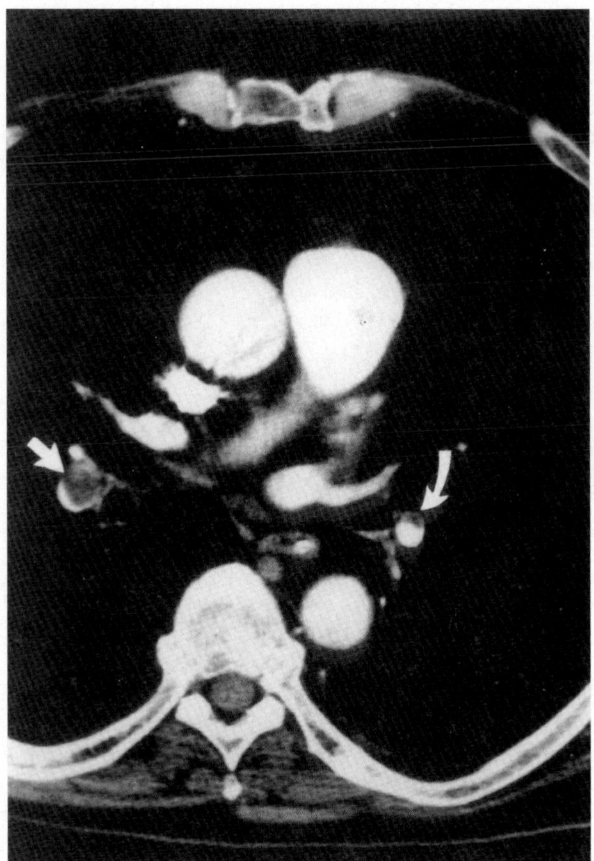

Figure 11-11. Bilateral filling defects in the opacified lower lobe pulmonary arteries, central on the right (*straight arrow*) and peripheral on the left (*curved arrow*). (From Grenier PA, Beigelman C: Spiral computed tomographic scanning and magnetic resonance angiography for the diagnosis of pulmonary embolism. Thorax 53(Suppl 2):S25, 1998.)

CT is used extensively in gynecologic oncology. In general, it is more useful to the clinician in staging than in diagnosis (Fig. 11-13). CT is superior to ultrasound in the diagnosis of retroperitoneal and intraperitoneal metastases. The lower limit of detectable intraperitoneal implants is between 1 and 5 mm. Nelson and coworkers summarized several studies and found a detection rate of 50% to 60% of intraperitoneal disease. Often a CT scan helps in the initial evaluation of a pelvic neoplasm. Although imperfect, CT scans are a valuable noninvasive technique to screen for retroperitoneal metastatic disease. A CT scan is able to identify an enlarged lymph node when it reaches a diameter of 1.5 to 2 cm. Unfortunately, there are many false-negative results.

In patients with ovarian carcinoma, the primary use of CT scans is in evaluating the extent of the disease. The CT is helpful

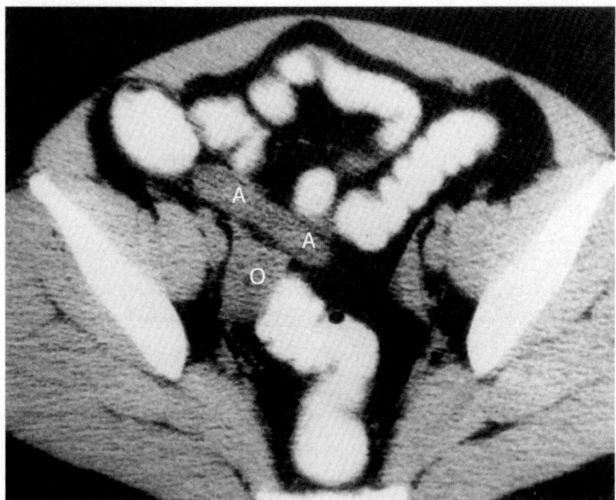

Figure 11-12. Computed tomography scan of a 54-year-old woman with an inflamed appendix (A) adjacent to the right ovary (O). (From Rao PM, Feltmate CM, Rhea JT, et al: Helical computed tomography in differentiating appendicitis and acute gynecologic conditions. Obstet Gynecol 93:417, 1999).

Figure 11-13. Stage IIB cervical carcinoma. CT scan through bladder (B) and uterine corpus (U). Right obturator lymph node metastasis (*arrow*), 2 cm in diameter, and left ovarian endometrioma (E) confirmed at laparotomy. (From Walsh JW, Goplerud DR: Prospective comparison between clinical and CT staging in primary cervical carcinoma. AJR 137:1000, 1981. © Copyright 1981 by the American Roentgen Ray Society. Reprinted with permission from the American Journal of Roentgenology.)

in that it reduces the need for multiple tests. An abdominal pelvic CT may serve to replace an intravenous pyelogram (IVP), barium enema, and liver and spleen scan to assess metastatic disease. It is an excellent technique to discern collections of ascites (Fig. 11-14). CT scans give further information of retroperitoneal involvement and ureteral obstruction. A scan may miss small areas of metastatic spread, especially along serosal surfaces. If the area of carcinoma is less than 5 mm in diameter and is on a visceral surface, it is unlikely to be visualized by this imaging technique. Studies are ongoing as to the use of CT to predict the success of cytoreduction surgery with ovarian malignancy.

CT scans have been used to diagnose other intraabdominal and pelvic problems in gynecology (Fig. 11-15). CT is valuable in identifying intraabdominal abscesses. In the postoperative patient with unexplained fever, CT is often helpful in assessing the abdomen and pelvis. CT scans also facilitate the drainage of abnormal fluid collections and are helpful in the evaluation of acute infection processes. After an abscess is localized, it may be possible to aspirate and drain using radiologic imaging techniques. Because of differences among fat, hair, and bone, CT is very accurate in the diagnosis of cystic teratoma. It is an excellent technique for confirming the diagnosis of ovarian vein thrombophlebitis (Fig. 11-16). When a linear mass is identified from the adnexal area to the vena cava or renal vein, the diagnosis is established, and appropriate medical therapy can be started.

The surface radiation dose for abdominal pelvic CT is about 2 rads and rarely as much as 10 rads. The dose to the midpelvis is approximately 50% of the surface dose. This radiation exposure is similar to that from a barium enema. Newer CT machines can vary the amount of radiation if there is a particular area of focus. One relative contraindication to the diagnostic use of

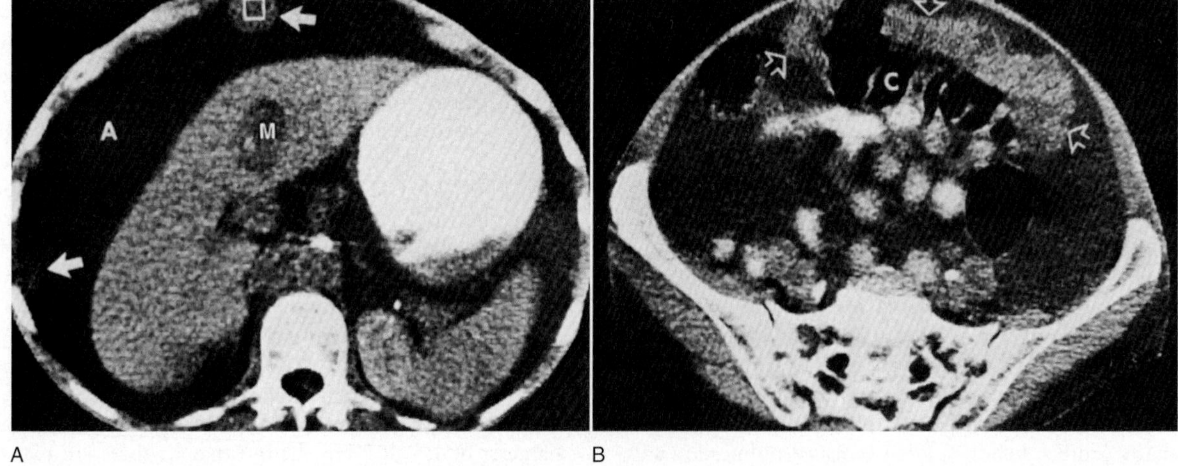

Figure 11-14. Metastatic ovarian carcinoma demonstrated by CT scan. **A,** Recurrent carcinoma is evident in this patient by ascites (A), liver metastases (M), and peritoneal metastatic implants (*arrows*). **B,** Omental metastases are also seen as a flattened mass (*arrows*) lying on top of transverse colon (C) in this patient. (From Federle MP: Female Patient 9:45, 1984.)

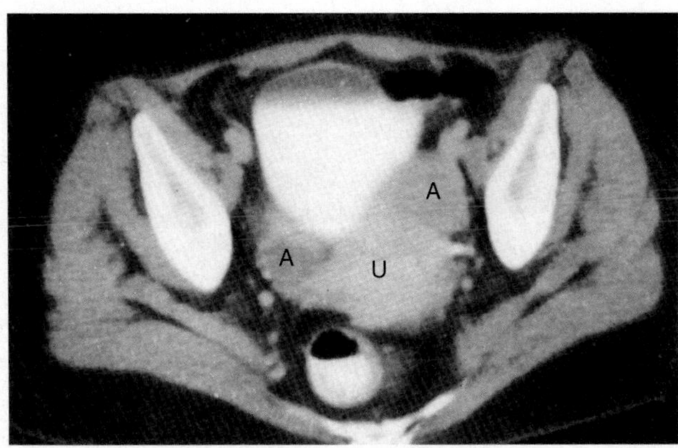

Figure 11-15. CT scan of patient with pelvic inflammatory disease with bilateral adnexal masses. A, tuboovarian abscesses; U, uterus. (From Gross BH, Moss AA, Mihara K, et al: Computed tomography of gynecologic diseases. AJR 141:771, 1983. © Copyright 1983 by the American Roentgen Ray Society. Reprinted with permission from the American Journal of Roentgenology.)

CT is the inability to tolerate the radiopaque contrast medium necessary for adequate visualization, usually secondary to allergic reactions to iodine.

In summary, CT scans are useful in evaluating pituitary tumors and in evaluating the spread of malignancy during the evaluation of a woman with a pelvic carcinoma.

MAGNETIC RESONANCE

MRI may be the greatest advance in radiology in the past four decades. The phenomenon of nuclear magnetic resonance was first discovered in 1945 and was renamed *magnetic resonance imaging* to avoid misinterpretation of the word *nuclear* by the public.

MRI is a technique that uses radio frequency nonionizing radiation and a varying magnetic field. The patient is placed within the machine, and a magnetic field is produced. The image depends on the resonant absorption and emission of radio waves by the atomic nuclei in the various tissues being observed. Because of their intrinsic magnetism, the nuclei act like small bar magnets and are influenced by the machine's magnetic field. The summation of the resonance of the vast number of atomic nuclei in a single thin slice of tissue provides the overall result. Resolution is 0.5 to 1 mm. The intensity of the image can be modified by varying the magnetic field.

Images are tomographic (in thin slices) and may be visualized in multiple planes, including coronal, sagittal, or transverse planes. This is particularly valuable in delineating pelvic structures that do not lie in perpendicular planes. The radio waves penetrate bone and air without attenuation. Thus MRI allows identification of soft tissue lesions inaccessible to other imaging techniques. Liquid and fat show up quite differently when different types of proton spin (T1 versus T2) are compared. Thus, unlike radiographs, in which tissue density determines the nature of the image, in an MRI the inherent type of tissue determines what the image looks like. The addition of computer analysis further increases MRI sensitivity by selecting and filtering out particular frequencies such as those from fat, thus allowing further delineation between types of tissue. These differences between MRI and CT are why many investigators believe that MRI examinations yield more information for the musculoskeletal system and pelvis than CT.

MRI uses nonionizing radiation. Extensive basic investigations have demonstrated no evidence of mutagenic effects in studies of bacteria, and no chromosomal changes were produced in human lymphocytes. No adverse or harmful effects have been reported from repetitive examinations. MRI is considered safe in pregnancy.

MRI can differentiate normal from malignant tissue and also can identify areas of abnormal tissue metabolism. MRI is most specific in the diagnosis of conditions associated with edema. Edema prolongs the spin–spin proton relaxation time (T2), thereby producing a stronger image. Investigators have discovered

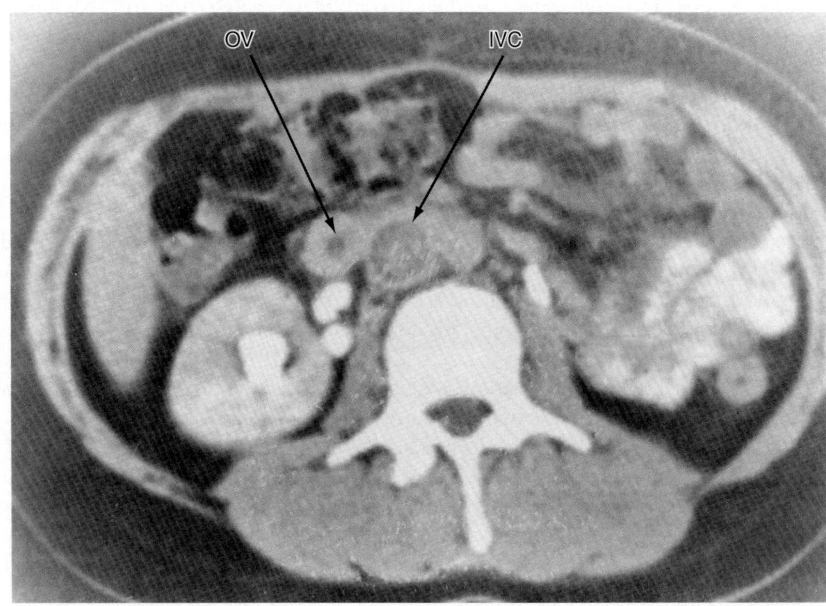

Figure 11-16. CT image of abdomen. Note thrombus within lumen of right ovary (OV) and inferior vena cava (IVC). Right ovarian vein is markedly enlarged. (From Angel JL, Knuppel RA: Computed tomography in diagnosis of puerperal ovarian vein thrombosis. Obstet Gynecol 63:62, 1984. Reprinted with permission from The American College of Obstetricians and Gynecologists.)

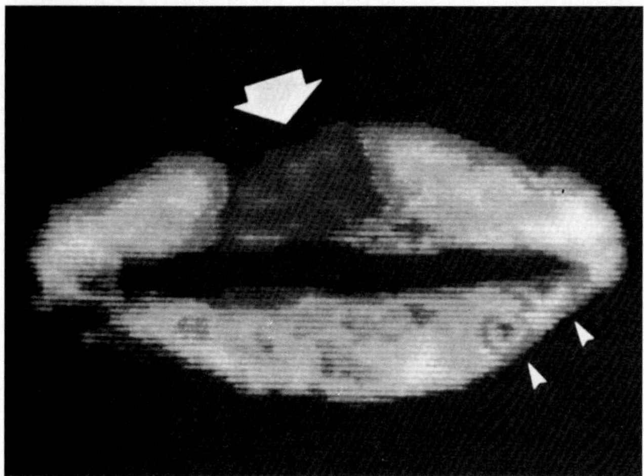

Figure 11-17. MRI of transverse slice of radical vulvectomy specimen. Large arrow indicates primary vulvar lesion; smaller arrows indicate two nodes containing metastatic disease that measured 0.7 and 1.0 cm in diameter. (From Mann WJ, Mendonca-Dias MH, Lauterbur PC, et al: Preliminary in vitro studies of nuclear magnetic resonance spin-lattice relaxation times and three-dimensional nuclear magnetic resonance imaging in gynecologic oncology. Am J Obstet Gynecol 148:93, 1984.)

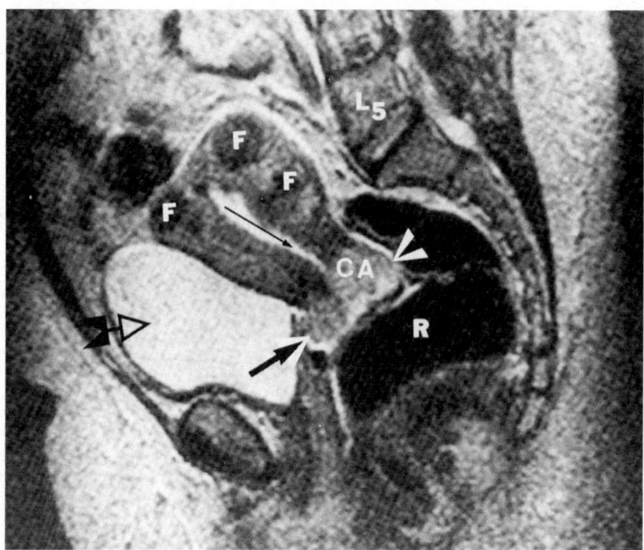

Figure 11-18. Sagittal MRI of woman with cervical cancer. Cancer (CA) is area of higher signal intensity within cervix (between *black arrows* on *white arrowheads*). Rectum (R) can be seen immediately posterior and inferior to enlarged cervical mass. Endometrial canal is slightly enlarged and contains fluid (*thin black arrow*). Three leiomyomata (F) can be seen scattered throughout myometrium. Bladder is seen internally as fluid-filled structure (*open arrowhead*). L5, fifth lumbar vertebra. Parameters for this examination were spin echo sequence of TR 2500/TE 80, 256 × 198 matrix, and 1 signal average. (Courtesy of Mark L. Schiebler, MD, University of North Carolina, Chapel Hill.)

significant prolonged proton relaxation times or spin lattice relaxation times (T1) for the atoms in most carcinomas.

In an early study of three-dimensional MRI, imaging could identify the exact area of a vulvar neoplasm (Fig. 11-17). MRI correctly identified microscopic tumor at the surgical margin of the vulvectomy incision. Because of the potential of the MRI examination to view the pelvis in any plane, it is an excellent modality for evaluating vaginal anatomy and congenital defects of the müllerian system. Chang and coworkers found MRI to have a 95% sensitivity and 90% specificity in evaluating vaginal malignancy. Several reports have documented the advantages of MRI in diagnosing and evaluating disease processes of adenomyosis, myomas, endometrial cancer (including myometrial invasion), and cervical carcinoma, both local and distant spread. Kinkel and colleagues, in their recent meta-analysis, concluded that MRI is superior to CT or ultrasound for the evaluation of endometrial cancer. Preoperative MRI was found to be 93% accurate in predicting ovarian malignancies in a study of 187 adnexal masses by Hricak and colleagues. MRI is more accurate than CT in evaluating the spread of uterine and cervical malignancy (Fig. 11-18). MRI has been employed to evaluate endometriosis and adnexal disease. However, selectivity should be exercised in choosing patients to undergo a preoperative MRI.

MRI has several distinct advantages over other forms of imaging. It does not use ionizing radiation; and therefore presents no known hazards. The X-ray photon has 10 billion times more energy than the radio frequency photon of MRI. Radio frequency electromagnetic radiation penetrates calcified material without significant attenuation. Unlike ultrasound, MRI can penetrate through gas, thus allowing visualization of the bowel and vagina. In addition, MRI does not require the use of radiopaque contrast agents required with CT scans. MRI uses gadolinium, a magnetically opaque contrast agent that is given intravenously. Gadolinium is rapidly dispersed into the interstitial spaces and is not nephrotoxic. Glucagon may be given prior to abdominopelvic MRI to decrease intestinal peristalsis.

One major limitation of MRI is patient acceptance. Many patients feel "trapped" in the machine. Meléndez and McCrank reviewed anxiety reactions associated with MRI examinations. They found that 4% to 30% of patients experienced some type of psychological problem, ranging from mild anxiety to severe apprehension necessitating discontinuation of the study. Most complaints focused on anxiety from the claustrophobic reactions and feelings of panic. The need for the patient to remain still for the long period of scanning contributed to the anxiety. The authors noted that most patients were fearful prior to the MRI examination. Techniques to alleviate anxiety include prescan education programs, music by earphones, antianxiety medications, hypnosis, relaxation techniques, and having family members present. Because patient compliance is essential for successful imaging, attention to patient anxiety prior to the study is important. Newer, "open" MRI scanners may induce much less anxiety. MRI should not be used in patients with cochlear implants or pacemakers. It is safe in women with IUDs, including copper-containing ones, and in patients with surgical clips and staples.

In summary, the applications of MRI are vast and MRI innovations are coming quickly. It is an imaging modality that uses nonionizing radio frequencies and magnetic fields to help differentiate types of tissue, penetrate bone, provide images in multiple planes, and can be used with a nontoxic contrast medium. However, MRI is not a screening tool. Examinations require good patient compliance and need to be individualized by the clinician and radiologist.

ENDOMETRIAL SAMPLING

Endometrial biopsy is one of the diagnostic tests most frequently performed by gynecologists. This rapid, safe, and inexpensive sampling of the endometrial lining is a common procedure in the clinical workup of women with abnormal vaginal bleeding. The renowned gynecologist Howard Kelly was an enthusiast for outpatient endometrial biopsy in the 1920s. Advances in the past 30 years have led to the development of instruments that abrade, scrape, brush, and aspirate the endometrium.

The older Randall and Novak curettes have long since been abandoned in favor of small easily used flexible catheters. There are many different models and modifications of devices used for endometrial sampling. Most instruments aspirate tissue from the endometrial lining following abrasion or scraping with a small curette or perforated cannula (Fig. 11-19). Most cannulas in current favor are 2 to 4 mm in diameter and are plastic. Aspiration of the endometrium is usually accomplished by a syringe. The thin, flexible polypropylene Pipelle cannula (Fig. 11-20) is as effective as rigid instruments in obtaining endometrial specimens, often with less discomfort. Most clinicians use the Pipelle as the instrument of first choice for endometrial sampling. Other flexible plastic cannulas are equally effective. A meta-analysis by Dijkhuizan and coworkers, and a systematic review by Clark and colleagues, found endometrial biopsy 99% sensitive in diagnosing endometrial cancer. The Pipelle cannula was notably effective. These reviews noted failure rates of the procedure to be approximately less than 8%. Negative findings with continued bleeding or nondiagnostic sampling requires follow-up with either repeat biopsy or more directed evaluation such as with hysteroscopically directed sampling.

Endometrial sampling is most frequently performed to evaluate dysfunctional uterine bleeding. Another indication for endometrial sampling is to investigate abnormal bleeding associated with increasing use of hormonal replacement therapy in postmenopausal women. Endometrial biopsy is the standard diagnostic test to confirm a chronic uterine infection such as endometritis. Less commonly, if pelvic tuberculosis is suspected, sampling of the endometrial lining is performed late in the menstrual cycle. This gives the pathologist the best opportunity to discover the classic giant cells and tubercles.

There are only a few contraindications to endometrial biopsy. Profuse bleeding is a relative contraindication. Endometrial biopsy should not be performed more than 14 to 16 days after ovulation because of the possibility of interfering with an early pregnancy. In contrast, endometrial biopsy 10 to 14 days following the temperature rise does not interfere with implantation during that cycle.

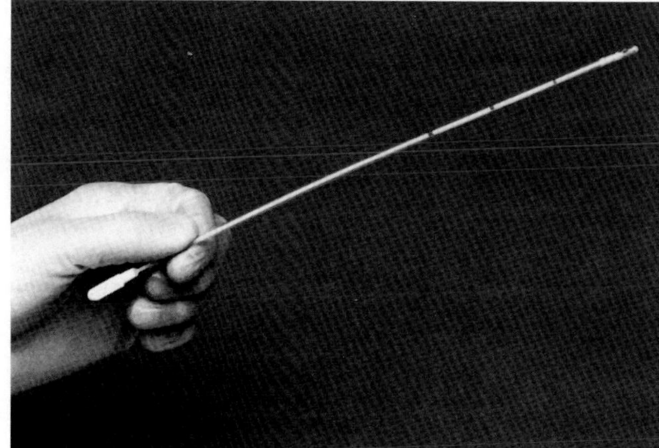

Figure 11-20. Pipelle endometrial suction curette. Note small diameter and flexible nature. Suction is produced by partly withdrawing inner stem.

Endometrial biopsy is performed on an outpatient basis. It is helpful to explain to the patient that she will experience uterine cramping during the short time that the biopsy instrument is inside the uterus. A bimanual examination is performed to note the size of the uterus and direction of the uterine cavity. A single-toothed tenaculum may be used to secure the anterior cervical lip. The exocervix is then cleaned of mucus and bacteria. Many physicians will cleanse the os with an iodine solution prior to sampling. When the indication for the biopsy is to evaluate abnormal bleeding, multiple areas of the endometrial cavity should be sampled. At least four separate areas should be abraded. If copious or necrotic tissue is discovered or the pathology report is inadequate, further evaluation is indicated.

The most frequent problem in performing endometrial sampling is cervical stenosis or spasm. When this is encountered, the optimal method to obtain pain relief and overcome resistance is a paracervical block with 1% lidocaine (Xylocaine). Occasionally the endocervical application of viscous 2–4% lidocaine may decrease discomfort. Zupi and coworkers have described the use of 5 mL of 2% mepivacaine injected transcervically into the uterus to reduce discomfort. Subsequently, the cervix can be dilated painlessly with narrow metal dilators, and the biopsy can be completed.

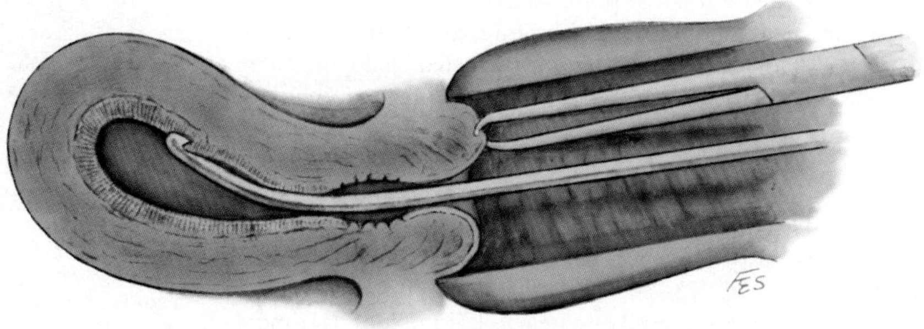

Figure 11-19. Office endometrial aspiration with 3-mm Randall suction curette. (From Copenhaver EH: Surgery of the Vulva and Vagina: A Practical Guide. Philadelphia, WB Saunders, 1981.)

Complications following endometrial biopsy are exceedingly rare. The major complication is uterine perforation, with an incidence of 1 or 2 cases per 1000. Infection and postprocedure hemorrhage are very rare. Some women develop a severe vasovagal reflex from instrumentation of the uterine cavity. This reflex can be diminished by either giving the patient intravenous atropine or performing a paracervical block. Some clinicians pretreat women with nonsteroidal antiinflammatory agents to decrease the pain associated with this procedure.

If abnormal perimenopausal or menopausal bleeding recurs following an endometrial biopsy, additional diagnostic procedures, such as hysteroscopy or ultrasound, should be performed. Feldman and colleagues evaluated 286 women with perimenopausal bleeding who had had a dilatation and curettage (D&C) or an endometrial biopsy. Nine of 86 (10.5%) who had negative findings initially, but continued to bleed, had carcinoma or complex hyperplasia on follow-up biopsy. In a retrospective review of 223 patients, Daniel and Peters found that 16% of tumors had a more advanced grade of endometrial carcinoma at hysterectomy than after office curettage. Thus lesions such as atypical hyperplasia warrant further evaluation. If a hysterectomy is performed, the uterus should be opened and evaluated.

In summary, the major advantages to the patient of the endometrial biopsy over D&C are convenience and cost savings. The clinical results obtained depend on two factors: the patient's acceptance and the physician's skill and perseverance. The patient's acceptance is higher with narrow cannulas made of plastic. Liberal use of paracervical block in difficult procedures allows the physician to be successful in obtaining tissue in more than 95% of cases. Routine preoperative endometrial biopsy in asymptomatic women undergoing hysterectomy is an unnecessary procedure and does not improve patient care.

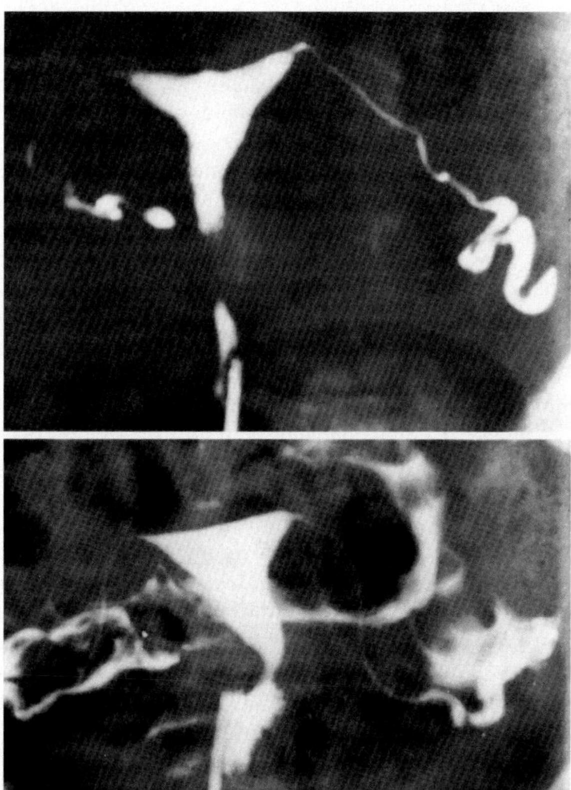

Figure 11-21. Two normal hysterosalpingograms. (Reprinted from Fertility and Sterility, 38, Soules MR, Spadoni LR, Oil versus aqueous media for hysterosalpingography: A continuing debate based on many opinions and few facts, 1. Copyright 1982, with permission from The American Society for Reproductive Medicine.)

HYSTEROSALPINGOGRAPHY

Hysterosalpingography (HSG) is a radiographic imaging technique in which the uterine cavity and the lumina of the fallopian tubes are visualized by injecting contrast material through the cervical canal. This test was first described by two investigators, Rubin and Cary, working independently in 1914. Recently though, advances in hysteroscopy and ultrasound have led to a substantial decrease in the use of HSG. The addition of image intensification with screen fluoroscopy provides more precise visualization and reduces radiation exposure. Spot films have limited value in evaluating infertile patients. HSG is a safe and rapid means of investigating abnormalities in the endometrial cavity and fallopian tubes (Fig. 11-21). Often an inference of abnormal function can be postulated from an abnormal HSG. These judgments should not be absolute; for example, approximately 15% of women who have "obstructed" fallopian tubes diagnosed by HSG subsequently become pregnant without further treatment. The cause of this false reading is thought to be tubal spasm.

The leading indications for HSG are primary and secondary infertility. This imaging technique gives evidence of endometrial irregularities, tubal patency, tubal mobility, and sometimes peritubal disease (Fig. 11-22). HSG has an approximate 83% specificity for evaluating tubal patency. Laparoscopy is a more sophisticated and accurate method of diagnosing tubal problems during an infertility investigation. Chromopertubation with an innocuous dye, such as indigo carmine, demonstrates tubal patency during laparoscopy. Comparative studies have documented that HSG discovers only 50% of the peritubal disease diagnosed by direct visualization via the laparoscope.

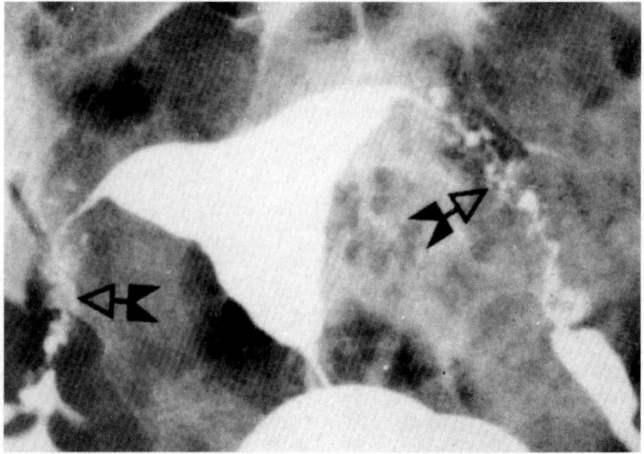

Figure 11-22. Hysterosalpingogram from patient with tubal endometriosis. Flecks of contrast material (*arrows*) are seen about isthmus without central linear pattern. Distal ends appear normally patient. (Reprinted from Fertility and Sterility, 40, Siegler AM, Hysterosalpingography, 139. Copyright 1983, with permission from The American Society for Reproductive Medicine.)

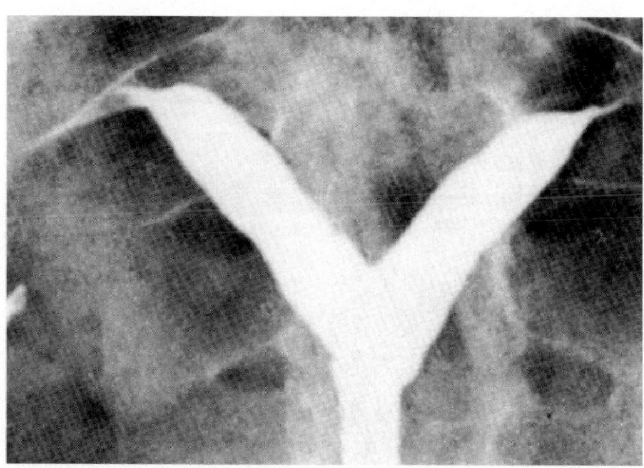

Figure 11-23. Hysterosalpingogram from 34-year-old nulliparous woman who had regular menses and no dysmenorrhea. V-shaped fundal defect with single cervix proved to be bicornuate uterus. (From Siegler AM: Hysterosalpingography. New York, Harper & Row, 1967.)

The study by Hutchinson of 409 infertile patients who had sequential HSG and laparoscopy under general anesthesia helped to define our understanding of tubal spasm. In this series, HSG showed 93 women to have blocked tubes, and 30 of these were patent by chromopertubation. Pain relief does not invariably alleviate tubal spasm. Tubal anomalies, including diverticula and accessory ostia, can be diagnosed by HSG. In summary, HSG is useful in diagnosing intrinsic disease of the fallopian tubes, whereas laparoscopy is more effective in identifying extrinsic disease.

Uterine cavity abnormalities, present in 10% of infertile women, may be discovered by HSG. Congenital müllerian anomalies, such as bicornuate, septate, arcuate, and T-shaped uteri (associated with in utero diethylstilbestrol exposure), may be diagnosed (Fig. 11-23). Pathology such as synechiae of the endometrial cavity may also be discovered (Fig. 11-24). Hysteroscopy is an alternative technique for evaluating intrauterine pathology. HSG is a basic tool in the evaluation of patients with poor reproductive histories. It may be applicable for women with repetitive second-trimester losses. Although HSG has been suggested as a technique for diagnosing an incompetent internal cervical os it is rarely used. The anatomic changes in the diameter of the internal os in the nonpregnant state have little predictive value for future competency in pregnancy.

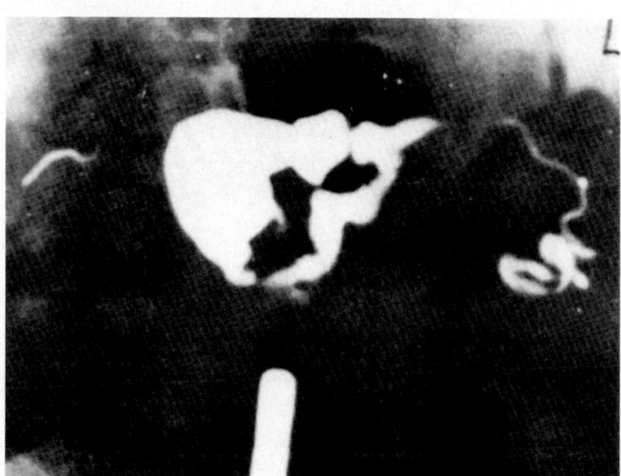

Figure 11-24. Hysterosalpingogram demonstrating intrauterine adhesions, grade 3, after repeated curettage for missed abortion. (Reprinted from Fertility and Sterility, 37, Schenker JG, Margalioth EJ, Intrauterine adhesions: An updated appraisal, 593. Copyright 1982, with permission from The American Society for Reproductive Medicine.)

Women with amenorrhea and a history of curettage who do not respond to a hormonal challenge should have an HSG or hysteroscopy. Uterine synechiae are identified by slowly injecting a water-soluble medium. If a woman has synechiae, tubal obstruction, and pelvic calcifications, a diagnosis of pelvic tuberculosis should be strongly suspected. HSG will also discover polyps or small submucous myomas in refractory cases of abnormal uterine bleeding.

Contraindications to HSG include the obvious: acute pelvic infection, active uterine bleeding, pregnancy, and allergy to iodine.

The choice of using a small Foley catheter or an adjustable rubber or plastic acorn and cannula for injection depends on physician preference. This decision does not seem to bias results as long as all air in the system is replaced by the liquid contrast medium. The choice of water-soluble versus oil-based contrast medium depends on the primary indication for the test and physician preference. Water-soluble iodine is preferred for documenting intrauterine filling defects and identifying the severity of mucosal damage in chronic tubal infection. Lipid-based material provides a more distinct and clearer radiographic image. Most investigators report that the pregnancy rate after HSG is two to three times greater with oil-soluble media. Watson and colleagues performed a meta-analysis of studies reporting the therapeutic effects of HSG contrast material. They reported a definite therapeutic effect and higher pregnancy rate with lipid-based or oil-soluble contrast. The effect was greatest in women with unexplained infertility. Researchers have speculated that the therapeutic effect may be secondary to a mechanical action on tubal epithelium, tubal debris, and tubal plugs or an inhibition of peritoneal macrophages. In contradistinction, Spring and coworkers reported from a multicenter randomized study of 666 women that there was no difference between the use of water-soluble or oil-soluble contrast media, or both, in rate of term pregnancies at one year.

The endpoint of a radiographic examination for tubal patency is either tubal filling with intraperitoneal spilling or increasing pelvic pain secondary to uterine distention associated with tubal obstruction. Tubal spasm may sometimes be overcome by glucagon (2 mg intravenously), which produces atony of smooth muscle. Glucagon is effective in about one of three women with tubal spasm.

Complications of HSG are rare but serious when they happen. Acute pelvic infection, serious enough to require hospitalization, develops in 0.3% to 3.1% of patients. This incidence of pelvic infection is directly related to the population studied, that is, more common in women with dilated tubes. The use of prophylactic antibiotics may reduce the incidence of acute infection following instrumentation of the uterus. As with any surgical procedure that invades the uterus, pelvic pain, uterine perforation, and vasovagal vasomotor reactions do occur. Allergic reactions, particularly to the iodine dye, are a possibility. Intravasation of the dye into the vascular system occurs with high

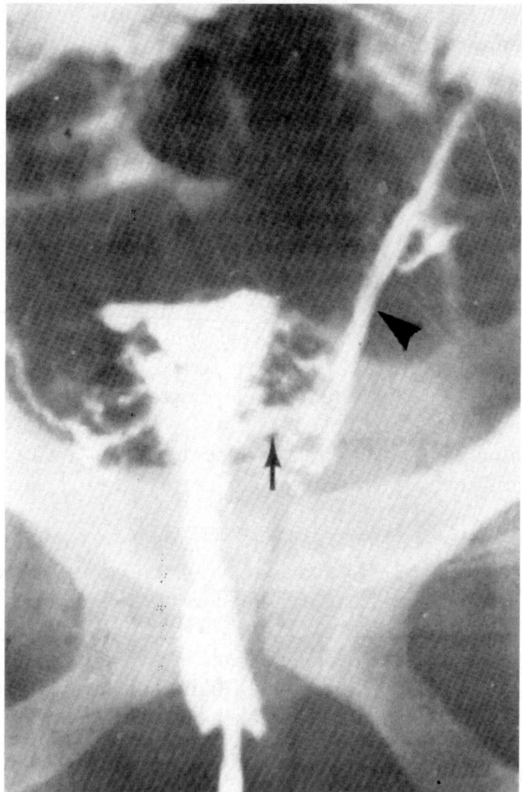

Figure 11-25. Hysterosalpingogram showing both lymphatic (*small arrow*) and venous (*large arrow*) intravasation. (Reprinted from Fertility and Sterility, 38, Soules MR, Spandoni LR, Oil versus aqueous media for hysterosalpingography: A continuing debate based on many opinions and few facts, 1. Copyright 1982, with permission from The American Society for Reproductive Medicine.)

injection pressures, partial perforation of the cannula, and endometrial defects associated with synechiae (Fig. 11-25). Embolic phenomena, pelvic peritonitis, and granuloma formation with oil-based dye are very rare complications.

In summary, HSG is a relatively safe imaging technique. Its major uses are in the evaluation of patients with infertility or poor pregnancy outcomes. The procedure can diagnose uterine and tubal abnormalities. Both oil- and water-based dyes are used. With a TV screen image intensifier, the average HSG takes 10 minutes to perform. This procedure involves approximately 90 seconds of fluoroscopic time and an average radiation exposure to the ovaries of 1 to 2 rad.

HYSTEROSCOPY

Hysteroscopy is the direct visualization of the endometrial cavity using an endoscope and a light source. The earliest hysteroscope was nothing more than a hollow tube with an alcohol lamp and mirror for a light source. In 1869, Pantaleoni reported the successful removal of an endometrial polyp through the scope. Modern hysteroscopes are modifications of cystoscopes with channels to introduce light via fiberoptics, uterine cavity distention media, and surgical instruments.

The popularity of hysteroscopy has been enhanced because it is a simple technique that can be performed in the office.

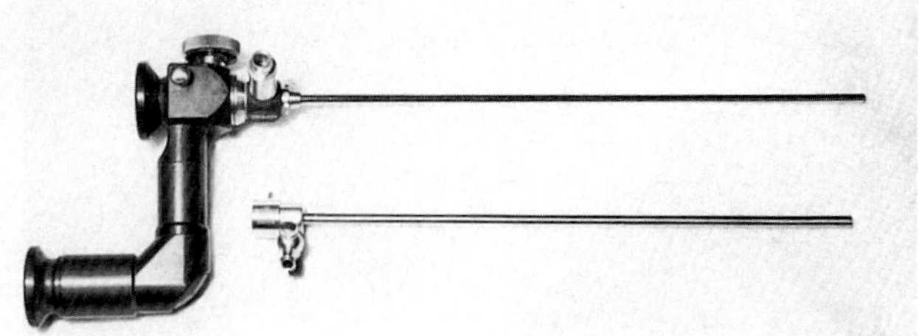

Figure 11-26. A 5-mm rigid hysteroscope (Storz Instruments).

Hysteroscopy has multiple indications, including diagnosis of recurrent abnormal bleeding, repetitive abortion, uterine synechiae, abnormal HSGs, and infertility. Operative procedures, which usually require local or regional anesthesia, performed under hysteroscopic guidance include location and removal of intact or fragmented IUDs, resection of submucous myomas, lysis of synechiae, incision of uterine septa, removal of endometrial polyps, and ablation of the endometrium.

Rigid hysteroscopes vary in diameter (Fig. 11-26). The smaller caliber scopes, 3 to 5 mm in diameter, are used for diagnostic purposes. Several are available that have views from 0 to 30°. Similar to that of a cystoscope, the outer sleeve of a rigid hysteroscope contains several channels that extend the full length of the instrument. Large scopes, with diameters of 8 to 10 mm, may be used for high flow of distending media and for moderate to complex procedures.

Flexible minihysteroscopic instruments and microendoscopes are convenient and very well tolerated in the office for diagnosis and simple operative procedures such as directed biopsies (Fig. 11-27). The narrower hysteroscopes, have diameters of 3 to 5 mm. Many clinicians suggest that patients take ibuprofen preoperatively.

The cavity of the uterus is a potential space. The success of hysteroscopy depends on the medium used to expand this space. The three most popular choices for diagnostic hysteroscopy are 32% dextran, which is highly viscous; 5% dextrose and water (D_5W), which has low viscosity; and carbon dioxide gas. Another common distending medium is 1.5% glycine. High-molecular-weight dextran (average molecular weight, 70,000 Da in 10%

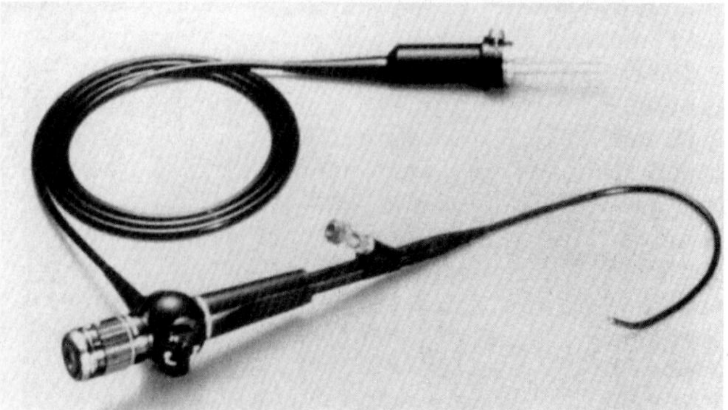

Figure 11-27. Small-size steerable fiberoptic hysteroscopes offer the advantage of entering hard-to-reach spaces within the uterus and likewise provide excellent operative access to all areas of the uterus. (From Baggish MS, Valle RF: Future of hysteroscopy. In Baggish MS, Barbot J, Valle RF [eds]: Diagnostic and Operative Hysteroscopy, 2nd ed. St. Louis, Mosby, 1999.)

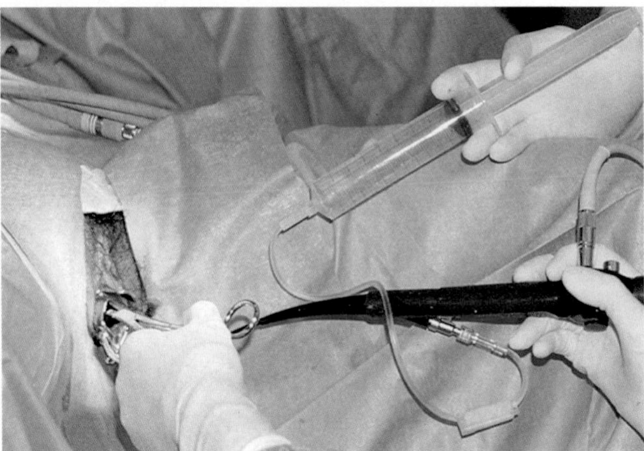

Figure 11-28. Flexible hysteroscopy. Uterine distention is maintained with normal saline or lactated Ringer's solution injected through intravenous extension tubing. (From Goldberg JM, Falcone T: Atlas of Endoscopic Techniques in Gynecology. London, WB Saunders, 2000, p 185.)

glucose) is preferred by the majority of investigators, especially if a surgical procedure is contemplated. This extremely viscous fluid is biodegradable, nontoxic, and nonconductive, and has good optical qualities. Most important, dextran is immiscible with blood, which helps to keep the field clear during intrauterine surgery. Dextran has two drawbacks: it is antigenic, and anaphylaxis has been reported. It also rapidly crystallizes; thus endoscopic instruments must be cleaned shortly after the procedure. Rare cases of pulmonary edema and coagulopathies from intravascular dextran have been reported. Carbon dioxide must be infused with special equipment that carefully limits flow to less than 100 mL/min and maintains the pressure at approximately 60 to 70 mm Hg. The major precaution with D_5W is the monitoring of total fluid intake so as not to produce water intoxication. In contrast, office hysteroscopy with the smaller flexible scopes most commonly incorporate the use of saline or lactated Ringer's solution for their ease of use and involve a short operating time (Fig. 11-28).

Diagnostic hysteroscopy is often performed as an office procedure. Unlike with larger rigid scopes, most patients will not require anesthesia. In selected patients, a local anesthetic may be applied to the endocervix, or a paracervical block may be used. Vaginal misoprostol (prostaglandin E_1) has also been used to aid in the transcervical passage of the hysteroscope. Anxious patients may be pretreated with alprazolam, diazepam, and/or nonsteroidal antiinflammatory agents. If extensive resections are anticipated via hysteroscopy, then the procedure is better performed on an outpatient basis in the surgical suite.

Hysteroscopy is ideal for directly visualizing and removing partially perforated or broken IUDs. Women with repetitive abortions should have a diagnostic hysteroscopic procedure. Congenital abnormalities that interfere with the success of early pregnancies, such as septa of the uterus, may be seen and removed (Fig. 11-29). Women with recurrent abnormal uterine bleeding may also benefit from this procedure. Often endometrial polyps or small submucous myomas are discovered and may be removed (Fig. 11-30). Women with persistent peri- or postmenopausal bleeding after a negative endometrial biopsy are also candidates for hysteroscopy. Focal lesions, particularly pedunculated structures, are frequently missed by endometrial biopsy or a D&C. The uterine synechiae of a woman with Asherman's syndrome can be cut with microscissors, reestablishing the endometrial cavity. Hysteroscopic metroplasty of intrauterine septa is safer with fewer complications than laparotomy.

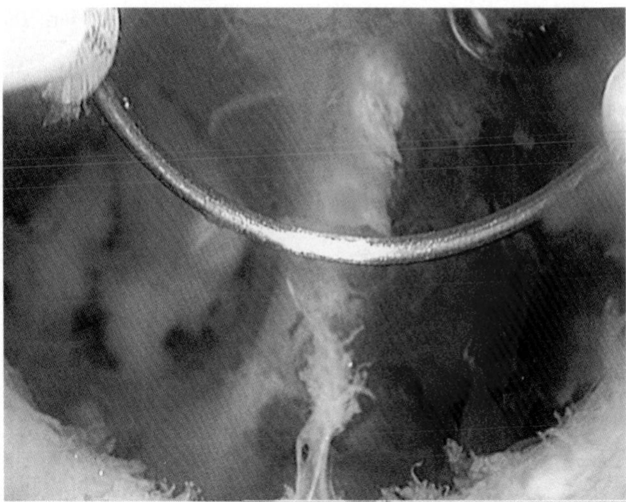

Figure 11-29. The loop is placed at the center of the apex of the septum. As the current is activated the loop is advanced toward the fundus in small increments always staying in the center of the septum. The septum separates as it is divided so that no tissue needs to be excised. (There are small endometrial fragments in the right cornua and a small clot adherent to the left aspect of the septum.) (From Goldberg JM, Falcone T: Atlas of Endoscopic Techniques in Gynecology. London, WB Saunders, 2000, p 194.)

Hysteroscopy is superior to HSG in discovering intrauterine disease. In comparative studies the use of hysteroscopy revealed synechiae, polyps, or myomas in 40% of patients with normal HSGs. These abnormalities were undetected and unsuspected using radiographic techniques. The false-positive rate of HSG is 33% compared with hysteroscopy. One in three women diagnosed as having an intrauterine filling defect by x-ray

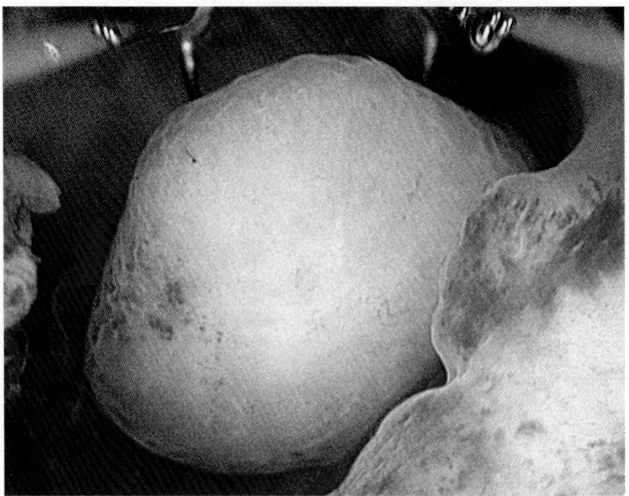

Figure 11-30. A uterine poly with the hysteroscopic resection tool behind the polyp. (From Goldberg JM, Falcone T: Atlas of Endoscopic Techniques in Gynecology. London, WB Saunders, 2000, p 187.)

imaging will have a normal cavity directly visualized with the hysteroscope.

The variety and extent of surgery performed transcervically with the hysteroscope have expanded significantly with technologic advances. Endoscopic procedures have progressed from snaring small polyps to complex myomectomies and ablating the entire endometrial lining.

Operative hysteroscopy may be performed with mechanical devices such as small operating scissors, electrocautery, and modified resectoscopes and lasers. Laser hysteroscopy with carbon dioxide or neodymium:yttrium-aluminum-garnet (Nd:YAG) lasers requires more expensive equipment and expertise. Laser hysteroscopy is significantly less popular and less advantageous than simpler techniques.

Submucous myomas may be removed with a modified urologic resectoscope using a cutting electric current and shaving the myoma until it is flat with the surrounding endometrial lining. Often an inflatable balloon is inserted into the uterine cavity and left for 12 to 24 hours, facilitating hemostasis. The pregnancy rate is as good or better with hysteroscopic myomectomy than with transabdominal myomectomy.

One technique for endometrial ablation utilizes a roller ball—a wire loop electrode to coagulate and thus destroy the endometrium (Fig. 11-31). In women with abnormal bleeding or menorrhagia who are poor surgical candidates or who wish to preserve their uterus, the endometrial lining may be ablated through the hysteroscope (Fig. 11-32). Hysterograms following treatment have demonstrated contraction, scarring, and dense adhesion formation. Long-term follow-up has documented that endometrial carcinoma may develop in residual foci of endometrium. Although lasers may also be used to produce ablation of the endometrium by photovaporizing the epithelium, laser photovaporization takes longer than electrode resection, and the equipment is more expensive.

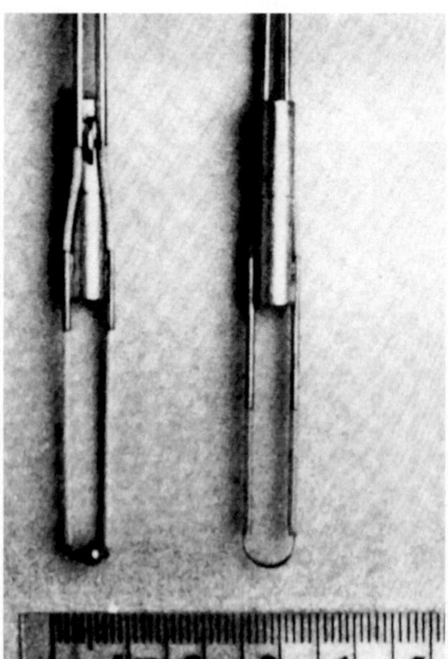

Figure 11-31. Ball-end and loop electrodes, side by side. Ball-end electrode is 2 mm in diameter, and the loop is 7 mm. (From Vancaillie TG: Electrocoagulation of the endometrium with the ball-end resectoscope. Obstet Gynecol 74:425, 1989.)

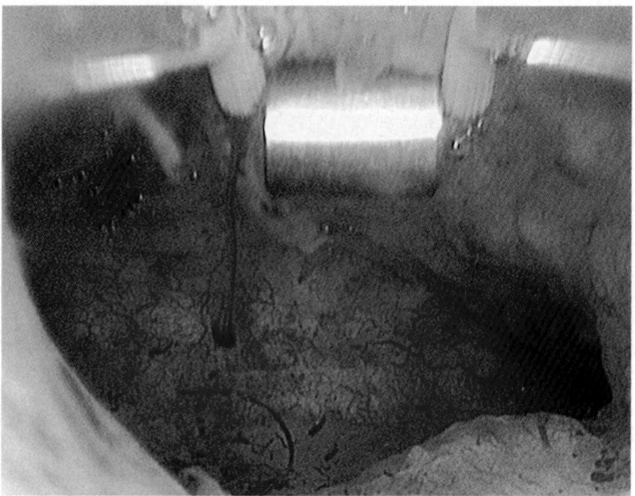

Figure 11-32. Endometrial cavity prior to ablation with a roller-ball. (From Goldberg JM, Falcone T: Atlas of Endoscopic Techniques in Gynecology. London, WB Saunders, 2000, p 197.)

Falloposcopy, also referred to as salpingograpy, is an innovation using an extension of hysteroscopy. This technique is used to evaluate the lumen of the fallopian tubes by cannulation with a flexible microendoscope through the hysteroscope. Falloposcopy is not as painful to the patient as hysterosalpingography and potentially provides more information about the fallopian tubes in the infertile patient. Several investigators have found it helpful in restoring tubal patency in the case of proximal occlusions. Hysteroscopic sterilization may be accomplished with plugs of the tubal ostia, chemical and cryoablation, or insertion of plugs or coils. The failure rate, safety, and acceptability have yet to be confirmed ion long-term studies. Several devices and protocols are currently available. No procedure is of yet reversible.

There are few contraindications to hysteroscopy. Acute pelvic infection is the leading one because of the potential of spreading the disease by the media used for uterine distention. Active bleeding is a relative contraindication. If the bleeding is brisk, the hysteroscopic procedure will be unsatisfactory. Pregnancy is a contraindication as is recent uterine perforation or cervical cancer.

Complications of hysteroscopy are noted in less than 2% of the procedures. Jansen and coworkers, using a large database of 136,000 hysteroscopies, noted the significant complication rate to be 0.28%. Complications include uterine perforation, pelvic infection, bleeding, and fluid overload from absorption of distending media. The potential complications of the distending media include anaphylaxis to dextran, circulatory overload with D_5W, pulmonary edema, coagulopathies, hyponatremia, and the potential of gas embolism with carbon dioxide. Monitoring of the patient's fluid status is important because of problems with absorption of distending media, leading to volume overload and electrolyte imbalance. Cardiac arrests have been reported with uterine insufflation with carbon dioxide when unmonitored amounts of gas were used. Thermal injury to surrounding organs may occur with deep resections or perforations with the electrocautery instrument. If injury or perforation is suspected during hysteroscopy, then intraperitoneal evaluation should be performed either by laparoscopy or celiotomy.

In summary, hysteroscopy is a simple technique for the diagnosis and treatment of intrauterine pathology. The indications for intrauterine surgery via the hysteroscope are expanding. Operative hysteroscopic costs vary and depend on the time involved and the specific procedure performed.

LAPAROSCOPY

Laparoscopy has radically changed the clinical practice of gynecology. As an outpatient surgical technique, laparoscopy provides a window to directly visualize pelvic anatomy as well as a technique for performing many operations with less morbidity than laparotomy (Fig. 11-33). Operative laparoscopy for complex surgeries is associated with as easier recovery and a shorter hospital stay.

Laparoscopy was first performed in the early 1900s. Two events of the early 1960s renewed interest in this surgical technique, the first being the development of fiberoptic cables and the second the change in society's attitude toward sterilization procedures. Patrick Steptoe is considered the "father" of modern laparoscopy for his work in the mid-1960s with laparoscopic sterilization. By the mid-1970s laparoscopy had been adopted as the method of choice for female sterilization.

The advantages of low cost, convenience, and shorter hospital stay are obvious when laparoscopy is compared with celiotomy (laparotomy). Minilaparotomy in an extremely thin woman may be competitive in time and cost to laparoscopy. However, if a woman is moderately obese, there is no comparison. Postoperative recovery time and the need for hospitalization time are also significantly less when compared with celiotomy. Laparoscopic visualization is excellent because the video camera and endoscope magnify the image.

There are multiple indications for laparoscopy, both diagnostic and therapeutic. The most common indication is female sterilization. Laparoscopy is an essential step in the diagnostic workup of a couple with infertility or a woman with chronic pelvic pain. In the past decade, gynecologists have progressed from using the laparoscope to perform such simple surgical tasks as tubal ligation to more complicated surgery, such as removal of ectopic pregnancies, and treatment of endometriosis, hysterectomy, node dissections, and urogynecologic procedures. The present indications for operative laparoscopy are almost identical to those for celiotomy.

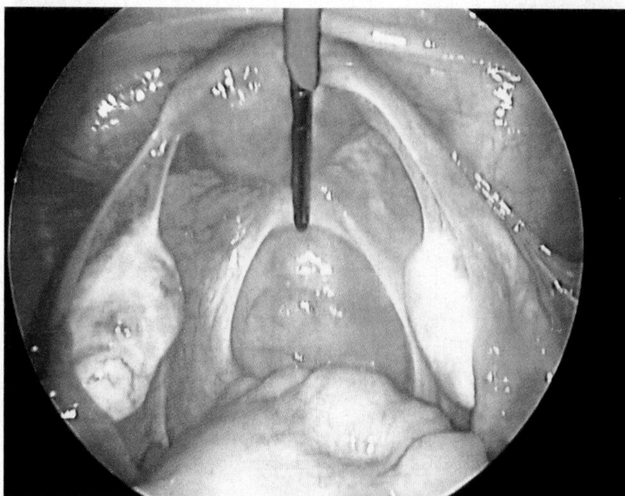

Figure 11-33. Laparoscopic view of normal pelvis in patient prior to tubal sterilization. (Courtesy of B. Beller, MD, Eugene, OR.)

Laparoscopy has made outpatient sterilization available to women throughout the world. Cumulative 10-year pregnancy rates vary between 8/1000 and 37/1000. Sterilization is accomplished with electric cauterization, or spring-loaded clips. Because of the serious complications with unipolar cautery, most cautery sterilization procedures are performed with bipolar coagulation of approximately 2 cm of the tube without division (Fig. 11-34). The clip should be placed on the narrow isthmus so the size of the appliance conforms to the diameter of the fallopian tube.

There are both diagnostic and therapeutic indications for laparoscopy in infertile women. Tubal patency and mobility can be directly observed via the laparoscope. Laparoscopy is able to confirm or rule out intrinsic pelvic disorders, such as endometriosis or chronic pelvic inflammatory disease. It is possible not only to describe and stage the extent of endometriosis or pelvic adhesions but also to treat them. Adhesions can be lysed, and areas of endometriosis can be ablated by electrocautery or laser (Fig. 11-35).

The management of pelvic pain has been dramatically changed by the laparoscope. The differential diagnosis of acute pain may be defined by direct visualization of the fallopian tubes, ovaries, and appendix. Several centers include laparoscopy in the management of acute pelvic infection, taking direct bacterial cultures of purulent material from the tubes. These direct transabdominal cultures have changed our opinions concerning the clinical management of polymicrobial pelvic infections. The enigma of chronic pelvic pain may be solved by the findings at laparoscopy and "pain mapping" (Fig. 11-36). Following the procedure, a plan for long-term management of the pain can be discussed with the patient.

The laparoscope is utilized for numerous other therapeutic indications. Intraperitoneal intrauterine devices are best retrieved with the laparoscope. Laparoscopic ovarian biopsy (for karyotyping in certain endocrine disorders) is possible. Lysis of adhesions, removal of ectopic pregnancies, and treatment of endometriosis are most frequently performed through the laparoscope. The laparoscope may be used to transform an abdominal hysterectomy into a vaginal hysterectomy, to laparoscopically assist vaginal hysterectomy, to sample lymph nodes, and to perform retropubic bladder suspensions. The limits and indications of surgical procedures via the laparoscope depend on the experience and judgment of the gynecologist. At some point, celiotomy is the more reasonable decision. We believe that a procedure should be performed through the laparoscope only if the gynecologist is prepared for the complications that might arise if that procedure were performed through a celiotomy.

Absolute contraindications to laparoscopy include intestinal obstruction, hemoperitoneum that produces hemodynamic instability, anticoagulation therapy, severe cardiovascular disease, and tuberculous peritonitis. Relative contraindications, in which each case must be individualized, include extensive obesity, large hiatal hernia, advanced malignancy, generalized peritonitis, and extensive intraabdominal scarring.

Laparoscopy may be performed under local, regional, or general anesthesia. For simple procedures, many prefer local

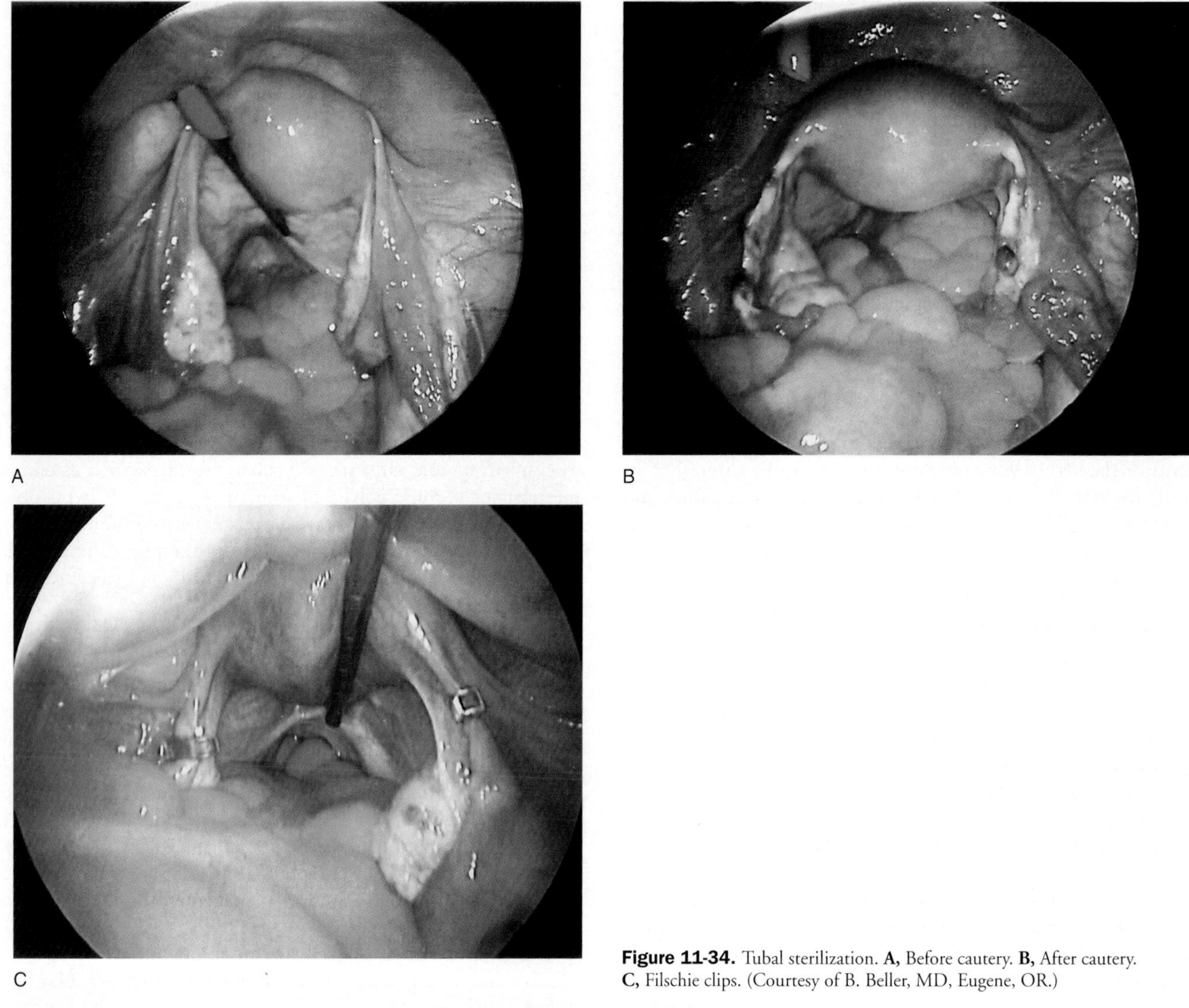

Figure 11-34. Tubal sterilization. **A,** Before cautery. **B,** After cautery. **C,** Filschie clips. (Courtesy of B. Beller, MD, Eugene, OR.)

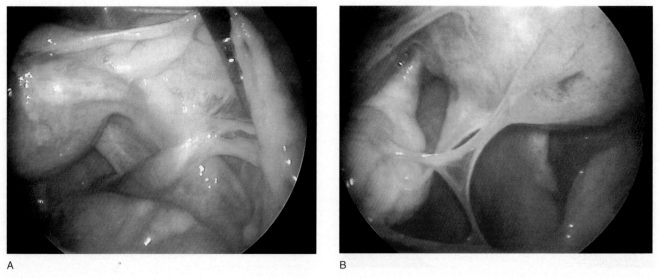

A

B

Figure 11-35. Pelvic adhesions in a patient with chronic pelvic pain and previous pelvic inflammatory disease. **A,** Right adnexae. **B,** Left adnexae. (Courtesy of B. Beller, MD, Eugene, OR.)

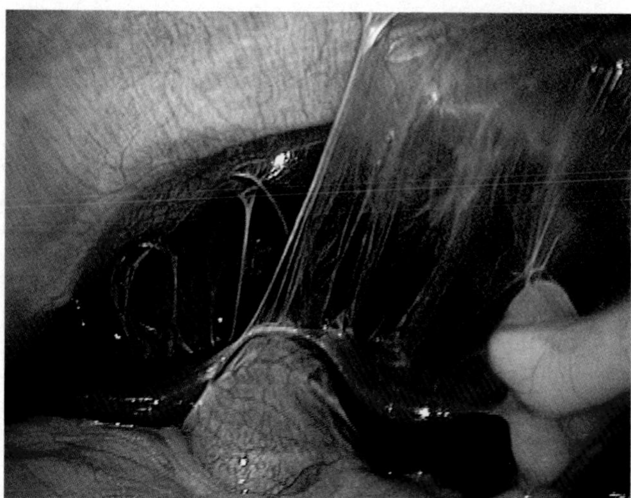

Figure 11-36. Fitz-Hugh-Curtis syndrome in a patient with previous pelvic inflammatory disease. (From Goldberg JM, Falcone T: Atlas of Endoscopic Techniques in Gynecology. London, WB Saunders, 2000, p 71.)

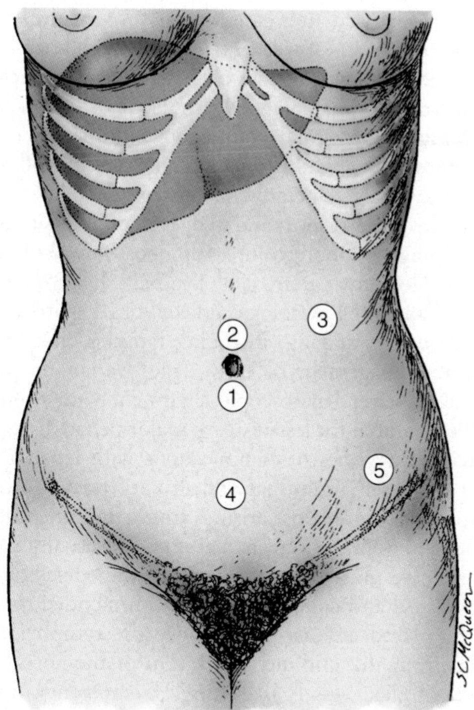

Figure 11-37. Usual sites for insertion of insufflating needle in laparoscopy: (1) infraumbilical fold, (2) supraumbilical fold, (3) left costal margin, (4) midway between umbilicus and pubis, and (5) left McBurney's point. (From Corson SL: Operating room preparation and basic techniques. In Phillips JM (ed): Laparoscopy. © Copyright 1977 by the Williams & Wilkins Co, Baltimore.)

anesthesia for its safety, with the addition of conscious sedation by intravenous medication. The risks associated with general anesthesia are one of the major hazards of laparoscopy. However, when operative laparoscopy is contemplated, general anesthesia is recommended. As Gomel has summarized, the requirements of operative laparoscopy include general anesthesia to ensure adequate muscle relaxation, patient comfort, and the ability to manipulate intraabdominal organs. The standard diagnostic laparoscope is 10 mm in diameter. Secondary puncture trochars vary from 5 mm (bipolar forceps), 7 or 8 mm in width (spring-loaded clip and Silastic band), to 10 mm for pouches to remove specimens. Newer "mini" and "micro" laparoscopes used primarily for diagnostic evaluation are as small as 2 mm in diameter. Most laparoscopes are 30 cm long and provide a field of vision of 60 to 75°. The inferior margin of the umbilicus is the preferred site of entry, as this is the thinnest area of the abdominal wall. Alternative sites are detailed in Figure 11-37. The choice of gas to develop the pneumoperitoneum depends on the choice of anesthesia. Nitrous oxide is preferable with local anesthesia, but carbon dioxide is the choice with general anesthesia. Nitrous oxide is nonflammable but does support combustion. Carbon dioxide quickly forms carbonic acid on the moist parietal peritoneal surface, which results in considerable discomfort to a patient without regional or general anesthesia.

Operative laparoscopy may be performed with mechanical instruments, including an extensive variety of scissors, scalpels, endoscopic syringes, manipulators, suture devices, electrocautery instruments (both unipolar and bipolar), suction, irrigation, and laser instruments. During operative laparoscopy, stabilization of the pelvic organs is essential, such as traction on the edges of an adhesion. Thus third and fourth puncture sites are often required. Because each puncture site is a potential gas leak, high-flow insufflation equipment is necessary. In addition, video cameras are employed so that both the surgeon and assistant can work effectively. Unlike the short time needed for diagnostic laparoscopy, operative laparoscopy may require several hours. Advantages of operative laparoscopy over celiotomy include decreased postoperative adhesion formation, decreased postoperative pain, shorter recovery time, and less, if any, hospital stay. Surgical risks from cardiac, pulmonary, and thromboembolic disease should be treated with the same cautions as a corresponding open procedure. These are presented in Chapter 24 (Preoperative Counseling and Management).

Laparoscopic treatment of ectopic pregnancy most often involves salpingotomy but also may include salpingectomy or an intraectopic injection of methotrexate (Fig. 11-38). HCG

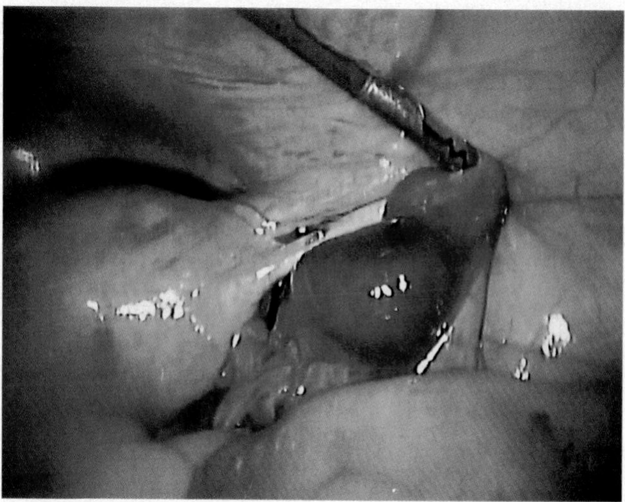

Figure 11-38. Ectopic pregnancy in the right fallopian tube. (Courtesy of B. Beller, MD, Eugene, OR.)

titers must be followed after conservative surgery until the titers fall to zero (usually 3 to 4 weeks) to ensure that all trophoblastic tissue has been removed. Tubal patency and subsequent pregnancy rates are comparable between laparoscopic techniques and celiotomy. Laparoscopic treatment of endometriosis includes lysis of adhesions, ablation of endometriomas, and removal of endometrial cysts. Operative laparoscopy has been used for myomectomy, ovarian biopsy and wedge resection-assisted hysterectomy, salpingo-oophorectomy, salpingostomy and fimbrioplasty, appendectomy, uterosacral ligament ligation, presacral neurectomy, and urogynecologic procedures. Laparoscopy may be used for cancer staging, including lymphadenectomy. The laparoscopic management of early stage ovarian neoplasms is controversial. Newer laparoscopic alignment with robotics has opened the potential for less-invasive major pelvic dissection.

The major categories of complications with laparoscopy are laceration of vessels, intestinal and urinary tract injuries, and cardiorespiratory problems arising from the pneumoperitoneum. Since abdominal wall hematomas are usually subfascial in location, care must be taken to avoid the epigastric vessels. For safety, Hurd and colleagues have recommended that lateral trochars be placed at least 5 cm above the symphysis and at least 8 cm from the midline. Laceration of the aorta, inferior vena cava, or iliac vessels is a surgical emergency. Intestinal injuries may be produced by the Veress needle or the trochar. Complications increase with the age of the patient and the complexity of the procedure. Several studies have evaluated the incidence of complications with operative laparoscopy. The incidence of ureteral injuries vary from 1% to 4% with laparoscopic dissection of the cardinal ligaments. The overall rate of complications from large series of operative laparoscopy varies from 0.2% to 2%. Chandler and coworkers compiled data from a series of injuries due to abdominal entry and laparoscopic access injuries reported to large insurance data banks. The series included general surgery as well as gynecology from both the United States and other countries. Over a 20-year period, the data bank collected 594 reports of organ injury, 33% in gynecology patients. Importantly, 50% of bowel injuries were unrecognized for 24 hours or more. Sixty-five deaths were reported. Age older than 59 years and delayed diagnosis of injury were independently associated with mortality in this series.

Open laparoscopy may be used to avoid intestinal injury. Instead of blind entry into the peritoneal cavity, a small incision is made in the fascia and parietal peritoneum. The cone is placed in the abdominal cavity under direct visual control. The fascia is secured to the sleeve of the cone to obtain an airtight seal. Open laparoscopy reduces the incidence of both bowel and vascular trauma. It is the procedure of choice if the patient has a history of multiple abdominal operations.

Complications directly related to the pneumoperitoneum include pneumothorax, diminished venous return, gas embolism, and cardiac arrhythmias. It is important not to develop pressures greater than 20 mm Hg in establishing the pneumoperitoneum. High pressures impede venous return and limit excursion of the diaphragm. A rare but life-threatening complication of laparoscopy is gas embolism, which produces hypotension and the classical "mill wheel" murmur, which can be heard over the entire precordium. The patient with this complication should be turned on her left side and the frothy blood aspirated by a central venous catheter directed into the right side of the heart. Other rare complications include incisional hernias at the site of the 10-mm scope. This has been estimated to occur in 1 in 5000 procedures. Metastases from ovarian malignancies to the laparoscopic wound site are also a rare but real problem.

In summary, laparoscopy, more than any other advance, has changed the clinical practice of gynecology over the past 3½ decades. Today's OB/Gyn residents have a difficult time contemplating the practice of the specialty prior to the introduction of the "silver tube." Laparoscopy provides a window for the diagnosis of infertility, pelvic pain, ectopic pregnancy, abdominal and pelvic trauma, staging the extent of pelvic disease, and the visual diagnosis of abnormal anatomy. Therapeutic uses of the laparoscope vary from female sterilization to hysterectomy and node sampling.

KEY POINTS

- Measurement of diastolic and systolic velocities by Doppler ultrasound provide indirect indices of vascular resistance. Muscular arteries have high resistance. Newly developed vessels, such as those arising in malignancies, have little vascular wall musculature and thus have low resistance.
- Advantages of ultrasound include the real-time nature of the image, the absence of radiation, the ability to perform the procedure in the office during or immediately after a pelvic examination, and the ability to describe the findings to the patient while she is watching.
- Sonography has not been found to cause adverse clinical effects in humans with the energy levels used in diagnostic studies.
- Several sonographic characteristics of pelvic masses correlate with malignancy, including septations; internal papillations—echogenic structures protruding into the mass; loculations; solid lesions; cystic lesions with solid components; and smaller cysts adjacent to or part of the wall of the larger cyst-daughter cysts.
- Ultrasound evaluation of endometrial pathology involves measurement of the endometrial thickness or stripe. The normal endometrial thickness is 4 mm or less in a postmenopausal woman not taking hormones.
- An intrauterine pregnancy should be routinely visualized by endometrial ultrasound by 5 weeks after the last normal menstrual period.
- Helical CT is a modification of standard CT that uses movement of the patient combined with rotation of several radiographic registers in a spiraling fashion. Vascular images are of a high enough quality that in many centers, helical CT has replaced pulmonary angiography and ventilation-perfusion scans.

KEY POINTS *Continued*

- CT is useful in discovering the extension of pelvic cancer into the fat of the retroperitoneal space and the detection of enlarged lymph nodes.
- CT is the most accurate imaging modality in the diagnosis of appendicitis.
- The surface radiation dose from CT scan is between 2 and 10 rads. This radiation exposure is similar to that of a barium enema. Helical CT allows for variations of the radiation dose.
- MRI penetrates bone and air without attenuation. Therefore this technique allows identification of soft tissue disease inaccessible to other imaging techniques.
- Unlike radiographs, in which a tissue density determines the nature of the image, in MRI the inherent type of tissue determines the nature of the image.
- MRI has the capacity to differentiate normal from malignant tissue and also may identify areas of abnormal tissue metabolism.
- MRI uses radio frequency radiation, which is nonionizing.
- Techniques to alleviate the anxiety associated with MRI include prescan education programs, music by earphones, antianxiety medications, hypnosis, relaxation techniques, and the presence of family members.
- MRI should not be used in patients with cochlear implants or pacemakers. It is safe in women with IUDs, including ones containing copper, and safe in patients with surgical clips and staples. Advantages of MRI over CT include the use of noniodine-based contrast material and the ability to obtain images in multiple planes.
- The most frequent problem in performing endometrial sampling is cervical stenosis or spasm.
- Complications following endometrial biopsy are exceedingly rare. The major complication is uterine perforation, with an incidence of 1 to 2 per 1000.
- The diagnostic accuracy of endometrial biopsy is approximately 95% when compared with subsequent findings at hysterectomy.
- Fifteen percent of women who have obstructed fallopian tubes, as determined by HSG, subsequently become pregnant without further treatment.
- The leading indications for HSG are primary and secondary infertility. This imaging technique gives evidence of endometrial irregularities, tubal patency, tubal mobility, and sometimes peritubal disease.
- Acute pelvic infection develops in 0.3% to 3.1% of patients following HSG. As with any surgical procedure that invades the uterus, pelvic pain, uterine perforation, and vasovagal vasomotor reactions do occur. Allergic reactions, particularly to the iodine dye, are a possibility.
- Major indications for diagnostic hysteroscopy include abnormal uterine bleeding, infertility, and recurrent pregnancy loss.
- Operative hysteroscopy may be used to remove polyps, myomas, and synechiae. The endometrial lining may be ablated through the hysteroscope in women with abnormal bleeding or menorrhagia who are poor surgical candidates or who wish to retain their uterus.
- Dextran is an extremely viscous fluid used to distend the uterus during hysteroscopy. Dextran is nontoxic, nonconductive, and immiscible with blood.
- Hysteroscopy is superior to HSG in discovering and diagnosing intrauterine pathology.
- Complications of hysteroscopy include uterine perforation, pelvic infection, bleeding, and absorption of the distending media.
- There are both diagnostic and therapeutic indications for laparoscopy in infertile women. Tubal patency and mobility can be directly observed via the laparoscope. It is possible not only to describe and stage the extent of endometriosis or pelvic adhesions but also to treat them. Adhesions can be lysed, and areas of endometriosis can be ablated by electrocautery or laser.
- The enigma of chronic pelvic pain may be solved by the findings at laparoscopy and "pain mapping." Following the procedure, a plan for long-term management of the pain can be discussed with the patient.
- Absolute contraindications to laparoscopy include hemoperitoneum that has produced hemodynamic instability, anticoagulation therapy, advanced malignancy, large abdominal masses, severe cardiovascular disease, and tuberculous peritonitis.
- Patients with ectopic pregnancies treated by laparoscopic salpingotomy should have serial HCG titers until the titers fall to zero.
- Major complications of laparoscopy are laceration of vessels, intestinal and urinary tract injuries, and cardiorespiratory problems arising from the pneumoperitoneum.
- The incidence of complications with operative laparoscopy varies from 0.2% to 2%.
- Laparoscopy provides a window for the diagnosis of infertility, pelvic pain, ectopic pregnancy, abdominal and pelvic trauma, staging the extent of pelvic disease, and the visual diagnosis of abnormal anatomy. Therapeutic uses of the laparoscope vary from female sterilization to hysterectomy and node sampling.

BIBLIOGRAPHY

Albers JR, Hull SK, Wesley RM: Abnormal uterine bleeding. Am Fam Physician 69:1915, 2004.

Alborzi S, Dehbashi S, Khodaee R: Sonohysterosalpingographic screening for infertile patients. Int J Gynecol Obstet 82:57, 2003.

American College of Obstetricians and Gynecologists: Operative laparoscopy. ACOG Educ Bull 239:1, 1997.

American College of Obstetricians and Gynecologists: Saline infusion sonohysterography. ACOG Technology Assessment 102:659, 2003.

American College of Obstetricians and Gynecologists: Practice Bulletin No. 14: Management of anovulatory bleeding. ACOG compendium 434, 2004.

Baggish MS, Barbot J, Valle RF: Diagnostic and Operative Hysteroscopy: A Text and Atlas, 2nd ed. Chicago, Mosby, 1999.

Bateman BG, Kolp LA, Hoeger K: Complications of laparoscopy-operative and diagnostic. Fertil Steril 66:30, 1996.

Batra N, Khunda A, O'Donovan PJ: Hysteroscopic myomectomy. Obstet Gynecol Clin North Am 31:669, 2004.

Berridge DL, Winter TC: Saline infusion sonohysterography: Technique, indications, and imaging findings. Ultrasound Med 23:97, 2004.

Bettocchi S, Nappi L, Ceci O, et al: Office hysteroscopy. Obstet Gynecol Clin North Am 31:641, 2004.

Breitkopf DM, Frederickson RA, Snyder RR: Detection of benign endometrial masses by endometrial stripe measurement in premenopausal women. Obstet Gynecol 104:120, 2004.

Brooks PG: Hysteroscopic surgery using the resectoscope: Myomas, ablation, septae and synechiae: Does pre-operative medication help? Clin Obstet Gynecol 35:249, 1992.

Brooks SE: Preoperative evaluation of patients with suspected ovarian cancer. Gynecol Oncol 55:S80, 1994.

Carter J, Saltzman A, Hartenbach E, et al: Flow characteristics in benign and malignant gynecologic tumors using transvaginal color flow Doppler. Obstet Gynecol 83:125, 1994.

Castelbaum AJ, Wheeler J, Coutifaris CB, et al: Timing of the endometrial biopsy may be critical for the accurate diagnosis of luteal phase deficiency. Fertil Steril 61:443, 1994.

Chandler JG, Corson SL, Way LW: Three spectra of laparoscopic entry access injuries. J Am Coll Surg 192:478, 2001.

Chang YCF, Hricak H, Thurnher S, et al: Vagina: Evaluation with MR imaging. Part II. Neoplasms. Radiology 169:175, 1988.

Check JH, Chase JS, Nowroozi K, et al: Clinical evaluation of the Pipelle endometrial suction curette for timed endometrial biopsies. J Reprod Med 34:218, 1989.

Childers JM, Aqua KA, Surwit EA, et al: Abdominal-wall tumor implantation after laparoscopy for malignant conditions. Obstet Gynecol 84:765, 1994.

Clark TJ, Voit D, Gupta JK, et al: Accuracy of hysteroscopy in the diagnosis of endometrial cancer and hyperplasia: A systematic quantitative review. JAMA 288:1610, 2002.

Cooper JM: Hysteroscopic sterilization. Clin Obstet Gynecol 35:282, 1992.

Cooper JM, Brady RM: Hysteroscopy in the management of abnormal uterine bleeding. Obstet Gynecol Clin North Am 26:217, 1999.

Corson SL, Brooks PG, Soderstrom RM: Gynecologic endoscopic gas embolism. Fertil Steril 65:529, 1996.

Daniel AG, Peters WA III: Accuracy of office and operating room curettage in the grading of endometrial carcinoma. Obstet Gynecol 71:612, 1988.

Daniel JF, Kurtz BR, Ke RW: Hysteroscopic endometrial ablation using the rollerball electrode. Obstet Gynecol 80:329, 1992.

De Kroon CD, de Bock GH, Dieben SEM, et al: Saline contrast hysterosonography in abnormal uterine bleeding: A systematic review and meta-analysis. Br J Obstet Gynaecol 110:945, 2003.

De Kroon CD, Jansen FW, Louwé LA, et al: Technology assessment of saline contrast hysterosonography. Am J Obstet Gynecol 188:945, 2003.

Dijkhuizen FPHLJ, Brölmann HAM, Potters AE, et al: The accuracy of transvaginal ultrasonography in the diagnosis of endometrial abnormalities. Obstet Gynecol 87:345, 1996.

Dijkhuizen FPHLJ, Mol BWJ, Brolmann HAM, et al: The accuracy of endometrial sampling in the diagnosis of patients with endometrial carcinoma and hyperplasia—A meta-analysis. Cancer 89:1765, 2000.

Dunphy B, Taenzer P, Bultz B, et al: A comparison of pain experienced during hysterosalpingography and in-office falloposcopy. Fertil Steril 62:67, 1994.

Edelman RR, Warach S: Magnetic resonance imaging. Part I. N Engl J Med 328:708, 1993.

Edelman RR, Warach S: Magnetic resonance imaging. Part II. N Engl J Med 328:785, 1993.

Eltabbakh GH, Piver MS, Hempling RE, Recio FO: Laparoscopic surgery in obese women. Obstet Gynecol 94:704, 1999.

Emanuel MH, Verdel MJ, Wamsteker K, Lammes FB: A prospective comparison of transvaginal ultrasonography and diagnostic hysteroscopy in the evaluation of patients with abnormal uterine bleeding: Clinical implications. Am J Obstet Gynecol 172:547, 1995.

Epstein E, Valentin L: Managing women with post-menopausal bleeding. Best Pract Res Clin Obstet Gynecol 18:125, 2004.

Farquhar C, Ekeroma A, Furness S, et al: A systematic review of transvaginal ultrasonography, sonohysterography and hysteroscopy for the investigation of abnormal uterine bleeding in premenopausal women. Acta Obstet Gynecol Scand 82:493, 2003.

Feldman S, Shapter A, Welch WR, Berkowitz RS: Two-year follow-up of 263 patients with post/perimenopausal vaginal bleeding and negative initial biopsy. Gynecol Oncol 55:56, 1994.

Forstner R, Chen M, Hricak H: Imaging of ovarian cancer. J Magn Reson Imaging 5:606, 1995.

Gleeson NC, Nicosia SV, Mark JE, et al: Abdominal wall metastases from ovarian cancer after laparoscopy. Am J Obstet Gynecol 169:522, 1993.

Goldstein SR: Postmenopausal endometrial fluid collections revisited: Look at the doughnut rather than the hole. Obstet Gynecol 83:738, 1994.

Goldstein SR: Saline infusion sonohysterography. Clin Obstet Gynecol 39:248, 1996.

Goodman SB, Rein MS, Hill JA: Hysterosalpingography contrast media and chromotubation dye inhibit peritoneal lymphocyte and macrophage function in vitro: A potential mechanism for fertility enhancement. Fertil Steril 59:1022, 1993.

Goodrich MA, Webb MJ, King BF, et al: Magnetic resonance imaging of pelvic floor relaxation: Dynamic analysis and evaluation of patients before and after surgical repair. Obstet Gynecol 82:883, 1993.

Gupta JK, Chien PF, Voit D, et al: Ultrasonographic endometrial thickness for diagnosing endometrial pathology in women with postmenopausal bleeding: a meta-analysis. Acta Obstet Gynecol Scand 81:799, 2002.

Hardacre JM, Talamini MA: Pulmonary and hemodynamic changes during laparoscopy—Are they important? Surg 127:241, 2000.

Härkki-Siren P, Sjöberg J, Kurki T: Major complications of laparoscopy: A follow-up Finnish study. Obstet Gynecol 94:94, 1999.

Hatasaka H: The evaluation of abnormal uterine bleeding. Clin Obstet Gynecol 48:258, 2005.

Honoré GM, Holden AEC, Schenken RS: Pathophysiology and management of proximal tubal blockage. Fertil Steril 71:785, 1999.

Hricak H, Chen M, Coakley FV, et al: Complex adnexal masses: Detection and characterization with MR imaging-multivariate analysis. Radiol 214:39, 2000.

Hricak H, Quivey JM, Campos Z, et al: Carcinoma of the cervix: predictive value of clinical and magnetic resonance (MR) imaging assessment of prognostic factors. Int J Radiat Oncol Biol Phys 27:791, 1993.

Hulka JF: Textbook of Laparoscopy, Philadelphia, WB Saunders, 1998.

Hurd WW, Bude RO, DeLancey JOL, Newman JS: The location of abdominal wall blood vessels in relationship to abdominal landmarks apparent at laparoscopy. Am J Obstet Gynecol 171:642, 1994.

Hutchinson CJ: Laparoscopy and hysterosalpingography in the assessment of tubal patency. Obstet Gynecol 49:325, 1977.

Israel R, March CM: Hysteroscopic incision of the septate uterus. Am J Obstet Gynecol 149:66, 1984.

Istre O, Skajaa K, Schjoensby AP, Forman A: Changes in serum electrolytes after transcervical resection of endometrium and submucous fibroids with use of glycine 1.5% for uterine irrigation. Obstet Gynecol 80:218, 1992.

Jansen FW, Vredevoogd CB, Van Ulzen K, et al: Complications of hysteroscopy: A prospective, multicenter study. Obstet Gynecol 96:266, 2000.

Karande VC, Pratt DE, Rabin DS, Gleicher N: The limited value of hysterosalpingography in assessing tubal status and fertility potential. Fertil Steril 63:1167, 1995.

Karlsson B, Granberg S, Wikland M, et al: Transvaginal ultrasonography of the endometrium in women with postmenopausal bleeding—A Nordic multicenter study. Am J Obstet Gynecol 172:1488, 1995.

Keltz MD, Olive DL, Kim AH, Arici A: Sonohysterography for screening in recurrent pregnancy loss. Fertil Steril 67:670, 1997.

Kinkel K, Kaji Y, Yu KK, et al: Radiologic staging in patients with endometrial cancer: A meta-analysis. Radiol 212:711, 1999.

Kurjak A, Shalan H, Kupesic S, et al: An attempt to screen asymptomatic women for ovarian and endometrial cancer with transvaginal color and pulsed Doppler sonography. J Ultrasound Med 13:295, 1994.

Langer RD, Pierce JJ, O'Hanlan KA, et al: Transvaginal ultrasonography compared with endometrial biopsy for the detection of endometrial disease. N Engl J Med 337:1792, 1997.

Leonard F, Lecuru F, Rizk E, et al: Perioperative morbidity of gynecological laparoscopy: A prospective monocenter observational study. Acta Obstet Gynaecol Scand 79:129, 2000.

Levine D: Gynaecologic ultrasound. Clin Radiol 53:1, 1998.

Lindequist S, Rasmussen F, Torp HH, et al: Diagnostic quality in hysterosalpingography: Comparison between iodixanol and iotrolan. Acta Radiol 39:730, 1998.

Magos A, Chapman L: Hysteroscopic tubal sterilization. Obstet Gynecol Clin North Am 31:705, 2004.
Maly Z, Riss P, Deutinger J: Localization of blood vessels and qualitative assessment of blood flow in ovarian tumors. Obstet Gynecol 85:33, 1995.
March CM: Hysterectomy. J Reprod Med 37:293, 1992.
Marsh F, Duffy S: The technique and overview of flexible hysteroscopy. Obstet Gynecol Clin North Am 31:655, 2004.
Maruri F, Azziz R: Laparoscopic surgery for ectopic pregnancies: technology assessment and public health implications. Fertil Steril 59:487, 1993.
Mayo-Smith WW, Lee MJ: MR imaging of the female pelvis. Clin Radiol 50:667, 1995.
McBean JH, Gibson M, Brumsted JR: The association of intrauterine filling defects on hysterosalpingogram with endometriosis. Fertil Steril 66:522, 1996.
McCall JL, Sharples K, Jadallah F: Systematic review of randomized controlled trials comparing laparoscopic with open appendectomy. Br J Surg 84:1045, 1997.
McGonigle KF, Shaw SL, Vasilev SA, et al: Abnormalities detected on transvaginal ultrasonography in tamoxifen-treated postmenopausal breast cancer patients may represent endometrial cystic atrophy. Am J Obstet Gynecol 178:1145, 1998.
Meléndez JC, McCrank E: Anxiety-related reactions associated with magnetic resonance imaging examinations. JAMA 270:745, 1993.
Mihm LM, Quick VA, Brumfield JA, et al: The accuracy of endometrial biopsy and saline sonohysterography in the determination of the cause of abnormal uterine bleeding. Am J Obstet Gynecol 186:858, 2002.
Mirhashemi R, Harlow BL, Ginsburg ES, et al: Predicting risk of complications with gynecologic laparoscopic surgery. Obstet Gynecol 92:327, 1998.
Montz FJ, Holschneider CH, Munro MG: Incisional hernia following laparoscopy: A survey of the American Association of Gynecologic Laparoscopists. Obstet Gynecol 84:881, 1994.
Mouton WG, Bessell JR, Otten KT, Maddern GJ: Pain after laparoscopy. Surg Endosc 13:445, 1999.
Nelson BE, Rosenfield AT, Schwartz PE: Preoperative abdominopelvic computed tomographic prediction of optimal cytoreduction in epithelial ovarian carcinoma. J Clin Oncol 11:166, 1993.
Nelson RC, Chezmar JL, Hoes MJ, et al: Peritoneal carcinomatosis: preoperative CA with intraperitoneal contrast material. Radiology 182:133, 1992.
Nunley WC Jr, Bateman BG, Kitchin JD III, et al: Intravasation during hysterosalpingography using oil-base contrast medium—A second look. Obstet Gynecol 70:309, 1987.
O'Connell LP, Fries MH, Zeringue E, Brehm W: Triage of abnormal postmenopausal bleeding: A comparison of endometrial biopsy and transvaginal sonohysterography versus fractional curettage with hysteroscopy. Am J Obstet Gynecol 178:956, 1998.
Pabuccu R, Atay V, Orhon E, et al: Hysteroscopic treatment of intrauterine adhesions is safe and effective in the restoration of normal menstruation and fertility. Fertil Steril 68:1141, 1997.
Papaioannou S, Afnan M, Sharif K: The role of selective salpingography and tubal catheterization in the management of the infertile couple. Curr Opin Obstet Gynecol 16:325, 2004.
Patel VH, Somers S: MR imaging of the female pelvis: Current perspective and review of genital tract congenital anomalies, and benign and malignant diseases. Crit Rev Diagn Imaging 36:417, 1997.
Pellerito JS, McCarthy SM, Doyle MB, et al: Diagnosis of uterine anomalies: Relative accuracy of MR imaging, endovaginal sonography, and hysterosalpingography. Radiology 183:795, 1992.
Pennehouat G, Risquez F, Naouri M, et al: Transcervical falloposcopy: Preliminary experience. Hum Reprod 8:445, 1993.
Perdigon PL: Imaging techniques for diagnosis of serious intraabdominal and pelvic infections. Prim Care Update Ob/Gyn 6:115, 1999.
Peterson HB, Xia Z, Hughes JM, et al: The risk of pregnancy after tubal sterilization: Findings from U.S. Collaborative Review of Sterilization. Am J Obstet Gynecol 174:1161, 1996.
Porpora MG, Gomel V: The role of laparoscopy in the management of pelvic pain in women of reproductive age. Fertil Steril 68:765, 1997.
Preutthipan S, Herabutya Y: A randomized controlled trial of vaginal misoprostol for cervical priming before hysteroscopy. Obstet Gynecol 94:427, 1999.
Prömpeler HJ, Madjar H, Sauerbrei W, et al: Diagnostic formula for the differentiation of adnexal tumors by transvaginal sonography. Obstet Gynecol 89, 428, 1997.
Rabin JM, Spitzer M, Dwyer AT, et al: Topical anesthesia for gynecologic procedures. Obstet Gynecol 73:1040, 1989.
Rao PM, Feltmate CM, Rhea JT, et al: Helical computed tomography in differentiating appendicitis and acute gynecologic conditions. Obstet Gynecol 93:417, 1999.
Rasmussen F, Lindequist S, Larsen C, Justesen P: Therapeutic effect of hysterosalpingography: Oil- versus water-soluble contrast media-a randomized prospective study. Radiology 179:75, 1991.
Rock JA, Warshaw JR: The history and future of operative laparoscopy. Am J Obstet Gynecol 170:7, 1994.
Romano F, Cicinelli E, Anastasio PS, et al: Sonohysterography versus hysteroscopy for diagnosing endouterine abnormalities in fertile women. Int J Gynecol Obstet 45:253, 1994.
Schutter E, Kenemans P, Sohn C, et al: Diagnostic value of pelvic examination, ultrasound, and serum CA 125 in postmenopausal women with a pelvic mass. Cancer 74:1398, 1994.
Shalev E, Yarom I, Bustan M, et al: Transvaginal sonography as the ultimate diagnostic tool for the management of ectopic pregnancy: Experience with 840 cases. Fertil Steril 69, 62, 1998.
Sironi S, Colombo E, Villa G, et al: Myometrial invasion by endometrial carcinoma: Assessment with plain and gadolinium-enhanced MR imaging. Radiology 185:207, 1992.
Sladkevicius P, Valentin L, Marsál K: Endometrial thickness and Doppler velocimetry of the uterine arteries as discriminators of endometrial status in women with postmenopausal bleeding: A comparative study. Am J Obstet Gynecol 171:722, 1994.
Spreafico C, Frigerlo L, Lanocita R, et al: Color-Doppler ultrasound in ovarian masses: Anatomo-pathologic correlation. Tumori 79:262, 1993.
Spring DB, Barkan HE, Pruyn SC: Potential therapeutic effects of contrast materials in hysterosalpingography: A prospective randomized clinical trial. Radiol 214:53, 2000.
Suh-Burgmann EJ, Goodman A: Surveillance for endometrial cancer in women receiving tamoxifen. Ann Intern Med 131:127, 1999.
Sultana CJ, Easley K, Collins RL: Outcome of laparoscopic versus traditional surgery for ectopic pregnancies. Fertil Steril 57:285, 1992.
Swart P, Mol BWJ, van der Veen F, et al: The accuracy of hysterosalpingography in the diagnosis of tubal pathology: a meta-analysis. Fertil Steril 64:486, 1995.
Swayne LC, Love MB, Karasick SR: Pelvic inflammatory disease: Sonographic-pathologic correlation. Radiology 151:751, 1984.
Tahir MM, Bigrigg MA, Browning JJ, et al: A randomized controlled trial comparing transvaginal ultrasound, outpatient hysteroscopy and endometrial biopsy with inpatient hysteroscopy and curettage. Br J Obstet Gynaecol 106:1259, 1999.
Timbos-Kemper TCM, Veering BT: Anaphylactic shock from intracavitary 32% dextran-70 during hysteroscopy. Fertil Steril 51:1053, 1989.
Togashi K, Nishimura K, Sagoh T, et al: Carcinoma of the cervix: Staging with MR imaging. Radiology 171:245, 1989.
Troiano RN, McCarthy S: Magnetic resonance imaging evaluation of adnexal masses. Semin Ultrasound CT MR 15:38, 1994.
Tulandi T, Bugnah M: Operative laparoscopy: Surgical modalities. Fertil Steril 63:237, 1995.
Valle RF: Office hysteroscopy. Clin Obstet Gynecol 42:276, 1999.
Van Den Bosch T, Vandendael A, Van Schoubroeck D, et al: Combining vaginal ultrasonography and office endometrial sampling in the diagnosis of endometrial disease in postmenopausal women. Obstet Gynecol 85:349, 1995.
Van den Bosch T, Van Schoubroeck D, Ameye L, et al: Ultrasound assessment of endometrial thickness and endometrial polyps in women on hormonal replacement therapy. Am J Obstet Gynecol 188:1249, 2003.
Venezia R, Zangara C, Knight C, Cittadini E: Initial experience of a new linear everting falloposcopy system in comparison with hysterosalpingography. Fertil Steril 60:771, 1993.
Vercellini P, Rossi R, Pagnoni B, Fedele L: Hypervolemic pulmonary edema and severe coagulopathy after intrauterine dextran instillation. Obstet Gynecol 79:838, 1992.
Watson A, Vandekerckhove P, Lilford R, et al: A meta-analysis of the therapeutic role of oil soluble contrast media at hysterosalpingography: A surprising result? Fertil Steril 61:470, 1994.
Wieser F, Kurz C, Wenzl R, et al: Atraumatic cervical passage at outpatient hysteroscopy. Fertil Steril 69:549, 1998.
Witz CA, Silverberg KM, Burns WN, et al: Complications associated with the absorption of hysteroscopic fluid media. Fertil Steril 60:745, 1993.

Woodward PJ, Gilfeather M: Magnetic resonance imaging of the female pelvis. Semin Ultrasound, CT, MR 19:90, 1998.
Wortman M, Daggett A: Hysteroscopic endomyometrial resection: A new technique for the treatment of menorrhagia. Obstet Gynecol 83:295, 1994.
Yaziciogulu HF: A clear hysteroscopic view and the use of other diagnostic modalities in addition to hysteroscopy to achieve better diagnostic accuracy. Am J Obstet Gynecol 176:950, 1997.
Zanetta G, Vergani P, Lissoni A: Color Doppler ultrasound in the preoperative assessment of adnexal masses. Acta Obstet Gynecol Scand 73:637, 1994.
Zupi E, Luciano AA, Valli E, et al: The use of topical anesthesia in diagnostic hysteroscopy and endometrial biopsy. Fertil Steril 63:414, 1995.

PART III

GENERAL GYNECOLOGY

Congenital Abnormalities of the Female Reproductive Tract 12

Anomalies of the Vagina, Cervix, Uterus, and Adnexa

Vern L. Katz and Gretchen M. Lentz

KEY TERMS AND DEFINITIONS

Accessory Ovary. Excess ovarian tissue near a normally placed ovary and connected to it.

Ambiguous Genitalia. Developmental anatomic modification of the external genitalia, which makes specific determination of sex difficult.

Androgen Resistance Syndrome. A group of conditions in which inadequate testosterone levels reach target tissues. The most common is an X-linked condition of a testosterone receptor defect in a 46,XY individual with testes and normal male testosterone levels. These individuals have no uterus, a normal female phenotype, and scanty body hair. The old name, *testicular feminization,* is no longer used.

Arcuate Uterus. A minimum septate uterus; of minimal clinical significance.

Bicornuate Uterus. A partial lack of fusion of two uterine corpora. A single cervix is present.

Didelphic Uterus. Complete duplication of the uterus and cervix without fusion of the two cavities. One fallopian tube joins each fundal cavity. This condition may be associated with a septate vagina.

Hermaphrodite. An individual with both testicular and ovarian tissue in either the same or opposite gonads.

Hematocolpos. Distention of an obstructed vagina (caused by imperforate hymen or transverse septum) with blood and blood products.

Hydrocolpos. Distention of an obstructed vagina (caused by imperforate hymen or transverse septum) with fluid.

Labial Fusion. Fusion of the labia minora in the midline, closing the introitus.

Mayer–Rokitansky–Küster–Hauser Syndrome (MRKH syndrome). A 46,XX female with müllerian failure (agenesis), usually showing absence of all or most of the vagina, cervix, uterus, and fallopian tubes.

Mucocolpos. A vagina blocked by an imperforate hymen or transverse septum and filled with mucus.

Ovotestes. Gonads that contain both ovarian and testicular remnants.

Pseudohermaphrodite. An individual with chromosomes of one sex, XX or XY, but external genitalia that is of the opposite sex or is ambiguous.

Recurrent Miscarriage. The loss of three or more pregnancies before 20 weeks' gestation. Functionally, however, many physicians will do a workup for repetitive spontaneous abortion after two or more pregnancy losses.

Rudimentary Uterine Horn. A structure that develops from one müllerian duct and does not communicate with the uterine cavity. The contralateral fallopian tube communicates with the uterine cavity. The ipsilateral fallopian tube communicates with that horn.

Septate Uterus. The presence of a septum that separates the uterine cavity either partially or completely into two separate cavities.

Supernumerary Ovary. The presence of a third ovary separated from the normally situated ovaries.

Unicolic (Unicornuate) Uterus. A uterus and cervix that develop from a single müllerian duct joined at the top of the fundus by only one fallopian tube. It represents complete arrest of one müllerian duct.

Vaginal Agenesis. Absence of the vagina.

Congenital abnormalities of the female reproductive tract are common. They can be caused by genetic errors or by teratologic events during embryonic development. Minor abnormalities may be of little consequence, but major abnormalities may lead to severe impairment of menstrual and reproductive functions. This chapter categorizes a number of such abnormalities and discusses diagnosis and treatment. Most studies find the incidence of müllerian anomalies to occur in 1% to 3% of women. Anomalies present at varying times in a woman's life, from birth, before puberty, with the onset of menses, and during pregnancy with adverse pregnancy outcomes. Because of the profound psychological effects such abnormalities can cause, the gynecologist must approach the problems of genital and müllerian anomalies with sensitivity and with a wide perspective of the effects they have on the woman.

EXAMINATION OF THE NEWBORN FOR AMBIGUOUS GENITALIA

The first major diagnostic decision of the obstetrician with respect to the newborn is gender assignment. In most cases the designation is clear. However, in approximately 1 in 14,000 newborns ambiguous genitalia will be found. This is a serious problem for the infant, the physician, and the parents. Females (individuals with XX karyotypes) and masculinized external genitalia are identified as female pseudohermaphrodites (Table 12-1). The most common cause is congenital adrenal hyperplasia. The timing of antenatal (embryonic) exposure to androgen influences the degree of masculinization (Fig. 12-1). The vaginal septum separates from the urogenital sinus at about 12 weeks. Androgen exposure after that point presents primarily with clitoral hypertrophy. The female who has been androgenized may appear similar to the male pseudohermaphrodite suffering from incomplete androgen resistance syndrome. Also, some vulvar abnormalities may resemble partial androgenization. It is therefore appropriate to systematically evaluate the newborn's genitalia to make the appropriate gender assignment, and when necessary perform imaging studies, chromosomal evaluations, serum electrolytes, and steroid assessment. Until 10 years ago gender was assigned primarily on the principal of "phallic adequacy," with neonates with ambiguous phallus being assigned female gender. This principle has fallen into disfavor, and full evaluation with appropriately timed corrective measures and procedures is now the desired approach.

The first and probably most important aspect of the examination of the neonate is inspection. The physician should systematically observe the newborn's perineum, beginning with the mons pubis. The clitoris should be noted for any obvious enlargement, the opening of the urethra should be identified, and the labia should be gently separated to see if the introitus can be visualized. If the labia are fused, this maneuver will be impossible. Palpation of the inguinal area and labia for testes is important at this point. At times the labia are joined by filmy adhesions; these generally separate in later childhood or respond

Table 12–1 Classification of Female Pseudohermaphroditism

I. Androgen-Induced
 A. Fetal Source
  1. Congenital adrenal hyperplasia
   a. Virilism only, defective adrenal 21-hydroxylation (CYP21)
   b. Virilism with salt-losing syndrome, defective adrenal 21-hydroxylation (CYP21)
   c. Virilism with hypertension, defective adrenal 11β-hydroxylation (CYP11B1)
   d. Virilism with adrenal insufficiency, deficient 3β-HSD 2 (HSD3B 2)
  2. P450 aromatase (CYP19) deficiency
  3. Glucocorticoid receptor gene mutation
 B. Maternal source
  1. Iatrogenic
   a. Testosterone and related steroids
   b. Certain synthetic oral progestagens and rarely diethylstilbestrol
  2. Virilizing ovarian or adrenal tumor
  3. Virilizing luteoma of pregnancy
  4. Congenital virilizing adrenal hyperplasia in mother*
 C. Undetermined source
  1. ?Virilizing luteoma of pregnancy
II. Non–Androgen-Induced Disturbances in Differentiation of Urogenital Structures

*In pregnant patient whose disease is poorly controlled or who are noncompliant, especially during the first trimester.
From Grumbach MM, Hughes IA, Conte FA: Disorders of sex differentation. In Larsen RP, Kronenberg HM, Melmed S, Polonsky KS (eds): Williams Textbook of Endocrinology, 10th ed. Philadelphia, Saunders, 2003, p 916.

to the application of estrogen cream when necessary. If it is possible to separate the labia, the hymen may be observed. Generally, it is partially perforate, revealing the entrance into the vagina. Posteriorly the labia fuse in the midline at the posterior fourchette of the perineum. Posterior to the perineal body the rectum can be visualized, and it should be tested to be sure that it is perforate. Meconium staining about the rectum is evidence for perforation. If there is doubt, the rectum may be penetrated with a moistened cotton-tipped swab.

If the labia are fused and the clitoris is not enlarged, other abnormalities may also be present, such as abnormalities of the abdominal wall or skeletal system. Thus, the infant should be carefully assessed for other anomalies. An enlarged clitoris and fused labia are evidence of androgen effect and may imply congenital adrenal hyperplasia, maternal ingestion of androgens,

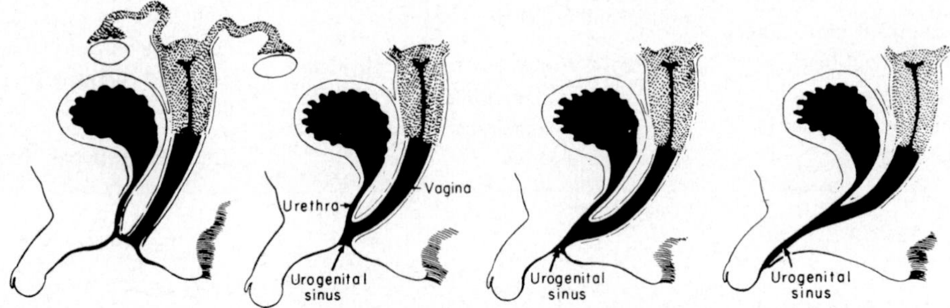

Figure 12-1. Female pseudohermaphroditism induced by prenatal exposure to androgens. Exposure after 12th fetal week leads only to clitoral hypertrophy (diagram on left). Exposure at progressively earlier stages of differentiation (depicted from left to right) leads to retention of the urogenital sinus and labioscrotal fusion. If exposure occurs sufficiently early, the labia fuse to form a penile urethra. (From Grumbach MM, Hughes IA, Conte FA: Disorders of sex differentiation. In Larsen RP, Kronenberg HM, Melmed S, Polonsky KS [eds]: Williams Textbook of Endocrinology, 10th ed. Philadelphia, WB Saunders, 2003, p 916.)

or increased natural androgen production. A bifid clitoris may be present; this anomaly is usually associated with extrophy of the bladder. In such cases, anterior rotation and shortening of the vagina with fused labia is usually present.

In most instances, inspection is all that is necessary. On the rare occasions when the physician needs to examine the vagina or see the cervix of the newborn, an endoscope, such as a pediatric cystoscope, may be used. The hymen is generally perforate and will accept this instrument. If there is any difficulty, ultrasound may be preferable.

If labial fusion is noted, the physician should palpate the groins and labial folds for evidence of gonads. Gonads palpable in the inguinal canal, labioinguinal region, or labioscrotal folds are almost always testes. Thus, such a finding implies a male with ambiguous genitalia rather than a virilized female. Conversely, an infant with ambiguous genitalia but without palpable testes in the scrotum is likely to be a virilized female, most often the result of congenital adrenal hyperplasia. Rectal examination may make it possible to palpate a cervix and uterus, thus helping in the sex assignment. Ultrasound should be strongly considered for verification and evaluation.

Perineal and Vaginal Defects

Clitoral Anomalies

The clitoris is generally 1 to 1.5 cm long and 0.5 cm wide in the nonerect state. The glans is partially covered by a hood of skin. The urethra opens near the base of the clitoris. Abnormalities are unusual, although the clitoris may be enlarged because of androgen stimulation. In such circumstances the shaft of the clitoris may be quite enlarged, and partial development of a penile urethra may have occurred (Fig. 12-2). Extreme cases of androgen stimulation are generally associated with fusion of the labia. These findings occur in infants with congenital adrenal hyperplasia and in those exposed in utero to exogenous or endogenous androgens (Fig. 12-3). Similar in appearance, males with androgen insensitivity syndrome have underdeveloped male external genitalia and a very small phallus that appears as clitoral hypertrophy (Fig. 12-4).

Bifid clitoris (Fig. 12-5) is usually seen in association with extrophy of the bladder. Extrophy of the bladder occurs rarely (1 per 30,000 births) and has a male predominance (3:1). However, when it occurs in females, it is often associated with bifid clitoris. Stanton noted that 43% of 70 female patients with bladder extrophy had associated reproductive tract anomalies. These included vaginal anomalies and müllerian duct fusion problems. In such cases, an anterior rotation and shortening of the vagina with labial fusion is quite common.

Labial Fusion

Labial fusion may occur without clitoromegaly. The resultant ambiguous genitalia implies a form of hermaphroditism. The term *hermaphrodite* is derived from the child of the Greek gods Hermes and Aphrodite, Hermaphroditus, who was part man and part nymph. A true hermaphrodite has both ovarian (including follicular elements) and testicular tissue, either in the same or opposite gonads. The term *pseudohermaphroditism* applies to individuals with a pure XX or XY karyotype but with external genitalia of the opposite sex or ambiguous genitalia. True hermaphroditism is extremely rare in North and South America, but more common (though still very rare) in Africa.

Although labial fusion may result from exposure to exogenous androgens or be associated with defects of the anterior abdominal wall, by far the most common cause is congenital adrenal hyperplasia. The most common form of congenital

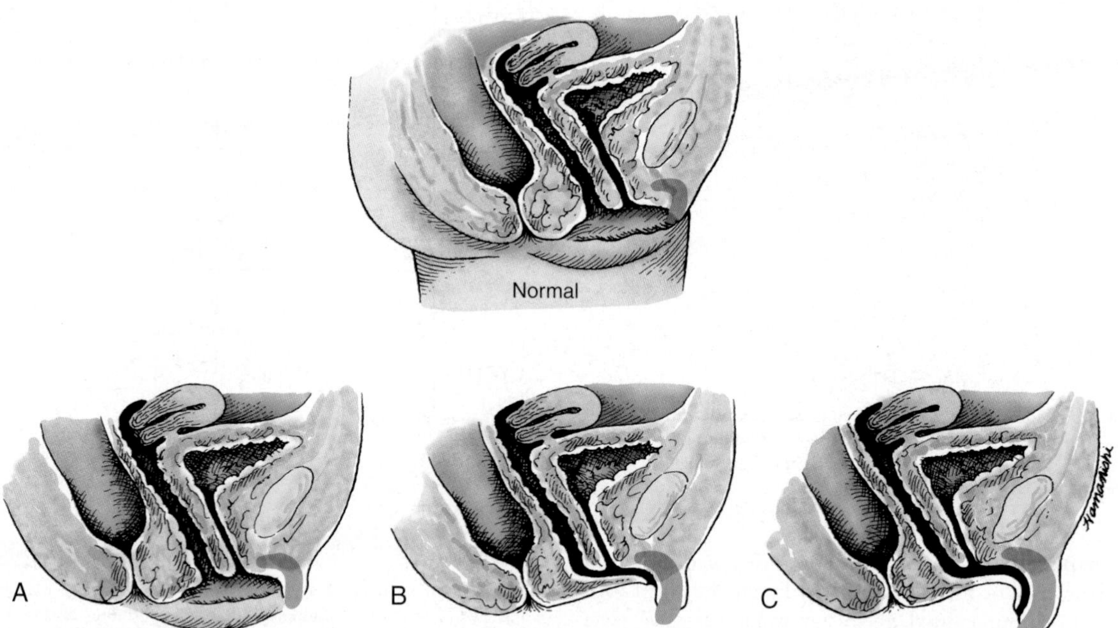

Figure 12-2. Sagittal views of genital deformities seen in female infants who are masculinized. **A,** Minimal masculinization with slight enlargement of the clitoris. **B,** Labial fusion and more marked enlargement of the clitoris. **C,** Complete labial fusion, enlargement of the clitoris, and formation of a partial penile urethra. (Modified from Verkauf BS, Jones HW Jr: Masculinization of the female genitalia in congenital adrenal hyperplasia: Relationship to the salt losing variety of the disease. South Med J 63:634, 1970.)

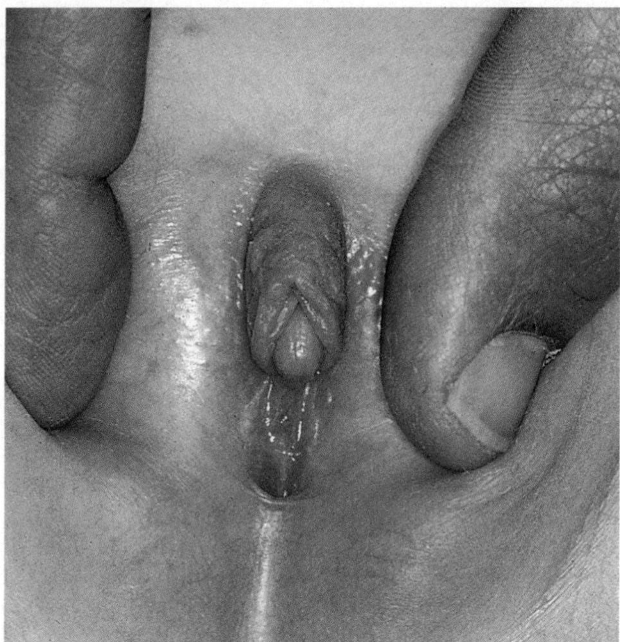

Figure 12-3. Clitoromegaly with posterior labial fusion in a child with congenital adrenal hyperplasia. (From McKay M: Vulvar manifestations of skin disorders. In Black M, McKay M, Braude P, et al [eds]: Obstetric and Gynecologic Dermatology, 2nd ed. Edinburgh, Mosby, 2003, p 120.)

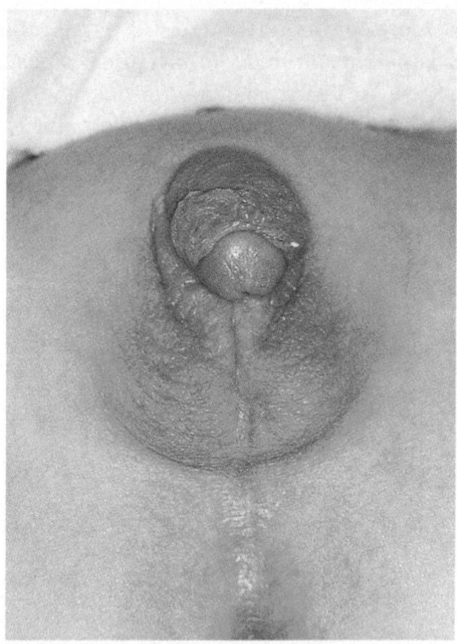

Figure 12-4. Ambiguous genitalia in an XY child with partial androgen insensitivity. (From McKay M: Vulvar manifestations of skin disorders. In Black M, McKay M, Braude P, et al [eds]: Obstetric and Gynecologic Dermatology, 2nd ed. Edinburgh, Mosby, 2003, p 121.)

adrenal hyperplasia is caused by an inborn error of metabolism involving deficiency of the enzyme 21-hydroxylase (Fig. 12-6). This condition is transmitted as an autosomal recessive gene coded on chromosome 6. Because of the absence of 21-hydroxylase, the major biosynthetic pathway to cortisol is blocked. 17-OH-progesterone is produced instead. This is converted to the androgen androstenedione. The fetal hypothalamic–

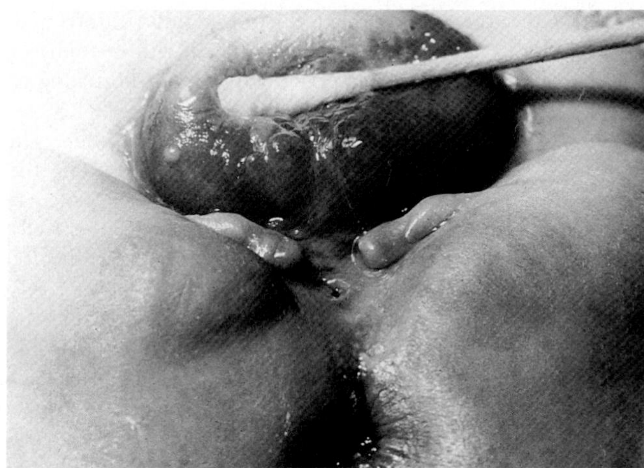

Figure 12-5. An example of a bifid clitoris in an infant with extrophy of the bladder. (Courtesy of Julian Ansell, MD.)

pituitary axis senses inadequate levels of cortisol and secretes excess adrenocorticotropic hormone (ACTH), which leads to increasing levels of androstenedione and fetal masculinization. Homozygous individuals occur with an incidence from 1 per 490 to 1 per 67,000 in the population, depending on the geographic location. Screening programs have noted the incidence to be approximately 1 in 14,000 births. Heterozygotic carriers are present in the population in a frequency ranging from 1 per 20 to 1 per 250.

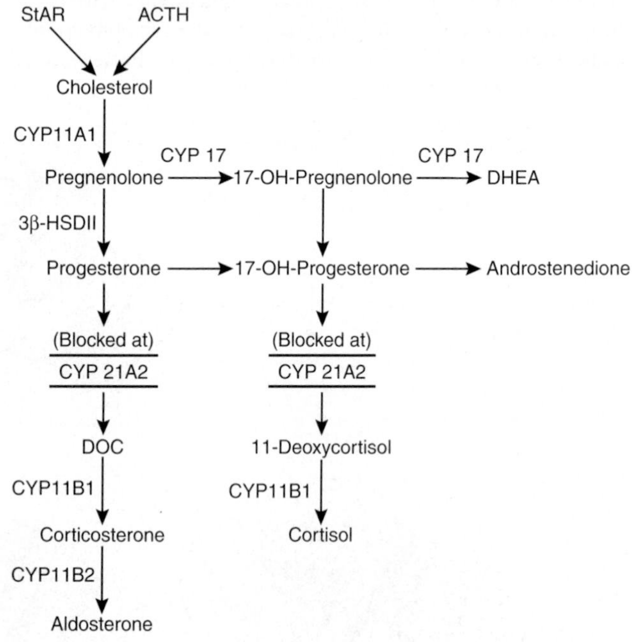

Figure 12-6. Steroid pathway in congenital adrenal hyperplasia with absence of 21 hydroxylase. ACTH, adrenocorticotropic hormone; 3β-HSDII, 3β-hydroxysteroid dehydrogenase; DHEA, dehydroeipandrosterone; DOC, deoxycorticosterone. (From Grumbach MM, Hughes IA, Conte FA: Disorders of sex differentiation. In Larsen RP, Kronenberg HM, Melmed S, Polonsky KS [eds]: Williams Textbook of Endocrinology, 10th ed. Philadelphia, WB Saunders, 2003, p 533)

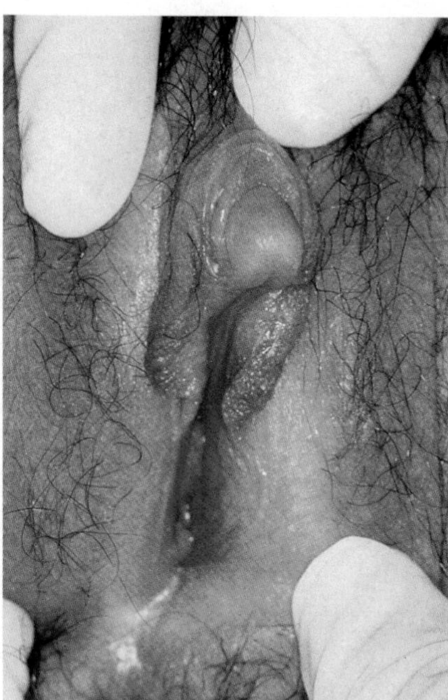

Figure 12-7. Eleven-year-old girl with clitoromegaly and thick genital hair, who presented with facial hair and was found to have 21-hydroxylase deficiency. (From McKay M: Vulvar manifestations of skin disorders. In Black M, McKay M, Braude P, et al [eds]: Obstetric and Gynecologic Dermatology, 2nd ed. Edinburgh, Mosby, 2003, p 120)

Two other less common enzyme defects, also transmittable as autosomal recessive traits, may produce similar abnormal findings: the 11-hydroxylase deficiency and the 3β-hydroxysteroid dehydrogenase deficiency. These two as well as 21-hydroxylase deficiency may cause ambiguous genitalia with masculinized females.

Congenital adrenal hyperplasia may be demonstrated at birth by the presence of ambiguous genitalia in genetic females or present later in childhood. A significant proportion (≤75%) of newborns with this condition are at risk for the development of a life-threatening neonatal adrenal crisis as a result of sodium loss because of absent aldosterone. For milder disease, a delayed diagnosis may result in accelerated bone maturation, leading ultimately to short stature. The development of premature secondary sexual characteristics in males and further virilization in females may also occur (Fig. 12-7)

In 1977, Pang and colleagues described a reliable and valid screening test employing capillary blood obtained by heel prick of infants that allowed for the radioimmunoassay determination of 17-hydroxyprogesterone in the serum. This test has been used in screening newborns for 21-hydroxylase deficiency, particularly in known high-risk populations, such as Alaskan native populations (Table 12-2). Using an elution technique employing a 3-mm filter paper disk to study the presence of 17-hydroxyprogesterone in capillary blood of these day-old newborns, these authors determined levels in normal infants to be less than 40 pg/3-mm disk. Affected infants had 17-OH-progesterone levels of 57 to 980 pg/disk. At the time of this publication 43 of 50 states in the United States have mandatory neonatal screening.

Treatment of congenital adrenal hyperplasia involves replacement of cortisol. This suppresses ACTH output and therefore decreases the stimulation of the cortisol-producing pathways of the adrenal cortex. Many of the infants affected with in utero androgenization may need corrective surgery. Initial corrective surgeries on the children may need follow-up vaginoplasty as teenagers because of vaginal stenosis. Almost all females with ambiguous genitalia should have ongoing psychological support and counseling because of the profound issues raised about identity with this diagnosis. In future pregnancies, the mother may be treated with dexamethasone for transplacental suppression of fetal pituitary until gender is diagnosed by either chorionic villus sampling (CVS) or amniocentesis.

Table 12–2 Incidence of Classic Congenital Virilizing Adrenal Hyperplasia (CYP21 Deficiency) after Screening

Population	Number of Newborns Screened	Newborns Affected/ Live Births	Incidence by Case Survey
Alaska	1131	1/282	1/490
La Réunion, France	31,472	1/3147	
Rome, Italy	22,400	1/5,600	
Lille (Lyon), France	199,624	1/11,090	1/23,000
Illinois	357,825	1/11,928	1/15,000 Wisconsin 1/40,000 USA
Sweden	370,000	1/12,758	
Portugal	100,000	1/14,285	
Emilia–Romagna, Italy	73,000	1/14,600	
Scotland	119,960	1/17,137	1/20,907
Washington	255,527	1/18,251	1/15,000 Wisconsin
New Zealand	168,965	1/18,773	
Japan	585,000	1/20,892	1/43,674

From Grumbach MM, Hughes IA, Conte FA: Disorders of sex differentiation. In Larsen RP, Kronenberg HM, Melmed S, Polonsky KS (eds): Williams Textbook of Endocrinology, 10th ed. Philadelphia, Saunders, 2003, p 918. Reprinted by permission of the publisher from Pang S, Clark A: Newborn screening, prenatal diagnosis, and prenatal treatment of congenital adrenal hyperplasia due to 21-hydroxylase deficiency. Trends Endocrinol Metab 1:302, 1990. Copyright 1990 by Elsevier Science Publishing Co., Inc.

Imperforate Hymen

The hymen represents the junction of the sinovaginal bulbs with the urogenital sinus and is composed of endoderm from the urogenital sinus epithelium. The hymen opens normally during embryonic life to establish a connection between the lumen of the vaginal canal and the vestibule. If this perforation does not take place, the hymen is imperforate (Fig. 12-8). The incidence is thought to be approximately 1 in 1000 live-born females. Several variations exist of partial hymeneal perforation (Fig. 12-9), many of which requires surgical correction.

It is rare to make the diagnosis of imperforate hymen before puberty, at which point primary amenorrhea is the major symptom. Occasionally in childhood a hydrocolpos or mucocolpos may occur. This is caused by a collection of secretions behind the hymen, which in rare cases may build up to form a mass that obstructs the urinary tract. If discovered, the hymen should be incised to release the build-up. At puberty the patient may expeience cyclic cramping but no menstrual flow. Over time the patient may develop a hematocolpos and a hematometrium. In more advanced cases the fallopian tubes may be distended with menstrual flow, and the flow may back up through the tubes and form endometrial implants in the peritoneal cavity. Quite surprisingly, many patients are free of symptoms.

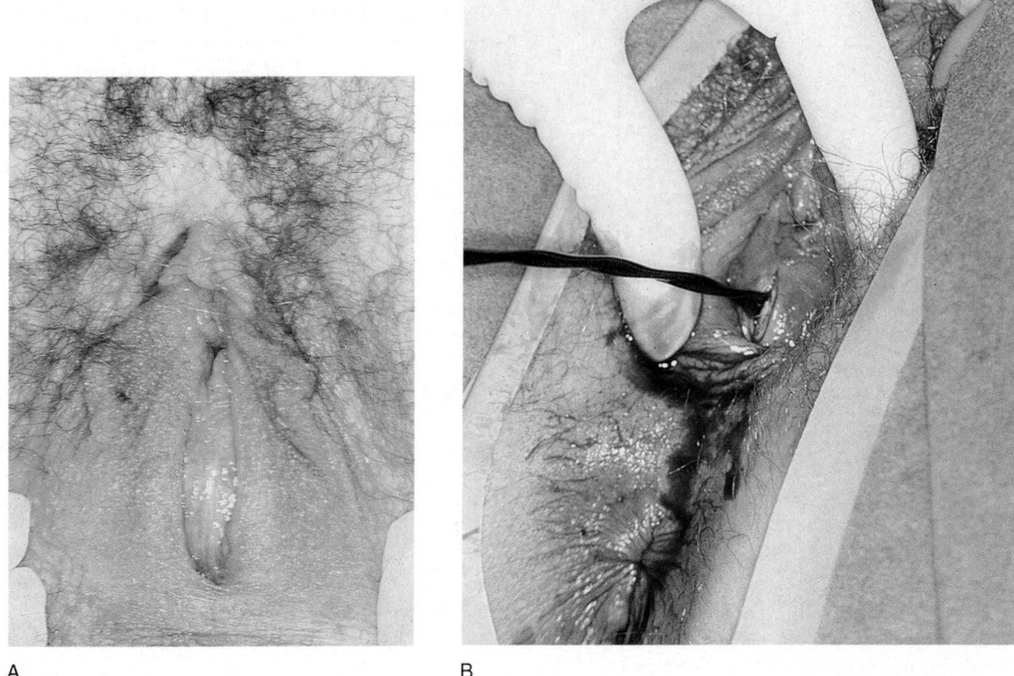

Figure 12-8. **A,** Imperforate hymen in a 13-year-old who presented with an acute abdomen. The vagina was distended by hematocolpos, with surgical incision (**B**) old blood was released. (From McKay M: Vulvar manifestations of skin disorders. In Black M, McKay M, Braude P, et al [eds]: Obstetric and Gynecologic Dermatology, 2nd ed. Edinburgh, Mosby, 2003, p 122.)

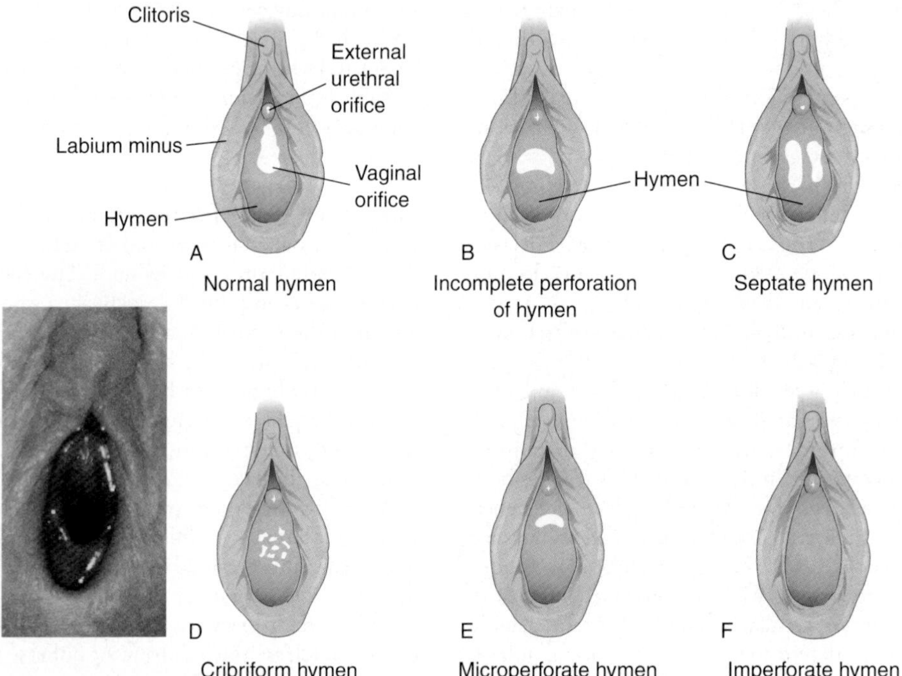

Figure 12-9. Congenital anomalies of the hymen. (From Moore KL, Persaud TVN: The Developing Human, 7th ed. Philadelphia, WB Saunders, 2003, p 322.)

The diagnosis can be determined by history and by the presence of a bulging membrane at the introitus. Therapy consists of a cruciate incision into the hymen extending to the 10, 2, and 6 o'clock positions. In the rare case of a thick and dense hymen a triangular section may be excised. Hemostasis is secured by fine suture, and evolution to normal usually occurs rapidly. This disease is thought to be a sporadic anomaly, though familial cases, as well as a case of autosomal dominant inheritance have been noted.

Vaginal Agenesis

Vaginal agenesis is usually associated with the Mayer–Rokitansky–Küster–Hauser syndrome (MRKH) (Fig. 12-10). This syndrome is characterized by congenital absence of the vagina and uterus, although small masses of smooth muscular material resembling a rudimentary bicornuate uterus are not uncommon. The syndrome occurs in approximately 1 in 5000 women. These individuals have a 46,XX karyotype. The disorder seems to be an accident of development and not an inherited condition.

Complete vaginal agenesis is discovered in 75% of patients with Mayer–Rokitansky–Küster–Hauser syndrome. Approximately 25% of patients have a short vaginal pouch. Some women may have rudimentary uterine horns, and case reports have been published documenting myomas as well as adenomyosis in the uterine tissue. Approximately 5% may have small amounts of endometrium with an epithelial lining, and rarely menstruation occurs, giving rise to monthly cyclic cramping. The ovaries in women with MRKH are normal, and the fallopian tubes are usually present. The differential diagnosis of vaginal agenesis includes transverse vaginal septum, cervical agenesis, and androgen insensitivity syndrome.

The androgen insensitivity syndrome comprises several genetic abnormalities centering on faulty androgen receptors. The syndrome until recently was termed *testicular feminization syndrome.* These individuals have a 46,XY karyotype. Because the developing fetus cannot sense any testosterone, the external genitalia are feminized, vaginal agenesis or the presence of a short pouch vagina is usually found. These patients have undescended testicles. The müllerian structures have resolved because the testes make antimüllerian hormone. Wolffian duct tissue exists instead. The individuals usually exhibit minimal pubic hair after puberty. After the growth spurt, the testes should be removed to prevent the development of gonadoblastoma. The ovaries of the patient with MRKH syndrome are normal and should not be removed.

Up to 50% of women with müllerian agenesis have concurrent urinary tract anomalies. Phelan and coworkers reported that of 72 patients with vaginal agenesis, 25% had urologic abnormalities noted on intravenous pyelography. A later study by Baramki demonstrated that 40% of 92 patients had urologic abnormalities. One study described a 12% incidence of skeletal anomalies, usually involving congenital fusion or absence of vertebrae in these patients. These and other studies indicate the need for imaging of the urinary tract in women with MRKH.

Diagnosis of MRKH syndrome is demonstrated by the presence of primary amenorrhea at the time of puberty, physical examination that demonstrates the absence of a vaginal opening or the presence of a short vaginal pouch, and failure to palpate a uterus on rectal examination, coupled with the finding of a normal karyotype. Although ultrasound examination may verify the presence of normal ovaries and the absence of the uterus, magnetic resonance imaging offers an excellent alternative for visualizing congenital anomalies of the internal reproductive organs and is currently the modality of choice for women with müllerian agenesis. Laparoscopic examination may be performed when the diagnosis is not clear or when there is some concern over the presence of functioning uterine tissue. In most cases, however, laparoscopic diagnosis is not necessary.

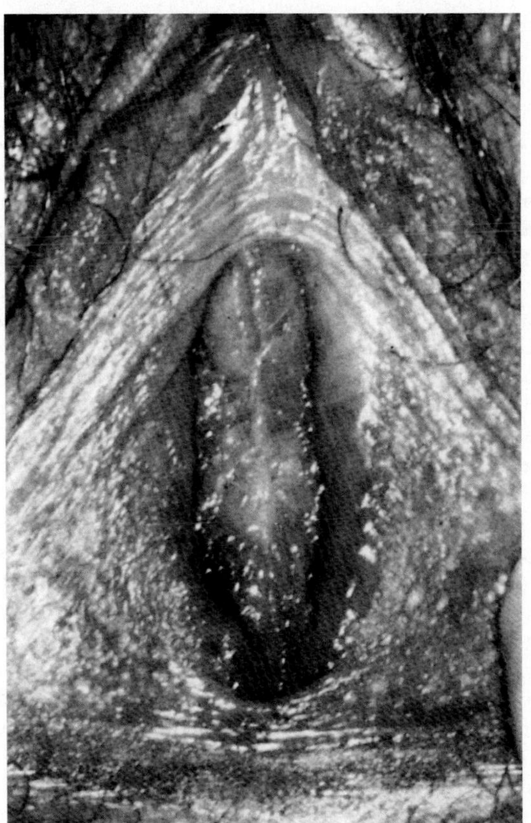

Figure 12-10. External genitalia of patient with congenital absence of vagina. (From Baramki TA: Treatment of congenital anomalies in girls and women. J Reprod Med 29:376, 1984.)

Therapy involves the creation of a vagina when the patient wishes to become sexually active. There are multiple therapeutic choices. The first, which is time consuming but nonsurgical, requires the use of progressive vaginal dilators. This can best be accomplished in a well-motivated, mature patient over a period of several months. Functioning vaginas have been achieved in many patients in this manner.

Using the concept of vaginal dilators, Ingram devised a useful technique. He used three sets of Lucite dilators. The first set contains 10 that are 1.5 cm in diameter and that increase in length from 1.5 to 10 cm; the second set contains 5 dilators that are 2.5 cm in diameter and that increase in length from 3 to 10 cm; and the third set has 8 dilators, 3.5 cm in diameter and from 3 to 10 cm long. A racing bicycle seat is mounted on a stool and is used to maintain dilator pressure on the introital dimple just posterior to the urethra. The patient holds the dilators in place with a pad or girdle and works through the three sets in progressive fashion, considering length and width as tolerated. The bicycle seat allows continuing pressure against the dilator; pressure is continued for 15 to 30 minutes at a time for a total of at least 2 hours a day. The patient may read or do other activities while sitting. It generally takes 4 to 6 months to develop an adequate neovagina by this technique.

Surgical reconstruction of the vagina has many variations to the technique. The operations, for the most part, develop the potential space between the bladder and the rectum and replaced this space with a stent utilizing tissue, most commonly a split-thickness skin graft or synthetic materials. The latter procedure, developed by Abbe-McIndoe, is easy to perform but must be done only when the patient will use the vagina frequently. If she does not and she fails to leave a plastic mold in place, the neovagina will frequently shrivel, scar, and become nonfunctional. Möbus and colleagues reported that in 24 patients who had undergone operative development of a neovagina, 20 of the 24 were found to be leading a healthy sexual life with unimpaired emotional and sexual responsiveness. They stressed that early and regular postoperative coitus was important for long-term success and was superior to the wearing of a stent. Thus, the timing of the operation to coincide with the opportunity for coitus is important.

An alternative procedure was devised by Williams. This procedure utilizes labial skin and results in a vaginal pouch whose axis is directly posterior. Although it is not as anatomically similar to a normal vagina as is the result of the McIndoe procedure, it does produce a functioning vaginal pouch and is well received by patients. Eventually, a normal vaginal axis is reported to develop.

Vecchietti developed a laparoscopic procedure for producing a neovagina. Sutures are placed laparoscopically in the peritoneal fold between the bladder and rudimentary uterus. A cutting edge needle then perforates the pseudohymen and an olive is attached to the suture and pulled tightly against the perineum. The sutures (two) are then fixed to a traction device on the anterior abdominal wall and graduated traction applied for 6 to 8 days. The olive is then removed and the patient uses vaginal dilators until sexual intercourse begins 10 to 15 days later. Several authors have reported good success with this procedure.

Transverse Vaginal Septum

The müllerian ducts join the sinovaginal bulb at a point known as the *müllerian tubercle.* Canalization of the müllerian tubercle and sinovaginal bulb is necessary to give a normal vaginal lumen. If the area of junction between these structures is not completely canalized, a transverse vaginal septum will occur (Fig. 12-11). This may be partial or complete and generally lies at the junction of the upper third and lower two thirds of the vagina (Fig. 12-12). It occurs in about 1 per 75,000 females. Partial transverse vaginal septa have been reported in diethylstilbestrol (DES)-exposed females. In the prepubertal state, diagnosis is generally not made unless there is the development of a mucocolpos or mucometrium behind the septum. In these girls an unexplained abdominal mass forms. At puberty, however, if the septum is complete, hematocolpos and hematometrium may occur in a fashion similar to that seen in the imperforate hymen, except that there is no bulging at the introitus. The patient complains of primary amenorrhea with cyclic cramping. The patient with an incomplete transverse septum may bleed somewhat but will still develop hematocolpos and hematometrium over time and may also complain of foul-smelling vaginal discharge.

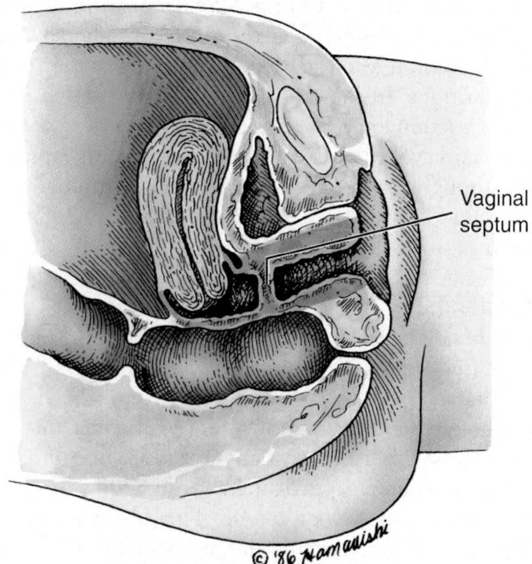

Figure 12-11. Diagram of transverse vaginal septum.

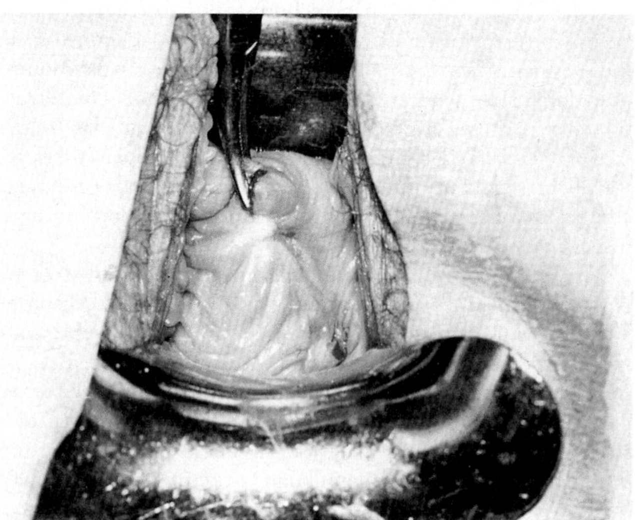

Figure 12-12. Patient with complete transverse vaginal septum.

The septum is often thin, generally less than 1 cm thick; however, many septa will be as thick as 2 cm. If an opening is noted, it may be expanded by manual dilation or simple incision, with suturing of the edges of the vagina on either side. In cases of a thick septum, the two areas of the vagina may be quite distant. In such cases excision may require the implantation of a split-thickness skin graft in a fashion similar to the Abee-McIndoe procedure. Most all women with congenital müllerian anomalies should have psychological counseling made available.

Longitudinal septa of the vagina will be discussed with duplication of the uterus and cervix.

Vaginal Adenosis

In the female exposed to DES in utero the junction between the müllerian ducts and the sinovaginal bulb may not be sharply demonstrated. If müllerian elements invade the sinovaginal bulb, remnants may remain as areas of adenosis in the adult vagina. They are generally palpated submucosally, although they may be observable at the surface.

Abnormalities of the Cervix and Uterus

Embryologic Considerations

Between the third and fifth weeks of gestation the metanephric ducts develop and join the cloaca. By the fifth week two bilateral ureteric buds develop from the mesonephric ducts near the distal ends (see Chapter 1, Fertilization and Embryogenesis). These grow cephalad toward the mesonephric mass. The müllerian or paramesonephric duct forms from a cleft between the mesonephros and the newly forming gonad. These ducts develop caudally just lateral to and intimately associated with the mesonephric ducts. The fate of all of these various embryonic elements is closely entwined. Damage to one usually affects the others. The paramesonephric ducts grow caudally, meet in the midline, and descend into the pelvis, reaching the urogenital sinus at an elevation known as the *müllerian tubercle.*

Musset analyzed 133 cases of genitourinary malformation and described a three-stage process for fusion of the two müllerian ducts into the uterus and cervix. The first stage is described as short, taking place at the beginning of the tenth week. The medial aspect of the more caudal portions of the two ducts fuse, starting in the middle and proceeding simultaneously in both directions. In this way a median septum is formed. The second stage continues from the tenth to the thirteenth week and occurs because of a rapid cell proliferation and the filling in of the triangular space between the two uterine cornua. In this way a thick upper median septum is formed. This is wedgelike and gives rise to the usual external contour of the fundus. At the same time the lower portion of the median septum is resorbed, unifying the cervical canal first and then the upper vagina. The third stage lasts from the thirteenth to about the twentieth week. In this stage the degeneration of the upper uterine septum occurs, starting at the isthmic region and proceeding cranially to the top of the fundus. In this way a unified uterine cavity is formed.

The vagina develops from a combination of the müllerian tubercles and the urogenital sinus. Cells proliferate from the upper portion of the urogenital sinus to form solid aggregates known as the *sinovaginal bulbs.* These cell masses develop into a cord, the vaginal plate, which extends from the müllerian ducts to the urogenital sinus. This plate canalizes, starting at the hymen, which is where the sinovaginal bulb attaches to the urogenital sinus, and proceeding cranially to the developing cervix, which has by this time already canalized. The process is completed at about the 21st week of intrauterine life.

Toaff and colleagues noted that the type of abnormality of the uterus depends on a teratogenic process active at a specific stage in the embryonic development. Most symmetrical communicating uteri such as uterine didelphys are associated with a normal urinary system, indicating that normal growth of the two mesonephric ducts had taken place before the fusion problem occurred. Interestingly, almost all patients with communicating uteri with atretic hemivagina have ipsilateral renal agenesis. Similarly, in patients with anomalies in which a hemicervix is absent, ipsilateral renal agenesis occurs. Toaff and colleagues inferred that an early teratogenic process active during the fourth week of gestation resulted in arrested growth of one mesonephric duct, agenesis of the ureteric bud, and therefore renal agenesis.

Genetic Studies of Müllerian Fusion Difficulties

Elias and associates reviewed the cases of sisters, mothers, and aunts of 24 women with known müllerian fusion abnormalities. Only 1 sister out of 37 (2.7%) was found to have a similar abnormality. No such abnormalities were found among 24 mothers, 45 maternal aunts, or 50 paternal aunts. Though the data in this study were accumulated by history and medical records, and not by direct uterine examination, Elias and associates concluded that the major genetic transmission mechanism is most likely polygenic or multifactorial. However, since that review, familial clusters have been reported.

Incidence

It is difficult to estimate the incidence of uterine fusion anomalies because the data in most reports are derived from case studies rather than from evaluation of the general population. The incidence is reported as 0.1% in retrospective studies and from 2% to 3% in observations of uteri at the time of delivery. Most uteri in the latter study, however, fit into the category of arcuate uterus or subseptate uterus. Lin and coworkers, summarizing the literature, reported the distribution of congenital uterine abnormalities to be bicornuate uterus 37%, arcuate and incomplete septum 28%, complete septum 9%, didelphic uterus 11%, and unicornuate 4%.

Symptoms and Signs

Complete duplication of the vagina, uterus, and cervix may be asymptomatic until the woman begins to menstruate. Frequently, the earliest symptom brought to the attention of the gynecologist is the fact that tampons do not obstruct menstrual flow. What occurs is that the patient inserts a tampon into one vagina but the other vagina is still open. The second most common way the diagnosis is made is by observation at the time of the first pelvic examination.

Obstructive vaginal anomalies often lead to cyclic pain at the time of menstruation or to the presence of a mucus-filled or blood-filled mass in the vagina. This may be mistaken for a paravaginal tumor.

A noncommunicating uterine horn becomes symptomatic in one of two fashions. The first may be a mass or pain that is exacerbated at the time of menses. This may be occasionally associated with symptoms and signs of endometriosis in a teenage woman. Along these lines, the early onset of signs and symptoms of endometriosis should alert the physician to the possibilities of uterine malformation. A mass is often noted on physical examination or seen with ultrasound.

The second way such a problem may present is as an ectopic pregnancy. Because sperm may migrate through the patent horn and because the rudimentary horn may have a normal tube attached to it, pregnancy can occur in a rudimentary horn. Because such horns are frequently small the pregnancy usually leads to rupture or pain.

A common presenting symptom is repetitive reproductive loss particularly in the early second trimester. Interestingly, didelphic uteri are usually not associated with this problem. Uterine anomalies and recurrent miscarriage is discussed in Chapter 16 (Spontaneous and Recurrent Abortion). Musset estimated that abnormalities of the uterus may occur in as many as 15% to 25% of women with a history of recurrent miscarriage. Makino and colleagues studied 1200 women with recurrent loss with hysterosalpingography and found that 188 had congenital uterine anomalies (15.7%). Most patients with pregnancy loss, however, had a variation of septate uterus. Metroplasty may lead to successful pregnancy outcomes in as much as 80%. A review by Homer and associates found a total of 658 women experiencing 1062 pregnancies, of which 88% ended in miscarriage and 9% in preterm delivery prior to treatment. Of the 491 pregnancies experienced by these women after hysteroscopic metroplasty, 80% ended in full-term deliveries, and only 14% were aborted and 6% were preterm. It is important to thoroughly evaluate such patients before exposing them to an operative procedure, since other problems may cause pregnancy loss.

Uterine dysfunction and abnormal uterine activity are complicating problems seen in labor in women with septate and bicornuate uteri. Likewise, breech presentations and transverse lies occur more commonly in women with such abnormal uteri as well.

Diagnosis

Diagnosis of a uterine anomaly may be indicated by a history, suggested by physical examination and confirmed with imaging. Several imaging modalities may be used, including sonohysterography hysterosalpingography, and hysteroscopy (Fig. 12-13). Ultrasound is a reasonable diagnostic procedure but should not be considered diagnostic until supplementary studies are performed. Magnetic resonance imaging is also appropriate, and many radiologists feel it is the modality of choice since the urinary tract may be evaluated simultaneously. Laparoscopy or laparotomy may be useful in rare cases. Evaluation of the urinary tracts is indicated in most cases particularly if there is a history of recurrent infection or if pelvic surgery is indicated.

Specific Anomalies

Absence of cervix and uterus. As discussed earlier, in many women with müllerian agenesis, the cervix and uterus are often not completely absent; the fallopian tubes and possibly some fibrous tissue are usually present. Absence is associated with urinary tract anomalies up to 50% of the time.

Unicornuate uterus. Destruction of one müllerian duct may occur for various reasons in the embryonic period. It is often related to lack of development of the mesonephric system on one side associated with lack of the appropriate development of the müllerian system. When this is the case, there is almost always a missing kidney and ureter on the same side. A single cervix and a single horn of the uterus with the fallopian tube of the side entering it are seen. The ovary may be present on the opposite side. Such a uterus usually supports a pregnancy. Unicornuate uterui are often not diagnosed unless the patient is evaluated with a hysterosalpingogram or is subjected to an operative procedure. In a review of 31 patients, Buttram found a 48% spontaneous abortion rate, a 17% prematurity rate, and a 40% live birth rate in patients with this anomaly.

Moutos and colleagues studied 29 women with unicornuate uteri and 25 women with didelphic uteri. Twenty women with unicornuate uteri produced a total of 40 pregnancies, and 13 women with didelphic uteri produced a total of 28 pregnancies. There was a 33% spontaneous abortion rate in the unicornuate group and a 23% rate in the didelphic group. The unicornuate group produced 9% preterm deliveries, 58% full-term deliveries, and 61% had living children. The didelphic group produced 32% preterm deliveries, 45% full-term deliveries, and 60% had living children. None of these differences were statistically different.

Anomalies of lateral fusion of müllerian ducts. Partial or complete duplication of the vagina, cervix, and uterus may be seen clinically. These may be classified as didelphic, which

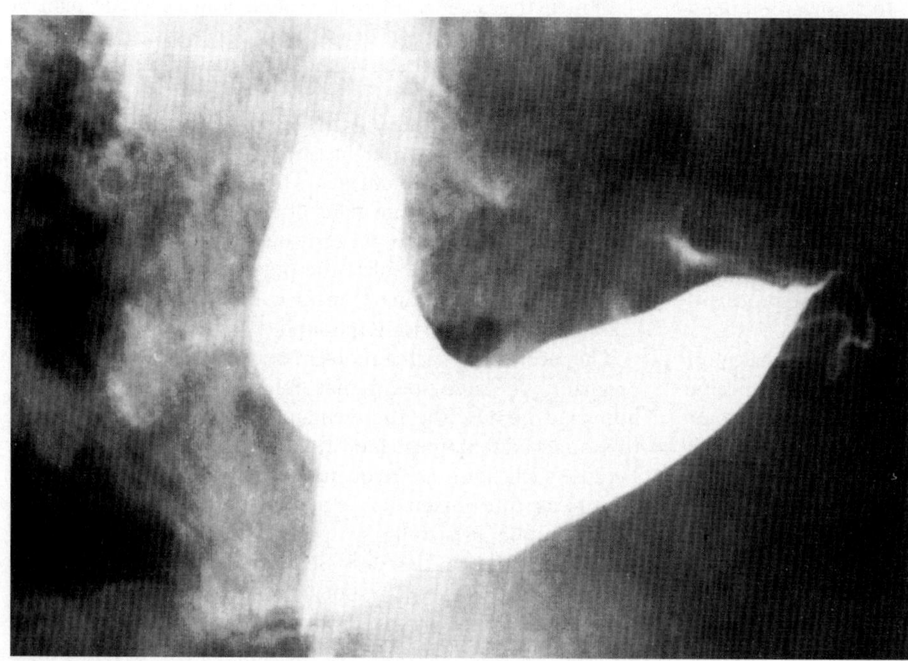

Figure 12-13. Hysterosalpingogram of bicornuate uterus seen in patient with repetitive abortions.

may involve a complete duplication of the vagina, uterus, and cervix; bicornuate, which consists of a single-chamber vagina and cervix with a complete or partial septate uterus and two uterine bodies (Fig. 12-14); septate, in which the uterus appears as a single organ but contains a midline septum that is either partial or complete; or arcuate, which demonstrates a small septate indentation at the upper end of the fundus.

Toaff and colleagues reviewed the subgroup of malformed uteri that includes duplication of the vagina, cervix, and uterus with communication between the horns. Nine subcategories have been described and are depicted in Figure 12-15. Some involve septate uteri and others didelphic uteri. Some involve obstructive areas of the vagina. Because of the structural differences the clinical findings may be quite different from case to case.

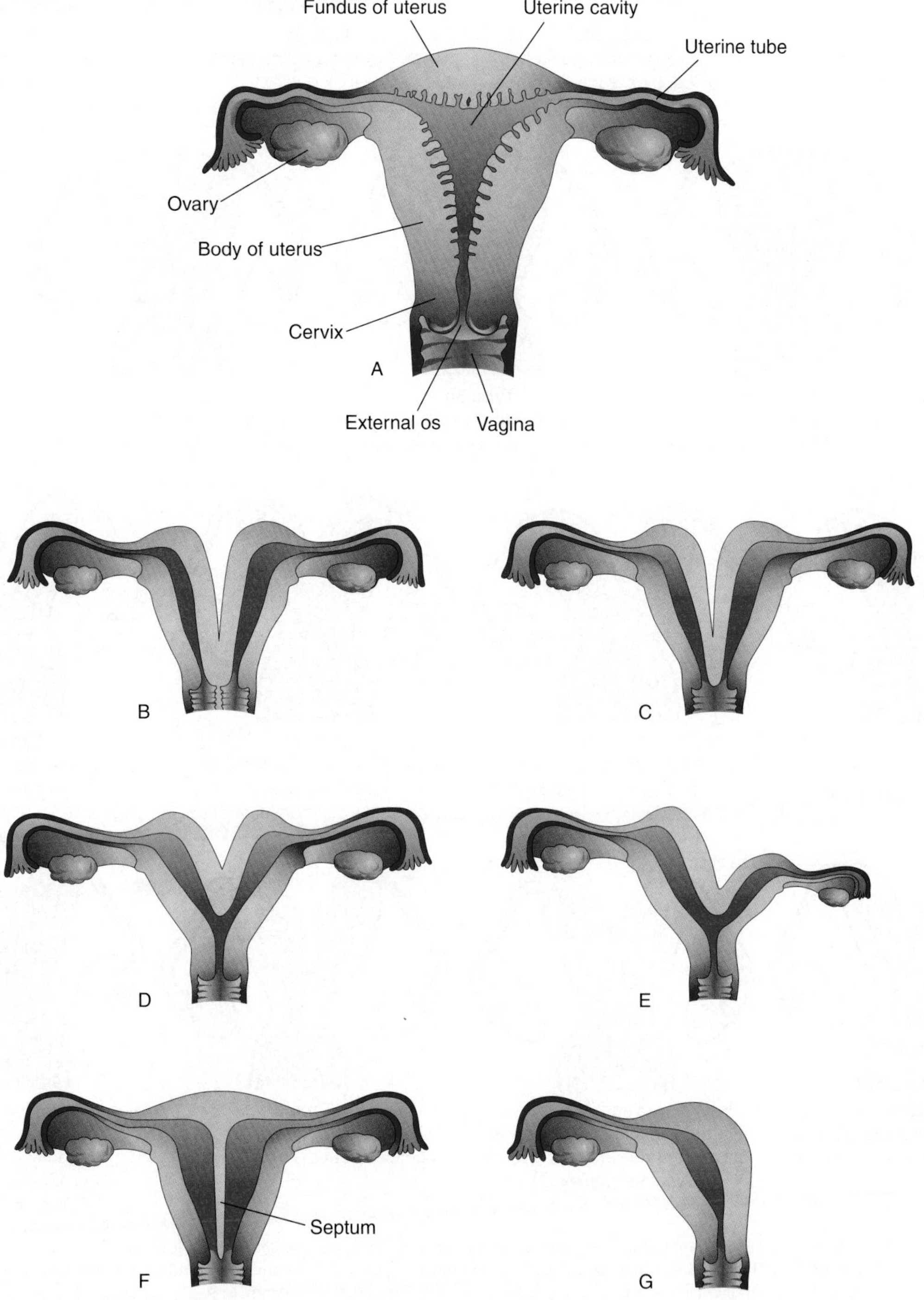

Figure 12-14. Various types of uterine anomalies. **A,** Normal uterus and vagina. **B,** Double uterus (uterus didelphys) and double vagina. **C,** Double uterus with single vagina. **D,** Bicornuate uterus. **E,** Bicornuate uterus with a rudimentary left horn. **F,** Septate uterus. **G,** Unicornuate uterus. (From Moore KL, Persaud TVN: The Developing Human, 7th ed. Philadelphia, WB Saunders, 2003, figure 13-43, p 321.)

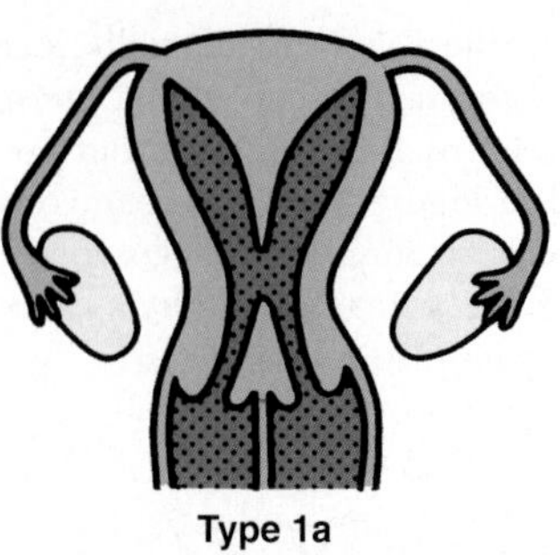

Type 1a
Uterus communicans septus, cervix duplex, vagina septa

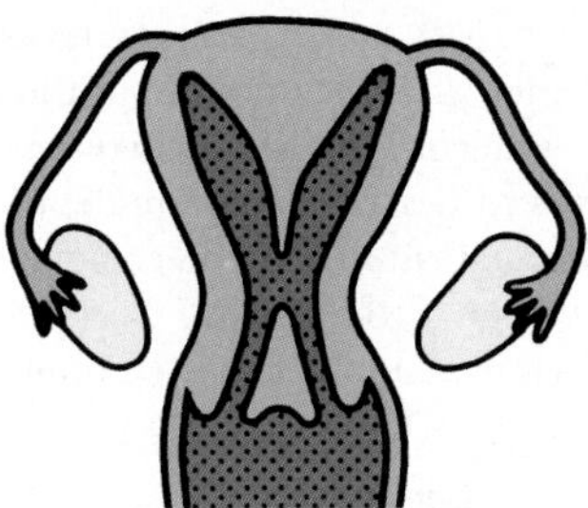

Type 1b
Uterus communicans septus, cervix duplex, vagina simplex

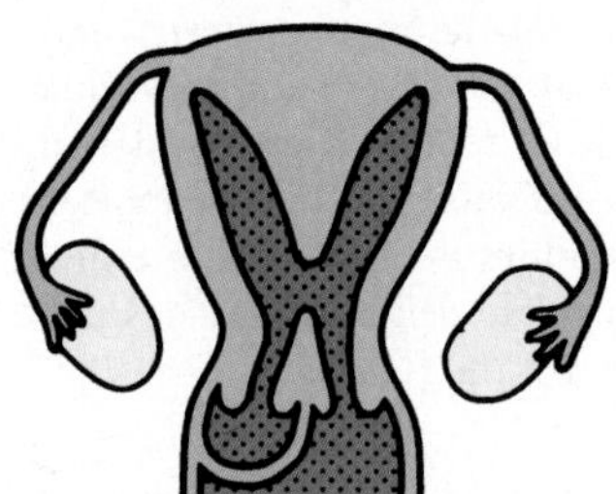

Type 2a
Uterus communicans septus, cervix duplex, vagina septa unilateralis atretica

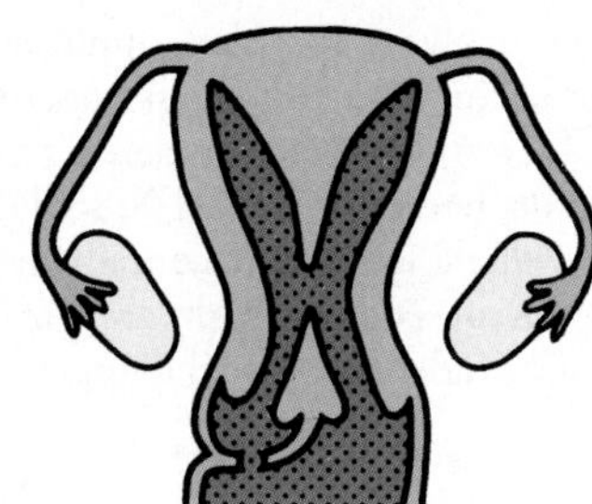

Type 2b
Uterus communicans septus, cervix duplex, vagina septa unilateralis atretica with vagino-vaginal fistula

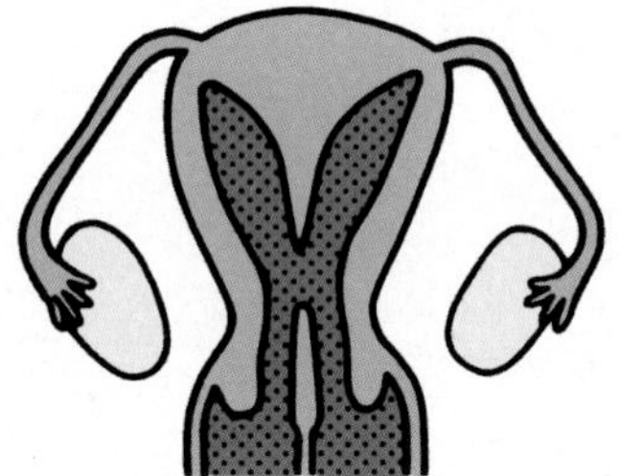

Type 3a
Uterus communicans septus, cervix septa, vagina septa

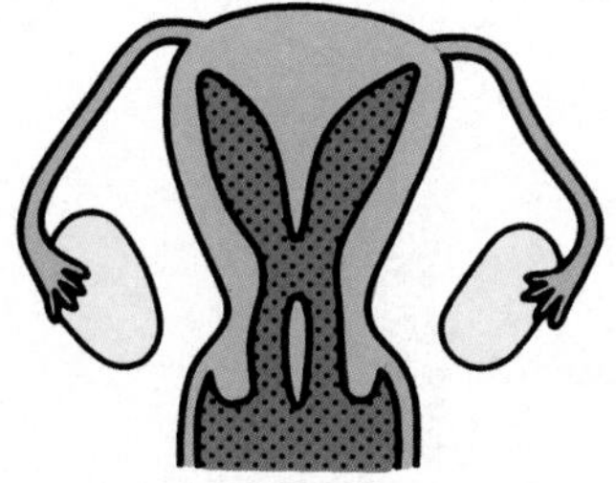

Type 3b
Uterus communicans septus, cervix septa, vagina simplex

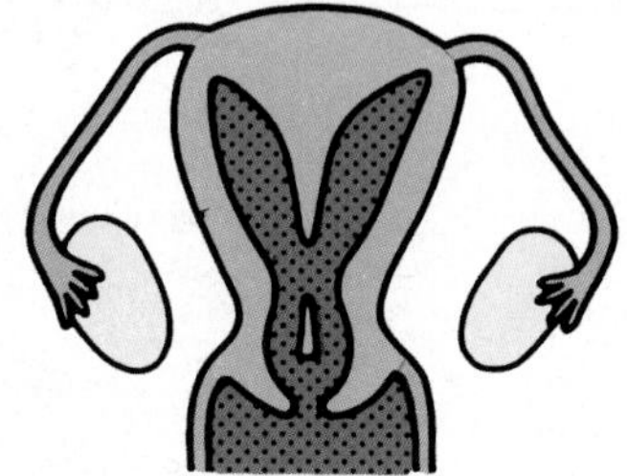

Type 3c
Uterus communicans septus, cervix subsepta, vagina simplex

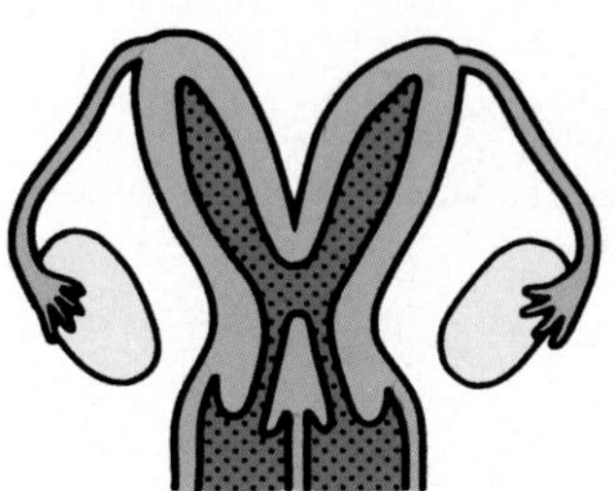

Type 4a
Uterus communicans bicornis, cervix duplex, vagina septa

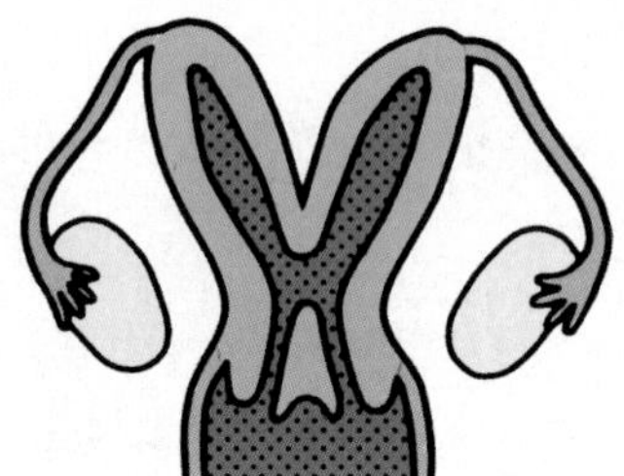

Type 4b
Uterus communicans bicornis, cervix duplex, vagina simplex

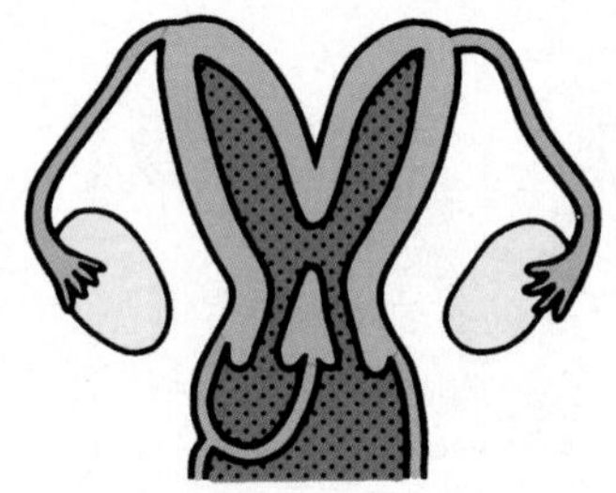

Type 5a
Uterus communicans bicornis, cervix duplex, vagina septa unilateralis atretica

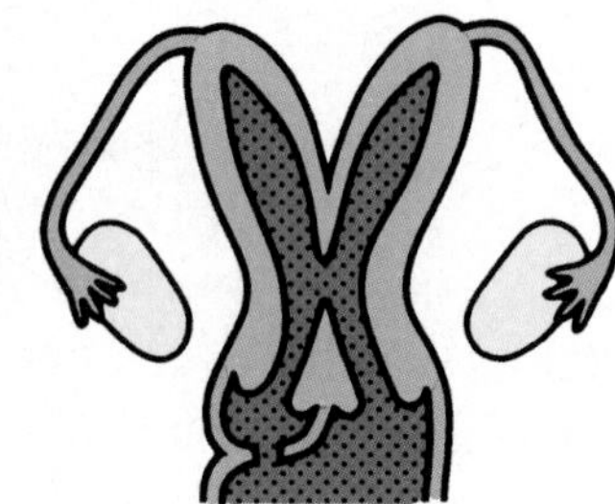

Type 5b
Uterus communicans bicornis, cervix duplex, vagina septa unilateralis atretica with vagino-vaginal fistula

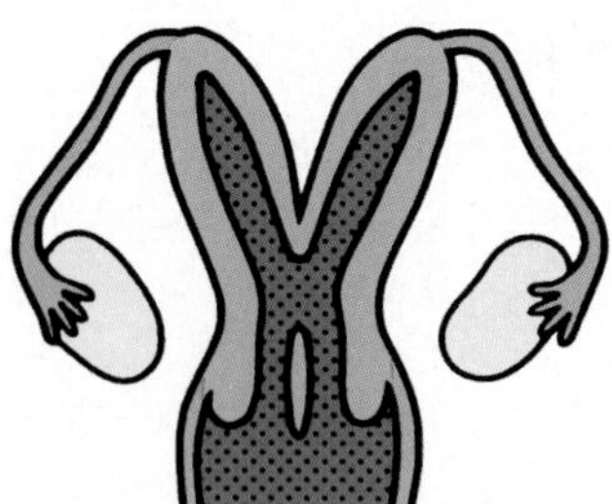

Type 6
Uterus communicans bicornis, cervix septa, vagina simplex

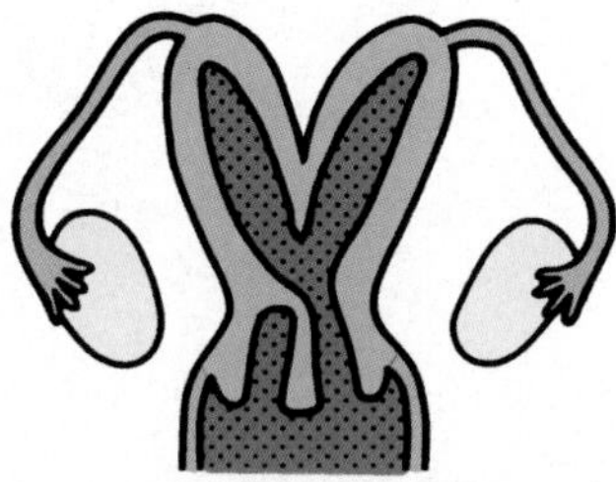

Type 7
Uterus communicans bicornis, cervix septa unilateralis atretica, vagina simplex

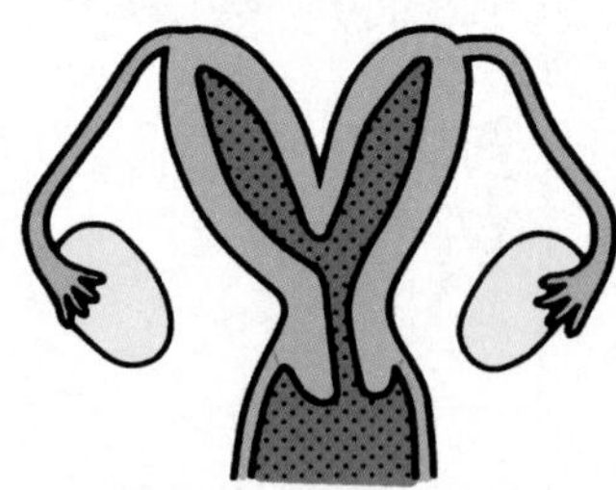

Type 8
Uterus communicans bicornis, hemicervix una, vagina simplex

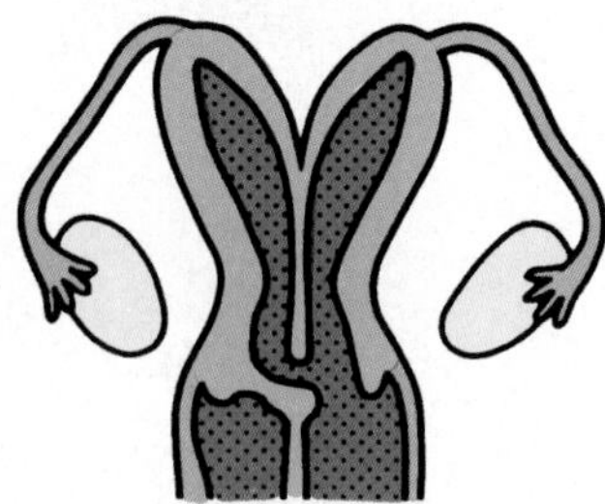

Type 9
Uterus bicornis, cervix communicans septa, unilateralis atretica, vagina septa

Figure 12-15. Morphologic classification of communicating uteri. All have an isthmic communication except type 9, which has a low cervical communication. (Reprinted from Fertility and Sterility, 41, Toaff ME, Lev-Toaff AS, Toaff R, Communicating uteri: Review and classification with introduction of two previously unreported types, 661. Copyright 1984, with permission from The American Society for Reproductive Medicine.)

Finally, obstructive varieties of duplication may be noted, again involving the uterus or the vagina.

Management

For patients with unobstructed abnormalities, therapy may be not needed. This is particularly true for women with unicornuate and didelphic uteri. On the other hand, septate uteri are frequently associated with reproductive wastage problems, and correction may be necessary to relieve these situations. A number of surgical corrective procedures are available. Patton and coworkers have emphasized that thorough evaluation is necessary prior to deciding on surgical treatment to establish the optimal strategy. Misdiagnosis of the anomaly is not uncommon.

Metroplasty was classically described by Strassman and involved the removal of the septum by a wedge incision and the reunification of the two cavities during laparotomy. However, a number of other means have been devised to eliminate the septum. Hysteroscopic resection is easier, in many cases safer, and is the treatment of choice for most women. Concurrent laparoscopy is used commonly to visualize the uterus during the procedure. This also allows for differentiation of a septate uterus from a bicornuate or didelphic uterus. An operating hysteroscope is then used to progressively cut the septum with scissors, until a cavity with normal-appearing contour is achieved.

Other means of dividing the septum may be utilized, including the use of a resectoscope. Vercellini and colleagues compared two groups of women, one which had the septum separated by microscissors and the other by resectoscope. They could find little difference in morbidity or outcome. Little or no bleeding generally occurs, since the septum is fibrous and poorly vascularized. After the operation some surgeons may insert an IUD for 30 days, and the patient may be treated with a conjugated estrogen (1.25 mg/day) for 1 month; other physicians prescribe slightly higher doses. This step has not been proved to be necessary and often can be withheld. This vaginal approach eliminates the need for an abdominal procedure and thus limits the risk of pelvic adhesions, which may interfere with fertility.

The surgical treatment of uterine septa because of primary infertility is controversial. Prophylactic cerclage of women with anomalies is not indicated. However, many clinicians recommend transvaginal ultrasound evaluation of the cervix in the second trimester in women with uterine anomalies for the evaluation of cervical incompetence.

Ovarian Abnormalities

Accessory Ovary and Supernumerary Ovary

In 1959 Wharton defined *accessory ovary* and *supernumerary ovary.* The former term is used when excess ovarian tissue is noted near a normally placed ovary and connected to it. Supernumerary ovary occurs when a third ovary is separated from the normally situated ovaries. Printz and associates pointed out that such ovaries may be found in the omentum or retroperitoneally, and Hogan and colleagues reported the presence of a dermoid cyst in a supernumerary ovary that occurred in the greater omentum. Wharton estimated that the occurrence of either accessory ovary or supernumerary ovary is quite rare, finding approximately 1 case of accessory ovary per 93,000 patients and 1 case of supernumerary ovary in 29,000 autopsies. In Wharton's review, 3 of 4 patients with supernumerary ovary and 5 of 19 patients with accessory ovary had additional congenital defects, most frequently abnormalities of the genitourinary tract.

Ovotestes

Ovotestes are present in individuals with ovaries that have an SRY antigen present. The majority are true hermaphrodites (quite rare). The degree to which müllerian and mesonephric development occurs depends on the amount of testicular tissue present in the ovotestes and the proximity to the developing duct system. Where a considerable amount of testicular tissue is present within the organ, there is a tendency for descent toward the labial scrotal area. Thus, palpation of the gonad in the inguinal canal or within the labial scrotal area is fairly common. Ovulation and menstruation may occur if the müllerian system is appropriately developed. In a similar fashion, spermatogenesis may occur as well. Where testicular tissue is present, there is an increased risk for malignant degeneration, and these gonads should be removed after puberty. Germ cell tumors, such as gonadoblastomas and dysgerminomas, have been reported in the ovarian portion of ovotestes.

KEY POINTS

- Gender identification in a newborn infant has tremendous emotional influence and should be performed prior to hospital discharge and as accurately as possible.
- Congenital adrenal hyperplasia is an autosomal recessive condition most commonly the result of an inborn error of metabolism involving the enzyme 21-hydroxylase. Homozygous individuals occur in 1 of every 490 to 67,000 births, average 1 in 14,000. Heterozygote carriers are present in 1 in 20 to 1 in 250 individuals. Differences depend on ethnic background of people tested.
- Up to 75% of females with ambiguous genitalia may develop a sodium wasting adrenal crisis.
- The hymen is the junction of the sinovaginal bulb with the urogenital sinuses and is derived from endoderm.
- Vaginal agenesis is most often associated with Mayer–Rokitansky–Küster–Hauser syndrome. Up to 50% of these women will have urologic abnormalities. Approximately one eighth will have skeletal abnormalities as well.
- Abnormalities of the uterus and cervix may be transmitted as a polygenic or multifactorial pattern of inheritance. They occur in about 2% to 3% of the female population.
- Up to 15% of women with histories of recurrent miscarriage may be found to have anomalies of the uterus.
- Pretherapy pregnancy wastage rates in women with some types of müllerian anomalies may be as high as 85% to 90%. After surgical repair the pregnancy efficiency rate may be as high as 80%.
- Accessory ovaries occur in approximately 1 per 93,000 patients. Supernumerary ovaries occur in approximately 1 of every 29,000 women.

BIBLIOGRAPHY

American Academy of Pediatrics, Committee on Genetics: Evaluation of the newborn with developmental anomalies of the external genitalia. Pediatrics 106:138, 2000.

Baramki TA: The treatment of congenital anomalies in girls and women. J Reprod Med 29:376, 1984.

Basile C, De Michele V: Renal abnormalities in Mayer–Rokitanski–Küster–Hauser syndrome. J Nephrol 14:316, 2001.

Beheshti M, Hardy BE, Churchill BM, et al: Gender assignment in male pseudo hermaphrodite children. Urology 22:604, 1983.

Buttram VC, Zanotti L, Acosta AA, et al: Surgical correction of septate uterus. Fertil Steril 25:373, 1974.

Committee on Adolescent Health Care: Nonsurgical diagnosis and management of vaginal agenesis. Int J Gynaecol Obstet 79:167, 2002.

Cruikshank SH, VanDrie DM: Supernumerary ovaries: Update and review. Obstet Gynecol 60:126, 1982.

Daaboul J, Frader J: Ethics and the management of the patient with intersex: A middle way. J Ped Endo Met 14:1575, 2001.

Daly DC, Walters CA, Soto-Albers CE, et al: Hysteroscopic metroplasty: Surgical technique and obstetric outcome. Fertil Steril 39:623, 1983.

Damiani D, Fellous M, McElreavey, et al: True hermaphroditism: Clinical aspects and molecular studies in 16 cases. Eur J Endo 136:201, 1997.

Dapunt O, Sölder E, Moncayo H, Hohn A: Results of the Strassmann operation at the Innsbruck University Gynecologic Clinic (1976–1991). Gynakol Geburtshilfliche Rundsch 32:134, 1992.

Doyle MB: Magnetic resonance imaging in müllerian fusion defects. J Reprod Med 37:33, 1992.

Dillon WP, Dewey M: A case of accessory ovary. Obstet Gynecol 58:660, 1981.

Edmonds DK: Congenital malformations of the genital tract and their management. Best Pract Res Clin Obstet Gynecol 17:19, 2003.

Edmonds DK: Vaginal and uterine anomalies in the pediatric and adolescent patient. Curr Opin Obstet Gynecol 13:463, 2001.

Elias S, Simpson JL, Carson SA, et al: Genetic studies in incomplete müllerian fusion. Obstet Gynecol 63:276, 1984.

Emans SJ, Grace E, Fleischnick E, et al: Detection of late onset 21-hydroxylase deficiency congenital adrenal hyperplasia in adolescents. Pediatrics 72:690, 1983.

Farkas A, Chertin B: Feminizing genitoplasty in patients with 46XX congenital adrenal hyperplasia. J Ped Endo Met 14:713, 2001.

Fedele L, Bianchi S, Tozzi L, et al: A new laparoscopic procedure for creation of a neovagina in Mayer–Rokitansky–Küster–Hauser syndrome. Fertil Steril 66:854, 1996.

Fedele L, Dorta M, Vercellini P, et al: Ultrasound in the diagnosis of subclasses of unicornuate uterus. Obstet Gynecol 71:274, 1988.

Fedele L, Ferranzzi E, Dorta M, et al: Ultrasonography in the differential diagnosis of "double" uteri. Fertil Steril 50:361, 1988.

Fleischnick E, Rum D, Alosco SM, et al: Extended MHC haplotypes in 21-hydroxylase deficiency congenital adrenal hyperplasia: Shared genotypes in unrelated patients. Lancet 1:152, 1983.

Gaucherand P, Awada A, Rudigoz RC, Dargent D: Obstetrical prognosis of the septate uterus: A plea for treatment of the septum. Eur J Obstet Gynecol Reprod Biol 54:109, 1994.

Greiss FC, Mauzy CH: Congenital anomalies in women: An evaluation of diagnosis, incidence, and obstetric performance. Am J Obstet Gynecol 82:330, 1961.

Hahn-Pedersen J, Larsen PM: Supernumerary ovary. Acta Obstet Gynecol Scand 63:365, 1984.

Hauser GA, Schreiner WE: Das Mayer–Rokitansky–Küster–Hauser syndrome Schweiz Med Wochenschr 91:381, 1961.

Hay D: Uterus unicornis and its relationship to pregnancy. J Obstet Gynaecol Br Emp 68:371, 1961.

Hogan ML, Barber DD, Kaufmann RH: Dermoid cyst in supernumerary ovary: The greater omentum: Report of a case. Obstet Gynecol 29:405, 1967.

Homer HA, Li T-J, Cooke ID: The septate uterus: A review of management and reproductive outcome. Fertil Steril 73:1, 2000.

Hughes IA: Congenital adrenal hyperplasia: 21-hydroxylase deficiency in the newborn and during infancy. Semin Reprod Med 20:229, 2002.

Hughes IA: Female development—all by default? N Engl J Med 351:8, 2004.

Ingram JM: The bicycle seat stool in the treatment of vaginal agenesis and stenosis: A preliminary report. Am J Obstet Gynecol 140:867, 1981.

Israel R, March CM: Hysteroscopic incision of the septate uterus. Am J Obstet Gynecol 149:66, 1984.

Kaufman RH, Noller K, Adam E, et al: Upper genital tract abnormalities and pregnancy outcome in diethylstilbestrol-exposed progeny. Am J Obstet Gynecol 148:973, 1984.

Kelalis P, King L, Bellman A: Clinical Pediatric Urology, 2nd ed, Philadelphia, WB Saunders, 1985.

Kirk EP, Chuong CJ, Coulam CB, Williams GJ: Pregnancy after metroplasty for uterine anomalies. Fertil Steril 59:1164, 1993.

Krege S, Walz KH, Hauffa BP, et al: Long-term follow-up of female patients with congenital adrenal hyperplasia from 21-hydroxylase deficiency, with special emphasis on the results of vaginoplasty. BJU Int 86:253, 2000.

Lachman MF, Berman MM: The ectopic ovary—A case report and review of the literature. Arch Pathol Lab Med 115:233, 1991.

Larsen PR, Kronenberg HM, Melmed S, Polonsky KS: Williams Textbook of Endocrinlology, 10th ed. Philadelphia, WB Saunders, 2003.

Lim YH, Ng SP, Jamil MA: Imperforate hymen: Report of an unusual familial occurrence. J Obstet Gynaecol Res 29:399, 2003.

Lin PC, Bhatnagar KP, Nettleton GS, et al: Female genitalia anomalies affecting reproduction. Fertil Steril 78:899, 2002.

Low Y, Hutson JM: Murdoch Childrens Research Institute Sex Study Group: Rules for clinical diagnosis in babies with ambiguous genitalia. J Paediatr Child Health 39:406, 2003.

MacLaughlin DT, Donahoe PK: Sex determination and differentiation. N Engl J Med 350:367, 2004.

Makino T, Umeuchi M, Nakada K, et al: Incidence of congenital uterine anomalies in repeated reproductive wastage and prognosis for pregnancy after metroplasty. Int J Fertil 37:167, 1992.

Maneschi F, Marana R, Muzil L, Mancuso S: Reproductive performance in women with bicornuate uterus. Acta Eur Fertil 24:117, 1993.

McIndoe A: Treatment of congenital absence and obliterative conditions of vagina. Br J Plast Surg 2:254, 1950.

Möbus V, Sachweh K, Knapstein PG, Kreienberg R: Women after surgically corrected vaginal aplasia: A follow-up of psychosexual rehabilitation. Geburtshilfe Frauenheilkd 53:125, 1993.

Moore KL, Persaud TVN: The Developing Human Clinically Oriented Embryology, 7th ed. Philadelphia, WB Saunders, 2003.

Moutos DM, Damewood MD, Schlaff WD, Rock JA: A comparison of the reproductive outcome between women with a unicornuate uterus and women with a didelphic uterus. Fertil Steril 58:88, 1992.

Muller U, Mayerova A, Debus B, et al: Correlation between testicular tissue and HY phenotype in intersex patients. Clin Genet 23:49, 1983.

Musset R: Classification globale des malformations uterines. Gynécol Obstét 66:145, 1967.

Nahum GG: Uterine anomalies—How common are they, and what is their distribution among subtypes. J Reprod Med 43:877, 1998.

Olive D, Henderson DY: Endometriosis and müllerian anomalies. Obstet Gynecol 69:412, 1987.

Palmer R: Anomalies uterines congenitales. In Boury-Heyler C, Maulbeon P, Rochet Y, et al: Uterus et Fécondité, vol 1. Paris, Masson, 1981.

Pang S, Murphey W, Levine LS, et al: A pilot newborn screening for congenital adrenal hyperplasia in Alaska. J Clin Endocrinol Metab 55:413, 1982.

Patton PE, Novy MJ, Lee DM, et al: The diagnosis and reproductive outcome after surgical treatment of the complete septate uterus, duplicated cervix and vaginal septum. Am J Obstet Gynecol 190:1669, 2004.

Phelan JT, Counseller VS, Greene LF: Deformities of the urinary tract with congenital absence of the vagina. Surg Gynecol Obstet 97:1, 1953.

Powell DM, Newman KD, Randolph J: A proposed classification of vaginal anomalies and their surgical correction. J Ped Surgery 30:271, 1995.

Printz JL, Choate JW, Townes PL, et al: The embryology of supernumerary ovaries. Obstet Gynecol 41:246, 1973.

Reiner WG: Assignment of sex in neonates with ambiguous genitalia. Curr Opin Pediatr 11:363, 1999.

Rock J, Azziz R: Genital anomalies in childhood. Clin Obstet Gynecol 30:682, 1987.

Semens JP: Congenital anomalies of the female genital tract: Functional classification based on a review of 56 personal cases and 5 unreported cases. Obstet Gynecol 19:328, 1962.

Simpson JL: Genetics of the female reproductive ducts. Am J Medical Genetics 89:224, 1999.

Stelling JR, Gray MR, Davis AJ, et al: Dominant transmission of imperforate hymen. Fertil Steril 74:1241, 2000.

Stikkelbroeck NM, Beerendonk CC, Willemsen WN, et al: The long term outcome of feminizing genital surgery for congenital adrenal hyperplasia: Anatomical, functional and cosmetic outcomes, psychosexual development, and satisfaction in adult female patients. J Pediatr Adolesc Gynecol 16:289, 2003.

Sultan C, Paris F, Jeandel C, et al: Ambiguous genitalia in the newborn. Semin Reprod Med 20:181, 2002.

Toaff ME, Lev-Toaff AS, Toaff R: Communicating uteri: Review and classification with introduction of two previously unrecorded types. Fertil Steril 41:661, 1984.

Troiano RN: Magnetic resonance imaging of Müllerian duct anomalies of the uterus. TMRI 14:269, 2003.

Usta IM, Awwad JT, Usta JA, et al: Imperforate hymen: Report of an unusual familial occurrence. Obstet Gynecol 82:655, 1993.

Valente S: Congenital vaginal malformation: Clinical experiences on vaginal agenesia. Clin Exp Obst Gyn 15:143, 1988.

Vecchietti G: Le neovagina dans le syndrome de Rokitansky–Küster–Hauser. Rev Med Suisse Romande 99:593, 1979.

Vercellini P, Vendola N, Colombo A, et al: Hysteroscopic metroplasty with resectoscope or microscissors for the correction of septate uterus. Surg Gynecol Obstet 176:439, 1993.

Warne SA, Wilcox DT, Creighton WS, et al: Long-term gynecological outcome of patients with persistent cloaca. J Urology 170:1493, 2003.

Wharton LR: Two cases of supernumerary ovary and one of accessory ovary within an analysis of previously reported cases. Am J Obstet Gynecol 78:1101, 1959.

Yordam N, Alikasifoglu A, Kandemir N, et al: True hermaphroditism: Clinical features, genetic variants and gonadal histology. J Pediatr Endo Metabolism 14:421, 2001.

Pediatric and Adolescent Gynecology 13

Gynecologic Examination, Infections, Trauma, Pelvic Mass, Precocious Puberty

Ann Jeanette Davis and Vern L. Katz

KEY TERMS AND DEFINITIONS

Adhesive Vulvitis. A self-limited condition in which denuded epithelium of the adjacent labia minora agglutinates and fuses the two labia together.

Adolescence. A transitional period of life during which an individual matures physiologically and occasionally psychologically from a child into an adult.

Labial adhesions. Agglutination of the adjacent labia minora from a denuded epithelium that fuses the two labia together.

Lichen Sclerosus Atrophicus. A skin dystrophy involving the labia seen typically in prepubertal children and postmenopausal women.

McCune-Albright Syndrome (Polyostotic Fibrous Dysplasia). A rare syndrome of café-au-lait spots, fibrous dysplasia, and lesions in the skull and long bones, accompanied by precocious puberty. The disorder is caused by a somatic mutation (thus noninherited) in neural crest cells with a mutation in the G protein system.

Puberty. The process of biologic and physical development after which sexual reproduction first becomes possible.

Urethral prolapse. Prolapse of the distal urethral mucosa seen typically in prepubertal children .

Vulvovaginitis. Inflammatory process involving the vulva and vagina.

Gynecologic diseases are uncommon in children, especially compared with the incidence and prevalence of diseases in women of reproductive age. This chapter considers gynecologic diseases of children from infancy through adolescence. Congenital anomalies, precocious development, and amenorrhea are covered in more detail in other chapters.

The evaluation of children's gynecologic problems involves considerations of physiology, psychology, and developmental issues that are different from those of adult gynecology. The evaluation of young females is age-dependent. For example, the physical presence of the mother often may facilitate examining a 4-year-old girl but may inhibit the cooperation of a 14-year-old adolescent. Thus, the gynecologic physical examination is performed differently in a prepubertal child than in an adolescent of reproductive age or a mature reproductive woman.

An outpatient visit by a prepubertal child to a gynecologist should be structured differently from a gynecologic visit by a woman of reproductive age. Considerable effort should be devoted to gaining the child's confidence and establishing rapport. If the interaction is poor during the first visit, the negative experience will detract from future physician–patient interactions. The pediatric gynecologic visit may be unique to both the child and the parent. Most pediatric visits are preventive in nature. However, the pediatric gynecologic visit is problem-oriented. This may create considerable and understandable anxiety in the child and parent. The vast majority of children's gynecologic problems are treated by medical rather than surgical means.

The most frequent gynecologic disease of children is *vulvovaginitis.* Vulvitis is generally the primary presenting problem, with vaginitis of secondary importance and symptomatology. Other common reasons for a pediatric gynecology visit include labial adhesions, vulvar lesions, suspicion of sexual abuse, and genital trauma.

Adolescence is the period of life during which an individual matures physiologically and begins to transition psychologically from a child into an adult. This period of transition involves important physical and emotional changes. Before puberty, the girl's reproductive organs are in a resting, dormant state. Puberty produces dramatic alterations in both the external and the internal female genitalia. Because the pubertal changes are frequently a cause of concern for adolescent females and their parents, the gynecologist must offer the adolescent female a kind, knowledgeable, and gentle approach. These interactions between the physician and the adolescent female will allow the physician an opportunity to educate the pubertal teenager about pelvic anatomy and reproduction.

GYNECOLOGIC EXAMINATION OF A CHILD

General Approach

A successful gynecologic examination of a child demands that the physician adapt an exam pace that conveys both gentleness and patience with the time spent and not seem to be hurried or rushed. One excellent technique is for the physician to sit, not stand, during the initial encounter. This conveys an unhurried approach. The ambiance of the examining room may decrease the anxiety of the child if familiar and friendly objects such as children's posters are present. Interruptions should be avoided. Speculums and instruments that might frighten a child or parent should be within drawers or cabinets and out of sight during the evaluation. If a child is scheduled to be seen in the middle of a busy clinic, the staff needs to be alerted that the pace and general routine will be different during her visit.

Performance of the Gynecologic Exam in a Child

The components of a complete pediatric examination include a history; inspection with visualization of the vulva, vagina, and cervix; and, if necessary, a rectal examination.

Obtaining a history from a child is not an easy process. Children are not skilled historians and will often ramble, introducing many unrelated facts. Much of the history must be obtained from the parents. However, young children can help define their exact symptomatology on direct questioning. While obtaining a history an opportunity exists to educate the child on vocabulary to describe the genital area. One way to describe genital area and breasts is to call them "private areas"—areas that are covered by your bathing suit. The exam also allows a period of opportunity to counsel children about potential sexual abuse. During the history and most of the general physical examination, the child should sit on the edge of the examination table.

After the history has been obtained, the parents and the child should be reassured that the examination will not hurt. It is important to give the child a sense that she will be in control of the examination process. A helpful technique is to place the child's hand on top of the physician's hand as the abdominal examination is being performed. This will give the child a sense of control as well as divert the child's attention if she is ticklish or is squirming. Emphasize that the most important part of the examination is just "looking" and there will be conversation during the entire process. To successfully examine a child, one needs the cooperation of the patient and a medical assistant such as a nurse.

A child's reaction will depend on her age, emotional maturity, and previous experience with health care providers. She should be allowed to visualize and handle any instruments that will be used. Many young children's primary contact with providers involves immunizations; children should be counseled and assured that this visit does not involve any "shots." It is also helpful to assure the adult that has accompanied the child that adult speculums are not part of the examination.

Occasionally it is best to defer the pelvic examination until a second visit. This is a difficult decision and is based on the extent of the child's anxiety in relation to the severity of the clinical symptoms. A physician may elect to treat the primary symptoms of vulvovaginitis for 2 to 3 weeks before searching for a foreign body. However, in the field of pediatric gynecology many errors are errors of omission rather than of commission.

A child should never be restrained for a gynecologic examination. Often reassurance and sometimes delay until another day are the best approach. Sometimes after performing the other elements of the general exam enough rapport has been established that the child will feel safe enough to allow a gynecologic examination. In rare circumstances it may be necessary to use continuous intravenous conscious sedation or general anesthesia to complete an essential examination. The most important technique to ensure cooperation is to involve the child as a partner. Children should ideally feel they are part of the exam rather than having an "exam done to them."

Draping for the gynecologic examination produces more anxiety than it relieves and is unnecessary in the preadolescent child. A handheld mirror may help in some instances when discussing specifics of genital anatomy. It is critical to have all tools, culture tubes, and equipments within easy reach during a pediatric genital examination. Children often cannot hold still for long intervals while instruments are being searched for.

The first aspect of the pelvic examination is evaluation of the external genitalia. An infant may be examined on her mother's lap. Young children may be examined in the frog leg position, and children as young as 2 to 3 years of age may be examined in lithotomy with use of stirrups. Lithotomy is generally used for girls 4 to 5 years of age and older.

Once the child is positioned the vulvar area and introitus should be inspected (Figs. 13-1 and 13-2) Many gynecologic conditions in children may be diagnosed by inspection. The introitus will gape open with gentle pressure downward and outward on the lower thigh or undeveloped thigh or labia majora area. (Fig. 13-3). Asking the child to pretend to blow out candles on a birthday cake may facilitate the process.

The second phase of the examination involves evaluation of the vagina. This can be accomplished without use of any insertion of instruments. One method is to utilize the knee chest position. (Fig. 13-4) The child lies prone and places her buttocks in the air with legs wide apart. The vagina will then fill with air, aiding the evaluation. The child is told to have her abdomen sag into the table. An assistant pulls upward and outward on the labia majora on one side while the examiner does the same with the nondominant hand on the contralateral labia. Then an otoophthalmoscope is used as a magnifying instrument and light source in the examiner's dominant hand. The otoophthal-

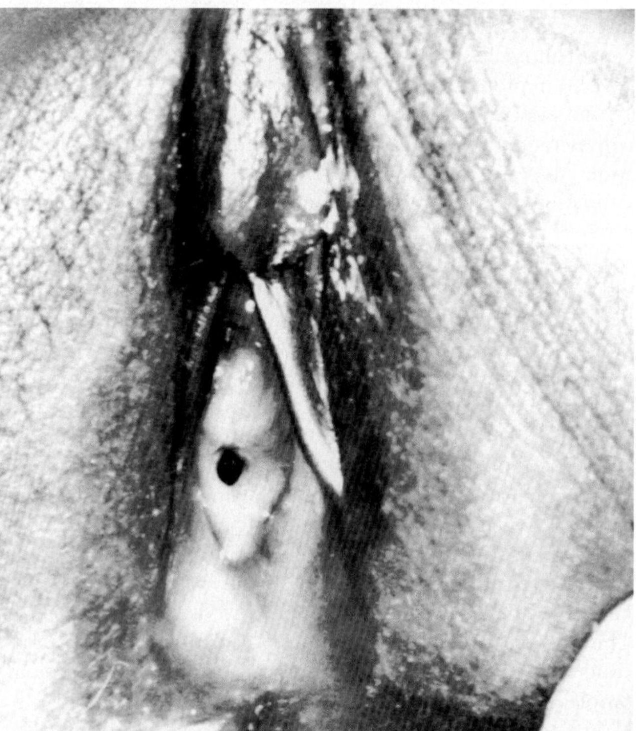

Figure 13-1. Appearance of normal external genitalia of a prepubertal female in the supine position using the lateral spread technique. (From Pokorny SF: Pediatric gynecology. In Stenchever MA [ed]: Office Gynecology, 2nd ed. St. Louis, Mosby, 1996.)

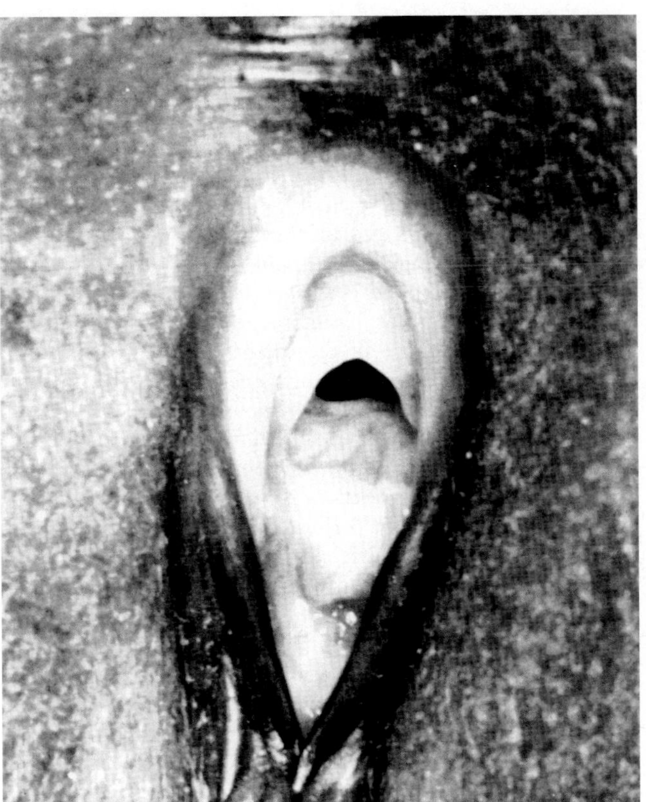

Figure 13-2. The same child shown in Figure 13-1 but in the knee-chest position. (From Pokorny SF: Pediatric gynecology. In Stenchever MA [ed]: Office Gynecology, 2nd ed. St. Louis, Mosby, 1996.)

moscope *is not* inserted into the vagina. A bright light helps to illuminate the upper vagina and cervix. The light is shone into the vagina as the examiner evaluates the vaginal walls through the otoophthalmoscope. The cervix appears as a transverse ridge or pleat that is redder than the vagina. This technique is generally successful in cooperative children unless there is a very high crescent-shaped hymen, in which case it is too difficult to shine the light into the small aperture at the vaginal introitus. Foreign

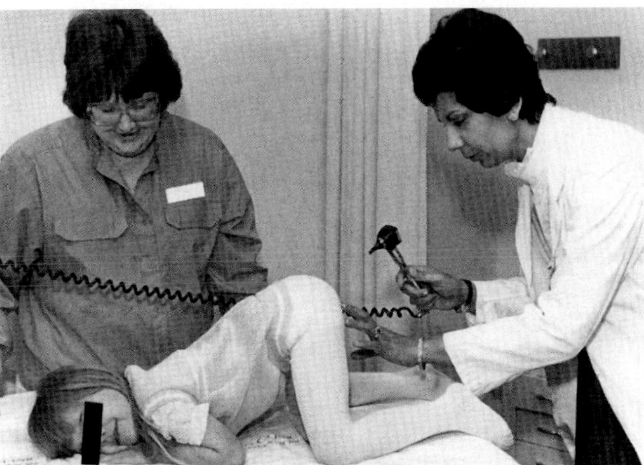

Figure 13-4. Knee-chest position used to examine child to visualize cervix and vagina. The otoscope head is usually longer than one shown in photograph. (From Gidwani GP: Approach to evaluation of premenarchal child with a gynecologic problem. Clin Obstet Gynecol 30:643, 1987.)

object and the cervix may be visualized using this technique. Following inspection of the vagina and cervix, vaginal secretions may be obtained for microscopic examination and culture.

Normal Findings: Hymen and Vagina of a Prepubertal Child

The hymen of a prepubertal child exhibits a diverse range of normal variations and configurations (Fig. 13-5). Hymens are often crescent-shaped but may be annular or ringlike in configuration. There are no reported cases of congenital absence of the hymen. A mounding of hymeneal tissue is often called a bump. Bumps are usually a normal variant and are often attached to longitudinal ridges within the vagina. Hymens in newborns are estrognenized, resulting in a thick elastic redundancy. Older unestrogenized girls will have thin nonelastic hymens. Prospective studies of hymens in children has demonstrated that complete transections of the hymeneal tissue between 3 o'clock and

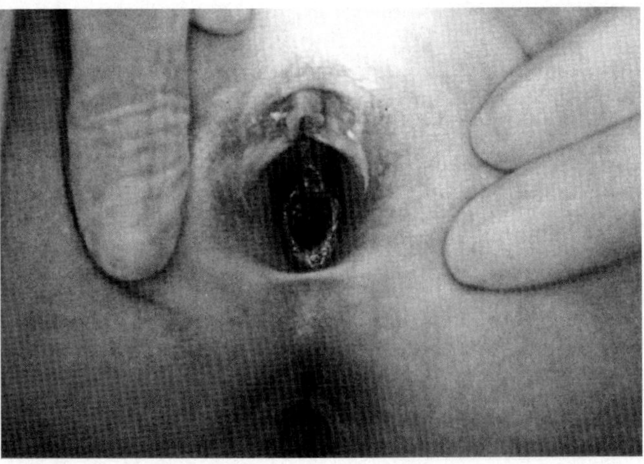

A

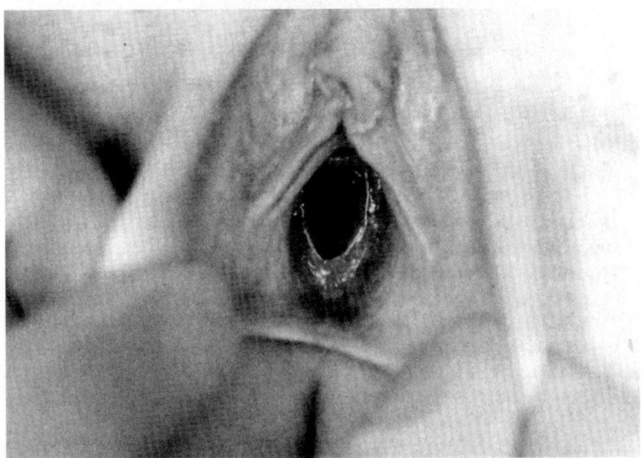

B

Figure 13-3. Examination of the vulva, hymen, and anterior vagina by gentle lateral retraction (**A**) and gentle gripping of the labia and pulling anteriorly (**B**). (From Emans SJ: Office evaluation of the child and adolescent. In Emans SJ, Laufer MR, Goldstein DP [eds]: Pediatric and Adolescent Gynecology, 4th ed. Philadelphia, Lippincott-Raven, 1998.)

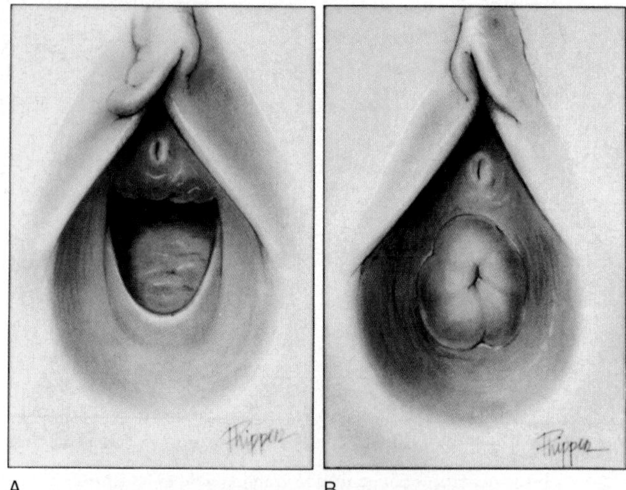

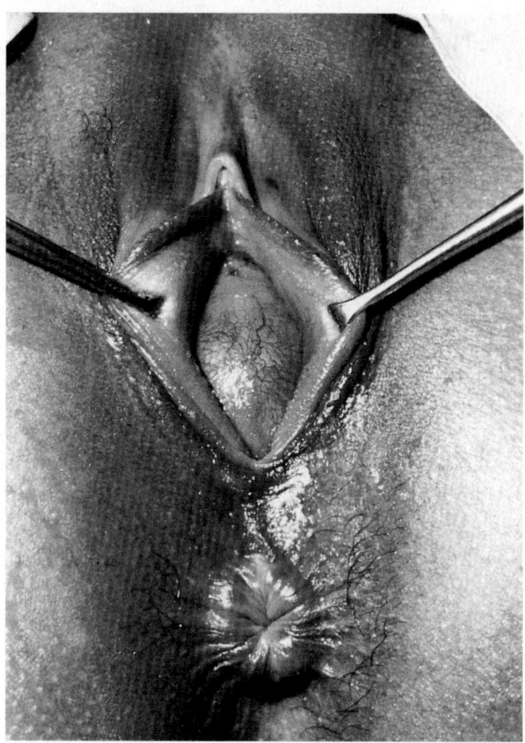

Figure 13-5. Types of hymens in prepubertal girls. **A,** Posterior rim of crescent-shaped hymen. **B,** Fimbriated, or redundant, hymen. **C,** Imperforate hymen. (From Pokorny SF: Configuration of the prepubertal hymen. Am J Obstet Gynecol 157:950, 1987.)

9 o'clock are not congenital but likely acquired. Noncongenital "bumps" may be present near hymeneal transections. The subject of hymens in relation to sexual abuse is covered later in this chapter.

The vaginal epithelium of the prepubertal child appears redder and thinner than the vagina of a woman in her reproductive years. The vagina is 4 to 6 cm long, and the secretions in a prepubertal child have a neutral or slightly alkaline pH. Recurrent vulvovaginitis, persistent bleeding, suspicion of a foreign body or neoplasm, and congenital anomalies may be indications for vaginoscopy. Introduction of any instrument into the vagina of a young child takes skillful patience. The prepubertal vagina is narrower, thinner, and lacking in the distensibility of the vagina of a woman in her reproductive years.

Vaginoscopy often requires a brief inhalation anesthesia but can be preformed in the office in very cooperative children in some circumstances. There are many narrow-diameter endoscopes that will suffice, including the Kelly air cystoscope, contact hysteroscopes, pediatric cystoscopes, small-diameter laparoscopes, plastic vaginoscopes, and special virginal speculums designed by Huffman and Pederson. The ideal pediatric endoscope is a cystoscope or hysteroscope because the accessory channel facilitates lavage of the vagina. A nasal speculum or otoscope is usually too short. Local anesthesia of the vestibule may be obtained with 2% topical viscous lidocaine (Xylocaine). The physician can divert the child's attention from the endoscope in the vagina by simultaneously gently compressing one of the patient's buttocks, an extinction technique. Vaginal evaluation should never be performed under duress or by force.

The last step in the pelvic examination is a rectal examination. This most distressing aspect of the examination may sometimes be omitted, depending on the child's symptoms. Common reasons to perform a rectal examination include genital tract bleeding, pelvic pain, and suspicion of a foreign body or pelvic mass. The child should be warned that the rectal examination will feel similar to the pressure of a bowel movement. The normal prepubertal uterus and ovaries are nonpalpable on rectal examination. The relative size ratio of cervix to uterus is 2 to 1 in a child, in contrast to the opposite ratio in an adult. Except for the cervix, any mass discovered on rectal examination in a prepubertal exam should be considered abnormal.

Examination of the Adolescent Female

The critical factors surrounding the pelvic examination of a female adolescent are different from those of examinations of children 2 to 8 years old. Many female adolescents do not want other observers in the examining room. In one study at a university hospital clinic, 24% of inner-city youths did not want a chaperon present. In many adolescent gynecology visits a full pelvic exam is unnecessary.

Adolescents often come for examinations with preconceived ideas that it will be very painful. Slang terminology for speculums among teens includes the threatening label "the clamp." Teens should be assured that although the exam may include mild discomfort it is not painful. Providers can counsel patients that they will inform them of each step in the process and then ask the teen if she is ready before performing each step. This places the teen in control of the tempo and allows her to anticipate the next element of the examination. Use of the "extinction phenomena" may be helpful. The examiner provides pressure lateral to the introitus on the perineum prior to insertion of the speculum.

Vulvovaginitis

Vulvovaginitis is the most common gynecologic problem in the prepubertal female. It is estimated that 80% to 90% of outpatient visits of children to gynecologists involve the classic symptoms of vulvovaginitis: introital irritation and discharge (Table 13-1).

Table 13-1 Clinical Features of Children Presenting with Vulvovaginitis

Features	Number	Percentage
Symptoms		
Itch	81	40
Soreness	108	54
Bleeding	37	19
Discharge	104	52
Signs		
Genital redness	167	84
Visible discharge	66	33
Perianal soiling	35	18
Specific skin lesion	28	14
None	5	2–4

From Pierce AM, Hart CA: Vulvovaginitis: Causes and management. Arch Dis Child 67:509, 1992.

The prepubertal vagina is neutral or slightly alkaline. With puberty the prepubertal vagina becomes acidic under the influence of bacilli dependant on a glycogenated estrogen-dependant vagina. Breast budding is a reliable sign that the vaginal pH is shifting to an acidic environment.

The severity of vulvovaginitis symptoms varies widely from child to child. The pathophysiology of the majority of instances of vulvovaginitis in children involves a primary irritation of the vulva with secondary involvement of the lower one third of the vagina. Most cases involve an irritation of the vulvar epithelium by normal rectal flora. This is referred to as nonspecific vulvovaginitis There may be a predisposing vulvar irritation secondary to a topical allergy, a vulvar irritant such as perfumed soaps or the tight seams of blue jeans, which creates denudation, allowing the rectal flora to easily infect the irritated epithelium. Cultures from the vagina return as normal rectal flora or *Escherichia coli*. In a primary care setting nonspecific vulvovaginitis accounts for the vast majority of vulvovaginitis cases.

There are both physiologic and behavioral reasons why a child is susceptible to vulvar infection. Physiologically, the child's vulva and vagina are exposed to bacterial contamination from the rectum more frequently than are the adult's. Because the child lacks the labial fat pads and pubic hair of the adult, when a child squats, the lower one third of the vagina is unprotected and open. There is no geographic barrier between the vagina and anus. The vulvar and vaginal epithelium lack the protective effects of estrogen and thus are sensitive to irritation or infection. The labia minora are thin and the vulvar skin is red because the abundant capillary network is easily visualized in the thin skin. The vaginal epithelium of a prepubertal child has a neutral or slightly alkaline pH, which provides an excellent medium for bacterial growth. The vagina of a child lacks glycogen, lactobacilli, and a sufficient level of antibodies to help resist infection. The normal vagina of a prepubertal child is colonized by an average of nine different species of bacteria: four aerobic and facultative anaerobic species and five obligatory anaerobic species.

A major factor in childhood vulvovaginitis is poor perineal hygiene (Table 13-2). This results from the anatomic proximity of the rectum and vagina coupled with the fact that following toilet training, most youngsters are unsupervised when they defecate. Many youngsters wipe their anus from posterior to anterior and thus inoculate the vulvar skin with intestinal flora. A minor vulvar irritation may result in a scratch–itch cycle, with the possibility of secondary seeding because children wash their hands infrequently. Children's clothing is often tight-fitting and nonabsorbent, which keeps the vulvar skin irritated, warm and moist, and prone to vulvovaginitis.

In some cases nonspecific vulvovaginitis may be caused by carrying viral infections from coughing into the hands directly to the abraded vulvar epithelium. Similarly, a child with an upper respiratory tract infection may autoinoculate her vulva, especially with group A β-hemolytic streptococci.

Table 13-2 Etiologic Factors of Premenarcheal Vulvovaginitis

Bacterial

A. Nonspecific
1. Poor perineal hygiene
2. Intestinal parasitic invasion with pruritus
3. Foreign bodies
4. Urinary tract infections with irritation

B. Specific

Bacterial
1. Group A: β-hemolytic streptococci
2. *Streptococcus pneumoniae*
3. *Haemophilus influenzae*/parainfluenzae
4. *Staphylococcus aureus*
5. *Neisseria meningitides*
6. *Escherichia coli*
7. *Shigella flexneri*/*sonnei*
8. Other enterics
9. *Neisseria gonorrhoeae*
10. *Chlamydia trachomatis*

Protozoal—*Trichomonas*

Mycotic
1. *Candida albicans*
2. Other

Helminthiasis—*Enterobius vermicularis*

Viral/Bacterial Systemic Illness
1. Chicken pox
2. Measles
3. Pityriasis rosea
4. Mononucleosis
5. Scarlet fever
6. Kawasaki disease

Other Viral Illnesses
1. Molluscum contagiosum in genital area
2. Condylomata acuminata
3. Herpes simplex-type II

Physical/Chemical Agents
1. Sandbox
2. Trauma
3. Bubble bath
4. Other

Allergic/Skin Conditions
1. Serborrhea
2. Lichen sclerosus
3. Psoriasis
4. Eczema
5. Contact dermatitis

Tumors

Other
1. Prolapsed urethra
2. Ectopic ureter

From Blythe MJ, Thompson L: Premenarchal vulvovaginitis. Indiana Med 86:237, 1993.

Vulvovaginitis in children may also be caused by specific pathogens. Cultures of the vaginal discharge may identify specific organisms such as group A or group B β-hemolytic streptococci, *Haemophilus. influenzae, Neisseria gonorrhoeae, Trichomonas vaginalis, Chlamydia trachomatis,* and *Shigella boydii.*

Pinworms are another cause of vulvovaginitis in prepubertal children. Approximately 20% of female children infected with pinworms (*Enterobius vermicularis*) develop vulvovaginitis. The classic symptom of pinworms is nocturnal vulvar and perianal itching. At night the milk-white, pin-sized adult worms migrate from the rectum to the skin of the vulva to deposit eggs. They may be discovered by means of a flashlight or by dabbing of the vulvar skin with clear cellophane adhesive tape. The tape is subsequently examined under the microscope.

Mycotic vaginal infections are not common in prepubertal children as the alkaline pH of the vagina does not support fungal growth. Mycotic vaginal infections may be seen in immunosuppressed prepubertal girls such as HIV patients or patients on chronic steroid therapy. Other specific causes of vulvovaginitis may include systemic diseases, chicken pox, and herpes simplex infection.

There is nothing specific about the symptoms or signs of childhood vulvovaginitis. Often the first awareness comes when the mother notices staining of the child's underwear or the child complains of itching or burning. There is a wide range in the quantity of discharge, from minimal to copious. The color ranges from white or gray to yellow or green. A discharge that is both bloody and purulent is likely not from vulvovaginitis but from a foreign body (see Prepubertal Bleeding without Puberty). A purulent bloody discharge can also be seen in patients with shigella vaginitis. The signs of vulvovaginitis are variable and not diagnostic, but include vulvar erythema, edema, and excoriation.

The differential diagnosis of persistent or recurrent vulvovaginitis not responsive to treatment should include considerations of a foreign body, primary vulvar skin disease, ectopic ureter, and child abuse. If the predominant symptom is pruritus, then pinworms or an irritant vulvitis are the most likely diagnosis. The vulvar skin of children may also be affected by systemic skin diseases, including lichen sclerosus, seborrheic dermatitis, psoriasis, and atopic dermatitis. The classic perianal "figure-8" or "hourglass" rash is indicative of lichens sclerosus. An ectopic ureter emptying into the vagina may only intermittently release a small amount of urine; thus this rare congenital anomaly should be considered in the differential diagnosis in young children.

Treatment of vulvovaginitis. The foundation of treating childhood vulvovaginitis is the improvement of local perineal hygiene. Both parent and child should be instructed that the vulvar skin should be kept clean, dry, and cool. For acute weeping lesions, wet compresses of Burow's solution should be prescribed. An alternative is a sitz bath containing 2 tablespoons of baking soda in the water. The child should be instructed to void with her knees spread wide apart and taught to wipe from front to back after defecation. Loose-fitting cotton undergarments should be worn. Chemicals that may be allergens or irritants, such as bubble bath, must be discontinued. Harsh soaps and chemicals should be avoided, and dryness of the vulva should be maintained with calamine lotion or a nonirritating cornstarch powder. Many episodes of childhood vulvovaginitis are cured solely by improved local hygiene. The vast majority of cases of persistent or recurrent nonspecific vulvovaginitis respond to a combination of topical creams, low-potency steroids, or oral antibiotics given for 10 to 14 days. If, however, the problem is hygiene, then broad-spectrum antibiotics will only offer temporary relief, and the problem is likely to recur. Relief of vulvar irritation may be facilitated by using a bland cream, such as zinc oxide creams or cod liver oil creams, both of which are readily available in the infant's sections of drug stores. They should be applied several times per day. Another approach is to utilize very low potency steroid creams which are available over the counter.

If the initial therapy is not successful oral antibiotics should be reconsidered. Vaginal cultures help to determine the choice of an oral broad-spectrum antibiotic. Dosage of the selected antibiotic depends on the child's weight. One method of obtaining a vaginal culture in children is to use a nasopharyngeal small swab moistened with nonbacterostatic saline. Pokorny has described another method for collecting fluid from a child's vagina using a catheter within a catheter. This easily assembled adaptation uses a No. 12 red rubber bladder catheter for the outer catheter and the hub end of an intravenous butterfly catheter for the inner catheter (Fig. 13-6). The outer catheter serves as an insulator, and the inner catheter is used to instill a small amount of saline and aspirate the vaginal fluid. The results of the vaginal culture may demonstrate normal flora or an overgrowth of a single organism that is a respiratory, intestinal, or sexually transmitted disease pathogen. The presence of any sexually transmitted organisms in a child is indication that sexual abuse may have taken place and appropriate referral and follow-up is necessary.

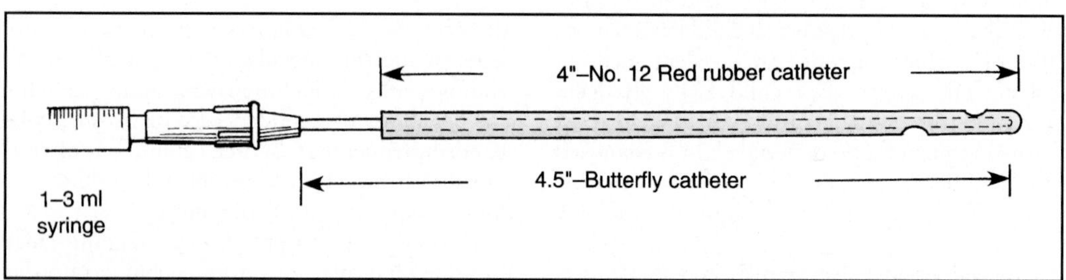

Figure 13-6. Assembled catheter within a catheter, as used to obtain samples of vaginal secretions from prepubertal patients. (Redrawn from Pokorny SF, Stormer J: Atraumatic removal of secretions from the prepubertal vagina. Am J Obstet Gynecol 156:581, 1987.)

Other Prepubertal Gynecologic Problems

Labial Adhesions (Adhesive Vulvitis)

Labial adhesions literally mean the labia minora have adhered or agglutinated together at the midline. Another term sometimes used to describe this condition is *adhesive vulvitis.* Denuded epithelium of adjacent labia minora agglutinates and fuses the two labia together, creating a "flat appearance" of the vulvar surface. A "tell-tale" somewhat translucent vertical midline line is visible on physical exam at the site agglutination. This thin, narrow line in a vertical direction is pathognomonic for adhesive vulvitis (Fig. 13-7). Labial adhesions are often partial and only involve the upper or lower aspects of the labia.

Inexperienced examiners may confuse labial adhesions for an imperforate hymen or vaginal agenesis. Although the physical exam findings are significantly different, all of these conditions may occlude the visualization of the vaginal introitus. In the patient with an imperforate hymen the labia minora appear normal like an upside down V, and no hymeneal fringe is visible at the introitus. In vaginal agenesis the hymeneal fringe is typically normal, but the vaginal canal ends blindly behind the hymeneal fringe.

Labial adhesions are most common in young girls between 2 and 6 years of age. Estrogen reaches a nadir during this time, predisposing the nonestrogenized labia to denudation (see Fig. 13-7). In one large study the average age of a child with agglutination of the labia was $2^1/_2$ years; 90% of cases appeared before age 6. There is considerable variation in the length of agglutination of the two labia minora. In the most advanced cases, there is fusion over both the urethral and the vaginal orifices. It is extremely rare for this fusion to be complete, and most children urinate through openings at the top of the adhesions even when the urethra cannot be visualized. However, the partially fused labia may form a pouch in which urine is caught and later dribbled, presenting as incontinence. Associated urinary infections have been reported.

No treatment is absolutely necessary or 'mandatory' for adhesive vulvitis unless the child is symptomatic. Symptoms include voiding difficulties, recurrent vulvovaginitis, discomfort from the labia pulling at the line of adhesions, and in rare cases bleeding from the line of adhesion pulling apart. Jenkinson and Mackinnon published results of a series of 10 girls who had no therapy and noted spontaneous separation of the adhesive vulvitis within 6 to 18 months. Attempts to separate the adhesions apart in the office by pulling briskly on the labia minora should not be done. It is very painful, and the raw edges are likely to readhese as the child will be reticent to allow application of medication after being subjected to this degree of pain. Some clinicians have also recommended placing local anesthetics on the adhesions and using swabs to tweeze them apart. Many adhesions that would resolve with this therapy are not symptomatic and may not require treatment. However, in rare cases this is appropriate if the local anesthesia (either lidocaine jelly or lidocaine/prilocaine) is successful in preventing discomfort.

The most commonly utilized treatment of this condition is topical estrogen cream dabbed onto the labia two times per day at the site of fusion. This will usually result in spontaneous separation, usually in approximately 2 weeks. In cases without resolution the clinician can reexamine the patient. If increased pigmentation is noted lateral to the midline line of agglutination the caregiver should be reinstructed to apply the cream to

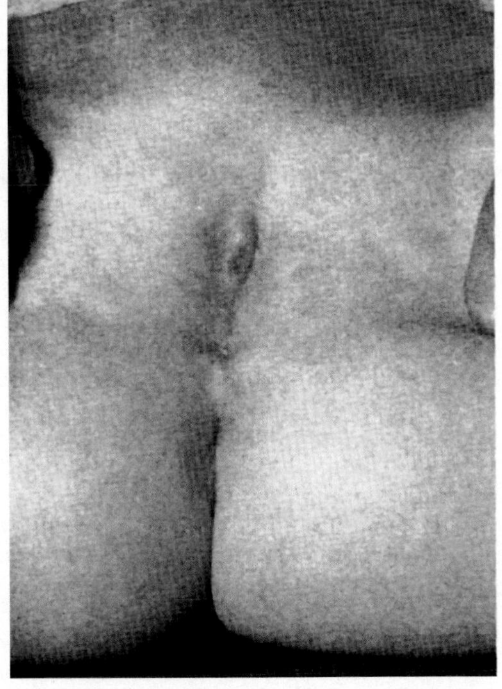

A

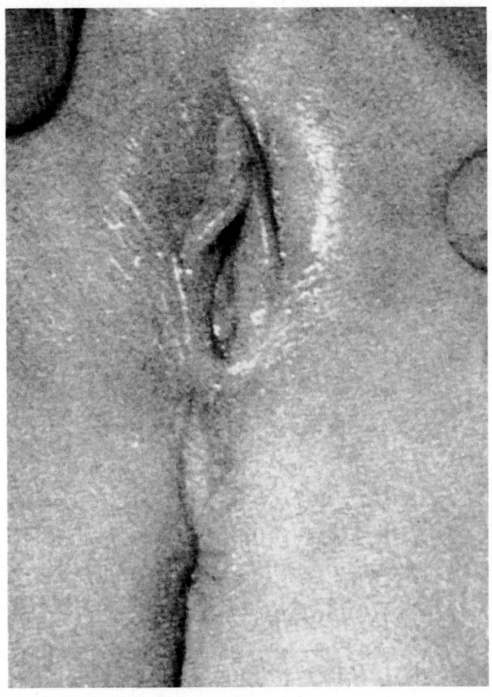

B

Figure 13-7. **A,** Labial adhesions in $2^1/_2$-year-old girl. Two tiny openings exist: one beneath clitoris and another near the middle of the line of fusion. **B,** Appearance in same child after 10 days of local application of estrogen ointment. (From Dewhurst CJ: Gynaecological Disorders of Infants and Children. Philadelphia, FA Davis, 1963.)

the line as the lateral pigmentation indicates the estrogen is being applied lateral to the actual adhesion.

Recurrent adhesive vulvitis occurs in one of five children. Once resolution has occurred reagglutination can often be prevented by applying a bland ointment (such as zinc oxide cream or petroleum jelly) to the raw epithelial edges for at least one month.

A familial form of true posterior labial fusion has been reported by several authors. Analysis of the pedigrees of these children suggests that this congenital defect may be an autosomal dominant trait with incomplete penetrance. McCann and colleagues (1988) reported the association between injuries of the posterior fourchette and labial adhesions in sexually abused children. Labial agglutination alone is so common that immediate suspicion of child abuse based solely on this finding in 2- to 6-year-olds is unwarranted. However, the combination of labial adhesions and scarring of the posterior fourchette especially in children with new-onset labial adhesions after age 6 should prompt the clinician to consider sexual abuse in the differential diagnosis.

Physiologic Discharge of Puberty

In the early stages of puberty, children often develop a physiologic vaginal discharge. This discharge is typically described as having a gray-white coloration although it may appear slightly yellow but is not purulent. The physiologic discharge represents desquamation of the vaginal epithelium. The estrogenic environment allows acid-producing bacilli to become part of the normal vaginal ecosystem. The acids the bacilli produce cause a desquamation of the prepubertal vaginal epithelium. When the physiologic discharge is examined with the microscope, sheets of vaginal epithelial cells are identified.

Clinically there is usually very little symptomatology associated with this discharge. Occasionally the thickness of the discharge causes the vulva to be "pasted" to undergarments and causes some symptoms of irritation and erythema. Usually the only treatment necessary is reassurance of both mother and child that this is a normal physiologic process that will subside with time. Symptomatic children maybe treated with sitz baths and frequent changing of underwear.

Urethral Prolapse

Prolapse of the urethral mucosa is not a rare event in children. The most common presentation is not urinary symptomatology but prepubertal bleeding. Often a sharp increase in abdominal pressure, such as coughing, precedes the *urethral prolapse.* On examination the distal aspect of urethral mucosa may be prolapsed along the entire 360° of the urethra (Fig. 13-8). This forms a red donut-like structure. The prolapse may be partial or incomplete, presenting as a ridge of erythematous tissue. It is critical to distinguish this from grapelike masses of sarcoma botryoides that originate from the vagina. Occasionally the prolapse becomes necrotic and blue-black in color.

Treatment is conservative and noninteventional. Many experts recommend application of various medications including estrogen creams and antibiotic ointments. Although such interventions appear appropriate, well-designed prospective studies have not been done to confirm they are therapeutic. Surgery is seldom necessary except in rare cases where necrosis is obviously present.

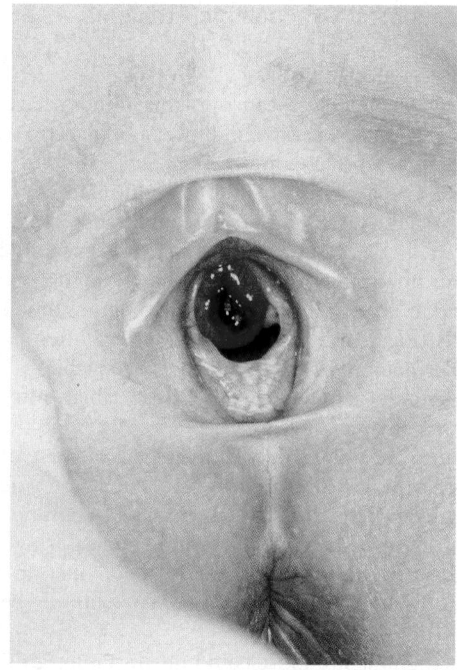

Figure 13-8. Prepubertal urethral prolapse with high crescent-shaped hymen.

Lichen Sclerosus

Lichen sclerosus (LS) formerly called *lichen sclerosus atrophicus,* is a skin dystrophy most commonly seen in postmenopausal women and prepubertal children. The cause is unclear although there is some evidence that it may be associated with autoimmune phenomena. This has not been confirmed by prospective studies. Histologically there is thinning of the vulvar epithelium with loss of the rete pegs. The most common symptoms are pruritus and vulvar discomfort. Other presentations may include prepubertal bleeding, constipation, and dysuria.

The appearance of LS varies, but lesions are always limited by the labia majora. If lesions go beyond the labia majora is unlikely to be LS. The lesion often appears in an hourglass or figure-8 formation involving the genital and perianal area (Fig. 13-9). The skin may be lichenified with a parchment-like appearance. Parents may note that the genital area appears "whitened." Pruritus is typical but not inevitable. In some cases the pruritus is so severe that patients have used hair brushes to scratch the area in an attempt to stop the pruritic sensation. Secondary changes may occur subsequent to the patient excoriating the area. When this occurs, there are often blood blisters and breaks in the integument. Patients with blood blisters may present with prepubertal bleeding.

Given the abnormal appearance of LS with secondary changes, clinicians unfamiliar with this skin dystrophy often arrive at the misdiagnosis of sexual abuse. However, clinicians experienced in pediatric or postmenopausal gynecology will usually have no difficulty arriving at the correct diagnosis. In cases where the diagnosis is unclear a small punch biopsy may confirm the diagnosis. Performing a biopsy in prepubertal children is often difficult. Many children will not tolerate a local injection, and holding down children to perform a biopsy is clearly not acceptable. General anesthesia is preferable in this

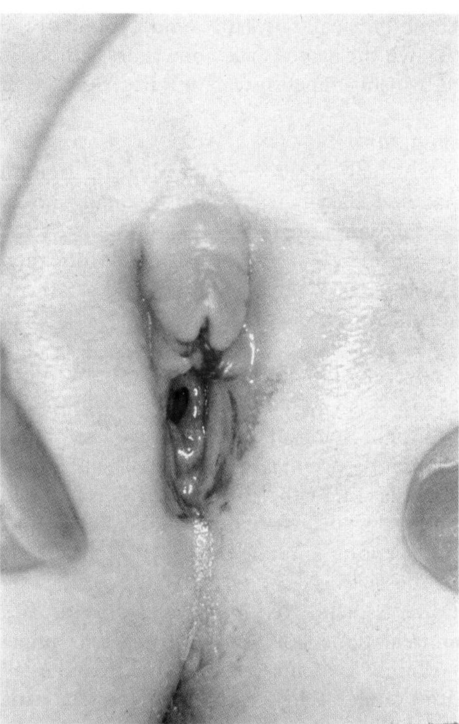

Figure 13-9. Lichen sclerosus atrophicus in prepubertal child with lichenification limited by labia majora and breaks in integument presenting as prepubertal bleeding.

situation. Some children will tolerate a biopsy using local anesthesia, and 1% lidocaine without epinephrine may be used.

The treatment of LS in children should always start with avoiding irritation or trauma to the genital epithelium. LS is a skin disorder in which lesions are most likely to occur in epithelium that is irritated. Children should be encouraged to avoid straddle activities such as bicycle or tricycle riding when symptomatic. Patients should clean the labia by soaking in sitz baths. Parents sometimes may assume lack of cleanliness is contributing to the disorder and scrub the area with soap, which may actually exacerbate the disease. Tight clothing such as blue jeans may also abrade and irritate the vulva.

In mature reproductive women clobetasol has become the treatment of choice. This powerful steroid is used for a short duration, given the serious complication of adrenal suppression. The safety of this medication has not been established in children younger than 12 years of age, and use in children is outside product labeling. However, clinicians have had success in treating LS with clobetasol in prepubertal children. Adrenal suppression with clobetasol is likely to be more common in diseases such as psoriasis and atrophic dermatitis in which larger surface areas of skin require treatment. If the clinician elects to use clobetasol in pediatric LS patients, the parents should be counseled regarding the labeling. Tapering the steroid level should be considered as soon as a response is seen or within a 2-week interval. The parents should apply the drug sparingly. Another approach is to reserve this potent steroid for patients in whom the conservative treatment of avoiding trauma and irritation with medium-potency local steroids have not cleared symptomatology.

Previously, many authors have asserted that LS improves with puberty. Though improvement and resolution occurs sometimes, many patients will continue to have symptoms or physical findings.

Prepubertal Bleeding without Secondary Signs of Puberty

Puberty in the female is the process of biologic change and physical development after which sexual reproduction becomes possible. This is a time of accelerated linear skeletal growth and development of secondary sexual characteristics, such as breast development and the appearance of axillary and pubic hair. The usual sequence of the physiologic events of puberty begins with breast development, the subsequent appearance of pubic and axillary hair, followed by the period of maximal growth velocity, and lastly, menarche. Menarche may occur before the appearance of axillary or pubic hair in 10% of normal females. Normal puberty occurs over a wide range of ages (see Chapters 4 and 38 [Reproductive Endocrinology and Primary and Secondary Amenorrhea and Precocious Puberty]). Precocious puberty is arbitrarily defined as the appearance of any signs of secondary sexual maturation at an early specific age more than 2.5 standard deviations below the mean. Precocious puberty is covered in detail in Chapter 38. A common clinical problem that is sometimes mistaken for precocious puberty is prepubertal bleeding in children without any other signs of puberty such as breast development (Table 13-3).

Vaginal Bleeding

The normal sequence of puberty is that thelarche precedes menarche. In children with prepubertal bleeding without breast budding there is almost never an endocrinologic cause, with the exception being a very rare presentation of McCune–Albright syndrome.

The differential diagnosis of vaginal bleeding without pubertal development includes foreign body, vulvar excoriation, lichen sclerosus, shigella vaginitis, separation of labial adhesions, trauma (abuse and accidental), urethral prolapse, and friable genital warts. Rare causes include malignant tumors (sarcoma botryoides and endodermal sinus tumors of the vagina) and an unusual presentation of McCune–Albright syndrome. Lists of the differential diagnosis of prepubertal bleeding often also include accidental estrogen exposure (for example from ingestion of a mother's birth control pills). However, in reality such

Table 13-3 Differential Diagnosis of Prepubertal Bleeding Without Any Breast Development

Foreign object
Genital trauma
Genital abuse
Lichen sclerosus
Infectious vaginitis (especially from *Shigella*)
Urethral prolapse
Breakdown of labial adhesions
Friable genital warts or vulvar lesions
Vaginal tumor
Rare presentation of McCune–Albright syndrome (typically have breast development)
Isolated menarche (controversial)

exposure would rarely provide enough endometrial stimulation to produce a withdrawal bleed without breast budding. Neonates may develop a white mucoid vaginal discharge or a small amount of vaginal spotting. Both conditions are secondary to exposure during pregnancy to the high levels of estrogen and are self-limited.

In a 20-year review of vaginal bleeding, 52 cases were identified in girls 10 years and younger from the Chelsea Hospital for Women in London. Genital tumors, precocious puberty, vulvar lesions, and urethral prolapse were the four leading causes in this series. This report was from a referral center and therefore may not truly represent the cases seen in the practitioner's office. The absence of sexual abuse in this study likely reflects referral patterns. However, it should be remembered that although the differential diagnosis of prepubertal bleeding includes sexual abuse, the vast majority of sexually abused children do not have prepubertal bleeding. In some settings, such as emergency departments, it is more likely that the cause of prepubertal bleeding is sexual abuse than in tertiary referral practice where the cause of the bleeding is often unclear to the referring physician.

Foreign Bodies

Symptoms secondary to a vaginal foreign body are responsible for approximately 4% of pediatric gynecologic outpatient visits. The vast majority of foreign bodies are found in girls between 3 and 9 years of age. The history is usually not helpful because an adult has not witnessed, nor does the child remember, putting a foreign object into the vagina. Many types of foreign bodies have been discovered; however, the most common are small wads of toilet paper. Other common foreign objects include small, hard objects such as hairpins, parts of a toy, tips of plastic markers, crayons, and sand or gravel. Some of these objects are not radiopaque. When small swabs are used to perform vaginal cultures the examiner may note an odd sensation of touching something other than vaginal mucosa. Objects such as coins and plastic toys are often easily visible on vaginal examination, especially in the knee-chest position. Foreign bodies may be inserted by children because the genital area is pruritic or when naturally curious children are exploring their bodies.

The classic symptom is a foul, bloody vaginal discharge. However, the discharge is often purulent and without blood. The natural history probably reflects the object initially causing irritation, creating a purulent discharge, and then as the object imbeds itself into the vaginal epithelium, bleeding and spotting may occur. There is often a lag between insertion of the object and the vaginal bleeding. Over time, the foreign body may become partially "buried" into the vagina, and difficult to remove without discomfort.

The presence of unexplained vaginal bleeding is one indication for a vaginoscopy. In children younger than 6 years of age this should be done expeditiously to rule out malignant vaginal tumors. If an object is seen on exam the clinician may be able, in a cooperative child, to either grasp the object with a forceps or wash the object out by irrigation. The catheter technique described previously may be utilized. (see Fig. 13-6). Often this is not possible because the child cannot cooperate or because a solid object is imbedded into the vaginal wall. In these cases the object can be removed at vaginoscopy.

Children who insert foreign objects often are "repeat performers." This may be secondary to pain or pruritus in the genital area, and the child uses the "object" (solid or toilet paper) to rub or scratch the genital area. Sometimes this possibility may be reduced by using wipes instead of toilet paper.

Shigella Vaginitis

Approximately half of all cases of shigella vaginitis present with prepubertal bleeding. There is generally no concurrent gastrointestinal symptomatology. Cultures for *Shigella* should be strongly considered in any child with no obvious cause for prepubertal bleeding. Rarely, vaginitis caused by other organisms can also present with prepubertal bleeding.

Rare Causes: Vaginal Tumors and McCune–Albright Syndrome

McCune–Albright syndrome is a rare somatic mutation that occurs during embryogenesis in neural crest cells. Since the mutation does not occur in the germline, it is not inherited. The mutation affects G protein receptors and has a quite variable expression, depending on how many early cells are affected (an example of mosaicism). The *GNAS1* gene is the affected area. The syndrome is manifested by the classic triad of café-au-lait spots, abnormal bone lesions, and precocious puberty. Most McCune–Albright patients present with prepubertal bleeding along with thelarche. Rarely a child may present with bleeding and no breast budding. Examination of the child with prepubertal bleeding should include examination of the skin for café-au-lait spots, and the historical intake should include queries about frequent bone fractures. In cases of unexplained prepubertal bleeding the possibility of McCune–Albright should be considered, and serial breast examinations may reveal breast budding.

Sarcoma Botryoides and Endodermal Sinus Tumors of the Vagina

Almost all cases of sarcoma botryoides of the vagina in prepubertal children occur prior to age 6, and endodermal sinus tumors occur prior to age 2. Although these tumors are extremely rare causes of prepubertal bleeding, they must be considered in every child. Both are aggressive malignancies and prompt diagnosis is critical. In young children with no evident cause of prepubertal bleeding a vaginoscopy should be done to rule out these malignancies.

Vaginoscopy for Prepubertal Bleeding without Signs of Puberty

Many times no clear cause of prepubertal bleeding is defined at vaginoscopy. In these cases there likely was a small foreign object that has been expelled from the vagina or disintegrated. Even though many vaginoscopies are negative, it is especially important for clinicians to perform them promptly in young prepubertal bleeders to exclude the rare but very aggressive vaginal malignancies.

ACCIDENTAL GENITAL TRAUMA

The usual cause of accidental genital trauma during childhood is a fall. Seventy-five percent of all accidental trauma to the vulva and vagina involves straddle injuries. Obviously, sexual abuse is an important consideration in the differential diagnosis. Sexual abuse is discussed later in this chapter.

Vulvar Trauma: Lacerations and Straddle Injury

One of the most common causes of genital trauma in a child is a straddle injury. This problem occurs when a child stands, or hovers, with her legs apart over a hard object, and then falls with the perineum against the object. Common straddle injuries in children occur on playground climbing structures such as a monkey bar, or fence rails. A straddle injury generally results in unilateral and superficial injury and very rarely involves the hymen. In two separate series involving a total of over 130 children with straddle injuries only 3 had hymeneal transection. In cases of hymeneal transection with a history of straddle injury, sexual abuse should be strongly considered. In the rare cases where the hymen is transected from accidental trauma there is usually a history of a penetrating injury such as falling onto a stick horse or broom.

If hymeneal transection has occurred the examiner must confirm that the object has not penetrated into the vaginal wall which could result in a dangerous hematoma, perforation into the cul-de-sac, or perforation of the abdominal cavity with potential visceral damage. A vaginoscopy or laparoscopy (or both) is generally required to rule out these possibilities. Perforations into the abdomen may not result in significant vaginal bleeding.

In children presenting with trauma and genital bleeding the examiner must first ascertain the site, extent, and amount of bleeding. Viscous lidocaine or a longer acting topical agent such as lidocaine/prilocaine should be applied and allowed appropriate time to provide anesthesia. Then the area can be gently washed by irrigating with sterile warmed water onto the labial area. Typical lacerations may involve denudation around the urethra or labia. The posterior fourchette is less commonly involved. Children with vulvar trauma should have a booster injection of tetanus toxoid if the last immunization was more than 5 years before the trauma.

Lacerations that are superficial (equivalent to first-degree obstetric lacerations) generally do not require repair in contrast to deeper lacerations. Often superficial lacerations can be adequately treated by applying oxidized cellulose or similar products to stop the bleeding. Slightly deeper lacerations can be repaired with small Steristrips. In some deeper lacerations one well-placed suture will stop substantial bleeding. This scenario is typical of lacerations on the inferior aspect of the labia minora. Placement of the suture may be aided by injection of lidocaine in cooperative children.

General anesthesia is usually required for diagnosis and treatment of extensive lacerations and deep lacerations in children unable to tolerate repair in the office or emergency department. During this anesthesia the laceration should be irrigated and débrided, the vessels ligated, and the injuries repaired. Occasionally it is necessary to perform laparoscopy or an exploratory celiotomy for a suspected retroperitoneal hematoma or intraabdominal injury.

Vulvar Hematomas

If the vulva strikes a blunt object, a hematoma usually results. If the object is sharp, such as a fence post, the injury may be a laceration with the potential for penetration of the perineum and injury to internal pelvic organs. Other common causes of vulvar and vaginal trauma include sexual abuse, automobile and bicycle accidents, kicks sustained in a fight, and self-inflicted wounds (Fig. 13-10).

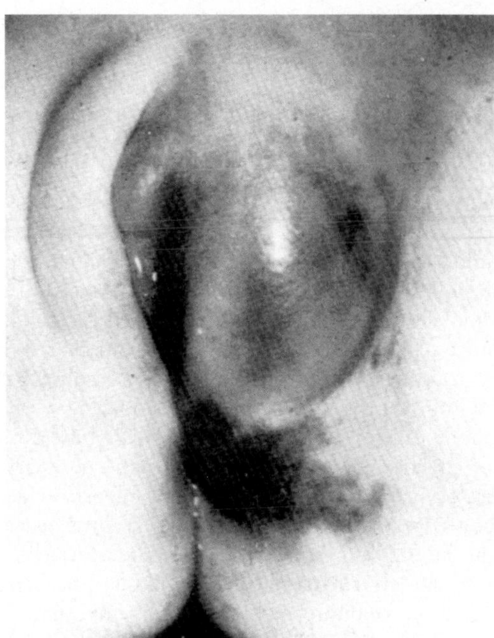

Figure 13-10. Vulvar hematoma resulting from a kick in a 2-year-old child. (From Huffman JW: The Gynecology of Childhood and Adolescence, 2nd ed. Philadelphia, WB Saunders, 1981.)

The size of vulvar and vaginal hematomas varies widely. Initially there is bleeding into the loose connective tissue. When the pressure from the expanding hematoma exceeds the venous pressure, in most cases the hematoma will stop growing. In the vast majority of cases surgical exploration should be avoided. It is rare to find a specific vessel to ligate except in cases where the hematoma is literally expanding over 1 to 2 minutes of observation, which likely represents a very rare arterial laceration. The extent of the hematoma should be determined by both visualization and palpation. The treatment of nonexpanding vulvar hematomas is observation by serial examinations and the use of an ice pack or ice sitz bath.

Sexual Abuse

Sexual abuse in reproductive women is covered in Chapter 10 (Rape, Incest, and Domestic Violence). This chapter contains information specifically related to sexual abuse in the prepubertal child. For a detailed and complete description of evaluation and treatment of the potentially sexually abused child, practitioners should refer to the American Academy of Pediatrics guidelines for the evaluation of child sexual abuse.

Scope of the Problem

Unfortunately, sexual abuse of children is extremely common in the United States. Approximately 20% girls are involved in some type of sexual activity during childhood. Although abduction cases with subsequent sexual abuse by a person unknown to the family attract national media coverage, this scenario is very rare. Most perpetrators are male acquaintances known and trusted by the families. Fathers are responsible approximately 21% of the time and other male relatives 19% of the time. It is often not appreciated that mothers are involved 4% to 8% of the time. Babysitting is a common modus operendi for abusers to gain access to children.

History in Sexual Abuse

There are two situations in which health care providers need to garner information regarding potential sexual abuse. One is the child or family that presents with potential sexual abuse as the chief complaint. The other situation is when the child is seen for another complaint, such as a purulent discharge, but the provider considers the possibility of sexual abuse based on historical information or physical examination.

Telephone calls regarding potential sexual abuse are a challenge for practitioners. Urgent evaluation is necessary if the abuse has occurred within 72 hours (for forensic evidence), if the child is currently in a danger of repeated abuse or self-harm, or obvious injuries such as lacerations require treatment. If none of these criteria are encountered, the child and her family can be evaluated on a nonurgent basis. This is important, because specially trained personnel should become involved as soon as possible in these situations. In many settings these children can be referred to a sexual abuse team on a nonemergency basis. In settings where teams are not available it is critical that practitioners be aware of other community resources.

If at all possible, it is usually ideal that the child and family be interviewed separately by a qualified mental health provider (such as a social worker or psychologist) who is experienced in evaluating sexual abuse. Guidelines have been published on appropriate interviewing of children who may be victims of sexual abuse. Often state departments of children's services or the social work department of the community hospital can refer providers to appropriate mental health providers. Unless there are compelling medical reasons, this interview should be performed prior to a genital examination. There are several reasons for this recommendation. First latency age children may not be able to separate the exam from touching involved in abuse, making the history more difficult to obtain. Second in the vast majority of abused children the exam is completely normal. It is important that families not rely on an exam to decide whether to seek counseling or intervention that would keep their child safe. Although providers should ask relevant questions, the more complete interview by an experienced mental health provider minimizes repetitive questioning of the child. The interview may also allow rapport to begin between the mental health professional doing the interview and the family so that the relationship can transit into therapy if indicated.

Practitioners may also consider sexual abuse based on historical complaints or physical examination findings. In this situation it is critical for the provider to query the guardian or parent in a nonthreatening manner. The approach should be "we are all on the same team and we both want to ensure the safety of your child." Queries directed to the child should be open-ended and nonjudgmental.

Legal Issues in Reporting Possible Sexual Abuse

Providers must be aware of their state's laws and how to file a report alleging sexual abuse. Every state requires that suspected and known child abuse be reported. The word *suspected,* however, deserves definition. Isolated complaints that may be associated with sexual abuse (e.g., nightmares or genital bleeding) do not require a report.

Clinicians may suspect sexual abuse based on a variety of historical complaints and physical exam findings. Consideration to other causes of these complaints and findings is also critical. For example in children who present with genital bleeding, the differential diagnosis may also include urethral prolapse, foreign bodies, and lichen sclerosus, vaginal tumors, or nonabusive trauma.

If a provider is unsure if a report is required he or she should discuss the situation with local child protective services. These agencies can help providers avoid filing vague unnecessary reports, which clog the services of overburdened state agencies. They can also aid in filing reports in borderline cases that justify exploration to obtain safety of children. In addition discussion with agencies may help protect providers from prosecution for failure to report. It is important to document discussions in patient charts. Guidelines have been developed by the American Academy of Pediatrics regarding appropriate filing of abuse reports. Providers should not be hesitant to file because of fear of liability for an alleged false report. Although suits have been flied against physicians, states generally ensue immunity, and, as of 1999, no such suits have been successful.

Physical Examination and Evaluation for Sexually Transmitted Infections

The exam of a potentially sexually abused child should include a general exam. Attention should be directed at evaluating skin for bruising, lacerations, or trauma. Parents or concerned adults should be counseled that a genital exam in children who have been abused is usually normal. Physical evidence is present in less than 5% of children. The genital exam should be carried out as described earlier in this chapter.

In situations in which abuse has occurred within 72 hours careful collection of forensic evidence is important. Collection of all clothing and undergarments is critical. Motile sperm will be present in the prepubertal vagina for approximately 8 hours, and nonmotile sperm for approximately 24 hours. Since prepubertal children do not have cervical mucous, sperm do not exist for the longer durations seen in reproductive females within the cervical canal. "Rape" kits will also often include testing for a protein specific to the prostate. Vaginal specimens may be obtained by using small swabs within the vagina, similar to the method described for obtaining vaginal cultures.

Given that only approximately 5% of abused children acquire a STI (sexually transmitted infection), providers must decide when STI testing is indicated. Both gonorrhea and chlamydia cause a vaginitis not a cervicitis in prepubertal children, so a vaginal culture should be done. In the United States a vaginal culture for gonorrhea and chlamydia, not DNA testing should be performed as recommended by the Centers for Disease Control and Prevention. Since nonculture methods are not labeled for use in children, positive testing may not be admissible in court. Testing in prepubertal children is also influenced by typical incubation intervals of STIs. If a child was abused in an isolated incident, an STI may not be found on testing immediately after the abuse.

In children presenting in nonacute presentations the provider must decide whether to perform testing for STIs. It is very

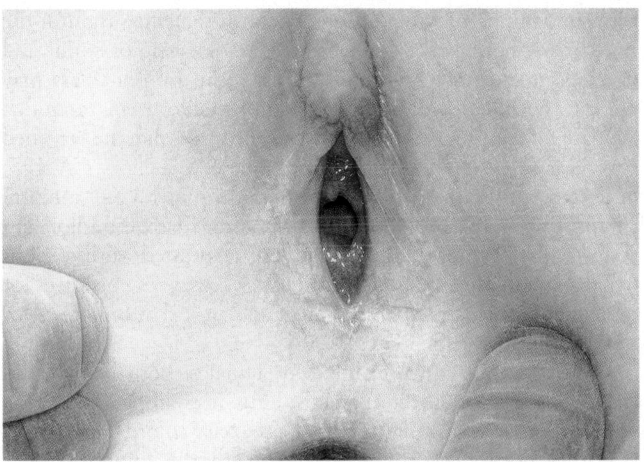

Figure 13-11. Hymenal bump along side of an incomplete transection of the hymen at approximately 7 to 8 o'clock.

rare for a child to have gonorrhea or chlamydia without a vaginal discharge. Standards of care regarding this issue may differ in various locations.

Hymens in the Evaluation of Sexual Abuse

There is a general misunderstanding regarding the significance of hymeneal changes. The transverse diameter of the hymen was previously used as a marker of abuse. However, it is now clear that there is significant variation in children, and the state of the hymen it is not a reliable marker of abuse. Complete transections of the hymen and clefts that extend to the junction of the hymen between 3 o'clock and 9 o'clock are not congenital, but if present could be from abuse or a child inserting an object. Controversies exist as to the significance of incomplete transections (Fig. 13-11).

Genital Warts

Human papillomavirus (HPV) the causative agent of genital warts may be transmitted to children from the maternal genital tract at delivery or by sexual or nonsexual transmission after birth. The incubation interval from transmission to the presence of visible genital warts has not been defined in children; however, it appears likely that most warts appearing prior to approximately 2 years of age are from maternal–child transmission. If the child is 2 years of age or older, serious consideration should be given to the possibility of sexual transmission. (See previous section on sexual abuse in this chapter). However, genital warts "discovered" in a 3-year-old may have been present for some time prior to being noticed. This is particularly a problem in the perianal area, which may not be examined carefully even in children undergoing a cursory genital exam as part of well-child annual care.

Approximately half of lesions will regress over 5 years. Expectant management is reasonable, but parents may prefer treatment. Treatment in children is difficult. Caustic treatments such as trichloroacetic acid are painful even if children are pretreated with local anesthesia. Topical imiquimod cream is labeled for use in children 12 years and older. If imiquimod cream is accidentally carried by the child to the cornea it could cause damage to the eye. Laser treatment is an option for significant wart tissue, but must be performed under an inhalation anesthesia and can be associated with significant postoperative pain.

The Ovary and Adnexa in Pediatric and Adolescent Gynecology: Cysts, Tumors, and Torsion

Most ovarian masses in this age group are functional ovarian cysts, and if a tumor is present is most often a benign teratoma (dermoid). Malignancies can, however, occur and are most often of germ cell origin, but can also be sex cord tumors such as a graunulosa cell malignancy.

Physiologic and functional cysts of the ovaries are from gonadotropin stimulation of the follicles. They may present in the fetus, newborn, infant, at puberty, and in adolescence. The appropriate management may depend on the age and on the appearance of the cyst on ultrasound. Cysts of follicular development will be clear without significant solid components and almost always are less than 7 to 10 cm in size.

Corpus luteum cysts are often more complex than other follicular cysts. Management is similar to that in mature reproductive women, and observation is warranted unless signs of malignancy are present. Consideration should be given to dermoids and the possibility of germ cell tumors if a mass has both solid and cystic components. In rare cases of intersex such as mixed gonadal dysgenesis suspicion of malignancy should be high. A rare presentation of hypothyroidism is pediatric ovarian cysts.

Prenatal Ovarian Cysts

Obstetric ultrasound of a female fetus occasionally demonstrates a simple abdominal cyst. Before a diagnosis of an ovarian cyst is made, it is critical to exclude urinary or gastrointestinal anomalies. Fetal malignancy is quite rare. The management of fetal ovarian cysts is essentially expectant. Cysts rarely may undergo torsion in the fetus, producing fetal ascites and rarely distress. This is extremely uncommon. If torsion does occur, autoinfarction is possible. The end product is unilateral agenesis of an ovary, and sometimes the tube. Again, this is rare. Cysts greater than 9 cm should be managed with cesarean section. Cyst aspiration could avoid the complication of silent ovarian torsion; however, the risks do not justify the complications, unless the fetus is very immature and in significant stress from the mass. With expectant management, approximately 90% will resolve within 3 months after birth.

Torsion may be more common prenatally than postnatally although spontaneous resolution may also be more common. The relative rarity of congenital absence of one ovary makes it likely that untwisting occurs. The incidence of congenital unilateral ovarian agenesis is only 1 in approximately 11,000 females. Ovarian malignancy is extremely rare in this age group and is not a consideration in the therapeutic approach.

Neonatal Ovarian Cysts

Simple cystic ovarian masses in newborns and neonates can be followed expectantly. Parents should be given ovarian torsion warnings, and if the infant presents with acute vomiting or abdominal pain she should be immediately evaluated for ovarian torsion. Repeat serial ultrasonography should be performed approximately monthly until the cyst resolves. Almost all will resolve if they do not undergo torsion. Malignancy is not a consideration in newborns in the therapeutic approach. Aspiration is a possibility for large cysts.

Ovarian Cysts in Children and Adolescents

The management of cystic ovarian structures in children and adolescents should also be expectant unless they are extremely large, in which case the possibility of functional cysts becomes more unlikely. Many times physiologic and functional cysts are discovered on an abdominal ultrasound performed for complaints such as abdominal pain. Often the presence of a cyst is incidental and unrelated to the complaint. However, in patients with pain the possibility of ovarian torsion should be entertained. Pain from ovarian cysts generally stems from three sources: (1) expansion of the ovarian cortex (which is typically during the growth phase of follicles and lasts less than 72 hours), (2) peritoneal bleeding from rupture (particularly common in bleeding disorders and patients on warfarin [Coumadin]), and (3) ovarian torsion. Ovarian cysts should be suspected in cases of chronic pelvic abdominal pain.

Ovarian Tumors in Childhood and Adolescents

Various tumors, both benign and malignant, can be seen in the childhood and adolescent years. These should always be considered, particularly in patients with solid ovarian masses or cystic and solid components on ultrasound. The diagnosis should also be considered in patients with presumed functional ovarian cysts that do not resolve during serial monitoring.

Germ cell tumors are the most common gynecologic neoplasm in this age group, and fortunately most are benign ovarian teratomas. The most common malignant germ cell tumor is the dysgerminoma followed by endodermal sinus tumors. These tumors are covered in detail in Chapter 33 (Neoplastic Diseases of the Ovary), but several issues are especially pertinent to children and adolescents.

Bilaterality is seen in 10% to 15% of dysgerminomas, but is rare in all of the other germ cell tumors of the ovary except for immature teratomas. Sex cord tumors, such as granulosa and thecal cell tumors, can also be seen in this age group and are often steroid-producing Rare tumors such as gonadoblastomas, a germ cell and sex cord tumor, are seen in patients with intersex disorders such as mixed gonadal dysgenesis.

Recurrent abdominal pain is a frequent complaint of grammar school age children and this common symptom occasionally is the presenting problem with ovarian neoplasia. The young child does not differentiate lower abdominal pain from pelvic pain. Because of the small size of the preadolescent female pelvis, the ovaries are abdominal organs. Thus, increasing abdominal girth is a frequent symptom associated with ovarian enlargement. The most common clinical manifestation of an ovarian tumor is lower abdominal pain or the presence of a mass. Some ovarian tumors in children produce only vague discomfort, such as abdominal fullness or bloating. However, adnexal masses in children are more frequently associated with acute complications, such as torsion, hemorrhage, and rupture, than are similar tumors in adults.

Ovarian tumors constitute approximately 1% of all neoplasms in premenarcheal children. Ultrasound, abdominal computed tomography (CT), or magnetic resonance imaging (MRI) may be utilized in the evaluation of a possible pelvic mass or abdominal pain of uncertain origin in children. Abdominal ultrasonography may be used to establish that the origin of the mass is in the pelvis, whether the mass is cystic or solid, and the presence of ascites. Calcifications in an ovarian mass may appear toothlike, indicating a diagnosis of ovarian teratoma. As part of the preoperative workup, the child may be screened for elevated serum levels of tumor markers such as CA 125, α-fetoprotein, human chorionic gonadotropin (HCG), inhibin, carcinoembryonic antigen, lactate dehydrogenase, estradiol, and testosterone; tumor markers that are associated with various ovarian neoplasms seen in girls. HCG may be positive for either the α or β subunit, so a pregnancy test that only tests for the β subunit is inadequate.

Ovarian tumors in preadolescent females, both benign and malignant, are usually unilateral. Thus it is imperative to be conservative in managing the opposite ovary in order to protect potential future fertility. During surgery the opposite ovary should be carefully inspected and palpated. It is unnecessary and potentially harmful to perform a biopsy on a normal-appearing contralateral ovary in a preadolescent female. Appropriate exceptions to this rule include consideration of performing a wedge biopsy in patients with dysgerminoma or a immature teratoma—malignancies in which bilaterality is not as rare.

Children with suspected ovarian cancer should be referred to specialists who are up to date on current data from the Pediatrics Oncology Group or Gynecologic Oncology Group. First these groups will be skilled in getting their patients proper staging procedures including lymph node sampling and omentectomy. In addition, standard of care is for patients with nondysgerminomas, with a few exceptions, to receive postoperative adjuvant chemotherapy. Use of tumor markers to help differentiate patients with benign teratoma from malignancies is useful in triaging appropriate referrals. However, regardless of what the makers show, referral is prudent.

Approximately 75% to 85% of ovarian neoplasms that necessitate surgery in premenarcheal females are benign, and approximately 15% to 25% are malignant neoplasms. The risk is less in young children. In a review of ovarian masses in children Brown and coworkers reported that the risk of malignancy was only 3% up to age 8.

In summary, even though ovarian neoplasia is rare in children, this diagnosis must be considered in a young girl with abdominal pain and a palpable mass. The surgical therapy should have two goals: first, and most important, the appropriate surgical procedure including lymph nodes as necessary, and second preservation of future fertility. The traditional hysterectomy performed in adults with epithelial ovarian cancers is not necessary even in rare cases of bilateral childhood or adolescent ovarian malignancy. The uterus should be retained for fertility, which may be possible through artificial reproductive technology such as use of donor eggs.

Ovarian Torsion

Ovarian torsion is covered in more detail in Chapter 18 (Benign Gynecologic Lesions). Issues unique to children and adolescents are covered in this discussion. Torsion in prepubertal females may be secondary to a pelvic mass or due to mechanical factors that occur in the peripubertal interval. In early puberty the ovaries drop from their prepubertal position at the pelvic brim into the pelvis. This drop occurs under the influence of gonadotropins that surge at puberty. Some young women may have longer supportive ligaments, predisposing them to twisting.

Approximately two thirds of the time ovarian torsion occurs on the right side, increasing the likelihood of the process being confused with appendicitis. The sigmoid colon in the left lower quadrant helps prevent the left ovary from twisting.

Although both appendicitis and torsion can present with acute pain and rebound, the gradual progression of appendicitis is quite different from the acute severe pain of torsion. Nausea and emesis often ensue immediately with torsion, owing to the severity of the pain. Appendicitis tends to present with anorexia, which gradually worsens. The young girl with acute onset of pain and simultaneous emesis likely has ovarian torsion rather than appendicitis.

Approximately a third of ovarian torsion cases in children and adolescents are not associated with a predisposing ovarian mass such as a dermoid, large functional cyst, or malignancy. Nevertheless, even in children without an ovarian mass, after torsion the ovary will become swollen and enlarged as the lymphatic flow is blocked. In children and adolescents the differentiation between torsion and appendicitis is a common dilemma. Radiologic evaluation to rule out appendicitis may reveal a pelvic mass, and the appropriate diagnosis of torsion is defined. The presence of vascular flow in the ovary does not rule out torsion, and in fact many cases of surgically proven torsion will have had normal vascular flow on ultrasound evaluation.

KEY POINTS

- In the field of pediatric gynecology, most diagnostic errors result from errors of omission during the examination rather than errors of commission.
- It is important to give the child a sense that she will be in control of the examination process. Emphasize that the most important part of the examination is just "looking" and that there will be conversation during the entire process.
- Many gynecologic conditions in children can be diagnosed by inspection alone.
- The vaginal epithelium of the prepubertal child appears redder and thinner than the vaginal epithelium of a woman in her reproductive years. The prepubertal vagina is also narrower, thinner, and lacking in the distensibility of the vagina of a reproductively mature woman. The vagina of a child is 4 to 5 cm long and has a neutral pH.
- During the physical examination and rectal examination of the prepubertal child, no pelvic masses except the cervix should be palpable. The normal prepubertal uterus and ovaries are nonpalpable. The relative size ratio of cervix to uterus is 2 to 1 in a child.
- Many female adolescents do not want other observers in the examining room.
- It is estimated that 80% to 90% of outpatient visits of children to gynecologists involve the classic symptoms of vulvovaginitis: introital irritation and discharge.
- Positive identification of *Trichomonas* infection, gonorrhea, or chlamydia in a child with premenarcheal vulvovaginitis often indicates sexual molestation. However, many infants are infected with *Chlamydia trichomatis* during birth and remain infected for several years in the absence of specific antibiotic therapy.
- The major factor in childhood vulvovaginitis is poor perineal hygiene.
- A vaginal discharge that is both bloody and foul-smelling strongly suggests the presence of a foreign body.
- In the period from 6 to 12 months before menarche, children often develop a physiologic discharge secondary to the increase in circulating estrogen levels.
- The foundation of treating childhood vulvovaginitis is the improvement of local perineal hygiene.
- The vast majority of cases of persistent or recurrent nonspecific vulvovaginitis respond to improved hygiene and treatment of irritation due to trauma or irritating substances.
- The classic symptom of pinworms (*Enterobius vermicularis*) is nocturnal vulvar and perianal itching, the treatment for which is the antihelminthic agent mebendazole (Vermox).
- The most common vaginal foreign body in preadolescent females is a wad of toilet tissue.
- Persistent vaginal bleeding is an extremely rare symptom in a preadolescent female. However, it is important to do a thorough workup because of the serious sequelae of some of the causes of vaginal bleeding.
- Labial adhesions do not require treatment unless they are symptomatic or voiding is compromised. If necessary, small amounts of daily topical estrogen to the labia may be used for treatment.
- The usual cause of genital trauma during childhood is an accidental fall. The majority of such trauma involves straddle injuries.
- Accidental genital trauma often produces extreme pain and overwhelming anxiety for the child and her parents. Because of compassion and empathy, the gynecologist may underestimate the extent of the anatomic injuries. Thus, if in doubt, examine the child under general anesthesia.
- Small follicular cysts are common in preadolescent females and are usually self-limiting.
- Ovarian tumors constitute approximately 1% of all neoplasms in premenarcheal children. In preadolescent females, both benign and malignant ovarian tumors are usually unilateral. Biopsy of the contralateral ovary should be avoided. Possible exceptions to this rule are dysgerminomas and immature teratomas.
- Approximately 75% to 85% of ovarian neoplasms necessitating surgery are benign, with cystic teratomas being the most common.
- The most common malignancy in preadolescent females is a germ cell tumor.
- Even though ovarian neoplasia is rare in children, this diagnosis must be considered in a young girl with abdominal pain and a palpable mass. The surgical therapy should have two goals: removal of the neoplasm and preservation of future fertility.

BIBLIOGRAPHY

Recommended Reading

American College of Obstetricians and Gynecologists: Pediatric gynecologic disorders. ACOG Tech Bull 201:1, 1995.

Bacon JL: Prepubertal labial adhesions: Evaluation of a referral population. Am J Obstet Gynecol 187:327, 2002.

Guidelines for the evaluation of sexual abuse of children: Subject review. American Academy of Pediatrics Committee on child abuse and neglect. Pediatrics 103(1): 186, 1999.

Heger A, Tiscon L, Velasquez O, Bernier R: Children referred for possible sexual abuse: Medical findings in 2384 children. Child Abuse Negl 26:645, 2002.

Pokorny SF, Pokorny WJ, Kramer W: Acute genital injury in the prepubertal girl. Am J Obstet Gynecol 166:1461, 1992.

Valerie E, Gilchrist BF, Frischer J, et al: Diagnosis and treatment of ureteral prolapse in children. Urology 54:1082, 1999.

General References

Allen AL, Siegfried EC: The natural history of condyloma in children. J Am Acad Dermatol 39:951,1989.

Bagolan P, Girolandino C, Nahom A, et al: The management of fetal ovarian cysts. J Pediatr Surg 37:25, 2002.

Bell TA, Stamm WE, Wang S, et al: Chronic *Chlamydia trachomatis* infections in infants. JAMA 267:400, 1992.

Berenson AB, Heger AH, Hayes JM, et al: Appearance of the hymen in prepubertal girls. Pediatrics 89:387, 1992.

Blake J: Gynecologic examination of the teenager and young child. Obstet Gynecol Clin North Am 19:27, 1992.

Bonazzi C, Peccatori F, Colombo N, et al: Pure ovarian immature teratoma, a unique and curable disease: 10 years' experience of 32 prospectively treated patients. Obstet Gynecol 84:598, 1994.

Bond GR, Dowd MD, Landsman I, Rimsza M: Unintentional perineal injury in prepubescent girls: A multicenter, prospective report of 56 girls. Pediatrics 95:628, 1995.

Bridges NA, Cooke A, Healy MJR, et al: Standards for ovarian volume in childhood and puberty. Fertil Steril 60:456, 1993.

Brown MF, Hebra A, McGeehin K, Ross AJ III: Ovarian masses in children: A review of 91 cases of malignant and benign masses. J Pediatr Surg 28:930, 1993.

Bryant AR, Laufer MR: Fetal ovarian cysts. J Reprod Med 49:329, 2004.

Buchta RM: Use of chaperons during pelvic examinations of female adolescents. Am J Dis Child 141:666, 1987.

Capraro VJ: Pediatric gynecology. In Danforth DN (ed): Obstetrics and Gynecology, 4th ed. Philadelphia, Harper & Row, 1982.

Carpenter SE, Rock JA (eds): Pediatric and Adolescent Gynecology. New York, Raven, 1992.

Centers for Disease Control and Prevention: 2002 sexually transmitted diseases treatment guidelines. MMWR Recommend Rep 51(PR-6): 1, 2002.

Cohen HL, Eisenberg P, Mandel F, Haller JO: Ovarian cysts are common in premenarchal girls: A sonographic study of 101 children 2–12 years old. AJR 159:89, 1992.

Cronjé HS, Niemand I, Bam RH, Woodruff JD: Granulosa and theca cell tumors in children: A report of 17 cases and literature review. Obstet Gynecol Surv 53:240, 1998.

Cushing B, Giller R, Ablin A, et al: Surgical resection alone is effective treatment for ovarian immature teratoma in children and adolescents: A report of the Pediatric Oncology Group and the Children's Cancer Group. Am J Obstet Gynecol 181:353, 1999.

Dowd MD, Fitzmaurice L, Knapp J: The interpretation of urogenital findings in children with straddle injuries. J Pediatric Surg 29:7, 1994.

Ehren IM, Mahour GH, Isaacs H: Benign and malignant ovarian tumors in children and adolescents. Am J Surg 147:339, 1984.

Emans SJ, Goldstein DP: The gynecologic examination of the prepubertal child with vulvovaginitis: Use of the knee-chest position. Pediatrics 65:758, 1980.

Emans SJH, Laufter MR, Goldstein DP: Pediatric and Adolescent Gynecology, 4th ed. Philadelphia, Lippincott-Raven, 1998.

Emans SJ, Woods ER, Allred EN, Grace E: Hymenal findings in adolescent women: Impact of tampon use and consensual sexual activity. J Pediatr 125:153, 1994.

Farrington PF: Pediatric Vulvo-vaginitis. Clin Obstet Gynecol 40:135, 1997.

Freud E, Golinsky D, Steinberg RM, et al: Ovarian masses in children. Clin Pediatr 38:573, 1999.

Goff CW, Burke KR, Rickenback C, Buebendorf DP: Vaginal opening measurement in prepubertal girls. Am J Dis Child 143:1366, 1989.

Hairston L: Physical examination of the prepubertal girl. Clin Obstet Gynecol 40:127, 1997.

Hammerschlag MR: Sexually transmitted diseases in sexually abused children: Medical and legal implications. Sex Trans Inf 74:167, 1998.

Handley J, Dinsmore W, Maw R, et al: Anogenital warts in prepubertal children: Sexual abuse or not? Int J STD AIDS 4:271, 1993.

Huffman JW: The Gynecology of Childhood and Adolescence, 2nd ed. Philadelphia, WB Saunders, 1981.

Humel KP, Jenny C: Child sexual abuse. Pediatr Rev 17:236, 1996.

Jabra AA, Fishman EK, Taylor GA: Primary ovarian tumors in the pediatric patient: CT evaluation. Clin Imaging 17:199, 1993.

Jenkinson SD, Mackinnon AE: Spontaneous separation of fused labia minora in prepubertal girls. Br Med J 289:160, 1984.

Kao SCS, Cook JS, Hansen JR, Simonson TM: MR imaging of the pituitary gland in central precocious puberty. Pediatr Radiol 22:481, 1992.

King LR, Siegel MJ, Solomon AL: Usefulness of ovarian volume and cysts in female isosexual precocious puberty. J Ultrasound Med 12:577, 1993.

Klein VR, Willman SP, Carr BR: Familial posterior labial fusion. Obstet Gynecol 73:500, 1989.

Leung AKC, Robson WLM: Labial fusion and asymptomatic bacteriuria. Eur J Pediatr 152:250, 1993.

Leung AKC, Robson WLM, Tay-Uyboco J: The incidence of labial fusion in children. J Paediatr Child Health 29:235, 1993.

Liapi C, Evain-Brion D: Diagnosis of ovarian follicular cysts from birth to puberty: A report of twenty cases. Acta Paediatr Scand 76:91, 1987.

McCann J, Voris J, Simon M: Labial adhesions and posterior fourchette injuries in childhood sexual abuse. Am J Dis Child 142:659, 1988.

McCann J, Voris J, Simon M, Wells R: Comparison of genital examination techniques in prepubertal girls. Pediatrics 85:182, 1990.

McCrea RS: Uterine adnexal torsion with subsequent contralateral recurrence. J Reprod Med 25:123, 1980.

Meffert JJ, Davis BM, Grimwood RE: Lichen sclerosus. J Am Acad Derm 32:393, 1995.

Millar DM, Blake JM, Stringer DA, et al: Prepubertal ovarian cyst formation: 5 years' experience. Obstet Gynecol 81:434, 1993.

Muram D: Child sexual abuse—genital tract findings in prepubertal girls. I. The unaided medical examination. Am J Obstet Gynecol 160:328, 1989.

Muram D, Elias S: Child sexual abuse-genital tract findings in prepubertal girls. II. Comparison of colposcopic and unaided examinations. Am J Obstet Gynecol 160:333, 1989.

Muram D, Laufer MR: Limitations of the medical evaluation for child sexual abuse. J Reprod Med 44:993, 1999.

Mylonas L, Hansch S, Markmann S, et al: Unilateral ovarian agenesis: Report of three cases and review of the literature. Arch Gynecol Obstet 268:57-60, 2003.

Pacheco BP, Di Paola G, Ribas JMM, et al: Vulvar infection caused by human papilloma virus in children and adolescents without sexual contact. Adolesc Pediatr Gynecol 4:136, 1991.

Pokorny SF: Prepubertal vulvovaginopathies. Obstet Gynecol Clin North Am 19:39, 1992.

Pokorny SF: Long-term intravaginal presence of foreign bodies in children: a preliminary study. J Reprod Med 39:931, 1994.

Pokorny SF: Genital trauma. Clin Obstet Gynecol 40:219, 1997.

Robinson AJ: Sexually transmitted organism in children and child sexual abuse. Int J STD AIDS 9:501, 1998.

Sanfilippo JS (ed): Pediatric and Adolescent Gynecology. Philadelphia, WB Saunders, 1994.

Sankila R, Olsen JH, Anderson H, et al: Risk of cancer among offspring of childhood-cancer survivors. N Engl J Med 338:1339, 1998.

Shawis RN, El Gohary AE, Cook RCM: Ovarian cysts and tumors in infancy and childhood. Ann R Coll Surg Engl 67:17, 1985.

Siegel MJ: Pediatric gynecologic sonography. Radiology 179:593, 1991.

Siegel MJ, Carel C, Surratt S: Ultrasonography of acute abdominal pain in children. JAMA 266:1987, 1991.

Siegel MJ, Surratt JT: Pediatric gynecologic imaging. Obstet Gynecol Clin North Am 19:103, 1992.

Siegel RM, Schuber CJ, Myers PA, Shapiro RA: The prevalence of sexually transmitted diseases in children and adolescents evaluated for sexual abuse in Cincinnati: Rationale for limited STD testing in prepubertal girls. Pediatrics 1995; 96:1090.74:239.

Smith YR, Quint EH. Clobetasol proprionate in the treatment of premenarchal vulvar lichen sclerosus. Ob Gyn 98:588, 2001.

Stricker T, Navratil F, Sennhauser FH: Vulvovaginitis in prepubertal girls. Arch Dis Child 88:324, 2003.

Tanger J, Zelterman D, Ma W, Schwartz PE: Reproductive function after conservative surgery and chemotherapy for malignant germ cell tumors of the ovary. Obstet Gynecol 101:251, 2003.

Thorp JM, Wells SR, Droegemueller W: Ovarian suspension in massive ovarian edema. Obstet Gynecol 76:912, 1990.

U.S. Department of Health and Human Services, Administration on Children, Youth and Families. Eleven years of reporting: Child maltreatment 2000. Washington, DC, U.S. Government Printing Office, 2002.

Van Winter JT, Simmons PS, Podratz KC: Surgically treated adnexal masses in infancy, childhood, and adolescence. Am J Obstet Gynecol 170:1780, 1994.

Zalel Y, Piura B, Elchalal U, et al: Diagnosis and management of malignant germ cell ovarian tumors in young females. Int J Gynaecol Obstet 55:1, 1996.

Zanger G, Bonazzi C, Cantu M, et al. Survival and reproductive function after treatment of malignant germ cell ovarian tumors. J Clin Oncol 19:1015, 2001.

Zitsman JL, Cirincione E, Margossian H: Vaginal bleeding in an infant secondary to sliding inguinal hernia. Obstet Gynecol 89:840, 1997.

Family Planning 14

Contraception, Sterilization, and Pregnancy Termination

Daniel R. Mishell, Jr.

KEY TERMS AND DEFINITIONS

Contraception. The prevention of pregnancy.

Contraceptive Failure Rate. Pregnancy rates with various types of contraceptives at different intervals, usually years. This rate is frequently expressed as number of pregnancies per 100 women at 1 year or per 100 woman-years.

Contraceptive Patch. An adhesive matrix 20 cm^2 patch containing ethinyl estradiol and norelgestromin that is placed transdermally by the user. The steroids are delivered into the circulation for 1 week.

Contraceptive Ring. A flexible soft transparent ring-shaped device containing etonogestrel and ethinyl estradiol that is placed in the vagina. The steroids are delivered into the circulation at a constant rate for 3 weeks.

Emergency Contraception. Administration of steroids or insertion of a copper IUD within 3 to 7 days after a single episode of unprotected, midcycle sexual intercourse.

Induced Abortion. Intentional medical or surgical termination of pregnancy before 20 weeks' gestation. Also called elective pregnancy termination if performed for the woman's desires or therapeutic abortion if performed for reasons of maintaining the mother's health.

Intrauterine Device (IUD). A small device, usually made of plastic with or without copper or a progestin, placed into the endometrial cavity to provide an effective method of contraception. Also called intrauterine contraceptives (IUC) or intrauterine systems (IUS).

IUD Event Rates. Incidence of adverse events, such as expulsion, removal for medical reasons, and pregnancy, at various times after insertion of an IUD.

Implant. An ethylene vinyl acetate rod containing etonogestrel that is placed in the subcutaneous tissue of the upper arm and provides excellent contraceptive effectiveness for 3 years.

Life Table Method. An actuarial technique for determining rates of occurrence of events, such as pregnancy and discontinuation, at various intervals after starting any type of contraceptive.

Perfect Use Effectiveness. The rate of effectiveness when the contraceptive method is always used correctly. Previously called *method use.*

Natural Family Planning. Periodic abstinence from intercourse during the periovulatory time of the cycle. Also known as *rhythm.*

Microinsert. A device that is inserted transcervically through a hysteroscope into the proximal portion of the oviduct to provide permanent tubal occlusion.

Oral Contraceptive Steroids (OCs). Formulations of various synthetic progestins usually combined with a synthetic estrogen that are ingested orally to prevent conception. When the progestin is combined with an estrogen the formulation is called a combination oral contraceptive (COC). Oral progestin tablets without estrogen are called minipills.

Pearl Index. A nonactuarial method used for determining the pregnancy (failure) rate of any contraceptive technique:

$$\text{Pregnancy rate} = \frac{\text{No. of pregnancies} \times 1200}{\text{Woman-months of use}}$$

Progestin. A class of sex steroids having progestational activity. The terms *progestogen* and *gestagen* are synonymous.

Spermicide. A local contraceptive containing the surfactant nonoxynol 9, which is toxic to sperm.

Sterilization. Prevention of pregnancy by vasectomy or tubal interruption or blockage. This method of contraception should be considered permanent.

Typical Use Effectiveness. Overall effectiveness rate in actual use for a specific contraceptive method. Previously called *use effectiveness.*

Reversible contraception is defined as the temporary prevention of fertility and includes all the currently available contraceptive methods except sterilization. Sterilization should be considered a permanent prevention of fertility even though both vasectomy and tubal interruption can usually be reversed by a meticulous surgical procedure. The reversible methods are also called *active methods,* and sterilization is also called a *terminal method.* A perfect method of contraception for all individuals is not currently available and probably will never be developed. Each of the various methods of contraception currently available has certain advantages and disadvantages. Therefore, when giving advice about contraception, the clinician should explain to the couple the advantages and disadvantages of each method, so they will be fully informed and can rationally choose the method most suitable for them. Because no reversible contraceptive method other than the condom has yet been developed for use by the male, the contraceptive provider generally counsels the female partner and should inform her if there are medical reasons that contraindicate the use of certain methods and offer her alternatives.

CONTRACEPTIVE USE IN THE UNITED STATES

In 2001, there were about 6.4 million pregnancies in the United States. About two thirds of these pregnancies, 4.0 million, resulted in births of children, and about one fifth, 1.3 million, were terminated by elective abortion. The remainder ended in spontaneous abortion or ectopic pregnancy. According to Finer and Henshaw's review of the 2002 National Survey of Family Growth, about half of the 6.4 million pregnancies in that year were unintended and 42% of these unintended pregnancies were terminated by elective abortion. The remainder were frequently associated with unwanted children. According to the survey, about 48% of the women who had unintended pregnancies were using a method of contraception in the cycle in which they conceived. Unintended pregnancies are most likely to occur among young, unmarried, black and Latina women and women with low income. According to an analysis of the 2002 National Survey of Family Growth, the latest survey to be analyzed, of the 61.5 million women of reproductive age in the United States in 2002, 38 million, 62% were using a method of contraception. Among the group using no method of contraception, about 3% had a prior hysterectomy and 9% were pregnant or trying to conceive. About 18% either were not sexually active or were having infrequent episodes of coitus. A total of 7.4% of women of reproductive age were sexually active and not using a method of contraception. Of the reproductive-age women, nearly 23% used sterilization as their contraceptive method: 16.7% by female methods and 5.7% by vasectomy (Table 14-1). Almost 19% used oral contraceptives, and the partners of 11% used the male condom. The progestin injection was used by 3%, the diaphragm by 0.2%, periodic abstinence by 1%, withdrawal by 2.5%, and the IUD by about 1%. Thus, of women using contraception, about 70% used very effective methods, including sterilization, oral contraceptives, injection, and IUD, and 30% used less-effective methods.

CONTRACEPTIVE EFFECTIVENESS

It is difficult to determine the actual effectiveness of a contraceptive method because of the many factors that affect contraceptive failure. The terms *method effectiveness* and *use effectiveness* (or *method failure* and *patient failure*) were previously used to describe conception occurring while the contraceptive method

Table 14–1 Number of Women 15–44 Years of Age and Percent Distribution (with Standard Error) by Current Contraceptive Status and Method: United States, 1982, 1995, and 2002

	YEAR OF SURVEY		
Contraceptive Status and Method	**1982**	**1995**	**2002**
	NUMBER IN THOUSANDS		
All Women	54,099	60,201	61,561
	PERCENT DISTRIBUTION (WITH STANDARD ERROR)		
Total	100.0	100.0	100.0
Using Contraception (Contraceptors)	55.7 (1.0)	64.2 (0.6)	61.9 (0.8)
Female sterilization	12.9 (0.6)	17.8 (0.4)	16.7 (0.6)
Male sterilization	6.1 (0.4)	7.0 (0.3)	5.7 (0.4)
Pill	15.6 (0.8)	17.3 (0.4)	18.9 (0.7)
Implant, Lunelle, or Patch*	NA	0.9 (0.1)	0.8 (0.1)
3-month injectable (Depo-Provera)	NA	1.9 (0.1)	3.3 (0.3)
Intrauterine device (IUD)	4.0 (0.4)	0.5 (0.1)	1.3 (0.2)
Diaphragm	4.5 (0.4)	1.2 (0.1)	0.2 (0.1)
Condom	6.7 (0.6)	13.1 (0.4)	11.1 (0.5)
Periodic abstinence-calendar rhythm	1.8 (0.3)	1.3 (0.1)	0.7 (0.1)
Periodic abstinence-natural family planning	0.3 (0.3)	0.2 (0.1)	0.2 (0.1)
Withdrawal	1.1 (0.3)	2.0 (0.2)	2.5 (0.3)
Other methods†	2.7 (0.3)	1.1 (0.1)	0.6 (0.1)
Not Using Contraception	44.3 (1.0)	35.8 (0.6)	38.1 (0.8)
Surgically sterile—female (noncontraceptive)	6.3 (0.4)	3.0 (0.2)	1.5 (0.2)
Nonsurgically sterile—female or male	1.2 (0.3)	1.7 (0.2)	1.6 (0.2)
Pregnant or postpartum	5.0 (0.3)	4.6 (0.3)	5.3 (0.4)
Seeking pregnancy	4.2 (0.4)	4.0 (0.2)	4.2 (0.3)
Other Nonuse			
Never had intercourse or no intercourse in 3 months before interview	19.5 (0.8)	17.1 (0.5)	18.1 (0.7)
Had intercourse in 3 months before interview	7.4 (0.4)	5.2 (0.2)	7.4 (0.4)
All other nonuse‡	0.7 (0.3)	0.2 (0.0)	0.0 (0.0)

0.0 = Quantity greater than zero but less than 0.05.
NA—Data not available (method not available in the United States in that year).
*1995 percentage only includes Norplant implant.
†Includes Today sponge, cervical cap, female condom, and other methods.
‡Includes male sterility of unknown origin and other small groups, not shown separately.
NOTE: Percents may not add to 100 because of rounding.

was being used correctly or incorrectly. These terms have now been replaced by the terms *typical use* and *perfect use.* In general, methods used at the time of coitus, such as the diaphragm, condom, spermicides, and withdrawal, have much greater perfect use effectiveness than typical use effectiveness. There is less difference between perfect and typical use effectiveness among methods not related to the time of coitus, such as OCs, contraceptive patches, vaginal rings, implants, injections, and intrauterine devices. Because less motivation is required with these latter methods than with coitus-related methods, the noncoitus-related methods have greater typical use effectiveness than coitus-related methods. Women should be counseled that these four methods are the most effective reversible methods of contraception currently available. Women should always be informed about perfect use failure rates so that they know the percentage of contraceptive failure that will occur when each method is used correctly and consistently.

The overall value of the various contraceptive methods as used by a couple (correctly or incorrectly) over a specific period, sometimes called *extended use effectiveness,* is determined by calculating the actual effectiveness and the continuation rate. Actuarial methods should be used to determine the various contraceptive failure rates.

Even with use of these excellent statistical techniques, it is difficult to determine the effectiveness of a contraceptive method in actual practice. Most studies undertaken for this purpose are performed in carefully controlled clinical trials. During these studies, frequent contact with supportive clinic personnel results in lower failure rates and higher continuation rates than occur in general use. Furthermore, these clinical trials are infrequently performed in a comparative randomized manner. Therefore, clinicians cannot accurately compare results of a trial of one type of contraceptive method with those of another.

Several other factors also influence contraceptive failure rates. One of the most important is motivation. Contraceptive failure is more likely to occur in couples seeking to delay a wanted birth compared with those seeking to prevent any more births, especially for coitus-related methods. The woman's age has a strong negative correlation with failure of a contraceptive method, as does socioeconomic status and level of education. Failure rates for most methods usually are lower among populations of married rather than unmarried women. Failure rates reported in prospective studies are also consistently lower than those of retrospective interview studies because of recall bias. Finally, for all methods, failure rates are greater during the first year of use than in subsequent years, yet most studies report only first-year-use failure rates. Thus, many variables must be considered when evaluating the effectiveness of any method of contraception for an individual woman.

Trussell and coworkers calculated percentage failure rates with the first year of use for the various methods of contraceptives available in the United States (Table 14-2). The percentage of actual use failure rates for durations more than 1 year are available for certain methods of long-acting contraceptives. The failure rate for 5 years of use of the levonorgestrel intrauterine system in clinical trials is 1.1%. The cumulative failure rate of the copper T380 IUD was 1.0, 1.4, and 1.6 per 100 women after 3, 5, and 7 years of use, respectively, in a large World Health Organization (WHO) study and only rises to 1.7 per 100 women after 12 years of use.

The failure rate of all types of tubal sterilization is 1.31 after 5 years and 1.85 per 100 women after 10 years, being highest for tubal fulguration and lowest for segmental resection in the 10 years following the procedure. Clinicians counseling women about long-term failure rates should inform them about the increased incidence of ectopic pregnancies that occur when conception occurs using progestin-only methods, the IUD, and female sterilization.

Ectopic pregnancy rates for women conceiving while using these methods range from about 30% with tubal sterilization failure to 25% with implant failure and 5% with copper IUD failure.

CONTRACEPTIVE COST

In addition to preventing unwanted pregnancy, all contraceptive methods reduce health care costs. Trussell and colleagues developed an economic model to compare the effectiveness and costs per person of 15 methods of contraceptives, including both permanent and reversible methods. To determine effectiveness the model calculated the number of pregnancies avoided with typical use of each method of contraception compared with the number of pregnancies expected to occur if no contraceptive method was used by the woman. To determine the cost of each contraceptive, the direct medical costs of the method itself, costs due to mistimed pregnancies, as well as costs incurred or avoided by adverse and beneficial side effects of the contraceptive method, were calculated. The costs of unintended pregnancies because of method failure included the costs of term deliveries as well as spontaneous and induced abortion and ectopic pregnancies. Because the costs of unintended pregnancy when no method of contraception is used are substantial, use of all 15 contraceptives was less costly than use of no method. Costs were calculated for contraceptive use for 1 and 5 years' duration. Although male and female sterilization had high initial costs, they became very cost effective over time for couples who did not want more children. However, these data were calculated before the nearly 2% 10-year failure rate of tubal ligation reported by Peterson and associates was published. The most cost-effective method for 5 years of use were the copper T IUD, vasectomy, the progestin implant, and progestin injection (Fig. 14-1). Use of each of these methods for 5 years saved about $14,000 per person and prevented about 4.1 pregnancies per person. Barrier methods and periodic abstinence saved between $9000 and $12,000 over 5 years, and oral contraceptives prevented 4.1 pregnancies and saved nearly $13,000 per year. This study indicated that initial acquisition costs do not predict the economic value of various contraceptives and that the most effective contraception methods provided the greatest cost savings.

SPERMICIDES: FOAMS, CREAMS, AND SUPPOSITORIES

Spermicides consist of an active agent and a carrier. The carriers include gels, foams, creams, tablets, films, and suppositories. The active agent is a surfactant, usually nonoxynol 9, that immobilizes or kills sperm on contact by destroying the sperm cell

Table 14–2 Percentage of women experiencing an unintended pregnancy during the first year of typical use and the first year of perfect use of contraception and the percentage continuing use at the end of the first year, in the United States

	PERCENTAGE OF WOMEN EXPERIENCING AN UNINTENDED PREGNANCY WITHIN THE FIRST YEAR OF USE		
Method (1)	**Typical Use* (2)**	**Perfect Use† (3)**	**Percentage of Women Continuing Use at 1 Year‡ (4)**
No method§	85	85	42
Spermicides‖	29	18	43
Withdrawal	27	4	51
Periodic abstinence	25		
Calendar		9	
Ovulation method		3	
Symptothermal¶		2	
Postovulation		1	
Cap**			
Parous women	32	26	46
Nulliparous women	16	9	57
Sponge			
Parous women	32	20	46
Nulliparous women	16	9	57
Diaphragm**	16	6	57
Condom††			
Female (Reality)	21	5	49
Male	15	2	53
Combined pill and minipill	8	0.3	68
Ortho-Evra patch	8	0.3	68
NuvaRing	8	0.3	68
Depo-Provera	3	0.3	56
Lunelle	3	0.05	56
IUD			
ParaGard (copper T)	0.8	0.6	78
Mirena (levonorgesterel containing intrauterine system)	0.1	0.1	81
Norplant and Norplant-2	0.05	0.05	84
Female sterilization	0.5	0.5	100
Male sterilization	0.15	0.10	100

Emergency contraceptive pills: Treatment initiated within 72 hr after unprotected intercourse reduces risk of pregnancy by at least 75%.‡‡
Lactational amenorrhea method: A highly effective, *temporary* method of contraception.§§

*Among *typical* couples who initiate use of a method (not necessarily for the first time), the percentage who experience an accidental pregnancy during the first year if they do not stop use for any other reason. Estimates of the probability or pregnancy during the first year of typical use of spermicides, withdrawal, periodic abstinence, the diaphragm, the male condom, the pill and Depo-Provera are taken from the 1995 NFSG corrected for underreporting of abortion; see text for the derivation of estimates for the other methods.
†Among couples who initiate use of a method (not necessarily for the first time) and who use it *perfectly* (both consistently and correctly), the percentage who experience an accidental pregnancy during the first year if they do not stop use for any other reason. See text for the derivation of estimate for each method.
‡Among couples attempting to avoid pregnancy, the percentage who continue to use a method for 1 year.
§The percentages becoming pregnant in columns (2) and (3) are based on data from populations where contraception is not used and from women who cease using contraception in order to become pregnant. Among such populations, about 89% become pregnant within 1 year. This estimate was lowered slightly (to 85%) to represent the percentage who would become pregnant within 1 year among women now relying on reversible methods of contraception if they abandoned contraception altogether.
‖Foams, creams, gels, vaginal suppositories and vaginal film.
¶Cervical mucus (ovulation) method supplemented by calendar in the preovulatory and basal body temperature in the postovulatory phases.
**With spermicidal cream or jelly.
††Without spermicides.
‡‡The treatment schedule is one dose within 120 h after unprotected intercourse, and a second dose 12 h after the first dose. Both doses of Plan B can be taken at the same time. Plan B (1 dose is 1 white pill) is the only dedicated product specifically marketed for emergency contraception. The US Food and Drug Administration has in addition declared the following 18 brands of oral contraceptives to be safe and effective for emergency contraception: Ogestrel or Ovral (1 dose is 2 white pills), Alesse, Lessina, or Levlite, (1 dose is 5 pink pills), Levlen or Nordette (1 dose is 4 light-orange pills), Cryselle, Levora, Low-Ogestrel, or Lo/Ovral (1 dose is 4 white pills), Tri-Levlen or Triphasil (1 dose is 4 yellow pills), Portia, Seasonale, or Trivora (1 dose is 4 pink pills), Aviane (one dose is 5 orange pills), and Empresse (one dose is 4 orange pills).
§§However, to maintain effective protection against pregnancy, another method of contraception must be used as soon as menstruation resumes, the frequency or duration of breastfeeds is reduced, bottle feeds are introduced or the baby reaches 6 months of age.
From Trussell J: Contraceptive efficacy. In Hatcher RA, Trussell J, Stewart F, et al (eds): Contraceptive Technology, 18th rev ed. New York, Ardent Media, 2004.

membrane. Spermicides also provide a mechanical barrier and need to be placed into the vagina before each coital act. The pregnancy rate with use of these agents in the first year ranges from 18% with perfect use to 29% with typical use. Most spermicides are used in combination with a barrier contraceptive to increase effectiveness.

The contraceptive sponge, a cylindrical piece of soft polyurethane impregnated with 1 mg of nonoxynol 9, does not have to be inserted into the vagina before each act of intercourse and is effective for 24 hours. The pregnancy rate in the first year with this spermicide in nulliparous women ranges from 9% with perfect use to 16% with typical use and is higher in parous women.

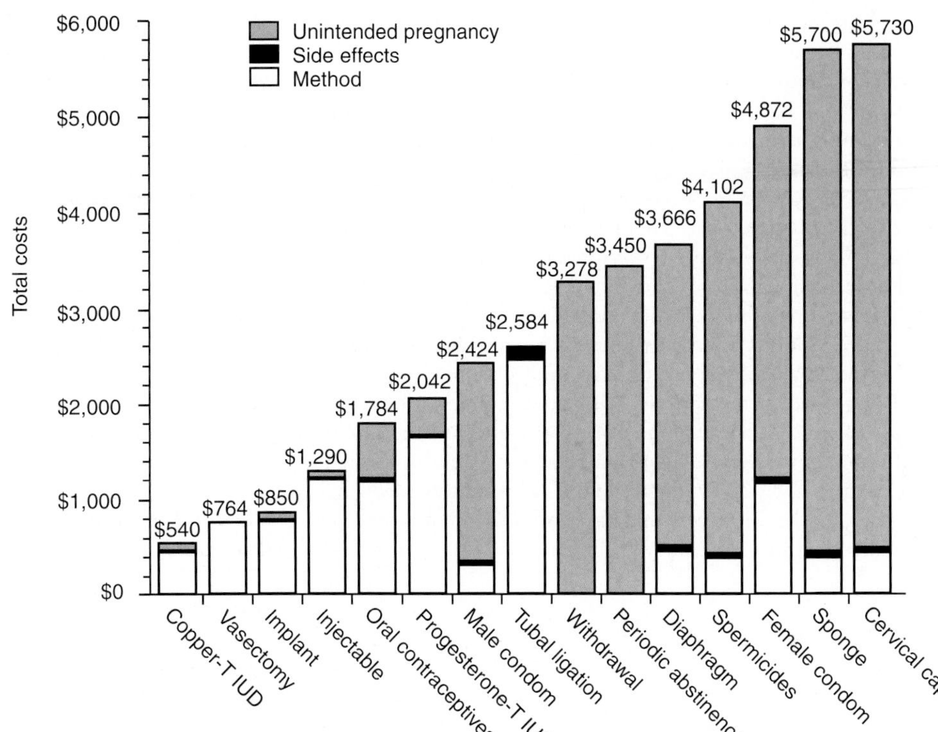

Figure 14-1. Five-year costs associated with contraceptive methods in the managed payment model. (From Trussell J, Leveque JA, Koenig JD, et al: The economic value of contraception: A comparison of 15 methods. Am J Public Health 85:494, 1995.)

Although a few early studies linked the use of a spermicide at the time of conception with an increased risk of some congenital malformations, these studies were probably flawed by recall bias. Several well-performed studies have shown no increased risk of congenital malformation in the newborns or karyotypic abnormalities in the spontaneous abortuses of women who conceived while using spermicides.

BARRIER TECHNIQUES

Diaphragm

A diaphragm must be carefully fitted by the health care provider. The largest size that does not cause discomfort or undue pressure on the vaginal mucosa should be used. After the fitting, the woman should remove the diaphragm and reinsert it herself. She should then be examined to make sure the diaphragm is covering the cervix. The diaphragm should be used with a spermicide and be left in place for at least 8 hours after the last coital act. If repeated intercourse takes place or coitus occurs more than 8 hours after insertion of the diaphragm, additional spermicide should be used. Although advisable, it may not be necessary to use a spermicide with the diaphragm, since it has not been conclusively demonstrated that pregnancy rates are lower when a spermicide is used with a diaphragm than when the diaphragm is used alone. The number of urinary tract infections in women who use diaphragms is significantly higher than in nonusers, probably because of the mechanical obstruction of the outflow of urine by the diaphragm. Diaphragm users should also be cautioned not to leave the device in place for more than 24 hours, as ulceration of the vaginal epithelium may occur with prolonged usage. One report, however, indicated that among a group of women who left the diaphragm in place without using spermicide, removing it only once daily to wash it before immediately reinserting it, as well as removing it during menses, the 12-month failure rate was only 2.8%. This rate was lower than the failure rate of 9.8% among a group of women who inserted the diaphragm with a spermicide in the usual manner only when having sexual intercourse and then leaving it in for 8 hours thereafter.

Data from the Oxford/Family Planning Association Contraceptive Study indicate that the diaphragm is an effective method of contraception in married, motivated women and that failure rates decline with increasing age and increasing duration of use. Analyses of data from two large clinical trials comparing use of the diaphragm with that of the cervical cap or sponge indicate that the failure rate during the first year of use for the diaphragm ranged from 12.5% to 17.1% among all users and was reduced to 4.3% to 5.3% with perfect use.

Cervical Cap

The cervical cap, a cup-shaped plastic or rubber device that fits around the cervix, has been used as a barrier contraceptive for decades, mainly in Britain and other parts of Europe.

There has been a recent resurgence of interest in the use of this older method, since the cervical cap can be left in place longer than the diaphragm and is more comfortable. The various types of caps are manufactured in different sizes and should be fitted to the cervix by a clinician. The cervical cap should not be left in place for more than 48 hours because of the possibility of ulceration, unpleasant odor, and infection.

One cervical cap is marketed in the United States. The cap should be left on the cervix for no more than 48 hours, and a spermicide should always be placed inside the cap before use. The marketed cap is manufactured in three sizes and requires more training than the diaphragm, both for the provider to fit it and for the user to place it correctly.

Failure rates with the cervical cap are similar to those observed with the diaphragm. In a large, randomized clinical trial of the cap and diaphragm, 1-year pregnancy rates were 17.4% for the cap and 16.7% for the diaphragm. Of the pregnancies with the cap, one third were method failures and two thirds were user-related failures. In other studies, pregnancy rates at 1 and 2 years with the use of the cervical cap ranged from 8% to 17% and 14% to 38%, respectively, with good continuation rates. Because of concern about a possible adverse effect of the cap on cervical tissue, the cervical cap should be used only by women with normal cervical cytology, and it is recommended that users have another cervical cytologic examination 3 months after starting to use this method.

Male Condom

Male condoms are made of three materials: latex, polyurethane, and animal tissue. Use of the latex male condom by individuals with multiple sex partners should be encouraged. The latex male condom is the most effective method of contraception to prevent transmission of sexually transmitted infections. Condoms made of animal tissue such as lamb cecum do not prevent transmission of sexually transmitted infections, but condoms made of polyurethane should prevent transmission of these organisms. The latex male condom should not be applied tightly. The tip should extend beyond the end of the penis by about half an inch to collect the ejaculate. Care must be taken upon withdrawal not to spill the ejaculate. When used by strongly motivated couples, the male condom is highly effective.

Barrier techniques are effective methods of contraception in women 30 years of age or older. In a U.S. study, the first-year failure rates for male condom use among women wishing no more pregnancies ranged between 3% and 6% when the woman was older than 30 but between 8% and 10% when the woman was younger than 25.

Female Condom

A female condom was approved for marketing in the United States in 1994. It consists of a soft, loose-fitting sheath and two flexible polyurethane rings. One ring lies inside the vagina at the closed end of the sheath and serves as an insertion mechanism and internal anchor. The outer ring forms the external edge of the device and remains outside the vagina after insertion, thus providing protection to the labia and the base of the penis during intercourse. The condom is prelubricated and is intended for one-time use only. Fitting by a health professional is not required.

Compared with the male condom, the female condom has the advantage of being able to be inserted prior to beginning sexual activity and to be left in place for a longer time after ejaculation has occurred. Because the female condom also covers the external genitalia, it should offer greater protection against the transfer of certain sexually transmitted organisms, particularly genital herpes. Because polyurethane is stronger than the latex used in male condoms, the female condom is less likely to rupture. In a multicenter clinical trial the cumulative pregnancy rates in U.S. centers at 6 months was 12.4%. The 6-month pregnancy rate with perfect use was 2.6%, indicating that the probable 1-year pregnancy rate with perfect use would be slightly more than 5%. The typical use failure rate at 1 year is estimated to be 21%. At the end of 6 months in the U.S. study about one third of the women had discontinued use of this method.

No data exist in which the effectiveness of the female condom for reducing sexual disease transmission is analyzed. Because polyurethane does not allow virus transmission it should reduce the risk of a woman acquiring HIV infection.

Barrier Techniques and Sexually Transmitted Infections

Barrier methods have the advantage of reducing the rate of transmission of sexually transmitted infections. Several studies have shown that spermicides reduce the frequency of clinical infection with sexually transmitted infections, both bacterial and viral. Several in vitro studies have demonstrated that latex condoms prevent the transmission of viruses, specifically the herpesvirus and the human immunodeficiency virus (HIV), as well as *Chlamydia trachomatis* bacteria, which is a frequent cause of salpingitis. Serial epidemiologic studies, both case-control and cohort, indicate that the use of the condom or diaphragm protects both men and women from clinically apparent gonorrheal infection.

An epidemiologic study of women with infertility caused by tubal obstruction found that the past use of barrier techniques protected women against tubal damage. The greatest protection occurred with the use of diaphragms or condoms in conjunction with spermicides. The incidence of cervical neoplasia was also markedly diminished among the female members of couples using condoms or diaphragms, probably because of the decreased transmission of human papillomavirus (HPV). This antiviral action may be the reason that women who use spermicides are only one third as likely to have cervical cancer as are members of a control group. Certain strains of this virus have been causally linked to the later development of cervical neoplasia. Unfortunately, the pregnancy failure rates of diaphragm or condom users are highest for persons younger than 25 years, those most likely to become infected with sexually transmitted diseases. Therefore, to prevent the transmission of these diseases as well as prevent unwanted pregnancy in this age group, the use of a barrier technique, together with one of the four most effective reversible methods of contraception, is advisable.

PERIODIC ABSTINENCE

The avoidance of sexual intercourse during the days of the menstrual cycle when the ovum can be fertilized is used by many highly motivated couples as a means of preventing pregnancy. Wilcox and colleagues reported that conception can only occur if coitus takes place during the 5 days preceding ovulation or the day of ovulation. Thus, if couples would only avoid coitus on these 6 days each month, conception would not occur. Because a woman cannot precisely determine when she will ovulate, four techniques of periodic abstinence have been utilized. The oldest of these is the calendar rhythm method. With this method, the period of abstinence is determined solely by calculating the length of the individual woman's previous menstrual cycle. The rationale for the rhythm method is based on three assumptions: (1) the human ovum is capable of being fertilized for only about 24 hours after ovulation, (2) spermatozoa retain their fertilizing ability for only about 48 hours after coitus, and (3) ovulation usually occurs 12 to 16 days (14 ± 2 days) before the onset of the subsequent menses. According to these assumptions, after the woman records the length of her cycles for several months, she establishes her fertile period by subtracting 18 days from the length of her previous shortest cycle and 11 days from her previous longest cycle. Then, in each subsequent cycle, the couple abstains from coitus during this calculated fertile period.

This method requires abstinence by the majority of women with regular menstrual cycles for nearly half the days of each cycle and cannot be used by women with irregular menstrual cycles. Although calendar rhythm is the most widely used technique of periodic abstinence, pregnancy rates are high, ranging from 14.4 to 47 per 100 woman-years, mainly because most couples fail to abstain for the relatively long periods required. The use of the calendar rhythm method by itself is currently not advocated or taught to couples who are interested in practicing periodic abstinence.

In the past two decades, new techniques have been developed whereby women rely on physiologic change during each cycle to determine the fertile period. The term *natural family planning* has been used instead of *rhythm* to describe these new techniques. They include the temperature method, the cervical mucus method, and the sympothermal method. Each of these techniques requires a great amount of motivation and training. In most reports of use of these methods pregnancy rates are relatively high and continuation rates are low.

The temperature method relies on measuring basal body temperature daily. The woman is required to abstain from intercourse from the onset of the menses until the third consecutive day of elevated basal temperature. Because abstinence is required for the entire preovulatory period in ovulatory cycles and for the entire cycle in anovulatory cycles, the temperature method alone is no longer commonly used.

The cervical mucus method requires that the woman be taught to recognize and interpret cyclic changes in the presence and consistency of cervical mucus; these changes occur in response to changing estrogen and progesterone levels. Abstinence is required during the menses and every other day after the menses ends, because of the possibility of confusing semen with ovulatory mucus, until the first day that copious, slippery mucus is observed to be present. Abstinence is required every day thereafter until 4 days after the last day when the characteristic mucus is present, called the "peak mucus day." In two well-designed, randomized clinical trials, the pregnancy rates for new users of this method in the first year after they completed a 3- to 5-month training period were 20% and 24%, with the discontinuation rates between 72% and 74%. In a five-country study of 725 highly motivated couples sponsored by the WHO, the typical use failure rate during the first year after the completion of three cycles of training was 19.6%, with a perfect use failure rate of 3.5%. Three fourths of these pregnancies resulted from conscious deviation from the rules of the method. The mean length of the fertile period in this study was 9.6 days, and abstinence was therefore required for about 17 days of each cycle. In this study the continuation rate after 1 year was high, 64.4%.

The sympothermal method, rather than relying on a single physiologic index, uses several indices to determine the fertile period—most commonly calendar calculations and changes in the cervical mucus to estimate the onset of the fertile period and changes in mucus or basal temperature to estimate its end. Because several indices need to be monitored, this method is more difficult to learn than the single-index methods, but it is more effective than the cervical mucus method alone. In two large, randomized studies comparing these methods, the pregnancy rates at the end of 1 year of use, after the training phase, were 10.9% and 19.8% with the symptothermal method, compared with 20% and 24% for the cervical mucus method. In addition, the continuation rate among the women who used the sympothermal method in these studies was higher after 1 year, about 50% in each study, than that among the women who used the cervical mucus method (26% and 40%).

The major reason for the lack of acceptance of natural family planning, as well as the relatively high pregnancy rates among users of these methods, is the need to avoid having sexual intercourse for a large number of days during each menstrual cycle. To overcome this problem, many women use barrier methods or spermicides during the fertile period. In a study of women who used the sympothermal method with barrier contraceptives or withdrawal during the fertile period, the failure rate during the first year was 9.9%, and the discontinuation rate was 33%.

Because the use of any method of contraception other than abstinence is unacceptable to some couples, simple, self-administered tests to detect hormonal changes have been developed to reduce the number of days of abstinence required in each cycle to a maximum of seven. Enzyme immunoassays for urinary estrogen and pregnandiol glucuronide have been developed. These assays can easily be used at home at minimal cost, and they require minimal time to perform. Such tests have to be performed by the woman for about 12 days each month, but they should reduce the number of days of abstinence required. It remains to be determined to what extent this aid to natural family planning will be used when it becomes generally available.

ORAL STEROID CONTRACEPTIVES

Oral steroid contraceptives (OCs) were initially marketed in the United States in 1960. Because of their extremely high rate of effectiveness and ease of administration, within a few years of their introduction they became the most widely used method of reversible contraception among both married and unmarried women. The major effect of the synthetic progestin component is to inhibit ovulation and produce other contraceptive actions such as thickening of the cervical mucus. The major effect of the synthetic estrogen is to maintain the endometrium and prevent unscheduled bleeding as well as inhibit follicular development. Most OC formulations contain a combination of a synthetic progestin and a synthetic estrogen in a single tablet. The initially marketed formulations of OCs contained 150 μg of the estrogen component, mestranol, and 9.85 mg of the progestin component, norethynodrel. With the high doses of steroids in the original formulations, minor side effects such as nausea, breast tenderness, and weight gain were common and frequently were of such magnitude as to cause discontinuation of use. During the past 46 years, many other formulations have been developed and marketed with steadily decreasing dosages of both the estrogen and progestin components. All the formulations initially marketed after 1975 contain less than 50 μg of ethinyl estradiol and 3 mg or less of several progestins. Use of these lower steroid dose formulations is associated with very low pregnancy rates, similar to those for formulations with higher doses of steroid, and a significantly lower incidence of severe adverse cardiovascular effects and minor adverse symptoms.

Because contraceptive steroid formulations with more than 50 μg of estrogen were associated with a greater incidence of adverse effects without greater efficacy, they are no longer marketed for contraceptive use in the United States, Canada, and Great Britain. Indications for prescribing formulations with 50 μg of estrogen are very uncommon.

Pharmacology

There are three major types of OC formulations: fixed-dose combination, combination phasic, and daily progestin. The combination formulations are the most widely used and are more effective than the daily progestin, also called the minipill. Fixed-dose products consist of tablets containing both an estrogen and progestin. In most formulations they are given continuously for 3 weeks. No steroids are given for the next 7 days, except for one formulation in which a low dose of estrogen is given for 5 additional days. After the steroid-free interval the active combination is given for an additional 3 weeks. Uterine bleeding usually occurs in the week when no steroid is ingested. Without estrogenic stimulation the endometrium usually begins to slough 1 to 3 days after stopping steroid ingestion. Withdrawal bleeding usually lasts 3 to 4 days, and uterine blood loss averages about 25 mL, less than the mean of about 35 mL that occurs during menses in a normal ovulatory cycle. Two recently introduced formulations provide active tablets for 24 days with 4 days inactive tablets. Another formulation provides active tablets for 84 days followed by 7 days without active tables to allow withdrawal bleeding.

The combination phasic formulations currently marketed contain two or three different amounts of the same estrogen and progestin. Each of the tablets containing one of these various dosages is given for intervals varying from 5 to 11 days during the 21-day medication period. These formulations have been described as biphasic or triphasic and are generally referred to as *multiphasic*. The rationale given for use of this type of formulation is that a lower total dose of steroid is administered without increasing the incidence of unscheduled uterine bleeding. However, there have been no published reports of comparative clinical trials in which multiphasic combinations have been shown to have significantly fewer adverse effects than fixed-dose combination formulations. The third type of contraceptive formulation, consisting of tablets containing a low does of progestin without any estrogen, are ingested once every day without a steroid-free interval.

All currently marketed formulations are made from synthetic steroids and contain no natural estrogens or progestins. There are two major types of synthetic progestins: derivatives of 19-nortestosterone and derivatives of 17α-acetoxyprogesterone. The latter group are C21 progestins, called *pregnanes,* and are structurally related to progesterone. Medroxyprogesterone acetate and megestrol acetate are C21 progestins marketed as tablets for noncontraceptive usage. In contrast to the 19-nortestosterone derivatives, when high dosages of the C21 progestins were given to female beagle dogs (an animal previously used for OC toxicology testing), the animals developed an increased incidence of mammary cancer. Because of this carcinogenic effect, oral contraceptives containing these progestins are no longer marketed despite the fact that the beagle, unlike the human, metabolizes C21 progestins to estrogen that then stimulates mammary nodules, which can become carcinogenic in this animal. An injectable contraceptive containing a C21 progestin, medroxyprogesterone acetate, is currently marketed in the United States and other countries.

The steroid structure of the 19-nortestosterone progestins more closely resembles testosterone than the C21 acetoxy progestins. Therefore, all progestational agents, except one, currently used in OCs have some degree of androgenic activity. The exception is a progestin called drosperinone, which is structurally related to spironolactone (Fig. 14-2). This progestin has antimineralcorticoid and antiandrogenic activity as well as progestational activity without androgenic activity. The 19-nortestosterone progestins used in OCs are of two major types: *estranes* and *gonanes.* Although the original estrane norethynodrel is no longer used in currently marketed OCs, other estranes, norethindrone and its derivatives with one or two acetates, norethindrone acetate and ethynodiol diacetate, are used in several marketed formulations (Fig. 14-3). Gonanes have greater progestational activity per unit weight than do estranes, and thus a smaller amount of the gonane type of progestin is used in OC formulations (Fig. 14-4). The parent compound of the gonanes is *dl*-norgestrel, which consists of both the dextro and levo isomers. Only the levo form is biologically active. Both *dl*-norgestrel and its active isomer levonorgestrel are present in several OC formulations. Three less androgenic derivatives of levonorgestrel, namely desogestrel, norgestimate, and gestodene, have also been synthesized. Formulations with each of these latter three progestins have been marketed in Europe for many

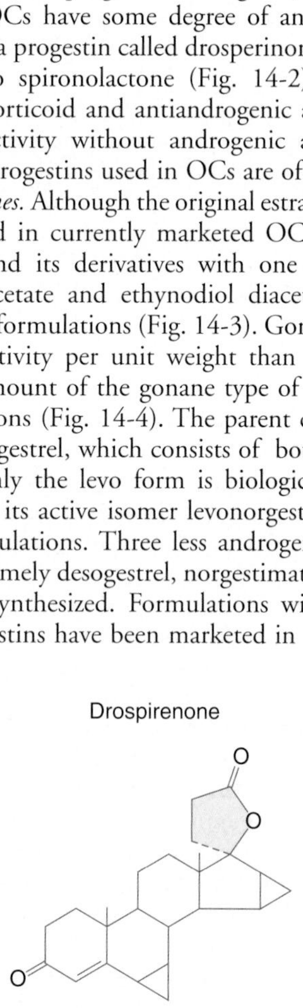

Drospirenone

O

O

O

Figure 14-2. Structural formulation of drosperinone.

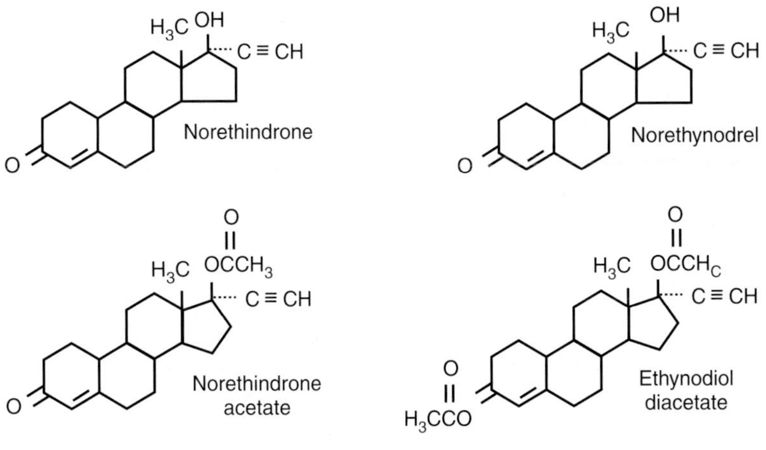

Figure 14-3. Chemical structures of the estrane progestins used in oral contraceptives.

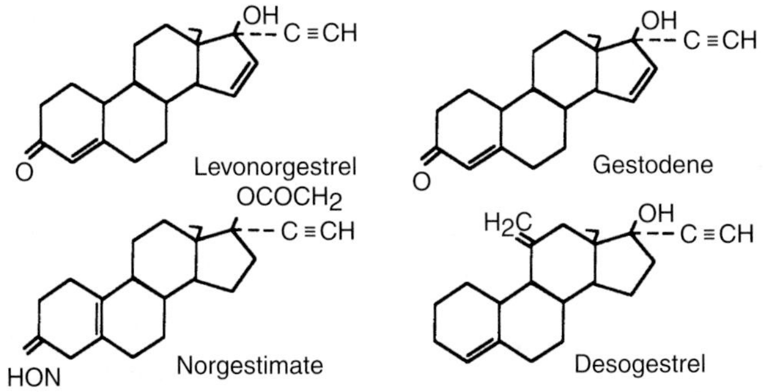

Figure 14-4. Chemical structure of the gonane progestins used in oral contraceptives.

years, and formulations with desogestrel and norgestimate, but not gestodene, have been marketed in the United States since 1992.

Except for two daily progestin-only formulations, the progestins are combined with varying dosages of two estrogens, ethinyl estradiol and ethinyl estradiol 3-methyl ether, also known as mestranol (Fig. 14-5). All the older higher dosage OC formulations contained mestranol, and this steroid is still present in some 50-μg formulations. All formulations with less than 50 μg of estrogen contain only the parent compound, ethinyl estradiol. In common usage formulations with 50 μg or more of estrogen (ethinyl estradiol or mestranol) have been termed *first-generation* OCs. Those with less than 50 μg of estrogen, 20 to 35 μg of ethinyl estradiol, are called *second-generation* products if they contain any progestin except the three newest levonorgestrel derivatives. Those formulations with desogestrel, norgestimate, and gestodene are called *third-generation* formulations. All the

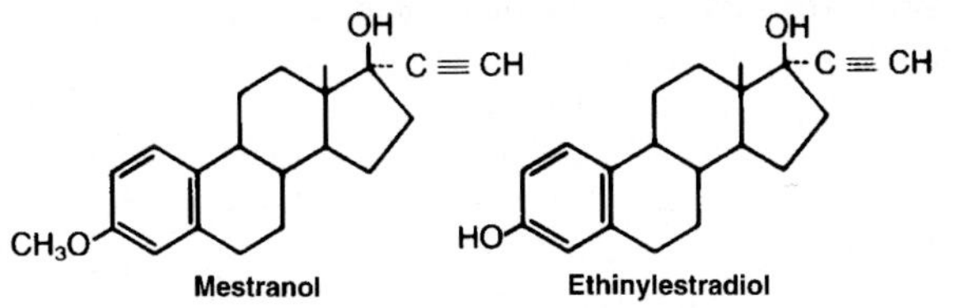

Figure 14-5. Structures of the two estrogens used in combination oral contraceptives.

synthetic estrogens and progestins in OCs have an ethinyl group at position 17. The presence of this ethinyl group enhances the oral activity of these agents, because their essential functional groups are not as rapidly metabolized as they pass through the intestinal mucosa and liver via the portal system, in contrast to what occurs when natural sex steroids are ingested orally. The synthetic steroids thus have greater oral potency per unit of weight than do the natural steroids. It has been estimated that ethinyl estradiol has about 100 times the potency of an equivalent weight of conjugated equine estrogen or estrone sulfate for stimulating synthesis of various hepatic globulins.

The various modifications in chemical structure of the different synthetic progestins and estrogens also affect their biologic activity. Thus, one cannot define the pharmacologic activity of the progestin or estrogen in a particular contraceptive steroid formulation based only on the amount of steroid present. The biologic activity of each steroid also has to be considered. Using established tests for progestational activity in animals, it has been found that a given weight of norgestrel is several times more potent than the same weight of norethindrone. Studies in humans, using delay of menses or endometrial histologic alterations such as subnuclear vacuolization as end points, also determined that norgestrel is about 10 times more potent than the same weight of norethindrone. Norethindrone acetate and ethynodiol diacetate are metabolized in the body to norethindrone and have equivalent potency per unit weight to the parent compound, norethindrone, whereas levonorgestrel is 10 to 20 times as potent. Each of the three most recently developed levonorgestrel derivatives has been shown in animal, but not human, studies to have similar or greater progestogenic potency than an equivalent weight of levonorgestrel, with less androgenic activity. The magnitude of difference in androgenic and progestational effects produced by each progestin is called *selectivity.*

The two estrogenic compounds used in OCs—ethinyl estradiol and its 3-methyl ether mestranol—also have different biologic activity in women. To become biologically effective, mestranol must be demethylated to ethinyl estradiol, because mestranol does not bind to the estrogen cytosol receptor. The degree of conversion of mestranol to ethinyl estradiol varies among individuals; some are able to convert it completely, whereas others convert only a portion of it. Thus, in some women, a given weight of mestranol is as potent as the same weight of ethinyl estradiol, and in other women it is only about half as potent. Overall, it has been estimated, using human endometrial response and effect on liver corticosteroid-binding globulin (CBG) production as end points, that ethinyl estradiol is about 1.7 times as potent as the same weight of mestranol. The biologic activity, as well as the quantity of both steroid components, need to be evaluated when comparing potency of the various formulations.

Radioimmunoassay methods have been developed to measure blood levels of these synthetic estrogens and progestins. Peak plasma levels of ethinyl estradiol are lower and occur later, about 2 to 4 hours, after ingestion of mestranol than after ingestion of ethinyl estradiol. The delay is due to the time necessary for mestranol to be demethylated to ethinyl estradiol in the liver.

When different doses of *dl*-norgestrel were administered to women, we found that the serum levels of levonorgestrel were related to the dosage. Peak serum levels were found 0.5 to 3 hours after oral administration, followed by a rapid, sharp decline (Fig. 14-6). However, 24 hours after ingestion, 20% to 25% of the peak level of levonorgestrel was still present in the serum. After 5 days of norgestrel administration, measurable amounts of levonorgestrel were present for at least the following 5 days.

Brenner and coworkers measured serum levels of levonorgestrel, follicle-stimulating hormone (FSH), luteinizing hormone (LH), estradiol (E_2), and progesterone 3 hours after ingestion of a combination OC containing 0.5 mg of *dl*-norgestrel and 50 μg of ethinyl estradiol in three women during two consecutive cycles, as well as during the intervening pill-free interval. Daily levels of levonorgestrel rose during the first few days of ingestion, plateaued thereafter, and declined after ingestion of the last pill. Nevertheless, substantial amounts of levonorgestrel remained in the serum for at least the first 3 to 4 days after the last pill was ingested. These steroid levels were sufficient to suppress gonadotropin release during the 1-week interval when no steroid was administered. Thus, follicle maturation, as evidenced by rising E_2 levels, did not occur during the week when no steroid was being ingested. When lower doses of steroids are administered, follicular growth but not ovulation may occur because of initiation of growth of the dominant follicle during the time that no steroid is being ingested. With the standard 21 days of hormone pills and 7 days of the hormone-free regimen, Sulak and associates reported that symptoms of pelvic pain, headache, breast tenderness, and bloating were all significantly more prevalent during the hormone-free days than when hormones were given. Shortening the hormone-free interval to 3 to 4 days with low-dose formulation should maintain sufficient circulating levels of exogenous steroids to inhibit follicular development and suppresses steroid synthesis and reduce side effects during the days when no hormones are given. Two formulations with 24 days of hormone pills followed by 4 days of no hormones have recently been marketed and others are undergoing clinical trials.

Accidental pregnancies occurring during OC use probably do not occur because of failure to ingest one to two pills more than a few days after a treatment cycle is initiated but rather because initiation of the next cycle of medication is delayed for a few days. Therefore, it is important that the pill-free interval is not extended more than 7 days. This is best accomplished by ingesting either a placebo or iron tablet daily during the steroid-free interval (the so-called 28-day package). Women should be advised that the most important pill to remember to take is the first one of each cycle.

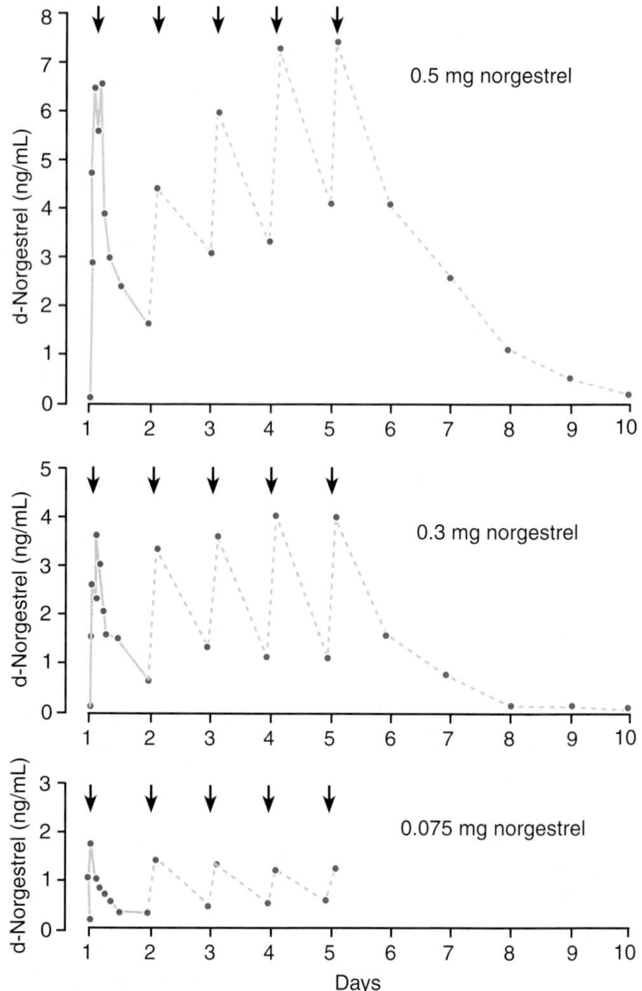

Figure 14-6. Serum levonorgestrel levels in three women at various times after ingestion of 0.5, 0.3, and 0.075 mg of *dl*-norgestrel once a day for 5 days. Arrows indicate days drug was ingested. (From Mishell DR Jr, Stanczyk F, Hiroi M, et al: Steroid contraception. In Crosignani PG, Mishell DR Jr [eds]: Ovulation in the Human. London, Academic Press, 1976.)

Physiology

Mechanism of Action

The estrogen–progestin combination is the most effective type of OC formulation because these preparations consistently inhibit the midcycle gonadotropin surge and thus prevent ovulation. The progestin-only formulations have a lower dose of progestin than do the combined agents and do not consistently inhibit ovulation. Both types of formulations also act on other aspects of the reproductive process. They alter the cervical mucus, making it thick, viscid, and scanty, which retards sperm penetration. They also alter motility of the uterus and oviduct, thus impairing transport of both ova and sperm. Furthermore, they alter the endometrium so that its glandular production of glycogen is diminished, and less energy is available for the blastocyst to survive in the uterine cavity. Finally, they may alter ovarian responsiveness to gonadotropin stimulation. With both types of formulations, neither gonadotropin production nor ovarian steroidogenesis is completely abolished. Levels of endogenous E_2 in the peripheral blood during ingestion of high-dose combination OCs are similar to those found in the early follicular phase of the normal cycle.

Contraceptive steroids prevent ovulation mainly by interfering with release of gonadotropin-releasing hormone (GnRH) from the hypothalamus. In rats and in a few studies in humans, this inhibitory action of the contraceptive steroids could be overome by the administration of GnRH. However, in the majority of other human studies, most women who had been ingesting combination OCs had suppression of the release of LH and FSH after infusion of GnRH, indicating that the steroids had a direct inhibitory effect on the pituitary and the hypothalamus.

It is possible that when hypothalamic inhibition is prolonged, the mechanism for synthesis and release of gonadotropins may become refractory to the normal amount of GnRH stimulation. However, in studies of a few OC users, after serial daily administration of GnRH, there was still a refractory response to a GnRH infusion. Thus, the combination contraceptive steroids probably do have a direct inhibitory effect on the gonadotropin-producing cells of the pituitary, in addition to affecting the hypothalamus. Direct pituitary inhibition occurs in about 80% of women ingesting high-dose combination OCs. Pituitary suppression is unrelated to the age of the woman or the duration of steroid use but is related to the potency of the formulation. The effect is more pronounced with formulations containing a more potent progestin and with those containing 50 μg or more of estrogen than with 30 to 35 μg of estrogen-containing formulations. It has not been demonstrated that the amount of pituitary suppression is related to the occurrence of amenorrhea after stopping OC use, but if there is a relationship, the lower dose formulations should be associated with a lower frequency of this entity. Some data show that the mean time to conception after discontinuation of OC use is shorter in women ingesting preparations with less than 50 μg of estrogen (4.01 cycles) than in those ingesting formulations with 50 μg of estrogen or more (4.79 cycles).

The daily progestin-only preparations do not consistently inhibit ovulation. They exert their contraceptive action via the other mechanisms listed earlier, but because of the inconsistent ovulation inhibition, their effectiveness is significantly less than that of the combination types of OCs. Because a lower dose of progestin is used in these formulations than in the combination tablets, it is important that these preparations be consistently taken at the same time of day to ensure that blood levels do not fall below the effective contraceptive level.

No significant difference in clinical effectiveness has been demonstrated among the various combination formulations currently available in the United States. As long as no tablets are omitted (perfect use), the pregnancy rate is about 0.3% at the end of 1 year with all marketed combination formulations.

Metabolic Effects

The synthetic steroids in OC formulations have many metabolic effects in addition to their contraceptive actions (Table 14-3). These metabolic effects can produce both the more common, less serious side effects, as well as the rare, potentially serious complications. The magnitude of these effects is directly related to the dosage and potency of the steroids in the formulations. Fortunately, in most instances the more common adverse effects are relatively mild. The most frequent symptoms produced by the estrogen component include nausea (a central nervous system effect), breast tenderness, and fluid retention (which usually does not exceed 3 to 4 pounds of body weight) caused by increased aldosterone synthesis and decreased sodium and fluid excretion. Minor, clinically insignificant changes in circulating vitamin levels also occurred after ingestion of the higher dosage OCs. These changes included a decrease in levels of the B complex vitamins and ascorbic acid and increases in levels of vitamin A. Even with use of the high-steroid-dose agents, dietary vitamin supplementation was not necessary, as the changes in circulating vitamin levels were small and clinically insignificant. Estrogen can also cause melasma, pigmentation of the malar eminences, to develop. Melasma is accentuated by sunlight and usually takes a long time to disappear after OCs are discontinued. The incidence of all these estrogenic side effects is much less with use of lower estrogen-dose formulations than that which occurred with use of high-estrogen-dose formulations. With high doses of estrogen OC usage was found to accelerate the development of the symptoms of gallbladder disease in young women but did not increase the overall incidence of cholelithiasis. The results of the large British Family Planning Association Study and a recent case-control study indicate that the use of high-dose OCs does not increase the incidence of gallbladder disease in women. When the data were stratified among women of different body weight or age, no increased risk of gallbladder disease was found in any subgroup. These results indicate that development of gallbladder disease is not a risk factor associated with OC use, even if these agents contain high doses of steroids and are used for more than 8 years.

It was previously postulated that high dosages of the synthetic estrogens could also produce changes in mood and depression brought about by diversion of tryptophan metabolism from its minor pathway in the brain to its major pathway in the liver. The end product of tryptophan metabolism, serotonin, is thus decreased in the central nervous system, and it was postulated that the resultant lowering of serotonin could produce depression in some women and sleepiness and mood changes in others. Analysis of the data from the Royal College of General Practitioners (RCGP) cohort study indicated that OC use was positively correlated with the incidence of depression, which in turn was directly related to the dose of estrogen in the formulation. In this study an increased incidence of depression was not found to occur among users of OCs containing less than 50 μg of estrogen. Data from postmenopausal women receiving estrogen therapy alone, as well as from estrogen–progestin sequential therapy, indicate that administration of physiologic doses of estrogen alone, which is less potent than the pharmacologic dose used in OCs, improves the mood of women, whereas the addition of a progestin increases the amount of depression, irritability, tension, and fatigue. These studies indicate that the progestin component of the agents may be the major cause of the adverse mood changes and tiredness observed in some women after ingestion of OCs, but it has not been definitely established which of the steroid components is the major factor in producing adverse mood changes. Possibly both are involved.

Table 14–3 Metabolic Effects of Contraceptive Steroids

	EFFECTS	
	Chemical	**Clinical**
Estrogen-Ethinyl Estradiol		
Proteins	↓	None
Albumin	↓	
Amino Acids	↑	None
Globulins		
Angiotensinogen		↑ Blood pressure
Clotting Factors		Hypercoagulability
Carrier proteins (CBG, TBG, SHBG, transferrin, ceroloplasmin)		None
Carbohydrate		
Plasma insulin	None	None
Glucose tolerance	None	None
Lipids		
Cholesterol	↑	None
Triglyceride	↑	None
HDL cholesterol	↑	? ↓ cardiovascular disease
LDL cholesterol	↓	? ↓ cardiovascular disease
Electrolytes		
Sodium excretion	↓	Fluid retention Edema
Vitamins		
B complex	↓	None
Ascorbic acid	↓	None
Vitamin A	↑	None
Other		
Breast	↑	Breast tenderness
Endometrial steroid receptors	↑	Hyperplasia
Skin	↓	Sebum production Facial pigmentation
Progestins—19-Nortestosterone Derivatives		
Proteins	↓SHBG	None
Carbohydrate		
Plasma insulin	↑	None
Glucose tolerance	↓	None
Lipids		
Cholesterol	↓	None
Triglyceride	↓	None
HDL cholesterol	↓	? ↓ Cardiovascular disease
LDL cholesterol	↑	? ↓ Cardiovascular disease
Other		
Nitrogen retention	↑	↑ Body weight
Skin-sebum production	↑	↑ Acne
CNS effects	↑	Nervousness, fatigue, depression
Endometrial steroid receptors	↓	No withdrawal bleeding

CBG, corticosteroid-binding globulin; HDL, high-density lipoprotein; LDL, low-density lipoprotein; SHBG, sex hormone-binding globulin; TBG, thyroxine-binding globulin.

The progestins, because they are structurally related to testosterone, also produce certain adverse androgenic effects. These include weight gain, acne, and a symptom perceived by some women as nervousness. Some women gain a considerable amount of weight when they take OCs, and this weight gain is believed to be produced by the anabolic effect of the progestin component. Although estrogens decrease sebum production, progestins increase it and can cause acne to develop or worsen. Thus, women who have acne should be given a formulation with a low progestin–estrogen ratio. Two formulations have been shown in randomized controlled trials to reduce acne to a greater extent than placebo. The treatment of acne is now an approved indication for use of these agents. The final symptom produced by the progestin component is failure of withdrawal bleeding or amenorrhea. Because the progestins decrease the synthesis of estrogen receptors in the endometrium, endometrial growth is decreased, and some women have failure of withdrawal bleeding. This symptom is not important medically, but since bleeding serves as a signal that the woman is not pregnant, it is desirable to have some amount of periodic withdrawal bleeding during the days she is not taking these steroids. The two steroid components can act together to produce irregular bleeding.

Unscheduled (breakthrough) bleeding (which is usually produced by insufficient estrogen, too much progestin, or a combination of both), as well as failure of withdrawal bleeding, can be alleviated by increasing the amount of estrogen in the formulation or by switching to a more estrogenic formulation. Many women taking OCs complain of an increased frequency of headaches. It has not been determined what is the exact relation, if any, between each of the steroids in OCs and the occurrence of headaches.

Protein

The synthetic estrogens used in OCs cause an increase in the hepatic production of several globulins. Progesterone and androgenic progestins do not affect the synthesis of globulins except that of sex hormone-binding globulin (SHBG). Synthesis of SHBG is reduced by androgens, including the androgenic progestins. Some of the globulins that are increased by ethinyl estradiol ingestion, such as factors V, VIII, X, and fibrinogen, enhance thrombosis, but another globulin, angiotensinogen, may be converted to angiotensin and increase blood pressure in some users. The circulating levels of each of these globulins are directly correlated with the amount of estrogen in the OC formulation. Epidemiologic studies have shown that the incidence of both venous and arterial thrombosis is also directly related to the dose of estrogen.

Although angiotensinogen levels are lower in women who ingest formulations with 30 to 35 μg of ethinyl estradiol than in those who ingest higher estrogen-dosage formulations, a slight but significant increase in mean blood pressure still occurs in women who ingest the lower dosage formulations and about 1 in 200 women will develop clinical hypertension. Thus, blood pressure should be monitored in all users of OCs. There is some indirect evidence that the progestin component may also raise blood pressure. However, women who receive progestins without estrogen do not have an increase in blood pressure over time, indicating that the estrogen component is the major cause of elevated blood pressure in a few users of OCs.

SHBG also binds circulating levels of estrogens and androgens. Progesterone is bound to corticosteroid-binding globulin but since the progestins used in oral contraceptives are 19-nortestosterone compounds, they are bound to SHBG. Estrogens increase SHBG levels, but androgens, including 19-nortestosterone derivatives, decrease SHBG levels. Thus, measurement of SHBG is one way to determine the relative estrogenic/androgenic balance of different OC formulations. Van der Vange and colleagues measured SHBG levels before and 6 months following ingestion of several OC formulations containing about the same amount of ethinyl estradiol. The greatest increase occurred with formulations containing cyproterone acetate (not used in OC formulations in the United States), desogestrel, and gestodene. SHBG increases of lesser magnitude occurred following ingestion of formulations containing low doses of norethindrone and levonorgestrel. Since SHBG binds endogenous testosterone and prevents it acting on the target tissue, formulations causing the greatest increase in SHBG should be associated with the least amount of androgenic effects. These formulations are particularly useful for treating women with symptoms of hyperandrogenism such as polycystic ovarian syndrome. The formulations with the antiandrogenic progestin, drosperinone, are also beneficial in treating women with hyperandrogenism.

Carbohydrate

The effect of OCs on glucose metabolism is mainly related to the dose, potency, and chemical structure of the progestin. Conflicting data exist as to whether the estrogen component affects carbohydrate metabolism. The estrogen may act synergistically with the progestin to impair glucose tolerance. In general the higher the dose and potency of the progestin, the greater the magnitude of impaired glucose metabolism. The amount of alteration appears to be greater with gonanes than with estranes. Several studies have shown that formulations with a low dose of progestin, including one containing levonorgestrel, do not significantly alter levels of glucose, insulin, or glucagon after a glucose load in healthy women or in those with a history of gestational diabetes. However, other studies indicate that the multiphasic formulations with norgestrel, but not those with norethindrone, produce some deterioration of glucose tolerance in normal women, as well as in those with a history of gestational diabetes. Some studies have shown increased levels of both glucose and insulin when glucose tolerance tests were administered to women ingesting desogestrel containing OCs.

Data from 20 years of experience using mainly high-dose formulations in the large RCGP cohort study indicated that there was no increased risk of diabetes mellitus developing among current OC users (relative risk [RR], 0.80) or former OC users (RR, 0.82) even among women who had used OCs for 10 years or more. More than 1 million woman-years of follow-up of OC users in the large Nurses Health Study cohort, which was initiated in 1976, were analyzed in 1992. Although type 2 diabetes mellitus developed in more than 2000 women, the risk was not increased among current OC users (RR, 0.71) and only marginally increased in past OC users (RR, 1.11) and occurred only among women who had used high-dose formulations many years previously, not for those who had used lower dose formulations. Kjos and coworkers followed a group of women with a history of gestational diabetes mellitus for several years after the end of the pregnancy. Three years after delivery women ingesting low-dose norethindrone combination and low-dose levonorgestrel combination containing OCs had no greater risk of developing diabetes mellitus than the control group not taking OCs. When prescribing oral contraceptives for women with a history of glucose intolerance, it is probably preferable to use formulations with a low dose of a norethindrone-type progestin than a levonorgestrel type and to monitor glucose tolerance periodically.

Lipids

The estrogen component of OCs cause an increase in high-density lipoprotein (HDL) cholesterol, a decrease in low-density lipoprotein (LDL) levels, and an increase in total cholesterol and triglyceride levels. The progestin component causes a decrease in HDL and an increase in LDL levels while causing a decrease in both total cholesterol and triglyceride levels.

The older formulations with high doses of progestin had adverse effects upon the lipid profile although they also contained high doses of the synthetic estrogen. These progestin-dominant formulations produced a decrease in HDL cholesterol levels and an increase in LDL cholesterol levels. They also caused an increase in serum triglyceride because the estrogen has a greater effect on triglyceride synthesis than does the progestin. Short-term longitudinal studies of several phasic formulations containing levonorgestrel and norethindrone found that a significant increase in triglyceride levels still occurred but there was little change in either HDL cholesterol or LDL cholesterol levels, as

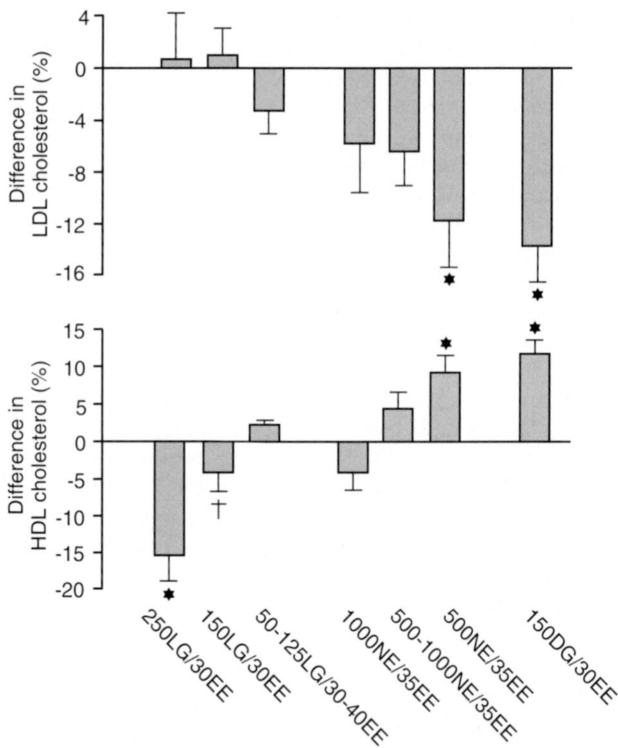

Figure 14-7. Percent differences in high-density lipoprotein (HDL) and low-density lipoprotein (LDL) cholesterol levels and in the incremental area for insulin in response to the oral glucose tolerance test (OGTT) between women taking one of seven combination oral contraceptives and those not taking oral contraceptives. The T bars indicate 1 SD. The asterisk ($p < 0.001$) and dagger ($p < 0.01$) indicate significant differences between users and nonusers in the mean values for the principal metabolic variables. (Modified from Godsland IF, Crook D, Simpson R, et al: The effects of different formulations of oral contraceptive agents on lipid and carbohydrate metabolism. N Engl J Med 323:1375, 1990. Copyright 1990 Massachusetts Medical Society. All rights reserved. Modified with permission.)

well as total cholesterol levels, because the effects of each steroid on lipid synthesis were offset by the other.

In a cross-sectional study in which lipid levels were measured in a large number of women ingesting several OC formulations and compared with non-OC users, Godsland and associates reported that there were insignificant differences in HDL and LDL cholesterol levels compared with non-OC users when low-dose monophasic and triphasic levonorgestrel and norethindrone formulations were ingested. The women ingesting formulations with only 0.5 mg of norethindrone or 150 μg of desogestrel had a significant increase in HDL cholesterol levels and a significant decrease in LDL cholesterol levels (Fig. 14-7). The three most

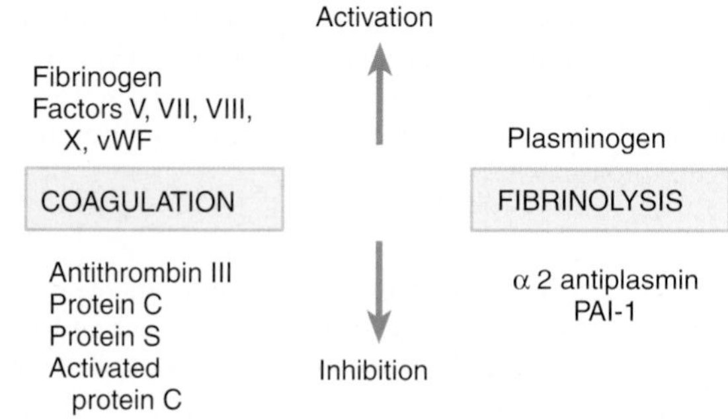

Figure 14-8. Factors involved in coagulation and fibrinolysis. PAI, plasminogen activator inhibitor; VwF, von Willibrand factor.

recently developed progestins derived from levonorgestrel have less androgenic activity than do the older progestins and, as such, when combined with an estrogen would be expected to have less adverse effect on lipid metabolism than on the older formulations. Speroff and colleagues in 1993 reviewed data from the published studies in which lipid levels were measured in women ingesting formulations with these three less androgenic progestins. They reported that with use of these formulations there was a significant increase in HDL cholesterol levels, a significant decrease in LDL cholesterol levels, little change in total cholesterol levels, and a substantial increase in triglyceride levels (Table 14-4). The long-term effect, if any, of these changes in lipid parameters remains to be determined.

Coagulation Parameters

The estrogen component of oral contraceptives increases the synthesis of several coagulation factors, including fibrinogen, which enhance thrombosis in a dose-dependent manner. The effect of OCs on parameters that inhibit coagulation, such as protein C, protein S, and antithrombin III, is less clear because of the diversity of techniques used to measure these parameters in different laboratories (Fig. 14-8). A similar lack of consistency occurs when parameters that enhance fibrinolysis (e.g., plasminogen) or inhibit fibrinolysis (e.g., plasminogen activator inhibitor-1) are measured in OC users. Changes in most of these coagulation parameters in OC users are very small, if they occur at all, and there is no evidence that these minor alterations in levels of coagulation parameters measured in the laboratory have any effect on the clinical risk of developing venous or arterial thrombosis. Nevertheless, if the woman has an inherited coagulation disorder (e.g., protein C, protein S, or antithrombin III deficiency or the more common activated protein C resistance), which increases her risk of developing thrombosis, her risk of

Table 14–4 Lipid Changes with Oral Contraceptives Containing New Progestins

		% CHANGE FROM BASELINE					
Progestin	***N***	**TG**	**C**	**LDL-C**	**HDL-C**	**Apo B**	**Apo A-1**
Desogestrel	608	29.3	2.8	−2.1	12.9	10.5	11.3
Gestodene	296	38.3	3.8	−2.5	8.1	16.0	7.1
Norgestimate	>2550	14.8	4.3	−0.2	9.9	5.3	7.3

Apo, apoprotein; C, total cholesterol; HDL-C, high-density lipoprotein cholesterol; LDL-C, low-density lipoprotein cholesterol; TG, triglyceride.
From Speroff L, DeCherney A, and the Advisory Board for the New Progestins: Evaluation of a new generation of oral contraceptives. Obstet Gynecol 81:1034, 1993.

developing thrombosis is increased severalfold if she ingests estrogen-containing oral contraception. Vandenbroucke and coworkers reported that the relative risk of developing deep venous thrombosis (DVT) among women with activated protein C resistance and OC use was increased 30-fold compared with non-OC users without the mutation. They estimated that the annual incidence of DVT in a woman of reproductive age with this genetic mutation was about 6 per 10,000 women if she did not take OCs and about 30 per 10,000 women if she took them. Currently, it is not recommended that screening for these coagulation deficiencies be undertaken before starting OC use because it is not cost effective unless the woman has a personal or family history of thrombotic events. However, if a woman has a known inherited or acquired thrombophilin, she should not take an estrogen-containing contraceptive. Progestins do not affect coagulation parameters.

Cardiovascular Effects

The cause of the increased incidence of both venous and arterial cardiovascular disease, including myocardial infarction, in users of OCs appears to be thrombosis and not atherosclerosis.

Venous Thromboembolism

Gerstman and colleagues analyzed the effect of OCs with different doses of estrogen on the incidence of venous thromboembolism (VTE) in a historical cohort study of more than 230,000 women age 15 to 44 in Michigan between 1980 and 1986. Among users of OC formulations with less than 50 μg of estrogen, the rate of VTE per 10,000 woman-years was 4.2; among users of formulations with 50 μg of estrogen, the rate was 7.0; and among users of formulations with greater than 50 μg of estrogen, the rate increased to 10.0 per 10,000 woman-years (Table 14-5). These data confirm earlier findings that indicate that the risk of VTE is directly related to the dose of estrogen in the formulation. The background rate of VTE in women of reproductive age is about 0.8 per 10,000 woman-years. An observational study by Farmer and Preston from nearly 700,000 women ages 14 to 45 years assessed the incidence of VTE events associated with pregnancy and exposure to combined OCs containing more than 20 μg but less than 50 μg of estrogen. The incidence of venous thromboembolic events among OC users was 3 per 10,000 woman-years, which was about four times the background rate but half the rate of 6 per 10,000 woman-years associated with pregnancy.

Table 14–5 Rates of Deep Venous Thromboembolic Disease in Oral Contraceptive Estrogen Dose-Refined Cohorts

Estrogen Defined-Cohorts (μg)	No. of Cases	Person-Years (× 10,000)	Rates/10,000 Person-Years
<50	53	12.7	4.2
50	69	9.8	7.0
>50	20	2.0	10.0
All	142	24.5	5.8

From Gerstman BB, Piper JM, Tomita DK, et al: Oral contraceptive estrogen dose and the risk of deep venous thromboembolic disease. Am J Epidemiol 133:32, 1991.

Numerous observational studies have been performed to determine the risk of VTE in users of OCs containing mainly less than 50 μg estrogen. An analysis of 220 articles published on this subject reported VTE risk was increased two- to threefold among women using combination OCs compared with women not using combination OCs.

Thus, use of OCs containing less than 50 μg of estrogen is associated with about a two- to threefold increased risk of VTE compared with a nonpregnant population not taking OCs but about a 50% reduction in risk of VTE compared with a pregnant or recently postpartum population. The increased risk of VTE is similar in women ingesting the same dose of progestin with 30 μg and 20 μg of estrogen. Thus, as stated in a WHO report, among users of combined oral contraceptive preparations containing less than 50 μg of ethinyl estradiol, the risk of venous thromboembolism is not related to the dose of estrogen.

Several observational studies reported that the risk of VTE among women ingesting low-estrogen-dose formulations containing desogestrel or gestodene was increased about 1.5 to 2.5 times that of women ingesting formulations containing less than 50 μg of estrogen and levonorgestrel. Because none of these studies were prospective clinical trials, controversy exists as to whether the increased risk of VTE was causally related to formulations containing these progestins or whether the increased risk was due to certain types of bias. Selection bias, diagnostic bias, and referral bias could have accounted for the differences, but a causal relation cannot be disproved. A recent study analyzing the risk of VTE with norgestimate-containing compounds reported that the increased risk of VTE in women using these formulations is similar to that of low-estrogen-dose levonorgestrel compounds.

Myocardial Infarction

Neither epidemiologic studies of humans nor experimental studies with subhuman primates have observed an acceleration of atherosclerosis with the ingestion of OCs. Nearly all the published epidemiologic studies indicate that there is no increased risk of myocardial infarction (MI) among former users of OCs. The incidence of cardiovascular disease is also not correlated with the duration of oral contraceptive use. Further data, which indicate that the increased risk of MI in OC users is due to thrombosis, not atherosclerosis, is provided by an angiographic study performed in 1982 by Engel and coworkers of young women who had an MI. In this study only 36% of users of OCs containing 50 μg ethinyl estradiol had evidence of coronary atherosclerosis compared with 79% of nonusers. A study with cynomolgus macaque monkeys found that the ingestion of an oral contraceptive containing high doses of norgestrel and ethinyl estradiol lowered HDL cholesterol levels significantly. However, after 2 years of ingesting this formulation and being fed an atherogenic diet, these animals had a significantly smaller area of coronary artery atherosclerosis than did a control group of female monkeys not ingesting OCs but fed the same diet. Another group of monkeys, who received levonorgestrel without estrogen, also had lowered HDL cholesterol levels. In this group, the extent of coronary atherosclerosis was significantly increased compared with that of the controls. The results of this study have since been confirmed in a larger study with two high-dose estrogen-progestin formulations. Both of these compounds lowered the HDL cholesterol levels by half and tripled the cholesterol/HDL cholesterol ratio. In this study, the mean extent of coronary artery plaque formation in the high-risk control group of female animals was more than 3 times greater than that found in animals ingesting a high-dose norgestrel + ethinyl estradiol compound and more than 10 times greater than that found in animals ingesting a high-dose ethynodiol diacetate + ethinyl estradiol compound with that of controls. These studies suggest that the estrogen component of OCs has a direct protective effect on the coronary arteries, reducing the extent of atherosclerosis that would otherwise be accelerated by decreased levels of HDL cholesterol.

The epidemiologic studies that reported an increased incidence of MI in older users of OCs were published in the late 1970s and thus used as a database women who only ingested formulations with 50 µg or more of estrogen. In these case-control and cohort studies, a significantly increased incidence of MI was found mainly among older users who had risk factors that caused arterial narrowing, such as preexisting hypercholesterolemia, hypertension, diabetes mellitus, or smoking more than 15 cigarettes a day.

Data accumulated during the first 10 years of the RCGP study (1968–1977), in which the majority of users ingested formulations with more than 50 µg of estrogen and high doses of progestin, showed that a significantly increased relative risk of death from circulatory disease occurred only among women older than 35 years of age who also smoked. A more recent analysis of data obtained during the first 20 years of this study (1968–1987) revealed that there was no significant increased relative risk of acute MI among current or former users of oral contraceptives who did not smoke any cigarettes (Table 14-6). Women who smoked and did not use OCs had a greater risk of MI than did nonsmokers whether or not they used OCs. Even though most of the women in this study used high-dose formulations, a significantly increased risk of MI with OC use compared with smokers not using OCs occurred only among both mild (<15 cigarettes per day) and heavy cigarette smokers; OC users who were heavy smokers had a greater relative risk than mild smokers. A case-control study analyzed the relation between OC use and the risk of MI among women admitted to a group of New England hospitals between 1985 and 1988. The relative risk of MI among current OC users was not significantly increased, RR 1.1 (confidence interval [CI], 0.4 to 3.1). Among women who smoked at least 25 cigarettes a day, current OC use increased the risk of MI 30-fold. Smoking alone, without use of OCs, increased the risk of MI about ninefold. The data indicate that cigarette smoking is an independent risk factor for MI,

Table 14–6 Relative Risk of Myocardial Infarction in Relation to Smoking and Oral Contraceptive Use (RCGP Study, 1968–1987) ($N = 158$)

	ORAL CONTRACEPTIVE USE		
Smoking	**Never (CL)**	**Previously (CL)**	**Current (CL)**
Never	1.0	1.1 (0.6–2.2)	0.9 (0.3–2.7)
<15 cig./day	2.0 (1.0–3.9)	1.3 (0.6–2.8)	3.5 (1.3–9.5)
≥15 cig./day	3.3 (1.6–6.7)	4.3 (2.3–8.0)	20.8 (5.2–83.1)

CL, confidence limits.

Modified from Croft P, Hannaford PC: Risk factors for acute myocardial infarction in women. BMJ 298:165, 1989.

but the use of high-dose OCs by cigarette smokers significantly enhances their risk of experiencing an MI, the two factors acting synergistically. Current or prior OC use is not associated with an increased risk of MI in nonsmokers.

The mechanism whereby cigarette smoking increases the risk of arterial thrombosis in OC users appears to be due to the effect of nicotine on the coagulation process. Although OCs increase the concentration of factors involved in producing blood coagulation, they also affect the activity of factors inhibiting coagulation. Notelovitz and colleagues found that smokers who ingested low-dose OCs had a significantly greater decrease in levels of endogenous coagulation inhibitors, mainly antithrombin III, than did OC users who did not smoke. Dynamic tests of coagulation and fibrinolysis by these investigators showed an altered procoagulant activity only among the OC users who also smoked. Mileikowsky and associates reported that platelet aggregation was increased only among OC users who also smoked and not among women who smoked and did not use OCs. This thrombotic effect was probably related to prostacyclin inhibition, as prostacyclin formation was reduced only among the women in the study who smoked and used OCs. The usual balance of prostacyclin and thromboxane is thus altered when OC users smoked, producing a relative excess of thromboxane. The results of this study therefore suggest that the synergistic effect of OCs and smoking on the effects of arterial thrombosis, such as MI and cerebral thrombosis, are produced by activation of the thromboxane A_2-mediated mechanism of platelet aggregation brought about by reduction of prostacyclin only during nicotine intake. Thus, former cigarette smokers do not have a risk of enhanced thrombosis, and nicotine administered in any form can increase the risk. Both the RCGP and WHO studies reported that the risk of MI in OC users was several-fold greater if they had hypertension than if they did not. Two large case-control studies in the United States have shown no significantly increased risk of MI in OC users. For many years in the United States OCs have not been prescribed to women with uncontrolled hypertension or those older than age 35 who smoked cigarettes. A WHO technical report stated that women who do not smoke, who have their blood pressure checked, and who do not have hypertension or diabetes are at no increased risk of MI if they use combined oral contraceptives regardless of their age.

Stroke

Although epidemiologic data from studies performed in the 1970s indicated that there was possibly a causal relation between ingestion of high-dose OC formulations and stroke, the data were conflicting, with some studies showing a significantly increased risk of ischemic stroke, others an increased risk of hemorrhagic stroke, and still others no significantly increased risk of either entity. Furthermore, as occurred with MI, the studies that did show a significantly increased risk of stroke in OC users indicated that the increased risk was mainly limited to older women who also smoked or were hypertensive (or both). The monkey study performed by Clarkson and coworkers revealed that the animals ingesting high-dose OCs, which lowered HDL cholesterol, had no greater extent of carotid artery atherosclerosis than did the control group of female animals. Epidemiologic studies consistently report that there is no increased risk of either ischemic or hemorrhagic stroke in past users of OCs compared to never users.

Data from the epidemiologic studies of OC use and cardiovascular disease performed in the 1960s and 1970s are not relevant to their current use, as the dose of both steroid components in the formulations now being marketed is markedly less, and women with cardiovascular risk factors such as uncontrolled hypertension are no longer receiving these agents. Furthermore, it is strongly recommended not to prescribe OCs to women older than age 35 who also smoke.

A nested case-control analysis by Hannaford and associates examined the data obtained between 1968 and 1990 during the RCGP Oral Contraception Study to determine the relationship between OC use and the risk of first-ever stroke, including the diagnosis of subarachnoid hemorrhage, cerebral hemorrhage, or ischemic stroke. Women using OCs containing a high estrogen dose (more than 50 mcg) had nearly a sixfold increase in the risk of stroke, whereas women ingesting OC formulations containing 30 to 35 μg estrogen did not have an increased risk. Similar data were reported from a WHO study. The risk of ischemic stroke among women ingesting OCs with 50 μg or more of estrogen was 5.3 compared with nonusers but only 1.5 (insignificant) in women ingesting OCs with less than 50 μg of estrogen. An analysis of strokes occurring in a large health maintenance organization in California from 1991 to 1994 by Pettiti and colleagues indicated that the users had no significant increase of either ischemic or hemorrhagic stroke with OC use. In this study the relative risk of ischemic stroke and hemorrhagic stroke for OC users was 1.18 and 1.13, respectively, compared with never users and past users. Another case study by Schwartz and coworkers analyzed these data as well as data from the state of Washington. The relative risk of ischemic and hemorrhagic stroke in OC users compared with nonusers was 1.4 and 1.3. Neither of these figures was statistically significant.

The results of these recent epidemiologic studies indicate that use of a low-dose estrogen–progestin OC formulation by nonsmoking women without risk factors for cardiovascular disease is not associated with an increased incidence of either MI or ischemic or hemorrhagic stroke. Smoking is a risk factor for arterial but not venous thrombosis. Combination OCs should not be prescribed to women older than the age of 35 who smoke cigarettes or use alternative forms of nicotine.

Reproductive Effects

In an attempt to determine whether the reproductive endocrine system recovers normally after cessation of OC therapy, Klein and Mishell measured serum levels of FSH, LH, E_2, progesterone, and prolactin in six women every day for 2 months after they discontinued use of high-dose OCs. Except for a variable prolongation of the follicular phase of the first postcontraceptive cycle, the patterns and levels of all of these hormones were indistinguishable from those found in normal ovulating subjects. In these six women, the initial LH peak occurred from 21 to 28 days after ingestion of the last tablet. These results indicate that after a variable, but usually short, interval after the cessation of oral steroids, their suppressive effect on the hypothalamic–pituitary–ovarian axis disappears. After the initial recovery, completely normal endocrine function occurs.

As previously mentioned the delay in the return of fertility is greater for women discontinuing use of OCs with 50 μg of estrogen or more than with those containing lower doses of estrogen. However, use of the low-dose formulations still causes a significant reduction in time to conception rates, with a mean of 5.88 cycles for OC users, compared with 3.18 cycles for women discontinuing other contraceptive methods. Among women stopping use of OCs in order to conceive, the reduced probability of conception compared with women stopping use of other methods is greatest in the first month after stopping their use and decreases steadily thereafter (Fig. 14-9). There is little, if any, effect of duration of OC use on the length of delay of subsequent conception but the magnitude of the delay to return of conception after OC use is greater among older primiparous women than among others.

Thus, for about 2 years after the discontinuation of contraceptives in order to conceive, the rate of return of fertility is lower for users of OCs than for women who have used barrier methods, but eventually the percentage of women who conceive after ceasing to use each of these contraceptive methods becomes the same. Thus, the use of OCs does not cause permanent infertility.

Because the resumption of ovulation is delayed for variable periods after OCs are stopped, it is difficult to estimate the expected date of delivery if conception takes place before spontaneous menses return. If conception occurs before resumption of spontaneous menses, gestational age should be estimated by serial sonography. Neither the rate of spontaneous abortion nor the incidence of chromosomal abnormalities in abortuses is increased in women who conceive in the first or subsequent months after ceasing to use OCs.

Several cohort and case-control studies of large numbers of babies born to women who stopped using OCs have been under-

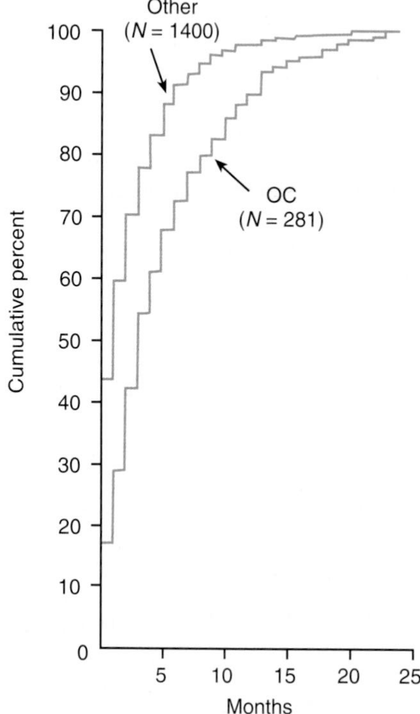

Figure 14-9. Cumulative conception rates for former oral contraceptive and other contraceptive users, Yale-New Haven Hospital 1980–1982. (Reprinted from Fertility and Sterility, 53, Bracken MB, Hellenbrand KG, Holford TR, Conception delay after oral contraceptive use: The effect of estrogen dose, 21. Copyright 1990, with permission from The American Society for Reproductive Medicine.)

taken. These studies indicate that these infants have no greater chance of being born with any type of birth defect than do infants born to women in the general population, even if conception occurred in the first month after the medication was discontinued. If OCs are accidentally ingested during the first few months of pregnancy, a large cohort study reported that there is no significantly increased risk of congenital malformations among the offspring of users overall or among those of nonsmoking users. Smokers who used OCs after conception had a threefold higher risk of delivering infants with anomalies than did the entire study group. Smoking by itself has been shown to have an adverse effect on reproductive outcome, increasing the risk of abortion. Although an increased risk of certain anomalies was reported in some case-control studies of women ingesting OCs after conception, the results could have been influenced by both recall bias and the confounding effect of smoking. A statement warning of a possible teratogenic effect of ingestion of OCs during pregnancy has been deleted from current product labeling for OCs.

Neoplastic Effects

OCs have been extensively used for more than 35 years, and numerous epidemiologic studies of both cohort and case-control design have been performed to determine the relation between use of these agents and the development of various types of neoplasms. Because as yet no elderly women have used OCs during their early reproductive years, the studies thus far published usually restrict the analysis to women younger than 65 years of age. The most comprehensive of these studies is an analysis of a large number of U.S. women from several geographic areas ages 20 to 54 with cancer initially diagnosed between 1980 and 1983 and an appropriate control group. This study, the Cancer and Steroid Hormone (CASH) study, was performed by the U.S. Centers for Disease Control and Prevention. Because hormones are mainly considered to be promoters, not initiators, of cancers, any adverse oncologic effects of these steroids should show a dose response, as demonstrated by an increased risk occurring with increased duration of use.

Breast Cancer

In 1996 a large, international collaborative group reanalyzed the entire worldwide epidemiologic data that had investigated the relation between risk of breast cancer and use of OCs. Analysis was performed on data from 54 studies performed in 25 countries, involving more than 53,000 women with breast cancer and more than 100,000 controls. The analysis indicated that while women took OCs they had a slightly increased risk of having breast cancer diagnosed (RR 1.24 [CI 1.15–1.30]). The magnitude of risk of having breast cancer diagnosed declined steadily after stopping OCs so there was no longer a significantly increased risk 10 or more years after stopping their use (RR 1.01 [CI 0.96–1.05]) It is of interest that the cancers diagnosed in women taking OCs were less advanced clinically than occurred in the nonusers. The risk of having breast cancer that had spread beyond the breast compared with a localized tumor was significantly reduced (RR 0.88 [CI 0.81–0.95]) in OC users compared with nonusers. The group concluded that these results could be explained by the fact that breast cancer is diagnosed earlier in OC users than in nonusers or could be due to biologic effects of the oral contraceptives. It was also found that women who had stopped using OCs more than 10 years earlier and developed breast cancer were significantly less likely to have nonlocalized disease than were women of similar age who had never used OCs. This reanalysis found that the risk of breast cancer diagnosis was not significantly altered by duration of oral contraceptive use, parity or family history of breast cancer. In this reanalysis 89% of the women with breast cancer initiated use of oral contraceptives before 1975 when formulations containing less than 50 μg of estrogen initially became available. Therefore, the data in this reanalysis are not relevant to breast cancer risk with OCs containing a low dose of estrogen. More recent data indicate there is a lack of association between OC use and increased breast cancer risk in users overall as well as those women with an increased risk of developing breast cancer.

A population-based case-control study by the National Institute of Child Health and Human Development Women's Contraceptive and Reproductive Experience (Women's CARE) analyzed the effect of OCs on breast cancer in women ages 35 to 64. The investigators interviewed 4575 women with breast cancer and 4682 controls between 1994 and 1998 and found there was no increased risk of breast cancer in current OC users (odds ratio [OR] 1.0, CI 0.8–1.3) and past users (OR .09, CI 0.8–1.0) compared with women who had never use OCs. There were also no significant difference in OC and breast cancer risk according to duration of OC use, age of first and last OC use, estrogen dose, and family history of breast cancer (Table 14-7). Marchbanks and the other investigators concluded that these data provide strong evidence that current or former use of OCs does not increase the risk of breast cancer in women ages 35 to 64. Another large case-control study performed in the United States, Canada, and Australia by Milne and colleagues analyzed women with breast cancer diagnosed before age 40 between 1992 and 1998. In this study there were 44 *BRCA-1* carriers, 36 *BRCA-2* carriers, and 1073 noncarriers. Like the Women's CARE study, this analysis showed no increased risk of breast cancer in *BRCA-1* or *BRCA-2* carriers or noncarries with OC use. The OR for OC ever use more than 1 year and breast cancer in noncarriers was 0.93 (CI 0.6 9–1.24), whereas for first OC use after 1975 the OR for OC use and breast cancer was 0.74 (CI 0.55–0.99) compared with never use or OC use less than 1 year. The OR for OC use and breast cancer in *BRCA-1* carriers was 0.22 (CI 0.10–0.49) and for *BRCA-2* carriers was 1.02 (CI 0.34–3.09) compared with no OC use or OC use less than 1 year. The results of these two studies indicate that women who use OCs with less than 50 μg of estrogen do not have an increased risk of developing breast cancer while they are taking OCs or after stopping OC use at least up to age 65. The risk of developing breast cancer with OC use is not changed in women with high risk of developing breast cancer, including women with an immediate family history of breast cancer and those with *BRCA-1* and *BRCA-2* mutations.

Cervical Cancer

The epidemiologic data regarding the risk of invasive cervical cancer as well as cervical intraepithelial neoplasia and OC use is conflicting. Confounding factors, such as the woman's age at first sexual intercourse, the number of sexual partners, exposure to human papillomavirus (HPV) (possibly greater among OC

Table 14–7 Risk of Breast Cancer According to the Use of Combination Oral Contraceptives*

Variable	Case Subjects (*N* = 4575)	Controls (*N* = 4682)	Odds Ratio (95% CI)
	NUMBER		
No use	1032	980	1.0
Any use	3497	3658	0.9 (0.8–1.0)
Current use†	200	172	1.0 (0.8–1.3)
Former use	3289	3481	0.9 (0.8–1.0)‡
Duration of use			
<1 yr	782	822	0.9 (0.8–1.1)
1 to <5 yr	1200	1280	0.9 (0.8–1.0)
5 to <10 yr	848	882	0.9 (0.8–1.0)
10 to <15 yr	426	466	0.8 (0.7–1.0)‡
≥15 yr	234	202	1.0 (0.8–1.3)
Age at first use			
<15 yr	72	79	0.9 (0.6–1.2)
15 to 19 yr	1239	1272	1.0 (0.8–1.1)
20 to 24 yr	1260	1369	0.9 (0.8–1.0)‡
25 to 29 yr	587	592	0.9 (0.8–1.1)
30 to 34 yr	209	239	0.8 (0.6–1.0)‡
35 to 39 yr	84	67	1.2 (0.8–1.6)
≥40 yr	38	35	1.0 (0.6–1.6)
Time since last use			
Current use	200	172	1.0 (0.8–1.3)
7 mo to <5 yr	165	207	0.7 (0.5–0.9)‡
5 to <10 yr	244	239	0.9 (0.8–1.2)
10 to <15 yr	426	418	0.9 (0.8–1.1)
15 to <20 yr	650	717	0.9 (0.7–1.0)
≥20 yr	1803	1899	0.9 (0.8–1.0)
High estrogen dose§			
Any use	1082	1265	0.8 (0.7–0.9)‡
Current use	7	10	0.7 (0.2–1.8)
Former use	1074	1255	0.8 (0.7–0.9)‡
Low estrogen dose			
Any use	1460	1560	0.9 (0.8–1.0)
Current use	183	160	1.0 (0.8–1.3)
Former use	1267	1398	0.9 (0.8–1.0)

*Odds ratios were derived by conditional logistic regression with the study site, race, and age (in five-year categories) as conditioning variables and were adjusted for menopausal status, age at menarche, age at menopause, number of term pregnancies, age at first term pregnancy, body-mass index, presence or absence of a family history of breast cancer, and use or nonuse of hormone-replacement therapy. Unknown oral-contraceptive formulations were classified as combination formulations. Missing values not included in one of the specified categories shown in Supplementary Appendix 1 were excluded. The reference group was the group of women who had never used oral contraceptives. Trend tests for the duration of use, age at first use, and time since last use were not significant at the 0.05 level. CI denotes confidence interval.

†Current use was defined as use of combination oral contraceptives within six months preceding the reference date.

‡The confidence interval does not include 1.0; some confidence limits were rounded to 1.0

§A high estrogen dose was defined as 50 μg or more of ethinyl estradiol or 75 μg or more of mestranol. A low estrogen dose was defined as less than 50 μg of ethinyl estradiol or less than 75 μg of mestranol.

From Marchbanks PA, McDonald JA, Wilson HG, et al: Oral contraceptives and the risk of breast cancer. N Engl J Med 346:2028, 2002.

users), cytologic screening (probably more frequent among OC users), and the use of barrier contraceptives or spermicides (primarily by women in the control group), as well as cigarette smoking (an independent risk factor for this disease), could account for the different results in different studies. In most of these studies statistical corrections were made for these confounding factors, and in many of them the control group did not use barrier methods of contraception. In 2002, the WHO commissioned a system review of published studies to determine the relation of hormonal contraceptives and cervical cancer. This review by Smith and colleagues in 2003 combined data from 28 studies, 4 cohort and 24 case-control, published between 1986 and 2002 which included data from 12,531 women with cervical cancer. The combined analysis found that the risk of cervical cancer, both invasive and in situ, increased with increasing duration of OC use, compared with the risk for those who had never used OCs. The summary relative risks for OC use of less than 5 years, 5 to 9 years, and 10 or more years were 1.1 (CI 1.1–1.2), 1.6 (CI 1.4–1.7), and 2.2 (1.9–2.4), respectively. The results were similar for squamous cell and adenocarcinoma as well as studies that adjusted for risk factors including HPV infection, number of sexual partners, cervical cytology screening, smoking, and use of barrier contraceptives.

There is no evidence that OC use alters the incidence or rate of the progression of cervical dysplasia to invasive cancer. Women with treated cervical dysplasia can use OCs.

Although it is uncertain whether OCs themselves increase the risk of cervical cancer, act as a cocarcinogen, or have no effect, users of OCs as a group are at high risk for cervical neoplasia and require at least annual screening of cervical cytology, especially if they have used OCs for more than 5 years.

Endometrial Cancer

Several case-control studies and cohort studies have examined the relation between OCs and endometrial cancer, and nearly all of these studies have indicated that the use of these agents has a protective effect against endometrial cancer, the third most common cancer among U.S. women. Women who use OCs for at least 1 year have an age-adjusted relative risk of 0.5 for development of endometrial cancer between ages 40 and 55 compared with nonusers. This protective effect is related to duration of use, increasing from a 20% reduction in risk with 1 year of use to a 40% reduction with 2 years of use to about a 60% reduction with 4 years of use. In Schlesselman's review of 10 studies of more than 1200 women with endometrial cancer, the risk of developing endometrial cancer was decreased by 54% with 4 years' use, 66% with 8 years' use, and 72% with 12 years' use (Fig. 14-10). This protective effect appears within 10 years of initial use and persists for at least 15 years after

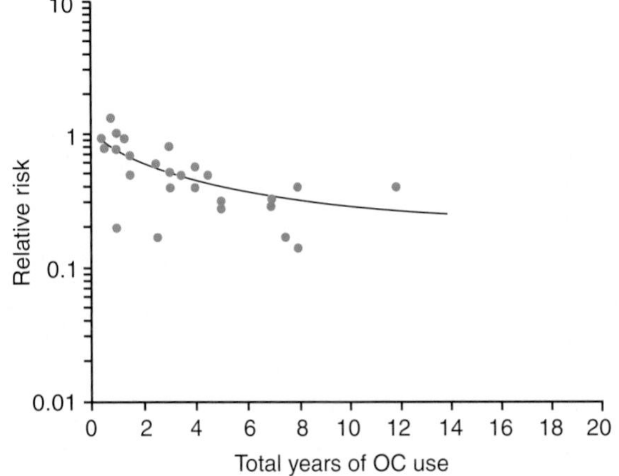

Figure 14-10. Relative risks of endometrial cancer by total years of oral contraceptive use. (From Schlesselman JJ: Net effect of oral contraceptive use on the risk of cancer in women in the United States. Obstet Gynecol 85:793, 1995.)

stopping use of OCs. In the study by Jick and associates of 142 cases of endometrial cancer among women 50 to 64 years of age the risk of endometrial cancer was decreased by 50% among former OC users compared with never users (RR 0.48, [CI 0.26–0.84]). The greatest protective effect is in nulliparous women (RR 0.2) or women of low parity, who are at greater risk of acquiring this disease. Voigt and coworkers reported the protective effect of OCs on endometrial cancer occurred with use of combination formulations with both high and low doses of progestin.

Ovarian Cancer

Numerous epidemiologic studies have consistently shown that more than 1 year of OC use reduces the risk of women developing ovarian cancer by about 30%, compared with women who never used OCs. In a review by Hankinson and associates of 20 epidemiologic studies, the summary relative risk of development of ovarian cancer among ever users of OCs was 0.64, a 36% reduction. OCs reduce the risk of the four main histologic types of epithelial ovarian cancer (serous, mucinous, endometrioid, and clear-cell) and the risk of both invasive ovarian cancers, as well as those with low malignant potential, is reduced. The magnitude of the decrease in risk is directly related to the duration of OC use, increasing from about a 40% reduction with 4 years of use, to a 53% reduction with 8 years of use, and a 60% reduction with 12 years of use (Fig. 14-11). Beyond 1 year there is about an 11% reduction in ovarian cancer risk for each of the first 5 years of use. The protective effect begins within 10 years of first use and continues for at least 30 years after the use of OCs ends. Studies by Ness and colleagues and Royar and coworkers found a similar level of protection with low-dose and high-dose formulations. The risk of developing ovarian cancer in the former study was 0.5 with use of low-estrogen/low-progestin formulations and 0.5 with high-estrogen/high-progestin formulations. In the latter study a similar 50% reduction in risk was reported for any type of formulation. OC use also reduces the risk of ovarian cancer in women with *BRCA-1* and *BRCA-2* mutations and with a family history of ovarian cancer to the same extent as in women without these risk factors. Two studies of OC use in women with the *BRCA* mutations found the risk of ovarian cancer is reduced by about 50% with OC use. As with endometrial cancer, the protective effect occurs mainly in women of low parity (≤4), who are at greatest risk for this type of cancer.

Liver Adenoma and Cancer

The development of a benign hepatocellular adenoma is a rare occurrence in long-term users of OCs, and the increased risk of this tumor was associated with prolonged use of high-dose formulations, particularly those containing mestranol. Although two British studies reported an increased risk of liver cancer among users of OCs, the number of patients was small and the results could have been influenced by confounding factors. The rate of death from the disease has remained unchanged in the United States over the past 25 years, a period when millions of women have used these agents. Data from a large, multicenter epidemiologic study coordinated by the WHO found no increased risk of liver cancer associated with OC users in countries with a high prevalence rate of this neoplasm. This study found no change in risk with increasing duration of use or time since first or last use.

Pituitary Adenoma

OCs mask the predominant symptoms produced by prolactinoma amenorrhea and galactorrhea. When OC use is discontinued, these symptoms occur, suggesting a causal relation. However, data from three studies indicate that the incidence of pituitary adenoma among users of OCs is not higher than that among matched controls.

Malignant Melanoma

Several epidemiologic studies have been undertaken to assess the relation of OC use and the development of malignant melanoma. A pooled analysis by Karagas and colleagues in 2002

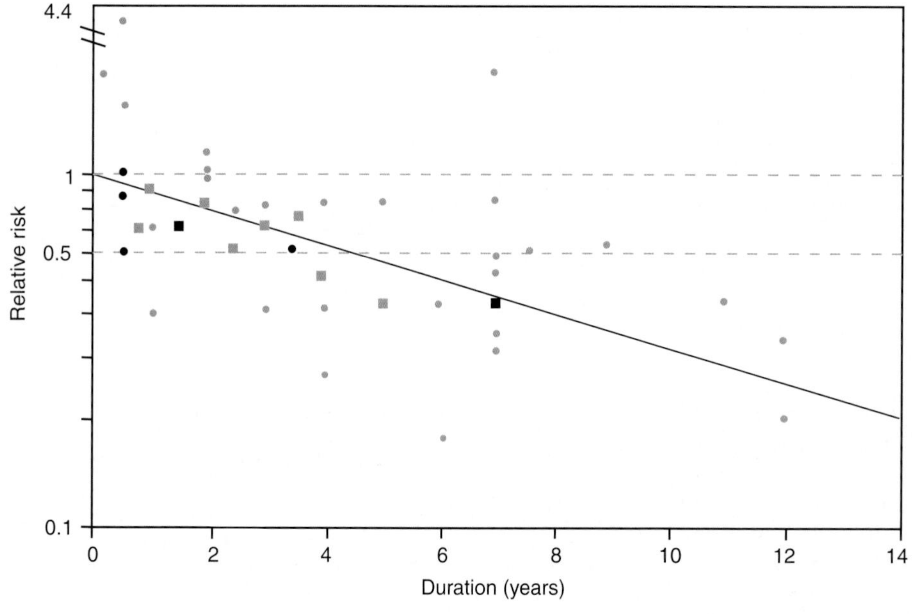

Figure 14-11. Relative risk of ovarian cancer associated with different durations of oral contraceptive use; findings of 15 studies. Study categories, indicating category weights ranging from smallest (weight in bottom 25% of range) to largest (weight in top 25% of range): blue circles = 1 (smallest); blue squares = 2; black circles = 3; black squares = 4 (largest). (From Hankinson SE, Colditz GA, Hunter DJ, Rosner B: A quantitative assessment of oral contraceptive use and risk of ovarian cancer. Obstet Gynecol 80:708, 1992.)

of 10 case-control studies found a pooled odds ratio of OC use more than 1 year compared with never use or use less than 1 year of 0.86 (CI 0.74–1.01). There was no relation of melanoma incidence and duration of OC use, current OC use, or years since last or first use with 2391 cases of melanoma. An analysis of the two large British cohort studies involving more than 40,000 women, which were initiated in 1968, reported that the adjusted RR of melanoma incidence developing in OC users was 0.92 and 0.85. The results of these large studies of long duration and the meta-analysis indicate that OC use does not alter the risk of development of malignant melanoma.

Colorectal Cancer

Several studies found that OC use reduces the risk of colorectal cancer. Fernandez and associates performed a meta-analysis of published studies of this relation. The pooled relative risk of OC ever use and colorectal cancer was 0.81 from eight case-control studies and 0.84 from four cohort studies. For colon cancer, the summary relative risk from 11 studies was 0.83 (CI 0.74–0.95) and for rectal cancer the summary relative risk from 6 studies was 0.74 (CI 0.59–0.93). Duration of use was not associated with decreased risk. Thus, OC use decreases the risk of developing both colon and rectal cancer.

Oral Contraceptive Use and Overall Mortality

In 1989 Vessey and colleagues reported the causes of mortality (through 1987) among OC users and nonusers enrolled in the Oxford Family Planning Association Cohort Study between 1968 and 1974. During this 20-year follow-up of 17,032 women, there were 238 deaths. The overall risk of death among the OC users was 0.9 (CI 0.7–1.2) compared with the women of similar age and socioeconomic status who used a diaphragm or condom for contraception. The risk of death from breast cancer in OC users compared with nonusers was 0.9 (CI 0.4–1.4), from cervical cancer 3.3 (CI 0.9–17.9), and from ovarian cancer 0.4 (CI 0.1–1.2). These cancer mortality rates are consistent with the other epidemiologic data reported earlier in this chapter. The death rate for circulatory disease was 1.5 (CI 0.7–3.0), and nearly all these deaths in OC users occurred in women who were also smokers. In 1994, Colditz and coworkers reported mortality rates among the 166,755 women enrolled in the Nurses Health Study in 1976 that were followed through 1980. A total of 2879 deaths occurred in this group of women, and the relative risk of death among ever users of OCs compared with never users was 0.93. There was no change in risk of death with long-term use. Among women who had used OCs for 10 or more years the relative risk of mortality was 1.06 compared with nonusers. There was no change in risk of deaths caused by cardiovascular disease or cancer. The risk of death from ovarian cancer was 0.79, from endometrial cancer 0.33, and from breast cancer 1.07. None of these differences were statistically significant. In 1999 Beral and colleagues reported mortality in the 25-year follow-up of the 46,000 women enrolled in the RCGP study. There were 1599 deaths reported. For current and recent (within 10 years) users, the risk of death from ovarian cancer was 0.2, cervical cancer 2.5, and cerebrovascular disease 1.9. Ten or more years after stopping OCs, mortality rates for all causes, as well as most specific causes, were similar in women who had and those who had not used OCs. The mortality rate for breast cancer was nearly identical in OC users and nonusers. It thus appears that high-dose OC use has no appreciable risk on overall mortality. With exclusive use of low-dose formulations given to women without cardiovascular risk factors who have frequent cervical cytologic screening, an overall beneficial effect on mortality with OC use may be expected.

Contraindications to Oral Contraceptive Use

OCs can be prescribed for the majority of women of reproductive age, because these women are young and generally healthy. However, there are certain absolute contraindications, including a history of vascular disease (thromboembolism, thrombophlebitis, atherosclerosis, and stroke) and systemic disease that may affect the vascular system (e.g., lupus erythematosus or diabetes with retinopathy or nephropathy). Cigarette smoking by OC users older than age 35 and uncontrolled hypertension are also contraindications. One of the contraindications listed in the product labeling is cancer of the breast or endometrium, although there are no data indicating that OCs are harmful to women with these diseases. Two other contraindications are undiagnosed uterine bleeding and elevated triglyceride levels.

Pregnant women should not ingest OCs, because it has been theorized that there is a masculinizing effect of the 19 norprogestins on the external genitalia of female fetuses. As mentioned earlier, concerns that OCs might produce other deleterious fetal effects, such as limb reduction and heart defects, have not proved valid. These concerns were raised by articles linking ingestion of any progestational agent in pregnancy to an increased incidence of congenital abnormalities. However, the major use of progestins in pregnancy had previously been for treatment of threatened abortion. Bleeding in pregnancy is itself associated with an increased incidence of anomalies. The incidence of birth defects has not decreased since the use of progestins for threatened abortion has been discontinued.

Women with functional heart diseases should not use OCs because the fluid retention they produce could result in congestive heart failure. There is no evidence, however, that individuals with asymptomatic mitral valve prolapse should not use OCs. Women with active liver disease should not take OCs. However, women who have recovered from liver disease, such as viral hepatitis, and whose liver function tests have returned to normal can safely take OCs.

Relative contraindications to OC use include heavy cigarette smoking younger than age 35, migraine headaches, undiagnosed causes of amenorrhea, and depression. About 20% of women have migraine headaches, and their frequency and severity can be worsened by OC use. There is no evidence that the risk of stroke is significantly increased in women with common migraine headaches who use OCs compared with non-OC users. Unless the women have aura or peripheral neurologic symptoms with the migraine headaches (classic migraine), OCs can be used. If fainting, temporary loss of vision or speech, or paresthesias develop in an OC user, the use of OCs should be stopped because of their hypercoaguable effect.

Since OC use may mask the symptoms produced by a prolactin-secreting adenoma amenorrhea and galactorrhea amenorrheic women should not receive OCs until the diagnosis for this symptom is established. If galactorrhea develops during OC use, OCs should be discontinued, and after 2 weeks a serum prolactin level should be measured. If elevated, further diagnostic evaluations are indicated. The presence of a prolactin-secreting macroadenoma, but not a microadenoma, is a contraindication for OC use. Use of OCs does not cause enlargement of prolactin-secreting pituitary microadenomas or worsen functional prolactinoma as was previously believed. Women with gestational diabetes can take low-dose OC formulations, because these agents do not affect glucose tolerance or accelerate the development of diabetes mellitus. Insulin-dependent diabetes without vascular disease is also not a contraindication for low-dose OC use.

Beginning Oral Contraceptives

Adolescents

In deciding whether a sexually active pubertal girl should use OCs for contraception, the clinician should be more concerned about compliance with the regimen than about possible physiologic harm. As long as she has demonstrated maturity of the hypothalamic–pituitary–ovarian axis with at least three regular, presumably ovulatory, menstrual cycles, it is safe to prescribe OCs without concern that their use will permanently alter future reproductive endocrinologic function. It is not necessary to be concerned about accelerating epiphyseal closure in the postmenarcheal female. Endogenous estrogens have already initiated the process a few years before menarche, and use of contraceptive steroids will not hasten it.

After Pregnancy

There is a difference in the relationship of the return of ovulation and bleeding between the postabortal woman and one who has had a full-term delivery. The first episode of menstrual bleeding in the postabortal woman is usually preceded by ovulation. After a full-term delivery, the first episode of bleeding is usually, but not always, anovulatory. Ovulation occurs sooner after an abortion, usually between 2 and 4 weeks, than after a full-term delivery, when ovulation is usually delayed beyond 6 weeks but may occur as early as 4 weeks in a woman who is not breast-feeding.

Thus, after spontaneous or induced abortion of a fetus of less than 12 weeks' gestation, OCs should be started immediately to prevent conception after the first ovulation. For women who deliver after 28 weeks and are not nursing, the combination pills should be initiated 2 to 3 weeks after delivery. If the termination of pregnancy occurs between 21 and 28 weeks, contraceptive steroids should be started 1 week later. The reason for delay in the latter instances is that the normally increased risk of thromboembolism occurring postpartum may be further enhanced by the hypercoagulable effects of combination OCs. Because the first ovulation is delayed for at least 4 weeks after a full-term delivery, there is no need to expose the woman to this increased risk.

Estrogen inhibits the action of prolactin in breast tissue receptors; therefore, the use of combination OCs (those containing both estrogen and progestin) diminishes the amount of milk produced by OC users who breast-feed their babies. Although the diminution of milk production is directly related to the amount of estrogen in the contraceptive formulation, only one study has been published in which the amount of breast milk was measured by breast pump in women using formulations with less than 50 μg of estrogen. In this study the use of this low dose of estrogen reduced the amount of breast milk. Thus, it is probably best for women who are nursing not to use combination OCs unless supplemental feeding is given to the infant.

Women who are breast-feeding every 4 hours, including during the night, will not ovulate until at least 10 weeks after delivery and thus do not need contraception before that time. Because only a small percentage of breast-feeding women will ovulate as long as they continue full nursing and remain amenorrheic, either a barrier method or a progestin-only OC can be used until menses resumes. Progestins do not diminish the amount of breast milk, and progestin-only OCs are effective in this group of women. Once supplemental feeding is introduced, ovulation can resume promptly and effective contraception is then needed. Combination OCs should be used once supplemental feeding is initiated.

Cycling Women

At the initial visit, after a history and physical examination have determined that there are no medical contraindications for OCs, the woman should be informed about the benefits and risks. For medicolegal reasons it is best to note on the patient's medical record that the benefits and risks have been explained to her.

Type of Formulation

In determining which formulation to use, it is best initially to prescribe a formulation with less than 50 μg of ethinyl estradiol, as these agents are associated with less cardiovascular risk as well as with fewer estrogenic side effects than formulations with 50 μg of estrogen. It would also appear reasonable to use formulations with the lowest androgenic potency of progestin, as there would be less androgenic metabolic and clinical adverse effects associated with their use. The development of multiphasic formulations has allowed the total dose of progestin to be reduced compared with some monophasic formulations, without increasing the incidence of breakthrough bleeding. However, several monophasic formulations have a lower total dose of progestin per cycle than the multiphasic formulations and the incidence of follicular enlargement is more frequent with multiphasic than with monophasic formulations.

The U.S. Food and Drug Administration (FDA) has stated that the product prescribed should be one that contains the least amount of estrogen and progestin that is compatible with a low failure rate and the needs of the individual woman. Because few randomized studies have been performed comparing the different marketed formulations, until large-scale comparative studies are performed, the clinician must decide on the formulation to use based on which has the least adverse effects among women in his or her practice. If estrogenic or progestogenic side effects occur with one formulation, a different agent with less estrogenic or progestogenic activity can be given.

The contraceptive formulations containing progestins and no estrogen have a lower incidence of adverse metabolic effects than do the combination formulations. Because the factors that predispose to thromboembolism are caused by the estrogen component, the incidence of thromboembolism in women ingesting these compounds is not increased. Furthermore, blood pressure is not affected, nausea and breast tenderness are eliminated, and milk production and quality are unchanged. Despite these advantages, these agents have the disadvantages of a high frequency of intermenstrual and other abnormal bleeding patterns (including amenorrhea) and a lower rate of effectiveness than the combined formulations. The failure rate of these preparations is higher than with the combined formulations, and a relatively high percentage of the pregnancies that do occur are ectopic. Since nursing mothers have reduced fertility and are amenorrheic, the major disadvantages of these preparations are minimized for these individuals. Furthermore, since milk production and quality are unaffected in contrast to the changes produced by combination pills, the formulations with only a progestin may be offered to these women while they are nursing. However, a small portion of these synthetic steroids have been detected in breast milk. The long-term effects (if any) of these progestins on the infant are not known, but none have been detected to date. A long-term follow-up study of breast-fed children whose mothers ingested 50 μg of estrogen in combined OCs while they were lactating revealed no difference in mean body weight or height up to 8 years of age compared with breast-fed children whose mothers did not ingest OCs. There was also no difference of occurrence of disease or in intellectual or psychological behavior between the two groups.

Follow-up

If a healthy woman has no contraindications to OC use, it is unnecessary to perform any laboratory tests, including cervical cytology, unless these are necessary for routine health maintenance. At the end of 3 months, the woman should be seen again; at this time a nondirected history should be obtained and the blood pressure measured. After this visit the woman should be seen annually, at which time a nondirected history should again be taken, blood pressure and body weight measured, and a physical examination (including breast, abdominal, and pelvic examination with cervical cytology) performed. It is important to perform annual cervical cytologic screening on OC users, as they are a relatively high-risk group for development of cervical neoplasia. The routine use of other laboratory tests is not indicated unless the woman has a family history of diabetes or vascular disease at a younger age. Routine use of these tests in women is not indicated because the incidence of positive results is extremely low. However, if the woman has a family history of vascular disease, such as MI occurring in family members younger than age 50, it would be advisable to obtain a lipid panel before OC use is started, as hypertriglyceridemia may be present and OC use will further raise triglycerides. Because the low-dose formulations do not adversely alter the lipid profile except for triglycerides it is not necessary to measure lipids, other than the routine cholesterol screening every 5 years, in women with no cardiovascular risk factors, even if they are older than 35. If the woman has a family history of diabetes or evidence of diabetes during pregnancy, a 2-hour postprandial blood glucose test should be performed before OCs are started, and if blood glucose is elevated, a glucose-tolerance test should be performed. If the woman has a history of liver disease, a liver panel should be obtained to make certain that liver function is normal before OCs are started.

Drug Interactions

Although synthetic sex steroids can retard the biotransformation of certain drugs (e.g., phenazone and meperidone) as a result of substrate competition, such interference is not important clinically. OC use has not been shown to inhibit the action of other drugs. However, some drugs can interfere clinically with the action of OCs by inducing liver enzymes that convert the steroids to more polar and less biologically active metabolites. Certain drugs (e.g., barbiturates, sulfonamides, cyclophosphamide, and rifampin) have been shown to accelerate the biotransformation of steroids in humans. Several investigators have reported a relatively high incidence of OC failure in women ingesting rifampin, and these two agents should not be given concurrently. The clinical data concerning OC failure in users of other antibiotics (e.g., penicillin, ampicillin, and sulfonamides), analgesics, and barbiturates are less clear. A few anecdotal studies have appeared in the literature, but reliable evidence for a clinical inhibitory effect of these drugs on OC effectiveness, such as occurs with rifampin, is not available. One study by Murphy and colleagues showed that when 2 g of tetracycline was given daily in divided doses the levels of both ethinyl estradiol and norethindrone in OC users were similar to those before antibiotic use. Women with epilepsy requiring medication probably should be treated with formulations containing 50 μg of estrogen, because a higher incidence of abnormal bleeding has been reported in these women with the use of lower dose estrogen formulations due to lower circulating levels of ethinyl estradiol brought about by the action of most antiepileptic medications.

Noncontraceptive Health Benefits

In addition to being one of the most effective method of contraception, OCs provide many other health benefits. Some are due to the fact that the combination OCs contain a potent, orally active progestin, as well as an orally active estrogen, and there is no time when the estrogenic target tissues are stimulated by estrogens without a progestin (unopposed estrogen).

Both natural progesterone and the synthetic progestins inhibit the proliferative effect of estrogen, the so-called antiestrogenic effect. Estrogens increase the synthesis of both estrogen and progesterone receptors, whereas progesterone decreases their synthesis. Thus, one mechanism whereby progesterone exerts its antiestrogenic effects is by decreasing the synthesis of estrogen receptors. Relatively little progestin is needed to exert this action, and the amount present in OCs is sufficient. Another way progesterone produces its antiestrogenic action is by stimulating the activity of the enzyme estradiol-17-β-dehydrogenase within the endometrial cell. This enzyme converts the more potent E_2 to the less potent estrone, reducing estrogenic action within the cell.

Benefits from Antiestrogenic Action of Progestins

As a result of the antiestrogenic action of the progestins in OCs, the height of the endometrium is less than in an ovulatory cycle, and there is less proliferation of the endometrial glands. These changes produce several substantial benefits for the OC user. One is a reduction in the amount of blood loss at the time of endometrial shedding. In an ovulatory cycle the mean blood loss during menstruation is about 35 mL, compared with

20 mL for women ingesting OCs. This decreased blood loss makes the development of iron deficiency anemia less likely for OC users than for nonusers. Data from the RCGP study showed that OC users were about half as likely to develop iron deficiency anemia as were controls. Moreover, the beneficial effect persisted to a similar degree in women who had previously used OCs and then stopped using them, probably because of an increase in the iron stores that remained for several years after the drug was discontinued.

Because OCs produce regular withdrawal bleeding, it would be expected that OC users would have fewer menstrual disorders than controls. The results of the RCGP study confirmed the fact that OC users were significantly less likely to have menorrhagia, irregular menstruation, or intermenstrual bleeding. Because these disorders are frequently treated by curettage or hysterectomy, OC users require these procedures less frequently than do nonusers.

Because progestins inhibit the proliferative effect of estrogens on the endometrium, as mentioned earlier, adenocarcinoma of the endometrium is significantly less likely to develop in women who use OCs.

Estrogen exerts a proliferative effect on breast tissue, which also contains estrogen receptors. Progestins may also inhibit the synthesis of estrogen receptors in this organ. Several studies have shown that OCs reduce the incidence of benign breast disease, and two prospective studies have indicated that this reduction is directly related to the amount of progestin in the compounds.

Data from the Oxford study indicate that current users of OCs have an 85% reduction in the incidence of fibroadenomas and 50% reductions in chronic cystic disease and nonbiopsied breast lumps, compared with controls using IUDs or diaphragms. The risk of development of these three diseases decreased with increased duration of OC use and persisted for about 1 year after discontinuation of OCs, after which no reduction in risk was observed. A large cohort study showed that long-term use of OCs was associated with a significant reduction in the diagnosis of benign breast disease of the proliferative type.

Benefits from Inhibition of Ovulation

Other noncontraceptive medical benefits of OCs result from their main action inhibition of ovulation. Some disorders, such as dysmenorrhea and premenstrual tension, occur much more frequently in ovulatory than in anovulatory cycles. In fact, inhibition of ovulation by exogenous steroids has been used for decades as therapy for severe dysmenorrhea. The RCGP study showed that OC users had 63% less dysmenorrhea and 29% less premenstrual tension than did controls. Another study indicated that OC users were less likely to have variation in the degree of feeling of well-being throughout the cycle than non-OC users.

Another potentially serious adverse effect of ovulatory menstrual cycles is the development of functional ovarian cysts—specifically, follicular and luteal cysts—that frequently require surgical management because of enlargement, rupture, or hemorrhage. When ovulation is inhibited, functional cysts do not usually develop. In a survey performed by the Boston Collaborative Drug Surveillance Program, less than 2% of women with a discharge diagnosis of functional ovarian cysts were taking OCs, in contrast to 20% of controls. However, 20% of women with nonfunctional cysts were taking OCs, an incidence similar to that observed in the controls. Although authors of one small case series postulated that the formation of functional ovarian cysts may be increased in users of multiphasic OCs, the rate of hospitalization for ovarian cysts in the United States has remained unchanged after the widespread use of multiphasic formulations.

Table 14–8 Rate Ratio Estimates for Functional Ovarian Cysts Comparing Each Oral Contraceptive Category with No Oral Contraception

	Rate Ratio*	95% Confidence Interval
No prescription	1.00	Reference category
Active prescription:		
Multiphasic	0.91	0.30–2.31
≤35 μg estrogen	0.52	0.17–1.33
>35 μg estrogen	0.24	0.01–1.34

*Rate ratios standardized to age distribution of index (i.e., "exposed") category.
From Lanes AF, Birmann B, Walter AM, Singer S: Oral contraceptive type and functional ovarian cysts. Am J Obstet Gynecol 166:956, 1992.

Lanes and colleagues studied the rate of functional cysts more than 2 cm in diameter by ultrasound, which required either hospitalization or outpatient surgery. They found that low-dose monophasic formulations resulted in about a 50% reduction in functional cysts, lower than the 75% reduction with high-dose formulations, whereas use of multiphasic formulations had only a slight reduction of ovarian cyst development (Table 14-8).

Another disorder linked to incessant ovulation is ovarian cancer. As mentioned earlier, the development of ovarian cancer is significantly reduced in OC users, with a duration-dependent decrease in risk.

Other Benefits

Several European studies, including the RCGP study, showed that the risk of development of rheumatoid arthritis in OC users was only about half that in controls. Another benefit is protection against salpingitis, commonly referred to as pelvic inflammatory disease (PID). At least 11 published epidemiologic studies have estimated the relative risk of PID developing among OC users. Seven of these studies compared OC use with nonuse of any other contraception. The relative risk of PID developing among OC users in most of these studies was about 0.5, a 50% reduction. It has been estimated that between 15% and 20% of women with cervical gonorrheal infection will develop salpingitis. In a Swedish study, all women with culture-proven cervical gonococcal infection had a diagnostic laparoscopy 1 day after hospital admission to determine whether salpingitis was present. Of those who used contraception other than the IUD and oral steroids, salpingitis developed in 15%; salpingitis developed in only about half as many, 8.8%, of those who used OCs. The results of this study indicate that OCs reduce the clinical development of salpingitis in women infected with gonorrhea. Although the incidence of cervical infection with *Chlamydia trachomatis* is increased in OC users compared with controls,

Wølner-Hanssen and coworkers reported that the incidence of chlamydial salpingitis in OC users was only half that of controls. This protection may be related to the decreased duration of menstrual flow, which permits a small number of organisms to ascend to the upper genital tract and allows the body's defenses to eliminate them more easily. One sequela of PID is ectopic pregnancy, an entity that has tripled in incidence in the past decade. OCs reduce the risk of ectopic pregnancy by more than 90% in current users and may reduce the incidence in former users by decreasing their chance of developing salpingitis.

Since the lower dose agents contain a progestin that inhibits estrogenic mitotic activity and also inhibits ovulation, the scope and magnitude of beneficial effects should be similar with all combination formulations currently marketed. It is unfortunate that the infrequent adverse effects of OCs have received widespread publicity, but the more common noncontraceptive health benefits have attracted little attention. In a study of women attending a Yale Health Center, about 80% of these well-educated women were unaware of these noncontraceptive health benefits. A nationwide survey sponsored by the American College of Obstetricians and Gynecologists also found that there was limited awareness of the noncontraceptive benefits of OCs by U.S. women, with less than half the women interviewed being aware of any benefit other than contraception.

There is also epidemiologic data that indicate that OCs reduce bone loss particularly in perimenopausal women with oligomenorrhea. Michaelsson and coworkers recently reported that OC use by women after the age of 40 decreased the risk of subsequent hip fracture. There are noncontraceptive health benefits associated with continuing OC use beyond age 40 into the perimenopausal years. There are limited data regarding metabolic risks of OC use by women older than 40, but Godsland and associates reported that there were no changes in cardiovascular risk markers with long-term OC use. Because the estrogen given for hormone replacement is not as thrombophilic as is the estrogen dose currently used in OCs, it is best to switch therapy at about age 50. To avoid discontinuing OC use when the woman is still ovulating, measurement of the FSH and E_2 levels on the last day of the pill-free interval provides information about ovarian follicular activity. If the FSH level is elevated and the E_2 level low, OCs may be discontinued and estrogen therapy begun.

LONG-ACTING CONTRACEPTIVE STEROIDS

To avoid contraceptive failure associated with the need to remember to take oral contraceptives daily, methods of administering contraceptive steroid formulations at infrequent intervals have been developed. To date, four types of long-acting steroids (injectable suspensions, subdermal implants, a contraceptive skin patch, and intravaginal ring) have been developed and are being used by women in the United States and elsewhere. The implant and progestin injections contain only a progestin without an estrogen, therefore, endometrial integrity is not maintained and uterine bleeding occurs at irregular and unpredictable intervals. Therefore, women wishing to use these methods need to be counseled beforehand about the development of irregular bleeding to enhance continuity of use.

Contraceptive Patch

A contraceptive skin patch with an area of 20 cm^2 has been marketed for several years. Each thin opaque matrix patch consists of three layers. These include an outer protective layer of polyester, an adhesive middle layer containing 75 μg ethinyl estradiol and 6.0 mg norelgestromin and a polyester release liner that is removed prior to placement on the skin. Norelgestromin is the active metabolite of the progestin norgestimate. Each patch delivering 150 μg norelgestromin and 20 μg ethinyl estradiol into the circulation each day at a fairly constant rate for at least 9 days. The woman applies one patch each week for 3 weeks and no patch for the following week to allow withdrawal bleeding. The patch may be applied to one of four anatomic sites: buttocks, upper outer arm, lower abdomen, or upper torso excluding the breasts. Following skin application both steroids appear in the circulation rapidly and reach a plateau within 48 hours. Mean serum levels of norelgestromin are between 600 and 800 pg/mL and for ethinyl estradiol are between 40 and 50 pg/mL. These steroid levels inhibit gonadotropin release and prevent ovulation. Contraceptive effectiveness and metabolic and clinical effects, including irregular bleeding, are similar to combination oral contraceptives. Efficacy may be less in women with body weight more than 90 kg. Rates of complete detachment of the patch from the skin are about 2%. The serum level area under the curve of ethinyl estradiol after patch application is higher than after ingestion of an oral contraceptive containing 30 μg ethinyl estradiol, but the peak levels of ethinyl estradiol are lower with the patch than the ring. The risk of venous thrombosis with this patch has been reported to be similar to that of women ingesting an oral contraceptive containing ethinyl estradiol and norgestimate.

Contraceptive Vaginal Ring

Steroids are also absorbed through the vaginal epithelium directly into the circulation. A flexible soft colorless ring-shaped device made of ethylene vinyl acetate copolymers with an outer diameter of 54 mm and a cross sectional diameter of 4 mm has been marketed for several years. Each ring contains 2.7 mg ethinyl estradiol and 11.7 mg etonogestrel. Etonogestrel (ENG) is the active metabolite of desogestrel. A ring is placed in the vagina for 21 days and then removed for 7 days to allow withdrawal bleeding. After this week a new ring is inserted by the woman. Since the steroids act systemically, the ring comes in only one size and does not have to be fitted or placed in a certain location. Following insertion of the ring the mean daily release of etonogestrel is 120 μg and ethinyl estradiol is 15 mcg. Serum levels of each steroid rise rapidly and plateau a few days after ring insertion. Mean ENG levels range between 1300 to 1600 pg/mL and mean ethinyl estradiol levels between 17 and 19 pg/mL. Like oral contraceptives, the main mechanism of action is inhibition of gonadotropins and prevention of ovulation. Each ring delivers sufficient steroids to inhibit ovulation for 5 weeks. Despite the low amount of ethinyl estradiol delivered each day, bleeding control is good. Irregular bleeding while the ring is in place is uncommon, occurring in 2.6% to 6.4% of cycles. Withdrawal bleeding of 4.7 to 5.3 days duration is initiated a few days after the ring is removed and occurs in 98% of treatment cycles. The area under the curve of ethinyl estradiol with the ring is about half that of a combination oral contraceptive containing 30 μg of ethinyl estradiol. Contraceptive effectiveness as well as metabolic and clinical effects are similar to combination oral contraceptives. Ring expulsion is uncommon.

Injectable Suspensions

Three types of injectable steroid formulations are currently in use for contraception throughout the world. These include depomedroxyprogesterone acetate (DMPA), given in a dose of 150 mg intramuscularly (IM) or 104 mg subcutaneously (SC) every 3 months; norethindrone enanthate, given in a dose of 200 mg every 2 months; and several once-a-month injections of combinations of different progestins and estrogens. Only the first of these three types is currently available in the United States. Injectable contraceptives are a popular method of contraception worldwide. In the United States they are used by about 3% of women of reproductive age.

Medroxyprogesterone acetate (MPA) is a 17-acetoxyprogesterone compound and is the only progestin used for contraception that is a C-21 progesterone derivative.

The 17-acetoxyprogestins, which do not have androgenic activity and are structurally related to progesterone instead of testosterone, were used in oral contraceptive formulations about 30 years ago. Although approved for contraception in many western countries in the 1960s, regulatory approval for these agents in the United States was stopped when tests on beagle dogs showed that ingestion of oral contraceptives with 17-acetoxyprogestins was associated with an increased risk of mammary cancer. It was discovered later that unlike humans and other animals the beagle uniquely metabolizes 17-acetoxyprogestins to estrogen, which causes mammary hyperplasia. Thus, when MPA is ingested by the beagle, it behaves differently than it does in the human, where it is not metabolized to estrogen. After epidemiologic studies showed that DMPA does not increase the risk of breast cancer in humans, regulatory approval for marketing this agent as a contraceptive was obtained in the United States in 1992.

Depot Formulation of MPA

MPA is a 17-acetoxy-6-methylprogestin that has progestogenic activity in the human (Fig. 14-12). Since MPA is not metabolized as rapidly as the parent compound progesterone, it can be given in smaller amounts than progesterone, with an equivalent amount of progestational activity. DMPA, the long-acting injectable formulation of MPA, consists of a crystalline suspension of this progestational hormone. The original contraceptive dosage with the intramuscular formulation (IM DMPA) is 150 mg DMPA, this agent is given by injection deep into the gluteal or deltoid muscle, after which the progestin is released slowly into the systemic circulation. The area should not be massaged, so that the drug is released slowly into the circulation and maintains its contraceptive effectiveness for at least 4 months. The newer subcutaneous formulation contains 104 mg of DMPA in 0.65 mL of diluent and is injected into the subcutaneous tissue of the anterior thigh or abdominal wall.

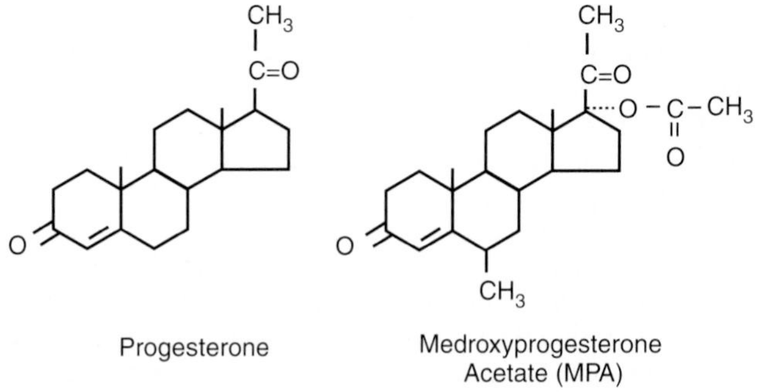

Figure 14-12. Comparative structures of progesterone and MPA.

DMPA is an extremely effective contraceptive. In a large WHO clinical trial studying use of IM DMPA, the pregnancy rate at 1 year was only 0.1%, and at 2 years the cumulative rate was 0.4%. Jain and colleagues reported the results of two interational large open-label phase 3 studies of SC-DMPA in which 1787 women were enrolled. The initial injection was given within 5 days thereafter of the onset of menses and every 91 + 7 days. A total of 16,023 woman-cycles of exposure were completed and no pregnancies occurred during the 1 year of the study. This study included a large number of overweight (BMI 25–30) and obese (BMI >30) women. In the American trial 44% of the women were overweight or obese and in the European/Asia trial, 27% of women were overweight or obese. This SC-DMPA, which delivers a lower total dose of MPA than IM DMPA, has a similar very high level of contraceptive effectiveness. Three mechanisms of action are involved. The major effect is inhibition of ovulation. Second, the endometrium becomes thin and does not secrete sufficient glycogen to provide nutrition for a blastocyst entering the endometrial cavity. Third, DMPA keeps the cervical mucus thick and viscous, so sperm are unlikely to reach the oviduct and fertilize an egg. With these multiple mechanisms of action, DMPA is one of the most effective reversible methods of contraception currently available.

Pharmacokinetics. MPA can be detected in the systemic circulation within 30 minutes after its IM injection. Although serum MPA levels vary among individuals, they rise steadily to contraceptively effective blood levels (>0.2 ng/mL) within 24 hours after both IM and SC injection.

The pattern of IM-MPA clearance from the circulation varies among different studies according to the type of assay used. After IM-DMPA was administered to three subjects, Ortiz and coworkers assayed blood MPA levels daily for 2 weeks, then three times a week for the next 3 months, and then weekly until MPA was undetectable. In two subjects MPA levels initially plateaued at 1.0 to 1.5 ng/mL for about 3 months, after which they declined slowly to about 0.2 ng/mL during the fifth month (Fig. 14-13). In a third subject, the blood levels were higher during the first month, then ranged between 1.0 and 1.5 ng/mL for the next 2 months, after which there was a further decline. MPA levels remained detectable in the circulation, above 0.2 ng/mL, for 7 to 9 months in all three subjects, after which it was not detectable. E_2 levels were found to be in the early to mid-follicular phase range, but consistently below 100 pg/mL during the first 4 months after injection. After 4 to 6 months, when

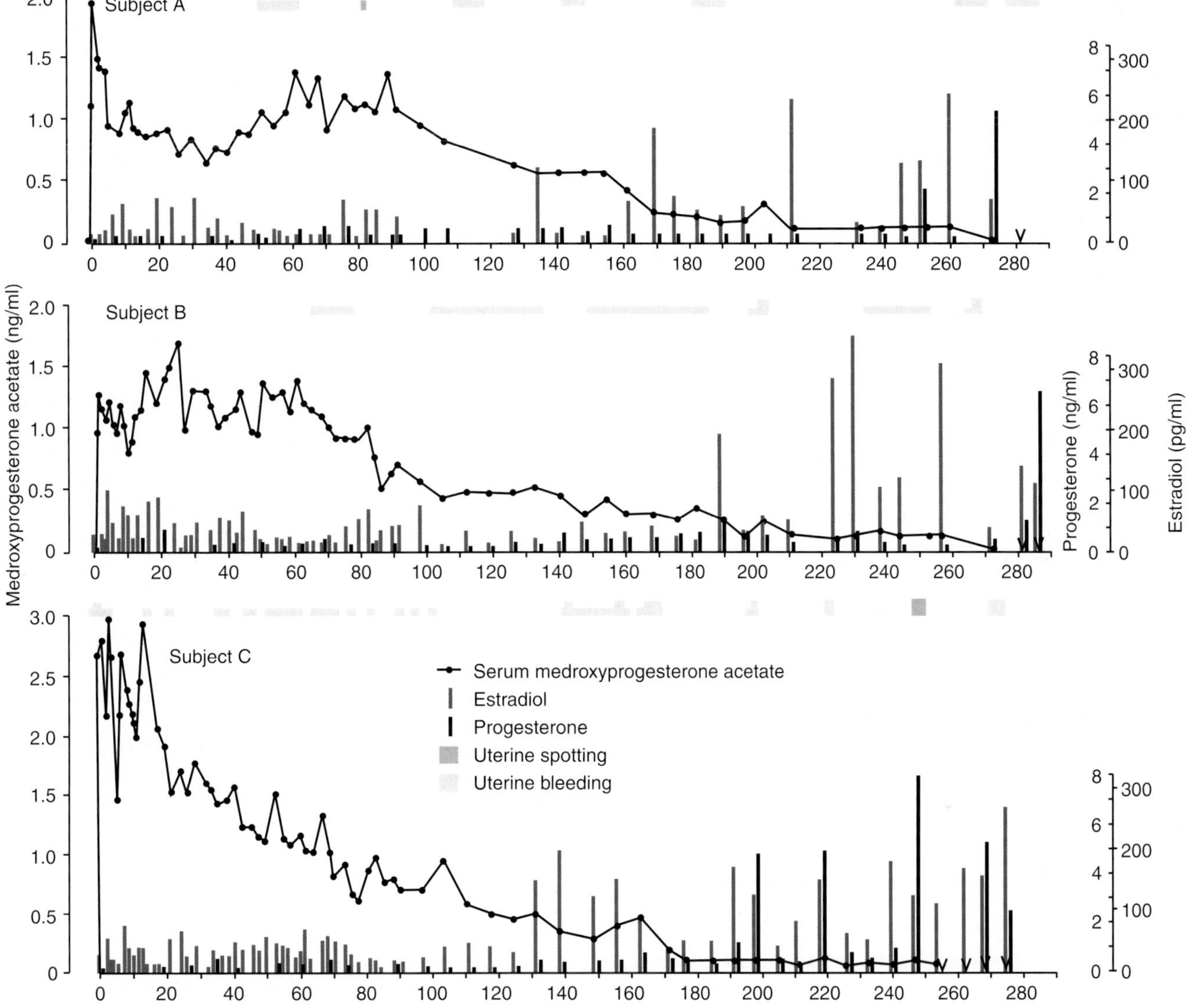

Figure 14-13. Serum MPA concentrations in three subjects during the first 24 hours after intramuscular injection of 150 mg of MPA. (From Ortiz A, Hiroi M, Stanczyk FZ, et al: Serum medroxyprogesterone acetate (MPA) concentrations and ovarian function following intramuscular injection of depo-MPA. J Clin Endocrinol Metab 44:32, 1977.)

MPA levels decreased to less than 0.5 ng/mL, E_2 concentrations rose to preovulatory levels, indicating follicular activity, but ovulation did not occur, as evidenced by persistently low progesterone levels. Return of follicular activity preceded the return of luteal activity by 2 to 3 months. This delay in resumption of luteal activity is probably due to the fact that the circulating MPA levels inhibit the positive feedback effect of the rise of E_2 on the hypothalamic–pituitary axis, which in the absence of MPA would stimulate the midcycle release of LH. The return of luteal activity in this study, indicated by a rise in serum progesterone levels, did not occur until 7 to 9 months after the injection, when the MPA levels were less than 0.1 ng/mL.

Following injections of SC-DMPA, absorption of MPA is rapid and rises above 0.2 ng/mL, the contraceptive effective level within 24 hours. Serum MPA levels peak about 8 days after the injection and gradually decline thereafter, but mean levels remain above 0.2 ng/mL (the contraceptively effective thresholds for about 4 months (Fig. 14-14).

Following injections of both IM-DMPA and SC-DMPA serum level of FSH, E_2, and progesterone are similar. FSH levels remain in the midfollicular range for 3 months without the midcycle FSH peak. E_2 levels remain suppressed and are similar to the levels on days 1 to 3 of a pretreatment control cycle (40 to 60 pg/mL). Progesterone levels are completely suppressed with both types of formulations. This ovarian follicular activity does occur after IM-DMPA and SC-DMPA, but ovulation is completely suppressed.

To obtain suppression of ovulation in the initial injection cycle, DMPA has to be administered within several days after the onset of menses. Siriwongse and coworkers reported that

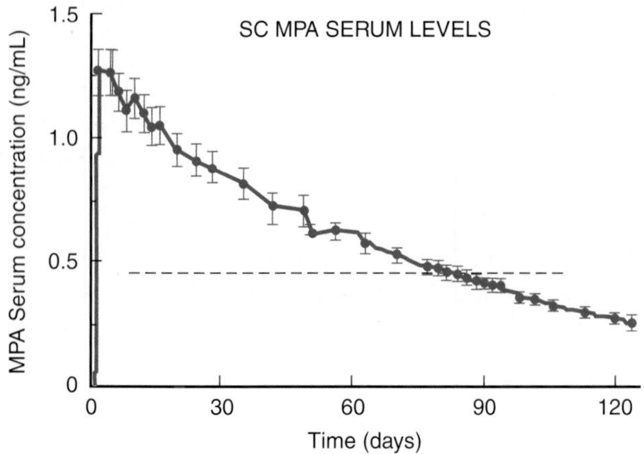

Figure 14-14. Serum medroxyprogesterone (MPA) levels after subcutaneous (SC) injection of an injection of depomedroxyprogesterone acetate.

when the drug was initially given on days 5 or 7 of the cycle none of the women ovulated but when it was given on day 9, 2 of 13 subjects had presumptive evidence of ovulation. The results of this study indicated that DMPA should be given no later than 7 days after the onset of menses to be effective in the first ovulatory cycle. The product labeling states that to ensure the woman is not pregnant at the time of the first injection, it must be given during the first 5 days of the cycle.

A cross-sectional study was performed by Mishell and associates on 121 women who received 150 mg of DMPA every 3 months for more than 1 year. An assay performed on a serum sample obtained on the day of the next scheduled injection showed marked differences in the E_2 levels, which varied from approximately 15 pg/mL to nearly 100 pg/mL (mean approximately 42 pg/mL) (Fig. 14-15). A similar range and mean value were also found among women who had been receiving DMPA for 1 to 2 years and those who had used it for 4 to 5 years. All these women had moist, well-rugated vaginas, and none stated that her breast size had decreased. None of the women complained of hot flushes. This use of contraceptive doses of DMPA does not decrease endogenous E_2 levels to the postmenopausal range and does not cause symptoms of estrogen deficiency.

Return of Fertility. Because of the lag time in clearing DMPA from the circulation after both IM-DMPA and SC-DMPA, resumption of ovulation is delayed for a variable period of time, which may last as long as 1 year after the last injection. In a recent study the median time for return to ovulation was 183 days for IM-DMPA and 212 days for SC-DMPA, a statistically insignificant difference. Women who wish to become pregnant and stop using DMPA should be informed that there will be a delay in the resumption of fertility until the drug is cleared from the circulation. After this initial delay, fecundity resumes at a rate similar to that found after discontinuing a barrier contraceptive (Fig. 14-16). Thus, use of DMPA does not prevent return of fertility; it only delays the time at which conception will occur. One year after the last DMPA injection, 94.7% of women receiving IM-DMPA and 97.4% of women receiving SC-DMPA had ovulated.

Because the half-life of the drug is constant, the return of fertility is not related to the number of injections that a woman receives. Schwallie and Assenzo reported that the median time to conception varied between 9 and 12 months after the last injection but did not differ according to the number of injections. With 10 or more injections, the median delay to the onset of fertility is similar to that in a woman who received only a few injections. Jain and colleagues reported that BMI and race did

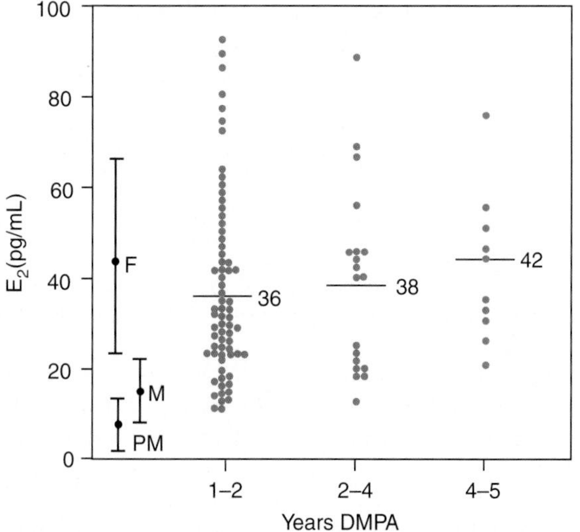

Figure 14-15. Serum estradiol (E_2) levels in 121 women who had used depomedroxyprogesterone acetate (DMPA) for contraception for more than 1 year. The horizontal bar in each time period represents the mean value. Vertical bars represent mean (λ) ± SD of serum estradiol levels in cycling women in the early follicular phase (F), normal males (M), and postmenopausal women (PM). (From Mishell DR Jr, Kharma KM, Thorneycroft IH, Nakamura RM: Estrogenic activity in women receiving an injectable progestogen for contraception. Am J Obstet Gynecol 113:372, 1972.)

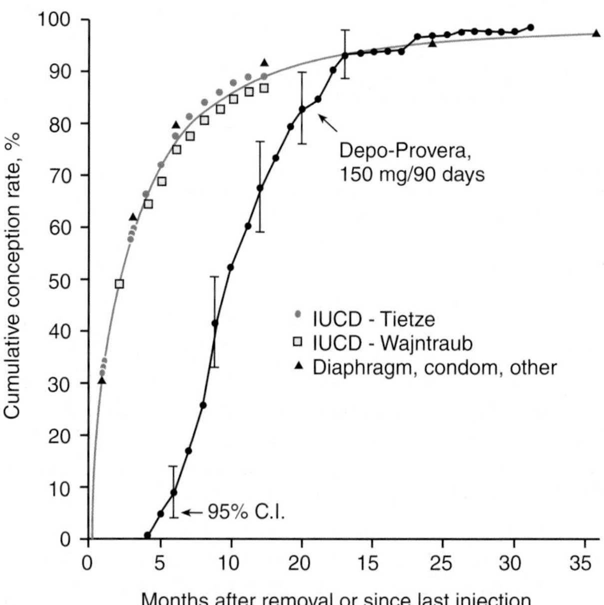

Figure 14-16. Cumulative conception rates of women who discontinued a contraceptive method to become pregnant. IUCD, intrauterine contraceptive device. (From Schwallie PC, Assenzo JR: The effect of depomedroxyprogesterone acetate on pituitary and ovarian function, and the return of fertility following its discontinuation: A review. Contraception 10(2):181, 1974.)

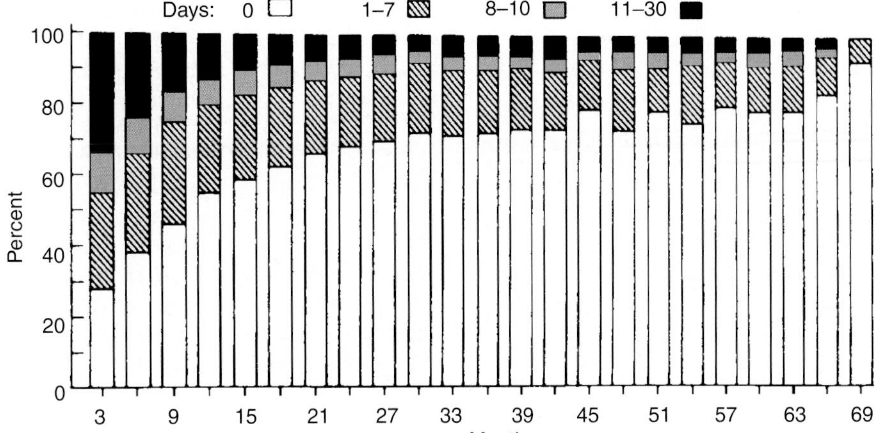

Figure 14-17. Percentage of patients with bleeding or spotting on days 0, 1–7, 8–10, or 11–30 per 30-day cycle while receiving injectable DMPA, 150 mg, every 3 months. (Reprinted from Fertility and Sterility, 24, Schwallie PC, Assenzo JR, Contraceptive use—efficacy study utilizing medroxyprogesterone acetate administered as an intramuscular injection once every 90 days, 331. Copyright 1973, with permission from The American Society for Reproductive Medicine.)

not affect the duration until ovulation resumed after an injection of SC-DMPA.

These investigators did find that the median time to conception after DMPA was discontinued varied according to body weight. As body weight increased, there was a similar concomitant increase in the median time to resumption of conception, most likely because the drug had been absorbed into adipose tissue and not cleared as rapidly.

Endometrial Changes. The histology of the endometrium at various intervals after starting DMPA was examined by Mishell and coworkers. Histologic examination of endometrial biopsies revealed three types of patterns: proliferative, quiescent, and atrophic. Secretory endometrium was not seen. Most of the women had a quiescent pattern, characterized by narrow, widely spaced glands and decidualization of the stroma.

Endometrial biopsies were performed at intervals of 1.5, 3, 6, 9, and 12 months after the first DMPA injection in a group of women receiving DMPA every 3 months. About half the biopsies showed that proliferative endometrium was present 6 weeks after the first injection. The percentage of women with proliferative endometrium then steadily declined, and after the second injection, less than 10% of the biopsy specimens showed proliferative tissue. The majority of the biopsy specimens showed a quiescent type of endometrium, but after 1 year of DMPA, about 40% of the specimens were characterized as atrophic.

Adverse Effects

Clinical. The major side effect of both IM-DMPA and SC-DMPA is complete disruption of the menstrual cycle. In the first 3 months after the first injection, about 30% of women are amenorrheic and another 30% to 40% have irregular bleeding and spotting occurring more than 11 days per month. The bleeding is usually light in amount and does not cause anemia to occur. As duration of therapy increases, the incidence of frequent bleeding steadily declines and the incidence of amenorrhea steadily increases, so that at the end of 1 year about 55% of women with both SC-DMPA and IM-DMPA are amenorrheic. After 2 years about 70% of the women treated with IM-DMPA are amenorrheic (Fig. 14-17). Women who use this method of contraception should be counseled that with time the irregular bleeding episodes will cease and amenorrhea will most likely occur.

After treatment with IM-DMPA is discontinued, about half of the women resume a regular cyclic menstrual pattern within 6 months and about three fourths have regular menses within 1 year. When bleeding does resume after the effect of the last injection is dissipated, it is initially regular in about half the women and irregular in the remainder. In a study involving 36 women who stopped using IM-DMPA, Gardner and Mishell reported that in the first 3 months, 27 women were amenorrheic, and 9 had irregular menses, which was usually characterized as spotting. During the next 3 months, about half the women began regular menses. The incidence of regular menses steadily increased, and 2 years after the last injection all the women were having regular menses or were pregnant. In this group of women, amenorrhea did not persist for more than 6 months after the last injection.

Weight Changes. In five cross-sectional studies, users of IM-DMPA weighed more than a comparison group not using hormonal contraceptives. Several longitudinal studies have indicated that IM-DMPA users gain between 1.5 and 4 kg in their first year of use and continue to gain weight thereafter. In the studies of SC-DMPA by Jain and colleagues the median weight change was an increase of 1.7 and 1.0 kg, respectively, after 1 year in the two groups. None of these studies included a control group so the weight could be due to factors other than DMPA use. In one retrospective, comparative, longitudinal study Moore and associates found no significant change in mean weight of DMPA, progestin implant, and oral contraceptive users. Thus, the effect among DMPA on body weight remains unclear. If DMPA users gain weight they should be counseled to decrease caloric intake and increase their exercise.

Mood Changes. The product labeling lists depression and mood changes as side effects of DMPA. Several studies, however, indicate that the incidence of depression and mood change in women using this method of contraception is less than 5%. No clinical trials with a comparison group not using DMPA have been performed to determine whether a causal relation between use of DMPA and development of depression exists.

Headache. Although development of headaches is the most frequent medical event reported by DMPA users and a common reason for discontinuation of its use, there are no comparative studies to indicate that use of DMPA increases the incidence or severity of tension or migraine headaches. Therefore, the presence of migraine headaches is not an absolute contraindication for use of DMPA. However, women should be counseled that if the frequency or severity of headaches increases after the injection is given it may be several months before the drug is cleared from the circulation. For this reason the presence of migraine headaches may be considered to be a relative contraindication for use of DMPA.

Metabolic Effects

Protein. Because DMPA does not increase liver globulin production as does the estrogen component of oral contraceptives (ethinyl estradiol), no alteration in blood-clotting factors or angiotensinogen levels is associated with its use. Thus, unlike OCs, DMPA has not been associated with an increased incidence of hypertension or thromboembolism. A WHO study reported that mean blood pressure measurements were unchanged in IM-DMPA users after 2 years of injections. In the 1-year studies of SC-DMPA there were no significant changes in blood pressure.

Carbohydrate. There have been two studies in which oral glucose tolerance tests have been performed on long-term IM-DMPA users and matched controls not using hormonal contraceptives. The mean glucose levels were slightly greater among the IM-DMPA users than among the controls in one, but not the other, study. Mean insulin levels were also higher. The slight deterioration in glucose tolerance among IM-DMPA users is probably not clinically significant and returns to normal after stopping use of IM-DMPA.

Lipids. Westhoff reviewed the findings of 11 studies that evaluated plasma lipids among groups of women using DMPA. Most of the studies were cross-sectional and compared lipid levels among DMPA users with women not using hormonal methods of contraception. There was little or no change in mean triglyceride and total cholesterol levels, but in all seven studies in which mean HDL cholesterol levels were measured, the levels were lower among the DMPA users. Of the five studies in which LDL cholesterol was measured, three noted an increase among the DMPA users. There are no studies in which the incidence of cardiovascular events among current or former long-term DMPA users was compared with the incidence among controls. Therefore, although the lipid changes with DMPA use are not beneficial, there is no evidence to date that they are associated with an acceleration of atherosclerosis.

Bone Loss. Several observational studies performed in several different countries with women of different ethnic groups indicate that the use of DMPA is associated with some degree of bone loss. The amount and location of the bone loss varied in the different studies, as well as the age groups most likely to experience this problem when using DMPA. Although there are scant data, the bone loss appears reversible after stopping use of DMPA. There are also no reports of an increased risk of fractures in DMPA users. It would appear useful to encourage calcium intake of 1500 mg/day in adolescent DMPA users. Measurement of bone mineral density is unnecessary because bone density increases after stopping DMPA.

Neoplastic Effects. Approval of DMPA for contraceptive use in the United States was delayed for many years because of concern about a causal relation between use of this agent and an increased risk of cervical, breast, and endometrial cancer. These concerns were raised because of studies showing an increased risk of abnormal cervical cytology in women using DMPA and studies reporting an increased risk of breast cancer in beagle dogs treated with DMPA and endometrial cancer in monkeys receiving long-term DMPA. These neoplastic concerns were found to be unwarranted as a result of several large epidemiologic studies, the majority of which were undertaken by the WHO. In the WHO studies the risk of neoplasia development among a large group of DMPA users in three countries (Kenya, Thailand, and Mexico) was investigated.

Breast Cancer. Two large case-control studies, the WHO study and a New Zealand study, indicated that the relative risk of developing breast cancer among all DMPA users was not significantly increased (RR of 1.2 [CI 0.96–1.15] and 1.0 [CI 0.8–1.3], respectively). When the data from these studies were pooled, the overall breast cancer risk among DMPA users was 1.1 (CI 0.97–1.4). In long-term users, that is, in those who had used the drug more than 5 years and those who had started use more than 14 years earlier, the risk of developing breast cancer was also not increased (RR of 1.0 [CI 0.70–1.5] and 0.89 [CI 0.6–1.3], respectively). However, among those women who had started use within the past 5 years and were mainly younger than age 35 there was a significant increased risk of developing breast cancer (RR 2.0 [CI 1.5–2.8]), similar to that found with use of oral contraceptives and women with first-term pregnancy at an early age. Thus, DMPA, like other contraceptive steroids, does not appear to change the overall incidence of developing breast cancer and women should be counseled accordingly.

Endometrial Cancer. A WHO case-control study found the risk of developing endometrial cancer to be significantly reduced among DMPA users (RR 0.21 [CI 0.06–0.79]). This reduction in risk persisted for at least 8 years after stopping use and was similar in magnitude to the protective effect observed with combination oral contraceptives.

Ovarian Cancer. In a WHO case-control study the risk of developing ovarian cancer among DMPA users was unchanged (RR 1.07 [CI 0.6–1.8]). These findings do not demonstrate a protective effect similar to that observed with oral contraceptives despite inhibition of ovulation with both agents. The lack of a protective effect observed with DMPA was probably due to the fact that in the countries studied DMPA was given only to multiparous women, women at low risk of developing epithelial ovarian cancer, who differ from the higher risk women of low parity taking oral contraceptives.

Cervical Cancer. In a large WHO case-control study the risk of developing invasive cancer of the cervix was not increased (RR 1.1 [CI 0.96–1.29]), similar to findings observed in a large case-control study in Costa Rica. Long-term use and a long time since first use were also not associated with a significant increase in risk of cervical cancer in these studies. The risk of developing cancer in situ was slightly increased in the WHO study (RR 1.4 [CI 1.2–1.7]), but not in the Costa Rica study (RR 1.0 [CI 0.6–1.8]) or two New Zealand studies investigating the risk of cancer dysplasia. Thus, the reports in which the neoplastic effects of DMPA on breast and reproductive tract neoplasia have been investigated are very reassuring.

Noncontraceptive Health Benefits. Cullins reported that there is good epidemiologic evidence that use of DMPA reduces the risk of developing iron deficiency anemia, PID, and endometrial cancer. It has a beneficial effect on hematologic

Noncontraceptive Health Benefits of Contraceptive Use of DMPA: Reduced Risk of the Following Disorders

Definite
Salpingitis
Endometrial cancer
Iron deficiency anemia
Sickle cell problems

Probable
Ovarian cysts
Dysmenorrhea
Endometriosis
Epileptic seizure
Vaginal candidiasis

parameters in women with sickle cell disease and reduces their incidence of clinical problems (see above box). DMPA also reduces seizure frequency in women with epilepsy and probably reduces the incidence of primary dysmenorrhea, ovulation pain, and functional ovarian cyst because it inhibits ovulation. DMPA also reduces the symptoms of endometriosis and in two small studies it reduced the incidence of vaginal candidiasis.

Clinical Recommendations. Women should be thoroughly counseled about the occurrence of abnormal bleeding and development of amenorrhea with use of DMPA prior to receiving the first injection. It has been shown that pretreatment counseling improves continuation rates. In addition, women should be counseled that the duration of action may last as long as 1 year following the last injection if they decide to discontinue use in order to become pregnant or because of side effects.

In cycling women the initial injection should be given no later than day 5 of the cycle to be certain to inhibit ovulation in the initial treatment cycle. Because of an absence of thrombogenic effects, the first injection should be given within 5 days postpartum in nonlactating women but for women who exclusively breast-feed their infants the product labeling states that the first injection should not be given until at least 6 weeks postpartum. DMPA does not affect the quantity or quality of breast milk or the health of children who breast-feed during its use. If a woman with lactational amenorrhea wishes to commence DMPA use and if a qualitative test for human chorionic gonadotropin (HCG) is negative, it is unlikely she is pregnant and therefore can receive the injection at that time. If concern about pregnancy exists, use of a barrier contraceptive should be advised for 2 additional weeks, at which time the assay for HCG should be repeated. If it is still negative, the injection can be given. A similar protocol can be utilized for the woman who has previously received DMPA but is delayed beyond 13 weeks in returning for her next injection and is still amenorrheic. If accidental pregnancy does occur in a woman receiving DMPA, there is no evidence that the agent is teratogenic or adversely affects the outcome of the pregnancy.

Norethindrone Enanthate

Norethindrone enanthate (NET-EN) is another injectable progestagen that has been approved for contraceptive use in more than 40 countries but not in the United States. It is administered in an oil suspension and thus has pharmacodynamics different from those of DMPA. Because of a shorter duration of action, it is recommended that NET-EN be given every 60 days for at least the first 6 months and no less often than every 12 weeks thereafter. The WHO recommends that the drug be given at intervals no shorter than 46 days and no longer than 74 days.

Progestin-Estrogen (Once Monthly) Injectable Formulations

Because the major reason for discontinuance of all progestin injectable contraceptives is menstrual irregularity, several combined progestin–estrogen injectables designed for once-a-month administration and production of regular withdrawal bleeding have been developed. They consist of a low dose of a long-acting progestin plus a small amount of an E_2 ester. Although many different formulations have been developed, currently four of them are most widely used. An injectable formulation containing 17α-hydroxyprogesterone caproate, 250 mg, and estradiol valerate, 5 mg, estimated to be used by at least 1% of all contraceptive users in China. A combination of dihydroxyprogesterone acetophenide, 150 mg, plus estradiol enanthate, 10 mg, is widely used in Mexico and other Latin American countries and is marketed under different brand names. The WHO has developed two formulations that are being used by several national family planning programs. A combination of MPA, 25 mg, and estradiol cypionate, 5 mg, is marketed as Cyclofem and also called Cycloprovera. This agent was approved for marketing in the United States with the name Lunelle, but is currently not being sold. The last compound is a combination of norethisterone enanthate, 50 mg, and estradiol valerate, 5 mg, called Mesigyna. Lunelle is formulated as a microcrystalline suspension given in 0.5 mL of an aqueous solution, and Mesigyna is formulated in 1 mL of an oil solution of castor oil and benzyl benzoate, 60:40. Both of these formulations are administered as deep IM injections into the deltoid, anterior thigh or gluteal muscle every 23 to 33 days (28 ± 5 days), with the first injection being given between 1 to 5 days after the onset of menses. The E_2 levels peak at 250 pg/mL 2 to 7 days after the injection and gradually decline thereafter reaching half the peak 8 days later at which time uterine bleeding usually occurs. E_2 levels fall to baseline about 2 weeks after the injection. MPA levels peak about 3 days after injection at 1.25 ng/mL. Levels decline slowly with a half-life of 14.7 days. Nondetectable levels are reached between 63 to 84 days. Steady-state conditions are reached after the first injection. Ovulation is inhibited for 63 to 112 days after the injection, after which there is a prompt return of fertility.

Newton and colleagues summarized the results of clinical trials with these compounds. The combined preparations offered better cycle control and less intermenstrual spotting than did the progestagen-only preparations of MPA and norethisterone enanthate. Amenorrhea rates were also lower with the combination injections, and about 85% of all cycles were regular following the first early bleed about 15 days after the first injection.

The results of five clinical trials with Mesigyna and Lunelle demonstrated a high level of effectiveness, with 12-month pregnancy rates of 0.4% or less for Mesigyna and 0.2% or less for Lunelle. Rates of discontinuation for amenorrhea varied between 0.8% and 4.2% for Mesigyna and 2.1% and 5.2% for Lunelle. Those for bleeding-related reasons were 5.4% to 12.0% with Mesigyna and 6.3% to 12.7% with Lunelle. The main bleeding disturbances were heavy, prolonged, and irregular bleeding.

Results of a 1-year nonrandomized U.S. study of Lunelle and a combination OC were reported by Kaunitz and coworkers. No pregnancies occurred in the 782 women accumulating 8008 woman-cycles of use with Lunelle. After 3 months regular menses occur in women treated with both the injection and OC, but bleeding irregularities were more common with the injection. Also women receiving the injection had more days of bleeding and spotting than those receiving the OCs as well as greater variability of cycle length. The WHO task force that studied Lunelle found no significant changes in the hemostatic parameters, lipid levels, or carbohydrate metabolism with Lunelle, and in clinical studies involving more than 12,000 women no venous or arterial cardiovascular events were recorded. Indications and contraindications for Lunelle are similar to oral contraceptives.

Subdermal Implants

Subdermal implants of capsules made of polydimethylsiloxane (Silastic) containing levonorgestrel for use as contraceptives were developed by the Population Council and patented with the name Norplant. Clinical trials of this long-acting, effective, reversible method of contraception were initiated in 1975. Norplant was approved by the FDA in 1990, and marketing in this country began in 1991, but this method of contraception is no longer sold in the United States. As with all steroid-containing Silastic devices, the rate of steroid delivery is directly proportional to the surface area of the capsules, whereas duration of action depends on the amount of steroid within the capsules. To produce effective blood levels of norgestrel, it was found necessary to use six capsules filled with crystalline levonorgestrel. The cylindrical capsules are 3.4 cm long and 2.4 mm in outer diameter, with the ends sealed with Silastic medical adhesive. Each capsule contains 36 mg of crystalline levonorgestrel for a total amount of 215 mg in each six-capsule set.

Insertion is performed in an outpatient setting, and the entire procedure takes about 5 minutes. After infiltration of the skin with local anesthesia, a 3-mm incision is made with a scalpel, usually in the upper arm, although the lower arm, the inguinal, scapular, and gluteal regions have also been used. When the capsules are inserted in any area of subcutaneous tissue, the steroid diffuses into the circulation at a relatively constant rate. The capsules are implanted into the subcutaneous tissue in a radial pattern through a 10- to 12-gauge trocar, and the incision is closed with adhesive. Sutures are not necessary. Because polydimethylsiloxane is not biodegradable, the capsules have to be removed through another incision when desired by the user or at the end of 5 years, which is the duration of maximal contraceptive effectiveness.

The removal process is, like the insertion procedure, performed in the clinic area, using local anesthesia and a small skin incision. Removal of Norplant is a more difficult process than insertion, because fibrous tissue develops around the capsule and must be cut prior to removing the capsules. It is important to insert the capsules superficially to enhance the ease of removal; deeply implanted capsules are more difficult to remove.

Manufacture of the capsules is complicated, and placing or removing six capsules creates some difficulties; therefore, norgestrel has been fabricated into solid rods that are a homologous mixture of Silastic and crystalline levonorgestrel covered with Silastic tubing. The rods are easier to manufacture, insert, and remove than the capsules. Because of different properties of diffusion, higher blood levels of norgestrel are achieved with a smaller total surface area of the rods. Thus, with two 4-cm covered rods with the same diameter as the capsules, the same release rate for norgestrel, about 50 μg/day, can be achieved as with placement of six 3-cm capsules. During a 5-year clinical study comparing rods and capsules, the serum norgestrel levels, bleeding patterns, and incidence of elevated progesterone levels were similar. A multicenter clinical study has confirmed these findings, and use of the two covered rods has been approved by the FDA for clinical use for 3 years. Nevertheless, the manufacturer has to date not decided to market the two-rod system, which is named Jadelle in the United States.

Single implants with other progestins have been manufactured and studied in clinical trials. These implants have a duration of action of 3 years, are extremely effective, and are much easier to insert and remove than the multiple levonorgestrel-releasing implants. A single ethylene vinyl acetate 4-cm long implant containing ENG (3-keto desogestrel) is only 2 mm in diameter and can be inserted through a trochar (Fig. 14-18). This implant is composed of a solid core of 40% ethylene vinyl acetate (EVA) with 60% crystals of the progestin etonogestrel, weighing 68 mg, imbedded within the core. The core is surrounded by a thin layer, 0.06 mm thick, of EVA that controls the rate of release of ENG. Etonogestrel is the active metabolite of desogestrel and has high progestational activity but weak androgenic activity. This implant should be inserted in the subcutaneous tissue of the nondominant arm about 6 to 8 cm above the elbow in the crease between the biceps and triceps muscles through the preloaded sterile applicator. No incision is necessary for insertion, but local anesthesia should be used. It is recommended that the implant is inserted during the first 5 days of the cycle. Removal of the implant is performed by making a 2-mm incision at the tip of the implant and pushing the rod until it pops out. Etonorgestrel is rapidly released from the implant, with about 60 μg/day being released during the first 2 months, which gradually declines to a release of 30 μg/day at

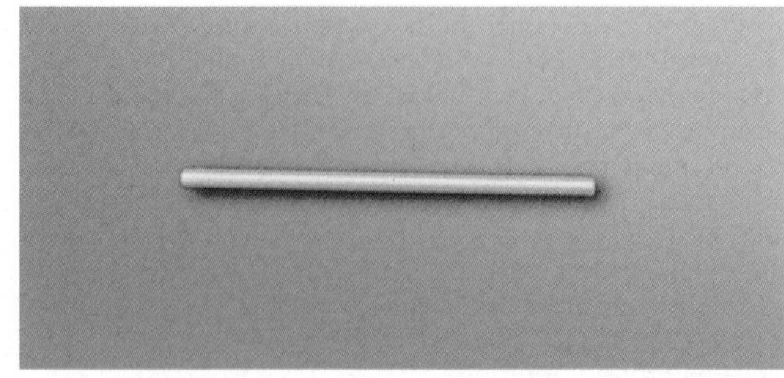

Figure 14-18. Contraceptive implant containing etonogestrel.

the end of the second year after insertion. Eight hours after insertion, ENG levels rise to a mean of 266 pg/mL, which is sufficient to inhibit ovulation. Maximum ENG levels reach a mean of 813 pg/mL about 4 days after insertion after which there is a gradual decline to a mean of 196 pg/mL after the first year and 156 pg/mL at the end of 3 years. Mean serum ENG levels are inversely related to body weight. When serum ENG levels are above 90 pg/mL ovulation is inhibited. Ovulation inhibition is the main mechanism of action of this implant together with thickening of the cervical mucus. Ovulation is inhibited for at least 30 months after insertion and no pregnancies were reported in clinical trials of nearly 2000 women with 7500 cycles of use. Following removal of the implant serum ENG levels decline rapidly and are undetectable within 1 week after removal. Ovulation resumes rapidly, and 90% of women ovulate within 1 month after removal and 90% resumed regular menses with 3 months.

During the first year after insertion of the implant serum E_2 levels are in the early follicular phase range (60 pg/mL) but rise to late follicular phase levels (80 to 100 pg/mL) in the second and third year after insertion. This implant does not result in a decrease of bone mineral density, even in women with amenorrhea.

In clinical trials continuation rates are high, with 50% to 80% of women continuing use until 2 years in different countries. Bleeding irregularities are the most common reason for discontinuation, accounting for about 60% of early removals. As with all progestin-only methods nearly all women have disruption of their regular bleeding pattern. Amenorrhea is common, occurring in about 20% of women and 27% have infrequent bleeding. About 12% of women have prolonged bleeding, and 6% frequent bleeding. There are no consistencies in the bleeding pattern of individual women. Although an increase in body weight is common in users of this implant, in one study the mean increase in weight was similar to a group of nonmedicated IUD users.

Acne develops in about 14% of women using the implant but accounts for only about 1% of premature removals. No clinically meaningful changes in carbohydrate or lipid metabolism occur with this implant.

EMERGENCY CONTRACEPTION

Various steroids and the copper IUD have been used for emergency contraception. The steroids are most effective if treatment is begun within 72 hours after an isolated midcycle act of coitus. Their effectiveness is less if more than one episode of coitus has occurred or if treatment is initiated later than 72 hours after coitus. The IUD is effective for 7 days after coitus.

It has been estimated that the clinical pregnancy rate after a single act of midcycle coitus without use of a contraceptive is about 8%.

A regimen of four tablets of ethinyl estradiol, 0.05 mg, and *dl*-norgestrel, 0.5 mg, combination oral contraceptive (Ovral), given in doses of two tablets 12 hours apart, was initially tested in Canada by Yuzpe.

Trussell and associates pooled the data from studies that were published between 1977 and 1993 involving 5226 women treated with this regimen. They calculated that the failure rate was 1.5% and that use of this regimen prevented about 75% of the expected pregnancies. The FDA approved a product containing four tablets of these contraceptive steroids (Preven) for emergency contraception but it is no longer marketed. Nevertheless, combinations of many other oral contraceptives that provide an equivalent dose of ethinyl estradiol and levonorgestrel can also be used. In one large Canadian study 30% of the subjects treated with this regimen reported having nausea without vomiting and another 20% had nausea with vomiting. These investigators included an antiemetic, a 50-mg tablet of dimenhydrinate, in the package and instructed the women to take it together with the second dose of contraceptive steroid if they experienced nausea after the first dose. They also reported that the time to onset of the subsequent menses was slightly shortened in the users of this regimen.

Ho and Kwan reported results of a randomized trial comparing the use of four tablets of ethinyl estradiol and levonorgestrel taken in divided doses 12 hours apart with a single tablet of 0.75 mg levonorgestrel taken initially and another one 12 hours later. Both regimens were ingested within 48 hours of unprotected intercourse. Failure rates of both regimens, about 2%, were similar, but there was significantly less nausea and vomiting with the progestin alone than with the one combined with estrogen. Subsequently, the WHO performed a randomized trial of the two regimens in about 2000 women in 21 centers. When given within 72 hours after a single act of unprotected sexual intercourse levonorgestrel alone was more effective, with a pregnancy rate of 1.1% and had fewer side effects than the estrogen–levonorgestrel combined oral contraceptive, which had a 3.2% pregnancy rate. The authors calculated that levonorgestrel prevented 85% of pregnancies compared with 57% for the combined OC. There were also fewer side effects of nausea and vomiting, dizziness, and fatigue with the levonorgestrel compound. Effectiveness was greater when the agents were given within 24 hours of sexual intercourse than when they were given in the subsequent 48 hours. In this study the earlier after intercourse treatment is given, the greater the efficacy with a downward gradient of efficacy from treatment within 24 hours to 44 to 72 hours. However, some degree of efficacy is still present when the progestin is given up to 120 hours after unprotected intercourse. A strip of two tablets of 0.75 mg levonorgestrel is marketed in several countries including the United States under a variety of brand names. In the United States it is called Plan B. It is believed that the main mechanism of action of high-dose progestin emergency contraception is inhibition of ovulation, but other mechanisms may be involved.

If the woman has a continuing need for contraception after the cycle in which any of these agents is used, one of the conventional methods should be prescribed.

Intrauterine insertion of a copper IUD within 5 to 10 days of midcycle coitus is a very effective method of preventing continuation of the pregnancy. Fasoli and coworkers summarized the results of four published studies in nine countries involving 879 women using the copper IUD. Only one pregnancy occurred, yielding a pregnancy rate of 0.1%. It is now estimated that more than 9400 postcoital copper IUD insertions have been performed with only 10 pregnancies, yielding a failure rate of less than 0.2%.

Glasier and associates have shown that mifepristone (also known as RU-486 and Mifeprex) is extremely effective when used as a postcoital contraceptive and is given as a single 600-mg dosage. Side effects were fewer and efficacy was similar to that with the use of two tablets of oral contraceptives taken 12 hours apart. A study by the WHO reported that use of a single tablet of 10 mg of mifepristone was an effective emergency contraceptive with a pregnancy rate of 1.2%.

INTRAUTERINE DEVICES

The main benefits of IUDs are (1) a high level of effectiveness, (2) a lack of associated systemic metabolic effects, and (3) the need for only a single act of motivation for long-term use. Despite these advantages only about 1% of women of reproductive age use the IUD for contraception in the United States, compared with 15% to 30% in most European countries and Canada. In contrast to other types of contraception, there is no need for frequent motivation to ingest a pill daily or to use a coitus-related method consistently. These characteristics, as well as the necessity for a visit to a health care facility to discontinue the method, account for the fact that IUDs have the highest continuation rate of all currently available reversible methods of contraception.

Unlike other contraceptives, such as the barrier methods, which rely on frequent use by the individual to be effective and therefore have higher typical failure rates than perfect failure rates, the IUD has similar rates of failure for typical or perfect use. First year failure rates with the copper T 380A IUD and the levonorgestrel releasing IUD (LNG-IUS) are less than 1%. Pregnancy rates are related to the skill of the clinician inserting the device. With experience, correct high-fundal insertion occurs more frequently, and there is a lower incidence of partial or complete expulsion, with resultant lower pregnancy rates. Furthermore, the annual incidence of accidental pregnancy decreases steadily after the first year of IUD use. The cumulative pregnancy rate after 12 years of use of the copper T 380A IUD is only 1.7% and after 5 years of the LNG-IUS is about 1.1%.

Table 14–9 Cumulative Discontinuation Rate for Copper T380A IUD

Event	YEARS SINCE INSERTION 3	5	7
Pregnancies	1.0	1.4	1.6
Expulsions	7.0	8.2	8.6
Medical removals	14.6	20.8	25.8
Nonmedical removals	13.8	25.6	34.4
Loss to follow-up	10.2	15.5	22.1
All discontinuations	32.2	46.7	56.3
Woman-months	38,571	56,010	67,885

Modified from World Health Organization: The TCu380A, TCu220C, multiload 250, and Nova TIUDS at 3, 5, and 7 years of use—Results from three randomized multicentre trials. Contraception 42:141, 1990.

The incidence of all major adverse events with IUDs, including pregnancy, expulsion, or removal for bleeding or pain, steadily decrease with increasing age. Thus, the IUD is especially suited for older parous women who wish to prevent further pregnancies (Tables 14-9 and 14-10).

Types of IUDs

In the past 35 years, many types of IUDs have been designed and used clinically. The devices developed and initially used in the 1960s were made of a plastic, polyethylene, impregnated with barium sulfate to make them radiopaque. In the 1970s, in order to diminish the frequency of the side effects of increased uterine bleeding and pain, smaller plastic devices covered with copper were developed and widely utilized. In the 1980s devices bearing a larger amount of copper, including sleeves on the horizontal arm, such as the copper T 380A and the copper T 220C, were developed, as well as the Multiload CU 250 and CU 375. These devices have a longer duration of high effectiveness and thus need to be reinserted at less frequent intervals than do the devices bearing a smaller amount of copper. The copper T 380A IUD is the only copper-bearing IUD currently

Table 14–10 Net Cumulative Termination Rates per 100 Each Year in 1821 Women Using a Levonorgestrel-Releasing Device (LNG-IUD) During 5 Years

	YEAR 1	2	3	4	5
Event	LNG-IUD	LNG-IUD	LNG-IUD	LNG-IUD	LNG-IUD
Pregnancy	0.1	0.1	0.2	0.3	0.3
Expulsion	3.4	4.2	4.8	4.9	4.9
Bleeding problems	5.8	8.3	9.6	10.3	10.9
Amenorrhea	1.5	2.9	3.6	4.2	4.3
Pain	1.6	2.8	3.4	3.9	4.2
Hormonal	2.3	4.8	6.4	7.6	8.4
PID	0.3	0.5	0.5	0.5	0.6
Other medical	2.7	3.6	4.8	5.5	5.8
Planning pregnancy	1.9	5.7	8.2	10.1	10.8
Other personal	0.6	1.5	2.0	2.3	2.9
Continuation	79.9	65.6	56.7	50.6	46.9

Modified from Andersson K, Odlind V, Rybo G: Levonorgestrel-releasing and copper-releasing (Nova T) IUDs during five years of use: A randomized comparative trial. Contraception 49:61, 1994.

marketed in the United States, but the Multiload CU 375 is widely used in Europe (Fig. 14-19).

Because of the constant dissolution of copper, which amounts daily to less than that ingested in the normal diet, all copper IUDs have to be replaced periodically. The copper T 380A is currently approved for use in the United States for 10 years and maintains its effectiveness for at least 12 years. At the scheduled time of removal, the device can be removed and another inserted during the same office visit.

Adding a reservoir of a progestin to the vertical arm also increases the effectiveness of the T-shaped devices. With the LNG-IUS, about 20 μg LNG is released into the endometrial cavity each day. This amount is sufficient to prevent pregnancy by thickening the cervical mucus and preventing transport of sperm into the endometrial cavity and oviducts (Fig. 14-20).

A large comparative trial of the copper T 380A and the LNG-IUS found that the effectiveness and continuation rates of both devices were similar. LNG-IUS has a high level of effectiveness for at least 5 years, with a cumulative pregnancy rate of 1.1%. This IUD also reduces menstrual blood loss and has been used therapeutically to treat excessive uterine bleeding.

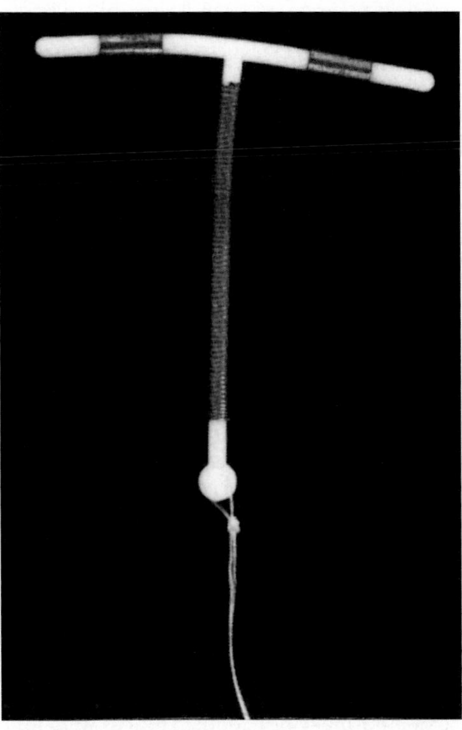

Figure 14-19. Intrauterine device currently being marketed in the United States—copper T 380A.

Mechanisms of Action

The main mechanism of contraceptive action of copper-bearing IUDs in the human is as a spermicide. This effect is caused by a local, sterile, inflammatory reaction produced by the presence of the foreign body in the uterine cavity. There is an approximate 1000% increase in the number of leukocytes in washings of the human endometrial cavity 18 weeks after the insertion

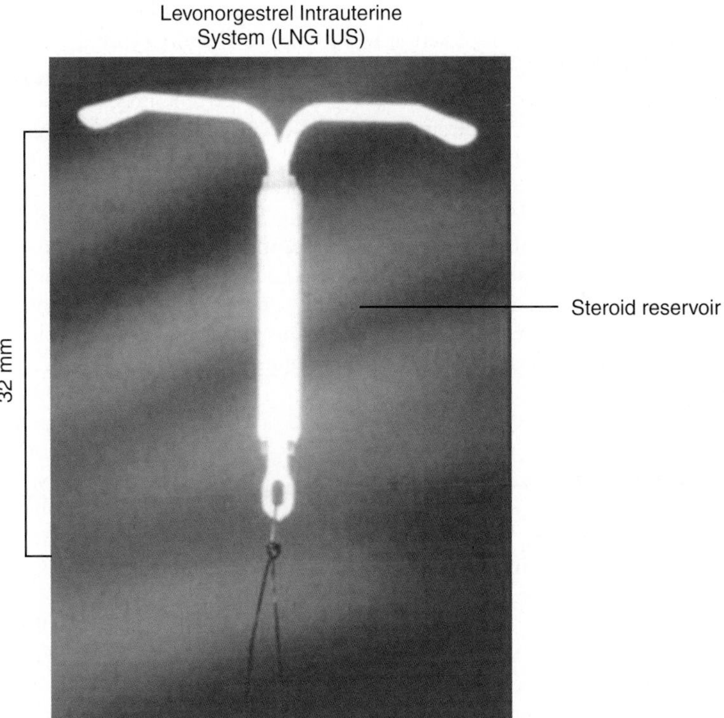

Figure 14-20. Levonorgestrel intrauterine system.

of an IUD compared with washings obtained before insertion. In addition to causing phagocytosis of spermatozoa, tissue breakdown products of these leukocytes are toxic to all cells, including spermatozoa. The amount of inflammatory reaction, and thus contraceptive effectiveness, is directly related to the size of the intrauterine foreign body. Copper markedly increases the extent of the inflammatory reaction, so this metal has been added to the small-sized frame of T-shaped devices. In addition, copper impedes sperm transport and viability in the cervical mucus. Since the copper T 380 has about twice as much copper surface area as the formerly marketed copper 7 IUD, the former IUD has a lower failure rate than the latter. Sperm transport from the cervix to the oviduct in the first 24 hours after coitus is markedly impaired in women wearing IUDs. Because of the spermicidal action of IUDs, very few, if any, sperm reach the oviducts, and the ovum usually does not become fertilized.

Further evidence for this spermicidal action of IUDs was reported by a group of investigators who performed oviductal flushing in 56 women wearing IUDs and 45 using no method of contraception who were sterilized by salpingectomy soon after ovulation. These women had unprotected sexual intercourse shortly before ovulation. Normally cleaving, fertilized ova were found in the tubal flushings of about half of the women not wearing IUDs, whereas no eggs that had the microscopic appearance of a normally developing embryo were found in the oviducts of the women wearing IUDs.

A long-term study of women wearing the copper T 380A IUD revealed that although the cumulative intrauterine pregnancy rate gradually increased with duration of IUD use, the ectopic pregnancy rate remained low and constant after the first year of use. If fertilization occurred frequently with IUD use and its main mechanism of action was to prevent uterine implantation of the blastocyst, the ectopic pregnancy rate would be expected to increase at a rate more rapidly than the intrauterine pregnancy rate, and this outcome did not occur. Thus, the principal mechanism of action of the copper T 380A IUD is as a spermicide, preventing fertilization of the ovum. The LNG-IUS, like the copper device, has a very low ectopic pregnancy rate. Therefore, fertilization does not occur and its main mechanism of action is also spermicidal.

On removal of the IUD, the inflammatory reaction rapidly disappears. Resumption of fertility following IUD removal is prompt and occurs at the same rate as resumption of fertility following discontinuation of the barrier methods of contraception. The incidence of full-term deliveries, spontaneous abortion, and ectopic pregnancies in conceptions occurring after IUD removal is the same as in the general non–contraceptive-using population.

Time of Insertion

Although it is widely believed that the optimal time for insertion of an IUD is during the menses, there are data indicating that the IUD can be safely inserted on any day of the cycle provided the woman is not pregnant. An analysis was made of 2-month event rates of about 10,000 women who had copper T 200s inserted on various days of the cycle. Differences in event rates with insertion occurring on different days of the cycle were small and of little clinical relevance. Therefore, the IUD can be inserted on any day of the cycle. Since bacteria are introduced into the endometrial cavity at the time of IUD insertion, it is preferable to insert the IUD after the menses cease to avoid providing a good environment for bacterial growth.

It has also been recommended that IUDs not be inserted until more than 2 to 3 months have elapsed after completing a full-term pregnancy. However, we analyzed event rates in our clinic among women who had copper T IUDs inserted between 4 and 8 weeks postpartum and more than 8 weeks postpartum. The 1- and 2-year event rates for all causes were similar for the two groups, indicating that copper T IUDs can be safely inserted at the time of the routine postpartum visit. No uterine perforations occurred in this series, in which the withdrawal technique of insertion was used. Although one report suggested that the uterine perforation rate was increased if the IUD is inserted when a woman is lactating, this finding has not been confirmed in several other studies.

The effect of breast-feeding on performance of the copper T 380A IUDs was evaluated from data obtained from a large, multicenter, clinical trial in which the device was inserted into 559 breast-feeding women and 590 nonbreast-feeding women, all of whom were at least 6 weeks postpartum. There were significantly fewer problems with pain and bleeding at the time of insertion in the group that was breast-feeding. The expulsion rate, which was low, and the continuation rate, which was high, were similar in the breast-feeding and nonbreast-feeding groups 6 months after insertion. Therefore, insertion of the IUD can be performed in postpartum women who are breast-feeding their infants, as well as in those who are not nursing at the time of the routine postpartum visit.

Adverse Effects

Incidence

In general, in the first year of use, copper IUDs have less than a 1% pregnancy rate, a 6% expulsion rate, and a 12% rate of removal for medical reasons, mainly bleeding and pain. The annual incidence of each of these events, especially expulsion, diminishes steadily in subsequent years.

In an ongoing WHO study of the copper T 380A, termination rates for adverse effects continued to decline annually following the first year after insertion for each of the 12 years in which sufficient data had been accumulated. In this study, the cumulative percentage discontinuation rate for pregnancy, bleeding and pain, and expulsion at the end of 7 years was 1.6, 22.7, and 8.6 per 100 women, respectively, and at the end of 12 years they were 1.7, 35.2, and 12.5 per 100 women (Table 14-11). In a large study of the LNG-IUS, Andersson and colleagues reported that termination rates at the end of 1 year for pregnancy, bleeding, and pain and expulsion were 0.1, 7.4, and 3.4 per 100 women, respectively. After 5 years the cumulative discomfort rate for pregnancy, bleeding, and pain and expulsion were 0.3, 15.1, and 4.9 per 100 women, respectively.

Uterine Bleeding

The majority of women discontinuing this method of contraception do so for medical reasons. Nearly all the medical reasons accounting for removal of copper-bearing IUDs involve one or more types of abnormal bleeding: heavy or prolonged menses

Table 14–11 Selected Cumulative Net Probabilities of Discontinuation (Standard Errors) per 100 Women Using Copper T 380A at 8, 10, and 12 Years of Use—WHO Study Excluding Chinese Centers

	8 years	10 years	12 years
Total pregnancies	1.7 (0.6)	1.7 (0.6)	1.7 (0.6)
Total medical removals	30.9 (1.8)	37.5 (2.2)	40.1 (2.4)
Total nonmedical removals	49.1 (2.0)	57.2 (2.1)	64.9 (2.2)
Continuation rate	19.3 (1.1)	12.6 (1.0)	7.9 (0.8)
Number of insertions	1195		
Number of women completing the interval	230	151	94
Woman-years experience	4947	5313	5537

Adapted from United Nations Development Programme/United Nations Population Fund/World Health Organization/World Bank, Special Programme of Research, Development and Research Training in Human Reproduction: Long-term reversible contraception: Twelve years of experience with the TCU 380A. Contraception 56:341, 1997.

or intermenstrual bleeding. The heavy bleeding may be produced by a premature and increased rate of local release of prostaglandins brought about by the presence of the intrauterine foreign body. The stimulation of uterine contractions by excessive levels of prostaglandins may prolong the duration of the menstrual flow, which is significantly longer in women wearing copper IUDs than in normally cycling women.

The amount of blood lost in each menstrual cycle is significantly greater in women using inert, as well as copper-bearing IUDs than in nonusers. The copper T 380A IUD is associated with about a 55% increase in menstrual blood loss (MBL). In contrast, with the LNG-IUS, the amount of blood loss is significantly reduced to about 5 mL/cycle and after 1 year 20% of women using this IUD are amenorrheic.

In a study of Swedish women in whom the copper T 380 was inserted, there was no significant change in mean measurements of several hematologic parameters, including hemoglobin, hematocrit, and erythrocyte count at 3, 6, and 12 months after IUD insertion compared with mean values before insertion.

A sensitive indicator of tissue iron stores is the serum ferritin level. In a study of women using the copper T 380A IUD there was no significant change in mean serum ferritin levels at 3, 6, and 12 months after IUD insertion. None of the women with low ferritin levels had a decrease in hemoglobin levels. They probably had an increase in intestinal iron absorption to compensate for the increased MBL as none of these women developed anemia. There is a significant reduction of MBL, about 60%, during the use of the LNG-IUS. This reduction is seen as early as 3 months after insertion and persists for the duration of use of the device. The reduction of MBL results in an improvement of blood hemoglobin levels. Thus, the LNG-IUS is useful in the prevention and the treatment of iron deficiency anemia and the depletion of iron stores by heavy MBL.

Excessive bleeding in the first few months following IUD insertion should be treated with reassurance and supplemental oral iron, as well as systemic administration of one of the prostaglandin synthetase inhibitors during menses. The bleeding usually diminishes with time, as the uterus adjusts to the presence of the foreign body.

Mefenamic acid ingested in a dosage of 500 mg three times a day during the days of menstruation has been shown to reduce MBL significantly in IUD users. If excessive bleeding continues despite this treatment, the device should be removed. After a 1-month interval, another type of device may be inserted if the woman still wishes to use an IUD for contraception. Consideration should be given to using the LNG-IUS, because this device is associated with less blood loss than the copper-bearing IUDs.

Perforation

Although uncommon, one of the potentially serious complications associated with use of the IUD is perforation of the uterine fundus. Perforation always occurs at the time of insertion. Sometimes only the distal portion of the IUD penetrates the uterine muscle at insertion. Then uterine contractions over the next few months force the IUD into the peritoneal cavity. IUDs correctly inserted entirely within the endometrial cavity do not wander through the uterine muscle into the peritoneal cavity. The incidence of perforation is generally related to the shape of the device or to the amount of force used during its insertion, as well as the experience of the clinician performing the insertion. Perforation of the uterus is best prevented by straightening the uterine axis with a tenaculum and then probing the cavity with a uterine sound before IUD insertion.

Perforation rates for the copper T 380A are only about 1 in 3000 insertions. Since the perforations occurring at the time of insertion are nearly always asymptomatic, the clinician should always suspect that perforation has occurred if the user cannot feel the appendage but did not observe that the device was expelled. One should not assume that an unnoticed expulsion has occurred when the appendage is not visualized. Sometimes the IUD is still in its correct position in the uterine cavity, but the appendage has been withdrawn into the cavity as the position of the IUD has changed. In this situation, after pelvic examination has been performed and the possibility of pregnancy excluded, the uterine cavity should be probed.

If the device cannot be felt with a uterine sound or biopsy instrument, a pelvic sonogram or radiograph should be obtained. If the device is not visualized with pelvic ultrasonography, a radiograph visualizing the entire abdominal cavity should be performed because IUDs that have been pushed through the uterus may be located anywhere in the peritoneal cavity, even in the subdiaphragmatic area.

Any type of IUD found to be outside the uterus, even if asymptomatic, should be removed from the peritoneal cavity because complications such as severe adhesions and bowel obstruction have been reported with intraperitoneal IUDs. Therefore, it is best to remove intraperitoneal IUDs shortly after the diagnosis of perforation is made. Unless severe adhesions have developed, most intraperitoneal IUDs can be removed by means of laparoscopy.

Perforation of the cervix has also been reported with devices having a straight vertical arm, such as the copper T. A plastic ball has been added to the distal vertical arm of the copper T 380A to reduce the rate of cervical perforation. When follow-up examinations are performed after IUD insertion, the cervix should be carefully inspected and palpated, because often perforations do not extend completely through the ectocervical epithelium. Cervical perforation is not a major problem, but devices that have perforated downward should be removed through the endocervical canal with uterine packing forceps. Their downward displacement is associated with reduced contraceptive effectiveness.

Complications Related to Pregnancy

Congenital Anomalies

When pregnancy occurs with an IUD in place, implantation takes place away from the device itself, so the device is always extraamniotic. Although there is a paucity of published data, so far there is no evidence of an increased incidence of congenital anomalies in infants born with a plastic, copper-bearing, or progestin-releasing IUD in utero.

Data from two studies of more than 300 babies conceived with a copper IUD in utero suggest that its presence does not exert a deleterious effect on fetal development or increase the risk of birth defects. Although relatively few infants have been born following gestation in a uterus containing the LNG-IUS, examination of these infants has revealed no evidence of cardiac or other anomalies.

Spontaneous Abortion

In all reported series of pregnancies with any type of IUD in situ, the incidence of fetal death was not significantly increased; however, a significant increase in spontaneous abortion has been consistently observed. If a woman conceives while wearing an IUD that is not subsequently removed, the incidence of spontaneous abortion is about 55%, approximately three times greater than would occur in pregnancies without an intrauterine IUD.

After conception, if the IUD is spontaneously expelled, or if the appendage is visible and the IUD is removed by traction, the incidence of spontaneous abortion is significantly reduced. In one study of women who conceived with copper T devices in place, the incidence of spontaneous abortion was only 20% if the device was removed or spontaneously expelled. This figure is similar to the normal incidence of spontaneous abortion and significantly less than the 54% incidence of abortion reported in the same study among women retaining the devices in utero. Thus, if a woman conceives with an IUD in place and wishes to continue the pregnancy, the IUD should be removed if the appendage is visible, to significantly reduce the chance of spontaneous abortion. If the appendage is not visible, blind probing of the uterine cavity may increase the chance of abortion, as well as sepsis. However, several recent reports indicate that with sonographic guidance it is possible during early gestation to remove intrauterine IUDs in the lower uterine cavity without a visible appendage and not adversely affect the outcome of the pregnancy.

Septic Abortion

If the IUD cannot be removed from the uterine cavity during early gestation, some evidence suggests that the risk of septic abortion may be increased if the IUD remains in place. Most of the evidence was based on data from women who conceived while wearing the shield type of IUD. This device, with its multifilament tail, was extensively used in the United States during the 1970s. The structure of the shield's appendage allowed vaginal bacteria to steadily enter the spaces between the filaments of the tail beneath the surrounding sheath. This action differs from the inability of bacteria to enter the monofilament tails or migrate along their surface through the cervical mucus barrier. During pregnancy, when the shield was drawn upward into the uterine cavity as gestation advanced, the bacteria in the tail string could exit into the uterine cavity and cause a severe and sometimes fatal uterine and systemic infection. This infection usually became manifest during the second trimester of pregnancy.

Although there is an increased risk of septic abortion if a patient conceived with a shield IUD in place, because of the structure of the shield's appendage, there is no conclusive evidence that IUDs with monofilament tail strings cause sepsis during pregnancy. In a British study, there was no significant difference in the incidence of septic abortion among women who conceived with an IUD in place and those who conceived while using other methods. In another study of 918 women who conceived with the copper T in situ, there were only two instances of septic abortion, both occurring in the first trimester. These data indicate that there is no increase in sepsis in pregnancy caused by the presence of an IUD except for the shield device. However, about 2% of all spontaneous abortions are septic, and the continued presence of an intrauterine IUD is associated with about a 50% risk of having a spontaneous abortion. Therefore, the overall incidence of septic abortion may be increased with any IUD in place because the incidence of spontaneous abortion is increased, not because the presence of the IUD increases the risk of sepsis by itself.

Ectopic Pregnancy

Because copper-bearing IUDs principally act by preventing fertilization through a cytotoxic effect on spermatozoa, the incidence of both ectopic pregnancy and intrauterine pregnancy are decreased with their use. The risk of the pregnancy being ectopic is increased about threefold from 1.4% to 6% if a woman becomes pregnant with a copper IUD in place than if she continues using no contraception method. However, because the copper T 380A IUD so effectively prevents all pregnancies, the estimated ectopic pregnancy rate is only 0.2 to 0.4 per 1000 woman-years. This rate is one tenth the rate in women using no contraception, 3 per 1000 woman-years. If a woman uses a copper T 380A IUD, her risk of having an ectopic pregnancy is reduced by 90% compared with use of no contraception.

In the 7-year WHO study of the copper T 380A IUD, the cumulative ectopic pregnancy rate at the end of 7 years was only 0.1 per 100 women. These data confirm that the copper T 380A reduces the risk of having both intrauterine and ectopic gestations. In Andersson's large study of 1821 women using the LNG-IUS, only five pregnancies occurred during 5 years' experience. Only one of these pregnancies was ectopic. Sivin estimated the ectopic pregnancy rate in women using this device was 0.2 per 1000 woman-years.

The increased risk of ectopic pregnancy for a woman who conceives while wearing an IUD is temporary and does not persist after removal of the IUD. In two large European studies women wishing to conceive after they had an ectopic pregnancy had a much greater chance of having a subsequent intrauterine pregnancy if they were using an IUD at the time of their ectopic pregnancy than were those who had an ectopic pregnancy and were not using an IUD.

Prematurity

In the previously cited study of conceptions occurring in the presence of copper T devices, the rate of prematurity among live births was four times greater when the copper T was left in place than when it was removed.

If a pregnant woman has an IUD in place and the device cannot be removed but she wishes to continue her gestation, she should be warned of the increased risk of prematurity, as well as that of spontaneous abortion and ectopic pregnancy. She should also be informed of the possible increased risk of septic abortion and advised to report promptly the first signs of pelvic pain or fever. There is no evidence that pregnancies with IUDs in utero are associated with an increased incidence of other obstetric complications. There is also no evidence that prior use of an IUD results in a greater incidence of complications in pregnancies occurring after its removal.

Infection in the Nonpregnant IUD User

In the 1960s, despite great concern among clinicians that use of the IUD would markedly increase the incidence of salpingitis, or PID, there was little evidence that such an increase did occur. During that decade the IUD was inserted mainly into parous women, and the incidence of sexually transmitted disease was not as high as occurred subsequently. In 1966 a study was performed in which aerobic and anaerobic cultures were made of homogenates of endometrial tissue obtained transfundally from uteri removed by vaginal hysterectomy at various intervals after insertion of the loop IUD. During the first 24 hours after IUD insertion, the normally sterile endometrial cavity was consistently infected with bacteria. Nevertheless, in 80% of uteri removed during the following 24 hours, the women's natural defenses had destroyed these bacteria and the endometrial cavities were sterile. In this study, when transfundal cultures were obtained more than 30 days after IUD insertion, the endometrial cavity, the IUD, and the portion of the thread within the cavity were always found to be sterile (Fig. 14-21). These findings indicate that development of PID more than a month after insertion of the IUD is due to infection with a sexually transmitted pathogen and is unrelated to the presence of the device.

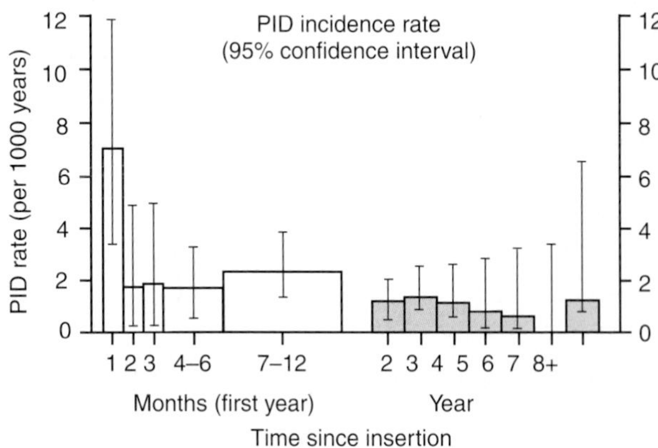

Figure 14-22. PID incidence by time since insertion. Incidence rate was estimated by the number of PID cases and years of exposure in each time interval. 95% confidence intervals were calculated from the Poisson distribution. (From Farley TM, Rosenberg MJ, Rowe PJ, et al: Intrauterine devices and pelvic inflammatory disease: An international perspective. Lancet 339:785, 1992.)

Results of a large multicenter clinical study coordinated by the WHO confirmed these findings. In this study of 22,908 women inserted with IUDs, the PID rate was highest in the first 3 weeks after insertion but remained lower and constant during the 8 years thereafter at 0.5 per 1000 woman-years (Fig. 14-22). An IUD should not be inserted into a woman who may have been recently infected with gonococci or *Chlamydia.* Insertion of the device will transport these pathogens from the cervix into the upper genital tract, where the large number of organisms may overcome the host defense and cause salpingitis. If there is clinical suspicion of infectious endocervicitis, cultures should be obtained and the IUD insertion delayed until the results reveal no pathogenic organisms are present. It does not appear to be cost effective to administer systemic antibiotics routinely with every IUD insertion, but the insertion procedure should be as aseptic as possible.

A randomized trial comparing use of azithromycin ingested just prior to IUD insertion with a placebo control reported no significant difference in the subsequent rate of pelvic inflammation. The rate was 0.1% in both study arms. In a study of the

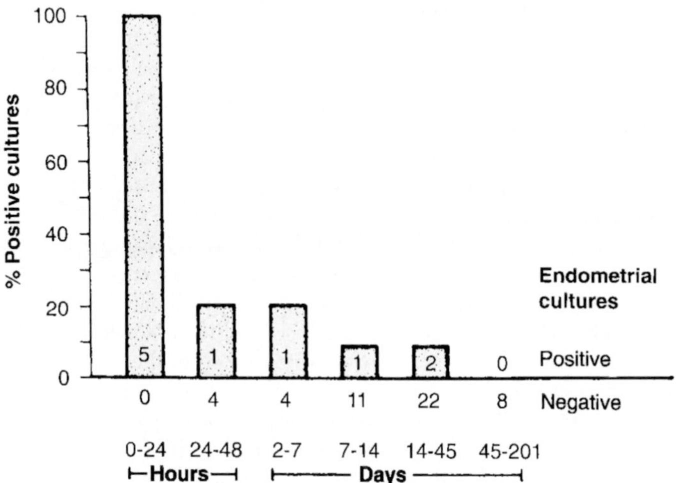

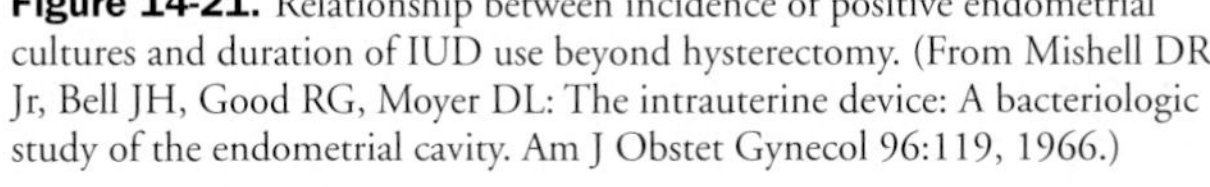
Figure 14-21. Relationship between incidence of positive endometrial cultures and duration of IUD use beyond hysterectomy. (From Mishell DR Jr, Bell JH, Good RG, Moyer DL: The intrauterine device: A bacteriologic study of the endometrial cavity. Am J Obstet Gynecol 96:119, 1966.)

Table 14-12 First-Year Event Rates per 100 Women for Copper T 380A

Event	1 Year Parous
Pregnancy	0.5
Expulsion	2.3
Bleeding/pain	3.4
Infection	0.3
Other medical	0.5
Planning pregnancy	0.6
Other personal	0.7

From Rosenberg MJ, Foldesy R, Mishell DR Jr, et al: Performance of the TCu 380A and Cu-Fix IUDs in an international randomized trial. Contraception 53:197, 1996.

copper T 380A IUD, the rate of removal because of infection during the first year of use was only 0.3% (Table 14-12).

Other epidemiologic studies have shown that the presence of an IUD with monofilament tail strings does not increase the incidence of PID after the insertion interval. One study determined the incidence of tubal infertility among former IUD users. It was reported that nulliparous women with a single sexual partner who had previously used an IUD had no increased risk of tubal infertility, whereas women with multiple sexual partners who used an IUD did have an increased risk of tubal infertility. Another study found that nulliparous women who used an IUD did not have an increased risk of tubal causes of infertility compared with non-IUD users.

Analysis of this large amount of data indicates that PID occurring more than a month following insertion of IUDs with monofilament tail strings is due to a sexually transmitted pathogen and not related to the presence of the IUD.

The increased risk of impairment of future fertility from PID developing in the first month after IUD insertion, as well as the possibility of ectopic pregnancy in the event of contraceptive failure, must be considered when deciding whether to use an IUD in a nulliparous woman, especially if she has multiple sexual partners. Contraceptive steroids reduce the risk of developing salpingitis in women infected with gonorrhea and should be offered to such women. However, for women with medical reasons for not using contraceptive steroids, the IUD is the only other effective reversible method of contraceptive and can be used. The use of condoms should be advised to reduce the risk of transmission of pathogens.

Symptomatic PID can usually be successfully treated with antibiotics without removing the IUD until the woman becomes symptom-free. For women with clinical evidence of a tuboovarian abscess, the IUD should be removed only after a therapeutic serum level of appropriate parenteral antibiotics has been reached, preferably after a clinical response has been observed. An alternative method of contraception should be substituted in women who develop PID with an IUD in place.

There is evidence that IUD users may have an increased risk for colonizing actinomycosis organisms in the upper genital tract. The relationship of actinomycosis to PID is unclear, as many women without IUDs have actinomycosis in their vagina and are asymptomatic. If actinomycosis organisms are identified on the routine examination of cervical cytology and the woman is asymptomatic, she may be treated with appropriate antimicrobial therapy to eradicate the organisms or followed without therapy. The IUD should not be removed from an asymptomatic woman who is colonized but not infected with actinomycosis. If pelvic infection is present, the woman should be treated with antibiotics and the IUD removed.

Contraindications

It is logical and consistent with good medical practice that IUDs not be inserted into women with the following seven conditions, which are listed as contraindications to IUD insertion in the United States: (1) pregnancy or suspicion of pregnancy, (2) acute PID, (3) postpartum endometritis or infected abortion in the past 3 months, (4) known or suspected uterine or cervical malignancy, (5) genital bleeding of unknown origin, (6) untreated acute cervicitis, and (7) a previously inserted IUD that has not been removed. However, little data are available to indicate that the complications of Wilson's disease, allergy to copper, and genital actinomycosis are true contraindications for insertion of copper-bearing IUDs and, because of the infrequency of these conditions, it is unlikely that data will ever become available.

The remaining contraindications for IUD use listed in the product labeling: abnormalities of the uterus resulting in distortion of the uterine cavity; history of PID; vaginitis, including bacterial vaginosis, until infection is controlled; patient or her partner has multiple sexual partners; and conditions associated with increased susceptibility to infections with microorganisms. These contraindications remain questionable because of the lack of clinical studies of IUD use in women with these conditions.

The reason why the IUD is stated to be contraindicated in women who have multiple sexual partners or whose partner has multiple sexual partners is unclear. Such women should be counseled to have their partners use condoms to protect against transmission of diseases and to use the IUD to effectively prevent pregnancy if they so desire.

Conditions previously believed to preclude IUD use but no longer considered to be contraindications include diabetes mellitus, valvular heart disease (including mitral valve prolapse), past history of ectopic pregnancy (except LNG-IUS), nulliparity, treated cervical dysplasia, irregular menses due to anovulation, breast-feeding, corticosteroid use, and age younger than 25.

Overall Safety

Several long-term studies have indicated that the IUD is not associated with an increased incidence of endometrial or cervical carcinoma and may actually be associated with a reduction in risk of developing these neoplasms during and following its use. The IUD is a particularly useful method of contraception for women who have completed their families and do not wish permanent sterilization and have contraindications to, or do not wish to use, other effective methods of reversible contraception. A recent analysis reported that after 5 years of use the IUD was the most cost-effective method of all methods of contraception, including sterilization (see Figure 14-1). Women in the United States who use an IUD have a higher level of satisfaction with their method of contraception than women using any of the other methods of reversible contraception.

STERILIZATION

In 2002 in the United States, sterilization of one member of a couple was the most widely used method of preventing pregnancy. The popularity of sterilization was greatest if (1) the wife was older than age 30, (2) the couple had been married more than 10 years, and (3) the couple desired no additional children. In contrast to the other methods of contraception, which are reversible or temporary, sterilization should be considered permanent. Although reanastomosis after vasectomy or tubal ligation is possible, the reconstructive operation is much more difficult than the original sterilizing procedure and the results are variable. Pregnancy rates after reanastomosis of the vas range from 45% to 60%, whereas those after oviduct reanastomosis range from 50% to 80%, depending on the amount of tissue damage associated with the original procedure, as well as the surgeon's technical competency. If women who have tubal sterilization wish to conceive, in vitro fertilization is now being performed more frequently than tubal reconstructive surgery.

Voluntary sterilization is legal in all 50 states, and the decision to be sterilized should be made solely by the individual in consultation with the provider. Because all currently available sterilization procedures require surgical techniques, individuals who request sterilization should be counseled regarding both the risks and the irreversibility of the procedures. It is advisable to inform the individual fully, and the spouse if possible, of the benefits and risks of these surgical procedures. In addition, it has been useful to have more than one counselor when sterilization is requested by a woman younger than age 25, as well as for all women without children.

The rationale for such careful scrutiny of younger candidates for sterilization is that they tend to change their minds more often, their attitudes may be less fixed, and they face a longer period of reproductive life during which divorce, remarriage, or death among their children can occur.

The most effective, least destructive method of tubal occlusion is the most desirable in younger women, since ovarian dysfunction and adhesion formation are diminished, and the incidence of successful reversal procedures is increased. The effective laparoscopic band techniques or the modified Pomeroy technique (also called partial salpingectomy) (Fig. 14-23) should be used in women younger than age 25. Reversal after this method of sterilization is followed by pregnancy in approximately 75% of women, a rate that is higher than that reported after most laparoscopic fulgurations, where more tube is destroyed. However, if pregnancy is desired after tubal occlusion, in vitro fertilization is recommended if there has been extensive tubal destruction by fulguration.

Male Sterilization

Sterilization in the male is performed by vasectomy, an outpatient procedure that takes about 20 minutes and requires only local anesthesia. The vas deferens is isolated and cut. The ends of the vas are closed, either by ligation or by fulguration; they are then replaced in the scrotal sac, and the incision is closed. Complications of vasectomy include hematoma (in up to 5% of the subjects), sperm granulomas (inflammatory responses to sperm leakage), and spontaneous reanastomosis. When the last occurs, it usually does so within a short time after the procedure. Usually about 14 to 20 ejaculations are required after the operation before the man is sterile. Although in the United States reversal requests range from 5% to 7% of men who had

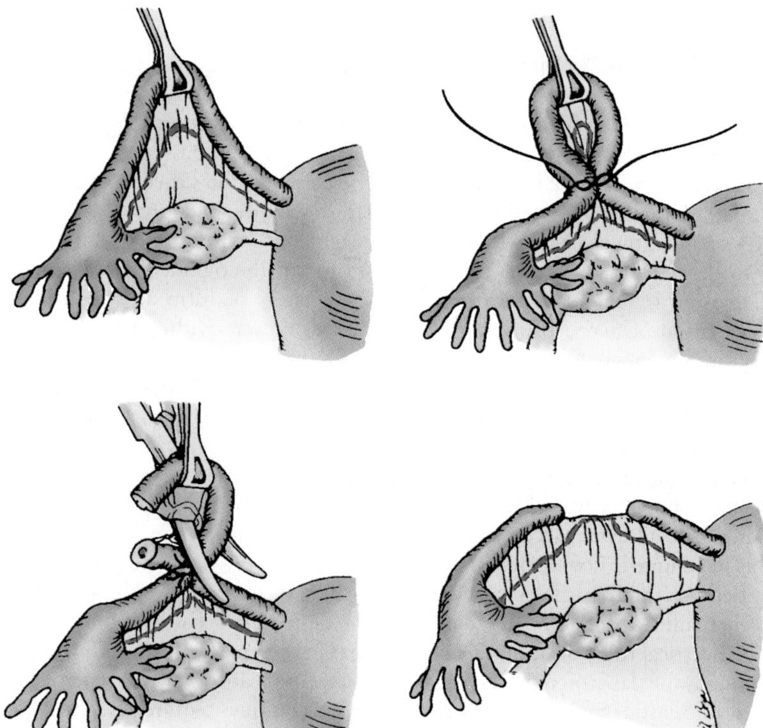

Figure 14-23. Modified Pomeroy technique of female sterilization. (From Sciarra JJ: Surgical procedures for tubal sterilization. In Sciarra JJ, Zatuchni GI, Daly MJ: Gynecology and Obstetrics, Vol 6. Philadelphia, Harper & Row, 1984.)

a vasectomy, vas reanastomosis is a difficult and meticulous procedure that has an optimal success rate of about 50%.

Female Sterilization

Sterilization of the female is more complicated, requiring a transperitoneal incision and usually general anesthesia. Postpartum sterilization is performed by making a small infraumbilical incision and performing either a Pomeroy or modified Irving-type of tubal ligation. These simple and rapid procedures can be performed either in the delivery room immediately after delivery or in the operating room the following day without prolonging the hospital stay. The same operative techniques can be used for female sterilization at times other than the puerperium, but additional techniques are also used for what has been termed *interval sterilization.* Ligation of the oviducts by the Pomeroy technique can be easily and rapidly performed through a small abdominal incision termed *minilaparotomy.* On occasion a colpotomy incision may also be used, but this incision is associated with a higher incidence of postoperative infection.

The development of fiberoptic light sources has made laparoscopy a popular gynecologic operative technique. By using various accessories in addition to the laparoscope, the operator can fulgurate and cut the oviducts without making an intraperitoneal incision other than one or two small punctures. Most gynecologists find the two-puncture technique for laparoscopy sterilization easier to learn and perform than the single-puncture technique. General anesthesia is usually employed for laparoscopic sterilization, but overnight hospitalization is unnecessary. Because the pregnancy rate after fulguration and transection is similar to that after fulguration alone, it is now recommended that the oviducts not be cut after fulguration. The incidence of complications after laparoscopic fulguration ranges from 1% to 6%; major complications (hemorrhage, puncture, or cautery of bowel) occur in about 0.6% of patients.

In an attempt to eliminate the problem of bowel injury, bipolar forceps were developed to replace the unipolar apparatus, which has a grounding plate attached to the patient through which the current passes. In the bipolar system the current passes from one prong of the forceps, through the tissue, to the other prong, producing a limited area of coagulation with destruction of a small segment of the oviduct. After coagulation, if division is to be performed, scissors are introduced to cut the oviduct. If division is not to be performed, some operators perform a coagulation of two or three contiguous burns on each oviduct to ensure adequate obliteration of the lumen. When the unipolar apparatus is used, a single 1-cm burn on each oviduct is sufficient. However, even with this small amount of coagulation, local tissue damage after unipolar coagulation is extensive, and attempts at reanastomosis have a very low rate of success. Because bipolar coagulation not only is safer but also is associated with a higher success rate after a reanastomosis procedure, this technique is now preferred.

Because of the problems of electrocoagulation, efforts have been made to develop safer methods that destroy less tissue. Nonelectrical tubal occlusion techniques that may be performed through the laparoscope are those using spring-loaded clips and the Silastic band (Falope Ring). All these techniques require a modification of the conventional laparoscope, as well as specialized training in their use. A microinsert device that is introduced transcervically through a hysteroscope and placed in the proximal portion of the oviduct to provide occlusion was approved for use in the United States in 2002. The device is 4 cm long and 2 mm in diameter and is made of a flexible stainless steel inner core, a dynamic outer coil made of nickel titanium alloy and a layer of polyethylene terephthalate fibers. The latter material causes tissue ingrowth and permanent tubal occlusion. A large multicenter study by Cooper and colleagues reported that bilateral placement of the microinserts occurred in 86% of initial procedures, which increased to 92% with an additional procedure. Uterine perforation and expulsion of the inserts occur in less than 3% of insertion procedures. A hysterosalpingogram is performed 3 months after insertion to document tubal occlusion. Following this documentation, effectiveness for preventing pregnancy in clinical trials is 99.8% at 3 and 4 years and 99.7% after 5 years of follow-up. Longer-term efficacy results are not yet available.

Female sterilization by surgical removal of a portion of the oviduct or mechanically occluding a portion of the lumen by clips, bands, or electrocoagulation was previously believed to be the most effective form of pregnancy prevention. This belief was based on studies that reported that failure rates during the first year of use of any type of reversible contraceptive were higher than the first-year failure rate of female sterilization. The results of a long-term study by Peterson and coworkers indicate that pregnancies continue to occur for many years after these sterilizations procedure. The failure rate increased from 0.55 per 100 women at 1 year to 1.31 at 5 years, and 1.85 10 years after the operation for all methods of tubal interruption, being higher for bipolar coagulation and spring clips and lower for partial salpingectomy. In women 18 to 27 years of age, 2.8% became pregnant 5 to 10 years after bipolar coagulation of the oviduct. There are several reversible methods of contraception, with failure rates similar to those of tubal sterilization. Cumulative 3-year failure rates with the single implant are less than 0.1%. The pregnancy rate after 10 years use of copper T 380 IUD is 1.7 per 100 users and is similar to female sterilization, 1.85 per 100 women. Furthermore, among women who become pregnant after female sterilization, about one third have ectopic pregnancies compared with 5% with the copper T 380 IUD. Because the copper T 380 IUD has an effective life span of 10 years, with a failure rate comparable to that of female sterilization and a lower ectopic pregnancy rate, as well as being less expensive, rapidly reversible and more convenient to use, it should be considered as an alternative to tubal sterilization.

INDUCED ABORTION

Induced abortion is one of the most common gynecologic operations performed in the United States and in many other countries. As determined by the landmark *Roe v. Wade* Supreme Court decision, the state may not interfere with the practice of abortion in the first trimester. In the second trimester, individual states may regulate abortion services in the interest of preserving the health of the woman.

From 1973 through 1980, the number of induced abortions performed annually in the United States steadily increased from 750,000 to about 1,600,000. The annual number of abortions stabilized at this figure from 1980 until 1990. Since 1990 there has been a gradual decline in the annual number of abortions performed in the United States, reaching 1.3 million in 2001. In 2001 the abortion ratio (number of abortions per 100 pregnancies) was 20, whereas the abortion rate (number of abortions per 1000 women ages 15 to 44) was 21. In the United States the abortion rates have declined gradually since 1980 but are higher than in all Western European countries and about one in five pregnancies in the United States are terminated by elective abortion. Approximately one third of abortions are performed in women younger than 20, another third in women age 20 to 24, and the remaining third among women ages 25 and older. Only one fourth of abortions are obtained by married women. Ninety percent of abortions are performed within the first 12 weeks of pregnancy, and about 50% of abortions are performed during the first 8 weeks of pregnancy. In the United States nearly all abortions are performed by various surgical techniques, whereas in Europe and a few U.S. centers many abortions are terminated with the use of drugs.

Methods

Three principal methods are used for elective abortion: transcervical evacuation, induction of labor, and major operations. Suction curettage is the predominant method of performing abortion in the United States, accounting for approximately 75% of all abortion procedures; the remainder are performed by dilation and evacuation (curettage techniques in the second trimester), labor induction, and major operations.

Curettage Methods

Curettage by vacuum aspiration is the predominant method of performing abortion in the first trimester. Very early in pregnancy, *endometrial aspiration,* also termed *menstrual extraction,* can be done with a small, flexible, plastic cannula without dilation or anesthesia. Abortions performed to terminate pregnancies with a gestational age of 8 weeks or more generally require dilation of the cervix and some type of anesthesia, either local or general.

Dilation of the cervix can be facilitated by use of osmotic dilators and administration of prostaglandins. The osmotic dilators are usually placed in the cervical canal for several hours or overnight to produce gradual dilation. Most commonly *Laminaria japonica,* made of seaweed sticks, are utilized. Synthetic osmotic dilators include a polyvinyl alcohol sponge impregnated with magnesium sulfate and a hygroscope plastic polymer. Use of such osmotic dilators in nulliparous women substantially reduces the risk of uterine trauma, such as perforation and cervical injury. In addition, administration of the prostaglandin and E_1 analogue misoprostol in a dosage of 400 μg given orally, vaginally, or bucally a few hours before vacuum aspiration reduces cervical trauma.

Dilation and evacuation (D&E) is the predominant method of abortion used beyond the first trimester. Because a greater amount of cervical dilation is usually needed, osmotic dilators are usually inserted for several hours or several days before the procedure. Although recent data are lacking, earlier studies indicated that D&E was substantially safer than induction of labor or major operations for abortions of 13 to 16 weeks' gestation. For later abortions, D&E and induction of labor appear to have comparable risks of morbidity and mortality, although the range of complications varies by technique. Disadvantages of D&E include the requirement of technical expertise, the emotional burden for participating physicians and medical personnel, and possible long-term deleterious effects upon the cervix. Advantages include less emotional stress for the woman, avoidance of the need for hospitalization, greater convenience, and lower cost than induction of uterine contractions.

Induction of Uterine Contractions

Second-trimester abortion is also performed by induction of uterine contractions. One technique uses instillation of hypertonic solution into the amniotic cavity. The solution most frequently used was hypertonic saline (2000 mL of 20% saline), although hypertonic glucose and urea were also employed. Uterine contractions usually began within 12 to 24 hours, and abortion occurred within a few hours thereafter. Use of an ancillary agent such as *Laminaria* or oxytocin facilitates the process. Uterine instillation of hypertonic solution is currently performed infrequently.

The most common method now used for medical termination in the second trimester is administration of prostaglandins. Prostaglandin E_2, administered as a vaginal suppository; a prostaglandin E_2 methyl analogue, misoprostol; given as tablets orally, bucally, or vaginally; and 15-methyl prostaglandin $E_2\alpha$, administered as an intramuscular injection, have all been used. These techniques have the advantage of easy administration. Each compound is given at 2- to 6-hour intervals until evacuation of the gestational material is achieved. Disadvantages include gastrointestinal side effects and, with the prostaglandin E_2 suppositories, hyperpyrexia. Jain and Mishell reported that the intravaginal placement of two 100-μg tablets of misoprostol every 12 hours was as successful as prostaglandin E_2, with fewer side effects and less cost. The success rate after 48 hours of treatment was nearly 90%. Dickenson and Evans compared 400 mg of misoprostol intravaginally every 6 hours with 400 mg of misoprostol orally every 3 hours for second-trimester pregnancy termination. Vaginal misoprostol was significantly more effective than oral misoprostol, 86% of women with vaginal misoprostol had delivered within 24 hours and 100% in 48 hours compared with 45% and 79%, respectively, with oral misoprostol. These same investigators compared 400 mg of misoprostol intravaginally every 6 hours with 200 mg intravaginally every 6 hours. The 400-mg dose was more effective and had a shorter induction to delivery interval than the 200-mg dose. At present, the preferred regimen of misoprostol for second-trimester pregnancy terminations is 400 mg intravaginally every 6 hours. This regimen appears to be safe in women with a prior cesarean delivery as uterine rupture is uncommon.

Major Operations

Hysterotomy and hysterectomy are infrequently used for performing abortion in the United States. Both procedures have a much higher risk of morbidity and mortality than do alternative methods. Hysterectomy should be reserved for those instances in which preexisting gynecologic pathology, such as carcinoma in situ of the cervix or large leiomyomata, also exist.

Pharmacologic Agents

Progesterone Antagonists. A few years ago Healy and coworkers synthesized a progestogenic steroid compound that had weak progestational activity but marked affinity for progesterone receptors in the endometrium. This compound, called RU-486,

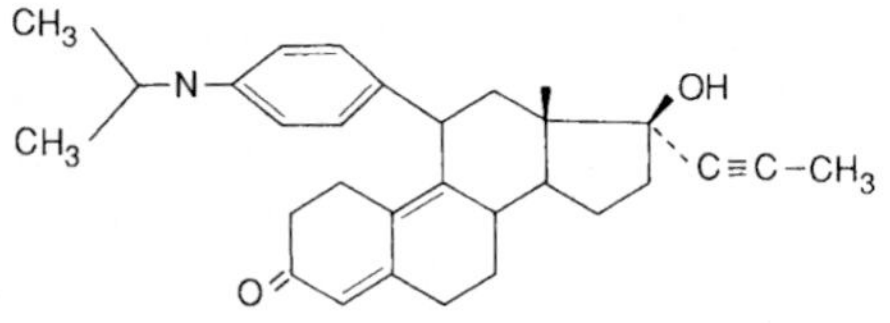

Figure 14-24. Molecular structure of RU-486. Molecular weight is 430, and empirical formula is $C_{29}H_{35}NO_2$. (Reprinted from Fertility and Sterility, 40, Healy DL, Baulieu EE, Hodgen GD, Induction of menstruation by an antiprogesterone steroid (RU 486) in primates: Site of action, dose-response relationships, and hormonal effects, 253. Copyright 1983, with permission from The American Society for Reproductive Medicine.)

or mifepristone (Fig. 14-24), because of its high receptor affinity prevents progesterone from binding to its receptors and thus inhibits the action of circulating progesterone on its target tissue. In clinical trials it was found that if a single 600-mg dose of RU-486 was administered orally in early pregnancy, prior to 7 weeks after the onset of the last menses, that about 85% of the pregnancies spontaneously terminated. When this treatment was combined with administration of a prostaglandin 36 to 48 hours later, the efficacy increased to 96%. However, side effects include nausea, vomiting, and abdominal pain. Two prostaglandin analogues, intramuscular sulprostone and vaginal gemeprost, were the agents initially used after mifepristone. Sulprostone is no longer marketed for this purpose, as three women who received this agent with mifepristone suffered an MI. Gemeprost is much more expensive than misoprostol, a prostaglandin analogue widely used to prevent peptic ulcer disease. Therefore, oral administration of misoprostol is now being used more extensively than gemeprost after mifepristone. Spitz and associates reported the results of a large multicenter study in the United States of first-trimester abortion using 600 mg mifepristone followed 48 hours later by 400 μg oral misoprostol. Success rates were 92% for pregnancies less than 49 days gestational age, 83% for pregnancies 50 to 56 days, and 77% for pregnancies 57 to 63 days (Table 14-13). The FDA approved this treatment regimen for elective termination of pregnancies of 49 days or less gestational age. The WHO reported that a 200-mg dose of mifepristone was as effective as a 600-mg dose when both doses were followed 48 hours later by 400 μg of misoprostol orally.

The results of a randomized trial with 400 mcg misoprostol given vaginally or orally found that when misoprostol is given vaginally instead of orally it is more effective and has fewer side effects. Schaff and colleagues reported that when 200 mg of mifepristone was followed by 800 mg of misoprostol placed intravaginally by the woman at home, 1, 2, or 3 days later in pregnancies of 56 or less days' gestational age, complete abortion rates were 98%, 98%, and 96%, respectively. This regimen reduces the cost of medical abortion as only one 200-mg tablet of mifepristone is used and one office visit is avoided. The main disadvantage of this medical abortifacient regimen is prolonged and sometimes heavy uterine bleeding that on occasion can cause anemia, necessitating a blood transfusion and possibly curettage. The mean duration of bleeding after administration of mifepristone is about 12 days when administered alone and 9 days when used with a prostaglandin.

Since mifepristone is unavailable in many countries, other pharmacologic agents have been used to terminate early gestation. Studies with 800 μg of misoprostol tablets placed in the vagina and moistened with saline for one, two, or three applications 24 hours apart report about a 90% effectiveness when given for a pregnancy of less than 8 weeks' gestational age. Side effects such as vomiting and diarrhea are frequent and can be lessened with use of prophylactic medications. Several investigators have administered methotrexate intramuscularly in a dosage of 50 mg/m^2 followed 3 to 7 days later by vaginal administration of 800 μg of misoprostol to groups of women with pregnancies less than 8 weeks' gestational age and found that about 90% of the pregnancies aborted. However, with this regimen only about two thirds of the women aborted within 1 day after receiving misoprostol. The mean time to abortion in the remainder was about 3 weeks. The mean length of time during which uterine bleeding occurred in the entire study group was more than 2 weeks. Because of these problems, as well as the need to determine the true incidence of side effects, this treatment regimen should be considered experimental and only used

Table 14-13 Results of Mifepristone and Misoprostol in Women Seeking Termination of Pregnancy.

Outcome	Pregnant ≤ 49 days (*N* = 827)	Pregnant 50 to 56 days (*N* = 678)	Pregnant 57 to 63 days (*N* = 510)
	NUMBER (PERCENT [95% CONFIDENCE INTERVAL])		
Success	762 (92 [90–94])	563 (83 [80–86])*	395 (77 [74–81])*†
After mifepristone alone	40 (5)	12 (2)‡	4 (0.8)*
Failure (need for surgical intervention)			
Medical indication for intervention	13 (2)	26 (4)‡	21 (4)‡
Patient's request for intervention	5 (0.6)	13 (2)	
Incomplete abortion	39 (5)	51 (8)‡	12 (2)‡
Ongoing pregnancy	8 (1)	25 (4)*	36 (7)
			46 (9)*§
Total	65 (8)	115 (17)*	115 (23)*†

*$p < 0.001$ for the comparison with the ≤49-days group.
†$p = 0.02$ for the comparison with the 50-to-56-days group.
‡$0.001 \leq p < 0.03$ for the comparison with the ≤49-days group.
§$p < 0.001$ for the comparison with the 50-to-56-days group.
From Spitz IM, Bardin CW, Benton L, Robbins A: Early pregnancy termination with mifepristone and misoprostol in the United States. N Engl J Med 338:1243, 1998. Copyright 1998 Massachusetts Medical Society. All rights reserved.

after an investigative protocol has been approved and the woman has signed an informed consent.

Ancillary Techniques

A qualitative assay for HCG should always be performed before an abortion is undertaken unless there is sonographic evidence of pregnancy. Performing a qualitative pregnancy test 2 weeks after the procedure will ensure that the pregnancy has been successfully aborted. In the first trimester, sonography should be done to determine gestational age when a substantial discrepancy occurs between the menstrual history and clinical examination; when uterine abnormalities, such as leiomyomata, are present; or when the presence of an ectopic gestation is suspected. Sonography should always be performed before initiating second-trimester abortions and has avoided the problem of misestimation of gestational age, which is an important cause of complications. Performing ultrasonography during a D&E may facilitate the procedure.

Complications

Elective abortion in the United States is a very safe operation. Complications are infrequent, and the overall mortality is less than 1 per 100,000 procedures. Two important determinants of complications are the gestational age and method of abortion chosen. When abortion is performed in pregnancies of 6 weeks' or less gestational age there are slightly higher complication rates than when the gestational age is between 7 and 10 weeks. Beyond 10 weeks, abortion complication rates increase progressively with gestational age. Suction curettage is the safest surgical method of abortion, followed by D&E, induction of labor, and major operations.

The most common complication is infection, and the routine use of perioperative antibiotic prophylaxis has been shown to reduce this risk. Other complications include hemorrhage, the consequences of uterine perforation, and anesthetic hazards.

KEY POINTS

- In 2002, of the 62 million women in the United States ages 15 to 44 years, approximately one third were not at risk for pregnancy, and 62%, 38 million, were using a method of contraception. About 7% of women of reproductive age were sexually active and not using any contraceptive.
- In 2001, there were about 6.4 million pregnancies in the United States. There were 4 million births and about 1.3 million elective abortions. Half of all pregnancies were unintended. About 20% of all pregnancies were electively terminated.
- Of women ages 15 to 44 in the United States in 2002, male and female sterilization were used by 22%, oral contraceptives by 19%, male condom by 11%, the progestin injection by 3%, and the IUD by 1.3%.
- Typical and perfect use failure rates in the first year of use range between 5% and 27% for coitus-related methods beween 0.3% and 8% for oral contraceptives (OCs) and 0.3% to 3% for the injection. The IUD and implants have typical use failure rates less than 1%.
- Contraceptive failure rates are increased in inverse relation to the user's age, level of education, and socioeconomic class.
- Pregnancy results from failure of spermicide use are not associated with an increased risk of fetal malformations.
- The active ingredient in spermicides is a surfactant, usually nonoxynol 9, which immobilizes or kills sperm on contact.
- Barrier techniques reduce the rate of transmission of sexually transmitted diseases, both bacterial and viral.
- The most effective type of periodic abstinence is the symptothermal method.
- OC formulations in the United States consist of varying dosages of one of the following progestins: estranes: norethindrone, norethindrone acetate, ethynodiol diacetate, or gonanes: norgestrel (or its active isomer, levonorgestrel), desogestrel, norgestimate, or a spironolactone derivative, drosperinone and either of two estrogens, ethinyl estradiol or ethinyl estradiol-3-methyl ether, also called *mestranol.*
- A given weight of norgestrel or the other gonanes has 5 to 10 times more progestational activity than the equivalent weight of norethindrone, whereas norethindrone acetate and ethynodiol diacetate are similar in potency to norethindrone.
- Metabolic effects of the estrogen component of OCs include an increase in serum globulins that have a thrombophilic effect and altering of the lipid profile to increase triglycerides and HDL cholesterol and lower LDL cholesterol.
- Metabolic effects of the progestin component of OCs include peripheral insulin resistance and lowering HDL cholesterol and raising LDL cholesterol.
- Ethinyl estradiol is approximately 1.7 times as potent as an equivalent weight of mestranol.
- No significantly increased risk of breast cancer occurs among current or former users of OC or in various high-risk subgroups of OC users.
- OC users have an increased risk of developing invasive cervical cancer, particularly adenocarcinoma, compared with users of no contraception, but a causal relation has not been established.
- The rate of return of fertility after stopping OCs is delayed, but eventually the percentage of women who conceive after stopping all methods of contraception, including OCs, is the same.
- Babies born to women who discontinue OCs or who conceive while ingesting OCs have no greater incidence of any type of birth defect.
- All OC formulations with less than 50 μg of estrogen increase the risk of venous thrombosis and embolism three- to fourfold.
- A significantly increased risk of developing MI occurs only in current OC users older than age 35 who smoke.
- Users of low-dose OCs do not have a significantly increased risk of developing ischemic or hemorrhagic stroke if they do not smoke or have hypertension.
- The cause of MI in older OC users who smoke is arterial thrombosis.

Continued

KEY POINTS *Continued*

- Adverse effects produced by the estrogenic component of OCs include nausea, breast tenderness, fluid retention, temporary increase in blood pressure, thrombosis, changes in mood, and chloasma. Progestins produce certain androgenic adverse effects, including weight gain, nervousness, depression, tiredness, and acne, as well as failure of withdrawal bleeding or amenorrhea.
- In an ovulatory cycle the mean blood loss during menstruation is approximately 35 mL, compared with 20 mL for women ingesting OCs.
- OC users are about half as likely to develop iron deficiency anemia as are control subjects.
- OC users are significantly less likely to develop menorrhagia, irregular menstruation, or intermenstrual bleeding than nonusers.
- The risk of developing endometrial cancer, as well as ovarian cancer, in OC users and former users is only half that in control subjects. OC users also have a 50% reduction in the incidence of benign breast disease.
- OC users have approximately 50% less dysmenorrhea and about 40% less premenstrual disorders than do control subjects.
- Functional ovarian cysts occur less frequently in OC users than in nonusers if they use monophasic, but not multiphasic, formulations.
- Prior use of OCs does not affect mortality rates in women.
- OCs reduce the clinical development of salpingitis (PID) in women infected with gonorrhea or *Chlamydia* by 50%, and the overall incidence of PID in OC users is reduced by 50%.
- OCs reduce the risk of ectopic pregnancy by more than 90% in women currently using them.
- There are three types of injectable contraception: depomedroxyprogesterone acetate (DMPA), norethindrone enanthate, and several progestin–estrogen combinations. All are very effective.
- Women using injectable DMPA (150 mg every 3 months) intramuscularly or 104 mg subcutaneously have a first-year pregnancy rate of 0.1%.
- Injectable DMPA is associated with loss of bone density that recovers after DMPA is stopped.
- Women treated with injectable progestins for contraception have complete disruption of the normal menstrual cycle and an irregular bleeding pattern that is usually followed by amenorrhea.
- The most effective method of emergency contraception is ingestion of two tablets of 750 μg of levonorgestrel taken 12 hours apart with a failure rate about 1%.
- The contraceptive patch is applied to the skin for seven days. Effectiveness and adverse effects are similar to OCs.
- The contraceptive vaginal ring is placed in the vagina for 3 weeks. Effectiveness and adverse effects are similar to OCs.
- The cumulative incidence of accidental pregnancy with the copper T 380A IUD is 1.6% after 7 years of use and 1.7% after 12 years of use. This IUD is approved for 10 years' use.
- The incidence of adverse events with IUDs steadily decreases with increasing age of the woman.
- The main mechanism of contraceptive action of the copper IUD is production of a local sterile inflammatory reaction of leukocytes, which destroys sperm and prevents fertilization.
- Resumption of fertility after IUD removal is not delayed and occurs at the same rate as resumption after discontinuation of use of mechanical contraceptive methods.
- A copper or progesterone-releasing IUD can be removed and a new one reinserted immediately afterward. The IUD can be safely inserted on any day of the cycle.
- In the first year of use, the copper T 380 IUD has approximately a 0.5% pregnancy rate, a 10% expulsion rate, and a 15% rate of removal for medical reasons, and the incidence of each of these events diminishes steadily in subsequent years.
- In women wearing a copper T IUD, 50 to 60 mL of blood is lost per cycle; with the levonorgestrel-releasing IUS, the amount of blood loss is about 5 mL per cycle.
- Mefenamic acid, 500 mg twice daily during menses, significantly reduces menstrual blood loss in IUD users.
- The fundal perforation rate with the copper T 380 IUD is about 1 per 3000 insertions.
- The incidence of congenital anomalies is not increased in infants born with any type of IUD in utero.
- If a woman conceives with an IUD in place and the IUD is not removed, the incidence of spontaneous abortion is about 55%, approximately three times greater than would occur without an IUD. If, after conception, the IUD is removed, the incidence of spontaneous abortion is reduced to about 20%.
- If a woman conceives with a copper IUD in place, her chances of having an ectopic pregnancy is about 5%, approximately 10 times greater than occurs in conceptions without an IUD.
- Women using a copper T 380 IUD have approximately a 90% lower overall risk of having an ectopic pregnancy than women using no method of contraception.
- The rate of prematurity among live births occurring with an IUD in utero is increased about two to four times.
- The overall risk of PID in users of IUDs with a monofilament tail string is increased only during the first 3 weeks after insertion.
- Pregnancy rates after reanastomosis of the vas range from 45% to 60%, whereas those after oviduct reanastomosis range from 50% to 80%.
- About 1% of sterilized women request reversal. In the United States approximately 7000 women request reversal each year.
- Usually about 15 to 20 ejaculations are required after vasectomy before a man is sterile.
- After vasectomy, two aspermic ejaculates are required before the male is considered sterile.

KEY POINTS *Continued*

- After sterilization by tubal interruption, the 1-year failure rate is 0.55 per 100 women, the 5-year failure rate is 1.31 per 100 women, and the 10-year failure rate is 1.85 per 100 women. About one third of the pregnancies are ectopic.
- Complication rates are three to four times higher for second-trimester abortions than for first-trimester abortions.
- The most effective medical means to terminate pregnancies less than 8 weeks' gestation is the combination of mifepristone followed by misoprostol, with a failure rate less than 5%.
- A single subdermally placed implant containing etonogestrel provides excellent contraceptive effectiveness for 3 years.
- A microinsert placed into the oviducts transcervically provides very effective permanent pregnancy prevention.

BIBLIOGRAPHY

Alvarez F, Gujiloff E, Brache V, et al: New insights on the mode of action of intrauterine contraceptive devices in women. Fertil Steril 49:768, 1988.

Anderson ABM, Haynes PJ, Guillebaud J, et al: Reduction of menstrual blood loss by prostaglandin synthetase inhibitors. Lancet 1:774, 1976.

Andersson K, Odlind V, Rybo G: Levonorgestrel-releasing and copper-releasing (Nova T) IUDs during five years of use: A randomized comparative trial. Contraception 49:56, 1994.

Austin H, Louv WC, Alexander WJ: A case-control study of spermicides and gonorrhea. JAMA 251:2822, 1984.

Back DJ, Breckenridge AM, Crawford FE, et al: The effects of rifampicin on the pharmacokinetics of ethinylestradiol in women. Contraception 21:135, 1980.

Backman T, Rauramo I, Jaakkola K, et al: Use of levonorgestrel-releasing intrauterine system and breast cancer. Obstet Gynecol 106:813, 2005.

Bahamondes L, Del Castillo S, Tabares G, et al: Comparison of weight increase in users of depot medroxyprogesterone acetate and copper IUD up to 5 years. Contraception 64:223, 2001.

Beral V, Hermon C, Kay C, et al: Mortality associated with oral contraceptive use: 25 year follow up of cohort of 46000 women from Royal College of General Practitioners' Oral Contraception Study. BMJ 318:96, 1999.

Bloemenkamp KWM, Rosendaal FR, Helmerhorst FM, et al: Enhancement of factor V Leiden mutation of risk of deep-vein thrombosis associated with oral contraceptives containing a third-generation progestagen. Lancet 346:1593, 1995.

Bokarewa MI, Falk G, Sten-Linder M, et al: Thrombotic risk factors and oral contraception. J Lab Clin Med 126:294, 1995.

Borgatta L, Burnhill MS, Tyson J, et al. Early medical abortion with methotrexate and misoprostol. Obstet Gynecol 97:11, 2001.

Borgatta L, Murthy A, Chuang C, et al. Pregnancies diagnosed during Depo-Provera use. Contraception 66:169, 2002.

Bracken MB, Vita K: Frequency of non-hormonal contraception around conception and association with congenital malformations in offspring. Am J Epidemiol 117:281, 1983.

Bracken MB, Hellenbrand KG, Holford TR: Conception delay after oral contraceptive use: The effect of estrogen dose. Fertil Steril 53:21, 1990.

Brenner PF, Goebelsmann U, Stanczyk FZ, Mishell DR Jr: Serum levels of ethinylestradiol following its ingestion alone or in oral contraceptive formulations. Contraception 22:85, 1980.

Brenner PF, Mishell DR Jr, Stanczyk FZ, et al: Serum levels of d-norgestrel, luteinizing hormone, follicle-stimulating hormone, estradiol, and progesterone in women during and following ingestion of combination oral contraceptives containing dl-norgestrel. Am J Obstet Gynecol 129:133, 1977.

Brinton LA, Reeves WC, Brenes MM, et al: Oral contraceptive use and risk of invasive cervical cancer. Int J Epidemiol 19:4, 1990.

Brinton LA, Vessy MP, Flavell R, et al: Risk factors for benign breast disease. Am J Epidemiol 113:203, 1981.

Brown JB, Blackwell LF, Billings JJ, et al: Natural family planning. Am J Obstet Gynecol 157:1082, 1987.

Castracane VD, Gimpel T, Goldzieher JW: When is it safe to switch from oral contraceptives to hormonal replacement therapy? Contraception 52:371, 1995.

Celentano DD, Klassen AC, Weisman CS, Rosenshein NB: The role of contraceptive use in cervical cancer: The Maryland cervical cancer case-control study. Am J Epidemiol 126:592, 1987.

Centers for Disease Control and Prevention: Combination oral contraceptives use and risk of endometrial cancer. JAMA 257:976, 1987.

Chasan-Taber L, Colditz GA, Willett WC, et al: A prospective study of oral contraceptives and NIDDM among U.S. women. Diabetes Care 20:330, 1997.

Chasan-Taber L, Willett WC, Manson JE, et al: Prospective study of oral contraceptives and hypertension among women in the United States. Circulation 94:483, 1996.

Chi IC, Potts M, Wilkens LR, et al: Performance of the copper T-380A intrauterine device in breast feeding women. Contraception 39:603, 1989.

Chow WH, Daling JR, Weiss NS, et al: IUD use and subsequent tubal pregnancy. Am J Public Health 66:131, 1986.

Clarkson TB, Shively CA, Morgan TM, et al: Oral contraceptives and coronary artery atherosclerosis of cynomolgus monkeys. Obstet Gynecol 75:217, 1990.

Coenen CMH, Thomas CMH, Borm GF, et al: Changes in androgens during treatment with four low-dose contraceptives. Contraception 53:171, 1996.

Coker AL, McCann MF, Hulka BS, Walter LA: Oral contraceptive use and cervical intraepithelial neoplasia. J Clin Epidemiol 45:1111, 1992.

Colditz GA for The Nurses' Health Study Research Group: Oral contraceptive use and mortality during 12 years follow-up: The Nurses' Health Study. Ann Intern Med 120:821, 1994.

Collaborative Group on Hormonal Factors in Breast Cancer: Breast cancer and hormonal contraceptives: Collaborative reanalysis of individual data on 53,297 women with breast cancer and 100,239 women without breast cancer from 54 epidemiological studies. Lancet 347:1713, 1996.

Collaborative Group on Hormonal Factors in Breast Cancer: Breast cancer and hormonal contraceptives: Further results. Contraception 54:1S, 1996.

Conant M, Hardy D, Sernatinger J, et al: Condoms prevent transmission of AIDS-associated retrovirus. JAMA 255:1706, 1986.

Conant MA, Spicer DW, Smith CD: Herpes simplex virus transmission: Condom studies. Sex Transm Dis 11:94, 1984.

Cooper JM, Carignan CS, Cher D, Kerin JF: Microinsert nonincisional hysteroscopic sterilization. Obstet Gynecol 102:59, 2003.

Craig S, Hepburn S: The effectiveness of barrier methods of contraception with and without spermicide. Contraception 26:347, 1982.

Creasy GW, for the Ortho EVRA/EVRA 002 Study Group: Efficacy and safety of a transdermal contraceptive system. Obstet Gynecol 98:799, 2001.

Creasy GW, for the Ortho EVRA/EVRA 004 Study Group: Evaluation of contraceptive efficacy and cycle control of a transdermal contraceptive patch vs an oral contraceptive: a randomized controlled trial. JAMA 285:2347, 2001.

Croft P, Hannaford PC: Risk factors for acute myocardial infarction in women. BMJ 298:165, 1989.

Cromer BA, Blair JM, Mahan JD, et al: A prospective comparison of bone density in adolescent girls receiving depot medroxyprogesterone acetate (Depo-Provera), levonorgestrel (Norplant), or oral contraceptives. J Pediatr 129:671, 1996.

Croxatto HB, and the Implanon Study Group: A multicentre efficacy and safety study of the single contraceptive implant implanon. Hum Reprod 14:976, 1999.

Cullins VE: Noncontraceptive benefits and therapeutic uses of depot medroxyprogesterone acetate. J Reprod Med 41(9):428, 1996.

Cundy T, Cornish J, Evans MC, et al: Recovery of bone density in women who stop using medroxyprogesterone acetate. BMJ 308:247, 1994.

Cundy T, Cornish J, Roberts H, et al. Menopausal bone loss in long-term users of depot medroxyprogesterone acetate contraception. Am J Obstet Gynecol 186:978, 2002.

Cundy T, Evans M, Roberts H, et al: Bone density in women receiving depot medroxyprogesterone acetate for contraception. BMJ 303:13, 1991.

Dickinson JE, Evans SF: A comparison of oral misoprostol with vaginal misoprostol administration in second-trimester pregnancy termination for fetal abnormality. Obstet Gynecol 101:1294, 2003.

Dickinson JE, Evans SF: The optimization of intravaginal misoprostol dosing schedules in second-trimester pregnancy termination. Am J Obstet Gynecol 186:470, 2002.

Doll H, Vessey M, Painter R: Return of fertility in nulliparous women after discontinuation of the intrauterine device: Comparison with women discontinuing other methods of contraception. Br J Obstet Gynecol 108:304, 2001.

Dong W, Colhoun HM, Poutler NR: Blood pressure in women using oral contraceptives: Results from the Health Survey for England 1994. J Hypertens 15:1063, 1997.

Dorflinger L: Relative potency of progestins used in oral contraceptives. Contraception 557:31, 1985.

El-Rafaey H, Rajasekar D, Abdalla M, et al: Induction of abortion with mifepristone (RU 486) and oral or vaginal misoprostol. N Engl J Med 332:983, 1995.

Engel HJ, Engel E, Lichtlen PR: Coronary atherosclerosis and myocardial infarction in young women: Role of oral contraceptives. Eur Heart J 4:1, 1983.

Farley TM, Rosenberg MJ, Rowe PJ, et al: Intrauterine devices and pelvic inflammatory disease: An international perspective. Lancet 339:785, 1992.

Farmer RDT, Preston NTD: The risk of venous thrombosis associated with low oestrogen oral contraceptives. J Obstet Gynecol 15:195, 1995.

Farr G, Gabelnlick H, Sturgen K, Dorflinger L: Contraceptive efficacy and acceptability of the female condom. Am J Public Health 84:1960, 1994.

Fasoli M, Parazzini F, Cecchetti G, et al: Post-coital contraception: An overview of published studies. Contraception 39:459, 1989.

Fernandez E, La Vecchia C, Balducci A, et al: Oral contraceptives and colorectal cancer risk: A meta-analysis. Br J Cancer 84:722, 2001.

Ferreira AE, Araujo MJ, Regina CH, et al: Effectiveness of the diaphragm, used continuously, without spermicide. Contraception 48:29, 1993.

Fihn SD, Latham RH, Roberts P, et al: Association between diaphragm use and urinary tract infection. JAMA 254:240, 1986.

Finer LB, Henshaw SK: Abortion incidence and services in the United States in 2000. Perspect Sex Reprod Health 35:6, 2003.

Finer LB, Henshaw SK: Disparities in rates of unintended pregnancy in the United States, 1994–2001. Perspect Sex Reprod Health 38(2):90, 2006.

Forman D, Vincent TJ, Doll R: Cancer of the liver and the use of oral contraceptives. BMJ 292:1357, 1986.

Gambacciani 1M, Spinetti A, Toponeco F, et al: Longitudinal evaluation of perimenopausal vertebral bone loss: Effects of a low-dose oral contraceptive preparation on bone mineral density and metabolism. Obstet Gynecol 83:392, 1993.

Gardner JM, Mishell DR Jr: Analysis of bleeding patterns and resumption of fertility following discontinuation of a long-acting injectable contraceptive. Fertil Steril 21:286, 1970.

Gerstman BB, Piper JM, Tomita DK, et al: Oral contraceptive estrogen dose and the risk of deep venous thromboembolic disease. Am J Epidemiol 133:32, 1991.

Gilbert A, Reid R: A randomized trial of oral versus vaginal administration of misoprostol for the purpose of mid-trimester termination of pregnancy. Aust N Z J Obstet Gynaecol 41:407, 2001.

Glasier A, Thong KJ, Dewar M, et al: Mifepristone (RU486) compared with high-dose estrogen and progestogen for emergency postcoital contraception. N Engl J Med 327:1041, 1992.

Godsland IF, Crook D, Wynn V: Clinical and metabolic considerations of long-term oral contraceptive use. Am J Obstet Gynecol 166:1955, 1992.

Godsland IF, Crook D, Simpson R, et al: The effects of different formulations of oral contraceptive agents on lipid and carbohydrate metabolism. N Engl J Med 323:1375, 1990.

Godsland IF, Crook D, Worthington M, et al: Effects of a low-estrogen, desogestrel-containing oral contraceptive on lipid and carbohydrate metabolism. Contraception 48:217, 1993.

Gray RH, Pardthaisong T: In utero exposure to steroid contraceptives and survival during infancy. Am J Epidemiol 134:804, 1991.

Hamoda H, Ashok PW, Flett GMM, et al. Medical abortion at 64 to 91 days of gestation: A review of 483 consecutive cases. Am J Obstet Gynecol 188:1315, 2003.

Hankinson SE, Colditz GA, Hunter DJ, et al: A quantitative assessment of oral contraceptive use and risk of ovarian cancer. Obstet Gynecol 80:708, 1992.

Hannaford P, Elliott A: Use of exogenous hormones by women and colorectal cancer: Evidence from the Royal College of General Practitioners' Oral Contraception Study. Contraception 71(2):95, 2005.

Hannaford PC, Croft PR, Kay CR: Oral contraception and stroke: Evidence from the Royal College of General Practitioners' Oral Contraception Study. Stroke 25:935, 1993.

Hannaford PC, Kay CR: Oral contraceptives and diabetes mellitus. BMJ 299:315, 1989.

Hannaford PC, Villard-Mackintosh L, Vessey MP, Kay CR: Oral contraceptives and malignant melanoma. Br J Cancer 63:430, 1991.

Harlap S, Shiono PH, Ramcharan S: Congenital abnormalities in the offspring of women who used oral and other contraceptives around the time of conception. Int J Fertil 30:39, 1985.

Healy DL, Baulieu EE, Hodgen GD: Induction of menstruation by an antiprogesterone steroid (RU 486) in primates: Site of action, dose-response relationships, and hormonal effects. Fertil Steril 40:253, 1983.

Helms SE, Bredle DL, Zajic J, et al: Oral contraceptive failure rates and oral antibiotics. J Am Acad Dermatol 36:705, 1997.

Ho PC, Kwan MSW: A prospective randomized comparison of levonorgestrel with the Yuzpe regimen in post-coital contraception. Hum Reprod 8:389, 1993.

Holt VL, Cushing-Haugen KL, Daling JR: Body weight and risk of oral contraceptive failure. Obstet Gynecol 99:820-827, 2002.

Hubacher D, Lara-Ricalde R, Taylor DJ, et al. Use of copper intrauterine devices and the risk of tubal infertility among nulligravid women. N Engl J Med 345:561, 2001.

Jain J, Dutton C, Nicosia A, et al: Pharmacokinetics, ovulation suppression and return to ovulation following a lower dose subcutaneous formulation of Depo-Provera®. Contraception 70:11, 2004.

Jain J, Jakimiuk AJ, Bode FR, et al: Contraceptive efficacy and safety of DMPA-SC. Contraception 70:269, 2004.

Jain JK, Mishell DR Jr: A comparison of misoprostol with and without laminaria tents for induction of second-trimester abortion. Am J Obstet Gynecol 175:173, 1996.

Janerich DT, Piper JM, Glebatis DM: Oral contraceptives and birth defects. Am J Epidemiol 112:73, 1980.

Jick H, Hanna MT, Stergachis A, et al: Vaginal spermicides and gonorrhea. JAMA 248:1619, 1982.

Jick SS, Walker AM, Jick H: Oral contraceptives and endometrial cancer. Obstet Gynecol 82:931, 1993.

Karagas MR, Stukel TA, Dykes J, et al: A pooled analysis of 10 case-control studies of melanoma and oral contraceptive use. Br J Cancer 86:1085, 2002.

Kaunitz AM, Carceau RJ, Cromie MA: Comparative safety, efficacy, and cycle control of Lunelle monthly contraceptive injection (medroxyprogesterone acetate and estradiol cypionate injectable suspension) and Ortho-Novum 7/7/7 oral contraceptive (norethindrone/ethinyl estradiol triphasic). Contraception 60:179, 1999.

Kimmerle R, Weiss R, Berger M, Kurz KH: Effectiveness, safety, and acceptability of a copper intrauterine device (CU Safe 300) in type 1 diabetic women. Diabetes Care 16:1227, 1993.

Kirton KT, Cornette JC: Return of ovulatory cyclicity following an intramuscular injection of medroxyprogesterone acetate (Provera®). Contraception 10:39, 1974.

Kjaer SK, Engholm G, Dahl C, et al: Case-control study of risk factors for cervical squamous-cell neoplasia in Denmark. III. Role of oral contraceptive use. Cancer Causes Control 4:513, 1993.

Kjos SL, Ballagh SA, LaCour M, et al: The copper T380A intrauterine device in women with type II diabetes mellitus. Obstet Gynecol 84:1006, 1994.

Kjos SL, Shoupe D, Douhan S, et al: Effect of low-dose oral contraceptives on carbohydrate and lipid metabolism in women with recurrent gestational diabetes: Results of a controlled randomized prospective study. Am J Obstet Gynecol 163:1822, 1990.

Klaus H: Natural family planning: A review. Obstet Gynecol Surv 37:128, 1982.

Klein TA, Mishell DR Jr: Gonadotropin, prolactin and steroid hormone levels after discontinuation of oral contraceptives. Am J Obstet Gynecol 127:585, 1977.

La Vecchcia C, Negri E, D'Avanzo B, et al: Oral contraceptives and noncontraceptive oestrogens in the risk of gallstone disease requiring surgery. J Epidemiol Community Health 46:234, 1992.

La Vecchia C. Oral contraceptives and ovarian cancer: An update, 1998–2004. Eur J Cancer Prev 15(2):117, 2006.

Lanes AF, Birmann B, Walter AM, Singer S: Oral contraceptive type and functional ovarian cysts. Am J Obstet Gynecol 166:956, 1992.

Le J, Tsourounis C: Implanon: A critical review. Ann Pharmacother 35:329, 2001.

Lee NC, Rubin GL: The intrauterine device and pelvic inflammatory disease revisited: New results from the women's health study. Obstet Gynecol 72:1, 1988.

Lidegaard Ø, Milsom I: Oral contraceptives and thrombotic diseases: Impact of new epidemiological studies. Contraception 53:135, 1996.

Lidegaard Ø, Edström B, Kreiner S: Oral contraceptives and venous thromboembolism: A five-year national case-control study. Contraception 65:187, 2002.

Lieu DFM, Ng CSA, Yong YM, et al: Long-term effects of depo-provera on carbohydrate and lipid metabolism. Contraception 31:51, 1985.

Linn S, Schoenbaum SC, Monson RR, et al: Lack of association between contraceptive usage and congenital malformations in offspring. Am J Obstet Gynecol 147:923, 1983.

Louik C, Mitchell AA, Werler MM, et al: Maternal exposure to spermicides in relation to certain birth defects. N Engl J Med 317:474, 1987.

Luyckx AS, Gaspard UJ, Romus MA, et al: Carbohydrate metabolism in women who used oral contraceptives containing levonorgestrel or desogestrel: A 6-month prospective study. Fertil Steril 45:635, 1986.

MacKay AP, Kieke BA Jr, Koonin LM, et al: Tubal sterilization in the United States, 1994–1996. Fam Plann Perspect 33:161, 2001.

Mäkäräinen L, van Beek A, Tuomivaara L, et al. Ovarian function during the use of a single contraceptive implant: Implanon compared with Norplant. Fertil Steril 69:714, 1998.

Marchbanks PA, McDonald JA, Wilson HG, et al: Oral contraceptives and the risk of breast cancer. N Engl J Med 346:2025, 2002.

Mattson RH, Rebar RW: Contraceptive methods for women with neurologic disorders. Am J Obstet Gynecol 168:2027, 1993.

Mattson RH, Cramer JA, Caldwell BVD, et al: Treatment of seizures with medroxyprogesterone acetate: Preliminary report. Neurology 34:1255, 1984.

Michaelsson K, Baron JA, Farahmand BY, et al: Oral-contraceptive use and risk of hip fracture: A case-control study. Lancet 353:1481, 1999.

Mileikowsky GN, Nadler JL, Huey F, et al: Evidence that smoking alters prostacyclin formation and platelet aggregation in women who use oral contraceptives, Am J Obstet Gynecol 159:1547, 1988.

Milne RL, Knight JA, John EM, et al: Oral contraceptive us and risk of early-onset breast cancer in carriers and noncarriers of BRCA1 and BRCA2 mutations. Cancer Epidemiol Biomarkers Prev 14:350, 2005.

Milson I, Anderson K, Jonasson K, et al: The influence of the Gyne-T 380A IUD on menstrual blood loss and iron status. Contraception 52:175, 1995.

Mishell DR Jr, Roy S: Copper intrauterine contraceptive device event rates following insertion 4 to 8 weeks postpartum. Am J Obstet Gynecol 143:29, 1981.

Mishell Dr Jr, Keltzky OA, Brenner PF, et al: The effect of contraceptive steroids on hypothalamic-pituitary function. Am J Obstet Gynecol 130:817, 1978.

Mishell DR Jr, Kharma KM, Thorneycroft IH, et al: Estrogenic activity in women receiving an injectable progestogen for contraception. Am J Obstet Gynecol 113:372, 1972.

Mishell DR Jr: Bell JH, Good RG, et al: The intrauterine device: A bacteriologic study of the endometrial cavity. Am J Obstet Gynecol 96:119, 1966.

Mishell DR Jr: Noncontraceptive benefits of oral contraceptives. J Reprod Med 38:1021, 1993.

Mohllajee AP, Curtis KM, Martins SL, Peterson HB: Hormonal contraceptive use and risk of sexually transmitted infections: A systematic review. Contraception 73(2):154, 2006.

Moore LL, Valuck R, McDougall C, et al: A comparative study of one-year weight gain among users of medroxyprogesterone acetate, levonorgestrel implants, and oral contraceptives. Contraception 52:215, 1995.

Moreno V, for the International Agency for Research on Cancer (IARC) Multicentric Cervical Cancer Study Group: Effect of oral contraceptives on risk of cervical cancer in women with human papillomavirus infection: The IARC multicentric case-control study. Lancet 359:1085, 2002.

Mosher WD, Martinez GM, Chandra A, et al: Use of contraception and use of family planning services in the United States: 1982–2002, Advance Data from Vital and Health Statistics, U.S. Department of Health and Human Services, Centers for Disease Control and Prevention, Number 350, December 10, 2004.

Mulders TMT, Dieben TOM: Use of the novel combined contraceptive vaginal ring NuvaRing for ovulation inhibition. Fertil Steril 75:865, 2001.

Murphy AA, Zacur HA, Charache P, Burkmand RT: The effect of tetracycline on levels of oral contraceptives. Am J Obstet Gynecol 164:28, 1991.

Naessen T, Olsson SE, Gudmundson J: Differential effects on bone density of progestogen-only methods for contraception in premenopausal women. Contraception 52:35, 1995.

Ness RB, Grisso JA, Klapper J, et al: Risk of ovarian cancer in relation to estrogen and progestin dose and use characteristics of oral contraceptives. Am J Epidemiol 152:233, 2000.

Ness RB, Grisso JA, Vergona R, et al: Oral contraceptives, other methods of contraception, and risk reduction for ovarian cancer. Epidemiology 12:307, 2001.

Newton JR, d'Arcangues C, Hall PE: Once-a-month combined injectable contraceptives. J Obstet Gynecol 14(Suppl 1):S1, 1994.

Notelovitz M, Levenson I, McKenzie L, et al: The effects of low-dose oral contraceptives on coagulation and fibrinolysis in two high-risk populations: Young female smokers and older premenopausal women. Am J Obstet Gynecol 152:995, 1985.

Ortiz A, Hiroi M, Stanczyk FZ, et al: Serum medroxyprogesterone acetate (MPA) concentrations and ovarian function following intramuscular injection of depo-MPA. J Clin Endocrinol Metab 44:32, 1977.

Pabinger I, Schneider B: Thrombotic risk of women with hereditary antithrombin III-protein C- and protein S-deficiency taking oral contraceptive medication: The GTH Study Group on Natural Inhibitors. Thromb Haemost 71:548, 1994.

Peipert JF, Gutmann J: Oral contraceptive risk assessment: A survey of 247 educated women. Obstet Gynecol 82:112, 1993.

Pelkman CL, Chow M, Heinbach RA, et al: Short-term effects of a progestational contraceptive drug on food intake, resting energy expenditure, and body weight in young women. Am J Clin Nutr 73:19, 2001.

Persson E, Holmberg K, Dahlgren S, et al: *Actinomyces israelii* in genital tract of women with and without intrauterine contraceptive devices. Acta Obstet Gynecol Scand 62:563, 1983.

Peterson HB, Xia Z, Hughes JM, et al: The risk of pregnancy after tubal sterilization: Findings from the U.S. Collaborative Review of Sterilization, Am J Obstet Gynecol 174:1161, 1996.

Petitti DB, Sidney S, Bernstein A, et al: Stroke in users of low-dose oral contraceptives. N Engl J Med 335:8, 1996.

Pirruccello Newhall E, Winikoff B: Abortion with mifepristone and misoprostol: Regimens, efficacy, acceptability and future directions. Am J Obstet Gynecol 183:S44, 2000.

Pituitary Adenoma Study Group: Pituitary adenomas and oral contraceptives: A multicenter case-control study. Fertil Steril 39:753, 1983.

Poulter NR, for the World Health Organization Collaborative Study of Cardiovascular Disease and Steroid Hormone Contraception: Venous thromboembolic disease and combined oral contraceptives: Results of international multicentre case-control study. Lancet 346:1571, 1995.

Poulter NR, for the World Health Organization Collaborative Study of Cardiovascular Disease and Steroid Hormone Contraception: Cardiovascular disease and use of oral and injectable progestogen-only contraceptives and combined injectable contraceptives: Results of an international, multicenter, case-control study,. Contraception 57:315, 1998.

Powell LMG, Mears BJ, Deber RB, Ferguson D: Contraception with the cervical cap: Effectiveness, safety, continuity of use, and user satisfaction. Contraception 33:215, 1986.

Rosenberg L, Palmer JR, Lesko SM, et al: Oral contraceptive use and the risk of myocardial infarction. Am J Epidemiol 131:1009, 1990.

Rosenberg L, Palmer JR, Rao RS, et al: Low-dose oral contraceptive use and the risk of myocardial infarction. Arch Intern Med 161:1065, 2001.

Rosenberg L, Palmer JR, Zauber AG: A case-control study of oral contraceptive use and invasive epithelial ovarian cancer. Am J Epidemiol 139:654, 1994.

Rosenberg MJ, Waugh MS, Stevens CM: Smoking and cycle control among oral contraceptive users. Am J Obstet Gynecol 174:628, 1996.

Rothman KJ, Louik C: Oral contraceptives and birth defects. N Engl J Med 299:522, 1978.

Roumen FJME, Apter D, Mulders TMT, et al: Efficacy, tolerability and acceptability of a novel contraceptive vaginal ring releasing etonogestrel and ethinyl oestradiol. Hum Reprod 16:469, 2001.

Rowe PJ, for United Nations Development Programme/United Nations Population Fund/World Health Organization: Long-term reversible contraception: Twelve years of experience with the Tcu380A and Tcu220C. Contraception 56:341, 1997.

Royar J, Becher H, Chang-Claude J: Low-dose oral contraceptives: Protective effect on ovarian cancer risk. Int J Cancer 95(6):370, 2001.

Ryden G, Fahraeus L, Molin L, et al: Do contraceptives influence the incidence of acute pelvic inflammatory disease in women with gonorrhea? Contraception 20:149, 1979.

Sandvei R, Ulstein M, Woolen AL: Fertility following ectopic pregnancy with special reference to previous use of an intrauterine contraceptive device (IUCD). Acta Obstet Gynecol Scand 66:131, 1987.

Schaff EA, Eisinger SH, Stadalius LS, et al: Low-dose mifepristone 200 mg and vaginal misoprostol for abortion. Contraception 59:1, 1999.

Schaff EA, Fielding SL, Westhoff C, et al: Vaginal misoprostol administered 1, 2 or 3 days after mifepristone for early medical abortion: A randomized trial. JAMA 284:1948, 2000.

Schlesselman JJ: Net effect of oral contraceptive use on the risk of cancer in women in the United States. Obstet Gynecol 85:793, 1995.

Scholes D, Lacroix AZ, Ott SM, et al: Bone mineral density in women using depot medroxyprogesterone acetate for contraception. Obstet Gynecol 93:233, 1999.

Schwallie PC, Assenzo JR: Contraceptive use: Efficacy study utilizing medroxyprogesterone acetate administered as an intramuscular injection once every 90 days. Fertil Steril 24:331, 1973.

Schwallie PC, Assenzo JR: The effect of depo medroxyprogesterone acetate on pituitary and ovarian function, and the return of fertility following its discontinuation: A review. Contraception 10(2):181, 1974.

Schwartz SM, Petitti DB, Siscovick DS, et al: Stroke and use of low-dose oral contraceptives in young women: A pooled analysis of two US studies. Stroke 29:2277, 1998.

Schwartz SM, Siscovick DS, Longstreth WT Jr, et al: Use of low-dose oral contraceptives and stroke in young women. Ann Intern Med 127:596, 1997.

Senanayake P, Kramer DG: Contraception and the etiology of pelvic inflammatory disease: New perspectives. Am J Obstet Gynecol 138:852, 1980.

Shalev E, Edelstein S, Engelhard J, et al: Ultrasonically controlled retrieval of an intrauterine contraceptive device (IUCD) in early pregnancy. J Clin Ultrasound 15:525, 1987.

Sidney S, Petitti DB, Quesenberry CP Jr, et al: Myocardial infarction in users of low-dose oral contraceptives. Obstet Gynecol 88:939, 1996.

Sidney S, Siscovick DS, Petitti DB, et al: Myocardial infarction and use of low-dose oral contraceptives: A pooled analysis of two US studies. Circulation 98:1, 1998.

Siriwongse T, Snidvongs W, Tantayaporn P, et al: Effect of depo-medroxyprogesterone acetate on serum progesterone levels when administered on various cycle days. Contraception 26:487, 1982.

Sivin I: Contraception with Norplant® implants. Hum Reprod 9:1818, 1994.

Sivin I: Dose- and age-dependent ectopic pregnancy risks with intrauterine contraception. Obstet Gynecol 78:291, 1991.

Skegg DC, Noonan EA, Paul C, et al: Depot medroxyprogesterone acetate and breast cancer: A pooled analysis of the World Health Organization and New Zealand studies. JAMA 273:799, 1995.

Skouby SO, Milsted-Pedersen L: Consequences of intrauterine contraception in diabetic women. Fertil Steril 42:468, 1984

Smith JS, Green J, Berrington de Gonzalez A, et al: Cervical cancer and use of hormonal contraceptives: A systematic review. Lancet 361:1159, 2003.

Spector TD, Romas E, Silman AJ: The pill, parity, and rheumatoid arthritis. Arthritis Rheum 33:782, 1990.

Speroff L, DeCherney A, and the Advisory Board for the New Progestins: Evaluation of a new generation of oral contraceptives. Obstet Gynecol 81:1034, 1993.

Spitz IM, Bardin CW, Benton L, Robbins A: Early pregnancy termination with mifepristone and misoprostol in the United States. N Eng J Med 338:1243, 1998.

Spitzer WO, Lewis MA, Heinemann LAJ, et al: Third generation oral contraceptives and risk of venous thromboembolic disorders: An international case-control study. BMJ 312:83, 1996.

Strom BL, Berlin JA, Weber AL, et al: Absence of an effect of injectable and implantable progestin-only contraceptives on subsequent risk of breast cancer. Contraception 69(5):353, 2004.

Sulak PJ, Kuehl TJ, Ortiz M, et al: Acceptance of altering the standard 21-day/7-day oral contraceptive regimen to delay menses and reduce hormone withdrawal symptoms. Am J Obstet Gynecol 186:1142, 2002.

Tatum HJ, Schmidt FH, Jain AK: Management and outcome of pregnancies associated with the Copper T intrauterine contraceptive device. Am J Obstet Gynecol 126:869, 1976.

The New Zealand Contraception and Health Study Group: Risk of cervical dysplasia in users of oral contraceptives, intrauterine devices or depot medroxyprogesterone acetate. Contraception 50:431, 1994.

Troisi RJ, Cowie CC, Harris MI: Oral contraceptive use and glucose metabolism in a national sample of women in the United States. Am J Obstet Gynecol 183:389, 2000.

Trussell J, Leveque JA, Koenig JD, et al: The economic value of contraception: A comparison of 15 methods. Am J Public Health 85:494, 1995.

Trussell J, Strickler J, Vaughan B: Contraceptive efficacy of the diaphragm, the sponge and the cervical cap. Fam Plann Perspect 25:100, 135, 1993.

Trussell J, Sturgen K, Strickler J, Dominik R: Comparative contraceptive efficacy of the female condom and other barrier methods. Fam Plann Perspect 26:66, 1994.

United Nations Development Programme/United Nations Population Fund/World Health Organization/World Bank, Special Programme of Research, Development and Research Training in Human Reproduction: Long-Term Reversible Contraception: Twelve years of experience with the TCU 380A. Contraception 56:341, 1997.

Van der Vange N, Blankenstein MA, Kloosterboer HJ, et al: Effects of seven low-dose combined oral contraceptives on sex hormone binding globulin, corticosteroid binding globulin, total and free testosterone. Contraception 41:345, 1990.

Van der Vange N, Kloosterboer HG, Haspels AA: Effect of seven low-dose combined oral contraceptive preparations on carbohydrate metabolism. Am J Obstet Gynecol 156:918, 1987.

Vandenbroucke JP, Koster T, Briet E, et al: Increased risk of venous thrombosis in oral-contraceptive users who are carriers of Factor V Leiden Mutation. Lancet 344:1453, 1994.

Vessey M, Painter R: Oral contraceptive use and benign gallbladder disease revisited. Contraception 50:167, 1994.

Vessey MP, Lawless M, McPherson K, et al: Fertility after stopping use of intrauterine contraceptive device. BMJ 286:106, 1983.

Vessey MP, Villard-Mackintosh L, McPherson K, et al: Mortality among oral contraceptive users: 20 year follow up of women in a cohort study. BMJ 299:1487, 1989.

Virutamasen P, Wongsrichanalai C, Tangkeo P, et al: Metabolic effects of depot medroxyprogesterone acetate in long-term users: A cross-sectional study. Int J Gynaecol Obstet 24:291, 1986.

Voigt LF, Deng Q, Weiss NS: Recency, duration, and progestin content of oral contraceptives in relation to the incidence of endometrial cancer. Cancer Causes Control 5:227, 1994.

von Hertzen H, for the Task Force on Postovulatory Methods of Fertility Regulation (World Health Organization, Geneva): Randomised controlled trial of levonorgestrel versus the Yuzpe regimen of combined oral contraceptives for emergency contraception. Lancet 352:428, 1998.

von Hertzen H, for the WHO Research Group on Post-Ovulatory Methods of Fertility Regulation: Low dose mifepristone and two regimens of levonorgestrel for emergency contraception: A WHO multicentre randomized trial. Lancet 360:1803, 2002.

von Hertzen H, for the World Health Organization Task Force on Post-ovulatory Methods of Fertility Regulation (World Health Organization, Geneva): Comparison of two doses of mifepristone in combination with misoprostol for early medical abortion: A randomized trial. Br J Obstet Gynaecol 107:524, 2000.

Walker GR, Schlesselman JJ, Ness RB: Family history of cancer, oral contraceptive use, and ovarian cancer risk. Am J Obstet Gynecol 186:8, 2002.

Walsh T, for the IUD Study Group: Randomised controlled trial of prophylactic antibiotics before insertion of intrauterine devices. Lancet 351:1005, 1998.

Warner P, Bancroft J: Mood, sexuality, oral contraceptives and the menstrual cycle. J Psychosom Res 32:417, 1988.

Weiderpass E, Adami H-O, Baron JA, et al: Use of oral contraceptives and endometrial cancer risk (Sweden). Cancer Causes Control 10(4):277, 1999.

Wenzl R, van Beek A, Schnabel P, Huber J: Pharmacokinetics of etonogestrel released from the contraceptive implant Implanon®. Contraception 58:283, 1998.

Westhoff C, Davis A: Tubal sterilization: Focus on the US experience. Fertil Steril 73:913, 2000.

Westhoff C, Kerns J, Morroni C, et al: Quick start: A novel oral contraceptive initiation method. Contraception 66:141, 2002.

Westhoff C: Depot medroxyprogesterone acetate contraception: Metabolic parameters and mood changes. J Reprod Med 41(Suppl 5):401, 1996.

White MK, Ory HW, Rooks JB, et al: Intrauterine device termination rates and the menstrual cycle day of insertion. Obstet Gynecol 55:220, 1980.

WHO Collaborative Study of Neoplasia and Steroid Contraceptives: Depot medroxyprogesterone acetate (DMPA) and risk of endometrial cancer. Int J Cancer 49:186, 1991.

WHO Collaborative Study of Neoplasia and Steroid Contraceptives: Depot medroxyprogesterone acetate (DMPA) and risk of epithelial ovarian cancer. Int J Cancer 49:191, 1991.

WHO Collaborative Study of Neoplasia and Steroid Contraceptives: Depot medroxyprogesterone acetate (DMPA) and risk of squamous cell cervical cancer. Contraception 45:299, 1992.

WHO Task Force on Postovulatory Methods of Fertility Regulation: Randomised controlled trial of levonorgestrel versus the Yuzpe regimen of combined oral contraceptives for emergency contraction. Lancet 352:428, 1998.

Wiebe E, Dunn S, Guilbert E, et al: Comparison of abortions induced by methotrexate or mifepristone followed by misoprostol. Obstet Gynecol 99:813, 2002.

Wilcox AJ, Weinberg CR, Baird DD: Timing of sexual intercourse in relation to ovulation: Effects on the probability of conception, survival of the pregnancy, and sex of the baby. New Engl J Med 333:1517, 1995.

Williams P, Johnson B, Vessey M: Septic abortion in women using intrauterine devices. BMJ 4:253, 1975.

Wilson JG, Brent RL: Are female sex hormones teratogenic? Am J Obstet Gynecol 141:567, 1981.

Wølner-Hanssen P, Svensson L, Mrdh PA, et al: Laparoscopic findings and contraceptive use in women with signs and symptoms suggestive of acute salpingitis. Obstet Gynecol 66:233, 1985.

World Health Organization (WHO): The TCu220C, multiload 250 and Nova T IUDs at 3.5 and 7 years of use: Results from three randomized multicentre trials. Contraception 42:141, 1990.

World Health Organization Collaborative Study of Cardiovascular Disease and Steroid Hormone Contraception: Venous thromboembolic disease and combined oral contraceptives: Results of international multicenter case-control study. Lancet 346:1575, 1995.

World Health Organization Collaborative Study of Cardiovascular Disease and Steroid Hormone Contraception: Effect of different progestagens in low-oestrogen oral contraceptives on venous thromboembolic disease. Lancet 346:1582, 1995.

World Health Organization Expanded Programme of Research, Development and Research Training in Human Reproduction Task Force on Long-Acting Systemic Agents for the Regulation of Fertility: Multinational comparative clinical evaluation of two long-acting injectable contraceptive steroids: Norethisterone enanthate and medroxyprogesterone acetate. Final report. Contraception 18:1, 1983.

World Health Organization: A prospective multicentre trial of the ovulation method of natural family planning. II. The effectiveness phase. Fertil Steril 36:591, 1981.

World Health Organization: Combined oral contraceptives and liver cancer. Int J Cancer 43:254, 1989.

Wright NH, Vessey MP, Kenward B, et al: Neoplasia and dysplasia of the cervix uteri and contraception: A possible protective effect of the diaphragm. Br J Cancer 38:273, 1978.

Yuzpe AA, Lancee WJ: Ethinylestradiol and dl-norgestrel as a postcoital contraceptive. Fertil Steril 28:932, 1977.

Breast Diseases 15

Diagnosis and Treatment of Benign and Malignant Disease

Fidel A. Valea and Vern L. Katz

KEY TERMS AND DEFINITIONS

Axillary Tail of Spence. A lateral projection of glandular tissue that extends from the upper, outer portion of the breast toward the axilla.

Cluster. A mammographic finding of five or more calcifications within a volume of 1 cm^3.

Cooper's Ligaments. Fibrous septa that extend from the skin through the breast to the underlying pectoralis fascia.

Cystosarcoma Phyllodes. Fibroepithelial breast tumors that are rare and may arise from fibroadenomas.

Digital Radiography. The technique by which X-ray photons are detected after passing through the breast tissue and the radiographic image is recorded electronically in a digital format and stored in a computer.

Fibroadenomas. Firm, freely mobile, solitary, solid, benign breast masses.

Fibrocystic Changes. General descriptive term that includes any change in contour of breast tissue. There is a wide spectrum and variation in clinical symptoms and palpable findings. Similarly, this term refers to a broad spectrum of benign histopathologic changes in the breast.

Intraductal Papilloma. Benign breast mass that is usually microscopic but may grow to 2 to 3 mm in diameter. The predominant symptom of an intraductal papilloma is spontaneous discharge from one nipple.

Lumpectomy. Conservative surgical procedure for breast carcinoma that involves removal of a wide margin of normal breast tissue surrounding a breast carcinoma less than 4 cm in diameter.

Modified Radical Mastectomy. An operation that includes removal of the breast and only the fascia over the pectoralis major muscle.

Montgomery Glands. Accessory glands located around the periphery of the areola. They represent an intermediate gland in between sebaceous glands and true mammary glands and as such can secrete milk.

Myoepithelial Cells. Specialized cells in the lactiferous ducts that are peripheral to epithelial cells, thus forming a double cellular layer in the ductal system. These cells are believed to be involved in the milk let-down phenomenon.

Paget's Disease. Rare breast carcinoma that has an innocent appearance and looks like eczema or dermatitis of the nipple.

Polymastia. More than two breasts.

Polythelia. More than two nipples.

Radical Mastectomy. An operation that includes en bloc removal of the breast, as well as underlying pectoralis major and pectoralis minor muscles.

Simple Mastectomy. An operation that includes removal of the breast without underlying muscle or fascial tissue.

Thermography. Potential technique to diagnose breast disease by directly measuring either cutaneous temperatures of the breast or infrared radiation from the breast by electronic detectors.

Virginal Hypertrophy of the Breasts. Rare condition in which there is massive hypertrophy of the breasts at puberty.

The importance of early detection and diagnosis of breast carcinoma cannot be overemphasized. Breast carcinoma is the most common malignancy of women and is one of the two leading causes of all cancer deaths in women. It is the number-one cause of death in women in their 40s. One in eight women (12.5% of American women) will develop carcinoma of the breast. Presently, the incidence of breast cancer in the United States is relatively stable. There has been an important reduction in breast cancer mortality in recent years. Since 1989, death rates from breast cancer have decreased an average of 1.8% per year. An increase in public awareness combined with recent improvements in mammography and newer imaging techniques have facilitated earlier detection of breast carcinoma. Combined with improvements in breast cancer therapy, improved survival rates are being reported. With the advent of chemoprevention in the high-risk woman, there is an opportunity to alter the natural course of the disease. The majority of women in whom breast cancer is diagnosed will not die of the disease.

The prognosis for and survival of a woman with breast carcinoma are improved by early discovery. Thus every gynecologist has an obligation to educate women concerning self-examination of the breast and to develop a routine for carefully screening women for breast disease. Detailed physical examination of the breast must be an integral step in evaluating every female patient.

Our culture attaches great significance to the female breast. An individual woman may react to the tremendous anxiety of suspected breast disease with behavior that varies from frequent visits to the physician for breast pain to denial of the presence of an obvious mass. The patient's description of her problem and her reactions to diagnoses and treatment must never be taken out of the context of this anxiety.

The major emphasis of this chapter is the epidemiology, detection, and diagnosis of breast carcinoma. Also, the chapter covers the chemoprevention of breast cancer as well as a discussion of benign breast diseases. Galactorrhea is presented in Chapter 39 (Hyperprolactinemia, Galactorrhea, and Pituitary Adenomas).

ANATOMY

The breasts are large, modified sebaceous glands contained within the superficial fascia of the anterior chest wall. A lateral projection of glandular tissue extends from the upper, outer portion of the breast toward the axilla and is called the *axillary tail of Spence.* The average weight of the adult breast is 200 to 300 g during the menstruating years. The mature breast consists of approximately 20% glandular tissue and 80% fat and connective tissue. The periphery of breast tissue is predominantly fat, and the central area contains more glandular tissue (Fig. 15-1).

The breast is composed of 12 to 20 lobes arranged in radial fashion from the nipple. Each lobe is triangular and has one central excretory duct that opens to the exterior at the nipple. Milk originates in the secretory cells of the alveoli. It is subsequently transported by the branching collecting ducts of the lobules into the lactiferous sinuses and terminally into the excretory ducts of each respective lobe of the breast. There is a wide range in number of lobules, between 10 and 100, in each lobe of the breast (Fig. 15-2). *Montgomery glands* are accessory glands located around the periphery of the areola. Because they are structurally intermediate between true mammary and sebaceous glands, they can secrete milk. Fibrous septa, *Cooper's ligaments,* extend from the skin to the underlying pectoralis fascia (Fig. 15-3). They are believed to offer support to the breast. Invasion of these ligaments by malignant cells produces skin retraction, which is a sign of advanced breast carcinoma.

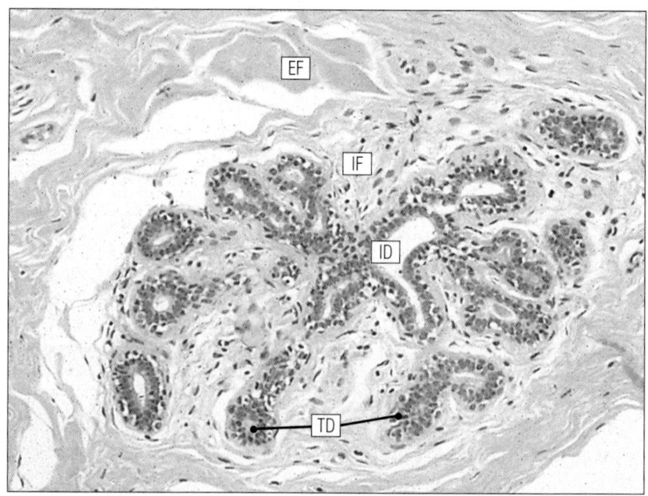

Figure 15-2. Histologic photograph of a mammary lobule. Note the ductal tissue surrounded by fibrous tissue. Terminal ductules (TD) surround the central ductule (ID). EF, extralobular fibrocollagenous tissue. (From Stevens A, Lowe J: Human Histology, 3rd ed. Philadelphia, Elsevier Mosby, 2005, p 390.)

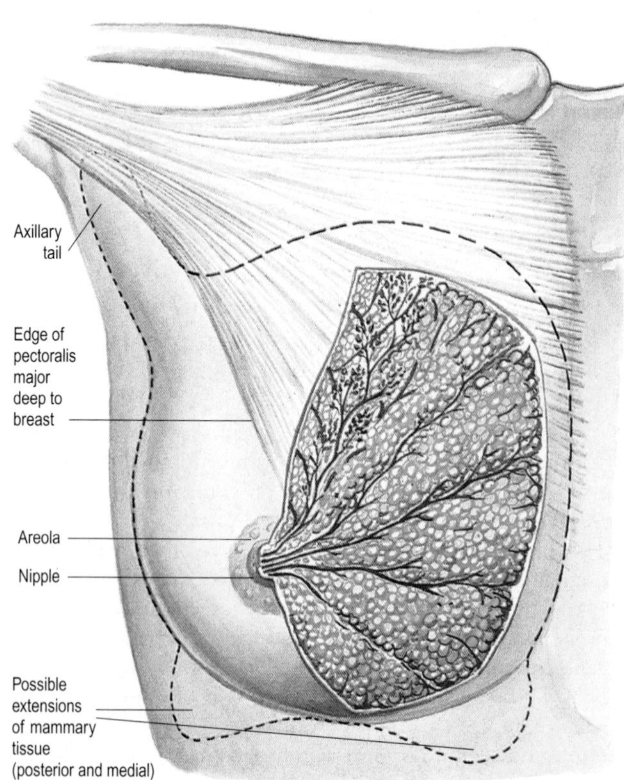

Figure 15-1. The structures of the breast. (From Shah P [ed]: Breast. In Standring S [ed]: Gray's Anatomy. London, Elsevier Churchill Livingstone, 2005, p 969, fig. 58.1A)

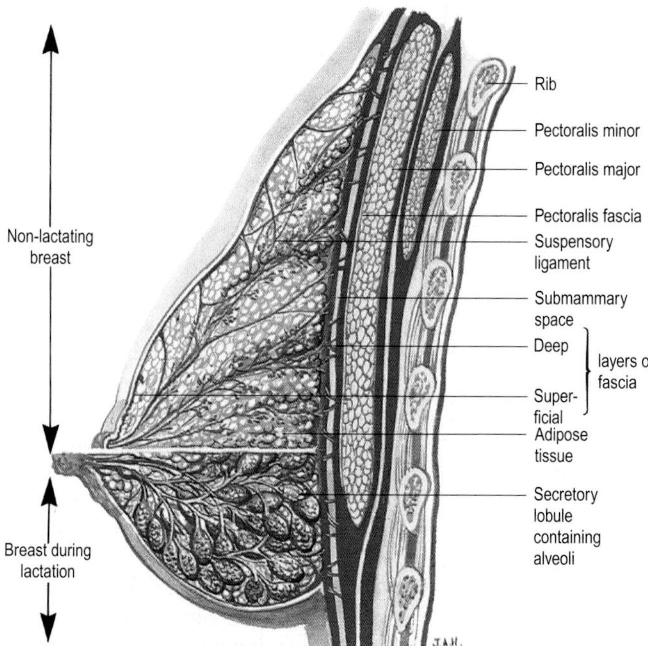

Figure 15-3. Lactating breast. (From Shah P [ed]: Breast. In Standring S [ed]: Gray's Anatomy. London, Elsevier Churchill Livingstone, 2005, p 969, fig. 58.1B.)

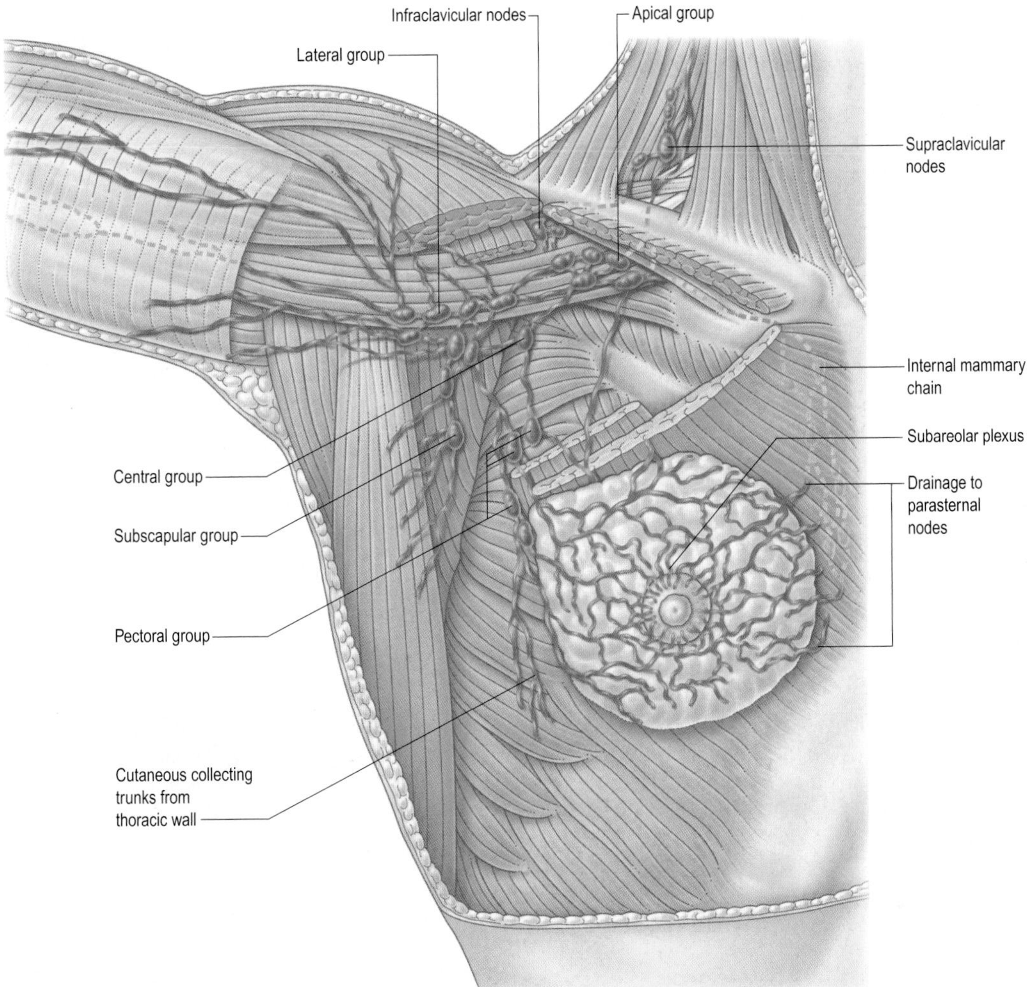

Figure 15-4. Lymph vessels of the breast and axillary lymph nodes. (From Shah P [ed]: Breast. In Standring S [ed]: Gray's Anatomy. London, Elsevier Churchill Livingstone, 2005, p 971, fig. 58.4.)

The lymphatic distribution of the breast is complex. Approximately 75% of the lymphatic drainage goes to regional nodes in the axilla. The axilla contains a varying number of nodes, usually between 30 and 60. Other metastatic routes include lymphatics adjacent to the internal mammary vessels. After direct spread into the mediastinum, lymphatic drainage may go to the intercostal glands, which are located posteriorly along the vertebral column, and to subpectoral and subdiaphragmatic areas (Fig. 15-4). Lymph drainage usually flows toward the most adjacent group of nodes. This concept represents the basis for sentinel node mapping in breast cancer. In most instances breast cancer spreads in an orderly fashion within the axillary lymph node basin based on the anatomic relationship between the primary tumor and its associated regional (sentinel) nodes. However, lymphatic metastases from one specific area of the breast may be found in any or all of the groups of regional nodes. In a large multicenter study, Krag and colleagues validated the use of sentinel node biopsy in women with breast cancer. All of the women studied had positive nodes. However, in only 3% of these women did the only positive node occur outside of the axilla. Metastases from one breast across the midline to the other breast or chest wall occur occasionally.

Breast tissue is sensitive to the cyclic changes in hormonal levels. The epithelium of the breast responds to fluctuating levels of estrogen and progesterone similar to other hormonally sensitive tissue. The stroma of the breasts and the myoepithelial cells of the breasts also respond to estrogen and progesterone. Women often experience breast tenderness and fullness during the luteal phase of the cycle. The average increase in volume of the premenstrual breasts is 25 to 30 mL, as measured by water displacement techniques. Premenstrual breast symptoms are produced by an increase in blood flow, vascular engorgement, and water retention. There is a corresponding enlargement in the lumina of ducts and an increase in ductal and acinar cellular secretory activity. During the follicular phase, there is parenchymal proliferation of the ducts. During the luteal phase, there is dilation of the ductal system and differentiation of the alveolar cells into secretory cells. The alveolar elements respond to both estrogen and progesterone. When menstruation begins, there is a regression of cellular activity in the alveoli and the ducts become smaller. Over time, the fibrous tissue surrounding the lobules increases in density and amount. In the postmenopausal woman, the breast lobules and ducts atrophy. The glandular components of the

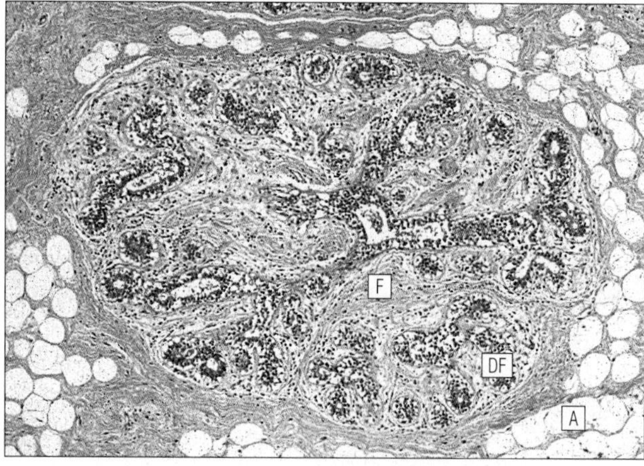

A

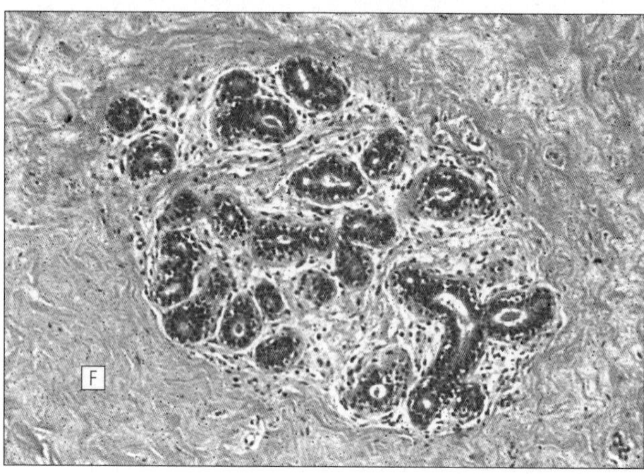

B

Figure 15-5. **A,** Micrograph showing normal breast tissue from a 23-year-old woman. At the center is a breast lobule in which the system of terminal ducts and ductules is embedded in loose intralobular fibrocollagenous stroma (F). There is a narrow surrounding zone of dense extralobular fibrocollagenous support tissue (DF), outside which is the soft adipose tissue (A) that forms the bulk of the breast. **B,** Micrograph showing normal breast tissue from a 43-year-old woman. As women age, the amount of fibrocollagenous tissue (F) in the breast increases, replacing some of the adipose tissue. The mammary lobules become enclosed in dense collagen. (From Stevens A, Lowe J: Human Histology, 3rd ed. Philadelphia, Elsevier Mosby, p 393.)

breast become replaced to varying degrees with adipose tissue (Fig. 15-5).

Accessory breasts or nipples can occur along the breast or milk lines, which run from the axilla to the groin. Supernumerary nipples (polythelia) or breasts (polymastia) are common anomalies (Fig. 15-6), which may be well developed and functional or rudimentary. They occur in approximately 1% to 2% of women of European descent and 5% to 6% of Asian women. Underdevelopment of one breast in relationship to the other is a common anomaly. In a recent study of 8408 mammograms, 3% were notable for asymmetrical volume reduction relative to the contralateral breast. This asymmetry represented a benign, normal variation unless an associated palpable abnormality was present. Massive hypertrophy of the breasts at puberty (virginal hypertrophy) is a rare occurrence that has a deeply disturbing effect on a teenager's self-image (Fig. 15-7). This condition is best managed by skillful cosmetic surgery.

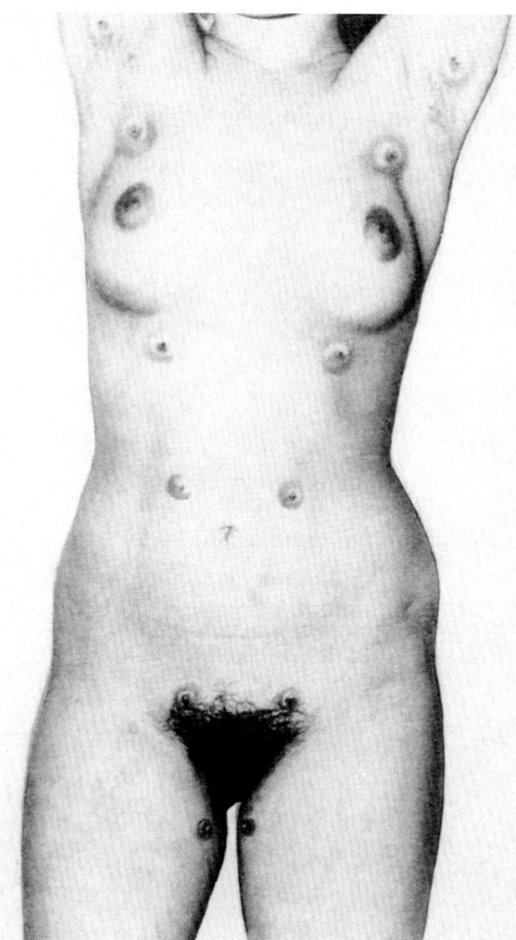

Figure 15-6. Extensive polythelia along the milk lines. (From Degrell I: Atlas of Diseases of the Mammary Gland. Basel, Switzerland, S Karger, 1976, p 41.)

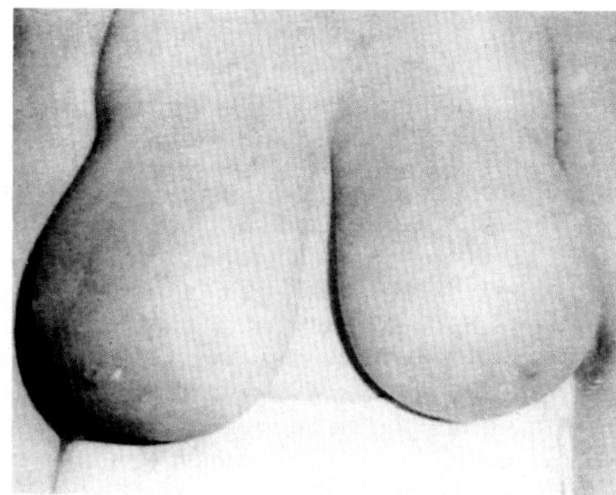

Figure 15-7. Virginal hypertrophy in a 13-year-old girl. (From Degrell I: Atlas of Diseases of the Mammary Gland. Basel, Switzerland, S Karger, 1976, p 46.)

BENIGN BREAST DISEASE

The classifications and terminologies of benign breast disease are confusing. Nevertheless, an understanding of these conditions is important. The symptomatology and physical findings of benign disease cause anxiety and fear in the patient, who often thinks the symptoms may be related to breast cancer. The common symptoms of breast disease (pain and tenderness) and the signs (a mass or nipple discharge) may result from either a benign or a malignant process. However, breast pain is a comparatively late symptom in women with breast carcinoma and is the sole presenting symptom in less than 10% of these women. During the second half of the menstrual cycle, the breasts increase in size, density, and nodularity. These three changes are often associated with increased sensitivity or pain.

Numerous epidemiologic studies have found an increased risk of developing breast carcinoma in women with benign breast disease with associated atypical epithelial hyperplasia. This risk varies from twofold to fivefold, depending on the degree of epithelial hyperplasia. The pathophysiology of the association between cellular atypia and subsequent carcinoma is straightforward and similar in concept to endometrial disease.

Dupont and Page performed the classic study on the relationship between benign breast disease and subsequent development of carcinoma. They followed more than 3000 women for at least 15 years after benign breast biopsy. The study population was divided into three groups of women according to histology of the original biopsy. The first group consisted of 70% of the women. Their biopsies revealed no proliferative changes, and their diagnoses included adenosis, apocrine metaplasia, duct ectasia, and mild epithelial hyperplasia. During the 15 years of follow-up, only 2% of these women developed breast carcinoma. The second group of women, 26%, had breast biopsies that demonstrated varying degrees of epithelial hyperplasia but without atypia. Of these women, 4% developed breast carcinoma during the 15 years; their relative risk was increased 1.6-fold. The last group consisted of the 4% of women with histology that demonstrated atypical ductal or lobular hyperplasia. Their relative risk was four to five times greater for developing malignancy; 8% developed carcinoma during the 15-year follow-up.

Fibrocystic Changes

Fibrocystic changes are the most common of all benign breast conditions. Often, clinicians use the nonspecific term *fibrocystic changes* to describe multiple irregularities in contour and cyclically painful breasts. The term *fibrocystic disease* is a misnomer and probably should not be used. This condition has a prolific terminology that includes over 35 different names, with mammary dysplasia and chronic cystic mastitis being the two most common. The exact incidence of fibrocystic changes is difficult to establish. Frantz and coworkers found histologic evidence of fibrocystic changes in 53% of "normal breasts" examined in a series of 225 autopsies. Clinical evidence of fibrocystic changes is discovered in breast examinations of approximately one in two premenopausal women.

Fibrocystic changes are believed to be an exaggeration of the normal physiologic response of breast tissue to the cyclic levels of ovarian hormones. However, no consistent abnormality of circulating hormone levels has been proven. The condition is most common in women between the ages of 20 and 50 and unusual after menopause unless associated with exogenous hormone use. Some postulate the cause to be a subtle imbalance

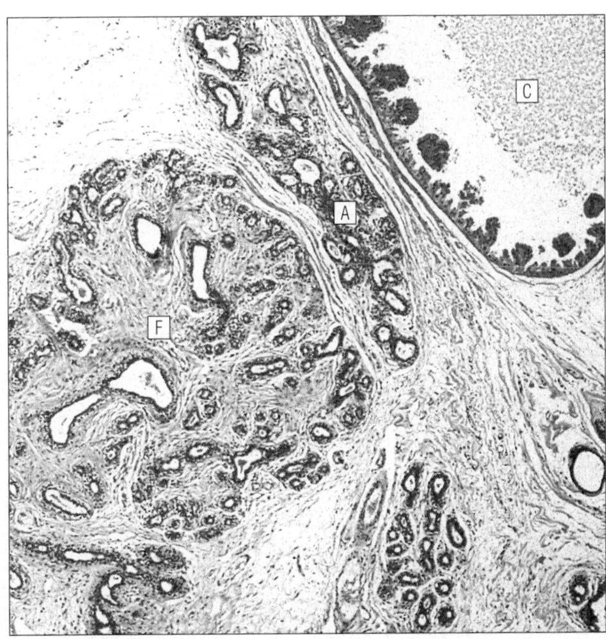

Figure 15-8. Fibrocystic changes from histologic Section. Note: Fibrosis (F), adenomatous changes with increased ductal tissue (A), and cysts (C). (From Stevens A, Lowe J: Human Histology, 3rd ed. Philadelphia, Elsevier Mosby, 2005, p 392.)

of the ratio of estrogen to progesterone. However, others have postulated that fibrocystic changes are secondary to increased daily prolactin production. Women with fibrocystic changes have enhanced prolactin production in response to thyroid-releasing hormone.

The classic symptom of fibrocystic changes is cyclic bilateral breast pain. The signs of fibrocystic change include increased engorgement and density of the breasts, excessive nodularity, rapid change and fluctuation in the size of cystic areas, increased tenderness, and occasionally spontaneous nipple discharge. Both signs and symptoms are more prevalent during the premenstrual phase of the cycle. The breast pain is bilateral, and it is often difficult for the patient to localize. The pain is most frequently located in the upper, outer quadrants of the breasts. Often the pain radiates to the shoulders and upper arms. Severe localized pain may occur when a simple cyst undergoes rapid expansion. The pathophysiology that produces these symptoms and signs includes cyst formation, epithelial and fibrous proliferation, and varying degrees of fluid retention (Fig. 15-8). The differential diagnosis of breast pain includes referred pain from a dorsal radiculitis or inflammation of the costal chondral junction (Tietze's syndrome). The latter two conditions have symptoms that are not cyclic and are unrelated to the menstrual cycle.

On physical examination the findings of excessive nodularity of fibrocystic changes have been described as similar to palpating the surface of a plateful of peas. Multiple solid areas are described as ill-defined thicknesses or areas of "palpable lumpiness" that are rubbery in consistency and may seem more two-dimensional than the three-dimensional mass usually associated with a carcinoma (Fig. 15-9). During palpation the larger cysts have a consistency similar to a balloon filled with water.

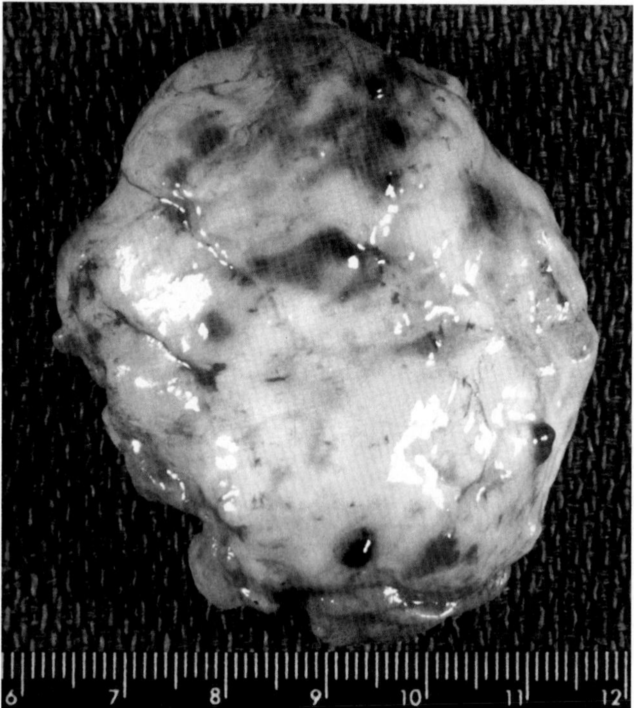

Figure 15-9. Breast biopsy from a 38-year-old woman demonstrating characteristic gross appearance of fibrocystic changes. Note multiple cysts interspersed between the dense fibrous connective tissue. (Courtesy of Fidel A. Valea, MD.)

There are three indistinct clinical stages, with each stage having predominant histologic findings. Clinically these stages have considerable overlap. The stages are described to allow understanding of the condition's natural history.

The first stage occurs in women in their 20s and is termed *mazoplasia* (mastoplasia). Breast pain is noted primarily in the upper, outer quadrants of the breast. The indurated axillary tail is in the most tender area of the breast. During this phase there is intense proliferation of the stroma.

The second clinical stage of *adenosis* occurs generally in women in their 30s. The breast pain and tenderness are premenstrual but less severe. Multiple small breast nodules vary from 2 to 10 mm in diameter. The histologic picture of adenosis demonstrates marked proliferation and hyperplasia of ducts, ductules, and alveolar cells.

The last stage is termed the *cystic* phase and usually occurs in women in their 40s. There is no severe breast pain unless a cyst increases rapidly in size. In this situation a woman experiences a sudden pain with point tenderness and discovers a lump. Cysts are tender to palpation and vary from microscopic to 5 cm in diameter. The cysts in fibrocystic changes often regress in size. The fluid aspirated from a large cyst is straw-colored, dark brown, or green, depending on the chronicity of the cyst.

Women with a clinical diagnosis of fibrocystic changes have a wide variety of histopathologic findings. The histology of fibrocystic changes is characterized by proliferation and hyperplasia of the lobular, ductal, and acinar epithelium. Usually proliferation of fibrous tissue occurs and accompanies epithelial hyperplasia. Many histologic variants of fibrocystic change have been described, including cysts (from microscopic to large, blue, domed cysts), adenosis (florid and sclerosing), fibrosis (periductal and stromal), duct ectasia, apocrine metaplasia, intraductal epithelial hyperplasia, and papillomatosis. Ductal epithelial hyperplasia and atypia and apocrine metaplasia with atypia are the most prominent histologic findings directly associated with the subsequent development of breast carcinoma. If these two conditions are discovered on breast biopsy, the chance of breast carcinoma in the future is approximately fivefold greater than in controls.

The proper management of fibrocystic changes, depending on the woman's age, includes appropriate imaging techniques, fine-needle aspiration cytology, and histologic evaluation with either a core needle or excision biopsy when indicated. If there is a persistent dominant mass or any uncertainty in the examination, a biopsy of the area should be performed to rule out a malignancy. There is a wide range of options for treating this condition. The treatment of fibrocystic change depends on the severity of symptoms and varies from mechanical support of the breast to extremely rare instances of surgical therapy for intractable pain. The vast majority of symptoms can be controlled by medical therapy. Initial therapy of fibrocystic changes consists of the patient wearing a "support" bra, which provides adequate support for the breasts both night and day. Diuretics during the premenstrual phase occasionally relieve breast discomfort. Minton has advocated advising patients to reduce their consumption of methylxanthines and tobacco. Methylxanthines are commonly found in coffee, tea, cola drinks, chocolate, and many nonprescription medications. Minton studied 106 women with clinical fibrocystic changes and found that in 68% the condition resolved and in another 24% the clinical symptoms improved by decreasing consumption of methylxanthines and nicotine. However, four recent case-control studies have found no association between caffeine or methylxanthine consumption and benign breast disease.

Oral contraceptives or supplemental progestins administered during the secretory phase of the cycle have both been used to treat fibrocystic change. Approximately 40% of women will have a recurrence of their symptomatology following discontinuation of oral contraceptives.

The drug of choice for severe symptoms is danazol. It is the only drug approved by the U. S. Food and Drug Administration for the treatment of mastalgia. Dosages of 100, 200, and 400 mg daily continuously for 4–6 months have been employed. Therapy should not continue more than 6 months because side effects are common, and the dosage should be tapered as described by Harrison in one report and Sutton in another. Danazol relieves breast symptoms and decreases nodularity of the breast in approximately 90% of patients. This effect lasts for several months after discontinuation of danazol. Patients who do not respond to danazol may receive a trial of bromocriptine or tamoxifen. Bromocriptine, an inhibitor of prolactin, is given continuously in a dosage of 5 mg daily. Tamoxifen is a synthetic antiestrogen commonly used as a chemotherapeutic agent for breast carcinoma. Tamoxifen competes with estradiol for estrogen receptors in the breast. Small clinical studies have documented a 70% relief of breast symptoms when tamoxifen is prescribed for fibrocystic changes. Women with cyclic breast pain seem to respond better than those with chronic mastalgia.

Severe cyclical mastalgia has been associated with abnormal levels of certain essential fatty acids. Gateley and associates report a 58% response rate with cyclical mastalgia and 38% response rate with noncyclic mastalgia using dietary supplementation of γ-linoleic acid with evening primrose oil.

On rare occasions a woman with severe fibrocystic changes is treated medically with gonadotropin-releasing hormone (GnRH) agonists or surgically by total mastectomy. Subcutaneous mastectomy produces a better cosmetic result. However, it does not remove all the breast tissue. Thus, if the surgery is being performed prophylactically, the risk of breast cancer remains. Indications for surgery include intractable pain not relieved by medical therapy or biopsy evidence of a precancerous lesion.

Fibroadenomas

Fibroadenomas are firm, rubbery, freely mobile, solid, usually solitary breast masses. They are the second most common type of benign breast disease. Fibroadenomas most frequently present in adolescents and women in their 20s. Typically the young woman discovers the painless mass accidentally while bathing. Growth of the mass is usually extremely slow but may be quite rapid. Fibroadenomas do not change in size with the menstrual cycle, and they do not produce breast pain or tenderness. Approximately 30% of fibroadenomas will disappear and 10% to 12% become smaller when followed for many years. Pathophysiologically, fibroadenomas should be considered as an abnormality of normal development rather than true neoplasm. However, the long-term risk of invasive breast cancer is approximately twice that for control patients. Women with fibroadenomas should be made aware of this risk and encouraged to maintain annual mammographic screening commencing at age 40.

The average fibroadenoma is 2.5 cm in diameter. Multiple fibroadenomas are discovered in 15% to 20% of patients. After surgical removal, fibroadenomas recur in approximately 20% of women.

Sometimes it is difficult to distinguish a fibroadenoma from a cyst. Mammography is rarely indicated in a woman younger than 35. However, ultrasound is helpful in differentiating a solid from a cystic mass. If the cause of the mass cannot be established by fine-needle aspiration, surgical removal is indicated. Regardless of age, any mass that rapidly increases in size should be removed, as should any solid mass in a woman older than 35. Fibroadenomas can be removed without difficulty under local anesthesia. They are rubbery in consistency, well circumscribed, and easily delineated from surrounding breast tissue (Fig. 15-10). Nonoperative management is appropriate for small fibroadenomas discovered in women younger than 35 if three separate clinical parameters support the diagnosis of fibroadenoma. The three parameters are clinical exam, imaging evaluation (either mammogram or ultrasound), and fine-needle aspiration cytology. The characteristic features of a fibroadenoma are found in approximately 95% of all fibroadenomas. Thus, conservative management can be considered with follow-up every 6 months. The only way to distinguish a fibroadenoma from a malignancy is with either a histologic or cytologic evaluation. Despite the option of conservative management of a fibroadenoma, most women usually prefer to have the lesion excised.

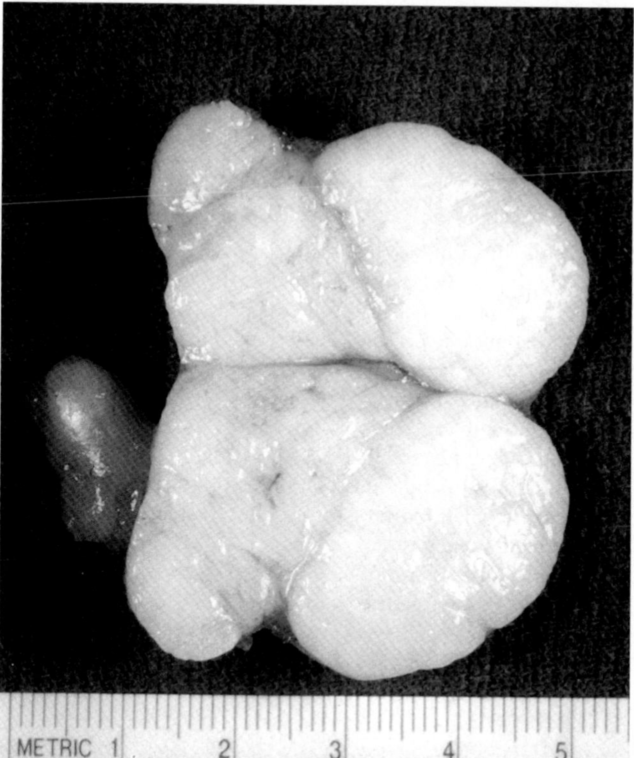

Figure 15-10. Classic fibroadenoma of the breast. (Courtesy of Fidel A. Valea, MD.)

Cystosarcoma Phyllodes

Cystosarcoma phyllodes are fibroepithelial breast tumors. However, microscopically, it is the hypercellularity of the connective tissue that is the distinctive characteristic of the tumor. Cystosarcoma phyllodes are rare in that they represent only 2.5% of fibroepithelial tumors and 1% of breast malignancies. They are the most frequent breast sarcoma. These rapidly growing tumors are most common in the fifth decade of life. In large series, the mean diameter of the tumor at time of diagnosis was approximately 5 cm. One in four of these tumors is malignant, yet only 1 out of 10 metastasizes. If metastatic disease is discovered, it is the stromal tissue that predominates. Differentiation of benign from malignant tumors by strict histologic criteria has resulted in poor correlation in some series. Recent studies using flow cytometry have improved on the predictive value in differentiating the biologic nature of the neoplasia. The treatment of a benign cystosarcoma phyllodes is excision of the mass, including a wide margin of normal tissue. Presence of microscopic tumor at the margins of the excised specimen is the major factor in predicting whether there will be a local recurrence of the tumor.

Intraductal Papilloma

The classical symptom of an intraductal papilloma is spontaneous bloody discharge from one nipple. This symptom usually appears in a woman in the perimenopausal age group. The discharge from the nipple is *spontaneous* and intermittent. The consistency of the discharge associated with an intraductal papilloma can be watery, serous, or serosanguineous. The amount of discharge varies from a few drops to several milliliters of fluid. Approximately 75% of intraductal papillomas are located beneath the areola. Often these tumors are difficult to palpate because they are small and soft. During examination of the breast, it is important to circumferentially put radial pressure on different areas of the areola. This technique helps to identify whether the discharge emanates from a single duct or multiple openings. When the discharge comes from a single duct, the differential diagnosis involves both intraductal papilloma and carcinoma. If multiple ducts are involved, the diagnosis of carcinoma is more likely. Radiologically, the involved duct may be identified by injecting contrast material into the duct with a small catheter (galactography). Intraductal papillomas are usually microscopic but may grow to 2 to 3 mm in diameter, extending radially from the alveolar margin. Treatment of an intraductal papilloma is excisional biopsy of the involved duct and a small amount of surrounding tissue. Although these tumors tend to regress in postmenopausal women and occasionally diminish in size in premenopausal women, they should be excised. In one series, women with a solitary papilloma showed an approximately twofold increased risk of subsequent development of carcinoma.

Nipple Discharge

Nipple discharge may be a complaint of women with either benign or malignant breast disease. Nipple discharge is a complaint of 10% to 15% of women with benign breast disease. However, nipple discharge is present in less than 3% of women with breast carcinoma. Leis reported a series of 7588 women with breast operations; 85% had a mass, and 7% had a chief complaint of discharge from the nipple. Of the 560 patients operated on for nipple discharge, 493 findings were benign and 67 malignant. If the nipple discharge is from a single duct, the chances of carcinoma are less (Table 15-1).

To be medically significant, discharge from the breast should be spontaneous and persistent in a nonlactating woman. Many normal women can express a few drops of sticky gray, green, or black viscous fluid. The importance of diagnosing the cause of *spontaneous* nonmilky discharge from the nipple is to rule out carcinoma. The color of the discharge does not differentiate a benign from a malignant process. Malignancies have been associated with clear, serous, serosanguineous, or bloody nipple discharges. Importantly, bloody discharge from the nipple, gross or microscopic, should be considered to be related to carcinoma until this diagnosis has been ruled out. Cytology of the discharge is important but often not diagnostic. Most series document a false-negative rate of approximately 20%. Therefore a negative cytologic finding should not deter surgical biopsy.

Before excisional biopsy a patient with a persistent discharge of any type should have mammography. In a young woman with a suspected intraductal papilloma, the involved duct, which is usually blue, and a small area of surrounding breast tissue can be removed. Table 15-2 documents that intraductal papillomas and fibrocystic changes are the two most common reasons for spontaneous nonmilky nipple discharge. In this series, 50 of 432 patients had a carcinoma diagnosed by breast biopsy.

Table 15-1 Causes of Single Duct Nipple Discharge in 170 Patients (Nottingham 1988)

Diagnosis	Number (%)
Duct papilloma	77 (45)
Benign disease (for example, duct ectasia)	80 (47)
Cancer in situ	2 (7)
No abnormality	1 (0.6)

From Chetty U: Nipple discharge. In Smallwood JA, Taylor I (eds): Benign Breast Disease. Baltimore, Urban & Schwarzenberger, 1990.

Fat Necrosis

Fat necrosis is rare but important because it is often confused with carcinoma. The patient presents with a firm, tender, indurated, ill-defined mass that may have an area of surrounding ecchymosis. Sometimes the area of fat necrosis liquefies and becomes cystic in consistency. Mammography may demonstrate fine, stippled calcification and stellate contractions. Occasionally there is skin retraction, which further confuses the prebiopsy diagnosis. The usual cause of fat necrosis is trauma. However, the majority of women do not remember the event that injured the breast. Treatment of fat necrosis is excisional biopsy. There is no relationship between fat necrosis and subsequent breast carcinoma.

BREAST CARCINOMA

Epidemiology

The cause of breast carcinoma is poorly understood despite extensive investigation. Epidemiologists have documented some risk factors that provide clues in understanding the pathophysiology of the disease's development in certain high-risk groups of women (Table 15-3). The risk factors can be divided into several categories: heredity, age, hormones, nutrition, demography, radiation, and previous breast disease. Generalizations concerning cause follow similar categories: genetic predisposition, environmental carcinogens, viral agents, and radiation exposure.

Three problems obscure a clear understanding of the risk factors of breast cancer. One is the long latency period before the development of clinically recognizable carcinoma. Second is the consideration of both the duration and the intensity of factors that may induce or promote cancer. For example, the peak incidence of breast carcinoma in Japanese women after the bombing of Hiroshima and Nagasaki occurred in women who were in the premenarcheal age group at the time of the atomic explosions. Subsequently these teenagers developed breast carcinoma in their mid-30s after the characteristic prolonged latency period. The *estrogen window hypothesis* suggests that the radiation (cancer inducer) acted with the background of the unopposed estrogen of adolescence (cancer promoter). Third, observational studies concentrating on a single risk factor often reach contrary conclusions.

Although there are limits in the clinical applicability of risk factors, selected women at increased risk may benefit from screening at more frequent intervals or consider some risk

Table 15-2 Relation Between Nipple Discharge and Diagnosis in 432 Operations from New York Medical College, 1960–1975

Discharge	Galactorrhea	Duct Ectasia	Infection	Intraductal Papilloma	Fibrocystic Disease	Cancer
Milky	2	0	0	0	0	0
Multicolored and sticky	0	46	0	0	0	0
Purulent	0	0	14	0	0	0
Watery	0	0	0	3	1	5
Serous	0	5	0	79	52	11
Serosanguineous	0	8	0	59	34	14
Sanguineous	0	6	0	45	28	20
Total	2	65	14	186	115	50

Reprinted from Pilnik S: Clinical diagnosis of benign breast diseases. J Reprod Med 22:286, 1979.

Table 15-3 Established and Probable Risk Factors for Breast Cancer

Risk Factor	Comparison Category	Risk Category	Typical Relative Risk
Family history of breast cancer	No first-degree relatives affected	Mother affected before the age of 60	2.0
		Mother affected after the age of 60	1.4
		Two first-degree relatives affected	4–6
Age at menarche	16yr	11 yr	1.3
		12 yr	1.3
		13 yr	1.3
		14 yr	1.3
		15 yr	1.1
Age at birth of 1st child	Before 20 yr	20–24 yr	1.3
		25–29 yr	1.6
		≥30 yr	1.9
		Nulliparous	1.9
Age at menopause	45–54 yr	After 55 yr	1.5
		Before 45 yr	0.7
		Oophorectomy before 35 yr	0.4
Benign breast disease	No biopsy or aspiration	Any benign disease	1.5
		Proliferation only	2.0
		Atypical hyperplasia	4.0
Radiation	No special exposure	Atomic bomb (100 rad)	3.0
		Repeated fluoroscopy	1.5–2.0
Obesity	10th percentile	90th percentile:	
		Age, 30–49 yr	0.8
		Age, ≥50 yr	1.2
Height	10th percentile	90th percentile:	
		Age, 30–49 yr	1.3
		Age, ≥50 yr	1.4
Oral contraceptive use	Never used	Current use*	1.5
		Past use*	1.0
Postmenopausal estrogen-replacement therapy	Never used	Current use all ages	1.4
		Age, <55 yr	1.2
		Age, 50–59 yr	1.5
		Age, 50–59 yr	1.5
Past use	1.0	Age, ≥60 yr	2.1
Alcohol use	Nondrinker	3 drinks/day	2.0

*Relative risks may be higher for women given a diagnosis of breast cancer before the age of 40.
Modified from Harris JR, Lippman ME, Veronesi U, Willett W: Breast cancer (1). N Engl J Med 327:319, 1992. Modified with permission.

reduction measures. Pharmacologic or surgical prophylaxis has been proven to significantly decrease the risk of developing breast cancer. Many risk factors are additive. Risk factors are estimates developed by epidemiologists that allow patients and physicians to consider the probability of developing the disease. They have been widely publicized in the lay press. The fact that has not been emphasized is that risk factors identify *only* 25% of women who will eventually develop breast carcinoma.

The United States has one of the highest rates of breast carcinoma in the world. Incidence rates increased gradually from 1940 to 1990. Subsequently, they appear to have remained stable. The stabilization of rates probably results from the increase in detection and screening that occurred in the 1980s. The specific risk to an American woman of developing a breast carcinoma is 1 in 8 (12.5%) during her entire lifetime. The lifetime risk for an American woman without a single risk factor is 1 in 17 (6%). Therefore the message concerning risk should be that every woman in the United States is at risk for breast carcinoma. The risk of breast carcinoma during a woman's lifetime is similar to the risk of lung cancer in a heavy smoker.

Approximately 5% to 10% of breast cancers have a familial or genetic link. Genetic predisposition to developing breast carcinoma has been recognized in some families. In these families breast cancer tends to occur at a younger age and there is a higher prevalence of bilateral disease. Recently, mutations in *BRCA* family of genes have been identified that confer a lifetime risk of breast cancer that approaches 85%. *BRCA1* and *BRCA2* genes are involved in the majority of inheritable cases of breast cancer. These genes function as tumor suppressor genes and several mutations have been described on each of these genes. *BRCA1* was mapped to chromosome 17, and in 1994 the DNA sequence of the gene was determined by Miki and colleagues. Although the lifetime risk of breast cancer is approximately 85%, the risk of ovarian cancer is variable depending on the location of the mutation. The average lifetime risk of ovarian cancer is approximately 40% to 50%. The *BRCA2* gene was mapped to chromosome 13, and the DNA sequence was determined by Schutte and coworkers in 1995. A woman with a *BRCA2* gene mutation has an 85% lifetime risk of breast cancer and a 15% to 20% lifetime risk of ovarian cancer. This mutation is also associated with male breast cancer, conferring a 5% to 10% lifetime risk for a male with the mutation. *BRCA3* gene has been recently mapped to chromosome 8, but the details of the clinical syndrome have not yet been described. Because of multiple mutations of each gene and the possibility of differing penetrance of the mutations, the most appropriate clinical use of this genetic information continues to be a matter of intense debate. Presently, management recommendations vary from earlier and increased interval screening tests to prophylactic measures such as chemoprevention with tamoxifen, mastectomy, and oophorectomy. A task force convened by the Cancer Genetics Studies Consortium in 1997 recommended breast self-examination beginning by age 20, annual or semiannual clinical examination beginning at age 25 to 35 years, and annual mammograms beginning at age 25 to 35 years. They made no recommendation for or against prophylactic surgery in these patients. Hartmann recently presented the Mayo Clinic experience with 28 patients who had a *BRCA* gene mutation and underwent prophylactic bilateral mastectomy. In this series, the risk reduction was estimated at 91%.

The frequency of breast carcinoma increases directly with the patient's age (see the following box and Fig. 15-11). Breast carcinoma is almost nonexistent before puberty; the incidence gradually increases during the reproductive years. Eighty-five percent of breast carcinoma occurs after age 40. After menopause the incidence of breast carcinoma increases directly with a woman's age.

The relationship between endogenous ovarian hormones and breast carcinoma has been studied extensively. Several clinical observations support the hypothesis that the risk of breast carcinoma is related to the intensity and duration of exposure to unopposed endogenous estrogen. Breast cancer is most unusual in the prepubertal female. Bilateral oophorectomy before age 35, without hormonal replacement, reduces the risk of breast carcinoma by 70%. Women have an incidence of breast carcinoma 100 times greater than that for men.

Risk by Age: A Woman's Risk of Developing Breast Cancer

By age 25	1 in 19,608
30	1 in 2525
35	1 in 622
40	1 in 217
45	1 in 93
50	1 in 50
55	1 in 33
60	1 in 24
65	1 in 17
70	1 in 14
75	1 in 11
80	1 in 10
85	1 in 9
Ever	1 in 8

Data from National Cancer Institute. Painter K: Factoring in cost of mammograms. USA Today, p 11D, December 5, 1996.

Obese women are at a higher risk for developing breast carcinoma during the postmenopausal years. The pathophysiology of this tendency is believed to be an increased amount of peripheral conversion of androstenedione to estrone and decreased levels of sex hormone-binding globulin. Marchant and coworkers described the increased risk associated with prolonged menstrual function. Women with spontaneous menopause before age 45 experience half the risk of developing breast carcinoma of women who are still menstruating at age 54. A similar study documented a twofold increased risk for women who menstruated for 40 years or longer contrasted with that for women who menstruated for 30 years or less.

Demographic data describe significant variations in the incidence of breast carcinoma from country to country. Women living in the United States have a much higher rate of breast carcinoma than women living in Africa, Asia, or the Middle East. The age-specific incidence of breast carcinoma in American women is six times greater than among women in Japan. Interestingly, studies of Japanese families who moved to the United States demonstrate that their rate of breast carcinoma becomes similar to that of American women after two generations. The demographic data were initially believed to be due to differences in total dietary fat and obesity. Epidemiologic studies performed within the same culture have demonstrated differences in incidences of breast cancer directly related to the amount of fat in the diet. However, recent epidemiologic studies, such as the Nurses' Health Study, failed to show any association between dietary fat and the risk of breast cancer. It is interesting to note that high consumption of olive oil modestly reduces breast cancer risk. Recently, the differences in breast cancer rates among the various groups is speculated to be due to caloric restriction in childhood. Dietary or lifestyle modification that shows the biggest reduction in risk is avoidance of weight gain in adulthood. Alcohol consumption has also been associated with breast cancer risk. Several studies have reported a 40% to 50% increase in the risk of developing breast cancer related to

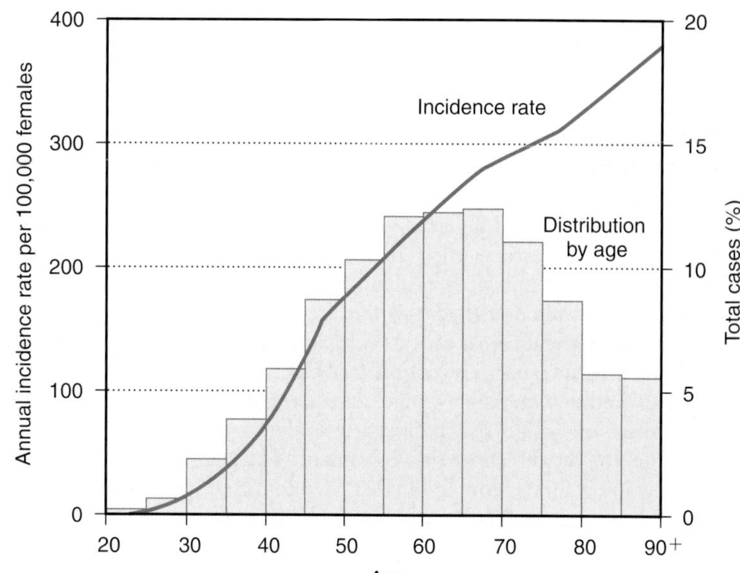

Figure 15-11. Incidence in the United States, by age, of female breast cancer. (From Seidman H, Mushinski MH: Breast cancer incidence, mortality, survival, and prognosis. In Feig SA, McLelland R [eds]: Breast Carcinoma: Current Diagnosis and Treatment. New York, Masson, 1983. © Copyright by American College of Radiology.)

alcohol consumption. Longnecker showed that the risk of breast cancer was strongly related to the amount of alcohol consumed and that even light drinking was associated with a 10% increase in risk. Zhang reported that light consumption of alcohol was not associated with an increased risk of breast cancer. At the present time the effects of light consumption of alcohol on breast cancer risk is uncertain.

Ionizing radiation is a definite risk factor because of the long-accepted relationship between radiation and malignant transformation. The experience of Japanese women who survived the atomic bomb has been discussed. There are small groups of women who received multiple radiation treatments for postpartum mastitis, irradiation of the thymus in infancy, or multiple fluoroscopic examinations during treatment for tuberculosis who have subsequently developed breast carcinoma at an increased rate. The data concerning relative risk of developing breast carcinoma are most consistent with a linear dose-response relationship.

Previous history of breast disease is an important risk factor. Although the risk varies between premenopausal and postmenopausal women with breast cancer, once the patient has developed carcinoma of one breast, her risk is approximately 1% per year of developing cancer in the other breast. As emphasized previously, the extent of epithelial hyperplasia and atypia in women with benign breast disease determines the magnitude of risk for developing carcinoma. Women with ovarian, endometrial, or colon carcinoma have a twofold to fourfold greater risk of also developing breast carcinoma.

The age at which a woman delivers her first child is more important as a risk factor than parity. If a woman's first term birth occurs before age 20, she has 50% less risk than a nulliparous woman. If the first full-term pregnancy occurs after age 35, the risk is 1.5 times greater than for women who have their first baby before age 26. For many years it was believed that nursing an infant offered a protective effect for the future development of breast neoplasia. Subsequent studies have documented that this finding may be confounded by parity, timing of first pregnancy, and the relative length of anovulation. Newcomb and colleagues reported that after adjusting for parity, age at first delivery, and other confounding factors lactation was associated with a slight reduction in the risk of breast cancer among premenopausal women compared with those who had never lactated (relative risk, 0.78 [95% CI, 0.6 to 0.91]). Reserpine, which elevates prolactin levels, has been shown not to be a risk factor.

There is no consensus on the association of exogenous estrogen administration, either as hormone replacement or in the form of oral contraceptives, and the risk of breast cancer. Numerous epidemiologic studies have failed to consistently demonstrate a detrimental effect of exogenous estrogen administration and breast cancer risk. Although some studies demonstrate a slight increased risk in the exogenous estrogen group, this risk is less than that associated with postmenopausal obesity or daily alcohol consumption. Recently, Schairer and colleagues concluded that current and recent users of an estrogen–progestin regimen had a higher increased risk of breast cancer than a patient using estrogen alone with relative risks of 1.4 (1.1 = 1.8) and 1.2 (1.0 = 1.4). This increase in relative risk was significant only in lean women. Estrogens are considered tumor promoters in respect to the pathophysiology of breast carcinoma rather than inducers or initiators of carcinoma. Thus any adverse effect should increase with duration of use, and a dose-response curve should be recognized. Some recently reported epidemiologic studies have found an elevated risk for subsets of women under age 45. However, no consistent evidence showed an increase in breast cancer risk through middle age, even in long-term oral contraceptive users or in women with a family history of breast carcinoma (see Chapters 13 [Pediatric and Adolescent Gynecology] and 42 [Menopause]). If there is an increased risk, it appears to be small compared with other risk factors. The decision to use postmenopausal hormone replacement in patients with risk factors should be individualized, and the patient should be informed of the risks and benefits so she can make an informed decision.

Prevention

Breast cancer risk reduction should be considered throughout a woman's life. Although there is no proven benefit for women with low to normal risk, lifestyle modifications such as weight control, avoidance of smoking, decreased alcohol consumption, and exercise are associated with good general health. Most importantly, women with a high risk of breast cancer have proven options that can decrease their risk of breast cancer. In the National Surgical Adjuvant Breast and Bowel Project (NSABP) B-14 trial, tamoxifen users had a significant decrease in the incidence of contralateral breast cancers compared with placebo. As a result, the Breast Cancer Prevention Trial (BCPT) was designed to assess whether tamoxifen would decrease the incidence of breast cancer in a high-risk population as determined by the Gail model for breast cancer risk assessment. The trial enrolled 13,388 women in a double-blinded, randomized, placebo-controlled trial to evaluate the effects of tamoxifen on risk reduction. The trial was closed prematurely because of a large discordance between the two groups. Tamoxifen significantly reduced the incidence of breast cancer in this population of patients by 49% compared with controls ($p < 0.00001$). It did not reduce the incidence of estrogen receptor-negative cancers.

Two other trials, the Royal Marsden Hospital trial and the Italian tamoxifen prevention study, failed to confirm this reduction in risk with prophylactic tamoxifen use. However, both studies were smaller and enrolled a lower risk population than the BCPT. Raloxifene, another selective estrogen receptor modulator, also reduces the relative risk. In a trial designed to test the efficacy of raloxifene on the prevention of bone fractures, 7705 postmenopausal women were treated with either raloxifene or a placebo. There was a 76% reduction in the incidence of breast cancer in the raloxifene group after 40 months of follow-up. As a result, the Study of Tamoxifen and Raloxifene (STAR) trial was designed and is currently enrolling women to determine which of the two drugs is superior in risk reduction. Until the results of the STAR trial are known, tamoxifen should be considered for breast cancer risk reduction in the high-risk patient according to the Gail model of breast cancer risk assessment. There is still no conclusive data on the use of tamoxifen in a population of patients with a *BRCA* gene mutation.

Surgical prophylaxis is another option for the woman who desires risk reduction. In a recent retrospective cohort of 639 patients, Hartmann was able to demonstrate a 90% risk reduction for the patient with a high risk of breast cancer after prophylactic bilateral mastectomy. In a follow-up study Hartmann was also able to demonstrate a similar risk reduction in a population of women with *BRCA* gene mutations. Although prophylactic bilateral mastectomy provides the greatest risk reduction it is usually reserved for the very high-risk patient because of the associated physiologic and complicated psychological consequences. Although most women who have undergone prophylactic bilateral mastectomy do not regret having undergone the procedure, approximately 5% to 20% report dissatisfaction according to Chlebowski.

Detection and Diagnosis

Detection of breast carcinoma is defined as the use of screening tests in asymptomatic women at periodic intervals to discover breast malignancies. The advantage of screening tests that facilitate early detection and diagnosis is reduced mortality because of smaller-sized cancers, more localized lesions, and a lower percentage of positive nodes. Established methods of detection include self-examination of the breasts, periodic examination by physicians, and mammography.

Physical examination and mammography are complementary procedures that must be considered together. Breast self-examination (BSE) has the major advantages of no cost to the patient and convenience. Diagnosis can be established only by biopsy or, sometimes, by fine-needle aspiration. Most importantly, a negative mammogram does not rule out breast carcinoma.

The kinetics of growth in breast carcinoma are important for understanding screening and detection. The average breast mass doubles in volume every 100 days and doubles in diameter every 300 days. A breast carcinoma grows for 6 to 8 years before reaching a diameter of 1 cm. In slightly less than another year the carcinoma will reach 2 cm in diameter. The mean diameter of a breast mass discovered by women who perform BSE at monthly intervals is 2 cm.

Greenwald and colleagues studied the results of BSE and of physician examination on the stage of breast carcinoma at initial diagnosis. Of 293 women with breast carcinoma, cancer was detected in clinical stage I in 54% when the detection method was routine physical examination, in 38% when the detection method was BSE, and in only 27% when the detection of the mass was accidental. In this study, only 50% of women who performed BSE did so on a monthly basis. These authors estimated that the breast cancer mortality rate might be reduced 19% by BSE and 24% by annual examination of the breasts by physicians.

In another study, Foster and Costanza determined the relationship between BSE and survival of breast cancer patients. Their study group included 1004 newly diagnosed invasive breast carcinoma in Vermont from July 1975 to December 1982. During this time, there was not widespread use of screening mammography in their state. The survival rate at 5 years was 75% for women who examined their own breasts versus 57% for women who did not examine their breasts. The authors concluded that in their population, BSE was responsible for earlier detection, improved survival, smaller tumor size, and fewer axillary node metastases. Their findings persisted after controlling the analysis for the potential bias of confounding variables, such as age, length-biased sampling, and lead-time bias.

In summary, present methods of screening for breast carcinoma are not ideal. Nevertheless, screening tests result in a reduction in mortality rate from breast cancer of approximately 25% to 30%.

Self-Examination of the Breasts

The majority of breast masses are initially discovered by the patient, either accidentally or during BSE. In a group of women having annual mammography and physical examinations by physicians, one of three carcinomas was discovered by the patients in the interval between professional detection methods. Even with widespread national publicity, approximately 50% of women do not perform monthly BSE. However, over 90% of women who regularly practice BSE were instructed in the techniques by their physicians. In Foster and Costanza's study of newly diagnosed carcinomas, 424 women performed BSE and 411 did not. The average size of the breast mass in women who performed BSE monthly was 2.1 cm. For those who performed BSE less than monthly, it was 2.4 cm; for the nonexaminers, 3.2 cm.

Although BSE has long been advocated, based on the studies cited here, its efficacy has been questioned because of the potential for bias. Several other studies have failed to show a benefit to BSE. In a recent case-controlled study within the Canadian National Breast Screening Study, Harvey demonstrated an odds ratio of 2.2 (95% CI 1.30 to 3.71) for cancer mortality or distant metastatic disease for women who omitted any part of the BSE. Although not conclusive, proficient BSE may reduce the risk of death from breast cancer.

The most effective teaching of BSE occurs in a one-to-one relationship. It is ideal to test the patient's ability to palpate masses in manufactured breast models. These models should contain masses with diameters as small as 0.3 to 0.5 cm.

Instructions for the patient concerning the techniques of breast self-palpation should emphasize timing, inspection, and palpation. The few days immediately after a menstrual period are the best time to detect changes in normal lumps or texture of the breasts. Postmenopausal women or women who have had a hysterectomy should be instructed to perform BSE on the same calendar days each month.

Women should be instructed that bilateral soft thickening and nodularity are normal physical findings. Palpation should begin in the shower, since many women have increased tactile sensitivity by using a "wet" technique. After the shower the woman should lie down, initially with one arm at her side and subsequently with the same arm underneath her head. She should be instructed to use the pads of her second, third, and fourth fingers to palpate the contralateral breast. Using the pads of her fingers, in a massaging motion with firm pressure, she should examine the entire breast and surrounding chest wall in a systematic fashion. One of the easier techniques to follow is to palpate the breasts in a clockwise fashion beginning at the nipple and gradually circumscribing larger circles. It is pragmatic not to include specific instructions for the woman to try to express secretions from her nipples.

Physical Examination

The ability to detect breast lumps varies widely from physician to physician. Fletcher and coworkers tested the physical examination techniques of 80 different physicians using manufactured breast models. The simulated breasts of the mannequins had a volume of 250 mL and the consistency of the breast tissue of a 50-year-old woman. The ability to detect the mass was directly related to the size of the mass; 87% of 1-cm, 33% of 0.5-cm, and 14% of 0.3-cm masses were discovered. The most disturbing finding was the wide range of detection rates among physicians, from 17% to 83%. In general, physicians with higher discovery rates spent more time performing the examination. The number of masses detected by a physician increased in those who used a consistent geometric pattern of examination with variable pressure exerted by the fingertips.

Although there has been widespread acceptance of physical exam as part of the screening for breast cancer, for ethical reasons there have not been randomized trials comparing physical exam to no screening. Several studies included the physical exam in addition to mammography, but only the Health Insurance Plan of New York (HIP) study demonstrated a significant reduction in breast cancer. Because 67% of the cancers in the HIP study group were detectable by physical exam, it was postulated that physical exam alone could have contributed to the reduction in breast cancer mortality. One randomized trial that compared physical exam with physical exam plus mammography for women over the age of 50 was the Canadian National Breast Screening Study II. Although there was no difference in mortality between the two groups, it generated interest in screening by physical exam. In a recent meta-analysis of clinical breast exam by Barton, there was indirect evidence of the effectiveness of the clinical exam. Clinical breast exam discovered approximately 15% to 20% of breast cancers that were missed by mammography.

A thorough breast examination by the physician should take 3 to 5 minutes to complete. This time is also an ideal opportunity to instruct the patient in the technique of BSE. A complete breast examination involves inspecting and palpating the breasts with the patient in the sitting as well as the supine position.

Initially, with a woman sitting on the examining table, the physician inspects the contour, symmetry, and vascular pattern of the breasts and the skin for irritation, retraction, or edema. It is important to have the patient place her arms above her head and subsequently place her hands on her hips. This sequence will contract the pectoralis muscles, which may allow the physician to visualize an abnormality. The patient in the sitting position is in the optimal position for the physician to determine the presence of adenopathy in the axilla (Fig. 15-12).

The woman's breasts should be subsequently examined with the woman in the supine position. It is important to examine both nipples for retraction, skin irritation, or a discharge. The areola should be compressed to identify any discharge. The normal breast has a small depression directly below the nipple. The skin of the breast is again carefully inspected for unusual vascular patterns, edema, erythema, or retraction.

Palpation is performed with both the woman's arms at her side and raised above her head and should not be limited to the breast tissue alone. A small pillow placed under the shoulder

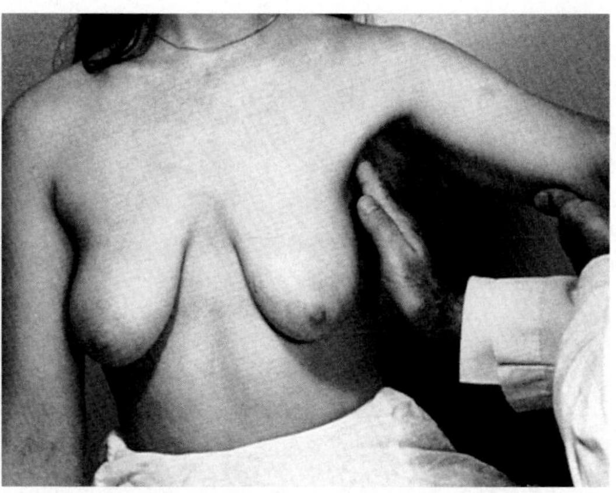

Figure 15-12. Examination of axilla in sitting position during breast examination. (From Marchant DJ: History, physical examination, and breast self-examination. Clin Obstet Gynecol 25:361, 1982.)

of the breast being examined often improves the examination. The examiner should palpate the axilla, the supraclavicular areas, and the adjacent chest wall. Palpation should use the pads of the first three fingers placed together, exerting firm but gentle pressure. Each physician determines his or her own systematic approach to examining all quadrants of the breast, the majority preferring concentric circles. It is very important that the physician draw a descriptive picture of any positive finding. This picture should include notations concerning the site, shape, size, consistency, and mobility of the mass. Special notation should be made as to whether the mass is tender and whether it is attached to skin or deep structures (Fig. 15-13). Physical examination is excellent as a screening procedure, but extremely poor in predicting the histopathology of the lesion. Studies have demonstrated that 30% to 40% of breast masses suspected by palpation to be malignant were found after biopsy to be benign. Conversely, 15% to 20% of benign-appearing masses during a physical examination subsequently are discovered by histopathology to be carcinoma.

Mammography

Mammography currently is the most practical method of detecting breast carcinoma at an early and highly curable stage, ideally discovering an occult cancer (<5 mm in diameter). The clinical advantages of discovering breast carcinoma during its earliest stage include higher percentage of localized disease, lower

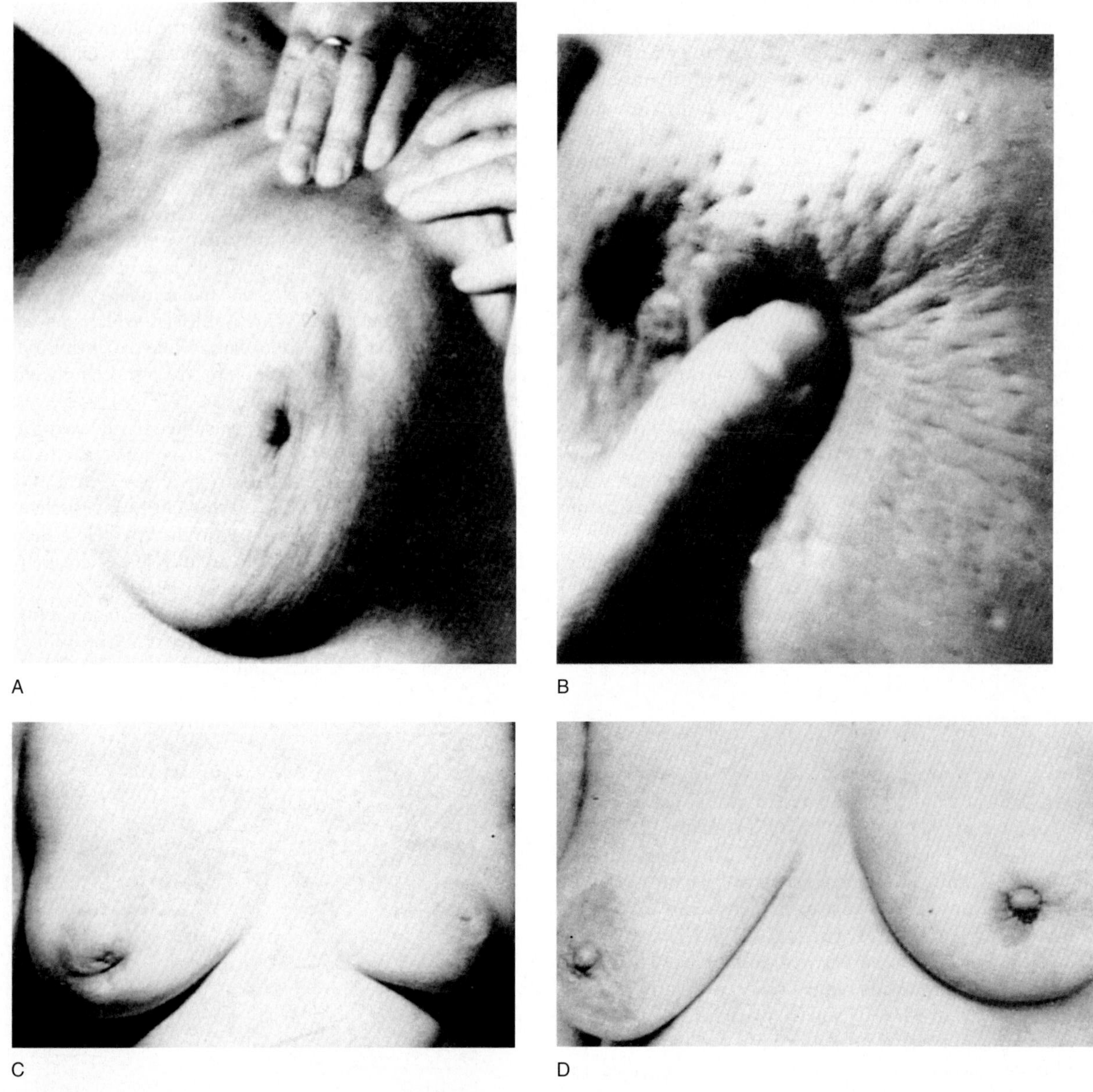

Figure 15-13. Signs of breast carcinoma. **A,** Retraction found during physical examination. **B,** Peau d'orange from underlying carcinoma. **C,** Retraction of right nipple. **D,** Retraction of left nipple from carcinoma. (From Degrell I: Atlas of Diseases of the Mammary Gland. Basel, Switzerland, S Karger, 1976, p 20.)

incidence of positive regional nodes, and reduced mortality. The 5-year survival rate for women whose breast cancer is believed to be localized to the breast with negative axillary nodes is approximately 85%. In contrast, the 5-year survival rate is only 53% when axillary nodes are positive. Ten-year survival statistics in women with negative nodes are approximately 74%, and 39% in women with positive nodes. Mammography is also the most accurate conventional method of detecting nonpalpable breast carcinoma. Therefore, with increasing emphasis on conservative surgery for early carcinomas, mammography will not only save lives but also conserve breasts. The number of women receiving screening mammography has increased dramatically over the past 10 years. Mammography is not as precise in younger women or in women with dense breasts secondary to fibroglandular tissue. Mammography is most sensitive in older women in which the majority of the breast is composed of fatty tissue.

Most physicians are able to consistently palpate breast masses when they are 1 cm in diameter or greater. Mammography may discover fine calcifications in breast neoplasms months to years before the carcinoma enlarges to a size that may be palpated on physical examination. Studying the kinetics of growth of breast cancer helps the clinician to appreciate why breast carcinoma is so often a systemic disease. Breast carcinoma must develop neovascularization to grow beyond 1–2 mm in diameter. Neovascularization provides the breast carcinoma the capability of metastasizing via the vascular system. It has been demonstrated that the development of angiogenesis as measured by microvessel density in histopathologic sections is the strongest independent predictor of relapse-free survival in women with node-negative breast cancer. The average breast carcinoma grows for 3 years, to enlarge from 1 mm to 1 cm.

Image quality in mammography has undergone major improvements since the 1980s. New equipment has decreased the radiation exposure associated with mammography by approximately one tenth. The vast majority of screening mammography in the mid-1990s was performed by dedicated mammographic equipment. Recently, there has been an increase in the routine use of grids and automatic exposure control. New film/screen combinations and improved film processing have facilitated superior images and sometimes reduced radiation dose. Conservative estimates are that 50 million American women should be screened by mammography each year. Restraints on the optimal use of mammography in identifying early breast carcinoma include a lack of properly trained and committed radiologists and the cost of the test. Mammography is a technically demanding procedure that requires an experienced and meticulous interpretation of the films, as well as correlation of the images with a thorough clinical examination. Elmore and colleagues reported the diagnostic consistency between pairs of radiologists in interpretation of mammograms. This consistency was moderate, with a median weight for percent of agreement at 78%. The frequency of the radiologists' recommendations for an immediate workup ranged from 74% to 96% in the woman with cancer and from 11% to 67% in the woman without cancer.

Historically, two landmark studies laid the foundation for the scientific credibility of mammography as a screening procedure. The first large, randomized control study was the HIP study, undertaken in the early 1960s. The HIP investigation involved yearly screening by both mammography and physical examination for 5 years. The women were followed for 10 to 14 years, and the study demonstrated a 30% reduction in mortality from breast carcinoma in the women who had annual mammography compared with the control group.

The second pivotal study was performed in 29 centers throughout the United States during the late 1970s. This immense undertaking was sponsored by the National Institutes of Health and was named the Breast Cancer Detection Demonstration Project (BCDDP). The BCDDP involved screening 275,000 women, and during the 5 years of the project, 3557 breast carcinomas were found, 42% discovered only by mammography.

The definite improvements in mammographic diagnosis over the 12-year interval between the two studies is documented by comparing their results. Cancer detection was approximately two times more frequent in the BCDDP study. In women ages 40 to 49, mammography found 39% of carcinomas in the HIP investigation, compared with 85% identified in the BCDDP project. Most important, in the detection of carcinoma less than 1 cm, the results were 36% in the BCDDP versus 8% in the HIP.

Present studies demonstrate that screening mammography reduces breast cancer mortality by approximately 33% in women 50 to 70 years of age. Even though screening mammography does not show a similar benefit for women 40 to 49 years of age, the most recent international randomized trials show about a 17% reduction in breast cancer mortality for women screened in this age group. Obviously, the sensitivity and specificity of a screening test are key factors in the success of the early detection of cancer.

Hormone replacement (HRT) may alter the effectiveness of mammographic screening. Lundström and coworkers demonstrated that an increase in mammographic density was much more common in women receiving continuous combination hormone replacement (52%) than women using cyclic (13%) and estrogen-only (18%) treatment. This was further substantiated by Greendale and colleagues, who noted an increase in mammographic density for patients on HRT. However, almost all the changes occurred within the first year of use. Laya and coworkers demonstrated that the specificity of mammography was significantly lower in current users of estrogen replacement therapy (82%), than in women who had never had estrogen replacement therapy (85%). Similarly, sensitivity also was significantly lower in current users (69%) versus 94% for never users. Thurfjell and colleagues did not detect any decrease in sensitivity of screening mammography in women currently using HRT, but there was some marginal decrease in specificity varying with the regimen and duration of treatment.

Present recommendations to detect breast cancer include encouraging all adult women to perform BSE monthly. The American Cancer Society recommends a clinical breast exam every 3 years for women younger than 40 and yearly for women older than 40 years of age. Because one third of breast carcinomas occur before age 50, increasing emphasis is being placed on early discovery in young women. After many years of debate there is consensus among the American Cancer Society, the American College of Radiology, and the American College of Obstetricians and Gynecologists that annual screening mammography should be offered to all women starting at the age of 40. There is a benefit to screening, although the reduction in mortality may not be as great for women age 40 to 49 years. In the United States more than 10,000 deaths occur each year in women who initially developed breast carcinoma between the ages of 40 and 49. Sickles and Kopans have reported that a meta-analysis of recent studies shows a 21% mortality reduction in women who have had mammographic screening compared with those in control groups. They further conclude that screening is at least as beneficial for women who are ages 40 to 49 as it is for those ages 50 to 64 years.

Obviously, many other nonscientific factors affect an individual physician's recommendations and an individual woman's decision. Among the more important of these are the cost of the test and the patient's anxiety regarding breast cancer. In addition, the anxiety related to false-positive mammograms can be an obstacle to screening. Elmore and colleagues performed a 10-year retrospective cohort study of breast cancer screening and discovered that over that time, one third of the women screened had additional evaluations because of abnormal screening tests. Multiple studies document that the primary barrier to mammographic screening is the lack of a strong recommendation from the woman's primary care physician. More frequent physical examinations and mammograms may be indicated, depending on individual risk factors and the finding of precursors of breast carcinoma.

Mammography is established as part of the diagnostic workup of women with breast symptoms. Often significant occult disease is identified in another quadrant of the same breast or in the contralateral breast. All patients with breast masses or persistent spontaneous nipple discharge should have mammograms of both breasts before biopsy. Mammography is also indicated in evaluating a breast mass the patient has found but that the physician cannot confirm by palpation. This technique is helpful in difficult clinical situations, such as the evaluation of large breasts or following augmentation mammoplasty. It is important to stress once again that mammography and physical examination are complementary procedures. One procedure does not replace the necessity of carefully performing the other.

Optimal identification of early breast carcinoma by mammography depends on a competent technician obtaining excellent images and the radiologist searching for subtle changes. For screening mammography, two views of each breast are performed: the mediolateral oblique (MLO) and the craniocaudal (CC). The MLO is the most effective single view because it includes the greatest amount of breast tissue and is the only view that includes all of the upper outer quadrant and axillary tail. Sickles emphasized the importance of firm breast compression of the breast during mammography for the following reasons (Fig. 15-14). First, it holds the breast still to prevent motion artifact. It brings the objects closer into view, thereby reducing the amount of blur. It also serves to separate overlapping tissues that can obscure an underlying lesion. Finally, it decreases the amount of radiation exposure by making the breast thinner and easier to penetrate with less radiation. Sickles further advocated the importance of side-by-side comparison of both breasts and evaluating current films with previous ones. This facilitates identification of the less classic, indirect signs of breast carcinoma, such as a single dilated duct with intraductal carcinoma, asymptomatic architectural distortion in dense breasts, and a developing density.

Breast cancer may be detected by visualizing clusters of fine calcifications, spiculations, or poorly defined multinodular masses with irregular contours, all characteristic of malignancy. Isolated clusters of tiny calcifications are the most common and

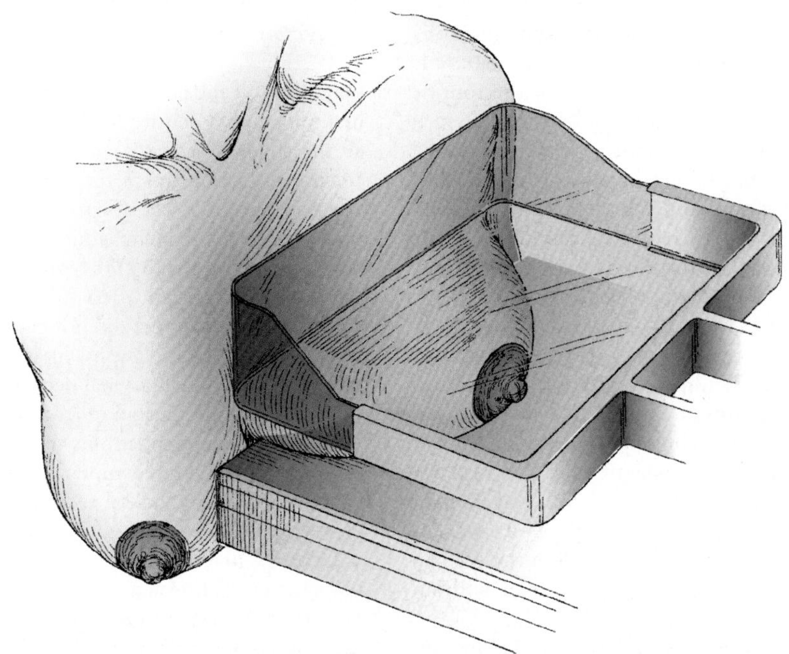

Figure 15-14. Mammography being performed with appropriate compression applied. (Redrawn from Wilson OL: Mammographic technique. In Parsons CA [ed]: Diagnosis of Breast Disease: Imaging, Clinical Features, and Pathology. London, Chapman & Hall, © Copyright, 1983, p 67.)

important diagnostic sign of an early carcinoma. Calcifications are often smaller than 0.5 mm in diameter and thus must be identified by a magnifying lens. The presence of five or more calcifications within a volume of 1 cm^3 is termed a *cluster.* Subsequent breast biopsies will find 25% of clusters associated with cancer and 75% with benign disease. Conversely, approximately 68% of occult breast carcinomas and 34% of palpable breast cancers demonstrate calcifications on mammographic examination.

Standardized terminology should be used to describe mammographic findings. As a result, the American College of Radiology Breast Imaging Reporting and Data System (BI-RADS) was devised to standardize mammographic terminology, reduce confusing interpretations, and facilitate the monitoring of outcomes. The report includes an overall assessment of the likelihood that the finding represents a malignancy. There are six assessment categories, each associated with a specific risk of cancer. In the conclusion of every mammogram report, the final assessment is provided to prevent confusion and to guide the referring health care professional as to a recommended plan of action.

Computer-aided diagnosis has been an area of active investigation in recent years. Delineation by computer program of microcalcifications and masses gives the radiologist a second opinion of the mammographic films. It has been long established that double reading of a mammographic study by two independent observers improves the breast cancer detection rate by approximately 10%. Obviously, it also increases the cost of screening. Computer-aided diagnosis shows promise of potentially detecting lesions that would not be identified by double reading.

The relationship between high levels of radiation and increased risk for breast carcinoma raises questions concerning the relative risk of the carcinogenic effect of mammography. The measured radiation dose to the breast by state-of-the-art mammography equipment is approximately 0.1 rad (0.001 Gy) for a two-view examination. Mettler and coworkers have summarized the recent literature regarding the benefits versus the risks from screening mammography. Their findings are that for a woman beginning annual screening at age 50 and continuing until age 75 the benefit exceeds the risk secondary to radiation by a factor of almost 100. For a high-risk woman who begins annual screening at age 35 the benefit–risk in reduced mortality is more than 25-fold (Table 15-4). Thus the benefits of screening far outweigh any possible radiation risk.

The incidence of breast carcinoma in the United States is 1000 cases per million women per year for women in their early 40s. In summary, the risk of radiation from mammography is negligible compared with the benefits of the discovery of early and potentially curable breast carcinoma.

Diagnostic mammography is a comprehensive radiologic examination that usually involves multiple individualized and specialized equipment and views. The extra views and magnification increase the sensitivity and specificity of the procedure. Often mammography is used to locate a breast lesion prior to open biopsy or to obtain stereotactic core biopsy during mammographic imaging. Although the primary role of mammography is to screen women with no symptoms or signs of breast cancer, mammography is also used diagnostically. The diagnostic follow-up to an abnormal screening mammogram is individualized depending on a woman's risk factors, physical examination, and age. The BI-RADS classification of screening mammograms can be helpful in assessing risk and devising a management plan (Fig. 15-15). Obviously, it is ideal to use nonsurgical methods to treat low-risk women and try to perform stereotactic or open biopsy depending on relative risk.

Table 15-4 Breast Cancer Benefit/Risk Ratio for a Woman Having Annual Mammography Beginning at Age 35

Age	Annual Baseline Breast Cancer Incidence/ 100,000	Fatal Radiation-Induced Cases	Fatal Cases Prevented by Mammography	Benefit/Risk Ratio
35	66	0	1.3	
36	66	0	1.3	
37	66	0	1.3	
38	66	0	1.3	
39	66	0	1.3	
40	129	0	12.9	>400
41	129	0	12.9	
42	129	0	12.9	
43	129	0	12.9	
44	129	0	12.9	
45	187	<0.1	18.7	352
46	187	<0.1	18.7	181
47	187	0.2	18.7	120
48	187	0.2	18.7	91
49	187	0.3	18.7	73
50	220	0.3	22	66
51	220	0.4	22	61
52	220	0.4	22	57
53	220	0.4	22	53
54	220	0.4	22	50
55	268	0.6	26.08	47
56	268	0.6	26.8	44
57	268	0.6	26.8	43
58	268	0.7	26.8	41
59	268	0.7	26.8	39
60	339	0.9	33.9	38
61	339	0.9	33.9	37
62	339	0.9	33.9	36
63	339	1	33.9	35
64	339	1	33.9	34
65	391	1.2	39.1	33
66	391	1.2	39.1	33
67	391	1.2	39.1	32
68	391	1.3	39.1	31
69	391	1.3	39.1	30
70	421	1.4	42.1	30
71	421	1.4	42.1	29
72	421	1.5	42.1	29
73	421	1.5	42.1	28
74	421	1.5	42.1	28
75	421	1.5	42.1	27

Tables assume reduction in mortality from breast cancer as a result of screening as follows: age 35–39, 5%; 40–49, 15%; and 50–75, 25%.

From Mettler FA, Upton AC, Kelsey CA, et al: Benefits versus risks from mammography: A critical reassessment. Cancer 77:903, 1996.

Ultrasound

Ultrasound has a definite role as a complementary procedure to other imaging techniques in the diagnosis of breast disease,

BI-RAD class	Description	Probability of malignancy (%)	Follow-up
0	Needs additional evaluation	1	Diagnostic mammogram, ultrasound
1	Normal mammogram	0	Yearly screening
2	Benign lesion	0	Yearly screening
3	Probably benign lesion	<2	Short-interval follow-up
4	Suspicious for malignancy	20	Biopsy
5	Highly suspicious malignancy	90	Biopsy
BI-RAD, Breast Imaging Reporting and Data Systems.			

Figure 15-15. BI-RAD classification of mammographic lesions. (From Pazdur R, Coia LR, Hoskins WJ, Wagman LD (eds): Cancer Management: A Multidisciplinary Approach, 4th ed. Melville, NY, Cligott Publishing Group, p 143.)

particularly in differentiating cystic from solid masses. It should not be used as a "screening test" except for women with very dense breasts who cannot be adequately screened with mammography. Ultrasound screening increased the detection of otherwise occult cancers by 37% in a recent study involving 3626 women age 42 to 67, with dense breasts and no visible abnormalities on mammography. In the general population the effectiveness of ultrasound "screening" is more limited. Sickles and colleagues reported a comparison study using state-of-the-art equipment. Mammography detected 62 of 64 (97%) carcinomas, whereas ultrasound diagnosed only 37 of 64 (58%). Only 8% of carcinomas smaller than 1 cm in diameter were discovered by ultrasound. The conclusion of this study was that the majority of breast carcinomas visualized by ultrasound can be palpated clinically and there was little use for the ultrasound as a screening tool. The primary advantage of ultrasound is the ability to produce images of breast tissue on multiple occasions without harmful effects. It is most useful in evaluating solitary masses greater than 1 cm in diameter. The greatest limitation of ultrasonography of the breast is the limited spatial resolution. Microcalcifications are not visualized because resolution of less than 2 mm is difficult with ultrasound. Whether it can distinguish benign from malignant lesions has been a topic of great debate. In one series, Stavros and coworkers described the sonographic evaluation of 750 solid breast nodules (palpable and nonpalpable) all of which had subsequent histologic confirmation. The negative predictive value of sonography was 99.5%. This is a higher negative predictive value than a BI-RAD 3 mammogram for which a 6-month follow-up is recommended. It can be used to evaluate mammographically detected lesions. A low-risk lesion according to strict sonographic criteria can either be aspirated or safely observed. When the lesion is believed to be intermediate risk it should undergo histologic evaluation because 10% to 15% will be malignant.

Ultrasonography of the breast is usually performed by a handheld, real-time, high-frequency probe. It is a highly operator- and reader-dependent test with a great deal of variation among different centers. Breast cancer is usually hypoechoic, and early cancers are difficult to distinguish from surrounding normal hypoechoic breast tissue. The most important use of ultrasound is to differentiate a cystic breast mass from a solid mass. The accuracy rate of ultrasound to diagnose a cystic mass is 96% to 100% and exceeds the combined accuracy of mammography and physical examination. Ultrasound may be used as a guide for needle aspiration, needle core biopsy, and in localization procedures. It has also been used to localize tumors intraoperatively without a guide wire with excellent success rates. In one series, pathologically negative margins were achieved in 97% of the cases by using sonography alone to localize the lesion intraoperatively. This imaging technique also may be useful in women with augmentation mammoplasty, in the differential diagnosis of masses in the dense breast tissue of younger women, evaluating a breast abscess, and possibly determining lymph node status in a woman with carcinoma. Although it can be used to evaluate the integrity of a silicone breast implant, most believe that MRI is better at detecting implant ruptures.

Duplex Doppler ultrasonography is a new technique; however, preliminary results do not demonstrate a high sensitivity or specificity.

In summary, ultrasound should not be used as a sole imaging technique for breast disease. Because of its lack of sensitivity and specificity for early breast carcinoma, it should not be used in an attempt to detect subclinical disease in the general population at this time.

Digital Radiography

Digital radiography is the technique by which X-ray photons are detected after passing through the breast tissue and the radiographic image is recorded electronically in a digital format and stored in a computer. Digital technology has multiple advantages compared with conventional mammography. Image acquisition, display, and storage are much faster, and image manipulation through adjustments in contrast, brightness, and electronic magnification of selected regions enables radiologists to obtain superior views. This technology makes it possible to subtract various layers of computerized imagery in order to examine suspicious areas and improve the ability to detect and diagnose breast carcinoma. Digital mammography is particularly helpful in screening women with very dense breasts and breast implants. With the ability to manipulate the images, digital mammography will reduce the number of women recalled for more images. Computer-aided diagnosis is also possible with this technique as well as the ability to transmit the image electronically. Because of low background "noise" and superior contrast capabilities, the final image is superior to conventional mammography.

The disadvantages of digital mammography include the high cost of the equipment, the limited image storage capacity, and the reduced spatial resolution due in part to inadequate resolution of current monitors. Although not yet FDA approved, there are several clinical trials underway designed to evaluate its utility as a screening test. The Department of Defense Digital Mammography Screening Trial is recruiting approximately 15,000 women to compare both conventional and digital mammography. The interim results revealed no difference in the number of cancers missed by either group. However, digital mammography is associated with a significantly lower recall rate (11.5% vs. 14.1%) and a higher rate of positive findings at the time of biopsy (43.3% vs. 23.7%). Although promising, for the near future the high cost per test will make it financially impractical to implement widespread digital radiography for screening purposes. This imaging technique will be the screening modality of the future, as it also requires less radiation exposure than modern mammographic equipment because of the increased quantum efficiency of the digital equipment.

Computed Tomography

Computed tomography (CT) has limited value when compared with mammography because of higher radiation dose and longer study times. The thickness of cross-sectional slices with CT misses the majority of areas of microcalcification. CT scans have demonstrated some preclinical cancers after injection with radiocontrast media. This imaging technique is excellent for studying the most medial and lateral aspects of the breast. It is sometimes used for preoperative wire location of a mass that is difficult to localize by mammography. However, the increased expense and radiation exposure virtually eliminate CT scans for screening programs.

Magnetic Resonance Imaging

Preliminary research studies using magnetic resonance imaging (MRI) in the workup of women suspected of having breast carcinoma are promising. Because of higher costs, this imaging technique will not be used in screening but as a diagnostic test. The ability of MRI to differentiate benign from malignant tissue may help to reduce the frequency of breast biopsy, especially in women with dense, fibroglandular breasts. MRI has been proven effective in detecting new tumors in patients with previous lumpectomy because it can accurately distinguish between scar tissue and cancerous lesions. This is best accomplished by the gadolinium-enhanced MRI. Other potential uses or indications for MRI are to improve imaging of structures close to the chest wall, to improve imaging of women with breast prosthesis, and to evaluate for prosthesis rupture. It is useful in the patient who presents with axillary adenopathy and no apparent mass in the breast. Because the average examination takes about 45 minutes to an hour, MRI will not be used in mass screening programs. MRI cannot identify microcalcifications. Another limitation of MRI is the loss of image quality with respiratory movements. Its role in the screening of very high-risk women is being evaluated.

Thermography

Thermography is unreliable as a screening technique for breast carcinoma or as a technique to determine women at increased risk for subsequent breast neoplasia. Lawson first described the elevation of skin temperature associated with breast carcinoma in 1956. Although thermography has been used clinically since that time, it has extremely high false-positive and false-negative rates.

Thermography is ineffective in detection of occult or preclinical cancers. This technique was initially included in the national multicenter breast cancer detection demonstration program. However, the detection rate with thermography was 42% as compared with 92% for mammography. The major fault of a normal thermography examination is the false sense of security engendered in the symptom-free woman. The addition of thermography to other established diagnostic methods increases costs without providing useful clinical information.

Transillumination

Transillumination, or dynamic optical breast imaging (DOBI), is a radiation-free technique that measures the light transmitted through breast tissue. The breast acts as a filter for the light; the hypothesis is that malignant tissue absorbs more infrared light than does benign tissue. Although this technique is inexpensive it is still experimental and unproven. To date, results of research studies using transillumination do not compare with results obtained with mammography.

Mammoscintigraphy (Scintimammography)

Mammoscintigraphy is a radionuclide imaging test for the detection of breast cancer. Technetium-99m sestamibi is a radiotracer with reported high sensitivity and high negative predictive value for breast cancer. It has a high diagnostic accuracy for the detection of breast cancer in all women, including women who may be unsuitable for conventional mammography. In a study designed to describe the diagnostic utility of mammoscintigraphy in women with a breast mass, Howarth and colleagues studied 115 patients and noted an overall sensitivity for the detection of breast cancer of 84% for scintimammography and 66% for conventional mammography. The specificity of scintimammography was also significantly better than conventional mammography, 84% and 67%, respectively. The high negative predictive value of this test for breast cancer potentially makes it an important adjunct to mammography by potentially reducing the number of biopsies performed for benign findings. Mammoscintigraphy is useful for locating tumors in the lateral areas of dense breasts as well as detecting metastatic disease in the lymph nodes of the axilla. Additional studies are needed before this test is widely accepted and its utility proven.

Other Imaging Techniques

There are several other imaging techniques that are currently being evaluated. Diffraction-enhanced imaging (DEI) is one such technique. With this technique an analyzing crystal is placed in the X-ray beam between the breast and an image-creating medium such as film or digital detector. The crystal diffracts the X-ray beam and produces two separate images, one based on standard radiograph and the other based on refraction. The result is an excellent quality image with superior tumor visibility. Digital thermal imaging is another new technique that uses the principles of thermography as well as digital technology to create an image base determined by temperature differences between the cancer and the normal breast. Microwave radiography is a portable, noninvasive adjuvant diagnostic approach that involves passive measurement of microwave emissions from breast tissue. All these techniques must undergo further appropriate testing to determine their safety and efficacy in the management of breast cancer.

Fine-Needle Aspiration

Fine-needle aspiration (FNA) of a breast mass is a well-established diagnostic test. It is a simple office-based procedure that is well accepted by women because it is sometimes less painful than a venipuncture. Most physicians do not use anesthesia, although some prefer to use a small amount of local anesthetic (1 mL of 1% lidocaine). The skin over the breast is the most sensitive area, but the breast tissue itself has few pain fibers. The anesthetic procedure has more disadvantages than advantages. The major disadvantage is that if excessive amounts of anesthetic are injected into the skin, or if a hematoma develops, the mass may be obscured and the accuracy of the FNA is decreased. However, an injection of local anesthesia into a small area of the skin will help to reduce the patient's anxiety. The skin is usually prepared for an FNA with either an alcohol or iodine solution. The slides for the aspirate should be properly labeled, or, preferably, a cytotechnologist should be available to process the slides and assess the adequacy of the specimen. The breast mass is secured with one hand and the other hand introduces a 20- or 22-gauge needle attached to a 10- or 20-mL syringe into the mass. If the mass is a cyst, one feels a "give" or reduced resistance after puncturing the cyst wall. It may be technically easier to manipulate the smaller needles without the syringe attached. Complete aspiration of all the fluid from the cyst is facilitated by negative pressure from the syringe and firm pressure on the cyst wall (Fig. 15-16). With withdrawal of the fluid the cyst wall collapses, and usually a residual mass cannot be palpated. After withdrawal of the needle, firm pressure is applied for 5 to 10 minutes to reduce the possibility of hematoma formation. Complications of needle aspiration are minimal, with hematoma formation being the only substantial one. Infection is very rare. The theoretic risk of spreading cancer along the needle track has not been substantiated. The relief of a patient's anxiety produced by successfully aspirating a newly discovered breast mass is most gratifying.

The color of the fluid obtained via aspiration varies from clear to grossly bloody. It is not uncommon to find yellow, brown, and even green fluid in a cyst. If the aspirated fluid is clear, it is not necessary to submit it for cytologic evaluation. One study in the literature documents no breast cancers discovered from almost 7000 consecutive nonbloody cyst aspirates. If the aspirated fluid is turbid or bloody, a sample should be placed on a cover slip and sent for cytologic interpretation and the mass should be further evaluated with a biopsy. Although bloody fluid is usually from a traumatic tap one must consider the possibility of a carcinoma.

No further workup is necessary if the aspirated fluid is clear and no residual mass is palpated immediately after the procedure and again 1 month later. However, if the mass remains after aspiration, a biopsy should be performed even if the cytologic analysis of the fluid was negative. A biopsy should be performed on cysts that recur within 2 weeks or that necessitate more than one repeat aspiration. Slightly less than 20% of cysts recur after a single aspiration and less than 10% recur after two aspirations. The percentage of false-positive, fine-needle aspirations is very rare, usually less than 2%.

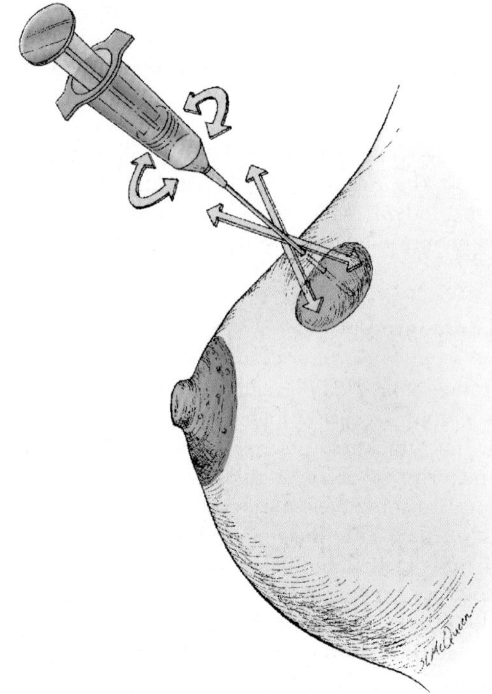

Figure 15-16. Needle biopsy and aspiration with negative pressure. Needle is rotated, moved back and forth, and slightly in and out to aspirate representative specimen. (From Vorherr H: Breast aspiration biopsy. Am J Obstet Gynecol 148:128, 1984.)

In the event that no fluid is obtained, the breast mass is probably solid and several passes are made through the mass with continuous suction from the syringe. Moving the needle within a single tract will give a satisfactory cellular yield in the majority of cases. The cellular specimen within the needle should be placed on a slide and fixed for analysis. Definitive diagnosis by open biopsy or core needle biopsy should be considered if there is the aspirate, mammogram, or physical exam are suggestive of cancer. This triple test has been advocated by many as a reliable alternative to biopsy. According to the National Cancer Institute's committee opinion on FNA, if the physical exam, imaging findings, and cytologic evaluation of the mass all confirm the same benign process, the mass can be followed. However, if any of these assessments is indicative of cancer, a biopsy should be performed. The false-negative rate of triple test diagnosis approaches that of surgical biopsy, and the false-positive rate is comparable to that for frozen section. Although optimal performance of FNA is operator-dependent, the results of the triple test for palpable masses have proven quite reliable. The sensitivity of FNA for palpable masses is approximately 90%, with a false-negative rate that varies from 0.7% to 22%. In experienced hands, the false-negative rate of FNA is approximately 3% to 10%. The major drawbacks of FNA are that it cannot distinguish invasive from noninvasive breast carcinoma and it is unable to confirm in histologic terms a definitive benign diagnosis.

Biopsy

The definitive diagnosis and ultimate foundation for treatment of breast carcinoma depends on histologic diagnosis of the biopsy material. Breast biopsy is one of the most common surgical procedures performed, but with the increasing acceptance of mammography and the development of less invasive procedures there has been a shift from the traditional open biopsy to the less invasive and more popular core-needle biopsy. The common indications for tissue biopsy include bloody discharge from the nipple, a persistent three-dimensional mass, or suggestive mammography. Nipple retraction or elevation and skin changes, such as erythema, induration, or edema, are also indications for breast biopsy. Obviously, the suspicious area must be sampled appropriately. This can be accomplished several ways.

Nonpalpable breast lesions are most commonly discovered through screening mammography, and they represent a large proportion of the suggestive areas investigated by biopsy. Although these lesions are relatively easy to identify, intraoperative localization and subsequent adequate excision can be very challenging. Until recently, the best available method was to perform a mammographically guided wire-localized excisional biopsy. With this method a wire is placed percutaneously in the vicinity of the abnormality by the radiologist, using mammogram guidance. Subsequently, the woman is taken to the operating suite where the surgeon uses the wire as a guide to excise the abnormal area. The specimen is removed with the wire in place and it is radiographed to confirm the removal of the abnormal area. More recently a needle is placed over the wire to help localize the lesion.

Mammographically guided wire-localized excisional biopsy is more invasive than the more widely accepted stereotactic core-needle biopsy. This latter procedure has changed dramatically how mammographically detected lesions are managed. The woman is placed prone on the stereotactic biopsy table with the breast in a dependent position. The breast is imaged, and the lesion is localized using computer-assisted positioning and targeting devices. A small nick is made in the skin and the core biopsy needle is advanced into the lesion. The lesion is sampled, and the "cores" of tissue are sent to pathology for histologic evaluation. Although this technique is very accurate, the finding of atypical hyperplasia or carcinoma in situ requires open wire-localized excisional biopsy to rule out an underlying invasive cancer. The false-negative rate for this procedure is less than 2%.

Palpable lesions can be evaluated by several techniques. The type of technique used depends on many factors, including the location and size of the lesion as well as patient and physician preference. Options include incisional or excisional biopsy, as well as core-needle biopsy. A small incisional biopsy may be appropriate for a large mass. However, it is important to obtain a large wedge of breast tissue so as not to miss an occult carcinoma identified by mammography. The intent of excisional biopsy is to remove the mass with a surrounding margin of normal tissue.

Today the majority of open breast biopsies are performed under local anesthesia on an outpatient basis. Twenty-five years ago, it was common practice to perform a biopsy, frozen section, and definitive surgery during the same operation. The modern two-step approach significantly decreases anxiety for the patient. The 1- to 2-week interval between biopsy and therapy gives the woman a chance to contemplate alternative choices in therapy. Cosmetic results are important, and the majority of biopsies can be performed with curvilinear incisions, often in the circumareolar area. An open biopsy should be performed using a cold knife rather than electrocautery. The use of electrocautery on the biopsy material may blur the margin of normal tissue around the tumor and cause abnormally low receptor levels. It is important to send the pathology laboratory a small sample (1 g of suggestive tissue) to determine the presence or absence of estrogen and progesterone receptors. These receptors are heat-labile, and therefore the tissue must be frozen within 30 minutes. The incidence of carcinoma in biopsies corresponds directly with the patient's age. Approximately 20% of breast biopsies in women age 50 are positive, and this figure increases to 33% in women age 70 or older.

Classification

Breast cancer is usually asymptomatic before the development of advanced disease. Breast pain is experienced by only 10% of women with early breast carcinoma. The classic sign of a breast carcinoma is a solitary, solid, three-dimensional, dominant breast mass. The borders of the mass are usually indistinct, which makes it difficult to define precisely the size of the mass. Often the mass is not freely mobile. Far-advanced local disease produces changes in the skin and nipples of the breast, including retraction, dimpling, induration, edema (peau d'orange), ulceration, and signs of inflammation.

The prognosis and treatment of breast carcinoma are primarily related to the stage of the disease and extent of spread to regional nodes. Variations in histologic types and degree of cellular atypia of breast cancer are of secondary importance. There have been numerous classifications of breast carcinoma that contain mixtures of both clinical and pathologic subgroups. The neoplasm is classified based on the predominant histologic cells; however, several cellular patterns may be found in any one tumor. A condensed classification is presented in Table 15-5. Most carcinomas originate in the epithelium of the collecting

Table 15-5 Simplified Classification of Breast Carcinoma

Type of Carcinoma	Percentage of All Cases Diagnosed
Ductal Carcinoma	
In situ	5
Infiltrating	80
Lobular Carcinoma	
In situ	3
Infiltrating	9
Inflammatory carcinoma	2
Paget's disease	1

ducts or terminal lobular ducts. Both in situ and invasive carcinoma have been described, often in the same quadrant of the breast. Bilateral breast carcinoma occurs in approximately 1% of all newly diagnosed cases. The prevalence of bilateral breast cancer is twofold greater in lobular neoplasia.

Intraductal carcinoma in situ is a disease in which the cellular abnormalities are limited to the ductal epithelium and have not penetrated the base membrane. It is most commonly discovered in perimenopausal and postmenopausal women. Intraductal carcinoma in situ is not usually detected by palpation because the disease does not produce a definitive mass. Mammography sometimes demonstrates the fine stippling of microcalcifications. The histologic diagnosis of intraductal carcinoma in situ includes a heterogeneous group of tumors with varying malignant potential. Literature reviews by Page and associates, among others, document carcinoma developing in approximately 35% of women with this disease within 10 years of initial diagnosis, usually in the same quadrant of the breast as the original biopsy. If the primary treatment is simple mastectomy, 5% to 10% of women will have a simultaneous invasive carcinoma in the same breast.

Lobular carcinoma in situ should not be treated as a cancer or as a precursor of breast cancer. It is considered to be a marker for an increased breast cancer risk. It does not have the same malignant potential as intraductal carcinoma in situ. However, it has a much greater tendency to be bilateral and to present as multifocal disease. Three of four patients are in the premenopausal age group. Lobular carcinoma in situ is not detected by palpation, and mammography shows no characteristic pattern. However, it should be considered as a major risk factor for the subsequent development of breast carcinoma. The latent period is longer than with intraductal carcinoma in situ; often more than 20 years will elapse before infiltrating carcinoma develops. Approximately 20% of women with this disease will develop invasive breast carcinoma during the remainder of their life. Interestingly, most of the subsequent carcinomas are ductal, not lobular (Table 15-6).

Table 15-6 Salient Characteristics of in Situ Ductal (DCIS) and Lobular (LCIS) Carcinoma of the Breast

	LCIS	DCIS
Age (years)	44–47	54–58
Incidence*	2%–5%	5%–100%
Clinical signs	None	Mass, pain, nipple discharge
Mammographic signs	None	Microcalcifications
Premenopausal	2/3	1/3
Incidence synchronous		
Invasive carcinoma	5%	2%–46%
Multicentricity	60%–90%	40%–80%
Bilaterality	50%–70%	10%–20%
Axillary metastasis	1%	1%–2%
Subsequent carcinomas:		
Incidence	25%–35%	25%–70%
Laterality	Bilateral	Ipsilateral
Interval to diagnosis	15–20 yr	5–10 yr
Histology	Ductal	Ductal

*Among biopsies of mammographically detected breast lesions.
From Frykberg ER, Ames FC, Bland KI: Current concepts for management of early (in situ and occult invasive) breast carcinoma. In Bland KI, Copeland EM (eds): The Breast. Philadelphia, WB Saunders, 1991, p 736.

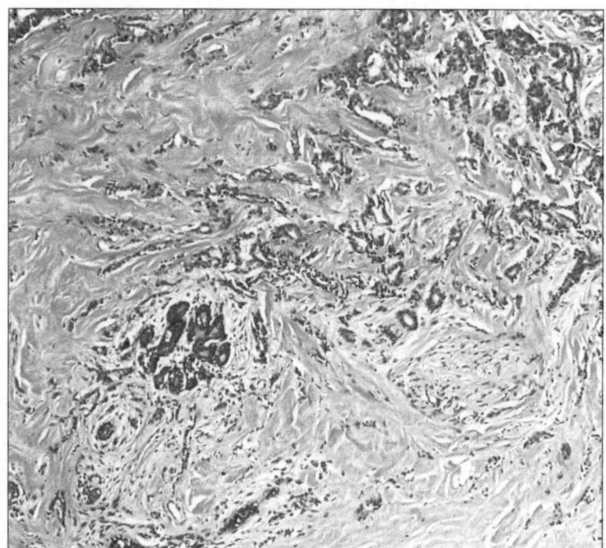

Figure 15-17. Invasive ductal carcinoma of the breast. Malignant cells are invading the fibrous tissue. (From Stevens A, Lowe J: Human Histology, 3rd ed: Philadelphia, Elsevier Mosby, 2005, p 392.)

Infiltrating ductal carcinoma is the most common breast malignancy. Histologically, nonuniform malignant epithelial cells of varying sizes and shapes infiltrate the surrounding tissue (Fig. 15-17). The degree of fibrous response to the invading epithelial cells determines the firmness to palpation and texture during biopsy. Often the stromal reaction may be extensive, thus the outdated term *cirrhosis carcinoma.* Approximately 10% of infiltrating ductal carcinomas are of a uniform histologic picture and are classified as medullary, colloid, comedo, tubular, or papillary carcinomas. In general the specialized forms are grossly softer, mobile, and well delineated. They are usually smaller and have a more optimistic prognosis than the more common nonhomogeneous variety. Medullary carcinomas are soft, with extensive stromal infiltration by lymphocytes and plasma cells. Colloid carcinomas have a similar soft consistency, with extensive deposition of extracellular mucin.

Infiltrating lobular carcinomas are characterized by the uniformity of the small, round neoplastic cells. Often the malignant epithelial cells infiltrate the stroma in a single-file fashion. This neoplasia tends to have a multicentric origin in the same breast and tends to involve both breasts more often than infiltrating ductal carcinoma. Histologic subdivisions of infiltrating lobular carcinoma include small cell, round cell, and signet cell carcinomas.

Inflammatory carcinomas comprise approximately 2% of breast cancers. This type is recognized clinically as a rapidly growing, highly malignant carcinoma. Infiltration of malignant cells into the lymphatics of the skin produces a clinical picture that simulates a skin infection. There is not a specific histologic cell type.

Paget's disease of the breast is rare, comprising slightly less than 1% of breast carcinomas (Fig. 15-18). This lesion has an innocent appearance and looks like eczema or a dermatitis of the nipple. The clinical picture is produced by an infiltrating ductal carcinoma that invades the epidermis. Paget's disease has an excellent prognosis.

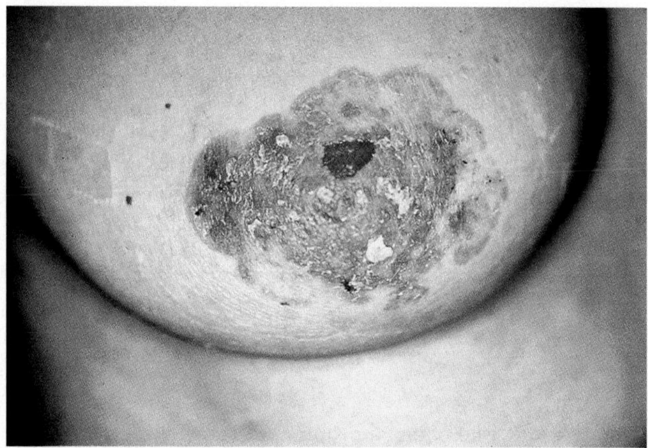

Figure 15-18. Paget's disease of the breast. Note the erythematous plaques around the nipple. (From Callen JP: Dermatologic signs of systemic disease. In Bolognia JL, Jorizzo JL, Rapini RP [eds]: Dermatology. Edinburgh, Mosby, 2003, p 714.)

Treatment

The treatment of breast carcinoma is complex, with many variables to consider. The most appropriate treatment varies from woman to woman. The four most important variables for treatment selection are the tumor's size; its inherent aggressiveness, as determined by the histology of the initial lesion; the presence of positive nodes; and the receptor status of the tumor. The TNM system is a widely recognized staging system based on both clinical and pathologic criteria (Table 15-7). When generalizations are offered concerning the preferred method of therapy, it is important to remember that breast carcinoma is a heterogeneous group of neoplasms. Unfortunately, neither clinical nor pathologic staging of the disease is nearly as precise as one would postulate in a carcinoma involving an external organ. Axillary nodes will be negative for metastatic disease at initial surgery in approximately 60% of women. However, approximately 25% of these women will develop recurrent carcinoma. Microscopic metastatic disease occurs early via both hematogenous and lymphatic routes. For example, 30% to 40% of women without gross adenopathy in the axilla will have positive nodes discovered during histologic examination. With the additional assessment tools of immunohistochemical staining for the presence of cytokeratin and serial sectioning of axillary nodes, 10% to 30% of women considered to have negative nodes by standard histologic analysis are found to be node-positive. Approximately two thirds of all women with breast carcinoma eventually develop distant metastatic disease regardless of the type of initial therapy.

It is important to understand the natural history of untreated breast carcinoma. In series of women refusing therapy, 20% will be alive at 5 years and 5% will be alive at 10 years. Breast carcinoma is a systemic disease that may recur many years, sometimes decades, after initial diagnosis. However, women with negative nodes have a 10-year survival rate of 75% (Table 15-8).

The major changes in management of breast carcinoma over the past two decades have resulted from changing concepts regarding the biology of the disease, with the understanding that many women with breast carcinoma have systemic disease

Table 15-7 TNM Staging of Breast Cancer

Primary Tumor (T)

TX	Primary tumor cannot be assessed
T0	No evidence of primary tumor
Tis*	Carcinoma in situ. Intraductal carcinoma, lobular carcinoma in situ, or Paget's disease of the nipple with no tumor
T1	Tumor is ≤2.0 cm in greater dimension
T1a	Tumor is ≤0.5 cm in greatest dimension
T1b	Tumor is >0.5 cm but not more than 1.0 cm in greatest dimension
T1c	Tumor is more than 1.0 cm but not more than 2.0 cm in greatest dimension
T2	Tumor is >2.0 cm but not more than 5.0 cm in greatest dimension
T3	Tumor is >5.0 cm in greatest dimension
T4	Tumor of any size with direct extension to chest wall or skin
T4a	Extension to chest wall
T4b	Edema (including peau d'orange) or ulceration of the skin of the breast or satellite skin nodules confined to the same breast
T4c	Both T4a and T4b above
T4d	Inflammatory carcinoma

Regional Lymph Node Involvement (N) (Clinical)

NX	Regional lymph nodes cannot be assessed (e.g., previously removed)
N0	No regional lymph node metastasis
N1	Metastasis to movable ipsilateral axillary lymph node(s)
N2	Metastasis to ipsilateral axillary lymph node(s) fixed to one another or the other structures
N3	Metastasis to ipsilateral mammary lymph node(s)

Distant Metastasis (M)

MX	Presence of distant metastasis cannot be assessed
M0	No distant metastasis
M1	Distant metastasis (includes metastasis to ipsilateral supraclavicular lymph node[s])

Stage Grouping

Stage 0	Tis	N0	M0
Stage I	T1	N0	M0
Stage IIa	T0	N1	M0
	T1	N1*	M0
	T2	N0	M0
Stage IIb	T2	N1	M0
	T3	N0	M0
Stage IIIa	T0	N2	M0
	T1	N2	M0
	T2	N2	M0
	T3	N1, N2	M0
Stage IIIb	T4	Any N	M0
	Any T	N3	M0
Stage IV	Any T	Any N	M1

Paget's disease associated with a tumor is classified according to the size of the tumor. Chest wall includes ribs, intercostal muscles, and serratus anterior muscle but not pectoral muscle.
*The prognosis of patients with pN1a is similar to that of patients with pN0.
From Eberlein TJ: Current management of carcinoma of the breast. Ann Surg 220:121, 1994.

at the time the diagnosis is initially established. The natural history of the majority of developing breast carcinomas results in years of growth of the neoplasm before discovery. Because occult vascular dissemination is likely to occur prior to diagnosis, treatment of breast carcinoma involves both local and systemic therapy. It is beyond the scope of this book to present the details of treatment of breast carcinoma. Thorough clinical and surgical staging is the cornerstone of any treatment plan. In the TNM classification, the tumor size and characteristics are

Table 15-8 Stages and Survival of Women with Breast Cancer

Clinical Staging (American Joint Committee)	Crude 5-Year Survival (%)	Range of Survival (%)
Stage I	85	82–94
Tumor < 2 cm in diameter		
Nodes, if present, not felt to contain metastases		
Without distant metastases		
Stage II	66	47–74
Tumor < 5 cm in diameter		
Nodes, if palpable, not fixed		
Without distant metastases		
Stage III	41	7–80
Tumor > 5 cm or,		
Tumor of any size with invasion of skin or attached to chest wall		
Nodes in supraclavicular area		
Without distant metastases		
Stage IV	10	—
With distant metastases		

Histologic Staging (NSABP)	CRUDE SURVIVAL (%)		5-Year Disease-Free Survival (%)
	5-Year	10-Year	
All patients	63.5	45.9	60.3
Negative axillary lymph nodes	78.1	64.9	82.3
Positive axillary lymph nodes	46.5	24.9	34.9
1–3 positive axillary lymph nodes	62.2	37.5	50.00
>4 positive axillary lymph nodes	32.0	13.4	21.1

NSABP, National Surgical Adjuvant Breast Project.
From Henderson IC, Canellos GP: Cancer of the breast: the past decade (first of two parts). N Engl J Med 302:18, 1980.

described (T), regional lymph node involvement is documented (N), and distant metastases are noted (M).

Veronesi and colleagues have listed the three major objectives of treating breast carcinoma: control of local disease, treatment of distant metastasis, and improved quality of life for women treated for the disease. There are several methods for controlling local disease. However, no difference in long-term survival rates has been documented, regardless of the extent of surgical therapy or aggressiveness of local radiotherapy. During the past 15 years, revolutionary changes have involved multiple therapeutic options in both local and systemic therapy for breast carcinoma. Women are assuming an increasingly active role in deciding their own treatment regimen. Breast conservation is a frequent choice for the control of local disease. Sentinel node resection is becoming standard practice in the treatment of early-stage breast cancer. Chemotherapy is used not only for patients with proved metastatic disease but also for women at high risk for the development of primary or recurrent disease. Recent emphasis on conservative surgery plus radiation therapy to control multifocal cancer in the same breast and on reconstructive surgery after mastectomy has improved the quality of life of women with breast carcinoma (Table 15-9).

Table 15-9 Ten-Year Disease-Free Survival Rates of Women with Breast Cancer

	Conservation Surgery and Radiation	Radical or Modified Radical Mastectomy Alone
Minimal breast cancer	92%	95%
Stage I	78%	80%
Stage II	73%	65%

Reprinted from Montague ED: Conservation surgery and radiation therapy in the treatment of operable breast cancer. Cancer 53:702, 1984

Surgical Therapy

The decision concerning appropriate therapy and extent of the surgical operation to treat breast carcinoma should be made by the woman in consultation with the surgeon, radiotherapist, and medical oncologist who will treat her. As emphasized, the size of the tumor, the initial extent of disease, virulence of the neoplasms, and presence of estrogen and progesterone receptors are the key medical factors in the decision. The initial size of the breast carcinoma is the single best predictor of the likelihood of positive axillary nodes. The presence and number of axillary node metastasis is the single best predictor of survival. Intensive discussions concerning breast reconstruction or external prostheses are important to help the woman contemplate the effects of surgery on body image. Morris and coworkers have studied the psychological and social adjustments to mastectomy in 160 women, who were followed at intervals of 3, 12, and 24 months after surgery. One in four women was still having problems with depression and associated marital and sexual problems 2 years after initial therapy.

Until approximately 25 years ago, radical mastectomy was the standard operation for carcinoma of the breast. Radical mastectomy was designed to control local disease by an extensive en bloc removal of the breast and underlying pectoralis major and pectoralis minor muscles and complete axillary dissection. It is a cosmetically disfiguring operation, leaving a major deformity of the chest wall. With an increased understanding that cancer of the breast is often a systemic disease, the therapeutic emphasis has changed to less radical surgery and increased use of radiotherapy and chemotherapy. It has also been recognized that often patients are not cured even with extensive local therapy. Thus protocols have been designed for more conservative approaches to local disease, and less radical operations have grown in popularity. The modified radical mastectomy removes the breast and only the fascia over the pectoralis major muscle. The pectoralis minor muscle may be removed to facilitate the axillary dissection. Simple mastectomy includes removal of the breast without underlying muscle tissue.

The primary therapy for the vast majority of women with stages I and II breast cancer is conservative surgery, which preserves the breast, followed by radiation therapy. Lazovich and coworkers reported that 60% of women with stage I and 39% of women with stage II breast carcinoma were treated with conservative surgery in a review of nine recent population-based cancer registries. Resection of a wider area of the breast than lumpectomy is referred to as *quadrantectomy.* The latter operation is more effective in preventing local recurrences. However, the cosmetic result is not as satisfactory. In trials with either lumpectomy or quadrantectomy without irradiation the rate of recurrence in the treated breast was approximately 40% compared with 10% when irradiation was given. Thus almost all women with conservative surgical therapy for invasive breast carcinoma receive radiotherapy. Interestingly, there was no definite difference in overall survival at 10 years. Radiotherapy may not be necessary in some selected instances in women older than age 55.

Veronesi and colleagues published a controlled study of 701 women with carcinomas measuring less than 2 cm in diameter without palpable axillary lymph nodes. The women were randomized preoperatively into two treatment groups. One group of 349 patients had radical mastectomy. The other group included 352 women who had excision of a quadrant of the breast to control the primary lesion, axillary dissection, and radiotherapy involving both external and interstitial sources. Five-year survival rates were virtually identical—90% in both groups. Five-year disease-free survival rates were similar, 83% and 84%. Fisher and associates, in the National Surgical Adjuvant Breast Project, have reported similar findings with breast carcinomas less than 4 cm, if the surgical margins were free of tumor. Three additional randomized prospective studies found no difference in therapeutic results contrasting conservative surgery and postoperative irradiation versus radical surgery for stage I or II breast carcinoma. These studies found local recurrence rates of 5% at 5 years and approximately 10% at 10 years. Radiotherapy was begun 1 to 2 weeks postoperatively and given for approximately 5 weeks. The radiotherapeutic dosage was 180 to 200 cGy/day for a total dose of approximately 5000 cGy.

Another conservative approach to the treatment of breast cancer involves the use of sentinel lymph node mapping as an alternative to axillary dissection. Although the presence of axillary node metastasis is an important prognostic factor for patients with breast cancer, there is a high incidence of chronic complications associated with axillary dissection. By injecting the primary tumor with radioactive colloid tracers and dyes, the surgeon can identify the first set of regional lymph nodes that receive lymphatic drainage from the tumor. These are termed *sentinel lymph nodes.* Subsequently, these nodes can be removed and the axillary dissection can be deleted if they are negative. In a large multiinstitutional trial, Krag and colleagues were able to identify the sentinel nodes in 93% of the cases. The accuracy of sentinel node mapping in this series for predicting the status of axillary nodes was 97%. The positive predictive value was 100% and the negative predictive value was 96%. Although sentinel lymph node mapping can accurately predict the status of the axillary nodes, the procedure can be technically challenging and the success rates vary according to the surgeon's expertise with the procedure.

It is important to offer every woman alternatives in treatment for stages I and II breast carcinoma. The cosmetic result obtained by lumpectomy and radiation therapy depends on the size and shape of the breast and the size of the initial tumor. For some women, mastectomy followed by reconstructive surgery may give a superior cosmetic result. Also, the management of the axillary nodes should be considered and the woman should be informed concerning all of her options.

Medical Therapy

Adjuvant systemic chemotherapy decreases the odds of dying from breast cancer during the first 10 years following diagnosis by approximately 25%. The two major factors in predicting the likelihood of systemic disease in breast carcinoma are the diameter of the primary tumor and the number of positive axillary nodes. Women whose initial tumor is less than 1 cm in diameter and who have negative axillary nodes have excellent disease-free survival, with a 10-year relapse rate of less than 10%. Multiple other determinations have been used as prognostic factors in clinical trials, including the presence of estrogen and progesterone receptors, the DNA content, mitotic index, growth rate measured by flow cytometry, epidermal growth factor receptor, overgrowth of the oncogene *erb*B-2 (HER-2 or *neu*) and the expression of various proteins such as heat shock proteins, collagenase type IV, and many others. The majority of breast carcinomas are adenocarcinomas. Nevertheless, they represent microscopically a heterogenous group of tumors. It is not established whether the response to chemotherapy of specific histologic subtypes differs because women in various chemotherapeutic studies have not been randomized according to histologic type.

The presence and concentration of receptors should be obtained at the initial diagnostic surgery, as receptor status may change after radiotherapy or chemotherapy. In general, receptor-positive tumors are usually better differentiated and exhibit a less aggressive clinical behavior, including a lower risk of recurrence and lower capacity to proliferate. When estrogen receptors are positive, approximately 60% of breast cancers will respond to hormonal therapy; an 80% response rate is noted when both estrogen and progesterone receptors are present. If estrogen receptors are negative, less than 10% of tumors respond to hormonal manipulation.

Hormonal therapy may include ablative surgery but is usually accomplished by drugs that change endocrine function by blocking receptor sites or blocking synthesis of hormones. In the past the most commonly used ablative surgery was bilateral oophorectomy in a premenopausal woman with breast carcinoma. Hormonal therapy is effective in producing a response in advanced metastatic carcinoma for approximately 1 year. Metastatic disease in soft tissue and bone is the most sensitive to hormonal manipulation. Tamoxifen, an oral antiestrogen, is an alternative to surgical castration and presently is the most frequently prescribed hormonal agent for breast carcinoma. Adrenalectomy or hypophysectomy has largely been replaced by medical adrenalectomy using aminoglutethimide in select cases. Medroxyprogesterone (Depo-Provera), androgens, danazol, and gonadotropin hormone-releasing hormone (GH-RH) agonists have also been used to treat breast carcinoma. Two endocrine agents used simultaneously do not produce better results than a single agent.

Adjuvant chemotherapy has produced positive responses and an increase in disease-free survival in many clinical studies. Initially, chemotherapy was selected to treat women with positive axillary nodes or remote disease. Chemotherapy has proved effective in shrinking measurable metastatic disease in both premenopausal and postmenopausal women.

The role for adjuvant therapy in the management of breast cancer continues to expand. Adjuvant chemotherapy has been shown to improve disease-free and overall survival in all patients with operable breast cancer with the exception of select node-negative patients with small (less than 1 cm) tumors that have no high-risk features. A recent update of the National Surgical Adjuvant Breast and Bowel Project (NSABP) B-20 trial indicated a significant advantage in the estrogen receptor-positive, node-negative patient who received chemotherapy in addition to tamoxifen. Even women in the postmenopausal age group with estrogen receptor-positive, node-negative breast cancers that traditionally would be treated with tamoxifen alone have been shown to benefit from the combination of chemotherapy and tamoxifen. Only limited data are available from randomized trials for women over the age of 70. In the absence of other comorbidities chemotherapy can be considered in this population of older women. The indications for adjuvant chemotherapy are summarized in Table 15-10. It is important to note that improvements in disease-free survival rates have not always been followed by similar improvements in overall survival rates.

It is firmly established that combinations of cytotoxic drugs are superior to a single agent. In the past, combinations included drugs such as cyclophosphamide, methotrexate, doxorubicin (Adriamycin), 5-fluorouracil, and vinblastine. Presently, it is believed that anthracycline-containing combinations are more effective than regimens that do not contain anthracyclines. Recently, paclitaxel has also become available for the treatment of breast cancer with very promising results. Preliminary results from a Cancer and Leukemia Group B (CALGB) study indicated that the addition of four cycles of paclitaxel to four cycles of the Adriamycin and cyclophosphamide regimen improved disease-free and overall survival rates in patients with node-positive breast cancer. Other drugs currently under investigation for the treatment of breast cancer include anthrapyrazoles, liposomal anthracyclines, and gemcitabine. The average total response rate to combined chemotherapy is 55%. Approximately 10% to 20% of women treated with combination chemotherapy experience a complete remission for about 18 months. The major short-term toxic effects of chemotherapy are alopecia and fatigue. Some women develop premature ovarian failure.

Tamoxifen has the greatest effect in postmenopausal women. As one would expect, tamoxifen is of greater benefit in women with tumors that have estrogen receptors than in tumors that are negative for estrogen receptors. There is no significant improvement in survival rates in patients with estrogen receptor-negative tumors. However, even in receptor-negative patients, 5 years of tamoxifen use will decrease the risk of a second primary or contralateral breast cancer by as much as 45%. Extending tamoxifen therapy beyond 5 years is not associated with further reduction in risk. Chronic tamoxifen therapy increases the prevalence of intrauterine polyps and endometrial hyperplasia and carcinoma. Recent clinical trials have investigated the use of extremely intensive chemotherapeutic regimens followed by transplantation of autologous bone marrow in women with advanced or recurrent disease. Obviously, this therapy is expensive, requires prolonged hospitalization, and has a mortality rate of approximately 15%. Some women have experienced complete remission for longer than 1 year, but to date there is no convincing evidence that high-dose chemotherapy is superior to conventional treatment. Its use should be limited to clinical trials until sufficient data support its efficacy.

Table 15-10 Indications for Adjuvant Systemic Therapy after Surgery in Women with Operable Breast Cancer

Type of Disease	Adjuvant Therapy Indicated*
Breast Cancer without Evidence of Invasion	
Noninvasive breast cancer (ductal or lobular carcinoma in situ)	None
Breast Cancer with Evidence of Invasion, but Negative Axillary Lymph Nodes	
Microinvasive breast cancer (< 1 mm in largest diameter)	None
Invasive ductal or lobular carcinoma < 1 cm in largest diameter	None
Invasive carcinoma < 3 cm in largest diameter with favorable histologic findings (pure tubular, mucinous, or papillary)	None
Invasive ductal or lobular carcinoma ≥ 1 cm in largest diameter	Chemotherapy, hormonal therapy, or both
Invasive carcinoma ≥ 3cm in largest diameter with favorable histologic findings (pure tubular, mucinous, or papillary)	Chemotherapy, hormonal therapy, or both
Invasive Breast Cancer with Positive Axillary Lymph Nodes	
All tumors, regardless of size or histologic findings	Chemotherapy, hormonal therapy, or both

*Chemotherapy consists of fluorouracil, doxorubicin, and cyclophosphamide (FAC); doxorubicin and cyclophosphamide (AC); or cyclophosphamide, methotrexate, and fluorouracil (CMF). Hormonal therapy consists of tomoxifen or ovarian ablation (either surgical or chemical).

From Hortobagyi GN: Treatment of breast cancer. N Engl J Med, 339:977, 1998.

KEY POINTS

- One out of eight women (12.5% of American females) develops carcinoma of the breast if she lives beyond age 90.
- The breast consists of approximately 20% glandular tissue and 80% fat and connective tissue.
- Lymph drainage of the breast usually flows toward the most adjacent group of nodes. This concept represents the basis for sentinel node mapping in breast cancer. In most instances, breast cancer spreads in an orderly fashion within

KEY POINTS *Continued*

the axillary lymph node basin based on the anatomic relationship between the primary tumor and its associated regional (sentinel) nodes.

- Numerous epidemiologic studies have found an increased risk of developing breast carcinoma in women with benign breast disease only if there is associated atypical epithelial hyperplasia. This risk varies from twofold to fivefold, depending on the degree of epithelial hyperplasia.
- Clinical evidence of fibrocystic changes is discovered in breast examination of approximately one in two premenopausal women.
- The classic symptom of fibrocystic changes is cyclic bilateral breast pain. The signs of fibrocystic changes include increased engorgement and density of the breasts, excessive nodularity, rapid change and fluctuation in the size of cystic areas, increased tenderness, and occasionally spontaneous nipple discharge.
- Fibroadenomas are most frequently present in adolescents and women in their 20s.
- Approximately 30% of fibroadenomas will disappear, and 10% to 12% become smaller after many years.
- Approximately 75% of intraductal papillomas are located beneath the areola. Often these tumors are difficult to palpate because they are small and soft.
- Nipple discharge is a complaint of 10% to 15% of women with benign breast disease. However, nipple discharge is present in less than 3% of women with breast carcinoma.
- The importance of determining the cause of *spontaneous* discharge from the nipple is to rule out carcinoma. The color of the nonmilky discharge does not differentiate a benign from a malignant process.
- Bloody discharge from the nipple, gross or microscopic, should be considered to be related to carcinoma until this diagnosis has been ruled out.
- Intraductal papilloma and fibrocystic changes are the two most common causes of spontaneous nonmilky nipple discharge.
- Fat necrosis caused by trauma may present as a firm, indurated, poorly defined mass that has a mammographic appearance of stippled calcifications.
- Risk factors identify only 25% of women who will eventually develop breast carcinoma.
- Approximately 5% to 10% of breast cancers have a familial or genetic link. Genetic predisposition to develop breast carcinoma has been recognized in some families. In these families breast cancer tends to occur at a younger age and there is a higher prevalence of bilateral disease.
- Mutations in *BRCA* family of genes have been identified that confer a lifetime risk of breast cancer that approaches 85%. *BRCA1* and *BRCA2* genes are involved in the majority of inheritable cases of breast cancer. These genes function as tumor suppressor genes, and several mutations have been described on each of these genes.
- The frequency of breast carcinoma increases directly with the patient's age; 85% occur after 40 years of age.
- Once a woman has developed carcinoma of one breast, her risk is approximately 1% per year of developing cancer in the other breast.
- Women with a high risk of breast cancer have proven options that can decrease their risk of breast cancer. Both tamoxifen and raloxifene significantly decrease the relative risk of developing breast carcinoma.
- Present methods of screening for breast carcinoma are not ideal. Nevertheless, screening tests result in a reduction of mortality from breast cancer of approximately 25% to 30%.
- Physical examination is excellent as a screening procedure but extremely poor in predicting the histopathology of the lesion. Studies have demonstrated 30% to 40% of breast masses suspected by palpation to be malignant were found after biopsy to be benign. Conversely, 15% to 20% of benign-appearing masses during a physical examination subsequently are discovered to be carcinoma by histopathology.
- The 5-year survival rate of a woman whose breast carcinoma is believed to be localized to the breast with negative axillary nodes is 85%. In contrast, the 5-year survival rate is only 53% when axillary nodes are positive.
- The number of women receiving screening mammography has increased dramatically over the past 10 years. Mammography is not as precise in younger women or in women with dense breasts secondary to fibroglandular tissue. Mammography is most sensitive in older women in which the majority of the breast is composed of fatty tissue.
- Present studies demonstrate that screening mammography reduces breast cancer mortality by approximately 33% in women 50 to 70 years of age.
- For screening mammography, two views of each breast are performed: the mediolateral oblique (MLO) and the craniocaudal (CC). The MLO is the most effective single view because it includes the greatest amount of breast tissue and is the only view that includes all of the upper outer quadrant and axillary tail.
- Mammographic signs of carcinoma include isolated clusters of fine, irregular calcifications or poorly defined masses with irregular contours.
- Double-reading of a mammographic study by two independent observers improves the breast cancer detection rate by approximately 10%. Obviously, it also increased the cost of screening. Computer-aided diagnosis shows promise of potentially detecting lesions that would not be identified by double-reading.
- The radiation dose to the breast by state-of-the-art mammography equipment is 0.1 rad (0.001 Gy) for a two-view examination.
- The most important use of ultrasound is to differentiate a cystic breast mass from a solid mass.
- Ultrasound should not be used as a sole imaging technique for breast disease. Because of its lack of sensitivity and specificity for early breast carcinoma, it should not be used in an attempt to detect subclinical disease.
- Digital technology has multiple advantages compared with conventional mammography. Image acquisition, display, and storage are much faster, and image manipulation through adjustments in contrast, brightness, and electronic magnification of selected regions enables radiologists to obtain superior views.

Continued

KEY POINTS *Continued*

- Digital technology makes it possible to subtract various layers of computerized imagery in order to examine suspicious areas and improve the ability to detect and diagnose breast carcinoma. Digital mammography is particularly helpful in screening women with very dense breasts and breast implants. With the ability to manipulate the images, digital mammography will reduce the number of women recalled for more images.
- The ability of MRI to differentiate benign from malignant tissue may help to reduce the frequency of breast biopsy, especially in women with dense, fibroglandular breasts. MRI has been proven effective in detecting new tumors in women with previous lumpectomy because it can accurately distinguish between scar tissue and cancerous lesions.
- If the aspirated fluid from a breast cyst is clear and no residual mass is palpated immediately after the procedure and again 1 month later, no further workup is necessary.
- Palpable lesions can be evaluated by several techniques. The type of technique used depends on many factors, including the location and size of the lesion as well as the patient's and physician's preference. Options include incisional or excisional biopsy, as well as core-needle biopsy.
- The incidence of carcinoma in biopsies corresponds directly with the patient's age. Approximately 20% of breast biopsies in women age 50 are positive, and this figure increases to 33% in women age 70 or older.
- Breast cancer is usually asymptomatic before the development of advanced disease. Breast pain is experienced by only 10% of women with early breast carcinoma.
- The classic sign of a breast carcinoma is a solitary, solid, three-dimensional, dominant breast mass. The borders of the mass are usually indistinct.
- Bilateral breast carcinoma occurs in approximately 1% of all newly diagnosed cases. The prevalence of bilateral breast cancer is twofold greater in lobular neoplasia.
- Infiltrating ductal carcinoma is the most common breast malignancy.
- Microscopic metastatic disease occurs early via both hematogenous and lymphatic routes. For example, 30% to 40% of women without gross adenopathy in the axilla will have positive nodes discovered during histologic examination. With the additional assessment tools of immunohistochemical staining for the presence of cytokeratin and serial sectioning of axillary nodes, 10% to 30% of patients considered to have negative nodes by standard histologic analysis are found to be node positive.
- Approximately two thirds of all women with breast carcinoma eventually develop distant metastatic disease regardless of the type of initial therapy.
- Three major objectives of treating breast carcinoma are control of local disease, treatment of distant metastasis, and improved quality of life for women treated for the disease.
- Breast conservation is a frequent choice for the control of local disease. Sentinel node resection is becoming standard practice in the treatment of early stage breast cancer. Chemotherapy is used not only for patients with proved metastatic disease, but also for women at high risk for the development of primary or recurrent disease.
- Recent emphasis on conservative surgery plus radiation therapy to control multifocal cancer in the same breast and on reconstructive surgery after mastectomy has improved the quality of life of women with breast carcinoma.
- The initial size of the breast carcinoma is the single best predictor of the likelihood of positive axillary nodes. The presence and number of axillary node metastasis is the single best predictor of survival.
- The primary therapy for the vast majority of women with stages I and II breast cancer is conservative surgery, which preserves the breast, followed by radiation therapy.
- Another conservative approach to the treatment of breast cancer involves the use of sentinel lymph node mapping as an alternative to axillary dissection.
- Adjuvant systemic chemotherapy decreases the odds of dying from breast cancer during the first 10 years following diagnosis by approximately 25%.
- When estrogen receptors are positive, approximately 60% of breast cancers will respond to hormonal therapy. If estrogen receptors are negative, less than 10% of tumors respond to a hormonal manipulation.
- Adjuvant chemotherapy has been shown to improve disease-free and overall survival in all patients with operable breast cancer with the exception of select node-negative patients with small (less than 1 cm) tumors that have no high-risk features.
- Approximately 10% to 20% of women treated with combination chemotherapy experience a complete remission for about 18 months.
- The major effect of multiagent systemic therapy has been on the disease-free interval rather than the effect on overall survival. In general, multiple-agent chemotherapy has greater effect than single-agent chemotherapy, especially in the premenopausal woman. Tamoxifen has the greatest effect in postmenopausal women.

BIBLIOGRAPHY

Key Reading

American Cancer Society: Cancer Facts & Figures—2000.

Baines CJ: Breast self-examination. Cancer 69:1942, 1992.

Colditz GA, Stampher MS, Willett WC, et al: Prospective study of estrogen replacement therapy and risk of breast cancer in postmenopausal women. JAMA 264:2648, 1990.

Colditz GA, Stampher MS, Willett WC, et al: Type of postmenopausal hormone use and risk of breast cancer: 12-year follow-up from the Nurses' Health Study. Cancer Causes Control 3:433, 1992.

Gail MH, Brinton LA, Byar DP, et al: Projecting individualized probabilities of developing breast cancer for white females who are being examined annually. J Natl Cancer Inst 81:1879, 1989.

Hoskins KF, Stopfer JE, Calzone KA, et al: Assessment and counseling for women with a family history of breast cancer: A guide for clinicians. JAMA 273:577, 1995.

Krag D, Weaver D, Ashikaga T, et al: The sentinel node in breast cancer. N Eng J Med 339:941, 1998.

Vorherr H: Breast aspiration biopsy. Am J Obstet Gynecol 148:127, 1984.

Key References

Barton MB, Harris R, Fletcher SW: Does this patient have breast cancer? The screening clinical breast examination: Should it be done? How? JAMA 282:1270, 1999.

Bassett LW, Gambhir S: Breast imaging in the 1990s. Semin Oncol 18:80, 1991.

Bassett LW, Giuliano AE, Gold RH: Staging for breast carcinoma. Am J Surg 157:250, 1989.

Berkel H, Birdsell DC, Jenkins H: Breast augmentation: A risk factor for breast cancer? N Engl J Med 326:1649, 1992.

Biro FM, Lucky AW, Huster GA, et al: Hormonal studies and physical maturation in adolescent gynecomastia. J Pediatr 116:450, 1990.

Black WC, Fletcher SW: Effects of estrogen on screening mammography: Another complexity. J Natl Cancer Inst 88:62, 1996.

Bland KI, Copeland EM III: Breast. In Schwartz SI, Shires GT, Spencer FE (eds): Principles of Surgery, 6th ed. New York, McGraw Hill, 1994, p 562.

Boothroyd A, Carty H: Breast masses in childhood and adolescence: A presentation of 17 cases and a review of the literature. Pediatr Radiol 24:81, 1994.

Bottels K, Chan JS, Holly EA: Cytologic criteria for fibroadenoma: A step wise logistic regression analysis. Am J Clin Pathol 89:707, 1988.

Brenner RJ, Bein ME, Sarti DA, Vinstein AL: Spontaneous regression of interval benign cysts of the breast. Radiology 193:365, 1994.

Burke W, Daly M, Garber J, et al: Recommendations for follow-up care of individuals with an inherited predisposition to cancer. JAMA 277:997, 1997.

Buzdar AU, Hortobagyi GN: Recent advances in adjuvant therapy of breast cancer. Semin Oncol 26 (Suppl 12):21, 1999.

Cant PJ, Madden MV, Coleman MG, and ent DM: Nonoperative management of breast mass diagnosed as fibroadenoma. Br J Surg 82:792, 1995.

Chlebowski RT: Reducing the risk of breast cancer. N Eng J Med 343:191, 2000.

Chua CL, Thomas A, Ng BK: Cystosarcoma phyllodes: A review of surgical options. Surgery 105:141, 1989.

Cummings SR, Eckert S, Krueger KA, et al: The effect of raloxifene on risk of breast cancer in postmenopausal women: Results from the MORE randomized trial. JAMA 281:2189, 1999.

Davis PL, Staiger MJ, Harris KB, et al: Breast cancer measurements with magnetic resonance imaging, ultrasonography, and mammography. Breast Cancer Res Treat 37:1, 1996.

Dershaw DD, Chaglassian TA: Mammography after prosthesis placement for augmentation or reconstruction mammoplasty. Radiology 170:69, 1989.

Dupont WD, Page DL: Risk factors for breast cancer in women with proliferative breast disease. N Engl J Med 312:136, 1985.

Dupont WD, Page DL, Parl FF, et al: Long-term risk of breast cancer in women with fibroadenoma. N Engl J Med 331:10, 1994.

Early Breast Cancer Trialists' Collaborative Group: Effects of adjuvant tamoxifen and of cytotoxic therapy on mortality in early breast cancer. N Engl J Med 319:1681, 1988.

Early Breast Cancer Trialists' Collaborative Group: Effects of radiotherapy and surgery in early breast cancer: An overview of the randomized trials. N Engl J Med 333:1444, 1995.

Eberlein TJ: Current management of carcinoma of the breast. Ann Surg 220:121, 1994.

Eklund GW, Cardenosa G, Parsons W: Assessing adequacy of mammographic image quality. Radiology 190:297, 1994.

Elmore JG, Barton MB, Moceri VM, et al: Ten-year risk of false positive screening mammograms and clinical breast examinations. N Engl J Med 338:1089, 1998.

Elmore JG, Wells CK, Lee CH, et al: Variability in radiologists' interpretations of mammograms. N Engl J Med 331:1493, 1994.

Feig SA: Age-related accuracy of screening mammography: How should it be measured? Radiology 214:633, 2000.

Feig SA, Ehrlich SM: Estimation of radiation risk from screening mammography: Recent trends and comparison with expected benefits. Radiology 174:638, 1990.

Fisher B, Costantino J, Redmond C, et al: Lumpectomy compared with lumpectomy and radiation therapy for the treatment of intraductal breast cancer. N Engl J Med 328:1581, 1993.

Fisher B, Bauer M, Margolese R, et al: Five-year results of a randomized clinical trial comparing total mastectomy and segmental mastectomy with or without radiation in the treatment of breast cancer. N Engl J Med 312:665, 1985.

Fisher B, Costantino J, Redmond C, et al: A randomized clinical trial evaluating tamoxifen in the treatment of patients with node-negative breast cancer who have estrogen-receptor-positive tumors. N Engl J Med 320:479, 1989.

Fisher B, Costantino JP, Wickerham DL, et al: Tamoxifen for the prevention of breast cancer: report of the National Surgical Adjuvant Breast and Bowel Project P-1 study. J Natl Cancer Inst 90:1371, 1998.

Fletcher SW, O'Malley MS, Bunce LA: Physicians' abilities to detect lumps in silicone breast models. JAMA 253:2224, 1985.

Folkman J: Angiogenesis and breast cancer. J Clin Oncol 12:441, 1994.

Foster RS, Costanza MC: Breast self-examination practices and breast cancer survival. Cancer 53:999, 1984.

Fowler PA, Casey CE, Cameron GG: Cyclic changes in composition and volume of the breast during the menstrual cycle, measured by magnetic resonance imaging. Br J Obstet Gynaecol 97:595, 1990.

Frantz VK, Pickren JW, Melcher GW, et al: Incidence of chronic cystic disease in so-called "normal breasts." Cancer 4:762, 1951.

Gasparini G, Harris AL: Clinical importance of the determination of tumor angiogenesis in breast carcinoma: Much more than a new prognostic tool. J Clin Oncol 13:765, 1995.

Gateley CA, Miers M, Mansel RE, Hughes LE: Drug treatments for mastalgia: 17 year experience in the Cardiff mastalgia clinic. J R Soc Med 85(1):12, 1992.

Greendale GA, Reboussin BA, Sie A, et al: Effects of estrogen and estrogen-progestin on mammographic parenchymal density. Ann Inter Med 130:262, 1999.

Greenlee RT, Murray T, Bolden S, Wingo PA: Cancer Statistics, 2000. CA Cancer J Clin 50:7, 2000.

Greenwald P, Nasca PC, Lawrence CE, et al: Estimated effect of breast self-examination and routine physician examinations on breast-cancer mortality. N Engl J Med 299:271, 1978.

Gusberg SB: The treatment of breast cancer: Should we play a role? Gynecol Oncol 49:277, 1993.

Harris JR, Lippman ME, Veronesi U, Willett W: Breast cancer: First of three parts. N Engl J Med 327:319, 1992.

Harris JR, Lippman ME, Veronesi U, Willett W: Breast cancer: Second of three parts. N Engl J Med 327:319, 1992.

Harris JR, Lippman ME, Veronesi U, Willett W: Breast cancer: Third of three parts. N Engl J Med 327:319, 1992.

Harris R, Leininger L: Clinical strategies for breast cancer screening: Weighing and using the evidence. Ann Intern Med 122:539, 1995.

Harrison BJ, Maddox PR, Mansel RE: Maintenance therapy of cyclical mastalgia using low-dose danazol. J R Coll Surg Edinb 34:79, 1989.

Hartmann LC, Schaid DJ, Sellers T, et al: Bilateral prophylactic mastectomy (PM) in BRCA1/2 mutation carriers. Proc Am Assoc Cancer Res 41:222, 2000. Abstract.

Hartmann LC, Schaid DJ, Woods JE, et al: Efficacy of prophylactic mastectomy in women with a family history of breast cancer. N Eng J Med 340:77, 1999.

Harvey BJ, Miller AB, Baines CJ, Corey PN: Effect of breast self-examination techniques on the risk of death from breast cancer. Can Med Assoc J 157:1205, 1997.

Hildreth NG, Shore RE, Dvoretsky PM, et al: The risk of breast cancer after irradiation of the thymus in infancy. N Engl J Med 321:1281, 1989.

Hindle WH, Alonzo LJ: Conservative management of breast fibroadenomas. 164:1647, 1991.

Hindle WH, Payne PA, Pan EY: The use of fine-needle aspiration in the evaluation of persistent palpable dominant breast masses. Am J Obstet Gynecol 168:1814, 1993.

Hortobagyi GN: Treatment of breast cancer. N Engl J Med 339:974, 1998.

Howarth D, Sillar R, Lan L, et al: Scintimammography: An adjunct test for the detection of breast cancer. Med J Aust 170:588, 1999.

Huang Z, Hankinson SE, Colditz GA, et al: Dual effects of weight and weight gain on breast cancer risk. JAMA 278:1407, 1997.

Kerlikowske K, Grady D, Rubin SM, et al: Efficacy of screening mammography: A meta-analysis. JAMA 273:149, 1995.

Kopans DB, Swann CA, White G, et al: Asymmetric breast tissue. Radiology 171:639, 1989.

Kornguth PJ, Rimer BK, Conaway MR, et al: Impact of patient-controlled compression on the mammography experience. Radiology 186:99, 1993.

Lancaster JM, Wiseman RW, Berchuck A: An inevitable dilemma: Prenatal testing for mutations in the BRCA1 breast-ovarian cancer susceptibility gene. Obstet Gynecol 87:306, 1996.

Land CE: Studies of cancer and radiation dose among atomic bomb survivors. JAMA 274:402, 1995.

Laya MB, Larson EB, Taplin SH, White E: Effect of estrogen replacement therapy on the specificity and sensitivity of screening mammography. J Natl Cancer Inst 88:643, 1996.

Layde PM, Webster LA, Baughman AL, et al: The independent associations of parity, age at first full-term pregnancy, and duration of breastfeeding with the risk of breast cancer. J Clin Epidemiol 42:963, 1989.

Lazovich D, Solomon CC, Thomas DB, et al: Breast conservation therapy in the United States following the 1990 National Institutes of Health Consensus Development Conference on the treatment of patients with early stage invasive breast carcinoma. Cancer 86:628, 1999.

Leis HP Jr: The significance of nipple discharge. In Schwartz GF, Marchant D (eds): Breast Disease, Diagnosis and Treatment, New York, Symposia Specialists, 1980, p 111.

Liljegren G, Holmberg L, Bergh J, et al: 10-year results after sector resection with or without postoperative radiotherapy for stage I breast cancer: a randomized trial. J Clin Oncol 17:2326, 1999.

Longnecker MP: Alcoholic beverage consumption in relation to risk of breast cancer: Meta-analysis and review. Cancer Causes Control 5:73, 1994.

Love RR, Mazess RB, Barden HS, et al: Effects of tamoxifen on bone mineral density in postmenopausal women with breast cancer. N Engl J Med 326:852, 1992.

Love SM, Gelman RS, Silen W: Fibrocystic "disease" of the breast-non-disease? N Engl J Med 307:1010, 1982.

Ludwig Breast Study Group: Prolonged disease-free survival after one course of perioperative adjuvant chemotherapy for node-negative breast cancer. N Engl J Med 320:491, 1989.

Lundström E, Wilczek B, von Palffy Z, et al: Mammographic breast density during hormone replacement therapy: Differences according to treatment. Am J Obstet Gynecol 181:348, 1999.

Marchant DJ, Kase NG, Berkowitz RL (eds): Breast Disease, New York, Churchill Livingstone, 1986, pp 6–7.

McGuckin MA, Cummings MC, Walsh MD, et al: Occult axillary node metastases in breast cancer: Their detection and prognostic significance. Br J Cancer 73:88, 1996.

Mettler FA, Upton AC, Kelsey CA, et al: Benefits versus risks from mammography: A critical reassessment. Cancer 77:903, 1996.

Meyer JE, Eberlein TJ, Stomper PC, et al: Biopsy of occult breast lesions: analysis of 1261 abnormalities. JAMA 263:2341, 1990.

Meyer JE, Frenna TH, Polger M, et al: Enlarging occult fibroadenomas. Radiology 183:639, 1992.

Miki Y, Swensen J, Shattuck-Eidens D, et al: A strong candidate for the breast and ovarian cancer susceptibility gene BRCA1. Science 266:66, 1994.

Miller AB, Baines CJ, To T, Wall C: Canadian National Breast Screening Study II: Breast cancer detection and death rates among women aged 50-59 years. Can Med Assoc J 147:1477, 1992.

Miller AB, Howe GR, Sherman GJ, et al: Mortality from breast cancer after irradiation during fluoroscopic examinations in patients being treated for tuberculosis. N Engl J Med 321:1285, 1989.

Minton JP: Methylxanthines in breast disease. In Schwartz GF, Marchant D (eds): Breast Disease, Diagnosis and Treatment, New York, Symposia Specialists, 1980, p 143.

Moffat CJC, Pinder SE, Dixon AR, et al: Phyllodes tumors of the breast: A clinicopathological review of thirty-two cases. Histopathology 27:205, 1995.

Monsonego J, Destable MD, Florent GDS, et al: Fibrocystic disease of the breast in premenopausal women: Histohormonal correlation and response to luteinizing hormone releasing hormone analog treatment. Am J Obstet Gynecol 164:1181, 1991.

Morris T, Greer HS, White P: Psychological and social adjustments to mastectomy. Cancer 40:2381, 1977.

Morrow M, Schmidt RA, Cregger B, et al: Preoperative evaluation of abnormal mammographic findings to avoid unnecessary breast biopsies. Arch Surg 129:1091, 1994.

Murad TM, Hines JR, Beal J, et al: Histopathological and clinical correlations of cystosarcoma phyllodes. Arch Pathol Lab Med 112:752, 1988.

National Cancer Institute Conference: The uniform approach to breast fine-needle aspiration biopsy. Am J Surg 174:371, 1997.

NCI Breast Cancer Screening Consortium: Screening mammography: a missed clinical opportunity? JAMA 264:54, 1990.

Newcomb PA, Storer BE, Longnecker MP, et al: Lactation and a reduced risk of premenopausal breast cancer. N Engl J Med 330:81, 1994.

Olivotto IA, Bajdik CD, Plenderleith IH, et al: Adjuvant systemic therapy and survival after breast cancer. N Engl J Med 330:805, 1994.

O'Malley MS, Fletcher SW: Screening for breast cancer with breast self-examination: A critical review. JAMA 257:2197, 1987.

Page DL, Dupont WD, Rogers LW, et al: Intraductal carcinoma of the breast: Follow-up after biopsy only. Cancer 49:751, 1982.

Painter K: Factoring in cost of mammograms. USA Today, Dec. 5, 1996, p 11D.

Palmer MD, DeRisi DC, Pelikan A, et al: Treatment options and recurrence potential for cystosarcoma phyllodes. Surg Obstet Gynecol 170:193, 1990.

Pisano E: Current status of full-field digital mammography. Radiology 214:26, 2000.

Powell DE, Stelling CB (eds): The Diagnosis and Detection of Breast Disease, St. Louis, Mosby-Year Book, 1994.

Powles T, Eeles R, Ashley S, et al: Interim analysis of the incidence of breast cancer in the Royal Marsden Hospital tamoxifen randomized chemoprevention trial. Lancet 352:98, 1998.

Recht A, Houlihan MJ: Axillary lymph nodes and breast cancer: A review. Cancer 76:1491, 1995.

Schairer C, Lubin J, Triosi R, et al: Menopausal estrogen and estrogen-progestin replacement therapy and breast cancer risk. JAMA 283:485, 2000.

Schutte M, Rozenblum E, Moskaluk CA, et al: An integrated high-resolution physical map of the DPC/BRCA2 region at chromosome 13q12. Cancer Res 55:4570, 1995.

Seitz S, Rohde K, Bender E, et al: Strong indication for a breast cancer susceptibility gene on chromosome 8p12-p22: Linkage analysis in German breast cancer families. Oncogene 14:741, 1997.

Shah AK, Girishkumar HT, Parithivel VS, et al: Stereotactic needle breast biopsy: A review of current status and practice. Prim Care Update Ob/Gyns 6:147, 1999.

Shapiro S: The call for change in breast cancer screening guidelines. Am J Public Health 84:10, 1994.

Shattuck-Eidens D, McClure M, Simard J, et al: A collaborative survey of 80 mutations in the BRCA1 breast and ovarian cancer susceptibility gene: Implications for presymptomatic testing and screening. JAMA 273:535, 1995.

Shimizu Y, Schull WJ, Kato H: Cancer risk among atomic bomb survivors: The RERF life span study. JAMA 264:601, 1990.

Sickles EA, Filly RA, Callen PW: Breast cancer detection with sonography and mammography: Comparison using state-of-the-art equipment. AJR 140:843, 1983.

Sickles EA, Kopans DB: Mammographic screening for women aged 40 to 49 years: The primary care practitioner's dilemma. Ann Intern Med 122:534, 1995.

Sigurdsson H, Baldetorp B, Borg A, et al: Indicators of prognosis in node-negative breast cancer. N Engl J Med 322:1045, 1990.

Speroff L: Postmenopausal hormone therapy and breast cancer. Obstet Gynecol 87:44S, 1996.

Stavros AT, Thickman D, Rapp CL, et al: Solid breast nodules: Use of sonography to distinguish between benign and malignant lesions. Radiology 196:123, 1995.

Strawbridge HTG, Bassett AA, Foldes I: Role of cytology in management of lesions of the breast. Surg Gynecol Obstet 152:1, 1981.

Sutherland HJ, Lockwood GA, Boyd NF: Ratings of the importance of quality of life variables: Therapeutic implications for patients with metastatic breast cancer. J Clin Epidemiol 43:661, 1990.

Sutton GLJ, O'Malley UP: Treatment of cyclical mastalgia with low dose short-term danazol. Br J Clin Pract 40:68, 1986.

Thurfjell EL, Holmberg LH, Persson IR: Screening mammography: Sensitivity and specificity in relation to hormone replacement therapy. Radiology 203:339, 1997.

Veronesi U, Maisonneuve P, Costa A, et al: Prevention of breast cancer with tamoxifen: Preliminary findings from the Italian randomized trial among hysterectomized women. Lancet 352:93, 1998.

Veronesi V, Sacozzi R, Del Vecchio M, et al: Comparing radical mastectomy with quadrantectomy, axillary dissection, and radiotherapy in patients with small cancers of the breast. N Engl J Med 305:6, 1981.

Walker MJ, Osborne MD, Young DC, et al: The natural history of breast cancer with more than 10 positive nodes. Am J Surg 169:575, 1995.

Weber BL: Genetic testing for breast cancer. Sci Am Sci Med Jan/Feb:12, 1996.

Wolf DM, Jordan C: Gynecologic complications associated with long-term adjuvant tamoxifen therapy for breast cancer. Gynecol Oncol 45:118, 1992.

Zhang Y, Kreger BE, Dorgan JF, et al: Alcohol consumption and risk of breast cancer: The Framingham study revisited. Am J Epidemiol 149:93, 1999.

Spontaneous and Recurrent Abortion 16

Etiology, Diagnosis, Treatment

Vern L. Katz

KEY TERMS AND DEFINITIONS

Anembryonic Gestation (Blighted Ovum). A gestational sac, on ultrasound, more than 17 mm in diameter without an embryo present. Sonographically, an embryo should be visualized in the uterine cavity beyond 43 days' gestational age.

Abortion. Termination of pregnancy before 20 weeks' gestation calculated from date of onset of last menses. An alternative definition is delivery of a fetus with a weight of less than 500 g. If abortion occurs before 12 weeks' gestation, it is called early; from 12 to 20 weeks it is called late.

Aneuploid Abortus. An abortus with the number of chromosomes less than or greater than the normal 46.

Anticardiolipin Antibody. An antiphospholipid antibody that is present in 5% to 15% of women with recurrent spontaneous abortion but in less than 2% of women with normal pregnancies.

Cerclage. A circular ligature used to treat the incompetent cervix. The suture is placed beneath the epithelium of the cervix at the level of the internal cervical os.

Complete Abortion. Spontaneous expulsion of all fetal and placental tissue from the uterine cavity before 20 weeks' gestation.

Conceptional Age. The duration of gestation from the date of conception.

Embryonic Death. Sonographic visualization of an embryo between 4 and 15 mm in length without cardiac activity.

Embryo. The human conceptus during the period of 35 to 70 days' gestational age.

Euploid Abortus. An abortus in which the chromosome complement is normal, 46,XX or 46,XY.

Fetus. The human conceptus during the period beyond 70 days' gestational age until delivery.

Gestational Sac. Fluid-filled structure in endometrial cavity. Earliest sonographic indicator of presence of intrauterine gestation.

Gestational Age. The duration of gestation from the date of onset of the last menstrual period before conception, usually considered to be 14 days longer than the conceptional age.

Incompetent Cervix (Cervical Incompetence). Condition whereby the internal cervical canal dilates without contractions, resulting in premature pregnancy loss.

Incomplete Abortion. Passage of some but not all fetal or placental tissue from the uterine cavity through the cervical canal before 20 weeks' gestation.

Induced Abortion. Intentional medical or surgical termination of pregnancy before 20 weeks' gestation. Also called elective pregnancy termination if performed for the woman's desires or therapeutic abortion if performed to maintain the woman's health.

Inevitable Abortion. Uterine bleeding from a gestation of less than 20 weeks accompanied by cervical dilation but without expulsion of any placental or fetal tissue through the cervix.

Intrauterine Fetal Death. Sonographic visualization of fetus more than 15 mm long, crown–rump length, without fetal heart activity.

Lupus Anticoagulant. An antibody directed against the negatively charged phospholipids of the prothrombin activator complex. This antibody prolongs the phospholipid-dependent coagulation tests in vitro. The presence of this antibody is associated with recurrent pregnancy loss.

Metroplasty. A surgical procedure to unify the endometrial cavity of a bicornuate uterus or remove the septum of a septate uterus.

Miscarriage. The loss of a pregnancy prior to 20 weeks—synonymous with spontaneous abortion.

Missed Abortion. Fetal death before 20 weeks' gestation without expulsion of any fetal or maternal tissue for at least 8 weeks thereafter.

Recurrent Spontaneous Abortion. (Recurrent Miscarriage) The loss of three or more pregnancies before 20 weeks' gestation. In practice it is advisable to perform a diagnostic evaluation for recurrent spontaneous abortion after two first-trimester pregnancy losses or one second-trimester loss.

Septic Abortion. Any type of abortion that is accompanied by uterine infection.

Spontaneous Abortion. Loss of a pregnancy at less than 20 weeks without medical intervention—synonymous with miscarriage.

Subchorionic Hematoma. Sonographically visible hematoma elevating the membranes surrounding the amniotic sac.

Threatened Abortion. Uterine bleeding from a gestation of less than 20 weeks without any cervical dilation or effacement.

Uterine Adhesions. Tissue within the uterine cavity that obliterates part or all of the endometrium. Also called uterine synechia.

Spontaneous abortion (SAB) is the loss of a pregnancy prior to 20 weeks' gestation. It has also been defined as the loss of a pregnancy prior to fetal viability outside of the womb. Viability is now in a gray area, beginning at approximately 23 weeks' gestation, although some states have defined viability as 22 weeks. Other definitions of SAB include the loss of a pregnancy less than or equal to 500 g. As medicine progresses, our definitions have evolved, and our terminology has evolved as well. As the word *abortion* has taken on a charged connotation in society, the synonym *miscarriage* has been substituted to an increasing extent for spontaneous abortion. Interestingly, the word *miscarriage* was noted in the *Oxford English Dictionary* to be first used as early as 1615 in the gynecologic context for pregnancy loss. In this chapter the terms *spontaneous abortion* and *miscarriage* will be used interchangeably. Similarly, the term *habitual abortion* has now been almost completely replaced by *recurrent miscarriage.*

Finally, it is important to understand the subtle distinctions between several terms used when discussing genetic issues: *congenital, inherited, genetic,* and *chromosomal.* These words are often used interchangeably; however, that can result in flawed interpretation of the literature. *Congenital* means present at birth. It does not infer whether or not a condition is inherited. *Inherited* means passed on from one or both parents. In other words, the parent(s) have a genetic change that can be passed to his/her offspring. *Genetic* means changes in the genes or chromosomes. Genetic changes can be sporadic events that are not inherited such as a "new mutation" or they can be inherited events such as cystic fibrosis. Another example is Down syndrome. If an individual has trisomy 21, it is not inherited. If a person has Down syndrome that resulted from a familial translocation, then it is inherited. *Chromosomal* problems are all genetic, but few are inherited. The only chromosomal problems that are inherited are the result of familial translocations.

Although quite common, affecting nearly 20% of all pregnancies, spontaneous abortions are still devastating for both the mother and her partner. The psychological effect of an unintended pregnancy loss cannot be overestimated. The social reaction, in contrast, is often destructive, and the response is often societal denial. Some of this reaction may be to avoid the "rubbing off of the bad luck." Common, seemingly polite responses such as, "You can have another" or "It was for the best" enforce a denial of the prosective mother's natural grieving process. For her the effect may be quite detrimental and long-lasting. It may also serve the purpose to set her apart, therefore lessening the perceived risk for others. The denial of a grieving response for a miscarriage may be present unknowingly among medical providers. In this setting, the denial is even worse. The loss of a pregnancy induces a high rate of depression and guilt. The role of the health provider is to assist the woman and the family through the process, and if possible find a scientific rationale or reason for the pregnancy loss. If appropriate, preventive measures should be offered for the future.

Historically, miscarriage has been treated differently in different cultures. Kueller and Katz described the finding of Greek and Roman burial urns in archaeologic excavations that were specifically used for the products of conception from miscarriage. Ritual purification has been described in Africa for women after miscarriage to prevent a recurrence of the pregnancy loss. Women in pre-Christian Europe and in the Middle East wore specialized amulets termed *eagle stones.* Eagle stones were hollow rocks with small pebbles inside the hollow that would rattle when shaken, symbolizing the pregnancy. These were worn to prevent pregnancy loss. Southern Asian cultures attributed spontaneous abortion to demons. The demon of Con Ranh, Kan Kamiak, and Kaure had to be exorcised to prevent recurrence of a miscarriage. In more modern times multiple medications, drugs, and vitamins have been suggested as treatment to prevent spontaneous abortion. Vitamin C and vitamin E deficiencies have been postulated to cause miscarriage. Even at present, magical thinking in the form of superstition persists in every modern subculture regarding the causes of pregnancy loss.

Physicians have often fallen into the medical confusion of mixing up association with cause and effect when working with women with spontaneous and recurrent miscarriage. The classic paradigm of this logic fallacy is the story of diethylstilbestrol (DES). From the 1940s until the early 1960s women were given the potent synthetic estrogen, stilbestrol (diethylstilbestrol), to prevent pregnancy loss. DES was prescribed as treatment based on the theory that estrogen levels were low in women who were aborting or had aborted. However, the estrogen levels were low as a result of the pregnancy loss, not as its cause. Unfortunately, tens of thousands of women received DES during early pregnancy. The DES did not prevent pregnancy loss, as was well documented, but the medication did cross the placenta and injure the developing genital tracts of both male and female fetuses. The subsequent generation, now almost through their reproductive years, have an excess of pregnancy loss themselves because of their mother's DES exposure.

Treatments such as DES for miscarriage stem from a laudable desire to prevent pain and help our patients. The psychological distress of patients with recurrent spontaneous abortion is one of desperation. The desire and the ability to reproduce are central to the status of human identity and feelings of self-worth for many. Patients and families will go to incredible lengths in hopes for any "miracle" to solve the problem of miscarriage.

In this chapter we will discuss the epidemiology of pregnancy loss and then review the etiology, diagnosis, and management of spontaneous abortion. Recurrent miscarriage may be caused by any factor that persists from one pregnancy to another, such as a balanced translocation or maternal thrombophilia, but is unlikely to be caused by an event such as a viral infection. The management of recurrent miscarriage is discussed throughout the chapter.

Spontaneous abortion needs to be viewed as a syndrome, as well as a spectrum. Loss in the embryonic period, less than 10 weeks, is in a continuum with a loss in the fetal period. However, as a syndrome there are multiple causes. The loss at less than 10 weeks is often due to a chromosomal abnormality, compared with a loss at 18 to 20 weeks, which will more often be from structural cervical or uterine problems. Additionally, many women have more than one cause for recurrent miscarriages. Importantly, for women who have miscarriages, a known etiology does not always cause pregnancy loss. Not all women with a particular problem will have a miscarriage in each pregnancy. For example, women with balanced translocations still have an almost 50% chance of a healthy live-born infant. In evaluating the medical literature, success of a treatment needs to account for the fact that most patients will have a successful pregnancy if no medical intervention is performed. Since 90%

of spontaneous miscarriages are nonrecurrent, doing nothing, as difficult as this may be from the psychological perspective, will often produce the best outcome. The skill and art of the practitioner must be used to teach and guide families through this time period with gentleness.

About 15% to 20% of all known human pregnancies terminate in clinically recognized abortion. However, the incidence of total human embryonic loss is estimated to be much higher. Wilcox and colleagues measured human chorionic gonadotropin (HCG) in daily urine samples of a group of 221 healthy women attempting to conceive. Of the 198 pregnancies that occurred, 22% ended before the pregnancy was clinically recognized and the total pregnancy loss, including clinically recognized abortions, was 31%. Because some fertilized ova do not implant and thus do not secrete detectable HCG and other abnormal pregnancies do not secrete sufficient intact HCG to be detectable by immunoassay, the rate of human pregnancy loss is probably much higher; it has been estimated to be as high as 70% (Table 16-1). Therefore, either the process of human reproduction is inefficient or pregnancy loss serves a particular biologic function. Most early pregnancy losses are the result of chromosomal or genetic abnormalities, the high frequency of abortion, as stated by Austin, is "an important and valuable provision of Nature...and...is in the best interests of the race," because "disadvantageous features from gene mutation are prevented from being incorporated into the overall hereditary pattern." However, this benefit does not alleviate the grief that women and their partner's and families feel. Thus the comment "it was for the best" should not be used in comforting or counseling patients.

Obtaining accurate data to determine the true incidence of clinical spontaneous abortion overall, as well as in particular subgroups of women, is difficult because of possible sources of bias produced by the selection process. Probably the most accurate data come from a study by Regan and coworkers. In this study 630 women who were contemplating pregnancy were interviewed before conception and examined by ultrasonography as soon as pregnancy was suspected and then serially throughout the first trimester. The overall incidence of spontaneous abortion was 12%, and half had occurred before 8 weeks' gestation. The abortion rate in primigravidas was only 5%, whereas it was 14% in multigravidas (Table 16-2). Women whose last pregnancy was successful also had a low abortion rate (5%), whereas women whose last pregnancy aborted had about a 20% abortion rate. The highest rate of abortion (24%) occurred in that group of women who had been pregnant in the past but in whom all the prior pregnancies had terminated in spontaneous abortion. This study indicates that reproductive history is the most relevant predictive factor for pregnancy, outcome in a subsequent pregnancy, and the risk of abortion in primigravidas, is less than previously believed.

Warburton and Fraser studied the incidence of abortion over a 10-year period in a group of more than 2000 women who had at least one pregnancy of at least 20 weeks' gestation. The overall incidence of clinical abortion was 14.7%, and the risk of a pregnancy terminating in spontaneous abortion increased with increasing parity, maternal age, and paternal age (Table 16-3). Each of these parameters was an independent risk factor for abortion, and this information has been confirmed in other studies. These investigators also found that in this group of women who had previously delivered at least one live-born infant, the incidence of clinical abortion was 12.3% if they had no prior abortion. After having one or more abortions, there was a 24% to 32% risk of abortion in successive pregnancies

Table 16-1 Life Table for Intrauterine Mortality in the Human (Per 100 Ova Exposed to Risk of Fertilization)

Week after Ovulation	Death (Expulsion of Dead Embryos)	Survivors
—	16 (not fertilized)	100.32
0	15 (failed to cleave)	84 (fertile)
1	27	69 (implanted)
2	5.0	42.32
6	2.9	37.32
10	1.7	34.12
14	0.5	32.42
18	0.3	31.92
22	0.1	31.62
26	0.1	31.52
30	0.1	31.42
34	0.1	31.32
38	0.2	31.32
Live births (including birth defects)		31.32
Natural wastage		69.32

From Léridon H: Intrauterine mortality. In Léridon H (ed): Human Fertility. Chicago, The Universtity of Chicago Press, 1977.

Table 16-2 Effect of Mother's Reproductive History on Risk of Spontaneous Abortion (*N* = 407)

History	Number of Patients	Number of Patients Aborting	Percentage
Last pregnancy aborted	214	40	19
Only abortions in the past	98	24	24
Only pregnancy aborted	59	12	20
Last pregnancy successful	95	5	5
All pregnancies successful	73	3	4
Only pregnancy successful	62	3	5
Termination of pregnancy	32	2	6
Primigravida	87	4	5
Total	407		

From Regan L, Braude PR, Trembath PL: Influence of past reproductive performance on risk of spontaneous abortion. BMJ 299:541, 1989.

Table 16-3 Relation of Abortion Frequency to Maternal and Paternal Age at Conception

Maternal Age	Percentage Abortion Frequency	Paternal Age	Percentage Abortion Frequency
<20	12.2	<20	12.0
20–24	14.3	20–24	11.8
25–29	13.7	25–29	15.7
30–34	15.5	30–34	13.1
35–39	18.7	35–39	15.8
40–44	25.5	40–44	19.5
44+	23.1		
Mean	14.7	Mean	14.7

From Warburton D, Frazer FC: Spontaneous abortion risks in man: Data from reproductive histories collected in a medical genetics unit. Am J Hum Genet 16:1, 1964.

Table 16-4 Overall Risk of Abortion, According to Age of Mother*

Age of Mother	Number of Pregnancies	Spontaneous Abortions (%)
-19	1105	10.8 (9.0–12.7)
20–29	13,173	9.7 (9.2–12.7)
30–34	3900	11.5 (10.6–12.6)
35–39	1299	21.4 (19.2–23.7)
40+	260	42.2 (35.1–47.4)
Overall	19,737	11.3 (10.9–11.8)

*The table is calculated from a 6.6% sample of the study pregnancies. Figures in brackets: 95% confidence limits χ^2 (trend) = 244; df = 1; $p < 0.0001$.
From Knudsen UB, Hansen V, Juul S, Secher NJ: Prognosis of a new pregnancy following previous spontaneous abortions. Eur J Obstet Gynecol Reprod Biol 39:31, 1991.

Table 16-5 Risk of Subsequent Pregnancy Ending in a Spontaneous Abortion*

Number of Previous Abortions	Number of Pregnancies Studied	Abortion Risk (%)
0	18,164	10.7 (10.3–11.2)
1	21,054	15.9 (15.4–16.4)
2	2,231	25.1 (23.4–27.0)
3	353	45.0 (39.8–50.4)
4	94	54.3 (43.7–64.4)
Overall	19,737	11.3 (10.9–11.8)

*The table is calculated from a 6.6% sample of the study pregnancies. Figures in parentheses: 95% confidence limits. χ^2 (trend) = 728; df = 1: $p < 0.001$.
From Knudsen UB, Hansen V, Juul S, Secher NJ: Prognosis of a new pregnancy following previous spontaneous abortions. Eur J Obstet Gynecol Reprod Biol 39:31, 1991.

that did not vary greatly with the number of abortions. These researchers also reported that a woman with multiple abortions has a tendency to abort at about the same gestational length.

Knudsen and associates reviewed the data for all patients admitted to hospitals in Denmark between 1980 and 1984. There were 33,900 spontaneous abortions during this 5-year period. The overall incidence of spontaneous abortion was 11.3%, which increased in women older than age 35. The abortion risk in women 35 to 40 was 21%, and for women older than 40 it was 42% (Table 16-4). The rate of spontaneous abortion also increased steadily with the number of prior abortions. The risk of abortion in women with no live births with one prior abortion was 13%. With two prior abortions it was 25%, with three it was 45%, and with four prior abortions the risk of abortion increased to 54% (Table 16-5). Several other studies have reported the chance of having a subsequent abortion after three prior abortions is about 50%. These figures obtained from clinical studies are much lower than the theoretical value of 84% for a similar population reported by Malpas using al assumptions.

About 80% of clinical abortions occur in the first trimester, with the incidence decreasing with increasing gestational age. Harlap and Shiono reported that the incidence of *clinical* abortion is relatively stable during each week of gestation before 12 weeks and declines steadily thereafter (Fig. 16-1). Goldstein followed a group of women with serial sonograms in early pregnancy. He reported that once an intrauterine gestational sac was visualized sonographically the rate of pregnancy loss between 4.5 and 8.5 weeks' gestational age was 11.5%. If the pregnancy was viable at 8.5 weeks' gestation, then no pregnancy loss occurred until beyond 15.5 weeks' gestation, when an additional 2.4% fetal deaths occurred. Thus the majority of pregnancy failure occurs in the embryonic period, and about two thirds of these are due to chromosomal abnormalities.

Several other studies also reported that when embryonic heart activity is present between 8 and 12 weeks' gestational age, the incidence of subsequent pregnancy loss is between 2% and 3%. However, when sonography is performed earlier in gestation, beginning between 5.5 and 6 weeks, the subsequent spontaneous abortion rate after embryonic heart activity is seen has

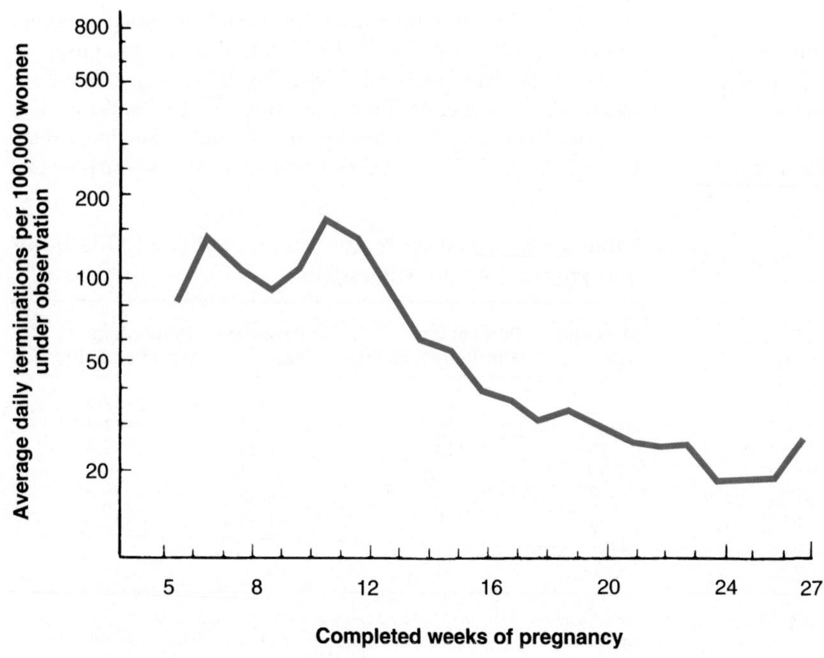

Figure 16-1. Spontaneous abortion by week of pregnancy. (From Harlap S, Shiono PH, Ramcharan S: A life table of spontaneous abortions and the effects of age, parity, and other variables. In Porter IH, Hook EB (eds): Human Embryonic and Fetal Death. New York, Academic Press, 1980.)

been reported to vary between 6% and 8%. There is an inverse relation between increasing length of gestational age between 5 and 8 weeks, in which embryonic heart activity is seen, and the risk of subsequent abortion. The later in early gestation that heart activity is seen, the lower the rate of subsequent abortion. The loss rate after visualization of embryonic heart activity, according to Siddiqi and coworkers, increases about two to three times when the woman is older than 34 compared with younger women. If uterine bleeding occurs when embryonic heart activity is present in the first trimester, the risk of abortion increases about threefold to about 15%, compared with pregnancies without uterine bleeding. Although spontaneous expulsion of the products of conception, clinical abortion, usually occurs between 8 and 12 weeks' gestational age, nearly all embryonic deaths take place several days or weeks prior to the initiation of uterine bleeding and cramping. Most losses are embryonic, not in the fetal period, which begins at approximately 10 weeks.

ETIOLOGY

The causes of spontaneous abortion can be divided into intrinsic abnormalities of the fetus (chromosomal, genetic, and structural) and those related to maternal conditions, including environmental exposures, diabetes, or thrombophilias. These categories overlap; for example, poorly controlled maternal diabetes may cause a lethal heart defect in the fetus.

Chromosomal

By far, the major cause of abortion is aneuploidy in the products of conception. Several large cytogenetic studies of tissue expelled from the uterus at the time of abortion confirm that the incidence of chromosomal anomalies varies between 50% and 60%. Samples of chorionic villi or tissue removed by curettage after nonviability confirmed sonographically, have documented a 70% to 85% rate of chromosomal abnormalities. The higher incidence of aneuploidy found in these recent studies may be due to several factors, including a greater yield of culturable material. Most of the analyses were performed from tissue obtained earlier in gestation. Finally, cytogenetic analysis of chorionic villi, not direct embryonic tissue, may have an increased aneuploid component. The incidence of chromosomal abnormalities in chorionic villi is higher than in fetal tissue.

The vast majority of the abnormal karyotypes in the gestational tissue are numeric abnormalities as a result of errors occurring during gametogenesis (chromosomal nondisjunction during meiosis), fertilization (triploidy as a result of digyny or diandry), or the first division of the fertilized ovum (tetraploidy or mosaicism). Only about 5% of the abnormal karyotypes of the gestations are abnormalities in the structure of individual chromosomes, particularly translocation.

In most surveys of chromosomal anomalies of abortuses the relative frequency of the different types of anomalies is similar. The most common type of anomaly is autosomal trisomy, which accounts for about half the abnormal karyotypes when cell cultures were used and about two thirds of the abnormal karyotypes when chorionic villi analysis was performed directly (Table 16-6). Trisomies of all autosomes except for autosome 1 have been reported after karyotyping of abortions, with trisomy 16 being the most common. About one third of all autosomal trisomies in abortuses are trisomy 16, with trisomy 22 the next most frequent. Many trisomies occurring in abortions have not been reported in live births, probably because the genotype is incompatible with fetal development.

The second most common chorionic abnormality is polyploidy, most frequently triploidy, and less commonly tetraploidy. Studies of chromosomes from miscarriage are derived primarily from placental tissue (chorionic villi) and thus may show more or skewed abnormalities versus embryonic karyotypes. However, these are the best data available, and in itself placental aneuploidy may still induce pregnancy loss. Polyploidy occurs in about 10% of the aneuploid abortions, and monosomy 45,X occurs in about 7% of the abnormal karyotypes in tissue examined by direct analysis. The survival rate of 45,X gestations is about 1 in 300.

To summarize, autosomal trisomy is the most common abnormal karyotype (50% to 65%), followed in decreasing frequency by monosomy 45,X (7% to 15%), triploidy (15%), tetraploidy (10%), and structural abnormalities (5%). The most common single chromosomal abnormality is monosomy 45,X. Karyotypes of abortuses of women who have had more than one abortion tend to be similar if the first abortus had either a normal karyotype or an autosomal trisomy. Except for monosomy, it is possible to estimate the parental origin of the chromosomal abnormality: Approximately 26% of fetal loss is caused by errors of maternal gametogenesis, 5% by errors of paternal gametogenesis, 4% by errors of fertilization, and 4% by errors of zygote division.

Multiple surveys have revealed no seasonal variability in the incidence of any type of chromosomal abnormality in abortions. Maternal age is directly related to the incidence of trisomies, mainly those in the D and G chromosome group. Maternal age has no effect on the incidence of the other chromosomal anomalies in abortions, although there is evidence

Table 16-6 Chromosome Results of 447 Abortuses

	Karyotyped (Banded)	Percentage of All Known Karyotype
Chromosomally Normal		
46,XY	111	24.8
46,XX	95	21.3
Total	206	46.1
Chromosomally Abnormal		
45,X	44	9.8
Primary autosomal trisomy	138	30.9
Double trisomy	7	1.7
Triple trisomy	1	0.4
Triploidy	29	6.5
Tetraploidy	8	1.8
Mosaicism	1	0.4
Structural rearrangement	11	2.5
Others (XXY, monosomy 21)	2	0.8
Total	241	53.9

From Kajii T, Ferrier A, Niikawa N, et al: Anatomic and chromosomal anomalies in 639 spontaneous abortuses. Hum Genet 55:87, 1980. With kind permission of Springer Science and Business Media.

Table 16-7 Frequency of Cytogenetic Diagnoses in 420 Miscarriages from 285 Couples with Recurrent Miscarriage

Diagnosis	No. of miscarriages	Frequency (%)
Euploid, female*	120	29
Euploid, male†	105	25
Trisomy 1	0	0
Trisomy 2	4	0.95
Trisomy 3	0	0
Trisomy 4	1	0.24
Trisomy 5	1	0.24
Trisomy 6	3	0.7
Trisomy 7	3	0.7
Trisomy 8	4	0.95
Trisomy 9	4	0.95
Trisomy 10	1	0.24
Trisomy 11	1	0.24
Trisomy 12	1	0.24
Trisomy 13	11	2.6
Trisomy 14	11	2.6
Trisomy 15	22	5.2
Trisomy 16	19	4.5
Trisomy 17	2	0.48
Trisomy 18	4	0.95
Trisomy 19	0	0
Trisomy 20	2	0.48
Trisomy 21	11	2.6
Trisomy 22	16	3.8
Double trisomy	9	2.1
Sex trisomy (47,XXY)	1	0.24
Monosomy X (45,X)	18	4.3
Monosomy X and trisomy 21	1	0.24
Triploidy	27	6.4
Tetraploidy	10	2.4
Unbalanced translocations	8	1.9
Total	420	100

*Consisting of 118 cases of 46,XX and two cases of balanced translocations.
†Consisting of 105 cases of 46,XY.
From Stephenson MD, Awartani KA, Robinson WP: Cytogenetic analysis of miscarriages from couples with recurrent miscarriage: A case control study. Hum Reprod 17:446–451, 2002.

that monosomy 45,X is associated with a younger maternal age than other aneuploid or euploid abortions. Recently, Kleinhaus and associates, reviewing a large cohort, noted paternal age to also contribute to miscarriage rates.

In contrast to the cause of a specific miscarriage, most causes of recurrent abortion are not chromosomal abnormalities. Stephenson and colleagues analyzed 420 karyotypes of aborted material from 285 couples with recurrent loss (Table 16-7). 66% of recurrent losses had normal cytogenetic evaluations, no different from controls. As would be predicted, advanced maternal age (older than 36) was associated with a significantly higher rate of aneuploidy. When this group of women was separated from the younger group of women, the younger women had a lower rate of aneuploid losses than controls (Table 16-8). In other words, in women younger than 36, recurrent loss was due primarily to causes other than chromosomal abnormalities. Several other recent studies by Sullivan and coworkers, Stern and associates, and Carp and colleagues have noted similar results. A small study, n = 24, of males from couples with recurrent loss found a slightly higher rate of sperm aneuploidy compared with the general population, RR 1.48 + 0.12. This finding would not necessarily translate into more aneuploid conceptus.

Abortion of chromosomally normal conceptuses tends to occur later in gestation than abortion of chromosomally abnormal embryos. The peak incidence of euploid abortion occurs at about 12 to 13 weeks of gestation. However, expulsion of the products of conception does not necessarily coincide with embryonic or fetal death. This is important because parents will equate the timing of miscarriage with the timing of embryonic or fetal death, and timing of the demise is helpful in evaluating cause.

The incidence of chromosomally normal abortions increases markedly after maternal age 35, rising to more than 30% of clinically recognized conceptions after age 40 (Fig. 16-2) Whether this increase in risk of abortion of euploid conceptions is the result of an increase in genetic abnormalities or abnormalities in the maternal environment or both has not been determined, but there is an increased incidence of both first- and second-trimester abortions after age 35, and uterine abnormalities generally are a cause of second-trimester abortion.

Greater than 98% of aneuploidy-related miscarriages occur spontaneously. However, a small proportion is due to balanced translocations in the parents. Tharapel and coworkers reviewed 79 studies of couples with two or more pregnancy losses, comprising a total of 8208 women and 7834 men. The composite prevalence of major chromosomal abnormalities in either parent was about 3%, five to six times higher than the general population.

Table 16-8 Comparison of Cytogenetically Abnormal Miscarriages Stratified by Maternal Age at Time of Miscarriage

Age (years)	Comparative Groups	Cytogenetically Abnormal Miscarriage	Trisomic	45,X	Polyploid	Others*	P
18–29	Recurrent miscarriage	29	16 (55)	5 (17)	8 (28)	0 (0)	NS
	Unselected population†	620	284 (45)	147 (24)	135 (22)	54 (9)	
30–35	Recurrent miscarriage	55	27 (49)	7 (13)	18 (33)	3 (5)	NS
	Unselected population†	331	219 (66)	39 (12)	62 (19)	11 (3)	
36–39	Recurrent miscarriage	64	45 (70)	6 (9)	8 (13)	5 (8)	NS
	Unselected population†	109	81 (74)	16 (15)	6 (5.5)	6 (5.5)	
≥40	Recurrent miscarriage	47	43 (91)	0 (6)	3 (2)	1	NS
	Unselected population†	55	50 (91)	1 (2)	3 (5)	1 (2)	
Total	Recurrent miscarriage	195	131 (67)	18 (9)	37 (19)	9 (5)	0.008
	Unselected population†	1115	634 (57)	203 (18)	206 (18)	72 (6)	

Values in parentheses are percentages.
*Including unbalanced translocations.
†Data from Hassold and Chiu (1985).
NS, not significant.
From Stephenson MD, Awartani KA, Robinson WP: Cytogenetic analysis of miscarriages from couples with recurrent miscarriage: A case control study. Hum Reprod 17:446–451, 2002.

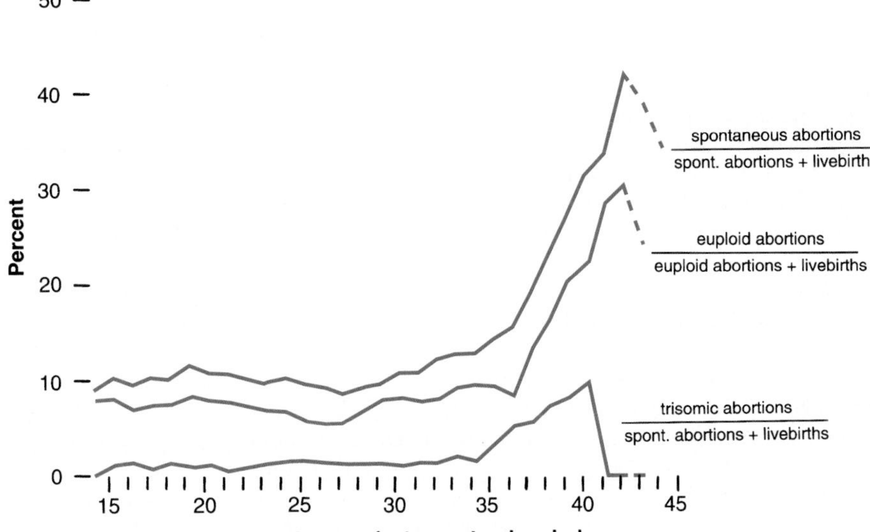

Figure 16-2. Estimated rates (%) of spontaneous abortion, euploid abortion, and trisomic abortion by maternal age for private and public patients combined. (*Broken line,* denominator less than 25.) (From Stein Z, Kline J, Susser E, et al: Maternal age and spontaneous abortion. In Porter IH, Hook EB (eds): Human Embryonic and Fetal Death, New York, Academic Press, 1980.)

Since this review, several large studies, including one from De Braekeleer and Dao, indicate that the prevalence of chromosomal abnormalities in one member of the couple may be as high as 5%. Abnormalities occur in the female parent about twice as frequently as in the male. About half of all chromosomal abnormalities are balanced reciprocal translocations, and one fourth are robertsonian translocations. About 12% are sex chromosomal mosaicism in the female, and the rest are inversions and other sporadic abnormalities. Thus, karyotypes of both members of the couple with two or more spontaneous abortions should be considered. If translocation is found in one parent, one would predict that about 80% of the couple's subsequent pregnancies will abort. In practice, the opposite is closer to the truth! A large study by Carp and colleagues found that the live birth rate was 45% in couples with recurrent loss due to a balanced translocation. Among 99 couples, there were 77 conceptions and 35 live births. If abortion does not occur in a subsequent pregnancy, fetal cytogenetic studies are indicated, because there is about a 5% incidence of unbalanced fetal karyotype in these gestations. Therefore, if an abnormal karyotype is found in one of the partners with recurrent abortion, genetic counseling is indicated. Use of donor gametes may be considered in subsequent pregnancy attempts. Recent data, however, suggest that it is not as indicated as patients may think. Similarly to Carp and colleagues, Stephenson and Sierra noted a 71% live birth rate in this population without artificial reproductive technology.

There are many possible causes for abortion of chromosomally normal conceptions. Simpson postulated that one cause might be a genetic abnormality, a mutation, or set of mutations. He based this assumption on the fact that about 2% of live births have a disorder involving a single gene mutation or polygenic inheritance, whereas only 0.5% of live births have a chromosomal abnormality. Thus, in humans, gene abnormalities are more common than are chromosomal abnormalities. The presumed defect could produce abortion by interfering with fetal metabolism or embryonic structural differentiation. At this time with the first full map of the human genome, investigators are beginning to look for genes that induce miscarriage in chromosomally anomalous conceptions. A different theory may involve a gene that may interfere with normal meiotic division. The theory is derived from several recent studies that have identified a small population of women with recurrent pregnancy loss who also have a skewed inactivation of one of their X chromosomes. According to the Lyon hypothesis, X inactivation should occur randomly. These women were noted to have more than 90% of one X chromosome inactivated. Theoretically, a gene on the X chromosome may be either overly suppressed or overly activated, thus affecting chromosomal replication. The women with disproportionate X inactivation have a significantly higher incidence of trisomy conceptuses.

Investigators have reported an increased incidence of histocompatibility locus antigen (HLA) sharing at the A, B, and DR locus among couples with recurrent abortion compared with controls. This has given rise to the theory that one cause of recurrent loss may be the absence of a maternal immunologic blocking factor normally produced in response to paternal antigens. Homozygosity for recessive major histocompatibility complex genes could be the responsible factor for the abortion. In several animal species, genes contributing to spontaneous abortion are located in the region of the chromosome that controls the major histocompatibility complex. In humans the histocompatibility complex is found in the HLA locus on chromosome 6. The sharing of the HLA antigens could be just the detectable marker for the segment of the chromosome that carries recessive genes that are potentially lethal. Some chromosomally normal couples who experience recurrent abortion, in addition to having increased sharing of HLA-A alleles, also have an increased incidence of the transferrin *C3* allele and a decreased frequency of the most common transferrin allele, *C1,* located on chromosome 3.

Environmental

In contrast to the frequent genetic causes of abortion, maternal or environmental causes are less common. Uterine abnormalities, either congenital or acquired, may not provide the optimal environment for nourishment and survival of the embryo and thus may cause the loss of a genetically normal embryo. Congenital uterine abnormalities can be divided into those brought about by abnormal uterine fusion, those produced by maternal DES ingestion, and those caused by abnormal cervical function. The last condition, the incompetent cervix, can also be acquired after mechanical cervical dilation. Uterine polyps or submucous myomas may be considered acquired.

Congenital Uterine Anomalies

Anomalies of Uterine Development

Anomalies of uterine development are relatively common, with the incidence reported in the literature ranging from about 1:200 to 1:600 women. Recent studies have found that some degree of uterine abnormalities, such as small septa, may occur in as many as 1 in 50 women. Overall, as much as 25% of women with anomalies of uterine fusion have problems with reproduction, recurrent abortion being the most serious. Although it has been stated that bicornuate and septate uteri are the anomalies most frequently associated with abortion, this belief has arisen from the fact that these anomalies can be corrected surgically and thus are more frequently reported as a cause of abortion before surgical correction. Uterine septa tend to cause more difficulties than bicornuate or didelphate uteri. In a study of all 182 women with uterine anomalies detected during an 18-year period at a large Finnish hospital, Heinonen and colleagues reported that the least common uterine anomaly, the unicornuate uterus, was associated with the greatest incidence of spontaneous abortion, about 50%. This incidence was higher than the 25% to 30% incidence of abortion that occurred in women with either a septate or bicornuate uterus. Salim and coworkers compared 509 women with unexplained recurrent loss to 1976 controls. Of the subject group 121 had uterine anomalies. When compared with women in the control group, the uterine distortions in the women with pregnancy loss were more complex, and the uterine volume was smaller.

Surgical correction of bicornuate and septate uteri is possible by using one of the transfundal metroplasty techniques originally described by Strassmann, Jones, or Tompkins, or by transcervical hysteroscopic resection of the uterine septum. The Strassmann technique of metroplasty was used for a bicornuate uterus, and the Jones and Tompkins techniques were used for resection of a uterine septum. In the series by Heinonen and colleagues, about one fifth of the women with bicornuate and septate uteri had a metroplasty performed, and the abortion rate declined from 84% to 12%. In other series the live birth rate increased from 7% to 76% after metroplastic unification of the uterine cavity. The treatment of uterine anomalies associated with recent pregnancy loss by these major surgical procedures has now been replaced by hysteroscopic resection of the uterine septum. When necessary, cervical cerclage may also be used. Sonographic measurements of cervical length help distinguish which patients may benefit from cerclage.

Hysteroscopic incision is the treatment of choice for women with a septate uterus and a history of pregnancy loss. March and Israel reported that it was possible to incise the septum, even those thicker than 1 cm, of all 82 women with recurrent abortion, using the hysteroscope. After this treatment the abortion rate declined from 95% to 13%. Bider and coworkers, among others, reported that when cervical cerclage was used to treat women with a bicornuate uterus and recurrent pregnancy loss the incidence of viable pregnancies markedly increased. In one series of 41 women with bicornuate uteri and recurrent abortion, 85% had a successful pregnancy outcome after cervical cerclage and in the other all 18 women had a term delivery following hysteroscopy.

Uterine Anomalies after DES

DES was prescribed to women throughout the 1950s and early to mid 1960s. Because it was withdrawn from the U.S. market in 1971, it is not a current cause of miscarriage, except in women at the end of their childbearing years. The issues of DES are presented not only for historical interest, but as a paradigm of medical management that evolved from the confusion between and association and an assumption of a cause-and-effect relationship. Comparative studies have shown that women exposed to DES during their fetal life have a significantly greater incidence of spontaneous abortion than do controls. Kaufman and colleagues reported that the percentage of first or all pregnancies in women exposed to DES that ended in spontaneous abortion was similar whether or not their hysterosalpingogram revealed abnormalities in the shape of the uterine cavity or intrauterine defects. One study noted that the endometrial cavity of women exposed to DES in utero had a significantly smaller surface area than normal, which could perhaps contribute to the increased spontaneous abortion rate in women exposed to DES in utero. No therapy, including cerclage, has been shown to significantly lower the abortion rate in women exposed to DES who have abnormalities of the uterine cavity and recurrent abortion unless they also have cervical incompetence. Because the length of gestation tends to increase with subsequent pregnancies among women who had fetal DES exposure, most of these women ultimately had a viable pregnancy.

Cervical Incompetence (Cervical Insufficiency)

Cervical incompetence is characterized by an asymptomatic dilation of the internal cervical os, leading to dilation of the cervical canal during the second trimester of pregnancy. The consequent lack of support of the fetal membranes leads to their prolapse and rupture, which is usually followed by expulsion of the fetus and placenta. The incidence of this problem was previously estimated to vary from 1 in 57 to 1 in 1730 pregnancies. The huge range of incidence speaks to the difficulty in diagnosis. Although excessive mechanical cervical dilation at the time of dilation and curettage was formerly the most common cause of this problem, since recognition of this syndrome, the use of excessive mechanical cervical dilation is now uncommon. Consequently, now the most common cause of cervical incompetence is believed to be a congenital defect in the cervical tissue, and the incidence of this disorder as a cause of recurrent abortion is infrequent because it is usually recognized after the first loss. In a series of 500 consecutive unselected women with recurrent abortion reported by Clifford and associates, none of the 176 women with late abortions had a history of cervical incompetence. Cervical incompetence is associated with the presence of uterine anomalies, particularly

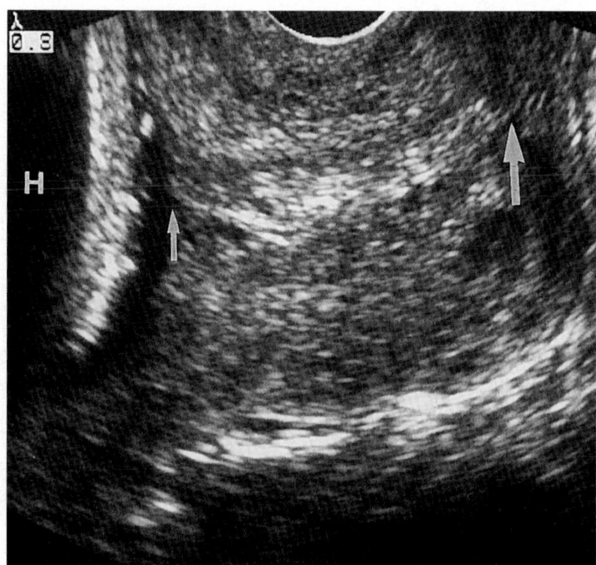

Figure 16-3. Transvaginal ultrasound of a normal appearing cervix, Large arrow to small area denotes canal from external os to internal os, respectively. H, fetal head. (From Fong KW, Farine D: Cervical incompetence and preterm labor. In Rumack CM, Wilson SR, Charboneau JW [eds]: Diagnostic Ultrasound, 2nd ed. St. Louis, Mosby, 1998.)

uterus didelphys, as well as with anomalies produced by fetal DES exposure.

There is no satisfactory test available for the diagnosis of cervical incompetence. Therefore the diagnosis is usually made by obtaining a history of second-trimester pregnancy loss accompanied by spontaneous rupture of the fetal membranes without preceding uterine contractions. Many times the patient will have mild contractions shortly before expelling the pregnancy or before an examination that finds the cervical dilatation to be advanced. Other times the cervix will be noted to be dilated at the time of a midtrimester ultrasound. If the history is equivocal, ultrasound measurements of cervical length as well as visualization of the internal os should be performed weekly from 16 to 23 weeks' gestation (Fig. 16-3). If the history is suggestive and the cervix shortens to less than 2 cm on transvaginal ultrasound, or a funnel forms in the internal os that measures more than 1 cm, a cerclage should be strongly considered. Normal cervical length is approximately 3.5 cm or greater (Fig. 16-4A and B).

The best treatment of cervical incompetence is placement of a concentric nonabsorbable suture as close to the level of the internal os as possible. If strict criteria are used to diagnose cervical incompetence, fetal survival rates after cerclage have been reported to increase from 20% to 80%. However, if the criteria for diagnosis are less certain, in several randomized clinical trials, there is only a slight increase in the incidence of term deliveries after cerclage is performed. It is recommended that the suture be placed electively between 10 to 14 weeks' gestation after major embryogenesis has been completed and the incidence of spontaneous abortion caused by genetic abnormalities has markedly lessened. An ultrasound examination should be performed before the cerclage is placed to document that a normal gestation is present. Occasionally, if there is a markedly shortened cervix or placement of a cerclage has failed to maintain the pregnancy, a transabdominal cerclage should be performed. If the suture is placed externally, it is usually removed at 38 weeks' gestation, and vaginal delivery is permitted to occur. If the suture is buried as in the Shirodkar procedure, then elective cesarean delivery may be considered.

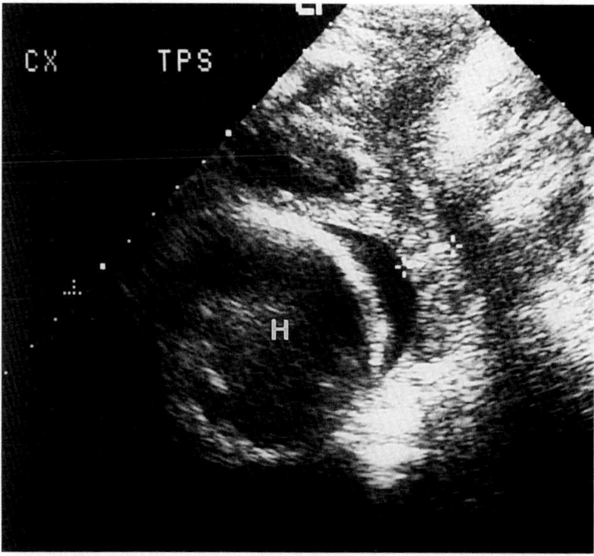

A

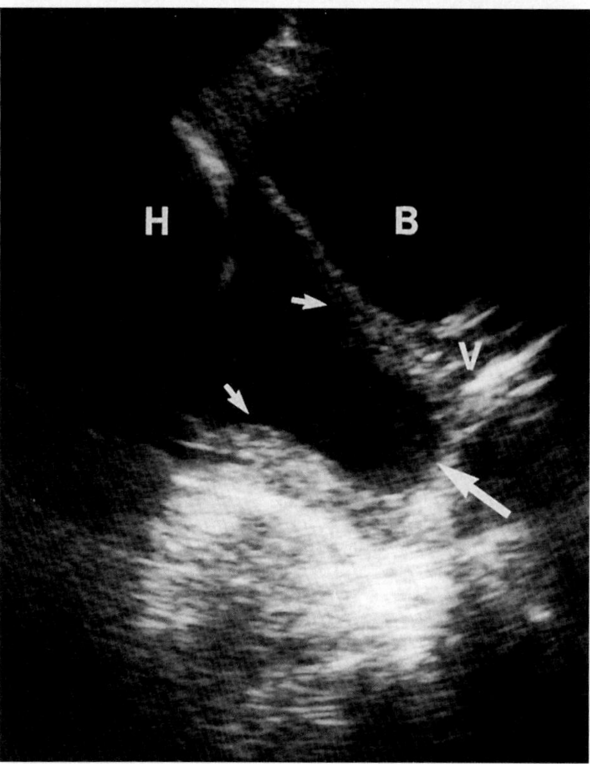

B

Figure 16-4. A, Cervical shortening, the cervix was measured as 15 mm. Cursors are on the cervix. **B,** Advanced funneling or herniation of the membranes into the canal. This view was seen on transabdominal scan (*small arrows,* internal os; *large arrow,* external os). B, maternal bladder; CX, cervix; H, fetal head; TPS, transperineal scan; V, vagina. (From Fong KW, Farine D: Cervical incompetence and preterm labor. In Rumack CM, Wilson SR, Charboneau JW [eds]: Diagnostic Ultrasound, 2nd ed. St. Louis, Mosby, 1998.)

Acquired Uterine Defects

Leiomyomas

Leiomyomas are very common benign uterine tumors that are present in about one third of women of reproductive age. Uterine leiomyomas, especially if they are submucosal, may be associated with repetitive abortion but overall are an uncommon cause. Although a causal relationship is difficult to establish, in a review of the literature, Buttram and Reiter reported that when myomectomy was performed for recurrent abortion in a total of 1941 women, the rate of spontaneous abortion was reduced from 41% to 19%. These data indicate that, on occasion, uterine leiomyomas are a cause of pregnancy loss. An important caution exists. Because myomas are present in greater than 30% of women, the presence of a myoma is not verification that the myoma has caused the miscarriage. Hysteroscopic findings of submucous myomas significantly distorting the uterine cavity are much more suggestive as a cause. Uterine polyps are a rare cause of abortion and are found and treated with the hysteroscope. The presentation is similar to that of submucous myomas. Intermenstrual spotting in this setting is an indication for hysteroscopy.

Intrauterine Adhesions

Adhesions in the uterine cavity can cause partial or complete obliteration of the endometrium, leading to menstrual abnormalities and amenorrhea, as well as being a cause of abortion. The latter is thought to be the result of insufficient endometrium to support adequate fetal growth. The major cause of adhesions is curettage of the endometrial cavity in association with a pregnancy or in the early puerperium (Table 16-9). In the series of March and Israel the most common antecedent factor was curettage for incomplete abortion. Curettage after a missed abortion or after postpartum hemorrhage is associated with a high incidence of subsequent intrauterine adhesion (IUA) formation. On occasion IUAs develop after a diagnostic curettage, as well as in women with genital tuberculosis. The diagnosis of IUA is usually made by the finding of filling defects seen at the time of hysterosalpingogram. The defects are typically irregular, with sharp contours and homogeneous opacity that persist in a series of films (Fig. 16-5). The diagnosis is best confirmed and treated by hysteroscopy (Fig. 16-6).

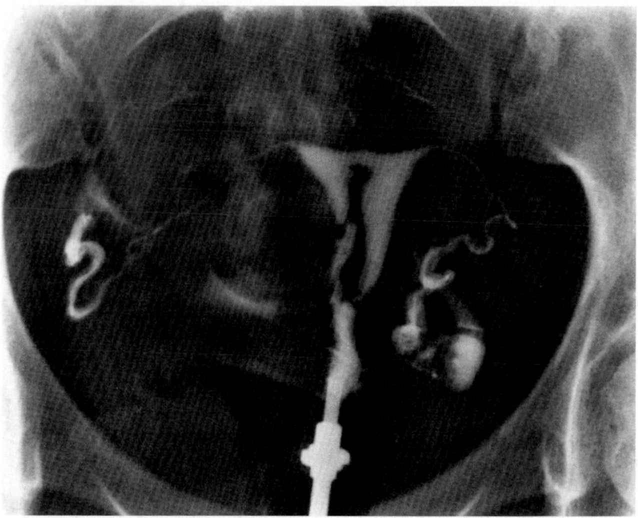

Figure 16-5. Endometrial adhesions. The patient was a 23-year-old gravida 5, para 0, spontaneous abortus 4, ectopic 1, with previous left linear salpingostomy, being evaluated for recurrent abortion. Irregular, linear filling defect represents adhesions between anterior and posterior walls of the endometrial cavity, extending from the internal os to a level near the fundus. (From Richmond JA: Hysterosalpingography. In Mishell DR Jr, Davajan V [eds]: Infertility, Contraception, and Reproductive endocrinology, 3rd ed. Oradell, NJ, Medical Economics Books, 1991. Reprinted with permission. All rights reserved.)

Table 16-9 Definite Causes of IUA in 1856 Cases

	Number of Cases	Percent
Trauma Associated with Pregnancy		
Curettage after abortion	1237	66.7
Spontaneous	544	
Induced	557	
Unknown	136	
Postpartum curettage	400	21.5
Cesarean section	38	2.0
Evacuation of hydatidiform mole	11	0.6
Trauma without Pregnancy		
Myomectomy	24	1.3
Diagnostic curettage	22	1.2
Cervical manipulation (biopsy, polypectomy, etc.)	10	0.5
Curettage because of menometrorrhagia	8	0.4
Insertion of IUD	3	
Insertion of radium	1	0.3
Without Known Trauma		
Postpartum; after abortion; others	28	1.5
Genital Tuberculosis	74	4.0
Total	1856	100.00

IUA, interuterine adhesion; IUD, intrauterine device.
Reprinted from Fertility and Sterility, 37, Schenker JG, Margalioth EJ, Intrauterine adhesions: An updated appraisal, 593. Copyright 1982, with permission from The American Society for Reproductive Medicine.

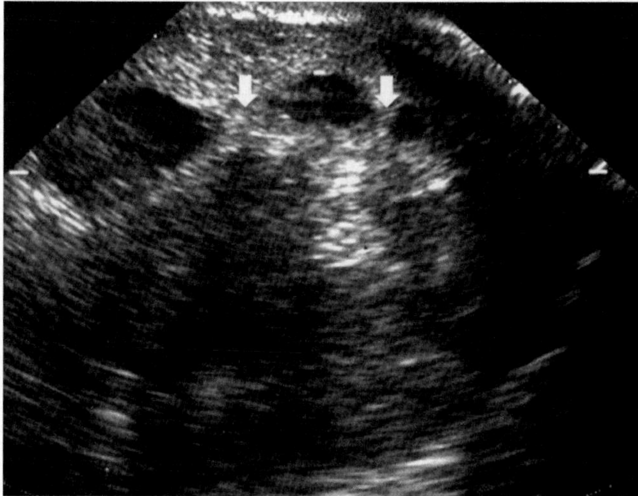

Figure 16-6. Sonohysterography of intrauterine adhesions (*arrows*). (From Goldberg JM, Falcone T: Atlas of Endoscopic Techniques in Gynecology. London, WB Saunders, 2000, p 27.)

The recommended treatment for IUA is lysis of the adhesions during hysteroscopy. After adhesion lysis, an IUD is usually placed in the cavity, and high-dose estrogen is administered for 60 days. Medroxyprogesterone acetate 10 mg per day is added for the last 5 to 10 days, and then the IUD is removed. To minimize the chances of development of IUA, curettage of the pregnant or recently pregnant uterus should be gentle and superficial and not extend deep into the muscle. Prophylactic antibiotics should be considered if there is any suggestion of infection or recent infection.

Endocrine Causes

Progesterone Deficiency

Maintenance of the endometrium for the first 7 weeks of gestation depends on progesterone produced by the corpus luteum. After this time the corpus luteum regresses, and progesterone synthesized by the trophoblast maintains the decidual tissue. Luteal progesterone synthesis depends on HCG produced by the trophoblast. When progesterone secretion from the corpus luteum is lower than normal or the endometrium has an inadequate response to normal circulating levels of progesterone, endometrial development may be inadequate to support the implanted blastocyst and may lead to spontaneous abortion. Investigators have reported that in conception cycles, midluteal peak progesterone levels in the circulation are always greater than 9 ng/mL.

Diagnosis of luteal insufficiency had also been made by performing histologic examination of the endometrium and finding a discrepancy of 3 days or more between the expected and actual endometrial dating pattern in at least two menstrual cycles. Several investigators using this method of diagnosis have reported luteal deficiency to occur in as many as one third of women with recurrent abortion, whereas others have reported it to be an uncommon cause of abortion. This discrepancy may have occurred because the precision of endometrial dating by histologic examination varies among different observers, and different criteria are used for determining the day of ovulation. Murray and colleagues at the University of North Carolina have pointed out the problems with endometrial biopsy in this setting. Fadare and Zheng reviewed more recent studies and advise that diagnosing by endometrial biopsy is of limited accuracy and value because of significant inter- and intraobserver variability.

Several investigators have treated women with recurrent loss and evidence of luteal deficiency with progesterone vaginal suppositories 25 mg twice daily or with intramuscular progesterone 12.5 mg/day beginning 3 days after ovulation and continuing throughout the first trimester. With this treatment, term pregnancy rates have been reported to range from 80% to 90%. However, no randomized clinical trials with a placebo control group have been undertaken to verify whether progesterone significantly reduces the incidence of abortion in women who have documented luteal insufficiency. Goldstein and coworkers performed a meta-analysis of randomized control trials of the use of progestational agents given to women in early pregnancy who had a history of two or more abortions without a specific diagnosis of luteal deficiency. There was no significant reduction in the rate of abortion with the use of progestational agents. Currently most investigators believe that luteal insufficiency is very rarely, if ever, the cause of recurrent spontaneous abortion. If it is the cause, then the losses would occur very early in the embryonic period. There is general skepticism as to whether administration of progesterone in the luteal phase of the cycle in which conception occurs, as well as during early pregnancy, is beneficial.

There is no evidence that administration of synthetic progestins, which themselves may be luteolytic, are of benefit in reducing the incidence of abortion. There is also no benefit to be derived by initiating progesterone therapy or administering exogenous HCG after the expected menstrual period is missed, especially if the woman develops symptoms of threatened abortion. Low progesterone levels at this gestational age are a result, not the cause, of the abortion. If progesterone deficiency is the cause of a pregnancy loss, the pregnancy is expelled very early in gestation, usually before the sixth week.

Thyroid Disease

Although older studies suggested that hypothyroidism may be a cause of abortion, three studies with large numbers of women with recurrent abortion, noted that only a few women in one of the studies were found to have abnormal thyroid function. Thus there is no definitive evidence that hypothyroidism is a cause of spontaneous abortion. There are, however, several studies that indicate that the presence of antithyroid antibodies is associated with pregnancy loss.

Stagnaro-Green and associates measured thyroglobulin and thyroid peroxidase antibodies in 552 unselected women in the first trimester of pregnancy. An antithyroid antibody was found in 20% of these women. Among the group of women in whom thyroid antibodies were detected, the spontaneous abortion rate was twice as high, 17% vs. 8.4% as that for women without the antibodies. Lejeune and colleagues measured these two antithyroid antibodies in 730 euthyroid women in early pregnancy and reported that one of these antibodies was present in 24% of women who had a first-trimester abortion but in only 5% of those with viable pregnancies.

Stagnaro-Green summarized several studies that have confirmed the association of antithyroid antibodies with recurrent first-trimester loss. The findings of these studies indicate that the presence of thyroid antibodies is a risk marker for abortion. Since the antibodies are found in euthyroid women it is likely that they are a marker for some type of immunologically mediated cause of abortion that is likely to reoccur. Intravenous immunoglobulin, heparin and aspirin, and thyroid supplementation have been used as treatments in women with these antibodies. Because of differences in design, the results of these studies cannot be summed. However, treatment with thyroid hormone was more effective than immunoglobulin, heparin, or aspirin in achieving successful pregnancy outcomes in subsequent gestations.

Diabetes Mellitus, Insulin Resistance, and Polycystic Ovary Syndrome

Uncontrolled diabetes mellitus has been associated with an increased miscarriage rate. The increased rate is due in part to structural anomalies in the fetus. Crane and Wahl found the incidence of spontaneous abortion to be similar in a group of women with either gestational diabetes (12.3%) or insulin-dependent diabetes (12.2%) and matched control groups (10.9% and 14.5%). Mills and colleagues performed a prospective study of insulin-dependent diabetic and nondiabetic women enrolled within 3 weeks of conception. The spontaneous abortion rate in both groups was 16%. However, a small group of women whose diabetes was not well controlled and who had elevated blood glucose and glycosylated hemoglobulin levels had a significantly increased risk of spontaneous abortion. Thus it appears that among women with diabetes and good control of blood glucose, diabetes is not a likely cause of abortion. However, diabetes without good metabolic control is associated with an increased risk of early pregnancy loss, with a direct correlation between the level of hemoglobin A_1 and the rate of abortion.

Recent evidence has supported the association of insulin resistance associated with polycystic ovary syndrome (PCOS) and spontaneous abortion. Women treated with metformin for insulin resistance associated with PCOS have a reduced incidence of pregnancy loss compared with controls. Similarly, Craig and coworkers noted an increased incidence of insulin resistance in a small cohort (n = 74) of women being evaluated for recurrent loss, compared with controls. Proposed mechanisms include not only the inherent metabolic problems associated with higher glucose levels and decreased insulin activity such as increased inflammatory mediators, but also increased levels of plasminogen activator inhibitor 1. This protein functions as a procoagulant and thrombophilic agent. Insulin resistance also induces a proinflammatory state.

The relationship of PCOS elevated luteinizing hormone (LH) levels and spontaneous abortion is an area of ongoing investigation. Homburg noted that about one third of women with POCS who conceive after undergoing ovulation induction have a spontaneous abortion—more than twice the incidence of spontaneous abortion of women with hypogonadotropic hypogonadism who conceive after ovulation induction. The incidence of spontaneous abortion was only increased in those women with PCOS who had elevations of follicular phase plasma LH levels, not those in whom the LH levels were in the normal range. Regan and associates prospectively measured follicular phase LH levels in a group of 193 women with regular menstrual cycles who were planning to become pregnant, the majority of whom had a history of one or more previous spontaneous abortions. Within 18 months 88% of women with normal LH levels (less than 10 IU/L) conceived, compared with 67% of women whose LH levels were elevated. These investigators found that of the women who conceived with elevated LH levels, 65% of the pregnancies ended in abortion, whereas only 12% of the pregnancies in women with normal LH levels aborted. Thus, if the LH levels were elevated on day 8 of the cycle, there was a significantly greater risk of the pregnancy ending in abortion, as well as a greater risk of infertility. These investigators concluded that hypersecretion of LH among women with and without PCOS is a cause of spontaneous abortion.

The mechanism whereby elevated LH levels are associated with miscarriage has not been determined. Clifford and colleagues studied a group of 500 consecutive women with recurrent spontaneous abortion who were referred to a special clinic to study this problem. Sonographic findings of polycystic ovaries were found in 56% of these women, but only 12% of them had elevated follicular phase serum LH levels. However, it was found that nearly 60% of the women with polycystic ovaries had elevated urinary LH levels. Urinary LH may be a more sensitive marker of LH hypersecretion than of serum LH since LH is secreted in a pulsatile manner. Clifford and colleagues performed a randomized controlled trial of women with recurrent abortion and elevated LH levels, comparing therapy of gonadotropin-releasing hormone (GnRH) analogues with no therapy. The viable birth rate was similar in the two groups, indicating that LH suppression with a GnRH analogue is not beneficial for improving live birth rates.

Immunologic Factors

The physiologic mechanisms by which the partially foreign fetal tissue is protected from the mother's immunologic system is poorly understood. The foreign antigens produced by the fetus initiate a rejection from the mother. Although some protection from this immunologic effect is offered by progesterone, in reality a complex biologic network prevents the fetus from being rejected. For 4 decades, investigators have postulated that abortion, and recurrent abortion, in particular may be associated with a failure of an immunologic suppression. Numerous studies have found differences in the immune mechanisms of couples with recurrent loss. However, to date, immunologic treatments have not been shown to be effective. The immunologic processes are complex, and the potential lesions and differences between the subset of recurrent aborters and controls are specific and very different in different subsets of patients. Some immunologic differences such as specific cytokines may be related to failures in organ systems other than the immunologic system. Treatments such as immunoglobulin or infusions of paternal antigens affect the maternal immunologic system on a broad front. In medicine, the more broad spectrum the treatment, the more numerous the additional affects. With broad-spectrum treatments of the immunologic system to prevent recurrent loss, some beneficial aspects may be affected.

It has also been postulated that if there is sharing of major histocompatability locus antigens (HLA) between the male and the female in the couple with recurrent abortion, then natural blocking factors would be less likely to develop and abortion would be more likely to occur. Numerous studies have investigated the degree of HLA sharing at several loci in groups of couples with recurrent abortion in whom no cause for the problem could be detected. Bellingard and colleagues, in addition to performing their own study, summarized the results of 23 previously published studies that investigated the degree of HLA sharing between spouses of couples with recurrent abortion. The findings were divided among the studies. HLA-A sharing was reported to be present in 11 and absent in 12 of the 23 studies, and HLA-B sharing was present in 10 but absent in 13 of the 23 studies. In the 17 studies in which HLA-DR sharing was investigated, 11 found sharing of this allele to be more frequent among couples with recurrent abortion of undetected cause than among controls. In their own study of women with three successive spontaneous abortions, Bellingard and colleagues found that the number of couples with HLA sharing in each of the three alleles was not significantly different among women with a known cause for their recurrent abortion and those with unexplained recurrent abortion, as well as a control group of parous women without spontaneous abortion.

In 1985 Mowbray and coworkers performed a randomized treatment trial in a group of women with recurrent abortion and no detectable antibody against paternal lymphocytes. In this study, women injected with paternal white cells had a significantly greater chance of a subsequent successful pregnancy (78%) than did those injected with their own white cells (37%). The investigators concluded that infusion of the foreign leukocytes increased maternal production of the blocking factors that would prevent rejection of the fetal tissues. However, in two subsequent studies performed by Cowchock and Smith, and by Hwang and associates, after paternal leukocytes were given to the female the outcome of the subsequent pregnancy was not related to the development of either maternal antipaternal antibodies or blocking factors. After the paternal white cell immunotherapy was performed, neither the formation of antipaternal antibodies nor blocking factors was associated with a decrease in the spontaneous abortion rate or an increase in term pregnancy rate compared with pregnancies after immunotherapy in which these factors did not substantially increase.

Several other aspects of the immune system have been investigated as potential causes of recurrent loss. One line of research involves the populations of lymphocytes in the deciduas compared with the peripheral maternal circulation. Normally, there are few B lymphocytes and neutrophils but a large proportion of natural killer cells in the deciduas. These proportions have been found (in some but not all studies) to be different in patients with unexplained recurrent loss than in controls. The frequency profiles of cytokines, including the interleukins, tumor necrosis factor, tumor necrosis factor, macrophage inhibiting cytokine, and the interferons, are also different in recurrent abortion patients and are influenced by the types of subpopulation of T helper cells in the decidua. These findings have led investigators to propose that immunoglobulin infusion may be helpful in blocking this abnormal immune response and augment a normal response. In a meta-analysis, Scott found no improvement in miscarriage rate with intravenous immunoglobulin therapy. He also analyzed paternal leukocyte infusion and found no benefits.

Since there are potential risks associated with leukocytic immunotherapy, including the possibility of virus transmission and the development of autoimmune disease, and therapy has not been shown to be effective, it is not cost-effective or necessary to perform HLA typing of the couple outside the investigational setting. Infusion of paternal leukocytes should only be performed under research protocols with informed consent, because the procedure has not been proven to be beneficial and has serious potential health risks. Infusions of immunoglobulin are similarly expensive and ineffective and should be used only as part of investigational protocols. Abnormal immune responses may eventually prove for some patients to be a cause of recurrent loss, but which patients and which therapies, are as of now unknown.

Celiac Disease

Celiac disease (sprue) is a systemic autoimmune disease caused by an allergy to gluten. Though in its most pronounced symptoms intestinal malabsorption occurs, most patients will have minimal gastrointestinal manifestations. When taking a history, questions of food intolerances are usually not included, and symptoms may be quite vague and nonspecific. For women with unexplained pregnancy loss, the history should include inquiry with open-ended questions about tolerance to wheat and gluten-containing foods such as pasta, as well as questions about family history of gluten intolerance.

A strong association has been documented with adverse pregnancy outcomes, including miscarriage and recurrent miscarriage and the antibodies of celiac disease. Antigliadin antibodies appear to be toxic to trophoblast. Suppression of the antibodies through dietary control has decreased the incidence of miscarriage. In the setting of an evaluation for miscarriage, any women with a personal or family history of celiac disease or gluten intolerance should be tested for antigliadin and antiendomysial antibodies. The prevalence of celiac disease in first-degree relatives of patients with sprue is 10%.

THROMBOPHILIA

An essential and vital component of a successful gestation is the healthy growth and development of the placental vasculature. The uteroplacental interface receives nearly 20% of maternal cardiac output. A self-protective physiologic adaptation is the increased thrombogenic characteristics of this interface. If the mother has a thrombotic tendency, a thrombophilia, the placenta may develop an overly thrombogenic microenvironment. This may lead to multiple small infarctions at the uteroplacental interface that interfere with placental function. All of the thrombophilias have been associated with miscarriage and adverse pregnancy outcomes, including recurrent miscarriage. Pregnancy, in general, is a time of increased coagulability. Estrogen increases several of the clotting factors (factors VIII, V, and fibrinogen) and induces a decline in thrombolytic factors, including protein S, activated protein C resistance, plasminogen activator inhibitor 1.

The incidence of thrombophilias, both acquired and inherited, is fairly large (>10% of the white population); thus it is difficult to equate the presence of a thrombophilia as a cause of an adverse pregnancy event. One of the most valuable clues that a thrombophilia led to a pregnancy loss may be found in the placental pathology. The theoretical mechanism that induces pathology in pregnancy is a vasculopathy in the placental bed. If placental vasculopathy is noted, then it is more likely that the thrombophilia is a cause of the miscarriage. Histologic findings include placental infarction, perivillous fibrin deposition, maternal floor infarction, and intervillous thrombosis. The findings, though, are nonspecific and variable. Heparin therapy has been noted to reduce the incidence of vasculopathy. Though the thrombophilias may induce a pregnancy loss at any time in gestation, a loss after a fetal heartbeat has been noted is considered stronger evidence of causality, since so many early first-trimester losses are related to aneuploidy. The following box lists thrombophilias that have been associated with pregnancy loss.

Thrombophilias are one of the most common inherited pathologies. Obviously, 10% of the population does not suffer with recurrent pregnancy loss. Thus, there are individual predilections and comorbidities in addition to the thrombophilias that induce pathology. As of yet, most of these cofactors have not been identified. Systematic reviews and meta-analyses of the

Thrombophilias Associated with Miscarriage

Antiphospholipid antibodies—anticardiolipin lupus anticoagulant
Antithrombin III deficiency
Elevated factor VIII levels
Factor V Leiden mutation
MTHFR mutations
Plasminogen activator inhibitor-1 deficiency
Protein C deficiency
Protein S deficiency
Prothrombin G20210A mutation

MTHFR, methylenetetrahydrofolate reductase.

thrombophilias indicate that there is an association between thrombophilias and miscarriage. Whether a thrombophilia is the cause of miscarriage in a specific patient, though, is much more difficult to determine. Cross-sectional and prospective studies show a much weaker association between thrombophilias and pregnancy loss. The composite epidemiologic studies to date emphasize the multifactorial nature of the association of thrombophilias (and other causes) and pregnancy loss. For example insulin resistance increases plasminogen activator 1. In the presence of PCOS with insulin resistance and the presence of factor V Leiden a woman may have a miscarriage. The combination of the two or more factors may be the problem. Similarly, studies of patients with multiple and more potent thrombophilias have found a stronger association with pregnancy loss.

Inherited Thrombophilias

Factor V Leiden is the most common inherited thrombophilia in whites. Up to 8% of some populations are heterozygous for this autosomal dominant mutation. The Leiden mutation is a substitution of glutamine for arginine at position 506 on the factor V protein. This mutation in factor V leads to a defect in binding with the activated protein C (APC) complex. Thus the factor V cannot be properly inhibited (Fig. 16-7).

The presence of factor V Leiden may be assessed directly with gene mutation analysis or indirectly by measuring APC resistance. APC resistance decreases in pregnancy as part of the thrombogenic changes. However, an APC resistance of less than 1.8 is pathognomonic for the heterozygous state of factor V Leiden mutation. An APC resistance of less than 1.4 usually

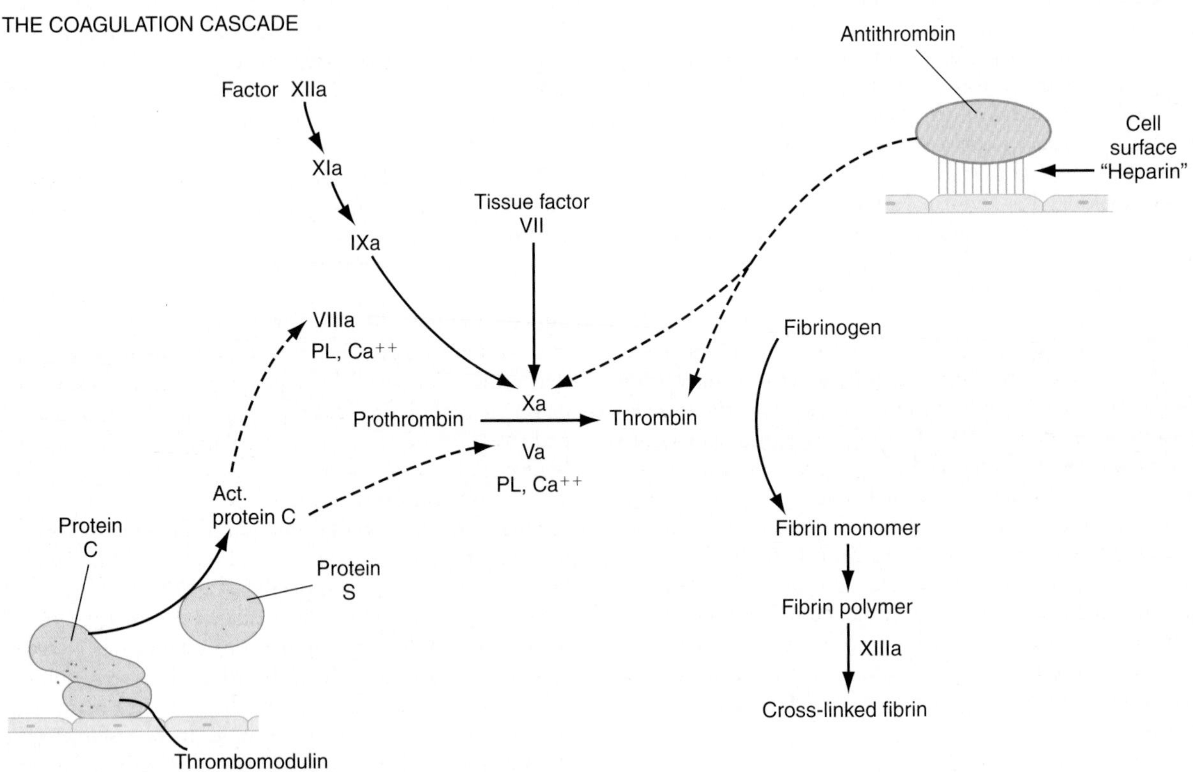

Figure 16-7. The coagulation cascade. Inhibitory steps and thrombolytic factor are marked with interrupted lines. The lowercase "a" denotes an activated factor. Ca, calcium; PL, phospholipid.

indicates the homozygous state. Patients who are homozygous for factor V Leiden have a >80% lifetime risk of thrombosis, as well as a significantly higher risk of adverse pregnancy outcomes, including recurrent miscarriage. Both the heterozygous and the homozygous state have been associated with miscarriage. Meta-analysis by Rey and coworkers noted a 2.01 relative risk (CI 1.13 to 3.58; Fig. 16-8) for early recurrent miscarriage, and a 7.83 RR (CI 2.83 to 21.67) of late recurrent loss. Kovalevsky and colleagues in their meta-analysis noted an odds ratio of 2.1, (CI 1.6 to 2.7) with factor V Leiden and recurrent pregnancy loss. Homozygosity for factor V Leiden is a greater risk of recurrent loss than the heterozygous state.

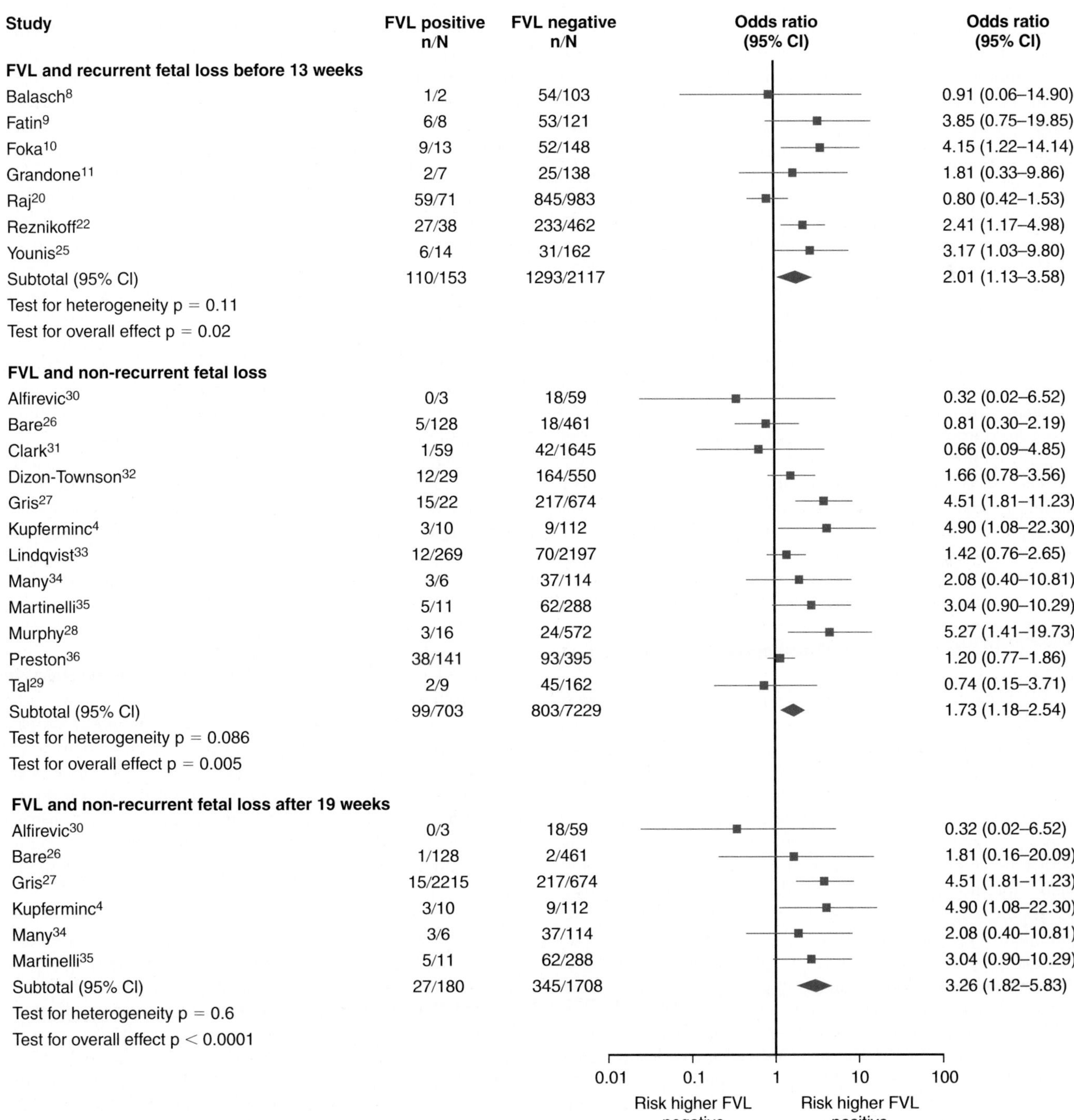

Study	FVL positive n/N	FVL negative n/N	Odds ratio (95% CI)
FVL and recurrent fetal loss before 13 weeks			
Balasch[8]	1/2	54/103	0.91 (0.06–14.90)
Fatin[9]	6/8	53/121	3.85 (0.75–19.85)
Foka[10]	9/13	52/148	4.15 (1.22–14.14)
Grandone[11]	2/7	25/138	1.81 (0.33–9.86)
Raj[20]	59/71	845/983	0.80 (0.42–1.53)
Reznikoff[22]	27/38	233/462	2.41 (1.17–4.98)
Younis[25]	6/14	31/162	3.17 (1.03–9.80)
Subtotal (95% CI)	110/153	1293/2117	2.01 (1.13–3.58)
Test for heterogeneity p = 0.11			
Test for overall effect p = 0.02			
FVL and non-recurrent fetal loss			
Alfirevic[30]	0/3	18/59	0.32 (0.02–6.52)
Bare[26]	5/128	18/461	0.81 (0.30–2.19)
Clark[31]	1/59	42/1645	0.66 (0.09–4.85)
Dizon-Townson[32]	12/29	164/550	1.66 (0.78–3.56)
Gris[27]	15/22	217/674	4.51 (1.81–11.23)
Kupferminc[4]	3/10	9/112	4.90 (1.08–22.30)
Lindqvist[33]	12/269	70/2197	1.42 (0.76–2.65)
Many[34]	3/6	37/114	2.08 (0.40–10.81)
Martinelli[35]	5/11	62/288	3.04 (0.90–10.29)
Murphy[28]	3/16	24/572	5.27 (1.41–19.73)
Preston[36]	38/141	93/395	1.20 (0.77–1.86)
Tal[29]	2/9	45/162	0.74 (0.15–3.71)
Subtotal (95% CI)	99/703	803/7229	1.73 (1.18–2.54)
Test for heterogeneity p = 0.086			
Test for overall effect p = 0.005			
FVL and non-recurrent fetal loss after 19 weeks			
Alfirevic[30]	0/3	18/59	0.32 (0.02–6.52)
Bare[26]	1/128	2/461	1.81 (0.16–20.09)
Gris[27]	15/2215	217/674	4.51 (1.81–11.23)
Kupferminc[4]	3/10	9/112	4.90 (1.08–22.30)
Many[34]	3/6	37/114	2.08 (0.40–10.81)
Martinelli[35]	5/11	62/288	3.04 (0.90–10.29)
Subtotal (95% CI)	27/180	345/1708	3.26 (1.82–5.83)
Test for heterogeneity p = 0.6			
Test for overall effect p < 0.0001			

Figure 16-8. Prevalence of factor V Leiden in women with fetal loss. (From Rey E, Kahn SR, David M, Shrier I: Thrombophilic disorders and fetal loss: A meta-analysis. Lancet 361:9018, 2003.) References cited in this figure are from the original source.

The second most common thrombophilia is the G20210A mutation in prothrombin. The prothrombin mutation is found in up to 5% of whites. It causes an excess concentration of prothrombin in the circulation. It confers a 2.56 relative risk (CI 1.04 to 6.29), for early pregnancy loss. Kovalesky and colleagues noted a 2.06 relative risk (CI 1.0 to 4.0). The prothrombin mutation is identified by gene analysis.

Less common thrombophilias include deficiencies in protein C (0.5% of the population for the heterozygous state), and protein S deficiency (0.5% of the population are heterozygous), and antithrombin-3 deficiency (approximately 0.05% of the population). All three of these proteins contribute to the thrombolytic pathway, and the homozygous states are not compatible with life. All three have been associated in cohort studies with an increased tendency for miscarriage and recurrent loss. Protein C and antithrombin-3 levels may be assessed in pregnancy. However, protein-S is an acute-phase reactant, decreasing with pregnancy, trauma, or surgery. Levels are significantly decreased by estrogen in general, and thus should be measured at least 6 to 8 weeks after a pregnancy. Elevated factor VIII, greater than 180% of normal, and plasminogen activator inhibitor deficiency (PAI-1) have also been associated with early pregnancy loss. Although fewer studies exist at this time, these compounds may be measured directly.

Treatment of the inherited thrombophilias involves subcutaneous heparin. Low-molecular-weight (LMW) heparin is preferable to unfractionated heparin. LMW heparin induces less osteoporosis, a much lower (almost absent) incidence of heparin-induced thrombocytopenia, and a decreased number of daily injections. Heparin is metabolized at an increased rate during pregnancy, and to achieve adequate levels of thromboprophylaxis throughout the day, every-8-hour injections are necessary with unfractionated heparin. LMW heparin, although often given once a day in the nonpregnant state, needs to be given at least every 12 hours during pregnancy. Doses are weight-dependent. Adequate prophylaxis to prevent pregnancy loss is an activated partial thromboplastin time (aPTT) of approximately 1.5 times normal for unfractionated heparin. LMW heparin does not induce changes in the aPTT, and is measured with an anti-Xa activity level. Many labs will just call this a LMW heparin level. Because of the increased metabolism in pregnancy, peak levels are not as helpful for LMW heparin during pregnancy, and trough levels may show a greater correlation with the appropriate levels. A trough level should be ordered 1 to 2 hours prior to the next dose. Anti-Xa activity levels of 0.18 to 0.2 are appropriate for thromboprophylaxis. Specific assays are calibrated for each LMW heparin. Thus, the assay for dalteparin is different from the assay for tinzaparin or enoxaparin. An antifactor Xa level of 0.2 corresponds approximately to a level of an aPTT of 1.5 times normal. Most investigators check platelets weekly in women on LMW heparin for 2 to 4 weeks, and then once in each trimester. Women taking unfractionated heparin need platelet levels checked weekly while they are on therapy. Once adequate dosing is obtained, levels should be checked each trimester. If a woman is being treated with therapeutic levels, for example for a homozygous state or for deep vein thrombosis (DVT), then levels of an aPTT on unfractionated heparin should be 2.5 to 3 times normal, or an anti-Xa activity trough level of 0.4. Bleeding tends to occur with levels greater than 0.8 to 1.0. Regional anesthesia should not be used within 24 hours of dosing of LMW heparin due to an increased incidence of epidural hematomas. All women on heparin should also receive vitamin D and calcium. Importantly for the gynecologist, these women should not be given estrogen-based contraception, nor should they receive estrogen replacement therapy, tamoxifen, raloxifene, or other selective estrogen receptor modulators (SERMs) without specific counseling.

Mild hyperhomocysteinemia is sometimes considered a thrombophilia. Homocysteine is an essential amino acid, which in excess may lead to damage to the vascular endothelium. Hyperhomocysteinemia may induce small clots as the vasculature repairs itself. Estrogen naturally decreases homocysteine levels, thus women with mild hyperhomocysteinemia rarely develop thrombosis prior to menopause. One of the enzyme systems that metabolizes homocysteine is methylenetetrahydrofolate reductase (MTHFR). Mutations in this enzyme can lead to higher levels of homocysteine, and thus blood clots. In the placental bed this is particularly significant, even though systemically it is rare for MTHFR to cause thrombosis during pregnancy. Mutations in the MTHFR enzyme occur in 10% to 15% of the white and Asian populations. With such a common frequency other cofactors, as yet unidentified, will contribute to the well-documented increase in miscarriage and recurrent miscarriage associated with MTHFR. Similar to the other thrombophilias, the MTHFR mutation is much less common in the population of African ancestry. Two mutations are commonly found in the enzyme, and either may lead to mild homocystinemia. However, the C677T mutation is significantly more problematic during pregnancy than the A1298C. Mild homocysteinemia is autosomal recessive. Even though the A1298C mutation is less of a problem, the compound heterozygous state for the two mutations is also associated with recurrent loss. Some patients refer to MTHFR as the "Monday, Thursday, Friday mutation."

Unlike the thrombophilias, though, mild homocystinemia may also induce pregnancy loss through a teratogenic effect. In some studies, up to 50% of open neural tube defects have been associated with homozygous MTHFR mutation. Complex cardiac disease in the fetus has also been associated with the homozygous state. During the investigation of miscarriage, gene mutation testing of MTHFR is recommended over homocystine levels since these levels vary throughout the menstrual cycle and with dietary influences. Additionally, most studies have evaluated the association of adverse outcomes with the mutation not with homocysteine levels.

The risk/benefit ratio strongly favors the treatment of this condition when it is found. To bolster enzyme activity, vitamin cofactors (4 mg of folic acid, 500 μg of vitamin B_{12}) should be given periconceptually and continued until regular menses have resumed. This treatment has been shown to not only decrease the rate of miscarriage, but also decrease the risk of pregnancy complications and congenital malformations. The treatment is continued postpartum to decrease the risk of thrombosis in the estrogen deplete puerperium. Women with MTHFR mutations may be given estrogen-based oral contraceptives and hormone replacement therapies, if appropriate, because of the beneficial effects of estrogen on homocysteine levels.

Antiphospholipid Antibodies

The first thrombophilias associated with adverse pregnancy outcomes were two antiphospholipid antibodies: the lupus anticoagulant (LAC) and the anticardiolipin antibody (ACA). Phospholipids are ubiquitous molecules that occur throughout the body and are found in almost all vasculature, particularly the placental vasculature. These antibodies react with proteins on the endothelium and induce platelet activation and thrombosis. The reaction induced by the antibody antigen complexes will induce both arterial and venous thrombosis. Alternative hypotheses for the deleterious effect of the antiphospholipid antibodies toward pregnancy include a specific reaction to exposed trophoblast in the placental vascular bed, which is cytotoxic.

Although these antibodies are associated with systemic lupus erythematosus and other collagen-vascular disorders, most women do not have clinical or subclinical lupus. Recurrent pregnancy loss, thrombosis, and the presence of antiphospholipid antibodies are necessary to make the diagnosis of antiphospholipid syndrome. However, most women will just manifest pregnancy loss and not yet have developed thromboses. Between 1% and 3% of the population will have low levels of immunoglobulin (Ig)M for ACA. Moderate to high levels of IgM or IgG are more significant in the setting of a patient with miscarriage. LAC is paradoxically named because it was first described in women with lupus. And in vitro, due to its binding with phospholipids, it will inhibit coagulation and increase the clotting time. In vivo, LAC is a strong procoagulant. To test for LAC pathologists use specifically prepared assays, such as the kaolin clotting time or the dilute Russell viper venom test. If blood does not clot, normal serum is added to assess if the result of the clotting is due to a deficiency of clotting factors. If the blood still fails to clot with normal serum being added, then LAC is suspected. Up to 2% of normal women will have low levels of the LAC. Because the Venereal Disease Research Laboratory (VDRL) test for syphilis uses a phospholipid assay, the presence of LAC may induce a false-positive VDRL. When specific tests for syphilis are used, the patient will test negative. Other antiphospholipid antibodies, include immunoglobulins that react against β-2 glycoprotein, phosphatidyl serine, phosphatidyl ethanolamine, and annexin-5. These antibodies may also induce pregnancy loss, but they are rare. The treatment of antiphospholipid syndrome in pregnancy is both 81 mg of aspirin daily, and prophylactic heparin. Glucocorticoid therapy is not effective. LMW heparin is given to achieve a trough level of 0.2 anti-Xa activity level. Women with a previous thrombosis and antiphospholipid antibodies are treated with full anticoagulation (trough of 0.4). Women with thrombosis and antiphospholipid antibodies have a near 100% risk of subsequent thrombosis. Thus, the recommendation is anticoagulation for the rest of her life. If a woman is contemplating pregnancy with the antiphospholipid syndrome, warfarin is usually stopped and heparin initiated to prevent warfarin embryopathy.

INFECTIONS

Numerous infectious agents present in the cervix, uterine cavity, or seminal fluid have been postulated to be etiologic factors for abortion. Although there is evidence that clinical endometritis caused by any infectious agent can produce an abortion, the evidence is unclear as to whether subclinical infections with certain microorganisms or viruses are a cause of spontaneous abortion. Most acute bacterial infections (e.g., *Staphylococcus, Streptococcus, Neisseria gonnorhoeae)* may cause a pregnancy loss. These agents are sporadic causes and are not etiologic agents of recurrent loss.

Although *Listeria monocytogenes* produces abortion in several animal species as well as humans in the second trimester, there is no evidence that it is an abortifacient in women in the first trimester. Rabau and David found no bacteriologic or serologic evidence of *Listeria* infection in 554 women who had aborted, including 74 with recurrent abortions, and Stray-Pedersen and colleagues were unable to isolate this organism from a group of 48 women with recurrent abortion. *Chlamydia trachomatis* is a common sexually transmitted pathogen, but there is no evidence that it causes abortion in asymptomatic women. Primary infections have been associated with pregnancy loss, but not recurrent loss.

Several authors have suggested that T strain mycoplasma, both *Ureaplasma urealyticum* and *Mycoplasma hominis,* can cause abortion. Data indicating that the first organism is a cause of abortion are stronger than for the latter. Stray-Pedersen and colleagues found that although the incidence of cervical colonization of *U. urealyticum* was similar in a group of women with recurrent abortion and controls, the incidence of endometrial colonization was significantly more common (28%) in the group with recurrent abortions than in the control group (7%). In this study the cultures were obtained at least 6 months after the last abortion, and there were no clinical or laboratory signs of infection in any of the women. These investigators could not correlate the presence of *M. hominis* in the uterus with an increased frequency of abortion. Stray-Pedersen and Stray-Pedersen reported that eradication of *U. urealyticum* in the endometrium by tetracycline treatment for 10 days resulted in a significantly lower subsequent abortion rate (19%). However, there are no randomized placebo-controlled clinical trials to prove that these organisms cause abortion and that treatment is effective. The parasite *Toxoplasma gondii* may infect the embryo and cause an abortion. However, it is difficult to document the presence of this organism before abortion occurs because there is a lack of correlation between serologic immunoassays for this organism and its detection in the endometrium by immunofluorescence.

Many viral agents may cause abortion if acquired as a primary infection in the first trimester; however, secondary infection does not cause pregnancy loss. Parvovirus B-19 may be embryotoxic in the first trimester, but is not a cause of recurrent loss. Similarly, infection from varicella, cytomegalovirus, and rubella may cause miscarriage, but are not a cause of recurrent loss. Primary infection with herpes simplex virus in the genital tract has been reported to cause abortion. Nahmias and coworkers reported that if genital herpes initially occurred in the first half of pregnancy, the abortion rate was about 34%. If pregnancy occurred within 18 months after initial detection of herpes infection, the abortion rate was 55%. Both these rates were significantly higher than the 11.5% abortion rate in the control population. Recurrent infection with herpes simplex does not cause loss.

ENVIRONMENTAL FACTORS

Smoking

In a retrospective study Kline and associates reported that women who smoked during pregnancy had a significantly greater chance of having a spontaneous abortion than did a control group (Table 16-10). For women who smoked more than 14 cigarettes per day the risk of having an abortion was 1.7 times greater than for women who did not smoke, but smoking less than this amount did not result in a significantly greater incidence of abortion. These investigators found that heavy smokers had an increased risk of aborting chromosomally normal embryos only. There was no increased risk of an aneuploid abortion in smokers. These data indicate that smoking acts as a toxic agent to destroy chromosomally normal fetuses.

Alcohol

Kline and associates also reported that drinking alcohol, acting independently from smoking, was a risk factor for abortion (Table 16-11). Women who drank alcohol at least 2 days a week had about a twofold greater risk of having an abortion than women who did not drink during pregnancy, with the risk increasing to threefold with daily ingestion of alcohol. As with smoking, an increased risk of abortion was confined to chromosomally normal embryos, indicating that drinking alcohol, like smoking, can act as a toxic agent on the normal embryo to cause its death. Harlap and Shiono found that even moderate drinking of alcohol increased the risk of second-, but not first-trimester pregnancy loss, confirming the toxic effect of alcohol on the embryo.

Coffee and Caffeine

Some epidemiologic data suggest that caffeine may be an independent risk factor for abortion. Because there may be a causal relation between these agents and abortion, women who become pregnant should limit their intake of caffeine. Recent studies suggest a threshold effect with more than two cups of coffee, or a 12-ounce cola drink. The risk of pregnancy loss increases beyond this limit.

Table 16-11 Frequency (%) of Alcohol Consumption Among Women Experiencing Spontaneous Abortions (Cases) and Women Delivering at 28 Weeks' Gestation or Later (Controls)

Frequency of Alcohol Consumption During Pregnancy	PERCENTAGE DISTRIBUTION						
	Cases		Controls		Adjusted Odds Ratio		95% Confidence Interval
Never	42.6		43.7		1.00		0.59–0.99
Twice a month and less	28.9		38.0		0.77		0.71–1.52
Less than twice a month	10.8	17.9	10.4	7.9	1.04	2.36	1.30–2.95
2–6 days a week	13.3		6.5		1.96		
Daily	4.5		1.4		3.00		1.39–6.49
Total	648						645

From Kline J, Stein Z, Susser M, et al: Environmental influences on early reproductive loss in a current New York City study. In Porter IH, Hook EB (eds): Human Embryonic and Fetal Death. New York, Academic Press, 1980.

Irradiation and Magnetic Fields

Animal studies have shown that ionizing radiation can produce congenital malformation, growth retardation, and embryonic death. These effects are dose-related, and there is a threshold dose below which an adverse effect does not occur. Although there is evidence in the human that high-energy radiation exposure is associated with teratogenic effects and growth retardation, there is no conclusive evidence that similar exposure increases the risk of spontaneous abortion.

Extrapolation from animal data indicates that the embryo is most sensitive to the lethal effect of irradiation during the day of implantation and a few days later (Table 16-12). The sensitivity decreases during the period of early embryogenesis, after which the minimum lethal dose (MLD) remains constant to term gestation. Brent reported that the MLD of irradiation to rats is 5 rads on the day of implantation. These data thus indicate that there is little likelihood that irradiation of less than 5 rads (severalfold greater than the amount used in nearly all diagnostic procedures) will cause an abortion in the human, even if it is administered during the time of implantation. Even exposures greater than 5 rads rarely causes pregnancy loss.

Table 16-10 Frequency (%) of Smoking Among Women Experiencing Spontaneous Abortions (Cases) and Women Delivering at 28 Weeks' Gestation or Later (Controls)

Number of Cigarettes Per Day	PERCENTAGE DISTRIBUTION				Adjusted Odds Ratio		95% Confidence Interval
	Cases		Controls				
None	62.0	37.9	69.8		1.00	1.28	—
1–13	20.5		20.5		1.07		0.80–1.42
14–80	17.4		10.2	30.2	1.73		1.23–2.43
Total	648		645				

From Kline J, Stein Z, Susser M, et al: Environmental influences on early reproductive loss in a current New York City study. In Porter IH, Hook EB (eds): Human Embryonic and Fetal Death. New York, Academic Press, 1980.

Table 16-12 Estimation of Abortigenic Hazards of X-Irradiation to Human Embryo from Animal Experiments

Stage of Human Gestation (Days)	Lethal Dose/50 (Rads)	MLD (Rads)
1	70–100	10
14	140	25
18	150	25
28	220	50
50	260	50
Late fetus to term	300–400	50

MLD, minimum lethal dose.
From Brent RL: Radiation-induced embryonic and fetal loss from conception to birth. In Porter IH, Hook EB (eds): Human Embryonic and Fetal Death. New York, Academic Press, 1980.

Exposure to magnetic fields induced by electric currents has not been associated with a significantly higher rate of miscarriage. Video display terminals and electric blankets are not harmful to a pregnancy.

Environmental Toxins

Though little valid information exists concerning the effect of environmental toxins on human abortion, several agents are deleterious, and recommendations are to avoid contact. Some, but not all, studies have shown an increased risk of abortion among women occupationally exposed to anesthetic gases. Most studies reporting such a relation are retrospective questionnaire studies of marginal validity. A well-done case-control study by Axelsson and Rylander indicated that the incidence of abortion in women exposed to anesthetic gases was not significantly increased. However, current practice is to adequately ventilate gases in hospitals and physician's and dental offices. Women exposed to anesthetic gases in veterinary offices should inquire about ventilation. Women exposed to chemotherapeutic agents, such as nurses and pharmacy technicians, may have an increased risk of miscarriage.

Information concerning a possible abortifacient effect after increased exposure to other environmental toxins is even less clear. Vianna and Polan reported that the entire population of women exposed to toxic chemical wastes in the Love Canal, New York, area had no significant excess of spontaneous abortions, although groups of women living in certain areas with a higher exposure may have had an increased risk of abortion. Heavy metals, lead, cadmium, mercury, and arsenic are embryotoxic. Women who drink well water and miscarry may have their water analyzed for inorganic content. Organic solvents, particularly those used in the computer industry are particularly worrisome. Organic pesticides are also well-known toxins.

Stress and Depression

Severe stress is a well-documented cause of pregnancy loss in the animal model, and anecdotally stress has been associated with pregnancy loss in humans. Older literature, from 75 to 150 years ago, proposed that emotional stress led to adverse pregnancy outcomes. Severe stress may lead to a higher incidence of late pregnancy outcomes, affecting uteroplacental function in some cases. However, stress has not been associated with early pregnancy loss. Women who receive counseling for depression associated with recurrent loss seem to have a higher successful pregnancy rate. Sugiura-Ogasawara and colleagues prospectively evaluated women with a psychological assessment for depression who had experienced two consecutive first-trimester losses. Depression was associated with a greater frequency of subsequent miscarriage. The interaction between stress, depression, and pregnancy outcome is complex. Currently, the relationship with pregnancy loss is equivocal at best.

DIAGNOSIS

Miscarriage is ultimately diagnosed through confirmation of a nonviable gestation. The types of abortion were originally described by the appearance of the patient when she presented to the physician. They include (1) threatened—bleeding with a viable pregnancy, (2) missed—nonviable intrauterine gestation less than 20 weeks with the cervical os closed; (3) incomplete—intrauterine gestation less than 20 weeks with the os open and some tissue already passed; (4) inevitable—if the cervix is open but no tissue is passed. (This is a misnomer, because in some circumstances a cerclage can be placed.); and (5) complete spontaneous abortion—passage of all the tissue and an empty uterus.

The diagnosis of abortion in any of these manifestations is made by physical examination usually augmented with ultrasound and HCG values. Throughout the assessment, the physician must give the highest levels of care and concern to the woman. The diagnostic time period is filled with intense anxiety. The caregiver's attitudes are often the most pronounced memory that the patient and her family take away from the experience.

In a healthy pregnancy, in early gestation, the HCG levels should rise in a predictable fashion. Levels may rise to 100,000 IU by week 10, and then fall. The proportionate rate of increase is most pronounced in the first 6 weeks' gestation, and then the rise is less rapid. Barnhart and coworkers performed a longitudinal evaluation of HCG levels. Of 861 observations in 287 subjects, HCG increased a mean of 50% in 24 hours, and 124% in 48 hours. In their study, the minimal increase for a viable pregnancy was 24% for a 24-hour period and 53% in 48 hours. The largest increase was 81%, and 330% at 24 and 48 hours, respectively. At a certain point, a viable pregnancy should be visualized by ultrasound in the uterus. The HCG at this point is called the "discriminatory zone," and approximates 1500 IU. After a level of 5000 IU ultrasound may be used without HCG levels for assessment of viability. A clinical caveat: conception is not always 14 days after the last menstrual period. Since conception is the variable, not last menstrual period, all worrisome ultrasounds should be reconfirmed 1 week later.

The first sonographic finding of a pregnancy is the gestational sac (Table 16-13). As Goldstein has stated this is a sonographic term, not a true anatomic delineation. The sac is an echolucent area in the uterus surrounded by echodense-

Table 16-13 Ultrasound Findings in Early Pregnancy

Ultrasound Findings	Gestational Age from LMP (days)	Approximate HCG (IU)	Approximate Risk of Miscarraige*
Gestational sac	23–29	1500	<12%
Yolk sac	32–45	5000	<9%†
Embryonic disk	35–45		<8%
Fetal cardiac activity	42 with CRL > 5 mm	13000–15000	<8%
Embryo 2 cm with heart rate	56		<2%

*If no vaginal bleeding.
†If the gestational sac is 10 mm.
CRL, crown–rump length; HCG, human chorionic gonadotropin; LMP, last menstrual period.

reactive endometrium (decidualized endometrium; Fig. 16-9). Intrauterine lucencies may be first visualized as early as 3 weeks after the last menstrual period, 1 week after conception, and may represent purely fluid in the secretory phase. In the interior of the sac is the developing fluid-filled chorionic sac. With visualization of the chorionic sac with secondary echoes, a true gestational sac may be defined. If the fluid is endometrial secretions it is considered a pseudogestational sac. The first fetal structure that may be visualized on ultrasound is the yolk sac (Fig. 16-10).

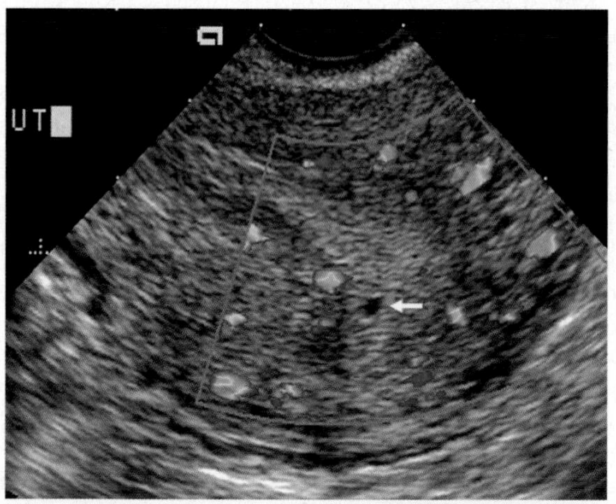

A

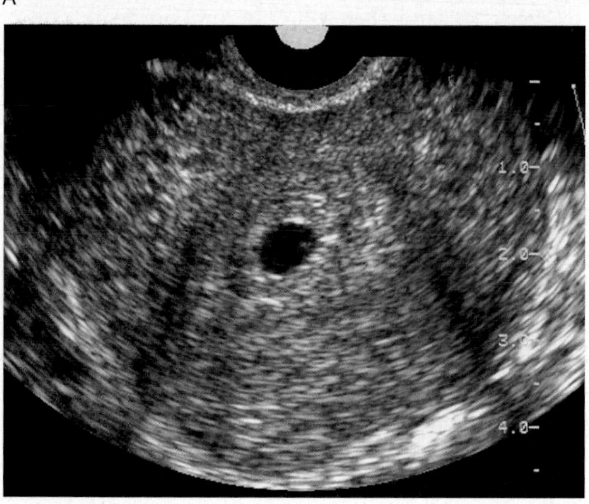

B

Figure 16-9. **A,** Ultrasound at 33 weeks with small sac *(arrow).* **B,** Endovaginal ultrasound 6 days later of a gestational sac, with mildly increased decidual reaction surrounding the echolucent sac, UT, uterus. (From Lyons EA, Levi CS, Dashefsky SM: The first trimester. In Rumack CM, Wilson SR, Charboneau JW [eds]: Diagnostic Ultrasound, 2nd ed. St. Louis, Mosby, 1998.)

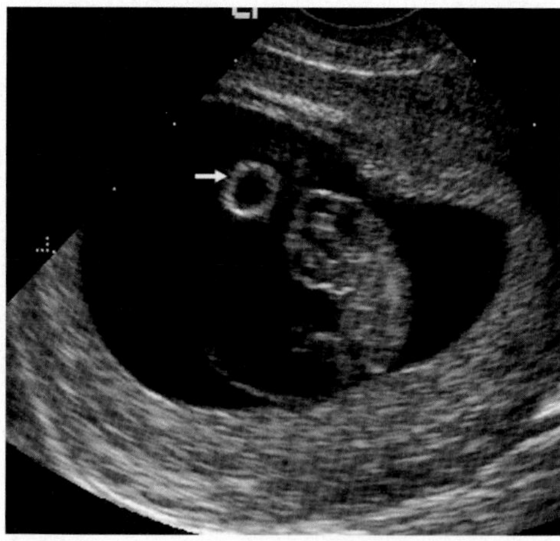

Figure 16-10. Normal yolk sac in a 9-week embryo. Arrow points to yolk sac. (From Lyons EA, Levi CS, Dashefsky SM: The first trimester. In Rumack CM, Wilson SR, Charboneau JW [eds]: Diagnostic Ultrasound, 2nd ed. St. Louis, Mosby, 1998.)

A distorted or large yolk sac is associated with pregnancy loss. The yolk sac should be seen within 1 week of visualization of the gestational sac and when the yolk sac is 1 cm in diameter.

The embryonic disk is notable as a thickening on the yolk sac as early as a few days after the yolk sac appears. An embryonic disk should be visualized by approximately 5 to 6 weeks' gestational age. Cardiac activity should be seen a few days afterward, and any time the embryo is greater than 1 cm in length. When the HCG concentration is more than 13,000 mIU/mL, the gestational sac should be more than 18 mm in diameter and an embryo with embryonic heart activity should be visualized in a normal gestation. If the gestational sac is more than 18 mm in diameter and no embryo is seen, an anembryonic gestation is present (Fig. 16-11). The earliest cardiac activity has been noted is 5 weeks after the last menstrual period in a 28-day cycle. Cardiac activity should always be noted by 6 weeks (4 weeks after conception). Initially, the fetal heart rate should be in the 80 to 110 beats per minute (bpm) range, and will then often increase into the 180 to 220 bpm range for the first few months of pregnancy, but by 12 weeks should return to 110-160 bpm.

If any findings are equivocal, whether gestational sac, yolk sac, or cardiac activity, the exam should be repeated most often in 1 week. Occasionally couples will request rechecking within a shorter time period. For an embryo larger than 1.5 to 2 cm, if there is no heart beat in 48 hours, it may be adequate to reevaluate in a shorter time. For gestational sacs without embryonic poles, 1 week is preferable.

Several sonographic parameters found in an early gestation are predicators of a viable birth. If embryonic heart activity is seen at 6 weeks' gestational age, the chance of spontaneous abortion is about 7%. If heart activity is still present after 8 weeks' gestation, the chance of spontaneous abortion falls to about 2%. Several studies have noted that an abnormal heart

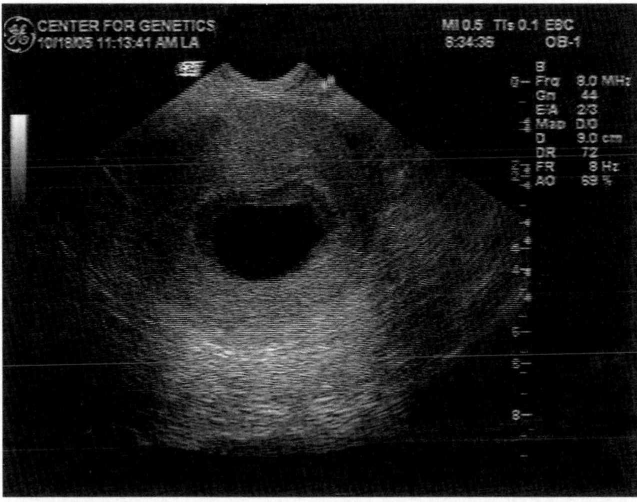

Figure 16-11. Anembryonic gestation in an 8-week pregnancy—empty sac. This has also been referred to as a blighted ovum, although the term is a misnomer.

rate, either above or below the expected rate for a gestational age, is a finding associated with a poor outcome.

Sonographic predictors of viable birth have less prognostic value among couples with recurrent spontaneous abortion because the pregnancy loss in those instances is more likely due to maternal disorders instead of problems with the gestation. Opsahl and Pettit and Stern and Coulam have reported that in contrast to the 7% abortion rate found after embryonic heart activity in all gestations when embryonic heart activity was seen in early gestation, among women with recurrent abortion the subsequent abortion rate was between 22% and 30%. Opsahl and Pettit also reported that if the difference in diameter between the gestational sac and crown–rump length was more than 8 mm in normal gestations, the spontaneous abortion rate was only 5%, but among women with recurrent abortion, the spontaneous abortion rate was 20%.

Threatened Abortion

It has been estimated that bleeding occurs during the first 20 weeks of pregnancy in about 30% to –40% of human gestations, with about half of these pregnancies ending in spontaneous abortion. The risk of abortion is greater among those women who bleed for 3 or more days (24%) than among those who bleed only 1 or 2 days (7%). Women with gestational bleeding who do not abort have a minimally increased incidence of complications of pregnancy, including a slightly increased incidence of fetal anomalies and preterm birth. To determine the prognosis of the pregnancy in a woman with threatened abortion, ultrasound is the primary diagnostic modality.

The sonogram of women who present with bleeding in the first trimester may demonstrate a lucency behind the brighter placental disk. Such anomalies can be seen in 20% of women with threatened miscarriage. Subchorionic hematoma have minimal clinical significance, and most women may be assured that things will most likely continue as long as the heart rate appears appropriate.

There have been several reports of ultrasonographic studies of groups of women with threatened abortion. In about two thirds of such pregnancies a live fetus is present, and about 85% of these fetuses subsequently are delivered and survive. Of the one third of women with a threatened abortion who do not have a live fetus present, about half have an anembryonic gestation, with the remainder being about equally divided between embryonic death and incomplete abortion, with an occasional molar gestation. Siddiqi and colleagues reported that even if embryonic heart activity is visualized early in gestation, the risk of the pregnancy ending in spontaneous abortion was increased about threefold if uterine bleeding occurred, from 5% without bleeding to 16% with bleeding.

In a patient bleeding during the first half of pregnancy the diagnosis of inevitable abortion is strengthened if the bleeding is profuse and associated with uterine cramping pains. Women with threatened abortion who do not abort usually do not have cramps.

Missed Abortion

The diagnosis of missed abortion is suspected clinically when the uterus fails to continue to enlarge with or without uterine bleeding or spotting. Typically after an episode of bleeding subsides, a continuous brown vaginal discharge is noted. When a dead fetus is retained in the uterus beyond 5 weeks after fetal death, consumptive coagulability with resultant hypofibrogenemia may occur. This condition is self-limited, resolving in 1 to 2 weeks. The incidence of this condition is correlated with both the length of gestation and the duration of fetal death: It is uncommon in gestations of less than 16 to 18 weeks. With the use of ultrasonography the term *missed abortion* is less relevant because the diagnosis of anembryonic gestation or fetal death can be easily determined without delay.

Septic Abortion

Infection occurs in about 1% to 2% of all spontaneous abortions, with the incidence increasing if the abortion has been induced by a nonsterilized instrument. All women with uterine bleeding or spotting during the first half of pregnancy accompanied by clinical signs of infection must be considered to have a septic abortion if no obvious source of infection outside the genital tract is evident.

Septic abortions can be threatened, inevitable, or incomplete. The infection frequently spreads from the endometrium through the myometrium to the parametrium and sometimes to the peritoneum. Thus, in addition to endometritis, parametritis and peritonitis frequently occur in women with septic abortions. In addition to an elevated temperature and leukocytosis, lower abdominal tenderness, cervical motion tenderness, and a foul uterine discharge are signs of septic abortion. The cause of the infection is usually polymicrobial, with *Escherichia coli* and other aerobic gram-negative rods frequently involved. Group B β-hemolytic streptococci, anaerobic streptococci, *Bacteroides* sp., and on occasion *Clostridium perfringens* are other organisms that can cause septic abortion. Because endotoxins can be released from the gram-negative bacilli, endotoxic shock may accompany septic abortion, particularly if it is caused by insertion of nonsterile agents into the uterine cavity.

TREATMENT

Threatened Abortion

Although some physicians recommend that women with threatened abortion restrict their physical activities or stay at bed rest, there is no evidence that these measures or any active medical therapy improves the prognosis of threatened abortion. Nevertheless, restriction of excessive physical activity and avoidance of coitus is commonly suggested until the bleeding ceases Women should be advised that such measures are primarily for comfort, not for true prevention. Treatment with natural progesterone, synthetic progestins, or HCG was previously advocated, but there is no evidence that such therapy improves the prognosis. Because such treatment may increase the probability of having a missed abortion, the use of this or any type of hormonal therapy is contraindicated. If the woman is Rh negative, Rh immune globulin should be given.

If bleeding increases, and is accompanied by uterine cramps, it is likely that the abortion is becoming inevitable and the woman should be examined in a medical facility. Uterine sonography will often aid in predicting the outcome. Once an intrauterine gestation is verified, serial HCG values have minimal value in management.

When the diagnosis of a nonviable pregnancy is made, a thorough discussion with the patient and her support person should be undertaken. If a photograph of the ultrasound can be obtained, it should be offered. The patient's medical history, social history, and physical examination should be obtained. Several factors from the history and physical will influence the next steps in management. The decision of how to proceed further is not only part of the management of the products of conception, but is also the first step in grieving and resolution. A patient's personal feelings about the pregnancy, as well as her cultural preferences will influence whether she chooses an immediate dilation and curettage, expectant management, or opts for medical therapy. If there is no evidence of infection and no medical risk factors, such as cardiac disease, all three options may be acceptable.

Some couples will request combinations of expectant management with an endpoint at which if there has not been passage of tissue, the woman will have a uterine evacuation. Multiple studies, from several countries, have compared expectant, surgical, and medical management. None of the three options is superior. Surgical complications such as perforation are obviously increased with dilation and curettage. However, heavy bleeding has been shown in some studies to occur more commonly with expectant management. Most all studies document that if women are given the choice of how to deal with the miscarriage, her psychological health is improved. Older texts from the 1940s through the mid 1990s recommend surgical evacuation due to theoretical risks of infection and bleeding. These issues are not as much of a problem currently, for most patients.

Studies of expectant management show that 50% to 70% of women will initially elect to wait for spontaneous miscarriage after a diagnosis of a missed abortion has been confirmed. In cases of incomplete abortion, up to 95% of women will complete the abortion spontaneously. For a missed abortion, 25% to 85% of women will complete the abortion spontaneously within 2 weeks. de Waard and colleagues noted that 37% of women aborted within 7 days. They recommend offering intervention at 7 to 14 days in women who choose expectant management. In their evaluation of 136 women, they found strong preferences by women for whatever choice that woman might make. When expectant management is elected, the patient should be given warnings about infection and severe bleeding, and a return appointment should be made for 10 to 14 days later.

Protocols for medical management commonly employ the prostaglandin E1 analogue, misoprostol. Most patients (80% to 95%) will completely pass an early or mid first-trimester pregnancy loss after one to two doses. Longer gestations are associated with higher rates of incomplete passage, necessitating a sharp curettage. Misoprostol is given orally or vaginally. The vaginal route is preferable, because serum levels peak and drop quickly with an oral route of administration. With vaginal application, serum levels remain higher for a longer period of time. Importantly, gastrointestinal side effects, including nausea, vomiting, and diarrhea, are more common with oral administration. 600 μg every 12 hours for four doses is most commonly prescribed. Barnhart and coworkers, evaluated HCG and progesterone levels in women with pregnancies that aborted prior to 11 weeks who had chosen medical management with E1. The investigators found, as would be expected, that the absolute levels of HCG and progesterone were not related to the success of medical management. Rather, a drop of 80% over the first 48 hours in hormone levels was associated with a 90% success. These authors used 800 μg of E1 To date, no dosing protocol has been noted superior for medical management of abortion. Many clinicians offer a pretreatment dose of an antiemetic.

Several studies including that by Chung and associates have shown that evacuation of retained products of conception after an incomplete abortion can be accomplished with the use of misoprostol. Thus curettage or vacuum aspiration is not needed. Mifepristone given 24 to 48 hours prior to misoprostol will increase successful passage of a fetus that is 9 to 14 weeks' gestation. Unfortunately, this medication is often difficult to obtain.

Recommendations for surgical versus medical management should be based partially on the size of the intrauterine contents. Many 9- to 10-week pregnancies by gestational age may be only 6 to 8 weeks by size, after ultrasound evaluation. A pregnancy of 11 or more weeks' gestation that presents as a missed or incomplete miscarriage is best handled surgically, because of the increased bleeding. Practitioners skilled in surgical uterine evacuation may perform dilation and evacuation up to 20 weeks. Those practitioners less experienced in uterine surgical evacuation of a second-trimester gestation, may opt for induction of labor. Prostaglandin E1 is used in an inpatient setting for patients with larger uteri with older gestation pregnancies. Prostaglandin E1, 600 to 800 μg, is administered every 8 to 12 hours. Cervical ripening prior to induction is helpful. Adequate analgesia in these situations is essential.

In all cases of intervention, medical or surgical, prophylactic antibiotics should be considered for patients with cardiac indications. Additionally, women with bacterial vaginosis would receive antibiotics with anaerobic coverage. For the patient with an incomplete abortion and signs of infection, perioperative broad-spectrum antibiotics should be given. Rh immune globulin also should be given to all Rh-negative women.

In the treatment of incomplete abortion with surgical evacuation, deep curettage should be avoided to prevent the subsequent development of uterine adhesions. After the procedure the vital signs and amount of vaginal bleeding should be monitored, after which the woman may be discharged home to remain at rest for 24 hours and avoid intercourse for 2 weeks. Oral ergonovine maleate, 0.2 mg, may be administered every 6 hours for 1 to 2 days. If necessary, iron sulfate, 300 mg, should be administered until hemoglobin levels return to normal and tissue iron stores are replenished.

Septic Abortion

Septic abortion is a potentially fatal condition, with an estimated fatality rate of 0.4 to 0.6/100,000 spontaneous abortions. All women with the diagnosis of septic abortion should have a complete blood count, urinalysis, chemistry, and electrolyte panel obtained. In addition, a specimen of the uterine discharge should be sent to the laboratory for culture and sensitivity. A Gram stain of the discharge may be performed in the admitting area. If the woman is seriously ill, blood cultures, a chest radiograph, and tests of blood coagulability should be obtained. Antibiotics should be administered intravenously, and the uterine contents evacuated. It is best to use broad-spectrum antibiotic therapy, including an agent that will be effective against anaerobic bacteria. After adequate blood levels of antibiotics are obtained, usually within 2 hours, the uterus should be evacuated as described previously.

If the uterus is larger than 14 weeks' gestation and the cervix is closed (threatened septic abortion), management is more difficult. The uterine cavity needs to be evacuated to provide drainage of the infected material. This can be performed by curettage, dilation and evacuation, or through the administration of oxytocics or prostaglandins. Sometimes it is necessary to perform a hysterectomy if the sepsis is severe and the uterus cannot be evacuated through the cervical canal. All women with septic abortions need to be closely monitored for stability of vital signs and urinary output. If signs of septic shock should develop, a central venous pressure catheter should be placed and additional cardiorespiratory support provided.

Follow-Up Care

An essential aspect of the care of women with spontaneous miscarriage is the follow-up visit. At this time the patient should be asked open-ended questions about her experience and thoughts. Multiple studies have noted patient's anger and difficulty with the health care system during the time of a miscarriage. Dealing with those frustrations will improve interactions in the future and may also decrease the risk of depression after the loss. Grieving and depression are significant issues after miscarriage. Open-ended questions are the best way to assess a patient's mood and status. Many women experience guilt after miscarriage, believing that the loss was something that they caused by some action that they performed. Counseling regarding this guilt is quite important. The guilt is sometimes brought on by ambivalence, since miscarriage often occurs during the time when the woman is unsure about the pregnancy. Grieving is quite normal, and should never be dismissed with rationalizations such as, "it is for the best" or "you can always get pregnant again." One study found that 80% of women had some guilt associated with a particular act or habit that is perceived as causing the miscarriage. These issues should be addressed. In addition, an investigation into the cause of miscarriage, whether productive or not, decreases the feelings of self-blame and guilt. Some women develop physical symptomatology with grieving that may mimic symptoms of depression, such as fatigue, anorexia, sleeplessness, and sometimes somatic symptoms such as headache and back pain.

As many as 30% of women will suffer from depression after miscarriage. If symptoms of depression are apparent, then counseling and therapy with antidepressants should be pursued. A study by Craig and colleagues found that 7.4% of women with recurrent miscarriage were suffering from severe depression. Thirty-three percent had some aspects of clinical depression and anxiety, and greater than 50% had psychological symptoms that warranted a diagnosis. Treatment for depression is often given for 6 months, with patient reassurance. Even without symptoms of depression the patient should be advised that if such symptoms develop she and her family should return. Staff should be advised that when patients call for advice after a miscarriage they might be calling with a disguised plea for help. Open-ended questions, such as "are things going as you expected?" are helpful in assessing a patient's mental state. Any unusual answer should prompt a request for the patient to come in to the office.

Five percent to 20% of women may develop transient symptoms of thyroid disease after a pregnancy loss. These women have a risk of thyroid disease over the next 5 years. The symptoms should be treated with thyroid replacement for low thyroid, and antithyroid medications for hyperthyroid symptoms. Treatment is usually continued for 6 to 9 months, at which point the patient is reevaluated. A free thyroxine level should be obtained.

Also, at the follow-up visit an assessment is given as to potential causes of miscarriage and possible explanations. Any testing can be ordered after two or more miscarriages. Workup is initiated for a cause of recurrent loss. Nikcevic and coworkers noted that an investigation into the cause of the miscarriage decreased the incidence of self-blame.

Future pregnancy planning is also discussed at this visit. Most couples will have resumed sexual activity. If another pregnancy is not desired prior to a year, hormonal-based contraception may be given if appropriate. If pregnancy is desired in less than a year, then barrier methods may be preferable since it is preferable to have two or three normal cycles before trying to conceive again. Couples should wait for 3 to 6 months after a pregnancy before trying to conceive again, as some literature has suggested a slightly increased risk of early miscarriage with short interpregnancy intervals.

Assessment of general health needs are also performed at this time, including such issues as Pap smear, a mammogram if necessary, iron supplementation, vaccines, and other age-appropriate issues.

RECURRENT MISCARRIAGE

Recurrent miscarriage has been defined as three spontaneous losses. The calculated probability of a woman's having three consecutive spontaneous abortions is about 0.3% to 0.4%, but the actual incidence is reported to range from 2% to 5% of couples. Approximately 60% of the time, a cause for the recurrent losses can be determined.

The abortuses of women who have three or more abortions are more likely to be chromosomally normal (80% to 90%) than those of women with a single spontaneous abortion. Women with recurrent abortions also have a tendency to abort later in gestation, indicating that maternal or environmental factors are a more likely cause of repeated pregnancy loss. Recurrent abortion has been called *habitual abortion.* As well as being pejorative, this term implies that every subsequent pregnancy in these women will end in an abortion; therefore, *recurrent miscarriage* is now the preferred term. Clifford and associates reported the pregnancy outcome of 201 women with a history of unexplained recurrent abortion who received no pharmacologic therapy for the subsequent pregnancy. The abortion rate in the subsequent pregnancy was 29% and 27% for those with three or four prior abortions, respectively, and 44% and 53% for those with five or six or more prior abortions, respectively. Overall nearly 70% of the women had a viable birth in their subsequent pregnancy without treatment. Brigham and colleagues followed 325 couples with recurrent loss in which thrombophilia and other causes had been excluded. They found that 75% of couples had a successful outcome in the subsequent pregnancy. One conclusion that falls out from such studies is that any potential therapeutic agents should have a placebo control arm to determine true efficacy.

Couples with recurrent abortion require careful, sympathetic care by the practitioner. Psychological counseling is often beneficial. Patients with recurrent loss suffer what has been termed *strain trauma.* The trauma of a single loss produces an emotional shock that is usually healed with grieving. Avoidance behaviors of activities and associations, such as the physician's office, are employed as defenses. However, in situations of repetitive emotional shocks, a strain trauma may develop in which the woman or the couple not only grieve each loss, but are constantly afraid of the pain of a new loss. For many women with recurrent miscarriage, this emotional trauma is magnified because they feel helpless to prevent a recurrence. The practitioner needs to express sympathy and continued understanding as counseling is performed and a diagnostic regimen is outlined. The practitioner's staff needs to be attuned to theses issues as well.

There is no need to wait for a woman to have three first-trimester abortions with their accompanying emotional trauma before beginning a diagnostic evaluation. Because one early abortion is relatively common, it is recommended that diagnostic evaluation be initiated after a woman has had two first-trimester abortions. Not uncommonly a history may elicit a particular line of investigation that should be initiated even after one loss. If a pregnancy loss occurs in the second trimester, the cause is more likely to recur. Thus a diagnostic evaluation should be considered after a woman has had only one second-trimester loss.

The evaluation for women with recurrent miscarriage starts with a history and physical examination with pertinent questions regarding cervical incompetence, abnormal exposures, gastrointestinal diseases, family history of miscarriages or birth defects, a family history of unusual thrombosis, and open-ended questions that explore the patient's ideas about causation. Laboratory evaluation should be pointed toward clues from the history. Any history suggestive of thyroid disease may prompt studies for a thyroid-stimulating hormone (TSH) and antithyroid antibodies. Other studies should include a thrombophilia profile, a complete blood count, evaluation for PCOS. If all these tests are normal an evaluation of the uterine cavity by hysterogram, sonohysterography, or hysteroscopy should be considered. Keltz an coworkers and other investigators, have reported that sonohysterography is a very sensitive, specific, and accurate screening method for assessing abnormalities in the uterine cavity of women with recurrent miscarriage. If no abnormalities are found, a karyotype of the husband and wife should be performed after three miscarriages to determine if a chromosomal anomaly exists. It is not necessary to obtain endometrial bacteriologic cultures or perform HLA typing of the woman and her partner.

If any of these tests reveals an abnormality that can be corrected with appropriate surgical or medical therapy as described, such therapy should be initiated. If a chromosomal abnormality is found, genetic counseling is indicated. Some individuals recommend that prophylactic antibiotic treatment be given to the woman and her partner in the conception cycle or that progesterone supplementation be given to all women with recurrent abortion in the first trimester of pregnancy. Neither of these modalities has been demonstrated to improve the outcome of the pregnancy.

If no diagnosis is obtained, the couple should be counseled regarding the probability of abortion in a subsequent pregnancy as described earlier. Pelvic sonography should be performed initially after HCG levels reach 1500 mIU/mL, at which time a gestational sac should be visualized. The sonogram should be repeated 2 weeks later, when an embryo with normal cardiac activity should be seen. These findings are reassuring, both to the woman and to the clinician, but are of less prognostic value to couples with recurrent abortion than to the rest of the population.

Three studies have demonstrated that extensive counseling and emotional support throughout early gestation results in significantly greater live birth rates than when only routine care is given. Stray-Pederson and Stray-Pederson reported that when a group of women with a history of unexplained recurrent abortion were given extensive antenatal counseling and psychological support, the live birth rate was 86%. Liddell and colleagues also reported that when a program of focused emotional support and close supervision was given to a group of 42 women with unexplained recurrent abortion, the live birth rate was 86%. Clifford and associates reported that women with unexplained recurrent miscarriage given supportive care early in pregnancy had a 74% viable birth rate without other therapy. When only routine antenatal care was given to a similar group of women, the live birth rate in these three reports was between 33% and 51%, significantly less. Thus, intensive psychological support during early pregnancy appears to be very beneficial for improving the prognosis of couples with recurrent abortion whose cause remains undetermined.

If a woman does abort, she should be offered cytogenetic evaluation of the conceptus and pathologic examination of the deciduas and placenta. These findings will be informative about the cause of the loss and may direct further management. For example, if pronounced placental vasculopathy is noted, a more extensive workup for the less common thrombophilias could be undertaken. In any case, the possibility of having an explanation is a tool in dealing with the grief of repetitive losses.

KEY POINTS

- About 15% to 20% of all human pregnancies end in a clinically recognized miscarriage.
- In the human, the total embryonic loss before 12 weeks' gestation is about 30%.
- About 80% of abortions occur in the first trimester, with the incidence decreasing with increasing gestational age.
- If embryonic cardiac activity is seen sonographically at 6 weeks' gestation, then the subsequent abortion rate is about 6% to 8%. If the embryo is viable at 8 weeks, then the subsequent abortion rate is only about 2% 3%.
- The risk of a pregnancy terminating in spontaneous abortion increases independently with increasing parity, maternal age, and paternal age.
- The risk of abortion occurring when embryonic heart activity is seen early in pregnancy is increased if uterine bleeding is present and when the maternal age is over 35. Women with multiple abortions have a tendency to abort at about the same gestational age.
- For a woman with a reproductive history of three pregnancies terminating in abortion with no live births, her chance of having an abortion in a subsequent pregnancy is about 50%; if she has had at least one live birth and three spontaneous abortions, the chance that her next pregnancy will terminate in abortion is only about 30%.
- The major cause of abortion is chromosomal. The incidence of chromosomal anomalies in abortuses is about 50% when tissue culture is performed but is as high as 85% with direct cytogenetic analysis of chorionic villous tissue.
- Only about 5% of the abnormal karyotypes of abortuses are structural abnormalities of the chromosomes, such as translocation.
- Autosomal trisomy is the most common abnormal karyotype (50%), followed in decreasing frequency by monosomy 45,X (20%), triploidy (15%), tetraploidy (10%), and structural abnormalities (5%).
- The most common single chromosomal abnormality is monosomy 45,X.
- It is neither cost-effective nor necessary to perform HLA typing of both partners of the couple that has experienced recurrent abortions.
- Thrombophilias occur in up to 10% of the white population and may be associated with pregnancy loss.
- Lupus anticoagulant is found in about 10% of women with recurrent spontaneous abortion of undetermined cause, and anticardiolipin antibody is found in about 5% of these women.
- Karyotypes of abortuses of women who have had more than one abortion tend to be similar if the first abortus had either a normal karyotype or an autosomal trisomy.
- Maternal age is directly related to the incidence of trisomic abortions.
- Monosomy 45,X abortion is associated with a younger maternal age rather than other aneuploid or euploid abortions.
- Abortion of chromosomally normal conceptuses is found to occur later in gestation than abortion of chromosomally abnormal conceptuses does, with the peak incidence of euploid abortion being about 12 to 13 weeks of gestation; the peak incidence of aneuploid abortions is about 11 weeks.
- The incidence of chromosomally normal abortions increases markedly after a maternal age of 35, rising to more than 30% of clinically recognized conceptions after age 40.
- About 20% to 25% of women with anomalies of uterine fusion have problems with reproduction, with recurrent abortion being the most serious.
- The least common uterine anomaly, the unicornuate uterus, is associated with the greatest incidence of spontaneous abortion, about 50%.
- Women with either a septate or bicornuate uterus have a 25% to 30% incidence of spontaneous abortion.
- Women with recurrent abortion as a result of bicornuate and septate uteri have a decline in the abortion rate from about 88% to 15% after surgical correction.
- In women with an incompetent cervix the rate of fetal survival increases from about 20% to 80% after cerclage.
- Spontaneous and induced abortions cause about two thirds of intrauterine adhesions.
- Diabetes, if well controlled by diet, oral medications, or insulin, is not a cause of abortion, whereas if uncontrolled, it is a potential cause.
- PCOS has been associated with pregnancy loss.
- In women who smoke more than 14 cigarettes per day the risk of having an abortion is 1.7 times greater than in women who do not smoke.
- Smoking and drinking alcohol introduce toxic agents that can destroy chromosomally normal fetuses.
- Women who drink alcohol at least 2 days a week have about a twofold greater risk of having an abortion.
- Irradiation of less than 5 rads will not cause an abortion in the human.

Continued

KEY POINTS *Continued*

- Threatened abortion occurs in about 30% to 40% of human gestations, with only about half of these pregnancies ending in spontaneous abortion.
- The prevalence of major chromosomal abnormalities present in either partner of a couple with two or more pregnancy losses is about 3%, five to six times higher than in the general population. Abnormalities occur in the female parent about twice as frequently as the male, with balanced reciprocal translocations occurring in half of these individuals.
- About 1% of all spontaneous abortions become infected.
- The expected probability of a woman's having three consecutive abortions is about 0.3% to 0.4%, but the actual incidence is reported to range from 0.4% to 0.8%.
- The abortuses of women who have had three or more abortions are more likely to be chromosomally normal (80% to 90%) than those of women with a single spontaneous abortion.
- Women with recurrent abortions have a tendency to abort later in gestation, with two thirds of such abortions occurring beyond 12 weeks' gestation, indicating that maternal or environmental factors are a more likely cause of repeated pregnancy loss.
- A diagnostic evaluation may be considered after a woman has had only one second-trimester spontaneous abortion or two first-trimester abortions.
- In most individuals with an early abortion, levels of HCG will rise at a slower rate than normal, plateau, and then decline.
- Maternal immunization with paternal white cells has not been proven to increase the incidence of live births. This therapy has risks and should be considered to be experimental.
- Hypothyroidism has not been shown to be a cause of abortion, but women who have an abortion are more likely to have antithyroid antibodies indicative of a possible immunologic problem.
- Women with elevated follicular phase LH levels, with and without polycystic ovaries, are more likely to have an abortion than are women with normal LH levels.
- With use of the vaginal probe a gestational sac should be seen when HCG levels reach 1500 mIU/mL.
- About two thirds of pregnancies in women with threatened abortion have a live embryo or fetus present, and about 85% of these will survive.
- Three studies have shown that intensive supportive care in early pregnancy of women with recurrent spontaneous abortion yields viable pregnancy rates of 70% to 80%, significantly higher than occurs with routine prenatal care.

BIBLIOGRAPHY

Achiron R, Tadmor O, Mashiach S: Heart rate as a predictor of first-trimester spontaneous abortion after ultrasound-proven viability. Obstet Gynecol 78:330, 1991.

Al-Sebai MAH, Kingsland CR, Diver M, et al: The role of a single progesterone measurement in the diagnosis of early pregnancy failure and the prognosis of fetal viability. Br J Obstet Gynaecol 102:364, 1995.

Althuisius SM, Dekker GA, Hummel P, et al: Cervical incompetence prevention randomization cerclage trial: Emergency cerclage with bed rest versus bed rest alone, Twenty-third Annual Meeting of the Society for Maternal-Fetal Medicine, 2003.

Ankum WM, deWard, MW, Bindels, PJE: Management of spontaneous miscarriage in the first trimester: An example of putting informed shared decision making into practice. BMJ 322:1343, 2001.

Axelsson G, Rylander R: Exposure to anaesthetic gases and spontaneous abortion: Response bias in a postal questionnaire study. Int J Epidemiol 11:250, 1982.

Backos M, Rai R, Baxter N, et al: Pregnancy complications in women with recurrent miscarriage associated with antiphospholipid antibodies treated with low dose aspirin and heparin. Br J Obstet Gynaecol 106:102, 1999.

Bagratee JS, Khullar V, Regan L, et al: A randomized controlled trial comparing medical and expectant management of first trimester miscarriage. Hum Reprod 19:266, 2004.

Balasch J, Font J, Lopez-Soto A, et al: Antiphospholipid antibodies in unselected patients with repeated abortion. Hum Reprod 5:43, 1990.

Ballen AH, Tan SL, Jacobs HS: Hypersecretion of luteinising hormone: A significant cause of infertility and miscarriage. Br J Obstet Gynaecol 100:1082, 1993.

Barnes AB, Colton T, Gundersen J, et al: Fertility and outcome of pregnancy in women exposed in utero to diethylstilbestrol. N Engl J Med 302:609, 1980.

Barnhart KT, Bader T, Huang X, et al: Hormone pattern after misoprostol administration for a nonviable first-trimester gestation. Fertil Steril 81:1099, 2004.

Barnhart KT, Sammel MD, Chung K, et al: Decline of serum human chorionic gonadotropin and spontaneous complete abortion: Defining the normal curve. Am Col Obstet Gyn 104:975, 2004.

Barnhart KT, Sammel MD, Rinaudo PF, et al: Symptomatic patients with an early viable intrauterine pregnancy: HCG curves redefined. Am Col Obstet Gyn 104.1:50, 2004.

Barranger E, Gervaise A, Doumerc S, et al: Reproductive performance after hysteroscopic metroplasty in the hypoplastic uterus: A study of 29 cases. BJOC 109:1331, 2002.

Batzer FR, Schlaff S, Goldfarb AF, et al: Serial β-subunit human chorionic gonadotropin doubling time as a prognosticator of pregnancy outcome in an infertile population. Fertil Steril 35:307, 1981.

Beever CL, Stephenson MD, Penaherrera S, et al: Skewed X-chromosome inactivation is associated with trisomy in women ascertained on the basis of recurrent spontaneous abortion or chromosomally abnormal pregnancies. Am J of Hum Genet 72:399, 2003.

Bellingard V, Hedon B, Eliaou JF, et al: Immunogenetic study of couples with recurrent spontaneous abortions. Eur J Obstet Gynecol Reprod Endocrinol 60:53, 1995.

Berry CW, Brambati B, Eskes TKAB, et al: The Euro-Team early pregnancy (ETEP) protocol for recurrent miscarriage. Hum Reprod 10:1516, 1995.

Bider D, Kokia AE, Seidman DS, et al: Cervical cerclage for anomalous uteri. J Reprod Med 37:138, 1992.

Boué J, Boué A, Lazar P: Retrospective and prospective epidemiological studies of 1500 karyotyped spontaneous human abortions. Teratology 12:11, 1975.

Brenner B: Inherited thrombophilia and pregnancy loss. Best Pract Res Clin Haematol 16.2:311, 2003.

Brenner B: Thrombophilia and pregnancy loss. Thromb Res 108:197, 2003.

Brent RL: Radiation-induced embryonic and fetal loss from conception to birth. In Porter IH, Hook EB (eds): Human Embryonic and Fetal Death. New York, Academic Press, 1980.

Brigham SA, Conlon C, Farquharson RG: A longitudinal study of pregnancy outcome following idiopathic recurrent miscarriage. Hum Reprod 14.11:2868, 1999.

Bromley B, Harlow BL, Laaboda LA, Benacerraf BR: Small sac size in the first trimester: A predictor of poor fetal outcome. Radiology 178:375, 1991.
Bussen S, Steck T: Thyroid autoantibodies in euthyroid non-pregnant women with recurrent spontaneous abortions. Hum Reprod 10:2938, 1995.
Buttram VC, Gibbons WE: Müllerian anomalies: A proposed classification (an analysis of 144 cases). Fertil Steril 32:40, 1979.
Buttram VC Jr, Reiter RC: Uterine leiomyomata: Etiology, symptomatology, and management. Fertil Steril 36:433, 1981.
Cacciatore B, Tiitinen A, Stenman UH, Ylostalo P: Normal early pregnancy: Serum HCG levels and vaginal ultrasonographic findings. Br J Obstet Gynaecol 97:899, 1990.
Cahill DJ: Managing spontaneous first trimester miscarriage. BMJ 322:1315, 2001.
Carp H, Toder V, Aviram A, et al: Karyotype of the abortus in recurrent miscarriage. Fertil Steril 75.4:678, 2001.
Carp H, Feldman B, Oelsner G, et al: Parental karyotype and subsequent live births in recurrent miscarriage. Fertil Steril 81.5:1296, 2004.
Carrell DT, Wilcox AL, Lowy L, et al: Elevated sperm chromosome aneuploidy and apoptosis in patients with unexplained recurrent pregnancy loss. Am Coll Obstet Gyn 101.6:1229, 2003.
Cashner KA, Christopher CR, Dysert GA: Spontaneous fetal loss after demonstration of a live fetus in the first trimester. Obstet Gynecol 70:827, 1987.
Cervical Insufficiency. ACOG Practice Bulletin No. 48 102.5:1091, 2003.
Chaouat G: Should we re-examine the status of lymphocyte alloimmunization therapy for recurrent spontaneous abortion. AJRI 50:433, 2003.
Chipchase J, James DE: Randomised trial of expectant versus surgical management of spontaneous miscarriage. Br J Obstet Gynecol 104:840, 1997.
Christiansen OB, Mathiesen O, Husth M, et al: Prognostic significance of maternal DR histocompatibility types in Danish women with recurrent miscarriages. Hum Reprod 8:1843, 1993.
Christiansen OB, Mathiesen O, Husth M, et al: Placebo-controlled trial of active immunization with third party leukocytes in recurrent miscarriage. Acta Obstet Gynecol Scand 73:261, 1994.
Chung T, Leung P, Cheung LP, et al: A medical approach to management of spontaneous abortion using misoprostol: Extending misoprostol treatment to a maximum of 48 hours can further improve evacuation of retained products of conception in spontaneous abortion. Acta Obstet Gynecol Scand 76:248, 1997.
Chung TKH, Lee DTS, Cheung LP, et al: Spontaneous abortion: a randomized, controlled trial comparing surgical evacuation with conservative management using misoprostol. Fertil Steril 71:1054, 1999.
Clifford K, Rai R, Regan L: Future pregnancy outcome in unexplained recurrent first trimester miscarriage. Hum Reprod 12:387, 1997.
Clifford K, Rai R, Watson H, Regan L: An informative protocol for the investigation of recurrent miscarriage: Preliminary experience of 500 consecutive cases. Hum Reprod 9:1328, 1994.
Clifford K, Rai R, Watson H, et al: Does suppressing luteinising hormone secretion reduce the miscarriage rate? Results of a randomised controlled trial. BMJ 312:1508, 1995.
Condous G: The management of early pregnancy complications. Best Pract Res Clin Obstet Gynecol 18.1:37, 2004.
Copumans ABC, Huijgens PC, Jakobs C, et al: Haemostatic and metabolic abnormalities in women with unexplained recurrent abortion. Hum Reprod 14:21, 1999.
Coughlin LB, Roberts D, Haddad NG, et al: Medical management of first trimester miscarriage (blighted ovum and missed abortion): Is it effective. J Obstet Gynecol 24.1:69, 2004.
Coulam CB: Immunologic tests in the evaluation of reproductive disorders: A critical review. Am J Obstet Gynecol 167:1844, 1995.
Coulam CB, Krysa L, Stern JJ, Bustillo M: Intravenous immunoglobulin for treatment of recurrent pregnancy loss. Am J Reprod Immunol 34:333, 1995.
Cowchock FS, Reece EA, Balaban D, et al: Repeated fetal losses associated with antiphospholipid antibodies: A collaborative randomized trial comparing prednisone with low-dose heparin treatment. Am J Obstet Gynecol 166:1318, 1992.
Cowchock FS, Smith JB: Fertility among women with recurrent spontaneous abortions: The effect of paternal cell immunization treatment. Am J Reprod Immunol 33:176, 1995.
Craig LB, Ke RW, Kutteh WH: Increased prevalence of insulin resistance in women with a history of recurrent pregnancy loss. Fertil Steril 78.3:487, 2002.
Craig M, Tata P, Regan L: Psychiatric morbidity among patients with recurrent miscarriage. J Psychosom Obstet Gyn 23:157, 2002.
Crane JP, Wahl N: The role of maternal diabetes in repetitive spontaneous abortion. Fertil Steril 36:477, 1981.
Daya S, Gunby J: The recurrent miscarriage immunotherapy trialists group: the effectiveness of allogeneic leukocyte immunization in unexplained primary recurrent spontaneous abortion. Am J Reprod Immunol 32:294, 1994.
Daya S, Gunby J, Clark DA: Intravenous immunoglobulin therapy for recurrent spontaneous abortion: A meta-analysis. Am J Reprod Immunol 39:69, 1998.
De Braekeleer M, Dao TN: Cytogenetic studies in couples experiencing repeated pregnancy losses. Hum Reprod 5:519, 1990.
Deleze M, Alarcon-Segovia D, Valdes-Macho E, et al: Relationship between antiphospholipid antibodies and recurrent fetal loss in patients with systemic lupus erythematosus and apparently healthy women. J Rheumatol 16:768, 1989.
de Waard MW, Vos J, Bonsel GJ, et al: Management of miscarriage: A randomized controlled trial of expectant management versus surgical evacuation. Hum Reprod 17.9:2445, 2002.
de Waard MW, Bindels PJE, Vos J, et al: Patient preferences for expectant management versus surgical evacuation in first-trimester uncomplicated miscarriage. J Clin Epidemiol 57:167, 2004.
Dickey RP, Olar TT, Taylor SN, et al: Relationship of small gestational sac-crown-rump length differences to abortion and abortus karyotypes. Obstet Gynecol 79:554, 1992.
Dickey RP, Gasser RF, Olar TT, et al: The relationship of initial embryo crown-rump length to pregnancy outcome and abortus karyotype based on new growth curves for the 2-31 mm embryo. Hum Reprod 9:366, 1994.
Eliakim R, Sherer DM: Celiac disease: Fertility and pregnancy. Gynecol Obstet Invest 51:3, 2001.
Empson M, Lassere M, Craig JC, Scott JR: Recurrent pregnancy loss with antiphospholipid antibody: A systematic review of therapeutic trials. Obstet Gynecol 99:135, 2002.
Fadare O, Zheng W: Histologic dating of the endometrium: Accuracy, reproducibility, and practical value. Adv Anat Pathol 12:39, 2005.
Fraser EJ, Grimes DA, Schulz KF: Immunization as therapy for recurrent spontaneous abortion: a review and meta-analysis. Obstet Gynecol 82:854, 1993.
Frost M, Condon JT: The psychological sequelae of miscarriage: A critical review of the literature, Aust NZ J Psychiatry 30:54, 1996.
Glueck CJ, Wang P, Fontaine RN, et al: Plasminogen activator inhibitor activity: An independent risk factor for the high miscarriage rate during pregnancy in women with polycystic ovary syndrome. Metabolism 48.12:1589, 1999.
Goldstein P, Berrier J, Rosen S, et al: A meta-analysis of randomized control trials of progestational agents in pregnancy. Br J Obstet Gynaecol 96:265, 1989.
Goldstein SR: Embryonic ultrasonographic measurements: Crown-rump length revisited. Am J Obstet Gynecol 165:497, 1991.
Goldstein SR: Significance of cardiac activity on endovaginal ultrasound in very early embryos. Obstet Gynecol 80:670, 1992.
Goldstein SR: Embryonic death in early pregnancy: A new look at the first trimester. Obstet Gynecol 84:294, 1994.
Goldstein SR, Wolfson R: Endovaginal ultrasonographic measurement of early embryonic size as a means of assessing gestational age. J Ultrasound Med 13:27, 1994.
Goldstein SR: Sonography in early pregnancy failure. Clinical Obstet Gyn 37.3:681, 1994.
Greenland H, Ogunbiyi I, Bugg G, et al: Medical treatment of miscarriage in a district general hospital is safe and effective up to 12 weeks' gestation. Curr Med Res Opin 19.8:699, 2003.
Gudnason V, Stansbie D, Scott J, et al: C677T (thermolabile alanine/valine) polymorphism in methylenetetrahydrofolate reductase (MTHFR): Its frequency and impact on plasma homocysteine concentration in different European populations. Atherosclerosis 136:347, 1998.
Hall RCW, Beresford TP, Quinones JE: Grief following spontaneous abortion. Psychiatr Clin North Am 10:405, 1987.
Hankey GJ, Elkelboom JW: Homocysteine and vascular disease. Lancet 354:407, 1999.
Harlap S, Shiono PH: Alcohol, smoking, and incidence of spontaneous abortions in the first and second trimester. Lancet 2:173, 1980.

Heinonen PK, Saarikoski S, Pystynen P: Reproductive performance of women with uterine anomalies. Acta Obstet Gynecol Scand 61:157, 1982.
Hill LM, Guzick D, Fries J, Hixson J: Fetal loss rate after ultrasonically documented cardiac activity between 6 and 14 weeks, menstrual age. J Clin Ultrasound 19:221, 1991.
Homburg R: Pregnancy complications in PCOS. Best Pract Res Clin Endocrinol Metab 20:281, 2006.
Hwang JL, Hsieh CY, Ho HN, et al: The role of blocking factors and antipaternal lymphocytotoxic antibodies in the success of pregnancy in patients with recurrent spontaneous abortion. Fertil Steril 58:691, 1992.
Illeni MT, Marelli G, Parazzini F, et al: Immunotherapy and recurrent abortion: A randomized clinical trial. Hum Reprod 9:1247, 1994.
Immunotherapy for recurrent miscarriage. The Cochrane Database of Systematic Review Online (Scott JR: Reviewer) September 2002.
Jablonowska B, Selbing A, Palfi M, et al: Prevention of recurrent spontaneous abortion by intravenous immunoglobulin: A double-blind placebo-controlled study. Hum Reprod 14:838, 1999.
Jeng GT, Scott JR, Burmiester LF: A comparison of meta-analytic results using literature vs individual patient data. JAMA 274:830, 1995.
Jin K, Ho H-N, Speed TP, Gill TJ III: Reproductive failure and the major histocompatibility complex. Am J Hum Genet 56:1456, 1995.
Jivraj S, Rai R, Underwood J, Regan L: Genetic thrombophilic mutations among couples with recurrent miscarriage. Hum Reprod 21:1161, 2006.
Kajii T, Ferrier A, Niikawa N, et al: Anatomic and chromosomal anomalies in 639 spontaneous abortuses. Hum Genet 55:87, 1980.
Katz VL, Kuller JA: Recurrent miscarriage. Am J Perinatol 11.6:386, 1994.
Kaufman RH, Noller K, Adam E, et al: Upper genital tract abnormalities and pregnancy outcome in diethylstilbestrol-exposed progeny. Am J Obstet Gynecol 148:973, 1984.
Keltz MD, Olive DL, Kim AH, et al: Sonohysterography for screening in recurrent pregnancy loss. Fertil Steril 67:670, 1997.
Khamashta MA, Cuadrado MJ, Mudic F, et al: The management of thrombosis in the antiphospholipid-antibody syndrome. N Engl J Med 332:993, 1995.
Kilpatrick DC, Liston WA: Influence of histocompatibility antigens in recurrent spontaneous abortion and its relevance to leukocyte immunotherapy. Hum Reprod 8:1645, 1993.
Kimball AC, Kean BH, Fuchs F: The role of toxoplasmosis in abortion. Am J Obstet Gynecol 111:219, 1971.
Kiprov DD, Nachtigall RD, Weaver RC, et al: The use of intravenous immunoglobulin in recurrent pregnancy loss associated with combined alloimmune and autoimmune abnormalities. Am J Reprod Immunol 36:228, 1996.
Kleinhaus K, Perrin M, Friedlander Y, et al: Paternal age and spontaneous abortion. Obstet Gynecol 108:369, 2006.
Kline J, Shrout P, Stein ZA, et al: Drinking during pregnancy and spontaneous abortion. Lancet 2:176, 1980.
Kline J, Stein ZA, Susser M, et al: Smoking: A risk factor for spontaneous abortion. N Engl J Med 297:793, 1977.
Kovalevsky G, Gracia CR, Berlin JA et al. Evaluation of the association between hereditary thrombophilias and recurrent pregnancy loss. Arch Int Med 164:558, 2004.
Knudsen UB, Hansen V, Juul S, Secher NJ: Prognosis of a new pregnancy following previous spontaneous abortions. Eur J Obstet Gynaecol 39:31, 1991.
Kumar KSD, Govindaiah V, Naushad SE, et al: Plasma homocysteine levels correlated to interactions between folate status and methylene tetrahydrofolate reductase gene mutation in women with unexplained recurrent pregnancy loss. J Obstet Gyn 23.1:55, 2003.
Kwak-Kim JYH, Chung-Bang HS, Ntrivalas EI, et al: Increased T helper 1 cytokine responses by circulating T cells are present in women with recurrent pregnancy losses and in infertile women with multiple implantation failures after IVF. Hum Reprod 18:767, 2003.
Laboda LA, Estroff JA, Benacerraf BR: First trimester bradycardia: a sign of impending fetal loss. J Ultrasound Med 8:561, 1989.
Laird SM, Tuckerman EM, Cork BA, et al: A review of immune cells and molecules in women with recurrent miscarriage. Hum Reprod Update 9:163, 2003.
Lee TS, Cheung LP, Haines CJ, et al: A comparison of the psychologic impact and client satisfaction of surgical treatment with medical treatment of spontaneous abortion: A randomized controlled trial. Am J Obstet Gyn 185:953, 2001.
Lejeune B, Grun JP, DeNayer P, et al: Antithyroid antibodies underlying thyroid abnormalities and miscarriage or pregnancy induced hypertension. Br J Obstet Gynaecol 100:669, 1993.
Li TC, Spring PG, Bygrave C, et al: The value of biochemical and ultrasound measurements of predicting pregnancy outcome in women with a history of recurrent miscarriage. Hum Reprod 13:3525, 1998.
Liddell HS, Pattison NA, Zanderigo A: Recurrent miscarriage: Outcome after supportive care in early pregnancy. Aust N Z J Obstet Gynaecol 31:320, 1991.
March CM, Israel R: Gestational outcome following hysteroscopic lysis of adhesions. Fertil Steril 36:455, 1981.
March CM, Israel R: Hysteroscopic management of recurrent abortion secondary to septate uterus. Am J Obstet Gynecol 156:834, 1987.
Marietta M, Facchinetti F, Sgarbi L, et al: Elevated plasma levels of factor VIII in women with early recurrent miscarriage. J Thromb Haemost 1:2536, 2003.
Martinelli P, Troncone R, Paparo F, et al: Coeliac disease and unfavourable outcome of pregnancy. Gut 46:332, 2000.
Marzuseh K, Dietl J, Klein R, et al: Recurrent first trimester spontaneous abortion associated with antiphospholipid antibodies: A pilot study of treatment with intravenous immunoglobulin. Acta Obstet Gynecol Scand 74:922, 1996.
Mills JL, Simpson JL, Driscoll SG, et al: Incidence of spontaneous abortion among normal women and insulin-dependent diabetic women whose pregnancies were identified within 21 days of conception. N Engl J Med 319:1618, 1988.
Montoro M, Collea JV, Frasier D, et al: Successful outcome of pregnancy in women with hypothyroidism. Ann Intern Med 94:31, 1981.
Mowbray JF, Gibbings C, Liddell H, et al: Controlled trial of treatment of recurrent spontaneous abortion by immunisation with paternal cells. Lancet 1:941, 1985.
MRC/RCOG Working Party on Cervical Cerclage: Final report of the Medical Research Council/Royal College of Obstetricians and Gynaecologists multicentre randomised trial of cervical cerclage. Br J Obstet Gynaecol 100:516, 1993.
Murray MJ, Meyer B, Zaino RJ, et al: A critical analysis of the accuracy, reproducibility, and clinical utility of histologic endometrial dating in fertile women. Fertil Steril 81:1333, 2004.
Muttukrishna S, Jauniaux E, Greenwold N, et al: Circulating levels of inhibin A, activin A and follistatin in missed and recurrent miscarriages. Hum Reprod 17:3072, 2002.
Nahmias AJ, Josey WE, Nain ZM, et al: Perinatal risk associated with maternal genital herpes simplex virus infection. Am J Obstet Gynecol 110:825, 1971.
Nazari A, Check JH, Epstein RH, et al: Relationship of small-for-dates sac size to crown-rump length and spontaneous abortion in patients with a known date of ovulation. Obstet Gynecol 78:369, 1991.
Ness RB, Grisso JA, Hirschinger N, et al: Cocaine and tobacco use and the risk of spontaneous abortion. N Engl J Med 340:333, 1999.
Ngai SW, Chan YM, Tang OS, et al: Vaginal misoprostol as medical treatment for first trimester spontaneous miscarriage. Hum Reprod 16:1496, 2001.
Nelen WLDM, Blom HJ, Steegers EAP, et al: Homocysteine and folate levels as risk factors for recurrent early pregnancy loss. Obstet Gyn 95:519, 2000.
Nikcevic AV, Tunkel SA, Kuczmierczyk AR, et al: Investigation of the cause of miscarriage and its influence on women's psychological distress. Br J Obstet Gyn 106:808, 1999.
Ogasawara M, Aoyama T, Kajiura S, et al: Are serum progesterone levels predictive of recurrent miscarriage in future pregnancies? Fertil Steril 68:806, 1997.
Ohno M, Maeda T, Matsunobu A: A cytogenetic study of spontaneous abortions with direct analysis of chorionic villi. Obstet Gynecol 77:394, 1991.
Opsahl MS, Pettit DC: First trimester sonographic characteristics of patients with recurrent spontaneous abortion. J Ultrasound Med 12:507, 1993.
Out HJ, Bruinse HW, Derksen RHWM: Antiphospholipid antibodies and pregnancy loss. Hum Reprod 6:889, 1991.
Parazzini F, Chatenoud L, DiCintio E, et al: Coffee consumption and risk of hospitalized miscarriage before 12 weeks of gestation. Hum Reprod 13:2286, 1998.
Pattison NS, Chamley LW, McKay EJ, et al: Antiphospholipid antibodies in pregnancy: Prevalence and clinical associations. Br J Obstet Gyneacol 100:909, 1993.

Pedersen JF, Mantoni M: Prevalence and significance of subchorionic hemorrhage in threatened abortion: A sonographic study. Am J Roentgenol 154:535, 1990.

Perino A, Vassiliadis A, Vucetich A, et al: Short-term therapy for recurrent abortion using intravenous immunoglobulins: Results of a double-blind placebo-controlled Italian study. Hum Reprod 12:2388, 1997.

Philipp T, Philipp K, Reiner A, et al: Embryoscopic and cytogenetic analysis of 233 missed abortions: Factors involved in the pathogenesis of developmental defects of early failed pregnancies. Hum Reprod 18:1724, 2003.

Poland BJ, Miller JR, Jones DC, et al: Reproductive counseling in patients who have had a spontaneous abortion. Am J Obstet Gynecol 127:685, 1977.

Portnoi MF, Joye N, Van Den Akker J, et al: Karyotypes of 1142 couples with recurrent abortion. Obstet Gynecol 72:31, 1988.

Pratt DE, Karande V, Kaberlein G, et al: The association of antithyroid antibodies in euthyroid nonpregnant women with recurrent first trimester abortions in the next pregnancy. Fertil Steril 60:1001, 1993.

Proctor JA, Haney AF: Recurrent first trimester pregnancy loss is associated with uterine septum but not with bicornuate uterus. Fertil Steril 80.5:1212, 2003.

Quere I, Bellet H, Hoffet M, et al: A woman with five consecutive fetal deaths: case report and retrospective analysis of hyperhomocystenemia prevalence in 100 consecutive women with recurrent miscarriages. Fertil Steril 69:152, 1998.

Rabau E, David A: *Listeria monocytogenes* in abortion. J Obstet Gynaecol Br Comm 70:481, 1963.

Rai R, Backos M, Elgaddal S, et al: Factor V Leiden and recurrent miscarriage-prospective outcome of untreated pregnancies. Hum Reprod 17:442, 2002.

Rai R, Clifford K, Regan L: The modern preventative treatment of recurrent miscarriage. Br J Obstet Gynaecol 103:106, 1996.

Rai R, Cohen H, Dave M, et al: Randomised controlled trial of aspirin and aspirin plus heparin in pregnant women with recurrent miscarriage associated with phospholipid antibodies (or antiphospholipid antibodies). BMJ 314:253, 1997.

Rai R, Regan L: Recurrent miscarriage. Lancet 368(9535):601, 2006.

Rai R, Regan L, Hadley E, et al: Second-trimester pregnancy loss is associated with activated protein C resistance. Br J Haematol 92:489, 1996.

Rai RS, Clifford K, Cohen H, Regan L: High prospective fetal loss rate in untreated pregnancies of women with recurrent miscarriage and antiphospholipid antibodies. Hum Reprod 10:3301, 1995.

Rai RS, Regan L, Clifford K, et al: Antiphospholipid antibodies and β_2-glycoprotein-I in 500 women with recurrent miscarriage: Results of a comprehensive screening approach. Hum Reprod 10:2001, 1995.

Regan L, Braude PR, Trembath PL: Influence of past reproductive performance on risk of spontaneous abortion. Br Med J 299:541, 1989.

Regan L, Owen EJ, Jacobs HS: Hypersecretion of luteinising hormone, infertility, and miscarriage. Lancet 336:1141, 1990.

Rey E, Kahn SR, David M, Shrier I. Thrombophilic disorders and fetal loss: A meta-analysis. Lancet. 361: 9018. 2003.

Reznikoff-Etievant MF, Cayol V, Zou GM, et al: Habitual abortions in 1678 healthy patients: Investigation and prevention. Hum Reprod 14:2106, 1999.

Ridker PM, Miletich JP, Buring JE, et al: Factor V Leiden mutation as a risk factor for recurrent pregnancy loss. Ann Intern Med 128:1000, 1998.

Roberts JM, Laros RK: Hemorrhagic and endotoxic shock: A pathophysiologic approach to diagnosis and management. Am J Obstet Gynecol 110:1041, 1971.

Sachs ES, Jahoda MGJ, Van Hemel JO, et al: Chromosome studies of 500 couples with two or more abortions. Obstet Gynecol 65:375, 1985.

Salim R, Regan L, Woelfer B, et al: A comparative study of the morphology of congenital uterine anomalies in women with and without a history of recurrent first trimester miscarriage. Hum Reprod 18.1:162, 2003.

Sargent IL, Wilkins T, Redman CWG: Maternal immune responses to the fetus in early pregnancy and recurrent miscarriage. Lancet 2:1099, 1988.

Sarig G, Younis JS, Hoffman R, et al: Thrombophilia is common in women with idiopathic pregnancy loss and is associated with late pregnancy wastage. Fertil Steril 77:342, 2002.

Sbracia M, Mastrone M, Scarpellini F, Grasso JA: Influence of histocompatibility antigens in recurrent spontaneous abortion couples and on their reproductive performances. Am J Reprod Immunol 35:85, 1996.

Scarpellini F, Mastrone M, Sbracia M, Scarpellini L: Serum CA 125 and first trimester abortion. Int J Gynaecol Obstet 49:259, 1995.

Schats R, Jansen CAM, Wladimiroff JW: Embryonic heart activity: Appearance and development in early human pregnancy. Br J Obstet Gyneacol 97:989, 1990.

Sebire NJ, Backos M, El Gaddal S, et al: Placental pathology, antiphospholipid antibodies, and pregnancy outcome in recurrent miscarriage patients. Obstet Gyn 101:258, 2003.

Shakar K, Ben-Eliyahu S, Loewenthal R, et al: Differences in number and activity of peripheral natural killer cells in primary versus secondary recurrent miscarriage. Fertil Steril 80:368, 2003.

Siddiqi TA, Caligaris JT, Miodovnik M, et al: Rate of spontaneous abortion after first trimester sonographic demonstration of fetal cardiac activity. Am J Perinatol 5:1, 1988.

Silver RK, MacGregor SN, Sholl JS, et al: Comparative trial of prednisone plus aspirin versus aspirin alone in the treatment of anticardiolipin antibody-positive obstetric patients. Am J Obstet Gynecol 169:1411, 1993.

Simpson JL: Genes, chromosomes, and reproductive failure. Fertil Steril 33:107, 1980.

Smith A, Gaha TJ: Data on families of chromosome translocation carriers ascertained because of habitual spontaneous abortion. Aust N Z J Obstet Gynaecol 30:57, 1990.

Smith JB, Cowchock FS: Immunological studies in recurrent spontaneous abortion: Effects of immunization of women with paternal mononuclear cells on lymphocytotoxic and mixed lymphocyte reaction blocking antibodies and correlation with sharing of HLA and pregnancy outcome. J Reprod Immunol 14:99, 1988.

Stagnaro-Green A, Glinoer D: Thyroid autoimmunity and the risk of miscarriage. Best Pract Res Clin Endocrinol Metab 18:167, 2004.

Stagnaro-Green A, Roman SH, Cobin RH, et al: Detection of at-risk pregnancy by means of highly sensitive assays for thyroid autoantibodies. JAMA 264:1422, 1990.

Stein Z, Kline J, Susser E, et al: Maternal age and spontaneous abortion. In Porter IH, Hook EB (eds): Human embryonic and Fetal Death. New York, Academic Press, 1980.

Stephenson MD, Awartani KA, Robinson WP: Cytogenic analysis of miscarriages from couples with recurrent miscarriage: A case-control study. Hum Reprod 17:446, 2002.

Stephenson MD, Sierra S: Reproductive outcomes in recurrent pregnancy loss associated with a parental carrier of a structural chromosome rearrangement. Hum Reprod 21:1076, 2006.

Stern JJ, Coulam CB: Mechanism of recurrent spontaneous abortion. I. Ultrasonographic findings. Am J Obstet Gynecol 166:1844, 1992.

Stern JJ, Dorfman AD, Gutierrez-Najar AJ: Frequency of abnormal karyotypes among abortuses from women with and without a history of recurrent spontaneous abortion, Fertility and Sterility 65:250-3, 1996.

Stray-Pedersen B, Stray-Pedersen S: Etiologic factors and subsequent reproductive performance in 195 couples with a prior history of habitual abortion, Am J Obstet Gynecol 148:140, 1984.

Stray-Pedersen B, Eng J, and Reikvam TM: Uterine T-mycoplasma colonization in reproductive failure, Am J Obstet Gynecol 130:307, 1978.

Strobino BA and Pantel-Silverman J: First-trimester vaginal bleeding and the loss of chromosomally normal and abnormal conceptions, Am J Obstet Gynecol 157:1150, 1987.

Sugiura-Ogasawara M, Furukawa TA, Nakano Y, et al: Depression as a potential causal factor in subsequent miscarriage in recurrent spontaneous aborters, Human Reproduction 17.10:2580-84, 2002.

Sullivan AE, Silver RM, LaCoursiere DY, et al: Recurrent fetal aneuploidy and recurrent miscarriage, Obstet Gyn 104:784-8, 2004.

Tadmor OP, Achiron R, Rabinowiz R, et al: Predicting first-trimester spontaneous abortion: ratio of mean sac diameter to crown-rump length compared to embryonic heart rate, J Reprod Med 39:459, 1994.

Tang OS, Lau WNT, Ng EHY, et al: A prospective randomized study to compare the use of repeated doses of vaginal with sublingual misoprostol in the management of first trimester silent miscarriages, Human Reproduction 18.1:176-81, 2003.

Tharapel AT, Tharapel SA, and Bannerman RM: Recurrent pregnancy losses and parental chromosome abnormalities: a review, Br J Obstet Gynaecol 92:899, 1985.

The German RSA/IVIG Group: Intravenous immunoglobulin in the prevention of recurrent miscarriage, Br J Obstet Gynaecol 101:1072, 1994.

The Recurrent Miscarriage Immunotherapy Trialists Group L worldwide collaborative observational study and meta-analysis on allogenic leukocyte

immunotherapy for recurrent spontaneous abortion, Am J Reprod Immunol 32:55, 1994.
Tho PT, Byrd TR, and McDonough PG: Etiologies and subsequent reproductive performance of 100 couples with recurrent abortion, Fertil Steril 32:389, 1979.
Tulppala M, Palosuo T, Ramsay T, et al: A prospective study of 63 couples with a history of recurrent spontaneous abortion: contributing factors and outcome of subsequent pregnancies, Hum Reprod 8:764, 1993.
Vianna NJ and Polan AK: Incidence of low birth weight among Love Canal residents, Science 226:1217, 1984.
Warburton D and Fraser FC: Spontaneous abortion risks in man: data from reproductive histories collected in a medical genetics unit, Am J Hum Genet 16:1, 1964.
Watson H, Kiddy DS, Hamilton-Fairley D, et al: Hypersecretion of luteinizing hormone and ovarian steroids in women with recurrent early miscarriage, Hum Reprod 8:829, 1993.
Wilcox AJ, Weinberg CR, O'Connor JF, et al: Incidence of early loss of pregnancy, N Engl J Med 319:189, 1988.
Wilson R, Ling LH, MacLean MA, et al: Thyroid antibody titer and avidity in patients with recurrent miscarriage, Fertil Steril 71:558, 1999.
Wong KS, Ngai CSW, Yeo ELK, et al: A comparison of two regimens of intravaginal misoprostol for termination of second trimester pregnancy: a randomized comparative trial, Hum Reprod 15:709, 2000.
World Health Organisation Task Force on Post-ovulatory Methods of Fertility Regulation. Special Programme of Research, Development and Research Training, World Health Organisation, Geneva: Comparison of two doses of mifepristone in combination with misoprostol for early medical abortion: a randomised trial. Br J Obstet Gynaecol 107:524, 2000.
Yamada H, Kishida T, Kobayashi N, et al: Massive immunoglobulin treatment in women with four or more recurrent spontaneous primary abortions of unexplained aetiology, Hum Reprod 13:2620, 1998.
Zalanyi S: Vaginal misoprostol alone is effective in the treatment of missed abortion, Br J Obstet Gynaecol 105:1026, 1998.
Zhang J, Gilles JM, Barnhart K, et al: A comparison of medical management with misoprostol and surgical management for early pregnancy failure, N Engl J Med 353:761, 2005.

Ectopic Pregnancy 17

Etiology, Pathology, Diagnosis, Management, Fertility Prognosis

Rogerio A. Lobo

KEY TERMS AND DEFINITIONS

Abdominal Pregnancy. Pregnancy that develops in any portion of the peritoneal cavity. It usually occurs after a secondary implantation of the trophoblast after tubal abortion (secondary abdominal pregnancy). A primary abdominal pregnancy is one that implants directly into the peritoneal cavity.

Arias-Stella Reaction. Hypersecretory appearance of endometrial glands. The cells demonstrate hyperchromatism, pleomorphism, increased mitotic activity, and hypertrophy.

Cervical Pregnancy. Pregnancy developing in the cervical canal below the level of the internal os.

Chronic Ectopic Pregnancy. Ectopic gestational tissue in the peritoneal cavity after tubal abortion or rupture. It produces chronic symptoms of lower abdominal pain and usually forms adhesions to bowel and peritoneum.

Cornual Pregnancy. Pregnancy developing in one horn of a bicornuate uterus.

Culdocentesis. Aspiration of fluid in cul-de-sac (pouch) of Douglas via a needle placed through the vagina.

Decidual Cast. Sloughing of nearly all of the decidua lining the endometrial cavity.

Ectopic Pregnancy. Pregnancy that develops after implantation of the blastocyst anywhere other than the endometrium lining the uterine cavity.

Hemoperitoneum. Blood in the peritoneal cavity. The blood from a ruptured ectopic pregnancy initially clots and then lyses so that hemoperitoneum is a combination of blood clots and hemorrhagic fluid that will not clot.

Heterotopic Pregnancy. Combined intrauterine and extrauterine pregnancy.

Interstitial Pregnancy. Pregnancy developing in the interstitial portion of the oviduct.

Ovarian Pregnancy. Pregnancy developing in the ovary. For the diagnosis to be made, the following four characteristics must be fulfilled: (1) the tube on the affected side should be intact, (2) the gestational site must occupy the normal position of the ovary, (3) the gestational site must be connected to the uterus by the ovarian ligament, and (4) histologically identified ovarian tissue must be present in the sac wall.

Persistent Ectopic Pregnancy. Continued growth of viable trophoblastic tissue after conservative treatment of an unruptured ectopic pregnancy; manifestations include HCG titers that do not decline or pelvic pain (or both).

Ruptured Ectopic Pregnancy. Ectopic pregnancy that has eroded through the tissue in which it has implanted, (producing hemorrhage from exposed vessels.

Salpingitis Isthmica Nodosa (Tubal Diverticulum). Direct invasion of the tubal muscularis by the tubal epithelium for varying distances between the lumen and the serosa.

Salpingostomy. Surgical incision of the oviduct, which is followed by removal of a tubal pregnancy for the purpose of retaining the oviduct. After hemostasis is achieved, the incision is left open.

Salpingotomy. Surgical incision of the oviduct, followed by removal of a tubal pregnancy and closure of the incision.

Tubal Abortion. Tubal pregnancy that has extruded out of the fimbrial end of the oviduct.

Tubal Pregnancy. Pregnancy occurring in the oviduct in the ampulla, fimbria, or isthmus. Pregnancy in the oviduct is the most common site of ectopic pregnancy.

Unruptured Tubal Gestation. Tubal pregnancy that has not yet eroded through the wall of the oviduct.

Ectopic pregnancy was probably first described in AD 963 by Albucasis, an Arab writer. In 1876, before the initiation of surgical therapy, the mortality rate from ectopic pregnancy was estimated to be 60%. The first successful operative treatment of ectopic pregnancy was performed in 1883 by Lawson Tait in England. In 1887, he reported that he had performed salpingectomy on four women with ectopic pregnancy and that they all survived.

EPIDEMIOLOGY

The incidence of ectopic pregnancy is expressed in different ways in the literature. The common characteristic used is the number of recognized conceptions, with the incidence expressed as the number of ectopic pregnancies per 1000 conceptions. Other characteristics include the number of women of reproductive age, expressed as the number of ectopic pregnancies per

10,000 women age 14 to 44, and the number of total births expressed as the number of ectopic pregnancies per 1000 births.

It would be best to be able to calculate the incidence of ectopic pregnancies per 1000 total conceptions; however, because most spontaneous abortions and many elective abortions are not reported, the denominator is always smaller than the actual number, yielding a spuriously increased incidence. Nevertheless, since an unknown number of ectopic pregnancies remain asymptomatic and thus are not reported, the numerator is also lower. Thus the true incidence of ectopic pregnancies per 1000 total conceptions can never be accurately calculated. The incidences reported in the literature, however, are good approximations and, since the same methodology is used, can be validly compared.

The incidence of ectopic pregnancy varies among different countries, with rates as high as 1 in 28 and 1 in 40 pregnancies reported in Jamaica and Vietnam. In the United States in 1989 the annual ectopic pregnancy rate per 10,000 women age 15 to 44 was 15.5, similar to that in Finland but higher than the rate in France.

During the past 40 years, the incidence of ectopic pregnancy has been steadily increasing in the United States, as well as in most European countries. In the United States, between 1970 and 1989 there was a fivefold increase in the annual number of women hospitalized for ectopic pregnancies (from 17,800 to 88,400), and there was a tripling of the rate per 1000 pregnancies (from 4.5 to 16.0). Since 1987 there has been an increasing trend toward treating ectopic pregnancy on an ambulatory basis without overnight hospitalization. With earlier detection of ectopic pregnancy a steadily increasing percentage of women with this problem are now being treated before tubal rupture occurs by outpatient laparoscopic procedures or by medical treatment with methotrexate. An analysis of both hospital discharge data, as well as an ambulatory medical care survey, revealed that the estimated number of hospitalizations for ectopic pregnancy in the United States declined from nearly 90,000 in 1989 to about 45,000 in 1994. However, in 1992 about half of all women with ectopic pregnancy in the United States were treated as outpatients, and the estimated number of total ectopic pregnancies in this year was 108,000, for a rate of 19.7 per 1000 reported pregnancies. Thus in the United States in 1992 about 2 of every 100 women who were known to conceive had an ectopic gestation. This increased incidence of ectopic pregnancy is thought to be due to two factors: (1) the increased incidence of salpingitis, due to increased infection with *Chlamydia trachomatis* or other sexually transmitted pathogens, and (2) improved diagnostic techniques, which enable diagnosis of unruptured ectopic pregnancy to be made with more precision and earlier in gestation before asymptomatic resolution of the pregnancy could occur.

There is a marked increase in the rate of ectopic pregnancy with increasing age when calculated as incidence per 1000 reported conceptions. In the United States the rate increased from 6.6 in women age 15 to 24 years to 21.5 in those age 35 to 44 years. However, when the number was calculated per 10,000 women age 15 to 44, the rate of ectopic pregnancy was lowest in the older group, reflecting the lower total number of pregnancies in this age group. These data indicate that the incidence rate of ectopic pregnancy should be calculated using total pregnancies as the denominator to determine the actual risk for a woman exposed to pregnancy. Because of the lower pregnancy rate in older women, overall only about 11% of ectopic pregnancies in the United States occur in women age 35 to 44, whereas more than half, 58%, occur in women age 25 to 34.

Most ectopic pregnancies occur in multigravid women. Only 10% to 15% of ectopic pregnancies occur in nulligravid women, whereas more than half occur in women who have been pregnant three or more times.

In the United States the rates of ectopic pregnancy are similar in each section of the country, but the rates are higher for nonwhite than white women. About 3% of all reported pregnancies in nonwhite women age 35 to 44 in the United States were ectopic.

MORTALITY

Even with the increased use of surgery and blood transfusions and earlier diagnosis, ectopic pregnancy remains a major cause of maternal death in the United States today. In 1988 there were 44, and in 1989 there were 34 deaths from complications related to ectopic pregnancy in the United States. Ectopic pregnancy is the most common cause of maternal death in the first half of pregnancy. Although the percentage of all maternal deaths in the United States that are the result of ectopic pregnancy increased from 8% in 1970 to 13% in 1989, the percentage of ectopic pregnancies that become fatal has decreased. The overall death-to-case rate of ectopic pregnancy has decreased 10-fold, from 35 per 10,000 women with ectopic pregnancy in 1970 to 3.8 in 1989. The death-to-case rate is similar in all age groups but is four times higher in blacks and other nonwhites than in white women. Because the incidence of ectopic pregnancy is also higher in blacks in the United States, a pregnant black woman is about five times more likely to die of ectopic pregnancy than a white woman. Ectopic pregnancy is the most common single cause of all maternal deaths among black women, causing about one fifth of such deaths. Unmarried women of all races have a 1.7 times greater chance of dying of ectopic pregnancy than married women do. Overall risk of death from ectopic pregnancy is about 10 times greater than the risk of childbirth and more than 50 times greater than the risk of legal abortion.

Atrash and colleagues studied the clinical aspects of deaths resulting from ectopic pregnancy in the United States from 1979 to 1982. They found that blood loss was the major cause of death (88%), with infection (3%) and anesthesia complications (2%) much less common. Dorfman and coworkers reported that about 80% of these gestations were in the oviduct itself, and the other 20% were interstitial or abdominal gestations. Because the overall incidence of ectopic pregnancy occurring in these latter locations is slightly less than 4%, interstitial and abdominal ectopic pregnancies have about a five times greater risk of being fatal than those pregnancies located in the portion of the tube distal to the uterus. About three fourths of the women with fatal ectopic pregnancies initially developed symptoms and died in the first 12 weeks of gestation. Of the remaining one fourth who developed symptoms and died after the first trimester, 70% had interstitial or abdominal pregnancies. Patient delay in consulting a physician after development of symptoms accounted for one third of the deaths, whereas treatment delay resulting from misdiagnosis contributed to the death in half. More than half of the women died of hemorrhage without emergency surgery. The most common misdiagnoses were intestinal disorders and intrauterine pregnancy (IUP).

ETIOLOGY

The major cause of ectopic pregnancy is salpingitis. Its morphologic sequelae account for about half of the initial episodes of ectopic pregnancy. Although other morphologic factors have been identified as a cause of ectopic pregnancy, in the majority of the remaining first episodes no such factor can be identified. Thus in about 40% of instances the cause cannot be determined and is presumed to be a physiologic disorder that results in delay of passage of the embryo into the uterine cavity so it remains in the oviduct at the gestational age (7 days) when implantation occurs. Ovulation from the contralateral ovary has been implicated as a cause of delay of blastocyst transport, and Breen reported contralateral ovulation to occur in about one third of tubal gestations treated by laparotomy. However, Saito and associates observed that the portion of the tube where implantation occurred in women with ectopic pregnancies was similar whether the corpus luteum was ipsilateral or contralateral to the pregnancy. If transmigration was a factor, they hypothesized that there would be a greater incidence of distal tubal pregnancies with ovulation in the contralateral ovary. Furthermore, women who have an ipsilateral oophorectomy together with salpingectomy for ectopic pregnancy have a repeat ectopic pregnancy rate similar to the rate in those who do not have the ovary removed. For these reasons it is unlikely that transmigration of the ovum from the opposite ovary is a common cause of ectopic pregnancy.

A more likely physiologic cause is hormonal imbalance, as elevated circulating levels of either estrogen or progesterone can alter normal tubal contractility. An increased rate of ectopic pregnancies has been reported in women who conceive with physiologically and pharmacologically elevated levels of progestogens. The latter condition can be produced locally with a progesterone-releasing IUD, as well as systemically with progestin-only oral contraceptives. Iatrogenic, physiologically increased levels of estrogen and progesterone occur after ovulation induction with either clomiphene citrate or human menopausal gonadotropins, and an increased rate of ectopic pregnancies has been reported in women conceiving after each of these treatment modalities.

Another probable cause is an abnormality of embryonic development. Stratford examined 44 human conceptuses from ectopic gestations by microdissection and histologic sections and found that about two thirds were abnormal and half had gross structural abnormalities. These types of abnormalities could interfere with normal tubal transport. Elias and colleagues, using cell culture technique, reported that the chromosomal complement of ectopic gestations was similar to that of intrauterine gestations of comparable gestational age. However, Karikoski and coworkers, using DNA flow cytometry, found aneuploidy to be present in one third of tubal gestations. These investigators suggested that this high incidence of chromosomal abnormalities could be a factor causing ectopic implantation. Inherited genetic abnormalities are most probably not a cause of ectopic pregnancy, because there is no increased incidence among first-degree relatives. Several epidemiologic studies indicate that cigarette smoking is associated with about a twofold increased risk of ectopic pregnancy, even when the data were controlled for the presence of other risk factors. The risk of ectopic pregnancy was directly related to the number of cigarettes smoked per day, with a fourfold increased risk noted among women who smoked 30 or more cigarettes per day (Fig. 17-1). Risk factors for ectopic pregnancy, presented as odds ratios and attributable risk are depicted in Table 17-1.

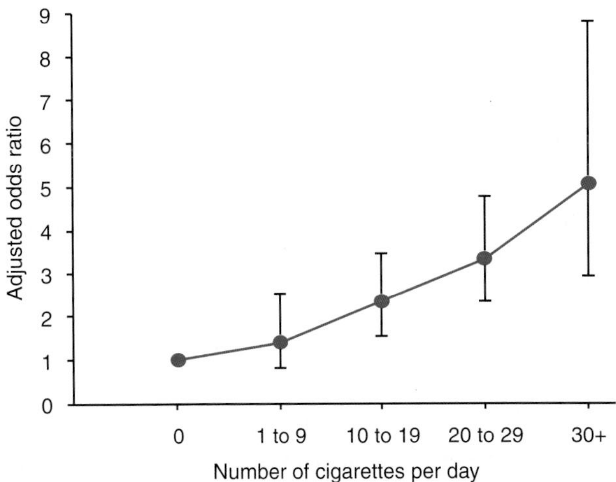

Figure 17-1. Dose response curve for smoking and ectopic pregnancy among women with no prior spontaneous abortion, adjusted for maternal age and race. (From Handler A, Davis F, Ferre C, Yeko T: The relationship of smoking and ectopic pregnancy. Am J Public Health 79:1239, 1989.)

Table 17-1 Odds Ratios for Ectopic Pregnancy (Compared with Women with Recent Successful Pregnancies) and the Attributable Risks Associated with Different Risk Factors

	Odds Ratio	Attributable Risk*
History of genital infection		0.18†
Probable salpingitis	2	
Confirmed salpingitis	3.5	
History of tubal surgery	3.5	0.18†
Smoking		0.35
Exsmoker	1.5	
1–9 cigarettes per day	2	
10–19 cigarettes per day	3	
≥20 cigarettes per day	4	
Age (years)		0.14
30–39	1.5	
≥40	3	
Obstetric history		
Spontaneous abortion	3	0.07
Elective abortion	2	0.03
IUD history	1.5	0.05
Previous infertility	2.5	0.18
All factors, taken together		0.76

Odds ratios for EP (compared with deliveries) and attributable risks of the principal risk factors.

*From Auvergne registry data (Bouyer J, Coste J, Shojaei T, et al: Risk factors for ectopic pregnancy: A comprehensive analysis based on a large case-control, population-based study in France. Am J Epidemiol 157:185, 2003.)

†Risk attributable to history of genital infection and tubal surgery together is 0.33.

IUD, intrauterine device.

From Fernandez H, Gervaise A: Ectopic pregnancies after infertility treatment: Modern diagnosis and therapeutic strategy. Hum Reprod Update 10:503, 2004.

The major causes of ectopic pregnancy will be discussed in more detail later.

Tubal Pathology

The permanent agglutination of the plicae (folds) of the endosalpinx produced by salpingitis can allow normal passage of the smaller sperm, but prevent normal transport of the larger morula. The morula can be trapped in blind pockets formed by adhesions of the endosalpinx. In their 20-year longitudinal study, Weström and colleagues found that nearly half (45.3%) of the women with ectopic pregnancy had a clinical history or histologic findings of a prior episode of acute salpingitis. This figure is in close agreement with the 40% incidence of histologic evidence of prior salpingitis found by several groups of investigators in the pathologic review of oviducts removed from women with ectopic pregnancy (Fig. 17-2).

Weström and colleagues prospectively followed 900 women age 15 to 34 who had laparoscopically confirmed diagnosis of acute salpingitis and found that the subsequent ectopic pregnancy rate was 68.8 per 1000 conceptions, yielding a sixfold increase in the risk of ectopic pregnancy after acute salpingitis compared with a control group of women without prior clinical evidence of salpingitis. The risk that the first pregnancy after acute salpingitis would be ectopic increased both with the number of episodes of infection and with increasing age of the women at the time of infection.

In two histopathologic studies of oviducts removed from women with ectopic pregnancy, Majmudar and coworkers and Green and Kott found that about half contained lesions of salpingitis isthmica nodosa (SIN) when numerous sections of the tube were examined. In their control groups only 5% of oviducts had SIN. SIN was defined as the microscopic presence of tubal epithelium within the myosalpinx or beneath the tubal serosa (Fig. 17-3). With serial sectioning it has been determined that SIN is actually a diverticulum or intrauterine extension of the tubal lumen (Fig. 17-4). Associated histologic evidence of chronic salpingitis was seen in only 6% of the oviducts in the first series, indicating that SIN was not necessarily the result of infection. These findings are in agreement with those of Persaud, who observed tubal diverticula (histologically similar to SIN) in the isthmus and proximal ampulla of half of the oviducts removed for tubal pregnancy. In both these series the tubal pregnancy usually implanted in a portion of the tube distal to the SIN, indicating that mechanical entrapment of the morula is not the mechanism whereby SIN causes tubal gestation. These investigators postulated that SIN itself or associated tubal anomalies may be responsible for dysfunction of the tubal transport mechanism without anatomic obstruction.

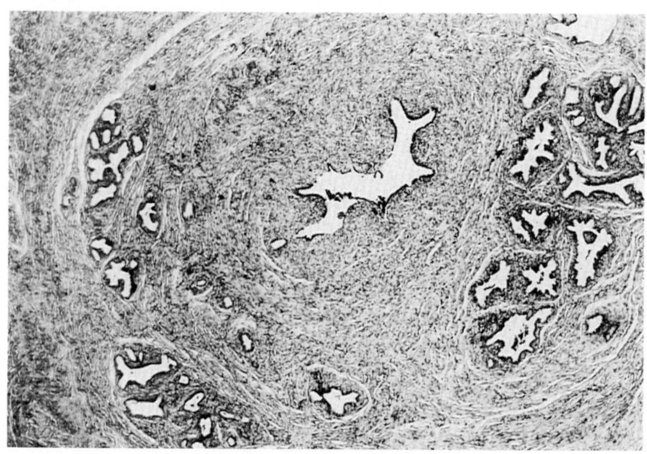

Figure 17-3. Microscopic section of fallopian tube showing typical lesion of salpingitis isthmica nodosa. Multiple glandular inclusions of tubal mucosa are seen in myosalpinx without continuity with luminal epithelium. (H&E, ×12.) (From Majmudar B, Henderson PH III, Semple E: Salpingitis isthmica nodosa: A high-risk factor for tubal pregnancy. Obstet Gynecol 62:73, 1983. Reprinted with permission from The American College of Obstetricians and Gynecologists.)

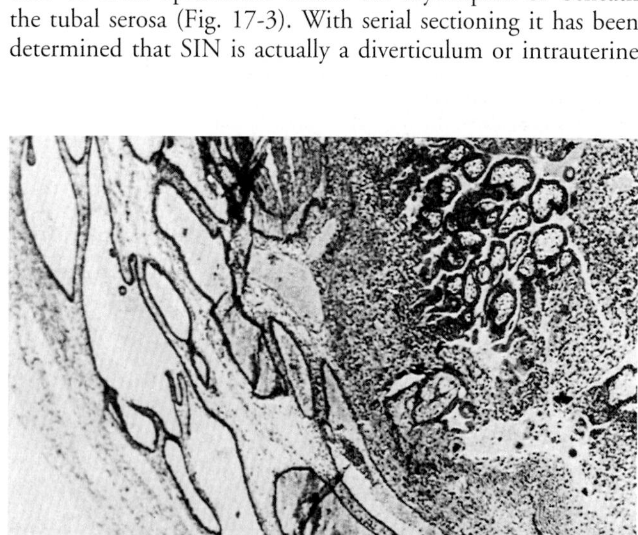

Figure 17-2. Tubal pregnancy with placental villi and trophoblastic cells to the right and wall of the tube to the left showing marked degree of follicular salpingitis. (Original magnification, ×70.) (From Bone NL, Greene RR: Histologic study of uterine tubes with tubal pregnancy. A search for evidence of previous infection. Am J Obstet Gynecol 82:1166, 1961.)

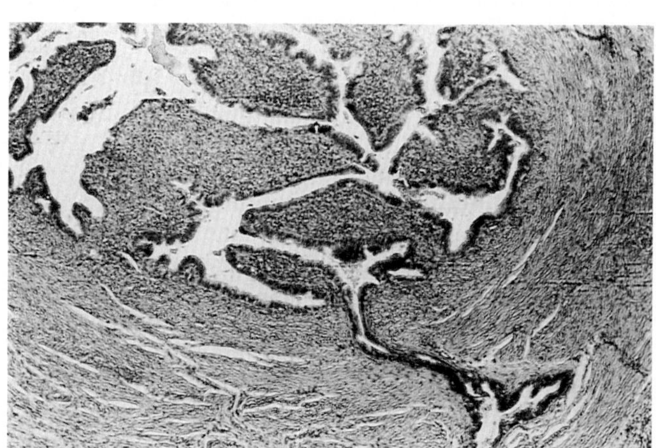

Figure 17-4. Tubal mucosa showing its actual extension into myosalpinx. (H&E, ×12.) (From Majmudar B, Henderson PH III, Semple E: Salpingitis isthmica nodosa: A high-risk factor for tubal pregnancy. Obstet Gynecol 62:73, 1983. Reprinted with permission from The American College of Obstetricians and Gynecologists.)

It is likely that adhesions between the tubal serosa and bowel or peritoneum may interfere with normal tubal motility and cause ectopic pregnancy because, as reported in two series respectively, 17% to 27% of women with ectopic pregnancy have had previous abdominal surgical procedures not involving the oviduct. On the other hand, neither endometriosis nor congenital anomalies of the tube have been associated with an increased incidence of ectopic pregnancy.

An operative procedure on the oviduct itself is a cause of ectopic pregnancy whether the oviduct is morphologically normal, as occurs with sterilization procedures, or abnormal, as occurs with postsalpingitis reconstructive surgery. The incidence of ectopic pregnancy occurring after salpingoplasty or salpingostomy procedures to treat distal tubal disease ranges from 15% to 25%, probably because the damage to the endosalpinx remains. The rate of ectopic pregnancy after reversal of sterilization procedures is lower, about 4%, because the tubes have not been damaged by infection.

Women who have had a prior ectopic pregnancy, even if treated by unilateral salpingectomy, are at increased risk for having a subsequent ectopic pregnancy. Of women who conceive after having one ectopic pregnancy, about 25% of subsequent pregnancies are ectopic. In two large series of women with ectopic pregnancy, 7% had a history of a prior ectopic pregnancy.

Herbst and associates, as well as others, have shown that the incidence of ectopic gestation is significantly greater (four to five times) in women who have been exposed to diethylstilbestrol (DES) in utero than in a control group. In various series the rate of ectopic pregnancy in such women is about 4% to 5%. Kaufman and colleagues reported that among women exposed to DES whose hysterosalpingograms demonstrated abnormalities in the uterine cavity, the ectopic pregnancy rate was 13%.

Contraception Failure

For several decades sterilization has been the most popular method of contraception used by couples in the United States. Since the development of laparoscopic surgery, female tubal sterilization is performed about twice as frequently as vasectomy. In a recent analysis of the long-term risk of pregnancy after tubal sterilization reported by Peterson and coworkers, it was found that within 10 years after the procedure the cumulative life table probability of pregnancy was 1.85%. The 10-year failure rate after bipolar coagulation of the oviducts was 2.48%, which rose to 5.43% if the sterilization procedure was performed when the woman was younger than 28 years of age. These investigators reported that for all 143 pregnancies occurring after tubal sterilization, 43, or 32.9%, were ectopic pregnancies.

Several investigators have reported that if pregnancy occurred after tubal sterilization by laparoscopic fulguration without concomitant transection, the ectopic pregnancy rate was about 50%. McCausland hypothesized that with the extensive tissue destruction caused by electrocoagulation, a uteroperitoneal fistula could develop that would allow sperm to pass into the distal segment of the oviduct and fertilize the egg (Fig. 17-5). Such fistulas were demonstrated radiographically by Shah and associates in 11% of 150 women after laparoscopic electrocoagulation and demonstrated histologically by McCausland, who called the process endosalpingosis or endosalpingoblastosis. McCann and Kessel also reported a 50% ectopic pregnancy rate after failure of laparoscopic electrocoagulation after failure of sterilization with metal clips or silicone rings. Peterson and colleagues reported that within 10 years after the sterilization procedure twice as many women sterilized by bipolar coagulation had ectopic pregnancies than those sterilized with metal clips or silicone bands. The ectopic pregnancy rate after bipolar coagulation sterilization was 1.7%.

With the marked increase in use of female sterilization techniques, failure of sterilization is becoming a more common cause of ectopic pregnancy. In contrast to a large series of ectopic pregnancies in the United States in the 1950s and 1960s in which only 0.6% of women with ectopic pregnancy had a prior tubal sterilization, Brenner and coworkers reported that 3% of 300 ectopic pregnancies occurring in 1976 to 1977 were the result of tubal sterilization failure. The incidence is probably even greater at present because tubal sterilization failure occurs throughout a woman's reproductive life. Peterson and colleagues reported that among women sterilized younger age 28, 2.8% became pregnant between 5 and 10 years after the procedure. Because about one third of pregnancies that occur after tubal sterilization are ectopic, women should be counseled that if they do not experience the expected menses at any time following tubal sterilization before menopause, a test to detect human chorionic gonadotropin (HCG) should be performed rapidly, and if they are pregnant a diagnostic evaluation to exclude the presence of ectopic pregnancy is necessary.

As summarized by Tatum and Schmidt, pregnancies occurring as a result of failure of certain contraceptive methods have a greater chance of being ectopic than among women becoming pregnant who were not using contraception. Although women who become pregnant while using diaphragms or combination oral contraceptives do not have an increased chance of having an ectopic pregnancy, women who become pregnant while using a Copper T380 IUD or progestin-only oral contraceptives have about a 5% chance of having an ectopic pregnancy. The incidence of ectopic pregnancy in women who become pregnant with the progesterone-releasing IUD is even higher, about

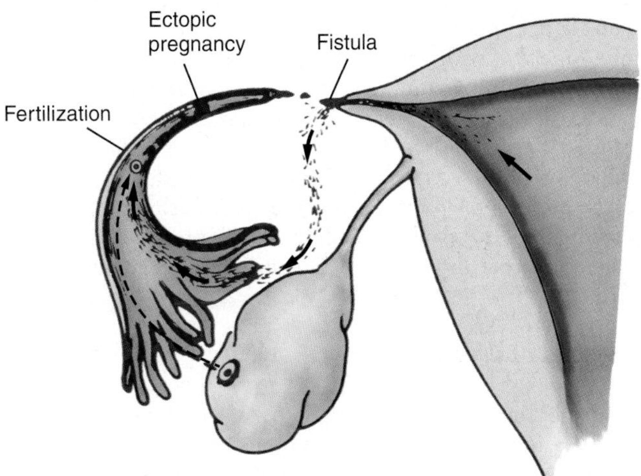

Figure 17-5. Mechanism of ectopic pregnancy after sterilization. (From Corson SL, Batzer FR: Ectopic pregnancy. A review of the etiologic factors. J Reprod Med 31:78, 1986.)

23%. Women using these methods of contraception who elect to have their pregnancies terminated should have a histologic examination of the tissue removed from the uterine cavity to be certain the pregnancy was intrauterine. If no chorionic villi are observed, a diagnostic evaluation to detect ectopic pregnancy should be performed.

Women using any type of contraception have a significantly decreased chance of having an ectopic pregnancy compared with sexually active, non–contraceptive users. Thus women who use any of the most effective reversible contraceptive methods are about 90% less likely to have an ectopic pregnancy than if they are sexually active and use no method of contraception. However, because the progesterone-releasing IUD inhibits tubal contractions and has a higher failure rate than the copper IUD, women who use this method of contraception have about twice the risk of ectopic pregnancy (7.5 per 1000 woman-years) than women who use no method of contraception (3.5 per 1000 woman-years).

Hormonal Alterations

As occurs with exogenous progesterone administration, if increased levels of exogenous or endogenous estrogens are present shortly after the time of ovulation, the incidence of ectopic pregnancy is increased. Morris and Van Wagenen reported that 3 of 30 pregnancies were ectopic in women receiving postovulatory high-dose estrogen to prevent pregnancy. Several investigators have reported that the ectopic pregnancy rate is about 1.5% for conceptions that occur after ovulation has been induced with clomiphene citrate. The ectopic rate in pregnancies occurring after ovulation is induced with human menopausal gonadotropin (HMG) has been reported to range between 3% and 4%. McBain and associates reported that if the urinary estrogen excretion during HMG therapy exceeded 200 μg/day, and conception occurred the ectopic pregnancy rate was 12.5%. Fernandez and colleagues in a case-control study found the risk of ectopic pregnancy was increased about fourfold among ovulatory women treated with controlled ovarian hyperstimulation, either clomiphene citrate, HMG, or a combination of both, for the treatment of unexplained infertility. These reports indicate that increased levels of estrogen, as well as of progesterone, interfere with tubal motility and increase the chance of ectopic gestation. Ectopic gestations occur in about 5% of pregnancies that develop after in vitro fertilization and embryonic transfer. The reason for this increased incidence is likely due to one or more of several factors: increased sex steroid hormone levels, presence of proximal tubal disease, flushing an embryo directly into the oviduct, and increased probability of early diagnosis before an asymptomatic tubal abortion could occur.

Previous Abortion

Although some studies have suggested that a prior induced abortion increases the risk of ectopic pregnancy, Levin and colleagues showed that when statistical techniques were used to control the effects of other risk factors, the history of one prior induced abortion did not significantly increase the risk of ectopic pregnancy (Table 17-2). In this study, the risk for ectopic pregnancy doubled if a woman had had two or more prior induced abortions, which (although not significant) indicates a possible association between multiple induced abortions and subsequent ectopic gestation, probably related to postabortal infection. A more recent study by Holt and coworkers, using a different type of control group, reported no significantly increased incidence of ectopic pregnancy in women having one prior abortion (RR = 0.9) or two or more prior abortions (RR = 1.2).

Table 17-2 Standardized* Relative Risks of Ectopic Pregnancy and 95% Confidence Intervals According to Selected Characteristics

History Characteristic	Relative Risk	95% Confidence Interval
One induced abortion	1.3	0.6–2.7
Two or more induced abortions	2.6	0.9–7.4
Ectopic pregnancy	7.7	1.9–31.5
Pelvic infection	7.5	3.5–16.0
Pelvic operation	2.6	1.4–4.6

*Standardized using the multiple logistic regression model.
From Levin AA, Schoenbaum SC, Stubblefield PG, et al: Ectopic pregnancy and prior induced abortion. Am J Public Health 72:253, 1982.

PATHOLOGY

Most ectopic pregnancies occur in the oviduct. In Breen's series 97.7% of the ectopic pregnancies were tubal, 1.4% were abdominal, and less than 1% were ovarian or cervical (Fig. 17-6). The majority of tubal gestations, 81%, were located in the ampullary portion of the oviduct, being about equally divided between the distal and middle third of the tube. About 12% of tubal gestations occur in the isthmus and 5% in the fimbrial region. Although Breen considered pregnancies located in the cornual area of the uterus to be uterine in origin, they are in fact pregnancies implanted in the interstitial portion of the oviduct. About 2% of all ectopic pregnancies are interstitial and are frequently associated with severe morbidity, because they become symptomatic later in gestation than do other tubal pregnancies, are difficult to diagnose, and frequently produce massive hemorrhage when they rupture (Fig. 17-7). A true cornual pregnancy is one located in the rudimentary horn of a bicornuate uterus, and this occurrence is quite rare. In a review of 240 true cornual pregnancies reported by O'Leary and O'Leary, about 90% of them ruptured with massive hemorrhage.

About 1 in 200 ectopic pregnancies are true ovarian pregnancies that fulfill the four criteria originally described by Spiegelburg:

1. The tube and fimbria must be intact and separate from the ovary.
2. The gestational sac must occupy the normal position of the ovary.
3. The sac must be connected to the uterus by the ovarian ligament.
4. Ovarian tissue should be demonstrable in the walls of the sac.

Many women with ovarian pregnancies are believed clinically to have a ruptured corpus luteum cyst. In Hallatt's series of 25

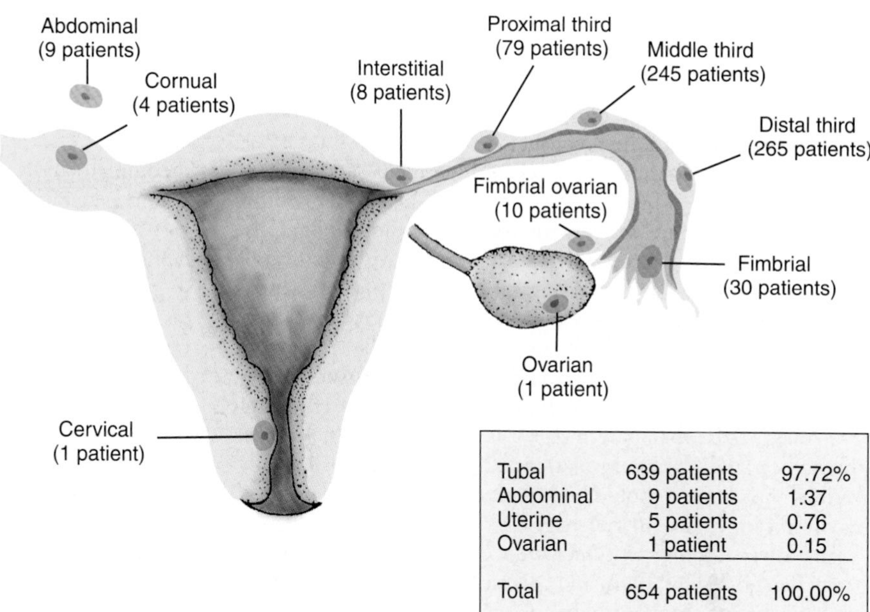

Tubal	639 patients	97.72%
Abdominal	9 patients	1.37
Uterine	5 patients	0.76
Ovarian	1 patient	0.15
Total	654 patients	100.00%

Figure 17-6. Anatomic site of ectopic pregnancy. (From Breen JL: A 21 year survey of 654 ectopic pregnancies. Am J Obstet Gynecol 106:1004, 1970.)

primary ovarian pregnancies, the correct diagnosis was made during the surgical procedure in only 28%. In his series the hemorrhagic mass was always located adjacent to the corpus luteum, never within it. Ovarian pregnancy is also associated with profuse hemorrhage, with 81% of Hallatt's cases having a hemoperitoneum greater than 500 mL. Nevertheless, most can be successfully treated by ovarian resection and not oophorectomy.

Most abdominal pregnancies occur secondary to tubal abortion with secondary implantation in the peritoneal cavity (Fig. 17-8). On rare occasions a primary abdominal pregnancy may occur. For the latter diagnosis to be made the following three criteria originally set forth by Studdiford must be present: (1) the tubes and ovaries must be normal, with no evidence of recent or past injury; (2) there must be no evidence of a uteroplacental fistula; and (3) the pregnancy must be related

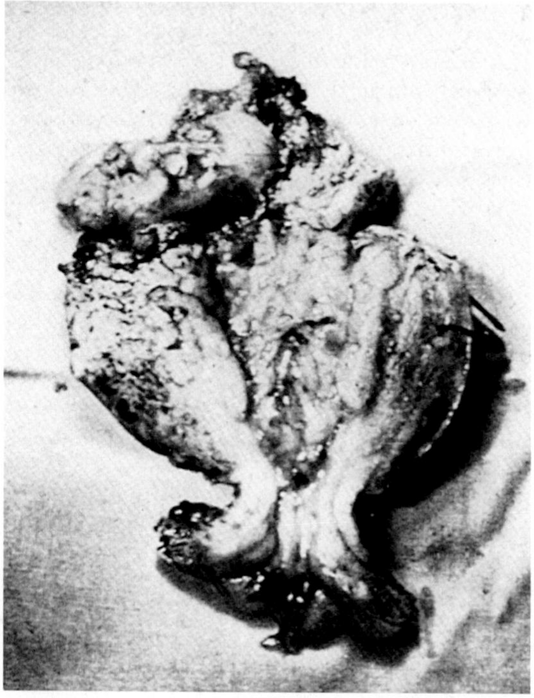

Figure 17-7. Anterior view of uterus that has been opened with an anterior Y incision, showing conceptus replaced in the site it had formerly occupied in cornual bed. (From Kalchman GG, Meltzer RM: Interstitial pregnancy following homolateral salpingectomy. Report of 2 cases and a review of the literature. Am J Obstet Gynecol 96:1139, 1966.)

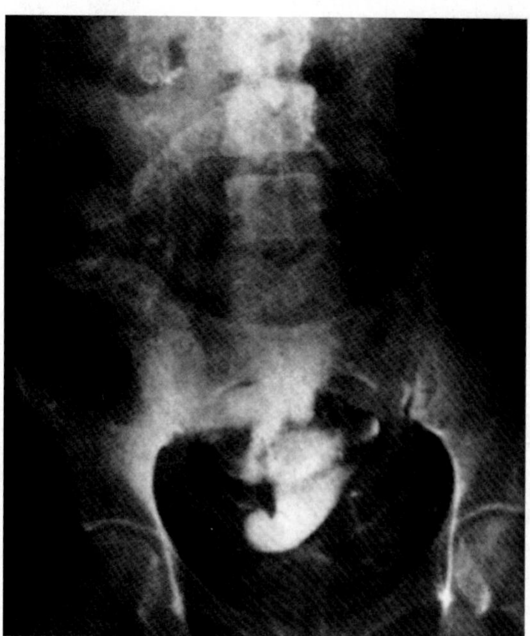

Figure 17-8. Hysterosalpingography demonstrating size of uterus and fetus, which is located outside of uterus. (From Clark JF, Guy RS: Abdominal pregnancy. Am J Obstet Gynecol 96:511, 1966.)

only to the peritoneal surface and early enough in gestation to eliminate the possibility of secondary implantation after primary tubal nidation. An unusual type of primary abdominal pregnancy may implant in the spleen or liver and produce massive intraperitoneal hemorrhage.

The prognosis for fetal survival in abdominal pregnancy is poor, found to be 11% by Clark and Guy. Diagnosis is difficult, but has become easier with the use of ultrasonography. Once the diagnosis is established, a laparotomy with removal of the fetus should be performed immediately to prevent a possible fatal hemorrhage. On occasion, when the placenta is tightly adherent to bowel and blood vessels, it should be left in the abdominal cavity. In such instances the placental tissue usually resorbs, but symptoms of abdominal pain and intermittent fever may persist for many months as a result of partial bowel obstruction and abscess formation. Thus, when it is surgically feasible, the placenta should be entirely removed. Partial removal may result in massive hemorrhage.

The four pathologic criteria for the diagnosis of cervical pregnancy as reported by Rubin and colleagues are (1) cervical glands must be present opposite the placental attachment, (2) the attachment of the placenta to the cervix must be intimate, (3) the placenta must be below the entrance of the uterine vessels or below the peritoneal reflection of the anteroposterior surface of the uterus, and (4) fetal elements must not be present in the corpus uteri (Fig. 17-9).

The clinical criteria for the diagnosis of cervical pregnancy described by Paalman and McElin are (1) uterine bleeding after amenorrhea without cramping pain, (2) a softened cervix that is disproportionately enlarged to a size equal to or larger than

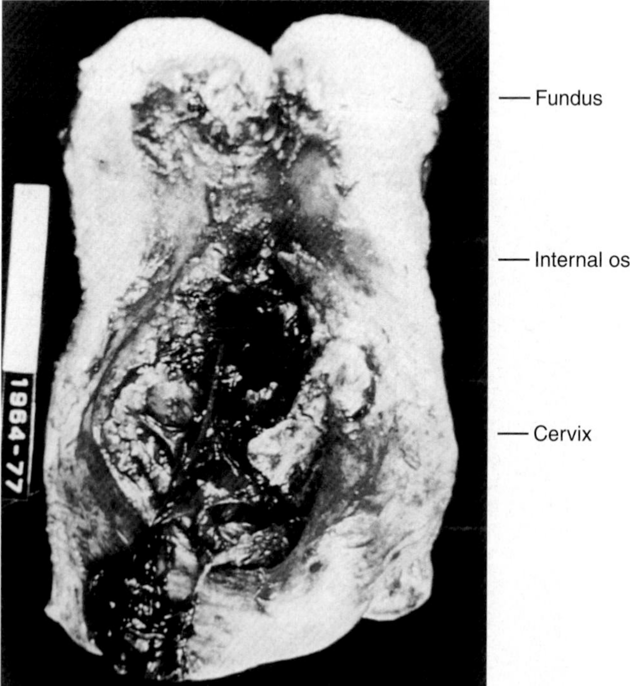

Figure 17-9. Cervical pregnancy, 10 weeks' gestation. (From Parente JT, Ou CS, Levy J: Cervical pregnancy analysis: A review and report of five cases. Obstet Gynecol 62:79, 1983. Reprinted with permission from The American College of Obstetricians and Gynecologists.)

the corpus, (3) complete confinement and firm attachment of the products of conception to the endocervix, and (4) a snug internal os.

Most cervical pregnancies occur after a previous sharp uterine curettage. The differential diagnosis is difficult and includes incomplete abortion, placenta previa, carcinoma of the cervix, and degenerative leiomyoma. Although this entity was previously associated with a high mortality because of massive hemorrhage, currently, with better methods of diagnosis and modern techniques of treatment, death is rare. More than half of the women with cervical pregnancy require a hysterectomy for treatment, and it is nearly always necessary if the pregnancy has advanced more than 18 weeks' gestational age. Even if a hysterectomy is not performed, the prognosis for future fertility is poor.

There have been several case reports in which cervical pregnancy was successfully treated by systemic methotrexate. Other case reports have shown that after angiographic uterine artery embolization evacuation of the pregnancy can be easily performed transcervically with minimal blood loss. Frates and coworkers reported that transvaginal ultrasound-guided injections of potassium chloride directly into the embryonic gestational sac of six cervical pregnancies successfully terminated the pregnancies. Local injection of methotrexate, with or without uterine artery embolization, has also been used to successfully treat cervical ectopic pregnancy.

Another uncommon form of ectopic gestation is combined intrauterine and extrauterine (heterotopic) pregnancy (94% tubal and 6% ovarian). With the use of mathematic calculation the incidence of this entity has previously been estimated to be either 1 in 16,000 or 1 in 30,000 pregnancies. However, a review of the recent experience at one institution by Reece and colleagues revealed that 1 of 8000 pregnancies was combined intrauterine and extrauterine, and 1 of 70 ectopic pregnancies was associated with an IUP. Bello and associates estimated that the incidence of heterotopic pregnancy may be as high as 1 of 4000 pregnancies. Combined intrauterine and extrauterine pregnancy may be more common after pharmacologic ovulation induction with the subsequent increase in multiple ovulation. With the increased use of ovulation-inducing agents, as well as an increased incidence of salpingitis, combined intrauterine and extrauterine pregnancy now occurs more frequently than previously estimated. In several large series, the incidence of heterotopic pregnancy ranges from 1% to 3% of all pregnancies occurring after in vitro fertilization. The incidence was higher when tubal damage was present or four or more embryos were transferred. Heterotopic pregnancy should be suspected when any of the following clinical criteria are present: (1) a fundus compatible with gestational age estimated by date of onset of last menses in a woman believed to have an ectopic gestation; (2) two corpora lutea seen at the time of laparotomy or laparoscopy and an enlarged, soft, and globular uterus; (3) the absence of withdrawal bleeding and the presence of pregnancy symptoms after excision of an ectopic pregnancy; (4) hemoperitoneum after the termination of an IUP; and (5) the combination of abdominal pain, adnexal mass with pain and tenderness, peritoneal irritation, and a uterus enlarged more than 8 weeks' gestational age.

A chronic ectopic pregnancy occurs when the intraperitoneal hemorrhage associated with tubal abortion or rupture is relatively minor and ceases spontaneously, but the ectopic gestation neither resolves completely nor implants and continues to develop as an abdominal pregnancy. The trophoblast continues to secrete HCG in small amounts, with the circulating levels less than 1000 mIU/mL in 50% and less than 100 mIU/mL in 20%. In the series of Cole and Corlett, about 6% of all surgically treated ectopic pregnancies in one institution were classified as chronic. The most common (72%) gross pathologic finding was dense adhesions produced by the inflammatory response to the trophoblast. These adhesions attach omentum and bowel to the site of the ectopic pregnancy. In one third of the cases a collection of clotted blood or old hematoma was present. Cole and Corlett reported that because of the extensive disease it was necessary to perform a hysterectomy in 25% and an oophorectomy in 60% of women with a chronic ovarian ectopic pregnancy.

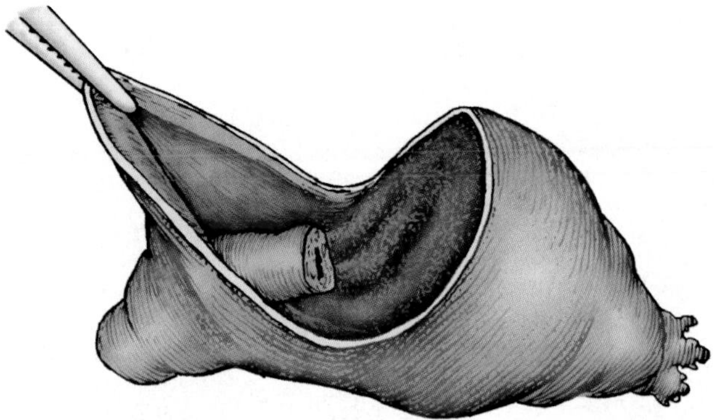

Figure 17-11. Artist's rendition of dissected ampullary ectopic pregnancy showing space between tube and peritoneum, revealed when blood clots and placenta were removed. Toward fimbriated end, no dissection was performed and external appearance is that of dilated tube. (From Budowick M, Johnson TRB, Genadry R, et al: The histopathology of the developing tubal ectopic pregnancy. Fertil Steril 34:169, 1980. Reproduced with permission of the publisher, The American Fertility Society.)

HISTOPATHOLOGY

When the morula implants in the oviduct, it does not grow mainly in the tubal lumen as has been assumed for many years. In a review of the pathology of tubal gestation, Budowick and coworkers found that after implanting on the mucosa of the endosalpinx, the trophoblast invades the lamina propria and then the muscularis of the oviduct and grows mainly between the lumen of the tube and its peritoneal covering (Fig. 17-10). Growth occurs both parallel to the long axis of the oviduct and circumferentially around it. As the trophoblast invades vessels, retroperitoneal tubal hemorrhage occurs that is mainly extraluminal but may extrude from the fimbriated end and create a hemoperitoneum before tubal rupture (Fig. 17-11).

The stretching of the peritoneum covered by this hemorrhage results in episodic pain before the final perforation into the peritoneal cavity. Rupture occurs when the serosa is maximally stretched, producing necrosis secondary to an inadequate blood supply.

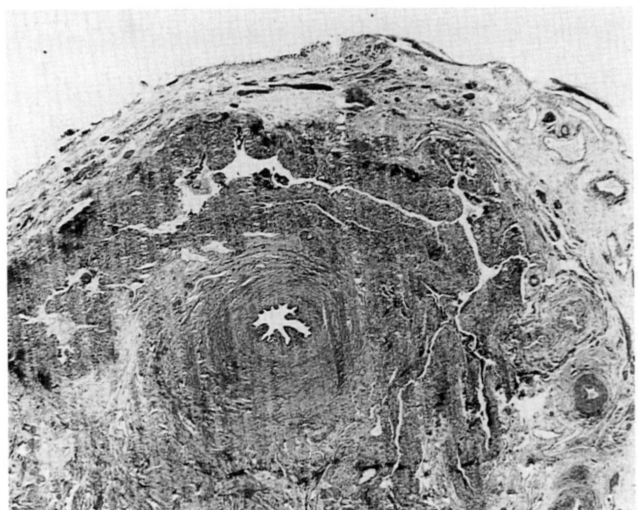

Figure 17-10. Low-power photograph showing tube almost completely surrounded by cleftlike space. Closer inspection revealed that cleft was produced by trophoblast that had implanted elsewhere, perforated wall of tube, and was dissecting along broad ligament between tube and peritoneum. (Reprinted from Fertility and Sterility, 34, Budowick M, Johnson TRB, Genadry R, et al, The histopathology of the developing tubal ectopic pregnancy, 169. Copyright 1980, with permission from The American Society for Reproductive Medicine.)

Hemoperitoneum is nearly always found in advanced ruptured ectopic pregnancy other than that which is cervical in origin. Usually there is a combination of clotted and unclotted blood in the peritoneal cavity. The unclotted blood does not clot on removal from the peritoneal cavity because it originates from lysis of blood that has previously coagulated, similar to what occurs during menstrual bleeding. The hematocrit value of this nonclotting blood is nearly always greater than 15%, such a finding being reported in 98% of specimens obtained by culdocentesis in the series of ectopic pregnancies reported by Brenner and associates. At the time of laparotomy for a ruptured ectopic pregnancy, about half of the women have less than 500 mL of hemoperitoneum, one quarter between 500 and 1000 mL, and one fifth more than 1000 mL.

When the oviduct is removed and examined histologically, inflammatory cells are nearly always seen. These include plasma cells, lymphocytes, and histiocytes. The presence of chorionic villi, which are frequently degenerated or hyalinized, as well as nucleated red cells, establish the diagnosis of ectopic pregnancy. Decidual reaction in the tube is uncommon.

Because of limited space or inadequate nourishment, the trophoblastic tissue of most ectopic pregnancies does not grow as rapidly as that of pregnancies within the uterine cavity. As a result, HCG production does not increase as rapidly as in a normal pregnancy, and although steroid production of the corpus luteum is initiated, elevated progesterone levels cannot be maintained. Thus initially the endometrium becomes decidualized because of continued progesterone production by the corpus luteum. Sometimes the secretory cells of the endometrial glands become hypertrophied with hyperchromatism, pleomorphism, and increased mitotic activity, as originally described by Arias-Stella (Fig. 17-12). The Arias-Stella reaction can be confused with neoplasia, but it is not unique for ectopic pregnancy, because it can occur with IUP, as well as after ovarian stimulation with clomiphene citrate. In a histologic study of the endometrium in 84 women with ectopic pregnancies, Ollendorff and Felgin found that about 40% had secretory

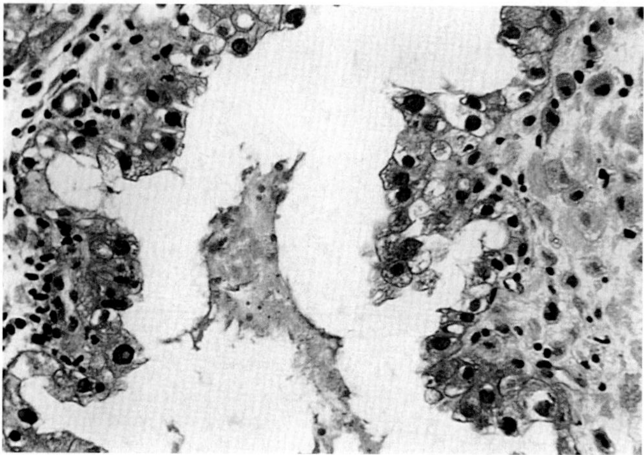

Figure 17-12. Arias-Stella reaction. (From DeCherney AH, Maheux R: Modern management of tubal pregnancy. Curr Probl Obstet Gynecol 6:2, 1983.)

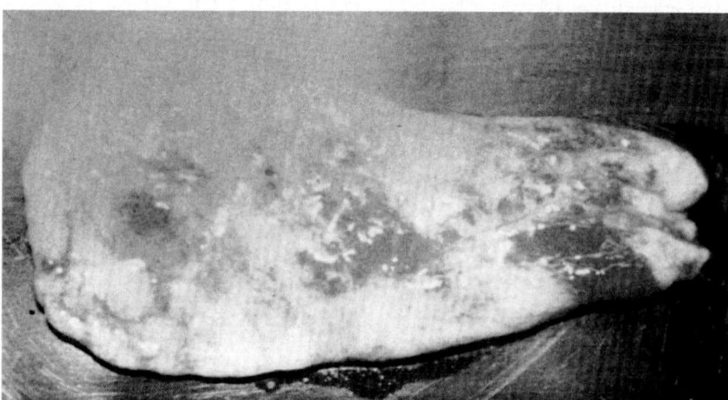

Figure 17-13. Decidual cast. (From DeCherney AH, Maheux R: Modern management of tubal pregnancy. Curr Probl Obstet Gynecol 6:2, 1983.)

endometrium, with the remainder being about equally divided among proliferative endometrium, decidual reaction, and Arias-Stella reaction. When progesterone levels fall as a result of insufficient daily increase of HCG, endometrial integrity is no longer maintained, and it sloughs, producing uterine bleeding. Sometimes nearly all the decidua is passed through the cervix intact, producing a decidual cast that may be clinically confused with a spontaneous abortion (Fig. 17-13).

SYMPTOMS

Among women with risk factors for ectopic pregnancy, with the use of early hormonal testing and vaginal sonography, it is now frequently possible to establish the diagnosis of ectopic pregnancy before symptoms develop. However, when the gestational age increases and intraperitoneal bleeding occurs from extrusion of blood through the fimbrial end of the oviduct or from tubal rupture, symptoms develop. It is important to be aware of the symptoms of ectopic gestation because this potentially fatal condition can occur in any sexually active woman of reproductive age whether or not she is using contraceptives or has undergone tubal sterilization.

Table 17-3 Symptoms of Ectopic Pregnancy

Symptoms	Percentage of Patients with Symptom
Abdominal pain	90–100
Amenorrhea	75–95
Vaginal bleeding	50–80
Dizziness, fainting	20–35
Urge to defecate	5–15
Pregnancy symptoms	10–25
Passage of tissue	5–10

From Weckstein LN: Current perspective on ectopic pregnancy. Obstet Gynecol Surv 40:259, 1985.

The most common symptoms of ectopic pregnancy are abdominal pain, absence of menses, and irregular vaginal bleeding (Table 17-3). Abdominal pain is nearly a universal symptom of intraperitoneal bleeding but its characteristics are similar with different causes of bleeding. Before rupture occurs, the pain may be characterized as only a vague soreness or be colicky in nature. Its location may be generalized, unilateral, or bilateral. Shoulder pain occurs in about one fourth of women with ruptured ectopic pregnancy as a result of diaphragmatic irritation from the hemoperitoneum. During rupture of the oviduct the pain usually becomes intense. Syncope occurs in about one third of women with tubal rupture. Other symptoms that occur following tubal rupture include dizziness and an urge to defecate.

The majority of women with ectopic pregnancy fail to have menses at the expected time but have one or more episodes of irregular vaginal bleeding when the decidual endometrial tissue is sloughed. The interval of amenorrhea is usually 6 weeks or more. The bleeding is usually characterized as spotting but may simulate menstrual bleeding. It is rarely as heavy as that which occurs in spontaneous abortion. About 5% to 10% of women with an advanced ectopic pregnancy will note passage of a decidual cast.

SIGNS

The most common presenting sign in a woman with symptomatic ectopic pregnancy is abdominal tenderness, which, together with adnexal tenderness elicited at the time of the bimanual pelvic examination, is present in nearly all women with an advanced or ruptured ectopic pregnancy (Table 17-4). It is possible to palpate an adnexal mass in half of the women,

Table 17-4 Signs of Ectopic Pregnancy

Sign	Percentage of Patients with Sign
Adnexal tenderness	75–90
Abdominal tenderness	80–95
Adnexal mass*	50
Uterine enlargement	20–30
Orthostatic changes	10–15
Fever	5–10

*20% present on the side opposite the ectopic pregnancy.
From Weckstein LN: Current perspective on ectopic pregnancy. Obstet Gynecol Surv 40:259, 1985.

and about one third have some degree of uterine enlargement that is nearly always smaller than a normal 8-week intrauterine gestation except when an interstitial gestation is present. Tachycardia and hypotension can occur after rupture if blood loss is profuse, but temperature elevation is an uncommon finding, being present in only about 5% to 10% of women with tubal rupture, and is rarely greater than 38°C.

DIAGNOSIS

Laboratory Tests

A hematocrit of less than 30% is found in about one fourth of women with ruptured ectopic pregnancy at the time of rupture. About half have a normal leukocyte count, with a mild elevation of 10,000 to 15,000/mm^3 in one third and a greater elevation in one fifth.

HCG is present in the circulation of nearly every woman with an ectopic gestation, but the levels are lower than 3000 mIU/mL in about half. The incidence of positive qualitative pregnancy tests depends on the sensitivity of the assay. With use of the sensitive enzyme-linked immunosorbent assays (ELISA), more than 90% of women with an ectopic pregnancy will have a positive pregnancy test. This incidence increases to nearly 100% if a radioimmunoassay for HCG is used.

Differential Diagnosis of Symptomatic Ectopic Pregnancy

The diagnosis is usually obvious for women with the classic symptoms of ruptured ectopic pregnancy: a history of irregular bleeding followed by sudden onset of pain and syncope accompanied by signs of peritoneal irritation. However, before rupture the symptoms and signs are nonspecific and may also occur with other gynecologic disorders. Entities frequently confused with ectopic pregnancy include salpingitis, threatened or incomplete abortion, ruptured corpus luteum, appendicitis, dysfunctional uterine bleeding, adnexal torsion, degenerative uterine leiomyoma, and endometriosis.

In the series of Brenner and associates, about 50% of the women with ruptured ectopic pregnancy had at least one consultation with a physician without the condition being correctly diagnosed before admission to a health care facility, where the correct diagnosis was made. About 33% of the women were seen once, 11% twice, and the remainder three to five times before the diagnosis was made. Other studies have confirmed that there is a high frequency of misdiagnosis and physician delay in determining that an ectopic pregnancy is present. Because of the possibility of a fatal outcome from undiagnosed ruptured ectopic pregnancy, it is essential that the diagnosis of ectopic pregnancy be considered in any woman of childbearing age with abdominal pain and irregular uterine bleeding even if she has had a previous tubal sterilization procedure or is using an effective method of reversible contraception.

Ectopic pregnancy should be suspected in any woman who develops the symptoms listed earlier, particularly if she has previously had a pelvic operation, especially tubal surgery, either a tubal reconstructive procedure or a sterilization procedure. Other risk factors include one or more episodes of salpingitis, a previous ectopic gestation, current use of a progesterone-releasing IUD, use of a progestin-only oral contraceptive, use of pharmacologic methods of ovulation induction, and a history of infertility. In any woman with the symptoms of ectopic gestation the diagnosis is facilitated by a quantitative assay for HCG and pelvic ultrasonography and can be established by laparoscopy or laparotomy. Culdocentesis and measurement of serum progesterone levels may also be of assistance, although culdocentesis is infrequently used currently since the advent of sensitive ultrasonography.

Procedures Used to Aid the Diagnosis of Severely Symptomatic Ectopic Pregnancy

Culdocentesis

Prior to the development of pelvic sonography with a vaginal transducer, the finding of nonclotting blood at the time of culdocentesis, especially if the hematocrit was above 15%, was of great assistance in establishing the diagnosis of ruptured ectopic pregnancy. With the use of pelvic sonography, the presence of intraperitoneal fluid can be easily visualized, so it is unnecessary to perform a culdocentesis.

Laparoscopy

A definitive diagnosis of ectopic pregnancy can nearly always be made by direct visualization of the pelvis with laparoscopy. However, sometimes because of hemoperitoneum, adhesions, or obesity, it is difficult to visualize the pelvic organs. In a study by Samuellson and Sjovall, 4 of 166 ectopic pregnancies were not visualized by the laparoscopist, and 6 of 120 women with an IUP were thought to have ectopic pregnancies. Thus there is a 2% to 5% chance of a false-positive or false-negative diagnosis with laparoscopy.

Procedures Used for the Diagnostic Evaluation of the Asymptomatic or Mildly Symptomatic Woman with Suspected Ectopic Pregnancy

Human Chorionic Gonadotropin

Although a negative qualitative urine test for HCG does not rule out ectopic pregnancy, if a sensitive serum immunoassay is negative, the diagnosis is unlikely. If β-HCG is not detected with use of radioimmunoassay of serum, the diagnosis of ectopic pregnancy can, with a rare exception, be ruled out. Although about 85% of women with ectopic pregnancy have serum HCG levels lower than those seen in normal pregnancy at a similar gestational age, a single quantitative HCG assay cannot be used to diagnose ectopic pregnancy because the actual dates of ovulation and conception are not known for most women. Even if the date of ovulation is known, 2.5% of women with normal gestations will have HCG levels lower than the normal 95% confidence limits. Furthermore, low HCG levels are also found in women with various stages of spontaneous abortion, conditions that must be considered in the differential diagnosis. Intact HCG and free β-HCG levels were measured in a large group of women in early pregnancy who presented with symptoms of ectopic pregnancy. Although mean levels of intact

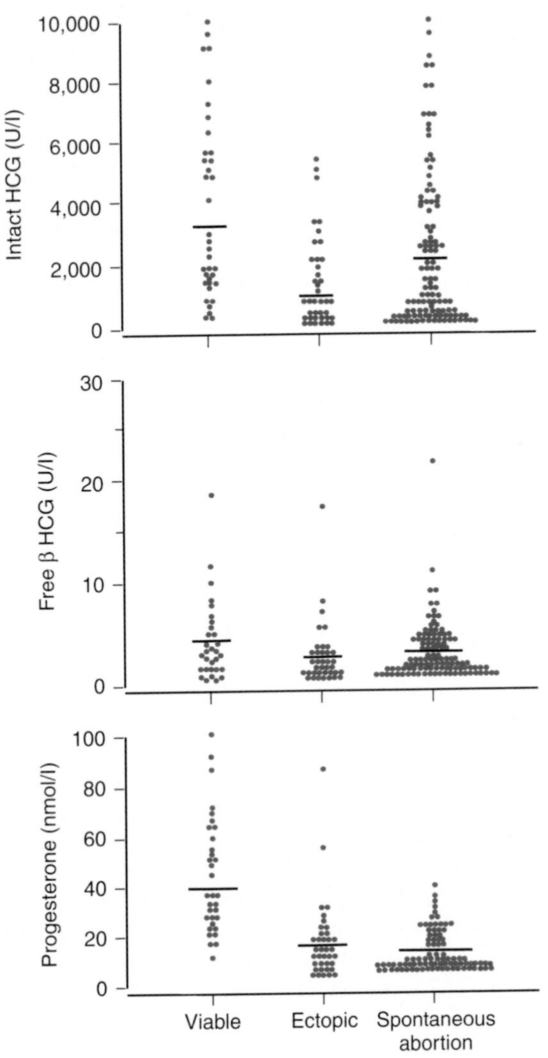

Figure 17-14. The distribution of serum concentrations of progesterone, intact human chorionic gonadotropin (HCG) and free β-HCG in viable and ectopic pregnancies and spontaneous abortions. Means are indicated by horizontal bars (—). (From Ledger WL, Sweeting VM, Chatterjee S: Rapid diagnosis of early ectopic pregnancy in an emergency gynaecology service—are measurements of progesterone, intact and free beta human chorionic gonadotrophin helpful? Hum Reprod 9:157, 1994.)

HCG and free β-HCG were significantly lower in the group of women with ectopic pregnancy and those who aborted than in those with viable intrauterine pregnancies, the individual HCG levels among the three conditions overlapped too much to devise a cut-off level for diagnostic purposes (Fig. 17-14).

In normal pregnancies in early gestation the levels of circulating HCG double about every 2 days. Levels should double in two thirds of women with normal pregnancies in 2 days and in all women in 3 days (Table 17-5). In abnormal pregnancies, ectopic gestations, and those destined to abort, HCG levels usually do not increase at the same rate. Kadar and colleagues reported that if the percentage increase in HCG during a 2-day period is less than 66%, the chance that the woman has an abnormal pregnancy is high. In their series only 15% of normal pregnancies failed to have this amount of increase, whereas only 13% of ectopic pregnancies had this normal rate of increase.

Table 17-5 Lower Normal Limits of Percentage Increase of Serum HCG during Early Pregnancy

Sampling Interval (Days)	Increase in HCG (%)
1	29
2	66
3	114
4	175
5	255

From Kadar N, Caldwell BV, Romero R: A method of screening for ectopic pregnancy and its indications. Obstet Gynecol 58:162, 1981. Reprinted with permission from The American College of Obstetricians and Gynecologists.

Cartwright and DiPietro reported that when serial HCG measurements were performed before surgical excision of an ectopic pregnancy in 25 women 20 had a plateau or decrease in HCG levels during a 2-day or longer duration before surgical excision (Fig. 17-15).

Romero and coworkers reported that 90% of women with ectopic pregnancies had one of two main patterns of serial HCG values. About half had falling HCG levels, and the other half had a subnormal rate of increase with a slope of less than 0.11 (corresponding to a 66% increase in 48 hours and a 114% increase in 3 days). Thus the sensitivity of measuring serial HCG levels to diagnose ectopic pregnancy compared with a normal IUP is 90%. However, the false-positive rate of intrauterine pregnancies with a subnormal slope was 12.5%. Kratzer and Taylor reported similar results when comparing the rates of HCG increase in ectopic and intrauterine pregnancies. Lindblom and associates refined this technique by plotting the slope of the rise of serial β-HCG levels against the initial level and reported that the positive predictive value for the diagnosis of ectopic pregnancy was 95% compared with IUP. Gronlund and Marushak measured two serum HCG levels at intervals of more than 2 days in 21 women with ectopic pregnancy and compared the median slope with that of 39 women with normal intrauterine pregnancies of less than 8 weeks' gestational age. The median slopes of increase were significantly different, with very little overlap. An increase of 1000 mIU/mL of HCG in 2 days was able to differentiate between an ectopic and a normal pregnancy, with a predictive value of 90%, sensitivity of 86%, and specificity of 93% (Fig. 17-16). These studies indicate that serial measurements of HCG are of great assistance in the early diagnosis of unruptured ectopic pregnancy. However, a differentiation between ectopic pregnancies and impending spontaneous abortion cannot be made with this technique because the rate of increase of HCG in women with an ectopic pregnancy is similar to that found in women with an impending intrauterine abortion.

Progesterone

Since a single HCG determination does not provide sufficient information to diagnose ectopic pregnancy because of the inability to determine gestational age with precision, and serial determinations require a 2- to 3-day delay, a single serum progesterone measurement in early gestation has been found by several groups to be of great use in differentiating an ectopic from an intrauterine gestation. Several investigators have shown

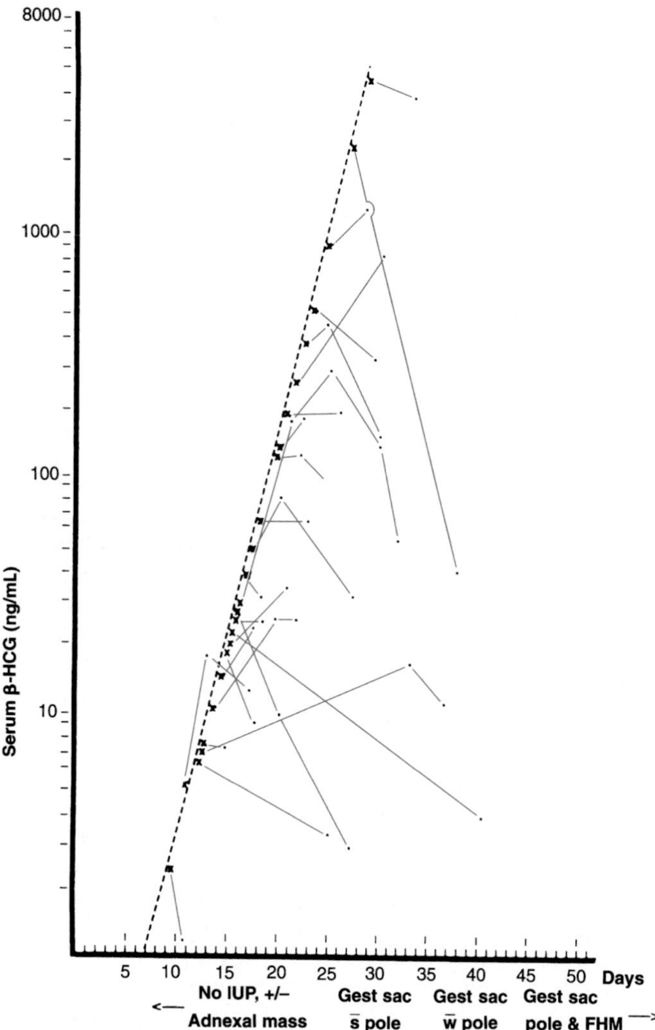

Figure 17-15. Serial quantitated serum β-human chorionic gonadotropin (β-HCG) levels for 25 patients with ectopic pregnancy. Broken line represents average HCG progression for first 30 days of normal pregnancy, with corresponding sonographic findings below. Each patient's first determined value is arbitrarily placed on standard line. FHM, fetal heart motion; Gest sac, gestational sac; IUP, intrauterine pregnancy; s̄ pole, without; w̄ pole, with. (From Cartwright PS, DiPietro DL: Ectopic pregnancy: changes in serum human chorionic gonadotropin concentration. Obstet Gynecol 63:76, 1984. Reprinted with permission from The American College of Obstetricians and Gynecologists.)

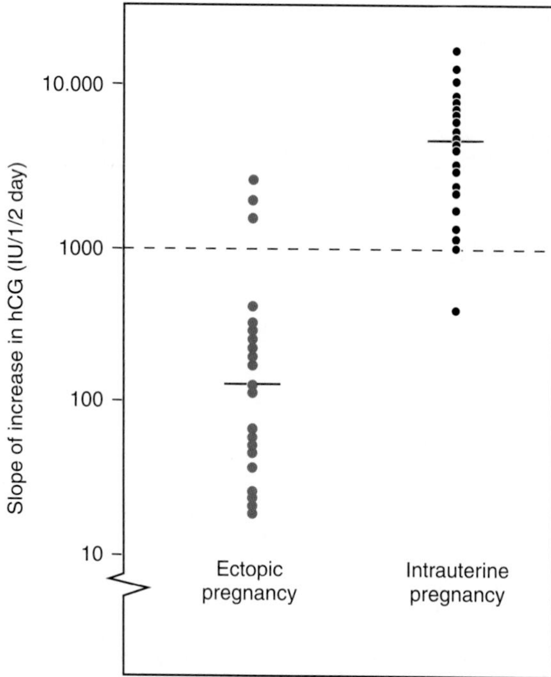

Figure 17-16. The slope of human chorionic gonadotropin (HCG) rise in patients with ectopic (N = 2) and intrauterine pregnancy (N = 29). Solid lines are median slopes. Dotted line at 980 IU/1/2 days. (From Gronlund B, Marushak A: Serial human chorionic gonadotrophin determination in the diagnosis of ectopic pregnancy. Aust N Z J Obstet Gynaecol 33:312, 1993.)

that when an ectopic pregnancy is present the corpus luteum does not secrete as much progesterone as occurs in normal pregnancies with similar levels of HCG. Stern and colleagues prospectively measured progesterone, as well as HCG, in serum samples at 4, 5, and 6 weeks of known gestational age from a group of women with infertility or a history of recurrent abortion who conceived. They found that in the women with ectopic pregnancies, mean serum progesterone levels were significantly lower at each of these gestational ages than in the women with intrauterine gestations whether or not these gestations subsequently aborted or continued to viability (Table 17-6) They also reported that at 4 weeks' gestation a threshold progesterone level of 5 ng/mL was able to differentiate ectopic from intrauterine gestations, with a sensitivity of 100% and a specificity of 97%. At 5 weeks' gestation the threshold level of progesterone increased to 10 ng/mL and at 6 weeks to 20 ng/mL, but the sensitivity and specificity of the use of serum progesterone measurement to differentiate ectopic from intrauterine gestations decreased as the gestational age increased.

Ledger and colleagues also found a significant difference in mean progesterone levels between women in early pregnancy with a viable intrauterine gestation and those with an ectopic gestation or those who had a spontaneous abortion (see Figure 17-14). Hahlin and coworkers found that in a group of women presenting with symptoms of ectopic pregnancy no woman with a viable IUP had progesterone levels less than 30 nM/L (10 ng/mL), whereas 88% of ectopic pregnancies and 83% of spontaneous abortions had progesterone values less than this amount.

Stovall and associates measured both HCG and serum progesterone levels in more than 1000 women in the first trimester of pregnancy. They found that all those women with a serum progesterone level less than 5 ng/mL had either an ectopic gestation or a nonviable intrauterine gestation, whereas 97% of women with a serum progesterone level above 25 ng/mL had a viable intrauterine gestation. They calculated that a single progesterone level of less than 15 ng/mL was as sensitive and more specific than lack of a rise of 66% of two HCG levels measured 48 hours apart for the detection of an abnormal pregnancy. This same group showed that the probability of an ectopic or abnormal IUP decreased with rising progesterone levels, with less than a 10% likelihood of an abnormal pregnancy occurring with the progesterone level above 17.6 ng/mL (Fig. 17-17). O'Leary and colleagues reported that a combination of HCG less than 3000 IU/L and a progesterone less than

Table 17-6 Mean Progesterone Concentrations Obtained at Weeks 4, 5, and 6 of Gestation from Women Whose Pregnancies Subsequently Terminated in Live Births, Spontaneous Abortions, or Ectopic Pregnancies

	PROGESTERONE CONCENTRATIONS AT DIFFERENT GESTATIONAL AGES (Weeks) (Mean ± SEM, ng/mL)				
Pregnancy Outcome	***n***	**4**	**5**	**6**	**Mean All Gestations**
Live birth	242	35.5 ± 6.2	31.0 ± 6.0	27.5 ± 5.3	31.2 ± 5.9
Spontaneous abortion	81	32.9 ± 4.62	23.9 ± 2.8	23.3 ± 2.6	26.7 ± 3.0
Ectopic	15	*1.9 ± 0.9	*11.9 ± 1.4	*7.0 ± 3.3	*7.0 ± 2.9

*Significantly lower than other values in same column ($P = 0.0005$).
From Stern JJ, Voss, F, Coulam, CB: Early diagnosis of ectopic pregnancy using receiver-operator characteristic curves of serum progesterone concentrations. Hum Reprod 8:775, 1993.

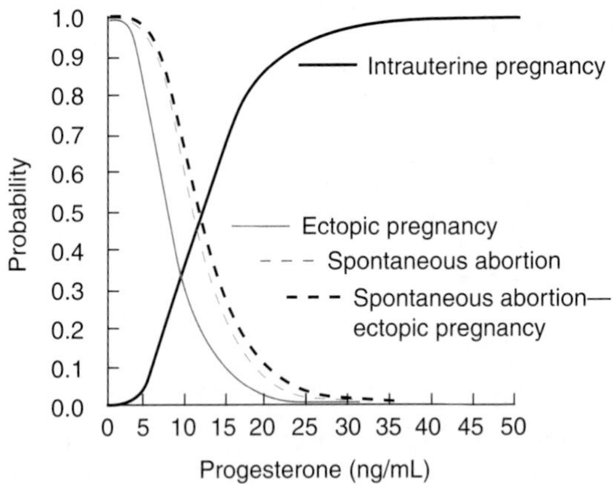

Figure 17-17. Predicted pregnancy outcome versus progesterone concentrations. The probability of ectopic pregnancy and spontaneous abortion decreases with rising progesterone levels, forming a negative-sloping sigmoid-shaped curve, a mirror image of the intrauterine pregnancy curve, with its slope decreasing sharply at approximately 5 ng/mL (15.9 nmol/L) and increasing sharply at approximately 17 ng/mL (54.1 nmol/L). (Reprinted from Fertility and Sterility, 66, McCord ML, Arheart KL, Muram D, et al, Single serum progesterone as a screen for ectopic pregnancy: exchanging specificity and sensitivity to obtain optimal test performance, 513. Copyright 1996, with permission from The American Society for Reproductive Medicine.)

13 ng/mL predicted an abnormal gestation, either ectopic pregnancy or nonviable intrauterine gestation, in 97% of women.

Sauer and coworkers reported that measurement of pregnanediol glucuronide in a single random urine specimen by a rapid enzyme immunoassay was also very useful in differentiating ectopic from IUP when a level of 9 μg/mL was used to discriminate the two entities. In their study, this single rapid assay was as effective as measurement of serum progesterone in distinguishing ectopic from intrauterine pregnancies between 5 and 8 weeks from the onset of the last menses.

Ultrasonography

With the use of abdominal ultrasonography, Kadar and colleagues reported in 1981 that if the HCG level was greater than 6500 mIU/mL and no gestational sac was seen in the uterus, nearly all the women had an ectopic pregnancy. However, this technique was not clinically useful, because about 90% of women with ectopic pregnancies had HCG levels below this threshold.

Development of the transvaginal transducer probes with 5.0- to 7.0-MHz scanning frequency has enabled more precise imaging of the pelvic organs in early pregnancy than is possible with transabdominal ultrasonography. With these probes it is usually possible to identify an intrauterine gestational sac when the HCG level reaches 1500 mIU/mL and always possible to identify a gestational sac in the uterus when the HCG level exceeds 2000 mIU/mL (First International Reference Preparation [1st IRP], now called the Third International Standard), about 5 to 6 weeks after the last menses. Kadar and colleagues reported that in both singleton and multiple gestations a gestational sac should always be seen sonographically beyond 24 days after conception, 38 days' gestational age. Because combined extrauterine and IUP is a rare event, the finding of an intrauterine gestational sac should nearly always exclude the presence of an ectopic pregnancy. When a gestational sac is not present and the HCG level is more than 1500 mIU/mL, a pathologic pregnancy, either an ectopic or a nonviable intrauterine gestation, is most likely present and should be suspected. Usually an adnexal mass or a gestational saclike structure can be identified in the oviduct when an ectopic pregnancy is present that produces levels of HCG above 2500 mIU/mL (Fig. 17-18).

Thus diagnostic criteria for the ultrasonographic diagnosis of ectopic pregnancy with the use of a vaginal probe include the detection of a complex or cystic adnexal mass or visualization of an embryo in the adnexa, or the absence of an intrauterine gestational sac when the gestational age is known to be more than 38 days, or the HCG level is above a certain threshold, usually between 1500 and 2500 mIU/mL.

About two thirds of women presenting with symptoms of ectopic pregnancy have HCG levels above 2500 mIU/mL,

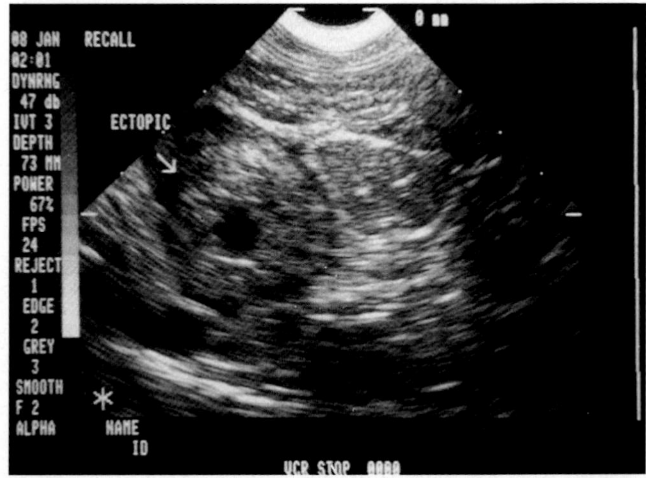

Figure 17-18. Ultrasound of ectopic pregnancy. (Photo courtesy of Advanced Technology Laboratories, Bothell, WA, 1991.)

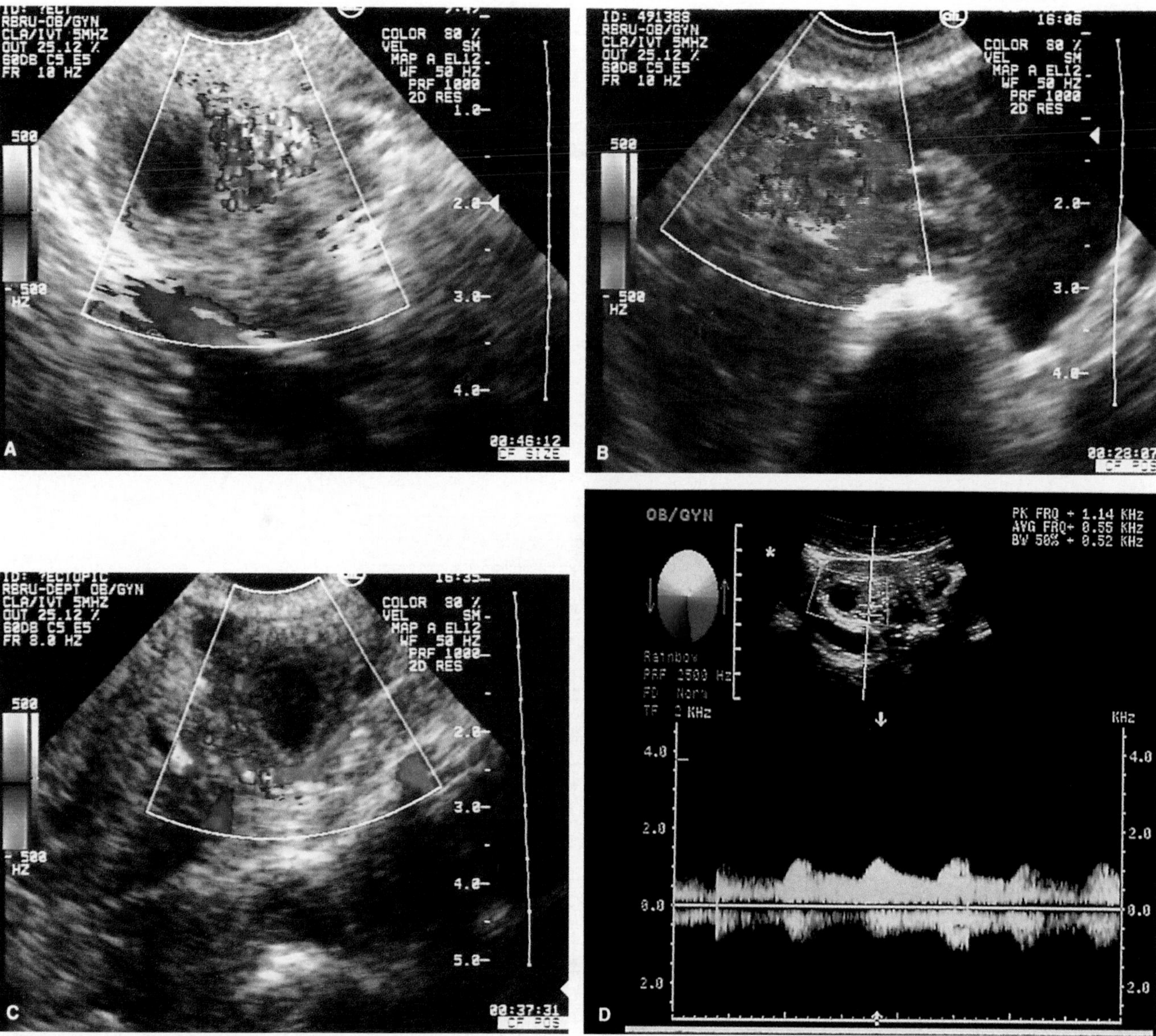

Figure 17-19. Ectopic pregnancy showing enhanced blood flow using color Doppler.

and when this occurs, the diagnosis of ectopic pregnancy can usually be made sonographically. For the other one third with lower HCG levels, unless a gestational sac is evident on ultrasonography, other diagnostic techniques, such as measurement of a serum progesterone level and serial HCG determination, should be performed. Repeat ultrasonographic examinations at 3- to 5-day intervals are often helpful in establishing a correct diagnosis.

Several investigators have shown that with the use of endovaginal color Doppler flow imaging it is possible to establish the diagnosis of ectopic pregnancy with greater sensitivity and specificity than with ordinary endovaginal sonography. With endovaginal color flow imaging of the pelvic structures in the presence of an ectopic pregnancy, about a 20% difference in the degree of tubal blood flow between the adnexae has been found compared with less than an 8% difference with intrauterine gestations. Use of endovaginal color flow compared with routine transvaginal sonography increased the sensitivity of the diagnosis of ectopic pregnancy from 71% to 95%, with a specificity of 96% to 100% in various studies (Fig. 17-19).

Dilation and Curettage

When serum HCG levels are more than 1500 mIU/mL, the gestational age exceeds 38 days, or the serum progesterone level is less than 5 ng/mL and no intrauterine gestational sac is seen with vaginal ultrasonography, a curettage of the endometrial cavity with histologic examination of the tissue removed, by frozen section if desired, can be undertaken to determine if any gestational tissue is present. Spandorfer and coworkers reported that frozen section was 93% accurate in identifying chorionic villi. If no chorionic villi are visualized in the removed tissue, a presumptive diagnosis of ectopic pregnancy can be made and treatment undertaken. A recent analysis by Ailawedi suggested that performing a dilatation and curettage in this setting results in less complications and is at least as cost-effective as the empiric use of methotrexate.

Diagnostic Evaluation of Women with Suspected Ectopic Pregnancy

Flow sheets have been developed by several authors to aid the clinician in establishing the diagnosis of an asymptomatic or mildly symptomatic ectopic pregnancy. They involve the use of vaginal probe pelvic ultrasonography, measurements of serial quantitative HCG and single serum progesterone levels, and uterine curettage (Fig. 17-20). These diagnostic aids are of particular use when following an asymptomatic woman with risk factors for ectopic pregnancy, beginning shortly after conception. Performing a quantitative HCG assay twice weekly and calculating the rate of increase, measuring serum progesterone levels at 4, 5, and 6 weeks' gestational age; and performing serial ultrasonography beginning 3 weeks after ovulation will help to establish the diagnosis of ectopic pregnancy before tubal rupture. The combination of these two techniques is particularly applicable for stable women treated in institutions with adequate facilities for ultrasound and rapid serial quantitative β-HCG assays. If a woman with or without risk factors for ectopic pregnancy develops mild symptoms consistent with an ectopic gestation and is hemodynamically stable, vaginal sonography, measurement of serum progesterone and serial HCG levels, as well as uterine curettage, if indicated, will aid in establishing the diagnosis. The use of a quantitative serum HCG assay and transvaginal sonography enables the diagnosis of ectopic gestation in hemodynamically stable women to be made with a sensitivity of 97% to 100% and a specificity of 95% to 99% (Fig. 17-21).

If a woman develops symptoms of a ruptured ectopic pregnancy that are of sufficient hemodynamic severity to require emergency care, a sensitive qualitative pregnancy test and vaginal sonography are usually all the diagnostic aids necessary to

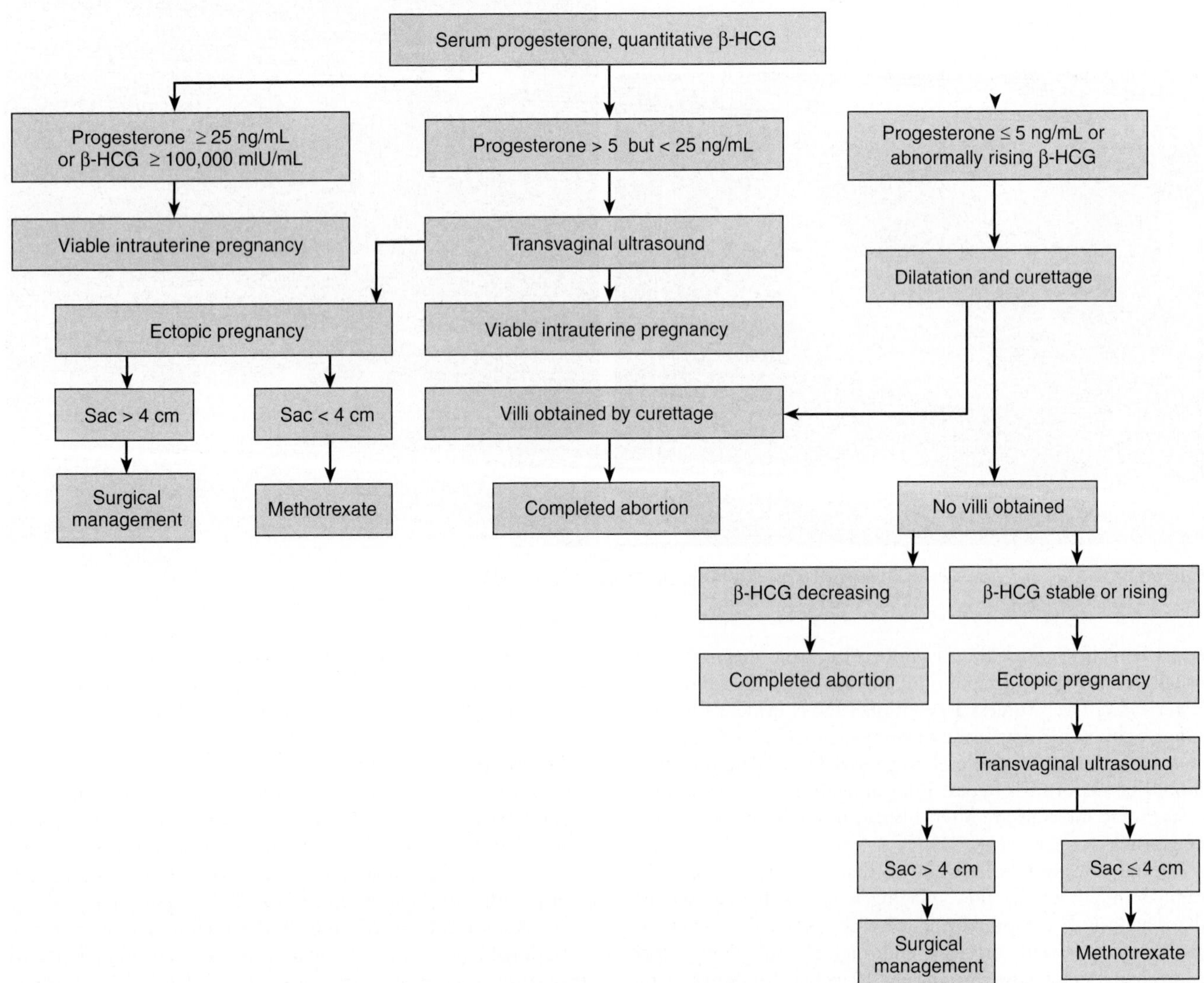

Figure 17-20. Algorithm for the diagnosis of unruptured ectopic pregnancy without laparoscopy. Progesterone measurements increase the sensitivity of the algorithm by screening large numbers of patients inexpensively during the first trimester of pregnancy. Definitive diagnosis is made by transvaginal ultrasound or uterine curettage and does not depend on the serum progesterone concentrations obtained during screening. β-HCG, β-human chorionic gonadotropin. (From Buster JE, Carson SA: Ectopic pregnancy: New advances in diagnosis and treatment. Curr Opin Obstet Gynecol 7:168, 1995.)

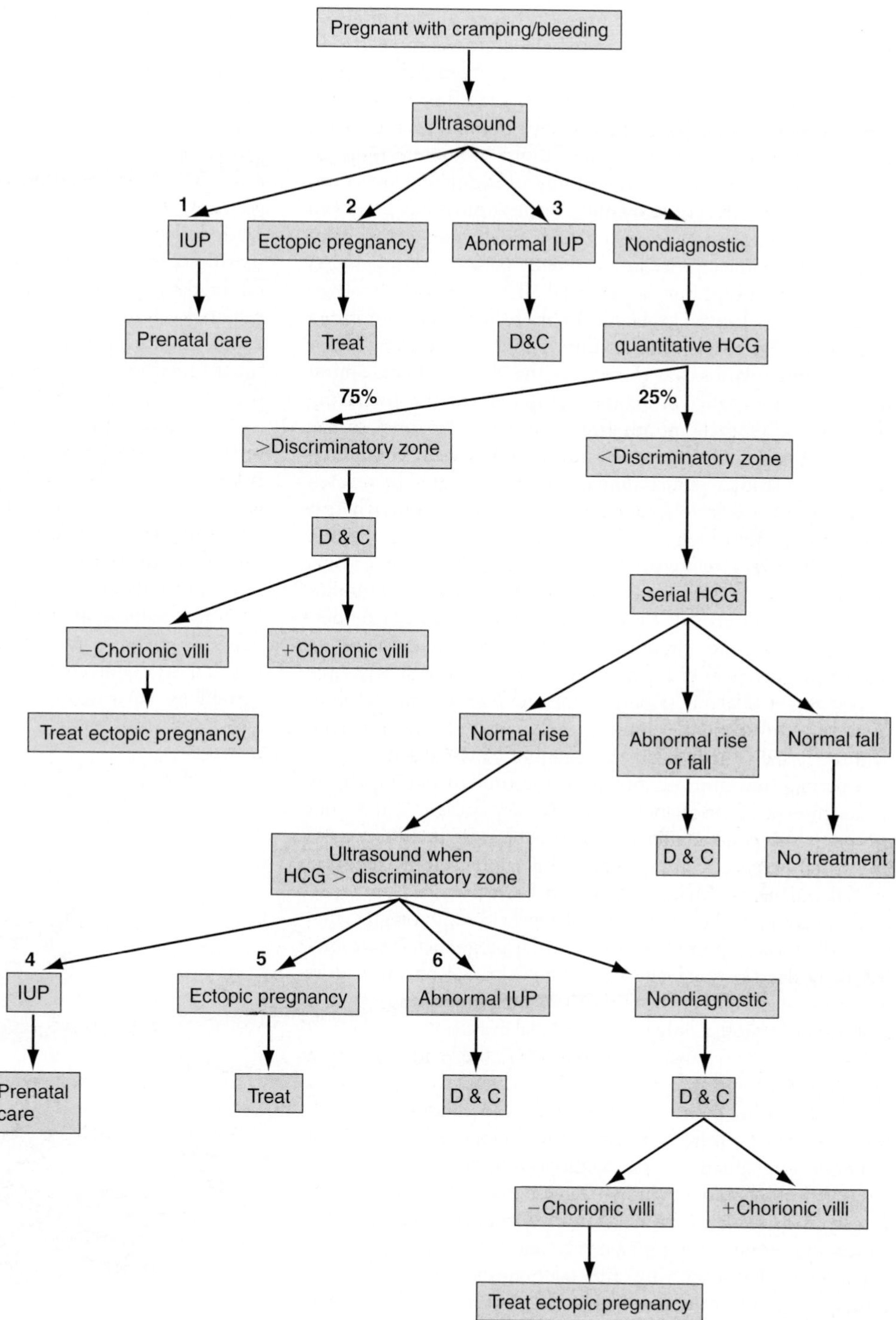

Figure 17-21. Sample schematic of strategy 1. Numbers refer to probabilities. D&C, dilatation and curettage; IUP, intrauterine pregnancy. (From Gracia C, Barnhart KT: Diagnosing ectopic pregnancy. Obstet Gynecol 97:465, 2001.)

establish the diagnosis. If vaginal sonography is not immediately available, culdocentesis may be performed. If HCG is present and peritoneal fluid is seen sonographically, it is most likely that an ectopic pregnancy is present, and laparoscopy should be performed. If peritoneal fluid is observed sonographically or nonclotting blood is obtained by culdocentesis, and a qualitative HCG assay is negative, the diagnosis of ruptured corpus luteum is likely and a laparoscopy should be performed.

MANAGEMENT

Surgical Therapy

The treatment of ectopic gestations in uncommon locations other than the oviduct was discussed earlier in the chapter (see Pathology section). An interstitial pregnancy usually becomes symptomatic at a late gestational age and is usually large. It may therefore require hysterectomy, although it can often be handled conservatively with a resection of the cornual region of the uterus. Nearly all ruptured ectopic pregnancies require surgical treatment, which can be either a radical or a conservative procedure. Radical operation consists of salpingectomy with or without accompanying oophorectomy or hysterectomy. A conservative procedure, salpingostomy or segmental resection, does not remove the entire oviduct. If the rupture has produced extensive damage to the oviduct or if no further pregnancies are desired, a radical procedure is usually performed; otherwise, a conservative procedure is preferred. It was previously advocated that an elective ipsilateral oophorectomy be performed in a woman wishing future fertility. The theoretical reason for this recommendation was to increase the chance of conception and reduce the chance of another ectopic pregnancy by having ovulation occur each month from the ovary proximal to the remaining tube. Results from various studies yield conflicting data. Some studies report similar conception rates in women treated with salpingectomy and salpingo-oophorectomy, whereas others report both higher and lower pregnancy rates in women having the ovary removed. However, the subsequent ectopic pregnancy rate in these studies was not decreased when oophorectomy was performed. An oophorectomy should not be performed under most circumstances. If a woman develops an ectopic pregnancy after tubal sterilization, it is usually advisable to perform a bilateral salpingectomy to prevent the development of a subsequent ectopic pregnancy in the contralateral oviduct. Usually the fistulous tract cannot be visualized.

A cornual resection performed at the time of salpingectomy for an interstitial pregnancy is unnecessary because it does not prevent a subsequent interstitial pregnancy. Of the 75 cases of interstitial pregnancy after homolateral salpingectomy reported by Kalchman and Meltzer, 20% had been preceded by a cornual resection. In Hallatt's series of repeat ectopic pregnancies, 8 of 10 ruptured homolateral interstitial pregnancies were preceded by deep cornual resection. Thus cornual resection does not prevent a subsequent interstitial pregnancy, and, if it is performed, it should only be a superficial excision.

Conservative treatment (not removing the oviduct) for an unruptured ectopic pregnancy is the method frequently used for women who desire future fertility. No randomized trials have compared future fertility or the incidence of ectopic or intrauterine pregnancies after salpingostomy or salpingectomy. However, observational studies suggest that when conservative surgery is correctly performed for an unruptured ectopic pregnancy, the repeat ectopic pregnancy rate is not increased compared with that occurring after salpingectomy, whereas the subsequent live birth rate is increased. In the large review by Yao and Tulandi of women with an ectopic pregnancy attempting to conceive after salpingostomy, 60% had a IUP and 15% an ectopic pregnancy. After salpingectomy 38% had an IUP and 10% an ectopic pregnancy. Therefore for hemodynamically stable women who wish to preserve fertility and have an unruptured tubal pregnancy, laparoscopic salpingostomy should be performed. The conservative surgical techniques used include salpingotomy (in which the tubal incision is closed primarily), salpingostomy (in which the tubal incision is allowed to close by secondary intention), fimbrial evacuation, and partial salpingectomy, also called segmental resection of the portion of the oviduct containing the ectopic pregnancy. Fimbrial evacuation of the gestational products by digital expression or blunt curettage traumatizes the endosalpinx and is associated with a high rate of recurrent ectopic pregnancy (24%), about twice as high as the rate after salpingectomy. In addition, this procedure may not remove the entire tubal gestation, and another operative procedure may be required a few days later. The best results of conservative operation occur after salpingotomy or salpingostomy. The latter technique is used more frequently in the United States (Fig. 17-22). Tulandi and Guralnick reported that the 2-year cumulative rates of IUP after salpingotomy and salpingostomy were similar, about 45%, but the 1-year rates were twice as great when salpingostomy was performed (45% vs. 21%), indicating that there is a more rapid return of normal tubal function when the incision heals by secondary intention than when it is sutured (Fig. 17-23).

These techniques can be used to treat the vast majority of unruptured tubal pregnancies. When the unruptured pregnancy is small (<5 cm), it is preferable to perform the salpingostomy with a laparoscopic procedure, using delicate technique under the principals of microsurgery. Vermesh and associates performed a prospective randomized trial using either laparoscopy or laparotomy for the treatment of unruptured ectopic gestation by linear salpingostomy. They found both techniques to be safe and effective, but the estimated blood loss and length of hospital stay and cost were all significantly less in the group treated by laparoscopy and recovery was faster. It was found

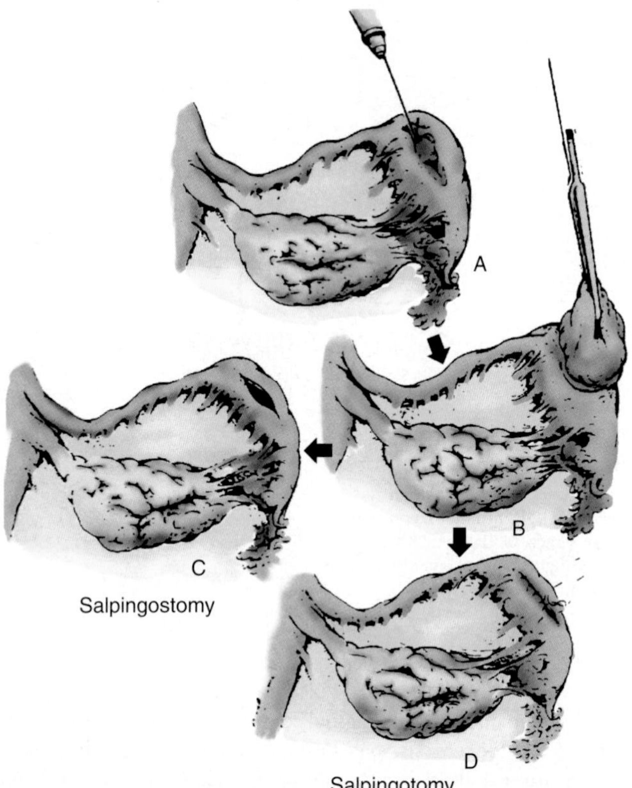

Figure 17-22. **A,** Incision is made into the antimesenteric border of the fallopian tube. **B,** Ectopic pregnancy is gently removed from within the fallopian tube. **C,** Salpingostomy site is allowed to heal by secondary intention. **D,** Salpingotomy is completed by primary closure. (From Leach RE, Ory SJ: Modern management of ectopic pregnancy. J Reprod Med 34:325, 1989.)

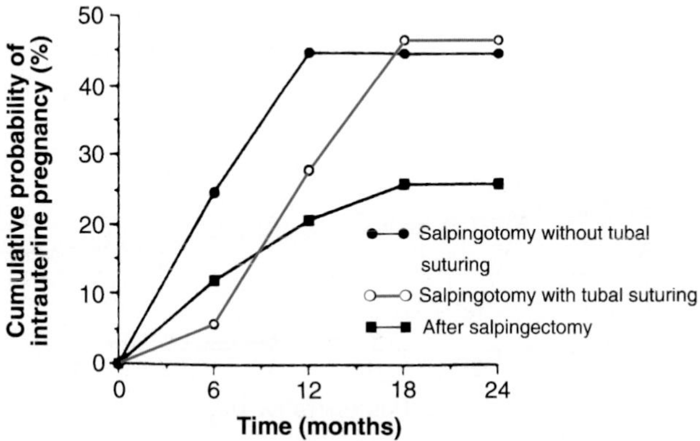

Figure 17-23. Cumulative probability of intrauterine pregnancy after conservative surgical treatment of tubal ectopic pregnancy by salpingotomy without tubal suturing, salpingotomy with tubal suturing, and after salpingectomy. (Reprinted from Fertility and Sterility, 55, Tulandi T, Guralnick M, Treatment of tubal ectopic pregnancy by salpingotomy with or without tubal suturing and salpingectomy, 53. Copyright 1991, with permission from The American Society for Reproductive Medicine.)

following a randomized trial of these two techniques by Lundorff and colleagues that significantly more subsequent pelvic adhesion formation occurred when ectopic pregnancies were treated by laparotomy than by laparoscopy. However, the risk of persistent ectopic pregnancy (PEP) in several series has been found to be significantly greater if the salpingostomy is performed laparoscopically rather than by laparotomy. Seifer and coworkers reported that the incidence of PEP was 16% following laparoscopic salpingostomy but only 2% when a laparotomy was performed—an eightfold increase with the former technique. If hemostasis cannot be maintained after a salpingostomy, which frequently occurs for those unruptured pregnancies located in the isthmus, a segmental resection of the oviduct can be performed and a reanastomosis done at a later time. Timonen and Nieminen reported that women who had a segmental reection had a lower subsequent full-term pregnancy rate (17%) than did women who had salpingectomy (29%). Therefore it is recommended that a partial salpingectomy be performed only if it is not technically possible to do a salpingostomy and the contralateral oviduct is absent or irrevocably damaged.

In his review of the conservative management of ectopic gestation, Vermesh presented a useful flow sheet developed to guide the clinician (Fig. 17-24).

Persistent Ectopic Pregnancy

With increasing use of conservative surgical treatment instead of salpingectomy for the treatment of ectopic pregnancy, the entity of PEP is becoming more common. Manifestations of PEP include either acute abdominal symptoms or persistent or rising HCG levels (or both) after conservative treatment of an unruptured ectopic gestation. The overall mean incidence of PEP after linear salpingostomy is about 5%, being higher when the procedure is performed laparoscopically and lower when performed by laparotomy. After fimbrial expression or tubal abortion the incidence of persistence ranges from 12% to 15%.

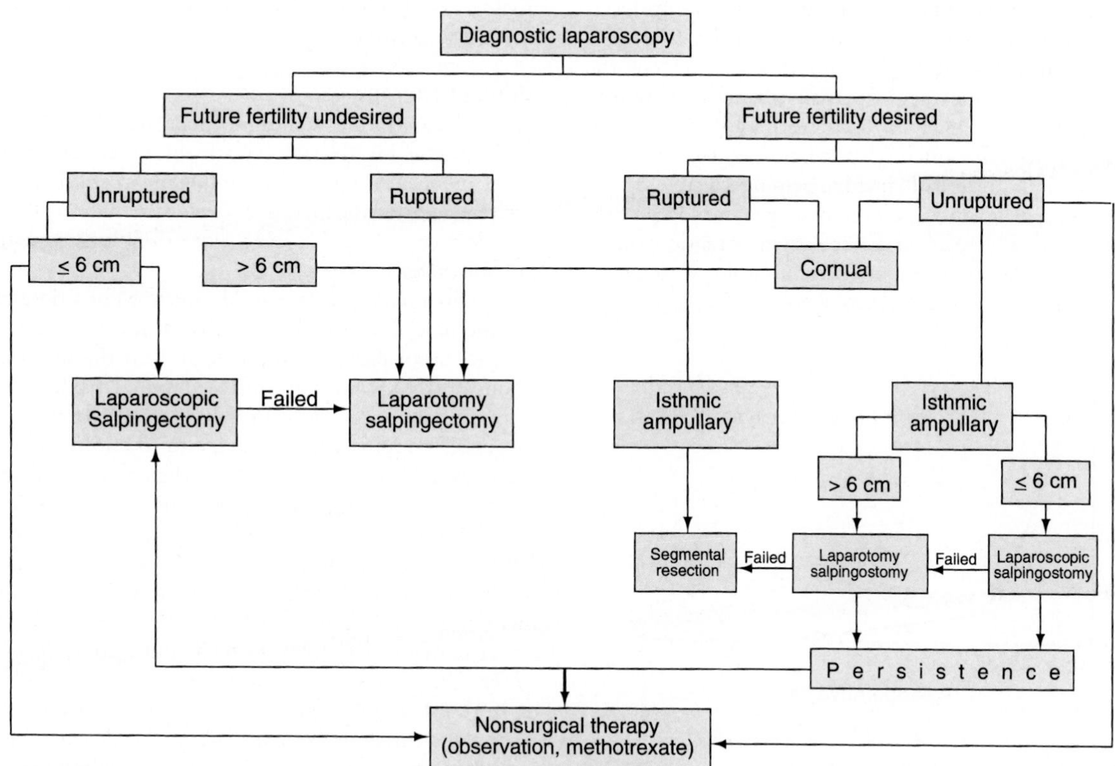

Figure 17-24. Algorithm of conservative management of ectopic gestation. (Reprinted from Fertility and Sterility, 51, Vermesh M, Conservative management of ectopic gestation, 559. Copyright 1989, with permission from The American Society for Reproductive Medicine.)

Stock reviewed the histologic findings of five women with persistent ectopic gestation treated by subsequent salpingectomy. He observed that in all five instances the implantation sites in the oviduct were medial to the original salpingostomy incision site. The original incision was made over the maximally dilated area of the tube, which contained blood clots and some gestational tissue, but some gestational tissue remained medial to the incision.

Persistent ectopic pregnancy is uncommon when the preoperative HCG level is below 3000 mIU/mL. When preoperative HCG levels are greater than 3000 mIU/mL, the incidence of PEP has been reported to range from about 22% to 42%. If the HCG level is above 1000 mIU/mL 7 days after surgery or is more than 15% of the original level at this time, PEP is nearly always present. If the day 7 HCG level is under 1000 mIU/mL or less than 15% of the initial value, PEP is very unlikely. Vermesh and associates measured both HCG and progesterone levels preoperatively and every 3 days after conservative tubal surgery for an unruptured ectopic gestation in a group of 114 women. Of this group, 6 (5.3%) had PEP. All six had an initial sharp drop in HCG levels to 25% of the pretreatment levels 6 days after surgery, similar to the remainder of the group who did not have PEP. After 6 days, titers of the former group plateaued or rose slightly (Fig. 17-25). Progesterone levels showed the same type of pattern (Fig. 17-26).

Based on these data, PEP is presumed to be present if a day 9 serum HCG level is more than 10% of the initial level or a day 9 serum progesterone level is higher than 1.5 ng/mL. It is now recommended that after linear salpingostomy either HCG or progesterone levels be measured initially on day 6 postoperatively and at 3-day intervals thereafter. Increasing levels of either of these hormones beyond day 6 or a day-6 level of HCG more than 1000 mIU/mL or more than 15% of the original value are all indicators of persistent ectopic gestation. Because tubal rupture is likely to occur with PEP, it is best to treat the entity before this emergency situation occurs.

Methods used to treat PEP include salpingectomy, salpingostomy, methotrexate, or expectant management. Expectant management is usually reserved for the asymptomatic woman whose HCG titers plateau but do not rise. Surgical management, should be utilized for those women who develop symptoms

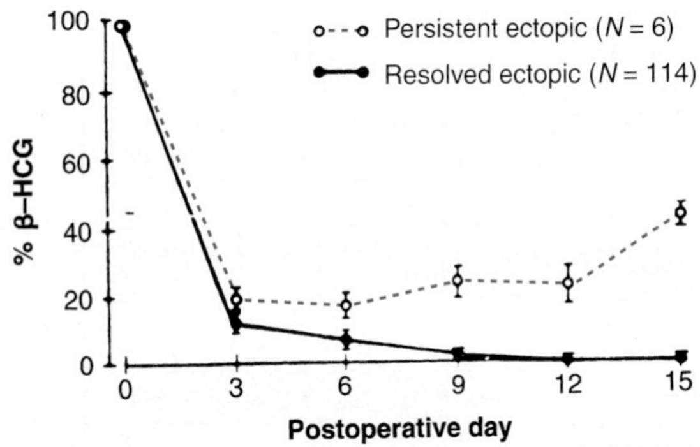

Figure 17-25. Serum β-human chorionic gonadotropin (β-HCG) patterns in persistent and resolved ectopic gestations after conservative surgery. (Reprinted from Fertility and Sterility, 50, Vermesh M, Silva PD, Rosen GF, et al, Persistent tubal ectopic gestation: Patterns of circulating beta-human chorionic gonadotropin and progesterone, and management options, 584. Copyright 1988, with permission from The American Society for Reproductive Medicine.)

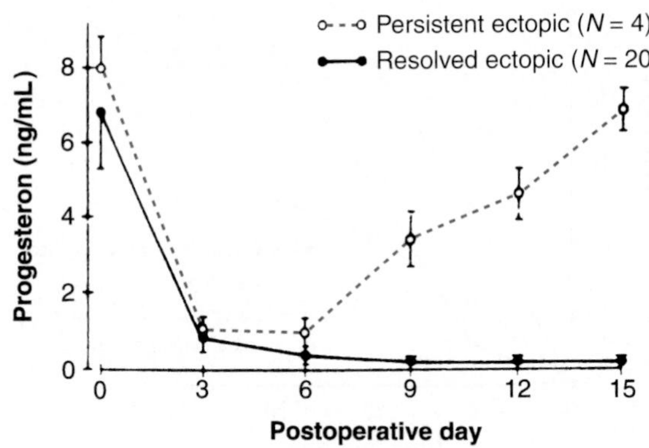

Figure 17-26. Serum progesterone patterns in persistent and resolved ectopic gestations after conservative surgery. (Reprinted from Fertility and Steriulity, 50, Vermesh M, Silva PD, Rosen GF, et al, Persistent tubal ectopic gestation: patterns of circulating beta-human chorionic gonadotropin and progesterone, and management options, 584. Copyright 1988, with permission from The American Society for Reproductive Medicine.)

of persistent lower abdominal pain. The remaining women with PEP are best treated with methotrexate. A single dose of 50 mg/m^2 of methotrexate is usually sufficient to cause resolution of PEP. Hoppe and coworkers used this therapy in 19 consecutive women with PEP, and all had resolution of the PEP. Graczykowski and Mishell performed a randomized trial in which a single dose of methotrexate or placebo was given within 24 hours after salpingostomy. The use of methotrexate reduced the risk of developing PEP by nearly 90%. The prophylactic use of a single dose of methotrexate may be considered in women unable or unwilling to have serial HCG measurements made after salpingostomy.

Medical Therapy

In 1982 Tanaka and colleagues reported the successful use of methotrexate for the sole treatment of an unruptured interstitial pregnancy, and in the following year Miyazaki and coworkers reported the first series of women with small, unruptured ectopic pregnancies that were successfully treated with systemic methotrexate.

Initially methotrexate was administered at a dose of 1 mg/kg on alternate days for four to five doses, with administration of citrovorum factor (reduced folate) on the intervening days. About 20% of women so treated developed side effects such as stomatitis or abnormal liver function tests. Stovall and associates suggested stopping the methotrexate when the HCG levels fell more than 15% in 48 hours or when four doses of the drug had been given. With this regimen only 29% of women received four doses of the drug and only 8% experienced side effects. By 1995, as reviewed by Buster and Carson, 11 series involving 262 women treated with this regimen had been published and there was a cumulative 94% success rate, with subsequent evidence of tubal patency in 82% and fertility in 66% (Table 17-7). These rates are similar to those reported with treatment of unruptured tubal pregnancy by salpingostomy. In a more recent meta-analysis by Barnhart and colleagues involving 26 published studies, the overall success of methotraxate was 89%. However, multidose regimens were more successful while having more side effects. Using single-dose therapy, it was recently described that the strongest predictor for failure of single-dose

Table 17-7 Outcome of Various Methods Used to Treat Unruptured Ectopic Pregnancy Since 1980

Therapy	Reports	*n*	Success (%)	Tubal Patency (%)	Total Fertility (%)	Intrauterine Pregnancy (%)	Ectopic Pregnancy
Laparoscopic salpingostomy	23	1218	95	81	74	61	13
Variable = dose methotrexate	12	262	94	82	63	59	7
Single = dose methotrexate	4	228	90	81	69	61	8
Direct tubal injection of methotrexate	11	295	83	88	82	78	4
Expectant management	11	216	61	100	NA	NA	NA

Adapted from Carson SA, Buster JE: Ectopic pregnancy. N Engl J Med 329: 1174, 1993. Copyright 1993 Massachusetts Medical Society. All rights reserved. Adapted with permission.

methotraxate therapy is the presence of a yolk sac on ultrasound. Also in this study by Bixby and coworkers, the average HCG level in the failure group (27%) was 3282 mIU/mL. Therefore, if only single-dose methotrexate therapy is the desired goal, the ideal candidate should have HCG levels which are lower (in the range of 1500 mIU/mL). Success may be accomplished with multidose regimens in patients with higher levels of HCG, as described later.

Criteria believed necessary for methotrexate treatment of asymptomatic or mildly symptomatic unruptured ectopic pregnancy include diameter of the gestational mass, as measured sonographically, to be less than 4 cm, and no clinical evidence of active bleeding or tubal rupture. It has been estimated that with monitoring early in gestation at least one third of women with ectopic pregnancies will satisfy these criteria and can be treated medically instead of surgically. In addition there should not be sonographic evidence of intraperitoneal fluid outside the pelvic cavity and no evidence of hepatic, hematologic, or renal disease.

Other regimens have subsequently been utilized for administration of methotrexate both locally and systemically. In 1993 Stovall and Ling reported their experience with use of a single dose of systemic methotrexate (50 mg/m^2) without the use of citrovorum. In four series of 228 women treated with this regimen 90% resolved without surgery. Of this group 10% required a second dose of methotrexate because HCG levels did not fall sufficiently. About 85% of patients treated with methotrexate have a transient rise in HCG level between 1 and 4 days after treatment. Between 4 and 7 days after methotrexate is administered the HCG levels should fall at least 15%. If this amount of decrease does not occur or there is less than a 15% decrease in HCG levels in each subsequent week, an additional dose of methotrexate should be given for a maximum of three doses. If after three doses of methotrexate HCG levels do not decline by 15% weekly, a surgical procedure should be performed. Saraj and associates reported that serum progesterone levels fall more rapidly than HCG levels after methotrexate, and a progesterone level of less than 1.5 ng/mL was an excellent predictor of resolution of the ectopic pregnancy. The rates of tubal patency and subsequent fertility with the single-dose regimen were similar to those with the multiple-dose regimen. Because of the need for surgical treatment in a higher percentage of the women treated with a single dose rather than with multiple doses of methotrexate, some investigators still advocate that use of the intermittent regimen is preferable. To reduce the incidence of tubal rupture with systemic methotrexate it is advisable to perform only a single bimanual pelvic examination before and after initiating treatment. Between 3 and 7 days after initiating therapy severe pelvic pain lasting up to 12 hours frequently occurs. This symptom, probably caused by tubal abortion, needs to be differentiated from the symptoms of tubal rupture. Serial monitoring of vital signs and measurement of hematocrit levels are helpful. If the woman remains hemodynamically stable and the pain disappears, a tubal abortion has probably taken place and no further therapy is necessary. Lipscomb and colleagues analyzed predictors of success in 350 women treated with methotrexate. A total of 30 women (9%) were treatment failures. There were no significant differences between women treated successfully and failures regarding age, parity, volume of the ectopic mass, or presence or absence of free peritoneal fluid. The mean HCG and progesterone level as well as frequency of cardiac activity were lower in the successfully treated group than the failures. If the initial HCG titer was less than 5000 mIU/mL the success rate was more than 90%; if it was more than 15,000 mIU/mL the success rate was only 68% (Table 17-8).

An intermediate dose regimen (between multidose and single dose) has recently been suggested for use in women with higher levels of HCG, thus improving efficacy but reducing the side effects of multidose therapy. Here the standard dose (50 mg/m^2) is given initially and repeated after 4 days without citrovorum. Although an attractive option, there are no real data as yet using this regimen.

There have been two randomized trials comparing the results of systemic methotrexate with laparoscopic salpingostomy for the treatment of unruptured ectopic pregnancy. In a Dutch

Table 17-8 Success Rates of Methotrexate Treatment in Women with Ectopic Pregnancies as a Function of Their Initial Serum Chorionic Gonadotropin Concentrations

Serum Chorionic Gonadotropin Concentrations (mIU/ml)	Success Number	Failure Number	Success Rate (95% CI)* Percent
<1000	118	2	98 (69–100)
1000–1999	40	3	93 (85–100)
2000–4999	90	8	92 (86–97)5
5000–9999	39	6	87 (79–98)5
10,000–14,999	18	4	82 (65–98)5
=15,000	15	7	68 (49–88)5

*CI denotes confidence interval. Treatment was successful in 320 women and failed in 30.

study, a similar degree of success was achieved with each treatment methodology. In the group treated medically, 14% required surgical intervention; in the group treated surgically, 20% required methotrexate treatment for persistent ectopic pregnancy.

In another study by Saraj and associates, 2 of 38 women treated with methotrexate required subsequent surgery, and 3 of 37 treated by salpingostomy required medical treatment for persistent ectopic pregnancy. Resolution following salpingostomy was more rapid than after methotrexate. The mean time to disappearance occurred about 20 days after salpingostomy and 27 days after methotrexate.

To avoid the toxicity of systemic methotrexate administration, a smaller dose of the drug has been administered directly into the oviduct with either laparoscopic or sonographic visualization. In the summary by Buster and Carson, of 11 series involving 295 women treated with tubal injection of methotrexate, only 83% had successful resolution of the ectopic pregnancy, but subsequent tubal patency rates were 88% and fertility rates were 82% (see Table 17-7).

Because of the lower success rate and need for direct needle placement with local injection, most clinicians are now using systemic methotrexate. There have also been several reports of direct intratubal injection of other substances, including potassium chloride, hypertonic glucose, and prostaglandins, but use of these agents is generally less successful than methotrexate.

Expectant Management

In 1955 Lund reported a series of 119 women with unruptured tubal pregnancy treated expectantly with only bed rest and frequent observation while hospitalized. Of these, 68 (57%) were eventually discharged without the need for a surgical procedure, but about 60% of them required hospitalization for more than 1 month. The remainder had a tubal rupture or required operative intervention for other reasons. The subsequent fertility rates were similar in the group treated surgically and those treated expectantly. In 1982 Mashiach and colleagues reported that if at the time of the initial laparoscopy a small unruptured tubal pregnancy was found and if serial HCG levels subsequently fell, it was possible to avoid surgical therapy, although they performed a repeat laparoscopy before discharge.

Other investigators subsequently reported similar results. In published reports of 347 women with ectopic pregnancy treated expectantly, since 1980 the success rate was 69%, with a high subsequent tubal patency rate (see Table 17-7). Trio and coworkers, using multivariate analysis, reported that an initial HCG titer of less than 1000 mIU/mL and a decrease in HCG levels between the initial serum sample and one obtained a few days later were each independent predictors of successful spontaneous resolution while sonographic visualization of an ectopic gestational sac was not an independent predictor of failure. In their series of 49 women managed expectantly, 88% of those with an initial HCG level less than 1000 mIU/mL had successful resolution.

Korhonen and associates measured serial HCG levels before and during outpatient expectant management of a group of 118 women with ectopic pregnancies. This group comprised one fourth of all the women with the diagnosis of ectopic pregnancy seen at their institution during 3 years. Initially their median gestational age was 44 days, and the median HCG level was 374 mIU/mL. Spontaneous resolution occurred in two thirds of the 118 women (16% of the entire group of women with ectopic pregnancies). If the initial HCG level was less than 200 mIU/mL, the rate of successful spontaneous resolution was 88%. When the initial HCG level was more than 2000 mIU/mL, the rate of spontaneous resolution was only 25%. When spontaneous resolution occurred, HCG levels declined to undetectable levels in 4 to 67 days, with a mean of 20 days. A distinct difference in the rate of decline of HCG levels in those who did and did not require surgery was not observed until 7 days after the initial examination (Fig. 17-27). If HCG levels had not fallen more than two thirds of the initial level in 7 days, two thirds of this group of women needed surgical treatment for either rising HCG levels, clinical symptoms, or sonographic findings of intraperitoneal bleeding. Atri and colleagues reported that when serial sonography is performed some of the tubal pregnancies can increase in size and become more vascular as they resolve. While knowledge of these facts is important, if an unruptured ectopic pregnancy is diagnosed by β-HCG and ultrasound, it is still preferable to treat with methotrexate or perform laparoscopy, depending on the clinical situation as discussed earlier.

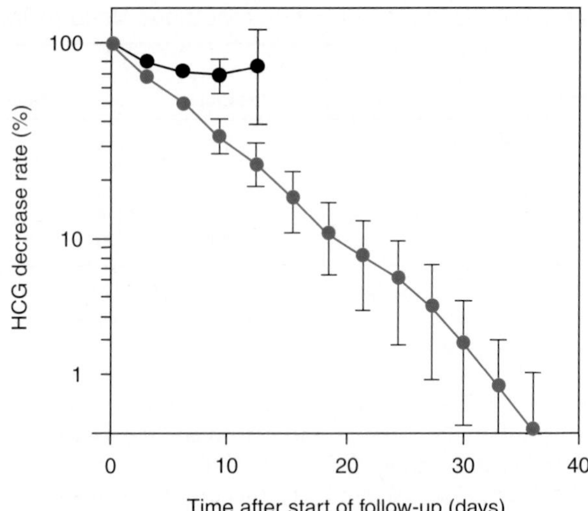

Figure 17-27. Mean value and 95% confidence limits for ratio of serum human chorionic gonadotropin (HCG) concentrations to starting value during expectant management in patients with a spontaneous resolution *(blue circles)* and in those later treated by laparoscopy *(black circles)*. The two group diverged at 7 days. (Reprinted from Fertility and Sterility, 61, Korhonen J, Stenman UH, Ylöstalo P, Serum human chorionic gonadotropin dynamics during spontaneous resolution of ectopic pregnancy, 632. Copyright 1994, with permission from The American Society for Reproductive Medicine.)

Rh Factor

It is recommended that all Rh-negative, unsensitized women with ectopic pregnancies receive Rh immunoglobulin at a dosage of 50 μg if the gestation is of less than 12 weeks' duration and 300 μg if it is beyond 12 weeks. However, Grimes and colleagues have reported that because most of their hospitalizations were unscheduled and not preceded by Rh screening, the majority of women with ectopic pregnancies in the United States who are Rh-negative do not receive Rh(D) immunoglobulin.

1. Calculate the score (number of points) for each risk factor:

Age (years)	Points	Smoking (cig/d)	Points	Other factors	Points YES	Points NO
<35	0	0	0			
35–39	3	1–20	2	EP history	10	0
40	6	>20	4	Endometriosis	9	0
				History of infection [1]	8	0
				Clomiphene	7	0
				Tubal surgery	4	0

[1] Salpingitis history (confirmed or not), and/or positive serology for *Chlamydia trachomatis* (1/64)

2. Add the points and read the absolute risk of EP according to the number of points

0	2	4	6	8	10	12	14	16	18	20	22	24	26	28	30	32	34	36	38	40	42	44	46	48
1%	2%	2%	3%	5%	7%	11%	15%	21%	28%	37%	47%	57%	66%	74%	81%	87%	91%	93%	96%	97%	98%	99%	99%	99%

For example, a woman aged 36 years, smoking 25 cigarettes/day, with an EP history and a pregnancy induced by clomiphene would have a score of 3 + 4 + 10 + 7 = 24, for an EP risk of 57%.

Figure 17-28. Ectopic pregnancy (EP) risk scale. (From Coste J, Bouyer J, Fernandez H, Job-Spira N: Predicting the risk of extra-uterine pregnancy. Construction and validation of a French risk scale. Contacept Fertil Sex 26:643, 1998.)

The magnitude of the risk of sensitization is unknown but is estimated to vary from nil at 1 month to about 9% at 3 months' gestation. Because of the potential benefits and lack of risk, this treatment should be utilized in all Rh-negative, unsensitized women with ectopic pregnancy.

THE DIAGNOSIS IN WOMEN WITH A HISTORY OF INFERTILITY

In women with a history of infertility, the diagnosis of ectopic pregnancy has been subjected to a risk-scoring assessment according to data by Coste (Fig. 17-28). In this scenario, methotrexate therapy is preferred unless the ectopic pregnancy involves a known hydrosalpinx, in which case salpingectomy should be preferred. The Cochran database has shown that methotrexate therapy is equivalent to laparoscopic surgery. A particular concern in the infertility patient is the occurrence of heterotopic pregnancy, occurring in 1% to 3% of patients, which limits the approach to surgical intervention.

PROGNOSIS FOR SUBSEQUENT FERTILITY

If a woman wishes to conceive after having an ectopic pregnancy, three possibilities exist. She may remain infertile. She may conceive and have an intrauterine gestation (with a viable birth or spontaneous abortion), or she may conceive and have an ectopic gestation. Overall the subsequent conception rate in women following all ectopic pregnancies is about 60%, with the other 40% remaining infertile. About one third of the pregnancies occurring after the initial ectopic pregnancy are another ectopic pregnancy and one sixth are spontaneous abortions. Therefore, only about half the pregnancies are viable and only one third of all women with an ectopic pregnancy have a subsequent live birth. However, these overall figures are modified by several factors, particularly age, parity, history of infertility, evidence of contralateral tubal disease, whether the ectopic pregnancy is ruptured or intact, and use of an intrauterine device (IUD) at the time of the ectopic gestation. The subsequent fertility rate is significantly higher in parous women younger than age 30. However, if the ectopic pregnancy occurs in a woman's first pregnancy, her overall subsequent conception rate is only about 35%, being lower with a history of infertility and higher with no such history. On the other hand, women with high parity (more than three births) who develop an ectopic pregnancy have a relatively high rate, about 80%, of subsequent conception. The subsequent conception rate is lower in women who have a history of salpingitis, as well as those who have visual evidence of pathologic changes in the opposite oviduct as a result of previous salpingitis. Several studies have reported that women who were using an IUD at the time of ectopic pregnancy have normal rates of subsequent fertility and no increased risk of a subsequent ectopic pregnancy. Future fertility is significantly higher in women who have an unruptured tubal pregnancy than in those with tubal rupture so that early diagnosis is desirable. In the report of Sherman and coworkers only 65% of women with a ruptured ectopic pregnancy subsequently conceived, whereas the conception rate in women with an unruptured tubal pregnancy was 82%.

In two large groups of women with unruptured ectopic pregnancy treated by conservative surgery, Langer and associates and Pouly and colleagues reported a high incidence of subsequent fertility (80% to 86%) and a low incidence of subsequent ectopic pregnancy (11% to 22%). The IUP rates were 64% to 70%. In both series the IUP rates were highest (82% to 86%) in women with no history of infertility or gross evidence of prior salpingitis. The IUP rates were significantly lower (41% to

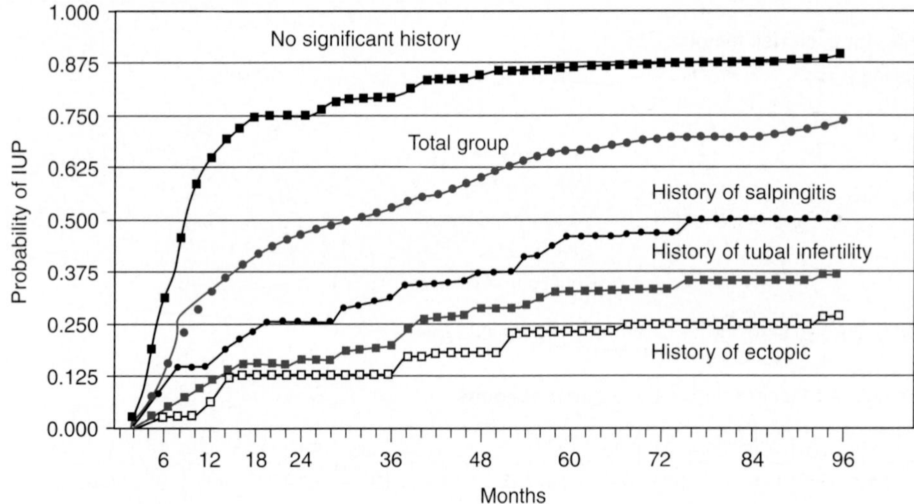

Figure 17-29. Cumulative pregnancy rate according to the patients' history. IUP, intrauterine pregnancy.

56%) in women with these problems. Sherman and coworkers and Tuomivaara and Kauppila reported that among women with a normal contralateral tube and no history of infertility, pregnancy rates were similar whether salpingectomy or salpingostomy was performed. However, in the group of women with evidence of prior tubal infection or a history of infertility, subsequent intrauterine conception rates were higher when they were treated with salpingostomy (73% to 76%) than with salpingectomy (43% to 44%). Most studies in the literature indicate that the overall subsequent ectopic pregnancy rate is similar among women treated radically or conservatively, and these two studies indicate that conservative surgery is most beneficial for women with evidence of contralateral tubal damage or peritubal adhesions, or history of infertility.

Vermesh and Presser analyzed the reproductive outcome for 3 years in a group of 60 women with unruptured tubal pregnancy treated by salpingostomy who were randomized to have the procedure performed by laparoscopy or laparotomy. At the end of 3 years 74% and 86%, respectively, had conceived after each procedure. The women treated by laparoscopy conceived sooner than those treated by laparotomy, and there were more ectopic pregnancies in the latter group. Overall, 68% and 71% of women in the two groups, respectively, had an IUP, and 5% and 19%, respectively, had an ectopic pregnancy.

Pouly and colleagues attempted to provide criteria for treating women with an unruptured ectopic pregnancy to determine whether a salpingostomy or salpingectomy should be performed to enhance the rate of subsequent pregnancy and decrease the rate of subsequent ectopic pregnancy. In this study the future fertility rate was lower in nulliparous than in parous women only if the former had a history of infertility. Future fertility or chance of subsequent ectopic pregnancy was unaffected by the size of the ectopic gestation or its location. A history of prior abdominopelvic surgery or use of an IUD also did not affect the risk of future fertility or subsequent ectopic pregnancy. Although the presence of adnexal adhesions increased the rate of infertility, it did not affect the risk of recurrence of ectopic pregnancy.

However, a history of infertility (particularly resulting from tubal disease), previous salpingitis, a prior ectopic pregnancy, or the presence of only one oviduct were each independent factors that decreased the rate of subsequent fertility and also increased the risk of subsequent ectopic pregnancy (Fig. 17-29). These authors suggested that if more than one of these factors were present it was preferable to perform a salpingectomy than salpingostomy, since 80% of the recurrent ectopic pregnancies occurred in the same tube as the initial ectopic pregnancy.

The rate of repeat ectopic pregnancies after a single ectopic pregnancy ranges from 8% to 27%, with a mean of about 20%. Since the overall pregnancy rate is in the 60% to 80% range, about one of three to four conceptions after an ectopic pregnancy is a repeat ectopic pregnancy. Women with an ectopic pregnancy who become pregnant again should be monitored by sonography early in pregnancy because of the high incidence of another ectopic pregnancy as well as spontaneous abortion. Only about one of three nulliparous women who have had an ectopic pregnancy ever conceives again (35%), and about one third of these conceptions are an ectopic pregnancy, for an overall rate of 13%. Skeldestad and coworkers followed up on 697 women with an ectopic pregnancy if they conceived again. The reported ectopic pregnancy rate was 21%, the viable birth rate was about 55%, and the spontaneous abortion rate was about 25%. Risk factors for a repeat ectopic pregnancy were ectopic pregnancy as first pregnancy, age younger than 25, evidence of tubal infection, and history of infertility (Table 17-9). With two ectopic pregnancies the subsequent fertility rate is decreased even further. If a woman has two consecutive ectopic pregnancies treated by salpingostomy, about half will subsequently conceive, but as reported by Vermesh and Presser the majority of them will be a repeat ectopic pregnancy. Therefore it is probably better to perform in vitro fertilization if a woman has two consecutive ectopic pregnancies in order to enhance the possibility of a viable pregnancy and reduce the risk of having a third ectopic pregnancy.

Several reports have covered the use of conservative surgery, either salpingostomy or salpingotomy, in women with an

Table 17-9 Odds of Repeat Ectopic Pregnancy in Subsequent Pregnancies

	Adjusted OR	95% CI
Pregnancy Order		
1st subsequent	11.8	2.0, 68.0
2nd subsequent	3.0	0.5, 21.1
3rd or more subsequent	1.0	Reference
Repeat Ectopic Pregnancy		
1 repeat (2nd) ectopic pregnancy	9.5	2.5, 36.6
No repeat (1st) ectopic pregnancy	1.0	Reference
Status at Index Ectopic Pregnancy		
Age (yr)		
=24	3.1	1.1, 8.9
=25	1.0	Reference
Infectious Pathology*		
Yes	2.7	1.5, 5.0
No	1.0	Reference
Have Started Infertility Work-Up		
Yes	2.3	1.0, 5.1
No	1.0	Reference
Conceived with Intrauterine Device in Situ at Index Pregnancy		
Yes	0.4	0.1, 0.9
No	1.0	Reference

*Defined as either adhesions or macroscopic damage to the contralateral tube or both.
CI, confidence interval; OR, odds ratio.
From Skjeldestad FE, Hadgu A, Eriksson N: Epidemiology of repeat ectopic pregnancy: A population-based prospective cohort study. Obstet Gynecol 91(1):129–135, 1998. Reprinted with permission from the American College of Obstetricians and Gynecologists.

Table 17-10 Results of Conservative Surgery for Tubal Pregnancy in Women with a Solitary Tube

Author	Year	Number of Patients Desiring Pregnancy	IUP	EUP
Henri-Suchet et al	1979	14	8	2
DeCherney et al	1982	12	6	2
Langer et al	1982	8	5	2
Valle and Lifchez	1983	11	11	0
Oelsner et al	1986	21	10	9
Pouly et al	1986	24	11	7
Total		90	51 (57%)	22 (24%)

Reprinted from Fertility and Sterility, 51, Vermesh M, Conservative management of ectopic gestation, 559. Copyright 1989, with permission from The American Society for Reproductive Medicine.

unruptured tubal pregnancy in the only remaining oviduct. In the great majority of the subjects the other oviduct had been removed because of another ectopic gestation. Of 90 women so treated in six different centers, the conception rate was 81%, with an IUP rate of 57% (Table 17-10). About one fourth of the women who conceived had a subsequent ectopic gestation, similar to the rate among all ectopic pregnancies. Thus conservative surgery or medical therapy may be performed when an unruptured ectopic pregnancy occurs in the only remaining oviduct.

KEY POINTS

- The annual ectopic pregnancy rates in the United States are about 1.5 per 1000 women ages 15 to 44.
- In the United States in 1992 about 2 of every 100 women who were known to conceive had an ectopic gestation.
- In the United States the rate of ectopic pregnancy increased from 6.6 per 1000 conceptions in women ages 15 to 24 to 21.5 per 1000 conceptions in those ages 25 to 34.
- Only 10% to 15% of ectopic pregnancies occur in nulligravid women, and more than half of the ectopic pregnancies occur in women who have been pregnant three or more times.
- Nonclotting blood is obtained by culdocentesis in more than 90% of ruptured ectopic pregnancies.
- About 85% of women with an ectopic pregnancy have serum HCG levels lower than those seen in normal pregnancy at a similar gestational age.
- In women with an ectopic gestation, about 90% have an abnormal pattern of serial HCG levels. Half of these have falling levels and half have a subnormal increase.
- Laparoscopy has a 2% to 5% misdiagnosis rate (false-positive or false-negative) for ectopic pregnancy.
- Ultrasonography with a vaginal probe allows visualization of an intrauterine gestation when the HCG level is between 1500 and 2500 mIU/mL, depending on the transducer.
- Criteria for the ultrasonographic diagnosis of ectopic pregnancy with use of currently available vaginal transducers include the finding of an adnexal mass or the absence of a gestational sac when the HCG level is above a certain threshold (about 1500 to 2500 mIU/mL).
- About two thirds of women with symptomatic ectopic pregnancy have HCG levels above 2500 mIU/mL and thus can be reliably diagnosed by ultrasonography.
- Similar subsequent conception rates and ectopic pregnancy rates occur in women with an ectopic pregnancy treated with salpingectomy or salpingo-oophorectomy.
- Cornual resection does not prevent a subsequent interstitial pregnancy.
- If the ectopic pregnancy has produced rupture of the oviduct or has involved the entire oviduct or if no further pregnancies are desired, salpingectomy is the treatment of choice.
- When an unruptured ectopic pregnancy is present, the repeat ectopic pregnancy rate with salpingostomy is not increased compared with salpingectomy, whereas the subsequent live birth rate is increased if the other tube is grossly abnormal or if there is a history of infertility.
- Fimbrial evacuation of the gestational products by digital expression has about twice the rate of recurrent ectopic pregnancy as treatment by salpingectomy.
- It is recommended that all Rh-negative unsensitized women with ectopic pregnancies receive Rh immunoglobulin.

Continued

KEY POINTS *Continued*

- Overall the subsequent conception rate in women with an ectopic pregnancy is about 60%. A little less than half of these pregnancies terminate in another ectopic pregnancy or spontaneous abortion; so only about one third of women with an ectopic pregnancy have a subsequent live birth.
- If the ectopic pregnancy occurs in a woman's first pregnancy, her chance of subsequent conception is only about 35%.
- The subsequent conception rate following an ectopic pregnancy is lower in women who have a history of salpingitis, as well as in those who have gross evidence of damage in the opposite oviduct caused by previous salpingitis.
- Future fertility is significantly higher among women who have an unruptured tubal pregnancy than in those with a ruptured ectopic pregnancy.
- Conservative tubal surgery is most beneficial in women with evidence of contralateral tubal damage or peritubal adhesions or a history of infertility.
- About one of four conceptions after an ectopic pregnancy is a repeat ectopic pregnancy.
- About one third of nulliparous women with an ectopic pregnancy have a subsequent ectopic pregnancy.
- In women with one remaining oviduct when an unruptured ectopic pregnancy is treated by salpingostomy, the conception rate is 81%, with an IUP rate of 56% and a subsequent ectopic gestation rate of 24%.
- The overall risk of ectopic pregnancy after tubal sterilization failure is about 30%, reaching 50% if the sterilization technique was bilateral tubal fulguration.
- The incidence of heterotopic ectopic pregnancy is about 1% of all pregnancies occurring after in vitro fertilization.
- If the HCG level is less than 3000 mIU/mL and the progesterone level is less than 12 ng/mL, the likelihood of ectopic pregnancy or nonviable intrauterine gestation is 97%.
- If the serum progesterone level is less than 5 ng/mL, the pregnancy is nonviable, whether in an ectopic or intrauterine location.
- All women with a serum progesterone level more than 25 ng/mL have a viable intrauterine gestation.
- With a gestational age more than 38 days or a serum HCG level more than 2500 mIU/mL, if an intrauterine gestation is present it should be visualized sonographically.
- The diagnosis of an asymptomatic ectopic pregnancy can usually be made with the use of vaginal probe pelvic sonography, serial HCG levels, or a serum progesterone measurement.
- The overall incidence of persistent ectopic pregnancy after conservative tubal surgery is about 5%, being higher when the procedure is performed laparoscopically than by laparotomy.
- The incidence of persistent ectopic pregnancy increases when the preoperative serum HCG is more than 3000 mIU/mL and can be diagnosed by a finding of an HCG level above 1000 mIU/mL or a decrease of HCG above 15% of the preoperative level 7 days after the salpingostomy.
- Asymptomatic persistent ectopic pregnancy can be treated expectantly or with methotrexate.
- The best medical treatment of unruptured ectopic pregnancy is to give methotrexate in a single intramuscular dose of 50 mg/m^2 without citrovorum factor.
- With monitoring in early gestation, at least one third of women with ectopic pregnancies can be treated medically.
- Expectant management of unruptured ectopic pregnancy can be used if the size of the tubal mass is less than 3 cm and the initial HCG level is less than 1000 mIU/mL without a rise in levels in 2 days.
- The HCG level should fall at least 15% between days 4 and 7 after the methotrexate injection and at least 15% weekly thereafter.
- The best predictor of successful treatment of ectopic pregnancy with methotrexate is the initial HCG level. If the level is less than 5000 mIU/mL the success rate is 90%.
- Factors that increase the risk of ectopic pregnancy after consecutive tubal surgery include a history of infertility, previous salpingectomy or a prior ectopic pregnancy, and the presence of only one oviduct.

BIBLIOGRAPHY

Ailawad M, Lorch SA, Barnhart KT: Cost-effectiveness of presumptively medical treating women at risk for ectopic pregnancy compared with first performing a dilatation and curettage. Fertil Steril 83(2):376, 2005.

Aleem FA, DeFazio M, Gintautas J: Endovaginal sonography for the early diagnosis of intrauterine and ectopic pregnancies. Hum Reprod 5:755, 1990.

Ankum WM, Van der Veen F, Hamerlynck JVThH, Lammes FB: Laparoscopy: A dispensable tool in the diagnosis of ectopic pregnancy. Hum Reprod 8:1301, 1993.

Ankum WM, Van der Veen F, Hamerlynck JVThH, Lammes FB: Transvaginal sonography and human chorionic gonadotrophin measurements in suspected ectopic pregnancy: A detailed analysis of a diagnostic approach. Hum Reprod 8:1307, 1993.

Atrash HK, Friede A, Hogue CJ: Ectopic pregnancy mortality in the United States, 1970–1983. Obstet Gynecol 70:817, 1987.

Atri M, Bret PM, Tulandi T: Spontaneous resolution of ectopic pregnancy: Initial appearance and evolution at transvaginal US. Radiology 186:83, 1993.

Atri M, Bret PM, Tulandi T, Senterman MK: Ectopic pregnancy: evolution after treatment with transvaginal methotrexate. Radiology 185:749, 1992.

Barnhart K, Gosman G, Ashby R, Sammel M: The medical management of ectopic pregnancy: A meta-analysis comparing "single dose" and "multidose" regimens. Obstet Gynecol 101(4);778, 2003.

Barnhart K, Mennuti MT, Benjamin I, et al: Prompt diagnosis of ectopic pregnancy in an emergency department setting. Obstet Gynecol 84:1010, 1994.

Barnhart K, Sammel MD, Chung K, Zhou L, et al: Decline of serum human chorionic gonadotropin and spontaneous complete abortion: Defining the normal curve. Obstet Gynecol 104(5 Pt 1):975, 2004.

Bello GV, Schonholz D, Moshirpur J, et al: Combined pregnancy: The Mount Sinai experience. Obstet Gynecol Surv 10:603, 1986.

Bengtsson G, Brytman I, Thorburn J, Lindblom B: Low-dose oral methotrexate as second-line therapy for persistent trophoblast after conservative treatment of ectopic pregnancy. Obstet Gynecol 79:589, 1992.

Bixby S, Tello R, Kuligowska E: Presence of a yolk sac on transvaginal sonography is the most reliable predictor of single-dose methotrexate treatment failure in ectopic pregnancy. J Ultrasound Med 24(5):591-8.

Breen JL: A 21-year survey of 654 ectopic pregnancies. Am J Obstet Gynecol 106:1004, 1970.

Brenner PF, Roy S, Mishell DR Jr: Ectopic pregnancy: A study of 300 consecutive surgically treated cases. JAMA 243:673, 1980.

Budowick M, Johnson TRB, Genadry R, et al: The histopathology of the developing tubal ectopic pregnancy. Fertil Steril 34:169, 1980.

Buster JE, Carson SA: Ectopic pregnancy: new advances in diagnosis and treatment. Curr Opin Obstet Gynecol 7:168, 1995.

Cacciatore B, Korhnone J, Stenman UH, Ylöstalo P: Transvaginal sonography and serum HCG in monitoring of presumed ectopic pregnancies selected for expectant management. Ultrasound Obstet Gynecol 5:297, 1995.

Cacciatore B, Stenman UH, Ylöstalo P, et al: Diagnosis of ectopic pregnancy by vaginal ultrasonography in combination with a discriminatory serum HCG level of 1000 IU/1 (IRP). Br J Obstet Gynaecol 97(10):904, 1990.

Canis M, Savary D, Pouly J-L, Wattiez A, Mage G. Grossesse extra-uterine: Criteres de choix du traitement medical ou du traitement chirurgical. J Gynecol Obstet Biol Reprod 32(Suppl.):3S54-3S63, 2003.

Carson SA, Buster JE: Ectopic pregnancy. N Engl J Med 329:1174, 1993.

Cartwright PS, DiPietro DL: Ectopic pregnancy: Changes in serum human chorionic gonadotropin concentration. Obstet Gynecol 63:76, 1984.

Centers for Disease Control and Prevention: Ectopic pregnancy—United States, 1988–1989. MMWR Morb Mortal Wkly Rep 41(Suppl 32): 591, 1992.

Centers for Disease Control and Prevention: Ectopic pregnancy—United States, 1990–1992. MMWR Morb Mortal Wkly Rep 44(Suppl 3):47, 1996.

Clark JF, Guy RS: Abdominal pregnancy. Am J Obstet Gynecol 96:511, 1966.

Clausen I: Conservative versus radical surgery for tubal pregnancy: A review. Acta Obstet Gynecol Scand 75:8, 1996.

Cole T, Corlett R Jr: Chronic ectopic pregnancy. Obstet Gynecol 59:63, 1982.

Corson SL, Batzer FR: Ectopic pregnancy: A review of the etiologic factors. J Reprod Med 31:78, 1986.

Cosin JA, Bean M, Grow D, et al: The use of methotrexate and arterial embolization to avoid surgery in a case of cervical pregnancy. Fertil Steril 67:1169, 1997.

Coste J, Bouyer J, Fernandez H, Job-Spira N: Predicting the risk of extra-uterine pregnancy. Construction and validation of a French risk scale. Contracept Fertil Sex 26:643, 1998.

DeCherney AH, Kase N: The conservative surgical management of unruptured ectopic pregnancy. Obstet Gynecol 54:451, 1979.

DeCherney AH, Maheux R: Modern management of tubal pregnancy. Curr Probl Obstet Gynecol 6:1, 1983.

DeCherney AH, Romero R, Naftolin F: Surgical management of unruptured ectopic pregnancy. Fertil Steril 35:21, 1981.

Delke I, Veridiano NP, Tancer ML: Abdominal pregnancy: Review of current management and addition of 10 cases. Obstet Gynecol 60:200, 1982.

Di Marchi JM, Kosasa TS, Kobara TY, Hale RW: Persistent ectopic pregnancy. Obstet Gynecol 70:555, 1987.

Dimitry ES, Margara R, Subak-Sharpe R, et al: Nine cases of heterotopic pregnancies in 4 years of in vitro fertilization. Fertil Steril 53:107, 1990.

Dorfman SF, Grimes DA, Cates W Jr, et al: Ectopic pregnancy mortality—United States, 1979 to 1980: Clinical aspects. Obstet Gynecol 64:386, 1984.

Dudley PS, Heard MJ, Sangi-Haghpeykar H, et al: Characterizing ectopic pregnancies that rupture despite treatment with methotrexate. Fertil Steril 82(5):1374, 2004.

Elias S, LeBeau M, Simpson JL, et al: Chromosome analysis of ectopic human conceptuses. Am J Obstet Gynecol 141:698, 1981.

Emerson DS, Cartier MS, Altieri LA, et al: Diagnostic efficacy of endovaginal color Doppler flow imaging in an ectopic pregnancy screening program. Radiology 183:413, 1992.

Fernandez H, Baton C, Benifla JL, et al: Methotrexate treatment of ectopic pregnancy: 100 cases treated by primary transvaginal injection under sonographic control. Fertil Steril 59:773, 1993.

Fernandez H, Coste J, Job-Spira N: Controlled ovarian hyperstimulation as a risk factor for ectopic pregnancy. Obstet Gynecol 78:656, 1991.

Fernandez H, Lellaidier C, Thouvenez V, Frydman R: The use of a pretherapeutic, predictive score to determine inclusion criteria for the on-surgical treatment of ectopic pregnancy. Hum Reprod 6:995, 1991.

Fernandez H, Olivenes F, Pauthier S, et al: Ultrasound-guided injection of methotrexate versus laparoscopic salpingotomy in ectopic pregnancy. Fertil Steril 63:25, 1995.

Frates MC, Benson CB, Doubilet PM, et al: Cervical ectopic pregnancy: results of conservative treatment. Radiology 191:773, 1994.

Gaetano V, Henno D: Combined pregnancy: The Mount Sinai experience. Obstet Gynecol Surv 41:603, 1986.

Glock JL, Johnson JV, Brumsted JR: Efficacy and safety of single-dose systemic methotrexate in the treatment of ectopic pregnancy. Fertil Steril 62:715, 1994.

Goldner TE, Lawson HW, Xia Z, Atrash HK: Surveillance for ectopic pregnancy—United States, 1970–1989. MMWR 42(Suppl 6):73, 1993.

Graczykowski JW, Mishell DR Jr: Methotrexate prophylaxis for persistent ectopic pregnancy after conservative treatment by salpingostomy. Obstet Gynecol 89:118, 1997.

Green LK, Kott ML: Histopathologic findings in ectopic tubal pregnancy. Int J Gynecol Pathol 8:255, 1989.

Grimes DA, Geary FH Jr, Hatcher RA: Rh immunoglobulin utilization after ectopic pregnancy. Am J Obstet Gynecol 140:246, 1981.

Gronlund B, Marushak A: Serial human chorionic gonadotrophin determination in the diagnosis of ectopic pregnancy. Aust N Z J Obstet Gynaecol 33:312, 1993.

Gruft L, Bertola E, Luchini L, et al: Determinants of reproductive prognosis after ectopic pregnancy. Hum Reprod 9:1333, 1994.

Hagstrom HG, Hahlin M, Bennegard-Eden B, et al: Prediction of persistent ectopic pregnancy after laparoscopic salpingostomy. Obstet Gynecol 84:798, 1994.

Hahlin M, Wallin A, Sjoblom P, Lindblom B: Single progesterone assay for early recognition of abnormal pregnancy. Hum Reprod 5:662, 1990.

Hajenius PJ, Mol BWJ, Ankum WM, et al: Clearance curves of serum human chorionic gonadotrophin for the diagnosis of persistent trophoblast. Hum Reprod 10:683, 1995.

Hallatt JG: Primary ovarian pregnancy: a report of twenty-five cases. Am J Obstet Gynecol 143:55, 1982.

Handler A, Davis F, Ferre C, Yeko T: The relationship of smoking and ectopic pregnancy. Am J Public Health 79:1239, 1989.

Hay DL, de Crespigny LC, McKenna M: Monitoring early pregnancy with transvaginal ultrasound and choriogonadotrophin levels. Aust N Z J Obstet Gynaecol 29:165, 1989.

Herbst AL, Hubby MM, Azizi F, et al: Reproductive and gynecologic surgical experience in diethylstilbestrol-exposed daughters. Am J Obstet Gynecol 141:1019, 1981.

Holt VL, Daling JR, Voigt LF, et al: Induced abortion and the risk of subsequent ectopic pregnancy. Am J Public Health 70:1234, 1989.

Hoppe DE, Bekkar BE, Nager MD: Single-dose systemic methotrexate for the treatment of persistent ectopic pregnancy after conservative surgery. Obstet Gynecol 83:51, 1994.

Ichinoe K, Wake H, Shinkai N, et al: Nonsurgical therapy to preserve oviduct function in patients with tubal pregnancies. Am J Obstet Gynecol 156:484, 1987.

Job-Spira N, Bouyer J, Pouly JL, et al: Fertility after ectopic pregnancy: First results of a population-based cohort study in France. Hum Reprod 11:99, 1996.

Johnson MR, Riddle AF, Irvine R, et al: Corpus luteum failure in ectopic pregnancy. Hum Reprod 8:1491, 1993.

Kadar N, Bohrer M, Kemmann E, Shelden R: The discriminatory human chorionic gonadotropin zone for endovaginal sonography: a prospective, randomized study. Fertil Steril 61:1016, 1994.

Kadar N, Caldwell BV, Romero R: A method of screening for ectopic pregnancy and its indications. Obstet Gynecol 58:162, 1981.

Kalchman GG, Meltzer RM: Interstitial pregnancy following homolateral salpingectomy. Am J Obstet Gynecol 196:1139, 1966.

Karikoski R, Aine R, Heinonen PK: Abnormal embryogenesis in the etiology of ectopic pregnancy. Gynecol Obstet Invest 36:158, 1993.

Kaufman RH, Noller K, Adam E, et al: Upper genital tract abnormalities and pregnancy outcome in diethylstilbestrol-exposed progeny. Am J Obstet Gynecol 148:973, 1984.

Kirchler HC, Seebacher S, Alge AA, et al: Early diagnosis of tubal pregnancy: Changes in tubal blood flow evaluated by endovaginal color Doppler sonography. Obstet Gynecol 82:561, 1993.

Korhonen J, Stenman UH, Ylöstalo P: Serum human chorionic gonadotropin dynamics during spontaneous resolution of ectopic pregnancy. Fertil Steril 61:632, 1994.

Kratzer PG, Taylor RN: Corpus luteum function in early pregnancies is primarily determined by the rate of change of human chorionic gonadotropin levels. Am J Obstet Gynecol 163:1497, 1990.

Langer R, Raszier A, Ron-El R, et al: Reproductive outcome after conservative surgery for unruptured tubal pregnancy: A 15-year experience. Fertil Steril 53:227, 1990.

Ledger WL, Sweeting VM, Chatterjee SP: Rapid diagnosis of early ectopic pregnancy in an emergency gynaecology service: Are measurements of progesterone, intact and free β human chorionic gonadotrophin helpful? Hum Reprod 9:157, 1994.

Levin AA, Schoenbaum SC, Stubblefield PG, et al: Ectopic pregnancy and prior induced abortion. Am J Public Health 72:253, 1982.

Lindblom B, Hahlin M, Lundorff P, Thorburn J: Treatment of tubal pregnancy by laparoscopy-guided injection of prostaglandin Fa_2. Fertil Steril 54:404, 1990.

Lindblom B, Hahlin M, Sjöblom P: Serial human chorionic gonadotropin determinations by fluoroimmunoassay for differentiation between intrauterine and ectopic gestation. Am J Obstet Gynecol 161:397, 1989.

Lipscomb GH, Bran D, McCord ML, et al: Analysis of three hundred fifteen ectopic pregnancies treated with single-dose methotrexate. Am J Obstet Gynecol 178:1354, 1998.

Lobel SM, Meyerovitz MF, Benson CC, et al: Preoperative angiographic uterine artery embolization in the management of cervical pregnancy. Obstet Gynecol 766:938, 1990.

Luc Pouly J, Canis M, Chapron C, et al: Multifactorial analysis of fertility after conservative laparoscopic treatment of ectopic pregnancy in a series of 223 patients. Fertil Steril 56:543, 1991.

Lund J: Early ectopic pregnancy. J Obstet Gynaecol Br Emp 62:70, 1955.

Lundorff P, Hahlin M, Sjöblom P, Lindblom B: Persistent trophoblast after conservative treatment of tubal pregnancy: prediction and detection. Obstet Gynecol 77:129, 1991.

Lundorff P, Thorburn J, Hahlin M, et al: Adhesion formation after laparoscopic surgery in tubal pregnancy: A randomized trial versus laparotomy. Fertil Steril 55:911, 1991.

Majmudar B, Henderson PH III, Semple E: Salpingitis isthmica nodosa: A high-risk factor for tubal pregnancy. Obstet Gynecol 62:73, 1983.

Makinen JI, Salmi TA, Nikkanen VPJ, Koskineew EYJ: Encouraging rates of fertility after ectopic pregnancy. Int J Fertil 34:46, 1989.

Marchbanks PA, Annegers JF: Risk factors for ectopic pregnancy: population based study. JAMA 259:1823, 1988.

Mashiach S, Carp HA, Serr DM: Nonoperative management of ectopic pregnancy: A preliminary report. J Reprod Med 1:127, 1982.

Matthews CP, Coulson P, Wild RA: Serum progesterone levels as an aid in the diagnosis of ectopic pregnancy. Obstet Gynecol 68:390, 1986.

McBain JC, Evans JH, Pepperell RJ, et al: An unexpectedly high rate of ectopic pregnancy following the induction of ovulation with human pituitary and chorionic gonadotrophin. Br J Obstet Gynaecol 87:5, 1980.

McCann MF, Kessel E: International experience with laparoscopic sterilization: Follow-up of 8500 women. Adv Planned Parent 12:199, 1978.

McCausland A: Endosalpingosis ("endosalpingoblastosis") following laparoscopic tubal coagulation as an etiologic factor of ectopic pregnancy. Am J Obstet Gynecol 143:12, 1982.

McCord ML, Arheart KL, Muram D, et al: Single serum progesterone as a screen for ectopic pregnancy: Exchanging specificity and sensitivity to obtain optimal test performance. Fertil Steril 66:513, 1996.

Mitra AG, Harris-Owens M: Conservative medical management of advanced cervical ectopic pregnancies. Obstet Gynecol Surv 55(6):385, 2000.

Miyazaki Y, Shrina Y, Wake N, et al: Studies on nonsurgical therapy of tubal pregnancy. Acta Obstet Gynaecol Jpn 35:489, 1983.

Molloy D, Hynes J, Deambrosis W, et al: Multiple-sited (heterotopic) pregnancy after in vitro fertilization and gamete intrafallopian transfer. Fertil Steril 53:1068, 1990.

Morris JM, Van Wagenen G: Interception: the use of postovulatory estrogens to prevent implantation. Am J Obstet Gynecol 115:101, 1973.

Nakajima ST, Nason FG, Badger GJ, Gibson M: Progesterone production in early pregnancy. Fertil Steril 55:516, 1991.

Nieuwkerk P, Hajenius P, Van der Veen, F, et al: Systemic methotrexate therapy versus laparoscopic salpingostomy in tubal pregnancy. Part II. Patient preferences for systemic methotrexate. Fertil Steril 70(3): 518, 1998.

Niles JH, Clark JJ: Pathogenesis of tubal pregnancy. Am J Obstet Gynecol 105:1230, 1969.

O'Leary JL, O'Leary JA: Rudimentary horn pregnancy. Obstet Gynecol 22:371, 1963.

O'Leary P, Nicols C, Feddema P, et al: Serum progesterone and human chorionic gonadotrophin measurements in the evaluation of ectopic pregnancy. Aust NS J Obstet Gynaecol 36:319, 1996.

Ollendorff BA, Felgin MD: The value of curettage in the diagnosis of ectopic pregnancy. Am J Obstet Gynecol 157:71, 1987.

Ory SJ: New options for diagnosis and treatment of ectopic pregnancy. JAMA 267(4):534, 1992.

Paalman RJ, McElin TW: Cervical pregnancy. Am J Obstet Gynecol 77:1261, 1959.

Pansky M, Golan A, Bukovsky I, Caspi E: Nonsurgical management of tubal pregnancy. Am J Obstet Gynecol 164:888, 1991.

Parente JT, Ou CS, Levy J: Cervical pregnancy analysis: a review and report of five cases. Obstet Gynecol 62:79, 1983.

Parker J, Bisits A: Laparoscopic surgical treatment of ectopic pregnancy: Salpingectomy or salpingostomy? Aust N Z J Obstet Gynaecol 37:115, 1997.

Parker J, Permezel M, Thompson D: Review of the management of ectopic pregnancy in a major teaching hospital: Laparoscopic surgical treatment and persistent ectopic pregnancy. Aust N Z J Obstet Gynaecol 34:575, 1994.

Pellerito JS, Taylor KJ, Quedens-Case C, et al: Ectopic pregnancy: evaluation with endovaginal color flow imaging. Radiology 183:407, 1992.

Persaud V: Etiology of tubal ectopic pregnancy. Obstet Gynecol 36:257, 1970.

Peterson HB: Extratubal ectopic pregnancies. J Reprod Med 31:108, 1986.

Peterson HB, Xia Z, Hughes JM, et al for the U.S. Collaborative Review of Sterilization Working Group: The risk of pregnancy after tubal sterilization: Findings from the U.S. Collaborative Review of Sterilization. Am J Obstet Gynecol 174:1161, 1996.

Peterson HB, for the US Collaborative Review of Sterilization Working Group: The risk of ectopic pregnancy after tubal sterilization. N Engl J Med 336:762, 1997.

Pouly JL, Canis M, Chapron C, et al: Multifactorial analysis of fertility after conservative laparoscopic treatment of ectopic pregnancy in a series of 223 patients. Fertil Steril 56:453, 1991.

Pouly JL, Mahnes H, Mage G, et al: Conservative laparoscopic treatment of 321 ectopic pregnancies. Fertil Steril 46:1093, 1986.

Ransom MX, Garcia AJ, Bohrer M, et al: Serum progesterone as a predictor of methotrexate success in the treatment of ectopic pregnancy. Obstet Gynecol 83:1033, 1994.

Reece EA, Petrie RH, Sirmans MF, et al: Combined intrauterine and extrauterine gestations: A review. Am J Obstet Gynecol 146:323, 1983.

Risquez F, Reidy J, Forman R, et al: Transcervical cannulation of the fallopian tube for the management of ectopic pregnancy: prospective multicenter study. Fertil Steril 58:1131, 1992.

Romero R, Kadar H, Castro D, et al: The value of serial human chorionic gonadotropin testing as a diagnostic tool in ectopic pregnancy. Am J Obstet Gynecol 155:392, 1986.

Rose PG, Cohen SM: Methotrexate therapy for persistent ectopic pregnancy after conservative laparoscopic management. Obstet Gynecol 76:947, 1990.

Rosenberg P, Chevret S, Camus E, et al. Medical treatment of ectopic pregnancies: A randomized clinical trial comparing methotrexate-mifepristone and methotrexate-placebo. Hum Repro 18:1802, 2003.

Rubin GL, Peterson HB, Dorfman SF, et al: Ectopic pregnancy in the United States 1970 through 1978. JAMA 249:1725, 1983.

Saito M, Koyama T, Yaoi Y, et al: Site of ovulation and ectopic pregnancy. Acta Obstet Gynecol Scand 54:227, 1975.

Samuellson S, Sjovall A: Laparoscopy in suspected ectopic pregnancy. Acta Obstet Gynecol Scand 51:31, 1972.

Saraj AJ, Wilcox JG, Najmabadi S, et al: Resolution of hormonal markers of ectopic gestation: A randomized trial comparing single-dose intramuscular methotrexate with salpingostomy. Obstet Gynecol 92:989, 1998.

Sauer MV, Vermesh M, Anderson R, et al: Rapid measurement of urinary pregnanediol glucuronide to diagnose ectopic pregnancy. Am J Obstet Gynecol 159:1531, 1988.

Seifer DB, Gutmann JN, Grant WD, et al: Comparison of persistent ectopic pregnancy after laparoscopic salpingostomy versus salpingostomy at laparotomy for ectopic pregnancy. Obstet Gynecol 81:378, 1993.

Shah A, Courney NG, Cunanan RG: Pregnancy following laparoscopic tubal electrocoagulation and division. Am J Obstet Gynecol 1129:459, 1977.

Shalev E, Romano S, Peleg D, et al: Spontaneous resolution of ectopic tubal pregnancy: Natural history. Fertil Steril 63:15, 1995.

Sherman D, Langer R, Sadovsky G, et al: Improved fertility following ectopic pregnancy. Fertil Steril 37:497, 1982.

Sivin I: Copper T IUD use and ectopic pregnancy rates in the United States. Contraception 19:151, 1979.

Skjeldestad FE, Hadgu A, Eriksson N: Epidemiology of repeat ectopic pregnancy: A population-based prospective cohort study. Obstet Gynecol 91:129, 1998.

Spandorfer SD, Menzin AW, Barnhart KT, et al: Efficacy of frozen-section evaluation of uterine curettings in the diagnosis of ectopic pregnancy. Am J Obstet Gynecol 175:603, 1996.

Spandorfer SD, Sawin SW, Benjamin I, Barnhart KT: Postoperative day 1 serum human chorionic gonadotropin level as a predictor of persistent ectopic pregnancy after conservative surgical management. Fertil Steril 68:430, 1997.

Spiegelburg O: Zur Canistik den ovarial-schwangenschaft. Arch Gynek 13:73, 1878.

Stern JJ, Voss F, Coulam CB: Early diagnosis of ectopic pregnancy using receiver-operator characteristic curves of serum progesterone concentrations. Hum Reprod 8:775, 1993.

Stock RJ: Persistent tubal pregnancy. Obstet Gynecol 77:267, 1991.

Stovall TG, Ling F, Kellerman AL, Buster JE: Outpatient chemotherapy of unruptured ectopic pregnancy. Fertil Steril 51:435, 1989.

Stovall TG, Ling FW: Single-dose methotrexate: An expanded clinical trial. Am J Obstet Gynecol 168:1759, 1993.

Stovall TG, Ling FW, Anderson RN, Buster JE: Improved sensitivity and specificity of a single measurement of serum progesterone over serial quantitative beta-human chorionic gonadotrophin in screening for ectopic pregnancy. Hum Reprod 7:723, 1992.

Stovall TG, Ling FW, Carson SA, Buster JE: Serum progesterone and uterine curettage in differential diagnosis of ectopic pregnancy. Fertil Steril 67:456, 1992.

Stovall TG, Ling FW, Cope BJ, Buster JE: Preventing ruptured ectopic pregnancy with a single serum progesterone. Am J Obstet Gynecol 160:1425, 1989.

Stovall TG, Ling FW, Gray LA, et al: Methotrexate treatment of unruptured ectopic pregnancy: A report of 100 cases. Obstet Gynecol 77:749, 1991.

Stratford B: Abnormalities of early human development. Am J Obstet Gynecol 107:1223, 1970.

Studdiford WE: Primary peritoneal pregnancy. Am J Obstet Gynecol 44:487, 1942.

Tanaka T, Hayashi H, Kutsuzawa T, et al: Treatment of interstitial ectopic pregnancy with methotrexate: Report of a successful case. Fertil Steril 37:851, 1982.

Tatum HJ, Schmidt FH: Contraceptive and sterilization practices and extrauterine pregnancy: A realistic perspective. Fertil Steril 28:407, 1977.

Timonen S, Nieminen U: Tubal pregnancy, choice of operative method of treatment. Acta Obstet Gynecol Scand 46:327, 1967.

Trio D, Lapinski RH, Strobelt N, et al: Prognostic factors for successful expectant management of ectopic pregnancy. Fertil Steril 63:469, 1995.

Tulandi T, Falcone T, Atri M, et al: Transvaginal intratubal methotrexate treatment of ectopic pregnancy. Fertil Steril 58:98, 1992.

Tulandi T, Guralnick M: Treatment of tubal ectopic pregnancy by salpingotomy with or without tubal suturing and salpingectomy. Fertil Steril 55:53, 1991.

Tummon IS, Nisker JA, Whitmore NA, et al: Transferring more embryos increases risk of heterotopic pregnancy. Fertil Steril 61:1065, 1994.

Tuomivaara L, Kauppila A: Radical or conservative surgery for ectopic pregnancy? A follow-up study of fertility of 323 patients. Fertil Steril 50:580, 1988.

Vermesh M: Conservative management of ectopic gestation. Fertil Steril 51:559, 1989.

Vermesh M, Presser SC: Reproductive outcome after linear salpingostomy for ectopic gestation: A prospective 3-year follow-up. Fertil Steril 57:682, 1992.

Vermesh M, Silva PD, Rosen GF, et al: Management of unruptured ectopic gestation by linear salpingostomy: A prospective, randomized clinical trial of laparoscopy versus laparotomy. Obstet Gynecol 73:400, 1989.

Vermesh M, Silva PD, Rosen GF, et al: Persistent tubal ectopic gestation: Patterns of circulation β-human chorionic gonadotropin and progesterone and management options. Fertil Steril 50:584, 1988.

Weckstein LN: Current perspective on ectopic pregnancy. Obstet Gynecol Surv 40:259, 1985.

Weckstein LN, Boucher AR, Tucker H, et al: Accurate diagnosis of early ectopic pregnancy. Obstet Gynecol 65:393, 1985.

Weström L, Bengtsson LPH, and Mårdh PA: Incidence, trends and risks of ectopic pregnancy in a population of women. Br Med J 282:15, 1981.

Wong YH, Liang EY, Lau, KY: A cervical ectopic pregnancy managed by medical treatment and angiographic embolization. Aust NZ J Obstet Gynecol 39(4):493, 1999.

Yao M, Tulandi T: Current status of surgical and nonsurgical management of ectopic pregnancy. Fertil Steril 67:421, 1997.

Yeko TR, Gorrill MJ, Hughes LH, et al: Timely diagnosis of early ectopic pregnancy using a single blood progesterone measurement. Fertil Steril 48:10, 1987.

Ylöstalo P, Cacciatore B, Sjoberg J, et al: Expectant management of ectopic pregnancy. Obstet Gynecol 80:345, 1992.

Benign Gynecologic Lesions 18

Vulva, Vagina, Cervix, Uterus, Oviduct, Ovary

Vern L. Katz

KEY TERMS AND DEFINITIONS

Adenomyoma. An isolated area of endometrial glands and stroma in the uterine musculature that can be identified grossly.

Adenomyosis. The growth of endometrial glands and stroma into the uterine myometrium to a depth of at least 2.5 mm from the basalis layer of the endometrium.

Allodynia. Hyperesthesia and pain induced by a nonpainful stimuli such as a cotton-tipped applicator.

Brenner Tumor. A small, smooth, solid fibroepithelial tumor of the ovary. It may be benign or malignant.

Degeneration of a Myoma. The process by which a myoma outgrows its blood supply and begins to necrose centrally. Forms of degeneration include hyaline, myxomatous, calcific, cystic, fat, and red degeneration.

Dermoid (Benign Cystic Teratoma). A benign germ cell tumor that contains well-differentiated derivatives of all three germ cell layers.

Dysontogenetic Cysts. Thin-walled cysts of embryonic origin.

Endometrial Polyp. A localized outgrowth of endometrial glands and stroma projecting beyond the surface of the endometrium and including a vascular stalk.

Follicular Hematoma. Follicular cysts filled with blood, usually from hemorrhage in the vascular theca zone.

Gartner's Duct Cysts. Cysts primarily of mesonephric origin found laterally in the vagina.

Hematometra. A uterus distended with blood, secondary to partial or complete obstruction of any portion of the lower genital tract.

Hidradenitis Suppurativa. A chronic infection involving skin, subcutaneous tissue, and apocrine glands.

Hidradenoma. A rare, small, benign vulvar tumor originating from apocrine sweat glands.

Hydatid Cysts of Morgagni. Pedunculated paratubal cysts found near the fimbriae of the oviduct.

Hydrometra. A collection of clear fluid in the uterine cavity.

Hyperreactio Luteinalis. Multiple theca lutein cysts causing bilateral ovarian enlargement during pregnancy.

Intravenous Leiomyomatosis. An extremely rare condition in which benign smooth muscle fibers invade and slowly grow into the venous channels of the pelvis.

Itch–Scratch Cycles. Repetitive cycles of itching leading to scratching. The scratching leads to excoriation, irritation, and healing, with subsequent irritation and itching.

Leiomyoma (Myoma or Fibroid). A benign tumor of muscle cell origin found in any tissue that contains smooth muscle.

Leiomyomatosis Peritonealis Disseminata. A benign disease with multiple small nodules over the surface of the pelvis and abdominal peritoneum, grossly mimicking disseminated carcinoma or sarcoma.

Lichenification. Changes in the skin from chronic irritation, characterized by whiteness, thickening, and leathery appearance.

Luteoma of Pregnancy. A rare, specific, benign, hyperplastic reaction of ovarian theca lutein cells during pregnancy.

Meigs' Syndrome. The constellation of symptoms of ascites and hydrothorax associated with a benign ovarian fibroma, resolving after the removal of the tumor.

Nabothian Cysts. Cervical retention cysts lined by endocervical-type columnar cells.

Parasitic Myoma. A myoma that outgrows its uterine blood supply and obtains a secondary blood supply from another organ, such as the omentum.

Prominence or Tubercle of Rokitansky. The protrusion of solid elements of a dermoid into the cyst cavity.

Pruritus. A symptom of intense itching with an associated desire to scratch.

Pyometra. A collection of pus in the uterine cavity.

Struma Ovarii. A specialized ovarian teratoma that consists of thyroid tissue as a major or exclusive component. Rarely, it may produce sufficient thyroid hormone to induce hyperthyroidism.

Submucosal Myoma. A myoma located immediately below the endometrial lining.

Subserosal Myoma. A myoma found just beneath the serosa of the uterus.

Syringoma. A benign tumor of the eccrine sweat glands.

Vulvodynia. A term describing chronic vulvar discomfort.

This book is divided primarily into chapters that deal with benign diseases and chapters that deal with malignant ones. For the clinician, however, the difference is not always clear. As in many areas of medicine, gynecologic problems do not fall into definitive categories, and those that include malignant disease often overlap with those that include benign disease. When the diagnosis from the history, physical examination, and laboratory tests is clear, management is usually self-evident. When a specific diagnosis is unclear, tissue biopsy is appropriate. This chapter deals primarily with benign lesions; however, the symptoms and differential diagnoses of these lesions have definite overlap with those of malignant disease. Thus, the clinical approach to many problems must be broad and not so focused as to prematurely exclude dangerous pathologies within the differential diagnosis, though they may be less common.

The discussions in this chapter are arranged anatomically, beginning with the vulva and subsequently covering the vagina, cervix, uterus, oviducts, and ovaries. This chapter does not attempt to be encyclopedic; rather, lesions have been selected based on their clinical importance and prevalence. Therefore, extremely rare lesions such as glomus tumors of the vulva or papillomas of the cervix have been omitted. Because several non-neoplastic abnormalities and lesions present in ways similar to those of benign tumors, this chapter also discusses entities that are not specifically abnormal growths. Clinical problems such as torsion of the ovary, lacerations of the vagina, and hematomas of the vulva are examples of common conditions included in this chapter.

The successful clinician must use both deductive and inductive reasoning in solving a problem. To have mastered both these techniques, he or she not only must be adept at history taking and physical examination but also must be able to form a complete list of possible lesions that may be involved in the patient's complaint. An understanding of the problems discussed in this chapter will be helpful in that endeavor.

VULVA

Urethral Caruncle

A urethral caruncle is a small, fleshy outgrowth of the distal edge of the urethra. The tissue of the caruncle is soft, smooth, friable, and bright red and initially appears as an eversion of the urethra (Fig. 18-1). Urethral caruncles are generally small, single, and sessile, but may be pedunculated and grow to be 1 to 2 cm in diameter. They occur most frequently in postmenopausal women and must be differentiated from urethral carcinomas. Urethral caruncles are believed to arise from an ectropion of the posterior urethral wall associated with retraction and atrophy of the postmenopausal vagina. The growth of the caruncle is secondary to chronic irritation or infection. Histologically the caruncle is composed of transitional and stratified squamous epithelium with a loose connective tissue. Often the submucosal layer contains relatively large dilated veins. Caruncles are frequently subdivided by their histologic appearance into papillomatous, granulomatous, and angiomatous varieties. They are often secondarily infected, producing ulceration and bleeding. If the diagnosis of a urethral caruncle is entertained in a child, most likely the correct diagnosis is urethral prolapse (Fig. 18-2).

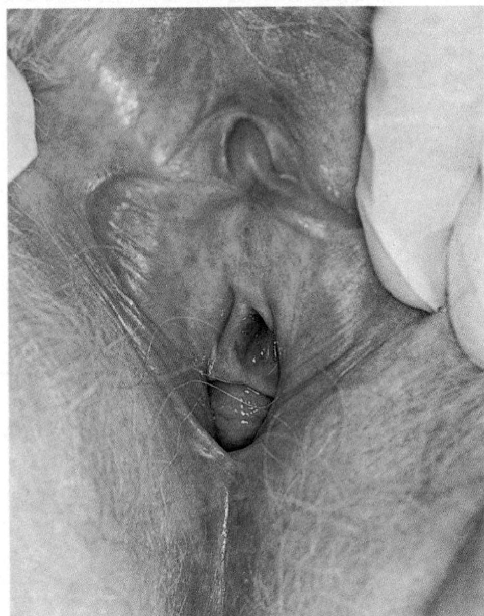

Figure 18-1. Urethral caruncle. Red popular lesion at the base of the meatus in a postmenopausal woman. (From Fisher BK, Margesson LJ: Genital Skin Disorders: Diagnosis and Treatment. St. Louis, Mosby, 1998.)

The symptoms associated with urethral caruncles are variable. Many women are asymptomatic, whereas others experience dysuria, frequency, and urgency. Sometimes the caruncle produces point tenderness after contact with undergarments or during intercourse. Ulcerative lesions usually produce spotting on contact more commonly than hematuria.

The differential diagnosis of urethral caruncles includes primary carcinoma of the urethra and prolapse of the urethral

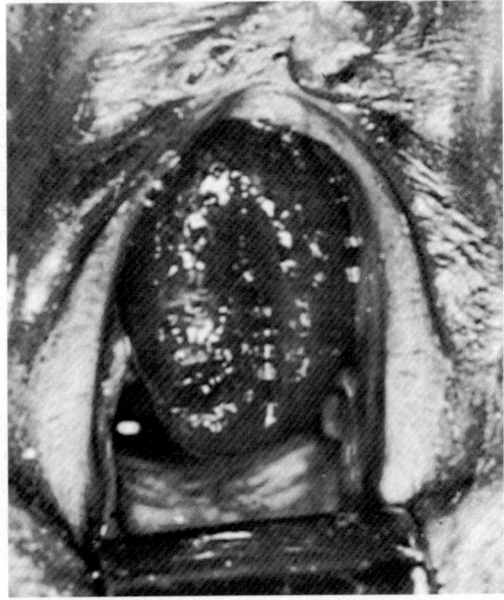

Figure 18-2. Prolapse of urethral mucosa in 7-year-old child. Edematous red collar of tissue surrounds urethral meatus. (From Kaufman RH: Solid tumors. In Kaufman RH, Faro S [eds]: Benign Diseases of the Vulva and Vagina, 4th ed. St. Louis, Mosby–Year Book, 1994.)

mucosa. Although urethral caruncles are not a precursor for urethral carcinoma, grossly the two are often confused. Marshall and colleagues reported a series of 394 urethral tumors. A clinical diagnosis of urethral caruncle was made in 376 of these women. Histologic examination of biopsy material demonstrated urethral carcinoma in nine patients in their series. Approximately 1 in 40 women with a clinical diagnosis of urethral caruncle has a malignant urethral neoplasm. Urethral carcinoma is primarily a disease of elderly women. The majority of urethral carcinomas are of squamous cell origin. Most of these rare carcinomas arise from the distal urethra. The symptoms of a urethral carcinoma include bleeding, urinary frequency, and dysuria, and the signs include a mass protruding from the urethra, with associated tenderness and induration of the urethra.

The diagnosis of a urethral caruncle is established by biopsy under local anesthesia. Initial therapy is oral or topical estrogen and avoidance of irritation. If the caruncle does not regress or is symptomatic, it may be destroyed by cryosurgery, laser therapy, fulguration, or operative excision. Following operative destruction, a Foley catheter should be left in place for 48 to 72 hours. Follow-up is necessary to ensure that the patient does not develop urethral stenosis. Often the caruncle may recur. Small, asymptomatic urethral caruncles do not need treatment.

Urethral prolapse is predominantly a disease of the premenarcheal female, although it does occur in postmenopausal women. Patients may have dysuria; however, the majority are asymptomatic. The annular rosette of friable, edematous, prolapsed mucosa does not have the bright-red color of a caruncle and is not as circumscribed in gross configuration. It may be ulcerated with necrosis or grossly edematous. Therapy of a prolapsed urethra is hot sitz baths and antibiotics to reduce inflammation and infection. Topical estrogen cream is sometimes an effective treatment. In rare cases it may be necessary to excise the redundant mucosa.

Cysts

The most common large cyst of the vulva is a cystic dilation of an obstructed Bartholin's duct. Approximately 2% of new gynecologic patients present with an asymptomatic Bartholin's duct cyst. Treatment is not necessary in women younger than 40 unless the cyst becomes infected or enlarges enough to produce symptoms. A more complete discussion of Bartholin's duct cysts and abscesses is included in Chapter 22 (Infections of the Lower Genital Tract). Occasionally the ducts of mucous glands of the vestibule are occluded. The resulting cysts may be clear, yellow, or blue. Similar small mucous cysts occur in the periurethral region. Wolffian duct cysts or mesonephric cysts are rare, but when they do occur, they are found near the clitoris and lateral to the hymeneal ring. These cysts have thin walls and contain clear serous fluid.

Skene's duct cysts are rare, usually small, and may present with symptoms of discomfort or be found on routine examination. These cysts arise secondary to infection and scarring of the small ducts. The differential includes urethral diverticula. Clinically, physical compression of the cyst, unlike compression of a urethral diverticula, should not produce fluid from the urethral meatus. Imaging studies may also assist in establishing the diagnosis. Asymptomatic cysts in premenopausal women may be managed conservatively. Treatment is excision with careful dissection to avoid urethral injury.

The most common small vulvar cysts are epidermal inclusion cysts or sebaceous cysts. Because these cysts cannot be differentiated grossly and since a continuing controversy exists with respect to their histogenesis, these two cysts are discussed together in this chapter. However, epithelial cysts are discovered much more frequently than sebaceous cysts. Epithelial cysts are located immediately beneath the epidermis. Most commonly they are discovered on the anterior half of the labia majora. These cysts are usually multiple, freely movable, round, slow growing, and nontender. They are firm to shotty in consistency, and their contents are usually under pressure. Grossly, they are white or yellow, and the contents are caseous, like a thick cheese. Local scarring of the adjacent skin sometimes occurs when rupture of the contents of the cyst produces an inflammatory reaction in the subcutaneous tissue.

An inclusion cyst may develop following trauma when an infolding of squamous epithelium has occurred beneath the epidermis in the site of an episiotomy or obstetric laceration. Most inclusion cysts of the vagina are directly related to previous trauma, whereas most inclusion cysts of the vulva are not related to trauma. Alternative theories of histogenesis include embryonic remnants and occlusion of pilosebaceous ducts of sweat glands. The histology of these cysts is characterized by an epithelial lining of keratinized, stratified squamous epithelium with a center of cellular debris that grossly resembles sebaceous material. Most vulvar epidermal cysts do not have sebaceous cells or sebaceous material identified on microscopic examination. Usually there are multiple cysts, with the vast majority being less than 1 cm in diameter. These cysts are asymptomatic unless they are secondarily infected. Large epidermal cysts may be confused with fibromas, lipomas, and hidradenomas.

Most of these cysts require no treatment. If the cyst becomes infected, treatment consists of heat applied locally and incision and drainage. Cysts that become recurrently infected or produce pain should be excised when the acute inflammation has subsided.

Nevus

A nevus, commonly referred to as a *mole,* is a localized nest or cluster of melanocytes. These undifferentiated cells arise from the embryonic neural crest and are present from birth. Many nevi are not recognized until they become pigmented at the time of puberty. Vulvar nevi are one of the most common benign neoplasms in females. As with nevi in other parts of the body, they exhibit a wide range in depth of color, from blue to dark brown to black, and some may be amelanotic. The diameter of most nevi ranges from a few millimeters to 2 cm. Grossly, a benign nevus may be flat, elevated, or pedunculated. Other pigmented lesions in the differential diagnosis include hemangiomas, endometriosis, malignant melanoma, vulvar intraepithelial neoplasia, and seborrheic keratosis.

Vulvar nevi are generally asymptomatic. Most women do not closely inspect their vulvar skin and are unaware of biologic changes in gross appearance of these lesions. Histologically the lesions are subdivided into three major groups: junctional, compound, and intradermal nevi (Fig. 18-3).

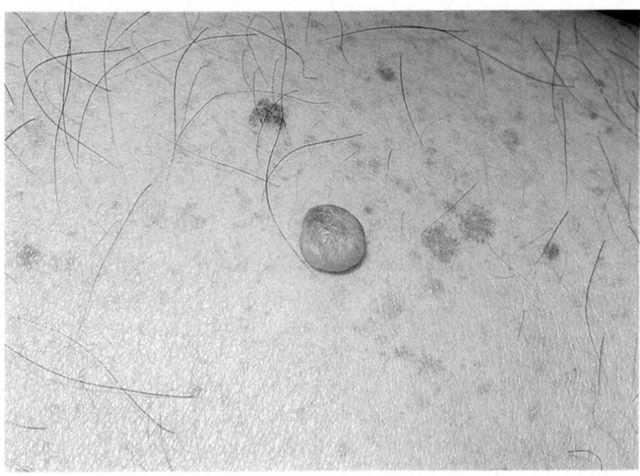

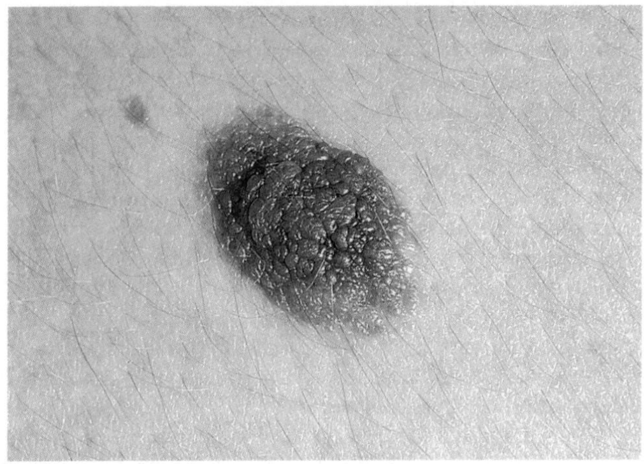

Figure 18-3. Vulvar nevi. **A,** Dome-shaped intradermal nevus. **B,** Compound nevus with irregular pigmentation. (From Fisher BK, Margesson LJ: Genital Skin Disorders: Diagnosis and Treatment. St. Louis, Mosby, 1998.)

Although the vulvar area contains approximately 1% of the skin surface of the body, 5% to 10% of all malignant melanomas in women arise from this region. The biologic reasons for this discrepancy are unknown. Speculation includes the hypothesis that junctional activity is common in vulvar nevi, and the many irritants to which vulvar skin is exposed may lead to malignancy. It is estimated that 50% of malignant melanomas arise from a preexisting nevus. The majority of women who develop melanomas are in their 50s. Family history of melanoma is one of the strongest risk factors for the disease.

Ideally, all vulvar nevi should be excised and examined histologically. Special emphasis should be directed toward the flat junctional nevus and the dysplastic nevus for they have the greatest potential for malignant transformation (Fig. 18-4).

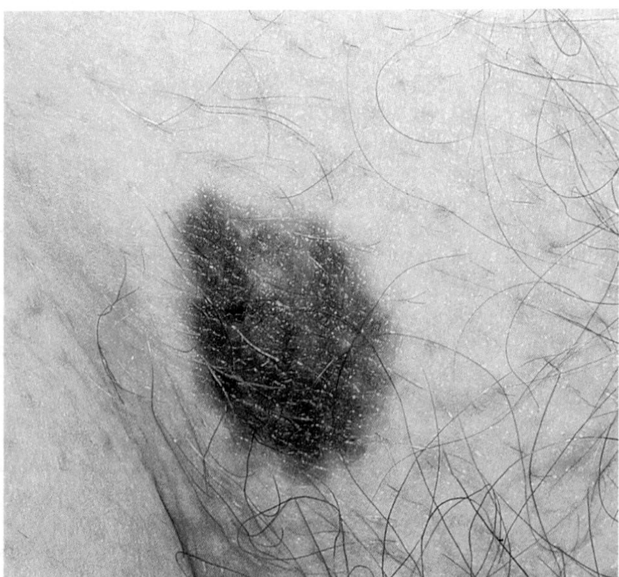

Figure 18-4. Suprapubic dysplastic nevus with an irregular shape, reddish hue to the edges, and indistinct margins. (From Fisher BK, Margesson LJ: Genital Skin Disorders: Diagnosis and Treatment. St. Louis, Mosby, 1998.)

The lifetime risk of a woman developing melanoma from a congenital junctional nevus that measures greater than 2 cm in diameter is estimated to be approximately 10%. The lifetime risk of a melanoma forming in women with dysplastic nevi is 15 times that of the general population. The dysplastic nevus is characterized by being more than 5 mm in diameter, with irregular borders and patches of variegated pigment. Removal may be accomplished with local anesthesia or coincidentally with obstetric delivery or gynecologic surgery. Proper excisional biopsy should be three-dimensional and adequate in width and depth. Approximately 5 to 10 mm of normal skin surrounding the nevus should be included, and the biopsy should include the underlying dermis as well. Some patients are reluctant to have a "normal"-appearing nevus removed. Nevi that are raised or contain hair rarely undergo malignant change. However, if they are frequently irritated or bleed spontaneously, they should be removed. Recent changes in growth or color, ulceration, bleeding, pain, or the development of satellite lesions mandate biopsy. The characteristic clinical features of an early malignant melanoma may be remembered by thinking ABCD: *asymmetry, border* irregularity, *color* variegation, and a *diameter* usually greater than 6 mm.

Hemangioma

Hemangiomas are rare malformations of blood vessels rather than true neoplasms. Vulvar hemangiomas frequently are discovered initially during childhood. They are usually single, 1 to 2 cm in diameter, flat, and soft, and they range in color from brown to red or purple. Histologically, the multiple channels of hemangiomas are predominantly thin-walled capillaries arranged randomly and separated by thin connective tissue septa. These tumors change in size with compression and are not encapsulated. Most hemangiomas are asymptomatic; occasionally they may become ulcerated and bleed.

There are at least five different types of vulvar hemangiomas. The strawberry and cavernous hemangiomas are congenital defects discovered in young children. The strawberry hemangioma is usually bright red to dark red, is elevated, and rarely increases in size after age 2. Approximately 60% of vulvar hemangiomas discovered during the first years of life spontaneously regress in size by the time the child goes to school. Cavernous hemangiomas are usually purple in color and vary in size, with the larger lesions extending deeply into the subcutaneous tissue. These hemangiomas initially appear during the first few months of life and may increase in size until age 2. Similar to strawberry hemangiomas, spontaneous resolution generally occurs before age 6. Senile or cherry angiomas are common small lesions that arise on the labia majora, usually in postmenopausal women. They are most often less than 3 mm in diameter, multiple, and red-brown to dark blue. Angiokeratomas are approximately twice the size of cherry angiomas, are purple or dark red, and occur in women between the ages of 30 and 50. They are noted for their rapid growth and tendency to bleed during strenuous exercise. In the differential diagnosis of an angiokeratoma is Kaposi's sarcoma and angiosarcoma. Pyogenic granulomas are an overgrowth of inflamed granulation tissue. These lesions grow under the hormonal influence of pregnancy, with similarities to lesions in the oral cavity. Pyogenic granulomas are usually approximately 1 cm in diameter and may be mistaken clinically for malignant melanomas, basal cell carcinomas, vulvar condylomas, or nevi. Treatment of pyogenic granulomas involves wide and deep excision to prevent recurrence.

The diagnosis is usually established by gross inspection of the vascular lesion. Asymptomatic hemangiomas and hemangiomas in children rarely require therapy. In adults, initial treatment of large symptomatic hemangiomas that are bleeding or infected may require subtotal resection. When the differential diagnosis is questionable, excisional biopsy should be performed. A hemangioma that is associated with troublesome bleeding may be destroyed by cryosurgery or use of an argon laser. Cryosurgical treatment usually involves a single freeze/thaw cycle repeated three times at monthly intervals. Obviously, if the histologic diagnosis is questionable, any bleeding vulvar mass should be treated by excisional biopsy so that the definitive pathologic diagnosis can be established. Surgical removal of a large, cavernous hemangioma may be technically quite difficult. Lymphangiomas of the vulva do exist but are extremely rare.

Another rare malformation is the vulvar venous malformation. These lesions may become symptomatic at any age, and are relatively prone to thrombosis. Venous malformations are different from vulvar varicosities which are exacerbated with pregnancy and tend to regress postpartum. Marrocco-Trischitta and coworkers reported on the successful use of sclerotherapy for the malformations, after venography and Doppler ultrasound verified the diagnosis.

Fibroma

Fibromas are the most common benign solid tumors of the vulva. They are more frequent than lipomas, the other common benign tumors of mesenchymal origin. Fibromas occur in all age groups and most commonly are found in the labia majora (Fig. 18-5). However, they actually arise from deeper connective tissue. Thus they should be considered as dermatofibromas. They grow slowly and vary from a few centimeters to one gigantic vulvar fibroma reported to weigh more than 250 pounds. The majority are between 1 and 10 cm in diameter. The smaller fibromas are discovered as subcutaneous nodules. As they increase in size and weight, they become pedunculated. Smaller fibromas are firm; however, larger tumors often become cystic after undergoing myxomatous degeneration. Sometimes the vulvar skin over a fibroma is compromised by pressure and ulcerates.

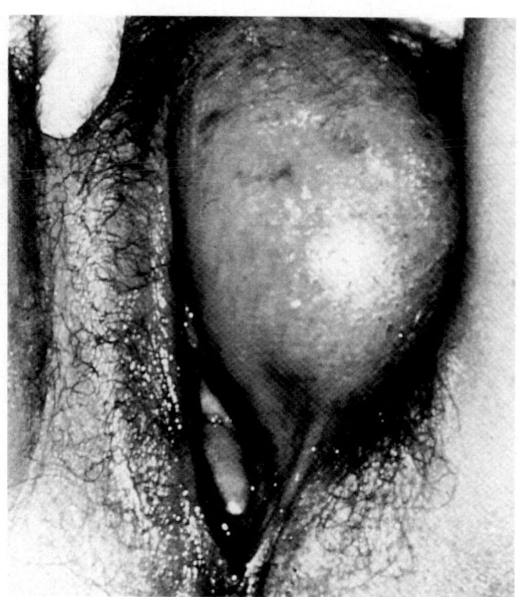

Figure 18-5. Vulvar fibroma, which is the most common benign solid tumor of the vulva. (From Friedrich EG [ed]: Vulvar Disease, 2nd ed. Philadelphia, WB Saunders, 1983.)

Fibromas have a smooth surface and a distinct contour. On cut surface the tissue is gray-white. Fat or muscle cells microscopically may be associated with the interlacing fibroblasts. Fibromas have a low-grade potential for becoming malignant. Smaller fibromas are asymptomatic; larger ones may produce chronic pressure symptoms or acute pain when they degenerate. Treatment is operative removal if the fibromas are symptomatic or continue to grow. Occasionally they are removed for cosmetic reasons.

Lipoma

Lipomas are benign, slow-growing, circumscribed tumors of fat cells arising from the subcutaneous tissue of the vulva (Fig. 18-6). Lipomas of the vulva are similar to lipomas of other parts of the body. When discovered they are softer and usually larger than fibromas. The majority of lipomas in the vulvar region are smaller than 3 cm in diameter. The largest vulvar lipoma reported in the literature weighed 44 pounds. Lipomas are the second most frequent benign vulvar mesenchymal tumor. Because of the fat distribution of the vulva, most lipomas are discovered in the labia majora and are superficial in location. They are slow growing, and their malignant potential is extremely low.

When a lipoma is cut, the substance is soft, yellow, and lobulated. Histologically, lipomas are usually more homogeneous

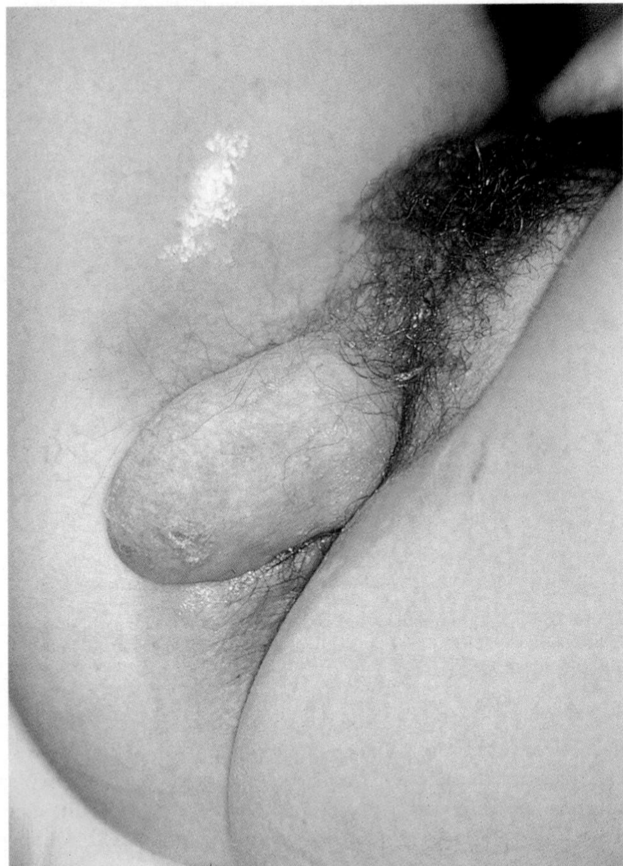

Figure 18-6. Skin-colored pedunculated lipoma of labium major observed in a 15-year-old. (From Fisher BK, Margesson LJ: Genital Skin Disorders: Diagnosis and Treatment. St. Louis, Mosby, 1998.)

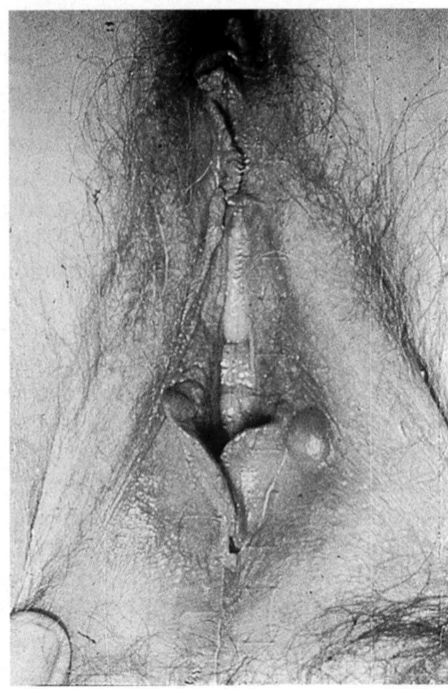

Figure 18-7. Hidradenoma. (From Shea CH, Stevens A, Dalziel KL, Robboy SJ: The vulva: Cysts, neoplasms, and related lesions. In Robboy SJ, Anderson MC, Russell P [eds]: Pathology of the Female Reproductive Tract. Edinburgh, Churchill Livingstone, 2002.)

than fibromas. Prominent areas of connective tissue occasionally are associated with the mature adipose cells of a true lipoma. Unless extremely large, lipomas do not produce symptoms. Excision is usually performed to establish the diagnosis, although smaller tumors may be followed conservatively.

Hidradenoma

The hidradenoma is a rare, small, benign vulvar tumor that originates from apocrine sweat glands of the inner surface of the labia majora and nearby perineum (Fig. 18-7). Occasionally, they may originate from eccrine sweat glands. For unknown reasons, they are discovered exclusively in white women between the ages of 30 and 70, most commonly in the fourth decade of life. These tumors have not been reported prior to puberty. Hidradenomas may be cystic or solid. In a review by Woodworth and colleagues 55% were cystic. Whereas 38% originated from the labia majora, 26% arose from the labia minora. Approximately 50% of hidradenomas are less than 1 cm in diameter.

These tumors are well defined and usually sessile, pinkish-gray nodules not larger than 2 cm in diameter. In most cases the surface epithelium is white, but occasionally necrosis of a central indented area occurs, with a protrusion of reddish-brown granulation tissue. These latter lesions may be confused with pyogenic granulomas.

These tumors have well-defined capsules. These papillary tumors arise deep in the dermis. Histologically, because of its hyperplastic, adenomatous pattern, a hidradenoma may be mistaken at first glance for an adenocarcinoma. On close inspection, however, although there is glandular hyperplasia with numerous tubular ducts, there is a paucity of mitotic figures and a lack of significant cellular and nuclear pleomorphism (Fig. 18-8). Hidradenomas are generally asymptomatic. However, they may cause pruritus or bleeding if the tumor undergoes necrosis. Excisional biopsy is the treatment of choice.

Syringoma

The syringoma is a very rare, cystic, asymptomatic, benign tumor that is an adenoma of the eccrine sweat glands. It appears as small subcutaneous papules, less than 5 mm in diameter, that are either skin-colored or yellow and that may coalesce to form cords of firm tissue. In the vulvar area, these asymptomatic papules are usually located in the labia majora. Identical tumors are often found in the eccrine glands of the eyelids. This tumor is usually treated by excisional biopsy or cryosurgery. The most common differential diagnosis is Fox–Fordyce disease, a condition of multiple retention cysts of apocrine glands accompanied by inflammation of the skin. The latter disease often produces intense pruritus, while syringoma is generally asymptomatic. Fox–Fordyce disease is treated by oral or topical estrogens and topical retinoic acid.

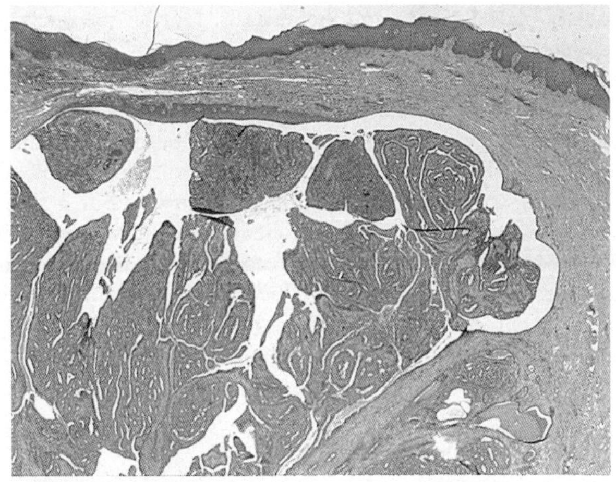

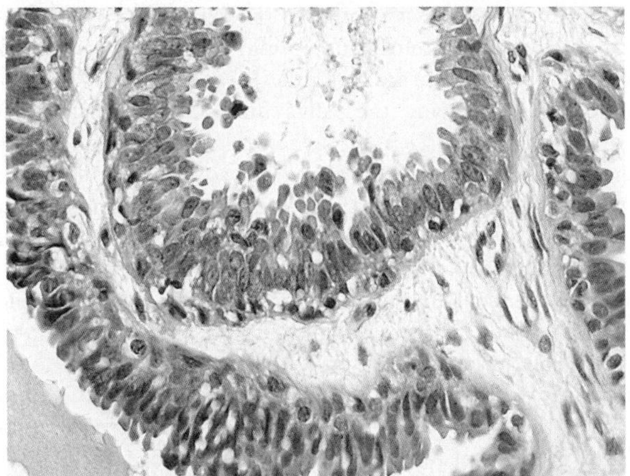

Figure 18-8. Histology, low-, and high-power micrographs of hidradenoma. (From Clement PB, Young RH: Atlas of Gynecologic Surgical Pathology. Philadelphia, WB Saunders, 2000.)

Endometriosis

Endometriosis of the vulva is rare. Only 1 in 500 women with endometriosis will present with vulvar lesions. The firm, small nodule or nodules may be cystic or solid and vary from a few millimeters to several centimeters in diameter. The subcutaneous lesions are blue, red, or purple, depending on their size, activity, and closeness to the surface of the skin. The gross and microscopic pathologic picture of vulvar endometriosis is similar to endometriosis of the pelvis (see Chapter 19, Endometriosis). Vulvar adenosis may appear similar to endometriosis. The former condition occurs after laser therapy of condylomata acuminata.

Endometriosis of the vulva is usually found at the site of an old, healed obstetric laceration, episiotomy site, an area of operative removal of a Bartholin's duct cyst, or along the canal of Nuck. The pathophysiology of development of vulvar endometriosis may be secondary to metaplasia, retrograde lymphatic spread, or potential implantation of endometrial tissue during operation. Paull and Tedeschi documented 15 cases of vulvar endometriosis they believed were associated with prophylactic postpartum curettage of the uterus to prevent postpartum bleeding. In their series there was not a single case of vulvar endometriosis in 13,800 deliveries without curettage, but 15 cases of vulvar endometriosis were associated with 2028 deliveries with prophylactic curettage. In general, symptoms do not appear for many months following implantation.

The most common symptoms of endometriosis of the vulva are pain and introital dyspareunia. The classic history is cyclic discomfort and an enlargement of the mass associated with menstrual periods. Treatment of vulvar endometriosis is by wide excision or laser vaporization depending on the size of the mass. Recurrences are common following inadequate operative removal of all the involved area.

Granular Cell Myoblastoma

Granular cell myoblastoma is a rare, slow-growing, solid vulvar tumor. The tumor originates from neural sheath (Schwann) cells and is sometimes called a *schwannoma.* These tumors are found in connective tissues throughout the body, most commonly in the tongue, and occur in any age group. Approximately 7% of solitary granular cell myoblastomas are found in the subcutaneous tissue of the vulva. Twenty percent of multiple granular cell myoblastomas are located in the vulva. The tumors are usually located in the labia majora, but occasionally involve the clitoris.

These tumors are subcutaneous nodules, usually 1 to 5 cm in diameter. They are benign but characteristically infiltrate the surrounding local tissue. The tumors are slow growing, but as they grow, they may cause ulcerations in the skin. The overlying skin often has hyperplastic changes that may look similar to invasive squamous cell carcinoma. Grossly, these tumors are not encapsulated. The cut surface of the tumor is yellow. Histologically, there are irregularly arranged bundles of large, round cells with indistinct borders and pink-staining cytoplasm. Initially the cell of origin was believed to be striated muscle; however, electron microscopic studies have demonstrated that this tumor is from cells of the neural sheath.

The tumor nodules are painless. Treatment involves wide excision to remove the filamentous projections into the surrounding tissue. If the initial excisional biopsy is not adequate and aggressive enough, these benign tumors tend to recur. Recurrence occurs in approximately one in five of these vulvar tumors. The appropriate therapy is a second operation with wider margins, since these tumors are not radiosensitive.

von Recklinghausen's Disease

The vulva is sometimes involved with the benign neural sheath tumors of von Recklinghausen's disease (generalized neurofibromatous and café-au-lait spots). The vulvar lesions of this disease are fleshy, brownish red, polypoid tumors. Approximately 18% of women with von Recklinghausen's disease have vulvar involvement. Excision is the treatment of choice for symptomatic tumors.

Other Abnormal Tissues Presenting as Vulvar Masses

The differential diagnosis of vulvar masses includes a large array of rare lesions and aberrant tissues, including leiomyomas, squamous papillomas, sebaceous adenomas, dermoids, accessory breast tissue and müllerian or wolffian duct remnants, epidermal inclusion cysts, sebaceous cysts, mucous cysts, and skin diseases such as seborrheic keratosis, condylomata acuminata, and molluscum contagiosum. Some of these diseases are discussed in this chapter, others in Chapter 22 (Infections of the Lower Genital Tract).

Hematomas

Hematomas of the vulva are usually secondary to blunt trauma such as a straddle injury from a fall, an automobile accident, or a physical assault. Traumatic injuries producing vulvar hematomas have been reported secondary to a wide range of recreational activities, including bicycle, motorcycle, and go-cart riding; sledding; water skiing; cross-country skiing; and amusement park rides (Fig. 18-9). Spontaneous hematomas are rare and usually occur from rupture of a varicose vein during pregnancy or the postpartum period.

The management of nonobstetric vulvar hematomas is usually conservative unless the hematoma is greater than 10 cm in diameter or is rapidly expanding. The bleeding that produces a vulvar hematoma is usually venous in origin. Therefore it may be controlled by direct pressure. Compression and application of an ice pack to the area are appropriate therapy. If the hematoma continues to expand, operative therapy is indicated in an attempt to identify and ligate the damaged vessel. Often identification of the "key responsible vein" is a futile operative procedure. However, obvious bleeding vessels are ligated, and a pack is placed to promote hemostasis. During the operation careful inspection and, if needed, endoscopy is performed to rule out injury to the urinary bladder and rectosigmoid.

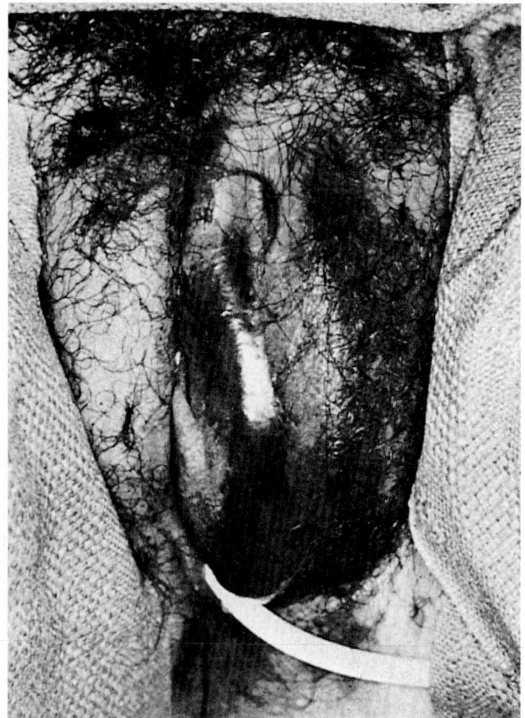

Figure 18-9. Vulva hematoma from straddle injury that produced urethral obstruction. (From Naumann RO, Droegemueller W: Unusual etiology of vulvar hematomas. Am J Obstet Gynecol 142:358, 1982.)

The majority of small hematomas regress with time. However, a "chronic expanding hematoma" may become particularly problematic. The most familiar clinical example of this type of problem is the chronic subdural hematoma, but a similar situation may accompany vulvar hematomas. The underlying pathophysiology is the repetitive episodes of bleeding from capillaries in the granulation tissue of the hematoma, which result in a chronic, slowly expanding vulvar mass. Treatment of a chronic expanding hematoma is drainage and débridement.

DERMATOLOGIC DISEASES

The skin of the vulva is similar to the skin over any surface of the body and is therefore susceptible to any generalized skin disease or involvement by systemic disease. The most common skin diseases involving the vulva include contact dermatitis, neurodermatitis, psoriasis, seborrheic dermatitis, cutaneous candidiasis, and lichen planus. The majority of vulvar skin problems are red, scalelike rashes, and the woman's primary complaint is of pruritus. The diagnosis and treatment of these lesions are often obscured or modified by the environment of the vulva. The combination of moisture and heat of the intertriginous areas may produce irritation; maceration; and a wet, weeping surface. Patients will commonly apply ointments and lotions, which may produce secondary irritation. Therefore, it is important that the gynecologist examine the skin of the entire body, because the patient may have more classic lesions of the dermatologic disease in another location. The skin of the vulva is susceptible to acute infections produced by *Streptococcus* or *Staphylococcus,* such as folliculitis, furunculitis, impetigo, and a special chronic infection, hidradenitis suppurativa.

The nonspecific symptom complex of vulvar pruritus and burning is presented next as an introduction to the discussion of dermatologic diseases of the vulva.

Pruritus

Pruritus the single most common gynecologic problem, is a symptom of intense itching with an associated desire to scratch and rub the affected area. Not uncommonly, secondary vulvar pain develops in association or subsequent to pruritus. In some women pruritus becomes an almost unrelenting symptom, with the development of repetitive "itch-scratch" cycles. The itch-scratch cycle is a complex of itching leading to scratching, producing excoriation and then healing. The healing skin itches, leading to further scratching. Pruritus is a nonspecific symptom. The differential diagnosis includes a wide range of vulvar diseases, including skin infections, sexually transmitted diseases, specific dermatosis, vulvar dystrophies, lichen sclerosus, premalignant and malignant disease, contact dermatitis, neurodermatitis, atrophy, diabetes, drug allergies, vitamin deficiencies, pediculosis, scabies, psychological causes, and systemic diseases such as leukemia and uremia.

The management of pruritus involves establishing a diagnosis, treating the offending cause, and improving local hygiene.

For successful treatment the itch–scratch cycle must be interrupted before the condition becomes chronic, resulting in *lichenification* of the skin, lichen simplex chronicus. During the latter process the skin becomes white, thickened, and "leathery." The resulting dry, scaly skin frequently cracks, forms fissures, and becomes secondarily infected, thus complicating the treatment. Chapter 30 (Neoplastic Diseases of the Vulva) discusses vulvar dystrophies.

Vulvar Pain Syndrome—Vulvar Vestibulitis and Dysesthetic Vulvodynia

Vulvar pain is one of the most common gynecologic problem, with as many as 15% of women having had chronic severe pain during their lifetimes. The disease has a wide spectrum of symptomatology as well as causes. The differential diagnosis of vulvodynia also includes neurologic diseases, especially of the nerve roots; herpes simplex infection; vulvar vestibulitis and vulvar dysesthetia; contact dermatitis; and psychogenic causes. Chronic pain may be designated as vulvodynia, once the diagnosis of infection, invasive disease, or inflammation have been excluded. Severe chronic pain can be socially debilitating, and these patients have a wide spectrum of associated affective symptomatology, as well. Women with primary symptoms of vulvar pain, vulvodynia, have greater psychologic distress than women who have other vulvar problems. These psychologic concerns must be addressed as part of the therapeutic management.

The terminology for the syndrome of chronic vulvar pain is continually evolving. The terms vulvar pain syndrome, vulvodynia, and vulvar vestibulitis are often used interchangeably. Vulvar pain syndrome is described as the triad of severe pain to touch, localized to the vaginal vestibule and dyspareunia; pain and tenderness localized only to the vestibule; and mild to moderate erythema. Vulvar pain syndrome is further subdivided into two categories: vulvar vestibulitis and dysesthetic vulvodynia. The two conditions have a significant amount of overlap, although probably different causes.

Vulvar vestibulitis is somewhat of a misnomer, since it is not inflammation. It involves the symptom of allodynia, which is hyperesthesia, a pain that is related to nonpainful stimuli. The diagnostic maneuver to establish the allodynia is to lightly touch the vulvar vestibule with a cotton-tipped applicator. If this produces pain, it is consistent with allodynia. Erythema is not always present, but when present, is confined to the vulvar vestibule (Fig. 18-10). Additionally, patients with vestibulitis experience intolerance to pressure in the vulvar region. The intolerance to pressure may be caused by tampon use, sexual activity, or tight clothing. The pain is described as raw and burning. It is not a spontaneous pain; it is invoked. However, it is severe in nature. Some authors have suggested that symptoms be present for at least 6 months prior to establishing the diagnosis. The symptoms may appear around the time of first intercourse, or within the next 5 to 15 years. Studies of women with vulvar vestibulitis have found no increased incidence of sexual abuse compared with controls.

Vulvar dysesthesia is a nonlocalized pain that is constant (not provoked by touch), mimicking a neuralgia. Allodynia is rarely noted, and erythema is also much less common than in vulvar vestibulitis. Women with vulvar dysesthesia are more often perimenopausal or postmenopausal. Dyspareunia is currently present, but has usually not been present prior to the development of dysesthesia. Similar to women with vulvar

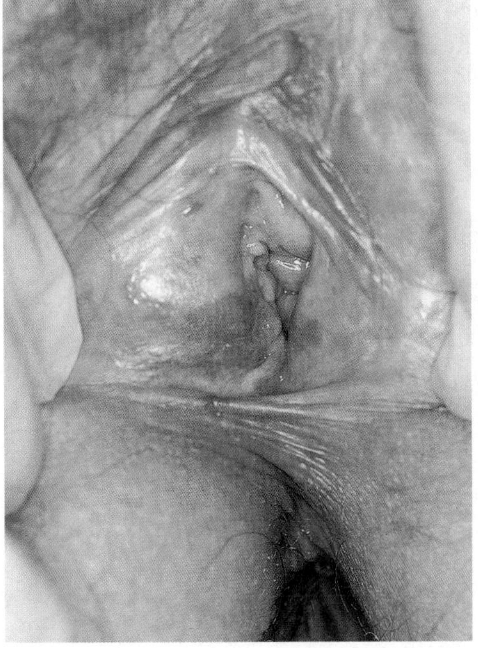

A

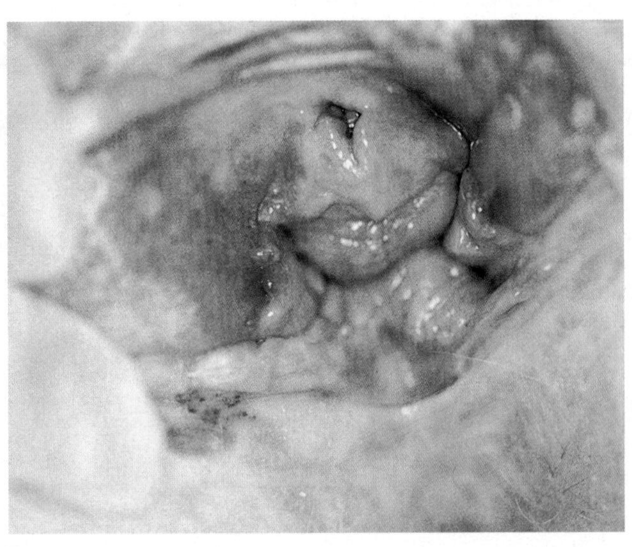

B

Figure 18-10. Vulvar vestibulitis. **A,** Redness localized to the right Bartholin's duct opening and, below it, vulvar vestibulitis. **B,** Discrete localized periglandular erythema in vulvar vestibulitis in a 60-year-old woman. (From Fisher BK, Margesson LJ: Genital Skin Disorders: Diagnosis and Treatment. St. Louis, Mosby, 1998.)

Table 18-1 Evaluation of Patients with Vulvar Pain

Examination of vulva for abnormal redness, erosions, crusting, ulceration, hypopigmentation
Cotton swab test to identify areas of pain on pressure (e.g., vestibule)
Sensory neurologic examination for allodynia and symmetrical sensation
Examination for vaginal redness, erosions, pallor, dryness
Biopsy of specific skin findings for evaluation by dermatopathologist
Microscopic evaluation of vaginal secretions for yeast, pH, increased white blood cells
Culture for *Candida* (exclusive of *C albicans*) and bacteria (especially group B *Streptococcus*)
Evaluation for depression and impact on quality of life
Classification of vulvar vestibulitis syndrome or dysesthetic vulvodynia

vestibulitis, there is not an increased history of sexual abuse compared with controls. Women with dysesthesia have been noted to have an increased incidence of chronic interstitial cystitis.

In general, both groups of women have an increased incidence of atopy. In some, a history of inflammation from topical agents may be elicited. These agents have usually either been self-prescribed or prescribed by a professional to treat initially what seems to be infection. Patients are often depressed and anxious, but this is thought to be a secondary reaction to the chronic pain. An outline for evaluation of these patients is presented by Edwards (Table 18-1). Prior to the diagnosis, she has suggested the exclusion of infection from atypical *Candida,* which can be diagnosed by culture, as well as exclusion of infection by group B *Streptococcus.*

The therapeutic approach for these two conditions emphasizes a sensitivity to the debilitating social aspects of the problem. Similar to other chronic pain syndromes, tricyclic antidepressants have been found to be helpful. Gabapentin has been suggested, and found to be successful in several series. Biofeedback has also produced relief. Zoenoun and coworkers, reported on 61 women treated successfully for vulvar vestibulitis with 5% lidocaine ointment nightly for a period of 6 to 8 weeks. In the past, women with refractory vulvar vestibulitis have been treated with surgical removal of the vulvar vestibule, and reapproximation of tissue. The surgery is difficult, with a significant complication rate, but results are generally good. Traas and colleagues reported on 126 women with vulvar vestibulitis. In their series, the complication rate was 39%; 89% of women felt that the surgery improved their condition enough to recommend it to other women. Importantly, 30% of women will have spontaneous relief of their symptoms without any treatment. There are currently very few, if any, randomized trials supporting treatment that would guide the clinician, and thus a series of treatments and a combination of treatments seem to be the best approach.

Contact Dermatitis

The vulvar skin, especially the intertriginous areas, is a frequent site of contact dermatitis. The vulvar skin is more reactive to exposure by irritants than other skin areas such as the extremities. Contact dermatitis may be one of two basic pathophysiologic processes: a primary irritant (nonimmunologic) or a definite allergic (immunologic) origin. Substances that are irritants produce immediate symptoms such as a stinging and burning sensation when applied to the vulvar skin. The symptoms and signs secondary to an irritant disappear within 12 hours of discontinuing the offending substance. In contrast, allergic contact dermatitis requires 36 to 48 hours to manifest its symptoms and signs. Often the signs of allergic contact dermatitis persist for several days despite removal of the allergen. Commonly, biologic fluids such as urine and feces cause irritation of the vulvar skin. Rarely, some women will be allergic to latex or semen. The majority of chemicals that produce hypersensitivity of the vulvar skin are cosmetic or therapeutic agents, including vaginal contraceptives, lubricants, sprays, perfumes, douches, fabric dyes, fabric softeners, synthetic fibers, bleaches, soaps, chlorine, dyes in toilet tissues, and local anesthetic creams (Fig. 18-11). External chemicals that trigger the disease process must be avoided. Some of the most severe cases of contact dermatitis involve lesions of the vulvar skin secondary to poison ivy or poison oak. Women with a history of atopy or eczema are more prone to contact dermatitis and tend to be more sensitive to skin irritations.

Acute contact dermatitis results in a red, edematous, inflamed skin. The skin may become weeping and eczematoid. The most severe skin reactions form vesicles, and any stage may become secondarily infected. The common symptoms of contact dermatitis include superficial vulvar tenderness, burning, and pruritus. Chronic untreated contact dermatitis can evolve into a syndrome of lichenification, with the skin developing a leathery appearance and texture, *lichen simplex chronicus* (Fig. 18-12).

The foundation of treatment of contact dermatitis is to withdraw the offending substance. Sometimes the distribution of the vulvar erythema helps to delineate the irritant. For

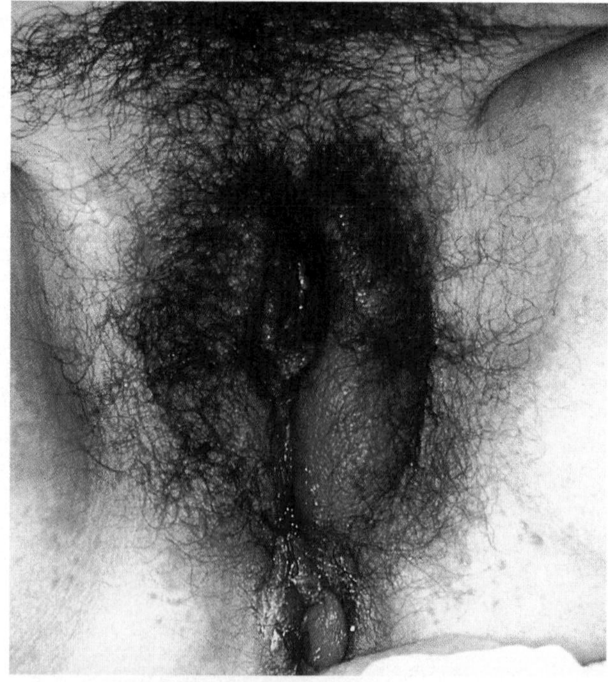

Figure 18-11. Acute contact dermatitis to chlorhexidine. Edema and erythema are present in areas where the antiseptic chlorhexidine solution was applied. (From Stevens A, Dalziel KL: Vulvar dermatoses. In Robboy SJ, Anderson MC, Russell P [eds]: Pathology of the Female Reproductive Tract. Edinburgh, Churchill Livingstone, 2002.)

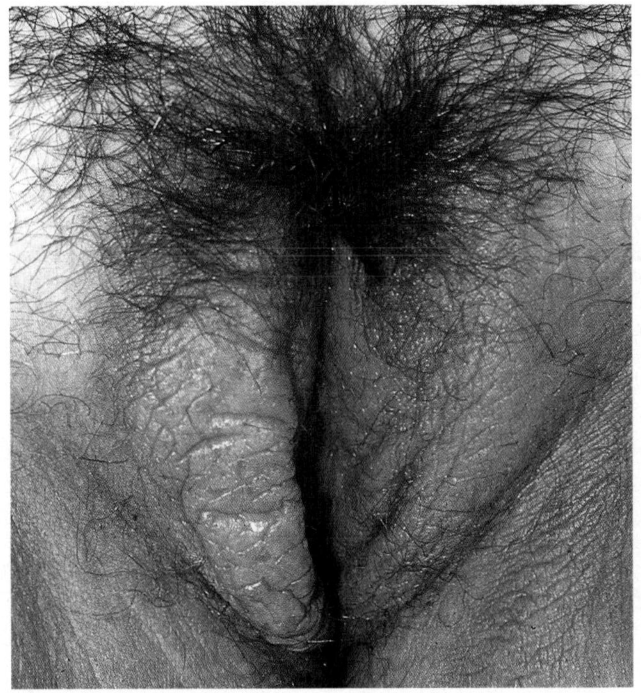

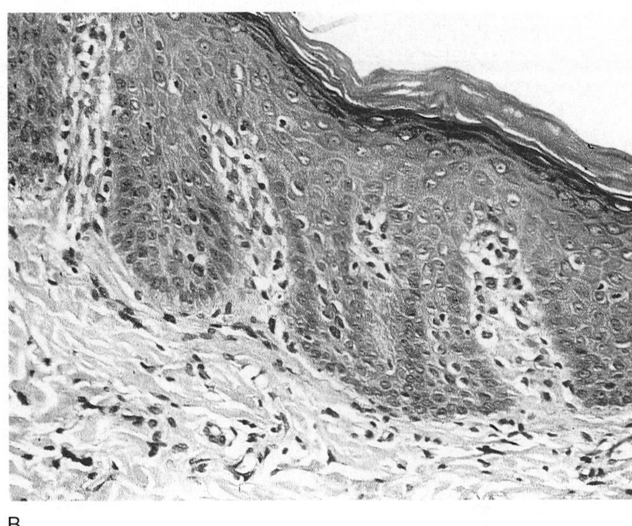

A B

Figure 18-12. **A,** Lichen simplex chronicus manifesting of the right labium majus. There is thickening and accentuation of skin markings, with surface excoriation due to recent scratching. **B,** Lichen simplex chronicus. The epidermis shows thickening of rete ridges, thickening of the granular layer and overlying hyperkeratosis. (From Stevens A, Dalziel KL: Vulvar dermatoses. In Robboy SJ, Anderson MC, Russell P [eds]: Pathology of the Female Reproductive Tract. Edinburgh, Churchill Livingstone, 2002.)

example, localized erythema of the introitus often results from vaginal medication, whereas generalized erythema of the vulva is secondary to an allergen in clothing. It is possible to use a vulvar chemical innocuously for many months or years before the topical vulvar "allergy" develops.

Initial treatment of severe lesions is with wet compresses of Burow's solution (diluted 1 to 20) for 30 minutes several times a day. This is followed by drying the vulva with cool air from a hair dryer. The vulvar skin should be kept clean and dry. Use of a lubricating agent such as petroleum jelly or Eucerin cream will reduce the pruritus by rehydrating the skin. Cotton undergarments that allow the vulvar skin to aerate should be worn, and constrictive, occlusive, or tight-fitting clothing such as pantyhose should be avoided. Vulvar dryness may be facilitated by using a nonmedicated cornstarch baby powder. Hydrocortisone (0.5% to 1%) and fluorinated corticosteroids (Valisone, 0.1%, or Synalar, 0.01%) as lotions or creams may be rubbed into the skin two to three times a day for a few days to control symptoms. Synthetic systemic corticosteroids (prednisone, starting with 50 mg/day for 7 to 10 days in a decreasing dose) are sometimes necessary for treatment of poison ivy and poison oak. Antipruritic medications, such as antihistamines, are not of great therapeutic benefit except as soporific agents.

Psoriasis

Psoriasis is a common, generalized skin disease of unknown origin. Generally, women develop psoriasis during their teenage years, with approximately 3% of adult women being affected. Approximately 20% of these have involvement of vulvar skin. The disease is chronic and relapsing, with an extremely variable and unpredictable course marked by spontaneous remissions and exacerbations. Twenty-five percent of women have a family history of the disease. Genetic susceptibility to develop psoriasis is believed to be multifactorial. Common areas of involvement are the scalp and fingernails. When psoriasis involves the vulvar skin, it produces both anxiety and embarrassment. Similar to candidiasis, psoriasis may be the first clinical manifestation of HIV infection.

Vulvar psoriasis usually affects intertriginous areas and is manifested by red to red-yellow papules. These papules tend to enlarge, becoming well-circumscribed, dull-red plaques (Fig. 18-13). Though the presence of classic silver scales and bleeding on gentle scraping of the plaques may help to establish the diagnosis, the scales are less common in the vulva than on other areas of the body.

With psoriasis on the vulvar region, the amount of scales is extremely variable and frequently absent. Under the influence of the moisture and heat of the vulva, vulvar psoriasis may resemble candidiasis. Importantly for the diagnosis, psoriasis does not involve the vagina. Sometimes dermatologists treat refractory cases of psoriasis with oral retinoids. The margins of psoriasis are more well defined than the common skin conditions in the differential diagnosis, including candidiasis, seborrheic dermatitis, and eczema. Initial treatment for mild disease is 1% hydrocortisone cream. If the patient has pain secondary to chronic fissures, more moderate disease, a 4-week course of a

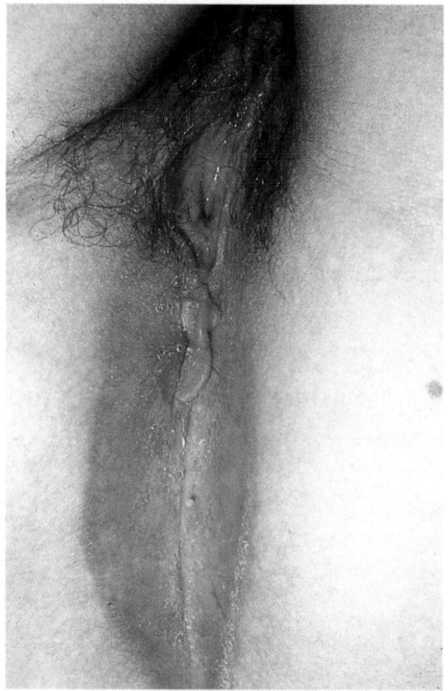

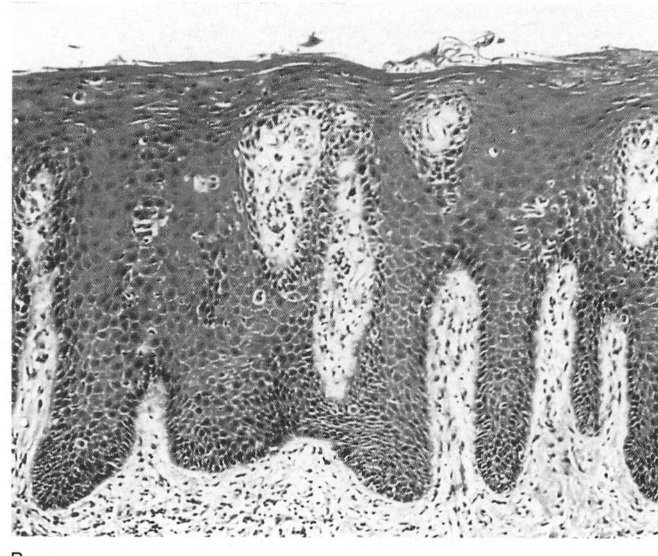

A B

Figure 18-13. **A,** Psoriasis of perineum and vulva. Flexural psoriasis often lacks the typical parakeratotic scale of psoriasis on other body sites. Painful erosion of the natal cleft is common. **B,** Psoriasis. There is psoriasiform hyperplasia of rete ridges with papaillary dermal edema and telangiectasia. The parakeratotic scale on the skin surface is not prominent in vulvar psoriasis. (From Stevens A, Dalziel KL: Vulvar dermatoses. In Robboy SJ, Anderson MC, Russell P [eds]: Pathology of the Female Reproductive Tract. Edinburgh, Churchill Livingstone, 2002.)

fluorinated corticosteroid cream should be given. If this treatment is not successful, a dermatologist should be consulted. Several newer antipsoriatric treatments may benefit this condition when it becomes moderate to severe. Systemic steroids often produce a rebound flare-up of the disease.

Seborrheic Dermatitis

Seborrheic dermatitis is a common chronic skin disease of unknown origin that classically affects the face, scalp, sternum, and the area behind the ears. Rarely, the mons pubis and vulvar areas may be involved. Vulvar lesions are pale to yellow-red, erythematous, and edematous, and they are covered by a fine, nonadherent scale that is usually oily. Excessive sweating and emotional tension precipitate attacks. The cause of the condition is most likely a yeast, *Pityrosporum ovale.* Approximately 2% to 4% of women have some form of the disease. The pruritus associated with seborrheic dermatitis varies from mild to severe. Treatment is similar to that for contact dermatitis, with hydrocortisone cream being the most effective medication. Refractory cases sometimes respond to topical ketoconazole cream. The differential diagnosis of seborrheic dermatitis includes psoriasis, cutaneous candidiasis, and contact dermatitis. Often it is difficult to differentiate between the cutaneous manifestations of psoriasis and seborrheic dermatitis. Clinically and pragmatically, the exact diagnosis is only of academic interest because the treatment is similar.

Lichen Planus

Lichen planus is an uncommon vulvovaginal dermatosis. Lichen planus is a unique, chronic eruption of shiny, violaceous papules. These tiny flat papules appear on flexor surfaces, mucous membranes, and vulvar skin in women older than 30 years of age. Most lesions are located on the inner aspects of the vulva, especially the labia minora and vestibule. Papules often develop in linear scratch marks. The lesions are intensely pruritic and usually painful. The initial onset usually follows a time of intense emotional stress. The disease presents most commonly as a hypertrophic, coalesced plaque similar to lichen sclerosis. Lichen sclerosis, though, does not involve the vagina, whereas lichen planus can. Additionally, lichen planus may also present as a potentially severe and deforming erosive vaginitis, which is extremely painful and debilitating (Fig. 18-14). This ulcerative vaginitis may be mistakenly treated as atrophic vaginitis.

The manifestation of symptoms include pruritus, and in the severe form, pain, burning, scarring, and eventually vaginal stenosis with loss of normal architecture. The cutaneous lesions of lichen planus tend to be self-limited. Often there is concomitant involvement of the oral mucous membranes, as well. The cause is thought to be an autoimmune phenomenon, which has been known to be initiated by certain drugs, including β-blockers, angiotensin-converting enzyme (ACE) inhibitors, and other medications. It may also arise spontaneously. Correct diagnosis is confirmed by a small punch biopsy of the vagina or vulva. Histologic findings (Fig. 18-15) include degeneration

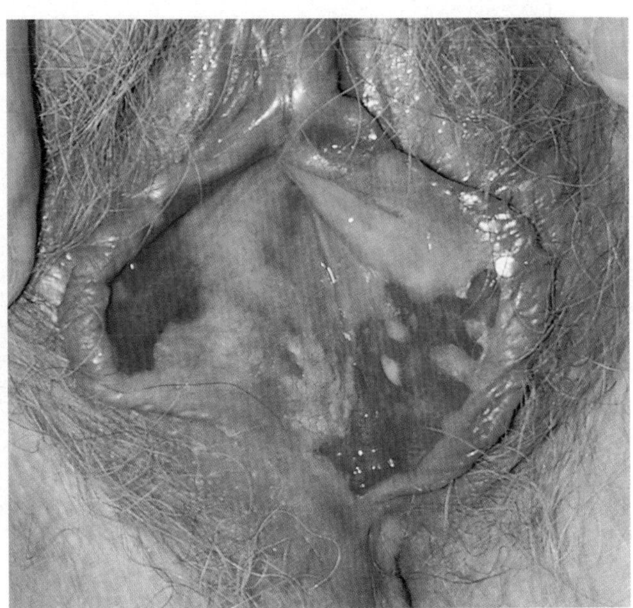

A

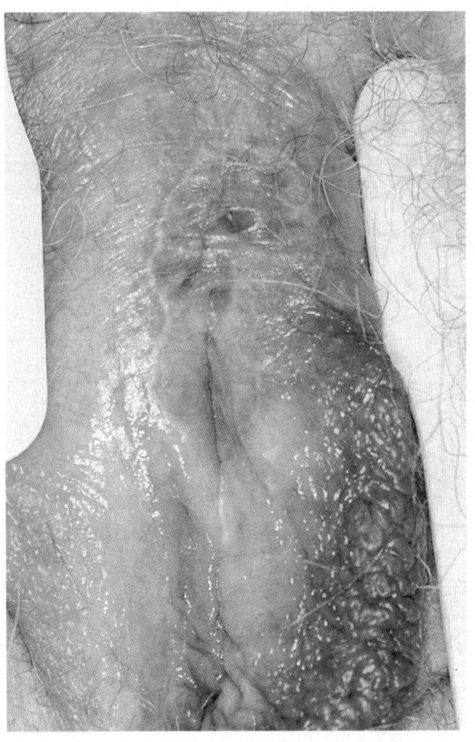

B

Figure 18-14. Lichen planus. **A,** Eroded ulcers in the vulva. **B,** Lacy reticulated pattern of lichen planus with periclitoral scarring in a 71-year-old woman who has had oral lichen planus for 10 to 15 years, cutaneous lichen planus of arms and legs for 18 months, and bouts of erosive vaginal lichen planus with scarring and partial vaginal stenosis. (From Fisher BK, Margesson LJ: Genital Skin Disorders: Diagnosis and Treatment. St. Louis, Mosby, 1998.)

of the basal layers, a lymphocytic infiltrate of the dermis, as well as epidermal acanthosis

This chronic disease tends to have spontaneous remissions and exacerbations that last for weeks to months. Treatment of local lesions is by use of a potent topical steroid cream such as clobetasol. If the patient is intensely symptomatic, oral steroids may be necessary. Dapsone for several months is sometimes effective in chronic resistant cases. Women with this condition should be monitored at periodic intervals because of an associated increased risk of developing vulvar carcinoma.

Figure 18-15. Lichen planus, histology. Note hyperkeratosis with extensive basal layer destruction and a dense lichenoid infiltrate at the dermoepidermal junction. (From Stevens A, Dalziel KL: Vulvar dermatoses. In Robboy SJ, Anderson MC, Russell P [eds]: Pathology of the Female Reproductive Tract. Edinburgh, Churchill Livingstone, 2002.)

Hidradenitis Suppurativa

Hidradenitis suppurativa is a chronic, unrelenting, refractory infection of the skin and subcutaneous tissue, primarily the apocrine glands. As the infection progresses over time, deep scars and pits are formed (Fig. 18-16). The patient undergoes great emotional distress as this condition is both painful and is associated with a foul-smelling discharge. The disease is primarily found in reproductive-aged women, tending to regress after menopause. The incidence varies in different populations. Current theories of the cause of this condition favor an inflammation beginning in the hair follicles (Fig. 18-17). The lesions involve the mons pubis, the genitocrural folds, and the buttocks. It may also involve the axilla. If treatment is unsuccessful with long-term antibiotic therapy and topical steroids, other medical therapies of the early stages of the disease include antiandrogens, isotretinoin, and cyclosporine. The early phase of the disease is infection of the follicular epithelium. Gradually a deep-seated chronic infection of apocrine glands develops, with occlusion of dilated ducts with inspissated keratin material. In the advanced stages, hidradenitis suppurativa progresses to multiple draining abscesses and sinuses. The diagnosis should be confirmed by

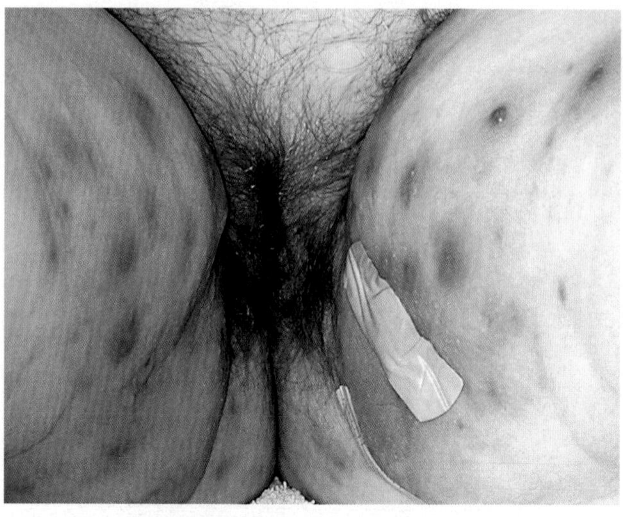

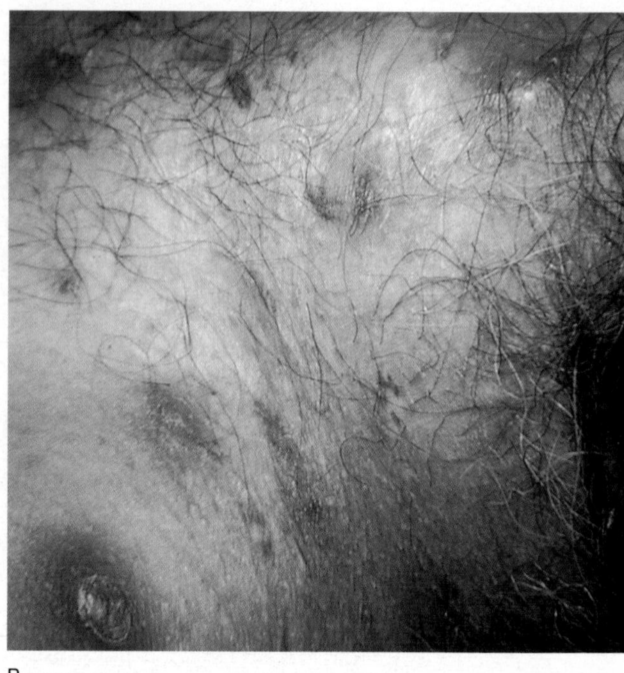

Figure 18-16. **A,** Multiple acneiform papules and nodules of hidradenitis suppurativa. **B,** Scars, nodules, and cysts in right inguinal area in hidradenitis suppurativa. (From Fisher BK, Margesson LJ: Genital Skin Disorders: Diagnosis and Treatment. St. Louis, Mosby, 1998.)

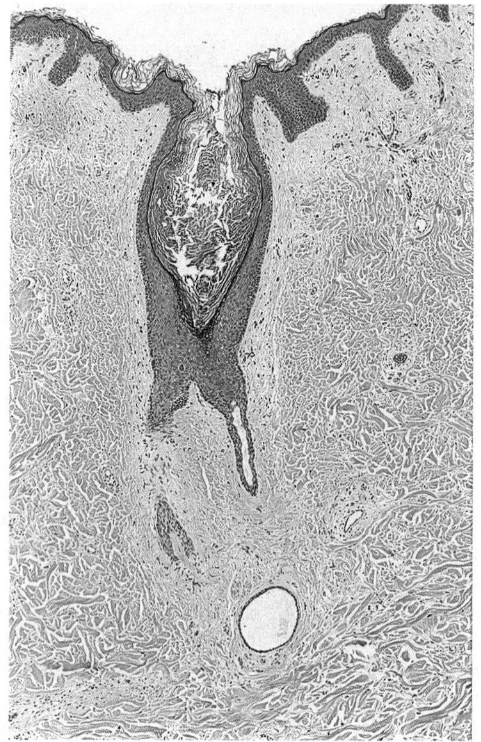

Figure 18-17. Hydradenitis suppurativa. Biopsy with follicular plugging and connection to dilated apocrine duct. (From Kelly P: Folliculitis and the follicular occlusion tetrad. In Bolognia JL, Jorizzo JL, Rapini RP [eds]: Dermatology. Edinburgh, Mosby, 2003.)

biopsy. The treatment of refractory cases is aggressive, wide operative excision of the infected skin. The differential diagnosis of hidradenitis suppurativa includes simple folliculitis, Crohn's disease of the vulva, and granulomatous sexually transmitted diseases.

Edema

Edema of the vulva may be a symptom of either local or generalized disease. Two of the most common causes of edema of the vulva are secondary reactions to inflammation or to lymphatic blockage. Vulvar edema is often recognized before edema in other areas of the female body is noted. The loose connective tissue of the vulva and its dependent position predispose to early development of pitting edema. Systemic causes of vulvar edema include circulatory and renal failure, ascites, and cirrhosis. Vulvar edema also may occur after intraperitoneal fluid is instilled to prevent adhesions or for dialysis. Local causes of vulvar edema include allergy, neurodermatitis, inflammation, trauma, and lymphatic obstruction caused by carcinoma or infection. Infectious diseases that are associated with vulvar edema include necrotizing fasciitis, tuberculosis, syphilis, filariasis, and lymphogranuloma venereum.

VAGINA

Urethral Diverticulum

A urethral diverticulum is a permanent, epithelialized, saclike projection that arises from the posterior urethra. Often they

Table 18-2 Location of the Ostium in 108 Female Patients with Diverticulum of the Urethra

Site	Number of Patients
Distal (external) third of the urethra	11
Middle third of the urethra	55
Proximal (inner) third of the urethra (including vesical neck) 18	18
Multiple sites	18
Unknown	6

From Lee RA: Diverticulum of the urethra: Clinical presentation, diagnosis, and management. Clin Obstet Gynecol 27:491, 1984.

Table 18-3 Final Diagnosis of Periurethral Mass and Frequency

Diagnosis	*N* (%)	95% Confidence Interval (%)
Urethral diverticulum	66 (84)	73, 91
Diverticulum with malignancy	4 (6)	2, 14.8
Vaginal cyst	6 (7)	3, 15
Leiomyoma	4 (5)	1, 12
Vaginal squamous cell carcinoma	2 (2.5)	0.03, 8.8
Etopic ureter	2 (2.5)	0.03, 8.8
Granuloma	1 (1)	0.03, 6.8

From Blaivas JG, Flisser AJ, Bleustein CB, Panagopoulos G: Periurethral masses: Diagnosis in a large series of women. Obstet Gynecol 103(5 Pt 1):842, 2004.

present as a mass of the anterior vaginal wall. It is a common problem, being discovered in approximately 1% to 3% of women. Blaivas and associates reported a series of 79 women referred to a urogynecology service because of periurethral masses (Table 18-2). Urethral diverticula accounted for 66/79 women (84%). Most urogynecologists have noted a decline in the prevalence of this condition during the past two decades. The majority of cases are initially diagnosed in reproductive-age females, with the peak incidence in the fourth decade of life. The symptoms of a urethral diverticulum are nonspecific and are identical to the symptoms of a lower urinary tract infection. To diagnose this elusive condition, one should suspect urethral diverticulum in any woman with chronic or recurrent lower urinary tract symptoms. The urologic aspects of this condition are discussed in Chapter 21 (Urogynecology). Histologically the diverticulum is lined by epithelium; however, there is a lack of muscle in the saclike pocket.

Urethral diverticula may be congenital or acquired. Few urethral diverticula are present in children; therefore it is assumed that most diverticula are not congenital. Huffman made the analogy that anatomically the urethra is similar to a tree with many stunted branches that represent the periurethral ducts and glands. It is assumed that the majority of urethral diverticula result from repetitive or chronic infections of the periurethral glands. The suburethral infection may cause obstruction of the ducts and glands, with subsequent production of cystic enlargement and retention cysts. These cysts may rupture into the urethral lumen and produce a suburethral diverticulum. Occasionally a suburethral diverticulum has associated stone formation in the dilated retention cyst. Urethral diverticula are small, from 3 mm to 3 cm in diameter. The majority of urethral diverticula open into the midportion of the urethra (Table 18-3). Occasionally, multiple suburethral diverticula occur in the same woman.

Classically, the symptoms associated with the urethral diverticulum are extremely chronic in nature and they have not resolved with multiple courses of oral antibiotic therapy. The most common symptoms associated with urethral diverticula are urinary urgency, frequency, and dysuria. Ginsburg and Genadry discovered that 90% of their patients had symptoms of chronic lower urinary tract infection as the presenting complaint. Approximately 15% of women with urethral diverticula experience hematuria. Other authors have stressed the three Ds associated with a diverticulum: *dysuria, dyspareunia,* and *dribbling* of the urine. Although for years, postvoiding dribbling has been termed a classic symptom of urethral diverticulum, it is reported by fewer than 10% of women with this condition. In Lee's series a palpable, tender mass was discovered in 56 of 108 patients. Ginsburg and Genadry found a palpable mass in 46 of 70 women with a urethral diverticulum. It is interesting that in most large series, approximately 20% of the women are asymptomatic. A classic sign of a suburethral diverticulum is the expression of purulent material from the urethra after compressing the suburethral area during a pelvic examination. Although the sign of producing a discharge by manual expression is very specific, its sensitivity is poor.

The foundation of diagnosing urethral diverticulum is the physician's awareness of the possibility of this defect occurring in women with chronic symptoms of lower urinary tract infection. Subsequently it is important to appreciate that a single diagnostic procedure may not identify the diverticulum. The two most common methods of diagnosing urethral diverticulum have been the voiding cystourethrography and cystourethroscopy. Approximately 70% of urethral diverticula will be filled by contrast material on a postvoiding radiograph with a lateral view. Cystourethroscopy will demonstrate the urethral opening of the urethral diverticulum in approximately 6 of 10 cases. Other diagnostic tests used to identify urethral diverticula include urethral pressure profile recordings, transvaginal ultrasound, computed tomography (CT) scans, magnetic resonance imaging (MRI), and positive-pressure urethrography. The latter test is done with a special double-balloon urethral catheter (Davis catheter) (Fig. 18-18). Classically, the recordings of the pressure profile of the urethra demonstrate a biphasic curve in a woman with a urethral diverticulum. No imaging modality has been shown to be superior to any other. If a woman has a urethral diverticulum and urinary incontinence, performing a stress urethral pressure profile will help to differentiate the etiology. The differential diagnosis includes Gartner's duct cyst, an ectopic ureter that empties into the urethra, and Skene's glands cysts.

Several different operations can correct urethral diverticula. Excisional surgery should be scheduled when the diverticulum is not acutely infected. Operative techniques can be divided into transurethral and transvaginal approaches, with most gynecologists preferring the transvaginal approach as described by Lee. The vast majority of diverticula enter into the posterior aspect of the urethra. Diverticula of the distal one third may be treated by simple marsupialization. Following operations, approximately 80% of patients obtain complete relief from symptoms. Some diverticula have multiple openings into the urethra. Complete excision of this network of fistulous connections is

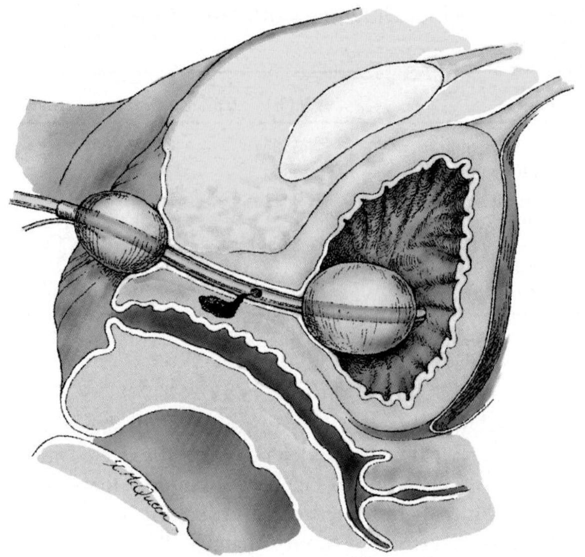

Figure 18-18. Double-balloon catheter in use for positive-pressure urethrography.

important. The recurrence rate varies between 10% and 20%, and many failures are due to incomplete surgical resection. The most serious consequences of surgical repair of urethral diverticula are urinary incontinence and urethrovaginal fistula. Postoperative incontinence usually follows operative repairs of large diverticula that are near the bladder neck. This incontinence may be secondary to damage to the urethral sphincter. The incidence of each of these complications is approximately 1% to 2%.

Inclusion Cysts

Inclusion cysts are the most common cystic structures of the vagina. In Deppisch's series of 64 women with cystic masses of the vagina, 34 had inclusion cysts. The cysts are usually discovered in the posterior or lateral walls of the lower third of the vagina. Inclusion cysts vary from 1 mm to 3 cm in diameter. Deppisch reported a mean diameter of 1.6 cm. Similar to inclusion cysts of the vulva, inclusion cysts of the vagina are more common in parous women. Inclusion cysts usually result from birth trauma or gynecologic surgery. Often they are discovered in the site of a previous episiotomy or at the apex of the vagina following hysterectomy.

Histologically, inclusion cysts are lined by stratified squamous epithelium. These cysts contain a thick, pale yellow substance that is oily and formed by degenerating epithelial cells. Often these cysts are erroneously called sebaceous cysts in the misbelief that the central material is sebaceous. Similar to vulvar inclusion cysts, the cause is either a small tag of vaginal epithelium buried beneath the surface following a gynecologic or obstetric procedure or a misplaced island of embryonic remnant that was destined to form epithelium.

The majority of inclusion cysts are asymptomatic. If the cyst produces dyspareunia or pain, the treatment is excisional biopsy.

Dysontogenetic Cysts

Dysontogenetic cysts of the vagina are thin-walled, soft cysts of embryonic origin. Whether the cysts arise from the mesonephros (Gartner's duct cyst), the perimesonephrium (müllerian cyst), or the urogenital sinus (vestibular cyst) is predominantly of academic rather than clinical importance. The cysts may be differentiated histologically by the epithelial lining (Fig. 18-19). Most mesonephric cysts have cuboidal, nonciliated epithelium. Most perimesonephric cysts have columnar, endocervical-like epithelium. Occasionally pressure produced by the cystic fluid produces flattening of the epithelium, which makes histologic diagnosis less reliable. Although most commonly single, dysontogenetic cysts may be multiple. The cysts are usually 1 to 5 cm in diameter and are usually discovered in the upper half of the vagina (Fig. 18-20). Sometimes multiple small cysts may present like a string of large, soft beads. A large cyst presenting at the introitus may be mistaken for a cystocele, anterior enterocele, or obstructed aberrant ureter. Approximately 1 in 200 females develop these cysts.

Embryonic cysts of the vagina, especially those discovered on the anterior lateral wall, are usually Gartner's duct cysts. In the embryo the distal portion of the mesonephric duct runs parallel with the vagina. It is assumed that a segment of this embryonic structure fails to regress, and the obstructed vestigial remnant becomes cystic. These cysts are most commonly found in the lower one third of the vagina.

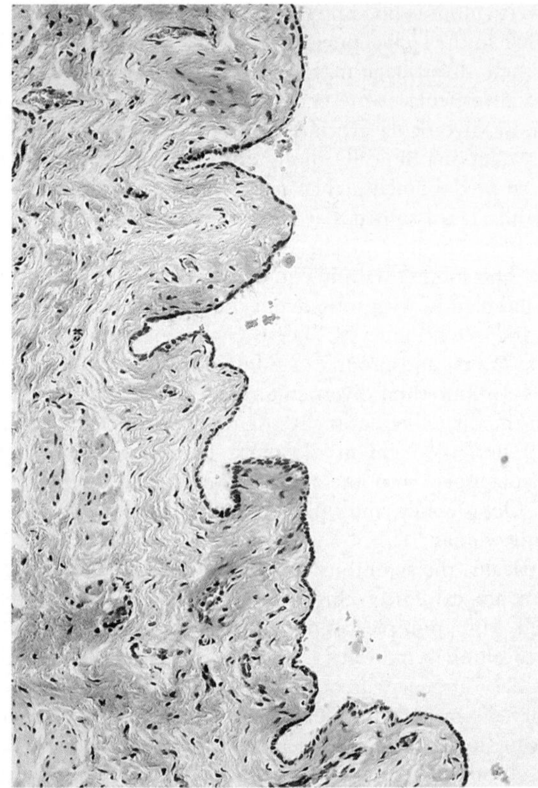

Figure 18-19. Histology of vaginal cyst. Gartner's duct cyst from the lateral vaginal wall. The cyst is lined by nonciliated cells. (From Clement PB, Young RH: Atlas of Gynecologic Surgical Pathology. Philadelphia, WB Saunders, 2000.)

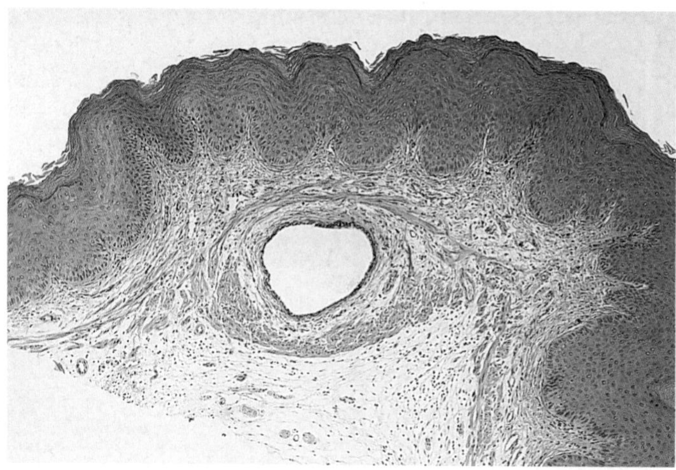
A

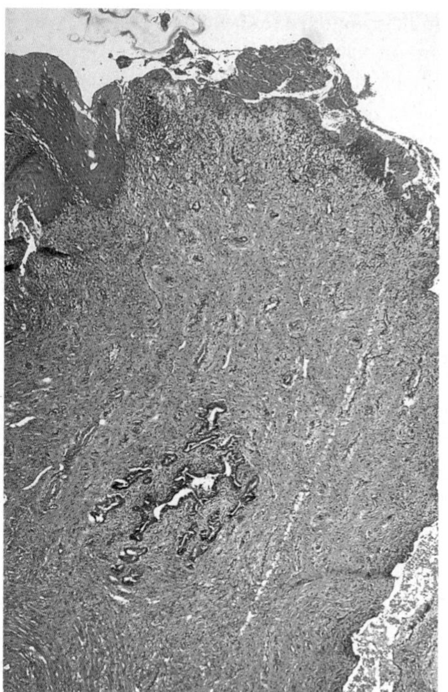
B

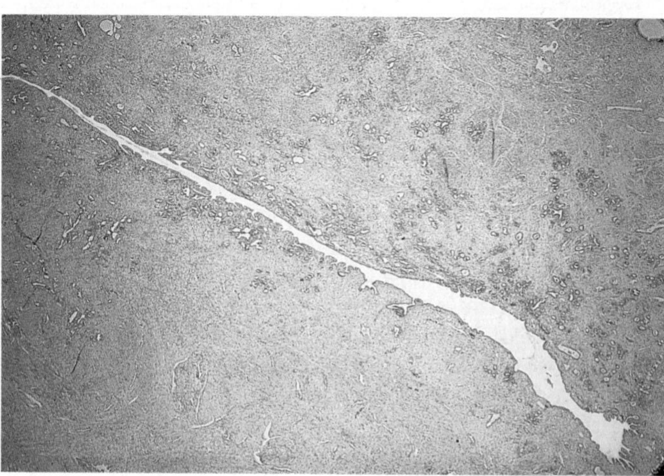
C

Figure 18-20. **A,** Normal mesonephric duct. On cross section it is a single duct in the submocosa surrounded by clusters of smooth muscle bands. **B,** Mesonephric duct. The mother duct, located deep in the wall of the vagina, is surrounded by smaller arborized offshoots. **C,** Elongated mesonephric duct. (From Robboy SJ, Anderson MC, Russell P, Morse A: The vagina. In Robboy SJ, Anderson MC, Russell P [eds]: Pathology of the Female Reproductive Tract. Edinburgh, Churchill Livingstone, 2002.)

Most of these benign cysts are asymptomatic, sausage-shaped tumors that are discovered only incidentally during pelvic examination. Small asymptomatic Gartner's duct cysts may be followed conservatively. Deppisch, in a series of 25 women undergoing operations for symptomatic dysontogenetic cysts, reported a wide range of symptoms, including dyspareunia, vaginal pain, urinary symptoms, and a palpable mass. Sometimes large cysts interfere with the use of tampons.

Operative excision is indicated for chronic symptoms. Rarely, one of these cysts becomes infected, and if operated on during the acute phase, marsupialization of the cyst is preferred. Excision of the vaginal cyst may be a much more formidable operation than anticipated. The cystic structure may extend up into the broad ligament and anatomically be in proximity to the distal course of the ureter.

Tampon Problems

The vaginal tampon has achieved immense popularity and ubiquitous use by women. It is not surprising that there are rare associated risks with tampon usage: vaginal ulcers, the "forgotten" tampon, and toxic shock syndrome. The latter, related to toxins elaborated by *Staphylococcus aureus,* is discussed in Chapter 22 (Infections of the Lower Genital Tract).

Wearing tampons for a few days has been associated with microscopic epithelial changes. The majority of women develop epithelial dehydration and epithelial layering, and some will develop microscopic ulcers. These minor changes take between 48 hours and 7 days to heal. In a study of colposcopic changes related to the tampon, Friedrich found serial changes of epithelial drying, peeling, layering, and ultimately microulceration. In his study, 15% of women wearing tampons only during the time of normal menstruation developed microulcerations. No clinical symptoms were associated with these microscopic changes. Theoretically, these microulcerations are a potential portal of entry for the HIV virus.

Barrett and colleagues were the first to describe large macroscopic ulcers of the vaginal fornix in four women who were tampon "abusers." Each of these young women wore vaginal tampons for prolonged lengths of time for persistent vaginal discharge or spotting, changing the individual tampon several times per day. The ulcers had a base of clean granulation tissue with smooth, rolled edges. Jimmerson and Becker found birefractal foreign body fragments in biopsy specimens (fibers from tampons) in the vaginal ulcers of 4 of 10 women. The pathophysiology of the ulcer is believed to be secondary to drying and pressure necrosis induced by the tampon. Obviously, many of these young women use tampons for the identical symptoms that are associated with a vaginal ulcer, that is, spotting and vaginal discharge. Often the intermenstrual spotting is believed to be breakthrough bleeding from oral contraceptives, and the possibility of a vaginal ulcer from chronic tampon usage is overlooked.

Vaginal ulcers are not uncommon secondary to several types of foreign objects, including diaphragms, pessaries, and medicated silicon rings. Management is conservative, because the ulcers heal spontaneously when the foreign object is removed. Any persistent ulcer should be biopsied to establish the cause.

A woman with a "lost" or "forgotten" tampon presents with a classic foul vaginal discharge and occasionally spotting. The tampon is usually found high in the vagina. The odor from a forgotten tampon is overwhelming. The woman should be treated with an antibiotic vaginal cream for the next 5 to 7 days.

Local Trauma

The most frequent cause of trauma to the lower genital tract of adult females is coitus. Approximately 80% of vaginal lacerations occur secondary to sexual intercourse. Other causes of vaginal trauma are straddle injuries, penetration injuries by foreign objects, sexual assault, vaginismus, and water-skiing accidents. The management of vulvar and vaginal trauma in children is discussed in Chapters 10 (Rape, Incest, and Domestic Violence) and 13 (Pediatric and Adolescent Gynecology).

The predisposing factors believed to be related to coital injury include virginity, the state of the postpartum and postmenopausal vaginal epithelium, pregnancy, intercourse after a prolonged period of abstinence, hysterectomy, and inebriation. Smith and colleagues reviewed 19 injuries from normal coitus; 12 of the women in his series were between the ages of 16 and 25 and 5 were older than 45. The most common injury is a transverse tear of the posterior fornix. Similar linear lacerations often occur in the right or left vaginal fornices. The location of the coital injury is believed to be related to the poor support of the upper vagina, which is supported only by a thin layer of connective tissue. The most prominent symptom of a coital vaginal laceration is profuse or prolonged vaginal bleeding. Many women experienced sharp pain during intercourse, and 25% noted persistent abdominal pain. The most troublesome but extremely rare complication of vaginal laceration is vaginal evisceration.

Often the history of the coital injury is not obtained, and, for personal reasons, the woman may even give misleading information. However, coital injury to the vagina should be considered in any woman with profuse or prolonged abnormal vaginal bleeding. Sensitive but thorough history regarding abuse is always appropriate.

Management of coital lacerations involves prompt suturing under adequate anesthesia. Secondary injury to the urinary and gastrointestinal tracts should be ruled out.

CERVIX

Endocervical and Cervical Polyps

Endocervical and cervical polyps are the most common benign neoplastic growths of the cervix. In an extensive series Farrar and Nedoss reported an incidence of endocervical polyps in 4% of gynecologic patients. Endocervical polyps are most common in multiparous women in their 40s and 50s. Cervical polyps usually present as a single polyp, but multiple polyps do occur occasionally. The majority are smooth, soft, reddish purple to cherry red, and fragile. They readily bleed when touched. Endocervical polyps may be single or multiple and are a few millimeters to 4 cm in diameter. The stalk of the polyp is of variable length and width (Fig. 18-21). Polyps may arise from either the endocervical canal (endocervical polyp) or ectocervix (cervical polyp). Endocervical polyps are more common than are cervical polyps. Often the terms *endocervical* and *cervical* polyps are used to describe the same abnormality. Polyps whose base is in the endocervix usually have a narrow, long pedicle and occur during the reproductive years, whereas polyps that arise from the ectocervix have a short, broad base and usually occur in postmenopausal women.

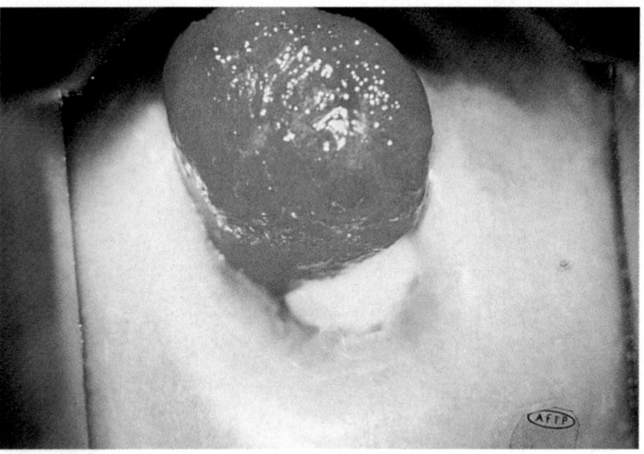

Figure 18-21. Cervical polyp. A large polyp protrudes from the external cervical os. The surface is red and rough, covered by endocervical epithelium. (From Anderson MC, Robboy SJ, Russell P, Morse A: The cervix—benign and non-neoplastic conditions. In Robboy SJ, Anderson MC, Russell P [eds]: Pathology of the Female Reproductive Tract. Edinburgh, Churchill Livingstone, 2002.)

The hypothesis of the origin of endocervical polyps is that they are usually secondary to inflammation or abnormal focal responsiveness to hormonal stimulation. Focal hyperplasia and localized proliferation are the response of the cervix to local inflammation. The color of the polyp depends in part on its origin, with most endocervical polyps being cherry red and most cervical polyps grayish white.

The classic symptom of an endocervical polyp is intermenstrual bleeding, especially following contact such as coitus or a pelvic examination. Sometimes an associated leucorrhea emanates from the infected cervix. Many endocervical polyps are asymptomatic and recognized for the first time during a routine speculum examination. Often the polyp seen on inspection is difficult to palpate because of its soft consistency.

Histologically the surface epithelium of the polyp is columnar or squamous epithelium, depending on the site of origin and the degree of squamous metaplasia (Fig. 18-22). The stalk is composed of an edematous, inflamed, loose, and richly vascular connective tissue. Six different histologic subtypes have been described: adenomatous, cystic, fibrous, vascular, inflammatory, and fibromyomatous. Greater than 80% are of the adenomatous

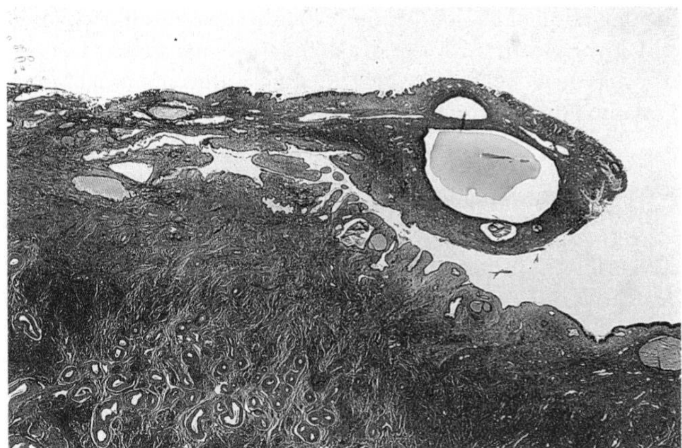

Figure 18-22. Cervical polyp. The stroma is fibromuscular and the base contains thick-walled blood vessels. Endocervical crypts, some dilated, are present within the polyp. (From Anderson MC, Robboy SJ, Russell P, Morse A: The cervix—benign and non-neoplastic conditions. In Robboy SJ, Anderson MC, Russell P [eds]: Pathology of the Female Reproductive Tract. Edinburgh, Churchill Livingstone, 2002.)

type. During pregnancy, focal areas of decidual changes may develop in the stroma. Often there is ulceration of the stalk's most dependent portion, which explains the symptom of contact bleeding. Malignant degeneration of an endocervical polyp is extremely rare. The reported incidence is less than 1 in 200. Considerations in the differential diagnosis include endometrial polyps, small prolapsed myomas, retained products of conception, squamous papilloma, sarcoma, and cervical malignancy. Microglandular endocervical hyperplasia sometimes presents as a 1- to 2-cm polyp. This is an exaggerated histologic response, usually to oral contraceptives.

Most endocervical polyps may be managed in the office by grasping the base of the polyp with an appropriately sized clamp. The polyp is avulsed with a twisting motion and sent to the pathology laboratory for microscopic evaluation. The polyp is usually friable. If the base is broad or bleeding ensues, the base may be treated with chemical cautery, electrocautery, or cryocautery. After the polyp is removed, endometrium should be evaluated in women older than 40 who have presented with abnormal bleeding, to rule out coexisting pathology. In one study by Pradhan and coworkers significant endometrial pathology was found in approximately 5% of asymptomatic women with endocervical polyps.

Nabothian Cysts

Nabothian cysts are retention cysts of endocervical columnar cells occurring where a tunnel or cleft has been covered by squamous metaplasia. These cysts are so common that they are considered a normal feature of the adult cervix. Many women have multiple cysts. Grossly, these cysts may be translucent or opaque whitish or yellow in color. Nabothian cysts vary from microscopic to macroscopic size, with the majority between 3 mm and 3 cm in diameter. Rarely, a woman with several large nabothian cysts may develop gross enlargement of the cervix. These mucous retention cysts are produced by the spontaneous healing process of the cervix. The area of the transformation zone of the cervix is in an almost constant process of repair, and squamous metaplasia and inflammation may block the cleft of a gland orifice. The endocervical columnar cells continue to secrete, and thus a mucous retention cyst is formed. Nabothian cysts are asymptomatic, and no treatment is necessary.

Lacerations

Cervical lacerations frequently occur with both normal and abnormal deliveries. Lacerations may occur in nonpregnant women with mechanical dilation of the cervix. Obstetric lacerations vary from minor superficial tears to extensive full-thickness lacerations at 3 and 9 o'clock, respectively, which may extend into the broad ligament. In gynecology the atrophic cervix of the postmenopausal woman predisposes to the complication of cervical laceration when the cervix is mechanically dilated for a diagnostic dilatation and curettage (D&C).

Acute cervical lacerations bleed and should be sutured. Cervical lacerations that are not repaired may give the external os of the cervix a fish-mouthed appearance; however, they are usually asymptomatic. The use of laminaria tents to slowly soften and dilate the cervix before mechanical instrumentation of the endometrial cavity has reduced the magnitude of iatrogenic cervical lacerations. Furthermore, the practice of routine inspection of the cervix, stabilized with one or more ring forceps, following every second- or third-trimester delivery has enabled physicians to discover and repair extensive cervical lacerations. Lacerations should be palpated to determine the extent of cephalad extension of the tear. Extensive cervical lacerations especially those involving the endocervical stroma may lead to incompetence of the cervix during a subsequent pregnancy.

Cervical Myomas

Cervical myomas are smooth, firm masses that are similar to myomas of the fundus (Figs. 18-23 and 18-24). A cervical myoma is usually a solitary growth in contrast to uterine myomas, which in general, are multiple. Depending on the series, 3% to

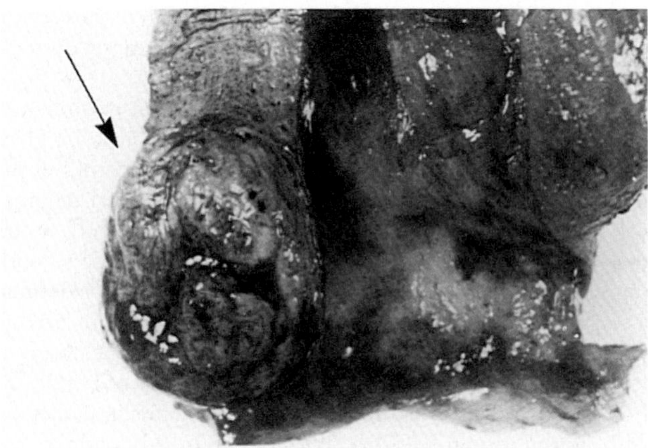

Figure 18-23. Leiomyoma (*arrow*), originating in cervix and dilating endocervical canal. It is soft, showing degenerative changes. (From Janovski NA [ed]: Color Atlas of Gross Gynecologic and Obstetric Pathology. New York, McGraw-Hill, 1969, p 71.)

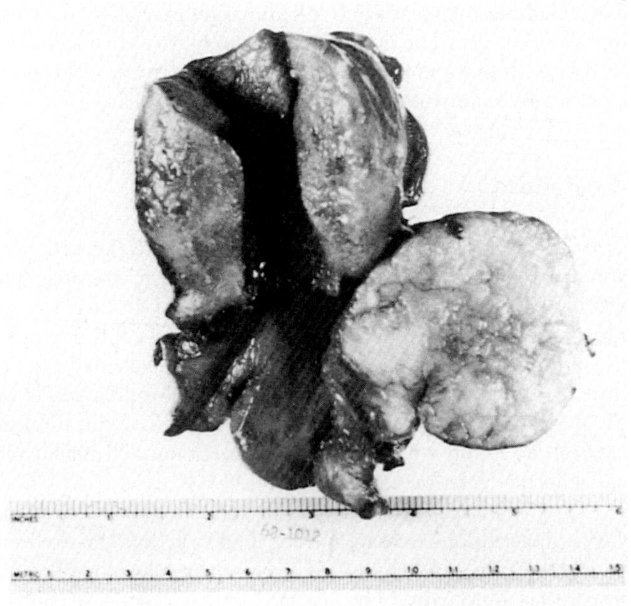

Figure 18-24. Leiomyoma of cervix most likely developing from lateral endocervix and protruding into broad ligament. Tumor is whitish, firm, and poorly encapsulated. (From Janovski NA [ed]: Color Atlas of Gross Gynecologic and Obstetric Pathology. New York, McGraw-Hill, 1969, p 69.)

8% of myomas are categorized as cervical myomas. Because of the relative paucity of smooth muscle fibers in the cervical stroma, the majority of myomas that appear to be cervical actually arise from the isthmus of the uterus.

Most cervical myomas are small and asymptomatic. When symptoms do occur, they are dependent on the direction in which the enlarging myoma expands. The expanding myoma produces symptoms secondary to mechanical pressure on adjacent organs. Cervical myomas may produce dysuria, urgency, urethral or ureteral obstruction, dyspareunia, or obstruction of the cervix. Occasionally a cervical myoma may become pedunculated and protrude through the external os of the cervix. These prolapsed myomas are often ulcerated and infected. A very large cervical myoma may produce distortion of the cervical canal and upper vagina. Rarely, a cervical myoma causes dystocia during childbirth.

The diagnosis of a cervical myoma is by inspection and palpation. Grossly and histologically, cervical myomas are identical to and indistinguishable from myomas of the corpus of the uterus. Occasionally the histologic picture of cervical myomas will demonstrate many hyalinized, thick-walled blood vessels that are postulated to be the source of the neoplastic smooth muscle tumor. This latter subtype of cervical myoma is termed a *vascular leiomyoma*. Management is similar to that of uterine myomas in that asymptomatic, small myomas may be observed for rate of growth. The occurrence and persistence of symptoms from a cervical myoma are an indication for medical therapy with gonadotropin-releasing hormone (GnRH) agonists or myomectomy or hysterectomy, depending on the patient's age and future reproductive plans. Treatment of cervical myomas that grow laterally may become a challenge if myomectomy is the operation of choice, because of both a complex blood supply and involvement with the distal course of the ureter. Cervical myomas may be treated by radiologic catheter embolization. Prolapsed uterine myomas are discussed later in this chapter.

Cervical Stenosis

Cervical stenosis most often occurs in the region of the internal os. Cervical stenosis may be divided into congenital or acquired types. The causes of acquired cervical stenosis are operative, radiation, infection, neoplasia, or atrophic changes. Cone biopsy and cautery of the cervix, either electrocautery or cryocoagulation, are the operations that most commonly cause cervical stenosis. Cervical stenosis may occur following loop electrocautery excision procedure (LEEP) procedures in women with low circulating estrogen levels such as secondary to periodic injections of medroxyprogesterone (Depo-Provera), postmenopausal women, and those who are breast-feeding.

The symptoms of cervical stenosis depend on whether the patient is premenopausal or postmenopausal and whether the obstruction is complete or partial. Common symptoms in premenopausal women include dysmenorrhea, pelvic pain, abnormal bleeding, amenorrhea, and infertility. The infertility is usually associated with endometriosis, which is commonly found in reproductive-age women with cervical stenosis. Postmenopausal women are usually asymptomatic for a long time. Slowly they develop a hematometra (blood), hydrometra (clear fluid), or pyometra (exudate).

The diagnosis is established by inability to introduce a 1- to 2-mm dilator into the uterine cavity. If the obstruction is complete, a soft, slightly tender, enlarged uterus is appreciated as a midline mass, and ultrasound examination demonstrating fluid within the uterine cavity. Management of cervical stenosis is dilation of the cervix with dilators under ultrasound guidance. If stenosis recurs, monthly laminaria tents may be used. Similarly, office follow-up and sounding of the cervix of women who have had a cone biopsy or cautery of the cervix is important to establish patency of the endocervical canal. Postmenopausal women with pyometra usually do not need antibiotics. After the acute infection has subsided, endometrial carcinoma and endocervical carcinoma should be ruled out by appropriate diagnostic biopsies. After cervical dilation it is often useful to leave a T tube or latex nasopharyngeal airway as a stent in the cervical canal for a few days to maintain patency. Two small series from Birmingham, England, and Syracuse, New York, reported the use of the CO_2 laser for treatment of cervical stenosis. In these series approximately 70% of patients were relieved of their cervical stenosis. The success of treatment depends on the proper use of the laser and the quality and quantity of residual columnar epithelium remaining in the endocervix.

UTERUS

Endometrial Polyps

Endometrial polyps are localized overgrowths of endometrial glands and stroma that project beyond the surface of the endometrium. They are soft, pliable and may be single or multiple.

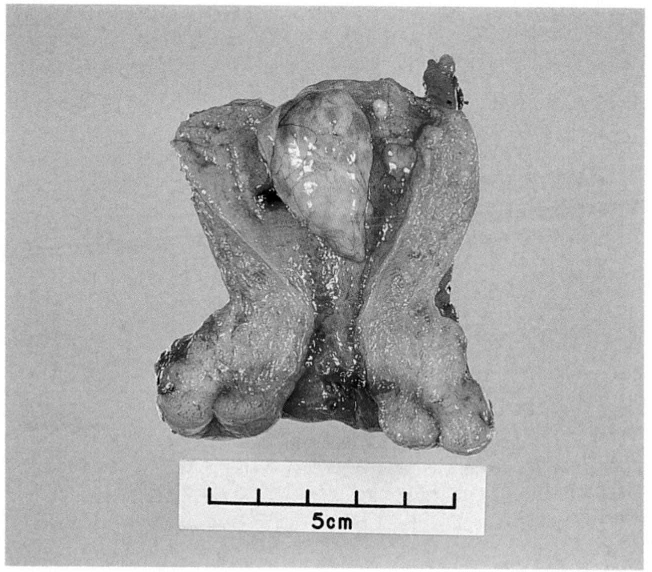

A

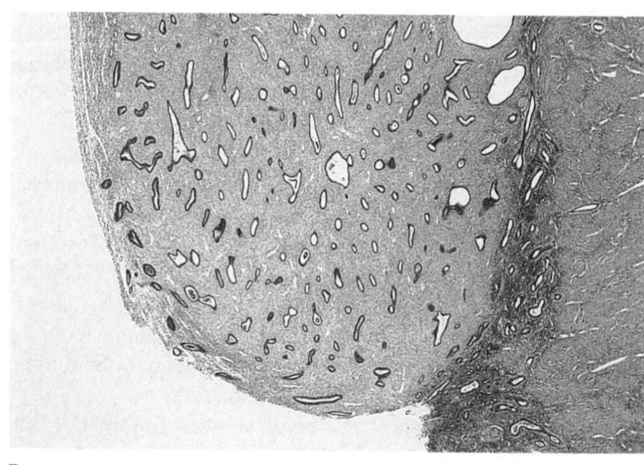

B

Figure 18-25. Endometrial polyp. **A,** Note cystic glands in the polyp. **B,** The fibrous stroma of the polyp contrasts with the cellular stroma of the adjacent endometrium. (From Anderson MC, Robboy SJ, Russell P, Morse A: Endometritis, metaplasias, polyps and miscellaneous changes. In Robboy SJ, Anderson MC, Russell P [eds]: Pathology of the Female Reproductive Tract. Edinburgh, Churchill Livingstone, 2002.)

Most polyps arise from the fundus of the uterus. *Polypoid hyperplasia* is a benign condition in which numerous small polyps are discovered throughout the endometrial cavity. Endometrial polyps vary from a few millimeters to several centimeters in diameter, and it is possible for a single large polyp to fill the endometrial cavity. Endometrial polyps may have a broad base (sessile) or be attached by a slender pedicle (pedunculated). In Novak and Woodruff's review of 1100 women with polyps, the growths were discovered in all age groups, with a peak incidence between the ages of 40 and 49. The prevalence of endometrial polyps in reproductive-age women is 20% to 25%. Endometrial polyps are noted in approximately 10% of women when the uterus is examined at autopsy. The cause of endometrial polyps is unknown. Because polyps are often associated with endometrial hyperplasia, unopposed estrogen may be one cause.

The majority of endometrial polyps are asymptomatic. Those that are symptomatic are associated with a wide range of abnormal bleeding patterns. No single abnormal bleeding pattern is diagnostic for polyps; however, menorrhagia, premenstrual and postmenstrual staining, and scanty postmenstrual spotting are the most common. Occasionally a pedunculated endometrial polyp with a long pedicle may protrude from the external cervical os. Sometimes large endometrial polyps may contribute to infertility.

Polyps are succulent and velvety, with a large central vascular core. The color is usually gray or tan but may occasionally be red or brown. Histologically, an endometrial polyp has three components: endometrial glands, endometrial stroma, and central vascular channels (Figs. 18-25 and 18-26). Epithelium must be identified on three sides, like a peninsula. Approximately two of three polyps consist of immature endometrium that does not respond to cyclic changes in circulating progesterone. This immature endometrium differs from surrounding endometrium and often appears as a "Swiss cheese" cystic hyperplasia during all phases of the menstrual cycle. The other one third of endometrial polyps consist of functional endometrium that will undergo cyclic histologic changes. The tip of a prolapsed polyp often undergoes squamous metaplasia, infection, or ulceration. The clinician cannot distinguish whether the abnormal bleeding originates from the polyp or is secondary to the frequently coexisting endometrial hyperplasia. Approximately one in four reproductive-age women with abnormal bleeding will have endometrial polyps discovered in her uterine cavity.

Malignant transformation in an endometrial polyp has been estimated to be as high as 0.5%. However, a population-based, case-control study from Sweden by Pettersson and associates

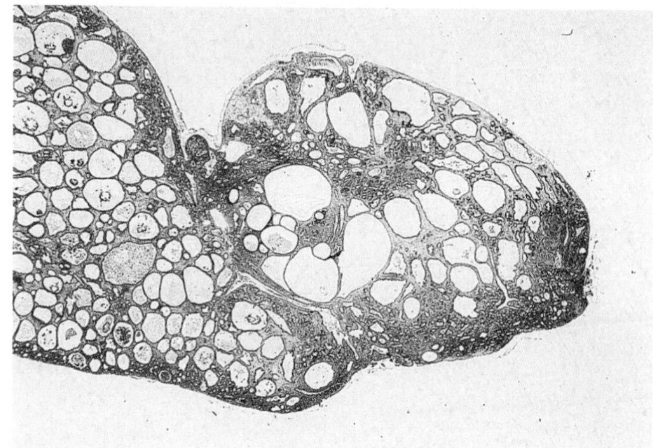

Figure 18-26. Endometrial polyp showing multiple cystic glands with flattened epithelial lining. (From Anderson MC, Robboy SJ, Russell P, Morse A: Endometritis, metaplasias, polyps and miscellaneous changes. In Robboy SJ, Anderson MC, Russell P [eds]: Pathology of the Female Reproductive Tract. Edinburgh, Churchill Livingstone, 2002.)

estimates that the increased risk of subsequent endometrial carcinoma in women with endometrial polyps is only twofold. This study provides a more realistic appraisal of the risk. Malignant change, when found in an endometrial polyp, is usually curable, and the endometrial carcinoma is most often of a low stage and grade. It is interesting that benign polyps have been found in approximately 20% of uteri removed for endometrial carcinoma. Unusual polyps have been described in association with chronic administration of the nonsteroidal antiestrogen tamoxifen. The endometrial abnormalities associated with chronic tamoxifen therapy include polyps, 20% to 35%; endometrial hyperplasia, 2% to 4%; and endometrial carcinoma, 1% to 2%. Bakour and colleagues from the U.K. reported on 67 women with polyps. The mean age was 54. Fifty-three of 62 (86%) of the polyps were benign, 7 of 62 (13%) were hyperplastic, and 2 of 62 (3%) were malignant. Another series from Goldstein and coworkers of 61 women with polyps found 54 of 61 (88%) to be benign and 3 of 61 (5%) to contain malignancy.

Because most endometrial polyps are asymptomatic, the diagnosis is not usually established until the uterus is opened following hysterectomy for other reasons. Endometrial polyps are often discovered by vaginal hydrosonography, hysteroscopy, or hysterosalpingography during the diagnostic workup of a woman with a refractory case of abnormal uterine bleeding or pelvic mass (Fig. 18-27). A well-defined, uniformly hyperechoic mass that is less than 2 cm in diameter, identified by vaginal ultrasound within the endometrial cavity, is usually a benign endometrial polyp (Fig. 18-28). DeWaay and colleagues evaluated 64 asymptomatic women with polyps over a $2^1/_2$-year period with hysterosonography. Four of seven women had regression of their polyps. Interestingly, at the second ultrasound, seven women had developed new polyps.

The optimal management of endometrial polyps is removal by hysteroscopy with D&C. Because of the frequent association of endometrial polyps and other endometrial pathology, it is important to examine histologically both the polyp and the associated endometrial lining. Polyps, because of their mobility, often tend to elude the curette. Postcurettage hysteroscopic studies have demonstrated that routine use of a long, narrow polyp forceps at the time of curettage at best results in discovery and removal of only approximately one in four endometrial polyps. The differential diagnosis of endometrial polyps includes submucous leiomyomas, adenomyomas, retained products of conception, endometrial hyperplasia, carcinoma, and uterine sarcomas.

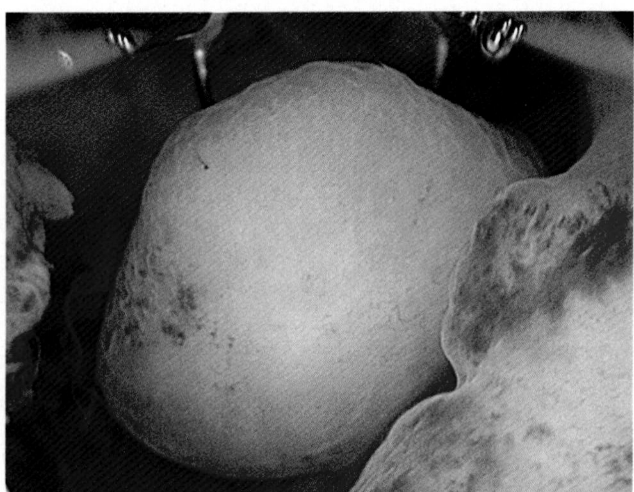

Figure 18-27. Endocervical polyp was seen at hysteroscopy. (From Goldberg JM, Falcone T: Atlas of Endoscopic Techniques in Gynecology. London, WB Saunders, 2000.)

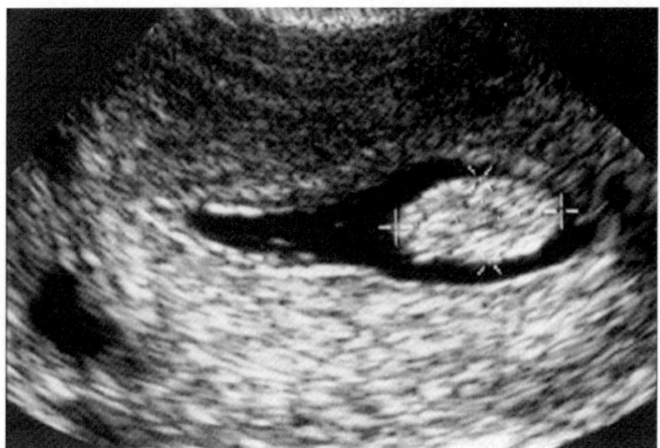

Figure 18-28. Sonohysterogram of an endometrial polyp. (From Goldberg JM, Falcone T: Atlas of Endoscopic Techniques in Gynecology. London, WB Saunders, 2000.)

Hematometra

A hematometra is a uterus distended with blood and is secondary to gynatresia, which is partial or complete obstruction of any portion of the lower genital tract. Obstruction of the isthmus of the uterus, cervix, or vagina may be congenital or acquired. The two most common congenital causes of hematometra are an imperforate hymen and a transverse vaginal septum. Among the leading causes of acquired lower tract stenosis are senile atrophy of the endocervical canal and endometrium, scarring of the isthmus by synechiae, cervical stenosis associated with surgery, radiation therapy, cryocautery or electrocautery, endometrial ablation, malignant disease of the endocervical canal.

The symptoms of hematometra depend on the age of the patient, her menstrual history and the rapidity of the accumulation of blood in the uterine cavity, and the possibility of secondary infection producing pyometra. Thus common symptoms of hematometra include primary or secondary amenorrhea and possibly cyclic lower abdominal pain. During the early teenage years the combination of primary amenorrhea and cyclic, episodic cramping lower abdominal pains suggests the possibility of a developing hematometra. Occasionally the obstruction is incomplete, and there is associated spotting of dark brown blood. Hematometra in postmenopausal women may be entirely asymptomatic. On pelvic examination a mildly tender, globular uterus is usually palpated. Ultrasound may be used to confirm the diagnosis.

The diagnosis of hematometra is generally suspected by the history of amenorrhea and cyclic abdominal pain. The diagnosis is usually confirmed by vaginal ultrasound or probing the cervix with a narrow metal dilator, with release of dark brownish black blood from the endocervical canal. Sometimes the blood retained inside the uterus becomes secondarily infected and has a foul odor.

Management of hematometra depends on operative relief of the lower tract obstruction. Treatment of congenital obstruction is discussed in Chapter 12 (Congenital Abnormalities of the Female Reproductive Tract). Appropriate biopsy specimens of the endocervical canal and endometrium should be obtained to rule out malignancy when the cause of hematometra is not obvious. If the uterus is significantly enlarged or if there is any suspicion that the retained fluid is infected, drainage should be accomplished first. Biopsy should be postponed for approximately 2 weeks to diminish the chances of infection or uterine perforation. Hematometra following operations or cryocautery usually resolves with cervical dilation. Rarely, a hematometra may form following a first-trimester abortion. This is treated by repeat suction aspiration of the products of conception that are blocking the internal os.

Leiomyomas

Leiomyomas, also called *myomas,* are benign tumors of muscle cell origin. These tumors are often referred to by their popular names, *fibroids* or *fibromyomas,* but such terms are semantic misnomers if one is referring to the cell of origin. Most leiomyomas contain varying amounts of fibrous tissue, which is believed to be secondary to degeneration of some of the smooth muscle cells.

Leiomyomas are the most frequent pelvic tumors and the most common tumor in women, with the highest prevalence occurring during the fifth decade of a woman's life. Estimates of the prevalence of myomas vary. A large population-based study from the Washington D.C. area, using transvaginal ultrasound, found myomas in more than 80% of African-American women and greater than 70% of white women, by age 50. More conservative estimates have found myomas in 30% to 50% of perimenopausal women. In general, a third of myomas will become symptomatic. Myomas are more prone to grow and become symptomatic in nulliparous women. Why some women develop myomas while others do not is unknown. Symptomatic uterine leiomyomas are the primary indication for approximately 30% of all hysterectomies. Outside the United States, fibroids have been noted to be the most common indication for a hysterectomy in Malaysia, France, Nigeria, and Japan.

Risk factors associated with the development of myomata include increasing age, early menarche, low parity, tamoxifen use, obesity, and in some studies a high-fat diet. Smoking has been found to be associated with a decreased incidence of myomata. African-American women have the highest incidence, while Hispanic and Asian women have similar rates to white women. There appears to be a familial tendency to develop myoma.

Although leiomyomas arise throughout the body in any structure containing smooth muscle, in the pelvis the majority are found in the corpus of the uterus. Occasionally, leiomyomas may be found in the fallopian tube or the round ligament, and approximately 5% of uterine myomas originate from the cervix. Myomas may be single but most often are multiple. They vary greatly in size from microscopic to multinodular uterine tumors that may weigh more than 50 pounds and literally fill the patient's abdomen. Initially most myomas develop from the myometrium, beginning as intramural myomas. As they grow, they remain attached to the myometrium with a pedicle of varying width and thickness. Small myomas are round, firm, solid tumors. With continued growth the myometrium at the edge of the tumor is compressed and forms a pseudocapsule. Although myomas do not have a true capsule, this pseudocapsule is a valuable surgical plane during a myomectomy.

Myomas are classed into subgroups by their relative anatomic relationship and position to the layers of the uterus (Fig. 18-29). The three most common types of myomas are intramural, subserous, and submucous, with special nomenclature for broad ligament and parasitic myomas (Fig. 18-30). Continued growth in one direction determines which myomas will be located just below the endometrium (submucosal) and which will be found just beneath the serosa (subserosal) (Fig. 18-31). Although only 5% to 10% of myomas become submucosal, they usually are the most troublesome clinically (Fig. 18-32). These submucosal tumors may be associated with abnormal vaginal bleeding or distortion of the uterine cavity that may produce infertility or abortion. Rarely, a submucosal myoma enlarges and becomes pedunculated. The uterus will try to expel it, and the prolapsed myoma may protrude through the external cervical os.

Subserosal myomas give the uterus its knobby contour during pelvic examination. Further growth of a subserosal myoma may lead to a pedunculated myoma wandering into the peritoneal

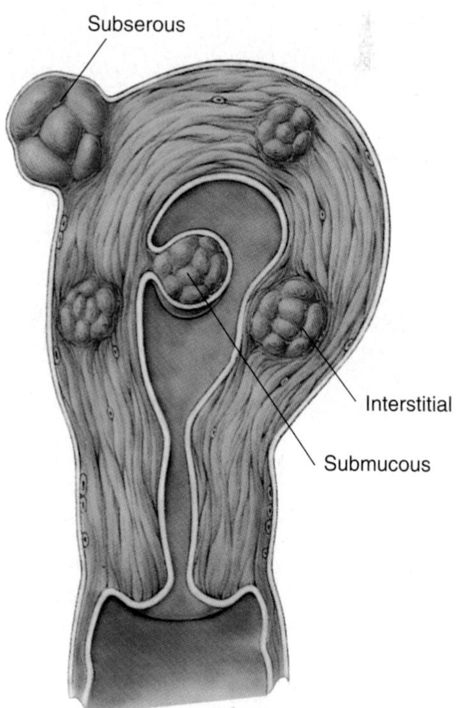

Figure 18-29. Drawing of cut surface of uterus showing characteristic whorl-like appearance and varying locations of leiomyomas. (From Novak ER, Woodruff JD [eds]: Novak's Gynecologic and Obstetric Pathology, 6th ed. Philadelphia, WB Saunders, 1967, p 215.)

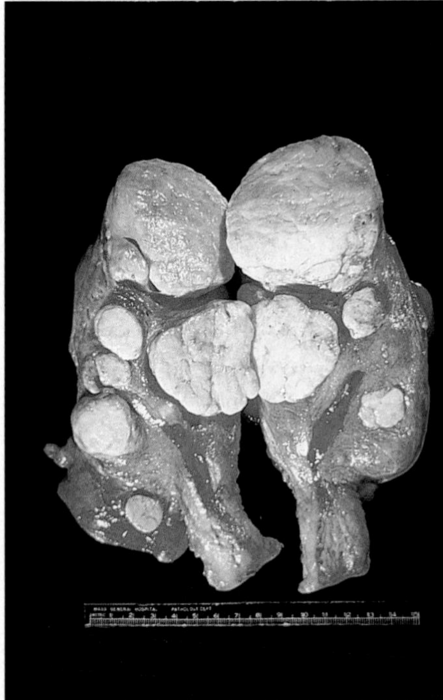

Figure 18-30. Multiple leiomyomas. These are predominantly intramural. The bulging cut surfaces are clearly shown. (From Anderson MC, Robboy SJ, Russell P: Uterine smooth muscle tumors. In Robboy SJ, Anderson MC, Russell P [eds]: Pathology of the Female Reproductive Tract. Edinburgh, Churchill Livingstone, 2002.)

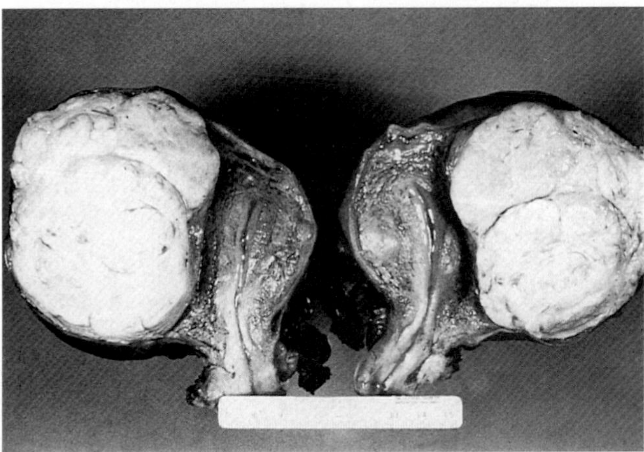

Figure 18-31. Large subserosal myoma. (Courtesy of William Droegemueller and Vern L. Katz.)

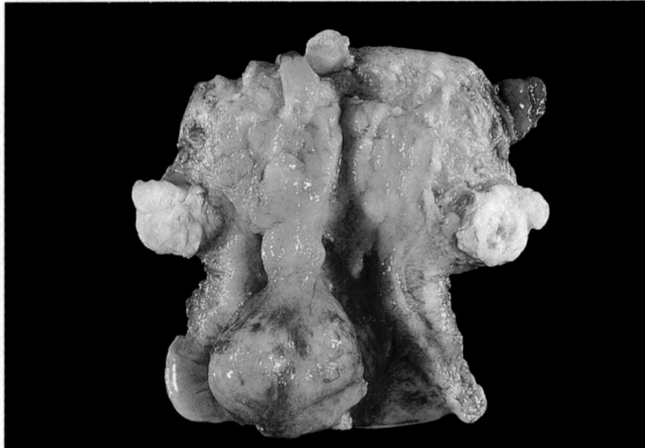

Figure 18-32. Uterus with multiple myomata, not the large central submucosal myoma. (From Voet RL: Color Atlas of Obstetric and Gynecologic Pathology. St. Louis, Mosby-Wolfe, 1997.)

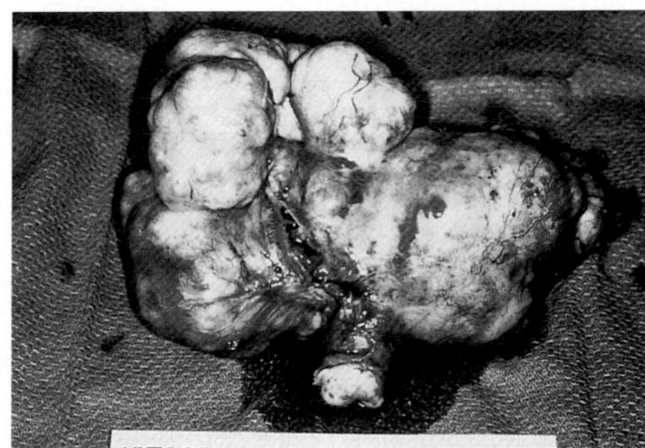

Figure 18-33. Hysterectomy specimen of myomatous uterus. (Courtesy of Vern L. Katz and William Droegemueller.)

cavity. This myoma may outgrow its uterine blood supply and obtain a secondary blood supply from another organ, such as the omentum, and become a parasitic myoma. Growth of a myoma in a lateral direction from the uterus may result in a broad ligament myoma (Fig. 18-33). The clinical significance of broad ligament myomas is that they are difficult to differentiate on pelvic examination from a solid ovarian tumor. Large, broad ligament myomas may produce a hydroureter as they enlarge.

Though the origin of uterine leiomyomas is incompletely understood, cytogenetic studies have yielded some clues to how and why myomas develop. Each tumor develops from a single muscle cell a progenitor myocyte, thus each myoma is monoclonal. Cytogenetic analysis has demonstrated that myomas have multiple chromosomal abnormalities. (Each myoma would have cells with the same abnormality.) The larger the myoma, the more an abnormal karyotype will be detected. Interestingly, the chromosomal anomalies of myomata have a remarkable clustering of changes. Twenty percent of abnormalities involve translocations between chromosomes 12 and 14. Seventeen percent involve a deletion of chromosome 7. Twelve percent involve a deletion of chromosome 12. The affected regions on chromosome 12 are also abnormal in many other types of solid tumors. The regions of chromosome 12 and 7 involve genes that may regulate growth-inducing proteins and cytokines, including transforming growth factor β (TGF-β) epidermal growth factor (EGF), insulin-like growth factors (IGF) 1 and 2, and platelet-derived growth factor (PDGF) (Fig. 18-34). Many of these cytokines have been found in significantly higher concentrations in myomas than in the surrounding myometrium. Current theory holds that the neoplastic transformation from normal myometrium to leiomyomata is the result of a somatic

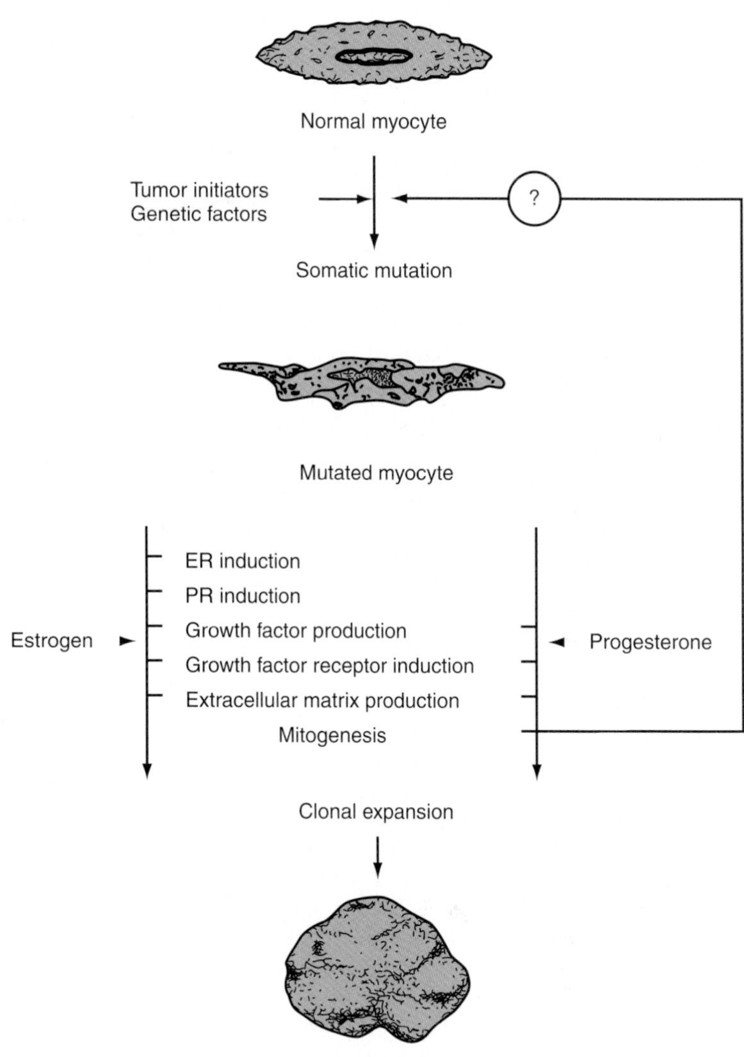

Figure 18-34. The initiation and growth of myomas likely involves a multistep cascade of separate tumor initiators and promoters. The initial neoplastic transformation of the normal myocyte involves somatic mutations. Although the initiators of the somatic mutations remain unclear, the mitogenic effect of progesterone may enhance the propagation of somatic mutations. Myoma proliferation is the result of clonal expansion and likely involves the complex interactions of estrogen, progesterone, and local growth factors. Estrogen and progesterone appear equally important as promoters of myoma growth. ER, estrogen receptor; PR, progesterone receptor. (Modified from Rein MS, Barbieri RL, Friedman AJ: Progesterone: A critical role in the pathogenesis of uterine myomas. Am J Obstet Gynecol 172:14, 1995).

mutation in the single progenitor cell. The mutation then affects cytokines that affect cell growth. Also, the growth may be influenced by relative levels of estrogen or progesterone. Both estrogen and progesterone receptors are found in higher concentrations in uterine myomas. There also appear to be similarities between fibroids and keloid formation.

Myomas are rare before menarche, and most myomas diminish in size following menopause with the reduction of a significant amount of circulating estrogen. Myomas often enlarge during pregnancy and occasionally enlarge secondary to oral contraceptive therapy. Medically induced hypoestrogenic states produce reductions in the size of myomas. Women who smoke cigarettes and are thus relatively estrogen-deficient have a lower incidence of myomas. Many women, though, have small myomas that do not grow under the influence of high circulating estrogen levels. Thus the relationship between estrogen and progesterone levels and myoma growth is complex.

Grossly, a myoma has a lighter color than the normal myometrium. On cut surface the tumor has a glistening, pearl-white appearance, with the smooth muscle arranged in a trabeculated or whorled configuration. Histologically there is a proliferation of mature smooth muscle cells. The nonstriated muscle fibers are arranged in interlacing bundles. Between bundles of smooth muscle cells are variable amounts of fibrous connective tissue, especially toward the center of any large tumor (Fig. 18-35). The amount of fibrous tissue is proportional to the extent of atrophy and degeneration that has occurred over time.

The eventual fate of some myomas is determined by their relatively poor vascular supply. This supply is found in one or two major arteries at the base or pedicle of the myoma. The arterial supply of myomas is significantly less than that of a similarly sized area of normal myometrium. Thus, with continued growth, degeneration occurs because the tumor outgrows its blood supply. The severity of the discrepancy between the myoma's growth and its blood supply determines the extent of degeneration: hyaline, myxomatous, calcific, cystic, fatty, or red degeneration and necrosis. The mildest form of degeneration of a myoma is hyaline degeneration (Fig. 18-36). Grossly, in this condition the surface of the myoma is homogeneous with loss of the whorled pattern. Histologically, with hyaline degeneration, cellular detail is lost as the smooth muscle cells are replaced by fibrous connective tissue. A recent interesting

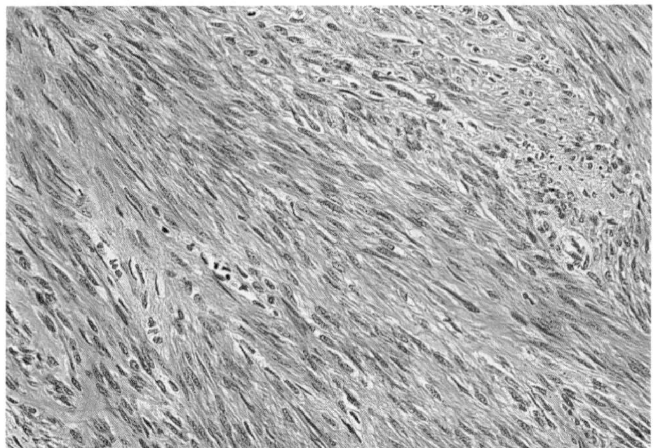

Figure 18-35. Leiomyoma. The smooth muscle cells are markedly elongated and have eosinophilic cytoplasm and elongated, cigar-shaped nuclei. The nuclei are uniform and mitotic figures absent or sparse. (From Anderson MC, Robboy SJ, Russell P: Uterine smooth muscle tumors. In Robboy SJ, Anderson MC, Russell P [eds]: Pathology of the Female Reproductive Tract. Edinburgh, Churchill Livingstone, 2002.)

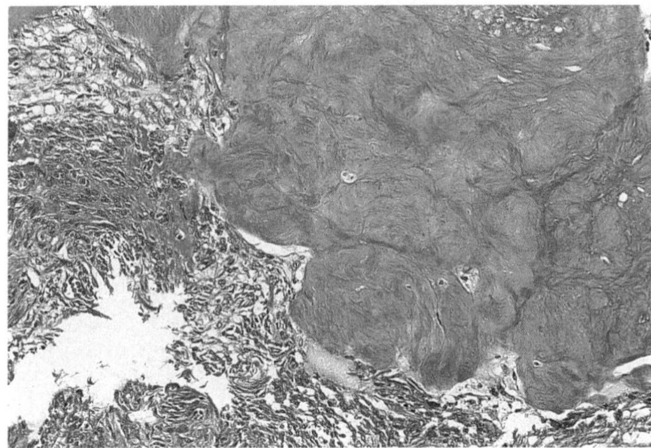

Figure 18-36. Hyaline degeneration is a leiomyoma. There is an eosinophilic ground-glass appearance. (From Anderson MC, Robboy SJ, Russell P: Uterine smooth muscle tumors. In Robboy SJ, Anderson MC, Russell P [eds]: Pathology of the Female Reproductive Tract. Edinburgh, Churchill Livingstone, 2002.)

study by Huang and colleagues using transvaginal color Doppler ultrasound documented that the intratumoral blood flow correlated with reduced tumor size and tumor volume, but did not correlate with angiogenesis or cell proliferation.

The most acute form of degeneration is red, or carneous, infarction (Fig. 18-37). This acute muscular infarction causes severe pain and localized peritoneal irritation. This form of degeneration occurs during pregnancy in approximately 5% to 10% of gravid women with myomas. The ultrasound appearance of painful myomas is one of mixed echodense and echolucent areas. Serial ultrasound examinations have also demonstrated that most (80%) myomas do not change size during pregnancy; if a change in size does occur, it is usually not associated with painful symptomatology. During pregnancy this complication should be treated medically, for attempts at operative removal may result in profuse blood loss. If the patient is not pregnant, acute degeneration is not a contraindication to myomectomy. The more advanced forms of degenerating myomas may become secondarily infected, especially when large necrotic areas exist. The histologic changes of degeneration are found more commonly in larger myomas. However, two thirds of all myomas show some degree of degeneration, with the three most common types being hyaline degeneration (65%), myxomatous degeneration (15%), and calcific degeneration (10%).

The literature emphasizes that the incidence of malignant degeneration is estimated to be between 0.3% and 0.7%. The term *malignant degeneration* is incorrect. It is unknown as to whether myomas degenerate into sarcomas. Given the very high prevalence of myomas, most investigators believe that sarcomas arise spontaneously in myomatous uteri. In a series of 1429 hysterectomies, in patients with a preoperative diagnosis of symptoms related to myomas, leiomyosarcomas were found

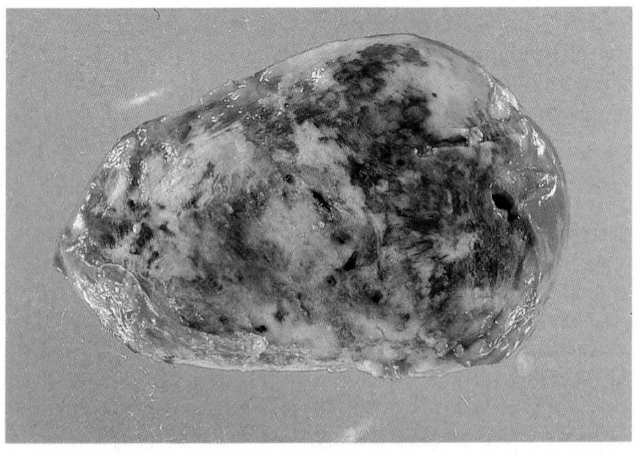

A

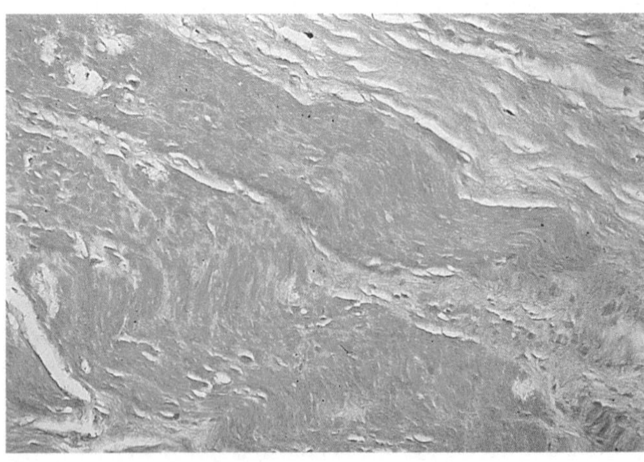

B

Figure 18-37. A, Gross view of an infracted leiomyoma. (From Anderson MC, Robboy SJ, Russell P: Uterine smooth muscle tumors. In Robboy SJ, Anderson MC, Russell P [eds]: Pathology of the Female Reproductive Tract. Edinburgh, Churchill Livingstone, 2002.) **B,** Red degeneration; the ghosts of the muscle cells and their nuclei remain. (From Voet RL: Color Atlas of Obstetric and Gynecologic Pathology. St. Louis, Mosby-Wolfe, 1997.)

histologically in 0.49%. The incidence increases in each advancing decade of life. The possibility of a uterine tumor being a leiomyoma sarcoma is 10 times greater in a woman in her 60s than in a woman in her 40s.

The most common symptoms related to myomas are pressure from an enlarging pelvic mass, pain including dysmenorrhea, and abnormal uterine bleeding. The severity of symptoms is usually related to the number, location, and size of the myomas. However, over two thirds of women with uterine myomas are asymptomatic.

One of three women with myomas experiences pelvic pain or pressure. Acquired dysmenorrhea is one of the most frequent complaints. Various forms of vascular compromise, either acute degeneration or torsion of the pedicle, produce severe pelvic pain. Mild pelvic discomfort is described as pelvic heaviness or a dull, aching sensation that may be secondary to edematous swelling in the myoma. An enlarged myoma or myomas often produce pressure symptoms similar to those of an enlarging pregnant uterus. Sometimes a woman will notice that her abdominal girth is increasing without appreciable change in weight. Alternatively, an anterior myoma pressing on the bladder may produce urinary frequency and urgency. In general, urinary symptoms are more common than rectal symptoms. Extremely large myomas and broad ligament myomas may produce a unilateral or bilateral hydroureter.

Abnormal bleeding is experienced by 30% of women with myomas. The most common symptom is menorrhagia, but intermenstrual spotting and disruption of a normal pattern are other frequent complaints. Wegienka and colleagues evaluated the bleeding pattern of 596 women with myomas. Compared with a control group, bleeding was more frequently described as gushing. Menses were longer in duration and heavier. In this study, symptoms of bleeding were related to the size of myomas. Interestingly, location of the myomas, submucous versus intramural, was not related to bleeding symptoms. The exact cause-and-effect relationship between myomas and abnormal bleeding is difficult to determine and is poorly understood. The explanation is straightforward when there are areas of ulceration over submucous myomas. However, ulceration is a rare finding. The most popular theory is that myomas result in an abnormal microvascular growth pattern and function of the vessels in the adjacent endometrium. The older theory that the amount of menorrhagia is directly related to an increase of endometrial surface area has been disproven. One of three women with abnormal bleeding and submucous myomas also has endometrial hyperplasia, which may be the cause of the symptom.

Occasionally, myomas are the only identifiable abnormality after a detailed infertility investigation. Because the data relating myomas to infertility are weak, myomectomy is indicated only in long-standing infertility and recurrent abortion after all other potential factors have been investigated and treated. Studies suggest that submucous myomas that distort the uterine cavity are the myomas that may affect reproduction. Successful full-term pregnancy rates of 40% to 50% have been reported following a myomectomy. The success of an operation is most dependent on the age of the patient, the size of the myomas, and the number of compounding factors that affect the couple's fertility.

Rapid growth of a uterine myoma after menopause is a disturbing symptom. This is the classic symptom of a leiomyosarcoma, and thus the patient should have a total abdominal hysterectomy so that the tissue may be examined histologically.

Rarely, a secondary polycythemia is noted in women with uterine myomas. This syndrome is related to elevated levels of erythropoietin. The polycythemia diminishes following removal of the uterus.

Clinically, the diagnosis of uterine myomas is usually confirmed by physical examination. Upon palpation, an enlarged, firm, irregular uterus may be felt. The three conditions that commonly enter into the differential diagnosis include pregnancy, adenomyosis, and an ovarian neoplasm. The discrimination between large ovarian tumors and myomatous uteri may be difficult on physical examination, because the extension of myomas laterally may make palpation of normal ovaries impossible during the pelvic examination. The mobility of the pelvic mass and whether the mass moves independently or as part of the uterus may be helpful diagnostically. Ultrasound is diagnostic. Submucosal myomas may be diagnosed by vaginal ultrasound, hysteroscopy, or occasionally as a filling defect on hysterosalpingography. Occasionally, an abdominopelvic radiograph will note concentric calcifications. There are several reports promoting CT and MRI studies of uterine myomas. However, these imaging techniques are more expensive than ultrasound. Until CT and MRI can distinguish between benign and malignant myomas, they will rarely be ordered in routine clinical management of myomas. MRI is helpful in differentiating adenomyosis or an adenomyoma from a single, solitary myoma, especially in a woman desiring preservation of her fertility. Serial ultrasound examinations have been used to evaluate progression in size of myomas or response to therapy. However, in a recent study Cantuaria and coworkers compared bimanual pelvic exam and ultrasound imaging prior to hysterectomy for uterine myomas. They found a strong correlation in determining the size of myoma between bimanual and ultrasound exams.

The management of small, asymptomatic myomas is judicious observation. When the tumor is first discovered, it is appropriate to perform a pelvic examination at 6-month intervals to determine the rate of growth. The majority of women will not need an operation, especially those women in the perimenopausal period, where the condition usually improves with diminishing levels of circulating estrogens.

Cases of abnormal bleeding and leiomyomas should be investigated thoroughly for concurrent problems such as endometrial hyperplasia. If symptoms do not improve with conservative management, operative therapy may be considered. The choice between a myomectomy and hysterectomy is usually determined by the patient's age, parity, and most important, future reproductive plans. Myomectomy is associated with longer hospital stays and more pelvic adhesions than hysterectomy. Studies suggest that myomectomy results in approximately 80% resolution of symptoms. Hysterectomy is associated with a greater than 90% patient satisfaction rate. Though, hysterectomy has a higher rate of urinary tract injuries, particularly abdominal hysterectomy. When myomectomies are performed to preserve fertility, care must be taken to avoid adhesions, which may compromise the goal of the operation. In the past, full-thickness myomectomies (surgeries that entered the endometrial cavity) were considered an indication for cesarean delivery prior to labor. Currently, most clinicians recommend strong consideration for cesarean section for all degrees of myomectomy other than removal of a pedunculated leiomyomata, or small hysteroscopic resection.

Classic indications for a myomectomy include persistent abnormal bleeding, pain or pressure, or enlargement of an asymptomatic myoma to more than 8 cm in a woman who has not completed childbearing. The causal relationship of myomas and adverse reproductive outcomes is poorly understood. Long-standing infertility or repetitive abortion directly related to myomas is rare. Contraindications to a myomectomy include pregnancy, advanced adnexal disease, malignancy, and the situation in which enucleation of the myoma would result in a severe reduction of endometrial surface so that the uterus would not be functional. The choice between the two operations is not always an easy one. To quote Richard TeLinde, "All indications and contraindications in medicine are relative, a fact that is especially true when one considers hysterectomy versus myomectomy."

Within 20 years of the myomectomy operation, one in four women subsequently has a hysterectomy performed, the majority for recurrent leiomyomas. Myomectomy may be performed in selected women using laparoscopic techniques. Hurst and associates have emphasized careful, multilayer closure and the use of ant-adhesive barriers. Some centers excise uterine myomas vaginally using an anterior or posterior colpotomy. They believe that vaginal myomectomy is an alternative surgical plan even in women with moderately enlarged tumors. Submucous myomas may be resected via the cervical canal using the hysteroscope. Although preliminary studies using laser surgery have been reported, most investigators advocate using an operative resectoscope. Three out of four women have long-term relief of their menorrhagia secondary to uterine myomas following hysteroscopic resection of the myomas.

The indications for hysterectomy for myomas are similar to indications for myomectomy, with a few additions. Some gynecologists selectively perform a hysterectomy for asymptomatic myomas when the uterus has reached the size of a 14- to 16-week gestation. The hypothesis is that most myomas of this size will eventually produce symptoms. However, it is impossible to predict which individual woman will develop symptoms. A previously mentioned indication for hysterectomy is rapid growth of a myoma after the menopause. Prolapse of a myoma through the cervix is optimally treated by vaginal removal and ligation of the base of the myoma, with antibiotic coverage. Hysteroscopic resection aids the transvaginal removal of a prolapsed myoma.

It is possible to treat leiomyomas medically by reducing the circulating level of estrogen and progesterone. GnRH agonists, medroxyprogesterone acetate (Depo-Provera), danazol, and the antiprogesterone RU 486 have undergone clinical trials. Recent studies in the past 10 years have emphasized the use of GnRH agonists, sometimes with add-back hormonal therapy, to treat myomas. Reduction in mean uterine volume and myoma size by 40% to 50% has been documented. However, individual responses vary greatly, from no response to an 80% reduction in uterine size. The vast majority of the reduction in size occurs within the first 3 months. After cessation of therapy, myomas gradually resume their pretreatment size. By 6 months after treatment, most myomas will have returned to their original size. During treatment, Doppler flow studies have demonstrated increased resistance in the uterine arteries and in the smaller arteries feeding the myoma. Also during treatment, the proliferative activity of the myoma and binding of epidermal growth factor is reduced. The use of suppressive therapy with GnRH agonists for women with large myomas, and those with anemia may reduce blood loss at the time of hysterectomy or myomectomy. The advantages and disadvantages of preoperative GnRH agonist therapy are listed in the following box.

Advantages and Disadvantages of Preoperative GnRH Agonist Treatment

Advantages Gained by Uterine-Fibroid Shrinkage
May allow vaginal hysterectomy
May decrease intraoperative blood loss
May allow Pfannenstiel incision
May facilitate endoscopic myomectomy

Advantages Gained by Induction of Amenorrhea
May correct hypermenorrhea–menorrhagia-associated anemia
May improve ability to donate blood
May decrease need for nonautologous blood transfusion
May atrophy endometrium, facilitating hysteroscopic resection of submucosal tumors

Disadvantages
Delay to final tissue diagnosis
Degeneration of some leiomyomas, necessitating piecemeal enucleation at myomectomy
Hypoestrogenic side effects (e.g., trabecular bone loss, vasomotor flushes)
Cost
Need to self-administer or receive injections in many cases
Vaginal hemorrhage in approximately 2% of patients

GnRH, gonadotropin-releasing hormone.
From Friedman AJ: Use of gonadotropin-releasing hormone agonists before myomectomy. Clin Obstet Gynecol 36:650, 1993.

Uterine myomas may also be treated with uterine artery embolization. Multiple embolic materials have been used including gelatin sponge (Gelfoam) silicone spheres, gelatin microspheres, metal coils, and polyvinyl alcohol (PVA) particles of various diameters. Postprocedural abdominal and pelvic pain is common for the first 24 hours and may last up to 2 weeks. Most patients remain overnight in the hospital for pain relief and observation; however, some women will go home a few hours after treatment. Fertility after arterial embolization is difficult to quantify. Higher than expected rates of intrauterine growth restriction, preterm delivery, and miscarriage have been reported. In general, women choosing a conservative approach to preserve fertility should have a surgical myomectomy rather than uterine artery embolization (UAE).

Complications of UAE include postembolization fever, sepsis from infarction of the necrotic myometrium (which may occur several weeks to a few months post procedure), and ovarian failure (up to 3% of cases in women younger than 45, and 15% in women older than 45). This is thought to occur from spread of emboli material into the ovarian circulation. There is, in general, a decreased ovarian reserve found in older women after

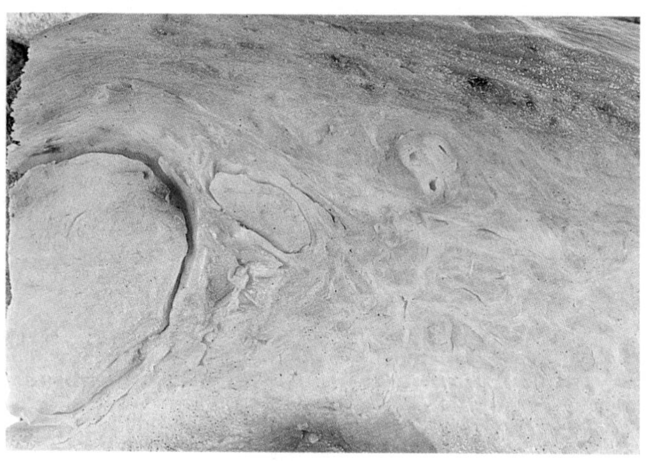

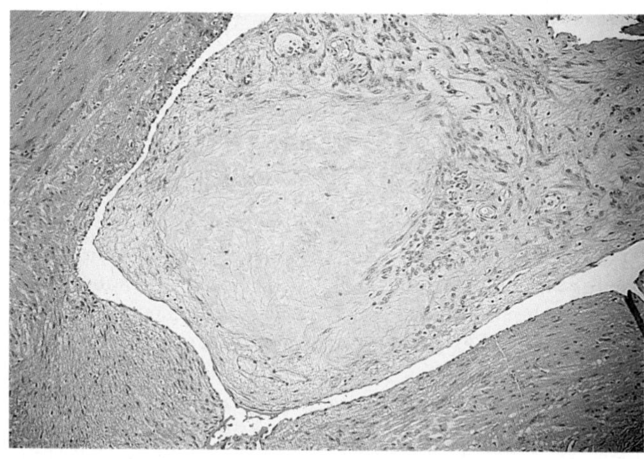

Figure 18-38. Intravenous leiomyomatosis. **A,** Tumor masses are present within distended blood vessels. **B,** This example shows hyaline degeneration of the intravascular element. (From Anderson MC, Robboy SJ, Russell P: Uterine smooth muscle tumors. In Robboy SJ, Anderson MC, Russell P [eds]: Pathology of the Female Reproductive Tract. Edinburgh, Churchill Livingstone, 2002.)

embolization. Amenorrhea may occur secondary to an endometrial hypoxic injury, as well. Rarely, necrosis of surrounding tissues may present as a complication of embolization.

Another complication of UAE is shedding of necrotic myomata or portions of myomata into the intrauterine cavity. Shedding may lead to infection or abdominal pain as the uterus tries to pass the material. This may require either a uterine curettage or hysteroscopic removal, although some authors have reported removing the necrotic material in the office. Because shedding of necrotic material is a relatively common complication, several authors have recommended that submucous myomata be removed hysteroscopically rather than attempted through UAE since these types of myomata are more prone to be shed into the uterine cavity.

Three associated but rare diseases should be noted: intravenous leiomyomatosis and leiomyomatosis peritonealis disseminata. *Intravenous leiomyomatosis* is a rare condition in which benign smooth muscle fibers invade and slowly grow into the venous channels of the pelvis (Fig. 18-38). The tumor grows by direct extension and grossly appears like a "spaghetti" tumor. Only 25% of tumors extend beyond the broad ligament; however, case reports exist of tumor growth into the vena cava and right heart. *Leiomyomatosis peritonealis disseminata* (LPD) is a benign disease with multiple small nodules over the surface of the pelvis and abdominal peritoneum. Grossly, LPD mimics disseminated carcinoma (Fig. 18-39). However, histologic examination demonstrates benign-appearing myomas (Fig. 18-40). This disorder is usually associated with a recent pregnancy. Estrogen and progesterone receptors should be ascertained when either of these conditions is diagnosed, as progestational therapy is often helpful in management. A rare autosomal syndrome of uterine and cutaneous leiomyomata and renal cell carcinoma also exists. Consideration should be given to renal evaluation in families with this history and with cutaneous leiomyomas.

In summary, leiomyomas are the most common tumor in women, and certainly one of the most common problems facing the gynecologist. Symptoms will present in 30% to 50% of women with myomata. Management is individualized to fit the patients' symptoms and reproductive desires.

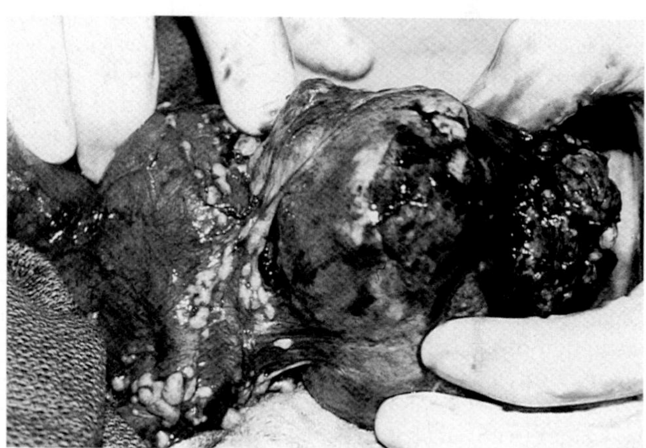

Figure 18-39. Photograph of leiomyomatosis peritonealis disseminate. (Courtesy of William Droegemueller and Vern L. Katz.)

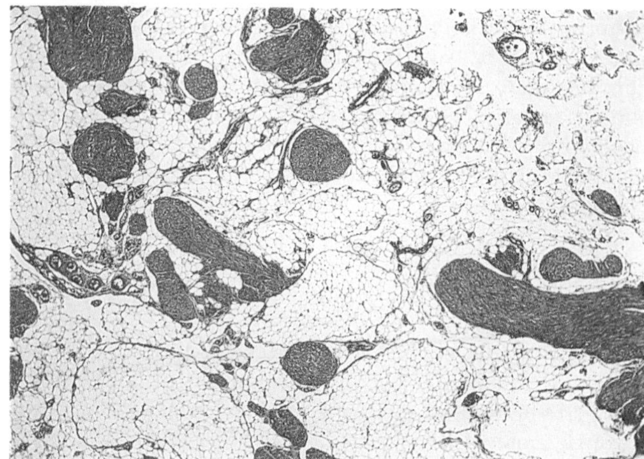

Figure 18-40. Peritoneal leiomyomatosis. Multiple tiny nodules of smooth muscle are scattered throughout the omentum. (From Anderson MC, Robboy SJ, Russell P: Uterine smooth muscle tumors. In Robboy SJ, Anderson MC, Russell P [eds]: Pathology of the Female Reproductive Tract. Edinburgh, Churchill Livingstone, 2002.)

ADENOMYOSIS

Adenomyosis has often been referred to as *endometriosis interna.* This term is misleading because endometriosis and adenomyosis are discovered in the same patient in less than 20% of women. More important, endometriosis and adenomyosis are most likely clinically different diseases. The only common feature is the presence of ectopic endometrial glands and stroma. Adenomyosis is derived from aberrant glands of the basalis layer of the endometrium. Therefore these glands do not usually undergo the traditional proliferative and secretory changes that are associated with cyclic ovarian hormone production. The disease is common and may be found in up to 60% of hysterectomy specimens in women in the late reproductive years. Most studies have documented an incidence closer to 30% with greater than 50 % of these women being relatively asymptomatic. The symptoms of menorrhagia and dysmenorrhea form a spectrum and are subjective, thus delineating an incidence of associated symptomatology with adenomyosis is problematic.

Adenomyosis is usually diagnosed incidentally by the pathologist examining histologic sections of surgical specimens. The frequency of the histologic diagnosis is directly related to how meticulously the pathologist searches for the disease. Adenomyosis is also a common incidental finding during autopsy. Serial histologic slides confirm the continuity of benign growth of the basalis layer of the endometrium into the myometrium. Thus the histogenesis of adenomyosis is direct extension from the endometrial lining.

The disease is associated with increased parity, and particularly uterine surgeries and traumas. The pathogenesis of adenomyosis is unknown but is theorized to be associated with disruption of the barrier between the endometrium and myometrium as an initiating step. Parazzini and colleageus noted a 1.7 RR (1.1–2.6) of a dilation and curettage with an SAB in women with adenomyosis versus control subjects. Other studies have found a higher rate of induced abortion with presumed curettage in women with adenomyosis versus controls. Panganamamula and associates noted the history of any prior uterine surgery to be a significant risk factor in a set of 412 women with adenomyosis, RR 1.37 (1.05–1.79). These studies and experimental work in animals strongly support the theory that trauma to the endometrial–myometrial interface as a significant factor in the etiology of this condition. However, since adenomyosis has been described well before uterine curettage, and may occur (though uncommonly) in nulliparous women, the full pathogenesis is yet to be determined.

Pathology

There are two distinct pathologic presentations of adenomyosis. The most common is a diffuse involvement of both anterior and posterior walls of the uterus. The posterior wall is usually involved more than the anterior wall (Fig. 18-41). The individual areas of adenomyosis are not encapsulated. The second presentation is a focal area or adenomyoma. This results in an asymmetrical uterus, and this special area of adenomyosis may have a pseudocapsule. Diffuse adenomyosis is found in two thirds of cases.

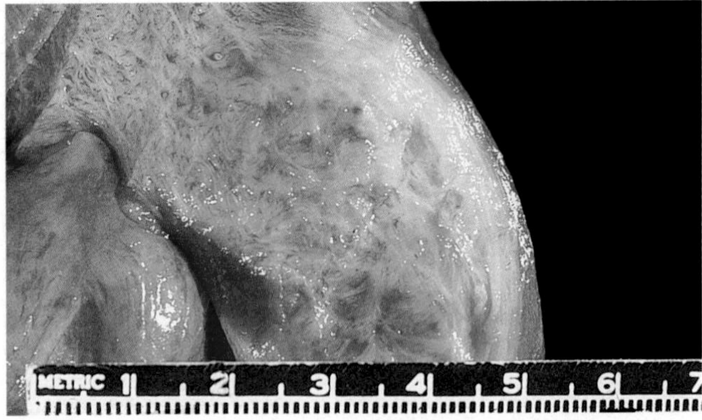

Figure 18-41. Adenomyosis. The myometrial wall is distorted and thickened by poorly circumscribed trabeculae that contain pinpoint hemorrhagic cysts. (From Anderson MC, Robboy SJ, Russell P: Uterine smooth muscle tumors. In Robboy SJ, Anderson MC, Russell P [eds]: Pathology of the Female Reproductive Tract. Edinburgh, Churchill Livingstone, 2002.)

In the more common, diffuse type of adenomyosis the uterus is uniformly enlarged, usually two to three times normal size. It is often difficult to distinguish on physical examination from uterine leiomyomas. However, the ultrasound appearance of leiomyomata helps to distinguish the two. Similarly on visual inspection the two entities are quite different. When the myometrium is transected by a knife, the cut surface protrudes convexly and has a spongy appearance. The cut surface of a uterus with adenomyosis is darker than the white surface of a myoma. Sometimes there are discrete areas of adenomyosis that are not densely encapsulated and contain small, dark cystic spaces. There is not a distinct cleavage plane around focal adenomyomas as there is with uterine myomas.

Histologic examination will note benign endometrial glands, and stroma are within the myometrium. These glands rarely undergo the same cyclic changes as the normal uterine endometrium. Studies have demonstrated both estrogen and progesterone receptors in tissue samples from adenomyosis.

The standard criterion used in diagnosis of adenomyosis is the finding of endometrial glands and stroma more than one low-powered field (2.5 mm) from the basalis layer of the endometrium. The small areas of adenomyosis have the same general appearance as the basalis layers of the endometrium. Histologically the glands exhibit an inactive or proliferative pattern. Rarely, one sees cystic hyperplasia or a pseudodecidual pattern. In general there is a lack of inflammatory cells surrounding the fossae of adenomyosis. Although the areas do not undergo full menstrual-type changes, bleeding may occur in these ectopic areas, as evidenced by both gross and microscopic findings. It is not unusual to see histologic variability in several different areas deep in the walls of the myometrium from the same uterus. Some fossae of adenomyosis undergo decidual changes either during pregnancy or during estrogen–progestin therapy for endometriosis. The reaction of the myometrium to the ectopic endometrium is hyperplasia and hypertrophy of individual muscle fibers (Figs. 18-41 and 18-42). Surrounding most foci of glands and stroma are localized areas of hyperplasia of the smooth muscle of the uterus. This change in the myometrium produces the globular enlargement of the uterus (see Fig. 18-42).

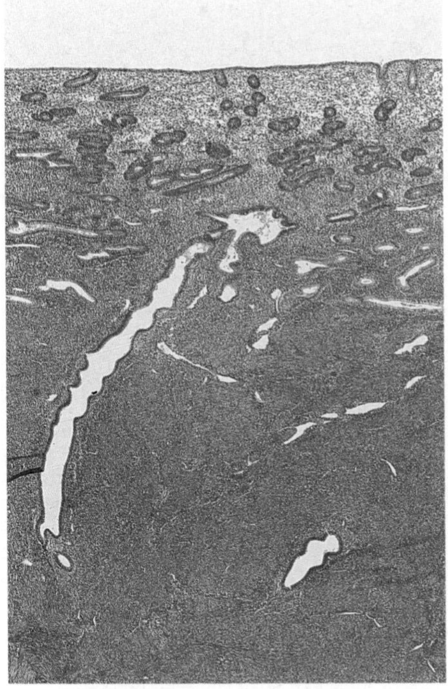
A

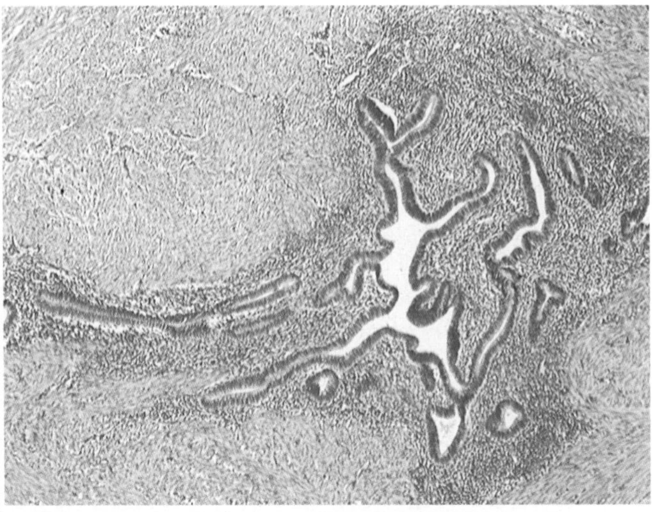
B

Figure 18-42. Adenomyosis, histologic appearance. **A,** Endometrial tissue infiltrates into the myometrium. **B,** The infiltrating islands of endometrium consist of both glands and stroma. The glands are inactive and of basal pattern. (From Anderson MC, Robboy SJ, Russell P: Uterine smooth muscle tumors. In Robboy SJ, Anderson MC, Russell P [eds]: Pathology of the Female Reproductive Tract. Edinburgh, Churchill Livingstone, 2002.)

Clinical Diagnosis

Over 50% of women with adenomyosis are asymptomatic or have minor symptoms that do not annoy them enough to seek medical care. They attribute the increase in dysmenorrhea or menstrual bleeding to the aging process and tolerate the symptoms. Symptomatic adenomyosis usually presents in women between the ages of 35 and 50. The severity of pelvic symptoms increases proportionally to the depth of penetration and the total volume of disease in the myometrium.

The classic symptoms of adenomyosis are secondary dysmenorrhea and menorrhagia. The acquired dysmenorrhea becomes increasingly more severe as the disease progresses. Occasionally the patient complains of dyspareunia, which is midline in location and deep in the pelvis. On pelvic examination the uterus is diffusely enlarged, usually two to three times normal size. It is most unusual for the uterine enlargement associated with adenomyosis to be greater than a 14-week-size gestation unless the patient also has uterine myomas. The uterus is globular and tender immediately before and during menstruation (Fig. 18-43). LevGur and colleagues evaluated the gynecologic histories of women with diffuse adenomyosis compared with women without such a history. In their series, the symptoms of dysmenorrhea and menorrhagia correlated with the amount of adenomyosis and the depth of myometrial invasion.

The diagnosis of adenomyosis is usually confirmed following histologic examination of the hysterectomy specimen. Frequently the clinical diagnosis is inaccurately assigned to the patient who has chronic pelvic pain. Traditionally the patient will have endometrial sampling to rule out other organic causes of abnormal bleeding. Many times adenomyosis is diagnosed retrospectively following a hysterectomy for other indications. Attempts have been made to establish the diagnosis preoperatively by transcervical needle biopsy of the myometrium. However, even with multiple needle biopsies, the sensitivity of the test is too low to be of practical clinical value. Adenomyosis may coexist with both endometrial hyperplasia and endometrial carcinoma. Approximately two of three women with adenomyosis have coexistent pelvic pathology, most commonly myomas but also endometriosis, endometrial hyperplasia, and salpingitis isthmica nodosa.

Ultrasound and MRI are useful to help differentiate between adenomyosis and uterine myomas in a young woman desiring future childbearing. Diagnosing adenomyosis by transvaginal ultrasonography has a reported sensitivity between 53% and 89% and a specificity of 50% to 89%. In some series, MRI is more sensitive, ranging between 88% and 93%, and has a higher specificity (66% to 91%) than ultrasonography in the diagnosis of adenomyosis. T2-weighted images are superior in making the diagnosis and documenting widened junctional zones. Findings of poorly defined junctional zone markings in the endometrial–myometrial interface helps confirm the diagnosis. Ascher and coworkers describe high signal intensity striations emanating from the endometrium and trailing into the myometrium as helpful findings. These bands most likely represent the glands and hypertrophied muscle of adenomyosis. MRI is clinically useful in differentiating adenomyosis from uterine leiomyoma, especially preoperatively in women who desire future fertility or who may choose uterine artery embolization for treatment of myomata. The success of uterine artery embolization for adenomyosis is unproven.

Management

There is no satisfactory proven medical treatment for adenomyosis. Occasionally, patients with adenomyosis are treated with GnRH agonists, cyclic hormones, or prostaglandin synthetase

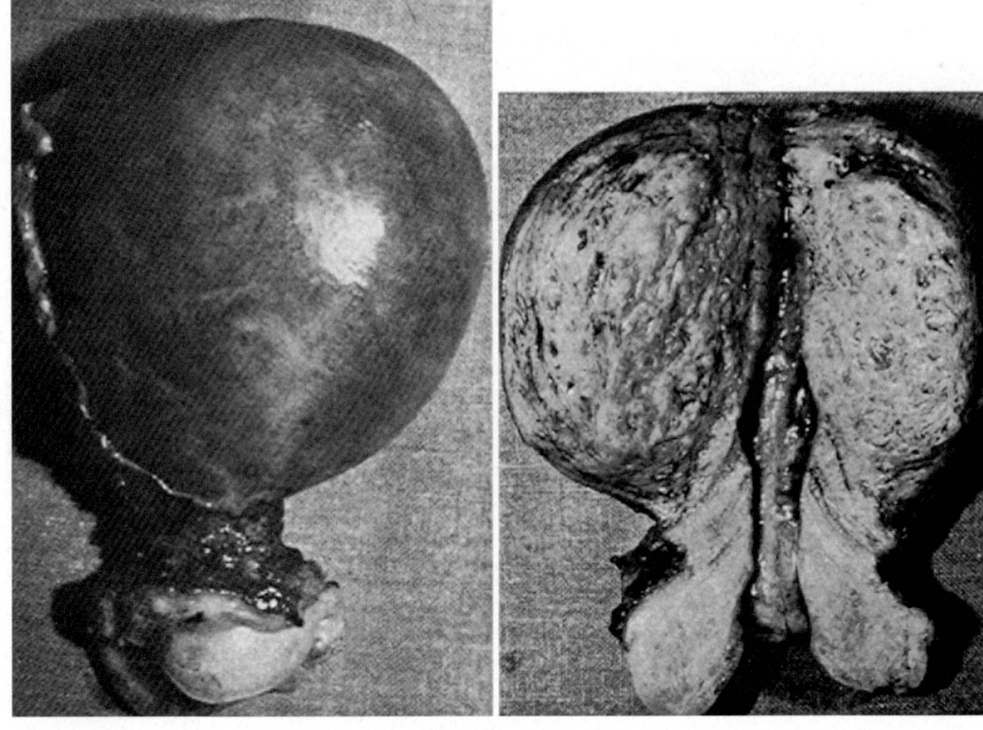

Figure 18-43. **A**, Hysterectomy specimen from 37-year-old woman showing adenomyosis. Note globular appearance of uterus. **B**, Bisection of posterior wall of uterus. (From Emge LA: The elusive adenomyosis of the uterus. Its historical past and its present state of recognition. Am J Obstet Gynecol 83:1551, 1962.)

inhibitors for their abnormal bleeding and pain. Hysterectomy is the definitive treatment if this therapy is appropriate for the woman's age, parity, and plans for future reproduction. Size of the uterus, degree of prolapse, and presence of associated pelvic pathology determine the choice of surgical approach. For the woman in her late 40s, the ovaries are often removed as a risk-reducing measure against ovarian carcinoma.

OVIDUCT

Leiomyomas

Both benign and malignant tumors of the oviduct are uncommon compared with other gynecologic neoplasms. Although these tumors are underreported, fewer than 100 women with myomas or leiomyomas of the oviduct are described in the literature. Tubal leiomyomas may be single or multiple and usually are discovered in the interstitial portion of the tubes. They usually coexist with the more common uterine leiomyomas. Myomas may originate from muscle cells in the walls of the tube or blood vessels or from smooth muscle in the broad ligament.

Leiomyomas of the tube present as smooth, firm, mobile, usually nontender masses that may be palpated during the bimanual examination. Similar to uterine myomas, they may be subserosal, interstitial, or submucosal. During laparoscopy the myomas appear as a spherical mass that protrudes from beneath the peritoneal surface. They vary from a few millimeters to 15 cm in diameter. Histologically they are identical to uterine leiomyomas.

The majority of the myomas of the oviduct are asymptomatic. Rarely, they may undergo acute degeneration or be associated with unilateral tubal obstruction or torsion. Treatment of a symptomatic tubal leiomyoma is excision.

Adenomatoid Tumors

The most prevalent benign tumor of the oviduct is the *angiomyoma* or *adenomatoid tumor.* (Fig. 18-44). They are small, gray-white, circumscribed nodules, 1 to 2 cm in diameter. These tumors are usually unilateral and present as small nodules just under the tubal serosa. These small nodules do not produce pelvic symptoms or signs. These benign tumors also are found below the serosa of the fundus of the uterus and the broad ligament. Microscopically they are composed of small tubules lined by a low cuboidal or flat epithelium. Histologic studies have established that the thin-walled channels that comprise these tumors are of mesothelial origin. (Fig. 18-45). These tumors do not become malignant; however, they may be mistaken for a low-grade neoplasm when initially viewed during a frozen-section evaluation.

Paratubal Cysts

Paratubal cysts are frequently incidental discoveries during gynecologic operations for other abnormalities. They are often multiple and may vary from 0.5 cm to more than 20 cm in diameter. The majority of cysts are small, asymptomatic, and

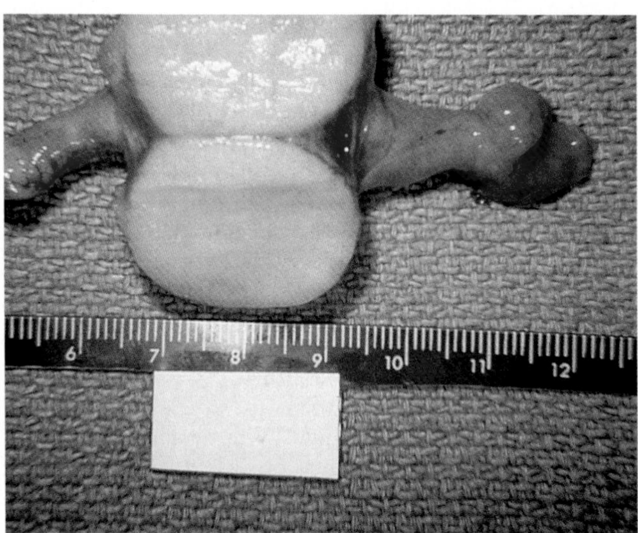

Figure 18-44. Adenomatoid tumor. (From Anderson MC, Robboy SJ, Russell P: The fallopian tube. In Robboy SJ, Anderson MC, Russell P [eds]: Pathology of the Female Reproductive Tract. Edinburgh, Churchill Livingstone, 2002.)

slow growing and are discovered during the third and fourth decades of life. When paratubal cysts are pedunculated and near the fimbrial end of the oviduct, they are called *hydatid cysts of Morgagni* (Figs. 18-46 and 18-47). Cysts near the oviduct may be of mesonephric, mesothelial, or paramesonephric origin. Sometimes the histologic differentiation is difficult because of mechanically produced changes in the cells that line the cyst. These cysts are translucent and contain a clear or pale yellow fluid.

The histogenesis of the majority of paratubal cysts had been believed to be from the mesonephric duct, with the cysts arising from the main duct or accessory tubules. These latter cysts often develop between the leaves of the broad ligament in the mesosalpinx, with the ovary being separate. However, a histologic study of 79 paratubal cysts by Samaha and Woodruff has documented that 60 of the cysts were of tubal origin. Thus the majority of grossly identified "paratubal cysts" are in reality accessory lumina of the fallopian tubes. The remaining 19 cysts

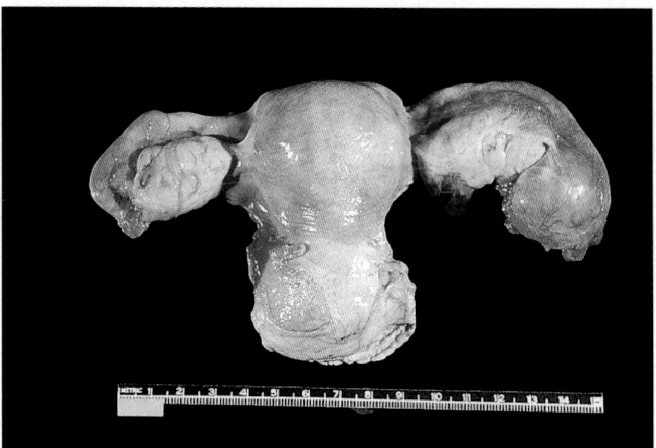

Figure 18-46. Broad ligament cyst. This parovarian, or paratubal cyst, is thin-walled and contains clear watery fluid. (From Anderson MC, Robboy SJ, Russell P: The fallopian tube. In Robboy SJ, Anderson MC, Russell P [eds]: Pathology of the Female Reproductive Tract. Edinburgh, Churchill Livingstone, 2002.)

in Samaha and Woodruff's series were of mesothelial origin. Paratubal cysts are thin-walled and smooth and contain clear fluid. Often there are multiple small cysts. These cysts are thin-walled and are filled with clear fluid. Occasionally there is a papillomatous proliferation on the internal wall of these cysts. Inflammatory cysts of the peritoneum may be found anywhere in the pelvis.

The majority of paratubal cysts are asymptomatic and are usually discovered incidentally during ultrasound or during gynecologic operations. When paratubal cysts are symptomatic, they generally produce a dull pain. During a pelvic examination it is difficult to distinguish a paratubal cyst from an ovarian mass. At operation the oviduct is often found stretched over a large paratubal cyst. The oviduct should not be removed in these cases, because it will return to normal size after the paratubal cyst is excised. Stein and associates recently reported a retrospective 10-year review of 168 women with parovarian tumors. Three low-grade malignant neoplasms were found in this series. These malignancies were in women of reproductive age who had cysts greater than 5 cm in diameter with internal papillary

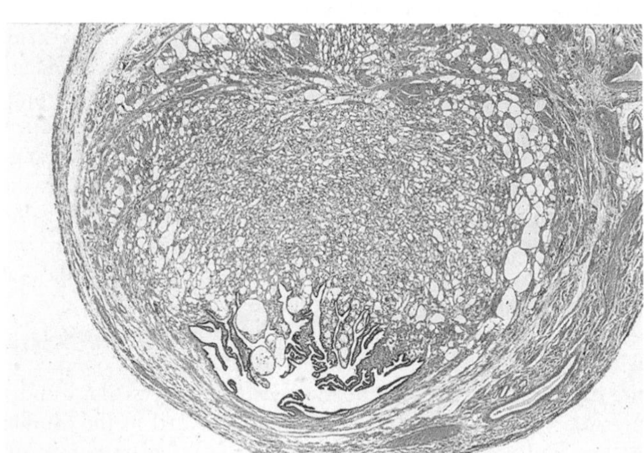

Figure 18-45. Adenomatoid tumor arising in the fallopian tube. (From Voet RL: Color Atlas of Obstetric and Gynecologic Pathology. St. Louis, Mosby-Wolfe, 1997.)

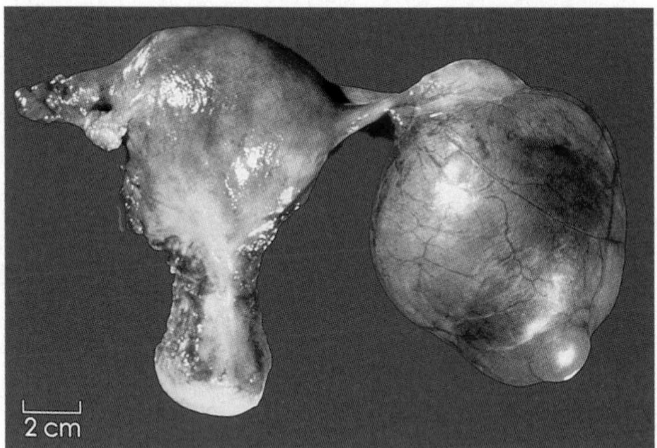

Figure 18-47. A nonneoplastic cyst with the broad ligament abuts the normal ovary. (From Clement PB, Young RH: Atlas of Gynecologic Surgical Pathology. Philadelphia, Saunders, 2000.)

projections. The authors cautioned that the differentiation between benign and malignant parovarian masses cannot be made by external examination of the cyst. The practice of aspirating cysts via the laparoscope should be limited to cysts that are completely simple and associated with normal cancer antigen-125 (CA-125) levels.

Paratubal cysts may grow rapidly during pregnancy, and most of the cases of torsion of these cysts have been reported during pregnancy or the puerperium. Treatment is simple excision.

Torsion

Acute torsion of the oviduct is a rare event; however, it has been reported with both normal and pathologic fallopian tubes. Pregnancy predisposes to this problem. Tubal torsion usually accompanies torsion of the ovary, as they have a common vascular pedicle. (See discussion of ovarian torsion later in this chapter.) Torsion of the fallopian tube is secondary to an ovarian mass in approximately 50% to 60% of patients. The right tube is involved more frequently than is the left (Fig. 18-48). The degree of tubal torsion varies from less than one turn to four complete rotations. Torsion of the oviduct is usually seen in women of reproductive age. However, it occurs also in preadolescent children, especially when part of the tube is enclosed in the sac of a femoral or inguinal hernia.

Tubal torsion may be divided into intrinsic and extrinsic causes. Prominent intrinsic causes include congenital abnormalities, such as increased tortuosity caused by excessive length of the tube, and pathologic processes, such as hydrosalpinx, hematosalpinx, tubal neoplasms, and previous operation, especially tubal ligation. Torsion of the fallopian tube following tubal ligation is usually of the distal end. Extrinsic causes of tubal torsion are ovarian and peritubal tumors, adhesions, trauma, and pregnancy.

The most important symptom of tubal torsion is acute lower abdominal and pelvic pain. The onset of this pain may be gradual or sudden, and the pain is usually located in the iliac fossa, with radiation to the thigh and flank. The duration of pain is generally less than 48 hours, and it is associated with

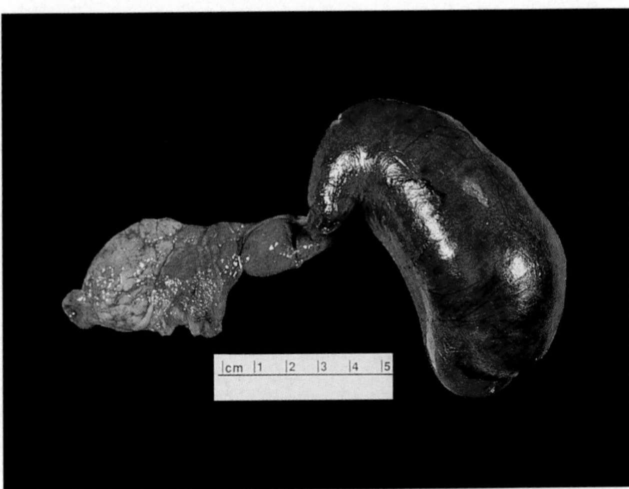

Figure 18-48. Hematosalpinx with torsion. (From Voet RL: Color Atlas of Obstetric and Gynecologic Pathology. St. Louis, Mosby-Wolfe, 1997.)

nausea and vomiting in two thirds of the cases. Usually, the pelvic pain, secondary to hypoxia, is so intense that it is difficult to perform an adequate pelvic exam. Unless there is associated torsion of the ovary, a specific mass is usually not palpable on pelvic examination.

The preoperative diagnosis of tubal torsion is made in less than 20% of reported cases. However, the number of cases diagnosed preoperatively has increased dramatically with the use of vaginal ultrasonography. Because of the severity of the pain, a wide differential diagnosis of abdominal and pelvic pathology must be considered. The differential diagnosis includes acute appendicitis, ectopic pregnancy, pelvic inflammatory disease, and rupture or torsion of an ovarian cyst.

Exploratory operation determines the extent of hypoxia and the choice of operative techniques. With tubal torsion, usually the tubes are gangrenous and must be excised. The twisted tube is usually filled with a bloody or serous fluid. It may be possible to restore normal circulation to the tube by manually untwisting it. The tube is usually sutured into a secure position to prevent recurrence.

OVARY

Functional Cysts

Follicular Cysts

Follicular cysts are by far the most frequent cystic structures in normal ovaries. The cysts are frequently multiple and may vary from a few millimeters to as large as 15 cm in diameter. A normal follicle may develop into a physiologic cyst. A minimum diameter to be considered as a cyst is generally considered to be between 2.5 and 3 cm. Follicular cysts are not neoplastic and are believed to be dependent on gonadotropins for growth. They arise from a temporary variation of a normal physiologic process. Clinically they may present with the signs and symptoms of ovarian enlargement and therefore must be differentiated from a true ovarian neoplasm. Functional cysts may be solitary or multiple. These cysts are found most commonly in young, menstruating women. Solitary cysts may occur during the fetal and neonatal periods and rarely during childhood, but there is an increase in frequency during the perimenarcheal period. Wolf coworkers studied 149 postmenopausal women and found simple cysts ranging in size from 0.4 to 4.7 cm in 15% of them. Large solitary follicular cysts in which the lining is luteinized are occasionally discovered during pregnancy and the puerperium. CA-125 may be used to evaluate such cysts in pregnancy. The values for CA-125 should be within the normal range past 12 weeks' gestation. Multiple follicular cysts in which the lining is luteinized are associated with either intrinsic or extrinsic elevated levels of gonadotropins. Interestingly, reproductive-age women with cystic fibrosis appear to have an increased propensity for developing individual follicular cysts.

Follicular cysts are translucent, thin-walled, and are filled with a watery, clear to straw-colored fluid. If a small opening in the capsule of the cyst suddenly develops, the cyst fluid under pressure will squirt out. These cysts are situated in the ovarian cortex, and sometimes they appear as translucent domes on the surface of the ovary. Histologically the lining of the cyst is usually composed of a closely packed layer of round, plump granulosa cells, with the spindle-shaped cells of the theca interna deeper in the stroma. In many cysts the lining of granulosa cells is difficult to distinguish, having undergone pressure atrophy. All that remains is a hyalinized connective tissue lining.

The temporary disturbance in follicular function that produces the clinical picture of a follicular cyst is poorly understood. Follicular cysts may result from either the dominant mature follicle's failing to rupture (persistent follicle) or an immature follicle's failing to undergo the normal process of atresia. In the latter circumstance the incompletely developed follicle fails to reabsorb follicular fluid. Some follicular cysts lose their ability to produce estrogen, and in others the granulosa cells remain productive, with prolonged secretion of estrogens. Occasionally, follicular cysts are better termed *follicular hematomas,* because blood from the vascular theca zone fills the cavity of the cyst.

The majority of follicular cysts are asymptomatic and are discovered during ultrasound imaging of the pelvis or a routine pelvic examination (Fig. 18-49). Because of their thin walls, these cysts may rupture during examination. The patient may experience tenesmus, a transient pelvic tenderness, deep dyspareunia, or no pain whatsoever. Rarely is significant intraperitoneal bleeding associated with the rupture of a follicular cyst. However, women who are chronically anticoagulated or those with von Willebrand's disease may bleed. Occasionally, menstrual irregularities and abnormal uterine bleeding may be associated with follicular cysts, which produce elevated blood estrogen levels. The syndrome associated with such follicular cysts consists of a regular cycle with a prolonged intermenstrual interval, followed by episodes of menorrhagia. Some women with larger follicular cysts notice a vague, dull sensation or heaviness in the pelvis.

The initial management of a suspected follicular cyst is conservative observation. The majority of follicular cysts disappear spontaneously by either reabsorption of the cyst fluid or silent rupture within 4 to 8 weeks of initial diagnosis. However, a persistent ovarian mass necessitates operative intervention to differentiate a physiologic cyst from a true neoplasm of the

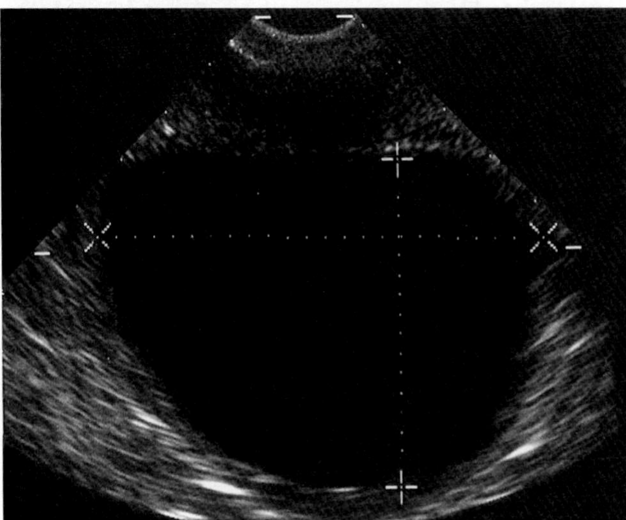

Figure 18-49. Ultrasound of simple follicular cyst. (From Goldberg JM, Falcone T: Atlas of Endoscopic Techniques in Gynecology. London, WB Saunders, 2000.)

ovary. There is no way to make the differentiation on the basis of signs, symptoms, or the initial growth pattern during early development of either process. Endovaginal ultrasound examination is helpful in differentiating simple from complex cysts and is also helpful during conservative management by providing dimensions to determine if the cyst is increasing in size. When the diameter of the cyst remains stable for greater than 10 weeks or enlarges, a neoplasia should be ruled out. Oral contraceptives may be prescribed for 4 to 6 weeks for young women with adnexal masses. This therapy removes any influence that pituitary gonadotropins may have on the persistence of the ovarian cyst. It also allows for several weeks of observation. In Spanos's series, 80% of cystic masses 4 to 6 cm in size disappeared during the time the patient was taking oral contraceptives. Steinkampf and colleagues performed a randomized prospective study of the effect of oral contraceptives on functional ovarian masses in women of reproductive age. Their study group consisted of women with infertility who had recently been treated by ovulation induction. In their series there was no difference in the rate of disappearance of functional ovarian cysts between the group that received oral contraceptives and the control group, perhaps because so many cysts will resolve spontaneously.

The evaluation of an asymptomatic cyst, found incidentally, is based on the principle that the cyst should be removed if there is any suspicion of malignancy. Suspicion may develop because of history, including family history, patient age, and other nongynecologic signs and symptoms. The size and physical characteristics of the cyst are as important as are other laboratory parameters. CA-125 is helpful in evaluating the adenexal mass in postmenopausal women. In premenopausal women, CA-125 is rarely helpful unless the mass is extremely suggestive of malignancy. Sonographic findings of concern include the presence of internal septations, thickness of the septations, bilaterality, solid elements, internal echoes, papulations or daughter cysts, and ascites or free fluid in the cul-de-sac. The appearance of the other ovary should be noted. Color Doppler indicating vascular resistance is advocated by some authors, but is neither sensitive nor specific enough to be used as a determining study. In most cases, simple small cysts may be observed. In general, complex cysts or persistent simple cysts larger than 10 cm should be evaluated. In women, with cysts in pregnancy, if the cyst is simple, with a normal CA-125 conservative management is acceptable. (CA-125 is generally not obtained in pregnant women with cysts less than 5 cm if they are simple.)

A cyst in a perimenopausal or postmenopausal woman should be removed if it is anything other than a simple cyst, if the CA-125 is abnormal (>35), or if the cyst is persistent or large (>10 cm). A small simple cyst in a perimenopausal or postmenopausal woman (<5 cm) with a normal CA-125 may be observed with regular reevaluation including ultrasound. Management of cysts between 5 and 10 cm that are otherwise not suggestive should be individualized. Ekerhovd and coworkers reported on 927 premenopausal women and 377 postmenopausal women with ovarian cysts. Of these women, 660 had unilocular simple cysts, 3 were borderline, and 4 were malignant (total of 1%). All of the borderline and malignant tumors were found in cysts greater than 7.5 cm. In women with cysts that had echodensity and papulations (644 women), 24 (3.7%) turned out to be borderline or malignant. Cysts that were multiseptate were not included in the study. All cysts with internal structures were excised, and had a much higher rate of malignancy. The authors, as well as others, have confirmed the recommendation that unilocular cysts less than 5 cm may be followed if there is no family history, a normal CA-125, or other significant findings.

In premenopausal women, operative management of non-malignant cysts is cystectomy, not oophorectomy. Many clinicians will manage simple cysts with the laparoscope. Since this procedure has an accompanying risk of spilling malignant cells into the peritoneal cavity if the cyst is an early carcinoma, strict preoperative criteria should be fulfilled before laparoscopy is attempted. These include the woman's age; size of the mass; and ultrasound characteristics, such as nonadherent, smooth, and thin-walled cysts, without papillae or internal echoes. (simple). DeWilde and associates reporting on a series of follicular cysts averaging 6 cm in diameter found that the recurrence rate following laparoscopic fenestration was approximately 2%. Higher rates of recurrence, up to 40%, have been reported for simple drainage of multiple types of benign cysts. The point being that drainage or fenestration is effective for follicular cysts and poorly effective for cystadenomas. When cysts are drained, it is essential to remember that cytologic examination of cyst fluid has poor predictive value and poor sensitivity in differentiating benign from malignant cysts. One recent report of fine-needle aspiration of ovarian cysts found sensitivity of 25%, specificity of 90%, false-positive rate of 73%, and false-negative rate of 12%. If there is any suspicion of malignancy, the cyst should be removed and histopathologic evaluation obtained.

Corpus Luteum Cysts

Corpus luteum cysts are less common than follicular cysts, but clinically they are more important. This discussion collectively combines corpus luteum cysts and persistently functioning mature corpora lutea (Fig. 18-50). Pathologists are sometimes able to make a distinction between a hemorrhagic cystic corpus luteum and a corpus luteum cyst, but at other times this difference cannot be established. All corpora lutea are cystic with gradual reabsorption of a limited amount of hemorrhage, which may form a cavity. Clinically, corpora lutea are not termed *corpus luteum cysts* unless they are a minimum of 3 cm in diameter. Corpus luteum cysts may be associated with either normal endocrine function or prolonged secretion of progesterone. The associated menstrual pattern may be normal, delayed menstruation, or amenorrhea.

Corpora lutea develop from mature graafian follicles. Intrafollicular bleeding does not occur during ovulation. However, 2 to 4 days later, during the stage of vascularization, thin-walled capillaries invade the granulosa cells from the theca interna. Spontaneous but limited bleeding fills the central cavity of the maturing corpus luteum with blood. Subsequently this blood is absorbed, forming a small cystic space. When the hemorrhage is excessive, the cystic space enlarges. If the hemorrhage into the central cavity is brisk, intracystic pressure increases and rupture of the corpus luteum is a possibility. If rupture does not occur, the size of the resulting corpus luteum cyst usually varies between 3 and 10 cm. Occasionally a cyst may be 11 to 15 cm in diameter. If a cystic central cavity persists, blood is replaced by clear fluid, and the result is a hormonally inactive corpus albicans cyst (Fig. 18-51). A corpus luteum of pregnancy is normally 3 to 5 cm in diameter with a central cystic structure, occupying at least 50% of the ovarian mass.

Most corpus luteum cysts are small, the average diameter being 4 cm. Grossly, they have a smooth surface and, depending on whether the cyst represents acute or chronic hemorrhage, are purplish red to brown. When a corpus luteum is cut, the convoluted lining is yellowish orange, and the center contains an organizing blood clot. Both the granulosa and the theca cells undergo luteinization. In chronic corpus luteum cysts the wall becomes gray-white, and the polygonal luteinized cells usually undergo pressure atrophy. Hallatt and colleagues reviewed 173 ruptured corpora lutea with hemoperitoneum. In

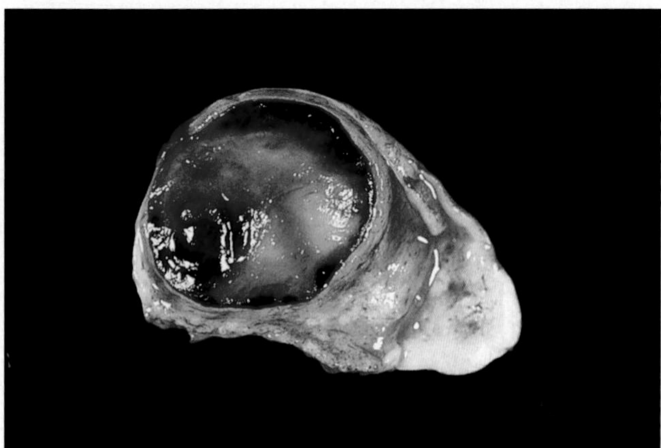

Figure 18-50. Hemorrhagic corpus luteum with an outer yellow rim and central hemorrhage. (From Voet RL: Color Atlas of Obstetric and Gynecologic Pathology. St. Louis, Mosby-Wolfe, 1997.)

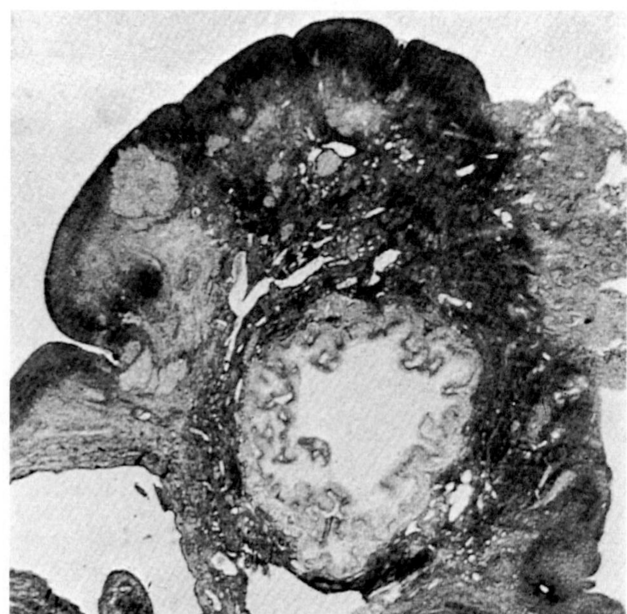

Figure 18-51. Corpus albicans cyst. Lining of cyst is composed of hyalinized connective tissue. (From Blaustein A: Nonneoplastic cysts of the ovary. In Blaustein A [ed]: Pathology of the Female Genital Tract. New York, Springer-Verlag, 1977, p 396.)

their institution the frequency of serious bleeding from a corpus luteum cyst compared with ectopic pregnancy was one in four.

Corpus luteum cysts vary from being asymptomatic masses to those causing catastrophic and massive intraperitoneal bleeding associated with rupture. Many corpus luteum cysts produce dull, unilateral, lower abdominal and pelvic pain. The enlarged ovary is moderately tender on pelvic examination. Depending on the amount of progesterone secretion associated with cysts, the menstrual bleeding may be normal or delayed several days to weeks with subsequent menorrhagia. Halban in 1915 described a syndrome of a persistently functioning corpus luteum cyst that has clinical features similar to an unruptured ectopic pregnancy. Halban's classic triad was a delay in a normal period followed by spotting; unilateral pelvic pain; and a small, tender, adnexal mass. This triad of symptomatology is similar to the triad of an anomalous period or delay in a normal period, spotting, and unilateral pelvic pain that is exhibited by the classic ectopic pregnancy. The differential diagnosis between these two conditions without a sensitive pregnancy test is difficult.

Corpus luteum cysts may cause intraperitoneal bleeding. The amount of bleeding varies from slight to clinically significant hemorrhage, necessitating blood transfusion. Internal bleeding often follows coitus, exercise, trauma, or a pelvic examination. However, episodes of bleeding usually do not recur, which differs from an ectopic pregnancy. Women with a bleeding diathesis or those undergoing chronic warfarin (Coumadin) therapy are especially prone to developing ovarian hemorrhage from a corpus luteum cyst. Bleeding occurs usually between days 20 and 26 of their cycle, and these women have a 31% chance for subsequent hemorrhage from a recurrent corpus luteum cyst. Oral contraceptives are sometimes used to suppress ovulation and avoid recurrent hemorrhage.

Hallatt and colleagues reported that sudden, severe, lower abdominal pain was a prominent symptom in women with hemoperitoneum caused by a ruptured corpus luteum cyst (Table 18-4). One of three women also noted unilateral cramping and lower abdominal pain for 1 to 2 weeks before overt rupture. The right ovary was the source of hemorrhage in 66% of their series. Tang and coworkers have also reported a right-sided predominance in the incidence of hemorrhage from corpus luteum cysts. They postulated that the difference is related to a higher intraluminal pressure on the right side because of the differences in ovarian vein architecture. Most ruptures occur between days 20 and 26 of the cycle, although in the series of Hallatt and colleagues 28% of the women had a delay in menses not explained by pregnancy (Table 18-5).

Table 18-4 Symptoms of 173 Women with Ruptured Corpus Luteum

	Number	Percent
Location		
Right ovary	114	66
Left ovary	56	32
Unknown	3	2
Abdominal pain	173	100
Onset with intercourse	29	17
Right ovary	21	72
Left ovary	8	28
Duration		
Less than 24 hours	94	54
1 to 7 days	40	23
Over 7 days	14	8
Unknown	25	15
Nausea or vomiting or diarrhea	60	35

From Hallatt JG, Steele CH Jr, Snyder M: Ruptured corpus luteum with hemoperitoneum: A study of 173 surgical cases. Am J Obstet Gynecol 149:6, 1984.

Table 18-5 Menstrual History in 173 Women with Ruptured Corpus Luteum

Last Menstrual Period to Operation	
Under 14 days	5
14 to 31 days (pregnant = 2)	77
31 to 60 days (pregnant = 15)	56
Over 60 days (pregnant = 10)	18
No menstrual period	14
Hysterectomy	5
Amenorrhea after oral contraceptives	5
Secondary amenorrhea	2
Menarche	1
Menopause	1
History of irregular menses	14
Unknown	3

From Hallatt JG, Steele CH Jr, Snyder M: Ruptured corpus luteum with hemoperitoneum: A study of 173 surgical cases. Am J Obstet Gynecol 149:6, 1984.

The differential diagnosis of a woman with acute pain and suspected ruptured corpus luteum cyst includes ectopic pregnancy, a ruptured endometrioma, and adnexal torsion. A sensitive serum or urinary assay for human chorionic gonadotropin (HCG) will help to differentiate a bleeding corpus luteum from ectopic pregnancy (see Chapter 17). Vaginal ultrasound is useful in establishing a preoperative diagnosis. Culdocentesis has been used in the past to establish the severity of the hemorrhage, but is rarely necessary today. If the hematocrit of the fluid obtained from the posterior cul-de-sac is greater than 15%, operative therapy becomes a necessity. Cystectomy is the operative treatment of choice, with preservation of the remaining portion of the ovary. In the series by DeWilde and associates reporting on persistent corpus luteum cysts treated by fenestration via the laparoscope, 6 of 44 (14%) recurred. Obviously, it was impossible for the authors to distinguish between a recurrent corpus luteum cyst and the development of a new corpus luteum. Unruptured corpus luteum cysts may be followed conservatively. Raziel and coworkers reported on a series of 70 women with ruptured corpora lutea. Ultrasonic evidence of large amounts of peritoneal fluid and severe pain were indications for operative intervention. In 12 of 70 patients with small amounts of intraperitoneal fluid and mild to moderate pain, observation alone was associated with resolution of symptoms.

Theca Lutein Cysts

Theca lutein cysts are by far the least common of the three types of physiologic ovarian cysts (Fig. 18-52). Unlike corpus luteum cysts, theca lutein cysts are almost always bilateral and produce moderate to massive enlargement of the ovaries. The individual cysts vary in size from 1 cm to 10 cm or more in diameter. These cysts arise from either prolonged or excessive stimulation of the ovaries by endogenous or exogenous gonadotropins or increased ovarian sensitivity to gonadotropins. The condition of ovarian enlargement secondary to the development

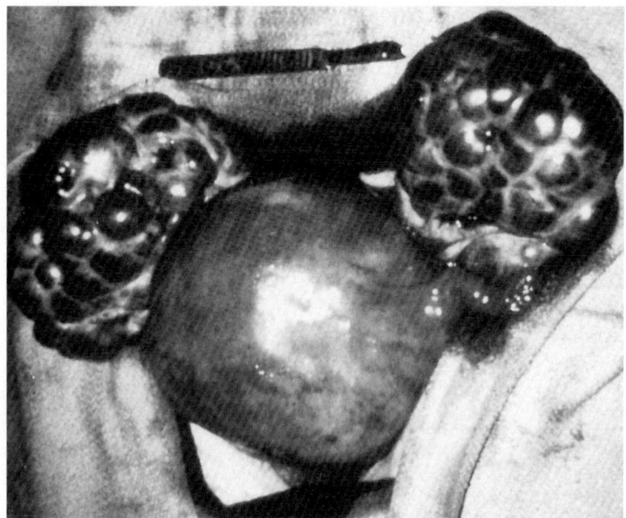

Figure 18-52. Bilateral theca lutein cysts. (Courtesy of Daniel R. Mishell, Jr., MD)

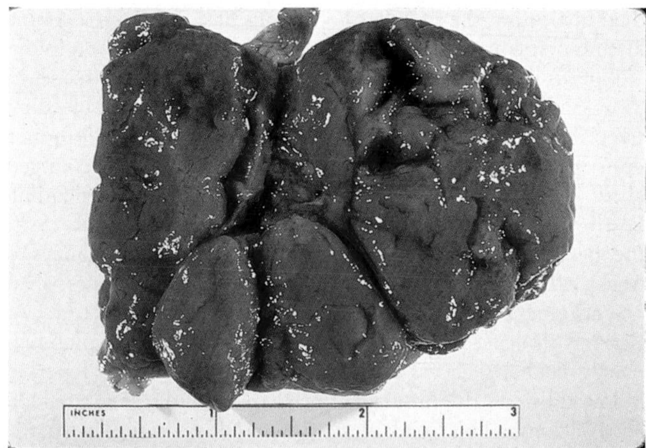

Figure 18-53. Luteoma of pregnancy with numerous solid brown nodules. (From Voet RL: Color Atlas of Obstetric and Gynecologic Pathology. St. Louis, Mosby-Wolfe, 1997.)

of multiple luteinized follicular cysts is termed *hyperreactio luteinalis.* Approximately 50% of molar pregnancies and 10% of choriocarcinomas have associated bilateral theca lutein cysts (Chapter 35, Gestational Trophoblastic Disease). In these patients the HCG from the trophoblast produces luteinization of the cells in immature, mature, and atretic follicles. The cysts are also discovered in the latter months of pregnancies often with conditions that produce a large placenta, such as twins, diabetes, and Rh sensitization. It is not uncommon to iatrogenically produce theca lutein cysts in women receiving medications to induce ovulation. Theca lutein cysts are occasionally discovered in association with normal pregnancy, as well as in newborn infants secondary to transplacental effects of maternal gonadotropins. Rarely, these cysts are found in young girls with juvenile hypothyroidism. Bakri and associates reported a case of theca lutein cysts in normal pregnancy that may have been associated with the patient's hypothyroidism. The authors speculated that similarities in the α-subunit of thyroid-stimulating hormone (TSH), HCG, and follicle-stimulating hormone (FSH) may have led to the ovarian enlargement.

Grossly the total ovarian size may be voluminous, 20 to 30 cm in diameter, with multiple theca lutein cysts. Bilateral ovarian enlargement is produced by multiple gray to bluish-tinged cysts. The bilateral enlargement is secondary to hundreds of thin-walled locules or cysts, producing a honeycombed appearance. Grossly the external surface of the ovary appears lobulated. The small cysts contain a clear to straw-colored or hemorrhagic fluid. Histologically the lining of the cyst is composed of theca lutein cells (paralutein cells), believed to originate from ovarian connective tissue. Occasionally there is also luteinization of granulosa cells. These voluminous and congested ovaries are slow growing. The vast majority of women with smaller cysts are asymptomatic. Generally only the larger cysts produce vague symptoms, such as a sense of pressure in the pelvis. Ascites and increasing abdominal girth have been reported with hyperstimulation from exogenous gonadotropins. Rarely, associated adnexal torsion may occur. Montz and colleagues, in reviewing the natural history of 102 women with theca lutein cysts, found that approximately 1% of patients experienced acute complications of either torsion or intraperitoneal bleeding. They also discovered that theca lutein cysts persisted in some women for weeks after HCG levels were nondetectable.

The presence of theca lutein cysts is established by palpation and often confirmed by ultrasound examination. Treatment is conservative because these cysts gradually regress. If these cysts are discovered incidentally at cesarean delivery, they should be handled delicately. No attempt should be made to drain or puncture the multiple cysts because of the possibility of hemorrhage. Bleeding is difficult to control in these cases because of the thin walls that comprise the cysts.

A condition related to theca lutein cysts is the *luteoma* of pregnancy. The condition is rare and not a true neoplasm but rather a specific, benign, hyperplastic reaction of ovarian theca lutein cells (Figs. 18-53 and 18-54). These nodules do not arise from the corpus luteum of pregnancy. Fifty percent of luteomas are multiple, and approximately 30% of those reported have

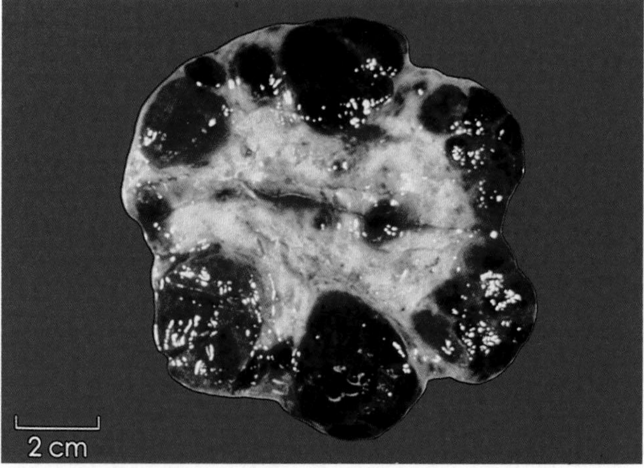

Figure 18-54. Luteoma with multiple reddish nodules. (From Clement PB, Young RH: Atlas of Gynecologic Surgical Pathology. Philadelphia, WB Saunders, 2000.)

bilateral nodules. In appearance they are discrete and brown to reddish brown and may be solid or cystic.

The majority of patients with luteomas are asymptomatic. The solid, fleshy, often hemorrhagic, nodules are discovered incidentally at cesarean delivery or postpartum tubal ligation. Most cases have been reported in multiparous African-American women. Masculinization of the mother occurs in 30% of cases, and masculinization of the external genitalia of the female fetus may sometimes occur. These tumors regress spontaneously following completion of the pregnancy.

Benign Neoplasms of the Ovary

Benign Cystic Teratoma (Dermoid Cyst, Mature Teratoma)

Benign ovarian teratomas are usually cystic structures that on histologic examination contain elements from all three germ cell layers. The word *teratoma* was first advanced by Virchow and translated literally means "monstrous growth." Teratomas of the ovary may be benign or malignant. Although *dermoid* is a misnomer, it is the most common term used to describe the benign cystic tumor, composed of mature cells, whereas the malignant variety is composed of immature cells (immature teratoma). *Dermoid* is a descriptive term in that it emphasizes the preponderance of ectodermal tissue with some mesodermal and rare endodermal derivatives. Malignant teratomas that are immature are usually solid with some cystic areas and histologically contain immature or embryonic-appearing tissue. (See Chapter 33 [Neoplastic Diseases of the Ovary] for further discussion of malignant teratomas.) Benign teratomas may contain a malignant component, usually in women older than 40. The malignant component is generally a squamous carcinoma and is found in less than 1% of cases. Nonovarian teratomas may arise in any midline structure of the body where the germ cell has resided during embryonic life.

Benign teratomas are among the most common ovarian neoplasms. They account for more than 90% of germ cell tumors of the ovary. These slow-growing tumors occur from infancy to the postmenopausal years. Depending on the series, dermoids represent 20% to 25% of all ovarian neoplasms and approximately 33% of all benign tumors, if follicular and corpus luteum cysts are excluded. Dermoids are the most common ovarian neoplasm in prepubertal females and are also common in teenagers. More than 50% of benign teratomas are discovered in women between the ages of 25 and 50 years. In the series of Lakkis and coworkers of 118 women with dermoids, 86% of the women were younger than 40 years of age, and 3.4% had recurrences (Fig. 18-55). Similarly, in the series by Comerci and colleagues of 573 tumors in 517 women the mean age was 32 years and 86% were younger than 43 years of age. With routine obstetric ultrasound, the mean age at diagnosis is expected to fall. In most large series of benign tumors in postmenopausal women, dermoids account for approximately 20% of the neoplasms.

Dermoids vary from a few millimeters to 25 cm in diameter. Comerci and colleagues reported a large tumor weighing 7657 g in a woman who was asymptomatic. However, 80% are less than 10 cm. These tumors may be single or multiple, with as many as nine individual dermoids having been reported in the same ovary. Benign teratomas occur bilaterally 10% to 15% of the time. Often, dermoid cysts are pedunculated. These cysts make the ovary heavier than normal, and thus they are usually discovered either in the cul-de-sac or anterior to the broad ligament. On palpation these tumors, which have both cystic and solid components, have a doughy consistency.

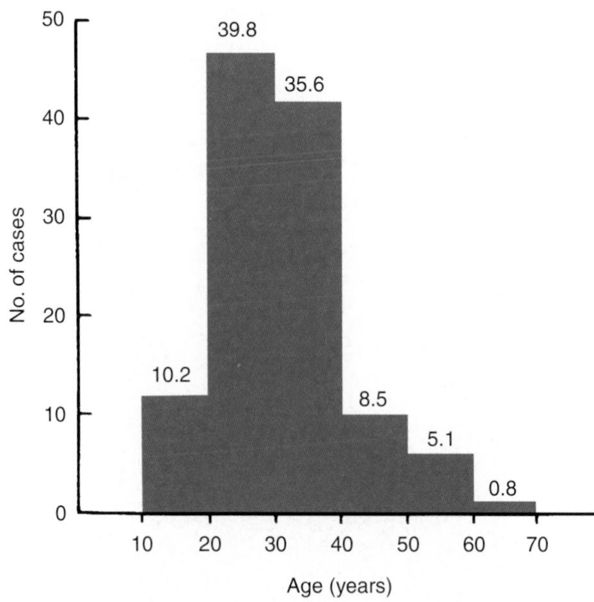

Figure 18-55. Age distribution of cystic teratomas. (From Lakkis WG, Martin MC, Gelfand MM: Benign cystic teratoma of the ovary: A 6-year review. Originally published in Canadian Journal of Surgery 28:444, 1985.)

The cysts are usually unilocular. The walls of the cyst are a smooth, shiny, opaque white color. When they are opened, thick sebaceous fluid pours from the cyst, often with tangled masses of hair and firm areas of cartilage and teeth (Figs. 18-56 and 18-57). The sebaceous material is a thick fluid at body temperature but solidifies when it cools in room air.

Benign teratomas are believed to arise from a single germ cell after the first meiotic division. Therefore they develop from totipotential stem cells, and they are neoplastic sequelae from a

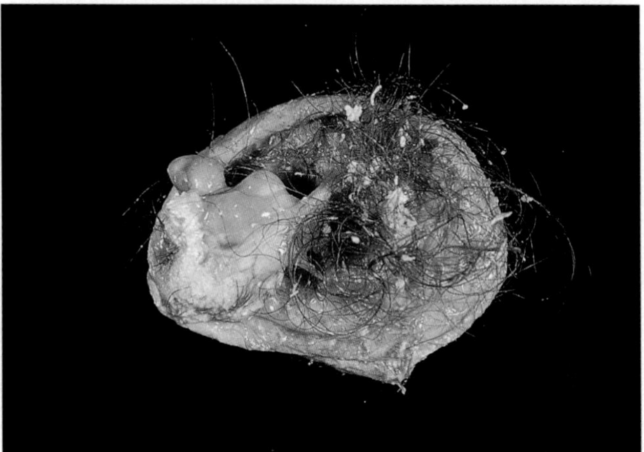

Figure 18-56. Mature cystic teratoma (dermoid cyst) filled with hair and keratinous debris with one solid nodular area (Rokitansky protuberance). (From Voet RL: Color Atlas of Obstetric and Gynecologic Pathology. St. Louis, Mosby-Wolfe, 1997.)

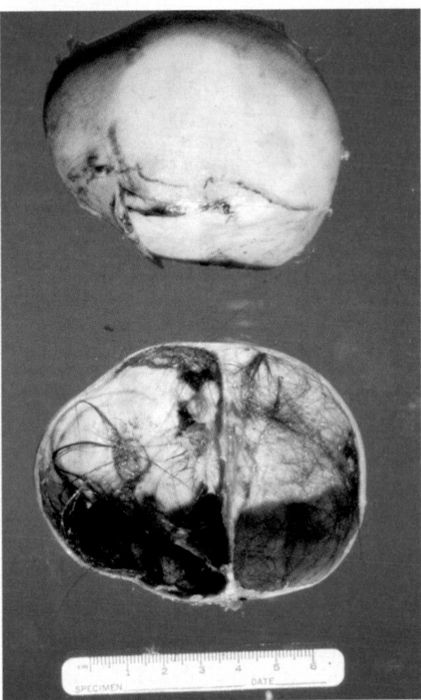

Figure 18-57. Bilateral mature cystic teratomas in pregnancy. The cyst is bilocular. Dermal papillae are noted. Teeth are also present in the left lobule. (From Russell P, Robboy SJ, Anderson MC: Germ cell tumors of the ovaries. In Robboy SJ, Anderson MC, Russell P [eds]: Pathology of the Female Reproductive Tract. Edinburgh, Churchill Livingstone, 2002.)

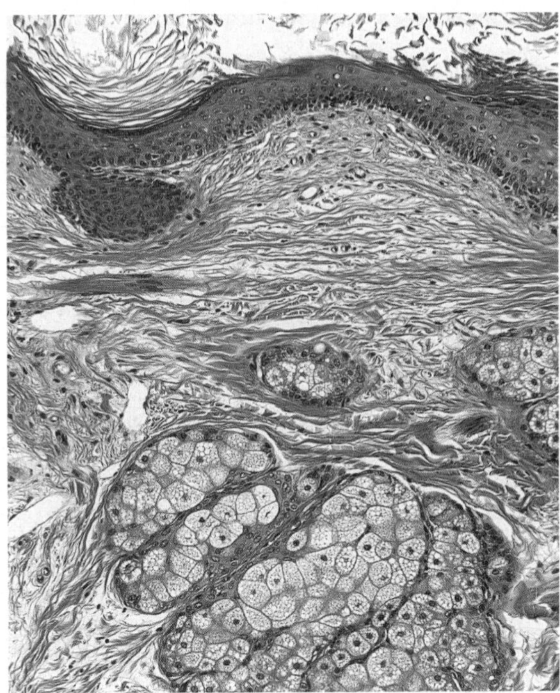

Figure 18-58. Mature cystic teratoma. This cyst is lined by mature epidermis and is subtended by connective tissue containing exuberant dermal appendages (pilosebaceous follicles). (From Russell P, Robboy SJ, Anderson MC: Germ cell tumors of the ovaries. In Robboy SJ, Anderson MC, Russell P [eds]: Pathology of the Female Reproductive Tract. Edinburgh, Churchill Livingstone, 2002.)

transformed germ cell. Dermoids have a chromosomal makeup of 46,XX. Linder and coworkers, in a series of experiments using chromosome banding techniques and electrophoretic variance, discovered that the chromosomes of dermoids were different from the chromosomes of the host. They postulated that dermoids began by parthenogenesis from secondary oocytes. An alternative hypothesis was that the dermoid resulted from fusion of the second polar body with the oocyte. The studies by Linder and coworkers ruled out the possibility that dermoids arise from somatic cells or from an oogonium before the first stage of meiosis. The first meiotic division occurs at approximately 13 weeks of gestation. Thus dermoids begin in fetal life sometime after the first trimester.

Histologically, benign teratomas are composed of mature cells, usually from all three germ layers (Fig. 18-58). A combination of skin and skin appendages, including sebaceous glands, sweat glands, hair follicles, muscle fibers, cartilage, bone, teeth, glial cells, and epithelium of the respiratory and gastrointestinal tracts, may be visualized. Teeth are predominantly premolar and molar forms. The fluid in dermoid cysts is usually sebaceous. Most solid elements arise and are contained in a protrusion or nipple (mamilla) in the cyst wall termed the *prominence* or *tubercle of Rokitansky.* This prominence may be visualized by ultrasound as an echodense region, thus aiding in the sonographic diagnosis. If malignancy occurs, it is most always found in this nest of cells. The wall of the cyst will often contain granulation tissue, giant cells, and pseudoxanthoma cells.

From 50% to 60% of dermoids are asymptomatic and are discovered during a routine pelvic examination, coincidentally visualized during pelvic imaging, or found incidentally at laparotomy. Presenting symptoms of dermoids include pain and the sensation of pelvic pressure. Specific complications of dermoid cysts include torsion, rupture, infection, hemorrhage, and malignant degeneration. Three medical diseases also may be associated with dermoid cysts: thyrotoxicosis, carcinoid syndrome, and autoimmune hemolytic anemia, the latter two being quite rare.

Adult thyroid tissue is discovered microscopically in approximately 12% of benign teratomas. *Struma ovarii* is a teratoma in which the thyroid tissue has overgrown other elements and is the predominant tissue (Fig. 18-59). Strumae ovarii comprise 2% to 3% of ovarian teratomas. These tumors are usually unilateral and measure less than 10 cm in diameter. Less than 5% of women with strumae ovarii develop thyrotoxicosis, which may be secondary to the production of increased thyroid hormone by either the ovarian or the thyroid gland.

Another rare finding with dermoids is the presence of a primary carcinoid tumor from the gastrointestinal or respiratory tract epithelium contained in the dermoid. One of three of these tumors is associated with the typical carcinoid syndrome even without metastatic spread. If the carcinoid is functioning, it may be diagnosed by measuring serum serotonin levels or urinary levels of 5-hydroxyindoleacetic acid. The autoimmune hemolytic anemia associated with dermoids is the rarest of the three medical complications.

Rupture or perforation of the contents of a dermoid into the peritoneal cavity or an adjacent organ is a potentially serious complication. The incidence varies between 0.7% and 4.6%. However, most series report less than 1%. Rupture is more common in pregnancy. If a rupture occurs during surgery, the abdomen should be copiously irrigated with saline, with careful

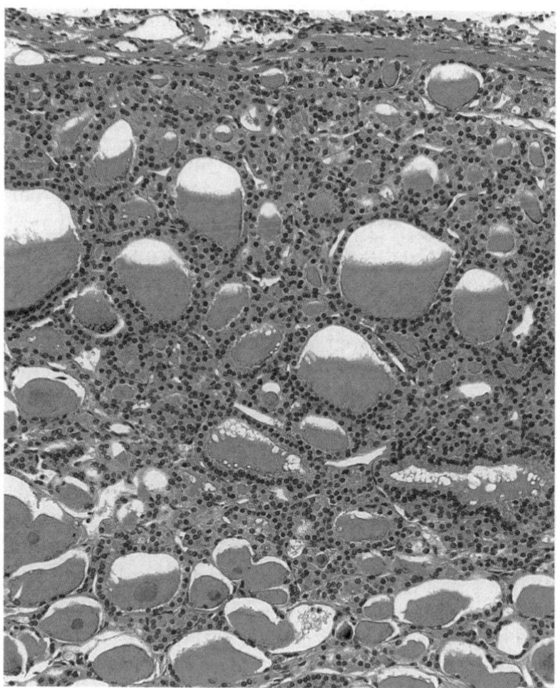

Figure 18-59. Struma ovarii. Variably sized banal thyroid follicles. (From Russell P, Robboy SJ, Anderson MC: Germ cell tumors of the ovaries. In Robboy SJ, Anderson MC, Russell P [eds]: Pathology of the Female Reproductive Tract. Edinburgh, Churchill Livingstone, 2002.)

removal of any particulate matter. Chemical peritonitis is reported in less than1% of ruptured dermoids. Rupture may occur either catastrophically, which produces an acute abdomen, or by a slow leak of the sebaceous material. The latter is clinically more common, with the sebaceous material producing a severe chemical granulomatous peritonitis. Waxman and Boyce warn that this possibility should be considered and a frozen section obtained so that the true diagnosis is established. Thus a young woman will not be mistakenly treated for suspected ovarian carcinoma with metastasis because of the identical gross appearance of a slow-leaking dermoid cyst. Infection, hemorrhage, and malignant degeneration are all unusual complications of dermoids, occurring in less than 1% of patients.

Torsion of a dermoid is the most frequent complication, occurring in 11% of the series by Pantoja and associates and 3.5% of the time in Comerci and colleague's series. Because of its weight, the benign teratoma is often pedunculated, which may predispose to torsion. Torsion is more common in younger women. Small dermoid cysts, less than 6 cm in diameter, grow slowly at an approximate rate of 2 mm per year.

The diagnosis of a dermoid cyst is often established when a semisolid mass is palpated anterior to the broad ligament. Approximately 50% of dermoids have pelvic calcifications on radiographic examination. Often an ovarian teratoma is an incidental finding during radiologic investigation of the genitourinary or gastrointestinal tract. Most dermoids have a characteristic ultrasound picture. These characteristics include a dense echogenic area within a larger cystic area, a cyst filled with bands of mixed echoes, and an echoic dense cyst. Laing and coworkers have found that only one of three dermoids has this "typical picture." In their series of 45 patients with 51 biopsy-proven dermoid cysts, 24% of the dermoid cysts were predominantly solid, 20% were almost entirely cystic, and 24% were not visible. Ultrasound has a more than 95% positive predictive value and a less than 5% false positive rate.

Operative treatment of benign cystic teratomas is cystectomy with preservation of as much normal ovarian tissue as possible. Laparoscopic cystectomy is an accepted approach. Rates of spillage are comparable to that from open laparotomy. However, adequate irrigation in such cases is essential and often more time-consuming. Many authors use a 10-cm diameter cutoff as the upper limit for a laparoscopic approach. If a teratoma is diagnosed incidentally during pregnancy, strong consideration should be given for removal in the second trimester. Dermoids have a higher incidence of torsion and potential for rupture during pregnancy. Though laparoscopy is safe during pregnancy, a small periumbilical minilaporortomy may be a faster, less traumatic approach. Reduced intraoperative time is an advantage during pregnancy. The treatment of a dermoid in pregnancy, as in the nonpregnant stated, is cystectomy, no matter the surgical approach.

Endometriomas

Endometriosis of the ovary is usually associated with endometriosis in other areas of the pelvic cavity. Approximately two out of three women with endometriosis have ovarian involvement. Interestingly, only 5% of these women have enlargement of the ovaries that is detectable by pelvic examination. However, because of the prevalence of the disease, endometriosis is one of the most common causes of enlargement of the ovary. Because most authors do not classify endometriosis as a neoplastic disease, the diagnosis of endometriosis may not be given due consideration in the differential diagnosis of an adnexal mass. Ovarian endometriosis is similar to endometriosis elsewhere and is described in greater detail in Chapter 19.

The size of ovarian endometriomas varies from small, superficial, blue-black implants that are 1 to 5 mm in diameter to large, multiloculated, hemorrhagic cysts that may be 5 to 10 cm in diameter (Fig. 18-60). Clinically, large ovarian endometriomas, greater than 20 cm in diameter, are extremely rare. Areas of ovarian endometriosis that become cystic are termed *endometriomas.* Rarely, large chocolate cysts of the ovary may reach

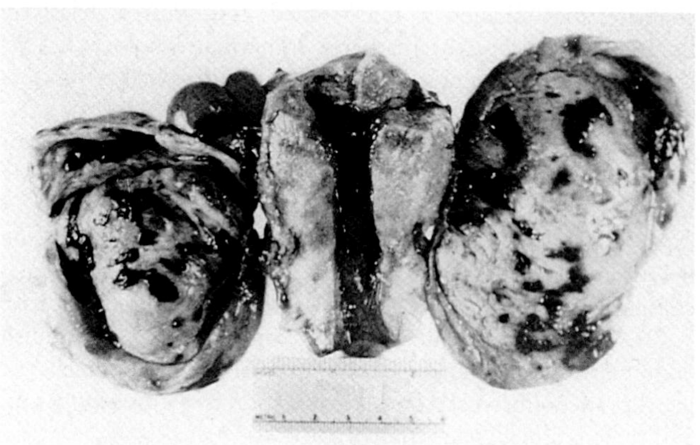

Figure 18-60. Endometriosis of ovaries. Wall of endometriotic cyst is thickened and fibrotic. Inner surface shows areas of dark brown discoloration. (From Janovski NA [ed]: Color Atlas of Gross Gynecologic and Obstetric Pathology. New York, McGraw-Hill, 1969, p 159.)

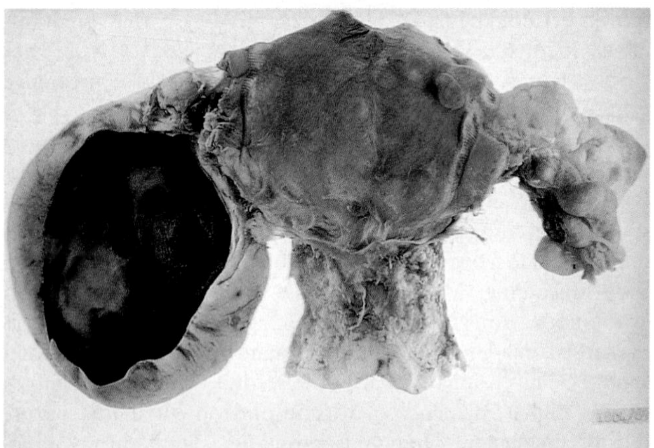

Figure 18-61. "Chocolate cyst" of ovary. The endometrioma is large, but has not yet completely replaced the ovary. (From Robboy SJ: Endometriosis. In Robboy SJ, Anderson MC, Russell P [eds]: Pathology of the Female Reproductive Tract. Edinburgh, Churchill Livingstone, 2002.)

15 to 20 cm (Fig. 18-61). Larger cysts are frequently bilateral. The surface of an ovary with endometriosis is often irregular, puckered, and scarred. Depending on their size, endometriomas replace a portion of the normal ovarian tissue.

Although most women with endometriomas are asymptomatic, the most common symptoms associated with ovarian endometriosis are pelvic pain, dyspareunia, and infertility. Approximately 10% of the operations for endometriosis are for acute symptoms, usually related to a ruptured ovarian endometrioma that was previously asymptomatic. Smaller cysts generally have thin walls, and perforation occurs commonly secondary to cyclic hemorrhage into the cystic cavity.

On pelvic examination the ovaries are often tender and immobile, secondary to associated inflammation and adhesions. Most commonly the ovaries are densely adherent to surrounding structures, including the peritoneum of the pelvic sidewall, the oviduct, the broad ligament, and sometimes the small or large bowel. Endometrial glands, endometrial stroma, and large phagocytic cells containing hemosiderin may be identified histologically (see Fig. 19-10). Pressure atrophy may lead to the loss of architecture of the endometrial glands. The ultrasound characteristics include a thick-walled cyst with a relatively homogeneous echo pattern that is somewhat echolucent. This appearance confers a greater than 95% positive predictive value in some studies.

The choice between medical and operative management depends on several factors, including the patient's age, future reproductive plans, and severity of symptoms. Medical therapy is rarely successful in treating ovarian endometriosis if the disease has produced ovarian enlargement. Often surgical therapy is complicated by formation of de novo and recurrent adhesions.

On pathologic examination, it is important to distinguish endometriosis from benign endometrial tumors, which are usually adenofibromas. The latter tumor is a true neoplasm, and there is a malignant counterpart.

Fibroma

Fibromas are the most common benign, solid neoplasms of the ovary. Their malignant potential is low, less than 1%. These tumors comprise approximately 5% of benign ovarian neoplasms and approximately 20% of all solid tumors of the ovary.

Fibromas vary in size from small nodules to huge pelvic tumors weighing 50 pounds. One of the predominant characteristics of fibromas is that they are extremely slow-growing tumors. The average diameter of a fibroma is approximately 6 cm; however, some tumors have reached 30 cm in diameter. In most series, less than 5% of fibromas are greater than 20 cm in diameter. The diameter of a fibroma is important clinically, because the incidence of associated ascites is directly proportional to the size of the tumor. Many ovarian fibromas are misdiagnosed and are believed to be leiomyomas prior to operation. Ninety percent of fibromas are unilateral; however, multiple fibromas are found in the same ovary in 10% to 15% of cases. The average age of a woman with an ovarian fibroma is 48. Thus this tumor often presents in a postmenopausal woman. The tumor arises from the undifferentiated fibrous stroma of the ovary. Bilateral ovarian fibromas are commonly found in women with the rare genetic transmitted basal cell nevus syndrome.

The pelvic symptoms that develop with growth of fibromas include pressure and abdominal enlargement, which may be secondary to both the size of the tumor and ascites. Smaller tumors are asymptomatic because these tumors do not elaborate hormones. Thus there is no change in the pattern of menstrual flow. Fibromas may be pedunculated and therefore easily palpable during one examination yet difficult to palpate during a subsequent pelvic examination. Sometimes on pelvic examination the fibromas appear to be softer than a solid ovarian tumor because of the edema or occasional cystic degeneration.

Meigs' syndrome is the association of an ovarian fibroma, ascites, and hydrothorax. Both the ascites and the hydrothorax resolve after removal of the ovarian tumor. The ascites is caused by transudation of fluid from the ovarian fibroma. Samanth and Black reported that the incidence of ascites was directly related to the size of the fibroma. Fifty percent of patients have ascites if the tumor is greater than 6 cm. However, true Meigs' syndrome is rare, occurring in less than 2% of ovarian fibromas. The hydrothorax develops secondary to a flow of ascitic fluid into the pleural space via the lymphatics of the diaphragm. Statistically the right pleural space is involved in 75% of reported cases, the left in 10%, and both sides in 15%. The clinical features of Meigs' syndrome are not unique to fibromas, and a similar clinical picture is found with many other ovarian tumors.

Grossly, fibromas are heavy, solid, well encapsulated, and grayish white. The cut surface usually demonstrates a homogeneous white or yellowish white solid tissue with a trabeculated or whorled appearance similar to that of myomas. The vast majority of fibromas are grossly edematous (Fig. 18-62). Less than 10% of fibromas have calcifications or small areas of hyaline or cystic degeneration. Histologically, fibromas are composed of connective tissue, stromal cells, and varying amounts of collagen interposed between the cells. The connective tissue cells are spindle-shaped, mature fibroblasts. They are arranged in an imperfect pattern. A few smooth muscle fibers may be occasionally identified. It is sometimes difficult to distinguish fibromas from nonneoplastic thecomas. Histologically the pathologist must differentiate fibromas from stromal hyperplasia, fibrosarcomas, and also look for epithelial elements of an associated Brenner tumor.

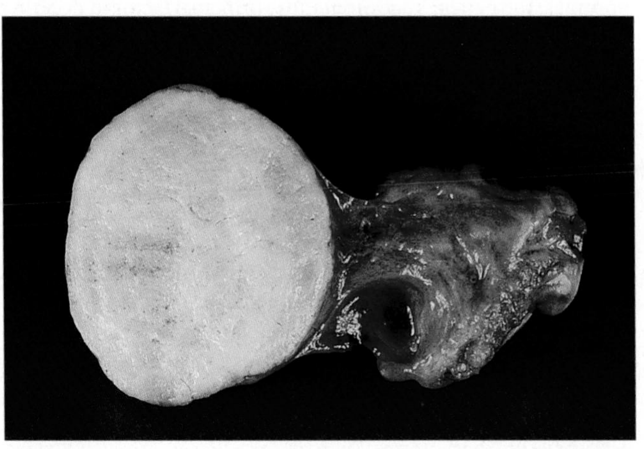

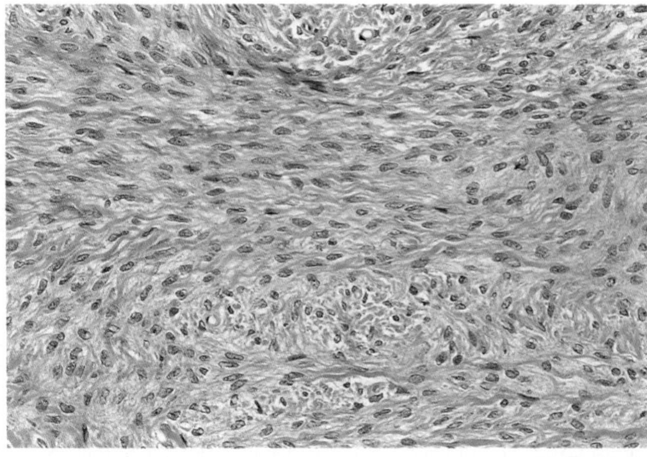

Figure 18-62. **A,** Fibroma of the ovary with a well circumscribed light tan mass. **B,** Histology of fibroma of the ovary, demonstrating bland fibrous differentiation. (From Voet RL: Color Atlas of Obstetric and Gynecologic Pathology. St. Louis, Mosby-Wolfe, 1997.)

The management of fibromas is straightforward because any woman with a solid ovarian neoplasm should have an exploratory operation soon after the tumor is discovered. Simple excision of the tumor is all that is necessary. Following excision of the tumor, there is resolution of all symptoms, including ascites. Because these tumors are frequently discovered in postmenopausal women, often a bilateral salpingo-oophorectomy and total abdominal hysterectomy are performed. Conversely, it is important to note that most women who preoperatively have the combination of a solid ovarian tumor and ascites are found to have ovarian carcinoma.

Transitional Cell Tumors-Brenner Tumors

Brenner tumors are rare, small, smooth, solid, fibroepithelial ovarian tumors that are generally asymptomatic. The semantic classification of neoplasms changes, and the current preferred term for benign Brenner tumor is *transitional cell tumor.* The benign, proliferative (low malignant potential), and malignant forms together comprise approximately 2% of ovarian tumors. These tumors usually occur in women ages 40 to 60 years. Approximately 30% of transitional cell tumors are discovered as small, solid tumors in association with a concurrent serous cystic neoplasia, such as serous or mucinous cystadenomas of the ipsilateral ovary. Some are microscopic, with the entire tumor contained in a single low-powered microscopic field, and others may reach a diameter of 20 cm; the majority are less than 5 cm in diameter. The tumor is unilateral 85% to 95% of the time.

The Brenner tumor was first described in 1898. In 1932, Robert Meyer postulated that it was a distinct, independent neoplasm from granulosa cell tumors. Since that time there has been a controversy in the gynecologic pathology literature as to the histogenesis of the neoplasm. Presently, most authorities accept the theory that most of these tumors result from metaplasia of coelomic epithelium into uroepithelium. Detailed three-dimensional histologic studies have demonstrated a downward growth in a cordlike fashion of epithelium from the surface of the ovary to deeper areas in the ovarian cortex. Others have postulated that sometimes the solid nests of epithelial cells of the tumor originate from the rete ovarii or Walthard rests. Shevchuk and coworkers, in an electron microscopy study, confirmed the histologic and ultrastructural similarity between epithelium in Brenner tumors and transitional epithelium. These authors argue that because of the histogenesis from coelomic inclusion cysts and also the mixture of müllerian-type epithelium in 30% of Brenner tumors, it might be appropriate to classify Brenner tumors in the epithelial group of ovarian neoplasms.

Approximately 90% of these small neoplasms are discovered incidentally during a gynecologic operation, although large tumors may produce unilateral pelvic discomfort. Postmenopausal bleeding is sometimes associated with Brenner tumors, as endometrial hyperplasia is a coexisting abnormality in 10% to 16% of cases. It is postulated that luteinization of the stroma produces estrogen with resulting hyperplasia. Recent reports by Moon and associates and Outwater and colleagues describe the CT and MRI characteristics of Brenner tumors of the ovary. The extensive fibrous content of these tumors results in lower signal intensity in T2-weighted images. During CT scanning, Brenner tumors characteristically demonstrate a finding of extensive amorphous calcification within the solid components of the ovarian mass.

Grossly, Brenner tumors are smooth, firm, gray-white, solid tumors that grossly resemble fibromas. Similar to fibromas, transitional cell tumors are slow growing. On sectioning, the tumor usually appears gray; however, occasionally there is a yellowish tinge with small cystic spaces (Fig. 18-63). Approximately 1% to 2% of these tumors undergo malignant change (Chapter 33, Neoplastic Diseases of the Ovary). Histologically, Brenner tumors have two principal components: solid masses or nests of epithelial cells and a surrounding fibrous stroma. The epithelial cells are uniform and do not appear anaplastic (Fig. 18-64). The histology and ultrastructure of the epithelial cells of a Brenner tumor are similar to transitional epithelium of the urinary bladder. The pale epithelial cells have a "coffee bean"-appearing nucleus, which is also described as a longitudinal groove in the cell's nucleus.

Electron microscopy has demonstrated that the longitudinal groove during routine microscopy is produced by prominent indentation of the nuclear membrane. An additional ovarian

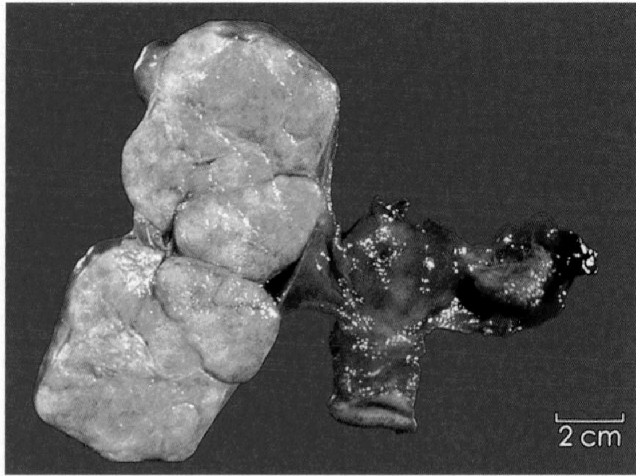

Figure 18-63. Brenner tumor. (From Clement PB, Young RH: Atlas of Gynecologic Surgical Pathology. Philadelphia, WB Saunders, 2000.)

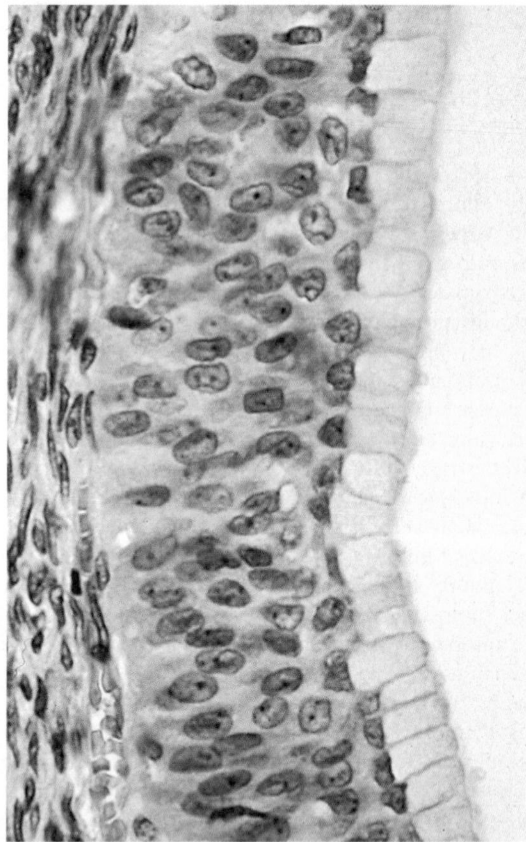

Figure 18-64. Benign Brenner tumor. A cyst in the Brenner tumor is lined by an inner layer of endocervical-type mucinous cells and an outer layer of stratified transitional cells, a few of which have grooved nuclei. (From Clement PB, Young RH: Atlas of Gynecologic Surgical Pathology. Philadelphia, WB Saunders, 2000.)

neoplasm is frequently found associated with Brenner tumors. Balasa and colleagues, in a review of 302 tumors, reported 100 other concurrent neoplasms, with the majority being serous and mucinous cystadenomas or teratomas.

Management of Brenner tumors is operative, with simple excision being the procedure of choice. However, as with ovarian fibromas, the patient's age often is the principal factor in deciding the extent of the operation.

Adenofibroma and Cystadenofibroma

Adenofibromas and cystadenofibromas are closely related. Both of these benign firm tumors consist of fibrous and epithelial components. The epithelial element is most commonly serous, but histologically may be mucinous and endometrioid or clear cell. They differ from benign epithelial cystadenomas in that there is a preponderance of connective tissue. Most pathologists emphasize that at least 25% of the tumor consists of fibrous connective tissue. Obviously, cystadenofibromas have microscopic or occasional macroscopic areas that are cystic. The varying degree of fibrous stroma and epithelial elements produces a spectrum of tumors, which have resulted in a confusing nomenclature with terms such as *papillomas, fibropapillomas,* and *fibroadenomas.*

Adenofibromas are usually small fibrous tumors that arise from the surface of the ovary. They are bilateral in 20% to 25% of women. They usually occur in postmenopausal women and are 1 to 15 cm in diameter. Grossly, they are gray or white tumors, and it is difficult to distinguish them from fibromas. Papillary adenofibromas, which project from the surface of the ovary, at first glance may appear to be external excrescences of a malignant tumor. Histologically, small precursors of adenofibromas are identified in many normal ovaries. Under the microscope, true cystic gland spaces lined by cuboidal epithelium are characteristic. However, differing from serous cystadenomas, the fibrous connective tissue surrounding the cystic spaces is abundant and is the predominant tissue of the tumor.

Smaller tumors are asymptomatic and are only discovered incidentally during abdominal or pelvic operations. Large tumors may cause pressure symptoms or, rarely, undergo adnexal torsion. Recently a small series of the MRI features of these tumors has been reported. Similar to Brenner tumors, the fibrous component produces a very low signal intensity on T2-weighted images. This interest in imaging results from an attempt to distinguish, prior to operation, whether a predominately solid ovarian mass is benign or malignant. Because adenofibromas are usually discovered in postmenopausal women, the treatment of choice is bilateral salpingo-oophorectomy and total abdominal hysterectomy. Because these tumors are benign and because malignant transformation is rare, simple excision of the tumor and inspection of the contralateral ovary is appropriate in younger women.

Torsion

Torsion of the ovary or both the oviduct and the ovary (adnexal torsion) is uncommon but an important cause of acute lower abdominal and pelvic pain. Torsion of the ovary may occur separately from torsion of the fallopian tube, but most commonly the two adnexal structures are affected together.

Adnexal torsion occurs most commonly during the reproductive years, with the average patient being in her mid-20s. Adnexal torsion is also a complication of benign ovarian tumors in the postmenopausal woman. Pregnancy appears to predispose women to adnexal torsion, with approximately one in five women being pregnant when the condition is diagnosed. Most susceptible are ovaries that are enlarged secondary to ovulation induction during early pregnancy. One series reported 4 cases of adnexal torsion in 648 pregnancies resulting from ovulation induction. The most common cause of adnexal torsion is ovarian enlargement by an 8- to 12-cm benign mass of the ovary. However, smaller ovaries may also undergo torsion. Ovarian tumors are discovered in 50% to 60% of women with adnexal torsion. Torsion of a normal ovary or adnexum is also possible and occurs more frequently in children. Hibbard reports that because of their relative prevalence, dermoids are the tumor most frequently reported in a series of women with adnexal torsion. However, the relative risk of adnexal torsion is higher with parovarian cysts, solid benign tumors, and serous cysts of the ovary. The right ovary has a greater tendency to twist (3 to 2) than does the left ovary. Torsion of a malignant ovarian tumor is comparatively rare.

Patients with adnexal torsion present with acute, severe, unilateral, lower abdominal and pelvic pain. Often the patient relates the onset of the severe pain to an abrupt change of position. A unilateral, extremely tender adnexal mass is found in more than 90% of patients. Approximately two thirds of patients have associated nausea and vomiting. These associated gastrointestinal symptoms sometimes lead to a preoperative diagnosis of acute appendicitis or small intestinal obstruction. Many patients have noted intermittent previous episodes of similar pain for several days to several weeks. The hypothesis is that previous episodes of pain were secondary to partial torsion, with spontaneous reversal without significant vascular compromise. With progressive torsion, initially venous and lymphatic obstruction occurs. This produces a cyanotic, edematous ovary, which on pelvic examination presents as a unilateral, extremely tender adnexal mass. Further progression of the torsion interrupts the major arterial supply to the ovary, resulting in hypoxia, adnexal necrosis, and a concomitant low-grade fever and leukocytosis. Fever is more common in women who have developed necrosis of the adnexa. Approximately 10% of women with adnexal torsion have a repetitive episode affecting the contralateral adnexum.

Most patients with adnexal torsion present with symptoms and signs severe enough to demand operative intervention (Fig. 18-65). Some authors have reported the successful use of Doppler ultrasound to evaluate ovarian arterial blood flow to help diagnose torsion. Abnormal color Doppler flow is highly predictive of torsion of the ovary. However, approximately 50% of women with surgically confirmed adnexal torsion will have a normal Doppler flow study. Increasingly, women with ovarian torsion are being treated via laparoscopic surgery. The most common gynecologic conditions that may be confused with adnexal torsion are a ruptured corpus luteum or an adnexal abscess. In recent series emphasizing the early diagnosis of adnexal torsion, conservative operative management has been possible in 75% of cases.

Because the majority of cases of adnexal torsion occur in young women, a conservative operation is ideal. The clinician should maintain a high index of suspicion for adnexal torsion so that early and conservative surgery is possible. Although salpingo-oophorectomy has been the routine treatment for ovarian torsion, many authors have reported large series of conservative management. Conservative surgery either through the laparoscope or via laparotomy entails gentle untwisting of the pedicle, possibly cystectomy, and stabilization of the ovary with sutures. McHutchison and colleagues have suggested the use of intravenous fluorescein intraoperatively with subsequent inspection of the untwisted ovary with an ultraviolet light to document vascular integrity. A recent review of the literature documented the risk of pulmonary embolus with adnexal torsion as approximately 0.2%. The risk was similar regardless of whether the condition was managed by conservative surgery with untwisting or adnexal removal without untwisting. With severe vascular compromise, the appropriate operation is unilateral salpingo-oophorectomy. The vascular pedicle should be clamped with care so as not to injure the ureter, which may be tented up by the torsion.

Ovarian Remnant Syndrome

Chronic pelvic pain secondary to a small area of functioning ovarian tissue following intended total removal of both ovaries is termed *ovarian remnant syndrome.* Most of the women who develop this condition had endometriosis or chronic pelvic inflammatory disease and extensive pelvic adhesions discovered

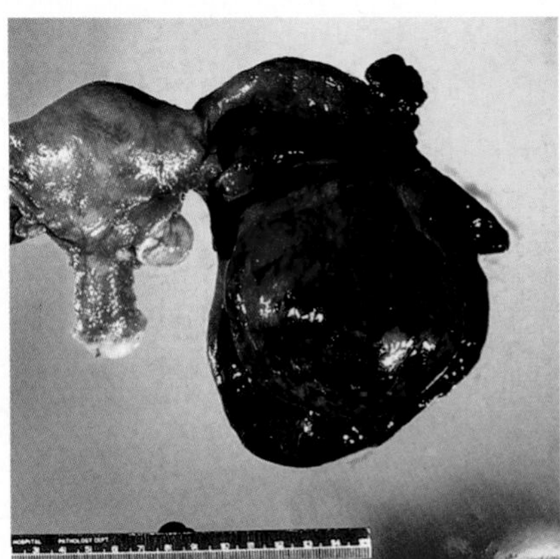

Figure 18-65. Adnexal torsion with hemorrhagic infarction. A benign cyst was found in the ovary. (From Clement PB, Young RH: Atlas of Gynecologic Surgical Pathology. Philadelphia, WB Saunders, 2000.)

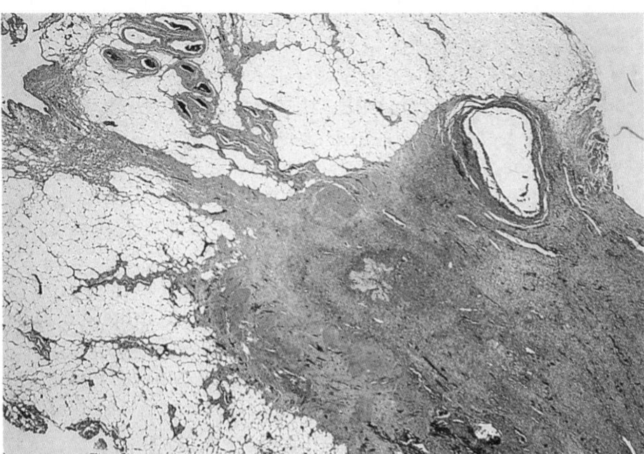

Figure 18-66. Ovarian remnant syndrome. Ovarian tissue that was left behind at the time of oophorectomy has regrown and is functional. (From Robboy SJ, Bentley RC, Russell P, Anderson MC: The peritoneum. In Robboy SJ, Anderson MC, Russell P [eds]: Pathology of the Female Reproductive Tract. Edinburgh, Churchill Livingstone, 2002.)

during previous surgical procedures. A more recently described risk factor is laparoscopic oophorectomy.

The chronic pelvic pain is usually cyclic and exacerbated following coitus. The masses are small, approximately 3 cm in diameter, and located in the retroperitoneal space immediately adjacent to either ureter. Histologically, the mass contains both ovarian follicles and stroma (Fig. 18-66). If the mass cannot be palpated during pelvic examination, imaging studies such as vaginal ultrasound or MRI are often helpful. Premenopausal levels of FSH or estradiol help to establish the diagnosis in a woman who has a history of a bilateral salpingo-oophorectomy. However, sometimes a small area of ovarian tissue does not produce enough circulating estrogen to suppress gonadotropins. Difficult cases have been diagnosed by challenging and stimulating the suspected ovarian remnant with either clomiphene citrate or a GnRH agonist.

Once the diagnosis is suspected, the most effective treatment is surgical removal of the ovarian remnant. The tissue should be removed by laparoscopy or laparotomy with wide excision of the mass using meticulous techniques so as to protect the integrity of the ureter. The recurrence rate is approximately 10%.

KEY POINTS

- Some urethral caruncles are asymptomatic; others cause dysuria, frequency, and urgency. In elderly women they must be differentiated from urethral carcinoma by biopsy. Treatment of urethral caruncles is topical or oral estrogen therapy.
- Physical compression of a Skene's duct cyst, unlike compression of a urethral diverticula, should not produce fluid from the urethral meatus.
- The majority of urethral carcinomas are of squamous cell origin. Most of these rare carcinomas arise from the distal urethra.
- Urethral prolapse is predominantly a disease of the premenarcheal female, although it does occur in postmenopausal women.
- The most common large cyst of the vulva is a cystic dilation of an obstructed Bartholin's duct. The most common small vulvar cysts are epidermal inclusion cysts or sebaceous cysts.
- The vulva contains 1% of the skin surface of the body, but 5% to 10% of all malignant melanomas in women arise from this region.
- Ideally, all vulvar nevi should be excised and examined histologically. Special emphasis should be directed toward the flat junctional nevus and the dysplastic nevus for they have the greatest potential for malignant transformation. The dysplastic nevus is characterized by being more than 5 mm in diameter, with irregular borders and patches of variegated pigment.
- Symptoms of an early malignant melanoma include *asymmetry, border* irregularity, *color* variegation, and a *diameter* usually greater than 6 mm (ABCD).
- Vulvar hemangiomas frequently are discovered initially during childhood. Approximately 60% of vulvar hemangiomas discovered during the first years of life spontaneously regress in size by the time the child goes to school.
- Fibromas are the most common benign solid tumors of the vulva. Lipomas are the second most frequent benign vulvar mesenchymal tumor.
- Hidradenomas are rare, small, benign, asymptomatic vulvar tumors originating from apocrine glands and are found in white women between 30 and 70 years of age.
- Endometriosis of the vulva is rare, with only 1 in 500 women with endometriosis having vulvar involvement.
- The most common symptoms of endometriosis of the vulva are pain and introital dyspareunia. The classic history is cyclic discomfort and an enlargement of the mass associated with menstrual periods.
- The management of nonobstetrical vulvar hematomas is usually conservative unless the hematoma is greater than 10 cm in diameter or rapidly increasing.
- The majority of vulvar skin problems are red, scalelike rashes, and the woman's primary complaint is of pruritus.
- Substances that are irritants produce immediate symptoms such as a stinging and burning sensation when applied to the vulvar skin. The symptoms and signs secondary to an irritant disappear within 12 hours of discontinuing the offending substance. In contrast, allergic contact dermatitis requires 36 to 48 hours to manifest its symptoms and signs. Often the signs of allergic contact dermatitis persist for several days despite removal of the allergen.
- The most common causes of vulvar contact dermatitis are cosmetic and local therapeutic agents. External chemicals that trigger the disease process must be avoided.
- Women usually develop psoriasis during their teenage years, with approximately 3% of adult women being affected. Approximately 20% of these have involvement of the vulvar skin.
- The margins of psoriasis are better defined than the common skin conditions in the differential diagnosis including candidiasis, seborrheic dermatitis, and eczema. Psoriasis does not involve the vagina, only the vulva.
- Lichen sclerosus does not involve the vagina, whereas lichen planus may involve the vagina.
- Hidradenitis suppurativa is a chronic, unrelenting, refractory infection of the skin and subcutaneous tissue. The diagnosis should be confirmed by biopsy.
- Urethral diverticula occur in approximately 1% to 3% of women.
- Classically, the symptoms associated with the urethral diverticulum are extremely chronic in nature and they have not resolved with multiple courses of oral antibiotic therapy.
- The two most common methods of diagnosing urethral diverticula are voiding cystourethrography and cystourethroscopy. Other diagnostic tests used to identify urethral diverticula include urethral pressure profile recordings, vaginal ultrasound, positive-pressure urethrography, and MRI.
- Embryonic cysts of the vagina, especially those on the anterior lateral wall, are usually Gartner's duct cysts. These cysts

KEY POINTS *Continued*

are most commonly found in the lower one third of the vagina.
- Prolonged tampon use may be associated with ulcerations of the vagina, discharge, and bleeding.
- Endocervical polyps are smooth, soft, red, fragile masses. They are found most commonly in multiparous women in their 40s and 50s.
- After the endocervical polyp is removed, endometrial sampling should be performed to diagnose a coexisting endometrial hyperplasia or carcinoma.
- Depending on the series, 3% to 8% of myomas are categorized as cervical myomas. Because of the relative paucity of smooth muscle fibers in the cervical stroma, the majority of myomas that appear to be cervical actually arise from the isthmus of the uterus.
- The causes of acquired cervical stenosis are operative, radiation, infection, neoplasia, or atrophic changes. Cone biopsy and cautery of the cervix, either electrocautery or cryocoagulation, are the operations that most commonly cause cervical stenosis.
- Endometrial polyps are noted in approximately 10% of women when the uterus is examined at autopsy. Approximately one in four women with abnormal bleeding will have an endometrial polyp.
- Malignant transformation of endometrial polyps has been estimated to occur in 0.5% of cases and is most often an endometrial carcinoma of low grade and stage.
- Hematometra in postmenopausal women is often asymptomatic. Appropriate biopsy specimens of the endocervical canal and endometrium should be obtained to rule out malignancy when the cause of hematometra is not obvious.
- Leiomyomas are the most frequent pelvic tumors, with the highest prevalence occurring during the fifth decade of a woman's life.
- Symptomatic uterine leiomyomas are the primary indication for approximately 30% of all hysterectomies.
- Five to 10% of myomas are submucosal, often presenting with symptoms of abnormal vaginal bleeding.
- The cause of uterine leiomyomas is incompletely understood. It is known that each tumor results from an original single muscle cell. Each individual uterine myoma is monoclonal. All the cells are derived from one progenitor myocyte.
- Acute muscular infarction, as is seen with red degeneration of a myoma, causes severe pain and localized peritoneal irritation.
- The majority of women with uterine myomas are asymptomatic, but one of three will experience pelvic pain, with dysmenorrhea being the most frequent complaint.
- Abnormal bleeding is experienced by 30% of women with myomas, with the most common symptom being menorrhagia, but intermenstrual spotting and disruption of the normal pattern are other frequent complaints.
- The management of women with small, asymptomatic myomas is conservative, and the majority of women will not need operations.
- Women with abnormal bleeding and leiomyomas should be investigated thoroughly for concurrent problems, such as endometrial hyperplasia.
- In comparison studies, the relative morbidity of abdominal hysterectomy and myomectomy is similar when one controls for uterine size.
- Classic indications for myomectomy include rapidly expanding pelvic mass, persistent abnormal bleeding, pain or pressure, or enlargement of an asymptomatic myoma to more than 8 cm in a woman who has not completed childbearing.
- Prolapse of a myoma through the cervix is optimally treated by vaginal removal and ligation of the base of the myoma.
- It is possible to treat leiomyomas medically by reducing the circulating level of estrogen and progesterone. Gonadotropin-releasing hormone (GnRH) agonists will reduce the mean uterine volume and myoma size by 40% to 50%. However, individual response varies greatly, from no response to an 80% reduction in uterine size. The vast majority of the reduction in size occurs within the first 3 months.
- The newest modality to manage uterine myomas is transcatheter uterine artery embolization as an ambulatory nonsurgical technique. Postprocedural abdominal and pelvic pain is common for the first 24 hours. Success rates in regard to decreasing menorrhagia and reduction in uterine size are promising.
- Adenomyosis is frequently asymptomatic. If multiple serial sections of the uterus are obtained, the incidence may exceed 60% in women 40 to 50 years of age.
- Pelvic MRI may be the most accurate imaging modality for adenomyosis.
- Symptomatic adenomyosis primarily occurs in parous women older than age 35. The classic symptoms are secondary dysmenorrhea and menorrhagia. The most common physical sign is a diffusely enlarged uterus, usually two to three times normal size.
- The severity of pelvic symptoms associated with adenomyosis increases proportionally to the depth of penetration and the total volume of disease in the myometrium.
- Adenomyosis rarely causes uterine enlargement greater than a size at 14 weeks' gestation unless there is concomitant uterine pathology.
- The most prevalent benign tumor of the oviduct is the angiomyoma or adenomatoid tumor. They are small, gray-white, circumscribed nodules, 1 to 2 cm in diameter.
- The main symptom of torsion of the tube is pain, usually located in the iliac fossa, with radiation to the thigh and flank. In two thirds of cases the pain is associated with nausea and vomiting.
- Follicular cysts are the most common cystic structures in normal ovaries. The cysts are frequently multiple and may vary from a few millimeters to as large as 15 cm in diameter.
- The initial management of a suspected follicular cyst is conservative observation. The majority of follicular cysts disappear spontaneously by either reabsorption of the cyst fluid or silent rupture within 4 to 8 weeks of initial diagnosis.

Continued

KEY POINTS *Continued*

- The practice of aspirating cysts via the laparoscope should be limited to cysts that are completely simple and associated with normal CA-125 levels.
- Corpus luteum cysts may be associated with either normal endocrine function or prolonged secretion of progesterone. The associated menstrual pattern may be normal, delayed menstruation, or amenorrhea.
- Women with a bleeding diathesis or taking warfarin (Coumadin) are especially prone to develop hemorrhage from rupture of a corpus luteum cyst. Bleeding occurs usually between days 20 to 26 of their cycle.
- The differential diagnosis of a woman with acute pain and a suspected ruptured corpus luteum cyst includes ectopic pregnancy, a ruptured endometrioma, and adnexal torsion.
- The treatment of unruptured corpus luteum cysts is conservative. However, if the cyst persists or intraperitoneal bleeding occurs, necessitating operation, the treatment is cystectomy.
- Drainage or fenestration is effective for follicular cysts and poorly effective for cystadenomas. They will tend to recur. When cysts are drained, it is essential to remember that cytologic examination of cyst fluid has poor predictive value and poor sensitivity in differentiating benign from malignant cysts.
- Theca lutein cysts arise from either prolonged or excessive stimulation of the ovaries by endogenous or exogenous gonadotropins or increased ovarian sensitivity to gonadotropins. The condition of ovarian enlargement secondary to the development of multiple luteinized follicular cysts is termed hyperreactio luteinalis. Approximately 50% of molar pregnancies and 10% of choriocarcinomas have associated bilateral theca lutein cysts.
- Benign ovarian teratomas vary from a few millimeters to 25 cm, may be single or multiple, and are bilateral 10% to 15% of the time.
- Dermoids are believed to arise during fetal life from a single germ cell. They are 46,XX in karyotype.
- Histologically, benign teratomas are composed of mature cells, usually from all three germ layers. Most solid elements arise and are contained in a protrusion or nipple (mamilla) in the cyst wall termed the prominence or tubercle of Rokitansky. This prominence may be visualized by ultrasound as an echodense region, thus aiding in the sonographic diagnosis.
- Although most dermoids are asymptomatic, torsion and rupture are two important complications.
- Operative treatment of benign cystic teratomas is cystectomy with preservation of as much normal ovarian tissue as possible.
- The most common symptoms associated with ovarian endometriosis are pelvic pain, dyspareunia, and infertility.
- Medical therapy is rarely successful in treating ovarian endometriosis if the disease has produced ovarian enlargement. Often, surgical therapy is complicated by formation of de novo and recurrent adhesions.
- Fibromas are the most common, benign, solid neoplasms of the ovary. They have a low malignant potential.
- Many ovarian fibromas are misdiagnosed and are believed to be leiomyomas prior to operation.
- Fibromas vary in size from small nodules to huge pelvic tumors weighing as much as 50 pounds. Ninety percent of fibromas are unilateral and have an average diameter of 6 cm.
- Fifty percent of patients with an ovarian fibroma will have ascites if the tumor is greater than 6 cm. The incidence of associated ascites is directly proportional to the size of the tumor.
- Transitional cell tumors (Brenner tumors) are small, smooth, solid, fibroepithelial tumors of the ovary. They usually occur in women between the ages of 40 and 60 and are predominantly unilateral.
- Adnexal torsion occurs most commonly in the reproductive years, with the average age of patients being in the mid-20s. Pregnancy predisposes to adnexal torsion.
- Ovarian tumors are discovered in 50% to 60% of women with adnexal torsion.
- Abnormal color Doppler flow is highly predictive of torsion of the ovary. However, approximately 50% of women with surgically confirmed adnexal torsion will have a normal Doppler flow study.
- The risk of pulmonary embolus with adnexal torsion as approximately 0.2%. The risk was similar regardless of whether the condition was managed by conservative surgery with untwisting or adnexal removal without untwisting.
- Chronic pelvic pain secondary to a small area of functioning ovarian tissue following intended total removal of both ovaries is termed *ovarian remnant syndrome.*

BIBLIOGRAPHY

Abulafia O, Sherer DM: Transcatheter uterine artery embolization for the management of symptomatic uterine leiomyomas. Obstet Gynecol Surv 54:745, 1999.

ACOG Committee Opinion: Vulvodynia. 345, 2006.

Aghajanian A, Bernstein L, Grimes DA: Bartholin's duct abscess and cyst: A case-control study. SMJ 87:26, 1994.

Ahnaimugan S, Asuen MI: Coital laceration of the vagina. Aust N Z J Obstet Gynaecol 20:180, 1980.

Al-Fozan H, Tulandi T: Factors affecting early surgical intervention after uterine artery embolization. Obstet and Gynecol Survey 57:810, 2002.

Al-Took S, Murray C, Tulandi T: Effects of pirfenidone and dermoid cyst fluid on adhesion formation. Fertil Steril 69:341, 1998.

Andersen PG, Christensen S, Detlefsen GU, Kern-Hansen P: Treatment of Bartholin's abscess: Marsupialization versus incision, curettage and suture under antibiotic cover. A randomized study with 6 months' follow-up. Acta Obstet Gynecol Scand 71:59, 1992.

Anderson M, Kutzner S, Kaufman RH: Treatment of vulvovaginal lichen planus with vaginal hydrocortisone suppositories. Obstet Gynecol 100:359, 2002.

Arnold LL, Ascher SM, Simon JA: Familial adenomyosis: A case report. Fertil Steril 61:1165, 1994.

Ascher SM, Arnold LL, Patt RH, et al: Adenomyosis: Prospective comparison of MR imaging and transvaginal sonography. Radiology 190:803, 1994.

Ascher SM, Jha RC, Reinhold C: Benign myometrial conditions: Leiomyomas and adenomyosis. TMRI 14:281-304, 2003.
Aungst M, Wilson M, Vournas K, et al: Necrotic leiomyoma and gram-negative sepsis eight weeks after uterine artery embolization. Am Col Obstet Gynecol 104:1161, 2004.
Axe S, Parmley T, Woodruff JD, et al: Adenomas in minor vestibular glands. Obstet Gynecol 68:16, 1986.
Baird DD, Dunson DB, Hill MC, et al: High cumulative incidence of uterine leiomyoma in black and white women: Ultrasound evidence. Am J Obstet Gynecol 188:100, 2003.
Bakour SH, Khan KS, Gupta JK: The risk of premalignant and malignant pathology in endometrial polyps. Acta Obstet Gynecol Scand 79:317, 2000.
Bakri YN, Bakhashwain M, Hugosson C: Massive theca-lutein cysts, virilization, and hypothyroidism associated with normal pregnancy. Acta Obstet Gynecol Scand 73:153, 1994.
Balasa RW, Adcock LL, Prem KA, et al: The Brenner tumor. Obstet Gynecol 50:120, 1977.
Baldauf JJ, Dreyfus M, Ritter J, et al: Risk of cervical stenosis after large loop excision or laser conization. Obstet Gynecol 88:933, 1996.
Barbieri RL: Ambulatory management of uterine leiomyomata. Clin Obstet Gynecol 42:196, 1999.
Barbieri RL, Dilena M, Chumas J, et al: Leuprolide acetate depot decreases the number of nucleolar organizer regions in uterine leiomyomata. Fertil Steril 60:569, 1993.
Baron JA, LaVecchia C, Levi F: The antiestrogenic effect of cigarette smoking in women. Am J Obstet Gynecol 162:502, 1990.
Barrett KF, Bledsoe S, Greer BE, et al: Tampon-induced vaginal or cervical ulceration. Am J Obstet Gynecol 127:332, 1977.
Bayer AI and Wiskind AK: Adnexal torsion: Can the adnexa be saved? Am J Obstet Gynecol 171:1506, 1994.
Bazot M, Cortez A, Sananes S, et al: Imaging of dermoid cysts with foci of immature tissue. J Comput Assist Tomogr 23:703, 1999.
Belardi MG, Maglione MA, Vighi S, di Paola GR: Syringoma of the vulva: a case report. J Reprod Med 39:957, 1994.
Bernardus RE, Van Der Slikke JW, Roex AJM, et al: Torsion of the fallopian tube: Some considerations on its etiology. Obstet Gynecol 64:675, 1984.
Bider D, Maschiach S, Dulitzky M, et al: Clinical, surgical and pathologic findings of adnexal torsion in pregnant and nonpregnant women. Surg Gynecol Obstet 173:363, 1991.
Birch HW, Sondag DR: Granular-cell myoblastoma of the vulva. Obstet Gynecol 18:443, 1961.
Blaivas JG, Flisser AJ, Bleustein CB, et al: Periurethral masses: Etiology and diagnosis in a large series of women. Am College Obstet Gynecol 103:842, 2004.
Blickstein I, Feldberg E, Dgani R, et al: Dysplastic vulvar nevi. Obstet Gynecol 78:968, 1991.
Boardman LA, Botte J: Recurrent vulvar itching. Am College Obstet Gynecol 105:1451, 2005.
Bornstein J, Zarfati D, Goldik Z, Abramovici H: Vulvar vestibulitis: physical or psychosexual problem? Obstet Gynecol 93:876, 1999.
Bradham DD, Stovall TG, Thompson CD: Use of GnRH agonist before hysterectomy: A cost simulation. Obstet Gynecol 85:401, 1995.
Broder MS, Goodwin S, Chen G, et al: Comparison of long-term outcomes of myomectomy and uterine artery embolization. Am College Obstet Gynecol 100:864, 2002.
Brosens I, Deprest J, Dal Cin P, Van Den Berghe H: Clinical significance of cytogenetic abnormalities in uterine myomas. Fertil Steril 69:232, 1998.
Brosens I, Johannison E, Dal Cin P, et al: Analysis of the karyotype and deoxyribonucleic acid content of uterine myomas in premenopausal, menopausal, and gonadotropin-releasing hormone agonist-treated females. Fertil Steril 66:376, 1996.
Burton CA, Grimes DA, March CM: Surgical management of leiomyomata during pregnancy. Obstet Gynecol 74:707, 1989.
Byun JY, Kim SE, Choi BG, et al: Diffuse and focal adenomyosis: MR imaging findings. Radiographics 19:S161, 1999.
Canis M, Mage G, Pouly JL, et al: Laparoscopic diagnosis of adnexal cystic masses: A 12-year experience with long-term follow-up. Obstet Gynecol 83:707, 1994.
Canis M, Mage G, Wattiez A, et al: Second-look laparoscopy after laparoscopic cystectomy of large ovarian endometriomas. Fertil Steril 58:617, 1992.
Cantuaria GHC, Angioli R, Frost L, et al: Comparison of bimanual examination with ultrasound examination before hysterectomy for uterine leiomyoma. Obstet Gynecol 92:109, 1998.
Carlson KJ, Nichols DH, Schiff I: Indications for hysterectomy. N Engl J Med 328:856, 1993.
Carneiro SJC, Gardner HL, Knox JM: Syringoma: three cases with vulvar involvement. Obstet Gynecol 39:95, 1972.
Carpenter TT, Walker WJ: Pregnancy following uterine artery embolisation for symptomatic fibroids: A series of 26 completed pregnancies. Int J Obstet Gynecol 112:321, 2005.
Carr BR, Marshburn PB, Weatherall PT, et al: An evaluation of the effect of gonadotropin-releasing hormone analogs and medroxyprogesterone acetate on uterine leiomyomata volume by magnetic resonance imaging: A prospective, randomized, double-blind, placebo-controlled, crossover trial. J Clin Endocrinol Metab 76:1217, 1993.
Caspi B, Appleman Z, Rabinerson D, et al: The growth pattern of ovarian dermoid cysts: A prospective study in premenopausal and postmenopausal women. Fertil Steril 68:501, 1997.
Caspi B, Lerner-Geva L, Dahan M, et al: A possible genetic factor in the pathogenesis of ovarian dermoid cysts. Gynecol Obstet Invest 56:2003-6, 2003.
Cin PD, Vanni R, Marras S, et al: Four cytogenetic subgroups can be identified in endometrial polyps. Cancer Res 55:1565, 1995.
Coates JB, Hales JS: Granular cell myoblastoma of the vulva. Obstet Gynecol 41:796, 1973.
Cohen LS, Valle RF: Role of vaginal sonography and hysterosonography in the endoscopic treatment of uterine myomas. Fertil Steril 73:197, 2000.
Cohen Z, Shinhar D, Kopernik G, Mares AJ: The laparoscopic approach to uterine adnexal torsion in childhood. J Pediatr Surg 31:1557, 2000.
Comerci JT Jr, Licciardi F, Bergh PA, et al: Mature cystic teratoma: A clinicopathologic evaluation of 517 cases and review of the literature. Obstet Gynecol 84:22, 1994.
Controversies and challenges in the modern management of uterine fibroids. BJOG 111:95, 2004.
Cramer SF, Robertson AL, Ziats NP, et al: Growth potential of human uterine leiomyomas: Some in vitro observations and their implications. Obstet Gynecol 66:36, 1985.
Danikas D, Goudas VT, Rao CV, Brief DK: Luteinizing hormone receptor expression in leiomyomatosis peritonealis disseminata. Obstet Gynecol 95:1009, 2000.
Davies A, Hart R, Magos AL: The excision of uterine fibroids by vaginal myomectomy: A prospective study. Fertil Steril 71:961, 1999.
DeCrespigny LC, Robinson HP, Davoren RAM, et al: The 'simple' ovarian cyst: Aspirate or operate? Br J Obstet Gynaecol 96:1035, 1989.
Deppisch LM: Cysts of the vagina. Obstet Gynecol 45:623, 1975.
DeWaay DJ, Syrop CH, Nygaard IE, et al: Natural history of uterine polyps and leiomyomata. Am College Obstet Gynecol 100:3, 2002.
DeWilde R, Bordt J, Hesseling M, et al: Ovarian cystostomy. Acta Obstet Gynecol Scand 68:363, 1989.
Dische FE, Ritche JM: Luteoma of pregnancy. J Pathol 100:77, 1970.
Dmochowski RR, Ganabathi K, Zimmern PE, Leach GE: Benign female periurethral masses. J Urol 152:1943, 1994.
Dottino PR, Levine DA, Ripley DL, Cohen CJ: Laparoscopic management of adnexal masses in premenopausal and postmenopausal women. Obstet Gynecol 93:223, 1999.
Dreyer L, Simson IW, Sevenster CBO, et al: Leiomyomatosis peritonealis disseminata: A report of two cases and a review of the literature. Br J Obstet Gynaecol 92:856, 1985.
Dubuisson JB, Lecuru F, Foulot H, et al: Myomectomy by laparoscopy: A preliminary report of 43 cases. Fertil Steril 56:827, 1991.
Duckman S, Suarez JR, Sese LQ: Giant cervical polyp. Am J Obstet Gynecol 159:852, 1988.
Dunnihoo DR, Wolff J: Bilateral torsion of the adnexa: A case report and a review of the world literature. Obstet Gynecol 64:55S, 1984.
Dunton CJ, Kautzky M, Hanau C: Malignant melanoma of the vulva: A review. Obstet Gynecol Surv 50:739, 1995.
Edwards L: New concepts in vulvodynia. Am J Obstet Gynecol 189:S24, 2003.
Eilber KS, Raz S: Benign cystic lesions of the vagina: A literature review. J Urol 170:717, 2003.
Ekerhovd E, Wienerroith H, Staudach A, et al: Preoperative assessment of unilocular adnexal cysts by transvaginal ultrasonography: A comparison between ultrasonographic morphologic imaging and histopatholigic diagnosis. Am J Obstet Gynecol 184:48, 2001.
Emanuel MH, Vamsteker K, Hart AAM, et al: Long-term results of hysteroscopic myomectomy for abnormal uterine bleeding. Obstet Gynecol 93:743, 1999.

Evans AT, Symmonds RE, Gaffey TA: Recurrent pelvic intravenous leiomyomatosis. Obstet Gynecol 57:260, 1981.
Farber EM, Nall L: Genital psoriasis. Cutis 50:263, 1992.
Farrar HK, Nedoss BR: Benign tumors of the uterine cervix. Am J Obstet Gynecol 81:124, 1961.
Fedele L, Bianchi S, Dorta M, et al: Transvaginal ultrasonography in the diagnosis of diffuse adenomyosis. Fertil Steril 58:94, 1992.
Fedele L, Bianchi S, Raffaelli R, et al: Treatment of adenomyosis-associated menorrhagia with a levonorgestrel-releasing intrauterine device, Fertil Steril 68:426, 1997.
Fedele L, Vercellini P, Bianchi S, et al: Treatment with GnRH agonists before myomectomy and the risk of short-term myoma recurrence. Br J Obstet Gynaecol 97:393, 1990.
Fischer G: Management of vulvar pain. Dermatol Ther 17:134, 2004.
Fischer G: The commonest causes of symptomatic vulvar disease: A dermatologist's perspective. Austl J Dermatol 57:12, 1996.
Fischer G, Spurrett B, Fischer A: The chronically symptomatic vulva: Etiology and management. Br J Obstet Gynaecol 102:773, 1995.
Flake GP, Andersen J, Dixon D: Etiology and pathogenesis of uterine leiomyomas: A review. Environ Health Perspect 111:1037, 2003.
Flierman PA, Oberye JJL, van der Hulst VPM, et al: Rapid reduction of leiomyoma volume during treatment with GnRH antagonist ganirelix. BJOG 112:638, 2005.
Foster DC: Vulvar disease. Am College Obstet Gynecol 100:145, 2002.
Friedel W, Kaiser IH: Vaginal evisceration. Obstet Gynecol 45:315, 1975.
Friedman AJ: Use of gonadotropin-releasing hormone agonists before myomectomy. Clin Obstet Gynecol 36:650, 1993.
Friedman AJ, Daly M, Juneau-Norcross M, Rein MS: Predictors of uterine volume reduction in women with myomas treated with a gonadotropin-releasing hormone agonist. Fertil Steril 58:413, 1992.
Friedman AJ, Haas ST: Should uterine size be an indication for surgical intervention in women with myomas? Am J Obstet Gynecol 168:751, 1993.
Friedman AJ, Hoffman DI, Comite F, et al: Treatment of leiomyomata uteri with leuprolide acetate depot: A double-blind, placebo-controlled, multicenter study. Obstet Gynecol 77:720, 1991.
Friedman RJ, Rigel DS, Kopf AW: Early detection of malignant melanoma: The role of physician examination and self-examination of the skin. CA 35:130, 1985.
Friedrich EG: Tampon effects on vaginal health. Clin Obstet Gynecol 24:395, 1981.
Friedrich EG, Wilkinson EJ: Vulvar surgery for neurofibromatosis. Obstet Gynecol 65:135, 1985.
Fong YF, Singh K: Medical treatment of a grossly enlarged adenomyotic uterus with the levonorgestrel-releasing intrauterine system. Contraception 60:173, 1999.
Gebauer G, Hafner A, Siebzehnrubl E, et al: Role of hysteroscopy in detection and extraction of endometrial polyps: Results of a prospective study. Am J Obstet Gynecol 184:59, 2001.
Gerber GS, Schoenberg HW: Female urinary tract fistulas. J Urol 149:229, 1993.
Gerrard ER, Lloyd K, Kubricht WS, et al: Transvaginal ultrasound for the diagnosis of urethral diverticulum. J Urol 169:1395, 2003.
Ginsburg D, Genadry R: Suburethral diverticulum: Classification and therapeutic considerations. Obstet Gynecol 61:685, 1983.
Goldberg J, Pereira L, Berghella V, et al: Pregnancy outcomes after treatment of fibromyomata: Uterine artery embolization versus laparoscopic myomectomy. Am J Obstet Gynecol 191:18, 2004.
Goldenberg M, Sivan E, Sharabi Z, et al: Outcome of hysteroscopic resection of submucous myomas for infertility. Fertil Steril 64:714, 1995.
Goldstein SR, Monteagudo A, Popiolek D, et al: Evaluation of endometrial polyps. Am J Obstet Gynecol 186:669, 2002.
Goodwin SC, McLucas B, Lee M, et al: Uterine artery embolization for the treatment of uterine leiomyomata midterm results. JVIR 10:1159, 1999.
Gordon JD, Hopkins KL, Jeffrey RB, Giudice LC: Adnexal torsion: color Doppler diagnosis and laparoscopic treatment. Fertil Steril 61:383, 1994.
Grimes DA, Hughs JM: Use of multiphasic oral contraceptives and hospitalizations of women with functional ovarian cysts in the United States. Obstet Gynecol 73:1037, 1989.
Guilbeault H, Wilson SR, Lickrish GM: Massive uterine enlargement with necrosis: An unusual manifestation of adenomyosis. J Ultrasound Med 13:326, 1994.
Haefner HK, Andersen F, Johnson MP: Vaginal laceration following a jet-ski accident. Obstet Gynecol 78:986, 1991.
Hallatt JG, Steele CH, Snyder M: Ruptured corpus luteum with hemoperitoneum: A study of 173 surgical cases. Am J Obstet Gynecol 149:5, 1984.
Hart WR: Paramesonephric mucinous cysts of the vulva. Am J Obstet Gynecol 107:1079, 1980.
Hartge P, Hayes R, Reding D, et al: Complex ovarian cysts in postmenopausal women are not associated with ovarian cancer risk factors. Am J Obstet Gynecol 183:1232, 2000.
Havrilesky LJ, Peterson BL, Dryden DK, et al: Predictors of clinical outcomes in the laparoscopic management of adnexal masses. Obstet Gynecol 102:243, 2003.
Herndon JH: Itching: The pathophysiology of pruritus. Int J Dermatol 14:465, 1975.
Higgins RV, Matkins JF, Marroum MC: Comparison of fine-needle aspiration cytologic findings of ovarian cysts with ovarian histologic findings. Am J Obstet Gynecol 180:550, 1999.
Hillis SD, Marchbanks PA, Peterson HB: Uterine size and risk of complications among women undergoing abdominal hysterectomy for leiomyomas. Obstet Gynecol 87:539, 1996.
Hirata JD, Moghissi KS, Ginsburg KA: Pregnancy after medical therapy of adenomyosis with a gonadotropin-releasing hormone agonist. Fertil Steril 59:444, 1993.
Hovsepian DM, Siskin GP, Bonn J, et al: Quality improvement guidelines for uterine artery embolization for symptomatic leiomyomata. Cardiovasc Intervent Radiol 27:307, 2004.
Huang SC, Yu CH, Huang RT, et al: Intratumoral blood flow in uterine myoma correlated with a lower tumor size and volume, but not correlated with cell proliferation or angiogenesis. Obstet Gynecol 87:1019, 1996.
Huddock JJ, Dupayne N, McGeary JA: Traumatic vulvar hematomas. Am J Obstet Gynecol 70:1064, 1955.
Huffman JW: The detailed anatomy of the paraurethral ducts in the adult human female. Am J Obstet Gynecol 55:86, 1948.
Hurst BS, Matthews ML, Marshburn PB: Laparoscopic myomectomy for symptomatic uterine myomas. Fertil Steril 83:1, 2005.
Innamaa A, Nunns D: The management of vulval pain syndromes. Hosp Med 66:23, 2005.
Iosif CS, Akerlund M: Fibromyomas and uterine activity. Acta Obstet Gynecol Scand 62:165, 1983.
Israel SL: The clinical similarity of corpus luteum cyst and ectopic pregnancy. Am J Obstet Gynecol 44:22, 1942.
Iverson RE Jr, Chelmow D, Strohbehn K, et al: Relative morbidity of abdominal hysterectomy and myomectomy for management of uterine leiomyomas, Obstet Gynecol 88:415, 1996.
Iverson RE Jr, Chelmow D, Strohbehn K, et al: Myomectomy fever: testing the dogma. Fertil Steril 72:104, 1999.
Jha RC, Takahama J, Imaoka I, et al: Adenomyosis: MRI of the uterus treated with uterine artery embolization. AJR 181:851, 2003.
Jimmerson SD, Becker JD: Vaginal ulcers associated with tampon usage. Obstet Gynecol 56:97, 1980.
Joura EA, Zeisler H, Bancher-Todesca D, et al: Short-term effects of topical testosterone in vulvar lichen sclerosus. Obstet Gynecol 89:297, 1997.
Kampraath S, Possover M, Schneider A: Description of a laparoscopic technique for treating patients with ovarian remnant syndrome. Fertil Steril 68:663, 1997.
Katz VL, Dotters DJ, Droegemueller W: Complications of uterine leiomyomas in pregnancy. Obstet Gynecol 73:593, 1989.
Kaufman RH, Faro S, Friedrich EG Jr, Gardner HL: Benign Diseases of the Vulva and Vagina, 4th ed. St. Louis, Mosby, 1994.
Kemmann E, Ghazi DM, Corsan GH: Adnexal torsion in menotropin-induced pregnancies. Obstet Gynecol 76:403, 1990.
Knudsen UB, Tabor A, Mosgaard B, et al: Management of ovarian cysts. Acta Obstet Gynecol Scand 83:1012, 2004.
Koonings PP, Grimes DA: Adnexal torsion in postmenopausal women. Obstet Gynecol 73:11, 1989.
Kruger E, Heller DS: Adnexal torsion: a clinicopathologic review of 31 cases. J Reprod Med 44:71, 1999.
Kupfer MC, Schiller VL, Hansen GC, Tessler FN: Transvaginal sonographic evaluation of endometrial polyps. J Ultrasound Med 13:535, 1994.
Kurjak A, Schulman H, Sosic A, et al: Transvaginal ultrasound, color flow, and Doppler waveform of the postmenopausal adnexal mass. Obstet Gynecol 80:917, 1992.

Kurman RJ (ed): Blaustein's Pathology of the Female Genital Tract, 4th ed. New York, Springer-Verlag, 1994.
Lafferty HW, Angiioli R, Rudolph J, Penalver MA: Ovarian remnant syndrome: Experience at Jackson Memorial Hospital, University of Miami, 1985 through 1993. Am J Obstet Gynecol 174:641, 1996.
Lahiti E, Vuopala S, Kauppila A, et al: Maturation of vaginal and endometrial epithelium in postmenopausal breast cancer patients receiving long-term tamoxifen. Gynecol Oncol 55:410, 1994.
Laing FC, Van Dalsem VF, Marks WM, et al: Dermoid cysts of the ovary: Their ultrasonographic appearances. Obstet Gynecol 57:99, 1981.
Lakkis WG, Martin MC, Gelfand MM: Benign cystic teratoma of the ovary: A 6-year review. Can J Surg 28:444, 1985.
LaMorte AI, Lalwani S, Diamond MP: Morbidity associated with abdominal myomectomy. Obstet Gynecol 82:897, 1993.
Lee RA: Diverticulum of the female urethra: Postoperative complications and results. Obstet Gynecol 61:52, 1983.
Lee RA: Diverticulum of the urethra: Clinical presentation, diagnosis, and management. Clin Obstet Gynecol 27:490, 1984.
Leibsohn S, d'Ablaing G, Mishell DR Jr, et al: Leiomyosarcoma in a series of hysterectomies performed for presumed uterine leiomyomas. Am J Obstet Gynecol 162:968, 1990.
Leppert PC, Catherin WH, Segars JH: A new hypothesis about the origin of uterine fibroids based on gene expression profiling with microarrays. Am J Obstet Gynecol 195:415, 2006.
Lethaby A, Vollenhoven B, Sowter M: Efficacy of pre-operative gonadotrophin hormone releasing analogues for women with uterine fibroids undergoing hysterectomy or myomectomy: A systematic review. BJOG 109:1097, 2002.
LevGur M, Abadi MA, Tucker A: Adenomyosis: Symptoms, histology, and pregnancy terminations. Obstet Gynecol 95:688, 2000.
LevGur M, Levie MD: The myomatous erythrocytosis syndrome: A review. Obstet Gynecol 86:1026, 1995.
Lewis FM: Vulvar lichen planus. Br J Dermatol 138:569, 1998.
Linder D, McCau BK, Hecht F: Parthenogenic origin of benign ovarian teratomas. N Engl J Med 292:63, 1975.
Lipitz S, Seidman DS, Menczer J, et al: Recurrence rate after fluid aspiration from sonographically benign-appearing ovarian cysts. J Reprod Med 37:845, 1992.
Loffer FD: Removal of large symptomatic intrauterine growths by the hysteroscopic resectoscope. Obstet Gynecol 76:836, 1990.
Luxman D, Bergman A, Sagi J, David MP: The postmenopausal adnexal mass: Correlation between ultrasonic and pathologic findings. Obstet Gynecol 77:726, 1991.
Maiman M, Seltzer V, Boyce J: Laparoscopic excision of ovarian neoplasms subsequently found to be malignant. Obstet Gynecol 77:563, 1991.
Mais V, Guerriero S, Ajossa S, et al: Transvaginal ultrasonography in the diagnosis of cystic teratoma.Obstet Gynecol 85:48, 1995.
Mann MS, Kaufman RH: Erosive lichen planus of the vulva. Clin Obstet Gynecol 34:605, 1991.
Marrocco-Trischitta MM, Nicodemi EM, Nater C, et al: Management of congenital venous malformations of the vulva. Obstet Gynecol 98:789, 2001.
Marshall LM, Spiegelman D, Barbieri RL, et al: Variation in the incidence of uterine leiomyoma among premenopausal women by age and race. Obstet Gynecol 90:967, 1997.
Marshall FC, Uson AC, Melicow MM: Neoplasms and caruncles of the female urethra. Surg Gynecol Obstet 110:723, 1960.
Matta WHM, Shaw RW, Nye M: Long-term follow-up of patients with uterine fibroids after treatment with the LHRH agonist buserelin. Br J Obstet Gynaecol 96:200, 1989.
McCausland AM: Hysteroscopic myometrial biopsy: Its use in diagnosing adenomyosis and its clinical application. Am J Obstet Gynecol 166:1619, 1992.
McCausland AM, McCausland VM: Frequency of symptomatic corneal hematometra and postablation tubal sterilization syndrome after total rollerball endometrial ablation: A 10-year follow-up. Am J Obstet Gynecol 186:1274, 2002.
McGovern PG, Noah R, Koenigsberg R, Little AB: Adnexal torsion and pulmonary embolism: Case report and review of the literature. Obstet Gynecol Surv 54:601, 1999.
McHutchison LLB, Koonings PP, Ballard CA, d'Ablaing G III: Preservation of ovarian tissue in adnexal torsion with fluorescein. Am J Obstet Gynecol 168:1386, 1993.
McKay M: Vulvar dermatoses. Clin Obstet Gynecol 34:614, 1991.
McLennan MT, Bent AE: Suburethral abscess: A complication of periurethral collagen injection therapy. Obstet Gynecol 92:650, 1998.
Meigs JV, Armstrong SH, Hamilton HH: A further contribution to the syndrome of fibroma of the ovary with fluid in the abdomen and chest, Meigs' syndrome. Am J Obstet Gynecol 46:19, 1943.
Meloni AM, Surti U, Contento AM, et al: Uterine leiomyomas: Cytogenetic and histologic profile. Obstet Gynecol 80:209, 1992.
Milingos S, Protopapas A, Drakakis P, et al: Laparoscopic treatment of ovarian dermoid cysts: Eleven years' experience. J Am Gynecol Laparosc 11:478, 2004.
Minke T, DePond W, Winkelmann T, Blythe J: Ovarian remnant syndrome: Study in laboratory rats. Am J Obstet Gynecol 171:1440, 1994.
Montz FJ, Schlaerth JB, Morrow CP: The natural history of theca lutein cysts. Obstet Gynecol 72:247, 1988.
Moon WJ, Koh BH, Kim SK, et al: Brenner tumor of the ovary: CT and MR findings. J Comput Assist Tomogr 24:72, 2000.
Moran O, Menczer J, Ben-Baruch G, et al: Cytologic examination of ovarian cyst fluid for the distinction between benign and malignant tumors. Obstet Gynecol 82:444, 1993.
Mulvaney NJ, Slavin JL, Östör AG, Fortune DW: Intravenous leiomyomatosis of the uterus: A clinicopathologic study of 22 cases. Int J Gynecol Pathol 13:1, 1994.
Murphy AA, Morales AJ, Kettel LM, Yen SSC: Regression of uterine leiomyomata to the antiprogesterone RU 486: Dose-response effect. Fertil Steril 64:187, 1995.
Mutter GL: Teratoma genetics and stem cells: A review. Obstet Gynecol Surv 42:661, 1987.
Naeyaert JM, Brochez L: Dysplastic nevi. N Engl J Med 249:23, 2003.
Nanda VS: Common dermatoses. Am J Obstet Gynecol 173:488, 1995.
Naumann RO, Droegemueller W: Unusual etiology of vulvar hematomas. Am J Obstet Gynecol 142:357, 1982.
Neuwirth RS: Urethral prolapse—a cause of vaginal bleeding in young girls. Obstet Gynecol 22:290, 1963.
Nezhat CH, Seidman DS, Nezhat FR, et al: Ovarian remnant syndrome after laparoscopic oophorectomy. Fertil Steril 74:1024, 2000.
Ngadiman S and Yang GCH: Adenomyomatous, lower uterine segment and endocervical polyps in cervicovaginal smears. Acta Cytol 39:643, 1995.
Nichols DH, Julian PJ: Torsion of the adnexa. Clin Obstet Gynecol 28:375, 1985.
NIH Consensus Development Panel on Early Melanoma: Diagnosis and treatment of early melanoma. JAMA 268:1314, 1992.
Niv J, Lessing JB, Hartuv J, Peyser MR: Vaginal injury resulting from sliding down a water chute. Am J Obstet Gynecol 166:930, 1992.
Novak ER, Woodruff JD (eds): Novak's Gynecologic and Obstetric Pathology with Clinical and Endocrine Relations, 8th ed. Philadelphia, WB Saunders, 1979.
Nucci MR, Young RH, Fletcher CDM: Cellular pseudosarcomatous fibroepithelial stromal polyps of the lower female genital tract: An underrecognized lesion often misdiagnosed as sarcoma. Am J Surg Pathol 24:231, 2000.
Oelsner G, Bider D, Goldenberg M, et al: Long-term follow-up of the twisted ischemic adnexa managed by detorsion. Fertil Steril 60:976, 1993.
Olive DL, Lindheim SR, Pritts EA: Non-surgical management of leiomyoma: impact on fertility. Current Opin Obstet Gynecol 16:239, 2004.
Outwater EK, Siegelman ES, Kim B, et al: Ovarian Brenner tumors: MR imaging characteristics. Magn Reson Imaging 16:1147, 1998.
Outwater EK, Siegelman ES, Talerman A, Dunton C: Ovarian fibromas and cystadenofibromas: MRI features of the fibrous component. J Magn Reson Imaging 7:465, 1997.
Outwater EK, Siegleman ES, Van Deerlin V: Adenomyosis: Current concepts and imaging considerations. AJR 170:437, 1998.
Paavonen J: Diagnosis and treatment of vulvodynia, Ann Med 27:175, 1995.
Paavonen J: Vulvodynia—a complex syndrome of vulvar pain, Acta Obstet Gynecol Scand 74:243, 1995.
Panganamamula UR, Harmanli OH, Isik-Akbay EF, et al: Is prior uterine surgery a risk factor for adenomyosis? Obstet Gynecol 104:1034, 2004.
Pantoja E, Rodriguez-Ibanez I, Axtmayer RW, et al: Complications of dermoid tumors of the ovary. Obstet Gynecol 45:89, 1975.
Parazzini F, Vercellini P, Panazza S, et al: Risk factors for adenomyosis. Hum Reprod 12:1275, 1997.
Parker MF, Conslato SS, Chang AS, et al: Chemical analysis of adnexal cyst fluid. Gynecol Oncol 73:16, 1999.

Parker WH, Berek JS: Management of selected cystic adnexal masses in postmenopausal women by operative laparoscopy: a pilot study. Am J Obstet Gynecol 163:1574, 1990.
Parker WH, Fu YS, Berek JS: Uterine sarcoma in patients operated on for presumed leiomyoma and rapidly growing leiomyoma. Obstet Gynecol 83:414, 1994.
Patrizi A, Neri I, Marzaduri S, et al: Syringoma: a review of twenty-nine cases. Acta Derm Venereol 78:460, 1998.
Paull T, Tedeschi LG: Perineal endometriosis at the site of episiotomy scar. Obstet Gynecol 40:28, 1972.
Payne JF, Robboy SJ, Haney AF: Embolic microspheres within ovarian arterial vasculature after uterine artery embolization. Obstet Gynecol 100:883, 2002.
Peckham EM, Maki DG, Patterson JJ, et al: Focal vulvitis: A characteristic syndrome and cause of dyspareunia. Am J Obstet Gynecol 154:855, 1986.
Peña JE, Ufberg D, Cooney N, Denis AL: Usefulness of Doppler sonography in the diagnosis of ovarian torsion. Fertil Steril 73:1047, 2000.
Peters WA, Thiagarajah S, Thornton WN: Ovarian hemorrhage in patients receiving anticoagulant therapy. J Reprod Med 22:82, 1979.
Peterson WF, Novak ER: Endometrial polyps. Obstet Gynecol 8:40, 1956.
Pettersson B, Adami HO, Lindgren A, et al: Endometrial polyps and hyperplasia as risk factors for endometrial carcinoma. Acta Obstet Gynecol Scand 64:653, 1985.
Platt LD, Agarwal SK, Greene N: The use of chorionic villus biopsy catheters for saline infusion sonohysterography. Ultrasound Obstet Gynecol 15:83, 2000.
Popp LW, Schwiedessen JP, Gaetje R: Myometrial biopsy in the diagnosis of adenomyosis uteri. Am J Obstet Gynecol 169:546, 1993.
Practice Committee of the American Society of Reproductive Medicine: Myomas and reproductive function, Fertil Steril 82:S111, 2004.
Pradhan S, Chenoy R, O'Brien PMS: Dilatation and curettage in patients with cervical polyps: A retrospective analysis. Br J Obstet Gynaecol 102:415, 1995.
Price FV, Edwards R, Buchsbaum HJ: Ovarian remnant syndrome: Difficulties in diagnosis and management. Obstet Gynecol Surv 45:151, 1990.
Pritts EA: Fibroids and infertility: A systematic review of the evidence. Obstet Gynecol Surv 56:483, 2001.
Propst AM, Thorp JM: Traumatic vulvar hematomas: Conservative versus surgical management. Southern Med J 91:144, 1996.
Rafla N: Vaginismus and vaginal tears, Am J Obstet Gynecol 158:1043, 1988.
Ravina JH, Vigneron NC, Aymard A, et al: Pregnancy after embolization of uterine myoma: Report of 12 cases. Fertil Steril 73:1241, 2000.
Raziel A, Ron-El R, Pansky M, et al: Current management of ruptured corpus luteum. Eur J Obstet Gynecol Reprod Biol 50:77, 1993.
Reed BD, Haefner HK, Harlow SD, et al: Reliability and validity of self reported symptoms for predicting vulvodynia. Obstet Gynecol 108:906, 2006.
Reid JD, Kommareddi S, Lankerani M, et al: Chronic expanding hematomas. JAMA 244:2441, 1980.
Rein MS, Barbieri RL, Friedman AJ: Progesterone: A critical role in the pathogenesis of uterine myomas. Am J Obstet Gynecol 172:14, 1995.
Rein MS, Friedman AJ, Stuart JM, et al: Fibroid and myometrial steroid receptors in women treated with gonadotropin-releasing hormone agonist leuprolide acetate. Fertil Steril 53:1018, 1990.
Reinhold C, Atri M, Mehio A, et al: Diffuse uterine adenomyosis: Morphologic criteria and diagnostic accuracy of endovaginal sonograph. Radiology 197:609, 1995.
Reinhold C, Tafazoli F, Mehio A, et al: Uterine adenomyosis: Endovaginal US and MR imaging features with histopathologic correlation. Radiographics 19:S147, 1999.
Reiter RC, Wagner PL, Gambone JC: Routine hysterectomy for large asymptomatic uterine leiomyomata: A reappraisal. Obstet Gynecol 79:481, 1992.
Ribeiro SC, Reich H, Rosenberg J, et al: Laparoscopic myomectomy and pregnancy outcome in infertile patients. Fertil Steril 71:571, 1999.
Richardson DA, Hajj SN, Herbst AL: Medical treatment of urethral prolapse in children. Obstet Gynecol 59:69, 1982.
Ridgeway LE: Puerperal emergency: Vaginal and vulvar hematomas. Obstet Gynecol Clin North Am 22:275, 1995.
Robboy SJ, Ross JS, Prat J, et al: Urogenital sinus origin of mucinous and ciliated cysts of the vulva. Obstet Gynecol 51:347, 1978.
Roberts DB: Necrotizing fasciitis of the vulva. Am J Obstet Gynecol 157:568, 1987.
Robson S, Kerin JF: Acute adnexal torsion before oocyte retrieval in an in vitro fertilization cycle. Fertil Steril 73:650, 2000.
Roehrborn CG: Long-term follow-up study of the marsupialization technique for urethral diverticula in women. Surg Gynecol Obstet 167:191, 1988.
Rulin MC, Preston AL: Adnexal masses in postmenopausal women. Obstet Gynecol 70:578, 1987.
Samaha M, Woodruff JD: Paratubal cysts: frequency, histogenesis, and associated clinical features. Obstet Gynecol 65:691, 1985.
Samanth KK, Black WC: Benign ovarian stromal tumors associated with free peritoneal fluid. Am J Obstet Gynecol 107:538, 1970.
Savelli L, DeIaco P, Santini D, et al: Histopathologic features and risk factors for benignity, hyperplasia, and cancer in endometrial polyps. Am J Obstet Gynecol 188:927-31, 2003.
Schindl M, Birner P, Obermair A, et al: Increased microvessel density in adenomyosis uteri. Fertil Steril 75:131, 2001.
Scialli AR, Jestila KJ: Sustained benefits of leuprolide acetate with or without subsequent medroxyprogesterone acetate in the nonsurgical management of leiomyomata uteri. Fertil Steril 64:313, 1995.
Scott RT, Beatse SN, Illinois EH, Snyder RR: Use of the GnRH agonist stimulation test in the diagnosis of ovarian remnant syndrome: A report of three cases. J Reprod Med 40:143, 1995.
Seoud M, Shamseddine A, Khalil A, et al: Tamoxifen and endometrial pathologies: A prospective study. Gynecol Oncol 75:15, 1999.
Shalev E and Peleg D: Laparoscopic treatment of adnexal torsion. Surg Gynecol Obstet 176:448, 1993.
Shevchuk MM, Fenoglio CM, Richart RM: Histogenesis of Brenner tumors. I. Histology and structure. Cancer 46:2607, 1980.
Siddall-Allum J, Rae T, Rogers V, et al: Chronic pelvic pain caused by residual ovaries and ovarian remnants. Br J Obstet Gynaecol 101:979, 1994.
Siegelman ES, Banner MP, Ramchandani P, Schnall MD: Multicoil MR imaging of symptomatic female urethral and periurethral disease. Radiographics 17:349, 1997.
Siegler AM, Camilien L: Adenomyosis. J Reprod Med 39:841, 1994.
Sims JA, Brzyski R, Hansen, Coddington CC III: Use of a gonadotropin releasing hormone agonist before vaginal surgery for cervical leiomyomas: a report of two cases. J Reprod Med 39:660, 1994.
Smart OC, MacLean AB: Vulvodynia. Cur Opin Obstet Gynecol 15:497, 2003.
Smith NC, Van Coeverden de Groot HA, Gunston KD: Coital injuries of the vagina in nonvirginal patients. S Afr Med J 64:746, 1983.
Soper DE, Patterson JW, Hurt WG, et al: Lichen planus of the vulva. Obstet Gynecol 72:74, 1988.
Sozen I, Arici A: Interactions of cytokines, growth factors, and the extracellular matrix in the cellular biology of uterine leiomyomata. Fertil Steril 78:1, 2002.
Spanos WJ: Preoperative hormonal therapy of cystic adnexal masses. Am J Obstet Gynecol 116:551, 1973.
Spies JB, Spector A, Roth AR, et al: Complications after uterine artery embolization for leiomyomas. Obstet Gynecol 100:873, 2002.
Steege JF: Ovarian remnant syndrome. Obstet Gynecol 70:64, 1987.
Stein AL, Koonings PP, Schlaerth JB, et al: Relative frequency of malignant parovarian tumors: Should parovarian tumors be aspirated? Obstet Gynecol 75:1029, 1990.
Steinauer J, Pritts EA, Jackson R, et al: Systematic review of mifepristone for the treatment of uterine leiomyomata. Obstet Gynecol 103:1331, 2004.
Steinkampf MP, Hammond KR, Blackwell RE: Hormonal treatment of functional ovarian cysts: A randomized prospective study. Fertil Steril 54:775, 1990.
Stewart DE, Reicher AE, Gerulath AH, Boydell KM: Vulvodynia and psychological distress. Obstet Gynecol 84:587, 1994.
Stewart EA, Morton CC: The genetics of uterine leiomyomata. Obstet Gynecol 107:907, 2006.
Stovall TG, Muneyyirci-Delale O, Summit RL, et al: GnRH agonist and iron versus placebo and iron in the anemic patient before surgery for leiomyomas: A randomized controlled trial. Obstet Gynecol 86:65, 1995.
Summitt RL Jr, Stovall TG: Urethral diverticula: Evaluation by urethral pressure profilometry, cystourethroscopy, and the voiding cystourethrogram. Obstet Gynecol 80:695, 1992.
Tang LCH, Cho HKM, Chan SYW, et al: Dextropreponderance of corpus luteum rupture. J Reprod Med 30:764, 1985.
Templeman CL, Fallat ME, Lam AM, et al: Managing mature cystic teratomas of the ovary. Obstet Gynecol Survey 55:738, 2000.

Tepper R, Zalel Y, Markov S, et al: Ovarian volume in postmenopausal women—suggestions to an ovarian size nomogram for menopause age. Acta Obstet Gynecol Scand 74:208, 1995.

Thomas R, Barnhill D, Bibro M, et al: Hidradenitis suppurativa: A case presentation and review of the literature. Obstet Gynecol 66:592, 1985.

Thorp JM Jr, Wells SR, Droegemueller W: Ovarian suspension in massive ovarian edema. Obstet Gynecol 76:912, 1990.

Traas MAF, Bekkers RLM, Dony JMJ, et al: Surgical treatment for the vulvar vestibulitis syndrome. Obstet Gynecol 107(Pt 2):256, 2006.

Tulandi T, Sammour A, Valenti D: Ovarian reserve after uterine artery embolization for leiomyomata. Fertil Steril 78:197, 2002.

Uduwela AS, Perera MAK, Aiqing L, et al: Endometrial-myometrial interface: relationship to adenomyosis and changes in pregnancy. Obstet Gynecol Survey 55:390, 2000.

Valente PT: Leiomyomatosis peritonealis disseminata. Arch Pathol Lab Med 108:669, 1984.

Van Bogaert LJ: Clinicopathologic findings in endometrial polyps,. Obstet Gynecol 71:771, 1988.

van der Putte SCJ: Mammary-like glands of the vulva and their disorders. Int J Gynecol Pathol 13:150, 1994.

Van Voorhis BJ, Schwaiger J, Syrop CH, Chapler FK: Early diagnosis of ovarian torsion by color Doppler ultrasonography. Fertil Steril 58:215, 1992.

Van Winter JT, Stanhope CR: Giant ovarian leiomyoma associated with ascites and polymyositis. Obstet Gynecol 80:560, 1992.

Varasteh NN, Neuwirth RS, Levin B, Keltz MD: Pregnancy rates after hysteroscopic polypectomy and myomectomy in infertile women. Obstet Gynecol 94:168, 1999.

Vercellini P, Crosignani PG, Mangioni C, et al: Treatment with a gonadotropin releasing hormone agonist before hysterectomy for leiomyomas: Results of a multicentre, randomised controlled trial. Br J Obstet Gynaecol 105:1148, 1998.

Vercellini P, Parazzini F, Oldani S, et al: Adenomyosis at hysterectomy: A study on frequency distribution and patient characteristics. Human Reprod 10:1160, 1995.

Vercellini P, Ragni G, Trespidi L, et al: Adenomyosis: A déjà vu? Obstet Gynecol Surv 48:789, 1993.

Vercellini P, Zàina B, Yaylayan L, et al: Hysteroscopic myomectomy: Long-term effects on menstrual pattern and fertility. Obstet Gynecol 94:341, 1999.

Villella J, Garry D, Levine G, et al: Postpartum angiographic embolization for vulvovaginal hematoma. J Reprod Med 46:65, 2001.

Visco A and Del Priore G: Postmenopausal Bartholin gland enlargement: a hospital-based cancer risk assessment. Obstet Gynecol 87:286, 1996.

Vollenhoven BJ, Shekleton P, McDonald J, et al: Clinical predictors for buserelin acetate treatment of uterine fibroids: A prospective study of 40 women. Fertil Steril 54:1032, 1990.

Walker WJ, Pelage JP: Uterine artery embolization for symptomatic fibroids: Clinical results in 400 women with imaging follow up. BJOG 109:1262, 2002.

Wallace EE, Vlahos NF: Uterine myomas: An overview of development, clinical features, and management, Obstet Gynecol 104:393-406, 2004.

Waxman M, Boyce JG: Intraperitoneal rupture of benign cystic ovarian teratoma. Obstet Gynecol 48:95, 1976.

Webb EM, Green GE, Scoutt LM: Adnexal mass with pelvic pain. Radiol Clin North Am 42:329, 2004.

Wegienka G, Baird DD, Hertz-Picciotto I, et al: Self-reported heavy bleeding associated with uterine leiomyomata. Obstet Gynecol 101:431, 2003.

Weissberg SM, Dodson MG: Recurrent vaginal and cervical ulcers associated with tampon use. JAMA 250:1430, 1983.

Weissman A, Barash A, Manor M, et al: Acute changes in endometrial thickness after aspiration of functional ovarian cysts. Fertil Steril 69:1142, 1998.

Wenström LV, Willén R: Vestibular nerve fiber proliferation in vulvar vestibulitis syndrome. Obstet Gynecol 91:572, 1998.

Wertheim I, Fleischhacker D, McLachlin CM, et al: Pseudomyxoma peritonei: A review of 23 cases. Obstet Gynecol 84:17, 1994.

Wolf SI, Gosnik BB, Feldesman MR, et al: Prevalence of simple adnexal cysts in postmenopausal women. Radiol 180: 65, 1991.

Wood C, Maher P, Hill D: Biopsy diagnosis and conservative surgical treatment of adenomyosis. Aust N Z J Obstet Gynaecol 33:319, 1993.

Woodworth H, Dockerty MB, Wilson RB, et al: Papillary hidradenoma of the vulva: A clinicopathologic study of 69 cases. Am J Obstet Gynecol 110:501, 1971.

Yeagley TJ, Goldberg J, Klein TA, et al: Labial necrosis after uterine artery embolization for leiomyomata. Obstet Gynecol 100:881, 2002.

Young SB, Rose PG, Reuter KL: Vaginal fibromyomata: two cases with preoperative assessment, resection, and reconstruction. Obstet Gynecol 78:972, 1991.

Zellis S, Pincus SH: Treatment of vulvar dermatoses. Semin Dermatol 15:71, 1996.

Zolnoun DA, Hartmann KE, Steege JF: Overnight 5% lidocaine ointment for treatment of vulvar vestibulitis. Obstet Gynecol 102:84, 2003.

Zweizig S, Perron J, Grubb D, Mishell DR Jr: Conservative management of adnexal torsion. Am J Obstet Gynecol 168:1791, 1993.

Endometriosis 19

Etiology, Pathology, Diagnosis, Management

Rogerio A. Lobo

KEY TERMS AND DEFINITIONS

Adenomyoma. An isolated area of endometrial glands and stroma in the uterine musculature that can be identified grossly.

Adenomyosis. The growth of endometrial glands and stroma into the uterine myometrium to a depth of at least 2.5 mm from the basalis layer of the endometrium.

Chocolate Cyst. A cystic area of endometriosis in the ovary.

Coelomic Metaplasia. The potential ability of coelomic epithelium to develop into several different histologic cell types.

Danazol. A synthetic steroid, an attenuated androgen, that is active when taken orally.

Dyschezia. Difficult or painful evacuation of feces from the rectum.

Endometrioma. An area of endometriosis that can be identified macroscopically, usually in the ovary.

Endometriosis. The presence and growth of glands and stroma identical to the lining of the uterus in an aberrant location.

GnRH Agonists. A group of synthetic hormones that suppresses gonadotrophin secretion, causing secondary diminution of ovarian steroidogenesis.

Retrograde Menstruation. The flow of menstrual blood, endometrial cells, and debris via the fallopian tubes into the peritoneal cavity.

ENDOMETRIOSIS

Endometriosis is a benign, but in many women, a progressive disease. The wide spectrum of clinical problems that occur with endometriosis has frustrated gynecologists, fascinated pathologists, and burdened patients for years. Although endometriosis was first described in 1860, the classic studies of Sampson in the 1920s were the first to emphasize the clinical and pathologic correlations of endometriosis. Even today, many aspects of the disease remain enigmatic.

By definition, endometriosis is the presence and growth of the glands and stroma of the lining of the uterus in an aberrant or heterotopic location. Adenomyosis is the growth of endometrial glands and stroma into the uterine myometrium to a depth of at least 2.5 mm from the basalis layer of the endometrium. Adenomyosis is sometimes termed *internal endometriosis*; however, this is a semantic misnomer because most likely they are separate diseases.

It is usually stated that the incidence of endometriosis has been increasing over the past 30 years. This "opinion" is secondary to an enlightened awareness of mild endometriosis as diagnosed by the increasing use of laparoscopy. During the past 10 years, diagnostic delay, the average time to the first diagnosis of the disease, has decreased dramatically. However, it has been estimated to take an average time of 11.7 years in the United States and 8 years in the United Kingdom. Evers has advanced a provocative hypothesis that endometrial implants in the peritoneal cavity are a physiologic finding secondary to retrograde menstruation, and their presence does not confirm a disease process. The prevalence of pelvic endometriosis in the general female population has been suggested to be 6% to 10%. The age-specific incidence or prevalence of endometriosis is not known and has only been estimated. Many patients are diagnosed incidentally during surgery performed for a variety of other indications. Conservative estimates find that endometriosis is present in 5% to 15% of laparotomies performed on reproductive-age females. The prevalence of active endometriosis is approximately 33% in women with chronic pelvic pain. The incidence of endometriosis is 30% to 45% in women with infertility. It must be emphasized that all studies of the prevalence of endometriosis are subject to selection bias and are dependent on the definition of "active disease."

The cause of endometriosis is uncertain and may involve retrograde menstruation, vascular dissemination, metaplasia, genetic predisposition, immunologic changes, and hormonal influences, as discussed later on. In addition, there is increasing evidence that environmental factors may also play a role, including exposure to dioxin and other endocrine disruptors. Clinically, it is most difficult to predict the natural course of endometriosis in any one individual. For example, the clinician is uncertain as to which woman with mild disease in her 20s will progress to severe disease at a later age.

The typical patient with endometriosis is in her mid-30s, is nulliparous and involuntarily infertile, and has symptoms of secondary dysmenorrhea and pelvic pain. The classic symptom of endometriosis is pelvic pain. However, in clinical practice the majority of cases are not "classic." The diagnosis and treatment of infertility associated with endometriosis is discussed in Chapter 41 (Infertility). Aberrant endometrial tissue grows under the cyclic influence of ovarian hormones and is particularly estrogen dependent; therefore the disease is most commonly found during the reproductive years. However, 5% of

Table 19-1 Endometriosis: A Disease of Clinical Contrasts

Characteristics	Contrasts
Benign disease	Locally invasive Widespread disseminated foci Proliferates in pelvic lymph nodes
Minimal disease	Severe pain
Many large endometriomas	Asymptomatic patient
Cyclic hormones cause growth	Continuous hormones reverse the growth pattern

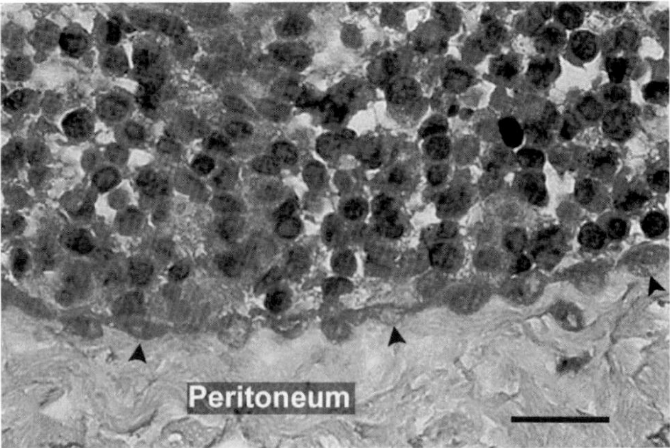

A

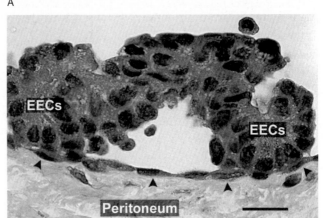

B

Figure 19-1. Attachment of endometrial stroma **(A)** and endometrial epithelium (EECs; **B**) to intact mesothelium. (From Strauss JF, Barbieri R: Yen & Jaffe's Reproductive Endocrinology, 5th ed. Philadelphia Saunders, 2004, pp 692–693.)

women with endometriosis are diagnosed following menopause. Postmenopausal endometriosis is usually stimulated by exogenous estrogen. Endometriosis in teenagers should be investigated for obstructive reproductive tract abnormalities that increase the amount of retrograde menstruation.

Endometriosis is a disease not only of great individual variability but also of contrasting pathophysiologic processes (Table 19-1). It is a benign disease, yet it has the characteristics of a malignancy—that is, it is locally infiltrative, invasive, and widely disseminating. Although the growth of ectopic endometrium is stimulated by physiologic levels of estrogen use of contraceptive steroids of various doses are usually beneficial for treatment. Another contrast often noted is the inverse relationship between the extent of pelvic endometriosis and the severity of pelvic pain. Women with extensive endometriosis may be asymptomatic, whereas other patients with minimal implants may have incapacitating chronic pelvic pain. However, as would be expected, women with deep infiltrating endometriosis, especially in retroperitoneal spaces, often experience severe episodes of pain. Finally, there is speculation as to the underlying pathophysiology that produces infertility in women with endometriosis.

Etiology

There are several theories to explain the pathogenesis of endometriosis. However, no single theory adequately explains all the manifestations of the disease. Most important, there is only speculation as to why some women develop endometriosis, and others do not. One popular theory is that there is a complex interplay between a dose-response curve of the amount of retrograde menstruation and an individual woman's immunologic response.

Retrograde Menstruation

The most popular theory is that endometriosis results from retrograde menstruation. Sampson suggested that pelvic endometriosis was secondary to implantation of endometrial cells shed during menstruation. These cells attach to the pelvic peritoneum and under hormonal influence grow as homologous grafts. Indeed, reflux of menstrual blood and viable endometrial cells in the pelvis of ovulating women has been documented. Endometriosis is discovered most frequently in areas immediately adjacent to the tubal ostia or in the dependent areas of the pelvis.

Endometriosis is frequently found in women with outflow obstruction of the genital tract. The attachment of the shed endometrial cells involves the expression of adhesion molecules and their receptors. This is thought to be an extremely rapid process as demonstrated in vitro (Figs. 19-1 and 19-2)

Metaplasia

In contrast to the theory of seeding from retrograde menstruation is the theory that endometriosis arises from metaplasia of the coelomic epithelium or proliferation of embryonic rests. The müllerian ducts and nearby mesenchymal tissue form the majority of the female reproductive tract. The müllerian duct is derived from the coelomic epithelium during fetal development. The metaplasia hypothesis postulates that the coelomic epithelium retains the ability for multipotential development. The decidual reaction of isolated areas of peritoneum during pregnancy is an example of this process. It is well known that the surface epithelium of the ovary can differentiate into several different histologic cell types. Endometriosis has been discovered in prepubertal girls, women with congenital absence of the uterus, and very rarely in men. These examples support the coelomic metaplasia theory.

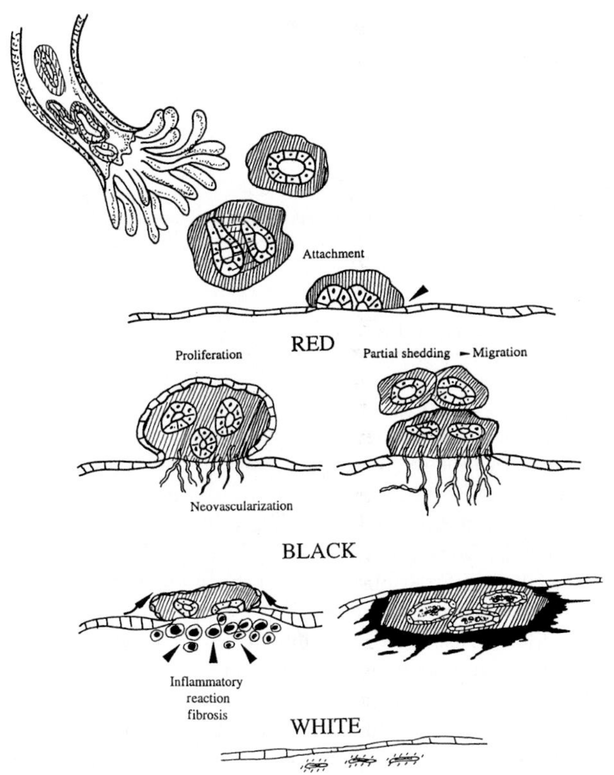

Figure 19-2. Proposed establishment of peritoneal endometriotic implants via retrograde menstruation, etc. (From Strauss JF, Barbieri R: Yen & Jaffe's Reproductive Endocrinology, 5th ed. Philadelphia Saunders, 2004, pp 692–693.)

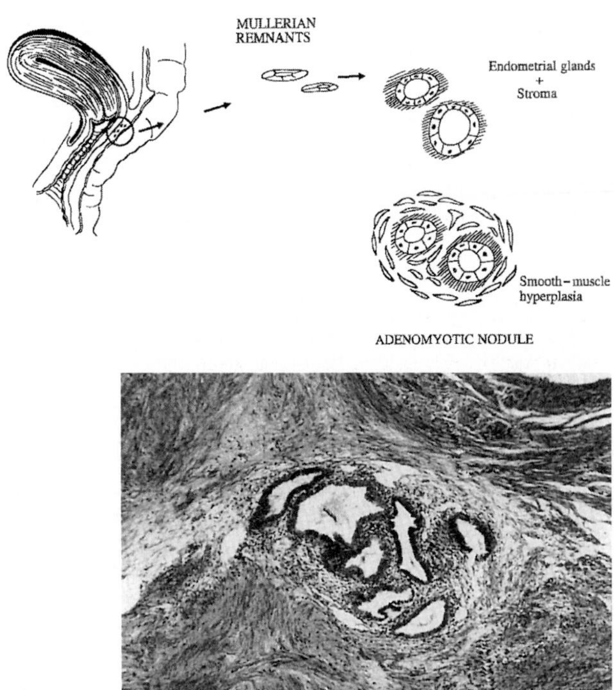

Figure 19-3. Proposed derivation of endometriotic lesion in the rectovaginal septum. (From Strauss JF, Barbieri R: Yen & Jaffe's Reproductive Endocrinology, 5th ed. Philadelphia Saunders, 2004, pp 692–693.)

Metaplasia occurs after an "induction phenomenon" has stimulated the multipotential cell. The induction substance may be a combination of menstrual debris and the influence of estrogen and progesterone. Batt and Smith have hypothesized that the histogenesis of endometriosis in peritoneal pockets of the posterior pelvis results from a congenital anomaly involving rudimentary duplication of the müllerian system. The peritoneal pockets that they describe are found in the posterior pelvis, the posterior aspects of the broad ligament, and the cul-de-sac of Douglas. Similarly, Nisolle and Donnez postulate that metaplasia of the coelomic epithelium that invaginates into the ovarian cortex is the pathogenesis for the development of ovarian endometriosis (Fig. 19-3).

Lymphatic and Vascular Metastasis

The theory of endometrium being transplanted via lymphatic channels and the vascular system helps to explain rare and remote sites of endometriosis, such as the spinal column and nose. Endometriosis has been observed in the pelvic lymph nodes of approximately 30% of women with the disease. Hematogenous dissemination of endometrium is the best theory to explain endometriosis of the forearm and thigh, as well as multiple lesions in the lung.

Iatrogenic Dissemination

Endometriosis of the anterior abdominal wall is sometimes discovered in women after a cesarean delivery. The hypothesis is that endometrial glands and stroma are implanted during the procedure. The aberrant tissue is found subcutaneously at the abdominal incision. Rarely, iatrogenic endometriosis may be discovered in an episiotomy scar.

Immunologic Changes

One of the most perplexing, unanswered questions concerning the pathophysiology of endometriosis is that some women with retrograde menstruation develop endometriosis, but the majority do not. Multiple investigations have suggested that changes in the immune system, especially altered function of immune-related cells, are directly related to the pathogenesis of endometriosis. Whether endometriosis is an autoimmune disease has been intensely debated for many years. Studies have demonstrated abnormalities in cell-mediated and humoral components of the immune system in both peripheral blood and peritoneal fluid. Depicted in Table 19-2 are various cytokines and growth factors that have been implicated in the pathogenesis of endometriosis.

Most likely the primary immunologic change involves an alteration in the function of the peritoneal macrophages so prevalent in the peritoneal fluid of patients with endometriosis. Halme and colleagues hypothesized that women who do not develop endometriosis have monocytic-type macrophages in their peritoneal fluid that have a short life span and limited function. Conversely, women who develop endometriosis have more peritoneal macrophages that are larger. These hyperactive cells secrete multiple growth factors and cytokines that enhance the development of endometriosis (Table 19-3). The attraction of leukocytes to specific areas is controlled by chemokines, which are chemotactic cytokines (Fig. 19-4). Changes in the

Table 19-2 Cytokines and Growth Factors in Peritoneal Fluid

Concentrations Increased in Endometriosis	
Complement	Badawy et al, 1984
Eotaxin	Hornung et al, 2000
Glycodelin	Koninckx et al, 1992
IL-1	Anderson and Hill, 1987
IL-6	Rier et al, 1994
IL-8	Ryan et al, 1995
MCP-1	Akoum et al, 1996
PDGF	Halme et al, 1988
RANTES	Khorram et al, 1993
Soluble ICAM-1	Daniel et al, 2000
TGF-β	Oosterlynck et al, 1994
VEGF	Shifren et al, 1996
Concentrations Unchanged in Endometriosis	
EGF	De Leon et al, 1986
Basic FGF	Huang et al, 1996
Interferon-γ	Khorram et al, 1993
IL-2	Keenan et al, 1995
IL-4	Gazvani et al, 2001
IL-12	Mazzeo et al, 1998
Concentrations Decreased in Endometriosis	
IL-13	McLaren et al, 1997

EGF, epidermal growth factor; FGF, fibroblast growth factor; ICAM, intercellular adhesion molecule; IL, interleukin; MCP, membrane cofactor protein; PDGF; platelet-derived growth factor; RANTES, regulated upon activation, normal T cell expressed and secreted; TGF, transforming growth factor; VEGF, vascular endothelial growth factor.
References are from the original source.
From McLaren J, Deatry G, Prentice A, et al: Decreased levels of the potent regulator of monocyte/macrophage activation, interleukin-13, in the peritoneal fluid of patients with endometriosis. Hum Reprod 12:1307, 1997.

Table 19-3 Candidate Genes and Susceptibility to Endometriosis

Cytochrome P450 1A1
N-acetyl transferase 2
Glutathione-*S* transferase M1, T1
Galactose-1-phosphate uridyl transferase
Estrogen receptor
Progesterone receptor
Androgen receptor
PTEN
p53
Peroxisome proliferator-activated receptor γ2 Pro-12-Ala allele

expression of integrins also may be an important local factor. Following the theory of different macrophage populations in endometriosis is the finding that the destroying of normally extruded endometrial cells in endometriosis may be deficient. Oosterlynck showed that natural killer (NK) cells have decreased cytotoxicity against endometrial and hematopoietic cells in women with endometriosis. Also, peritoneal fluid of women with endometriosis has less influence of NK activity than is found in fertile women without endometriosis.

Another attractive theory is the recent finding of a protein similar to haptoglobin in endometriosis epithelial cells called Endo 1. This chemoattractant protein-enhanced local production of interleukin-6 (IL-6) self perpetuates lesion/cytokine interactions. Further compounding the proliferative activity of endometriosis lesions are angiogenic factors that are increased in lesions. Here the expression of basic fibroblast factor, IL-6, IL-8,

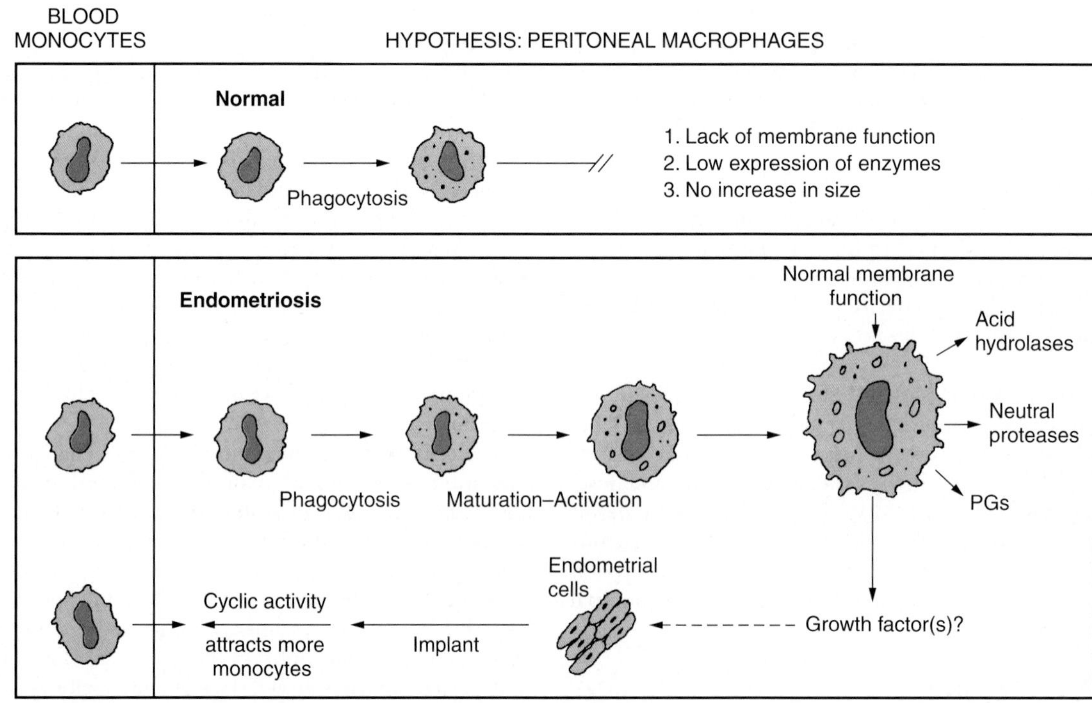

Figure 19-4. Hypothesis regarding pathophysiologic characteristics of human peritoneal macrophages in endometriosis. PG, prostaglandins. (Redrawn from Halme J, Becker S, Haskill S, et al: Altered maturation and function of peritoneal macrophages: Possible role in pathogenesis of endometriosis. Am J Obstet Gynecol 156:787, 1987.)

platelet-derived growth factor (PDGF), and vascular endothelial growth factor (VEGF) are all increased.

Steroid interactions also enhance the progression of disease. Estrogen production is enhanced locally, and there is evidence for up-regulation of aromatase activity and dysregulation of 17β-dehydrogenase activity, where there is a deficiency in 17β-dehydrogenase II activity. Enhanced aromatase activity appears to be the result of overexpression of the orphan nuclear receptor steroidogenic factor-1 (SF-1) in lesions. The local production of estrogen through aromatase activity explains why progression of lesions may occur even with ovarian suppression. Further, there is evidence for progesterone "resistance." This is occasioned by a dysregulation of the isoform B of the progesterone receptor in some endometriotic lesions. The latter propensity may be on a genetic basis as discussed later on. Autoimmunity may well exist in women with endometriosis, and although the finding of abnormalities of the histocompatibility locus antigen (HLA) system have not been consistent, there are reports of increased B and T cells, and serum immunoglobulin (IgG, IgA, and IgM) autoantibodies in endometriosis. A survey of the U.S. Endometriosis Association has provided suggestive evidence of the higher prevalence of other autoimmune diseases. The association of all these immune processes in the symptoms and signs of endometriosis is depicted in Figure 19-5.

Genetic Predisposition

Several studies have documented a familial predisposition to endometriosis with grouping of cases of endometriosis in mothers and their daughters. An investigation by Simpson and coworkers demonstrated a sevenfold increase in the incidence of endometriosis in relatives of women with the disease compared with controls. One of 10 women with severe endometriosis will have a sister or mother with clinical manifestations of the disease. Women who have a family history of endometriosis are likely to develop the disease earlier in life and to have more advanced disease than women whose first-degree relatives are free of the disease. Recent studies have identified deletions of genes, most specifically increased heterogenicity of chromosome 17 and aneuploidy, in women with endometriosis compared with controls. The expression of this genetic liability most likely depends on an interaction with environmental factors. Preliminary data suggest some bilateral ovarian endometrial cysts may arise independently from different clones.

Although no consistent abnormality has been found in women with endometriosis, there are several candidate genes. Table 19-4 provides a list of genes and gene products aberrantly expressed in endometriosis.

Several of these aberrantly expressed gene products, for example the matrix metalloproteinases (MMPs) and integrins, have important implications for endometrial lesion attachment and for implantation defects which may exist in infertile women with endometriosis. Reflux of MMPs into the peritoneal cavity at menstruation may contribute to peritoneal attachment in susceptible women.

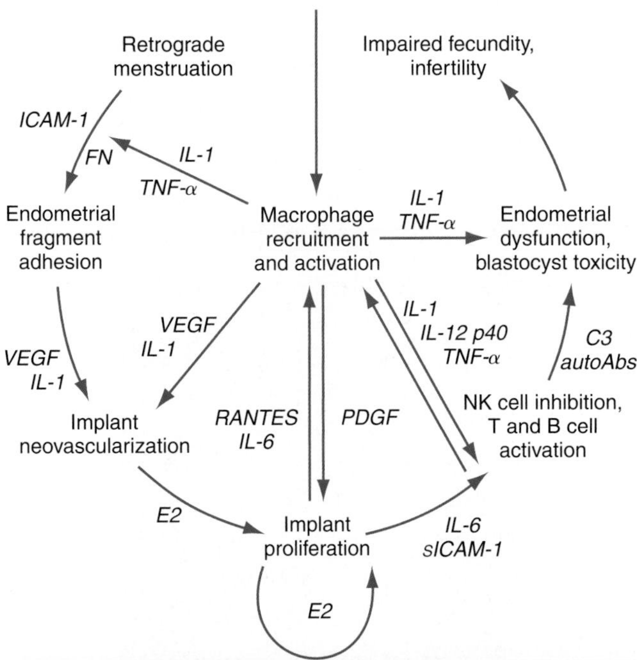

Figure 19-5. Schematogram depicting the network of chemokines, cytokines, and growth factors. ICAM, intercellular adhesion molecule; IL, interleukin; NK, natural killer; PDGF, platelet-derived growth factor; RANTES, regulated upon activation, normal T cell expressed and secreted; TNF, tumor necrosis factor; VEGF, vascular endothelial growth factor. (Modified from Taylor R, Hornung D, Mueller M, Lebovic DI: In Arici A (ed): Infertility and Reproductive Clinics of North America. Philadelphia, WB Saunders, 2002, pp 145–157.

Pathology

The majority of endometrial implants are located in the dependent portions of the female pelvis (Fig. 19-6). The ovaries are the most common site, being involved in two of three women with endometriosis. In most of these women the involvement is bilateral. The pelvic peritoneum over the uterus; the anterior and posterior cul-de-sac; and the uterosacral, round, and broad ligaments are also common sites where endometriosis develops. Pelvic lymph nodes are involved in 30% of cases (Fig. 19-7). The cervix, vagina, and vulva are other possible pelvic locations. Brosens and Brosens have emphasized the importance of distinguishing between superficial and deep lesions of endometriosis. Deep lesions, penetrations of greater than 5 mm, represent a

Table 19-4 Genes and Gene Products Aberrantly Expressed in Endometrium from Women with Endometriosis

Aromatase
Endometrial bleeding factor
Hepatocyte growth factor
17β-hydroxysteroid dehydrogenase
HOX A10
HOX A11
Leukaemia inhibitory factor
Matrix metalloproteinases 3, 7, and 11
Tissue inhibitors of metalloproteinases
Progesterone-receptor isoforms
Complement 3
Glutathione peroxidase
Catalase
Thrombospondin 1
Vascular endothelial growth factor
Integrin $\alpha_v\beta_3$
Glycodelin

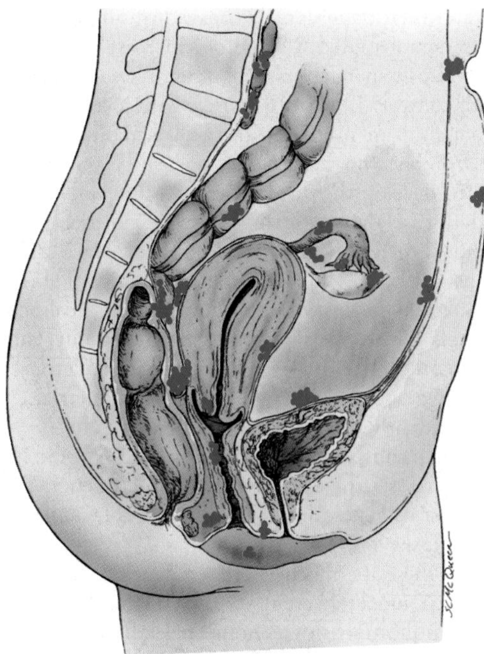

Figure 19-6. Common pelvic sites of endometriosis.

more progressive form of the disease. Distinguishing superficial implant lesions on peritoneal surfaces, including the ovary, from deep endometriotic ovarian cysts and cul-de-sac modules is important for therapy (discussed later on) in that these latter abnormalities may suggest different causes of the disease (e.g., metaplastia), which require a surgical approach.

Approximately 10% to 15% of women with advanced disease have lesions involving the rectosigmoid. Depending on the amount of associated scarring, endometriosis of the bowel may be difficult to differentiate grossly from a primary neoplasm of the large intestine. Endometriosis may be found in a wide variety of sites, including the umbilicus, areas of previous surgical incisions of the anterior abdominal wall or perineum, the bladder, ureter, kidney, lung, arms, legs, and even the male urinary tract (Table 19-5).

Gross pathologic changes of endometriosis exhibit wide variability in color, shape, size, and associated inflammatory and fibrotic changes. The visual manifestations of endometriosis in the female pelvis are protean and have many appearances. Increased awareness and anticipation have focused on the subtle lesions of endometriosis. Recently, clinicians closely inspect the

Table 19-5 Anatomic Distribution of Endometriosis

Common Sites	Rare Sites
Ovaries	Umbilicus
Pelvic peritoneum	Episiotomy scar
Ligaments of the uterus	Bladder
Sigmoid colon	Kidney
Appendix	Lungs
Pelvic lymph nodes	Arms
Cervix	Legs
Vagina	Nasal mucosa
Fallopian tubes	Spinal column

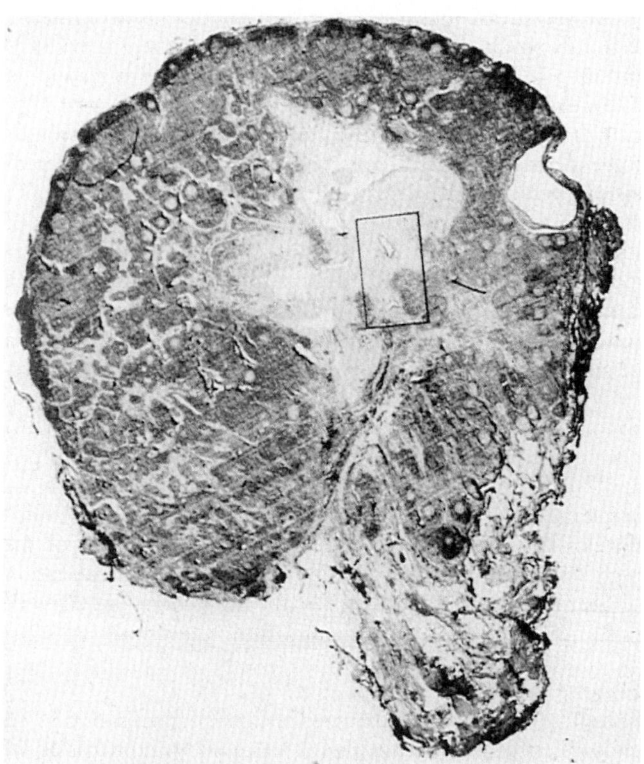

A

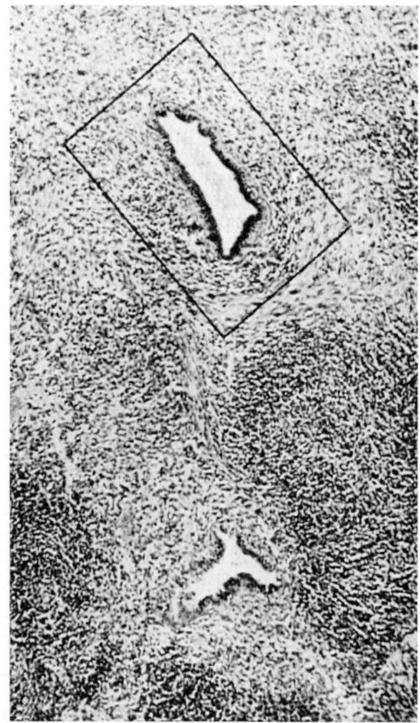

B

Figure 19-7. Endometriosis in right ureteral lymph node. **A,** Low-power view. **B,** Higher-power view showing two glands and surrounding stroma. (From Javert CT: Pathogenesis of endometriosis based on endometrial homeoplasia, direct extension exfoliation and implantation, lymphatic and hematogenous metastasism. Cancer 2:403, 1949.)

Table 19-6 Terminology Used to Describe Peritoneal Endometriosis

Powder-burn, puckered black lesions
Vascularized glandular papules
Vesicular lesions
Serous, surrounded by marked vascularization
Red hemorrhagic
Red, flamelike
Petechial peritoneum
Hypervascularized area
Discolored area
Yellow-brown
Blue
White
White scarring
Peritoneal defects
Cribriform peritoneal
Subovarian adhesions

From Brosens IA: Endometriosis: A disease because it is characterized by bleeding. Am J Obstet Gynecol 176:265, 1997.

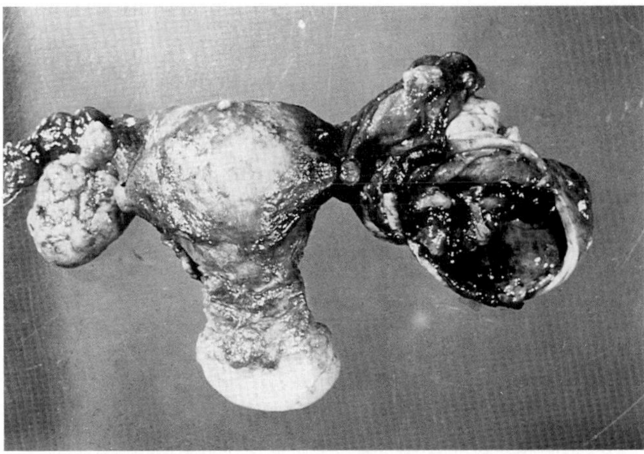

A

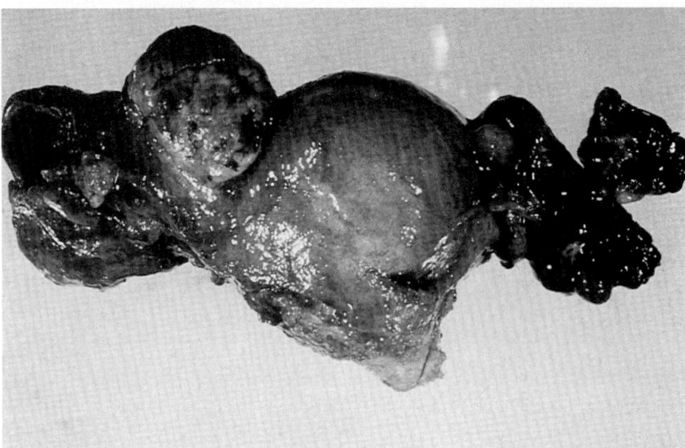

B

Figure 19-8. A, Total hysterectomy specimen from woman with endometriosis. Right ovary was partially destroyed by endometrioma. **B,** Anterior view of same specimen. Note small endometrial implants on surface of right ovary. (Courtesy of Fred Askin, MD.)

pelvic peritoneum to identify abnormal areas and small, nonhemorrhagic lesions. More emphasis has been placed on biopsy confirmation of endometriosis because of increasing awareness of subtle lesions. The gross appearance of the implant depends on the site, activity, relationship to the day of the menstrual cycle, and chronicity of the area involved. The color of the lesion varies widely and may be red, brown, black, white, yellow, pink, clear, or a red vesicle. The predominant color depends on the blood supply and the amount of hemorrhage and fibrosis. The color also appears related to the size of the lesion, degree of edema, and the amount of inspissated material (Table 19-6). Other peritoneal lesions that grossly appear similar to endometriosis, but on histologic examination are not, include necrotic areas of an ectopic pregnancy, fibrotic reactions to suture, hemangiomas, adrenal rest, Walthard's rest, breast cancer, ovarian cancer, epithelial inclusions, residual carbon from laser surgery, peritoneal inflammation, psammoma bodies, peritoneal reactions to oil-based hysterosalpingogram dye, and splenosis.

New lesions are small, bleblike implants that are less than 1 cm in diameter. Initially these areas are raised above the surrounding tissues. Red, blood-filled lesions have been shown, by histologic and biochemical studies, to be the most active phase of the disease (see Fig. 19-2). With time the areas of endometriosis become larger and assume a light or dark brown color, and they may be described as "powder burn" areas or "chocolate cysts." The older lesions are white, have more intense scarring, and are usually puckered or retracted from the surrounding tissue. White or mixed colored lesions are more likely to provide histologic confirmation of endometriosis. Also, the progression from red to white lesions also seems to correlate with age.

The pattern of ovarian endometriosis is also variable (Fig. 19-8). Individual areas range from 1 mm to large chocolate cysts greater than 8 cm in diameter. The associated adhesions may be filmy or dense. Larger cysts are usually densely adherent to the surrounding pelvic sidewalls or broad ligament.

The three cardinal histologic features of endometriosis are ectopic endometrial glands, ectopic endometrial stroma, and hemorrhage into the adjacent tissue (Figs. 19-9 and 19-10). Previous hemorrhage can be discovered by identifying large macrophages filled with hemosiderin near the periphery of the lesion. In the majority of cases the aberrant endometrial glands and stroma respond in cyclic fashion to estrogen and progesterone. These changes may or may not be in synchrony with the endometrial lining of the uterus. The ectopic endometrial stroma will undergo classic decidual changes similar to pregnancy when exposed to high physiologic or pharmacologic levels of progesterone.

In approximately 25% of the cases of endometriosis, viable endometrial glands and stroma cannot be identified. Repetitive episodes of hemorrhage may lead to severe inflammatory changes and result in the glands and stroma undergoing necrobiosis secondary to pressure atrophy or lack of blood supply. In these cases a presumptive diagnosis of endometriosis is made by visualizing the intense inflammatory reaction and the large macrophages filled with blood pigment.

The natural history of endometriosis is a subject of intense speculation. Spontaneous regression or disappearance of active disease is common. The pathophysiology of progression from subtle endometriosis to severe disease may be expected from the multiple mechanisms of potential disease acceleration discussed earlier, but in reality is not known.

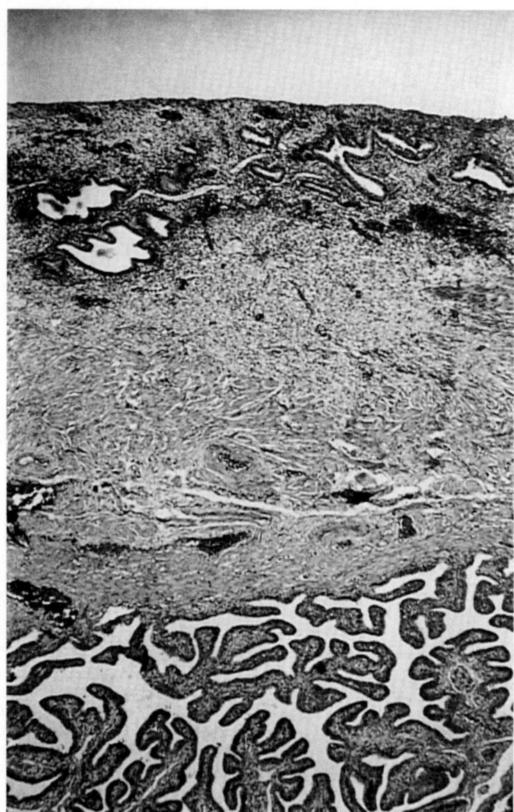

Figure 19-9. Endometriosis on fallopian tube. Serosa of tube is being invaded by glands and stroma. (Courtesy of Fred Askin, MD.)

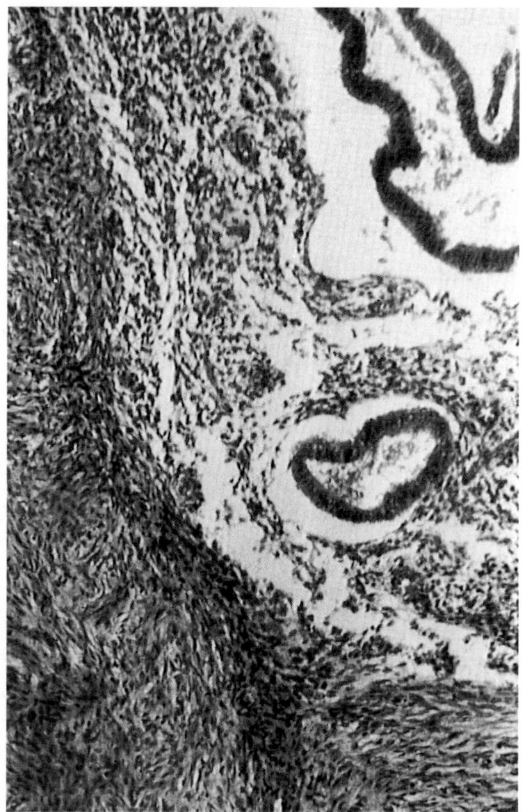

Figure 19-10. High-power view of endometrial glands in ovarian stroma. (Courtesy of Fred Askin, MD.)

Clinical Diagnosis

Symptoms

It is important to reemphasize that endometriosis has many different clinical presentations, with one in three women being asymptomatic. Most importantly, the disease has an extremely unpredictable course. The classic symptoms of endometriosis are cyclic pelvic pain and infertility. The chronic pelvic pain usually presents as secondary dysmenorrhea or dyspareunia (or both). Secondary dysmenorrhea usually begins 36 to 48 hours prior to the onset of menses. However, approximately one third of patients with endometriosis are asymptomatic, with the disease being discovered incidentally during an abdominal operation or visualized at laparoscopy for an unrelated problem. Conversely, endometriosis is discovered in approximately one of three women whose primary symptom is chronic pelvic pain.

Clinicians have appreciated the paradox that the extent of pelvic pain is often inversely related to the amount of endometriosis in the female pelvis. Women with large, fixed adnexal masses sometimes have minor symptoms, whereas other patients with only a few small foci with deep infiltration may experience moderate to severe chronic pain. Fedele and colleagues could find no correlation between the anatomic stage of the disease and the patient's perception of severity of pelvic pain. In their study, 124 women were staged according to the revised scoring system of the American Society of Reproductive Medicine. No relationship was found between stage of the disease and frequency or severity of pain symptoms.

The cyclic pelvic pain is related to the sequential swelling and the extravasation of blood and menstrual debris into the surrounding tissue. The chemical mediators of this intense sterile inflammation and pain are believed to be prostaglandins and cytokines. Infiltrative endometriosis, which involves extenive areas of the retroperitoneal space, often is associated with moderate to severe pelvic pain. Recently, studies of pain mapping by laparoscopy under minimal sedation have found that the pelvic pain arises from areas of normal peritoneum adjacent to areas of endometriosis.

Secondary dysmenorrhea is a common component of pain which varies from a dull ache to severe pelvic pain. It may be unilateral or bilateral and may radiate to the lower back, legs, and groin. Patients often complain of pelvic heaviness or a perception of their internal organs being swollen. Unlike primary dysmenorrhea, the pain may last for many days, including several days before and after the menstrual flow.

The dyspareunia associated with endometriosis is described as pain deep in the pelvis. The cause of this symptom seems to be immobility of the pelvic organs during coital activity or direct pressure on areas of endometriosis in the uterosacral ligaments or the cul-de-sac. Sometimes patients describe areas of point tenderness. The acute pain, experienced during deep penetration, may continue for several hours following intercourse.

Abnormal bleeding is a symptom noted by 15% to 20% of women with endometriosis. The most frequent complaints are premenstrual spotting and menorrhagia. Usually this abnormal bleeding is not associated with an anovulatory pattern.

On the other hand, patients with endometriosis frequently have ovulatory dysfunction. Approximately 15% of women with endometriosis have coincidental anovulation.

An increased incidence of first-trimester abortion in women with untreated endometriosis has been reported. However, recent epidemiologic studies question a true increased incidence and, if there is, raise serious doubt as to a cause-and-effect relationship.

Less common yet troublesome are the symptoms resulting from endometriosis influencing the gastrointestinal and urinary tracts. Cyclic abdominal pain, intermittent constipation, diarrhea, dyschezia, urinary frequency, dysuria, and hematuria are all possible symptoms. Bowel obstruction and hydronephrosis may occur. One rare clinical manifestation of endometriosis is catamenial hemothorax, bloody pleural fluid occurring during menses. Massive ascites is a rare symptom of endometriosis, but it is important because the disease process initially masquerades as ovarian carcinoma.

Signs

The classic pelvic finding of endometriosis is a fixed retroverted uterus, with scarring and tenderness posterior to the uterus. The characteristic nodularity of the uterosacral ligaments and cul-de-sac may be palpated on rectovaginal examination in approximately one third of women with the disease. Advanced cases have extensive scarring and narrowing of the posterior vaginal fornix. The ovaries may be enlarged and tender and are often fixed to the broad ligament or lateral pelvic sidewall. The adnexal enlargement is rarely symmetrical, as one might expect in some benign pelvic conditions. In one study of 561 women with ovarian endometriomas, bilateral cysts were observed in 158 (28%). In women with unilateral endometriomas, 63% were found in the left ovary.

Endometriosis is a disease that produces tenderness of the pelvic structures and scarring that restricts movement of the pelvic organs. Occasionally the physician discovers endometriosis in an old surgical incision or a site of a previous amniocentesis. Speculum examination may demonstrate small areas of endometriosis on the cervix or upper vagina. Lateral displacement or deviation of the cervix is visualized or palpated by digital exam of the vagina and cervix in approximately 15% of women with moderate or severe endometriosis. The diagnosis is straightforward if a patient presents with secondary dysmenorrhea, deep dyspareunia, and infertility and if during a pelvic examination the physician discovers a fixed posterior uterus, bilateral adnexal tenderness, and beading of the uterosacral ligaments. An experienced clinician may instruct the patient to return for a pelvic examination during the first or second day of her menstrual flow when the diagnosis of endometriosis is in doubt. This is the time of maximum swelling and tenderness in the areas of endometriosis. The diagnosis can be confirmed in most cases by direct laparoscopic visualization of endometriosis with its associated scarring and adhesion formation. In many patients it is discovered for the first time during an infertility investigation. Biopsy of selected implants gives confirmation of the diagnosis. However, sometimes the pathologist may be unable to find glandular elements and endometrial stroma in the biopsy specimens.

When laparoscopy is undertaken to establish the diagnosis of endometriosis, it is important to describe systematically the extent of the pathology (Figs. 19-11 and 19-12). In 1993, a committee of the American Society for Reproductive Medicine developed a detailed form to help the clinician document and assign numeric values illustrating the operative appearance of the disease including the most important features of endometriosis and pelvic pain (Fig. 19-13). The key elements of this

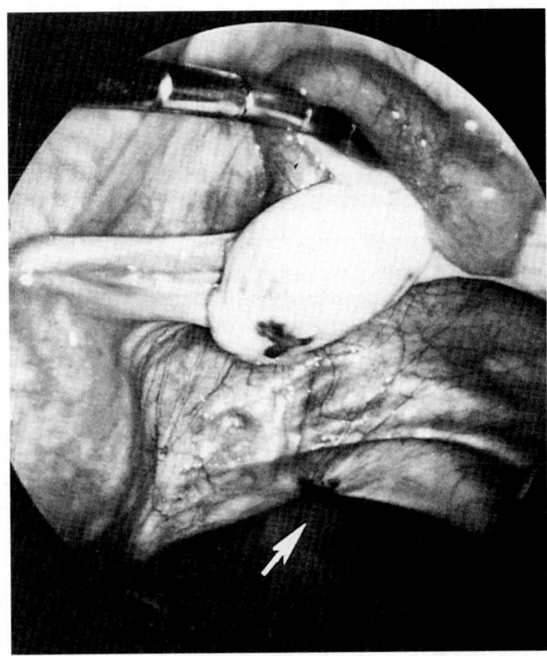

Figure 19-11. Laparoscopic view of ovarian and pelvic endometriosis. Tube is being elevated by a probe. Note the retracted area of the broad ligament around the endometriosis (*arrow*). (Courtesy of Jaroslav Hulka, MD, University of North Carolina, Chapel Hill.)

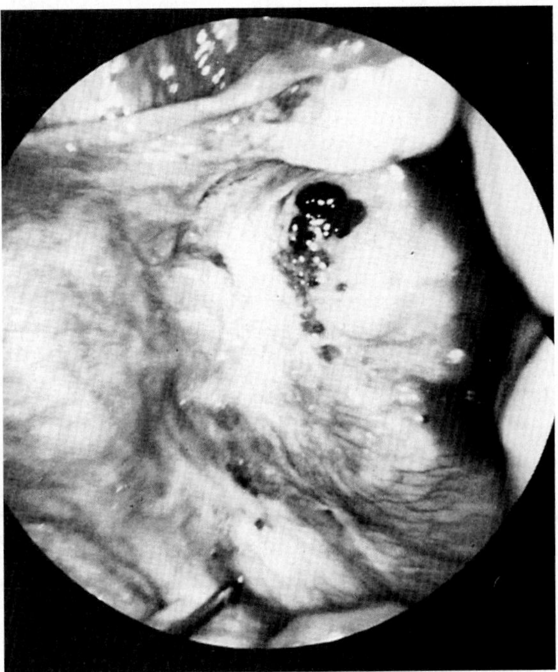

Figure 19-12. Laparoscopic view of endometriosis on the posterior leaf of the broad ligament and cul-de-sac. Note the many adhesions. (Courtesy of Jaroslav Hulka, MD, University of North Carolina, Chapel Hill.)

MANAGEMENT OF ENDOMETRIOSIS IN THE PRESENCE OF PELVIC PAIN
A Clinical Instrument to Document the Extent of Endometriosis and Pelvic Pain[1]

Patient's Name ____________________ Age ________ Date __________

PRE-OPERATIVE ASSESSMENT OF PELVIC PAIN

Complaints ____

____

Describe the patient's symptoms of pain quality and position, and any limitation caused by these symptoms. Abbreviate quality of pain as **A = mild, B = discomforting, C = distressing, D = horrible, E = excruciating**. On the anatomic drawings below, draw a **SOLID LINE** around the area(s) of pain described by the patient, and mark the most intense area(s) with an **X**.

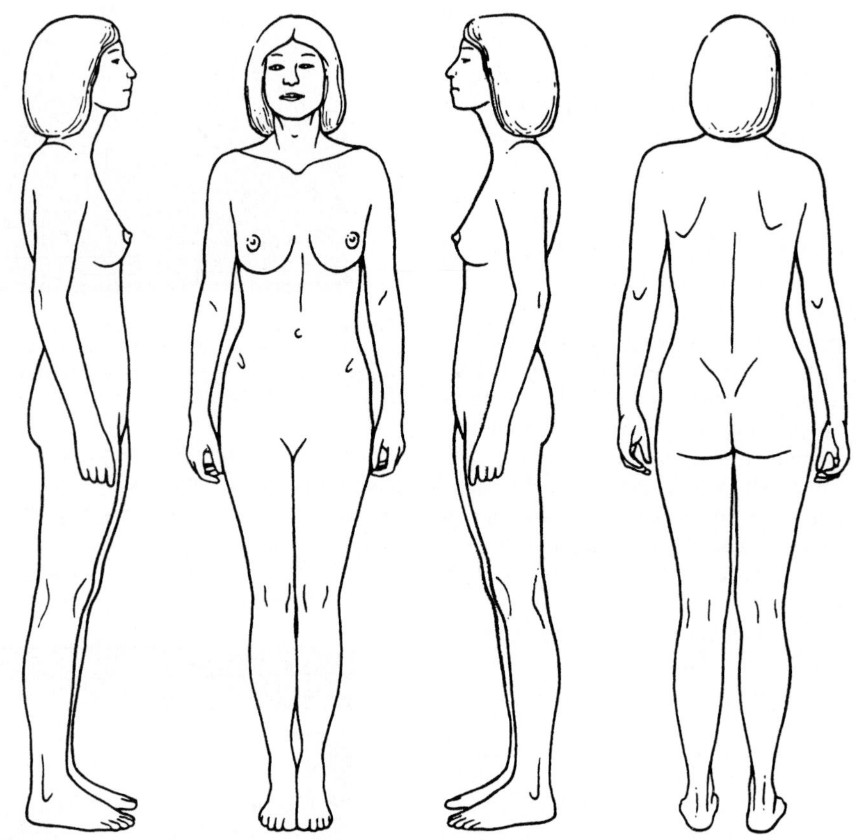

Physical findings ____

____

Identify the quality and site of tenderness caused by palpation, extent of nodularity, diffuse or focal distribution, and/or fixation of uterus/adnexa. On the anatomic drawings above, draw a **BROKEN LINE** around the area(s) of tenderness found on examination.

Adjuncts: [ ] IVP? [ ] BE? [ ] Sigmoidoscopy? [ ] Other? ____________________

____

[1]The association of pelvic pain and endometriosis remains enigmatic because the extent of disease by the previous AFS classifications does not dependably relate to the severity of pelvic pain or tenderness. This form was designed by the AFS Committee on Classification of Endometriosis to carefully document the location and intensity of pelvic pain and tenderness in addition to distribution of endometriosis and pelvic adhesions. Constant recording of this data will permit consistent management of the patient with endometriosis and pelvic pain, and facilitate clinical research.

A

Procedure ____

____

OPERATIVE DESCRIPTION OF PELVIC ADHESIONS

Describe the location, points of attachment and characteristics of adhesions. Abbreviate characteristics as **A = avascular/thin, T = thick/dense, B = band/string-like, S = sheet-like.** Draw a picture of these adhesions at the appropriate location in each quadrant.

IIa (Left lateral)

I (Anterior)

IIb (Right lateral)

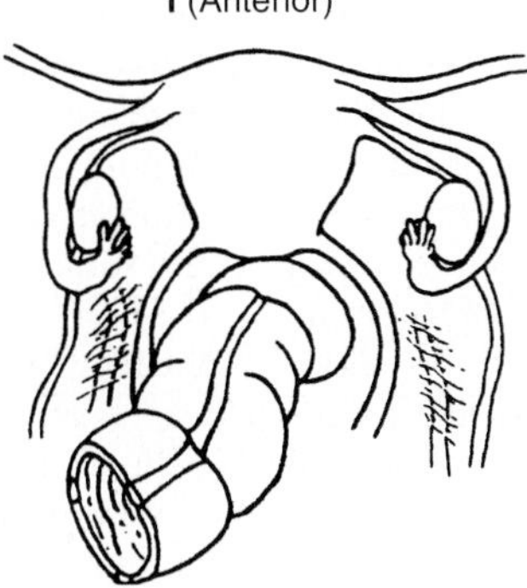

IV (Other sites)

III (Posterior)

OPERATIVE APPEARANCE OF THE DISTRIBUTION OF ENDOMETRIOSIS

After mobilizing the pelvic viscera, measure the size (mean diameter in millimeters) and depth of each visible lesion. Use a calibrated endoscopic probe, if necessary. Record the location, dimension, visual appearance and histologic confirmation of these lesions. Abbreviate the visual appearance as **C = clear, V = vesicles/blebs, P = pink, R = red/flame-like, B = black/blue, Y = yellow/brown, W = white, F = peritoneal fibrosis.** Document the site of each lesion by positioning the index number (No. on the table below) at the appropriate location in each quadrant.

IIa (Left lateral)

I (Anterior)

IIb (Right lateral)

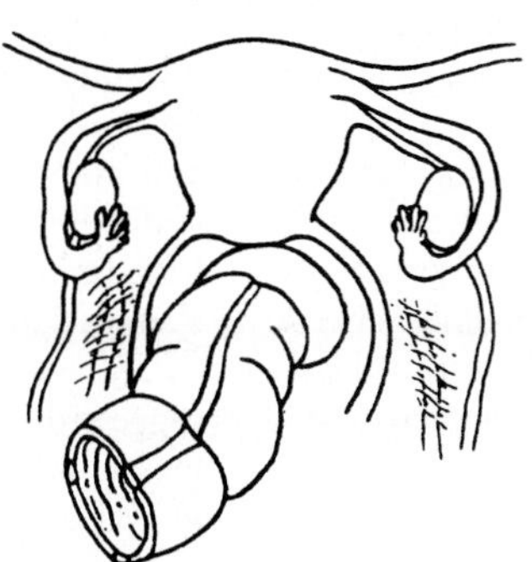

IVa (Other intra-abdominal sites)

IVb (Outside peritoneal cavity)

III (Posterior)

No.	Size in mm	Depth	Appearance	Histology	Location	No.	Size in mm	Depth	Appearance	Histology	Location
i.e.	*8 m*	*2 mm*	*F*	*Glands & stroma*	*III*						
1						11					
2						12					
3						13					
4						14					
5						15					
6						16					
7						17					
8						18					
9						19					
10						20					

Histology ____

Results ____

____

B

Figure 19-13. Form for the management of endometriosis in the presence of pelvic pain. (Reprinted from Fertility and Sterility, 60, The American Fertility Society, Management of endometriosis in the presence of pelvic pain, 953. Copyright 1993, with permission from The American Society for Reproductive Medicine.)

form and point-scoring system include a complete description of the location, width, and depth of the implants, and the presence and severity of adhesive disease by location thickness and points of attachment. An updated scoring system developed in 1996 by the American Society for Reproductive Medicine was designed primarily to record the progress of the disease in fertility patients. The focus here was intended to provide characterization of disease extent for fertility and not for pain assessment. Nevertheless, there are no data supporting this correlation of scoring with pregnancy rates. It is easy to combine this form with a numeric pain scale to periodically document specific pain symptoms and the physical findings of tenderness during pelvic exam (Fig. 19-14).

Ultrasound examination shows no specific pattern to screen for pelvic endometriosis but may be helpful in differentiating solid from cystic lesions and may help distinguish an endometrioma from other adnexal abnormalities. Since the lesions are vascular, increased Doppler flow may be demonstrated in endometriosis.

Magnetic resonance imaging (MRI) provides the best diagnostic tool for endometriosis but is not always a practical modality for its diagnosis. With a detection ratio and specificity of around 78% for implants, MRI for endometriosis has a reported sensitivity and specificity of approximately 91% to 95%. There is a characteristic hyperintensity on T1-weighted images and a hypointensity on T2-weighted images.

Although a benign disease, endometriosis exhibits characteristics of both malignancy and sterile inflammation. Therefore the common considerations in the differential diagnosis include chronic pelvic inflammatory disease, ovarian malignancy, degeneration of myomas, hemorrhage or torsion of ovarian cysts, adenomyosis, primary dysmenorrhea, and functional bowel disease.

Occasionally a large endometrioma of the ovary may rupture into the peritoneal cavity. This results in an acute surgical abdomen and brings into the differential diagnosis conditions such as ectopic pregnancy, appendicitis, diverticulitis, and a bleeding corpus luteum cyst. Studies have not demonstrated any temporal relationship between the timing of an endometrioma's acute rupture and the day of the menstrual cycle.

Natural History

Endometriosis is a chronic and sometimes progressive disease. The disease is usually first diagnosed in a woman during her mid to late 20s. The rate of progression of the disease varies widely from one patient to another. Serial pelvic examinations are a poor indicator of progression of the disease. Therefore the natural history of the disease is largely speculation. In some centers, second-look or reassessment laparoscopy is performed routinely. These limited studies have given insight into the success of therapy but have not been shown to be a benefit in women trying to conceive. Serum levels of cancer antigen-125 (CA-125) have been used as a marker for endometriosis. CA-125 levels are elevated in most patients with endometriosis and increases incrementally with advanced stages. However, assays for serum levels of CA-125 have a low specificity because they also increase with other pelvic conditions such as myomas, acute pelvic inflammatory disease, and the first trimester of pregnancy. Similarly, serum CA-125 levels have a low sensitivity for the diagnosis of early or minimal endometriosis. It is also useful for tracking the course of the disease with treatment.

Glycodelin, previously known as placental protein 14, has been shown to be elevated in endometriosis and is produced in endometriotic lesions. Levels also fall with removal of disease. However, because of great variability in levels, glycodelin has not proved to be useful clinically.

It would be optimal to identify women who are going to develop endometriosis. All we have currently is family history. However, the optimal preventive therapy for a young teenager not desirous of pregnancy until her late 20s is unknown. Clinical options include no treatment, continuous use of oral contraceptives, or cyclic oral contraceptive therapy. Controlled prospective studies are needed to answer the difficult clinical question of the best method to inhibit progression of the disease. Approximately 10% of teenagers who develop endometriosis have associated congenital outflow obstruction. Therefore teenagers with pelvic pain should be examined for this possibility.

At one time there was a general belief that pregnancy improved endometriosis. A careful study by McArthur and Ulfelder of external endometriosis, which could be observed throughout the pregnancy, discovered that this generalization was not invariably true. In some cases endometriomas rapidly increase in size during the first few weeks of pregnancy. In general, during the third trimester, symptoms are less severe and the size of the external lesions decreases. Clearly endometriosis and large endometriomas have been found at the time of cesarean section, although this is an unusual occurrence.

In the past few years, there has been the realization that endometriosis may be associated with ovarian cancer. Not only are lesions found at the time of diagnosis of ovarian cancer, but the risk of developing ovarian cancer may be increased fourfold in women with endometriosis. Loss of heterozygosity and mutations in suppressor genes, for example, *p53,* may explain this commonality. These findings warrant caution in the long-term follow-up of women who have extensive disease and ovarian endometriomas.

The association of other cancers with endometriosis, although suggested, has not been substantiated. However, cervical endometriosis is a particular condition that can produce abnormalities in cervical cytology.

Endometriosis is dependent on ovarian hormones to stimulate growth. With natural menopause, there is a gradual relief of symptoms. Following surgical menopause, areas of endometriosis rapidly disappear. However, it is important to note that 5% of symptomatic cases of endometriosis present after menopause. The vast majority of cases in women in their late 50s or early 60s are related to the use of exogenous estrogen.

Management

The two primary short-term goals in treating endometriosis are the relief of pain and promotion of fertility. The primary long-term goal in the management of endometriosis is attempting to prevent progression or recurrence of the disease process. Presently, there is a paucity of definitive, evidence-based literature on which to select the most appropriate method of treatment. The appropriate treatment for endometriosis varies widely because of the vast differences in the spectrum of clinical symptoms and in the extent of the disease from one woman to

Patient's name ____________________ Date ____________

Stage I (Minimal) - 1–5
Stage II (Mild) - 6–15
Stage III (Moderate) - 16–40
Stage IV (Severe) - > 40
Total ____________

Laparoscopy ______ Laparotomy ______ Photography ______
Recommended Treatment ____________________

Prognosis ____________

PERITONEUM	**ENDOMETRIOSIS**	< 1cm	1–3cm	> 3cm
	Superficial	1	2	4
	Deep	2	4	6
OVARY	R Superficial	1	2	4
	Deep	4	16	20
	L Superficial	1	2	4
	Deep	4	16	20

	POSTERIOR CULDESAC OBLITERATION	Partial	Complete
		4	40

OVARY	**ADHESIONS**	< 1/3 Enclosure	1/3–2/3 Enclosure	> 2/3 Enclosure
	R Filmy	1	2	4
	Dense	4	8	16
	L Filmy	1	2	4
	Dense	4	8	16
TUBE	R Filmy	1	2	4
	Dense	4*	8*	16
	L Filmy	1	2	4
	Dense	4*	8*	16

*If the fimbriated end of the fallopian tube is completely enclosed, change the point assignment to 16.
Denote appearance of superficial implant types as red [(R), red, red-pink, flamelike, vesicular blobs, clear vesicles], white [(W), opacifications, peritoneal defects, yellow-brown], or black [(B) black, hemosiderm deposits, blue]. Denote percent of total described as R ___%, W___ % and B___ %. Total should equal 100%.

Additional endometriosis: ____________________

Associated pathology: ____________________

To be used with normal tubes and ovaries

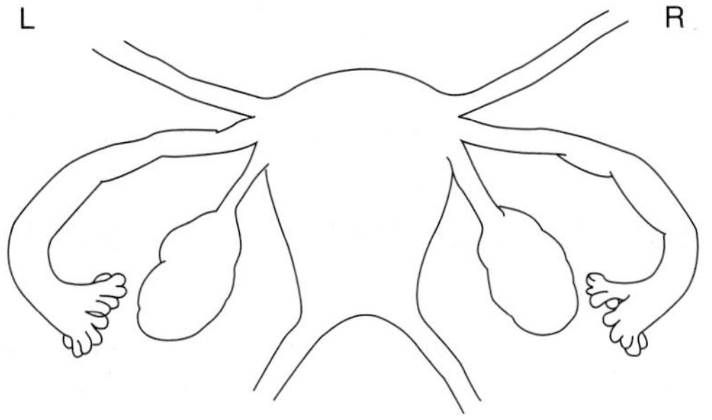

L R

To be used with abnormal tubes and/or ovaries

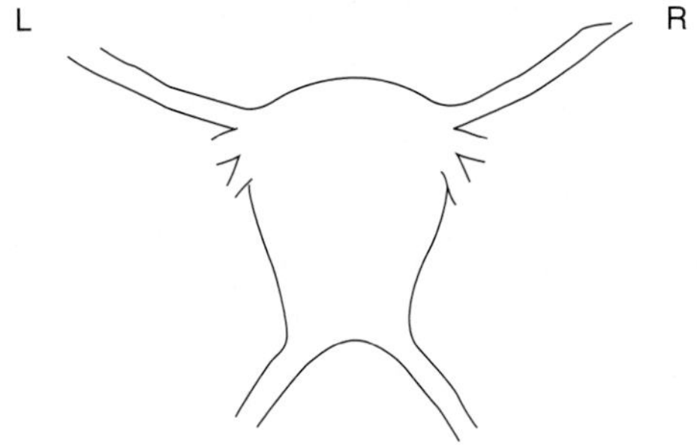

L R

Figure 19-14. Updated scoring system to record the progress of endometriosis in fertility patients. (Reprinted from Fertility and Sterility, 67, American Society for Reproductive Medicine, Revised American Society for Reproductive Medicine classification of endometriosis: 1996, 817. Copyright 1997, with permission from The American Society for Reproductive Medicine.)

another. Therefore the treatment plan must be individualized. Choice of therapy, for women whose primary symptom is pelvic pain, depends on multiple variables, including the patient's age, her future reproductive plans, the location and extent of her disease, the severity of her symptoms, and associated pelvic pathology. Most patients should undergo a diagnostic evaluation, which may necessitate a diagnostic laparoscopy to establish the nature and extent of endometriosis before embarking on prolonged therapy. However, if other gynecologic conditions such as chronic pelvic inflammatory disease or neoplasia have been ruled out, empiric medical therapy for 3 months with a gonadotropin-releasing hormone (GnRH) agonist is a reasonable option. Although pelvic pain may decrease, such therapy has not been thought to help diagnostically.

Treatment of endometriosis can be medical, surgical, or a combination of both. Most of the sex steroids, alone or in combination, have been tried in clinical studies to suppress the growth of endometriosis. Optimal regression secondary to medical treatment is observed in small endometriomas that are less than 1 to 2 cm in diameter. Response in larger areas of endometriosis may be minimal with medical therapy. A poor therapeutic result may be governed by the reduction of blood supply to the mass caused by surrounding scar tissue.

Surgical therapy is divided into conservative and definitive operations. Conservative surgery involves the resection or destruction of endometrial implants, lysis of adhesions, and attempts to restore normal pelvic anatomy. Definitive surgery involves the removal of both ovaries, the uterus, and all visible ectopic foci of endometriosis.

Medical Therapy

The primary goal of the hormonal treatment of endometriosis is induction of amenorrhea. Recurrent bleeding in the ectopic implants is one of the most important pathophysiologic processes to interrupt. Brosens has advanced the hypothesis that endometriosis is a physiologic process unless recurrent bleeding in the ectopic implants produces progressive disease and symptoms. Therefore, he postulates that effective medical therapy can be established by amenorrhea without the induction of hypoestrogenism. Recent clinical studies confirm that effective medical treatment can be achieved without the induction of severe hypoestrogenism. It is hoped that hormonal treatment will create an environment that will inhibit growth and promote regression of the disease. Medical therapy is very effective in relieving pain while the patient is taking medication. However, symptoms often recur several months after discontinuing therapy. Both clinical symptomatology and findings on second-look laparoscopy have demonstrated that clinical improvement correlates directly with establishment of amenorrhea. The choice of medical therapy for the individual patient depends on the clinician's evaluation of adverse effects, side effects, cost of therapy, and expected patient compliance. The clinical effectiveness, as measured by relief of symptoms and recurrence rates of current medical therapies, are similar. The recurrence rate following medical therapy is 5% to 15% in the first year and increases to 40% to 50% in 5 years. Obviously the chance of recurrence is directly related to the extent of initial disease. In summary, medical therapy usually suppresses symptomatology and prevents progression of endometriosis, but it does not provide a long-lasting cure of the disease. The recurrence rate in women who initially had minimal disease is approximately 35% while in those women whose initial disease was severe the rate is approximately 75%. The only two approved therapies for endometriosis are danazol and GnRH agonists.

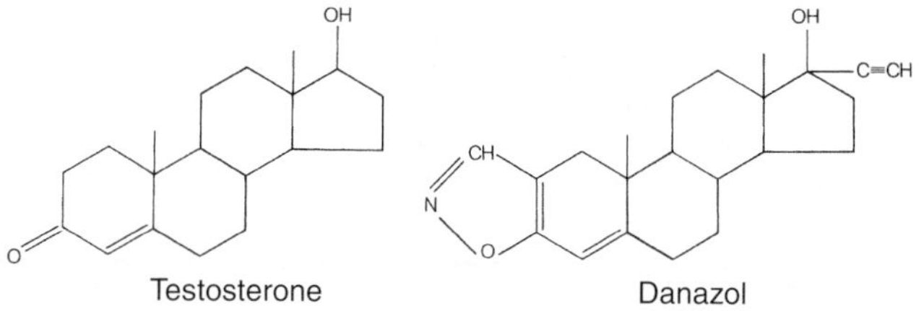

OH OH C≡CH CH N O O Testosterone Danazol

Figure 19-15. Chemical structures of danazol and testosterone.

Danazol. Danazol was approved by the Food and Drug Administration in the mid-1970s for the treatment of endometriosis. In recent years clinicians are less likely to prescribe danazol and most frequently select GnRH agonists, progestogens, or oral contraceptives as their drugs of choice for medical therapy of endometriosis. Danazol also may be prescribed for women with benign cystic mastitis, menorrhagia, and hereditary angioneurotic edema. Danazol is an attenuated androgen that is active when given orally. Chemically it is a synthetic steroid that is the isoxazole derivative of ethisterone (17-α-ethinyltestosterone) (Fig. 19-15). Danazol produces a hypoestrogenic and hyperandrogenic effect on steroid-sensitive end organs. The drug is mildly androgenic and anabolic. Many of danazol's side effects are directly related to these two properties. The androgenic effects of testosterone are approximately 200 times greater than those of danazol.

Danazol binds to androgen and progesterone receptors and also binds to sex hormone-binding globulin. The latter effect results in a threefold increase in endogenous free testosterone levels. Danazol directly inhibits several steroidogenic enzymes in both the ovary and the adrenal gland, thus reducing circulating steroid levels. In vitro and in vivo studies have shown that danazol may also modulate immunologic function through an effect on macrophages or T lymphocytes.

Danazol induces atrophic changes in the endometrium of the uterus and similar changes in endometrial implants (Fig. 19-16). An endometrial biopsy performed after several weeks of therapy shows endometrial atrophy with few glands and an inactive stroma. It would be difficult to differentiate the biopsy of a young woman taking danazol from the biopsy of a postmenopausal woman.

The standard prescribed dosage of danazol is 400 to 800 mg/day for approximately 6 months. The half-life of this oral drug is between 4 and 5 hours. Therefore, for the 800-mg dosage regimen, it is best to recommend one tablet four times a day rather than two tablets in the morning and two at night. Prescribing danazol 200 mg every 6 hours results in mean serum estradiol (E_2) concentrations that are 40% lower than with the alternative regimen, 400 mg twice a day. Traditionally the drug is started on the fifth day after the onset of menses. The length of therapy of oral danazol should be individualized, depending partly on the stage of endometriosis. Women should use mechanical contraceptives for the first month, as danazol has produced female pseudohermaphroditism in a developing fetus. If one is certain the patient is not pregnant, danazol is begun on the first day of the menstrual bleeding. By starting the hormone

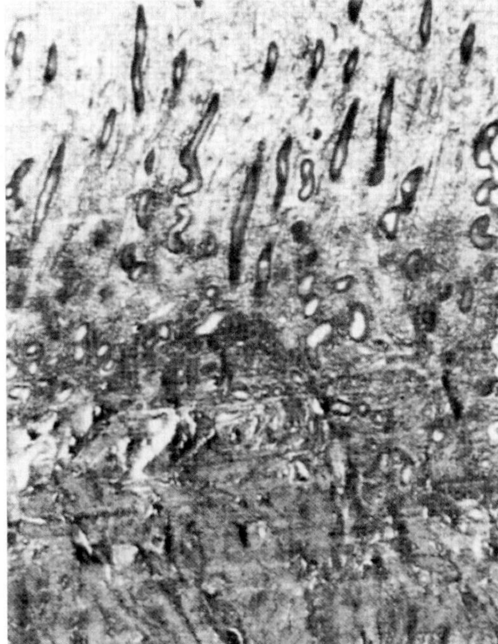

A

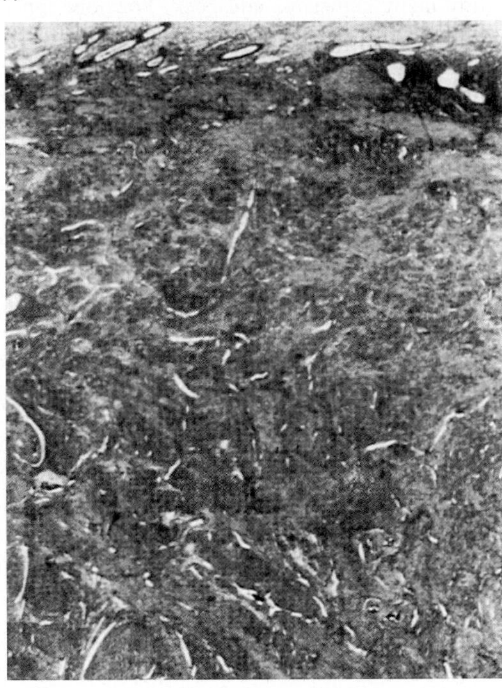

B

Figure 19-16. **A,** Untreated endometrium. **B,** Endometrium after 4 months treatment with danazol. (Reprinted from Fertility and Sterility, 22, Greenblatt RP, Dmowski WP, Mahesh VB, Scholer HFL, Clinical studies with an antigonadotropin—Danazol, 108. Copyright 1971, with permission from The American Society for Reproductive Medicine.)

earlier in the cycle, the patient will experience less breakthrough bleeding during the first 4 to 6 weeks.

Many investigators have reduced the total daily dosage of the drug down to 200, and even 100 mg of danazol daily. Because the relief of the symptoms is directly related to the incidence of amenorrhea, the lower dosages of danazol are not as effective but may be tried. However, women with an atrophic endometrium may experience breakthrough bleeding.

Table 19-7 Adverse Reactions to Danazol (800 mg/day)

Androgenic Action	
Acne	17%
Edema	6%
Weight gain	5%
Hirsutism	6%
Voice changes	3%
Antiestrogenic Action	
Flushes and sweats	15%
Uterine spotting	10%
Decrease in breast size	5%
Change in libido	3%–5%
Atrophic vaginitis	3%
Idiopathic Drug Reactions	
Gastrointestinal disturbances	8%
Weakness, dizziness	8%
Muscle cramps	4%
Skin rashes	3%
Headaches	2%
Sleep disturbances	Uncommon

From Luciano AA: Contemp OB/GYN 19:228, 1982. Modified from Greenblatt R (ed): Recent Advances in Endometriosis: Proceedings of a Symposium, Augusta, GA, March 5–6, 1975. Bridgewater, NJ, Excerpta Medica, 1976, p 368.

Side effects of the hormonal changes are encountered by 80% of patients taking danazol. Approximately 10% to 20% of women discontinue the drug because of side effects. Virtually all of the symptoms disappear on cessation of drug therapy. However, there are scattered reports of deepening of the voice that did not resolve after discontinuation. Symptoms that have been related to danazol therapy are listed in (Table 19-7). Danazol is metabolized in the liver with cleavage of the isoxazole ring. Mild elevation in serum liver enzyme levels has been reported in women treated for endometriosis, and women who take danazol for longer than 6 months should have serum liver enzyme determinations. An androgenic effect on lipids occurs, with reduction in high-density lipoprotein (HDL) cholesterol and triglycerides and an increase in low-density lipoprotein (LDL) cholesterol.

The standard length of treatment with danazol is 6 to 9 months. Approximately three of four patients note significant improvement in their symptoms, and about 90% have objective improvement discovered at second-look laparoscopy. The uncorrected fertility rate following danazol therapy is approximately 40%. Unfortunately, 15% to 30% of women will have recurrence of symptoms within 2 years following therapy.

Several randomized, double-blind clinical studies have compared the therapeutic effectiveness of danazol with GnRH agonists. The results do not show significant differences between the efficacies of these two drugs.

GnRH Agonists

Multiple GnRH agonists have been developed and approved for the treatment of endometriosis. Representative agonists are leuprolide acetate (Lupron, injectable), nafarelin acetate (Synarel, intranasal), and goserelin acetate (Zoladex, subcutaneous implant). The usual dose of leuprolide acetate is 3.75 mg intramuscularly once per month or 11.25 mg depot injection every 3 months. Nafarelin acetate nasal spray is given in a dose of one spray (200 μg) in one nostril in the morning and one spray (200 μg) in the other nostril in the evening up to a maximum of 800 μg daily. Goserelin acetate is given in a dosage of 3.6 mg every 28 days in a biodegradable subcutaneous implant.

Studies have determined the dose-response curve of the GnRH agonists, establishing the optimal dose to produce sufficient down-regulation and desensitization of the pituitary to produce extremely low levels of circulating estrogen and amenorrhea. Chronic use of GnRH agonists produces a "medical oophorectomy." A dramatic reduction occurs in serum estrone, E_2, testosterone, and androstenedione to levels similar to the hormonal levels in oophorectomized women. The total serum estrone and estradiol levels and the free serum E_2 concentration are 25% to 50% of those measured in women taking danazol chronically for endometriosis.

GnRH agonists have no effect on sex hormone-binding globulin. Thus the androgenic side effects from danazol caused by the increase in free serum testosterone are not observed. Similarly, no significant changes occur in total serum cholesterol, HDL, or LDL levels during therapeutic periods of as long as 6 months. Endometrial samples obtained after several months of chronic agonist therapy demonstrated either atrophic or early proliferative endometrium.

The side effects associated with GnRH agonist therapy are primarily those associated with estrogen deprivation, similar to menopause. The three most common symptoms are hot flushes, vaginal dryness, and insomnia. A decrease in bone mineral content has been demonstrated in the trabecular bone of the lumbar spine by quantitative computer tomography. This decrease in bone density is not seen in the compact bone of the distal radius. There is a decrease in measured bone mass of 2% to 7% during a 6-month course of agonist therapy. However, it has been established that the decrease in bone density associated with 6 months of therapy with GnRH agonist completely recovers between 12 and 24 months after discontinuing therapy.

The clinical response to agonist therapy depends on when the therapy is initiated in regard to the menstrual cycle. If agonist therapy is begun during the follicular phase, an agonist phase results in an initial rapid rise in FSH and E_2 for approximately 3 weeks. FSH levels fall to basal levels by the third to fourth week of therapy. E_2 levels rapidly decline after 21 days of therapy. The expected LH surge does not occur, and serum progesterone levels do not become elevated. Amenorrhea is induced within 6 to 8 weeks. In contrast, beginning agonist therapy during the luteal phase, or if artificially manipulated by the concurrent administration of oral progestogen, serum E_2 levels are suppressed to those postoophorectomy within 2 weeks. Amenorrhea is induced in 4 to 5 weeks. It is important to ensure that the patient is not pregnant when beginning GnRH agonist therapy during the luteal phase.

GnRH agonist therapy results in amelioration of symptomatology in 75% to 90% of patients with endometriosis, depending on the extent of the disease in the study group. Growth of endometriosis is arrested, diminished, or eliminated. The greatest therapeutic effects are seen in patients whose areas of endometriosis are less than 1 cm in diameter. In comparison studies, the results of GnRH agonist therapy are directly comparable with those obtained with danazol.

Ovarian function will return to normal in 6 to 12 weeks after 6 months of GnRH agonist therapy. Large ovarian endometriomas and severe adhesive disease have not responded to hormonal therapy. The primary advantage of GnRH agonists over danazol is better patient compliance. Most patients find the side effects of GnRH agonists more tolerable.

Currently many clinicians "add-back" hormone replacement therapy with dosages similar to menopausal therapy in combination with chronic GnRH agonist regimens. The clinical hypothesis is that the add-back medication will reduce or eliminate the vasomotor symptoms and vaginal atrophy and also diminish or overcome the demineralization of bone. Barbieri has suggested that there is a therapeutic window that he estimates is a circulating level of approximately 30 pg/mL of E_2. He postulates that this level of E_2 is enough to protect the body from substantial bone loss and is not high enough to interfere with the inhibition of growth of endometriosis (Fig. 19-17). Multiple randomized series have demonstrated that add-back therapy does not interfere in the effectiveness of agonists to relieve the pelvic pain from endometriosis. The majority of studies have also demonstrated no diminished therapeutic efficacy when add-back therapy is initiated simultaneously with the GnRH agonist. Some clinicians additionally give bisphosphonates and calcium with the low-dose progestins and estrogen. Add-back regimens not only reduce or eliminate adverse clinical and metabolic side effects associated with hypoestrogenism, but also facilitate safe and effective prolongation of GnRH agonist

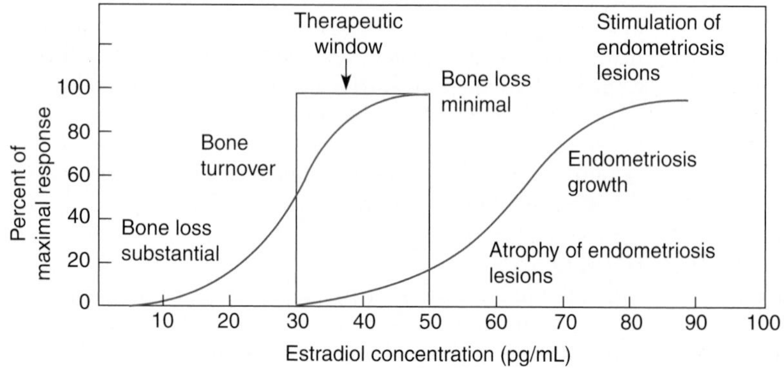

Figure 19-17. Estradiol therapeutic window. The concentration of estradiol required to cause growth of endometriosis lesions may be greater than the concentration required to stabilize bone mineral density. (From Barbieri RL: Hormone treatment of endometriosis: The estrogen threshold hypothesis. Am J Obstet Gynecol 166:740, 1992.)

therapy for up to 12 months Additional agents which have been used for add back therapy are tibolone and raloxifene.

For women not wishing to conceive, who predominantly have pain and no indication for surgery (which may include failed medical therapy), stopping and starting various treatments and interchanging them is a reasonable approach to control symptoms.

Oral Contraceptives. Kistner was the first to popularize the continuous use of high-dosage, combination oral contraceptives for endometriosis. In the late 1950s very large doses of norethynodrel with mestranol daily was given to produce amenorrhea and a "pseudopregnancy." Most of the published studies involved the first-generation, high-estrogen-content oral contraceptives. However, more recent reports have established that the present low-estrogen monophasic combination pills, specifically the ones with a relatively high progestin potency, are equally effective when used in a continuous fashion. Over the past 30 years, the most economical regimen for the treatment of women with mild or moderate symptoms of endometriosis has been continuous daily oral contraceptives for 6 to 12 months.

The regimen is started by a single daily monophasic oral contraceptive tablet beginning on the third day of the patient's period and the pills are taken continuously. Doses have been increased to deal with breakthrough bleeding. As in other hormonal regimens for endometriosis, amenorrhea is the desired endpoint. The optimal regimen is the lowest daily dose of steroids that will produce amenorrhea in the individual patient. Most patients are able to maintain the amenorrhea for 6 to 9 months, using at most three to four contraceptive tablets a day. It is necessary to emphasize to the patient the importance of continuous rather than intermittent oral contraceptive therapy.

The initial histologic response is similar to that of normal pregnancy, with an increase in vascularity and edema in the endometrial implants. This transient growth phase may cause an acute exacerbation of the clinical symptoms. Occasionally, large ovarian endometriomas rupture, resulting in an acute surgical abdomen during the first 6 weeks of oral contraceptive therapy. During prolonged therapy the endometrial glands atrophy and the stroma undergoes a marked decidual reaction. Some smaller endometriomas (<1 to 2 cm) can undergo necrobiosis and resorption.

The most common side effects of inducing amenorrhea with oral contraceptives include weight gain and breast tenderness. Approximately one in three women discontinue this therapy because of side effects.

The results of continuous oral contraceptive therapy include a decrease in symptomatology in approximately 80% of patients during therapy.

NSAIDs

NSAIDs are beneficial for pain relief and as concomitant therapy may improve the bleeding control of patients on oral contraceptives. There may also be a direct therapeutic value in endometriosis. Although cyclooxygenase-2 (Cox-2) inhibitors are now infrequently used because of cardiovascular concerns in older individuals, this therapy for endometriosis has a rationale in that lesions of endometriosis have been found to express high levels of Cox-2. In summary, antiinflammatory agents may be beneficial for pain relief as well as potentially for the treatment of endometriosis particularly when other suppressive therapy cannot be used.

Other hormonal treatments. For women who cannot tolerate the high dosage of estrogen in the pseudopregnancy regimen or who have a contraindication to estrogen therapy, treatment with progestins only has been successful. Medroxyprogesterone (Provera), 30 mg orally per day or depomedroxyprogesterone (Depo-Provera) in a dosage of 150 mg intramuscularly every 3 months to a maximum of 200 mg every month, will produce a prolonged amenorrhea. The medication is most appropriate for the older woman who has completed childbearing. The time of resumption of ovulation following discontinuation of injectable medroxyprogesterone is prolonged and extremely variable. Some women will not ovulate for more than a year after their last injection. Therefore this form of therapy should not be prescribed for a young woman who is contemplating pregnancy in the near future. Oral medroxyprogesterone in a dosage of 30 mg/day is an alternative mode of therapy, as is norethindrone acetate (10 to 40 mg) daily. This more androgenic progestogen, although quite effective, has a similar symptom profile to that for continuous medroxyprogesterone.

The most prominent side effects while taking medroxyprogesterone are breakthrough spotting or bleeding. Approximately 40% of patients develop abnormal bleeding associated with high-dose progestin therapy. If there is no contraindication to estrogen, this symptom can be alleviated by small doses of oral estrogen. Many women find unacceptable the changes in mood, depression, and irritability produced by high-dose progestogens.

Gestrinone is a progestogen originally developed as a once-a-week oral contraceptive. Recently, this drug has undergone clinical trials for endometriosis with dosages ranging from 2.5 to 7.5 mg/week. Gestrinone acts as an agonist–antagonist of progesterone receptors and an agonist of androgen receptors and also binds weakly to estrogen receptors. At completion of therapy in a randomized trial, a tendency for prolonged pain relief was observed for gestrinone when compared with GnRH agonist.

There are several other potential agents for use based on in vitro evidence of altered expression in endometriosis as reviewed earlier. These include Cox-2 inhibitors; aromatase inhibitors (which have been successfully used in some women); and peroxisome proliferator-activated receptor (PPAR)-ligands, which has been shown to inhibit macrophage action in mice. Additionally, targeting haptoglobin (because of structural similarity to Endo-1, which is a novel chemoattractant product of endometriosis epithelial cells) or MMPs, as well as tumor necrosis factor-β (TNFβ) and VEGF all have had some experimental support. Use of antiprogestogens, specifically RU 486 and mifepristone, has revealed beneficial effects in humans but may have limited use because of antiglucocorticoid effects. Among estrogen receptor modulators, tamoxifen may worsen the situation, and raloxifene may be neutral or beneficial. An antiinflammatory immunomodulator, pentoxifylline, has been shown to be beneficial as well.

Finally, refinement of existing therapies may be beneficial. GnRH antagonists may be more beneficial because of lack of an agonistic "flare" effect and a more suitable therapeutic window in estrogen levels. Delivering progestogens or danazol locally (intrauterine or vaginally) may also enhance effectiveness.

Surgical Therapy

The choice between medical treatment to suppress endometriosis and surgical therapy to remove lesions depends on the patient's age, symptomatology, and reproductive desires. Surgical therapy often occurs concurrently when a laparoscopy is performed to establish the diagnosis of the disease. Obviously, surgical therapy is the only option for failed medical therapy. Because endometriosis is a puzzling disease, with great individual variation in its natural course, many therapeutic regimens exist, and individualized treatment is necessary.

Surgery has been the foundation of treatment for women with moderate or severe endometriosis especially those with adhesions and when the disease involves nonreproductive organs. A surgical approach is mandatory in cases involving acute rupture of large endometriomas, ureteral obstruction, compromise in intestinal function or for large ovarian endometriomas.

Laparoscopy is employed frequently for both diagnostic and therapeutic reasons. The major advantage of treating endometriosis with the laparoscope, using surgical instruments, the laser, or electrocautery, is that patients may be treated at the time of diagnosis. Depending on the operative technique chosen, endometriosis is coagulated, vaporized, or resected. Surgical treatment for endometriosis should mainly be carried out via laparoscopy rather than by laparotomy because of a shorter recovery period and reduction in the extent of subsequent adhesions.

Adhesions in the pelvis have varying characteristics. They may be minimal or extensive, filmy or dense, and avascular or vascular. If the laser is used, the surgeon must adjust spot size, power setting (watts), and time of application to control depth of penetration. The laser is preferable to electrocautery when endometriosis is adjacent to the ureter, bladder, or bowel because the depth of penetration can be controlled. Follow-up studies have documented pain improvement in 70% to 80% of patients treated via the laparoscope.

In a prospective randomized trial, Sutton demonstrated efficiency of laser laparoscopy over expectant management after diagnostic laparoscopy. Pain decreased by 62.5% compared with 22.6% with expectant management, and pain relief continued in 55% of women over 72 months. The median time to pain recurrence after surgery has been estimated to be 20 months. It has been suggested that photosensitization of lesions in endometriosis may also add some therapeutic value although this approach is still considered experimental.

The surgical difficulties in treating invasive carcinoma and endometriosis are similar. The infiltrative nature of both disease processes and the associated scarring result in a loss of cleavage planes and results in difficult dissections. Technically it is easier to palpate rather than visualize the extent of the infiltrative process of endometriosis. Special care must be taken not to injure the bladder or bowel during excision of areas impinging on these structures.

Conservative surgery has as its goal the removal of all macroscopic, visible areas of endometriosis with preservation of ovarian function and restoration of normal pelvic anatomy. Conservative operations include removal or destruction of implants, removal of endometriomas, lysis of adhesions, appendectomy, and sometimes presacral neurectomy. Throughout these procedures the surgeon observes the principles of microsurgery and plastic surgery, including minimal and gentle handling of tissues, avoiding hypoxia of the peritoneum, and attempting to restore the pelvic anatomy to normal. Approximately one in four women will have a second operation for a recurrence of endometriosis. Laparoscopy has been proven to be as effective and reliable as laparotomy in the treatment of ovarian endometriomas. The rate of recurrence is directly dependent on the duration of follow-up and is highest in women with stage 4 disease and a history of previous surgery for endometriosis. Recent studies have documented that excision of an ovarian endometrioma is associated with a lower reoperation rate than using a fenestration technique, and both are superior to cyst aspiration alone.

If the patient has midline pain, such as dysmenorrhea or dyspareunia, occasionally a presacral neurectomy or resection of the uterosacral ligaments may be performed. Ablation of the uterosacral nerves when performed via the laparoscope is called laser uterosacral nerve ablation (LUNA). This procedure is less frequently performed today due to questionable efficacy and concerns of surgical complications. A successful presacral neurectomy relieves only midline pain and does not diminish pain in other areas of the pelvis.

Somewhere between conservative and definitive surgery for endometriosis there is a place for total abdominal hysterectomy with ovarian preservation of one or both ovaries. This operation is selected for women who have completed childbearing and are in their late 20s or 30s. It is interesting that without repetitive episodes of retrograde menstruation, the endometriosis remains quiescent in the majority of these women. Approximately one out of three women develop recurrent symptoms, and they subsequently have a second operation involving oophorectomy.

Definitive surgical treatment is reserved for patients with far-advanced disease and for whom future fertility is not a consideration. Patients with pain that continues after medical and conservative surgery are treated by definitive surgery. Definitive surgery involves total abdominal hysterectomy, bilateral salpingo-oophorectomy, and the removal of all visible endometriosis. If the surgery was not complete because of the extensiveness of the disease, it is best to treat a premenopausal woman with progestogens or continuous oral contraceptive therapy for approximately 6 to 12 months before beginning cyclic hormonal therapy.

Medical therapy and surgical therapy are often performed in combination for advanced stages of the disease. Clinicians debate the advantages of either preoperative or postoperative medical therapy. Presently many surgeons favor preoperative medical treatment followed by surgery in women with extensive disease. It is postulated that preoperative therapy facilitates the subsequent operative procedure although this perception is not evidence-based. Depending on the extensiveness of disease and the success of surgery, medical therapy postoperatively may also be considered.

Photodynamic therapy for endometriosis is undergoing preliminary trials as mentioned earlier. This procedure involves intravenous injection of a special dye that is concentrated in areas of endometriosis. A laser light produces a photochemical reaction to destroy the areas.

If a patient has recurrent symptoms following definitive surgery for endometriosis and has not been taking exogenous estrogen, it is possible that she has a remnant of residual ovary, which can be diagnosed by measuring serum gonadotropin levels. If the follicle-stimulating hormone (FSH) and luteinizing hormone (LH) levels are not in menopausal range, some viable ovarian tissue remains, usually in the retroperitoneal space. Operative management is the preferred method of treatment for persistent pelvic pain secondary to retroperitoneal remnants of active ovarian tissue. In rare instances, when recurrent operative procedures fail to relieve the symptoms of recurrent endometriosis, it is appropriate to ablate the remnants using external radiotherapy with a total dose of 10 to 20 Gy.

Most surgeons routinely remove the appendix when performing surgery for endometriosis not related to infertility. In a series of more than 100 consecutive patients with endometriosis, 13% had histologic evidence of endometriosis in the appendix. This involvement could be discovered by gross examination in only 60% of patients.

Therapy for Fertility

Medical therapy cannot be first-line treatment for endometriosis because suppression of ovulation interferes with the ability to conceive. Occasionally as an adjunct, more prolonged (than usual) GnRH agonist therapy may be used before in vitro fertilization (IVF). In this section surgical options will be considered.

It is clear that for symptomatic women with ovarian endometriomas, laparoscopic surgical excision should be undertaken. However, in cases of extensive pelvic disease where in vitro fertilization/embryo transfer (IVF-ET) is a necessary approach, and when pelvic pain is not a significant issue, the removal of endometriomas is of no benefit. Size comes into play as well for purposes of IVF-ET; if all visible normal ovarian tissue is replaced by endometriomas surgical excision may be necessary. Otherwise for small lesions (>2 cm) follicle aspiration can be accomplished avoiding the endometriomas. In general, the presence of endometriomas tends to decrease the number of oocytes aspirated but may not impair oocyte or embryo quality.

There has long been a debate as to whether treating mild endometriotic lesions or implants would improve fertility. Two prospective randomized trials have provided some guidance. Data from the Canadian and Italian studies both suggest that the pregnancy rates are improved with implant ablation (Fig. 19-18). Thus one additional pregnancy may be expected for eight surgical procedures. The way these data should be extrapolated into practice is that if a laparoscopy is being performed in a woman wishing to conceive, visible lesions should be ablated if technically possible rather than ignoring them.

Apart from the mechanical factors (endometriomas, adhesions, fibrosis) affecting pregnancy rates, in endometriosis, macrophage and cytokine abnormalities are thought to play a significant role in inhibiting fertility (see Fig. 19-5). These factors may affect oocyte quality, fertilization, and embryo quality as well as endometrial receptivity. Therefore, in addition to ablating lesions when present, several strategies have been devised to enhance fecundity. Controlled ovarian stimulation and intrauterine insemination, an approach to enhance fecundity in women with unexplained infertility, has been found to be beneficial in women with endometriosis. Finally, if IVF-ET is undertaken (because of mechanical factors or with other failed approaches), although pregnancy rates are generally favorable, one meta-analysis has suggested that the pregnancy rates are lower than for

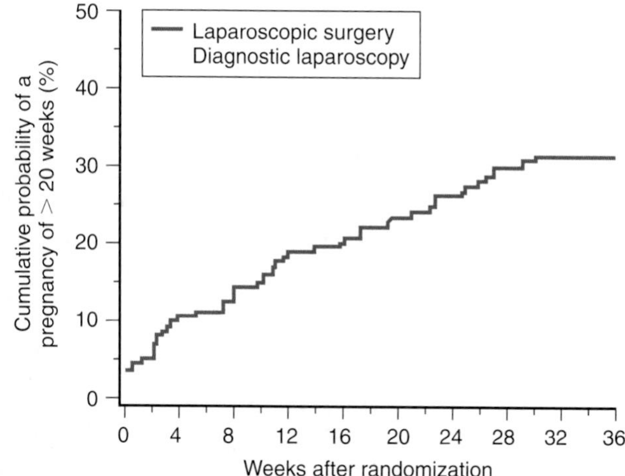

Figure 19-18. Cumulative probability of pregnancy in 36 weeks following laparoscopy with or without (diagnostic) surgical ablation of endometriosis. (Modified from Marcoux S, Maheux R, Berube S, et al: Laparoscopic surgery in infertile women with minimal or mild endometriosis. N Engl J Med 337:217–222, 1997. Copyright 1997 Massachusetts Medical Society. All rights reserved. Modified with permission.)

women with tubal disease alone (Odds ratio: 0.56) (Fig. 19-19). Although this reemphasizes the pathophysiologic consequences of having endometriosis (described earlier), this lower success rate should not preclude carrying out this treatment; young patients with tubal disease usually carry the best prognosis for pregnancy with IVF-ET.

Gastrointestinal Tract Endometriosis

The frequency of gastrointestinal tract involvement in series of women with histologically proven endometriosis varies from 3% to 34%. Most large series document a frequency of approximately 5%. Implants that involve the gastrointestinal tract are the most common site of extrapelvic endometriosis. The severity and extent of involvement of the bowel by ectopic endometrium varies from the incidental finding of a spot on the serosa of the bowel to obstruction of the rectosigmoid. In most cases the implants do not produce clinical symptoms. In the majority of cases, endometriosis of the gastrointestinal tract involves the sigmoid colon and the anterior wall of the rectum (Fig. 19-20). An important clinical marker is the finding that women with endometriosis of the ovaries have an increased frequency of extensive, invasive disease of the large intestine.

Endometriosis of the appendix is fairly common. The incidence in patients with pelvic endometriosis is reported between 1% and 13% (Fig. 19-21). Endometriosis of the appendix is usually an incidental pathologic finding. It is not clinically important because pathophysiologically the aberrant endometrium in the appendix wall does not produce symptoms.

Endometriosis of the small bowel is rare. Approximately 200 cases of endometriosis of the ileum have been reported in the literature. This is a troublesome process because of the high incidence of associated small bowel obstruction.

Classic symptoms of endometriosis of the large bowel include cyclic pelvic cramping and lower abdominal pain and rectal pain with defecation, especially during the menstrual period.

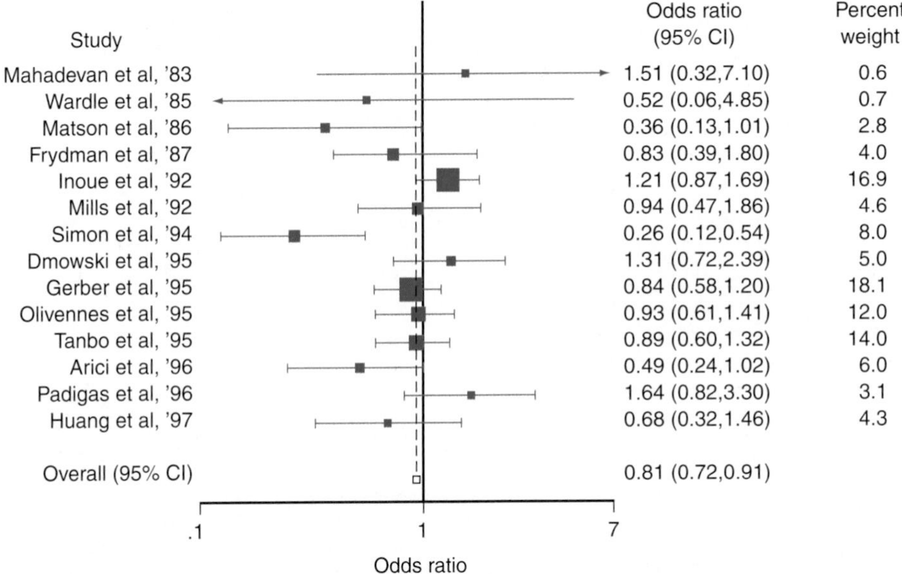

Figure 19-19. Unadjusted meta-analysis of 14 studies comparing pregnancy by in vitro fertilization in endometriosis patients versus tubal factor infertility controls. Horizontal bars depict study-specific 95% confidence intervals, and solid squares indicate weighting in the meta-analysis. References are from the original source. (Modified from Fertility and Sterility, 77, Barnhart K, Dunsmoor-Su R, Coutifaris C, Effect of endometriosis on in vitro fertilization, 1148. Copyright 2002, with permission from The American Society for Reproductive Medicine.)

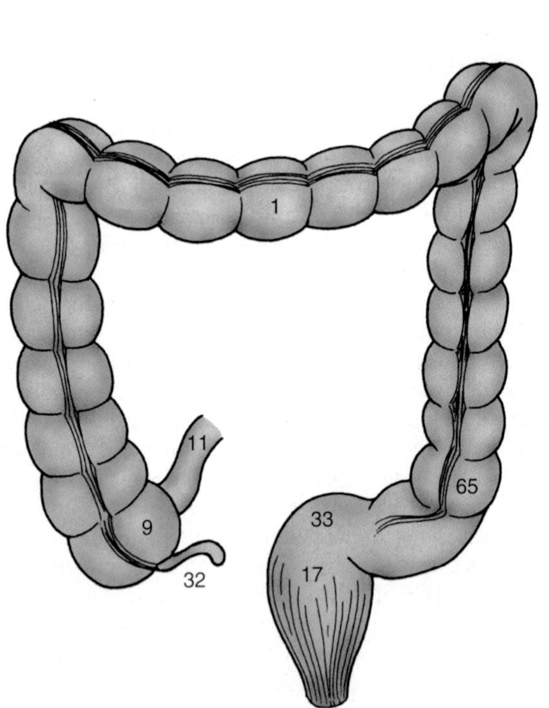

Figure 19-20. Locations of 168 bowel lesions found in 163 patients with endometriosis of the bowel. (Redrawn from Weed JC, Ray JE: Endometriosis of the bowel. Obstet Gynecol 69:727, 1987.)

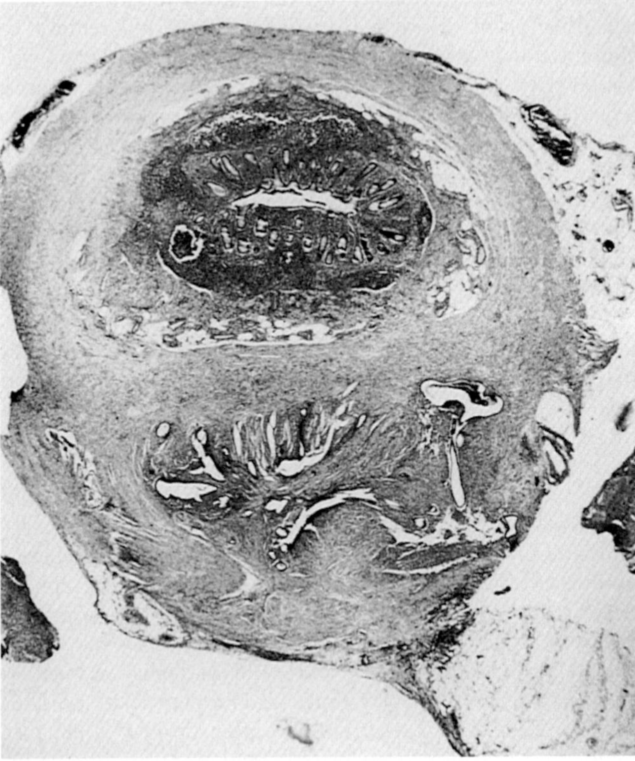

Figure 19-21. Cross section of appendix showing lumen of bowel and island of endometriosis. (From Dougherty CM: Surgical Pathology of Gynecologic Disease. New York, Harper & Row, 1968, p 636.)

Table 19-8 Preoperative Symptoms in 130 Patients Undergoing Colorectal Resection for Endometriosis

Symptom	No. of Patients	(%)
Pelvic pain	111	(85)
Rectal pain	68	(52)
Cyclic rectal bleeding	24	(18)
Diarrhea	55	(42)
Constipation	53	(41)
Diarrhea and constipation	18	(14)
Dyspareunia	83	(64)

From Bailey HR, Ott MT, Hartendorp P: Aggressive surgical management for advanced colorectal endometriosis. Dis Colon Rectum 37:747, 1994.

Associated with the abdominal and pelvic pain is a change in bowel function, diarrhea or constipation (or both) (Table 19-8). Mathias and colleagues have demonstrated a consistent and distinct dysfunction of the enteric nervous system, which they believe is the primary cause of the abnormalities of bowel function in women with endometriosis. It is difficult to differentiate the symptoms associated with endometriosis from the constellation of symptoms associated with inflammatory disease of the colon or malignancy. Women with a gastrointestinal malignancy usually experience intermittent rather than cyclic intestinal bleeding. Early diagnosis of gastrointestinal endometriosis demands a high index of suspicion by the physician. The initial clue to the diagnosis of the patient with multiple symptoms is the cyclic nature of these symptoms. Bowel resection is indicated for obstruction of the bowel or with extensive lesions in which malignancy may not be ruled out. On pathologic examination the aberrant endometrial glands and stroma penetrate the serosa of the bowel and muscularis. It is unusual for endometriosis to involve the submucosa of the bowel. However, studies have demonstrated that 25% to 35% of women with advanced endometriosis of the large bowel experience episodic rectal bleeding from endometriosis extending into the submucosa.

Diagnosis of endometriosis invading the rectosigmoid is usually suspected by palpation of a pelvic mass or "rectal shelf" on rectovaginal examination. Sigmoidoscopy usually demonstrates absence of a mucosal lesion in addition to fixation and immobility of the anterior rectal wall. Donnez and coworkers speculate that endometriosis of the rectovaginal septum is a disease process more closely related to foci of adenomyosis than endometriosis. They postulate that the nodules originate from müllerian rests in the rectovaginal space. Colonoscopy and an air-contrast barium enema are important steps in suspected cases, since they help to establish the differential diagnosis and the degree of obstruction. There is no specific radiologic appearance for endometriosis. However, a filling defect and absence of a mucosal lesion with the presence of extramucosal involvement are usually demonstrated. The definitive diagnosis and differentiation of endometriosis from carcinoma of the bowel may be delayed until a frozen section is obtained during exploratory surgery.

The treatment of endometriosis of the gastrointestinal tract is dependent on the extent and severity of symptoms. Endocrine therapy is not recommended for advanced cases. The importance of preoperative preparation of the bowel should not be forgotten. Surgical procedures vary from superficial excision of the endometriosis to bowel resection with anastomosis.

Urinary Tract Endometriosis

Endometriosis in the female pelvis occasionally produces dysfunction in adjacent pelvic organs. Approximately 10% of women with endometriosis have involvement of the urinary tract by implants of endometriosis and associated retroperitoneal fibrosis. In most cases an incidental finding of aberrant endometrial glands and stroma is discovered on the bladder peritoneum and anterior cul-de-sac. The most serious consequence of urinary tract involvement is ureteral obstruction, which occurs in about 1% of women with moderate or severe pelvic endometriosis. The pathogenesis of endometriosis of the bladder is controversial. Interestingly, approximately 50% of women with endometriosis of the urinary tract have a history of previous pelvic surgery. The lesions may develop from implanted endometrium during cesarean delivery or may be an extension from adenomyosis of the anterior uterine wall.

Patients with endometriosis involving the urinary tract have nonspecific clinical presentations. Hematuria and flank pain are experienced by less than 25% of women. One of three women with documented complete ureteral obstruction secondary to endometriosis has no pelvic symptoms whatsoever. The clinical challenge is to diagnose minimal ureteral obstruction at an early stage, before loss of renal function. The obstruction is almost always in the distal one third of the course of the ureter. The importance of an imaging study to diagnose ureteral compromise in all women with retroperitoneal endometriosis cannot be overemphasized.

Endometriosis of the bladder is discovered most often in the region of the trigone or the anterior wall of the bladder. Bladder endometriosis produces midline, lower abdominal, and suprapubic pain, dysuria, and, occasionally, cyclic hematuria. Treatment of endometriosis of the peritoneum over the bladder can be accomplished by medical or surgical means. Ureteral obstruction may be intrinsic, from active endometriosis, or extrinsic, from long-standing fibrotic reactions to retroperitoneal inflammation. Extrinsic endometriosis is three to five times more common than the intrinsic form. There are few reports of endometriosis of the ureter responding to danazol or GnRH agonists. However, long-term follow-up with serial ultrasound imaging or intravenous pyelograms must be undertaken to ensure that the disease process does not recur.

Surgical therapy is preferred for ureteral obstruction secondary to endometriosis. The operations are rare and should be individualized. However, operative removal of the uterus and both ovaries and the relief of urinary obstruction by ureterolysis or by ureteroneocystostomy are the most common choices. If ureterolysis is the operation chosen, peristalsis in the involved segment of the ureter should be observed, along with adequate resection of the endometriosis and surrounding inflammation in the retroperitoneal space. Ureteroneocystostomy has the advantage of bypassing the urinary obstruction and making it technically easier to resect the area of endometriosis and associated retroperitoneal fibrosis.

INFERTILITY KEY POINTS

- Laparoscopic ablation of endometriosis lesions is beneficial for infertile couples.
- The presence of endometriosis decreases the success of IVF-ET by as much as 20%.

KEY POINTS

- Endometriosis is a benign, usually progressive, and sometimes recurrent disease that invades locally and disseminates widely.
- Endometriosis is present in 5% to 15% of celiotomies performed on women of reproductive age.
- The incidence of endometriosis is 30% to 45% in women with infertility.
- Approximately 5% of women with endometriosis are diagnosed following menopause. Postmenopausal endometriosis is usually secondary to the use of exogenous estrogen.
- Possible causal factors of endometriosis include retrograde menstruation, coelomic metaplasia, vascular metastasis, immunologic changes, iatrogenic dissemination, and a genetic predisposition.
- Some postulate that there is a complex interplay between a dose-response curve of the amount of retrograde menstruation and an individual woman's immunologic response.
- One of 10 women with severe endometriosis will have a sister or mother with clinical manifestations of endometriosis.
- The ovaries are the most common site, being involved in two of three women with endometriosis. The pelvic peritoneum over the uterus; the anterior and posterior cul-de-sac; and the uterosacral, round, and broad ligaments are also common sites where endometriosis develops. Pelvic lymph nodes are involved in 30% of cases.
- Grossly, endometriosis appears in many forms, including red, brown, black, white, yellow, pink, or clear vesicles and lesions. Biopsy is important in establishing the diagnosis.
- Red, blood-filled lesions have been shown, by histologic and biochemical studies, to be the most active phase of endometriosis.
- Three cardinal features of microscopic endometriosis are ectopic endometrial glands, ectopic endometrial stroma, and hemorrhage into the adjacent tissue.
- Viable endometrial glands and stroma cannot be identified on pathologic examination in approximately 25% of cases of endometriosis.
- Classic symptoms of endometriosis are cyclic pelvic pain and infertility. However, approximately one third of patients with endometriosis are asymptomatic.
- Endometriosis is discovered in approximately one of three women whose primary symptom is chronic pelvic pain.
- Secondary dysmenorrhea usually begins 36 to 48 hours prior to the onset of menses. Unlike primary dysmenorrhea, the pain may last for many days, including several days before and after the menstrual flow.
- The most prominent pelvic sign of endometriosis is a fixed, retroverted uterus with scarring and tenderness posterior to the uterus. The characteristic nodularity of the uterosacral ligaments and cul-de-sac of Douglas may be palpated on rectovaginal examination.
- Serum CA-125 levels have a low sensitivity for the diagnosis of early or minimal endometriosis.
- Approximately 10% of teenagers who develop endometriosis have associated congenital outflow obstruction.
- The two primary short-term goals in treating endometriosis are the relief of pain and promotion of fertility. The primary long-term goal in the management of a woman with endometriosis is attempting to prevent progression or recurrence of the disease process.
- Recurrent bleeding in the ectopic implants is one of the most important pathophysiologic processes to interrupt.
- Optimal regression secondary to medical treatment is observed in small endometriomas that are less than 1 to 2 cm in diameter.
- The choice of medical therapy for the individual patient depends on the clinician's evaluation of adverse effects, side effects, cost of therapy, and expected patient compliance. The recurrence rate following medical therapy is 5% to 15% in the first year and increases to 40% to 50% in 5 years.
- The side effects of danazol are related to its androgenic and anabolic properties, as well as to the "pseudomenopause" produced by the drug.
- Approximately three of four women note significant improvement in symptoms following danazol therapy. Unfortunately, 15% to 30% of women will have a recurrence of symptoms within 2 years following completion of medical therapy.
- With chronic administration of GnRH agonists, specific suppression of gonadotropin secretion occurs, with secondary diminution of ovarian steroidogenesis. The GnRH agonists bind with receptors for a prolonged time and induce protracted periods of down-regulation.
- GnRH agonists produce a "medical oophorectomy" without the side effects of danazol on steroid-sensitive target organs.
- The side effects associated with GnRH agonist therapy are primarily those associated with estrogen deprivation, similar to menopause. The three most common symptoms are hot flushes, vaginal dryness, and insomnia. A decrease in bone mineral content of trabecular bone has been demonstrated in the cortical bone on the lumbar spine by quantitative computed tomography.

KEY POINTS *Continued*

- It has been established that the decrease in bone density associated with 6 months of therapy with GnRH agonist completely recovers between 12 and 24 months after discontinuing therapy.
- Initial clinical response to GnRH agonist therapy depends on when the therapy is begun in relation to the menstrual cycle.
- Many clinicians "add-back" very low doses of estrogen, low doses of progestins, or both in combination with chronic GnRH agonist therapy.
- Laparoscopy is employed frequently for both diagnostic and therapeutic reasons. The major advantage of treating endometriosis with the laparoscope, using surgical instruments, laser, or electrocautery, is that patients may be treated at the time of diagnosis.
- The goals of conservative surgery for endometriosis include removal of macroscopic endometriosis, lysis of adhesions, and restoration of normal anatomy.
- Classic symptoms of endometriosis of the large bowel include cyclic pelvic cramping and lower abdominal pain and rectal pain with defecation, especially during the menstrual period.
- The pathogenesis of endometriosis of the bladder is controversial. Interestingly, approximately 50% of women with endometriosis of the urinary tract have a history of previous pelvic surgery.
- Endometriosis of the bladder is discovered most often in the region of the trigone or the anterior wall of the bladder. Bladder endometriosis produces midline, lower abdominal, and suprapubic pain, dysuria, and, occasionally, cyclic hematuria.
- Surgical therapy is preferred for ureteral obstruction secondary to endometriosis.
- Adenomyosis is frequently asymptomatic. If multiple serial sections of the uterus are obtained, the incidence may exceed 60% in women 40 to 50 years of age.
- Symptomatic adenomyosis primarily occurs in parous women older than age 35. The classic symptoms are secondary dysmenorrhea and menorrhagia. The most common physical sign is a diffusely enlarged uterus, usually two to three times normal size.
- The severity of pelvic symptoms associated with adenomyosis increases proportionally to the depth of penetration and the total volume of disease in the myometrium.
- Adenomyosis rarely causes uterine enlargement greater than a size at 14 weeks' gestation unless there is concomitant uterine pathology.

BIBLIOGRAPHY

Adamson GD: Diagnosis and clinical presentation of endometriosis. Am J Obstet Gynecol 162:568, 1990.

American Fertility Society: Management of endometriosis in the presence of pelvic pain. Fertil Steril 60:952, 1993.

American Society for Reproductive Medicine: Revised American Society for Reproductive Medicine classification of endometriosis: 1996. Fertil Steril 67:817, 1997.

Arnold LL, Ascher SM, Simon JA: Familial adenomyosis: A case report. Fertil Steril 61:1165, 1994.

Ascher SM, Arnold LL, Patt RH, et al: Adenomyosis: Prospective comparison of MR imaging and transvaginal sonography. Radiology 190:803, 1994.

Bailey HR, Ott MT, Hartendorp P: Aggressive surgical management for advanced colorectal endometriosis. Dis Colon Rectum 37:747, 1994.

Barbieri RL: Gonadotropin-releasing hormone agonists: Treatment of endometriosis. Clin Obstet Gynecol 36:636, 1993.

Barbieri RL: Hormone treatment of endometriosis: The estrogen threshold hypothesis. Am J Obstet Gynecol 166:740, 1992.

Barbieri RL, Gordon AC: Hormonal therapy of endometriosis: the estradiol target. Fertil Steril 56:820, 1991.

Barlow D: Today's treatments: How do you choose? Int J Gynaecol Obstet 64:S15, 1999.

Barnhart K, Dunsmoor-Su R, Courtifaris C: Effect of endometriosis on in vitro fertilization. Fertil Steril 77:1148, 2002.

Bateman BG, Kolp LA, Mills S: Endoscopic versus laparotomy management of endometriomas. Fertil Steril 62:690, 1994.

Batt RE, Smith RA: Embryologic theory of histogenesis of endometriosis in peritoneal pockets. Obstet Gynecol Clin North Am 16:15, 1989.

Berga SL: A skeleton in the closet? Bone health and therapy for endometriosis revisited. Fertil Steril 65:702, 1996.

Bergqvist A: Different types of extragenital endometriosis: A review. Gynecol Endocrinol 7:207, 1993.

Bergqvist A: Extragenital endometriosis: A review. Eur J Surg 158:7, 1992.

Bird CC, McElin TW, Manalo-Estrella P: The elusive adenomyosis of the uterus-revisited. Am J Obstet Gynecol 112:583, 1972.

Blumenkrantz MJ, Gallagher N, Bashore RA, et al: Retrograde menstruation in women undergoing chronic peritoneal dialysis. Obstet Gynecol 57:667, 1981.

Bozdech JM: Endoscopic diagnosis of colonic endometriosis. Gastrointest Endosc 38:568, 1992.

Brinton L, Gridley G, Persson I, et al. Cancer risk after a hospital discharge diagnosis of endometriosis. Am J Obstet Gynecol 176:572, 1997.

Brosens IA: New principles in the management of endometriosis. Acta Obstet Gynecol Scand 159:S18, 1994.

Brosens IA: Endometriosis—a disease because it is characterized by bleeding. Am J Obstet Gynecol 176:263, 1997.

Brosens IA, Brosens JJ: Redefining endometriosis: Is deep endometriosis a progressive disease? Hum Reprod 15:1, 2000.

Brosens JJ, Barker FG: The role of myometrial needle biopsies in the diagnosis of adenomyosis. Fertil Steril 63:1347, 1995.

Busacca M, Marana R, Caruana P, et al: Recurrence of ovarian endometrioma after laparoscopic excision. Am J Obstet Gynecol 180:519, 1999.

Byun JY, Kim SE, Choi BG, et al: Diffuse and focal adenomyosis: MR imaging findings. Radiographics 19:S161, 1999.

Candiani GB, Fedele L, Vercellini P, et al: Presacral neurectomy for the treatment of pelvic pain associated with endometriosis: A controlled study. Am J Obstet Gynecol 167:100, 1992.

Candiani GB, Fedele L, Vercellini P, et al: Repetitive conservative surgery for recurrence of endometriosis. Obstet Gynecol 77: 421, 1991.

Cedars MI, Lu JKH, Meldrum DR, et al: Treatment of endometriosis with a long-acting gonadotropin-releasing hormone agonist plus medroxyprogesterone acetate. Obstet Gynecol 75:641, 1990.

Chyishima F, Hayakawa S, Sugita K, et al. Increased expression of cyclooxygenase-2 in local lesions of endometriosis patients. Am J Reprod Immunol 48:50, 2002.

Cornillie FJ, Oosterlynck D, Lauweryns JM, et al: Deeply infiltrating pelvic endometriosis: Histology and clinical significance. Fertil Steril 53:978, 1990.

Coronado C, Franklin RR, Lotze EC, et al: Surgical treatment of symptomatic colorectal endometriosis. Fertil Steril 53:411, 1990.

Crosignani PG, Vercellini P: New clinical guidelines are needed for the treatment of endometriosis. Hum Reprod 9:2205, 1994.
Darrow SL, Selman S, Batt RE, et al: Sexual activity, contraception, and reproductive factors in predicting endometriosis. Am J Epidemiol 140:500, 1994.
Dawood MY: Impact of medical treatment of endometriosis on bone mass. Am J Obstet Gynecol 168:674, 1993.
Dawood MY, Lewis V, Ramos J: Cortical and trabecular bone mineral content in women with endometriosis: Effect of gonadotropin-releasing hormone agonist and danazol. Fertil Steril 52:21, 1989.
Dawood MY, Obasiolu CW, Ramos J, Khan-Dawood FS: Clinical, endocrine, and metabolic effects of two doses of gestrinone in treatment of pelvic endometriosis. Am J Obstet Gynecol 176:387, 1997.
Dawood MY, Ramos J, Khan-Dawood FS: Depot leuprolide acetate versus danazol for treatment of pelvic endometriosis: Changes in vertebral bone mass and serum estradiol and calcitonin. Fertil Steril 63:1177, 1995.
Deaton JL, Gibson M, Blackmer KM, et al. A randomized, controlled trial of clomiphene citrate and intrauterine insemination in couples with unexplained infertility or surgically corrected endometriosis. Fertil Steril 54:1083, 1990.
Dickinson CJ: Could tight garments cause endometriosis? B J Obstet Gynaecol 106:1003, 1999.
D'Hooghe T, Cunco S, Nugent N, et al. Recombinant human TNF binding protein-1(r-hTBP-1) inhibits the development of endometriosis in baboons: A prospective, randomized, placebo- and drug-controlled study. Fertil Steril 76 (Suppl 3):S1 (Abst), 2001.
D'Hooghe TM, Bambra CS, Raeymaekers BM, Koninokx PR: Serial laparoscopies over 30 months show that endometriosis in captive baboons (*Papio anubis, Papio cynocephalus*) is a progressive disease. Fertil Steril 65:645, 1996.
diZerega GS: Contemporary adhesion prevention. Fertil Steril 61:219, 1994.
Dinulescu DM, Ince TA, Quade BJ, et al: Role of K-ras and Pten in the development of mouse models of endometriosis and endometrioid ovarian cancer. Nat Med 11:63, 2005.
Dlugi AM, Miller JD, Knittle J, et al: Lupron depot (leuprolide acetate for depot suspension) in the treatment of endometriosis: A randomized, placebo-controlled, double-blind study. Fertil Steril 54:419, 1990.
Dmowski WP: Danazol-induced pseudomenopause in the management of endometriosis. Clin Obstet Gynecol 31:829, 1989.
Dmowski WP, Gebel HM, Braun DP: The role of cell-mediated immunity in pathogenesis of endometriosis. Acta Obstet Gynecol Scand 159:7, 1994.
Dochi T, Lees B, Sidhu M, Stevenson JC: Bone density and endometriosis. Fertil Steril 61:175, 1994.
Dodin S, Lemay A, Maheux R, et al: Bone mass in endometriosis patients treated with GnRH agonist implant or danazol. Obstet Gynecol 77:410, 1991.
Donnez J: Today's treatments: medical, surgical and in partnership. Int J Gynaecol Obstet 64:S5, 1999.
Donnez J, Nisolle M, Gillerot S, et al: Rectovaginal septum adenomyotic nodules: A series of 500 cases. Br J Obstet Gynaecol 104:1014, 1997.
Evers JLH: Endometriosis does not exist; all women have endometriosis. Hum Reprod 9:2206, 1994.
Farquhar C, Sutton C: The evidence for the management of endometriosis. Curr Opin Obstet Gynecol 10:321, 1998.
Fedele L, Arcaini L, Vercellini P, et al: Serum CA-125 measurements in the diagnosis of endometriosis recurrence. Obstet Gynecol 72:19, 1988.
Fedele L, Bianchi S, Marchini M, et al: Superovulation with human menopausal gonadotropins in the treatment of infertility associated with minimal or mild endometriosis: A controlled randomized study. Fertil Steril 58:28-31, 1992.
Fedele L, Bianchi S, Zanconato G, et al: Use of a levonorgestrel-releasing intrauterine device in the treatment of rectovaginal endometriosis. Fertil Steril 75:485, 2001.
Fedele L, Bianchi S, Bocciolone L, et al: Pain symptoms associated with endometriosis. Obstet Gynecol 79:767, 1992.
Fedele L, Bianchi S, Raffaelli R, et al: Treatment of adenomyosis-associated menorrhagia with a levonorgestrel-releasing intrauterine device. Fertil Steril 68:426, 1997.
Fedele L, Bianchi S, Viezzoli T, et al: Gestrinone versus danazol in the treatment of endometriosis. Fertil Steril 51:781, 1989.
Fedele L, Marchini M, Bianchi S, et al: Endometrial patterns during danazol and buserelin therapy for endometriosis: Comparative structural and ultrastructural study. Obstet Gynecol 76:79, 1990.
Fedele L, Parazzini F, Bianchi S, et al: Stage and localization of pelvic endometriosis and pain. Fertil Steril 53:155, 1990.
Fedele L, Piazzola E, Raffaelli R, Bianchi S: Bladder endometriosis: Deep infiltrating endometriosis or adenomyosis? Fertil Steril 69:972, 1998.
Fong YF, Singh K: Medical treatment of a grossly enlarged adenomyotic uterus with the levonorgestrel-releasing intrauterine system. Contraception 60:173, 1999.
Friedman AJ, Hornstein MD: Gonadotropin-releasing hormone agonist plus estrogen-progestin "add-back" therapy for endometriosis-related pelvic pain. Fertil Steril 60:236, 1993.
Friedman AJ, Juneau-Norcross M, Rein MS: Adverse effects of leuprolide acetate depot treatment. Fertil Steril 59:448, 1993.
Fujii S: Secondary müllerian system and endometriosis. Am J Obstet Gynecol 165:219, 1991.
Gannon MJ, Brown SB: Photodynamic therapy and its applications in gynaecology. Br J Obstet Gynecol, 106:1246, 1999.
Garcia-Velasco JA, Mahutte NG, Corona J, Zuniga V, et al. Removal of endometriomas before in vitro fertilization does not improve fertility outcomes: A matched, case-control study. Fertil Steril 81(5):1194, 2004.
García-Velasco JA, Arici A: Chemokines and human reproduction. Fertil Steril 71:983, 1999.
Gehr TWB, Sica DA: Case report and review of the literature: Ureteral endometriosis. Am J Med Sci 294:346, 1987.
Gestrinone Italian Study Group: Gestrinone versus a gonadotropin-releasing hormone agonist for the treatment of pelvic pain associated with endometriosis: A multicenter, randomized, double-blind study. Fertil Steril 66:911, 1996.
Giudice L, Kao, LC: Endometriosis. Lancet 364:1789, 2004.
Graham B, Mazier WP: Diagnosis and management of endometriosis of the colon and rectum. Dis Colon Rectum 31:952, 1988.
Guerrieros S, Mais V, Ajossa S, et al: Transvaginal ultrasonography combined with CA-125 plasma levels in the diagnosis of endometrioma. Fertil Steril 65:293, 1996.
Guilbeault H, Wilson SR, Lickrish GM: Massive uterine enlargement with necrosis: An unusual manifestation of adenomyosis. J Ultrasound Med 13:326,1994.
Halme J, Becker S, Haskill S: Altered maturation and function of peritoneal macrophages: Possible role in pathogenesis of endometriosis. Am J Obstet Gynecol 156:783, 1987.
Halme J, White C, Kauma S, et al: Peritoneal macrophages from patients with endometriosis release growth factor activity in vitro. J Clin Endocrinol Metab 66:1044, 1988.
Han AC, Hovenden S, Rosenblum NG, Salazar H: Adenocarcinoma arising in extragonadal endometriosis: An immunohistochemical study. Cancer 83:1163, 1998.
Hastings JM, Licence DR, Burton GJ, et al. Soluble vascular endothelial growth factor receptor 1 inhibits edema and epithelial proliferation induced by 17 beta-estradiol in the mouse uterus. Endocrinology 144:326, 2003.
Henzl MR: Gonadotropin-releasing hormone and its analogues: From laboratory to bedside. Clin Obstet Gynecol 36:617, 1993.
Henzl MR, Corson SL, Moghissi K, et al: Administration of nasal nafarelin as compared with oral danazol for endometriosis: A multicenter double-blind comparative clinical trial. N Engl J Med 318:485, 1988.
Hirata JD, Moghissi KS, Ginsburg KA: Pregnancy after medical therapy of adenomyosis with a gonadotropin-releasing hormone agonist. Fertil Steril 59:444, 1993.
Hornstein MD, Gleason RE, Barbieri RL: A randomized double-blind prospective trial of two doses of gestrinone in the treatment of endometriosis. Fertil Steril 53:237, 1990.
Hornstein MD, Hemmings R, Yuzpe AA, Henrichs WL: Use of nafarelin versus placebo after reductive laparoscopic surgery for endometriosis. Fertil Steril 68:860, 1997.
Hornstein MD, Thomas PP, Gleason RE, Barbieri RL: Menstrual cyclicity of CA-125 in patients with endometriosis. Fertil Steril 58:279, 1992.
Hornstein MD, Surrey ES, Weisberg GW, et al: Leuprolide acetate depot and hormonal add-back in endometriosis: A 12-month study. Obstet Gynecol 91:16, 1998.
Hornung D, Waite LL, Ricke EA, et al. Nuclear peroxisome proliferator-activated receptors alpha and gamma have opposing effects on monocyte chemotaxis in endometriosis. J Clin Endocrinol Metab 86:3108, 2001.
Hoshiai H, Ishikawa M, Sawatari Y, et al: Laparoscopic evaluation of the onset and progression of endometriosis. Am J Obstet Gynecol 169:714, 1993.

Ishimaru T, Masuzaki H: Peritoneal endometriosis: Endometrial tissue implantation as its primary etiologic mechanism. Am J Obstet Gynecol 165:210, 1991.

Israel R: Pelvic endometriosis. In Mishell DR, Davajan V, Lobo RA (eds): Infertility, Contraception and Reproductive Endocrinology, 3rd ed. Oradell, NJ, Medical Economics Books, 1990.

Jain S, Dalton ME: Chocolate cysts from ovarian follicles. Fertil Steril 72:852, 1999.

Javert CT: Pathogenesis of endometriosis based on endometrial homeoplasia, direct extension exfoliation and implantation, lymphatic and hematogenous metastasism. Cancer 2:399, 1949.

Jiang X, Morland S, Hitchcock A, et al. Allelotyping of endometriosis with adjacent ovarian carcinoma reveals evidence of a common lineage. Cancer Res 58:1707, 1998.

Jimbo H, Hitomi Y, Yoshikawa H, et al: Clonality analysis of bilateral ovarian endometrial cysts. Fertil Steril 72:1142, 1999.

Jones K, Haines P, Sutton C. Long-term follow-up of a controlled trial of laser laparoscopy for pelvic pain. JSLS 5:111, 2001.

Joseph J, Sahn SA: Thoracic endometriosis syndrome: New observations from an analysis of 110 cases. Am J Med 100: 164, 1996.

Kane C, Drouin P: Obstructive uropathy associated with endometriosis. Am J Obstet Gynecol 151:207, 1985.

Kauma S, Clark MR, White C, et al: Production of fibronectin by peritoneal macrophages and concentrations of fibronectin in peritoneal fluid from patients with or without endometriosis. Obstet Gynecol 72:13, 1988.

Kauppila A: Changing concepts of medical treatment of endometriosis. Acta Obstet Gynecol Scand 72:324, 1993.

Kennedy SH, Williams IA, Brodribb J, et al: A comparison of nafarelin acetate and danazol in the treatment of endometriosis. Fertil Steril 53:998, 1990.

Kettel L, Murphy A, Morales A, et al. Preliminary report on the treatment of endometriosis with low-dose mifepristone (RU 486). Am J Obstet Gynecol 178:1151, 1998.

Kettel LM, Murphy AA, Morales AJ, et al: Treatment of endometriosis with the antiprogesterone mifepristone (RU 486). Fertil Steril 65:23, 1996.

Kettel LM, Murphy AA, Mortola JF, et al: Endocrine responses to long-term administration of the antiprogesterone RU 486 in patients with pelvic endometriosis. Fertil Steril 56:402, 1991.

Kinkel K, Chapron C, Balleyguier C, et al: Magnetic resonance imaging characteristics of deep endometriosis. Hum Reprod 14:1080, 1999.

Kistner RW: Conservative management of endometriosis. J Lancet 79(5):179, 1959.

Kitawaki J, Kusuki I, Koshiba H, et al: Detection of aromatase cytochrome P-450 in endometrial biopsy specimens as a diagnostic test for endometriosis. Fertil Steril 72:1100, 1999.

Klein RS, Cattolica EV: Ureteral endometriosis. Urology 13:477, 1979.

Knapp VJ: How old is endometriosis? Late 17th- and 18th-century European descriptions of the disease. Fertil Steril 72:10, 1999.

Koninckx PR: Is mild endometriosis a disease? Is mild endometriosis a condition occurring intermittently in all women? Hum Reprod 9:2202, 1994.

Kosugi Y, Elias S, Malinak LR, et al: Increased heterogeneity of chromosome 17 aneuploidy in endometriosis. Am J Obstet Gynecol 180:792, 1999.

Koutsilieris M, Akoum A, Lazure C, et al: N-terminal truncated forms of insulin-like growth factor binding protein-3 in the peritoneal fluid of women without laparoscopic evidence of endometriosis. Fertil Steril 63:314, 1995.

Kupker W, Felberbaum RE, Krapp M, et al. Use of GnRH antagonists in the treatment of endometriosis. Reprod Biomed Online 5:12-16, 2002.

Langlois NEI, Park KGM, Keenan RA: Mucosal changes in the large bowel with endometriosis: A possible cause of misdiagnosis of colitis? Hum Pathol 25:1030, 1994.

Letterie GS, Stevenson D, Shah A: Recurrent anaphylaxis to a depot form of GnRH analogue. Obstet Gynecol 78:943, 1991.

Leyendecker G: Endometriosis is an entity with extreme pleomorphism. Hum Reprod 15:4, 2000.

Lim YT, Schenken RS: Interleukin-6 in experimental endometriosis. Fertil Steril 59:912, 1993.

Ling FW, Pelvic Pain Study Group: Randomized controlled trial of depot leuprolide in patients with chronic pelvic pain and clinically suspected endometriosis. Obstet Gynecol 93:51, 1999.

Low WY, Edelmann RJ, Sutton C: Short term psychological outcome of surgical intervention for endometriosis. Br J Obstet Gynaecol 100:191, 1993.

Luciano AA, Turksoy RN, Carleo J: Evaluation of oral medroxyprogesterone acetate in the treatment of endometriosis. Obstet Gynecol 72:323, 1988.

Luster AD: Chemokines-chemotactic cytokines that mediate inflammation. N Engl J Med 338:436, 1998.

MacDonald SR, Klock SC, Milad MP: Long-term outcome of nonconservative surgery (hysterectomy) for endometriosis-associated pain in women <30 years old. Am J Obstet Gynecol 180:1360, 1999.

Mahmood TA, Templeton AA, Thomson L, Fraser C: Menstrual symptoms in women with pelvic endometriosis. Br J Obstet Gynaecol 98:558, 1991.

Mahnke JL, Dawood MY, Huang JC: Vascular endothelial growth factor and interleukin-6 in peritoneal fluid of women with endometriosis. Fertil Steril 73:166, 2000.

Marcoux S, Maheux R, Berube S, et al. Laparoscopic surgery in infertile women with minimal or mild endometriosis. N Engl J Med 337:217, 1997.

Mathias JR, Franklin R, Quast DC, et al: Relation of endometriosis and the neuromuscular disease of the gastrointestinal tract: new insights. Fertil Steril 70:81, 1998.

McArthur JW, Ulfelder H: The effect of pregnancy upon endometriosis. Obstet Gynecol Surv 20:709, 1965.

McCausland AM: Hysteroscopic myometrial biopsy: Its use in diagnosing adenomyosis and its clinical application. Am J Obstet Gynecol 166:1619, 1992.

Meek SC, Hodge DD, Musich JR: Autoimmunity in infertile patients with endometriosis. Am J Obstet Gynecol 158:1365, 1988.

Miller JD, Shaw RW, Casper RFJ: Historical prospective cohort study of the recurrence of pain after discontinuation of treatment with danazol or a gonadotropin-releasing hormone agonist. Fertil Steril 70:283, 1998.

Moen MH, Magnus P: The familial risk of endometriosis. Acta Obstet Gynecol Scand 72:560, 1993.

Moghissi KS: Gonadotropin-releasing hormones: Clinical applications in gynecology. J Reprod Med 35:1097, 1990.

Moghissi KS: Treatment of endometriosis with estrogen-progestin combination and progestogens alone. Clin Obstet Gynecol 31:823, 1989.

Moghissi KS, Schlaff WD, Olive DL, et al: Goserelin acetate (Zoladex) with or without hormone replacement therapy for the treatment of endometriosis. Fertil Steril 69:1056, 1998.

Mol BWJ, Bayram N, Lijmer JG, et al: The performance of CA-125 measurement in the detection of endometriosis: A meta-analysis. Fertil Steril 70:1101, 1998.

Myers WC, Kelvin FM, Jones RS: Diagnosis and surgical treatment of colonic endometriosis. Arch Surg 114:169, 1979.

Nafarelin European Endometriosis Trial Group: Nafarelin for endometriosis: A large-scale, danazol-controlled trial of efficacy and safety, with 1-year follow-up. Fertil Steril 57:514, 1992.

Namnoum AB, Hickman TN, Goodman SB, et al: Incidence of symptom recurrence after hysterectomy for endometriosis. Fertil Steril 64:898, 1995.

Nelson JR, Corson SL: Long-term management of adenomyosis with a gonadotropin-releasing hormone agonist: A case report. Fertil Steril 59:441, 1993.

Newfield R, Spitz I, Isacson CV, et al. Long-term mifepristone (RU-486) therapy resulting in massive benign endometrial hyperplasia. Clin Endocrinol (Oxf)54:399, 2001.

Nishida M: Relationship between the onset of dysmenorrhea and histologic findings in adenomyosis. Am J Obstet Gynecol 165:229, 1991.

Nisolle M, Donnez J: Peritoneal endometriosis, ovarian endometriosis, and adenomyotic nodules of the rectovaginal septum are three different entities. Fertil Steril 68:585, 1997.

Olive DL, Henderson DY: Endometriosis and müllerian anomalies. Obstet Gynecol 69:412, 1987.

Oosterlynck DJ, Meuleman C, Sobis H, et al: Angiogenic activity of peritoneal fluid from women with endometriosis. Fertil Steril 59:778, 1993.

Oosterlynck DJ, Meuleman C, Waer M, et al: Transforming growth factor-activity is increased in peritoneal fluid from women with endometriosis. Obstet Gynecol 83:287, 1994.

Outwater EK, Siegleman ES, Van Deerlin V: Adenomyosis: Current concepts and imaging considerations. AJR 170:437, 1998.

Pabuccu R, Onalan G, Goktolga U, Kucuk T, et al. Aspiration of ovarian endometriomas before intracytolasmic sperm injection. Fertil Steril 82(3):705, 2004.

Parazzini F, Fedele L, Busacca M, et al: Postsurgical medical treatment of advanced endometriosis: Results of a randomized clinical trial. Am J Obstet Gynecol 171:1205, 1994.

Patel A, Thorpe P, Ramsay JWA, et al: Endometriosis of the ureter. Br J Urol 69:495, 1992.
Popp LW, Schwiedessen JP, Gaetje R: Myometrial biopsy in the diagnosis of adenomyosis uteri. Am J Obstet Gynecol 169:546, 1993.
Propst AM, Storti K, Barbieri RL: Lateral cervical displacement is associated with endometriosis. Fertil Steril 70:568, 1998.
Prystowsky JB, Stryker SJ, Ujiki GT, et al: Gastrointestinal endometriosis. Arch Surg 123:855, 1988.
Ramey JW, Archer DF: Peritoneal fluid: Its relevance to the development of endometriosis. Fertil Steril 60:1, 1993.
Redwine DB: Is "microscopic" peritoneal endometriosis invisible? Fertil Steril 50:665, 1988.
Redwine DB: Ovarian endometriosis: A marker for more extensive pelvic and intestinal disease. Fertil Steril 72:310, 1999.
Reimnitz C, Brand E, Nieberg RK, et al: Malignancy arising in endometriosis associated with unopposed estrogen replacement. Obstet Gynecol 71:444, 1988.
Reinhold C, Atri M, Mehio A, et al: Diffuse uterine adenomyosis: Morphologic criteria and diagnostic accuracy of endovaginal sonograph. Radiology 197:609, 1995.
Reinhold C, Tafazoli F, Mehio A, et al: Uterine adenomyosis: Endovaginal US and MR imaging features with histopathologic correlation. Radiographics 19:S147, 1999.
Rivlin ME, Krueger RP, Wiser WL: Danazol in the management of ureteral obstruction secondary to endometriosis. Fertil Steril 44:274, 1985.
Rivlin ME, Miller JD, Krueger RP, et al: Leuprolide acetate in the management of ureteral obstruction caused by endometriosis. Obstet Gynecol 75:532, 1990.
Rock JA: Endometriosis and pelvic pain. Fertil Steril 60:950, 1993.
Rock JA, Truglia JA, Caplan RJ, Zoladex Endometriosis Study Group: Zoladex (goserelin acetate implant) in the treatment of endometriosis: A randomized comparison with danazol. Obstet Gynecol 82:198, 1993.
Rock JA, Zoladex Endometriosis Study Group: The revised American Fertility Society classification of endometriosis: reproducibility of scoring. Fertil Steril 63:1108, 1995.
Rolland R, van der Heijden PFM: Nafarelin versus danazol in the treatment of endometriosis. Am J Obstet Gynecol 162:586, 1990.
Rose PG, Alvarez B, MacLennan GT: Exacerbation of endometriosis as a result of premenopausal tamoxifen exposure. Am J Obstet Gynecol 183:507, 2000.
Rovati V, Faleschini E, Vercellini P, et al: Endometrioma of the liver. Am J Obstet Gynecol 163:1490, 1990.
Ryan IP, Taylor RN: Endometriosis and infertility: New concepts. Obstet Gynecol Surv 52:365, 1997.
Saleh A, Tulandi T: Reoperation after laparoscopic treatment of ovarian endometriomas by excision and fenestration. Fertil Steril 72:322, 1999.
Sampson JA: Peritoneal endometriosis due to menstrual dissemination of endometrial tissue into peritoneal cavity. Am J Obstet Gynecol 14:422, 1927.
Schenken RS: Gonadotropin-releasing hormone analogs in the treatment of endometriosis. Am J Obstet Gynecol 162:579, 1990.
Schenken RS, Guzick DS: Revised endometriosis classification: 1996. Fertil Steril 67:815, 1997.
Seltzer VL, Benjamin F: Treatment of pulmonary endometriosis with a long-acting GnRH agonist. Obstet Gynecol 76:929, 1990.
Shah M, Tager D, Feller E: Intestinal endometriosis masquerading as common digestive disorders. Arch Intern Med 155:977, 1995.
Shaw RW: A risk benefit assessment of drugs used in the treatment of endometriosis. Drug Saf 11:104, 1994.
Shaw RW, Zoladex Endometriosis Study Team: An open randomized comparative study of the effect of goserelin depot and danazol in the treatment of endometriosis. Fertil Steril 58:265, 1992.
Siegler AM, Camilien L: Adenomyosis. J Reprod Med 39:841, 1994.
Simpson JL, Elias S, Malinak LR, et al: Heritable aspects of endometriosis. Am J Obstet Gynecol 137:327, 1980.
Spitzer M, Benjamin F: Ascites due to endometriosis. Obstet Gynecol Survey 50:628, 1995.
Stahl C, Grimes EM: Endometriosis of the small bowel: Case reports and review of the literature. Obstet Gynecol Surv 42:131, 1987.
Stripling MC, Martin DC, Chatman DL, et al: Subtle appearance of pelvic endometriosis. Fertil Steril 49:427, 1988.
Suginami H: A reappraisal of the coelomic metaplasia theory by reviewing endometriosis occurring in unusual sites and instances. Am J Obstet Gynecol 165:214, 1991.
Surrey ES and the Add-Back Consensus Working Group: Add-back therapy and gonadotropin-releasing hormone agonists in the treatment of patients with endometriosis: Can a consensus be reached? Fertil Steril 71:420, 1999.
Surrey ES, Gambone JC, Lu JKH, et al: The effects of combining norethindrone with a gonadotropin-releasing hormone agonist in the treatment of symptomatic endometriosis. Fertil Steril 53:620, 1990.
Surrey ES, Voigt B, Fournet N, Judd HL: Prolonged gonadotropin-releasing hormone agonist treatment of symptomatic endometriosis: The role of cyclic sodium etidronate and low-dose norethindrone "add-back" therapy. Fertil Steril 63:747, 1995.
Sutton C: Laser treatment of endometriosis. Practitioner 237:601, 1993.
Sutton C, Ewen S, Whitelaw N, et al: Prospective, randomized double-blind, controlled trial of laser laparoscopy in the treatment of pelvic pain associated with minimal, mild, and moderate endometriosis. Fertil Steril 62:696, 1994.
Suzuki T, Izumi S, Matsubayashi H, Awaji H, et al: Impact of ovarian endometrioma on oocytes and pregnancy outcome in in vitro fertilization. Fertil Steril 83:908, 2005.
Tahara M, Matsuoka T, Yokoi T, et al: Treatment of endometriosis with a decreasing dosage of a gonadotropin-releasing hormone agonist (nafarelin): A pilot study with low-dose agonist therapy ("draw-back" therapy). Fertil Steril 73:799, 2000.
Takahashi K, Okada S, Okada M, et al: Magnetic resonance imaging and serum Ca-125 in evaluating patients with endometriomas prior to medical therapy. Fertil Steril 65:288, 1996.
Takayama K, Zeitoun K, Gunby RT, et al: Treatment of severe postmenopausal endometriosis with an aromatase inhibitor. Fertil Steril 69:709, 1998.
Thomas EJ: Endometriosis, 1995-confusion or sense? Int J Gynecol Obstet 48:149, 1995.
Thomas WW, Hughes LL, Rock J: Palliation of recurrent endometriosis with radiotherapeutic ablation of ovarian remnants. Fertil Steril 68:938, 1997.
Torkelson SJ, Lee RA, Hidahl DB: Endometriosis of the sciatic nerve: A report of two cases and a review of the literature, Obstet Gynecol 71:473, 1988.
Treloar SA, O'Connor DT, O'Connor VM, Martin NG: Genetic influences on endometriosis in an Australian twin sample. Fertil Steril 71:701, 1999.
Troiano RN, Taylor KJW: Sonography guided therapeutic aspiration of benign-appearing ovarian cysts and endometriomas. AJR 171:1601, 1998.
Tsudo T, Harada T, Iwabe T, et al: Altered gene expression and secretion of interleukin-6 in stromal cells derived from endometriotic tissues. Fertil Steril 73:205, 2000.
Tummon IS, Asher LJ, Martin JS, et al: Randomized controlled trial of superovulation and insemination for infertility associated with minimal or mild endometriosis. Fertil Steril 68:8, 1997.
Urbach DR, Reedijk M, Richard CS, et al: Bowel resection for intestinal endometriosis. Dis Colon Rectum 41:1158, 1998.
Vercellini P, Aimi G, De Giorgi O, et al: Is cystic ovarian endometriosis an asymmetric disease? Br J Obstet Gynaecol 105:1018, 1998.
Vercellini P, Aimi G, Panazza S, et al: A levonorgestrel-releasing intrauterine system for the treatment of dysmenorrhea associated with endometriosis: A pilot study. Fertil Steril 72:505, 1999.
Vercellini P, Cortesi I, Crosignani PG: Progestins for symptomatic endometriosis: A critical analysis of the evidence. Fertil Steril 68:393, 1997.
Vessey MP, Villard-Mackintosh L, Painter R: Epidemiology of endometriosis in women attending family planning clinics. Br Med J 306:182, 1993.
Vignali M, Infantino M, Matrone R, et al: Endometriosis: Novel etiopathogenetic concepts and clinical perspectives. Fertil Steril 78:665, 2002.
Waller KG, Shaw RW: Gonadotropin-releasing hormone analogues for the treatment of endometriosis: Long-term follow-up. Fertil Steril 59:511, 1993.
Weed JC, Ray JE: Endometriosis of the bowel. Obstet Gynecol 69:727, 1987.
Wheeler JM, Malinak LR: Recurrent endometriosis: Incidence, management, and prognosis. Am J Obstet Gynecol 146:247, 1983.
Wheeler JM, Malinak LR: The surgical management of endometriosis. Obstet Gynecol Clin North Am 16:147, 1989.
Wild RA, Hirisave V, Bianco A, et al: Endometrial antibodies versus CA-125 for the detection of endometriosis. Fertil Steril 55:90, 1991.
Witz C, Thomas M, Montoya-Rodriguez I, et al: Short-term culture of peritoneum explants confirms attachment of endometrium to intact peritoneal mesothelium. Fertil Steril 75:385, 2001.

Wolf GC and Singh KB: Cesarean scar endometriosis: a review, Obstet Gynecol Surv 44:89, 1989.

Worthington M, Irvine LM, Crook D, et al: A randomized comparative study of the metabolic effects of two regimens of gestrinone in the treatment of endometriosis. Fertil Steril 59:522, 1993.

Yang J, Van Dijk-Smith JP, Van Vugt DA, et al: Fluorescence and photosensitization of experimental endometriosis in the rat after systemic 5-aminolevulinic acid administration: A potential new approach to the diagnosis and treatment of endometriosis. Am J Obstet Gynecol 174:154, 1996.

Yu J, Grimes DA: Ascites and pleural effusions associated with endometriosis. Obstet Gynecol 78:533, 1991.

Anatomic Defects of the Abdominal Wall and Pelvic Floor 20

Abdominal and Inguinal Hernias, Cystocele, Urethrocele, Enterocele, Rectocele, Uterine and Vaginal Prolapse, and Rectal Incontinence: Diagnosis and Management

Gretchen M. Lentz

KEY TERMS AND DEFINITIONS

Abdominal Wall Hernia. An outpouching of peritoneum, with or without intra-abdominal contents, through weak areas of the abdominal wall. Also called a ventral hernia.

Anal Incontinence. Incontinence of gas or fecal material via the anus, which can be due to damage to the anal sphincter at the time of vaginal delivery with or without neuronal injury.

Anal Manometry. A commonly used test that objectively assesses the resistance to spontaneous defecation provided by the anorectal sphincter mechanism and the sensory capabilities of the rectum to provide a feeling of imminent defecation.

Cystocele. Protrusion of the bladder into the vagina, signifying the relaxation of fascial supports of the bladder.

Descensus of Cervix and Uterus (Prolapse, Procidentia). Protrusion of the cervix and uterus into the barrel of the vagina.

- **First Degree.** Prolapse into the upper vagina.
- **Second Degree.** Prolapse to or near the introitus.
- **Third Degree.** Prolapse through the introitus.

Dovetail Sign. Loss of anterior perianal folds indicating a defect in the external anal sphincter (EAS) or chronic third degree laceration.

Electromyography (EMG). Evaluates the bioelectrical action potentials that are generated by depolarization of skeletal striated muscle. EMG evaluation consists of systematic examination of spontaneous activity, recruitment patterns, and the waveform of the motor unit action potentials (MUAP).

Endoanal Ultrasound. Allows a circumferential viewing of the internal and external anal sphincters to assess for defects that may contribute to anal incontinence.

Enterocele. Herniation of the pouch of Douglas (cul-de-sac) between the uterosacral ligaments into the rectovaginal septum; usually contains small bowel.

Fecal Incontinence. The inability to defer the elimination of stool until there is a socially acceptable time and place to do so. Damage to the anal sphincter during vaginal delivery is the most common cause in women.

Femoral Hernia. A hernia that occurs through the femoral triangle. The hernia sac passes beneath the inguinal ligament through Hesselbach's triangle (an area bounded laterally by the inferior epigastric artery, inferiorly by the inguinal ligament, and medially by the lateral margin of the rectus sheath).

Incarcerated Hernia. A hernia whose contents cannot be reduced readily.

Incisional Hernia. A hernia that occurs in a surgical incision.

Inguinal Hernia. A hernia that occurs through the inguinal canal.

Pessary. A prosthesis inserted into the vagina to help support pelvic structures.

Pudendal Nerve Terminal Motor Latencies (PNTML). Nerve conduction studies that measure the time from stimulation of a nerve to a response in the muscle it innervates.

Rectoanal Inhibitory Reflex (RAIR). A reflex response to increased pressure in the rectum from gas or stool. Normally, the internal anal sphincter relaxes to allow a sampling of the rectal contents by the anal canal to determine if the contents are gas or stool and whether it is an appropriate time to defecate or pass flatus.

Rectocele. Protrusion of the rectum into the vagina, signifying a relaxation of rectal supports.

Reducible Hernia. A hernia whose contents can be reduced from the sac.

Sliding Hernia. A hernia in which the organ protruding makes up a portion of the wall of the hernia sac.

Spigelian Hernia. A rare hernia at a point where the vertical linea semilunaris joins the lateral border of the rectus muscle.

Strangulated Hernia. A hernia whose contents are incarcerated and whose blood supply to the content's structures is compromised.

Umbilical Hernia. A hernia protruding through the umbilicus.

Urethrocele. Protrusion of the urethra into the vagina, signifying loss of fascial supports of the urethra.

Vaginal Vault Prolapse. Loss of apical support of the vaginal tube.

Ventral Hernia. Ventral hernias are defects in the abdominal wall and include incisional, umbilical, epigastric, or spigelian.

The structural supports of the abdomen and pelvis are susceptible to a number of stresses. In the female these supports are affected by congenital anatomic weaknesses, the stresses of childbearing, injury, surgical damage, and straining. In addition, a combination of chronic stresses, such as lifting heavy objects, chronic cough, straining at stool, or activities that require frequent stretching, plus the aging process, may make older women more susceptible to such abnormalities. This chapter considers hernias of the abdominal wall and pelvic region, as well as conditions that are a result of the loss of pelvic supports. In addition it considers the causes, diagnosis, and treatment of rectal incontinence.

ABDOMINAL WALL HERNIAS

The abdominal wall is made up of the following structures beginning externally: skin; subcutaneous connective tissue; external oblique, internal oblique, and transversus abdominis muscles with their investing fascia; and parietal peritoneum. The rectus abdominis muscles run longitudinally in the midline from the xiphoid to the pubic symphysis. The investing fasciae of the external oblique, internal oblique, and transversus abdominis muscles completely encase the rectus abdominis muscles cephalad to the semilunar line. Caudally from the semilunar line the muscle is completely behind the aponeurosis of the fasciae of these muscles and lies directly on the peritoneum (Fig. 20-1). Normally the investing fasciae join in the midline after surrounding the rectus abdominis muscles.

In the male the descent of the testes from their original retroperitoneal site to the scrotum necessitates passing through the abdominal wall to the inguinal region. At the level of the transversalis fascia where the descent begins, the internal inguinal ring is formed. The medial margin of this ring is defined by the inferior epigastric artery as it courses from the external iliac artery medially and superiorly into the rectus sheath. The inguinal canal runs from the internal inguinal ring obliquely downward, emerging through the external inguinal ring and opening in the external oblique aponeurosis just above the pubic spine and then continuing into the scrotum. This allows for passage of the testes and for the presence of part of the spermatic cord.

In the female the round ligament courses in the same direction but ends short of the labia. An inguinal hernia, that is, a bulge of peritoneum through the internal inguinal ring and into the inguinal canal, is less common in the female than in the male and is frequently identified after stretching of the abdominal wall during or after pregnancy. It may be related to a congenital weakness of this area. Occasionally a femoral-type groin hernia may develop. In this case the defect in the transversalis fascia occurs in Hesselbach's triangle, which is an area bounded laterally by the inferior epigastric artery, inferiorly by the inguinal ligament, and medially by the lateral margin of the rectus sheath (Fig. 20-2). The hernia sac passes under the inguinal ligament into the femoral triangle rather than coursing through the inguinal canal. Femoral hernias are more common in females than in males.

The hernia is said to be *reducible* if the contents can be returned to the abdominal cavity. If the contents cannot be reduced, the hernia is said to be incarcerated. An incarcerated hernia may be acute, accompanied by pain, or may be longstanding and asymptomatic. If the blood supply to the incarcerated structure is compromised, the hernia is said to be *strangulated.* Because the hernia sac is primarily prolapsed peritoneum, the hernia itself is not strangulated but only its contents.

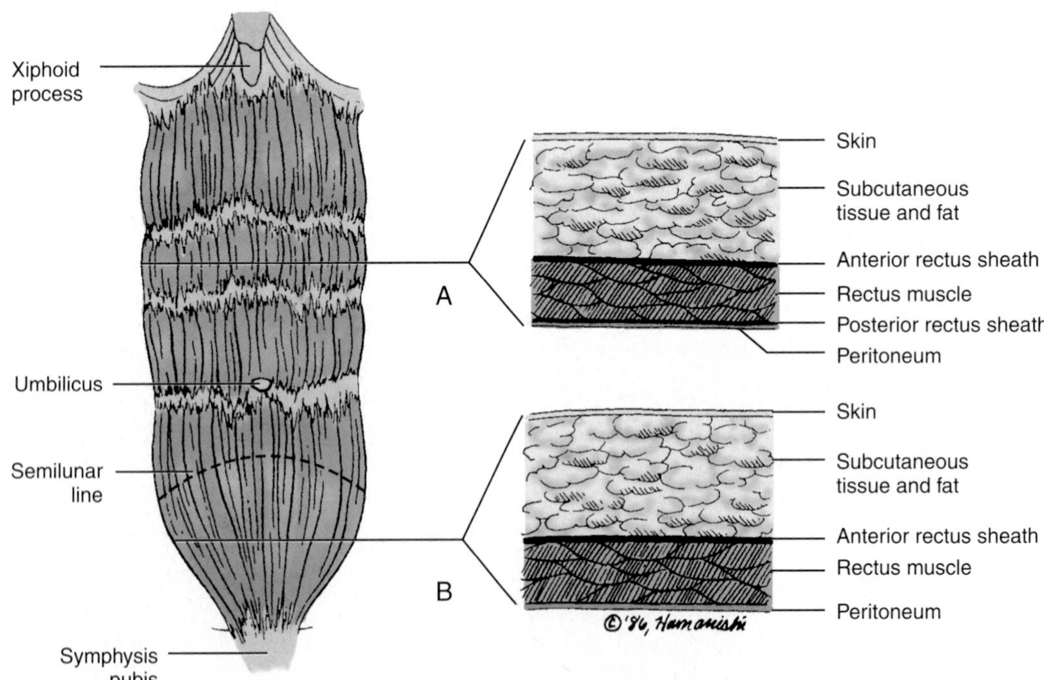

Figure 20-1. Graphic representation of layers of the abdominal wall. **A,** Above semilunar line. **B,** Below semilunar line.

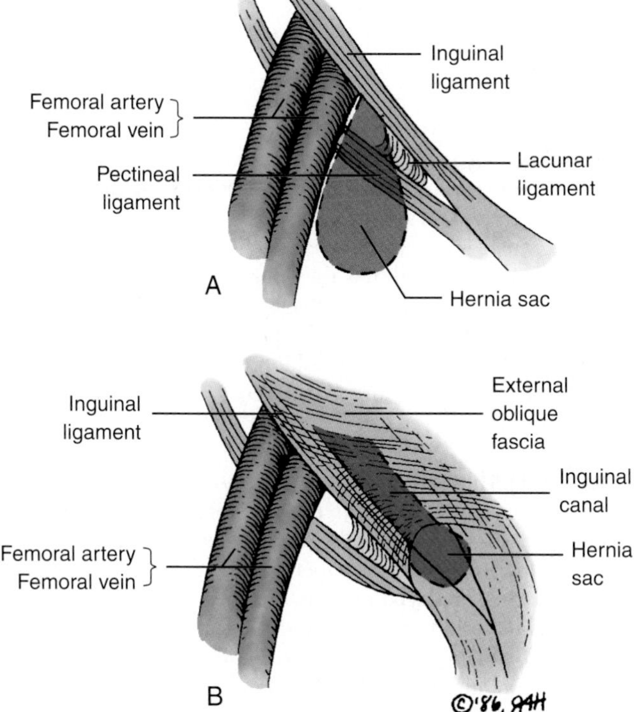

Figure 20-2. Graphic representation of right femoral **(A)** and right inguinal **(B)** hernias in the female.

On rare occasions a portion of the wall of the hernia sac is composed of an organ such as the sigmoid colon or the cecum. In these instances the hernia is called a *sliding hernia.*

A ventral hernia occurs in the abdominal wall away from the groin. Examples include umbilical hernias, which are caused by congenital relaxation of the umbilical ring, and incisional hernias, which are herniations through separation of fascial planes after operative incision. Two special ventral hernias include the epigastric hernia, which occurs in a defect of the linea alba above the umbilicus, and the rare spigelian hernia, which is a herniation at a point where the vertical linea semilunaris joins the lateral border of the rectus muscle.

Incisional hernias generally involve the separation of the fascia of the abdominal wall with the hernia sac palpated beneath the skin and subcutaneous tissue. The sac wall is composed of peritoneum.

Because the umbilicus consists of a fusion of skin, fascia, and peritoneum, an umbilical hernia generally occurs because the fascial ring is grossly separated, allowing the hernia sac to protrude. This occurs most frequently in obese women. The hernia sac itself is made up of peritoneum and subcutaneous tissue beneath the skin (Fig. 20-3).

Etiology

Hernias may be the result of a congenital malformation. The umbilical hernia is the best example. Before 10 weeks' gestation the abdominal contents are partially herniated through the umbilicus into the extra embryonic coelomic cavity. However, after

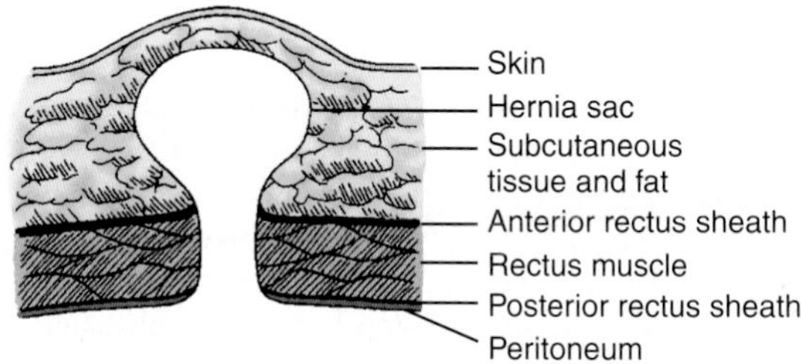

Figure 20-3. Graphic representation of umbilical hernia.

10 weeks the viscera normally return to the abdominal cavity, and the defect in the abdominal wall closes during subsequent fetal growth. Generally at birth only the space occupied by the umbilical cord remains patent. After the cutting of the cord the area heals so that the skin in the area of the umbilicus fuses above the closed fascial layer. Some infants at birth will show a small umbilical hernia, but in most instances the fascial defect closes during the first 3 years of life. If it does not close, an umbilical hernia will form. In rare cases the abdominal wall closure process is less complete, leading to an omphalocele, which is a hernia sac at the umbilicus covered only by peritoneum and including bowel and other abdominal contents. Omphaloceles are usually seen in infants with other malformations and possibly chromosome anomalies, such as trisomy 13.

Black infants have umbilical hernias more often than do white infants. Occasionally, umbilical hernias occur in adults after the distention of the abdominal cavity with pregnancy or with ascites.

Inguinal hernias are more common in males than in females. Femoral hernias occur primarily in females. Hernias that occur in adults are often associated with trauma or injury. In many instances the hernia bulge develops slowly after years of heavy labor. It is likely that a congenital anatomic defect was always present but became exaggerated over time, leading to the development of a hernia. Zimmerman and Anson thought that such lesions resulted from inadequate muscle support at the lower area of the inguinal canal, primarily caused by a defect in the internal oblique muscle. Stretching of this area in pregnancy may initiate a hernia, but other factors, such as chronic cough caused by smoking or chronic respiratory disease, may be responsible.

Incisional hernias generally occur because of poor healing of the fascia. This may be secondary to poor nutrition, infection, or necrosis of the fascia secondary to suturing. It may also occur because absorbable suture loses its tensile strength before healing is complete. Stress and strain secondary to chronic cough or retching in the postoperative period may contribute to the process. Emergency surgery increases the risk of incisional hernia. Other conditions that inhibit wound healing include obesity, smoking, connective tissue disorders, and immunosuppressant medications.

Symptoms and Signs

Bulges in the abdominal wall lead to the discovery of most ventral or groin hernias in women, either by a physician at the time of physical examination or by the patient. These hernias are generally symptom free. Occasionally, excessive straining or trauma will be implicated, and the patient may experience a feeling of tearing of tissue. Frequently the bulges are noted during an increase in intraabdominal pressure, such as with pregnancy or ascites. Most hernias are asymptomatic, but in some cases, particularly with larger ones, there may be aching or discomfort. Should intraabdominal organs move into the sac, the patient may experience some discomfort. Organs that strangulate within the sac cause acute pain and discomfort. Incarcerated organs may give nonspecific visceral pain, which is most likely the result of mesenteric stretching.

In cases where a hernia exists but no contents are within the sac, physical examination reveals a weakening at the site of the hernia. It is often possible to feel the "ring" of the hernia as one palpates the defect through the skin and subcutaneous tissue. The patient's straining will generally accentuate the hernia, making it more palpable and visible. In the case of inguinal and femoral hernias it may be necessary for the patient to be standing for one to palpate the hernia.

When there are intraabdominal contents within the hernia sac, the hernia is more easily palpated. The physician should then decide, based on his or her attempts to gently milk the contents from the sac back through the defect ring, whether the contents are reducible. For a hernia that does not reduce easily but in which there is no evidence of vascular compromise it is sometimes useful to apply ice packs to the abdomen in the area of the incarcerated hernia before additional attempts are made to reduce it. In cases of strangulated hernia, evidence of devitalization of an organ, such as fever, leukocytosis, and evidence for an acute abdomen, may be noted.

Management

Nonoperative management of hernias of the ventral wall and groin in women is often feasible. Umbilical hernias in little girls will generally close by age 3 or 4 years and rarely become incarcerated. An incisional hernia, if not too large, can frequently be managed by a corset, which prevents it from becoming incarcerated. Unincarcerated groin hernias are often small and become uncomfortable only with an increase in intraabdominal pressure, such as occurs with pregnancy. Many authors advocate repair, however, because the small neck of these hernias may make incarceration more likely. With pregnancy the opportunity for incarceration is reduced because the increasing size of the uterus pushes bowel contents away from the area of the herniation. Trusses and other supports are generally difficult to fit and are of little value in women.

Larger hernias, hernias that continuously contain intraabdominal contents, hernias that cause continuing discomfort, and those that have been incarcerated should be repaired. Some general principles of operative repair can be stated. The first principle involves the anatomy of the hernia. The hernia almost always consists of a sac of peritoneum with a narrow neck and a fascial defect of some sort. In rare instances, if a peritoneal sac is broad based, it may be possible to simply reduce the sac through the fascial defect without opening it and then to repair the fascial defect. However, if a narrow-necked sac exists, it must be dissected free of the fascial defect, emptied of its contents, and then excised and sutured at the neck (base). The fascial defect is then mobilized completely to remove stress and scarring, and it is closed with permanent suture. In some cases the fascial defect may be large and the degree of mobilization that is required may be impossible. In such instances, patching with inert material, such as polyester fiber (Mersilene) mesh, may be necessary. Mesh repairs have become the preferred technique for incisional hernias because the recurrence rate is lowered.

The second principle involves management of the contents of the hernia sac. Usually the hernia sac reduces with ease, but if intraabdominal contents are fixed to the sac wall by adhesions, the sac must be opened and the adhesions carefully separated. Care must be taken not to damage the organs or their blood supply. When these organs are reduced from the sac, the sac may be handled in the usual fashion. When incarceration has occurred, the organs must be inspected for viability before replacement.

Umbilical Hernia

A curved incision is made at the inferior margin of the umbilicus (Fig. 20-4). The umbilicus is dissected free of the sac and reflected upward. The sac is then dissected free of the fascial defect and either reduced or excised, depending on the circumstances. The fascial edges are freshened and either closed by direct approximation anterior to posterior using nonabsorbable sutures or mobilized and closed in a "vest over pants" manner, suturing the anterior edge to the posterior edge in an overlapping fashion. Studies have not shown that either of these closures is superior to the other, and the approach taken generally is the one that best fits the circumstances. The umbilicus is then tacked to the fascial defect and the skin margin approximated. Large defects may require mesh placement to avoid tension on the closure.

Incisional Hernia

Repair of an incisional hernia can be accomplished by incising the skin through the old scar or via a parallel incision and dissecting through the subcutaneous tissue to identify both margins of the separated fascial defect. The peritoneum of the hernia sac is then isolated, dissected free of the margins, and reduced in the most appropriate fashion, with the surgeon exercising care not to damage any organs that may be fixed in the sac by adhesions. The fascial edges are then mobilized completely and closed with a mass suture technique. Outcome studies show a sutured repair is more likely to result in a recurrence than a mesh repair. Sutured repair may be adequate for small hernias and when the risk of using a mesh prosthesis is unacceptable. Laparoscopic repairs appear to reduce perioperative complications and recurrence risk although larger randomized trials are needed to confirm this.

Prevention of incisional hernias bears mention since 10% to 15% of abdominal incisions will develop a hernia. Preventing wound infection with appropriate antibiotic prophylaxis if indicated and careful surgical technique is worthwhile since the hernia rate increases to 23% with postoperative wound infection. A meta-analysis of abdominal fascial closure concluded a continuous nonabsorbable suture closure resulted in significantly lower rates of incisional hernia.

Groin Hernia

To repair an inguinal or femoral hernia, an incision is made above the inguinal ligament, usually parallel to its medial

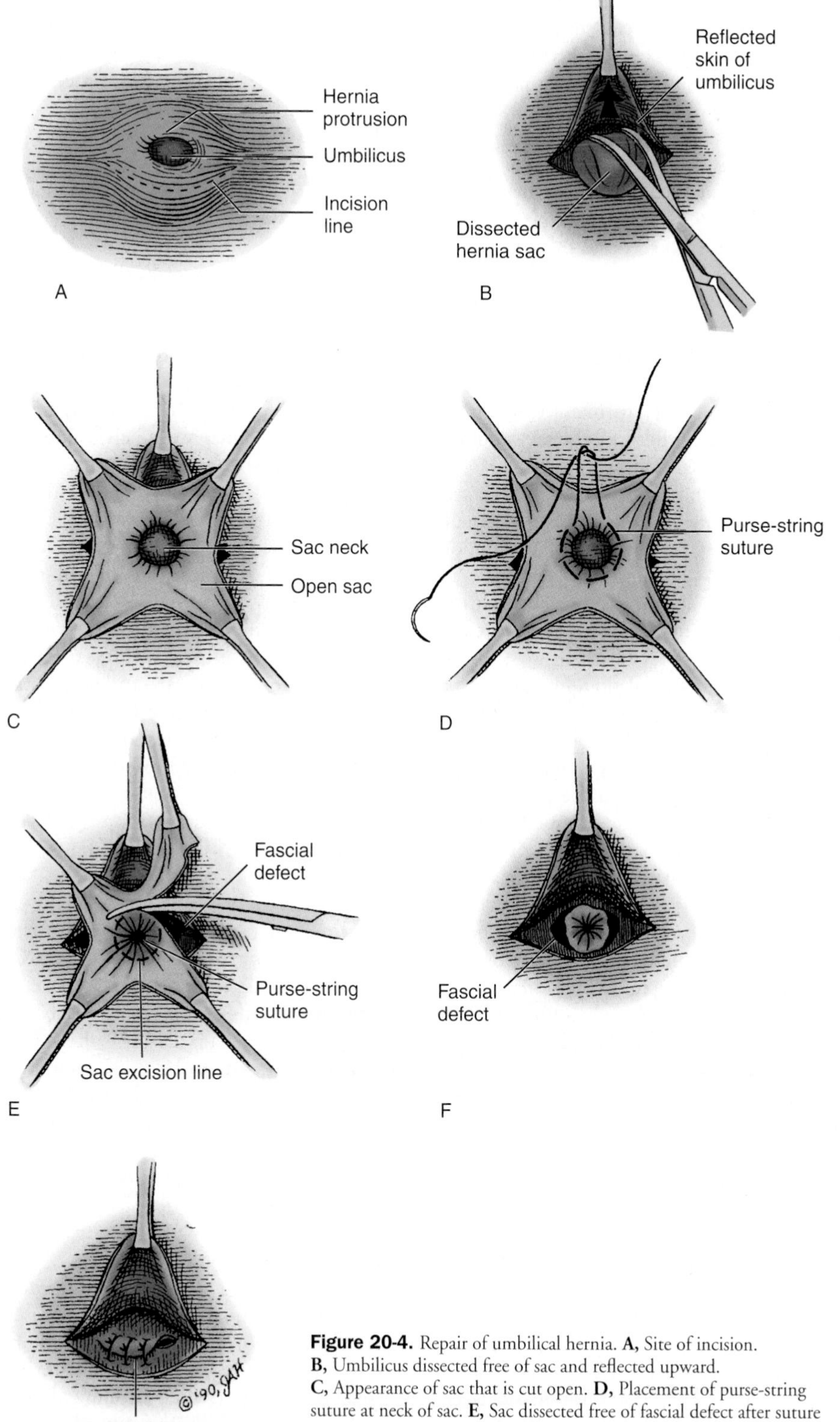

Figure 20-4. Repair of umbilical hernia. **A,** Site of incision. **B,** Umbilicus dissected free of sac and reflected upward. **C,** Appearance of sac that is cut open. **D,** Placement of purse-string suture at neck of sac. **E,** Sac dissected free of fascial defect after suture is tied. **F,** Appearance of fascial defect after sac excised. **G,** Fascial defect closed; umbilicus will be tacked to it.

portion. Subcutaneous tissue is separated, and the aponeurosis of the external oblique muscle is exposed. The external oblique is then incised from above down through the external inguinal ring, with the surgeon taking care to avoid the ilioinguinal nerve, which is frequently adherent to the external ring. The sac is identified and by careful dissection excised down to its emergence through the transversalis fascia. The sac is opened, and the intraperitoneal contents are reduced. The surgeon should place his or her finger through the sac neck into the peritoneal cavity and palpate the structures immediately within to be sure that there are no other hernia sacs protruding, particularly into the femoral canal. The sac neck is then ligated and transfixed away from the ring, often to Cooper's ligament. The transversalis fascia is approximated with nonabsorbable suture. The external oblique aponeurosis is then closed with nonabsorbable suture, and the skin and subcutaneous tissue are closed. Occasionally on opening the external oblique aponeurosis, only a mass of fat is found. In such instances the diagnosis of a hernia was made in error and no sac is present. Often, however, there is both fat and a sac, and the surgeon must be careful to determine the contents of the inguinal canal.

Femoral Hernia

When the sac is protruding beneath the inguinal ligament and through the femoral canal, an attempt may be made to reduce it from above. Frequently it is necessary to incise the inguinal ligament to free up the sac neck. In either case the sac should be ligated at its base, with the surgeon making sure that its contents are not damaged and that they are reduced. The sac, as in all cases, is generally handled by excising excess peritoneum and placing a purse-string suture of absorbable material about the base. Although it is probably not necessary to repair the inguinal ligament, most surgeons will do so. To prevent recurrent hernia in the transversalis fascia, the sac neck is sutured to Cooper's ligament beneath the inguinal ligament. To support the transversalis fascia repair, the external oblique aponeurosis is sutured over the transversalis fascia for extra support, all with interrupted, nonabsorbable suture material.

Recently, many groin hernias have been repaired laparoscopically. This may be carried out both in the preperitoneal space and intraperitoneally. In most instances a mesh patch is placed across the defect and fixed with either staples or sutures. Although many different materials may be utilized, Mersilene mesh seems to be popular and safest. Intraperitoneal exploration by laparoscopy often makes it possible to see a small hernia developing on the opposite side, which can also be fixed. In a study of 79 patients undergoing a repair of inguinal hernia, Panton and Panton determined that 25% were found to have a hernia on the contralateral side. Operative complications occur in 5% 10% of patients and include lateral thigh paresthesia, inferior epigastric artery injury, enterotomy from adhesiolysis, bowel obstruction secondary to herniation through trocar sites, and bladder injury. Recurrence rates are reported as 1% to 2% in most studies.

DISORDERS OF PELVIC SUPPORT

Pelvic organ prolapse (POP) is a condition characterized by the failure of various anatomic structures to support the pelvic viscera. POP is common in parous women, with a lifetime prevalence of 30% to 50%, although many are asymptomatic. Racial prevalence data from urogynecologic referral clinics find no significant difference in the presence or severity of POP in blacks versus whites. Pelvic support structures are often weakened by childbirth, other pelvic trauma, stress and strain, and the aging process. Abnormalities that result from these relaxation problems include urethrocele, cystocele, rectocele, enterocele, and uterine prolapse (descensus of the cervix and uterus). If a hysterectomy has been performed, prolapse of the vagina may also be a problem. It is unusual to have only one of these conditions. In most cases the relaxation affects all the support structures of the pelvis. Frequently, relaxation of the urethra, the bladder neck, and the bladder (urethrocele, cystocele) is associated with urinary incontinence, which is discussed in Chapter 21 (Urogynecology).

Pathophysiology

The pathophysiology of POP is probably multifactorial. Bump and Norton outlined a useful concept in looking at risk factors as either predisposing, inciting, promoting, or decompensation events (Fig. 20-5). Much research has been reported recently on the use of magnetic resonance imaging (MRI) for evaluating healthy female pelvic anatomy and anatomic variations to compare to women with pelvic floor dysfunction. Hoyte and colleagues used three-dimensional color thickness mapping to compare the levator ani of 30 women: 10 asymptomatic, 10 with urodynamic stress incontinence, and 10 with POP. Thicker, bulkier levator ani muscles were found in the asymptomatic women. Loss of levator muscle bulk was found in women with POP and stress incontinence. Theoretical explanations for these findings include muscle atrophy from denervation from childbirth injuries or muscle wasting from muscle insertion detachment also from childbirth, and possibly age and hormonal status (Fig. 20-6). Imaging is not usually necessary in women with prolapse, but current research in this area is furthering our understanding of support defects.

Urethrocele and Cystocele

Attenuation or rupture of the pubovesicle cervical fascia for any reason may allow the descent of the urethra (urethrocele), bladder neck, or bladder (cystocele) into the vaginal canal. Often only a cystocele is present (Fig. 20-7), and generally in these cases the patient is continent. When a urethrocele is present as well, the woman usually suffers from stress incontinence. Urethroceles seem to be more common in women with wide subpubic arches (gynecoid type), which allow the full force of the fetal head against this area during descent in labor. Narrower arches, such as those associated with the android or anthropoid pelvic types, seem to protect this region from the descent of the fetal head.

Symptoms and Signs

Symptoms of POP are often not specific to the area that is prolapsing. However, in general, symptoms and signs of urethrocele and cystocele consist of a sensation of fullness, pressure or vaginal bulge and at times a feeling that organs are falling out, occasional urgency, and often a feeling of incomplete emptying with voiding. The patient and the physician note a soft, bulging mass of the anterior vaginal wall. In some patients this mass must be replaced manually before the patient can void. Strain or cough accentuates the bulge. The mass may descend to or beyond the introitus. Although urethroceles and cystoceles almost always occur in parous women, they have been noted in nulliparous women who have poor structural supports. This is particularly true in women who have congenital malformations

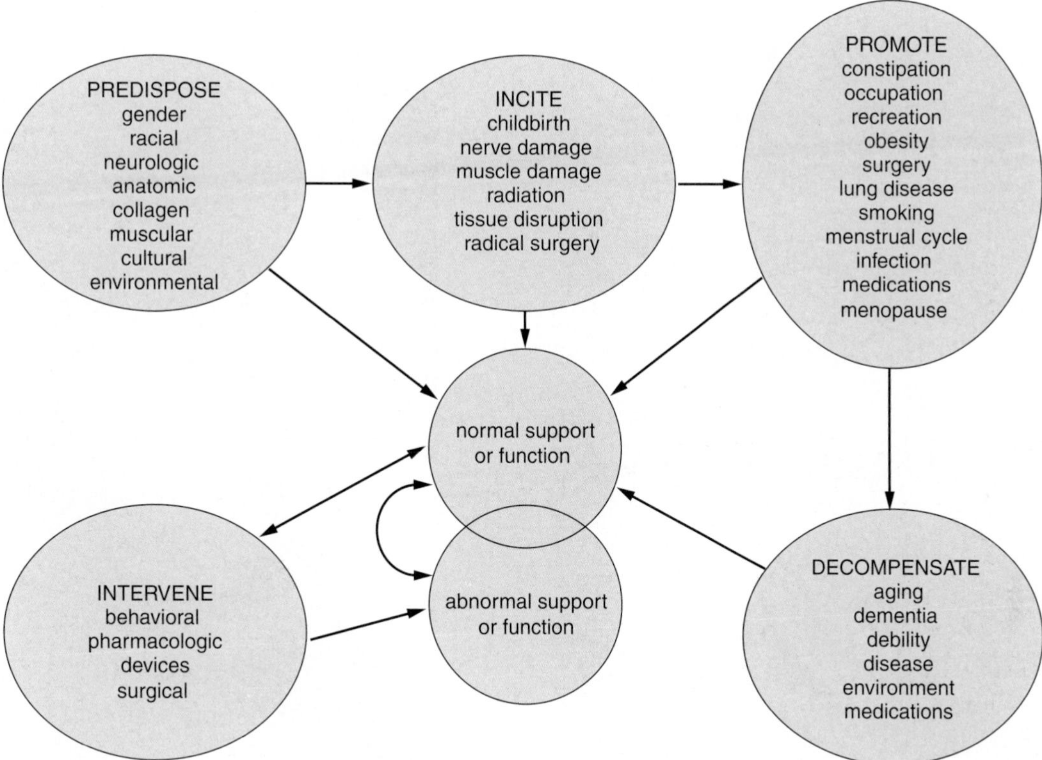

Figure 20-5. Model for the development of pelvic floor dysfunction in women. (From Bump RC, Norton PA: Epidemiology and natural history of pelvic floor dysfunction. Obstet Gynecol ClNA 25(4):723, 1998.)

or weaknesses of the endopelvic connective tissue and musculature of the pelvic floor. Most parous women demonstrate some degree of cystocele, and when asymptomatic, they do not require therapy.

Women with prolapse often have other urinary symptoms. Some women have stress incontinence due to urethral hypermobility. Others are continent despite lack of urethral support. Another group of women may have occult or latent stress incontinence because their continence depends on urethral kinking or obstruction from severe prolapse.

Diagnosis

The urethrocele and the cystocele are best demonstrated with a patient in the lithotomy position. A retractor or posterior wall blade of a Graves speculum is used to depress the posterior wall. The patient is then asked to strain, and the degree of the cystocele or urethrocele is noted. The physician should palpate the bladder neck and note whether it is well supported. Generally, if the supports of the bladder neck are adequate, the urethra is adequately supported. If a cystocele and a urethrocele are present, it invariably follows that the bladder neck is not supported. The examination for cystocele and urethrocele is best performed with the bladder at least partially filled (100–250 mL).

Urethroceles must be differentiated from inflamed and enlarged Skene's glands and urethral diverticula. Cystoceles must be differentiated from bladder tumors and bladder diverticula, both of which are rare but may occur. Urethroceles and cystoceles are generally soft, pliable, and nontender. Although diverticula may be reducible, a sensation of a mass is usually present. Inflamed Skene's glands are generally tender, and it may be possible to express pus from the urethra when they are palpated. Pus may be expressed also in the presence of a diverticulum of the urethra. In such cases gonococcal and chlamydial infections should be considered.

Management

Treatment of urethroceles and cystoceles may be nonoperative or operative. Nonoperative treatment consists of supporting the herniation of the bladder into the vagina with the use of the Smith-Hodge, ring, or inflatable pessary (see Fig. 20-15) or even with the intermittent use of a large tampon. Kegel exercises (see Chapter 21, Urogynecology) help to strengthen the pelvic floor musculature and thereby may relieve some of the pressure symptoms produced by the cystocele. While there is no direct evidence that pelvic floor muscle training prevents or treats POP, it may be beneficial and it is effective for concomitant symptoms of urinary and fecal incontinence. Women who have performed Kegel exercises on their own and have not improved, may still benefit from working with a physical therapist. In an older woman the use of estrogen vaginal cream may improve vaginal atrophy and patient comfort if the prolapsed vaginal mucosa is irritated or ulcerated.

A younger woman with a large cystocele should be encouraged to avoid operative repair until she has completed her family. Occasionally the abnormality is so uncomfortable that repair must be performed before childbearing is complete. If this is the case, cesarean delivery should be considered for subsequent pregnancies.

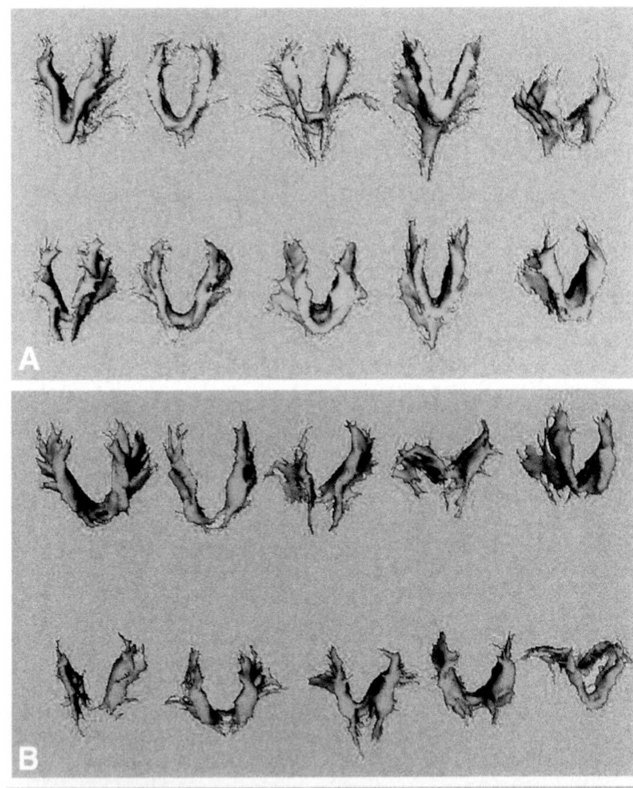

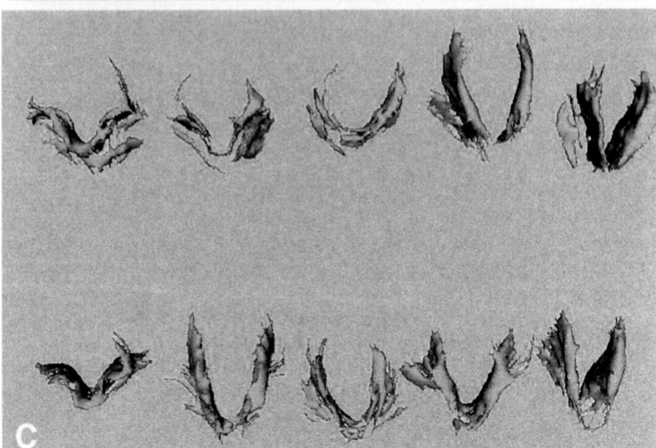

Figure 20-6. Color images of reconstructed levator ani muscles from three subject groups: Asymptomatic group **(A)**, GSI group **(B)**, prolapse group **(C)**. (From Hoyte L, Jakab M, Warfield SK: Levator ani thickness variations in symptomatic and asymptomatic women using magnetic resonance-based 3-dimensional color mapping. Am J Obstet Gynecol 191:856, 2004.)

Operative repair of a cystocele is generally performed in conjunction with the repair of all other pelvic support defects. It is unusual for anterior supports of the vagina to relax without an accompanying relaxation of the posterior wall. Repair therefore usually consists of an anterior and posterior colporrhaphy. If uterine descensus is noted, this must also be treated. Frequently an enterocele accompanies a cystocele and rectocele and where present must be excised and repaired. These problems are discussed later in this chapter.

Anterior wall repair (colporrhaphy) is performed by incising the vaginal epithelium transversally just above the anterior lip

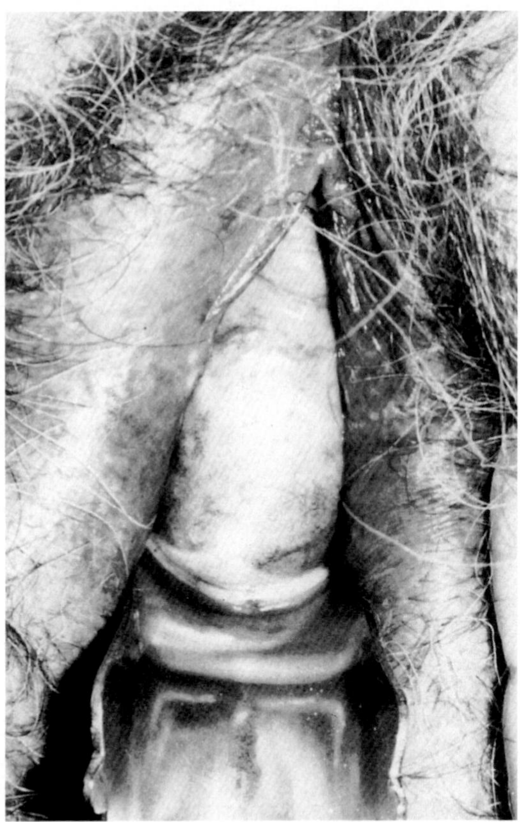

Figure 20-7. Cystocele.

of the cervix in the region of the bladder reflection (Fig. 20-8). If the woman has undergone a hysterectomy in the past, the incision may be made approximately 1 to 1.5 cm anterior to the vaginal scar. The vagina is then incised longitudinally from the transverse incision to the level of the bladder neck. If no urethrocele is present, this incision is sufficient. If a urethrocele is present, the incision must be continued under the urethra as well. The longitudinal incision is made by separating the vaginal wall from the underlying tissue progressively, using Metzenbaum scissors. When the longitudinal incision is complete, the cut edge of the vagina is held under tension and the pubocervical fascia that is attached is separated from it by blunt and sharp dissection. This is repeated on each side. At this point the bladder is free of the pubocervical fascia, which is itself free of the vaginal wall. The surgeon then places a suture over the bladder neck (Kelly stitch), bringing together the pubocervical fasciae on either side. The stitch should be placed in such a fashion that the pubocervical fascia is sutured as far away from the cut edge as possible and parallel to the previous incision. A similar stitch is taken on the opposite side, and the suture tied. Most appropriate for this closure is 0 or 2-0 polyglycol suture. With the bladder neck well identified and supported, the pubocervical fascia is then closed with progressive similar stitches to completely imbricate the fascia over the bladder. If the urethrocele is present, similar sutures are also placed over the urethra. (Additional procedures to correct stress incontinence are discussed in Chapter 21, Urogynecology.) After the imbrication of the pubocervical fascia is completed, the vaginal edges are trimmed

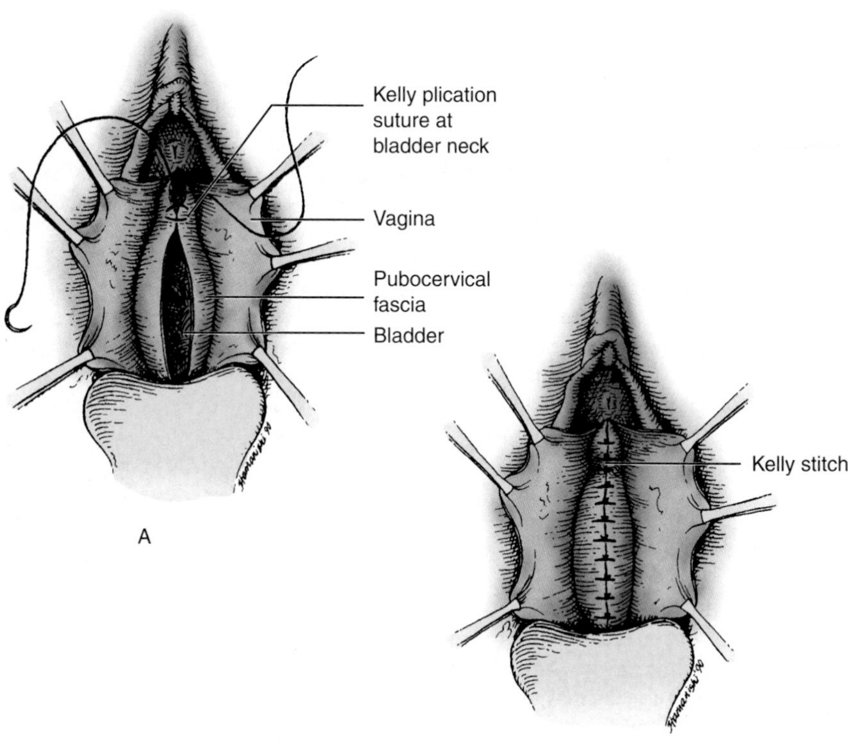

Figure 20-8. Cystourethrocele repair. **A,** The placement of Kelly stitch in the pubocervical fascia at the junction of the urethra with the bladder neck. **B,** The repair of the cystocele as the pubocervical fascia is sutured. Thus the cystocele is plicated. (Redrawn from Symmonds RE: Relaxation of pelvic supports. In Benson RC [ed]: Current Obstetric and Gynecologic Diagnosis and Treatment, 5th ed. Los Altos, CA, Lange Medical, 1984.)

and the vagina closed with a row of interrupted 2-0 polyglycol or catgut sutures. Addition of graft materials to the repair has been studied, and small randomized trials of polyglactin mesh (Vicryl) suggest modest improvements in success rates. However, to date, there is no long-term evidence proving graft materials improve outcomes and many graft complications have been reported.

Postoperatively the bladder should be drained for about 2 to 3 days. There are several ways to accomplish this. The first is to leave a No. 16 Foley catheter in place for 2 to 3 days, remove the catheter on the second to third day, and allow the patient to try to void. After voiding of at least 200 mL the patient should be catheterized for the presence of residual urine or alternatively, a bladder ultrasound can estimate residual volume. If residual urine is found in a quantity of more than 150 mL on two successive voidings or if the amount voided is less than 200 mL, the physician should consider replacing the catheter for 24 to 48 hours. If residual urine amounts are less than 150 mL on two consecutive voidings, no further steps are necessary. Occasionally, after an anterior repair, voiding does not occur after 5 days of bladder drainage. At that point the patient may require catheterization for 24 to 48 hours longer, or she may be treated with a Foley catheter in place for continuous drainage for a week, to be rechecked for voiding and residual urine as an outpatient in 1 week. It is rarely necessary to treat the patient with antibiotics during this period; however, lower urinary tract infections are common and should be treated as they occur. In some patients who have had chronic urinary tract infections, prophylactic antibiotics, such as a sulfa preparation or nitrofurantoin can be administered.

Alternatives to the above-mentioned regimen include suprapubic catheter drainage or teaching the patient clean intermittent self-catheterization (CISC). With a suprapubic catheter, the drainage tube can be clamped, allowing the patient to void when she can and allowing residual urine measurements to be taken. The suprapubic technique is simple to use and seems to have a lower incidence of infection than does transurethral catheterization, but patients may complain of extravasation of urine around the site and occasionally of hematoma formation. CISC can be threatening for patients to learn, but once learned, many patients prefer not having an indwelling catheter and can measure their own postvoid residual urine volumes. CISC is generally not necessary if short periods of catheterization are anticipated. The surgeon should decide which method is best suited to the needs of his or her institution and develop a system that the surgeon and nursing team understand and can follow.

Postoperatively it is important to emphasize to the patient that heavy lifting, straining, or prolonged periods of standing should be avoided for 3 months. The healing process is slow, and the tissue is generally weak initially. Complete healing should be ensured before the tissue is stressed by normal activities.

Kohli and coworkers studied the recurrence rate of cystocele in 27 patients who underwent anterior colporrhaphy for symptomatic cystocele and 40 patients who underwent anterior colporrhaphy and needle suspension for cystocele and genuine stress incontinence. Recurrence of the cystocele occurred in 2 of the 27 cystocele patients and 13 of the 40 cystoceles with genuine stress incontinent patients in an average of 13 months. They speculated that the increased recurrency rate was due to the retropubic dissection necessary for the needle suspension. It is possible that the incontinent patients in the latter group suffered from a different pathologic problem such as nerve damage, collagen defect, and so on, and that this may have been responsible for the poorer outcome.

Certainly, recurrent anterior vaginal wall prolapse remains as the most frustrating problem for the gynecologic surgeon and patients. In fact, George R. White was quoted in 1909 saying, "Ahlfet states that the only problem in a plastic gynecology left unsolved by the gynecologist is that of permanent cure of cystocele." It is still the problem of the current century with reported failure rates of 0 to 20% for anterior colporrhaphy. The reintroduction of the paravaginal repair by Richardson brought hopes of reducing the recurrence of cystoceles. However, studies show failure rates of 3% to 14%, and controlled studies reporting long-term outcomes are lacking. So, when POP repair is planned vaginally, anterior colporrhaphy is still indicated for cystocele correction. If stress incontinence is also present, a specific repair is indicated besides the anterior colporrhaphy. A Cochrane database review found evidence from six trials that an open abdominal retropubic bladder neck suspension was significantly more effective than anterior repair for urinary incontinence (18% failure rate vs. 45%).

Rectocele

Symptoms and Signs

The patient with a rectocele often complains of a heavy or "falling out" feeling in the vagina. She may complain of constipation and occasionally may need to splint the vagina with her fingers to effect a bowel movement. She may also have a feeling of incomplete emptying of the rectum at the time of the bowel movement.

Diagnosis

A rectocele may be identified by retracting the anterior vaginal wall upward with one-half of a Graves or Pederson speculum and again having the patient strain. The rectum will bulge into the vagina, and this bulge may protrude through the introitus (Fig. 20-9). The physician should then place one finger in the rectum and one in the vagina and palpate the hernia. Often the rectovaginal septum is paper-thin, and the rectocele can be palpated to its upper margin. If an enterocele is present, it may be possible to differentiate it from the rectocele by having the patient strain. Frequently, however, the diagnosis of a small enterocele is established only at the time of operation.

Management

Nonoperative management of a rectocele is similar to that mentioned for a cystocele. Pessaries, Kegel exercises, and estrogen may be useful in the appropriate situations. Gastrointestinal symptoms must be thoroughly evaluated including screening for colorectal cancer if appropriate. If constipation and straining are issues, a dietary fiber and fluid intake review should be obtained. At least 20 g of fiber, six to eight glasses of fluid, regular exercise, and allowing time for defecation after meals can be recommended to regulate bowel habits as first-line therapy.

Operative management of a rectocele (posterior colporrhaphy) is generally performed at the time of an anterior colporrhaphy with or without enterocele repair or operation for descensus. Most women with rectoceles also have gaping vaginas and weakness in their perineal body. Therefore as part of a rectocele repair a perineorrhaphy is performed as well. The surgeon should estimate at the time of starting the posterior repair what degree of perineorrhaphy he or she wishes to perform. The margins of the perineum to be narrowed are generally marked by placing Allis clamps at their extreme at the introital opening (Fig. 20-10). The tissue of the introitus is then incised between these clamps, and the vaginal wall is separated from the underlying tissue and rectum in a progressive manner longitudinally in the midline, beginning at the introital incision and being carried forward to the apex of the vagina above the limit of the rectocele. This is done by progressive separation and incision using the Metzenbaum scissors in a fashion similar to that described for cystocele repair.

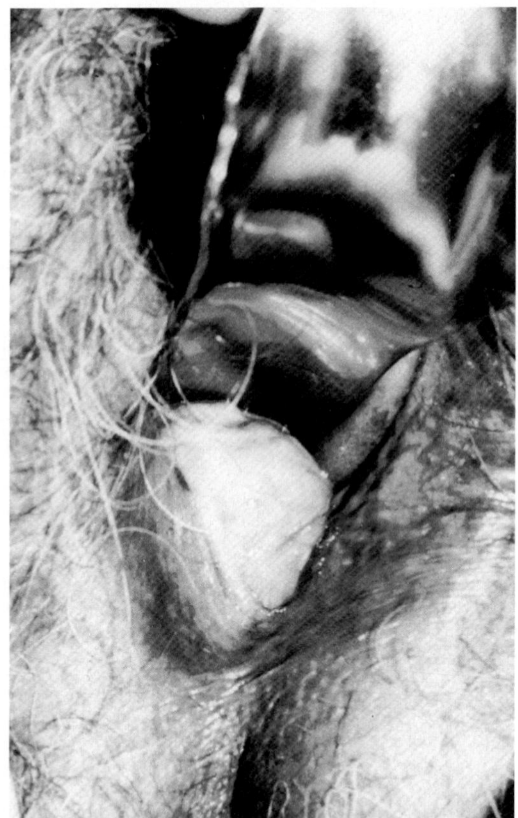

Figure 20-9. Rectocele.

When the vaginal wall is completely incised, the edges are grasped and placed under tension, and the perirectal connective tissue is separated from the vaginal mucosa by blunt and sharp (if necessary) dissection. This is carried out bilaterally until it is possible for the operator to palpate the perirectal space on each side. The operator then places a finger of his or her nondominant hand into the rectum using a double-gloved technique while an assistant picks up perirectal tissue on either side. The operator then places a delayed absorbable suture into the perirectal tissue on either side. Approximately three to five of these stitches are placed, and these are held without tying. The operator should use his or her finger in the rectum to ensure that no suture is placed into the rectum. The perirectal tissue usually includes portions of the levator ani muscles. When the sutures are tied, these tissues are interposed between rectum and vagina, thereby reducing the rectocele. These sutures also serve to tack the vagina to the levator ani area, thereby, it is hoped, avoiding future vaginal prolapse if a hysterectomy has also been performed. However, if vaginal vault prolapse is also present,

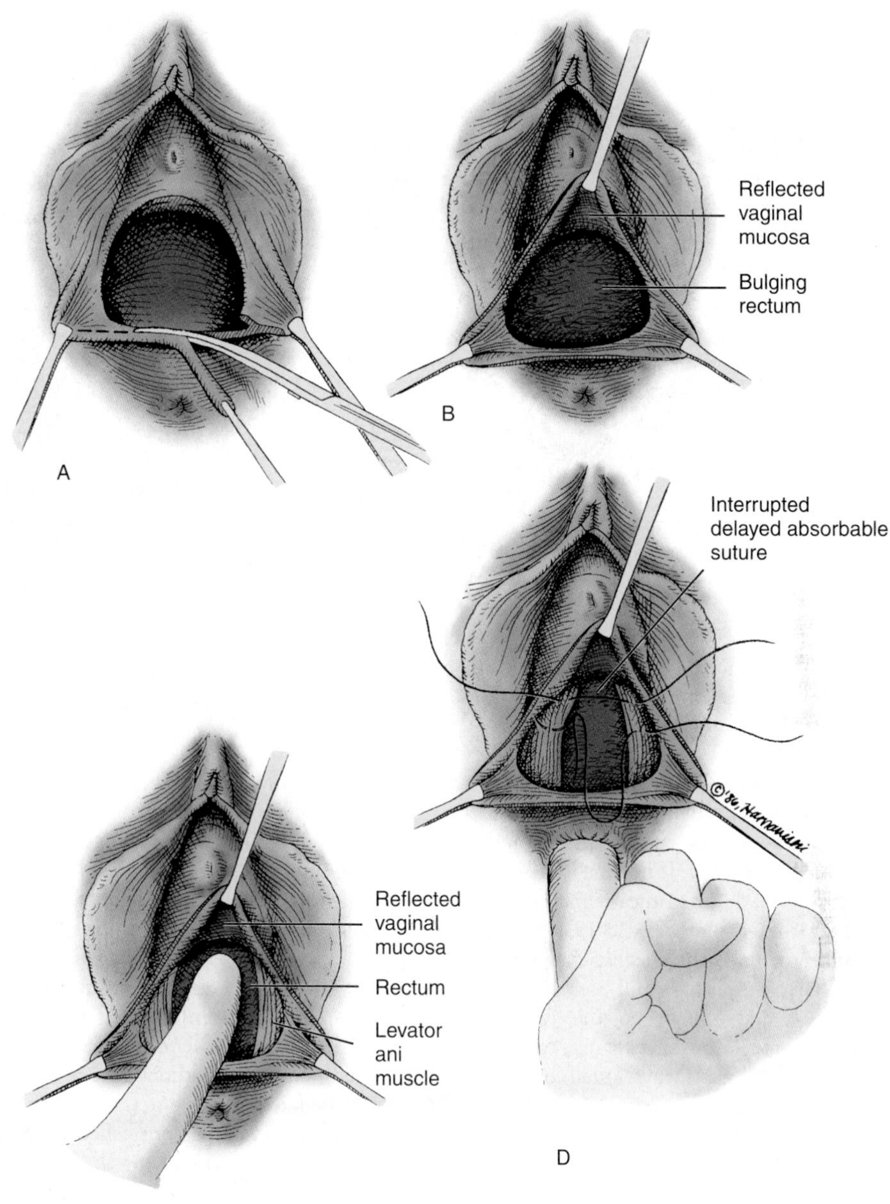

Figure 20-10. Repair of rectocele. **A,** Placement of Allis clamps at margins of perineal incision; perineal incision is being made. **B,** Reflected vaginal mucosa with rectum bulging. **C,** Depression of rectum identifying margins of levator ani muscle. **D,** Placement of sutures in perirectal tissue and levator ani bundles.

a separate repair is indicated for support of the vaginal apex and this is discussed later. The vaginal edges are then trimmed and the vagina closed with a row of either continuous or interrupted absorbable suture.

Attention is then turned to the perineorrhaphy when there is perineal muscle separation, which is closed in the following fashion. Polyglycol sutures are placed in the lateral margins of the transverse incision, essentially bringing bulbocavernosal and superficial perineal muscles together from either side to the midline. The operator should be sure that the bulbocavernosal muscle insertions are included in the sutures by pulling on the suture and noting whether the tension identifies the muscle bundles. The remainder of the perineal incision is then closed with a row of 2-0 polyglycol sutures to the deep tissue, and the skin of the perineum is closed with either interrupted or continuous subcuticular suture of 3-0 chromic catgut or polyglycol.

Although anatomic position is often corrected by a posterior colporrhaphy, function may not. Defecatory problems may remain, so patients should be forewarned. Furthermore, dyspareunia can be a problem postoperatively, especially if levator ani plication is done. Levator ani plication may best be indicated in nonsexually active women because of possible vaginal narrowing and band formation, which may lead to dyspareunia.

Enterocele

Enteroceles frequently occur after an abdominal or vaginal hysterectomy and generally are the result of a weakened support for the pouch of Douglas. In the prevention of enteroceles, the uterosacral and cardinal ligaments are the most important support structures and should be incorporated into the vault

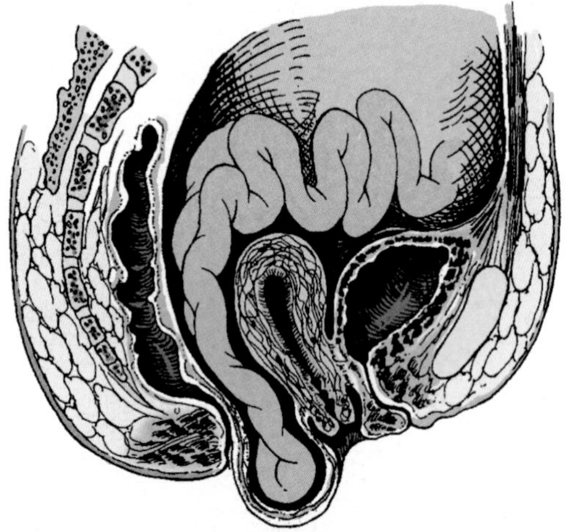

Figure 20-11. Enterocele and uterine prolapse. (Reproduced with permission from Symmonds RE: Relaxation of pelvic supports. In Benson RC [ed]: Current Obstetric and Gynecologic Diagnosis and Treatment, 5th ed. Los Altos, CA, Lange Medical, 1984.)

repair at the time of a hysterectomy and the ligaments from each side joined together.

Diagnosis

An enterocele is not always easy to diagnose. It is a true hernia of the peritoneal cavity emanating from the pouch of Douglas between the uterosacral ligaments and into the rectovaginal septum (Fig. 20-11). It may be noticed as a separate bulge above the rectocele, and at times it may be large enough to prolapse through the vagina (Fig. 20-12). If such is the case, it may be possible to make the specific diagnosis of enterocele by transilluminating the bulge and seeing small bowel shadows within the sac. It may also be possible to differentiate the enterocele from a rectocele by rectovaginal examination. The contents of an enterocele are always small bowel and may also include omentum. The contents may be easily reducible or may be fixed to the peritoneum of the sac by adhesions.

Management

Enteroceles may be reduced transabdominally as a primary procedure or at the time of other abdominal procedures. In the primary procedure the sac should be reduced upward if possible, and if the uterosacral ligaments are present, these may be brought together in the midline. If the uterosacral ligaments cannot be identified, as with large enteroceles after previously performed hysterectomy, the cul-de-sac may be obliterated by concentric purse-string sutures in the endopelvic fascia. Care must be taken to avoid damaging the ureters, rectum, and sigmoid colon. It is best to perform this procedure with permanent sutures. The enterocele has probably occurred because of weakening of pelvic floor structures. Therefore, for optimum results, repair of the lower pelvis using a vaginal approach is probably indicated, even though the enterocele is obliterated abdominally.

Repair of the enterocele can be carried out at the time of the posterior colporrhaphy. The sac will be visualized as the vagina is separated from the rectum. The sac must then be dissected

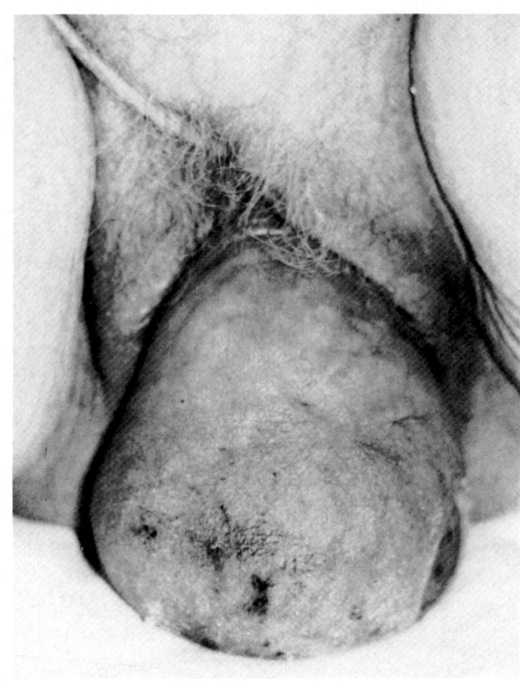

Figure 20-12. Elderly patient with vaginal prolapse who proved to have large enterocele with ulcers on the vagina.

free of underlying tissue and isolated at its neck. It should be opened to ensure that all contents are replaced. The neck of the hernia is then sutured with a purse-string 0 chromic or polyglycol suture ligature and the sac excised (Fig. 20-13).

It is important to support the neck of the enterocele sac as much as possible. Approximating the anterior and posterior vaginal connective tissue may be beneficial. Usually with an enterocele, support of the vaginal apex is indicated. If uterosacral ligaments can be identified or if they are present when a vaginal hysterectomy has been performed in association with an enterocele repair, they can be used in the repair. This can be accomplished by fixing the uterosacral ligaments to the peritoneum of the sac and the vaginal vault connective tissue using a suture of 0 polyglycol, beginning on one side of the vagina and continuing through the uterosacral ligament of that side, the peritoneum of the sac, and the uterosacral ligament and vagina of the opposite side. Multiple sutures can be placed if space allows. This technique was described by McCall and is often called the *McCall stitch.* It effectively shortens the cul-de-sac and supports the enterocele neck. If uterosacral ligaments cannot be identified, as is often the case if the uterus has been previously removed, the rectocele repair should be continued to the area of the enterocele sac neck to reinforce this area and support the cul-de-sac as high as possible. This usually involves the joining of the levator ani muscles up to the area of the enterocele sac.

Correctly repaired enteroceles usually will not recur. Enteroceles repaired without proper attention to ligation of the neck of the sac, closure of the anterior and posterior vaginal connective tissue, and without appropriate rectocele repair may recur. In such cases a subsequent operation with special attention to these surgical principles is indicated.

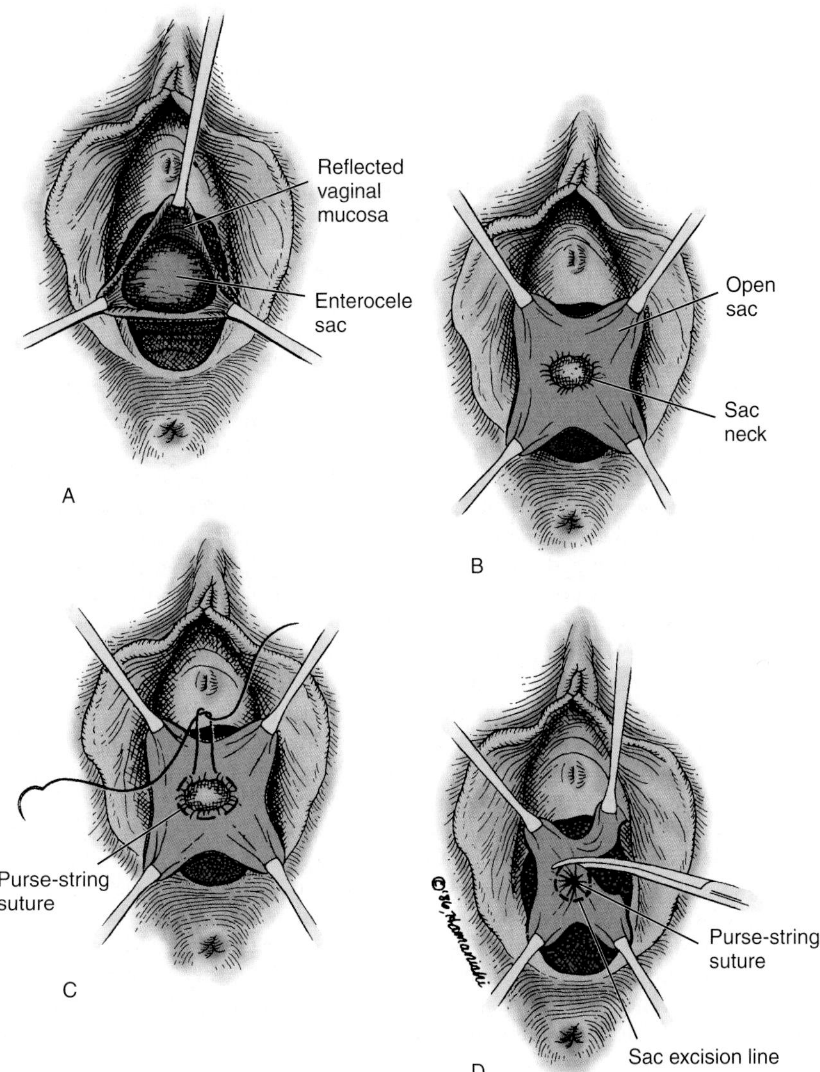

Figure 20-13. Repair of enterocele. **A,** Appearance of enterocele sac with vaginal wall reflected. **B,** Appearance of open enterocele sac with sac neck identified. **C,** Placing of purse-string suture at the neck of the enterocele sac. **D,** Excision of enterocele sac.

Uterine Prolapse (Descensus, Procidentia)

Descensus of the uterus and cervix into or through the barrel of the vagina is associated with injuries of the endopelvic fascia, including the cardinal and uterosacral ligaments, as well as injury to the neuromuscular unit with relaxation of the pelvic floor muscles, particularly the levator ani muscles. Occasionally, prolapse is the result of increased intraabdominal pressure, such as with ascites or large pelvic or intraabdominal tumors superimposed on poor pelvic supports. In some instances, sacral nerve disorders, especially injuries to S1 to S4, or diabetic neuropathy may be responsible. Using computed tomography, Sze and associates demonstrated that women with advanced genital prolapse had larger transverse inlet diameters, but not anterior–posterior diameters than do women without prolapse, suggesting an anatomic predisposition. Associated factors that increase tension on pelvic floor musculature, such as chronic respiratory disease including chronic bronchitis, asthma, and bronchiectasis, or severe obesity, may be associated. Congenitally damaged or relaxed pelvic floor supports may cause prolapse in young, nulliparous women. Most of the time, however, the patients are multiparous, with the prolapse being at least in part a result of childbirth trauma. Descensus is almost always associated with rectocele and cystocele and, at times, enterocele, supporting the concept of overall relaxation of the pelvic support structures.

A prolapse into the upper barrel of the vagina is called *first degree.* If the prolapse is through the vaginal barrel to the region of the introitus, it is *second degree.* If the cervix and uterus prolapse out through the introitus, it is called *third degree* or *total.* In total prolapse the vagina is everted around the uterus and cervix and completely exteriorized. When this occurs, the patient is in danger of developing dryness, thickening, and chronic inflammation of the vaginal epithelium. Stasis ulcers may result as edema and interference with blood supply to the vaginal wall occur. These ulcers rarely become cancerous, but biopsies should always be taken to ensure that they are not. In almost every case of acquired prolapse, the perineal supports are poor and the perineal body is damaged.

In 1996 a standardized terminology for the description of female pelvic organ prolapse and pelvic floor dysfunction was adapted by the International Continence Society, the American Urogynecologic Society, and the Society of Gynecologic Surgeons. This is an objective, site-specific system for describing, quantitating, and staging pelvic support and was developed to enhance both clinical and academic communication with respect to individual patients and populations of patients. The terminology replaces such terms as *cystocele, rectocele, enterocele,* and *urethrovesical junctions* with precise descriptions relating to specific anatomic landmarks. The first points are on the anterior vaginal wall and categorize anterior vaginal wall prolapse accordingly. Point Aa is a point located in the midline of the anterior wall 3 cm proximal to the urethral meatus and is roughly the location of the urethrovesical crease. Point Ba represents the most distal position of any part of the anterior vaginal wall. Point C represents either the most distal edge of the cervix or the leading edge of the vagina if a hysterectomy has been performed. Point D represents the location of the posterior fornix (pouch of Douglas) in a woman with a cervix. Point Bp is a point most distal of any part of the upper posterior vaginal wall, and point Ap is a point located in the midline of the posterior vaginal wall 3 cm proximal to the hymen. To record measurements, these points should be expressed in centimeters above or below the hymen. It is important for the examining individual to express the position and other circumstances of the examination (i.e., straining or not, patient flat on table or in examining chair, etc.). Figure 20-14 shows a diagram of the points and sites described earlier.

When the examination is recorded according to the anatomic points just cited, staging may be performed (listed in Table 20-1). These organizations hope that by using this system, a clearer understanding of a patient's prolapse will be achieved, and the transmittal of this information to others will be made more accurate. They also expect that this system will make it possible to standardize research information.

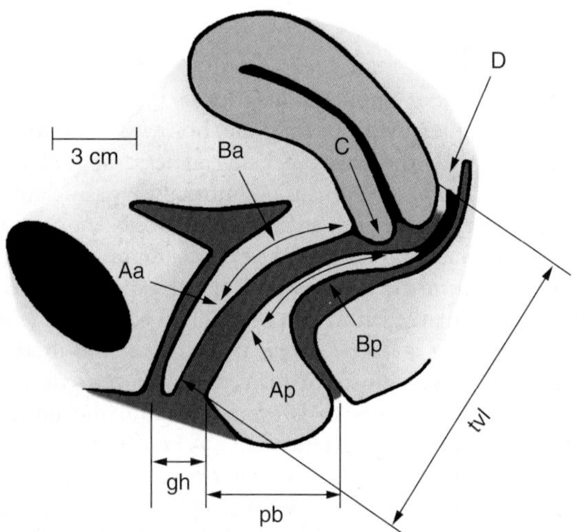

Figure 20-14. Quantitative description of pelvic organ prolapse six sites (points Aa, Ba, C, D, Bp, and Ap), genital hiatus (gh), perineal body (pb), and total vaginal length (tvl) used for pelvic organ support quantitation. (From Bump RC, Mattiasson A, Bo K: The standardization of terminology of female pelvic organ prolapse and pelvic floor dysfunction. Am J Obstet Gynecol 175:10, 1996.)

Table 20-1 Staging of Pelvic Floor Prolapse Using International Continence Society Terminology

Stage 0	No prolapse is demonstrated. Points Aa, Ap, Ba, and Bp are all at –3 cm and either point C or D is between total vaginal length –2 cm.
Stage I	Criteria for stage 0 are not met, but the most distal portion of the prolapse is >1 cm above the level of the hymen.
Stage II	The most distal portion of the prolapse is less or equal to 1 cm proximal or distal to the plane of the hymen.
Stage III	The most distal portion of the prolapse is >1 cm below the plane of the hymen, but protrudes no further than 2 cm less than the total vaginal length in centimeters.
Stage IV	Essentially complete eversion of the total length of the lower genital tract.

Symptoms and Signs

Major symptoms noted by patients with descensus are a feeling of heaviness, fullness, or "falling out" in the perineal area. In cases where the cervix and uterus are low in the vaginal canal, the cervix may be seen protruding from the introitus, giving the patient the impression that a tumor is bulging out of her vagina. Where total descensus has occurred, the patient is aware that a mass has actually prolapsed out of the introitus. Because prolapse almost always is related to anterior and posterior vaginal wall relaxation, symptoms that were reported earlier for cystocele and rectocele may be present as well.

It is not uncommon for the cervix or vaginal epithelium to become damaged or ulcerated, in which case the patient may report pain or vaginal bleeding. There is often discharge from the cervix and vagina when secondary infection occurs.

Management

Minimum prolapse does not require therapy unless the patient is very uncomfortable. Degrees of prolapse that place the cervix at or through the introitus probably cause greater discomfort and are usually more bothersome to the patient. Medical management of such conditions involves the use of a pessary, usually of the Smith-Hodge, donut, cube, or inflatable variety (Fig. 20-15). These require the replacement of the uterus and cervix to their usual position in the pelvis and then the institution of support using one of these devices. Pessaries are available in varying sizes and should be properly fitted to the patient. In general the perineum must be capable of holding the pessary in place, or the pessary will frequently fall out. There is currently no evidence from randomized controlled trials on pessary use to direct the selection of the device or to compare pessaries with other treatments or surgery. A recent prospective trial found 75% of 203 women fitted with a pessary successfully retaining the device at 2 weeks. Failure to retain the pessary was significantly associated with increasing parity and past hysterectomy. Forty-eight percent of the women completed a questionnaire at 4 months. The pessary reduced symptoms of POP including general symptoms of a vaginal bulge. It also relieved urinary symptoms such as voiding problems in 40% of women, urinary urgency in 38%, and urge incontinence in 29%. There was no improvement in stress urinary incontinence. Bowel symptoms improved as well.

Complications from vaginal pessaries are rare with proper use. This includes regular removal, cleaning, and replacement, as well

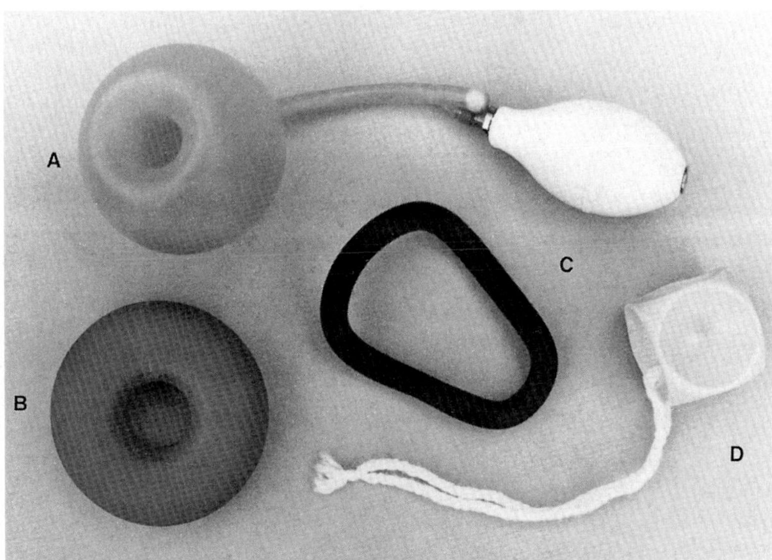

Figure 20-15. Examples of pessaries. **A,** inflatable; **B,** donut; **C,** Smith-Hodge; **D,** cube type.

as use of vaginal estrogen cream for postmenopausal women with vaginal atrophy. Complications include vaginal infections, bleeding, discomfort, vaginal erosion and ulceration, and impaction. More serious complications have been rarely reported.

If the patient is a young woman and pregnant, it is important to replace the uterus before it enlarges and becomes trapped in the lower pelvis or vagina. If this happens, edema may cause incarceration and even loss of blood supply to the uterus. In a postmenopausal woman, estrogen replacement for at least 30 days with vaginal estrogen cream may help improve the vitality of the vaginal epithelium, the cervix, and the vasculature of these organs, making fitting of a pessary or the operative procedure and the healing process more efficient. The patient should not undergo operation until all ulcers of the vagina and cervix are healed, because to do otherwise is to risk infection and breakdown of the repair.

Operative repair for prolapse of the uterus and cervix generally involves a vaginal hysterectomy with a vaginal vault suspension. The hysterectomy is performed carefully, isolating the uterosacral and cardinal ligaments so that they may be used in the support of the vaginal vault. The uterosacral ligaments should be sutured together so that the cul-de-sac is shortened or obliterated and the risk of a subsequent enterocele is lessened. Other vaginal vault suspension procedures can be used instead of the McCall type.

In some cases a vaginal hysterectomy is not advisable. These circumstances include previous intraabdominal operation for an inflammatory process, such as endometriosis or pelvic inflammatory disease. Where such is the case an abdominal hysterectomy may be performed, followed by a vaginal anterior and posterior colporrhaphy, if needed. Under these circumstances the cardinal and uterosacral ligaments should be treated as noted earlier. As an alternative, a laparoscopically assisted vaginal hysterectomy may be performed in such situations.

In some women the cervix is hypertrophied and elongated to the area of the introitus, but the supports of the uterus itself are good. A cystocele and rectocele may be present, and operative repair can consist of a Manchester (Donald or Fothergill) operation. This operation combines an anterior and posterior colporrhaphy with the amputation of the cervix and the use of the cardinal ligaments to support the anterior vaginal wall and bladder. Although it was suggested for repair in young women who wish to maintain their reproductive abilities, the loss of the cervix may interfere with fertility or lead to incompetence of the internal cervical os. The operation has value in elderly women with comorbid medical conditions who have an elongated cervix and well-supported uterus because it is technically easier and has a shorter operative time than the vaginal hysterectomy in such cases, and the entering of the peritoneal cavity is avoided.

Recently, in a retrospective chart analysis, Thomas and colleagues compared the data on 88 consecutive Manchester procedures to 105 randomly selected vaginal hysterectomy patients. All operations were performed at Mt. Sinai Hospital in New York between 1984 and 1988. Patients undergoing a Manchester procedure tended to be older and postmenopausal but were less likely to have significant medical illnesses than were patients who underwent vaginal hysterectomy. Operative time was shorter and blood loss less in patients undergoing a Manchester procedure, and long-term operative outcomes were similar for the two groups.

In elderly women who are no longer sexually active a simple procedure for reducing prolapse is a partial colpocleisis. The classic procedure was described by Le Fort (Fig. 20-16) and involves the removal of a strip of anterior and posterior vaginal wall, with closure of the margins of the anterior and posterior wall to each other. This procedure may be performed with or without the presence of a uterus and cervix, and when it is completed, a small vaginal canal exists on either side of the septum, which is produced by the suturing of the lateral margins of the excision. The line of dissection of the vaginal wall is carried to the level of the bladder neck anteriorly and to the reflection of bladder onto the cervix at the upper margin of the vagina. Posteriorly the dissection is carried from just inside the introitus to a position just posterior to the cervix. If a hysterectomy has been previously performed, the dissection may begin approximately 1 cm on either side of the vaginal scar. When the

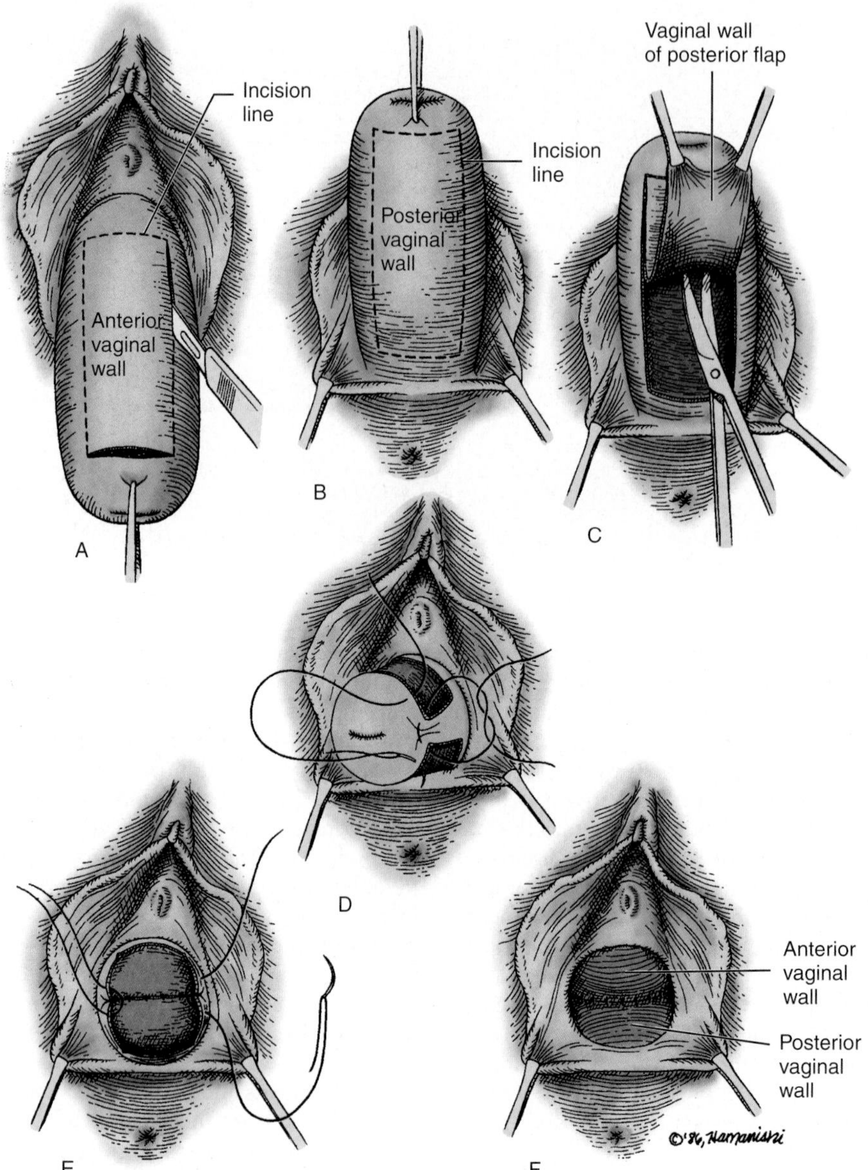

Figure 20-16. Le Fort procedure. **A,** Incision of anterior vaginal wall strip. **B,** Incision of posterior wall strip. **C,** Removal of vaginal strip. **D** and **E,** Placement of sutures. **F,** Appearance of vagina after procedure is completed but before perineorrhaphy is performed.

procedure is completed, the bladder neck is spared from any scarring, and urinary incontinence is generally avoided. Bladder neck plication may be carried out if the patient is incontinent. After healing of the plication a small introital area is noted; this has cosmetic benefits in older women. In addition, narrow canals are noted on each lateral vaginal wall. If the cervix and uterus are still present and intrauterine pathology occurs, bleeding along these canals could take place, alerting the physician to a potential problem.

The Goodall–Power modification of the Le Fort operation (Fig. 20-17) allows for the removal of a triangular piece of vaginal wall beginning at the cervical reflection or 1 cm above the vaginal scar at the base of the triangle, with the apex of the triangle just beneath the bladder neck anteriorly and just at the introitus posteriorly. The cut edge of vaginal wall making up the base of the triangle anteriorly is sutured to the similar wall posteriorly, and the vaginal incision is then closed with a row of interrupted sutures beginning beneath the bladder neck and carried side to side to the area of the introitus. This procedure works well for relatively small prolapses, whereas the Le Fort is best for larger ones.

When a colpocleisis is performed, if an enterocele is found when the vaginal wall is stripped away, the sac must be identified, its neck ligated, and the peritoneum of the sac excised to prevent recurrence of the enterocele behind the colpocleisis.

In most cases a perineorrhaphy is performed with a colpocleisis to reinforce the introitus.

Prognosis for a colpocleisis procedure to reduce the prolapse and prevent recurrence is generally excellent. Case series report 91% to 100% success rates. Ridley reports no prolapse recurrences in 58 patients unless an incomplete procedure was performed in an attempt to salvage vaginal depth and function. Three patients developed stress incontinence where none was present preoperatively.

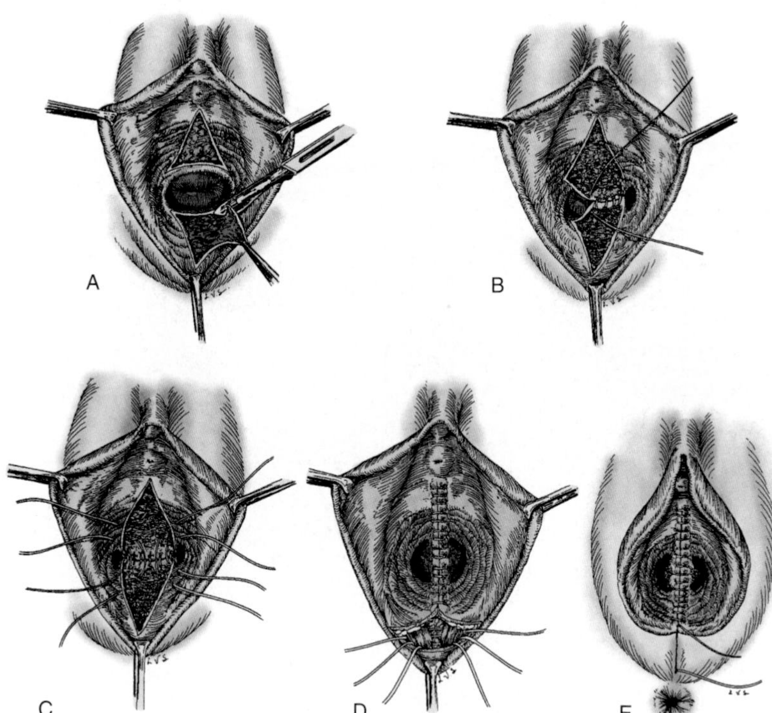

Figure 20-17. Goodall–Power modification of Le Fort operation. **A,** Representation of vaginal incision on anterior and posterior wall. **B,** Early placement of sutures. **C,** Later placement of sutures. **D,** Vaginal incision completely closed; perineorrhaphy being performed. **E,** Appearance at completion of procedure. (Reprinted with permission from Symmonds RE: Relaxation of pelvic supports. In Benson RC [ed]: Current Obstetric and Gynecologic Diagnosis and Treatment, 5th ed. Los Altos, CA, Lange Medical, 1984.)

Denehy and coworkers compared 25 elderly women (average age 82 years) in poor health and with a uterovaginal prolapse treated by colpocleisis with 42 women who also had a similar prolapse but were treated with vaginal hysterectomy, anterior colporrhaphy, and posterior colporrhaphy. Members of the vaginal hysterectomy group were considerably younger, with an average age of 66 (range 39–80). Average operating time for the Le Fort procedure was 75 minutes compared with 150 minutes for the vaginal hysterectomy. There was one postoperative death in the Le Fort group, but 19 of the 20 remaining Le Fort patients had excellent results for a follow-up of an average of 25 months (range 4–40 months). These authors performed Kelly urethral plication and posterior colpoperineoplasty in all patients as suggested earlier.

A special circumstance involves the treatment of women who wish to maintain their fertility despite the fact that they have a total uterine prolapse. Kovac and Cruikshank have demonstrated that uterosacral ligaments bilaterally could be sutured to the sacrospinus ligaments, thereby reversing the prolapse. In 19 such patients treated, 5 delivered a total of 6 babies (1 delivered twice).

Vaginal Apex Prolapse

Prolapse of the vaginal apex at some time remote to the performance of either abdominal or vaginal hysterectomy has been reported as occurring in 0.1% to 18.2% of patients. The prolapse may be total and may be accompanied by a cystocele, a rectocele, an enterocele, or some combination thereof. Occasionally the prolapse involves only one of those entities and not the entire vaginal apex. In a study in Munich, Richter reported that of 97 vaginal stump prolapses, 6.2% were cystocele only, 5.1% rectocele only, 9.3% primarily an enterocele type, and 72.2% of mixed type. Specific classification was not given for 7.2%.

Vaginal apex prolapse is probably the result of continuing pelvic support weakness and failure of the vaginal support structures, namely, the cardinal and uterosacral ligaments, to maintain their tone or attachment to the vagina.

Symptoms and Signs

Symptoms and signs of vaginal apex prolapse are similar to those delineated for descensus of the uterus. They include pelvic heaviness, backache, and a mass protruding through the introitus. At times, stress incontinence, urgency, frequency, dribbling, vaginal bleeding or discharge (if there is an ulcer), and, depending on the size of the mass, difficulty with sitting or walking may occur.

Diagnosis

Examination may help determine the contents of the herniation depending on where the vaginal scar is located in relation to the protruding mass and the extent to which the supports of the pelvis are lost. Rectovaginal examination is often helpful in delineating an enterocele from a rectocele.

Management

Although the management of descensus with the uterus present is uniformly agreed to be vaginal hysterectomy with vaginal vault suspension and if indicated, anterior and posterior colporrhaphy, there is much controversy over the appropriate procedure for vaginal apex prolapse. Nevertheless, certain principles and facts are important. The first is that the normal position of the vagina in the standing position is against the rectum and no more than 30° from the horizontal (Fig. 20-18). The second

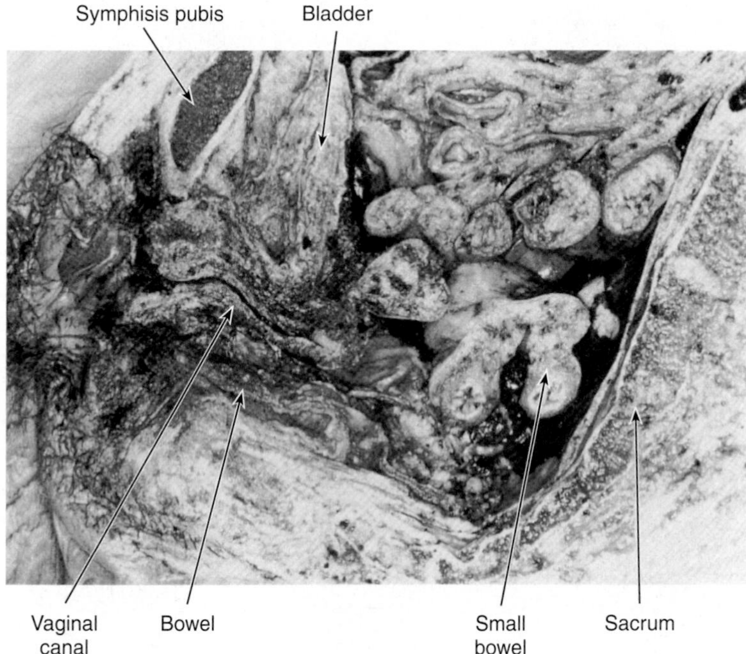

Figure 20-18. Pelvis of a dissected cadaver in supine position demonstrating vaginal canal orientation in the pelvis. (Courtesy of Richard Hebertson, MD.)

principle is that pelvic relaxation is a part of the problem and dictates that an existing cystocele, rectocele, or enterocele must be repaired as part of the procedure. The third principle acknowledges that the perineal body is almost always severely weakened in such patients and must therefore be reconstructed as well. Nonsurgical management, such as the use of pessaries, estrogen, and the healing of ulcers, should be used as appropriate. Pessaries, however, are rarely retained in such patients, and attempts to treat these patients nonsurgically are generally met with frustration.

The choices of operative procedures are many. These include those that use the abdominal route, the vaginal route, or some combination thereof. For the abdominal approach a variety of procedures have been tried. These include fixation of the vaginal vault to the anterior abdominal wall, to the lumbar spine, to the sacral promontory, to various tendonous lines in the musculature of the true pelvis, and to the sacrospinous ligament. The anterior abdominal wall fixation increases the diameters of the pouch of Douglas and frequently adds to the risk of subsequent enterocele development, often creating a recurrence in short order. Fixation to the lumbar spine or the sacral promontory is often difficult to achieve directly and requires the interposition of a different material. In the past, ox fascia lata, fascial aponeurosis from the patient, or inert materials such as Mersilene have been used. In such procedures it is important to cover the stent with peritoneum, thereby rendering it retroeritoneal to avoid troublesome adhesions and internal hernias at a future date. After such procedures the pouch of Douglas may still be large enough to allow an enterocele to develop. Fixation to various aspects of the pelvic wall or to the sacrospinous ligament has had encouraging degrees of success, the latter being the most successful. Using the sacrospinous ligament can frequently be accomplished vaginally. Randall and Nichols report excellent success with both abdominal and vaginal approaches. In 18 patients treated with fixation of the vaginal vault to the sacrospinous ligament via the vaginal route, all had successful outcomes.

Morley and DeLancey reported the results of 100 patients treated at the University of Michigan for vaginal vault prolapse or posthysterectomy enterocele with sacrospinous ligament suspension of the vaginal vault. Of 71 patients who were followed for 1 year or more, 64 (90%) had complete symptomatic relief, 10 had some asymptomatic relaxation of the vaginal walls, and 9 had either vaginal stenosis or stress incontinence. In addition, four patients developed cystoceles, and three had recurrent prolapse of the vagina. Other authors have reported equally encouraging results using this procedure.

Sze and Karram reviewed the literature on transvaginal vault prolapse repair in 1997. They compared the cumulative results for sacrospinus ligament fixation (n = 1062) and endopelvic fascia vault fixation (n = 322). Of the sacrospinus ligament fixation group, 193 (18%) developed recurrent relaxation, including 32 vault eversions, 81 anterior wall and 24 posterior wall prolapses, and 56 with other or multiple defects. Of the endopelvic fascia fixation groups, 34 (11%) developed recurrent relaxation, including 9 vault prolapses, 2 anterior and 11 posterior wall prolapses, and 12 developed other defects. Follow-up was from 1 to 12 years, and these authors concluded that the true efficacy of these procedures remains inconclusive.

Figure 20-19 depicts the fixation of the vaginal vault to the sacrospinous ligament and the direction of the vagina after the procedure. Miyazaki reports the use of an instrument, the Miya hook ligature carrier, to lessen the difficulty of placing a suture into the sacrospinous ligament. This is depicted in Figure 20-20. Some surgeons favor the use of this instrument in the performance of this procedure. Sharp has reported equally good results using an orthopedic instrument, the Shutt suture punch system, as an alternative to the Miya hook ligature carrier. Several special ligature carriers and autosuturing devices have also been

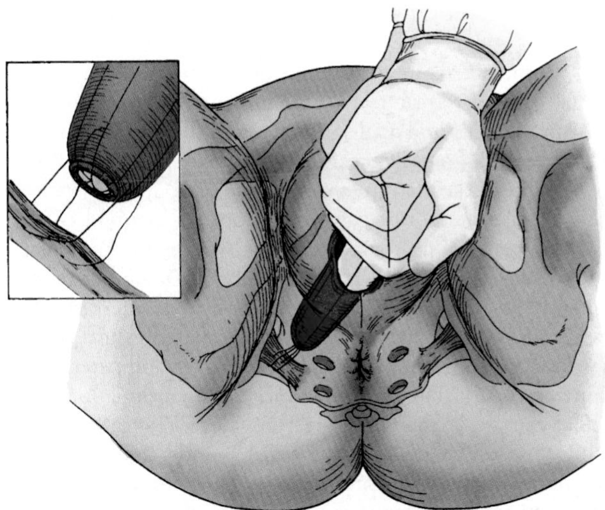

Figure 20-19. Sutures tied to bring the new vaginal apex into contact with the ligament and overlying muscle. Vaginal wall is advanced toward the sacrospinous ligament while tying sutures. A "suture bridge" is to be avoided. (Redrawn from Morley GW, DeLancey JOL: Sacrospinous ligament fixation for eversion of the vagina. Am J Obstet Gynecol 158:872, 1988.)

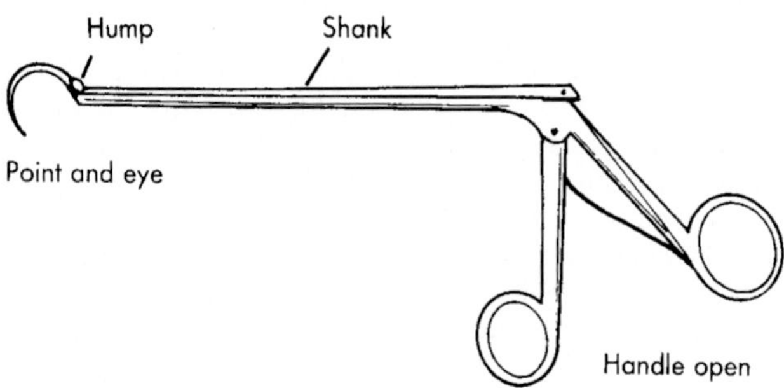

Figure 20-20. The Miya hook ligature carrier. (From Miyazaki FS: Miya hook ligature carrier for sacrospinous ligament suspension. Obstet Gynecol 70:286, 1987.)

found useful. It is likely that other instruments will be developed for this purpose.

A variety of vaginal procedures have been designed. The best success, however, occurs in procedures in which adequate vaginal length is maintained and the vagina is positioned against the rectum nearly parallel to the horizontal. Thornton and Peters reported on 41 women who underwent repair of vaginal apex, in which the vaginal approach was used with good, lasting success. Of these patients, 20 required a repair of an enterocele and a posterior repair, which especially detailed the attachment of the posterior wall of the vagina to the perirectal fascia and levator ani muscles. In addition, 21 patients underwent a repair of an enterocele with both an anterior and a posterior repair because a cystocele was believed to be a major part of their prolapse problem. Long-term follow-ups were effected, and the success rate was said to be excellent.

Richter and Albrich combined the repair of cystocele, rectocele, and enterocele where necessary with a unilateral or bilateral vaginal sacrospinal fixation procedure. They also stressed the importance of suturing the vagina in its physiologic position to the perirectal support tissue. The success in their group of 97 patients was also excellent, in that 61.7% of the patients had what were considered ideal results in long-term follow-up. There was a recurrence of cystocele in 14.8%, rectocele in 8.6%, and enterocele in 3.7%. Stress incontinence was reported in 3.7% of their patients and urgency incontinence in 2.5% with long-term follow-up. For operative procedures that fix the vaginal vault to an anterior structure (i.e., the anterior abdominal wall) an obliteration of the cul-de-sac must be carried out as part of the operative procedure to prevent enteroceles from forming.

An equally good technique (and possibly better than vaginal techniques) for suspending the vaginal vault is the fixation of the vault to the sacrum. This generally requires the use of a stent, which can be a fascial strip taken from the patient or an inert mesh such as Mersilene. The stent is sutured to the anterior and posterior upper vaginal vault and the opposite end to the ligamentum flavum of the sacral promontory or the anterior longitudinal ligament of the sacrum. Care must be taken to avoid the middle sacral artery and the plexus of veins in its vicinity. The stent should be made retroperitoneal by bringing the peritoneum in front of it. The procedure should also include an obliteration of the cul-de-sac. Snyder and Krantz reported on 147 patients undergoing abdominal sacral colpopexy using a Dacron graft and reported good long-term results. Four patients experienced a graft erosion and one patient a recurrent prolapse. Other authors have reported similarly good outcomes.

Few studies have been performed to attempt to compare the efficacy of vaginal versus abdominal repair of vault prolapse. Benson and associates performed a randomized trial of bilateral sacrospinous vault suspensions and paravaginal repair (n = 48) and colposacral suspension and paravaginal repair (n = 40). Surgical effectiveness as judged by recurrent prolapse was optimal in 29% of the vaginal and 58% of the abdominal group and was unsatisfactory leading to reoperation in 33% of the vaginal and 16% of the abdominal group.

If an abdominal sacrocolpopexy (ASC) is to be performed for treatment of POP, urinary continence must be considered. A multicenter 2006 trial by Brubaker and colleagues randomized 322 women with no stress incontinence symptoms to have a concomitant Burch colposuspension or not (controls). Three months after surgery, 24% of women in the Burch group and 44% of controls had stress incontinence, even though none reported stress incontinence preoperatively. Burch colposuspension significantly reduced postoperative stress incontinence when performed at the time of ASC, without an increase in other urinary problems.

In elderly women who are no longer sexually active, and particularly in those who have medical reasons to avoid a longer procedure, a Le Fort-type colpocleisis operation may be performed with excellent results. It is extremely important to identify and repair enteroceles in such women, but this can readily be done as part of the procedure. Perineorrhaphy should always be performed as part of any procedure to repair a vaginal apex prolapse.

The question of continuing sexual activity after vaginal vault repairs is obviously an important one. With an adequate vaginal operation (with the exception of colpocleisis), intercourse is achievable in most patients who wish to maintain this activity.

Weber and coworkers studied sexual function in 81 women who were sexually active before undergoing surgery for pelvic prolapse or urinary incontinence or both. All remained sexually active after surgery, but dyspareunia was likely to occur if a combination of the Burch procedure and posterior colporrhaphy was performed.

FECAL INCONTINENCE

Fecal incontinence is one of the most devastating of all physical disabilities. Yet, because of the social embarrassment and psychological effects, most patients fail to report their symptoms and many physicians do not ask. Therefore, the exact prevalence of this condition is unknown. Estimates range from 2% to 16% of community-dwelling women older than 64 years of age. Prevalence increases with age. Over 30% of women reporting urinary incontinence also report fecal incontinence, known as dual incontinence.

Anal incontinence is the inability to defer the elimination of stool or gas until there is a socially acceptable time and place to do so. Fecal incontinence is the inability to defer the elimination of stool. Because maintaining continence is a complex physiologic process that requires a person's ability to perceive the type of fecal bolus, store or retain when necessary, and to excrete when desirable, the loss of that ability is equally complex.

In the evaluation of anal incontinence, it is important for the physician to understand the patient's symptoms, type of loss (i.e., flatus or stool), frequency of incontinence, and effect on the quality of her life. Fecal incontinence affects each patient's life in a different manner. What may be acceptable for one patient may be intolerable to another. Evaluation and treatment should be directed by the severity of the patient's symptoms and the expected goals of therapy.

Physiology of Fecal Continence

Fecal continence requires normal stool consistency and volume, normal colonic transit time, a compliant rectum, innervation of the pelvic floor and anal sphincter, and the interplay between the puborectalis muscle, rectum, and anal sphincters. Loss of one or more of these abilities can lead to fecal incontinence.

As a bolus of stool or gas passes from the sigmoid colon to the rectal canal, receptors within the wall of the puborectalis sense the distention of the rectum. As long as the pressure in the anal canal is maintained at a higher level than the rectal pressure, continence is maintained. Anal canal pressure depends on a functional internal anal sphincter (IAS) and external anal sphincter (EAS). The IAS is a thickened continuation of the circular muscle of the colon and provides 75% to 85% of the resting tone of the anal canal. The IAS, under autonomic control, maintains the high-pressure zone or continence zone and along with the EAS keeps the anal canal closed. The shape of the combined IAS and EAS is nearly cylindrical as it encircles the anal canal. The sphincter complex averages 18.3 mm in thickness and 2.8 cm in length in the midline anteriorly. Fifty-four percent of the anterior thickness is attributable to the IAS and the remainder to the EAS. The EAS provides the voluntary squeeze pressure that prevents incontinence with increasing rectal or abdominal pressure. The EAS is innervated by the hemorrhoidal branch of the pudendal nerve from the S2 through the S4 nerve roots. Contraction of the EAS, either voluntarily or through a spinal reflex, doubles the anal canal pressure.

The third muscular component of the sphincter complex is the puborectalis muscle (Fig. 20-21). The puborectalis, part of the levator ani muscle complex, originates from the pubic bone on either side of the midline, passes beside the vagina and rectum, and fuses posteriorly behind the anorectal junction to

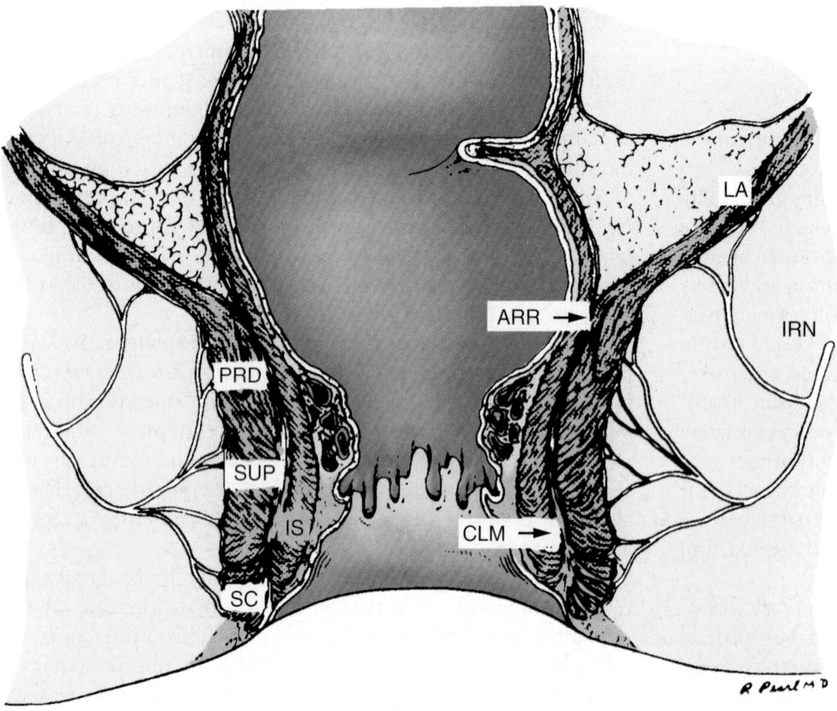

Figure 20-21. Coronal section of the anal canal and lower rectum. ARR, level of anorectal ring; CLM, conjoined longitudinal muscle; IRN, inferior rectal nerve; LA, levator ani muscles; PRD, puborectalis/deep external sphincter complex; SC, subcutaneous external sphincter. (From Pearl RK: In Smith L [ed]: Practical Guide to Anorectal Testing. New York, Igaku-Shoin, 1995.)

Table 20-2 Anal Incontinence: An Underrecognized, Undertreated Problem

Component	Function	Symptoms of Deficit
External anal sphincter	Provides emergency control for liquid stool and flatus	Fecal urgency; urge-related incontinence of liquid and flatus
Puborectalis	Maintains continence of solid stool	Incontinence of solid stool
Internal anal sphincter	Keeps anal canal closed at rest; allows sampling of stool content and enhances continence of liquid stool and flatus	Fecal soiling Incontinence of liquid stool and flatus
Anal sensation	Allows discrimination of gas, liquid, and solid stool Provides warning of impending incontinence	Fecal soiling Fecal leakage that is promptly halted by voluntary contraction or conscious detection
Colonic motility	Controls stool volume, consistency, and delivery rate to the rectum	Incontinence of liquid/loose stools during prolonged or severe diarrheal states
Rectal reservoir	Maintains adequate reservoir under low pressure	Incontinence of solid stool associated with sudden rectal distension Fecal urgency and urge-related incontinence

From Toglia M: Anal incontinence: An underrecognized, undertreated problem. Female Patient 21:27, 1996.

form the U-shaped sling that cradles the rectum while sending some fibers onto the walls of the anal canal. Unlike most other striated muscles, the puborectalis, like the EAS, maintains a constant muscle tone that is directly proportional to the volume of the rectal content and pressure, and relaxes at the time of defecation. Both the puborectalis and EAS contain a majority of type I, or slow twitch, muscle fibers, which are ideally suited to maintaining a constant contraction or tone. Each muscle group also contains a small proportion of type II, or fast twitch, fibers that allow for quick responses to rapid increases in intraabdominal pressure. The puborectalis is innervated by direct branches from S3 and S4 and, to a lesser degree, from the pudendal nerve. The constant contraction of the puborectalis creates a 90° angle between the rectum and anal canal. This angle, known as the anorectal angle, has been the source of much discussion and evaluation in determining its role in the maintenance of continence. Parks postulated that this angle creates a flap-valve effect that presses the anterior rectal wall down onto the upper anal canal and thereby prevents rectal contents from entering the anal canal when intraabdominal pressure is applied. The anterior rectal wall therefore acts as a plug. However, Bartolo found that when the anal sphincter was maximally stressed and the rectum was visualized radiographically, there was no contact between the rectal wall and anal canal. In addition, surgeries that try to recreate this angle in hopes of restoring continence have not proven effective.

When a bolus of stool or gas is sensed in the rectum, the IAS has a reflex relaxation that allows for colonic contents to be sampled by the anal canal to distinguish solid, liquid, and gas forms of fecal material. After the sampling, the IAS contracts and the fecal material is pushed back into the rectum. The reflex, known as the rectoanal inhibitory reflex, or RAIR, is absent in patients with Hirschprung's disease. This reflex can also be inhibited by chronic dilation of the anus with fecal impaction and lead to incontinence. If the impaction is cured, the reflex and anal tone can return to normal.

If the rectum has normal compliance and the person chooses to defer defecation, the IAS and EAS sphincters and the puborectalis remain contracted until the appropriate time to eliminate. As seen in Table 20-2, loss of any of these important components can lead to incontinence of flatus, liquid, or solid stool.

Etiology and Pathophysiology

There are many causes of fecal incontinence as seen in Table 20-3. One way to categorize the reasons for fecal incontinence is to separate the initial cause into those that start outside the pelvis with a normal pelvic floor from those that start with an abnormal pelvic floor. Causes that start outside the pelvis include all of the pathologies that cause diarrhea or increased intestinal motility, overflow incontinence from fecal impaction, and rectal neoplasms. Known or diagnosable neurologic conditions such as multiple sclerosis, diabetic neuropathy, trauma, or neoplasms in the spinal cord or cauda equina initially begin as pathologies outside of the pelvis and the pelvic floor is presumed normal. As these neuropathies progress, there is damage to the

Table 20-3 Common Causes of Fecal Incontinence

Obstetric injury
Disruption of internal anal sphincter
Disruption of external anal sphincter
Pelvic floor denervation
Trauma
Pelvic fracture
Accidental injury
Anorectal surgery
Rectovaginal fistula
Diarrheal states
Irritable bowel
Infectious diarrhea
Inflammatory bowel disease
Short-gut syndrome
Laxative abuse
Radiation enteritis
Rectal neoplasia
Rectal prolapse
Rectocele
Overflow
Impaction
Encopresis
Neurologic disease
Congenital anomalies (i.e., myelomeningocele)
Multiple sclerosis
Diabetic neuropathy
Neoplasms or injury of brain, spinal cord, cauda equina
Pudendal neuropathy (childbirth, chronic straining, perineal descent)
Congenital anomalies of anorectum pelvis

pelvic floor musculature or in rectal sensation, resulting in fecal incontinence.

Fecal incontinence secondary to an abnormal pelvic floor is due to congenital anorectal malformations, surgery, obstetric injury, aging, or pelvic floor denervation without a known neurologic disease. Historically, incontinence secondary to denervation has been designated as idiopathic and represents 80% of patients with fecal incontinence. Pelvic floor denervation has been studied extensively in the last 15 years in women with urinary and fecal incontinence as well as pelvic organ prolapse. Denervation may be secondary to vaginal delivery, chronic straining with constipation, rectal prolapse, or descending perineal syndrome. Histologic studies of the EAS and puborectalis show fibrosis, scarring, and fiber-type grouping consistent with nerve damage and reinnervation in women with idiopathic fecal incontinence. Electromyographic (EMG) studies have demonstrated reinnervation of the pelvic floor with increased fiber density and prolongation of nerve conduction on pudendal nerve terminal motor latency (PNTML) studies.

In healthy women, the most common cause of fecal incontinence is damage to the anal sphincters at the time of vaginal delivery with or without neuronal injury. This type of incontinence is often referred to as anal incontinence. Damage can occur by mechanical disruption or separation of the IAS or EAS (or both) or by damage to the muscle innervation by stretching or crushing the pudendal and pelvic nerves. Sultan and coworkers showed that 13% of primiparas and 23% of multiparas developed fecal incontinence or fecal urgency 6 weeks postpartum. By anal ultrasound, all but one of the women had evidence of anal sphincter disruption. The incidence of occult external anal sphincter disruption after vaginal delivery determined by endoanal ultrasound ranges from 11% to 35%. The chance of muscular injury is increased with midline episiotomy, instrumented delivery, and vaginal delivery of larger infants. Other risk factors include increasing maternal age, prolonged second stage (greater than 2 hours), and clinically diagnosed sphincter laceration at the time of delivery. The first vaginal delivery appears to have the greatest effect on pelvic floor function and risk of EAS disruption, but subsequent deliveries can increase the risk of permanent damage, especially in women with transient symptoms of fecal incontinence after their first delivery. Not all risk factors are known, and not all women are susceptible to pelvic floor and sphincter damage with vaginal delivery.

Detection of Fecal Incontinence

For fecal incontinence, even more than urinary incontinence, if the physician does not ask, the patient will not volunteer the information. Ideally, a question such as, "How often do you leak gas, liquid, or solid stool?" should be placed on the standard office intake questionnaire. Several reports have shown that twice as many patients complain of fecal or flatal incontinence when given written questionnaires rather than answering verbal questioning.

Since approximately 1 in 10 women will develop some fecal incontinence or fecal urgency after one vaginal delivery, it is especially important to incorporate open-ended questions concerning flatal or fecal incontinence as part of the 6-week postpartum visit. In addition, as women age, the chances of developing fecal incontinence increase, so it is also important to target older women for questioning.

Evaluation

Assessment of the patient with fecal incontinence must include a thorough history because the origin of the problem may be the single most important criterion of therapy.

The history should include onset, duration, severity of the condition, effect on the patient's daily activities, pad use, frequency of bowel movements, consistency of bowel movements, use of laxatives, fiber intake, and dietary habits. Specific questions concerning diarrhea, amount of flatus, the average number of stools per day, passage of mucus, and bloating should be asked. Physicians and patients define normal bowel function differently. Diarrhea may mean frequent bowel movements to one person but loose and watery bowel movements to another. It is best to have the patient quantitate the number of bowel movements and incontinent episodes and describe the stool consistency. A diary of bowel habits and incontinent episodes can be useful, and several standardized classification systems are available. Table 20-4 gives a frequently used scoring system developed by Jorge and Wexner. The patient circles the appropriate number on each line of the scale. The numbers are then added. A perfect score or 0 indicates no incontinence and a score of 20 indicates complete incontinence. The value of this scale is that it can be utilized before and after treatment to determine efficacy of the intervention. A standardized questionnaire should be used whenever possible to direct diagnosis and treatment and to assess treatment success.

The history should also identify specific complaints such as feelings of incomplete emptying, straining with bowel movements, fecal urgency, pain with defecation, and insensible loss of stool. It is important to determine if the patient senses the need to have a bowel movement or if she is unaware that she needs to defecate, but finds stool in her undergarments. A sensory impairment or hygiene problem is implied when stool leakage occurs without warning. If the patient is aware of impending incontinence, but cannot prevent the passage of stool, a motor impairment is suggested. Patients may have pseudoincontinence secondary to soiling from prolapsing hemorrhoids or rectovaginal or anovaginal fistulas.

Table 20-4 Continence Grading Scale

	FREQUENCY				
Type of Incontinence	**Never**	**Rarely**	**Sometimes**	**Usually**	**Always**
Solid	0	1	2	3	4
Liquid	0	1	2	3	4
Gas	0	1	2	3	4
Wears pad	0	1	2	3	4
Lifestyle alteration	0	1	2	3	4

0 = perfect, 20 = complete incontinence. Never = 0 (never); rarely = <1/month; sometimes = <1/week, ≥1/month; usually = <1/day, ≥1/week; always ≥ 1/day.
The continence score is determined by adding points from the above table, which takes into account the type and frequency of incontinence and the extent to which it alters the patient's life.
From Jorge JM, Wexner SD: Etiology and management of fecal incontinence. Dis Colon Rectum 36:77, 1993.

The review of systems should include abdominal pain or cramping, lower back or pelvic pain, any changes in pelvic or lower extremity sensation, or changes in sexual response. Changes in the neurologic function of the pelvis or lower extremities or a history of an acute onset of fecal incontinence should direct the physician to rule out a neurologic disease such as multiple sclerosis or a neoplasm of the brain or lumbar/sacral spinal cord.

Past medical history should include detailed history of vaginal deliveries, including birth weights, length of second stage, episiotomies or lacerations, and use of forceps. Any breakdown or complications of episiotomy healing should be noted. Past history of abdominal and pelvic surgeries or trauma to the back or pelvis should be reviewed. Details and operative reports of any anal dilatations, anal sphincterotomy, hemorrhoidectomy, rectovaginal fistula repairs, or posterior colporrhaphy should be obtained. Patients should also be questioned about previous evaluations and results of flexible sigmoidoscopy, colonoscopy, barium enemas. Any family history of colon cancer, inflammatory bowel disease, or familial polyposis should be elicited.

Many medications also affect bowel function. The patient should not only be asked about laxatives and bowel stimulants, but a complete list of all prescription and over-the-counter medications, as well as any dietary or herbal supplements should be reviewed. Many medications, including anticholinergics, antidepressants, iron, narcotics, nonsteroidals, and pseudoephedrine, can cause chronic constipation that may contribute to overflow incontinence or pelvic floor neuropathy secondary to straining.

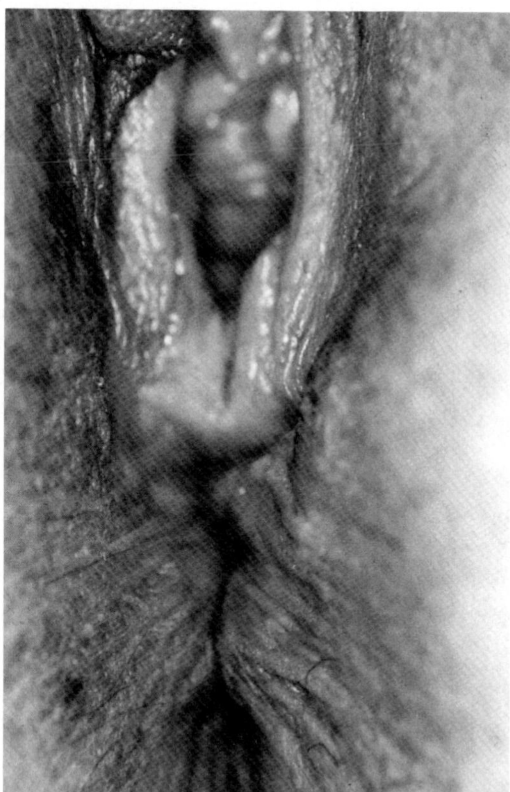

Figure 20-22. Perineum with chronic laceration of external anal sphincter (EAS). Inspection of the perineum shows the classic "dovetail" sign with loss of the anal skin creases anteriorly due to a chronic third-degree laceration of the EAS. Normally, with an intact sphincter, the skin creases are arranged radially around the anus. (From Stenchever MA, Benson JT [eds]: Atlas of Clinical Gynecology. New York, McGraw-Hill, 2000.)

Physical Examination

Undergarments or pads should be inspected for stool, mucus, blood, or pus. If material is found, the patient should be asked if this is her normal leakage. Physical examination begins with inspection of the perineum and anal region. Pruritus ani, or discoloration and irritation of the perianal skin, is commonly seen with fecal incontinence of liquid stool and chronic diarrhea. Perianal skin creases or folds should completely encircle the anus. Note the presence of protruding tissue around or from the anus and determine if there are external hemorrhoids or mucosal or full-thickness rectal wall prolapse. The dovetail sign or loss of anterior perineal folds indicates a defect in the EAS or chronic third-degree laceration (Fig. 20-22). Previous episiotomy, laceration, or surgical scars should be noted. The size of the genital hiatus and the presence of genital prolapse should be assessed as an indicator of pelvic floor neuromuscular function. The innervation of the EAS can be grossly tested by eliciting the clitoral–anal or bulbocavernosus reflex. Using a cotton swab, a gentle, quick touch beside the clitoris or over the bulbocavernosus muscle should elicit a contraction of the EAS. If intact, the reflex implies that the pudendal nerve afferents and the rectal or external hemorrhoidal branch of the pudendal efferent nerves are functional. Unlike males, who should always exhibit this reflex, about 10% of women lack this reflex naturally. However, if absent, and in the presence of fecal incontinence, further neurologic testing is indicated. Sensation in the S2 through S4 dermatomes should be screened by dull and pinprick discrimination when touching the perineum. Loss of sensation should direct the clinician to further neurologic or radiologic assessment of the nervous system.

Next, the patient should be asked to squeeze as if trying to not pass gas. Inspection of the perianal folds should be evaluated for a concentric contraction and some upward movement of the perineal body as she contracts the EAS and levator ani. Substitution with contraction of the buttocks, upper thighs, or abdomen should be noted. The patient should then be asked to bear down as if trying to have a bowel movement. She should be reassured that it is expected she may pass flatus during this part of the examination. The degree of perineal descent and any prolapse of the vagina, pelvic viscera, or rectum should be noted. If there appears to be any pelvic organ prolapse, the examination should be performed in the standing position or after straining on a commode to maximize the prolapse.

Rectal examination is used to assess both resting and squeeze tone of the anal canal. The resting tone of the anal canal is an indicator of IAS function. When asked to squeeze, a circumferential contraction and tightening should be felt. An upward movement of the rectum and posterior compartment of the pelvis should be seen as the levator ani muscles contract. As these muscles also play an important role in anal continence, palpation of the levators for strength and symmetry should be performed by palpating the muscles on each side of the vagina at the introitus.

In addition to assessing rectal tone, the anal canal and rectum should be palpated for masses and a dilated rectum or the presence of stool in the rectal vault. A chronically distended rectum, either with stool, a tumor, or an intussuscepting bowel, will disrupt the normal rectoanal inhibitory reflex that allows the highly sensitive anal canal to sample the stool contents by relaxing the IAS while time contracting the EAS to prevent incontinence. If this reflex is suppressed, the anal canal remains dilated, the EAS fatigues, and incontinence will occur.

While doing the rectal examination, the patient is also asked to strain to diagnose the presence of a rectocele, enterocele, rectal prolapse, or bowel intussusception. With a finger in the rectum the integrity of the rectovaginal septum, posterior vaginal wall, and perineal body can be assessed by palpating through the vagina via bimanual examination.

Testing

Clinical diagnosis based on physical examination and history alone will be accurate in a majority of patients. However, further evaluation, including radiologic and physiologic tests, have been shown in a prospective study at a tertiary colorectal referral clinic to alter the final diagnosis of the cause of fecal incontinence in 19% of cases. Which tests to consider should be based on history and physical examination, prior treatment, and proposed therapy. The algorithm outlined in Figure 20-23 recommends further evaluation based on history and the rectal tone. Normal rectal tone directs the clinician away from anal incontinence and toward a metabolic or colonic origin. Metabolic tests including thyroid-stimulating hormone and glucose should be checked.

Poor resting tone on rectal examination directs the clinician to a neuromuscular cause. A normal resting tone, with an anterior sphincter defect, indicates a chronic third-degree laceration of the EAS.

Evaluation or further testing is not only performed for diagnostic purposes, but also to determine which nonsurgical and surgical therapies are most likely to benefit the patient. In addition, certain tests, such as anal manometry or a sphincter ultrasound, can be used for baseline assessment for which post-treatment assessment or function can be compared. Whenever the patient's history does not match her physical examination, further testing should be considered. In addition, if the patient has had prior surgery, or has other pelvic floor dysfunction, testing before treatment, especially surgical, may help direct care. It is important to remember that the patient may have more than one cause or pathology contributing to her fecal incontinence such as pudendal neuropathy and an anal sphincter defect or irritable bowel in combination with a weakened pelvic floor (Table 20-5).

Diagnostic Procedures

Colonoscopy. A colonoscopy is indicated for any patient with chronic diarrhea to evaluate for inflammatory bowel disease and infectious diarrhea.

Transanal Ultrasound. Transanal ultrasound has significantly enhanced the ability to delineate defects of both the IAS and EAS. The integrity, thickness, and length of the IAS and EAS can be determined. The IAS is visible as a hypoechoic circle, and the EAS is seen as a hyperechoic circle (Fig. 20-24). Transanal ultrasound is most useful in evaluation of patients for chronic third-degree lacerations or occult sphincter tears. Knowing the boundaries of the sphincter defect and if both

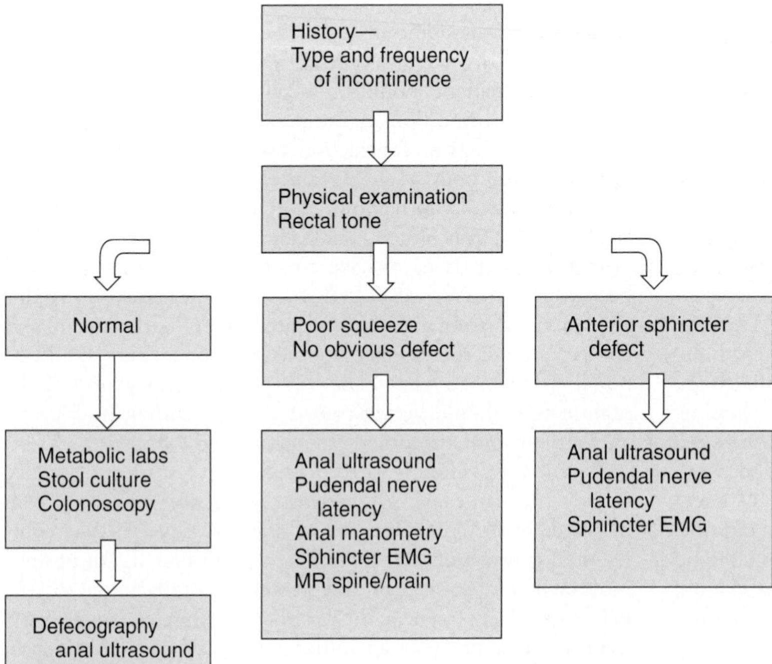

Figure 20-23. Evaluation of fecal incontinence. A detailed history differentiates incontinence of gas, liquid, or solid stool, along with frequency, onset, and effect on the patient's quality of life. The history should assess the possibility of Crohn's disease, ulcerative colitis, irritable bowel syndrome, radiation to the pelvis, neurologic diseases such as multiple sclerosis, and prior anorectal surgeries. A detailed obstetric history should include type of delivery, weight of largest infant, length of second stage, episiotomy or lacerations, and use of forceps or vacuum extraction. Rectal examination should assess resting and squeeze tone, presence of a rectocele or rectal mass, and fecal impaction. Inspection of the rectum and vagina should evaluate for a rectovaginal fistula, prolapsing hemorrhoids, or rectal prolapse. Further evaluation, including radiologic and physiologic tests, have been shown in a prospective study at a tertiary colorectal referral clinic to alter the final diagnosis of the cause of fecal incontinence in 19% of the cases. EMG, electromyography; MRI, magnetic resonance imaging. (Modified from Stenchever MA, Benson JT [eds]: Atlas of Clinical Gynecology. New York, McGraw-Hill, 2000.)

the EAS and IAS are disrupted can direct the surgeon at time of anal sphincteroplasty. Similar information can be obtained from EMG of the EAS when used to map the sphincter defect. In general, transanal ultrasound is less painful and better tolerated by the patient.

Anal Manometry. Anal manometry is a commonly used test that objectively assesses the resistance to spontaneous defecation provided by the anorectal sphincter mechanism and the sensory capabilities of the rectum to provide a feeling of

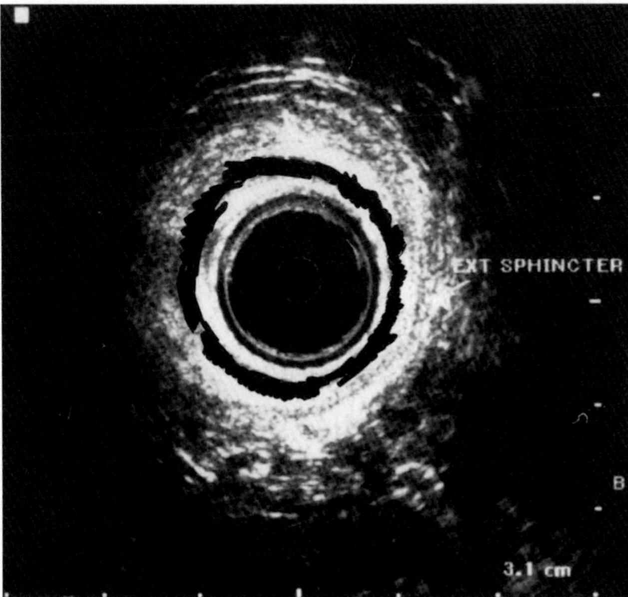

A

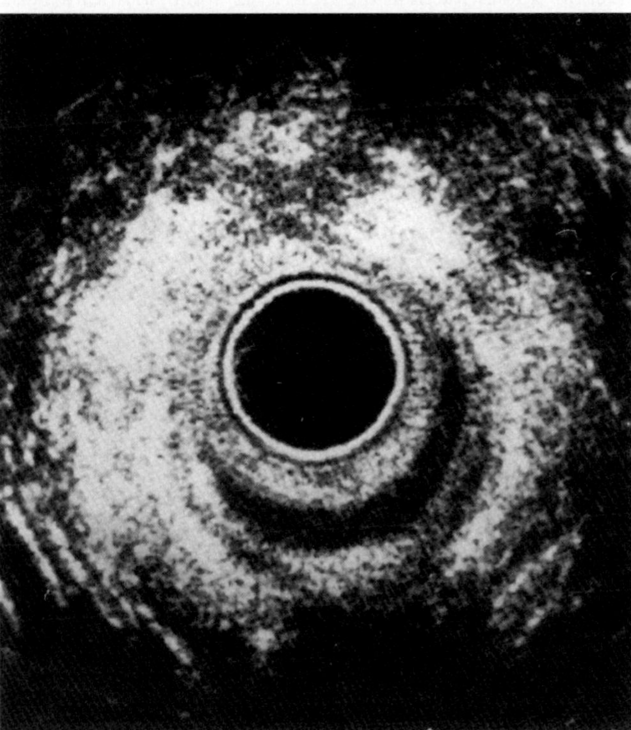

B

Table 20-5 Tests of Anorectal Function for Patients with Fecal Incontinence

Test	Measures	Indication
Anal manometry	Resting anal pressures	Low resting and squeeze pressure on rectal exam
	Maximum squeeze pressure	Prior radiation treatment
	Rectoanal inhibitory reflex	Fecal urgency
	Rectal sensation	Fecal impaction
Single-fiber EMG	Fiber density	Denervation
	Muscle activity	Reinnervation injury
		Map EAS defect
Pudendal nerve motor latency	Speed of signal along pudendal nerve	Pudendal nerve damage from childbirth or straining
Endoscopic ultrasound	IAS and EAS defect	Obstetric or traumatic sphincter injuries
Defecating proctogram	Movement of pelvic floor	Perineal descent
	Pelvic floor defects	Posterior compartment deficits

EAS, external anal sphincter; EMG, electromyogram; IAS, internal anal sphincter.

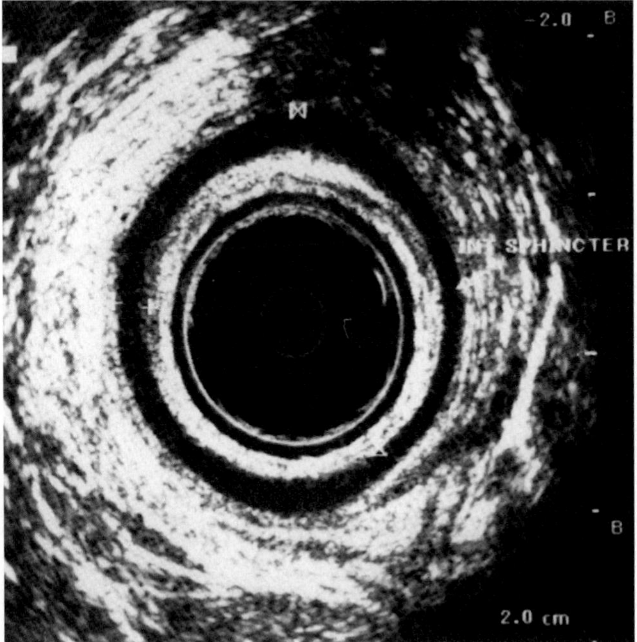

C

Figure 20-24. Anal ultrasound. **A,** Anal ultrasound has significantly enhanced the ability to delineate defects of the internal and external anal sphincters. The internal anal sphincter (IAS) is visible as a hypoechoic circle, and the external anal sphincter (EAS) is seen as a hyperechoic circle. Scarred areas have a homogeneous, gray appearance. Both IAS and EAS are intact. **B,** With the patient supine, a defect in the AIS from 3 o'clock to 9 o'clock and a defect at 12 o'clock in the EAS is shown. **C,** Again, with the vagina at the 12 o'clock position, there is an intact IAS and defect in the EAS. (From Stenchever MA, Benson JT [eds]: Atlas of Clinical Gynecology. New York, McGraw-Hill, 2000.)

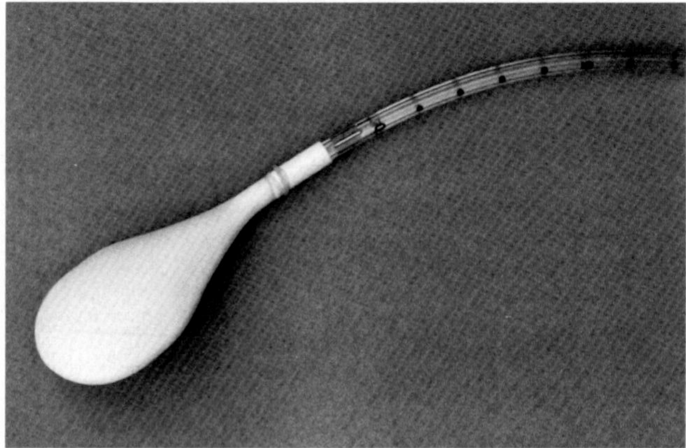

Figure 20-25. Anal manometer, a four-channel perfusion catheter with balloon tip. There are many different types and methods for performing anal manometry. A balloon or probe is inserted into the rectum, and a pressure transducer relays information to a recorder or computer. Important manometric parameters include sphincter length, resting and squeeze pressures, rectal sensation, and the presence of the anorectal inhibitory reflex (RAIR). The balloon is placed in the rectum and inflated by 10-cm^3 increments to determine rectal sensation and compliance. The presence of the RAIR is determined with balloon inflation and seeing the IAS relax and the EAS contract to allow for the "sampling" of rectal contents. The four radical ports are perfused with sterile water, and resting and squeeze pressures around the anal canal are measured at centimeter intervals along the anal canal. The catheter can be pulled at a constant rate to determine the length of the sphincter and "high pressure" or incontinence zone.

imminent defecation. Anal manometry is helpful for patients who have had prior surgery to the anorectal canal or radiation therapy that could have altered the rectal storage function. In patients who, by history, report a normal sensation to defecate, anal manometry has been largely replaced by transanal ultrasound and PNTML or sphincter EMG alone. Although these studies do not give information on rectal function, they are more accurate in assessing the neuromuscular function of the anal sphincters.

Anal manometry uses a rectal balloon to assess rectal sensation, rectal compliance, the rectoanal inhibitory reflex (RAIR), and maximal tolerable rectal volume (Fig. 20-25). The RAIR is a reflex response to increased pressure in the rectum from gas or stool. Normally, the IAS relaxes to allow a sampling of the rectal contents by the anal canal to determine if the contents are gas or stool and whether it is an appropriate time to defecate or pass flatus. At the same time, the EAS squeezes to prevent incontinence.

In addition to rectal function, resting and squeeze pressures in the anal canal are obtained by pulling a perfusion catheter with radial ports (four or eight) through the anal canal. The IAS contributes 80% of the resting pressure. Voluntary contraction of the EAS should double the resting pressure (Fig. 20-26). Although objective documentation is useful for diagnosis or preoperative baseline, normal resting and squeeze pressures can be accurately assessed on rectal examination by most experienced clinicians.

Electromyography. EMG is used for mapping of the EAS defect and for determining the presence and degree of neuropathy and denervation and reinnervation. EMG evaluates the bioelectrical action potentials that are generated by depolarization of skeletal striated muscle. EMG evaluation consists of systematic examination of spontaneous activity, recruitment patterns, and the waveform of the motor unit action potentials (MUAP).

Performance and interpretation of EMG of the EAS requires special training and experience. A needle electrode is inserted into the skeletal muscle of the EAS. First, spontaneous activity is heard and seen. Next, the patient voluntarily squeezes her pelvic floor and recruitment activity is recorded. Straining should decrease activity and coughing should increase recruitment. The final step in analysis is evaluation of the MUAP waveform. Following nerve damage, as seen with a vaginal delivery, reinnervation of the muscle fibers leads to a single motor unit innervating multiple muscle fibers. On single-fiber EMG the MUAPs have larger amplitudes, longer duration, and more phases or crossings of the baseline.

Pudendal Nerve Terminal Motor Latencies. Nerve conduction studies measure the time from stimulation of a nerve to a response in the muscle it innervates. The pudendal nerve terminal motor latency (PNTML) is determined by using a glove-mounted electrode known as a St. Mark's pudendal electrode, connected to a pulsed stimulus generator and, with the examiner's index finger in the vagina or anus, the pudendal nerve is stimulated at the ischial spine.

The latent period between the pudendal nerve stimulation and the electromechanical response of the muscle is measured. Normal PNTML is 2.0 + 0.2 msec. A normal PNTML is the

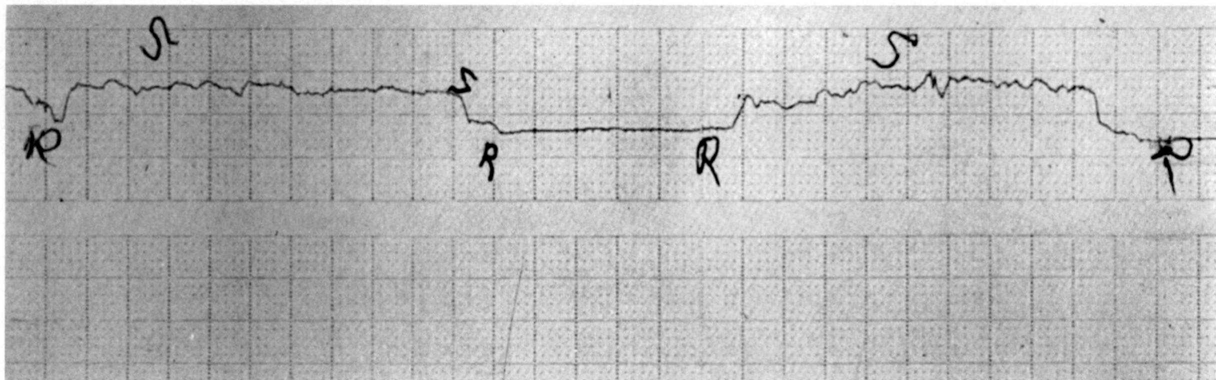

Figure 20-26. A single-channel recording of the resting pressure of the anal canal (R) and the squeeze pressure (S). The IAS contributes 80% of the resting pressure. Voluntary contraction or squeezing of the EAS should double the resting pressure.

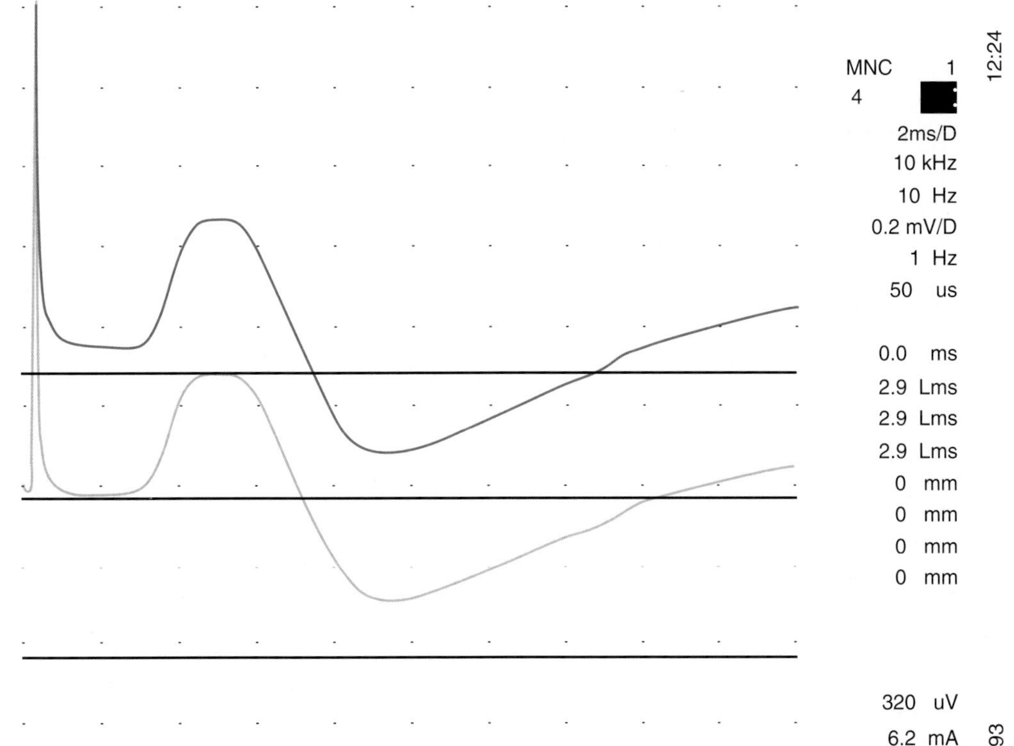

Figure 20-27. Pudendal nerve terminal motor latencies (PNTML). Normal bilateral PNTML have been shown to be 2.0 + 0.2 msec. The latency response is measured from the onset of the stimulus to the onset of the response in the external anal sphincter. A normal PNTML is the measurement of the fastest response of the pudendal nerve and does not necessarily mean the entire nerve is normal. Neither does an abnormal latency indicate abnormal muscle function. A damaged nerve can heal and reinnervate the muscle, and although the PNTML may be slightly prolonged, the muscle functions normally. (From Stenchever MA, Benson JT [eds]: Atlas of Clinical Gynecology. New York, McGraw-Hill, 2000.)

measurement of the fastest response of the pudendal nerve and does not necessarily mean the entire nerve is normal (Fig. 20-27). Prolonged PNTMLs have been found in patients with idiopathic fecal incontinence and in patients with rectal prolapse and may be predictive of continence following surgical repair.

PNTML measurement is particularly important in suspected neurogenic incontinence and prior to sphincter repair. PNTML has been found to be the most sensitive predictor of functional outcome of overlapping EAS repairs (Table 20-6). Gilliland and colleagues found in reviewing 100 patients at a median of 24 months after surgery that pudendal neuropathy was the only significant predictor of surgical success. Not patient age, parity, prior sphincteroplasty, cause or duration of incontinence, extent of EMG damage, size of the endoanal ultrasound defect, or pressures on anal manometry successfully predicted postoperative continence. However, 62% of 59 patients with bilaterally normal PNMTLs had a successful outcome compared with 1 of 12 patients with unilateral or bilateral prolonged PNMTLs (<0.01). The high failure rate seen with prolonged PNTML may occur for several reasons. First, prolongation of the PNTMLs is associated with increased mean fiber density of the EAS, resulting in a less efficient sphincter. Second, as the pudendal nerves also convey sensory nerve fibers from the levator muscles, the sensation of rectal distention may be diminished. Loss of rectal sensation leads to rectal distention and decreased anal resting tone leading to incontinence.

Defecography. Dynamic cystoproctography or defecography is an imaging technique that has been widely used in the evaluation of anorectal function and anatomy, dating back to the mid-1960s. Defecography may be used as an adjunct to physical

Table 20-6 Influence of Pudendal Neuropathy on Outcome after Sphincteroplasty Percentage Success

			% SUCCESS		
Author*	**Institution**	**Number of Patients**	**Patients without Neuropathy**	**Patients with Neuropathy**	***P* Value**
Lauberg et al, 1988	St. Marks	19	80	11	<0.05
Wexner et al, 1991	Cleveland Clinic, Florida	16	92	50	ns
Engel et al, 1994	St. Marks	55	not recorded	not recorded	ns
Simmang et al, 1994	Washington University	14	100	67	ns
Londono-Schimmer et al, 1994	St. Marks	94	55	30	<0.001
Sitzler and Thompson, 1996	St. Marks	31	67	63	ns
Felt-Bersma et al, 1996	Vrije University	18	not recorded	not recorded	ns
Sangwan et al, 1996	Lahey Clinic	15	100	14	<0.005
Gilliland et al, 1998	Cleveland Clinic, Florida	100	63	10	<0.01

NS, not significant.
*References are from the original source.
From Gilliland R, Altomare DF, Moreira H, et al: Pudendal neuropathy is predictive of failure following anterior overlapping sphincteroplasty. Dis Colon Rectum 41:1516, 1998.

examination in patients with chronic constipation and pelvic floor defects or hernias that may be contributing to their fecal incontinence. Intussusception or rectal prolapse can be seen on defecography along with rectoceles that do not empty at the time of defecation. Stool retained in the rectocele can cause chronic distention of the rectum and loss of rectal sensation. The loss of rectal sensation leads to chronic constipation or impaction, causing further neuromuscular damage to the pelvic floor and ultimately fecal incontinence. Perineal descent and the anorectal angle can be objectively measured using defecography.

Magnetic Resonance Imaging of the Anal Sphincters. Magnetic resonance imaging (MRI) of the anal sphincters has the ability to evaluate both muscular and connective tissue supports of the pelvis. Recent advances in MRI technologies using the endoanal coil, rapid sequencing, and cinematic display have replaced defecography in evaluation of the pelvic floor and defecation disorders in a few centers. Muscular defects along with POP and perineal descent can be assessed. Specialized dynamic MRI may replace defecography and transanal ultrasound in the future.

Transit Study. A transit study is used to evaluate colonic motility and is most often used in the evaluation of chronic constipation. For patients for whom fecal impaction or overflow incontinence is high on the differential, a transit study may be indicated. There are numerous variations of the study. The patient ingests a Sitzmark capsule containing 20 or 25 radiopaque rings. She does not take any laxatives or bowel stimulants. Five days after taking the capsule, an abdominal flat radiographic plate is obtained. Normally, 80% of the capsules should have been passed. Diffuse or global colon dysfunction is indicated if the rings are dispersed throughout the colon or segmental abnormalities can be seen if the rings are clustered in one area or trapped in a rectocele.

Treatment

Treatment of fecal incontinence includes medications, biofeedback, electrical stimulation, and surgery. Obstructive devices, including transanal plugs, have been marketed but are not widely used.

Fecal incontinence should, obviously, be treated based on diagnosis as in medications or surgery for inflammatory bowel disease or surgery for a neoplasm of the cauda equina. For patients with fecal incontinence associated with liquid or watery stools, dietary modifications and medications are the first line of therapy. Increasing dietary fiber with diet changes or bulking agents or fiber supplements such as methyl cellulose or psyllium helps to increase stool size. A larger more formed stool may improve rectal sensation and emptying. To slow intestinal transit and allow for increased water absorption, several medications (Table 20-7) are available. For some patients, a daily cleansing of the rectum with an enema allows for several hours of freedom from their incontinence.

Table 20-7 Medications for Treatment of Diarrhea

Drug	Dosage	Mechanism of Action
Loperamide	2 mg tid or 4 mg followed by 2 mg after loose BM Max 16 mg/day	Inhibits circular and longitudinal muscle contraction
Diphenoxylate with atropine	5 mg qid	Direct action of circular smooth muscle to decrease peristalsis
Hyoscyamine sulfate	25 mg qid	Anticholinergic
Alosetron	1 mg bid	5 HT_3 receptor antagonist
Cholestyramine	4 mg pack qd or bid	Binds bile acids after cholecystectomy

Biofeedback

For fecal incontinence, like urinary incontinence, biofeedback requires a motivated patient, a feedback device, and a planned exercise program. Although the patient may not perceive normal sensation or be able to contract her pelvic floor voluntarily, she must be neurologically intact in order to benefit from biofeedback. No correlation has been seen with premanometry testing as long as some neuromuscular function is present. About 60% to 70% of patients with fecal incontinence secondary to an abnormal pelvic floor will have a 90% reduction in incontinence with biofeedback.

Biofeedback of any type is founded on the patient hearing, seeing, or sensing a response from a planned exercise. A measuring device, either electrode or pressure transducer, is used transvaginally or transanally to record and give feedback to the patient on how she is squeezing the pelvic floor. She then uses this feedback to increase or lengthen the pelvic floor contraction. If the patient has incontinence secondary to a sensory deficit in the rectum, rectal balloons can be used to "retrain" the patient to perceive rectal distention while squeezing her external sphincter in response to rectal distention. The patient can be taught by a physical therapist who not only provides encouragement but also instructs on proper technique. Although initially labor-intensive, biofeedback has no side effects or morbidity and can be used in conjunction with other treatment modalities, including surgery. In addition, for patients with urinary and fecal incontinence, a single therapy may improve both conditions.

Electrical Stimulation Therapy

Functional electrical stimulation therapy has been shown to improve fecal incontinence in patients with a weakened pelvic floor who are unable to contract their EAS or puborectalis on command. Because of the expense, electrical stimulation is generally reserved for patients who are unable to respond to traditional biofeedback protocols. Both transvaginal and transrectal probes are available. Most protocols recommend high-frequency stimulation at a maximum tolerable stimulation of 50 MHz for 15 to 20 minutes twice a day. Response to therapy is usually seen in 6 weeks with maximum improvement by 12 weeks.

Preliminary reports indicate that using sacral nerve stimulation with implantable electrodes may provide an additional treatment modality for patients with fecal incontinence.

Surgery

Surgical management of fecal incontinence includes repair of rectal prolapse, anal sphincteroplasty, anal sphincter neomuscular flaps, and the implantation of artificial sphincters. Unfortunately, postanal repair or posterior levatorplasty has not

Table 20-8 Outcome after Sphincteroplasty

Author*	Institution	Number of Patients	Follow-up Period (mean [range]; months)	Success (%)	Improved (%)
Fang et al, 1984	Minnesota	76	35 (2–62)	82	89
Browning and Motson, 1988	St. Marks	83	39.2 (4–116)	78	91
Ctercteko et al, 1988	Cleveland Clinic, Ohio	44	50	75	
Laurberg et al, 1988	St. Marks	19	18 (median: 9–36)	47	79
Yoshioka and Keighley, 1989	Birmingham	27	48 (median: 16–108)		74.1
Wexner et al, 1991	Cleveland Clinic, Florida	16	10 (3–16)	76	87.5
Fleshman et al, 1991	Washington University	55	0 (12–24)	72	87
Simmang et al, 1994	Washington University	14	0 (6–12)	71	93
Engel et al, 1994	St. Marks	55	15 (6–36)	60.4	
Engel et al, 1994	Amsterdam	28	46 (median: 15–116)	75	
Londono-Schimmer et al, 1994	St. Marks	94	58.5 (median: 12–98)	50	75
Sitzler and Thompson, 1996	St. Marks	31	0 (1–36)	74	
Felt-Bersma et al, 1996	Vrije University	18	14 (3–39)		72
Oliveira et al, 1996	Cleveland Clinic, Florida	55	29 (3–61)	70.1	80
Nikiteas et al, 1996	Birmingham	42	38 (median: 12–66)	60	
Gilliland et al, 1998	Cleveland Clinic, Florida	100	24 (median: 2–96)	55	69

*References are from the original source.
From Gilliland R, Altomare DF, Moreira H, et al: Pudendal neuropathy is predictive of failure following anterior overlapping sphincteroplasty. Dis Colon Rectum 41:1516, 1998.

been shown to be effective in the treatment of fecal incontinence in most patients and will not be discussed.

Repair of rectal prolapse, either transrectally or transabdominally, restores continence in 50% of patients. Success depends on the neuromuscular function of the pelvic floor.

Overlapping anterior anal sphincteroplasty provides symptomatic control of incontinence in 60% to 80% of patients (Table 20-8). Patients who have both an anal sphincter defect and prolonged PNTML should be counseled that their chance of continence following surgery may be decreased. But unless there is absolutely no nerve function, surgical repair should be considered. Repair of an anal sphincter laceration includes not only repair of the EAS but identification and repair of any IAS defects. Since the IAS maintains the resting tone of the anus, it is important to restore sphincter integrity, especially for control of flatus.

The surgery is performed through a transperineal incision from 11 o'clock to 2 o'clock over the EAS defect. With a gloved hand in the rectum, the internal sphincter is identified and plicated in the midline with 3-0 prolonged absorbable sutures. Next, the ends of the EAS are identified. The use of a nerve stimulator can facilitate identification of the sphincter ends. The fibrous scar tissue at the ends of the sphincter is kept for added strength. The sphincter ends are dissected free to allow overlap in the midline without tension. The sphincter is then closed with 2-0 or 3-0 prolonged absorbable sutures by overlapping the sphincter ends (Fig. 20-28). The advantage of the overlapping sphincteroplasty over the traditional end-to-end repair is decreased tension to prevent separation of the suture line once anesthesia no longer prevents sphincter contraction.

When anal sphincter injury occurs at the time of vaginal delivery, the type of repair needed has been debated. To date according to only a few studies, there is no significant difference between end-to-end and overlapping anal sphincteroplasties. The outcome of anal sphincteroplasties after delivery is unacceptably poor, with 47% to 67% of women complaining of defecatory symptoms such as flatus incontinence, fecal urgency, and fecal incontinence. Although frank fecal incontinence is reported at a much lower rate of 2% to 9%, the other defecatory symptoms are nonetheless bothersome to women. Furthermore, endoanal ultrasound examinations after sphincteroplasty show persistent anatomic defects in 40% to 85% of repairs.

Because the outcome after anal sphincteroplasty is suboptimal, prevention emerges as an even more important consideration. Since vaginal childbirth injury to the anal sphincter is such a common cause of fecal incontinence, prevention should start here. Midline episiotomy has been shown repeatedly in studies to be strongly associated with anal sphincter damage. Avoidance of routine episiotomy and consideration of a mediolateral episiotomy when absolutely necessary could be beneficial in prevention efforts.

Neosphincters. There are basically two types of neosphincters: one using the patient's own skeletal muscle, usually the gracilis, and the other using an artificial Silastic cuff connected to a fluid reservoir to occlude the anal canal. The gracilis muscle wrap has been shown to have inconsistent results. Initially described by Pickrell and colleagues in 1952, the entire muscle is mobilized and its distal portion is wrapped snugly around the anus and anchored to the contralateral ischial tuberosity. Recently, the addition of chronic, low-frequency electrical stimulation of the nerve or muscle has been used to convert fatigue-prone type II muscle fibers to fatigue-resistant type I fibers. Once converted, the muscle may be continuously stimulated, resulting in prolonged closure of the anal canal. A report by Baeten and colleagues for the Dynamic Graciloplasty Therapy Study Group reported on 123 adults treated at 20 institutions with dynamic graciloplasty and found 63% of patients reported a 50% or greater improvement in incontinent events 1 year after surgery. Another 11% noted some improvement and 26% reported no improvement or worse. There was one surgery-related death and 74% of patients experienced an adverse event related to the treatment with 40% of patients requiring an additional surgery. Despite these frequent complications, most patients showed a significant improvement in quality of life following the surgery.

Artificial sphincters are indicated in patients with anal incontinence caused by neuromuscular disease or trauma.

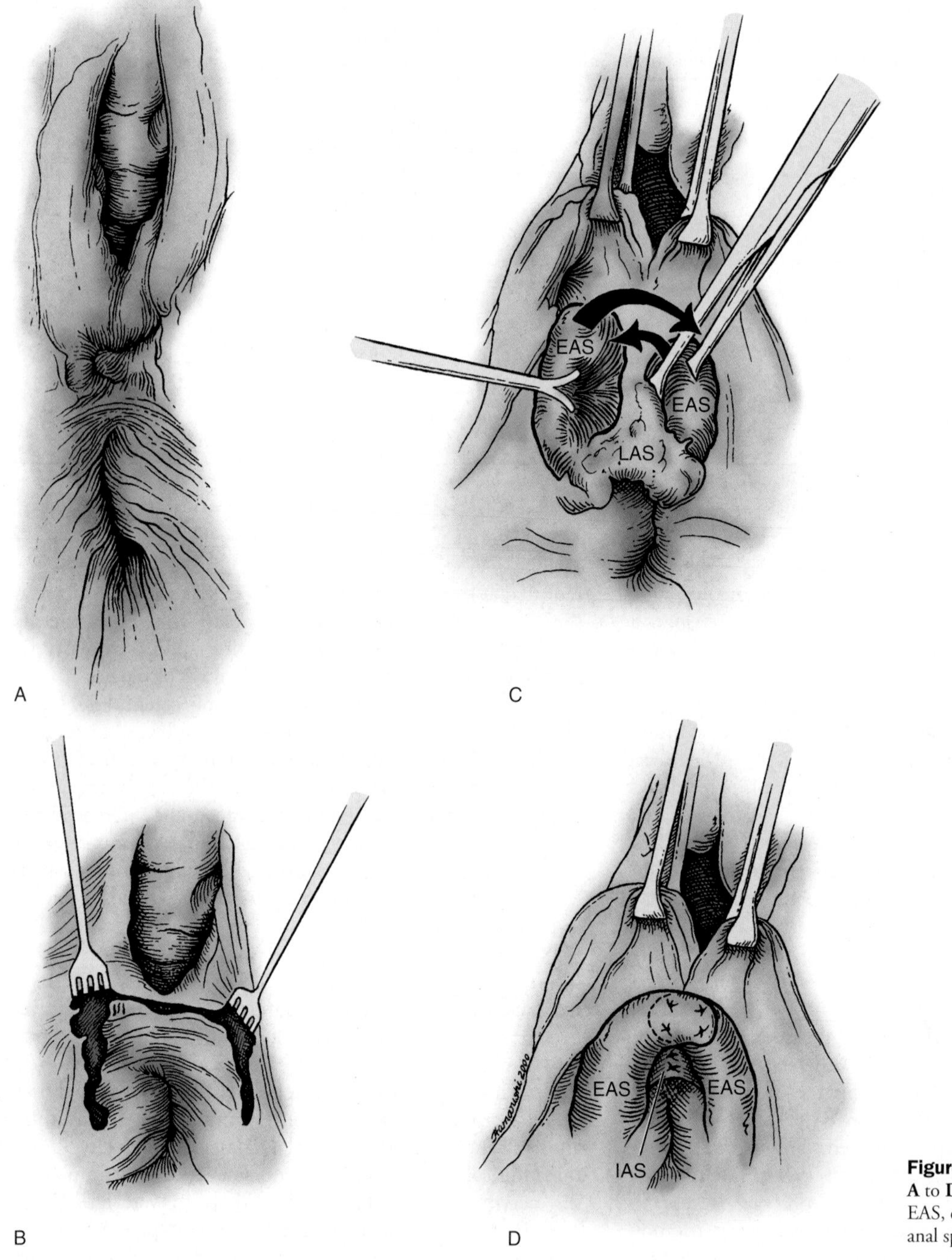

Figure 20-28. Sphincter drawing (4). **A** to **D,** Overlapping sphincteroplasty. EAS, external anal sphincter; IAS, internal anal sphincter.

Complications include infection and mechanical breakdown. Seventy-five percent success rates and 33% complication rates, similar to those for the muscle transpositions, have been reported.

RECTOVAGINAL FISTULAS

Although not a true source of fecal incontinence by definition, rectovaginal fistulas (RVF) are common enough complications of vaginal birth and gynecologic surgeries to be addressed under this heading. Any time a patient presents complaining of fecal or flatal incontinence, an RVF should be included in the differential diagnosis.

The causes of RVF, as seen in Table 20-9, include traumatic, inflammatory, and neoplastic origins, but obstetric injuries are, by far, the most common cause. It is estimated that 0.1% of vaginal births will result in an RVF.

A fistula occurring caudad or adjacent to the EAS is termed an anovaginal fistula and is managed differently from an RVF. Fistulas that occur more than 3 cm above the anal verge are true RVFs.

Most RVFs secondary to obstetric injury occur in the lower third of the vagina and may be associated with a sphincter

Table 20-9 Origin of Rectovaginal Fistula

Category	Condition	Mechanism
Traumatic		
Obstetric	Prolonged second stage of labor	Pressure necrosis of rectovaginal septum
	Midline episiotomy	Extension directed into rectum
	Perineal lacerations	
Foreign body	Vaginal pessaries	Pressure necrosis
	Violent coitus	Mechanical perforation
	Sexual abuse	Mechanical perforation
Iatrogenic	Hysterectomy	Injury to anterior rectal wall
	Stapled colorectal anastomosis	Staple line includes vagina
	Transanal excision of anterior rectal tumor	Deep margin of resection into vagina
	Enemas	Mechanical perforation
	Anorectal surgery such as incision and drainage of intramural abscesses	Mechanical perforation
Inflammatory	Crohn's disease	Transmural inflammation-perforation
	Pelvic radiation	Early-tumor necrosis
	Pelvic abscess	Late transmural inflammation
	Perirectal abscess	
Neoplastic	Rectal	Local tumor growth into neighboring structure
	Cervical	
	Uterine	
	Vaginal	
	Primary or recurrent tumors	

From Stenchever MA, Benson JT (eds): Atlas of Clinical Gynecology. New York, McGraw-Hill, 2000.

defect in the EAS. It is important to evaluate the EAS as outlined earlier with either a transanal ultrasound or EMG to map any defects prior to surgical treatment.

Fistulas secondary to surgical trauma, malignancy, or inflammatory process may occur anywhere along the vaginal wall, including the apex. If a fistula develops after a difficult surgery, such as following pelvic inflammatory disease, or after radiation, it is important to check for more than one fistula prior to repair. If the patient has a history of malignancy, examination with biopsy specimens should be performed to rule out cancer as the cause of the fistula.

Depending on the size and location of the fistula, the patient may be nearly asymptomatic or complain of a small amount of flatus passing into her vagina with a low, small fistula. With a large fistula, she may have formed stool coming through the vagina with every bowel movement, causing significant distress and hygiene problems.

Evaluation of a patient includes history and physical examination to determine cause. If there is suspicion of inflammatory bowel disease, a colonoscopy is warranted. A rectal examination is important to determine the integrity of the anal sphincters, the quality of the tissues surrounding the fistula, and to palpate for abscesses and other masses. Methylene blue mixed in lubricant can help identify the fistula. If still not identified, a dilute methylene blue enema with a tampon in the vagina may help in isolating the fistula. If the vaginal orifice is found, but not the rectal opening, insertion of an angiocath with a squirting of hydrogen peroxide can show bubbling on the rectal side.

An office anoscopy or proctoscopy may also help to evaluate the surrounding tissues. In general, a mature epithelialized fistula that is not infected is not painful on digital examination. If the exam in the office is not successful in locating the fistula or is too painful for the patient, she should be taken to the operating room for exam under anesthesia. If the fistula has still not been identified, filling the vagina with water and insufflating the rectum should produce bubbling in the vagina that can be traced to the opening. A barium enema may also be helpful for identifying high fistulas. A vaginogram using dilute barium solution may also help identify a fistula.

Surgical management of an anovaginal or anoperineal fistula is accomplished by opening of the fistula tract, curetting the tract, and leaving the tract open to heal secondarily. Excision of the tract and primary closure will result in recurrent fistula formation in most cases.

Many surgical procedures have been described for management of RVF. Regardless of the procedure chosen, basic surgical principles must be followed. The tissue must be healthy, well vascularized, and free of infection and induration. This may require waiting for up to 3 months following the original trauma or surgery for complete healing. If there is significant fecal contamination, prior radiation, or persistent abscess, a diverting colostomy should be considered. After a colostomy, a delay of 8 to 12 weeks is generally required for the inflammation and cellulites around the fistula to heal. At the time of repair, a Martius fat pad graft can be used to increase the vascular supply to the area. Preoperatively, the patient should have a complete mechanical bowel prep starting several days before the surgery to prevent liquid stool from contaminating the field. Some surgeons may place the patient on a liquid diet several days before surgery with no mechanical bowel prep except enemas until clear the night before surgery. The goal is to have no liquid stool in the rectum and to have her first postoperative bowel movement, several days after surgery, be soft, but formed. Antibiotic bowel prophylaxis is warranted.

Other surgical principles include excision of the entire fistulous tract, wide mobilization of the rectal tissue, and broad tissue-to-tissue closure without tension. The rectal side is the high-pressure side and requires the attention to repair. The vaginal side may be closed or left open to drain if indicated and should close spontaneously. A delayed-absorbable suture, such as a 3-0 Polysorb, is used on all layers. Permanent suture is not used.

Both transvaginal and transrectal repairs have been described, but gynecologists, generally, prefer the transvaginal approach. Depending on the location and the need to repair the anal sphincters, an uncomplicated fistula can be repaired similar to a fourth-degree laceration as a perineoproctotomy with layer closure. After cutting from the perineal body, through the sphincters and to the fistulous tract, care must be taken to excise the tract and any surrounding scar tissue. A two-layered closure of the rectum and anal canal is then performed as in a fourth-degree closure. Care should be given to closing the EAS.

To preserve an intact sphincter, the RVF can be cored out by placing a pediatric Foley transvaginally and filling the balloon on the rectal side and then using the Foley for traction by pulling upward. After excision, depending on the size, a small fistula can be closed with two-layer purse-string sutures or with an interrupted two-layer closure.

Transrectal repairs, preferred by many colorectal surgeons, generally involve the development of rectal mucosal flaps, mobilized and brought down or lateral to cover the excised fistula site. In 23 patients treated at the Cleveland Clinic with rectal advancement flaps, fistulas were successfully cured in 77% of the patients with obstetric or surgical injury and 60% of the patients with Crohn's disease.

Postoperatively, the patient's diet and medications should be managed to keep her bowel movements soft, but formed. In most cases, a clear liquid diet is continued for the first 3 days after surgery followed by a low-residue diet. Broad-spectrum antibiotics should be continued for 2 weeks.

Sitz baths, two or three times a day, followed by the use of a blow dryer or heat lamp, keeps the area clean and dry.

ACKNOWLEDGMENT

This chapter was extensively revised by Drs. Dee Fenner and Morton Stenchever in the previous edition, and I wish to express particular gratitude to them.

KEY POINTS

- Femoral hernias are more common in females than in males, whereas inguinal hernias are more common in males.
- Congenital fascial defects at the umbilicus generally close within the first 3 years of life.
- In the female, large hernias, hernias that continuously have intraabdominal contents, hernias that cause continuing discomfort, and hernias that have been incarcerated should be operatively repaired.
- In the repair of abdominal wall hernias, fascia should be sutured with nonabsorbable material.
- Urethroceles and cystoceles are more common in women with a gynecoid pelvis than in those with android or anthropoid types.
- Urinary incontinence is usually noted with loss of support of the urethra and bladder neck.
- After cystocele repair, bladder drainage for 1 to 5 days is generally necessary before normal voiding can be anticipated.
- Bladder drainage after cystocele repair may be with a transurethral or suprapubic catheter.
- When an enterocele is present, the sac must be dissected free and ligated at its neck to prevent recurrence.
- Descensus of the uterus and cervix is graded as first degree (prolapse into the upper vagina); second degree (prolapse to or near the introitus); and third degree, or complete (prolapse through the introitus).
- Prolapse of the vaginal apex at some time after hysterectomy has been reported in 0.1% to 18.2% of patients.
- Vaginal prolapse after hysterectomy includes a mixture of cystocele, rectocele, and enterocele in 72% of cases.
- Vaginal vault prolapse can be repaired abdominally or vaginally.
- Vaginal vault prolapse repair using fixation to the sacrospinous ligament will have a success rate approaching 100%, but recurrence rate necessitating reoperation may be as high as 33%.
- Estimates of fecal incontinence range from 2% to 16% of community-dwelling women older than 64 years of age.
- Over 30% of women reporting urinary incontinence also report fecal incontinence, known as dual incontinence.
- The IAS, under autonomic control, maintains the high-pressure zone or continence zone and, along with the EAS, keeps the anal canal closed.
- The EAS provides the voluntary squeeze pressure that prevents incontinence with increasing rectal or abdominal pressure. The EAS is innervated by the hemorrhoidal branch of the pudendal nerve from the S2 through the S4 nerve roots.
- Incontinence secondary to denervation has been designated as idiopathic and represents 80% of patients with fecal incontinence.
- A common cause of fecal incontinence is damage to the anal sphincter at the time of vaginal delivery with or without neuronal injury.
- The incidence of occult external anal sphincter disruption after vaginal delivery determined by endoanal ultrasound ranges from 11% to 35%. The chance of muscular injury is increased with midline episiotomy, instrumented delivery, and vaginal delivery of larger infants.
- Approximately 1 in 10 women will develop some fecal incontinence or fecal urgency after one vaginal delivery.
- At a tertiary colorectal referral clinic, a prospective study showed that further evaluation, including radiologic and physiologic tests, altered the final diagnosis or the cause of fecal incontinence in 19% of cases.
- Sixty to 70% of patients with fecal incontinence secondary to an abnormal pelvic floor will have a 90% reduction in incontinence with biofeedback.
- Overlapping anterior anal sphincteroplasty provides symptomatic control of incontinence in 60% to 80% of patients.
- It is estimated that 0.1% of vaginal births will result in a rectovaginal fistula.

BIBLIOGRAPHY

Key Readings

Bump RC, Mattiasson A, Bo K: The standardization of terminology of female pelvic organ prolapse and pelvic floor dysfunction. Am J Obstet Gynecol 175:10, 1996.

Engel AF, van Baal SJ, Brummelkamp WH: Late results of anterior sphincter plication for traumatic faecal incontinence. Eur J Surg 160:633, 1994.

Jackson SL, Weber AM, Hull TL, et al: Fecal incontinence in women with urinary incontinence and pelvic organ prolapse. Obstet Gynecol 89:423, 1997.

Jorge JM, Wexner SD: Etiology and management of fecal incontinence. Dis Colon Rectum 36:77, 1993.

McCall ML: Posterior culdeplasty-surgical correction of enterocele during vaginal hysterectomy: a preliminary report. Obstet Gynecol 10:595, 1957.

Maher CF, Qatawneh AM, Dwyer PL, et al: Abdominal sacral colpopexy or vaginal sacrospinous colpopexy for vaginal vault prolapse: A prospective randomized study. Am J Obstet Gynecol 190:20, 2004.

Olson AL, Smith VJ, Bergstrom JO, et al: Epidemiology of surgically managed pelvic organ prolapse and urinary incontinence. Obstet Gynecol 89:501, 1997.

Snooks SJ, Setchell M, Swash M, Henry MM: Injury to innervation of pelvic floor sphincter musculature in childbirth. Lancet 2:546, 1984.

Sultan AH, Kamm MA, Hudson CN, Bartram CI: Third degree obstetric anal sphincter tears: Risk factors and outcome of primary repair. BMJ 308:887, 1994.

General References

Adams E, Thomson A, Maher C, Hagen S: Mechanical devices for pelvic organ prolapse in women. (Cochrane Review). In The Cochrane Library, Issue 2, 2004. Oxford: Update Software.

Baden WR, Walker TA: Genesis of the vaginal prolapse. Clin Obstet Gynecol 15:1048, 1972.

Beecham CT: Classification of vaginal relaxation, Am J Obstet Gynecol 136:957, 1980.

Beecham CT, Beecham JB: Correction of prolapsed vagina or enterocele with fascia. Obstet Gynecol 42:542, 1973.

Benson JT, Lucente V, McCellan E: Vaginal versus abdominal reconstructive surgery for the treatment of pelvic support defects: A prospective randomized study with long-term outcome evaluation. Am J Obstet Gynecol 175:1418, 1996.

Birnbaum EH, Stamm L, Rafferty JF, et al: Pudendal nerve terminal motor latency influences: Surgical outcome and treatment of rectal diseases. Dis Colon Rectum 39:1215, 1996.

Bittner R, Sauerland S, Schmedt CG: Comparison of endoscopic techniques vs Shouldice and other open nonmesh techniques for inguinal hernia repair: A meta-analysis of randomized controlled trials. Surg Endosc 19:605, 2005.

Bo K: Can pelvic floor muscle training prevent and treat pelvic organ prolapse? Acta Obstet Gynecol Scand 85(3):263, 2006.

Brooks DC: A prospective comparison of laparoscopic and tension-free open herniorrhaphy. Arch Surg 129:361, 1994.

Brubaker L, Cundiff GW, Fine P, et al: Abdominal sacrocolpopexy with Burch colposuspension to reduce urinary stress incontinence. N Engl J Med 354:1557, 2006.

Bump RC: Racial comparisons and contrasts in urinary incontinence and pelvic organ prolapse. Obstet Gynecol 81:421, 1993.

Bump RC, Norton PA: Epidemiology and natural history of pelvic floor dysfunction. Obstet Gynecol Clin North Am 25:723, 1998.

Burrows LJ, Meyn LA, Walters MD, Weber AM: Pelvic symptoms in women with pelvic organ prolapse. Obstet Gynecol 104:982, 2004.

Clemons JL, Aguilar VC, Tillinghast TA, et al: Risk factors associated with an unsuccessful pessary fitting trial in women with pelvic organ prolapse. Am J Obstet Gynecol 190:345, 2004.

Clemons JL, Aguilar VC, Tillinghast TA, et al: Patient satisfaction and changes in prolapse and urinary symptoms in women who were fitted successfully with a pessary for pelvic organ prolapse. Am J Obstet Gynecol 190:1025, 2004.

Colombo M, Maggioni A, Zanetta G, et al: Prevention of postoperative stress incontinence after surgery for genitourinary prolapse. Obstet Gynecol 87:266, 1996.

Cundiff GW, Fenner D: Evaluation and treatment of women with rectocele: Focus on associated defecatory and sexual dysfunction [published erratum appears in Obstet Gynecol 105:222, 1005] Obstet Gynecol 104:1403, 2004.

Deans GT, Wilson MS, Royston CM, Brough WA: Recurrent inguinal hernia after laparoscopic repair: possible cause and prevention. Br J Surg 82:539, 1995.

Denehy TR, Choe JY, Gregori CA, Breen JL: Modified Le Fort partial colpocleisis with Kelly urethral plication and posterior colpoperineoplasty in the medically compromised elderly: A comparison with vaginal hysterectomy, anterior colporrhaphy, and posterior colpoperineoplasty, Am J Obstet Gynecol 173:1697, 1995.

Ellerkmann RM, Cundiff GW, Melick CF, et al: Correlation of symptoms with location and severity of pelvic organ prolapse. Am J Obstet Gynecol 185:1332, 2001.

Fernando RJ, Thakar R, Sultan AH, et al: Effect of vaginal pessaries on symptoms associated with pelvic organ prolapse. Obstet Gynecol 108:93, 2006.

FitzGerald MP, Brubaker L: Colpocleisis and urinary incontinence. Am J Obstet Gynecol 189:1241, 2003.

Glassow F: Inguinal and femoral hernia in women. Int Surg 57:34, 1972.

Glazener CM, Cooper K: Anterior vaginal repair for urinary incontinence in women. Cochrane Database Syst Rev CD001755, 2000.

Graham CA, Mallett VT: Race as a predictor of urinary incontinence and pelvic organ prolapse. Am J Obstet Gynecol 185:116, 2001.

Halverson K, McVay CB: Inguinal and femoral hernioplasty: a 22 year study of author's methods, Arch Surg 101:127, 1970.

Handa VL, Jones M: Do pessaries prevent the progression of pelvic organ prolapse? Int Urogynecol J Pelvic Floor Dysfunct 13:349, 2002.

Hendrix SL, Clark A, Nygaard I, et al: Pelvic organ prolapse in the Women's Health Initiative: Gravity and gravidity. Am J Obstet Gynecol 186:1160, 2002.

Hodgson NC, Malthaner RA, Ostbye T: The search for an ideal method of abdominal fascial closure: A meta-analysis. Ann Surg 231(3) 436, 2000.

Hoyte L, Jakab M, Warfield SK: Levator ani thickness variations in symptomatic and asymptomatic women using magnetic resonance-based 3-dimenstional color mapping. Am J Obstet Gynecol 191:856, 2004.

Jarvis SK, Hallam TK, Lujic S, et al: Peri-operative physiotherapy improves outcomes for women undergoing incontinence and or prolapse surgery: Results of a randomized controlled trial. Aust NZ J Obstet Gynaecol 45:300, 2005.

Kahn MA, Stanton SL: Posterior colporrhaphy: Its effect on bowel and sexual function. Br J Obstet Gynaecol 104:82, 1997.

Kammerer-Doak DN, Dorin MH, Rogers RG, Cousin MO: A randomized trial of Burch retropubic urethropexy and anterior colporrhaphy for stress urinary incontinence. Obstet Gynecol 93:75, 1999.

Kauppila O, Punnonen R, Teisala K: Operative technique for the repair of posthysterectomy vaginal prolapse. Ann Chir Gynaecol 75:242, 1986.

Kavic MS: Laparoscopic hernia repair: Three-year experience. Surg Endosc 9:12, 1995.

Keating JP, Stewart PJ, Eyers AA, et al: Are special investigations of value in the management of patients with fecal incontinence? Dis Colon Rectum 40:896, 1997.

Kobak WH, Rosenberger K, Walers MD: Interobserver variation in the assessment of pelvic organ prolapse. Int Urogynecol J Pelvic Floor Dysfunct 7:121, 1996.

Kohli N, Sze EHM, Roat TW, Karram M: Incidence of recurrent cystocele after anterior colporrhaphy with and without concomitant transvaginal needle suspension. Am J Obstet Gynecol 175:1476, 1996.

Kovac SR and Cruikshank SH: Successful pregnancies and vaginal deliveries after sacrospinous uterosacral fixation in five of nineteen patients. Am J Obstet Gynecol 168:1778, 1993.

Kuhn RJ, Hollyock VE: Observations on the anatomy of the recto-vaginal pouch and septum, Obstet Gynecol 59:445, 1982.

Lind LR, Choe J, Bhatia N: An in-line suturing device to simplify sacrospinous vaginal vault suspension. Obstet Gynecol 89:129, 1997.

McCormack K, Scott NW, Go PM, et al: Laparoscopic techniques versus open techniques for inguinal hernia repair. Cochrane Database Syst Rev CD001785, 2003.

Maher C. Baessler K, Glazener CMA, et al: Surgical management of pelvic organ prolapse in women (Cochrane Review). In The Cochrane Library, Issue 4, 2004. Oxford: Update Software.

Mant J, Painter R, Vessey M: Epidemiology of genital prolapse: Observations from the Oxford Family Planning Association Study. Br J Obstet Gynaecol 104:579, 1997.

Meeks GR, Washburne JF, McGehee RP, Wiser WL: Repair of vaginal vault prolapse by suspension of the vagina to iliococcygeus (prespinous) fascia, Am J Obstet Gynecol 171:1444, 1994.

Miyazaki FS: Miya hook ligature carrier for sacrospinous ligament suspension. Obstet Gynecol 70:286, 1987.

Morley GW, DeLancey JO: Sacrospinous ligament fixation for eversion of the vagina. Am J Obstet Gynecol 158:872, 1988.

Nichols DH: Transvaginal sacrospinous fixation. Pelvic Surgeon 1:10, 1981.

Novara G, Artibani W: Surgery for pelvic organ prolapse: current status and future perspectives. Curr Opin Urol 15(4):256, 2005.

Olsen AL, Smith VJ, Bergstrom JO, et al: Epidemiology of surgically managed pelvic organ prolapse and urinary incontinence. Obstet Gynecol 89:501, 1997.

Panton ON, Panton RJ: Laparoscopic hernia repair. Am J Surg 167:535, 1994.

Paraiso MF, Ballard LA, Walters MD, et al: Pelvic support defects and visceral and sexual function in women treated with sacrospinous ligament suspension and pelvic reconstruction. Obstet Gynecol 175:1423, 1996.

Paraiso MF, Walters MD, Rackley RR, et al: Laparoscopic and abdominal sacral colpopexies: A comparative cohort study. Am J Obstet Gynecol 192:1752, 2005.

Pasley WW: Sacrospinous suspension: A local practitioner's experience, Am J Obstet Gynecol 173:440, 1995.

Podratz KC, Ferguson LK, Hoverman VR, et al: Abdominal sacral colpopexy for posthysterectomy vaginal vault descensus. J Pelvic Surg 1:18, 1995.

Ramshaw BJ, Tucker JG, Mason EM, et al: A comparison of transabdominal preperitoneal (TAPP) and total extraperitoneal approach (TEPA) laparoscopic herniorrhaphies. Am Surg 61:279, 1995.

Randall CI, Nichols DH: Surgical treatment of vaginal inversion. Obstet Gynecol 38:327, 1971.

Richardson AC: The anatomic defects in rectocele and enterocele. J Pelv Surg 1:214, 1995.

Richter K: Massive eversion of the vagina: Pathogenesis, diagnosis and therapy of the "true" prolapse of the vaginal stump. Clin Obstet Gynecol 25:897, 1982.

Richter K, Albrich W: Long-term results following fixation of the vagina on the sacrospinal ligament by the vaginal root (vaginae fixatio sacrospinalis vaginalis). Am J Obstet Gynecol 141:811, 1981.

Ridley JH: Evaluation of the colpocleisis operation: a report of 58 cases. Am J Obstet Gynecol 113:1114, 1972.

Schlesinger RE: Vaginal sacrospinous ligament fixation with the Autosuture Endostitch device. Am J Obstet Gynecol 176:1358, 1997.

Schwartz SI, Shires GT, Spencer FC, Storer EH: Principles of Surgery, 4th ed. New York, McGraw-Hill, 1984.

Sharp TR: Sacrospinous suspension made easy. Obstet Gynecol 82:873, 1993.

Shull B, Benn SJ, Kuehl TJ: Surgical management of prolapse of the anterior vaginal segment: An analysis of support defects, operative morbidity, and anatomic outcome. Am J Obstet Gynecol 171:429, 1994.

Snyder TE, Krantz KE: Abdominal-retroperitoneal sacral colpopexy for the correction of vaginal prolapse. Obstet Gynecol 77:944, 1991.

Strohbehn K, Jakary JA, Delancey JO: Pelvic organ prolapse in young women. Obstet Gynecol 90:33, 1997.

Subak LL, Waejten LE, van den Eeden S, et al: Cost of pelvic organ prolapse surgery in the United States. Obstet Gynecol 98:646, 2001.

Sweiger M: Method for determining individual contributions of the voluntary and involuntary anal sphincter to resting tone. Dis Colon Rectum 22:415, 1979.

Swift SE: The distribution of pelvic organ support in a population of female subjects seen for routine gynecologic health care. Am J Obstet Gynecol 183:277, 2000.

Symmonds RE: Relaxation of pelvic supports. In Benson RC (ed): Current Obstetric and Gynecologic Diagnosis and Treatment, 5th ed. Los Altos, CA, Lange Medical, 1984.

Symmonds RE, Williams TJ, Lee RA, Webb MJ: Posthysterectomy, enterocele and vaginal vault prolapse. Am J Obstet Gynecol 140:852, 1981.

Sze EHM, Karram MM: Transvaginal repair of vault prolapse: A review. Obstet Gynecol 89:466, 1997.

Sze EHM, Kohli N, Miklos JR, et al: Computed tomography comparison of bony pelvic dimensions between women with and without genital prolapse. Obstet Gynecol 93:229, 1999.

Thakar R, Stanton S: Management of genital prolapse. BMJ 324:1258, 2004.

Thill RH, Hopkins WM: The use of Mersilene mesh in adult inguinal and femoral hernia repairs: A comparison with classic techniques. Am Surg 60:553, 1994.

Thomas AG, Brodman ML, Dottino PR, et al: Manchester procedure vs vaginal hysterectomy for uterine prolapse: A comparison. J Reprod Med 40:299, 1995.

Thornton WN Jr, Peters WA: Repair of vaginal prolapse after hysterectomy. Am J Obstet Gynecol 147:140, 1983.

Tucker JG, Wilson RA, Ramshaw BJ, et al: Laparoscopic herniorrhaphy: Technical concerns in prevention of complications and early recurrence. Am Surg 61:36, 1995.

Valaitis SR, Stanton SL: Sacrocolpopexy: A retrospective study of a clinician's experience. Br J Obstet Gynaecol 101:518, 1994.

Veronikis DK, Nichols DH: Ligature carrier specifically designed for transvaginal sacrospinous colpopexy. Obstet Gynecol 89:478, 1997.

Wake BL, McCormack K, Fraser C, et al: Transabdominal pre-peritoneal (TAPP) vs totally extraperitoneal (TEP) laparoscopic techniques for inguinal hernia repair. Cochrane Database Syst Rev CD004703, 2005.

Webb MJ, Aronson MP, Ferguson LK, Lee RA: Posthysterectomy vaginal vault prolapse: primary repair in 693 patients. Obstet Gynecol 92:281, 1998.

Weber AM, Richter HE: Pelvic organ prolapse. Obstet Gynecol 106:615, 2005.

Weber AM, Walters MD: Anterior vaginal prolapse: Review of anatomy and techniques of surgical repair. Obstet Gynecol 89:311, 1997.

Weber AM, Walters MD, Piedmonte MR: Sexual function and vaginal anatomy in women before and after surgery for pelvic organ prolapse and urinary incontinence. Am J Obstet Gynecol 182:1610, 2000.

Wexner SD, Marchetti F, Jagelman DG: The role of sphincteroplasty for fecal incontinence re-evaluated: A prospective physiologic and functional review. Dis Colon Rectum 34:22, 1991.

White GR: Cystocele. JAMA 853:1707, 1909.

Wilson DE, Noseworthy TW, Grace MG: Caremap management in low-severity surgery: A comparative trial. J Am Coll Surg 181:49, 1995.

Zacharin RF: Pulsion enterocele: review of functional anatomy of the pelvic floor. Obstet Gynecol 55:135, 1980.

Zimmerman LM, Anson BJ: The Anatomy of Surgery of Hernia. Baltimore, Williams & Wilkins, 1953.

FECAL INCONTINENCE

Aronson MP, Lee RA, Berquist TH: Anatomy of anal sphincters and related structures in continent women studied with magnetic resonance imaging. Obstet Gynecol 76:846, 1990.

Baeten CG, Bailey HR, Bakka A, et al: Safety and efficacy of dynamic graciloplasty for fecal incontinence: Report of a prospective, multicenter trial. Dynamic Graciloplasty Therapy Study Group. Dis Colon Rectum 43:743, 2000.

Bartolo DCC, Roe AM, Locke-Edmunds JC, et al: Flap-valve theory of anorectal continence. Br J Surg 73:1012, 1986.

Birnbaum EH, Stamm L, Rafferty JF, et al: Pudendal nerve terminal motor latency influences: surgical outcome in treatment of rectal prolapse. Dis Colon Rectum 39:1215, 1996.

Browning GG, Motson RW: Anal sphincter injury: management and results of Parks sphincter repair. Ann Surg 199:

Burhenne HJ: Intestinal evaluation study: A new roentgenologic technique. Radiol Clin 33:79, 1964.

Burnett SJD, Speakman CTM, Kamm MA, et al: Confirmation of endosonographic detection of external anal sphincter defects by simultaneous electromyographic mapping. Br J Surg 78:448, 1991.

Chen AS, Luchtefeld MA, Senagore AJ, et al: Pudendal nerve latency: Does it predict outcome of anal sphincter repair? Dis Colon Rectum 41:1005, 1998.

Ctercteko GC, Fazio VW, Jagelman DG, et al: Anal sphincter repair: A report of 60 cases and a review of the literature. Aust N Z J Surg 58:703, 1988.

Dhaenes G, Emblem R, Ganes T: Fibre density in idiopathic ano-rectal incontinence. Electromyogr Clin Neurophysiol 35:285, 1995.

Donnelly V, Fynes M, Campbell D, et al: Obstetric events leading to anal sphincter damage. Obstet Gynecol 92:955, 1998.

Eason E, Labrecque M, Wells G, Feldman P: Preventing perineal trauma during childbirth: A systematic review. Obstet Gynecol 95:464, 2000.

Engel AF, Kamm MA, Sultan AH, et al: Anterior anal sphincter repair in patients with obstetric trauma. Br J Surg 81:1231, 1994.

Fang DT, Nivatvongs S, Vermeulen FD, et al: Overlapping sphincteroplasty for acquired anal incontinence. Dis Colon Rectum 27:720, 1984.

Felt-Bersma RJ, Cuesta MA, Koorevaar M: Anal sphincter repair improves anorectal function and endosonographic image: A prospective clinical study. Dis Colon Rectum 39:878, 1996.

Fenner DE, Kriegshauser JS, Lee HH, et al: Anatomic and physiologic measurements of the internal and external anal sphincters in normal females. Obstet Gynecol 91:369, 1998.

Fitzpatrick M, Behan M, O'Connell PR, O'Herlihy C: A randomized clinical trial comparing primary overlap with approximation repair of third-degree obstetric tears. Am J Obstet Gynecol 183:1220, 2000.

Fitzpatrick M, Fynes M, Cassidy, et al: Prospective study of the influence of parity and operative technique on the outcome of primary anal sphincter repair following obstetrical injury. Eur J Obstet Gynecol Reprod Biol 89:159, 2000.

Fleshman JW, Dreznik Z, Fry RD, Kodner IJ: Anal sphincter repair for obstetric injury: Manometric evaluation of functional results. Dis Colon Rectum 34:1061, 1991.

Fleshman JW, Peters WR, Shemesh EI, et al: Anal sphincter reconstruction: Anterior overlapping muscle repair. Dis Colon Rectum 34:739, 1991.

Fynes MM, Donnelly V, Behan M, et al: Effect of second vaginal delivery on anorectal physiology and faecal incontinence: A prospective study. Lancet 354:983, 1999.

Gilliland R, Altomare DF, Moreira H Jr, et al: Pudendal neuropathy is predictive of failure following anterior overlapping sphincteroplasty. Dis Colon Rectum 41:1516, 1998.

Gosling JA, Dixson JS, Critchley HD, Thompson SA: A comparative study of the human external sphincter and periurethral levator ani muscles. Br J Urol 53:35, 1981.

Henry MM, Parks AG, Swash M: The pelvic floor musculature in the descending perineum syndrome. Br J Surg 69:470, 1982.

Howard D, DeLancey JO, Burney RE: Fistula-in-ano after episiotomy. Obstet Gynecol 93:800, 1999.

Jacobs PPM, Scheuer M, Kuijpers JHC, Vingerhoets MH: Obstetric fecal incontinence: Role of pelvic floor denervation and results of delayed sphincter repair. Dis Colon Rectum 33:494, 1990.

Jarrett ME, Mowatt G, Glazener CM, et al: Systematic review of sacral nerve stimulation for faecal incontinence and constipation. Br J Surg 91:1559, 2004.

Jensen LL, Lowry AC: Biofeedback: A viable treatment option for anal incontinence. Dis Colon Rectum 34:(Suppl)P6. Abstract, 1991.

Jones IT, Fazio VW, Jagelman DG: The use of transanal rectal advancement flaps in the management of fistulas involving the anorectum. Dis Colon Rectum 30:919, 1987.

Keating JP, Stewart PJ, Eyers AA, et al: Are special investigations of value in the management of patients with fecal incontinence? Dis Colon Rectum 40:896, 1997.

Khullar V, Damiano R, Toozs-Hobson P, Cardozo L: Prevalence of faecal incontinence among women with urinary incontinence. Br J Obstet and Gynaecol 105:1211, 1998.

Kiff ES, Barnes PRH, Swash M: Evidence of pudendal neuropathy in patients with perineal descent and chronic straining at stool. Gut 25:1279, 1984.

Kiff ES, Swash M: Slowed conduction in the pudendal nerves in idiopathic (neurogenic) faecal incontinence. Br J Surg 71:614, 1984.

Laurberg S, Swash M, Henry MM: Delayed external sphincter repair for obstetric tear. Br J Surg 75:786, 1988.

Law PJ, Kamm MA, Bartram CI: A comparison between electromyography and anal endosonography in mapping external anal sphincter defects. Dis Colon Rectum 33:370, 1990.

Leigh RJ, Turnberg LA: Faecal incontinence: The unvoided symptom. Lancet 1:1349, 1982.

Londono-Schimmer EE, Garcia-Duperly R, Nicholls RJ, et al: Overlapping anal sphincter repair for faecal incontinence due to sphincter trauma: Five year follow-up functional results. Int J Colorectal Dis 9:110, 1994.

MacArthur C, Bick DE, Keighley MRB: Faecal incontinence after childbirth. Br J Obstet Gynaecol 104:46, 1997.

Madoff RD, Baeten CGMI, Christiansen J, et al: Standards for anal sphincter replacement. Dis Colon Rectum 43:135, 2000.

Madoff RD, Williams JG, Caushaj PF: Fecal incontinence. N Engl J Med 326:1002, 1992.

Miller R, Orrom WJ, Cornes H, et al: Anterior sphincter plication and levatorplasty in the treatment of faecal incontinence. Br J Surg 75:1058, 1989.

Muller C, Belyaev O, Deska T, et al: Fecal incontinence: An up-to-date critical overview of surgical treatment options. Langenbecks Arch Surg 390:544, 2005.

Neill ME, Parks AG, Swash M: Physiological studies of the anal sphincter musculature in faecal incontinence and rectal prolapse. Br J Surg 68:531, 1981.

Neill ME, Swash M: Increased motor unit fibre density in the external anal sphincter muscle in anorectal incontinence: A single fibre EMG study. J Neurol Neurosurg Psychiatry 43:343, 1980.

Nelson R, Norton N, Cautley E, Furner S: Community-based prevalence of anal incontinence. JAMA 274:559, 1995.

Nikiteas N, Korsgen S, Kumar D, Keighley MR: Audit of sphincter repair: factors associated with poor outcome. Dis Colon Rectum 39:1164, 1996.

Obstetrics and gynecology clinics of North America: Bump RC, Cardiff GW (eds): Urogynecology and Pelvic Floor Dysfunction. Philadelphia, WB Saunders, 1998, p. 25.

Oliverira L, Pfeifer J, Wexner SD: Physiological and clinical outcome of anterior sphincteroplasty. Br J Surg 83:502, 1996.

Parks AG: Anorectal incontinence. Proc R Soc Med 68:681, 1975.

Parks AG, Swash M, Urich H: Sphincter denervation in anorectal incontinence and rectal prolapse. Gut 18:656, 1977.

Pescatori M, Anastasio G, Bottini C, Mentasti A: New grading and scoring for anal incontinence: Evaluation of 335 patients. Dis Colon Rectum 35:482, 1992.

Pickrell KL, Broadbent IR, Masters FW, Metzger JT: Constitution of a rectal sphincter and restoration of anal incontinence by transplanting the gracilis muscle. A report of four cases in children. Ann Surg 135:853, 1952.

Rasmussen OO, Puggaard L, Christiansen J: Anal sphincter repair in patients with obstetric trauma: Age affects outcome. Dis Colon Rectum 42:193, 1999.

Rieger NA, Schloithe A, Saccone G, Wattchow D: A prospective study of anal sphincter injury due to childbirth. Scand J Gastroenterol 33:950, 1998.

Rieger NA, Wattchow DA, Sarre RG, et al: Prospective trial of pelvic floor retraining in patients with fecal incontinence. Dis Colon Rectum 40:821, 1997.

Ryhammer AM, Bek KM, Laurberg S: Multiple vaginal deliveries increase the risk of permanent incontinence of flatus and urine in normal premenopausal women. Dis Colon Rectum 38:1206, 1995.

Sagar PN, Pemberton JH: Anorectal and pelvic floor function. Relevance of continence, incontinence, and constipation. Gastroenterol Clin North Am 25:163, 1996.

Signorello LB, Harlow BL, Chekos AK, Repke JT: Midline episiotomy and anal incontinence: retrospective cohort study. BMJ 320:86, 2000.

Simmang C, Birnbaum EH, Kodner IJ, et al: Anal sphincter reconstruction in the elderly: Does advancing age affect outcome? Dis Colon Rectum 37:1065, 1994.

Sitzler PJ, Thomson JP: Overlap repair of damaged anal sphincter: A single surgeon's series. Dis Colon Rectum 398:1356, 1996.

Smith ARB, Hosker GL, Warrell DW: The role of partial denervation of the pelvic floor in the aetiology of genitourinary prolapse and stress incontinence of urine: A neurophysiological study. Br J Obstet Gynaecol 96:24, 1989.

Snooks SJ, Swash M: Abnormalities of the innervation of the urethral striated sphincter in incontinence. Br J Urol 56:401, 1984.

Snooks SJ, Barnes PRH, Swash M: Damage to the innervation of the voluntary anal and periurethral sphincter musculature in incontinence: An electrophysiological study. J Neurol Neurosurg Psychiatry 47:1269, 1984.

Sultan AH, Kamm MA, Hudson CN, et al: Anal-sphincter disruption during vaginal delivery. N Engl J Med 329:1905, 1993.

Sultan AH, Nugent K: Pathophysiology and nonsurgical treatment of anal incontinence. Br J Obstet Gynaecol Suppl 1:84, 2004.

Swash M: Histopathology of pelvic floor muscles. In Henry MM, Swash M (eds): Coloproctology and the Pelvic Floor. London, Butterworths, 1985, p. 129.

Swash M, Snooks SJ, Henry MM: Unifying concept of pelvic floor disorders and incontinence. J R Soc Med 78:906, 1985.

Sweiger M: Method for determining individual contributions of voluntary and involuntary anal sphincters to resting tone. Dis Colon Rectum 22:415, 1979.

Taverner D, Smiddy FG: An electromyographic study of the normal function of the external anal sphincter and pelvic diaphragm. Dis Colon Rectum 2:153, 1959.

Tetzschner T, Sorensen M, Rasmussen OO, et al: Pudendal nerve damage increases the risk of fecal incontinence in women with anal sphincter rupture after childbirth. Acta Obstet Gynaecol Scand 74:434, 1995.

Toglia MR: Anal incontinence: An under recognized, under treated problem. Female Patient 21:27, 1996.

Toglia MR, DeLancey JOL: Anal incontinence and the obstetrician-gynecologist. Obstet Gynecol 84:731, 1994.

Varma A, Gunn J, Gardiner A, et al: Obstetric anal sphincter injury: Prospective evaluation of incidence. Dis Colon Rectum 42:1537, 1999.

Varma A, Gunn J, Lindow S, Duthie GS: Do routinely measured delivery variables predict anal sphincter outcome? Dis Colon Rectum 42:1261, 1999.

Venkatesh KS, Ramanujham PS, Larson DM, Haywood MA: Anorectal complications of vaginal delivery. Dis Colon Rectum 32:1039, 1989.

Wexner JJM: Etiology and management of fecal incontinence. Dis Colon Rectum 36:77, 1993.

Wexner SD, Marchett F, Jagelman DG: The role of sphincteroplasty for fecal incontinence reevaluated: A prospective physiologic and functional review. Dis Colon Rectum 34:22, 1991.

Womack NRT, Morrison JFB, Williams NS: Prospective study of the effects of postnatal repair in neurogenic faecal incontinence. Br J Surg 7:52, 1988.
Wong WD, Jensen LL, Bortolo DC, Rothenberger DA: Artificial anal sphincter. Dis Colon Rectum 39:1345, 1996.
Wunderlich M, Swash M: The overlapping innervation of the two sites of the external anal sphincter by the pudendal nerves. J Neurol Sci 5:109, 1983.
Yoshioka K, Keighley MR: Sphincter repair for fecal incontinence. Dis Colon Rectum 32:39, 1989.
Zetterstrom J, Lopez A, Norman M, et al: Anal sphincter tears at vaginal delivery: Risk factors and clinical outcome of primary repair. Obstet Gynecol 94:21, 1999.
Zetterstrom J, Mellgren A, Jensen LL, et al: Effect of delivery on anal sphincter morphology and function. Dis Colon Rectum 42:1253, 1999.

Urogynecology

21

Physiology of Micturition, Diagnosis of Voiding Dysfunction, and Incontinence: Surgical and Nonsurgical Treatment

Gretchen M. Lentz

KEY TERMS AND DEFINITIONS

Abdominal Leak Point Pressure. A test that measures the intravesical pressure necessary to overcome urethral resistance (urinary leakage) under increased abdominal pressure in the absence of a detrusor contraction.

Biofeedback. Information about a normally unconscious physiologic process presented to the patient or therapist as a visual, auditory, or tactile signal.

Chronic Retention of Urine. A nonpainful bladder, which remains palpable or percussable after the patient has passed urine.

Cystometry. Describes part of the urodynamic investigation assessing the filling phase of micturition.

Detrusor Overactivity Incontinence. Involuntary contraction of the bladder during bladder filling that is associated with urgency and leads to urine leakage.

Detrusor Pressure. Component of intravesical pressure created by forces in the bladder wall.

Extraurethral Incontinence. The loss of urine through channels other than the urethra.

Filling Cystometry. Method for measuring pressure–volume relationships of the bladder during filling.

Flow Rate. Volume of urine expelled via the urethra per unit time, expressed in milliliters.

Incontinence. The complaint of any involuntary loss of urine.

Interstitial Cystitis. A complex inflammatory condition of the bladder of poorly understood etiology and pathophysiology that is usually associated with altered epithelial permeability, mast cell activation, and an up-regulation of secondary afferent nerves. Falls under the global definition of painful bladder syndrome.

Intra-abdominal Pressure. Pressure surrounding the bladder.

Intravesical Pressure. Pressure within the bladder.

Intrinsic Sphincter Dysfunction. A form of stress urinary incontinence in which the defect is defined arbitrarily by a low urethral closure pressure or low Valsalva leak point pressure.

Kegel Exercises. Isometric contractions of the pubococcygeus muscles to improve control of continence.

Mixed Urinary Incontinence. The complaint of involuntary leakage associated with urgency and also with exertion, effort, sneezing, or coughing.

Osteitis Pubis. An inflammation of the periosteum of the pubic bone, often occurring after suprapubic urethral suspension procedures.

Osteomyelitis Pubis. An infection of the pubic bone, which may occur after pelvic operations.

Overactive Bladder. The symptom of urgency with or without incontinence usually with frequency and nocturia.

Painful Bladder Syndrome. A complaint of suprapubic pain related to bladder filling accompanied by other symptoms such as increased daytime and nighttime frequency, in the absence of proven urinary infection or other obvious pathology.

Pelvic Floor Training. Repetitive selective voluntary contraction and relaxation of specific pelvic floor muscles.

Reflex Incontinence. The involuntary loss of urine caused by abnormal reflex activity in the spinal cord in the absence of the sensation that is usually associated with the desire to micturate.

Residual Urine. Volume of urine remaining in the bladder immediately after completion of micturition.

Stress Urinary Incontinence. The symptom of involuntary urinary leakage on exertion or effort such as coughing, straining, exercising, or sneezing.

Trigone (Bladder). The area of the floor of the urinary bladder that forms a triangle with the urethral opening at the apex and the ureteral openings at the ends of the base.

Urethral Closure Pressure Profile. Subtraction of intravesical pressure from urethral pressure.

Urethral Pressure Profile. Intraluminal pressure along the length of the urethra with the bladder at rest.

Urethral Syndrome. An ill-defined inflammatory condition of the urethra in which bacterial cultures are found to be negative. In some cases, *Chlamydia* can be cultured.

Urge Urinary Incontinence. The involuntary loss of urine associated with a strong desire to void (urgency).

Urgency. The complaint of a sudden compelling desire to pass urine, which is difficult to defer.

Urodynamic Stress Incontinence. Condition of immediate involuntary loss of urine when intravesical pressure exceeds the maximum urethral pressure in the absence of detrusor activity. Replaces the term *genuine stress incontinence.*

The gynecologist frequently consults on and treats urologic problems in the female patient. Perhaps the most commonly seen of these problems involves infection and inflammation of the lower tract (urethritis and cystitis). However, many women suffer from some degree of urinary incontinence. In a telephone interview study of 851 women ages 18 and older selected at random in Australia, 267 (31%) stated that they had noted some degree of incontinence during the preceding 12 months, and 142 (12%) suffered two or more regular episodes of leakage per month. Daily incontinence was reported by 5%, and 2.3% were incontinent often or continuously.

This condition increases in incidence with age, and because the number of older women in our population is growing, it is likely that this problem will grow in magnitude with time. At a conference of the National Association of Retired People, Teasdale and colleagues learned (by questionnaire) that 33% of the total responders experienced some form of urinary incontinence. Women accounted for 75% of the respondents, representing 168 individuals. Of these, 118 complained of dribbling, 13 of spontaneous large losses of urine, and 37 of both dribbling and large losses. Of women older than age 60 who are not institutionalized, 15% to 30% report experiencing incontinence, with 25% to 30% of these reporting frequent episodes. Among older adults, only about 38% of women actually discuss incontinence with a physician.

Continence depends on a number of factors, including the neurologic control of micturition, the anatomic relationships of the urinary tract, and the specific effects of a number of systemic, infectious, and neoplastic conditions. This chapter considers the physiology of micturition and the diagnosis and treatment of pathologic entities that affect the female urologic system, and it offers suggestions on diagnosis and management of urinary incontinence.

PHYSIOLOGY OF MICTURITION

A number of factors are in play to maintain continence. The central nervous system (CNS) coordinates function of the lower urinary system through complex neural pathways. Basically these involve those that maintain a urethral closure mechanism and those that affect detrusor function. In the final analysis it is the balance between urethral closure and detrusor function that determines whether micturition occurs or continence is maintained.

The factors affecting the urethral closure mechanism primarily involve urethral tone and include the basic elasticity of the urethra, the presence of smooth and voluntary (striated) muscle, the vascular component supplying the urethra, and the presence of α receptors from the sympathetic nervous system, which when stimulated cause contraction of the urethral sphincter.

Bladder detrusor contractility is stimulated by the activity of the parasympathetic nervous system mediated through the neurotransmitter acetylcholine. This stimulates receptors in the bladder wall, which then activate detrusor contraction. Sympathetic nervous system β receptors within the bladder cause bladder relaxation when stimulated. Bladder contraction may also be affected by irritation and inflammation of the bladder wall, causing uncoordinated contractions.

The act of voiding is under the control of four basic autonomic and somatic nervous system feedback loops. The first loop (loop I) involves a circuit from the cerebral cortex to the brainstem, which inhibits micturition by modifying sensory stimuli emanating from loop II. Loop II, which originates in the sacral micturition center (S2 through S4) and the detrusor muscle wall itself, represents sensory fibers to the brainstem, where modulation of the stimuli by loop I takes place. If cerebral inhibition is not imposed (loop I), the stimuli are returned to the sacral micturition center as a response to the bladder filling, allowing activation of loop III. Loop III involves sensory flow from the bladder wall to the sacral micturition center with returning motor fibers to the urethral sphincter striated muscle, which allows the voluntary relaxation of the urethral sphincter as the detrusor contracts. Loop IV originates in the frontal lobe of the cerebral cortex and runs to the sacral micturition center and then to the urethral striated muscle, allowing urethral voluntary muscles to relax, and thus leading to the initiation of voiding. Figure 21-1 demonstrates these four loops as visualized by Williams and Pannill. Table 21-1 summarizes the important aspects of each loop as reviewed by Ostergard.

Both the parasympathetic and sympathetic nervous systems function with the CNS in these feedback loops via the pontine micturition center. Basically, the parasympathetic system is involved in the act of voiding via nuclei in S2 through S4 (micturition center). As mentioned earlier, the parasympathetic

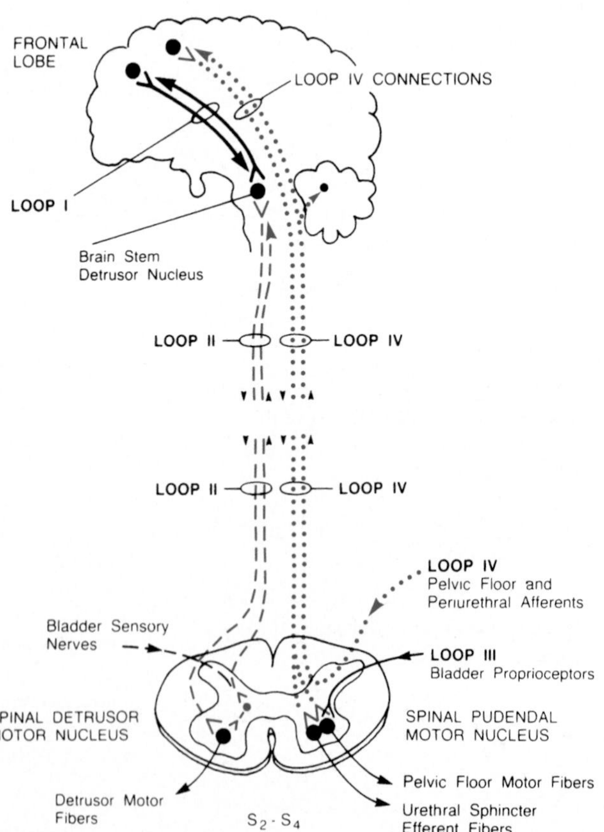

Figure 21-1. Central nervous system feedback loops. (From Williams ME, Pannill FC 3rd: Urinary incontinence in the elderly: Physiology, pathophysiology, diagnosis, and treatment. Ann Intern Med 97:895, 1982.)

Table 21-1 Neurologic Control of Micturition: Clinical Considerations on Central Nervous System Reflex Loops

Loop	Origin	Termination	Function	Associated Conditions
I	Frontal lobe	Brainstem	Coordinates volitional control of micturition	Parkinson's disease, brain tumors, trauma, cerebrovascular disease, MS, lower urinary tract disease
II	A. Brainstem B. Bladder wall	Sacral micturition center Brainstem	Detrusor muscle contraction to empty bladder	Spinal cord trauma, MS, spinal cord tumors
III	Sensory afferents of detrusor muscle	Striated muscle of urethral sphincter via pudendal motor neurons and sacral micturition center	Allows relaxation of urethral sphincter in synchrony with detrusor contraction	MS, spinal cord trauma or tumors, diabetic neuropathy, local urinary tract disease
IV	Frontal lobe	Pudendal nucleus	Volitional control of striated external urethral sphincter	Cerebral or spinal trauma or tumor, MS, cerebrovascular disease, lower urinary tract disease

MS, multiple sclerosis.
Modified from Ostergard DR: The neurological control of micturition and integral voiding reflexes. Obstet Gynecol Surv 34:417, 1979.

system mediates its activity through the neurotransmitter acetylcholine, directly stimulating muscarinic receptors in the bladder wall. This signal is transmitted via the pelvic nerve and causes the detrusor to contract. At the same time, the pontine micturition center (PMC) in the brain inhibits the sympathetic pathway as well as the somatic pathway to the urethra. This allows the urethra to relax so coordinated voiding can occur. The sympathetic system, on the other hand, basically acts to prevent micturition. Via this system norepinephrine is secreted, stimulating both α- and β-adrenergic receptors. The bladder contains primarily β receptors, stimulation of which causes relaxation of the detrusor muscle. The urethra contains primarily α receptors. Stimulation of these α receptors causes contraction of the urethral sphincter. Thus the overall effect is to prevent micturition (Fig. 21-2). Estrogen and progesterone receptors are present in the bladder and urethra although their role in affecting continence has not been fully elucidated. Many other neurotransmitters and receptors have been identified in the lower urinary tract, including dopamine, serotonin, nitric oxide, γ-aminobutyric acid (GABA), glutamine, and ATP.

Because the neurogenic control of micturition is so complex and depends on the interaction of so many factors, it is understandable that a host of general systemic diseases or diseases involving the nervous system may affect bladder control. These

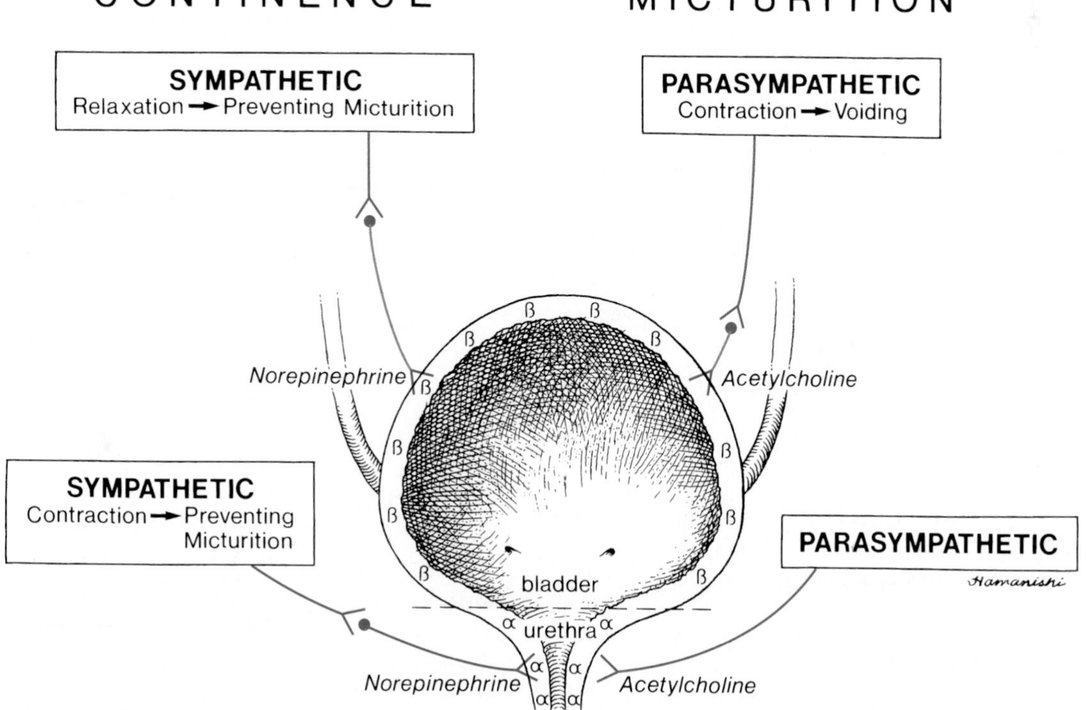

Figure 21-2. The innervation of the bladder and urethra. Parasympathetic fibers arising in S2 through S4 have long preganglionic fibers and pelvic ganglia close to the bladder and urethra. These parasympathetic fibers excrete acetylcholine. Sympathetic fibers that have long postganglionic fibers discharge norepinephrine to β receptors, primarily in the bladder, and α receptors, primarily in the urethra. (Redrawn and modified from Raz S: Pharmacological treatment of lower urinary tract dysfunction. Urol Clin North Am 5:323, 1978.)

Table 21-2 Some Common Drugs That Affect Continence and Micturition (See Appendix for Additional Information)

Drug	Action
Sympathetic (relaxes bladder; controls urethral sphincter)	
Dopamine	α-Adrenergic stimulator
Ethylphenylephrine	α-Adrenergic stimulator
Methamphetamine	α-Adrenergic stimulator
Norepinephrine	α-Adrenergic stimulator
Phenylephrine	α-Adrenergic stimulator
Albuterol	β-Adrenergic stimulator
Ethylnorepinephrine	β-Adrenergic stimulator
Isoproterenol	β-Adrenergic stimulator
Methoxyphenamine	β-Adrenergic stimulator
Terbutaline	β-Adrenergic stimulator
Parasympathetic (stimulates bladder contraction; relaxes urethral sphincter)	
Pilocarpine	Stimulates acetylcholine
Pralidoxime	Stimulates acetylcholine
Pyridostigmine	Stimulates acetylcholine
Sympathetic Blockers	
Guanethidine	Adrenergic blocker
Hydralazine	Adrenergic blocker
Methyldopa	Adrenergic blocker
Reserpine	Adrenergic blocker
Parasympathetic Blockers	
Anisotropine	Parasympathetic inhibitor
Atropine	Parasympathetic inhibitor
Clidinium	Parasympathetic inhibitor
Homatropine	Parasympathetic inhibitor
Papaverine	Parasympathetic inhibitor
Scopolamine	Parasympathetic inhibitor

include, but are not limited to, demyelinating diseases (such as multiple sclerosis), diabetes mellitus, vascular diseases, and CNS trauma and tumors. In addition, medications that have an effect on the CNS or autonomic nervous systems may affect bladder control. Compounds with atropine-like effects may interfere with the initiation of micturition, whereas those with cholinergic effects may cause bladder irritability (Table 21-2). An appendix at the end of this chapter contains an exhaustive list developed by Ostergard of agents that affect bladder function.

With the neurologic principles of micturition in mind, it is appropriate to assess other factors that may influence continence. Asmussen and Ulmsten noted that the bladder and the urethra are essentially a functional unit, with the bladder's subfunction to store urine and the urethra's to allow it to pass. For urine to pass through the urethra, the maximum urethral pressure must be lower than the intravesical pressure. Intravesical pressure depends on (1) the volume of fluid in the bladder, (2) the part of the intraabdominal pressure transmitted to the bladder, and (3) the tension in the bladder wall related to muscular and nervous system activity. The resting pressure in the bladder is between 20 and 30 cm H_2O.

The intraurethral pressure depends on (1) the striated muscle fibers of the urethral wall, (2) smooth muscle fibers of the urethral wall, (3) the vascular content of the urethral submucosal cavernous plexus, (4) the passive elasticity of the urethral wall, and (5) the part of the intraabdominal pressure transmitted to the urethra.

Anatomically, the exact border between the bladder and urethra is difficult to determine. The functional length of the urethra, however, is that part in which the urethral pressure exceeds the bladder pressure. Asmussen and Ulmsten have noted that the urethral closure pressure (UCP) is defined as the maximum urethral pressure minus the bladder pressure. For continence to be present the UCP must be greater than the bladder pressure. Urethral pressure varies with age, increasing up to the age of 20 and then gradually decreasing until menopause. However, after menopause the fall of this pressure is more rapid. Asmussen and Ulmsten have demonstrated that the highest pressure zone in the urethra is about midpoint in the functional urethral length, and Westby and coworkers have located this zone at about 0.5 cm proximal to the urogenital diaphragm. Most of the functional urethral length is, indeed, above the urogenital diaphragm (Fig. 21-3). Asmussen and Ulmsten and Gosling and associates have pointed out that the submucosal cavernous plexus of vessels, the bulk of the smooth and striated muscle, and the bulk of the autonomic nerve supply are most prominent in the area in which they record the maximum urethral pressure. Because the urethral pressure displays high-pressure zone oscillations that are synchronous with the heartbeat, the submucosal cavernous plexus is probably important in helping to maintain continence (Fig. 21-4). Indeed, this structure is under the control of estrogen. Enhorning and also Asmussen and Ulmsten have demonstrated that urethral pressure can

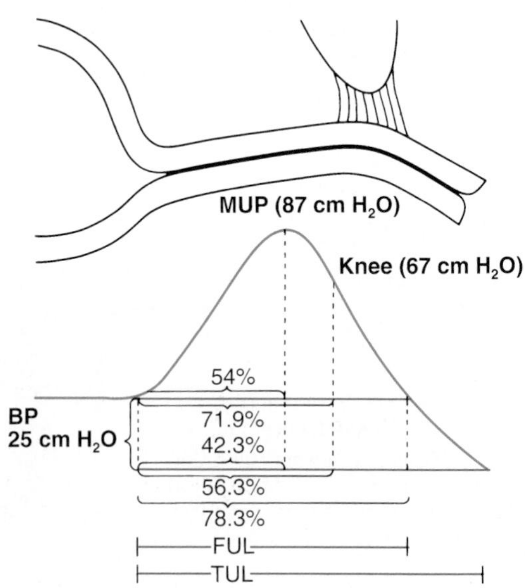

Figure 21-3. The location of maximum urethral pressure in relation to the urogenital diaphragm (average value of 25 normal women). Knee indicates the location of the urogenital diaphragm seen on X-ray film and transformed to the pressure curve. BP, blood pressure; MUP, maximal urethral pressure. (From Asmussen M, Ulmsten U: On the physiology of continence and pathophysiology of stress incontinence in the female. In Controversies in Gynecology and Obstetrics, Vol 10. Basel, Karger, 1983, pp 32–50.)

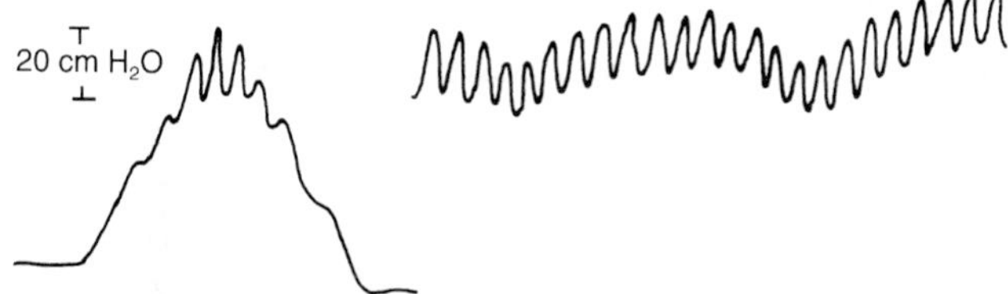

Figure 21-4. The maximum urethral pressure shows great variation synchronously with the heartbeat. Variations of 20 cm H_2O as shown in the curve are not uncommon. (From Asmussen M, Ulmsten U: On the physiology of continence and pathophysiology of stress incontinence in the female. In Controversies in Gynecology and Obstetrics, Vol 10. Basel, Karger, 1983, pp 32–50.)

oscillate as much as 25 cm H_2O in young women but seldom more than 5 cm H_2O in postmenopausal women. The cavernous plexus is thicker walled and less elastic in older women. Thus, not only is the epithelium of the bladder and the bladder neck dependent on hormone stimulation, but so probably is the vascular system of these areas.

Because the maximum urethral pressure area under normal circumstances lies above the urogenital diaphragm and because intraabdominal pressure likely affects both the bladder and this area of the urethra equally, if normal anatomic relationships are maintained, a sudden intraabdominal pressure increase should not, under normal circumstances, cause incontinence. On the other hand, if the functional urethra is displaced from its usual anatomic relationships, it may be excluded from the effect of increased intraabdominal pressure and therefore is susceptible to it. This problem will be addressed further in the discussion of stress incontinence.

DeLancey made some interesting observations on functioning periurethral anatomy by studying serial histologic sections of intact pelvic viscera and surrounding tissue, as well as by dissecting 22 fresh and embalmed cadavers. Because the length of the urethra varies from woman to woman, topography of urethral and paraurethral structures was expressed in terms of the location along the urethra using percentages of the total urethra. DeLancey considered the zero location as that point in which the urethra leaves the bladder lumen and the 100th percentile as that point in which the urethra terminates on the perineum. From the standpoint of functional anatomy there is excellent agreement among the measurements made from each of his specimens when percentiles were used. Table 21-3 depicts these anatomic relationships. It can be seen that the intramural urethra represents approximately 20% of the length of the urethra. The portion of the urethra encircled by striated urethral sphincter muscle and associated with the pubourethral ligament and vaginal levator attachment concerns the midurethra, that is, that portion which is from the 20th to 60th percentile along the total length. The 60th to 80th percentile of the urethral length passes through the urogenital diaphragm and is under the influence of the urethrovaginal sphincter muscles. Finally, the last 20%, or distal urethra, traverses the bulbocavernosus muscles. These urethral landmarks are depicted in Figure 21-5, which highlights the actual ranges and values found in DeLancey's study. The actual anatomic relationships are depicted in Figure 21-6. DeLancey's observations help to correlate the anatomic relationships to the physiologic observations that others have made.

Table 21-3 Topography of Urethral and Paraurethral Structures*

Approximate Location†	Region of the Urethra	Paraurethral Structures
0–20	Intramural urethra	Urethral lumen traverses the bladder wall
20–60	Midurethra	Striated urethral sphincter muscle Pubourethral ligament Vaginolevator attachment
60–80	Urogenital diaphragm	Compressor urethrae muscle Urethrovaginal sphincter muscle
80–100	Distal urethra	Bulbocavernosus muscle

*Smooth muscle of the urethra was not considered.
†Expressed as a percentile of total urethral length.
From DeLancey JOL: Correlative study of paraurethral anatomy. Obstet Gynecol 68:91, 1986. Reprinted with permission from The American College of Obstetricians and Gynecologists.

In a subsequent paper, DeLancey pointed out that additional anatomic factors might influence continence. Using serial histologic sections from 8 female cadavers and the dissections of 34 other cadavers, he noted that the proximal urethra gets added support because the anterior vagina is attached to the muscles of the pelvic diaphragm and to the arcus tendineus fasciae pelvis. Contraction of the pelvic diaphragm thus pulls the vagina against the posterior surface of the urethra, helping to close it. At rest the urethra is supported by both its attachment to the arcus tendineus fasciae pelvis and the tone of the pelvic diaphragm muscles. Two striated muscle arches, the compressor urethrae and urethrovaginal sphincter support the distal urethra in the region of the urogenital diaphragm. These muscles help to compress the distal urethra, helping to maintain continence during a cough. Collagen is extremely important in maintaining the strength of the support structures of the urethra and the vagina. Estrogen contributes directly to collagen synthesis and therefore may play a role in this aspect of continence.

The U.S. Department of Health and Human Services, Agency for Health Care Policy and Research published a clinical practice guideline on urinary incontinence in adults. The following box lists the currently known risk factors that are associated with incontinence, summarizing the work of several authors. Most of these have been alluded to in this chapter, but a few warrant specific mention. Bump and McClish compared risk factors and determinants of urodynamic stress incontinence between smokers and nonsmokers using a case-control method. Seventy-one smokers and 118 nonsmokers were compared following a complete urogynecologic evaluation. Smokers were found to have stronger urethral sphincters and generated greater increase in bladder pressure with coughing but had similar findings with respect to urethral mobility and pressure transmission ratios when compared with nonsmokers. Urodynamic stress incontinence developed in smokers despite their stronger urethral sphincter findings, probably due to more violent coughing leading to earlier development of anatomic and pressure transmission defects.

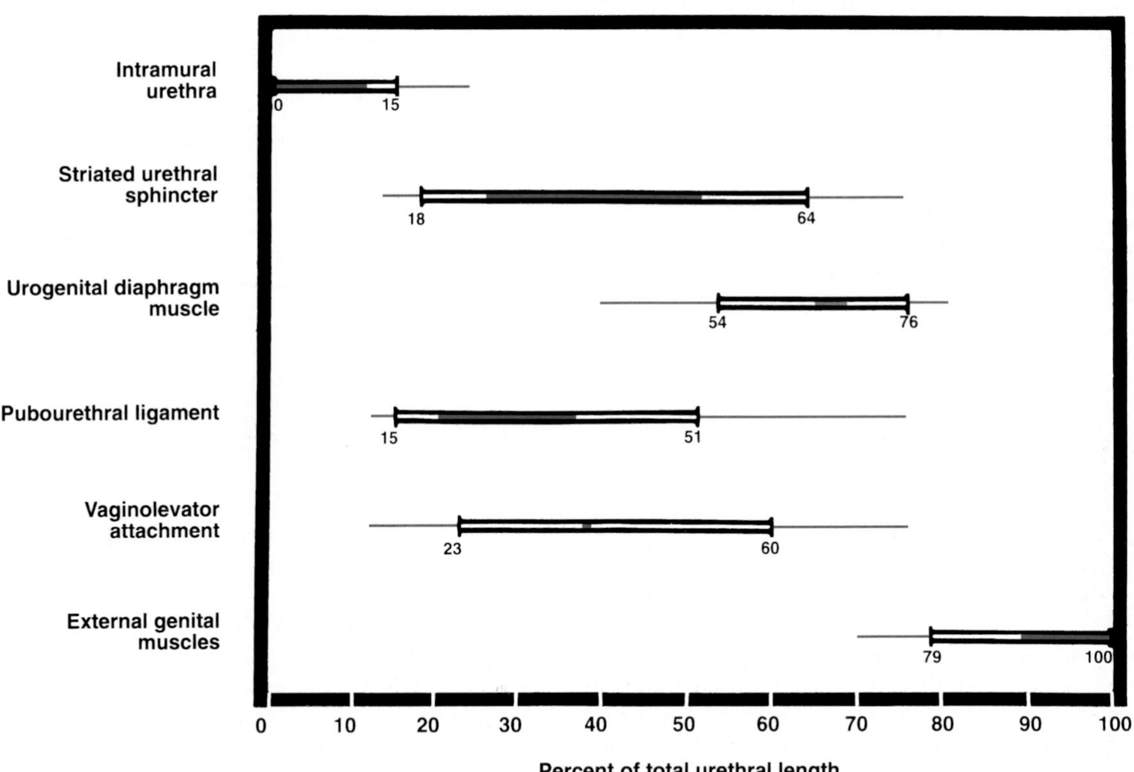

Figure 21-5. Average spatial distribution of paraurethral structures, as well as the range of values found. Urogenital diaphragm muscles are the compressor urethrae and urethrovaginal sphincter. (From DeLancey JOL: Correlative study of paraurethral anatomy. Obstet Gynecol 68:91, 1986. Reprinted with permission from The American College of Obstetricians and Gynecologists.)

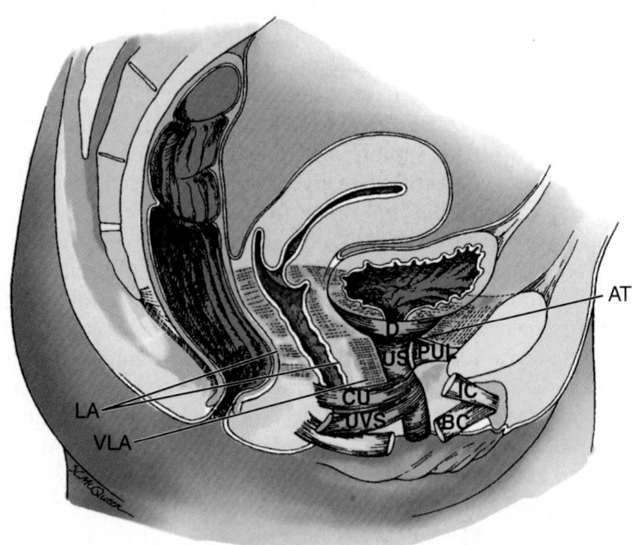

Figure 21-6. Interrelationships of approximate location of paraurethral structures. Levator ani muscles are shown as light lines running deep to the pelvic viscera. The vaginal levator attachment is shown as a darker area. AT, arcus tendineus fasciae pelvis; BC, bulbocavernosus muscle; CU, compressor urethrae; D, detrusor muscle; IC, ischiocavernosus muscle; LA, levator ani muscles; PUL, pubourethral ligament; US, urethral sphincter; UVS, urethrovaginal sphincter; and VLA, vaginal levator attachment. (Redrawn from DeLancey JOL: Correlative study of paraurethral anatomy. Obstet Gynecol 68:91, 1986. Reproduced with permission from The American College of Obstetricians and Gynecologists.)

A second area of interest involves racial differences with respect to the presence of urinary incontinence and other pelvic relaxation problems. Bump pointed out that black women with urinary incontinence have a different distribution of symptoms and have different reasons for their incontinence than do white women. The black women had a significantly lower prevalence of pure urodynamic stress incontinence than did the white women. These conclusions were based on a study of 200 consecutive women, 54 of whom were black, referred for evaluation of urinary stress incontinence or pelvic organ prolapse. The findings may possibly relate to a difference in collagen and connective tissue in individuals of the two races.

DIAGNOSTIC PROCEDURES

The clinical history is quite useful in the diagnosis of urinary incontinence. Several validated scales are available such as the Urogenital Distress Inventory (UDI), Incontinence Impact Questionnaire (IIQ), Bristol Female Lower Urinary Tract Questionnaire and King's Health Questionnaire although one has not become the preferred instrument. Useful testing can be done in the gynecologist's office without the need for sophisticated equipment. These procedures are described next and their benefits noted. Their description is followed by a discussion of more sophisticated diagnostic techniques requiring specialized equipment.

Factors Independently Associated with Urinary Incontinence in Women

Modifiable Factors	
Gynecologic	**Medications**
Cystocele	Diuretics
Uterine prolapse	Estrogen
Nonnormal gynecologic examination	Benzodiazepines
	Tranquilizers
Poor pelvic floor muscle contraction	Antidepressants
	Hypnotics
	Laxatives
Urologic and Gastrointestinal	Antibiotics
Recurrent urinary tract infections	
Dysuria	**Smoking**
Fecal incontinence	
Constipation	**High caffeine intake**
Bowel problems	
	Higher body mass index
Comorbid Diseases	
Diabetes	**Functional impairment**
Stroke	
Elevated systolic blood pressure	
Cognitive impairment	
Parkinsonism	
Arthritis	
Back problems	
Hearing and visual impairment	
Nonmodifiable Factors	
Gynecologic Factors	
Hysterectomy in older women	**Age**
Prolapse surgery	
	White race
Pregnancy-Related Factors	
Vaginal delivery	**Higher education**
Forceps delivery	
Cesarean section	**Childhood enuresis**
Increased parity	
Fetal birth weight	**Presence of two or more comorbid diseases**

From Holroyd-Leduc JM, Straus SE: Management of urinary incontinence in women. Clinical applications. JAMA 291: 996, 2004.

Urinalysis and Culture

A simple urinalysis and urine culture may give a great deal of information. The presence of white blood cells or red blood cells and bacteria in a catheterized or clean voided sample (in which the perineum around the urethra is appropriately prepared with an antiseptic solution) may suggest urethritis, a diverticulum that is infected, or cystitis. Their presence may also suggest an infection in the upper urinary tract, such as pyelonephritis. Chronic infection in the lower tract may be associated with urgency, frequency, dysuria, and even incontinence. In such instances the urinalysis and urine culture may be diagnostic. Several dipstick methods are available to detect bacteriuria and pyuria. The accuracy of these methods is quite variable, but they do have some use in screening patients who are incontinent or who have symptoms suggestive of infection. In most cases a culture should be obtained both to identify the specific organism involved and to verify the presence of an infection.

Test for Residual Urine

This simple procedure can be extremely helpful in the evaluation of a patient with pelvic organ prolapse, voiding problems, or chronic retention of urine. The patient is asked to void, and a catheter is inserted no more than 10 to 15 minutes thereafter. The urine remaining in the bladder is measured and may be sent for urinalysis and culture. Under normal circumstances the amount of residual urine should be less than 50 mL after the patient has voided at least 100 to 150 mL. Large amounts of residual urine suggest urinary retention resulting from inadequate bladder emptying. Reasonable accuracy of residual urine volume can also be obtained noninvasively by ultrasound. Handheld bladder scan ultrasound units are available, and patients prefer to avoid urethral catheterization.

Bladder Diary

Asking the patient to complete a bladder diary is a simple, inexpensive way to obtain information about the women's fluid intake, voiding habits, voided volumes, and incontinent episodes. An example diary form is shown in Figure 21-7. A 2006 systematic review concluded that a large proportion of cases of urodynamic stress incontinence could be correctly diagnosed in a primary care setting from the clinical history alone. The bladder diary appears to be the most cost-effective tool and is useful for diagnosing detrusor overactivity with reasonable sensitivity and specificity when used with the clinical history. The clinical stress test is effective in diagnosing stress incontinence (see later section).

Office Cystometrics

Bladder capacity and bladder function may be measured with sophisticated tools, which are discussed later. Nevertheless it is possible to gain a great deal of information about bladder capacity and bladder function with a relatively simple apparatus. If after a catheter is inserted to check for residual urine, the catheter is left in place and attached to a graduated Asepto syringe without bulb, it is possible to pour sterile saline (or sterile water) into the syringe and measure the amount of saline that first causes the patient to have the urge to void. This urge should normally occur after 150 to 200 mL of saline has been infused. However, normal women should be able to continue to maintain continence at that level, with a strong, normally uncontrollable urge to void usually occurring when 400 to 500 mL has been instilled. Thus a normal bladder first transmits an urge to void at 150 to 200 mL, and functional capacity is reached at 400 to 500 mL. Most women can maintain continence with larger volumes, but this is usually accomplished with a great deal of conscious effort.

Your Daily Bladder Diary

This diary will help you and your health care team. Bladder diaries help show the causes of bladder control trouble. The "Example" line (below) will show you how to use the diary.

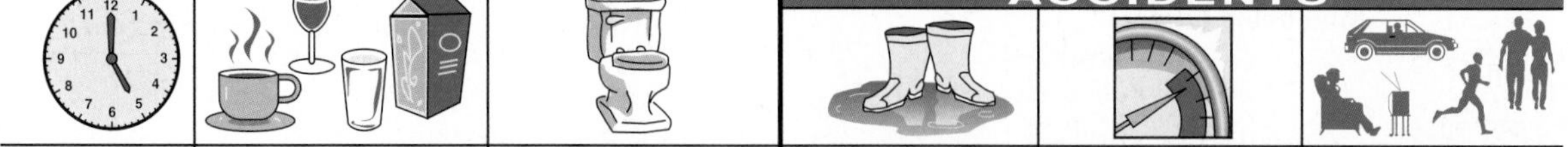

Time	Drinks		Urine		ACCIDENTS		
					Accidental leaks	Did you feel a strong urge to go?	What were you doing at the time? *Sneezing, exercising, driving, lifting, etc.*
	What kind?	*How many?*	*How many times?*	*How much? sm med lg*	*sm med lg*		
Example	coffee	2 cups	//	☐ ☒ ☐	☐ ☒ ☐	☒ Yes ☐ No	Running
6–7 am				☐ ☐ ☐	☐ ☐ ☐	☐ Yes ☐ No	
7–8 am				☐ ☐ ☐	☐ ☐ ☐	☐ Yes ☐ No	
8–9 am				☐ ☐ ☐	☐ ☐ ☐	☐ Yes ☐ No	
9–10 am				☐ ☐ ☐	☐ ☐ ☐	☐ Yes ☐ No	
10–11 am				☐ ☐ ☐	☐ ☐ ☐	☐ Yes ☐ No	
11–12 noon				☐ ☐ ☐	☐ ☐ ☐	☐ Yes ☐ No	
12–1 pm				☐ ☐ ☐	☐ ☐ ☐	☐ Yes ☐ No	
1–2 pm				☐ ☐ ☐	☐ ☐ ☐	☐ Yes ☐ No	
2–3 pm				☐ ☐ ☐	☐ ☐ ☐	☐ Yes ☐ No	
3–4 pm				☐ ☐ ☐	☐ ☐ ☐	☐ Yes ☐ No	
4–5 pm				☐ ☐ ☐	☐ ☐ ☐	☐ Yes ☐ No	
5–6 pm				☐ ☐ ☐	☐ ☐ ☐	☐ Yes ☐ No	
6–7 pm				☐ ☐ ☐	☐ ☐ ☐	☐ Yes ☐ No	

Your name: ______________________ **Date:** __________

Figure 21-7. Daily bladder diary. (From Vasavada SP, Appell R, Sand PK, et al [eds]: Female Urology, Urogynecology, and Voiding Dysfunction. New York, Marcel Dekker, 2005, p 127.)

Stress Test

If a bladder has been previously filled to measure capacity, it should then be emptied to about 250 mL of saline, or if the bladder is empty, 250 mL of saline should be instilled. The catheter is then removed, and the patient is asked to cough while in the recumbent position. If urine spurts from the urethral meatus, stress incontinence may be present. The bladder neck can be gently elevated with the finger or an instrument such as a Kelly clamp, and the patient can be asked to cough once again (Bonney test). Care should be taken not to compress the urethra, thereby mechanically occluding it. If urine no longer spurts from the urethra when the bladder neck is supported, this suggests that the bladder neck hypermobility may be responsible for the incontinence, and an appropriate operative repair could be expected to produce continence.

Migliorini and Glenning questioned the value of the Bonney test because they noted that a group of women with urethral sphincter weakness demonstrated by urodynamic studies were still incontinent even when the bladder neck was elevated. Bhatia and Bergman had previously reached a similar conclusion, stating that they believed the test restored continence by obstructing the urethra and urethrovesicle junction.

Because urine loss with cough should be immediate if stress incontinence is the problem, it may be possible to detect evidence of detrusor instability by observing the time of the spurt of urine in the stress test. Classically the detrusor reacts a few seconds after the stimulus; therefore a spurt that occurs after a delay after a cough suggests the presence of an involuntary detrusor contraction.

After the stress test is performed in a recumbent patient, it should be repeated with the patient standing. Frequently the patient will appear to be continent with stress while lying down but may demonstrate incontinence when the influence of gravity on the pelvic organs is brought into play in the standing position.

Thus with the urinalysis, urine culture, test for residual urine, bladder diary, information about the amount of urine required to cause the first urge to void, information concerning general bladder capacity, and the stress test in both the recumbent and the standing positions, the physician will have a great deal of information concerning the cause of the patient's urinary problem. More sophisticated urodynamic evaluations using specific and often costly equipment should be performed by individuals who are trained and experienced in these tests. A short discussion of these procedures and the equipment involved follows.

Urethroscopy

Urethroscopy is excellent for visualizing the urethra and therefore offers information about inflammatory processes within the urethra, urethral diverticula, other anatomic defects, and estrogenic effects and permits some estimate of urethral tone. The use of a gas medium such as carbon dioxide is appropriate for these studies. Although the equipment used for performing gas urethroscopy makes it possible to measure pressures within the urethra and the bladder, caution must be exercised because a rapid instillation of carbon dioxide into the lower urinary tract may stimulate detrusor contraction, which may in itself lead to reflex opening of the vesical neck, thus giving false information about the bladder neck and the urethral sphincter.

A variety of equipment is available for this procedure. Relatively inexpensive apparatuses can be used for urethroscopy, as well as for cystometry and uroflowmetry.

Cystoscopy and Urodynamics

Cystoscopy may be performed using a water system or a carbon dioxide gas system. The bladder may be visualized and the presence of inflammation or benign or malignant processes noted.

Urodynamic investigation attempts to measure bladder and urethral function as well as voiding function. Cystometry is the part of the urodynamic test that describes the filling phase of the micturition cycle. Pressure flow studies measure voiding in terms of detrusor and urethral function. In attempting to understand the basis of urinary stress incontinence, the practitioner must realize that what must be determined is the relationship between the simultaneous intraurethral and intravesical pressures (Fig. 21-8). For greatest accuracy, these must be measured with the patient in the standing and reclining positions, at rest and with straining. The ideal means of evaluating a patient for incontinence is to use a multichannel recorder that permits pressure determinations at two points within the urethra (proximal and midpoint to distal), one within the bladder, and one intraabdominally as recorded by an intrarectal sensor or by a sensor within the vagina if the vagina is in a relatively normal position (not prolapsed). Should intraabdominal stress be transmitted equally to the bladder and the urethra and should the intravesical pressure be less than the urethral closing pressure, one would expect closing pressure to be overcome and stress incontinence to be demonstrated if an intraabdominal pressure increase is transmitted to the bladder but not to the urethra.

Multichannel devices involve more expensive equipment and require continuous maintenance. It is possible to add a video urodynamic system to the multichannel recorders, making it possible via fluoroscopy to identify reflux into the ureters under pressure situations. The video system also makes it possible to actually observe the act of micturition, any anatomic changes, and the effect of stress. Because the data obtained by multichannel pressure recordings plus the ability to actually visualize the patient micturate offer the most accurate diagnostic information that the clinician can obtain, this technique is considered the standard against which other tests are measured.

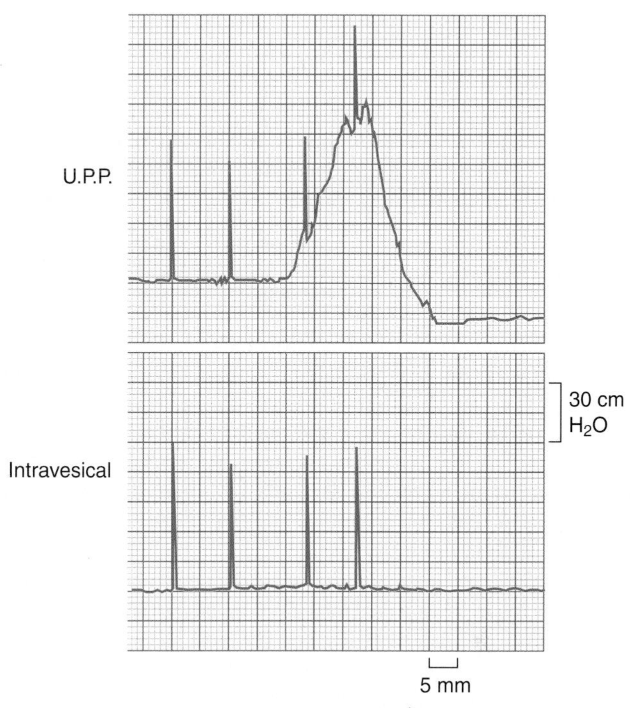

Figure 21-8. Simultaneous recordings of urethra and intravesical pressures during coughing. Stress produces a parallel increase of bladder and urethral pressure because the intraabdominal position of the bladder and proximal two thirds of the urethra are displayed. U.P.P, urethral pressure profile (From Raz S: Pharmacological treatment of lower urinary tract dysfunction. Urol Clin North Am 5:323, 1978.)

Cystometry is not always necessary for beginning a conservative treatment program for stress, urge, or mixed incontinence symptoms. However, if the diagnosis is unclear, the patient has failed conservative therapy, has had prior incontinence surgery, has voiding complaints, or has a complicated medical history (such as neurologic disease), then urodynamic testing is indicated.

INFECTIONS OF THE LOWER URINARY TRACT

Infections of the urethra and bladder are almost always associated with some combination of the following: frequency, urgency, dysuria, pyuria, hematuria, acute or chronic pelvic pain, backache, and at times fever. As many as 50% of all women develop urinary tract infections (UTIs) at some time during their life, and by age 70 as many as 10% of women will have chronic UTIs. At times incontinence is associated with acute and chronic infections. Although *Escherichia coli* is the cause of most of the infections, a myriad of organisms, including *Enterobacter, Klebsiella, Pseudomonas, Proteus, Streptococcus faecalis, Staphylococcus saprophyticus, Enterococcus,* and *Chlamydia* are often found. The presence of bacteria in the urine (bacteriuria) does not necessarily prove clinical infection. Bacteriuria is fairly common in women, especially older women. For instance, cumulative data from several studies suggest that 20% of women older than 65 years of age will demonstrate bacteriuria, but the percentage increases from about 15% in the 65- to 70-year group to 20% to 50% for women older than 80. Bacteriuria is quite common in women who are on chronic catheterization and in women in nursing homes who are chronically incontinent. Asymptomatic bacteriuria is no longer treated, even in the elderly, unless they are undergoing an invasive procedure.

The presence of at least 100,000 organisms per milliliter of urine is generally accepted as evidence for a clinical infection. In cases of urethritis and trigonitis the presence of as few as 100 organisms per milliliter may indicate an infection because of the dilution of bladder urine. White blood cells are always seen in the urine (pyuria) when UTI occurs, and red blood cells may be present in microscopic or macroscopic numbers. Hematuria is common in acute infections.

Many explanations have been offered as to why the female urinary tract is vulnerable to infection. These include the fact that the female urethra is short, thereby allowing easier access of bacteria to the bladder; the proximity of the vulva, vagina, and rectum to the opening of the urethra; the effects of sexual intercourse on the entrance of bacteria into the urethra and the lower urinary tract; and the effect of loss of estrogen on the reproductive tract of elderly women. To this list it is probably appropriate to add personal immunologic genetic variations that may make one woman more susceptible than other women to certain bacteria.

Additional circumstances that may be responsible for infections in women include the dilation of the urinary tract in pregnancy, urinary tract obstruction, ureteral reflux, and pelvic relaxation. Other causes of UTIs in both men and women are the need for frequent catheterization, instrumentation, and overdistention of the bladder in neurogenic conditions in which stasis becomes a problem. Refer to the section on acute cystitis in Chapter 22 (Infections of the Lower Genital Tract) for a more complete discussion.

Urethritis

Patients with urethritis generally have the typical findings of lower UTI, which include dysuria, frequency, and urgency. They often have a urethra that is tender to palpation. Under certain circumstances it may be possible to express pus from the urethra; this is particularly common in acute infections with the gonococcus or *Chlamydia.* In these situations the infection involves not only the urethra but also the periurethral glands. Frequently, significant pyuria is noted in a clean-catch urine sample, particularly that taken early in the voiding. The urine should be inspected, since *Trichomonas* infestation is occasionally noted in such instances. Herpes simplex virus has also been associated with urethritis.

Pus expressed from the urethra should be submitted for culture and for smear with Gram stain. Intracellular diplococci are suggestive of gonorrhea. *Neisseria gonorrhoeae* or *Chlamydia* is usually cultured in such situations. Nucleic acid amplification tests enable detection of both organisms. In particular, this is the preferred test for *C. trachomatis.* Urine obtained by the clean-catch method should also be cultured. Remember these are reportable diseases to the state health department.

If no specific organism is identified on smear, a broad-spectrum coverage such as a sulfa preparation or nitrofurantoin (Macrodantin), 50 or 100 mg three or four times a day, should be prescribed for 10 days. If *Chlamydia* is suspected doxycycline, 100 mg twice a day, should be prescribed for at least 7 days or azithromycin, 1 g orally in a single dose. If gonorrhea is diagnosed, the current recommended treatment consists of ceftriaxone 125 mg intramuscularly (single dose) or cefixime, 400 mg orally in a single dose. An alternative therapy is ofloxacin or levofloxacin orally. Penicillin is no longer the drug of choice because of the many penicillin-resistant strains of gonococcus now present. Resistance to fluoroquinolones is also spreading. Coinfections with *N. gonorrhoeae* and *C. trachomatis* are common, so dual therapy is often indicated.

Urethral Syndrome (Urethral Pain Syndrome)

The so-called *urethral syndrome* is poorly characterized but most reports suggest the same symptoms of dysuria, frequency, urgency, and pain that are seen with urethritis. In the case of urethral syndrome, however, the symptoms are generally of long standing, and no specific organism can be identified. The International Continence Society standardization report in 2002 added a new genitourinary pain syndrome category. It defined urethral pain syndrome as the "occurrence of recurrent episodic urethral pain usually on voiding, with daytime frequency and nocturia, in the absence of proven infection or other obvious pathology." Classically, urethroscopy has revealed a reddened, chronically inflamed urethra with spasm at the bladder neck. The prevalence of this condition is unknown but may affect as many as 20% to 30% of all women at one time or another. The cause is unknown, but there are many theories, including allergic, immunologic, infectious, neurologic, atrophic, and psychogenic causes. Some feel the problem resides in the paraurethral glands and that infection with such organisms as *Mycoplasma, Uroplasma,* or *Chlamydia* might be responsible. The incidence of these infections, however, has been about the same as in populations of women without the syndrome. Nevertheless, such organisms should be sought and eradicated with appropriate antibiotic therapy when they are found, since this may alleviate symptoms in such cases.

Gittes and Nakamura drew attention to the fact that the periurethral glands, analogous to the prostate in the male, might be inflamed clinically just as can the prostate. They suggested treating patients with urethral syndrome in the same fashion that men with prostatitis are treated. Baerheim and colleagues compared the success of treatment with antibacterial therapy in 51 patients with acute lower UTI and 58 patients with acute urethral syndrome and found improvement by 3 days in about half of each group.

Because the cause in most cases is unknown, various therapies have been devised with varying success. These include dilation of the urethra with progressive dilators, antispasmodics, estrogen (in postmenopausal women), and more recently, cryosurgery. Sand and coworkers, in a randomized cross-over trial, compared cryosurgery using a specially designed cryoprobe with dilation and massage of the urethra in 24 patients diagnosed as having the urethral syndrome. Of the patients first treated with cryosurgery, 91% achieved relief of their symptoms, compared with 33% of patients first treated with dilation and massage. When cross-over of the failures occurred, 75% of women treated with cryosurgery were relieved of symptoms, compared with none of the cryotherapy failures who were then treated with dilation and massage.

Patients diagnosed as having the urethral syndrome deserve a careful evaluation before specific therapy is determined. Most of the studies on urethral syndrome were published before 1990. Many reports indicate suprapubic pain is a feature with relief after voiding. Chronic urethral syndrome may be a subset of interstitial cystitis.

Cystitis

Cystitis is the most common bacterial infection seen in out-patient settings. The majority of acute UTIs show a clean-catch urine sample or catheterized specimen to have bacteria concentration of 100,000 or more per milliliter of urine when the patient suffers the symptoms of dysuria, frequency, urgency, and pain. Stamm and others have demonstrated that concentrations as low as 100 colonies per milliliter of urine can cause acute UTI symptoms. White blood cells are almost always seen in large numbers in the urine (pyuria), as are bacteria. Red blood cells are frequently present in microscopic numbers, but gross hematuria may occur as a result of extravasations of blood across dilated and inflamed capillaries. If the bladder is visualized, it is noted to be uniformly reddened and inflamed. Uncomplicated UTIs occur in healthy females with normal urinary function. UTIs are classified as complicated when there are comorbid conditions that require longer treatment courses, such as underlying urologic abnormalities, presence of a foreign body (catheter), urinary calculi, obstruction of urine flow, diabetes mellitus, spinal cord injury, pregnancy, or other illnesses. Acute uncomplicated UTIs can often be diagnosed successfully with symptom assessment and urine dipstick for leukocyte esterase, or microscopic unspun urine evaluation for pyuria, as the pathogens are predictable. Complicated UTIs often require urine culture. The Infectious Diseases Society of America (IDSA) and Council for Appropriate and Rational Antibiotic Therapy (CARAT) have evidence-based guidelines for treatment of UTIs. Where local *E. coli* bacterial resistance rates are less than 20%, trimethoprim–sulfamethoxazole (TMP-SMX) is recommended. If resistance is greater than 20%, a fluoroquinolone is advised. Three-day therapy is adequate for acute, uncomplicated UTIs. The resistance of *E. coli* to TMP-SMX has increased dramatically recently, so fluoroquinolone use has increased. Short course (3-day) therapy improves patient tolerability, compliance, and reduces costs. This treatment strategy results in greater than a 90% cure rate. If nitrofurantoin is used for mild to moderate symptoms of an uncomplicated UTI, at least 5 days of drug is recommended. Resistance rates of E. coli to nitrofurantoin have remained low. With uncomplicated UTIs, progression to pyelonephritis is an extremely rare event. For complicated UTIs, a 7- to 10-day course of a fluoroquinolone is recommended. If obtained, when results of the culture are reported, the antibiotic may be changed if the organisms noted are not sensitive to the antibiotic in use. The patient should remain well hydrated and should be encouraged to continue treatment even though symptoms generally disappear within 48 hours. Infections frequently recur and become chronic because they are not adequately eradicated. This may result from physician error (treating with too low a dose of antibiotic, the wrong antibiotic, or for too short a period of time) or patient error (not taking the medication as prescribed).

Recurrent infections of different organisms should alert the physician to the need for a more complete evaluation. However, intravenous pyelogram (seeking structural abnormalities of the bladder, kidney, or ureters) is rarely useful in otherwise healthy women. Occasionally, continuous antibiotic therapy at lower doses for more prolonged periods is necessary to ensure that the patient is no longer infected. Postmenopausal women with recurrent UTIs often benefit from vaginal estrogen therapy as this restores the acidic environment of the vagina and restores normal bacteria and lactobacillus. Raz and Stamm have shown significant reduction in recurrent UTIs in postmenopausal women using vaginal estrogen cream.

Frequent catheterizations or manipulation of the lower urinary tract often causes UTIs. An indwelling catheter for 24 hours leads to bacteriuria in as many as 50% of patients. When left in place for 96 hours, an indwelling catheter causes bacteriuria in nearly 100% of patients. Many physicians suggest prophylactic antibiotics in patients who must continue catheter use, but no good evidence supports this thesis. Certainly a patient with an indwelling catheter should be monitored for the possibility of UTIs, be kept well hydrated, and have a urine culture if symptoms occur. Postoperative and debilitated patients are at greatest risk.

While physicians commonly recommend preventative measures to their patients for preventing UTIs, studies do not support these practices. This includes wiping the rectum away from the urethra, voiding after intercourse, and drinking more fluid.

Painful Bladder Syndrome and Interstitial Cystitis

There is no consensus on how to define this condition. Interstitial cystitis (IC) is a complex inflammatory condition of the bladder. The etiology and pathophysiology is poorly understood and most likely multifactorial. It is usually associated with an altered epithelial permeability, mast cell activation, and an up-regulation of sensory afferent nerves. It is a common disease seen in females more often than males, but the incidence is really unknown, although it has been estimated to be as high as 500 per 100,000. Painful bladder syndrome is a more global definition adopted by the International Continence Society to deal with patients with pain syndromes of the lower urinary tract without evidence of bladder pathology. By definition, painful bladder syndrome (PBS) is the complaint of suprapubic pain related to bladder filling accompanied by other symptoms, such as daytime frequency and nocturia, in the absence of proven UTIs or other pathology.

Symptoms of IC are urgency, daytime and nighttime frequency, and bladder pain without evidence for infection. It is often confused with other bladder conditions, pelvic inflammatory disease, and endometriosis. The patient will usually void frequently and a voiding diary will often demonstrate frequent voiding of less than 150 mL each and with as many as 20 or more voidings per day. Sleep can be disrupted by frequent needs to void. On exam, suprapubic and anterior vaginal wall tenderness may be found.

On cystoscopy, the bladder frequently appears normal during filling, but with distention under anesthesia, characteristic petechial hemorrhages resembling glomeruli usually appear. Oozing of blood is often seen. However, glomerulations may be a nonspecific finding as they can be seen in asymptomatic women. This cystoscope finding is not diagnostic of IC. Hunner's ulcers are diagnostic of IC but are infrequently seen in women with bladder pain. If a biopsy under anesthesia is taken, ulcers with granulation tissue, mucosal hemorrhage, monocytic infiltration, and mast cells in the lamina propia and detrusor muscle are often seen. Parsons has proposed that the changes are related to a defective or altered glycosaminoglycan mucus layer, which results in altered bladder permeability. However, investigations to date do not show whether this alteration is cause or effect. Some authors feel that these changes are the result of an autoimmune disease. The presence of immunoglobulins and complement in the bladder wall and the increase in interleukin-6 in the urine of patients may support this. To date, there is no laboratory test or urine test that is diagnostic of IC. Although urodynamic testing may reveal these patients have early first sensation to void and low bladder capacities, there is no range in volume that is specific for IC. Parsons and associates developed the potassium sensitivity test (PST). The PST involves inserting a catheter into the bladder and instilling a saline solution followed by a potassium chloride solution. A positive PST test is noted if increased pain occurs with the potassium solution. In Parsons and associates' study in gynecologic offices, 244 women with pelvic pain, vulvodynia, or urgency/frequency syndrome diagnoses underwent the PST. Eighty-four percent of these women ($N = 206$) had genitourinary symptoms, and 88% had a positive PST compared with 76% without urinary symptoms. The International Consultation on Incontinence (ICI) stated in 2005 that these are "inadequate data to recommend using the PST for diagnosis" of IC.

Several symptoms indices are useful for evaluating women with painful bladder complaints although they were not developed for screening. The pain, urgency, frequency (PUF) scale (Table 21-4) and O'Leary-Sant scale both are helpful in characterizing the patient's complaints, especially in light of the lack of diagnostic tests. IC should be considered in the differential diagnosis of any female with chronic pelvic pain.

Many treatments are available, but few have been uniformly helpful. Patients are encouraged to see the problem as a chronic one that is not malignant and to try to reduce stress, encourage family support, and avail themselves of the writings and support of the Interstitial Cystitis Association. They should be instructed to avoid acidic, alcoholic, and carbonated beverages, spicy foods, coffee, tea, chocolate, tomatoes, vinegar, and artificial sweeteners, all of which have been associated with increased pain in patients with IC. Tobacco should be avoided as well. Bladder retraining to increase the interval between voiding may help and antidepressant medications may be useful in appropriate patients. The tricyclic antidepressants may be particularly helpful as they can inhibit the neural activation that leads to pain. Amitriptyline is not FDA-approved for IC but doses of 10 to 75 mg nightly showed pain relief in two thirds of women and decreases in urgency and frequency.

Standard medical therapy has included dimethyl sulfoxide (DMSO) bladder instillation often accompanied by heparin, steroids, or local anesthetics. DMSO is an antiinflammatory agent that acts as a bladder anesthetic, relaxes muscles, causes mast cell inhibition, and may dissolve collagen. Often DMSO is given as a single treatment followed by heparin therapy for up to 1 year.

Heparin has been used by bladder instillation for 1 hour, three times a week. Recently, a heparin analogue, pentosan polysulfate sodium (PPS, Elmiron), has been given 100 mg three times a day orally with some reported improvement. PPS is the only FDA-approved oral drug for IC and may help repair the glycosaminoglycan layer of the bladder epithelium. This drug can take 6 months to be effective, and improvements are modest; 38% of patients have a greater than 50% improvement at 12 weeks. Antihistamines such as hydroxyzine may be of benefit for patients with concurrent allergies and for decreasing mast cell degranulation. Hydrodistension of the bladder under anesthesia is therapeutic in 20% to 30% of patients and is sometimes done at the initial evaluation when performing cystoscopy to rule out other pathology. However, most experts do not use hydrodistension as a diagnostic criterion any longer since the findings of glomerulations are nondiagnostic. Three to six months of symptom improvement occurs with distension in responders.

Table 21-4 Pelvic Pain and Urgency/Frequency Patient Symptom Scale (PUF)

	0	1	2	3	4	Score
1. How many times do you go to the bathroom during the day	3–6	7–10	11–14	15–19	20+	
2. a. How many times do you go to the bathroom at night?	0	1	2	3	4+	
b. If you get up at night to go to the bathroom, does it bother you?	Never	Occasionally	Moderate	Severe		
3. Are you currently sexually active? Yes ______ No ______						
4. a. If you are sexually active, do you now or have you ever had pain or symptoms during or after sexual intercourse?	Never	Occasionally	Usually	Always		
b. If you have pain, does it make you avoid sexual intercourse?	Never	Occasionally	Usually	Always		
5. Do you have pain associated with your bladder or in your pelvis (vagina, labia, lower abdomen, urethra, perineum)?	Never	Occasionally	Usually	Always		
6. Do you still have urgency after you go to the bathroom?	Never	Occasionally	Usually	Always		
7. a. If you have pain, is it usually		Mild	Moderate	Severe		
b. Does your pain bother you?	Never	Occasionally	Usually	Always		
8. a. If you have urgency, is it usually		Mild	Moderate	Severe		
b. Does your urgency bother you?	Never	Occasionally	Usually	Always		
					Total score	

Since IC is a complex disease, it is best treated by experienced physicians with the expertise and patience to deal with the patient and her needs over a prolonged period of time. Usually, multiple interventions are necessary with a combination of behavioral changes, pelvic floor physical therapy, counseling, oral medications, and bladder instillations. Hormonal manipulation in premenopausal women with menstrual flares may provide benefit.

Urethral Diverticulum

Etiology

Urethral diverticula occur in perhaps as many as 1% to 6% of all women sometime during their lifetime. Age distribution in published reports ranges from 19 to 76 years, but the majority of diverticula seem to occur between the ages of 30 and 50. Andersen has suggested that the disease occurs more frequently in blacks, with a ratio perhaps as high as 6 to 1.

A variety of causes have been suggested, including congenital, acute and chronic inflammatory, and traumatic. The congenital theory stems from the fact that rare cases have been reported in children and neonates. Evidence for acute and chronic infection stems from the fact that several observers have noted infection and obstruction of periurethral glands, which result in the formation of retention cysts that, when repeatedly infected, may rupture into the lumen of the urethra and remain as an outpouching, giving rise to the diverticulum. Several authors have suggested that the gonococcus is the cause of this, but *E. coli* and other organisms have been found in such processes. Urethral trauma from multiple catheterizations or from childbirth has also been suggested as a causal factor. However, many women with diverticula have neither been catheterized nor given birth. The infectious origin is probably the most common and the prevalence in women with recurrent UTIs may be as high as 40%.

Symptoms and Signs

The classic description of symptoms in a patient with urethral diverticula include the three "Ds" of postvoid dribbling, dysuria, and dyspareunia. More common is complaints of frequency/urgency, dysuria, a history of recurrent UTI, dribbling, and incontinence. Occasionally, hematuria occurs. In a series reported from the Mayo Clinic, Lee noted that a palpable, tender, suburethral mass was present in 51 of 85 patients (60%) and that protrusion of the diverticulum from the vaginal introitus occurred in 4 patients. More recent reports suggest a tender mass is only found 35% of the time. Occasionally, patients have urinary stones within the diverticula or discharge or pus from the urethra.

Diagnosis

Diagnosis is generally suggested by physical examination. The anterior vaginal wall may be tender, or a cystic mass may be found about midurethra. Pus or cloudy urine may be expressed as the urethra and mass are massaged. A normal exam and nonclassic symptoms is often how a patient presents, which is why the diagnosis is often delayed. The double-catheter balloon technique, which essentially closes the urethra at each end and forces contrast medium into the diverticulum under pressure during cystogram, has been the gold standard. Now, MRI with cross-sectional imaging offers the most detailed anatomic study, which can also image diverticula that do not communicate with the urethra, as well as multiple outpouchings. Other tests are often still used, such as urethroscopy, voiding cystourethrogram, urodynamics (since 35% to 50% will have incontinence) transvaginal ultrasound, and virtual computed tomography (CT) urethroscopy.

Management

No treatment is indicated for asymptomatic urethral diverticula. Mild symptoms of frequency/urgency can be treated with anticholinergics and infections with antibiotics. Carcinoma has been reported in diverticula so caution is needed if no surgical therapy is planned. A variety of procedures have been suggested for the management of urethral diverticula. Lapides has suggested a technique for transurethral marsupialization that involves the resection of the roof of the diverticulum, using transurethral electrocautery. Essentially this technique enlarges the orifice of the diverticulum by incising its roof. Spence and Duckett reported a marsupialization technique in which the diverticulum was opened and sutured to the vaginal epithelial surface. Generally this leads to a fistula and requires secondary closure, making this technique useful in only rare circumstances. Diverticulectomy is the more common procedure done today.

A classic operative approach uses urethroscopy to identify the location of the diverticulum. It is important at this point to note the presence of multiple diverticula. In Lee's report from the Mayo Clinic the diverticulum was noted coming from the distal third of the urethra in only 10 of the 85 patients, whereas 38 patients demonstrated an origin from the middle third and 13 from the proximal third, including the bladder neck. Lee noted multiple diverticula in 18 of his 85 patients.

After the diverticulum is identified and evaluated, an incision is made in the anterior vaginal wall and the diverticulum is dissected free of the pubocervical fascia. The diverticulum's attachment to the urethra is noted, it is excised by sharp dissection, and the urethral wall is closed with a row of interrupted 4-0 catgut or polyglycol sutures. The closure line is generally in the longitudinal axis. Occasionally, however, a transverse closure is necessary because of the nature of the attachment. The pubocervical fascia is then reinforced with a row of 3-0 polyglycol reabsorbable interrupted sutures. Hemostasis is scrupulously secured with electrocautery, and the vaginal incision is closed with catgut or polyglycol sutures (Fig. 21-9).

Most diverticula emanate from the ventral wall of the urethra. Occasionally, however, the diverticulum is noted to be arising from the lateral wall of the urethra or even from the anterior wall. In such cases the dissection must be carefully carried to the base of the diverticulum and the procedure carried out as stated. In cases of diverticula arising from the dorsal wall of the urethra, it is appropriate to simply excise the diverticulum at its neck and allow the tissue of the urethra to retract. In all cases a No. 16 or 18 Foley catheter is left in place for 6 to 7 days.

Several nuances have been offered to make dissection and subsequent repair easier. One of these is placing a ureteral catheter into the diverticulum and allowing it to coil so that the diverticulum is more easily observable during dissection. Other surgeons have attempted to dilate the neck of the diverticulum before beginning the excision and occasionally have

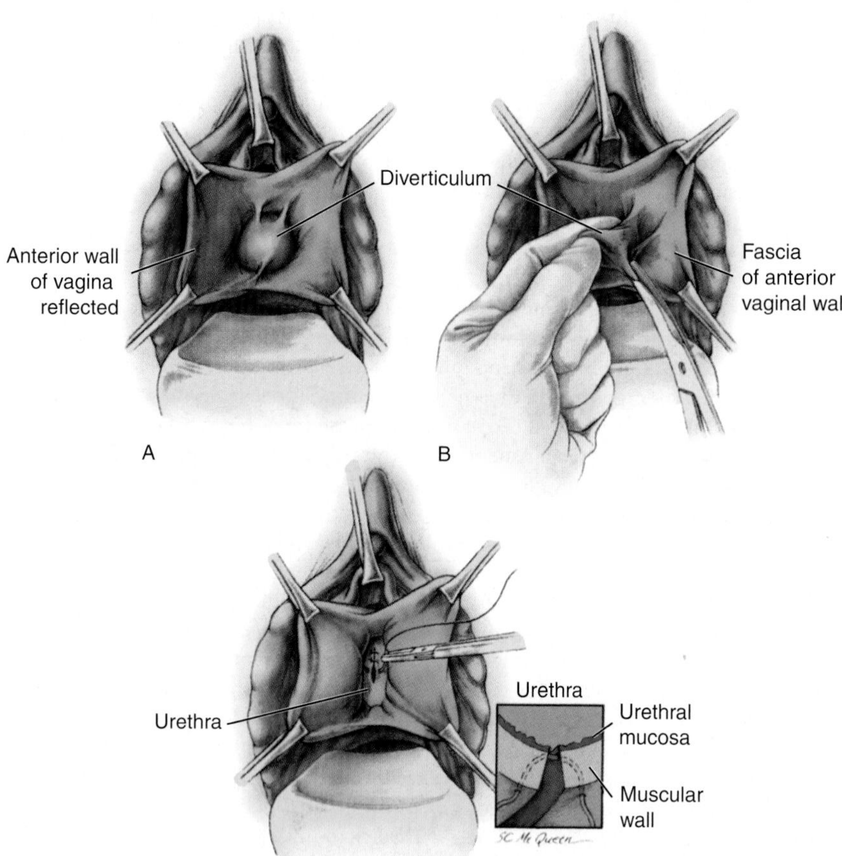

Figure 21-9. Resection of urethral diverticulum. **A,** Diverticulum exposed with vaginal lining and endopelvic fascia retracted. **B,** Fingers hold diverticulum on traction, which aids in dissection and identification of ostium. **C,** After complete resection of diverticulum, urethra is closed with fine, interrupted, extramucosal sutures. (Redrawn from Lee RA: Diverticulum of the female urethra: postoperative complications and results. Obstet Gynecol 61:52, 1983. Reprinted with permission from The American College of Obstetricians and Gynecologists.)

even tried to pack foreign substances such as gauze through the neck to make the dissection easier. Often a Martius flap is brought into the field between the periurethral fascial closure and vaginal wall. This is thought to prevent fistula formation.

Complications

Major complications of this procedure include urethrovaginal fistula formation, development of stress urinary incontinence, recurrence of the diverticulum, and stricture of the urethra.

In a study from the Mayo Clinic, MacKinnon and colleageus reported on 140 patients treated operatively, 7 of whom (5%) developed urethrovaginal fistulas. In Lee's report of a later study from the Mayo Clinic, only one patient developed a fistula. In another series, Spraitz and Welch, reporting on 94 patients repaired, found 4 with urethrovaginal fistulas. Fistula rates as high as 8.3% have been reported.

Recurrence of diverticula is reported in about 5% to 10% of patients in various series. If the diverticulum recurs within the first few months after operation, it may represent a second diverticulum that was overlooked or an inappropriate repair of the diagnosed diverticulum. If the diverticulum occurs after 1 year, it is probably a new lesion.

Stricture of the urethra has rarely been reported in any of the operative series. It is a theoretic possibility.

Other complications involve stress incontinence, which may be related to the dissection of the bladder neck away from its usual location, and the development of the urethral syndrome, probably caused by continuing inflammation and irritation. These conditions generally respond to appropriate specific therapy.

Urolithiasis

Urinary tract stones (renal or ureteral) may occur in patients of either sex and at any age. About 5% of women will develop a symptomatic stone by age 70. They may be related to metabolic abnormalities, such as gout or errors of calcium metabolism, but usually they relate to chronic infection and stasis of urine. Risk factors for calculi in women include pregnancy, during which time the urinary tract becomes dilated and stasis is more common; a history of kidney stones or family history, certain medications, excessive vitamin C intake, low calcium intake, chronic diarrhea and dehydration.

Symptoms occur most often when a stone passes from the kidney to the ureter. Pain occurs on the side of the stone and varies from a dull ache to severe paroxysms of pain called renal colic. Flank pain, lower abdominal and groin pain can occur, and the location can vary as the stone moves down the ureter with radiation of pain to the groin. Gross or microscopic hematuria is usually presents. CT scan has become the gold standard for diagnosis, particularly if the abdominal radiograph is normal. Ultrasound misses small stones but is recommended for pregnant women.

A variety of management techniques are available, including observation with pain medications and fluids awaiting spontaneous passage, endoscopic removal, surgical removal, and the destruction of the stone with the shockwave lithotripsy. The principal consideration, however, should be the correction of the basic problem that caused the stone.

STRESS INCONTINENCE

Stress incontinence occurs when increased intraabdominal pressure is not transmitted equally to the bladder and the functional urethra. If intraabdominal pressure plus bladder pressure is sufficient to overcome urethral closing pressure, incontinence will occur. One of the problems is the fact that the bladder neck, the base of the bladder, and the proximal urethra are no longer adequately supported. This may result from a separation of the supports that hold the upper vagina and urethra to the pubic symphysis, neuromuscular damage to the pelvic fascia and musculature secondary to childbearing or the aging process, from some sort of trauma, or from an altered connective tissue metabolism causing decreased collagen production. Because the proximal two thirds of the urethra normally is an intraabdominal structure, an increased intraabdominal pressure would normally be exerted against it as well as the bladder. However, with a change in the anatomic relationships of this portion of the urethra, its intraabdominal position may be lost, thereby making it bear the brunt of such pressure rather than allowing it this degree of protection.

Over the years urethral length has been implicated as a related factor in stress incontinence. Lapides and coworkers measured urethral length using calibrated intraurethral catheters before and after operative correction of stress incontinence and found the urethra was shorter in cases of incontinence. However, during their procedure, downward traction was exerted to give the most meaningful measurement. Because the bladder neck in such women frequently funnels, accuracy of the measurements by Lapides and coworkers has been considered suspect. Other studies by multiple investigators using bead-chain urethrocystography have failed to show any change in urethral length before or after standard repair procedures. Thus it seems that, except for the most unusual circumstances, anatomic urethral length is not a major factor in stress incontinence other than some healthy segment of urethra is needed to provide coaptation.

Urethral closure is another factor to consider in continence. This is affected by the mucosa and vasculature, the adjacent connective tissue structures, the striated and smooth muscles and the involuntary and voluntary muscle contractions that prevent incontinence in response to stress.

Jeffcoate and Roberts using urethrocystographic techniques in both continent and incontinent women first discussed the importance of a posterior urethrovesical angle in maintaining continence. They concluded that a normal posterior urethrovesical (PUV) angle of less than 120° was an important aspect of the continence mechanism, because such an angle was characteristically greater than 120° in patients suffering from stress incontinence. Several authors have verified this point since then. It has been noted that the relationship of the bladder neck and urethra to the pubic symphysis is not the major anatomic feature of the etiology of stress incontinence, because many patients with bladder descent but with a normal PUV angle were continent, whereas some incontinent women had bladders and urethras appropriately positioned to the pubic symphysis but had lost their PUV. Normal continent women demonstrate a bladder base nearly parallel to the horizontal in a standing position and have a sharply defined PUV angle of 90° to 100°. When such bladders are visualized by cystourethrography, it is noted that the angle is maintained even with cough, and funneling does not occur. Most women with stress incontinence usually demonstrate near complete loss of the PUV angle and funneling and posterior descent of the vesical neck.

In the past Green and others have attempted to grade the severity of stress incontinence by the amount of loss of PUV angle. They defined type I loss as showing complete or almost complete loss of PUV angle but with the angle of inclination to the vertical of the urethral axis as being normal (10° to 30°) or at least 45° in the lateral standing-straining configuration, as measured by urethrocystogram. They define a type II defect as representing loss of the PUV angle, with an abnormal angle of inclination to the vertical of the urethral axis generally of 45° 90°. In 1971 the concept of a saline-moistened cotton swab test was introduced to differentiate these two types of defects. This test involved placing a cotton swab into the urethra and observing the angle the urethra made with the horizontal in the relaxed and voiding positions. Montz and Stanton reevaluated the cotton swab test and discovered that 32% of patients with a positive test had either pure detrusor instability or pure sensory urgency after a complete urologic workup. Furthermore, 29% of the patients who had a negative test were finally diagnosed as having pure genuine stress incontinence. Although these authors noted that the cotton swab test was more likely to be positive in younger patients with a cystourethrocele who had undergone minimal bladder neck repair, they believed that the test was not sensitive enough to differentiate stress incontinence from other forms of incontinence and recommended that more sensitive and specific urodynamic investigations be carried out in incontinent women.

Other investigators have noted similar findings and have concluded that the cotton swab test suggests defects in the anterior vaginal wall supports but not a specific urologic diagnosis. The test also quantifies the mobility of the bladder neck and proximal urethra in both continent and incontinent women with and without pelvic support relaxation but offers no additional information about incontinence to that noted by history or physical examination.

A second test developed to help identify abnormalities of the bladder neck was the bead-chain cystourethrogram. This involved placing a sterile bead chain through the urethra into the bladder and radiographing the patient during the resting stage and during voiding. However, Fantl and coworkers demonstrated that 83 cystourethrograms interpreted by three radiologists using five specific radiologic landmarks failed to identify any agreement in interpretation, with a variation in interpretation of from 19.3% to 54.2%. Further, Fantl's group could find no statistically significant difference in the distribution of radiographic characteristics between patients with stress incontinence and detrusor instability.

Bladder neck funneling and position can be evaluated by perineal ultrasound, and this test may have many useful applications in the future. Ultrasound examination of the urethral sphincter may also be helpful in measuring length, thickness, and striated muscle volume. Athanasiou and associates using three-dimensional ultrasound have shown that women with stress urinary incontinence had significantly shorter, thinner, and smaller volumes of striated muscle in their urethras than did continent women of comparable ages and parity.

It is well accepted today that the degree of loss of PUV angle is not as critical as the position of the bladder neck within the abdominal cavity, and Green's classification is no longer used in most centers. In addition to the importance of the urethral sphincteric system to continence, the support system has been studied further. DeLancey's "hammock" theory explains the urethra sits on the endopelvic fascia and anterior vaginal wall. Because that support layer is attached to the pelvic wall via the arcus tendineus fascia pelvis and levator ani, when increased abdominal pressure occurs, the urethra is actually compressed. This maintains urethral closure pressures above increases in abdominal and bladder pressure and prevents urinary leakage (Fig. 21-10). Therefore stress incontinence may occur with injury or degeneration to either the urethral support system or the urethral sphincter mechanism or both. This theory alters the common thinking that the urethra is an intraabdominal organ and loss of support leads to incontinence because pressures are not transmitted equally to the urethra if it is displaced.

The possibility of trauma, by obstetric delivery or other traumatic experience, has been implicated in the cause of stress incontinence. Meyer and colleagues studied 149 patients during pregnancy and 9 weeks postpartum. They found that 36% of women who were delivered by forceps and 21% who delivered spontaneously suffered from urinary incontinence. Bladder neck mobility was significantly increased after all vaginal births, but bladder neck position at rest was only lowered in the forceps group. Women who underwent cesarean delivery were unaffected. DeLancey and coworkers have reported MRI images showing levator ani injuries in 10% to 15% of primiparous women. These injuries may lead to later pelvic floor dysfunction and incontinence although long-term follow-up studies are needed (Fig. 21-11). Considering other forms of pelvic floor training, Nygaard, female American Olympic athletes, could not find a difference between the low-impact (swimmers) and the high-impact (gymnasts and track and field performers) athletes with respect to the development of stress incontinence later in life.

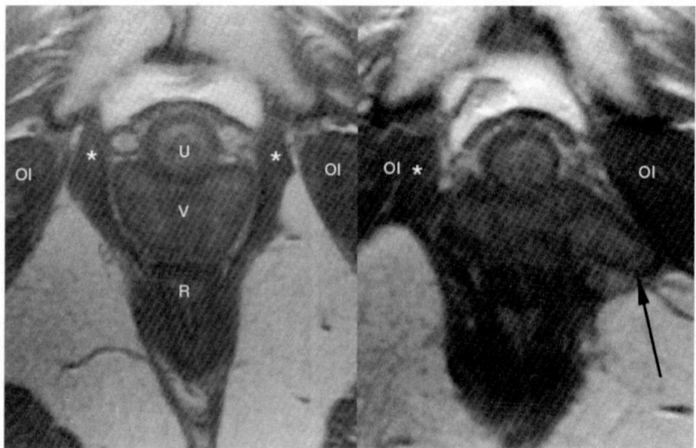

Figure 21-11. Axial magnetic resonance imaging scan at the level of the midurethra in a normal nullipara (*left*) and a woman 9 months after vaginal birth (*right*) in whom the pubovisceral portion of the levator ani muscle has been lost. The pubovisceral muscle (*) is seen between the urethra (U) and the obturator internus (OI) muscle in the normal woman but is missing in the woman on the right. R, rectum; V, vagina. (From Delancey JOL, Ashton-Miller JA: Pathophysiology of adult urinary incontinence. Gastroenterolgy 126(Suppl 1):S23, 2004.)

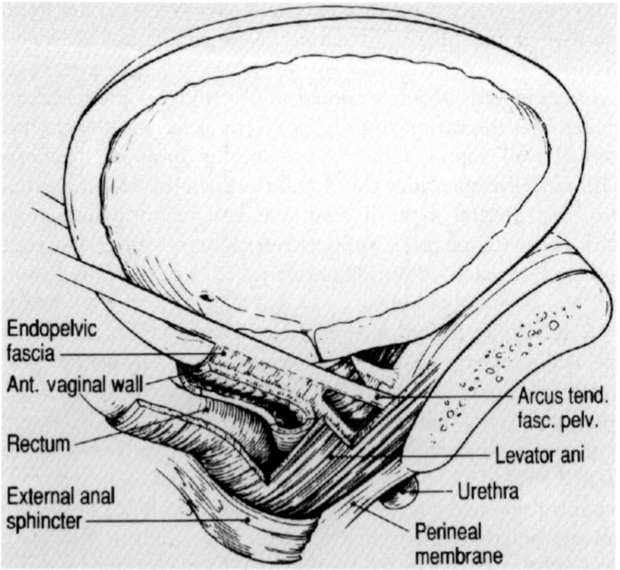

Figure 21-10. Lateral view of the components of the urethral support system. Note how the levator ani muscles support the rectum, vagina, and urethrovesical neck. Also note how the endopelvic fascia beside the urethra attaches to the levator ani muscle; contraction of the levator muscle leads to elevation of the urethrovesical neck. (From Delancey JOL, Ashton-Miller JA: Pathophysiology of adult urinary incontinence. Gastroenterolgy 126(Suppl 1):S23, 2004.)

Further Diagnostic Considerations

Confusion in diagnosis is commonly caused by the presence of a cystocele. A cystocele is a herniation of the bladder into the vagina and is visualized with the patient in the lithotomy position as a bulge of the anterior vaginal wall. Many patients with cystoceles, however, have well-supported bladder necks and are continent. At times the anatomic defect involves the urethra and the bladder neck as well, forming a cystourethrocele. In such cases, in addition to the presence of the cystocele, the bladder neck is also displaced. Whereas the patient with a cystocele sometimes has stress incontinence, the patient with the cystourethrocele frequently has stress incontinence.

Several authors have described the concept of leak point pressure tests. Instead of measuring the intravesical pressure needed to overcome passive urethral resistance, this test measures the intravesical pressure necessary to overcome urethral resistance under stress (cough or strain). Swift and Ostergard studied 108 consecutive patients prospectively using history, physical examination, cough stress test, and multichannel urodynamics. Sixty-five patients (60%) were found to have urodynamic stress incontinence. They noted that urine loss with cough during multichannel studies had a 91% sensitivity and 100% specificity, whereas positive stress leak point pressure determination had a 78% sensitivity and was 100% specific. They compared this with several other observations relating to stress urinary incontinence and concluded that urine loss with cough during multichannel urodynamics was the best examination for diagnosing urodynamic stress incontinence in their population. Sultana studied 56 women with urodynamic stress incontinence urodynamically and found that 40 subjects demonstrated a leak on Valsalva maneuver. In these, maximum urethral closure pressure and leak point pressures were related significantly ($P < 0.001$). This relationship was strongest between leak point pressures up to 120 cm H_2O and absolute vesical pressure with Valsalva rather than with the change in vesical pressure. The leak point pressure test has sensitivity for predicting low urethral pressure of 100%. Swift and Ostergard also demonstrated the use of this test in determining stress incontinence secondary to low pressure urethra.

Studies have reported many variations in techniques to measure leak point pressures. The International Continence Society defines an abdominal leak point pressure (ALPP) as the lowest of the intentional or actively increased intravesical pressure that provokes urinary leakage in the absence of a detrusor contraction. This increased pressure can result from a Valsalva maneuver or coughing. The ALPP has been used to separate urinary stress incontinence as either related to an anatomic defect (hypermobility of the urethra) or intrinsic sphincter deficiency. However, is has become clear there is significant overlap in these conditions and using a simple cut off of less than 60 cm H_2O to define intrinsic sphincter deficiency is too simplistic.

Management

Before considering the operative approaches to the treatment of stress incontinence, it is reasonable to discuss other means of management. The first of these is pelvic floor muscle training directed toward the strengthening of the levator ani and pubococcygeal muscles. This can be affected by isometric exercises as described by Kegel. Although a number of modifications of these exercises exist, one useful application is to teach the patient to contract these muscles for the count of 10, 5 to 10 times, and to repeat this series several times a day. Interestingly, Kegel in 1956 suggested that the patient contract her pubococcygeal muscles five times on waking, five times on rising, and five times every half hour throughout the day. The patient can be instructed on how to contract these muscles by being told to attempt to stop the urinary stream while she is voiding. After she learns which muscles to contract, she may perform the exercises at any time without any relationship to voiding. These exercises improve the muscular supports of the bladder neck, and in some cases this may be enough to overcome the anatomic weakness that led to the stress incontinence.

Several studies have been performed to demonstrate the ability of patients to overcome stress incontinence by performing pelvic floor exercises. Henalla and colleagues used a form of pelvic floor exercise under the direction of physical therapists in two different hospitals. Using a perineal pad weighing test to assess the quantity of urine lost during exercise before and after 3 months of therapy, they found that 67% of patients achieved either complete continence or a significant improvement of symptoms. Although the severity of the symptoms before therapy and the patient's age had no effect on outcome, the treatment was noted to be more effective when the symptoms were present for less than a year. Tchou and coworkers performed urodynamic evaluations on 14 patients before and after pelvic floor exercise therapy. Of these, nine experienced a reversion of their urinary stress test to negative, and all subjects reported an improvement in symptoms. Henalla and colleagues in a different study divided 104 patients with stress incontinence into four groups. The first group ($N = 26$) was treated with pelvic floor exercises; the second group ($N = 25$) was treated with a course of 10 interferential (electric current) treatments over a 10-week period (one per week); the third group ($N = 24$) was treated with vaginal conjugated estrogen cream, 2 g per night for 12 weeks (1.25 mg conjugated estrogen/2 g dose); and the fourth group ($N = 25$) was given no treatment and served as a control group. The groups were evaluated before and after therapy (after 3 months) with a perineal pad weighing test, and all 100 were available for questionnaire evaluation 9 months after therapy. A total of 65% (17) of the pelvic floor exercise group, 32% (8) of the interferential group, 12% (3) of the estrogen-treated group, and none of the controls were found either cured or improved.

The 2005 Cochrane Database review of pelvic floor muscle training analyzed 43 trials, although many trials were small and poorly controlled. Pelvic floor exercises were better than placebo or no treatment for women with stress or mixed incontinence. It is not clear that they help urge incontinence. There is insufficient evidence to know whether adding additional treatments, such as biofeedback or weighted vaginal cones, is beneficial. However, more intensive treatment strategies appeared to improve outcomes.

Many patients enjoy a prolonged relief even after stopping pelvic floor muscle exercise. Bø and Talseth studied 23 women who participated in a 6-month intensive pelvic floor muscle exercise routine and noted that 5 years later 75% demonstrated no leakage during a stress test and 70% were satisfied with their continence. Seventy percent of these patients were still exercising their pelvic muscles at least once a week and demonstrated pelvic floor muscle strength. Nygaard noted similar findings. These authors noted improvement of incontinence not only in patients with stress incontinence but also in those with urge and mixed urinary incontinence.

It is important to be sure that the patient is aware of how to perform the exercises correctly. In a study by Bump and coworkers in which 47 women were given either simple verbal or written instructions, 23 (49%) had an ideal Kegel effort signified by an increase in force of the urethral closure, and 12 subjects (25%) were performing the technique poorly and in such a way that incontinence might be promoted. These authors recommended a demonstration approach rather than a written or verbal approach.

A variation in pelvic muscle training is the use of vaginal cones. This involves a set of cones of increasing weight that require pelvic muscle contraction to hold them within the vagina. Peattie and associates demonstrated an improvement in 70% of 30 premenopausal women with stress incontinence after only 1 month of exercise. A correlation was noted between decreased urine loss and the ability to retain cones of increased weight. Other studies also show benefit of weighted vaginal cones over no treatment, but there is not evidence that cones are any better than pelvic muscle exercises.

Pelvic floor electrical stimulation has also been used and shown to be of value in improving pelvic floor muscle strength and decreasing symptoms of stress incontinence. Sand and colleagues conducted a multicenter prospective, randomized, double-blind placebo-controlled, 15-week trial comparing the use of pelvic floor stimulation with a sham device. Thirty-five women used the active unit, and 17 used the sham device. All were followed by urodynamic testing. Significant improvement from the baseline was found in the study patients but not in the controls, with respect to numbers of leakage episodes per day and per week, pad studies, and vaginal muscle strength.

In postmenopausal women, estrogen therapy may increase the vasculature and the tone of the bladder neck, thereby increasing urethral closing pressure and again overcoming the effects that have led to mild degrees of stress incontinence. Estrogen also has a positive effect on vaginal atrophy in women, and many observational studies have shown the combination of estrogen and Kegel exercises may occasionally be all that some women require to overcome their stress incontinence (see the following box). But, more recent randomized studies have called into question the effects of estrogen on incontinence. The Heart and Estrogen/Progestin Replacement Study (HERS) found the group of women taking combined hormone replacement actually reported worsened incontinence. Oral estrogen is no longer advised for stress incontinence. (See Estrogen and the Lower Urinary Tract section at the end of this chapter).

Other non-FDA drugs and combinations of drugs have been studied to determine whether nonoperative therapy could aid stress incontinent women. In a study of 30 stress incontinent women using clinical and urodynamic assessment, Kiesswetter and colleagues compared continence profiles after treatment with an α-adrenergic stimulant, midodrine; a cholinesterase inhibitor, distigmine bromide; a tricyclic antidepressant, imipramine; or an estriol, triodurin. In each case the patients were treated for 4 weeks and reevaluated. Finally, a suspensory sling operation was performed. After a successful sling operation the profile for continence as outlined by the authors increased 45% compared with an increase of 9% for midodrine, 8.9% for imipramine, and 7.9% for the combination of estriol and distigmine bromide. The urethral pressures showed an increase of mean value of 8.1% after operation, 8.3% after midodrine, 7.9% after imipramine, 3.5% after estriol, and 3.5% after distigmine bromide. The authors believed that estriol plus midodrine and estriol plus imipramine were favored subjectively by the patients over single-drug therapy, but little difference was noted in urodynamic assessment to show the advantage of one drug or combination over another. Although imipramine is a tricyclic antidepressant, it has α-adrenergic enhancement characteristics. Other α-adrenergic drugs such as phenylpropanolamine may be useful in treating stress incontinence because of their action on the α-receptors in the bladder neck and urethra, causing muscle contraction. Overall, there is limited benefit with drugs for treating stress incontinence and weak evidence to suggest adrenergic drugs are any better than placebo treatment. Table 21-5 is a summary by Corlett of classes of other agents that may affect urinary function or therapy.

Methods of Pelvic Muscle Strengthening

Kegel exercises
Isometric with vaginal cones (weights)
Electrical stimulation of pelvic floor

Before the 1950s the operative approach to treat stress incontinence primarily involved vaginal procedures, which included plication of the bladder neck (Kelly procedure) with anterior colporrhaphy to reduce a cystocele. However, after Green attempted to grade the degree of PUV angle loss in such patients, it was demonstrated by Bailey and others that the success rate using the vaginal approach varied according to the cause of the incontinence. Patients showing an almost complete loss of PUV angle had a 90% success rate when followed for 5 to 10 years after a bladder neck plication and anterior colporrhaphy, but only 50% of patients with lesser PUV angle loss remained continent over that period. However, after the introduction of suprapubic urethrovesical suspension operations, the 5-year cure rate for these latter patients surpassed 90% in most series. Bergman and Giovanni and Harris and coworkers have published data demonstrating that the retropubic urethropexy operations have a higher cure rate than do anterior colporrhaphies for stress incontinence when the patients are followed long term.

Table 21-5 Drugs with Possible Effects on the Lower Urinary Tract

Class	Possible Side Effects	Drug and Usual Indication	Action
Antihypertensives	Incontinence	Reserpine—hypertension Methyldopa—hypertension	Pharmacologic sympathectomy by depleting catecholamines
Dopaminergic agonists	Bladder neck obstruction	Bromocriptine—galactorrhea Levodopa—Parkinson's disease	Increased urethral resistance and decreased detrusor contractions
Cholinergic agonists	Decreased bladder capacity and increased intravesical pressure	Digitalis—cardiotropic	Increased bladder wall tension
Neuroleptics	Incontinence	Major tranquilizers: prochlorperazine, promethazine, trifluoperazine, chlorpromazine, haloperidol	Dopamine receptor blockade, with internal sphincter relaxation
β-Adrenergic agents	Urinary retention	Isoxsuprine—vasodilator Terbutaline—bronchodilator Ritodrine—tocolytic agent	Inhibited bladder muscle contractility
Xanthines	Incontinence	Caffeine	Decreased urethral closure pressure

From Corlett RC: Female Patient 10:20, 1985.

It thus seemed important to determine the type of anatomic defect the patient had and to design appropriate operative management. For the continent patient with a definite relaxation of the anterior vaginal wall and a bladder neck that is displaced into the lower pelvis, an anterior colporrhaphy with bladder neck plication is appropriate. This is frequently performed in conjunction with a vaginal hysterectomy if there is evidence for uterine prolapse, and a posterior colporrhaphy, because the support structures of both anterior and posterior vaginal walls were frequently relaxed in such patients. The decision of whether to perform a vaginal hysterectomy and posterior wall repair depends on the circumstances and does not modify the success rate of the anterior colporrhaphy. The anterior colporrhaphy is carried out by incising the vaginal mucosa in the midline and separating the pubocervical fascia from the vaginal mucosa by blunt and sharp dissection. The dissection is carried to the area of the bladder neck, and the first plication suture is placed on either side of the bladder neck using a 0 or 2-0 polyglycol suture. The slowly absorbable suture is ideal for this type of repair. Bladder plication is then continued from the area of the bladder neck to reduce an existing cystocele (Fig. 21-12).

Transvaginal needle suspensions (TVNS) were introduced in the late 1950s as a less invasive alternative to retropubic operations. Special needles were developed by Pereyra that could be used to guide sutures from the paravaginal tissue through the space of Retzius and suspended from the rectus fascia. Nonabsorbable material was used, and the suture was tied over the rectus fascia just above the bladder neck. This was carried out through a small suprapubic incision. Direct urethrocystoscopy helped avoid injuring the bladder neck during the needle placement. Stamey's 1973 modification of the Pereyra procedure used a small tube of Dacron material to buttress the suture, thereby keeping it from pulling through. Stamey reported about 3% of the patients in his series required a removal of the suprapubic suture because of pain or infection. Many other modifications of TVNS have been described and popularized.

In assessing the long-term success rate of the use of the modified Pereyra procedure in patients with recurrent stress urinary incontinence, Holschneider and colleagues studied 54 patients. These women were divided into two groups. Group 1 comprised those individuals with no risk factors, which include evidence for detrusor instability, low-pressure urethra, fibrotic urethra, a negative cotton swab test, and neurogenic incontinence. Group 2 comprised individuals who had such risk factors. Of the 38 patients in group 1, 81.6% demonstrated continence after a mean follow-up period of 36.3 months. On the other hand, the 16 patients in group 2 demonstrated only a 43.8% cure rate, and the mean time to the recurrence of incontinence in those who failed in this group was 6.8 months. These authors noted an intraoperative complication rate of 7.4% for both groups, with the complications involving suture in the bladder and hemorrhage, and a postoperative complication rate of 25.9%, in which infection most often was the complication. Also, 33.3% of these patients suffered late postoperative complications, which included detrusor instability and obstructive voiding dysfunction.

Several national and international organizations convened and reviewed the long-term success rates of incontinence operations when it became apparent that TVNS held up poorly after 2 to 3 years. Consensus statements suggested slings and retropubic suspensions have more durable results than TVNS or anterior repair for stress incontinence. TVNS have rapidly declined as a primary treatment option for stress incontinence, as have anterior repairs.

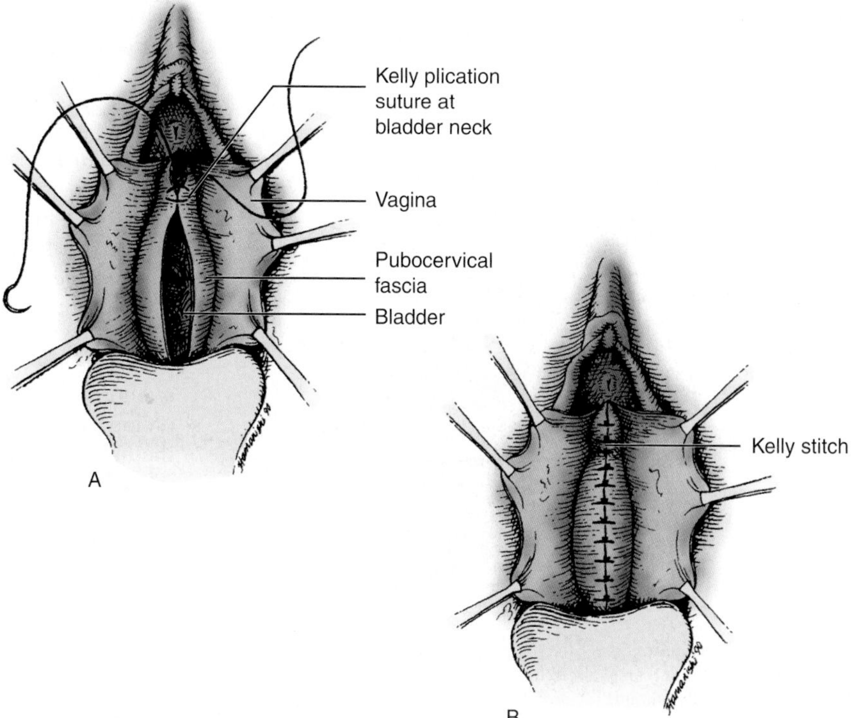

Figure 21-12. Cystourethrocele repair. **A,** Appearance of cystourethrocele after plication of bladder neck and repair of cystocele; cut edge of vagina is held apart above repair. **B,** Repair of vagina over cystocele is noted. (Redrawn from Symmonds RE: Relaxation of pelvic supports. In Benson RC [ed]: Current Obstetric and Gynecologic Diagnosis and Treatment, 5th ed. Los Altos, CA, Lange Medical, 1984.)

Appropriate therapy for patients with urodynamic stress incontinence, in most instances is a suprapubic approach or a vaginal sling. The Marshall–Marchetti–Krantz suprapubic urethrovesical suspension operation was first reported in 1949 and has been the mainstay of many surgeons attempting to alleviate stress incontinence in such patients. The procedure may be done by itself or in conjunction with other abdominal procedures, such as an abdominal hysterectomy. The space of Retzius is entered, the bladder neck is identified generally with a 30-mL bulb Foley catheter in the bladder, and the paravaginal tissue adjacent to the bladder neck is identified and sutured to the pubic symphysis using two or three interrupted sutures on each side of the bladder neck. Again, 0 or 2-0 polyglycol suture is ideal for this procedure, but some operators prefer nonabsorbable suture. The operator must be careful not to place undue stress on the bladder neck. Stress can generally be assessed by placing one hand in the vagina and palpating the tension on the bladder neck at the time the sutures are tied (Fig. 21-13). The patient is followed for 2 to 5 days with continuous catheter drainage. In most cases, after removal of the catheter, the patient will void. Occasionally, voiding is delayed and the patient may need to be discharged with an indwelling catheter in the bladder to be checked 1 week hence. It is usual to check a patient for residual urine after she voids; residuals of less than 100 to 150 mL, after the patient voids at least 200 mL, are considered acceptable. Larger residuals should signal continuing catheterization for 48 to 72 hours or the use of intermittent self-catheterization.

A rare (1% to 2%) but painful complication of the Marshall–Marchetti–Krantz procedure is osteitis pubis. This condition is an inflammatory reaction in the periosteum of the pubic bone more often associated with permanent suture material. This complication after suprapubic cystotomy was first reported in 1923 by Legueu and Rochet. The next year Beer described six patients with pubic symphysis periostitis after suprapubic procedures. Pain is the major symptom, but patients usually demonstrate a "waddling gait."

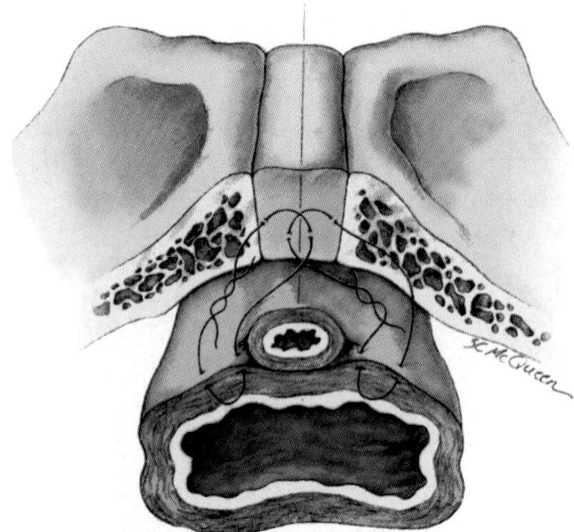

Figure 21-13. Demonstration of the relative position of a pair of sutures adjacent to the urethra securely placed into the pubic symphysis. (Redrawn from Buchsbaum HJ, Schmidt JD [eds]: Gynecologic and Obstetric Urology. Philadelphia, WB Saunders, 1982. Reprinted with permission.)

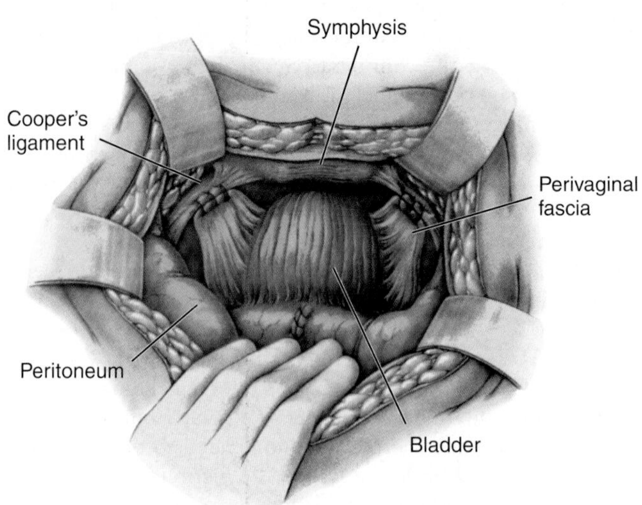

Figure 21-14. Burch procedure. The lateral edges of the vagina have been sutured to the Cooper's ligaments. (Redrawn from Burch JC: Urethrovaginal fixation to Cooper's ligament for correction of stress incontinence, cystocele, and prolapse. Am J Obstet Gynecol 81:281, 1961.)

Kammerer-Doak and coworkers reviewed the Mayo Clinic experience with 2030 Marshall–Marchetti–Krantz procedures performed between 1980 and 1994. There were 15 cases of osteitis pubis (0.74%) occurring an average of 69 days postoperative (range, 10–459 days). Conservative therapy relieved symptoms in 47% and seven of the remaining patients needed surgical intervention, including suture removal (57%) and symphyseal débridement (86%). In five cases bone cultures were positive.

It is important to differentiate this condition from true osteomyelitis. The latter condition, seen occasionally after radical pelvic operations and other pelvic procedures, involves infection of the bone and is often associated with positive blood cultures. Hoyme and associates reviewed this subject in relation to radical gynecologic operations. Treatment of osteomyelitis often involves prolonged antibiotic therapy and surgical débridement. Treatment of osteitis pubis includes antibiotics and analgesics and may require the removal of permanent sutures.

In 1961 Burch advocated a modification of the suprapubic bladder neck suspension by suspending the vaginal wall to Cooper's ligament (Fig. 21-14). The original description uses 2-0 chromic catgut sutures, but polyglycol or nonabsorbable sutures are more appropriate now. Postoperative care similar to that described for the Marshall–Marchetti–Krantz operation is appropriate. At times patients have difficulty voiding for prolonged periods, and the occasional patient may report that she needs to rise off the commode to a semistanding position to void.

Both the Marshall–Marchetti–Krantz and Burch procedures have their advocates. When properly performed, each procedure produces a long-term cure in more than 80% of patients with stress incontinence. Feyereisl and colleagues reported a long-term success rate of 81.6% in 87 women carefully evaluated preoperatively for stress urinary incontinence. Their follow-up was between 5 and 10 years. Colombo and coworkers performed a prospective randomized clinical trial using the Burch and

Marshall–Marchetti–Krantz procedures. The follow-up was 2 to 7 years. These authors reported subjective and objective cure rates of 92% and 80%, respectively, for the Burch procedure and 85% and 65%, respectively, for the Marshall–Marchetti–Krantz procedure. These differences were not statistically significant. In a recent Cochrane Database review of 39 trials of the Burch procedure, Lapitan and associates noted that the success rate reported varied from 85% to 90% at 1 year, and 70% were dry at 5 years. Other studies have shown a 69% success rate at 10 to 20 years. Frequently, failures can be resolved by performing the same procedure again, indicating that the problem was technical performance of the procedure rather than a failure of the type of procedure.

Herbertsson and Iosif studied 72 women who had undergone retropubic colpourethrocystopexy between 1979 and 1982 for stress incontinence. Follow-up urodynamic studies were performed in 1989 and 1990. The surgical cure rate was considered to be 90.3%, but five of the seven patients who were considered failures felt that their symptoms had improved. Thirty-eight of the patients were found on urodynamic studies to have an incompetent bladder neck. But 31 of these 38 patients were still continent. The authors concluded that this type of surgical approach to stress urinary incontinence was most appropriate.

The Burch procedure can also be performed laparoscopically. Saidi and colleagues have reported comparable 12-month cure rates in 70 patients undergoing laparoscopic procedures (91.4%) and 87 patients undergoing open procedures (92%). The laparoscopic procedures had a somewhat shorter operative time and a much shorter hospital stay. Ross followed 48 consecutive patients who underwent laparoscopic Burch procedures and found a cure rate of 93% and 89% at 1 and 2 years, respectively, using multichannel urodynamic studies. Further studies have not been large enough to clarify the proposed benefits and one randomized study found a higher 3-year failure rate compared with an open technique. With the introduction of minimally invasive vaginal midurethral slings, it is unclear what role laparoscopic Burch will serve.

Shull and Baden reported on 149 consecutive patients who were assessed anatomically and found to have a paravaginal defect causing stress urinary incontinence. In such cases they performed an abdominal repair in which the anterior vaginal wall was sutured with permanent suture to the white line bilaterally. In follow-up for as long as 48 months, 97% of the patients remained continent. However, 6% suffered vaginal cuff prolapse, 5% developed an enterocele in addition to cuff prolapse, and 5% redeveloped the cystocele after the operation. When, on anatomic examination, the paravaginal fascial defect is noted, this operation has good application as an alternative to other described procedures. It may also be utilized in conjunction with other procedures when multiple anatomic defects are identified. It can be performed abdominally or vaginally. Most surgeons do not perform a paravaginal defect repair as the sole operation for stress incontinence due to the paucity of studies. However, for anatomic correction of a paravaginal support defect, it may be useful.

The newer midurethral vaginal tape slings have quickly gained popularity for treating urodynamic stress incontinence surgically. The first to be introduced was the tension-free vaginal tape sling (TVT). This was developed based on the theory

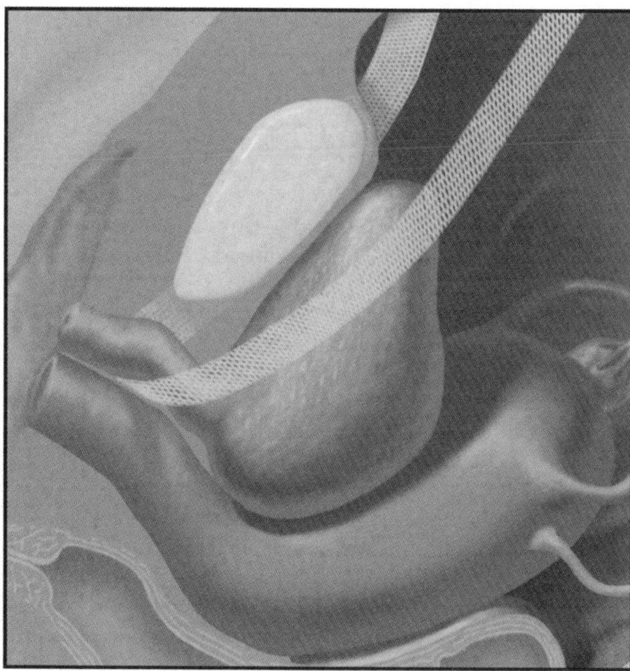

Figure 21-15. Tension-free vaginal tape (TVT) sling with Prolene mesh placed midurethrally without the need for fixation. (From Gynecare, a division of Ethicon. Somerville, NJ.)

that the tension on the pubourethral ligaments interacted with muscles of the pelvic floor and the suburethral vaginal support structure. Ulmsten and coworkers published a 1996 article on 75 women treated with a midurethral sling made of permanent mesh (Fig. 21-15). The sling was placed under local anesthesia with sedation. An 84% cure rate was reported, an additional 8% were improved and 8% failed. At 3 years after surgery, Ulmsten and coworkers reported an 86% cure rate. Many other authors from around the world published similar success rates. Studies in the elderly and obese populations also have similar success. Complications have included retropubic hematoma, bladder perforation, intraoperative bleeding, urinary retention, mesh exposure, and rare bowel and urethral injuries and vascular injury. Ward, Hilton, and the UK and Ireland TVT trial group have published a prospective, randomized study comparing TVT with Burch colposuspension for primary urodynamic stress incontinence. With very strict outcome data, the TVT procedure appears to be as effective as the Burch at 2 years, with 63% and 51% cured by objective outcome data, respectively.

Delorme introduced the transobturator approach in 2001 with the hope of avoiding vascular, bladder, and bowel injuries. Initial reports show similar success rates to the TVT but no long-term outcome data are available to date or direct comparison data.

Urethral Sphincter Dysfunction

Sand and associates offered some insight into why at least some retropubic urethropexy procedures fail. In a study of 86 patients who were evaluated preoperatively and postoperatively with urodynamic studies, they noted that in women younger than 50 years of age there was a significant risk of failure if the preoperative urethral closure pressure was less than 20 cm H_2O. Although low urethral closure pressure was found to be an independent risk factor in women younger than 50, it was not found to be so in women older than 50.

In 1981 McGuire noted the loss of intrinsic urethral tone in a number of women, particularly those with a history of pelvic trauma, radiation, underlying neurologic conditions, or scarring of the urethral sphincter. At first this was called type III incontinence but is currently referred to as *intrinsic sphincter deficiency (ISD)*. Currently, the two types of stress incontinence (hypermobility and ISD) are thought to be interdependent and not separate entities. However, it is still useful to consider a discussion of severe stress incontinence in women with a fixed and poorly functioning urethra.

Horbach and Ostergard retrospectively evaluated 263 consecutive patients undergoing a complete urodynamic evaluation because of urinary leakage. Intrinsic sphincter dysfunction was defined as maximum urethral closure of 20 cm H_2O or less in the sitting position at maximum cystometric capacity. One hundred and thirty-two women (50.2%) were found to have intrinsic sphincter dysfunction. Women in this group tended to be older and were more likely to have undergone a hysterectomy and at least one antiincontinence procedure compared with those women with continence problems who had normal urethral pressure. By multivariant analysis, they noted that age greater than 50 years was the only independent variable that could predict the presence of intrinsic sphincter dysfunction in women with stress urinary incontinence.

At present, treatment for urinary stress incontinence caused by intrinsic urethral dysfunction consists of one of the following: periurethral bulking substance injections, urethral sling procedure, or the use of an artificial sphincter device. A number of substances have been used for periurethral bulking injection. These have included the individual's blood or fat, polytetrafluoroethylene (Teflon), and more recently, bovine collagen. Injection of blood or fat has given only transient relief, and the use of Teflon has resulted in several complications, primarily caused by the wandering of the Teflon to distant sites. GAX-collagen has been used as a urethral bulking agent. This is a cross-linked glutaraldehyde bovine dermal collagen first used by Appell and colleagues, who reported a high success rate. This agent has a relatively high incidence of hypersensitivity reaction, and therefore the patient should be skin tested before its use. Without hypersensitivity it appears to be a relatively safe and minimally invasive means of closing the urethra, and centers are now using it for this purpose. It seems to have a positive effect for at least 2 years, and it is possible to reinject patients. Long-term follow-up has been disappointing, with a 26% success rate at 5 years. Part of the failure may result because collagen is biodegradable and not necessary durable. Permanent materials of silicone microimplants and pyrolytic zirconium oxide beads have been studied. Short-term success rates range widely from 33% to 60% for cure or improvement, but safety and durability are yet to be reported in the long run. Nonetheless, for elderly, unfit women and women who have failed other incontinence surgeries, an injectable material for stress incontinence might be an attractive option.

A variety of traditional sling procedures, including the use of fascia lata, anterior rectus fascia tissue, cadaveric fascia lata and inert materials such as Mersilene, can be used. These procedures mobilize the bladder neck, often by a vaginal or vaginal and abdominal approach, and allow the interposition of a strip of material under the proximal urethra surrounding the bladder neck, which is attached to the anterior rectus sheath. This creates support and compression to the urethra and prevents urethral movement during increased abdominal pressure. This procedure is generally effective in creating continence.

The surgeon must exercise care in determining the tension to be applied on the bladder neck when the sling is fixed. Making it too tight may interfere with voiding and may actually damage the bladder neck; making it too loose will abrogate its effectiveness. Generally with a No. 16 or 18 Foley catheter in the urethra it should be possible for the surgeon to judge the tension so that the sling fits comfortably against the urethra without compressing it. Concomitant cystoscopy may also be used.

Beck and coworkers reported their results in treating 170 patients over 22 years with a fascia lata sling procedure. These patients had undergone one or more unsuccessful attempts to correct their stress urinary incontinence. In all patients an intraurethral pressure of 80 to 90 cm H_2O was created at the site of the sling. Their success rate in curing the stress urinary incontinence was 98.2%, with 100% success noted in their last 148 cases. The most troublesome postoperative problem was delayed voiding, which averaged 59.6 days. Many other reports using other sling material show success rates (cure or improvement) of 86% to 92% with complications of urinary retention and de novo development of urgency.

Although an anterior rectus sheath fascial sling procedure is probably as effective as a Marshall–Marchetti–Krantz or Burch procedure, it involves a greater degree of dissection, as well as entry into the vagina with the potential risk of ascending infection. Thus sling procedures are generally reserved for patients with intrinsic sphincter deficiency or patients whose previous antiincontinence procedure failed. Fascia lata slings are being used by many surgeons and can be performed mostly vaginally in a relatively short operative time. Autologous fascia lata is more effective than irradiated and freeze-dried donor fascia lata, with the use of the latter type leading to a concern about graft degeneration and, thus, procedure failure.

The use of the artificial urinary sphincter may be a viable option for some women and will generally produce continence. Artificial urinary sphincters are generally placed by an abdominal and vaginal surgical approach. Expulsion and mechanical problems with these devices are potential side effects. The artificial sphincter consists of a cuff surrounding the urethra. The device is controlled by a pressure balloon placed in the space of Retzius. The patient controls the device by releasing pressure when she wishes to void and reestablishing pressure when she wishes to be continent. Diokno and coworkers reported a 91% success rate in 32 patients in whom they implanted the device. Other authors have reported similar results.

Table 21-6 summarizes the overall long-term cure and improvement rates in multiple studies published before 1995 as summarized by the U.S. Department of Health and Human Services, Agency for Health Care Policy and Research. Outcome reporting varies by study and the definition of cure has not been standardized so this cannot be considered a direct comparison of techniques. The newer midurethral slings are being studied for intrinsic sphincter deficiency.

Table 21-6 Treatment Outcome for Intrinsic Deficiency (Combined Multiple Studies)

Outcome	Collagen (%)	Sling (%)	Artificial Sphincter (%)
Cured	69	84	92
Improved	25	6	4
Cured or improved	94	95	96
Complications	—	31	32

Urodynamic Studies after Retropubic Urethropexy for Stress Incontinence

In a study of 29 women with stress incontinence investigated urodynamically before and after Marshall–Marchetti–Krantz operation by Beisland and colleagues, no major changes in the urethral pressure profile could be demonstrated. The authors did note a good correlation between clinical results and the changes in transmission of increased abdominal pressure to the urethra. The operative procedure did not seem to increase the urethral pressure. Those patients with low maximal urethral pressure preoperatively continued to have insufficient urethral sphincter function after the operation. Indeed the operation in some cases may have caused injury to the sphincter because of excessive dissection around the urethra.

In a study of 25 women after Burch colposuspension in which 88% had objective evidence of cure, an increase in voiding difficulty and urodynamic evidence of outflow obstruction was seen 6 months after the procedure. Beisland and colleagues also noted that the Burch procedure, like the Marshall–Marchetti–Krantz operation, does not induce any significant change in resting urethral profile; they believed the changes noted were probably a mechanical obstruction of the bladder neck.

Recently, van Geelen and associates investigated the urodynamic effects of both anterior repair and Burch procedures. There were no changes in resting urethral pressure profiles in either group of patients after surgery. Pressure transmission rates in the proximal urethra were increased in women treated successfully with the Burch procedure in supine, sitting, and standing positions, but in women unsuccessfully relieved of their incontinence, no significant increase in pressure transmission could be noted. In those women treated successfully with an anterior repair, a significant increase in pressure was observed in the midurethra in the sitting position and in the proximal urethra in the standing position. The authors concluded that the Burch procedure was more effective than an anterior repair in correcting urodynamic stress incontinence.

Some authors have suggested that the chance of curing urodynamic stress incontinence with a surgical procedure was increased by performing a hysterectomy as well. Van Geelen and associates did not note this in their study, and in a recent report by Langer and colleagues no differences were found in the cure rate of 45 patients, of whom 22 underwent a Burch procedure without hysterectomy and 23 underwent a Burch procedure with hysterectomy.

It is difficult to compare the results obtained in curing stress incontinence with different procedures. Differences in techniques and skills of operators and variations in patient selection methods make different procedures difficult to compare. In a large study reported by Park and Miller of 680 surgically treated patients, the Marshall–Marchetti–Krantz procedure and Kelly plication were noted to be equally successful in correcting stress incontinence after 3 years (69% and 66%, respectively). Patients who underwent the Pereyra procedure as their primary repair had a 41% success rate after 3 years. Still, the reader must remember that differences in the groups and in the skills of the surgeons involved may have played a role in the outcomes.

OVERACTIVE BLADDER

Walter and Olesen studied 303 patients complaining of urinary incontinence and discovered that 43% had stress incontinence, 21% urge incontinence, and 36% both urge and stress incontinence. Overactive bladder (OAB) is a relatively new term defined as the symptom of urgency with or without urge incontinence, usually with frequency and nocturia. Urgency is the complaint of a sudden compelling desire to pass urine, which is difficult to defer. Urge incontinence is the complaint of involuntary leakage of urine accompanied by or immediately preceded by urgency. This condition is generally chronic and is associated with an urgency–frequency problem often accompanied by painless urine loss. Generally a large volume of urine is lost; leakage may occur in any position and often with a change in position. Stress secondary to running, walking, coughing, sneezing, or laughing may trigger this type of incontinence, but it is generally delayed until several seconds after the stress has occurred. Stress incontinence frequently disappears during the night, but urge incontinence continues, often with nocturia. OAB occurs in approximately 17% of the population, and the incidence increases with age. OAB patients have lower quality of life than women with stress incontinence.

Detrusor overactivity is a urodynamic observation and the result of sudden, spontaneous detrusor contraction. It has previously been termed *detrusor dyssynergia, unstable bladder,* or *detrusor instability*. The term *idiopathic detrusor overactivity* is used as a urodynamic definition when there is no defined cause of the condition. If a neurologic disorder, such as stroke, Parkinson's disease, or other CNS pathology is present, the term *neurogenic detrusor overactivity* is appropriate. In the elderly, both urge incontinence and urgency can coexists with elevated residual urine. Dribbling often results. This condition is called detrusor hyperactivity with impaired contractile function (DHIC) and these two conditions may have different causal factors.

The loss of urine is probably triggered by sudden, uninhibited stimulation of receptors in the bladder wall. The problem may be caused by the breakdown of normal neurologic and inhibitory reflexes. A postal survey of 6000 women in a Washington State health maintenance organization estimated the prevalence of urinary incontinence to be 42% and major depression 3.7%. However, the depression rate was significantly higher in women with incontinence and in particular, women with moderate and severe incontinence (5.7% and 8.3%, respectively). It also differed by incontinence type (4.7% stress, 6.6% in urge/mixed). The study does not show one condition caused the other, but there is an increased odds of major depression in women with urinary incontinence so it is worth screening for depression in this population. It is possible that altered neurotransmitter function such as serotonin or norepinephrine, could alter bladder function, contributing to uninhibited detrusor contractions and urge incontinence.

Sands and colleagues reported a study of 86 women with urodynamic stress incontinence. Of these, 20 (23.3%) also had unstable detrusor function preoperatively. Of these 20, 11 (55%) had stable detrusor function after retropubic urethropexy, whereas 5 of the 66 (7.6%) patients who had stable detrusor function preoperatively developed unstable detrusors postoperatively. Overall, women with both stress incontinence and unstable detrusors experienced a cure rate of only 30% with surgery. No relationship could be found in preoperative symptoms, age, history of previous procedures, and cystometric parameters between those who were cured and those who were not. In addition, none of these criteria could predict which patient who was detrusor stable before surgery would develop instability after surgery. Risks of developing detrusor instability after surgery must be recognized and may require further medical therapy.

Diagnosis

A bladder diary like that shown in Figure 21-7 can be useful in making the diagnosis of OAB as the diary can document frequency (>8 daytime voids), nocturia (>1 night-time voids), and episodes of incontinence preceded by urgency. Additional information can be obtained about incontinence related to activity (stress incontinence), fluid intake, pad usage, and voided volumes (a measure of bladder capacity). The ideal diary length has yet to be established, but 2 to 7 days is generally recommended. Filling cystometry, which evaluates the pressure/volume relationship of the bladder, allows the detection of spontaneous involuntary detrusor contractions within the bladder, which are noted as the bladder fills. These techniques are also useful in detecting urodynamic stress incontinence in patients who have an urgency component to their incontinence. It is important that in such cases both problems be treated, or it is not likely that incontinence will be cured.

Management

Behavioral therapy and operative procedures may be used to treat OAB, but pharmacologic therapy remains first-line treatment. In those patients who have stress and urge incontinence, an operation may have a place in the specific therapy. However, if the major part of the problem seems to be urge incontinence, this should be treated first, because an operative procedure frequently may not be necessary. Likewise, patients who have undergone an operation for stress urinary incontinence and continue to be incontinent should be evaluated for detrusor overactivity. Bates and coworkers demonstrated that a high percentage of such failures would be found on urodynamic studies to have detrusor overactivity.

Because the majority of patients with detrusor overactivity have abnormal voiding habits, retraining or bladder drills may be of use. This should take the form of bladder retraining, which involves a programmed progressive lengthening of the period between voiding with or without the addition of biofeedback techniques. In a study Millard and Oldenburg demonstrated improvement in 74% of women with detrusor instability using such techniques. Cystometric studies performed on these patients revealed a reversion to stable bladder function. But compliance with bladder retraining by patients is often a problem. Visco and associates studied 123 women who were offered bladder retraining and found that 55% either never started treatment or were noncompliant. They noted that women who were given concurrent pharmacologic therapy had an 87% compliance rate, compared with a 53% rate for those who started training and did not complete it and who were not given medication. Other behavioral treatments such as scheduled voiding, fluid management, and a bedside commode may be particularly helpful in elderly women with OAB.

Pelvic floor muscle training is generally recommended as first-line treatment for stress incontinence symptoms and sometimes for mixed urinary incontinence. In a 2006 Cochrane Database review, the authors concluded that women with incontinence who did pelvic floor muscle training were more likely to report cure or improvement, although only about one less incontinence episode per day. Although women with urge incontinence may experience less benefit than women with stress incontinence, there did appear to be improvement and few adverse effects. Given the noninvasive nature of muscle training it makes sense as initial therapy for all urinary incontinence problems over a 3-month period.

Anticholinergic (antimuscarinic) drugs may be useful. Table 21-7 shows the currently available drugs. At times these medications in conjunction with bladder retraining have greater efficacy than either alone. Overall, in clinical studies, antimuscarinic drugs reduce incontinence episodes by 60% to 75%, but only 20% to 40% of patients have no incontinent episodes. Poor patient compliance is often found with these medications because of continued incontinence and anticholinergic side effects. The most common side effect is dry mouth. Flexible-dosing schedules of several drugs, changing to a different drug, or using the oxybutynin patch allows options to find a tolerable drug for this chronic condition. However, one recent report by Salvatore and colleagues found two thirds of women discontinued therapy within 4 months likely because they do not provide long-lasting symptom relief. Intravesical instillation of anticholinergic medication can provide an alternative delivery mechanism for women who fail or cannot tolerate oral therapy.

Table 21-7 Medications for Overactive Bladder

Drug	Dosage
Oxybutynin (Ditropan IR)*	5 mg bid, tid, or qid
Oxybutynin (Ditropan XL)†	5 mg or 10 mg qd
Tolterodine (Detrol IR)	2 mg or 4 mg
Tolterodine (Detrol LA)‡	4 mg qd
Oxybutynin transdermal (Oxytrol)	3.9 mg patch (twice/week)
Darifenacin (Enablex)	7.5 mg or 15 mg qd
Solifenacin (VESIcare)	5 mg or 10 mg qd
Trospium (Sanctura)	20 mg bid
Imipramine (Tofranil)§	25 mg or 50 mg qd to tid

*Intermediate-release (IR)
†Extended release (XL)
‡Long acting (LA)
§Off-label

Table 21-8 Effective Treatment Options for Women with Urinary Incontinence by Type of Incontinence

Treatment Option	Stress Incontinence	Urge Incontinence
Nonpharmacologic	Pelvic floor muscle training Bladder training Prompted voiding	Pelvic floor muscle training Bladder training Prompted voiding Electrical stimulation
Pharmacologic		Anticholinergic drugs (antimuscarinic) Tolerodine Oxybuynin
Surgical	Open retropubic colposuspension Suburethral sling procedure	

From Holroyd-Leduc JM, Straus SE: Management of urinary incontinence in women. Clinical applications. JAMA 291:996, 2004.

Women with intractable detrusor overactivity who have failed conservative treatment and medications have some new surgical options although most are not well studied. Botulinum toxin shows promise as an injectable medication into the bladder wall, but is not yet approved. Long-term efficacy data are not available. Reinjection is necessary. Sacral neuromodulation involves an implantable device, which chronically stimulates the sacral nerves and reduces symptoms. The FDA approved Interstim (Medtronic) in 1997. A 2006 retrospective study of 41 patients used a test stimulation. If the test showed a 50% improvement in urge incontinence symptoms, then the permanent stimulator was implanted. Ninety percent of the patients had a greater than 50% reduction in symptoms when assessed at 12 months. However, 29% of patients had some complication. This is a feasible option for some patients with refractory urge incontinence.

Table 21-8 summarizes the treatment options for the two most common types of urinary incontinence.

OTHER TYPES OF INCONTINENCE

Nocturnal enuresis is the complaint of loss of urine occurring during sleep. *Continuous urinary incontinence* is a term defined by the International Continence Society as the continuous leakage of urine where the patient does not describe urgency or activity associated with the leakage. *Extraurethral incontinence* is defined as the observation of urine leakage through channels other than the urethra, including urinary fistulas.

Chronic Retention of Urine

Overflow incontinence is the old term used to describe chronic retention of urine. It occurs when a bladder is overdistended because of its inability to empty. The problem may be caused by a neurologic disorder that interferes with normal bladder reflexes or by partial obstruction of the urethra. Typically the patient complains of voiding small amounts and still having the feeling that there is urine in the bladder. The bladder is nonpainful and may be palpable after the patient has voided. Typically, the retention of urine volume is more than 300 mL.

In addition, the patient frequently loses small amounts of urine without any control. This condition is commonly seen in patients with multiple sclerosis, diabetic neuropathy, and trauma or tumors of the central nervous system. A complete general medical and urologic workup is necessary to clarify the patient's condition. Therapy directed at the primary cause may be beneficial. Often the patient must be trained in techniques of intermittent self-catheterization.

ESTROGEN AND THE LOWER URINARY TRACT

Estrogen has long been known to play a role in the lower urinary tract function since estrogen and progesterone receptors are found throughout the vagina, bladder, and urethra. Estrogen seems to stimulate α receptors and may affect continence by increasing urethral resistance. Progestogens have been associated with increased bladder irritability. Estrogens have been prescribed for years for the treatment of stress incontinence, until controlled trials and the Hormones and Urogenital Therapy (HUT) Committee reported estrogen was not an efficacious treatment for stress incontinence. Estrogen does appear to be superior to placebo for urge incontinence, urgency frequency, and nocturia although the benefit may be due to treatment of vaginal atrophy rather than a specific bladder and urethral effect. Possible confounding effects of progestogens and the multitudes of different estrogen preparations, both oral and vaginal, hamper most of the studies. Low does of vaginal estrogens clearly benefit urogenital atrophy symptoms and likely reduces recurrent UTI symptoms.

KEY POINTS

- As many as 30% of all women may suffer from some degree of urinary incontinence during their lifetime.
- Continence is determined by the balance between those forces that maintain urethral closure and those that affect detrusor function.
- Parasympathetic nervous system activity via the neurotransmitter acetylcholine stimulates receptors in the bladder wall to activate detrusor contraction.
- Anticholinergic agents decrease detrusor activity.
- Sympathetic nervous system receptors in the bladder are mostly β receptors and when stimulated cause relaxation.
- Sympathetic nervous system receptors in the urethra are basically α receptors. Stimulation causes contraction.
- The highest pressure zone in the urethra is about midpoint in the functional urethra, which is roughly 0.5 cm proximal to the urogenital diaphragm.
- Resting pressure within the bladder is between 20 and 30 cm H_2O.

Continued

KEY POINTS *Continued*

- A normal bladder transmits a voiding urge at 150 to 200 mL volume, and functional capacity is generally 400 to 500 mL.
- About 50% of all women will develop urinary infections at some time in their life, and by age 70 as many as 10% of women will have chronic UTIs.
- Bacterial counts of 100,000 or greater per milliliter of urine usually indicate a UTI. *Escherichia coli* is the most common organism seen.
- Bacterial counts of 100 per milliliter may be seen in patients with urethritis and sometimes in women with acute UTIs.
- Interstitial cystitis is an inflammatory condition of the bladder that is not related to infection and is associated with altered epithelial permeability, mast cell activation, and an up-regulation of sensory afferent nerves.
- Some 1% to 6% of all women will suffer from urethral diverticula, with the majority of cases occurring between the ages of 30 and 50. Most urethral diverticula originate in the middle third of the urethra, but diverticula may occur from any area of the urethra and may be multiple.
- Urethral syndrome is an ill-defined condition and should not be diagnosed until all infectious organisms have been discounted. It has been renamed urethral pain syndrome.
- Some 75% to 80% of women with urinary incontinence suffer from stress incontinence.
- The long-term cure rate for Marshall–Marchetti–Krantz and Burch procedures is usually greater than 80% in properly selected patients. The newer midurethral slings appear to have similar efficacy for surgical treatment of stress incontinence.
- Osteitis pubis occurs in 1% to 2% of suprapubic suspension operations.
- Intrinsic urethral sphincter deficiency is seen in women older than 50 and in individuals with a history of urethral and bladder neck surgery or radiation. Intraurethral pressure is generally less than 20 cm H_2O.
- Intrinsic urethral sphincter dysfunction is best treated by periurethral collagen injection, a sling procedure, or instillation of an artificial urethral sphincter.
- About 20% of women with urinary incontinence suffer from detrusor overactivity. Behavioral changes and antimuscarinic medications are first-line treatment for this condition.
- An indwelling catheter left in place for more than 24 hours leads to bacteriuria in about 50% of cases and in nearly 100% after 96 hours.

BIBLIOGRAPHY

Key Readings

Abrams P, Cardozo L, Fall M, et al, for the Standardisation Sub-committee of the International Continence Society. The standardisation of terminology of lower urinary tract function: Report from the Standardisation Sub-committee of the International Continence Society. Neurourol Urodyn 21:167, 2002.

Bergman A, Giovanni E: Three surgical procedures for genuine stress incontinence: Five year follow-up of a prospective randomized study. Am J Obstet Gynecol 173:66, 1995.

Black NA, Downs SH: The effectiveness of surgery for stress incontinence in women: A systematic review. Br J Urol 78: 497, 1996.

Brubaker L, Cundiff GW, Fine P, et al: Abdominal sacrocolpopexy with Burch colposuspension to reduce urinary stress incontinence. N Engl J Med 354:1557, 2006.

Burgio KL, Goode PS, Locher JL, et al: Behavioral training with and without biofeedback in the treatment of urge incontinence in older women: A randomized controlled trial. JAMA 288:2293, 2002.

DeLancey JO: Structural aspects of the extrinsic continence mechanism. Obstet Gynecol 72:296, 1988.

DeLancey JOL, Ashton-Miller JA; Pathophysiology of adult urinary incontinence. Gastroenterology 126:1; S23, 2004.

Glazener CMA, Cooper K: Anterior vaginal repair for urinary incontinence in women. Cochrane Database Syst Rev CD001755, 2001.

Key References

Adatto K, Doebele K, Galland L, et al: Behavioral factors and urinary tract infections. JAMA 241:2535, 1979.

Andersen MTF: The incidence of diverticula in the female urethra. J Urol 98:96, 1967.

Appell RA, Macaluso JN, Deutsch JS, et al: Endourologic control of incontinence with GAX collagen: The LSU experience. J Endourol 6:275, 1992.

Arnold EP, Webster JR, Loose H, et al: Urodynamics of female incontinence: Factors influencing the results of surgery. Am J Obstet Gynecol 117:805, 1973.

Asmussen M, Ulmsten U: A new technique for measurement of the urethra pressure profile. Acta Obstet Gynecol Scand 55:167, 1976.

Asmussen M, Ulmsten U: Simultaneous urethrocystometry with a new technique. Scand J Urol Nephrol 10:7, 1976.

Athanasiou S, Khullar V, Boos K, et al: Imaging the urethral sphincter with three dimensional ultrasound. Obstet Gynecol 94:295, 1999.

Baerheim A, Digranes A, Hunskaar S: Equal symptomatic outcome after antibacterial treatment of acute lower urinary tract infection and the acute urethral syndrome in adult women. Scand J Prim Health Care 17:170, 1999.

Bailey KV: A clinical investigation into uterine prolapse with stress incontinence. Treatment by modified Manchester colporrhaphy. J Obstet Gynaecol Br Comm Part I, 61:291, 1954; Part II, 63:663, 1956; Part III, 70:947, 1963.

Barnett RM: The modern Kelly plication. Obstet Gynecol 34:667, 1969.

Bates CP, Loose H, Stanton SLR: The objective study of incontinence after repair operations, Surg Gynecol Obstet 136:17, 1973.

Beck RP, Maughan GB: Simultaneous intraurethral and intravesical pressure studies in normal women and those with stress incontinence. Am J Obstet Gynecol 89:746, 1964.

Beck RP, McCormick S, Nordstrom L: The fascia lata sling procedure for treating recurrent genuine stress incontinence of urine. Obstet Gynecol 72:699, 1988.

Beer E: Periostitis of the symphysis and descending rami of the pubes following suprapubic Operations. Int J Med 37:224, 1924.

Beisland HO, Fossberg E, Sander S: Urodynamic studies before and after retropubic urethropexy for stress incontinence in females. Surg Gynecol Obstet 155:333, 1982.

Bhatia NN, Bergman A: Urodynamic appraisal of the Bonney test in women with stress urinary incontinence. Obstet Gynecol 62:696, 1983.

Bhatia NN, Ostergard DR: Urodynamics in women with stress urinary incontinence. Obstet Gynecol 60:552, 1982.

Blaivas JG, Jocobs BZ: Pubovaginal fascial sling for the treatment of complicated stress urinary incontinence. J Urol 145:1214, 1991.

Bø K, Talseth T: Long-term effect of pelvic floor muscle exercise 5 years after cessation of organized training. Obstet Gynecol 87:261, 1996.

Bouchelouche K, Nordling J, Hald T, Bouchelouche P: The cysteinyl leukotriene D4 receptor antagonist montelukast for the treatment of interstitial cystitis. J Urol 166:1743, 2001.

Bump RC, Hurt WG, Fantl JA, Wyman JF: Assessment of Kegel pelvic floor muscle exercise performance after brief verbal instruction. Am J Obstet Gynecol 165:322, 1991.
Bump RC, McClish DM: Cigarette smoking and pure genuine stress incontinence of urine: A comparison of risk factors and determinants between smokers and nonsmokers. Am J Obstet Gynecol 170:579, 1994.
Bump RC: Racial comparisons and contrasts in urinary incontinence and pelvic organ prolapse. Obstet Gynecol 81:421, 1993.
Burch JC: Cooper's ligament urethrovesical suspension for stress incontinence. Am J Obstet Gynecol 100:764, 1968.
Burgio KL, Locher JL, Goode PS, et al: Behavioral vs drug treatment for urge urinary incontinence in older women: a randomized trial. JAMA 288:2293, 1995.
Burgio KL, Locher JL, Goode PS: Combined behavioral and drug therapy for urge incontinence in older women. J Am Geriatr Soc 48:370, 2000.
Burgio KL, Matthews KA, Engel BT, et al: Prevalence, incidence and correlates of urinary incontinence in healthy middle aged women. J Urol 146:1255, 1991.
Burton GA: A three-year randomized urodynamic study comparing open and laparoscopic colposuspension. Neurourol Urodynam 16:353, 1997.
Caputo RM, Benson JT: The Q-tip test and urethrovesical junction mobility. Obstet Gynecol 82:892, 1993.
Cardozo L, Lose G, McClish D, et al: A systematic review of estrogens for recurrent urinary tract infections: third report of the hormones and urogenital therapy (HUT) committee. Int Urogynecol J Pelvic Floor Dysfunct 12(1): 15, 2001.
Chapple CR, Martinez-Garcia R, Selvaggi L, et al., for the STAR Study Group. A comparison of the efficacy and tolerability of solifenacin succinate and extended release tolterodine at treating overactive bladder syndrome: results of the STAR trial. Eur Urol 48:464, 2005.
Cherney C, Boscia JA: Asymptomatic bacteriuria in the elderly. Geriat Med 7:46, 1988.
Colombo M, Milani R, Vitoello D, Maggioni A. A randomized comparison of Burch colposuspension and abdominal paravaginal defect repair for female stress urinary incontinence. Am J Obstet Gynecol 175(1):78, 1996.
Colombo M, Scalambrino S, Maggioni A, Milani R: Burch colposuspension versus modified Marshall-Marchetti-Krantz urethropexy for primary genuine stress urinary incontinence: A prospective, randomized clinical trial. Am J Obstet Gynecol 171:1573, 1994.
David RD, DeBlieux PMC, Press R: Rational antibiotic treatment of outpatient genitourinary infections in a changing environment. Am J Med 118:75, 2005.
DeLancey JO, Kearney R, Chou Q, et al: The appearance of levator ani muscle abnormalities in magnetic resonance images after vaginal delivery. Obstet Gynecol 101:46, 2003.
DeLancey JO: Correlative study of periurethral anatomy. Obstet Gynecol 68:91, 1986.
DeLancey JO: Structural support of the urethra as it relates to stress urinary incontinence: The hammock hypothesis. Am J Obstet Gynecol 170(6):1713, 1994.
DeLancey JO: The hidden epidemic of pelvic floor dysfunction: achievable goals for improved prevention and treatment. Am J Obstet Gynecol 192:1488, 2005.
Delorme E: Transobturator urethral suspension: Mini-invasive procedure in the treatment of stress urinary incontinence in women. Prog Urol 11(6):1306, 2001
Diokno AC, Brock BM, Brown HB, Herzog AR: Prevalence of urinary incontinence and other neurologic symptoms in the non-institutionalized elderly. J Urol 136:1022, 1986.
Diokno AC, Taub ME: Experience with the artificial urinary sphincter at Michigan. J Urol 116:496, 1988.
Dmochowski RR, Sand PK, Zinner NR, et al, for the Transdermal Oxybutynin Study Group: Comparative efficacy and safety of transdermal oxybutynin and oral tolterodine versus placebo in previously treated patients with urge and mixed urinary incontinence. Urology 62:237, 2003.
Dwyer PL, Teele JS: Prazosin: A neglected cause of genuine stress incontinence. Obstet Gynecol 79:117, 1992.
Enhorning G: Simultaneous recording of intravesical and intraurethral pressure. Acta Chir Scand Suppl 276:1, 1971.
Falconer C, Ekman G, Malmström A, and Ulmsten U: Decreased collagen synthesis in stress-incontinent women. Obstet Gynecol 84:583, 1994.
Fantl JA, Beachley MC, Bosch HA, et al: Bead-chain cystourethrogram: an evaluation. Obstet Gynecol 58:237, 1981.
Fantl JA, Cardozo L, McClish DK: Estrogen therapy in the management of urinary incontinence in postmenopausal women: A meta-analysis. First report of the Hormones and Urogenital Therapy Committee. Obstet Gynecol 83(1):12, 1994.
Feyereisl J, Dreher E, Haenggi W, et al: Long-term results after Burch colposuspension. Am J Obstet Gynecol 171:647, 1994.
Fitzgerald MP, Mollenhauer J, Bitterman P, Brubaker L: Functional failure of fascia lata allographs. Am J Obstet Gynecol 181:1339, 1999.
Fossberg E, Veisland HO, Lundgren RA: Stress incontinence in females: Treatment with phenylpropanolamine: A urodynamic and pharmacological evaluation. Urol Int 38:293, 1983.
Gillespie WA, Henderson EP, Linton KB, Smith PJB: Microbiology of the urethral (frequency and dysuria) syndrome: A controlled study with a 5-year review. Br J Urology 64:270, 1989.
Gittes RF, Nakamura RM: Female urethral syndrome. A female prostatitis? Invest J Med 164:435, 1996.
Gorton E, Stanton S, Monga A, et al: Periurethral collagen injection: A long-term follow-up study. BJU Int 84(9):966, 1999.
Gosling JA, Dixon JS, Critchley HO, and Thompson SA: Comparative studies of the human external sphincter and periurethral levator ani muscles. Br J Urol 53:35, 1981.
Grady D, Brown J. Vittinghoff E, et al: Postmenopausal hormones and incontinence: The Heart and Estrogen/Progestin Replacement Study. Obstet Gynecol 97:116, 2001.
Green TH Jr: Urinary stress incontinence differential diagnosis pathophysiology and management. Am J Obstet Gynecol 122:368, 1975.
Griffiths DJ, McCracken PN, Harrison GM, et al: Urge incontinence and impaired detrusor contractility in the elderly. Neurourol Urodyn 21:126, 2002.
Gupta K, Scholes D, Stamm WE: Increasing prevalence of antimicrobial resistance among uropathogens causing acute uncomplicated cystitis in women. JAMA 281:736, 1999.
Haeusler G, Leitich H, vanTrotsenburg M, et al: Drug therapy of urinary urge incontinence: A systematic review. Obstet Gynecol 100:1003, 2002.
Harris RL, Yancey CA, Wiser WL, et al: Comparison of anterior colporrhaphy and retropubic urethropexy for patients with genuine stress urinary incontinence. Am J Obstet Gynecol 173:1671, 1995.
Hay-Smith E, Dumoulin C: Pelvic floor muscle training versus no treatment, or inactive control treatments for urinary incontinence in women. Cochrane Database Syst Rev CD005654: 2006.
Hay-Smith EJC, Bo K, Berghmans LCM, et al: Pelvic floor muscle training for urinary incontinence in women. Cochrane Database Syst Rev CD005654, 2006.
Hay-Smith J, Herbison P, Ellis G, Morris A: Which anticholinergic drug for overactive bladder symptoms in adults. Cochrane Database Syst Rev CD005429:2005.
Hedlund H, Schultz A, Talseth T, Tonseth K, van der Hagen A: Sacral neuromodulation in Norway: clinical experience of the first three years. Scand J Urol Nephrol Suppl 210:87-95,2002.
Henalla SM, Hutchins CJ, Robinson P, MacVicar J: Nonoperative methods in the treatment of female genuine stress incontinence of urine. Br J Obstet Gynaecol 9:222, 1989.
Henalla SM, Kirwan P, Castleden CM, et al: The effect of pelvic floor exercises in the treatment of genuine urinary stress incontinence in women at two hospitals. Br J Obstet Gynaecol 95:602, 1988.
Henriksson L, Ulmsten U: Urodynamic evaluation of the effects of abdominal urethrocystopexy and vaginal sling urethroplasty in women with stress incontinence. Am J Obstet Gynecol 131:77, 1978.
Herbertsson G, Iosif CS: Surgical results and urodynamic studies 10 years after retropubic Colpourethrocystopexy. Acta Obstet Gynecol Scand 72:298, 1993.
Herbison P, Hay-Smith J, Ellis G, Moore K: Effectiveness of anticholinergic drugs compared with placebo in the treatment of overactive bladder: Systematic review. BMJ 326:841, 2003.
Hilton P, Stanton SL: A clinical and urodynamic assessment of the Burch colposuspension for genuine stress incontinence. Br J Obstet Gynaecol 90:934, 1983.
Hilton P, Stanton SL: Urethral pressure measurements by microtransducer: The results of symptom-free women and in those with genuine stress incontinence. Br J Obstet Gynaecol 90:919, 1983.
Hilton P, Stanton SL: Use of intravaginal oestrogen cream in genuine stress incontinence. Br J Obstet Gynaecol 90:940, 1983.

Hodgkinson CP, Ayers MA, Drukker BH: Dyssynergic detrusor dysfunction in the apparently normal female. Am J Obstet Gynecol 87:717, 1963.

Hodgkinson CP, Cobert N: Direct urethrocystommetry. Am J Obstet Gynecol 79:648, 1960.

Hodgkinson CP, Drukker BH, Hershey GJG: Stress urinary incontinence in the female. VIII. Etiology significance of the short urethra. Am J Obstet Gynecol 86:16, 1963.

Hodgkinson CP: Relationships of the female urethra and bladder in urinary stress incontinence. Am J Obstet Gynecol 65:506, 1953.

Holroyd-Leduc JM, Strauss SE: Management of urinary incontinence in women: Clinical applications. JAMA 291:996, 2004.

Holroyd-Leduce JM, Straus SE: Management of urinary incontinence in women. Scientific review. JAMA 291(8):986, 2004.

Holschneider CH, Solh S, Lebherz TB, Montz FJ: The modified Pereyra procedure in recurrent stress urinary incontinence: A 15-year review, Obstet Gynecol 83:573, 1994.

Holst K, Wilson PD: The prevalence of female urinary incontinence and reasons for not seeking treatment. N Z Med J 101:758, 1988.

Horbach NS, Ostergard DR: Predicting intrinsic urethral sphincter dysfunction in women with stress urinary incontinence. Obstet Gynecol 84:188, 1994.

Hoyme UB, Tamimi HK, Eschenbach DA, et al: Osteomyelitis pubis after radical gynecologic Operations. Obstet Gynecol 63:47S, 1984.

Huggins M, Bhaia NN, Ostergard DR: Urinary incontinence: Newer pharmacotherapeutic trends. Curr Opin Obstet Gynecol 15:419, 2003.

Interstitial Cystitis Association Website: *http://ichelp.org*.

Jackson S, Donovan J, Brookes, S, et al: The Bristol Female Lower Urinary Tract Symptoms questionnaire: Development and psychometric testing. Br J Urol 77(6):805, 1996.

Jeffcoate TNA, Roberts H: Observations of stress incontinence of urine. Am J Obstet Gynecol 64:721, 1952.

Jewart RD, Green J, Lu CJ, et al: Cognitive, behavioral, and physiological changes in Alzheimer disease patients as a function of incontinence and medications. Am J Geriatr Psychiatry 13:324, 2005.

Kammerer-Doak DN, Cornella JL, Margrina JF, et al: Osteitis pubis after Marshall-Marchetti-Krantz urethropexy: A pubic osteomyelitis. Am J Obstet Gynecol 179:586, 1998.

Karram MM, Bhatia NN: The Q-tip test: Standardization of the technique and its interpretation in women with urinary incontinence. Obstet Gynecol 71:807, 1988.

Karram MM, Rosenzweig BA, Bhatia NN: Artificial urinary sphincter for recurrent/severe stress incontinence in women: urogynecologic perspective. J Reprod Med 38:791, 1993.

Katchmen MG, Paul M, Christiaens T, et al: Duration of antibacterial treatment for uncomplicated urinary tract infection in women. (Review) Cochrane Collaboration, 2005.

Kegel AH: Stress incontinence of urine in women: Physiologic treatment. J Int Coll Surg 25:487, 1956.

Koziol JA: Epidemiology of interstitial cystitis. Urol Clin North Am 21:7, 1994.

Kujansuu E: The effect of pelvic floor exercises on urethral function in female stress incontinence and urodynamic study. Ann Chir Gynaecol 72:28, 1983.

Langer R, Ron-El R, Neuman M, et al: The value of simultaneous hysterectomy during Burch colposuspension for urinary stress incontinence. Obstet Gynecol 72:866, 1988.

Lapides J, Ajemian EP, Stewart BH, et al: Physiopathology of stress incontinence. Surg Gynecol Obstet 111:224, 1960.

Lapides J: Transurethral treatment of urethral diverticula in women. Trans Am Assoc Genitourin Surg 70:135, 1978.

Lapitan MC, Cody DJ, Grant AM: Open retropubic colposuspension for urinary incontinence in women. Cochrane Database Syst Rev 20(3):CD002912, 2005.

Latini JM, Alipour M, Kreder KJ: Efficacy of sacral neuromodulation for symptomatic treatment of refractory urinary urge incontinence. Urology 67(3):550, 2006.

Lee RA: Diverticulum of the female urethra: postoperative complications and results. Obstet Gynecol 61:52, 1983.

Lentz GM, Bavendam T, Stenchever MA, et al: Hormonal manipulation in women with chronic, cyclic irritable bladder symptoms and pelvic pain. Am J Obstet Gynecol 186(6):1268, 2002.

Lentz SS: Osteitis pubis: a review. Obstet Gynecol Surv 50:310, 1995.

Low JA: Clinical characteristics of patients with demonstrable urinary incontinence. Am J Obstet Gynecol 88:322, 1964.

MacKinnon M, Pratt JH, Pool TL: Diverticulum of the female urethra. Surg Clin North Am 39:953, 1959.

Marchetti AA, Marshall VF, Shultis LD: Simple vesicourethral suspension for stress incontinence of urine. Am J Obstet Gynecol 74:57, 1957.

Martin JL, Williams KS, Abrams KR, et al: Systematic review and evaluation of methods of assessing urinary incontinence. Health Technol Assess 10(6), 2006.

Matilla J: Vascular immunopathology in interstitial cystitis. Clin Immunol Immunopathol 23:648, 1982.

McGuire EJ: Urodynamic findings in patients after failure of stress incontinence operations. Prog Clin Biol Res 78:351, 1981.

McGuire EJ, Wang SC, Appell RA, et al: Treatment of urethral continence by collagen injection. J Urol 143:224A, 1990.

Melville JL, Delaney K, Newton K, Katon W: Incontinence severity and major depression in incontinent women. Obstet Gynecol 106:585, 2005.

Melville JL, Walker E, Katon W, et al: Prevalence of comorbid psychiatric illness and its impact on symptom perception, quality of life, and functional status in women with urinary incontinence. Am J Obstet Gynecol 187(1):80, 2002.

Meyer S, Schreyer A, DeGrandi P, Hohlfeld P: The effects of birth on urinary continence mechanisms and other pelvic floor characteristics. Obstet Gynecol 92:613, 1998.

Migliorini GR, Glenning PP: Bonney's test-fact or fiction? Br J Obstet Gynaecol 94:157, 1987.

Millard RJ, Oldenburg BF: The symptomatic urodynamic and psychodynamic results of bladder reeducation programs. J Urol 130:715, 1983.

Milsom I, Abrams P, Cardozo K. et al: How widespread are the symptoms of an overactive bladder and how are they managed? A population-based prevalence study. BJU Int 87:760, 2001.

Montz FJ, Stanton SL: Q-tip test in female urinary incontinence. Obstet Gynecol 67:258, 1986.

Muellner SR, Fleischner FG: Normal and abnormal micturition study of the bladder behavior by means of fluoroscopy. J Urol 61:233, 1949.

Nichols DH: A Mersilene mesh gauze hammock for severe urinary stress incontinence. Obstet Gynecol 41:88, 1973.

Norton P, Karram M, Wall L, et al: Randomized double-blind trial of terodiline in the treatment of urge incontinence in women, Obstet Gynecol 84:386, 1994.

Nygaard IE, Kreder KJ, Lepic MM, et al: Efficacy of pelvic floor muscle exercises in women with stress, urge, and mixed urinary incontinence. Am J Obstet Gynecol 174:120, 1996.

Nygaard IE: Does prolonged high-impact activity contribute to later urinary incontinence? A retrospective cohort study of female Olympians. Obstet Gynecol 90:718, 1997.

O'Leary MP: The interstitial cystitis symptom index and problem index. Urol 49:58, 1997.

Ostergard DR: The effect of drugs on the lower urinary tract. Obstet Gynecol Surv 34:424, 1979.

Ostergard DR: The neurologic control of micturition and integral voiding reflexes. Obstet Gynecol Surv 34:417, 1979.

Owens RG, Kohlt N, Wynne J, et al: Long term results of a fascia lata suburethral patch sling for severe stress urinary incontinence. J Pelvic Surg 5:196, 1999.

Park GS, Miller EJ Jr: Surgical treatment of stress urinary incontinence: a comparison of the Kelly plication, Marshall-Marchetti-Krantz, and Pereyra procedures. Obstet Gynecol 71:575, 1988.

Parmar MS: Kidney stones. Br Med J 328:1420, 2004.

Parsons CL, Benson G, Childs SJ, et al: A quantitatively controlled method to prospectively study interstitial cystitis and demonstrate the efficacy of pentosan polysulfate. J Urol 150:845, 1993.

Parsons CL: The therapeutic role of sulfated polysaccharides in the urinary bladder. Urol Clin North Am 21:93, 1994.

Parsons LL: Interstitial cystitis. In Kurol ED, McGuire EJ (eds): Female Urology. Philadelphia, Lippincott, 1994.

Patel AK, Chapple CR: Female urethral diverticula. Curr Opin Urol 16:248, 2006.

Peattie AB, Plevnik S, Stanton SL: Vaginal cones: A conservative method of treating genuine stress incontinence. Br J Obstet Gynaecol 95:1049, 1988.

Peeker R, Aldenborg F, Dahlstrom A, et al: Immunologic and neurobiologic characteristics support that interstitial cystitis is a heterogeneous syndrome. Urology 57(6 Suppl 1): 130, 2001.

Pereyra AJ, Lebherz TB: Combined urethrovesical suspension and vaginal urethroplasty for correction of stress incontinence. Obstet Gynecol 30:537, 1967.

Pereyra AJ: A simplified surgical procedure for the correction of stress incontinence in women. West J Surg 67:223, 1959.

Perez-Marrero R, Emerson LE, Feltis JT: A controlled study of dimethyl sulfoxide in interstitial cystitis. J Urol 140:36, 1988.

Raz R, Stamm WE: A controlled trial of intravaginal estriol in postmenopausal women with recurrent urinary tract infections. N Engl J Med 329(11):753, 1993.

Ronald A, Nicolle L, Stamm E, et al: Urinary tract infection in adults: Research priorities and strategies. Int J Antimicrob Agents 17:343, 2001.

Rosamilia A, Dwyer PL: Interstitial cystitis and the gynecologist. Obstet Gynecol Survey 53:309, 1998.

Ross JW: Multichannel urodynamic evaluation of laparoscopic Burch Colposuspension for genuine stress incontinence. Obstet Gynecol 91:55, 1998.

Rudd T: Urethral pressure profile in continent women from childhood to old age. Acta Obstet Gynecol Scand 59:331, 1979.

Saidi MH, Gallagher MS, Skop IP, et al: Extraperitoneal laparoscopic colposuspension: Short-term cure rate, complications, and duration of hospital stay in comparison with Burch Colposuspension. Obstet Gynecol 92:619, 1998.

Salvatore S, Khullar V, Cardozo L, et al: Long-term prospective randomized study comparing two different regimens of oxybutynin as a treatment for detrusor overactivity. Eur J Obstet Gynaecol Reprod Biol 119:237, 2005.

Sand PK, Bowen LW, Ostergard DR, et al: Cryosurgery versus dilation and massage for the treatment of recurrent urethral syndrome. J Repro Med 34:499, 1989.

Sand PK, Bowen LW, Ostergard DR, et al: The effect of retropubic urethropexy on detrusor stability. Obstet Gynecol 71:818, 1988.

Sand PK, Bowen LW, Panganiban R, Ostergard DR: The low pressure urethra as a factor in failed retropubic urethropexy. Obstet Gynecol 69:399, 1987.

Sand PK, Richardson DA, Staskin DR, et al: Pelvic floor electrical stimulation in the treatment of genuine stress incontinence: A multicenter, placebo-controlled trial. Am J Obstet Gynecol 173:72, 1995.

Sant GR, LaRock DR: Standard intravesicle therapies for interstitial cystitis. Urol Clin North Am 21:73, 1994.

Schaer GN, Koechli OR, Schuessler B, Haller U: Improvement of perineal sonographic bladder neck imaging with ultrasound contrast medium. Obstet Gynecol 86:950, 1995.

Schaer GN, Koechli OR, Schuessler B, Haller U: Perineal ultrasound for evaluating the bladder neck in urinary stress incontinence. Obstet Gynecol 85:220, 1995.

Schmidt RA, Jonas V, Oleson KA, et al: Sacral nerve stimulation for treatment of refractory urinary urge incontinence. Sacral Nerve Stimulation Study Group. J Urol 162:3562, 1999.

Shull BL, Baden WF: A six-year experience with paravaginal defect repair for stress urinary Incontinence. Am J Obstet Gynecol 160:1432, 1989.

Shumaker SA, Wyman JF, Uebersax JS, et al: Health-related quality of life measures for women with urinary incontinence: The Incontinence Impact Questionnaire and the Urogenital Distress Inventory. Continence Program in Women (CPW) Research Group. Qual Life Res 3(5);291, 1994.

Sjoberg B, Nyman CR: Hydrodynamics of micturition in stress incontinent women: comparisons of pressure and flow at different micturition volumes in stress incontinent and continent women. Scand J Urol Nephrol 16:1, 1982.

Smith CP, Nishiguchi J, O'Leary M, et al: Single-institution experience in 110 patients with botulinum toxin A injection into bladder or urethra. Urology 174(2):611, 2005.

Spence HM, Duckett JW Jr: Diverticulum of the female urethra: Clinical aspects and presentation of a simple operative technique for cure. J Urol 104:432, 1970.

Spraitz AF Jr, Welch JS: Diverticulum of the female urethra. Am J Obstet Gynecol 91: 1013, 1965.

Stamey TA: Endoscopic suspension of the vesical neck for urinary incontinence in females: Report of 203 consecutive cases. Ann Surg 192:465, 1980.

Stamm WE, Raz R: Factors contributing to susceptibility of postmenopausal women to recurrent urinary tract infections. Clin Infect Dis 28(4):723, 1999.

Staskin DR, MacDiarmid SA: Pharmacologic management of overactive bladder: Practical options for the primary care physician. Am J Med 119:245, 2006.

Staskin DR, MacDiarmid SA: Using anticholinergics to treat overactive bladder: The issue of treatment tolerability. Am J Med 119 (Suppl 3A):9S, 2006.

Sultana CJ: Urethral closure pressure and leak-point pressure in incontinent women. Obstet Gynecol 86:839, 1995.

Swift SE, Ostergard DR: A comparison of stress leak-point pressure and maximal urethral closure pressure in patients with genuine stress incontinence. Obstet Gynecol 85:704, 1995.

Swift SE, Ostergard DR: Evaluation of current urodynamic testing methods in the diagnosis of genuine stress incontinence. Obstet Gynecol 86:85, 1995.

Tchou DCH, Adams C, Varner RE, Denton B: Pelvic-floor musculature exercises in treatment of anatomical urinary stress incontinence. Phys Ther 68:652, 1988.

Te Linde RW: Urethral sling operation. Clin Obstet Gynecol 6:206, 1963.

Teasdale TA, Taffet GE, Luchi RJ, Adam E: Urinary incontinence in a community-residing elderly population. J Am Geriatr Soc 36:600, 1988.

Teichman JM: Clinical Practice. Acute renal colic from ureteral calculus. N Engl J Med 350:684, 2004.

Ulmsten U, Henriksson L, Johnson P, Varhos G: An ambulatory surgical procedure under local anesthesia for treatment of female stress incontinence. Int Urogynecol J 7:81, 1996.

U.S. Department of Health and Human Services, Public Health Service Agency for Health Care Policy and Research: Urinary Incontinence in Adults. April, 1995.

Van Geelen JM, Theeuwes AGM, Eskes TKAB, Martin CB Jr: The clinical and urodynamic effects of anterior vaginal repair and Burch colposuspension. Am J Obstet Gynecol 159:137, 1988.

Van Kerrebroeck P, Kreder K, Jonas U, et al., for the Tolterodine Study Group: Tolterodine once-daily: Superior efficacy and tolerability in the treatment of overactive bladder. Urology 57:414, 2001.

Vasavada SP, Appell RA, Sand PK, Raz, S: Female Urology, Urogynecology, and Voiding Dysfunction. New York, Marcel Dekker, 2005.

Vesey SG, Rivett A, O'Boyle PJ: Teflon injection in female stress incontinence: Effect on urethral pressure profile and flow rate. Br J Urol 62:39, 1988.

Visco AG, Weidner AC, Cundiff GW, Bump RC: Observed patient compliance with a structured outpatient bladder retraining program. Am J Obstet Gynecol 181:1392, 1999.

Walter S, Olesen KP: Urinary incontinence in genital prolapse in the female: Clinical urodynamic and radiologic examinations. Br J Obstet Gynaecol 89:393, 1982.

Walters MD, Diaz K: Q-tip test: A study of continent and incontinent women. Obstet Gynecol 70:208, 1987.

Walters MD, Shields LE: The diagnostic value of history, physical examination, and the Q-tip cotton swab test in women with urinary incontinence. Am J Obstet Gynecol 159:145, 1988.

Ward KL, Hilton P, UK and Ireland TVT Trial Group: A prospective multicenter randomized trial of tension-free vaginal tape and colposuspension for primary urodynamic stress incontinence: Two-year follow-up. Am J Obstet Gynecol 192:984, 2004.

Waxman JA, Sulak PJ, Kuehl TJ: Cystoscopic findings consistent with interstitial cystitis in normal women undergoing tubal ligation. J Urol 160:1663, 1998.

Weinberger MW, Ostergard DR: Long-term clinical and urodynamic evaluation of the polytetrafluoroethylene suburethral sling for treatment of genuine stress incontinence. Obstet Gynecol 86:92, 1995.

Westby M, Asmussen M, Ulmsten U: Localization of maximum intraurethral pressure related to urogenital diaphragm in the female subject as studied by simultaneous urethrocystommetry and voiding urethrocystography. Am J Obstet Gynecol 144:408, 1982.

Williams ME, Pannill FC: Urinary incontinence in the elderly. Ann Intern Med 97:895, 1982.

Wyman JF, Fantl JA, McClish DK, et al: Comparative efficacy of behavioral interventions in the management of female urinary incontinence. Continence Program for Women Research Group. Am J Obstet Gynecol 179:999, 1998.

Young SB, Rosenblatt PL, Pingeton DM, et al: The Mersilene mesh suburethral sling: A clinical and urodynamic evaluation, Am J Obstet Gynecol 173:1719, 1995.

APPENDIX Drugs That Affect Bladder Functions

Generic Name	Trade Name
Drugs affecting sympathetic nervous system	
Alpha-adrenergic blockers	
Azapetine	Ilidar
Dihydroergotoxine	Hydergine
Ergot alkaloids	—
Phenothiazines	(Various; see Drugs Affecting Autonomic Nervous System— Causing Retention)
Phentolamine	Regitine
Piperoxan	Benodaine
Tolazoline	Priscoline
Beta-adrenergic blockers	
Alprenolol	—
Butidrine	—
Butoxamine	—
Dichloroisoproterenol	Alderlin, Nethalide, Pronethalol
Isopropylmethoxamine	—
Ko692	—
LB-46	Prinololol
M 1999	Sotalol
Oxprenolol	—
Practolol	Eraldin
General adrenergic stimulators	
Adrenalone	Kephrine
Aminorex	—
—	Aranthol
Benzphetamine	Didrex
Chlorphentermine	Pre-Sate
Clortemine	Voranil
Cyclopantamine	Clopane
Deoxyepinephrine	Epinine
Dextroamphetamine	Dexedrine
Diethylpropion	Tenuate, Tepanil
Epinephrine	—
Ethylnorepinephrine	Bronkephrine
Fenfluramine	Pondimin
Hydroxyamphetamine	Paredrine
H1032	—
Isometheptene	Octin
Levamphetamine	Ad-Nil, Amodril, Cydril, Malgret
Mazindol	Sanorex
Mephentermine	Wyamine
Methamphetamine	Dexoxyn
Methylaminophetane	Oenethyl
Methylhexamine	Forthane
Naphazoline	Privine
Oxymetazoline	Afrin
Phedrazine	—
Phendimetrazine	Dietrol, Plegine
Phenmetrazine	Preludin
Phentermine	Ionamin, Wilpo
Pholedrine	Paredrinal
Propylhexedrine	Benzedrex
Pseudoephedrine	Sudafed, Ro-Fedrin
Racephedrine	—
Synephrine	—
Tenaphtoxaline	—
Tetrahydrozoline	Tyzine
Tramazoline	—
Tuaminoheptane	Taumine
Tymazoline	Pemazene
Xylometazoline	Otrivin
Alpha-adrenergic stimulators	
Amidephrine	—
Cyclopentamine	Clopane
Dopamine	Intropin
Etafedrine	—
Alpha-adrenergic stimulators—cont'd	
Ethylphenylephrine	Effortil
Hydroxyamphetamine	Paredrine
Metaraminol	Aramine
Methamphetamine	Desoxyn; Efroxine, Methedrine, Norodin, Synodroy
Methoxamine	Vasoxyl
Methylhexaneamine	Forthane
Nordefrin	Cobefrin
Norepinephrine	Levarterenol
Novadral	—
Phenylephrine	Neo-Synephrine, Isophrin, Synasal, Alconefrin Biomydrin, Isohalent Improved
Phenylpropylmethylamine	Vonedrine
Propylhexedrine	Benzedrex
Tyramine	—
Beta-adrenergic stimulators	
Albuterol	Proventil, Ventolin
Bamethan	—
Chlorprenaline	—
Dioxethedrine	—
Etafedrine	—
Ethylnorepinephrine	Butanefrine, Bronkephrine
Hydroxyephedrine	—
Isoethamine	—
Isoproterenol	Aludrine, Isuprel, Norisodrine
Methoxyphenamine	Orthoxine
Nylidrin	Arlidin
Protokylol	Caytine
Salbutanal	—
Soterenol	—
Terbutaline	Bricamyl
Adrenergic neuron blockers	
Alseroxylon	Rautensin, Rauwiloid
Bethanidine	Esbatal
Bretylium	Darenthin
Debrisoquin	Declinax
Deserpidine	Harmonyl
Guanadrel	—
Guanethidine	Ismelin
Guanoclor	Vatensol
Guanoxan	Envacar
Hydralazine	Apresoline
Methyldopa	Aldomet
Methyldopate	Aldomet Ester
Nialamide	—
Pargyline	Eutonyl
Prazosin	Minipress
Rauwolfia	Hyperloid, Raudixin, Rauja, Raulfin, Rautina, Rauval, Venibar
Rescinnamine	Cinatabs, Moderil
Reserpine	Lemiserp, Rau-Sed, Resercen, Reserpoid, Rolserp, Sandril, Serpasil, Sertina, Vio-Serpine
Syrosingopine	Singoserp
Tranylcypromine	—
Veratrum alkaloids	Unitensin, Veralba, Veriloid, Vertairs
Drugs affecting parasympathetic nervous system	
Stimulators	
Ambenonium	Mytelase
Carbachol	Carcholin, Isopto Carbachol
Echothioplate	Phospholine
Demecarium	Humorsol
Edrophonium	Tensilon
Isoflurophate	Floropryl

Drugs That Affect Bladder Functions—*cont'd*

Generic Name	Trade Name
Stimulators—cont'd	
Methacholine	Mecholyl
Pilocarpine	Pilocar
Pralidoxime	Protopam
Pyridostigmine	Mestinon
Inhibitors	
Adiphenine	Trasentine
Alverine	Prafenil, Spacolin
Anisotropine	Valpin
Atropine	—
Belladonna extract	—
Carbofluorene	Pavatrine
Clidinium	Librax, Quarzan
Cyclopentolate	Cyclogyl
Diphemanil	Prantal
Ethaverine	Ethaquin, Laverin, Neopavrin
Eucatropine	Euphthalmine
Glycopyrrolate	Robinul
Hexocyclium	Tral
Homatropine hydrobromide	—
Homatropine methylbromide	Homapin, Malcotran, Mesopin, Novatrin
Hyoscyamine sulfate	Levsin
Isometheptene	Isometene, Octin
Mepenzolate	Cantil
Methixene	Trest
Methscopolamine bromide	Pamine
Methylatropine nitrate (atropine methylnitrate)	Metropine
Oxyphenonium	Antrenyl
Papaverine	Cerespan, Pap-Kaps, Pavabid, Pavacap, Pavacen, Pavarine, Pavatest, Paveril, Vasal, Vaso-span
Pentapiperium	Quilene
Penthienate	Monodral
Pipenzolate	Piptal
Piperidolate	Dactil
Poldine	Nacton
Scopolamine	—
Thihexinol	Sorboquel
Thiphenamil	Trocinate
Tincture of belladonna	—
Tricyclamol	Elorine
Tridihexethyl	Pathilon
Tropicamide	Mydriacyl
Valethamate	Murel
Drugs affecting sympathetic and parasympathetic nervous system—ganglionic blockers	
Azamethonium	Pendiomid
Chlorisondamine	Ecolid
Hexamethonium	—
Mecamylamine	Inversine
Methaphan	Arfonad
Pentolium	Ansolysen
Sparteine	Spartocin, Tocosamine
Trimethidinium	Ostensin
Drugs affecting autonomic nervous system ***Causing retention***	
Acetophenazine	Tindal
Amitriptyline	Elavil
Amphotericin B	Fungizone
Benztropine	Cogentin
Biperiden	Akineton
Bromodiphenhydramine	Ambodryl
Brompheniramine	Dimetane
Butaperazine	Repoise
Carbinoxzmine	Clistin
Carphenazine	Proketazine
Causing retention—cont'd	
Chlorpheniramine	Chlor-Trimeton, Histaspan, Teldrin
Chlorphenoxamine	Systral, Phenoxene
Chlorpromazine	Thorazine
Chlorprothixene	Taractan
Cycrimine	Pagitane
Deanol	Deaner
Desipramine	Norpramin, Pertofrane
Dexbrompheniramine	Disomer
Dexchlorpheniramine	Polaramine
Dimethindene	Forhistal, Triten
Diphenhydramine	Benadryl
Diphenylpyraline	Diafen, Hispril
Doxepin	Adapin, Sinequan
Doxylamine	Decapryn
Droperidol	Inapsine
Ethopropazine	Parsidol
Fluphenazine	Prolixin, Permitil
Haloperidol	Haldol
Imipramine	Tofranil, Presamine
Isocarboxazid	Marplan
Mepazine	—
Mesoridazine	Serentil
Metaxalone	Skelaxin
Methapyrilene	Histadyl
Methdilazine	Tacaryl
Methylphenidate	Ritalin
Methysergide	Sansert
Molindone	Moban
Nortriptyline	Aventyl
Orphenadrine	Norflex
Perphenazine	Trilafon
Pheneizine	Nardil
Phenindamine	Thephorin
Piperacetazine	Quide
Pipradrol	Meratran
Prochlorperazine	Compazine
Procyclindine	Kemadrin
Promazine	Sparine
Promethazine	Phenergan
Protriptyline	Vivactil
Pyrilamine	—
Rotoxamine	Turiston
Thiopropazate	Dartal
Thioridazine	Mellaril
Thiothixene	Navane
Tranylcypromine	Parnate
Trifluoperazine	Stelazine
Triflupromazine	Vesprin
Trihexyphenidyl	Artane, Pipanol, Tremin
Trimeprazine	Temaril
Tripelennamine	Pyribenzamine
Tripolidine	Actidil
Causing miscellaneous urologic symptoms *Frequency*	
Dantrolene	Dantrium Triavil (mixture)
Iron Sorbitex	Jectofer Etrafon (mixture)
Incontinence	
Estrogens	—
Hydroxystilbamidine	—
Urgency	
Disodium Edetate	Endrate
Frequency, retention, and incontinence	
Levodopa	Bendopa, Dopar, Larodopa, Levodopa
Levopropoxyphene	Novrad

Combined Preparation Drugs

Drugs affecting sympathetic nervous system

Actified-C Expectorant
Acutuss
Acutuss Expectorant with Codeine
Aerolone Compound
Amesec
Amodrine
Asbron
Arycap
AyrLiquid
Bihisdin
Brondilate
Bronkometer
Bronkosol
Bronkotabs
Calcidrine Syrup
Cerose Expectorant
Chlor-Trimeton Expectorant with Codeine
Citra
Colrex Compund
Copavin
Copavin Compound
Coricidin Nasal Mist
Co-Xan
Dainite
Deinite-KI
Deltasmyl
Duo-Medihaler
Duovent
Dylephrine
Ephed-Organidin
Ephedrine and Chlorcyclizine
Ephedrine and Nembutal
Ephedrine and Seconal Sodium
Ephoxamine
Glynazan/EP
Hyadrine
Hydryllin with Racephedrine Hydrochloride
Iso-Tabs
Isuprel Compound
Lufyllin-EP
Marax
Neo-Vadrin
Norisodrine with Calcium Iodide
Novalene
NTZ
Numa
Orthoxine and Aminopylline
Pyracort
Quadrinal
Tedral
Tedral-25
Tedral Anti-H
Thalfed
Triaminicin

Drugs inhibiting sympathetic nervous system

Aldoclor
Aldoril
Butiserpazide
Diupres
Diutensen
Enduronyl
Esimil
Eutron
Exna-R
Hydromox-R
Hydropres
Maxitate with Rauwolfia
Metatensin
Naquival
Nyomin
Oreticyl
Protalba-R
Rautrax
Rawiloid + Veriloid
Regroton
Renese-R
Salutensin
Sandril with Pyronil
Serpasil-Esidrix
Singoserp-Esidrix

Drugs inhibiting parasympathetic nervous system

Belbarb
Belladenal
Bellergal
Butibel
Cantil with Phenobarbital
Chardonna
Combid
Daricon-PB
Donnatal
Donphen
Enarax
Histalet
Hybephen
Kinesed
Kolantyl
Levsin with Phenobarbital
Milpath
Nolamine
Pamine
Pathibamate
Pathilon with Phenobarbital
Phenobarbital and Belladonna
Probanthine with Dartal
Probanthine with Phenobarbital
Robinul-PH
Sidonna
Trasetine-phenobarbital
Valpin-PB

From Ostergard DR: The effect of drugs on the lower urinary tract. Obstet Gynecol Surv 34:424, 1979.

Infections of the Lower Genital Tract 22

Vulva, Vagina, Cervix, Toxic Shock Syndrome, HIV Infections

Linda O. Eckert and Gretchen M. Lentz

KEY TERMS AND DEFINITIONS

Bubo. An enlarged and inflamed lymph node, particularly in the axilla or groin, caused by infections such as plague, syphilis, gonorrhea, lymphogranuloma venereum, or tuberculosis.

Calymmatobacterium granulomatis. The gram-negative, nonmotile rod that causes granuloma inguinale.

Clue Cells. Epithelial cells with clusters of bacteria adherent to their external surfaces, obscuring their normal, fine border. They have a granular or stippled appearance and are associated with bacterial vaginosis.

Condyloma Acuminatum. A sexually transmitted viral disease of the vulva, vagina, cervix, and rectum caused by the human papillomavirus.

Condyloma Latum. The nonpainful large, raised, flattened, grayish white lesions of secondary syphilis, most often found on the vulva.

Dark-Field Microscopy. A technique used to identify the spirochetes of syphilis, *Treponema pallidum.*

Donovan Bodies. The pathognomonic clusters of dark-staining bacteria (bipolar in appearance) found in the cytoplasm of large mononuclear cells in patients with granuloma inguinale.

Groove Sign. A depression between groups of inflamed nodes producing a double genitocrural fold in patients with lymphogranuloma venereum.

Gumma. An infectious granuloma characteristic of late or tertiary syphilis.

Mucopurulent Cervicitis. This inflammatory condition is diagnosed by gross visualization of yellow mucopurulent material or the presence of 10 or more polymorphonucleocytes per high-powered field on Gram stain of the endocervix.

Nit. The egg of the crab louse.

Podophyllin. A topical resin mixed with benzoin and alcohol used to treat the lesions of condyloma acuminatum.

Prozone Phenomenon. A false-negative VDRL or RPR caused by an excess of anticardiolipin antibody in the serum.

Sexually Transmitted Disease (STD). A term used to describe an infection acquired primarily through sexual contact; venereal disease.

Toxin 1. The toxin involved in producing the signs and symptoms of toxic shock syndrome. It is a small protein with a molecular weight of 22,000. Its primary effects are the production of increased vascular permeability and profuse leaking of fluid from the intravascular space to the extravascular space.

Whiff Test. A test used clinically. The smell of vaginal discharge after the addition of 10% potassium hydroxide. A positive sample associated with either bacterial vaginosis or *Trichomonas* infections will give off a fishy or aminelike smell.

Word Catheter. A short catheter with an inflatable Foley balloon used to help develop a fistulous tract from a Bartholin duct to the vestibule.

The Centers for Disease Control and Prevention (CDC) regularly revises its treatment protocols for sexually transmitted diseases. The recommendations and medications in this edition are based on the 2006 CDC guidelines. Readers are urged to consult any updates in the CDC guidelines, since bacterial sensitivities and epidemiologic concerns may lead to changes in treatment protocols. The latest information may be found on the CDC Internet site: http://www.cdc.gov/.

The discussion of infectious diseases of the female genital tract is divided into two chapters. Infections involving the vulva, vagina, and cervix are discussed in this chapter, and infections involving the uterus, oviducts, and ovaries are discussed in Chapter 23 (Infections of the Upper Genital Tract). This separation has been made only to be similar to other chapters of the book and for clarity of presentation. The female genital tract has anatomic and physiologic continuity. Thus infectious agents that colonize and involve one organ often infect adjacent organs. To understand the pathophysiology and natural history of infectious diseases of the genital tract, one must keep this continuity in mind.

The symptoms caused by infections of the lower genital tract produce the most common conditions seen by gynecologists. Therefore the focus of this chapter is on clinical presentation and differential diagnosis of vulvitis, vaginitis, and cervicitis.

Toxic shock syndrome (TSS) and syphilis are discussed in this chapter also, although the most devastating pathologic processes from these diseases occur in sites other than the genital tract. Often they obtain entry into the body through the vulvar, rectal, vaginal, or cervical epithelium.

Many of the infections discussed in this chapter may be acquired through sexual contact and are termed sexually transmitted diseases (STDs). STDs often coexist—for example, vulvar herpes and condyloma acuminatum or infections of *Chlamydia trachomatis* and *Neisseria gonorrhoeae.* When one disease is suspected, appropriate diagnostic methods must be used to detect other infections. This principle cannot be overemphasized.

INFECTIONS OF THE VULVA

The skin of the vulva is composed of a stratified squamous epithelium containing hair follicles and sebaceous, sweat, and apocrine glands. The subcutaneous tissue of the vulva also contains specialized structures such as the Bartholin glands. Similar to skin elsewhere on the body, the vulvar area is subject to both primary and secondary infections. The three most prevalent primary viral infections of the vulva are herpes genitalis, condyloma acuminatum, and molluscum contagiosum. However, symptoms from secondary infections of the vulva caused by organisms that produce vulvovaginitis are among the most common of all gynecologic conditions. To understand the differential diagnosis of vulvar infections, one must consider that vulvar skin is also sensitive to hormonal, metabolic, and allergic influences.

Vulvar itching or burning of acute onset and short duration suggests infection or contact dermatitis. Approximately 10% of outpatient visits to gynecologists are for vulvar pruritus. The signs of erythema, edema, and superficial skin ulcers of the vulva also suggest infection. Skin fissures and excoriation may be signs of primary infection, may be caused by the patient's scratching as a result of irritation from a vaginal discharge, or may be the manifestation of a primary dermatologic disease.

Acute Bacterial Cystitis

It is estimated that 10% to 20% of adult women experience symptoms of dysuria and urinary frequency each year. An individual woman's lifetime risk of developing at least one urinary tract infection (UTI) is approximately 50%. The highest incidence of acute bacterial cystitis is found in women during their early 20s. Reproductive-age women are prone to ascending infections because of the shortness of the female urethra and the fact that the distal one third of the urethra is often colonized by bacteria from the vulvar vestibule. Independent risk factors for the development of acute bacterial cystitis include sexual intercourse, use of a vaginal diaphragm or spermicide in premenopausal women, previous UTI, and recent exposure to antibiotics. In postmenopausal women followed prospectively for 2 years, a history of six or more prior UTIs and insulin-treated diabetes were independent risk factors for cystitis, but sexual activity was not. In postmenopausal women, the lack of estrogenic effect on urovaginal epithelium and sometimes the presence of residual urine after voiding predisposes them to infection. Basic science studies have demonstrated that vaginal and uroepithelial cells have an increased susceptibility to adherence by *Escherichia coli* in some women.

Acute bacterial cystitis is characterized by multiple symptoms, including dysuria, urgency, and frequent voiding. It is usually abrupt in onset. Suprapubic tenderness is a specific sign for acute bacterial cystitis; however, it is not present in the majority of patients. The differential diagnosis of an adult woman with dysuria includes acute cystitis, acute urethritis, or vulvovaginitis. Table 22-1 lists characteristic features that help to differentiate the three most common causes of dysuria in adult women.

The patient's perception of the anatomic site of the dysuria may be helpful. Vulvovaginitis may be associated with "external" dysuria in contrast to a deeper "internal" dysuria associated with cystitis. In general, women with urethritis have more chronic symptoms, with a gradual onset and less urgency, than do women with acute bacterial cystitis. The most common pathogens causing acute urethritis are *C. trachomatis* and *N. gonorrhoeae.* Postmenopausal women may experience urethral symptoms related to estrogen deficiency without significant bacterial colonization of the bladder.

The most common cause of acute bacterial cystitis is ascending infection from the introitus and distal urethra. The pathogens most frequently involved in uncomplicated lower UTIs are *E. coli* (approximately 80%) and *Staphylococcus saprophyticus* (approximately 5% to 15%). Certain bacterial virulence factors provide a selective advantage to strains possessing them with regard to colonization and infection. There is increasing resistance of urinary tract pathogens with up to one third of bacterial isolates resistant to sulfanilamides, ampicillin, and first-generation cephalosporins. These agents should not be used for empiric therapy. A national study of antibiotic susceptibility patterns among acute bacterial cystitis isolates documented significant,

Table 22-1 Major Infectious Causes of Acute Dysuria in Women

Condition	Pathogen	Pyuria	Hematuria	Urine Culture* (cfu/mL)	Symptoms, Signs, and Factors
Cystitis	*Escherichia coli, Staphylococcus saprophyticus, Proteus* sp., *Klebsiella* sp.	Usually	Sometimes	10^2 to $\geq 10^5$	Abrupt onset, severe symptoms, multiple symptoms (dysuria, increased frequency and urgency), suprapubic or low back pain; suprapubic tenderness on examination
Urethritis	*Chlamydia trachomatis, Neisseria gonorrhoeae,* herpes simplex virus	Usually	Rarely	$<10^2$	Gradual onset, mild symptoms, vaginal discharge or bleeding (due to concomitant cervicitis), lower abdominal pain, new sexual partner; cervicitis or vulvovaginal herpetic lesions on examination
Vaginitis	*Candida* sp., *Trichomonas vaginalis*	Rarely	Rarely	$<10^2$	Vaginal discharge or odor, pruritus, dyspareunia, external dysuria, no increased frequency or urgency; vulvovaginitis on examination

*Values indicate colony-forming units (cfu) per milliliter of urine.
From Stamm WE, Hooton TM: Management of urinary tract infections in adults. N Engl J Med 329:1328, 1993.

geographic variation in prevalence of *E. coli* isolates resistant to trimethoprim/sulfamethoxazole. (TMP-SMX) The western United States has a high of 22% to a low of 10% in the northeast. Resistance to the fluoroquinolones remains well below 5% in most studies and prevalence of resistance to nitrofurantoin among *E. coli* is less than 5%, though often higher in non-*E. coli* pathogens.

Examination of strains of TMP-SMX resistant *E. coli* found 9.5% of these strains also resistant to ciprofloxacin. Overall, nitrofurantoin resistance was found in 1.9% of TMP-SMX resistant *E. coli* but in 10.4% of strains resistant to ciprofloxacin.

Resistance data for *S. saprophyticus* is more limited but studies have found 3% resistance to TMP-SMX with rare resistance to nitrofurantoin, cephalothin, and ciprofloxacin. Fosfomycin is less active *S. saprophyticus* and should not be used.

There are varying diagnostic steps in the laboratory workup of classic symptoms of acute cystitis. The first step is to demonstrate pyuria by microscopic examination of the urine. Pyuria is demonstrated in the vast majority of episodes of acute bacterial cystitis and gross hematuria identified in approximately 20%. Alternatively, the leukocyte esterase dipstick has a reported sensitivity of approximately 85% in the detection of white blood cells in the urine. In women with classic symptoms and confirmation of pyuria, it is not necessary to perform a urine culture. However, indications for urine cultures include patients with a complicated history (e.g., recent catheterization), UTI within the past month, urinary symptomatology that has been present more than 7 days, cystitis in a woman older than 65, pregnancy, or intercurrent diseases such as diabetes mellitus or immunosuppression.

To obtain accurate estimates of the number of bacteria per milliliter, it is important to culture the urine within 2 hours or to refrigerate the specimen until it is sent to the laboratory. The gold standard of more than 10^5 uropathogens per milliliter had been the criterion used to make the diagnosis of significant bacteriuria in asymptomatic women. However, bacterial concentrations of as few as 10^2 per milliliter are accepted as bacteriologic confirmation of cystitis in symptomatic women.

For the first episode of acute, uncomplicated cystitis the current treatment of choice is 3 days of oral therapy with TMP-SMX, trimethoprim alone, or one of the quinolones such as ciprofloxacin or norfloxacin (Table 22-2). Compared with the traditional 7 to 14 days of therapy, the advantages of 3-day therapy are simplicity, better patient compliance, lower cost, and reduction of side effects such as diarrhea and vaginitis. With appropriate antibiotic therapy it takes approximately 24 hours for the symptoms of acute bacterial cystitis to resolve. In a community where resistance to trimethoprim is greater than 25%, treatment with a quinolone such as 250 mg twice daily of ciprofloxacin is appropriate. Obviously standard empiric regimens for acute bacterial cystitis should be reassessed periodically because of changing patterns of resistance to antibiotics. When resistance of *E. coli* to a therapeutic agent (e.g., TMP-SMX) reaches 20%, that agent should no longer be used for empiric therapy. Women with chronic infections, systemic manifestations of infection, renal disease, anatomic abnormalities of the urinary tract, pregnancy, or diabetes mellitus should be given more prolonged oral therapy for a minimum of 7 to 14 days. Failure to respond necessitates quantitative culture of the urine for bacteria and also culture of the endocervix and urethra for chlamydia and gonorrhea organisms. In the past, single-dose therapy was a popular regimen because of the convenience and simplicity. However, the rates of recurrence and failure with single-dose therapy were found to be unacceptable.

Persistent or recurrent cystitis following the initial infection presents in approximately 20% of women (Fig. 22-1). It is important to differentiate whether the infection is a relapse or a reinfection. More than 90% of recurrences in young women are exogenous reinfection with new isolates arising from local flora. Behavioral modification has become popular for preventing recurrent acute cystitis. Possible modifications in lifestyle include discontinuing use of a diaphragm for contraception, increasing oral fluid intake, voiding frequently, voiding immediately after intercourse, double voiding. Studies do not clearly demonstrate cranberry juice consumption treats or prevents acute cystitis. Approximately 75% of episodes of acute bacterial infection in women with recurrent cystitis occur within 24 hours of coitus. These women are excellent candidates to be treated with prophylactic antibiotics. The type of prophylaxis depends on the individual patient's history whether broad-spectrum antibiotics are prescribed continuously, postcoitally, or when the patient believes she is developing an infection. The broad-spectrum antibiotics that are most commonly chosen for low-dose antibiotic prophylaxis are trimethoprim, TMP-SMX, nitrofurantoin, or a cephalosporin. Prophylaxis may be given for months without significant emergence of antibiotic-resistant bacteria.

Complicated lower UTIs are those caused by antibiotic-resistant bacteria and those infections that occur in women with anatomic or functional abnormalities of the urinary tract. Many different organisms can be cultured in complicated cystitis, including *E. coli, Enterococcus faecalis, Proteus mirabilis, Staphylococcus epidermidis, S. aureus, Klebsiella, Pseudomonas, Enterobacter,* and *Serratia.* The quinolones currently are the drugs of choice for empiric therapy of complicated cystitis, primarily because of their broad antibacterial spectrum.

Table 22-2 Recommended Three-Day Regimens for Acute Uncomplicated Cystitis in Young Women

Drug	Dosage
Trimethoprim/sulfamethoxazole	160/180 mg q12h
Trimethoprim	100 mg q12h
Quinolones	
Ciprofloxacin	250 mg q12h
Enoxacin	400 mg q12h
Lomefloxacin 4	400 mg q12h
Norfloxacin	400 mg q12h
Ofloxacin	200 mg q12h

From Sweet RL, Gibbs RS: Infectious Diseases of the Female Genital Tract, 3rd ed. Baltimore, Williams & Wilkins, 1995.

Infections of Bartholin's Glands

Bartholin's glands normally are two rounded, pea-sized glands deep in the perineum. They are located at the entrance of the vagina at 5 o'clock and 7 o'clock. A normal Bartholin's gland cannot be palpated. The Bartholin's ducts are approximately 2 cm in length, and they open in a groove between the hymen and

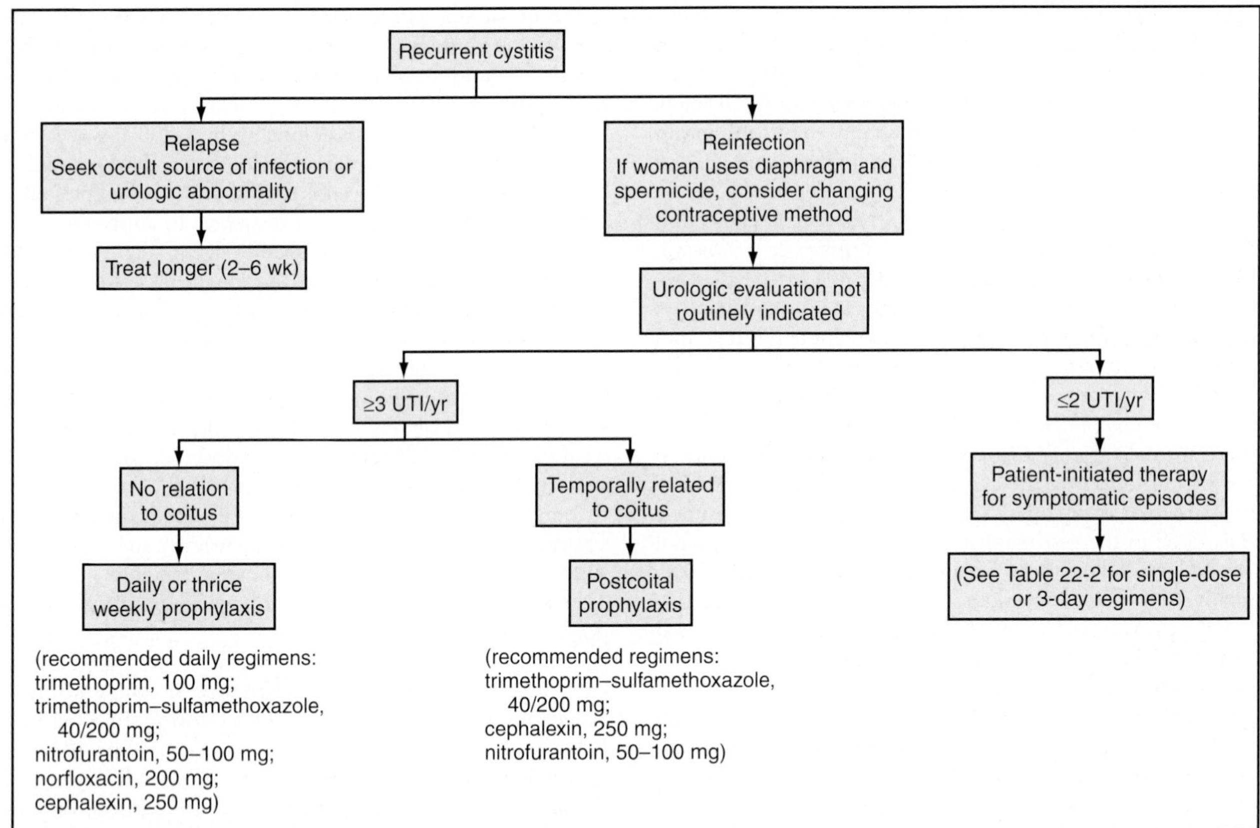

Figure 22-1. Strategies for managing recurrent cystitis in women. (From Stamm WE, Hooton TM: Management of urinary tract infections in adults. N Engl J Med 329:1328, 1993.)

labia minora in the posterior lateral wall of the vagina. Approximately 2% of adult women develop enlargements of one or both glands, of which there are three common causes. The most common cause is cystic dilation of Bartholin's duct (Fig. 22-2).

The cause of a Bartholin's duct cyst is obstruction of the duct secondary to nonspecific inflammation or trauma. Histologically, Bartholin's ducts are lined by transitional epithelium. These ducts are easily obstructed, usually near the distal orifice. Following obstruction, there is continued secretion of glandular fluid, which results in the cystic dilation. Years ago bilateral enlargement of Bartholin's glands was believed to be a pathognomonic sign of gonococcal infection. This is no longer true. Unilateral or bilateral Bartholin's gland infection in the majority of cases is not caused by a sexually transmitted disease. Lee and colleagues obtained bacterial cultures of fluid from Bartholin's duct cysts and abscesses. More than 80% of cultures from cysts were sterile, as were one in three cultures from Bartholin's abscesses. Brook reported positive cultures from 26 of 28 patients. He reported a total of 67 bacterial isolates, 43 of which were anaerobic and 24 of which were aerobic and facultative anaerobic organisms. In summary, positive cultures from Bartholin's gland abscesses are often polymicrobial and contain a wide range of bacteria similar to the normal flora of the vagina.

The differential diagnosis of Bartholin's gland cysts includes mesonephric cysts of the vagina and epithelial inclusion cysts. Mesonephric cysts are generally more anterior and cephalad in the vagina, whereas epithelial inclusion cysts are more superficial. Rarely, a lipoma, fibroma, hernia, vulvar varicosity, or hydrocele may be confused with a Bartholin's duct cyst. Bartholin's duct cysts are found in the labia majora, and the duct orifices are at the base of the labia minora just distal to the hymen.

Most women with Bartholin's duct cysts are asymptomatic. The cysts may vary from 1 to 8 cm in diameter, and they are usually unilateral, tense, and nonpainful. The majority of cysts are unilocular. However, occasionally in chronic or recurrent cysts there are multiple compartments.

An abscess of a Bartholin's gland tends to develop rapidly over 2 to 4 days. Symptoms include acute vulvar pain, dyspareunia, and pain during walking. Local symptoms of acute pain and tenderness are secondary to rapid enlargement, hemorrhage, or secondary infection. The signs are those of a classic abscess: erythema, acute tenderness, edema, and occasionally cellulitis of the surrounding subcutaneous tissue. Without therapy, most abscesses tend to rupture spontaneously by the third or fourth day.

The treatment of infections or enlargement of Bartholin's glands depends on their symptomatology. Asymptomatic cysts in women younger than 40 do not need treatment. The therapy for acute adenitis without abscess formation is broad-spectrum antibiotics and frequent hot sitz baths.

The treatment of choice for a symptomatic cyst or abscess is the development of a fistulous tract from the dilated duct to the vestibule. Simple incision and drainage of a Bartholin gland

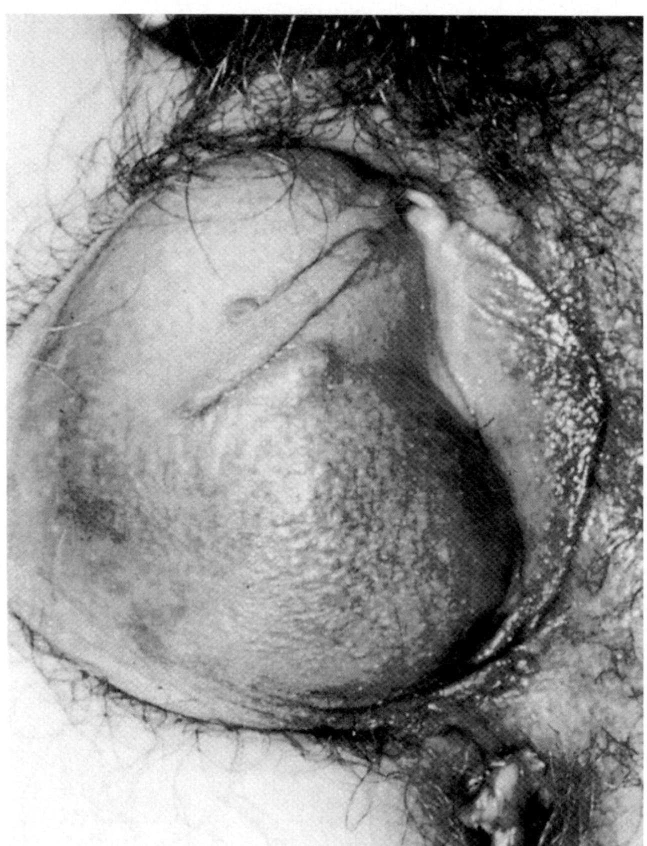

Figure 22-2. Bartholin's abscess. Mass is tender and fluctuant and is situated on lower lateral aspect of labium minus at 5 o'clock. (From Kaufman RH: Cystic tumors. In Kaufman RH, Faro S [eds]: Benign Diseases of the Vulva and Vagina, 4th ed. St. Louis, Mosby–Year Book, 1994.)

abscess are complicated by a tendency for the abscess to recur. The classic surgical treatment is to develop a fistulous tract to "marsupialize" the duct. After an elliptical wedge of tissue has been removed, the remaining edges of the duct or abscess are everted and sutured to the surrounding skin with interrupted sutures. This forms an epithelialized pouch that provides drainage for the gland. The recurrence rate following marsupialization is approximately 5% to 10%. An alternative surgical approach is to insert a Word catheter (a short catheter with an inflatable Foley balloon) through a stab incision into the abscess and leave it in place for 4 to 6 weeks (Fig. 22-3). During this period a tract of epithelium will form. All of the previously mentioned operations may be performed with local anesthesia. Antibiotics are not necessary unless there is an associated cellulitis surrounding the Bartholin gland abscess.

Biopsy for gland enlargement in women older than 40 is performed to exclude adenocarcinoma of Bartholin's gland. Excision of a Bartholin duct and gland is indicated for persistent deep infection or multiple recurrences of abscesses and may be performed for enlargement of the gland in women older than 40. Removal of a Bartholin gland for recurrent infection should be performed when the infection is quiescent. Because of the richness of the vascular supply to the region, including the vestibular bulbs directly below Bartholin's gland, excision is a more formidable task than one would expect. It is best to have either regional block or general anesthesia for excision. Removal of a Bartholin gland is often accompanied by morbidity, including intraoperative hemorrhage, hematoma formation, fenestration of the labia, postoperative scarring, and associated dyspareunia. Bartholin's gland secretions are not important for providing lubrication during sexual intercourse. Mucinous secretions from Bartholin's glands do provide moisture for the epithelium of the vestibule but are not important for vaginal lubrication.

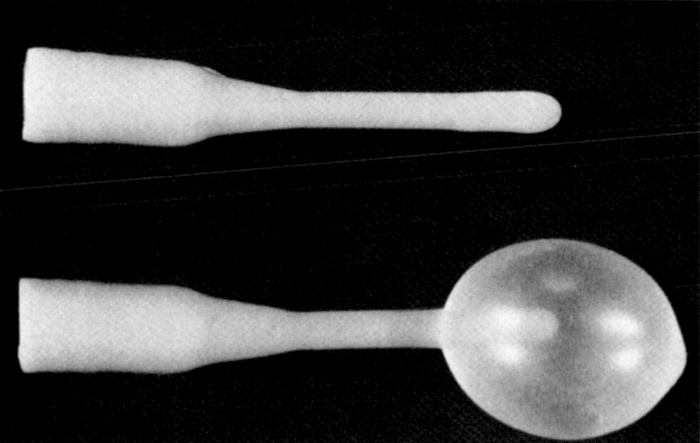

Figure 22-3. Word catheters before and after inflation. They are used to develop a fistula from Bartholin's cyst or abscess to vestibule. (From Friedrich EG: Vulvar Disease, 2nd ed. Philadelphia, WB Saunders, 1983.)

Pediculosis Pubis and Scabies

The skin of the vulva is a frequent site of infestation by animal parasites, the two most common being the crab louse and the itch mite. Ideally, early diagnosis and treatment are of the utmost importance in controlling parasitic infection.

Pediculosis pubis is an infestation by the crab louse, *Phthirus pubis.* The crab louse is also called the pubic louse and is a different species from the body or head louse. The louse is transmitted usually by close contact, although it may be acquired from towels or bedding. Lice in the pubic hair are the most contagious of all sexually transmitted diseases. It is estimated that over 90% of sexual partners are infected following a single exposure. *Phthirus pubis* is generally confined to the hairy areas of the vulva. It may occasionally be found in other areas such as the eyelids. The major nourishment of the louse is human blood. Body lice predominately infect schoolchildren and, secondarily, their mothers, by direct contact. Schools and playgrounds are the major reservoir. In contrast, pubic lice are typically transmitted by direct sexual contact. However, nonsexual transmission of pubic lice has been documented.

The louse's life cycle has three stages: egg (nit), nymph, and adult. The entire life cycle is spent on the host. Eggs are deposited at the base of hair follicles. The adult parasite is approximately 1 mm long and dark gray when its alimentary tract is not filled with blood (Fig. 22-4). Of clinical importance for diagnosis is the fact that the louse moves slowly.

The predominant clinical symptom of louse infestation is constant itching in the pubic area, which is secondary to allergic sensitization. It is estimated that it takes a minimum of 5 days

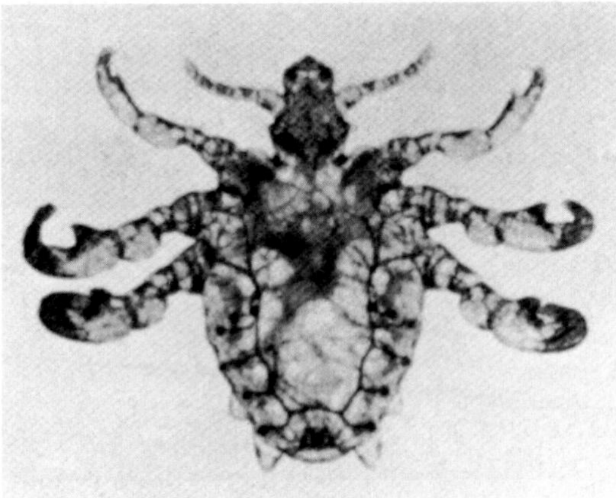

Figure 22-4. Pubic louse, *Phthirus pubis,* after blood meal. (From Billstein S: Human lice. In Holmes KK, Mårdh PA, Sparling PF, et al [eds]: Sexually Transmitted Diseases. New York, McGraw-Hill, 1984.)

following initial infection to develop allergic sensitization. Usually, initial sensitization takes several weeks to develop. The incubation period for pediculosis is approximately 30 days. Pruritus may occur within 24 hours after a reinfection. Examination of the vulvar area without magnification demonstrates eggs and adult lice and "pepper grain" feces adjacent to the hair shafts (Fig. 22-5). The tiny rough spots visualized with the naked eye are the alimentary tracts of lice filled with human blood. The vulvar skin may become secondarily irritated or infected by constant scratching. For definitive diagnosis one can make a microscopic slide by scratching the skin papule with a needle and placing the crust under a drop of mineral oil. The louse's body looks like that of a miniature crab with six legs that have claws on them.

Scabies is a parasitic infection of the itch mite, *Sarcoptes scabiei.* Epidemic outbreaks of scabies tend to occur approximately every 20 to 30 years. Similar to the crab louse, it is transmitted by close contact. Unlike louse infestation, scabies is an infection that is widespread over the body without a predilection for hairy areas. The adult female itch mite digs a burrow just beneath the skin. She lays eggs in this home during her life span of approximately 1 month. The adult itch mite is usually less than 0.5 mm long, approximately the size of a grain of sand. Unlike the crab louse, an itch mite travels rapidly over skin and may move up to 2.5 cm in 1 minute. Mites are able to survive for only a few hours away from the warmth of skin.

The predominant clinical symptom of scabies is severe but intermittent itching. Generally, more intense pruritus occurs at night when the skin is warmer and the mites are more active. Initial symptoms usually present approximately 3 weeks after primary infestation. Scabies may present as papules, vesicles, or burrows. However, the pathognomonic sign of scabies infection is the burrow in the skin. The burrow usually has the appearance of a twisted line on the skin surface, with a small vesicle at one end. Any area of the skin may be infected, with the hands, wrists, breasts, vulva, and buttocks being most commonly involved. A handheld magnifying lens is helpful for examining suspicious areas. Microscopic slides may be made by use of mineral oil and a scratch technique (Fig. 22-6). Mites lack lateral claw legs but have two anterior triangular hairy buds. Scabies

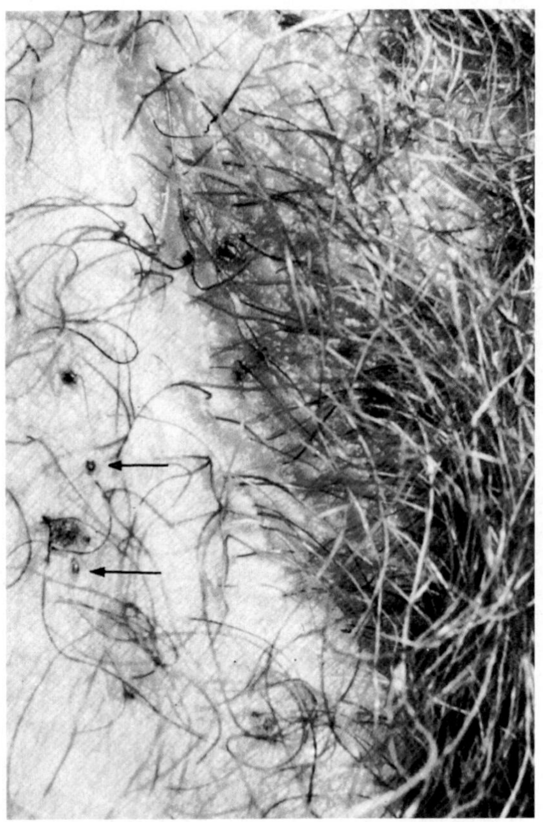

Figure 22-5. Crab lice and nits of pediculosis pubis *(arrows.)* (From Kaufman RH: Miscellaneous vulvar disorders. In Kaufman RH, Faro S [eds]: Benign Diseases of the Vulva and Vagina, 4th ed. St. Louis, Mosby–Year Book, 1994.)

has been termed the *great dermatologic imitator,* and the differential diagnosis includes virtually all dermatologic diseases that cause pruritus.

The treatment of pediculosis pubis or scabies involves an agent that kills both the adult parasite and the eggs. The therapy currently recommended by the CDC for pediculosis pubis involves the use of permethrin (Nix Creme), lindane (Kwell), or pyrethrins with piperonyl butoxide. Permethrin is available as a 1% cream rinse. It should be applied to affected areas and washed off after 10 minutes. Lindane 1% is recommended as a shampoo. It should be applied for 4 minutes to the affected area and subsequently thoroughly washed off. An alternative is pyrethrin with piperonyl butoxide applied to the affected area and washed off in 10 minutes. None of the regimens should be applied to the eyelids. Permethrin is more expensive than lindane, and it has less potential for toxicity in the event of inappropriate use. Seizures have been reported when lindane was applied immediately after a bath or in women with extensive dermatitis. Lindane is not recommended for pregnant or lactating women, or for children younger than age 2. Women should be reevaluated after 7 days if symptoms persist. Retreatment may be necessary if lice are found or if eggs are observed at the hair–skin junction.

The CDC recommendation for scabies is permethrin cream 5% applied to all areas of the body from the neck down and washed off after 8 to 14 hours or ivermectin 0.2 mg/kg orally, repeated in 2 weeks, if necessary. Alternative regimens include

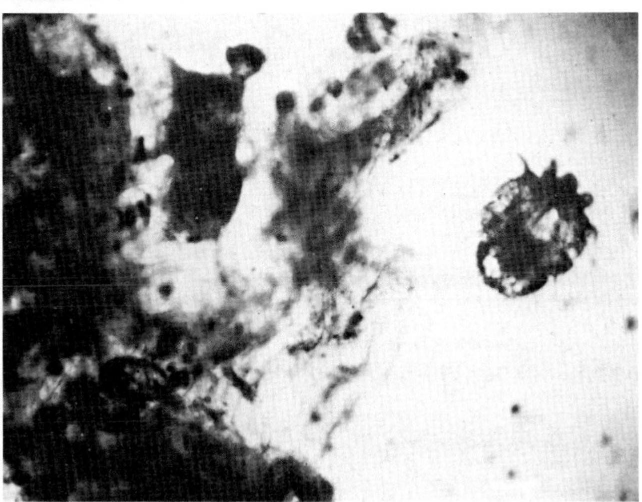

Figure 22-6. Skin scrapings of unexcoriated papules fortuitously disclose adults, larvae, eggs, and fecal pellets, any of which would be diagnostic of scabies. (From Orkin M, Howard IM: Scabies. In Holmes KK, Mårdh PA, Sparling PF, et al [eds]: Sexually Transmitted Diseases. New York, McGraw-Hill, 1984.)

lindane 1% 1 oz of lotion or 30 g of cream applied thinly to all areas of the body from the neck down and thoroughly washed off after 8 hours. Resistance to lindane has been reported in some parts of the United States. Patients with scabies have intense pruritus that may persist for many days following effective therapy. An antihistamine will help to alleviate this symptom. Similar to pediculosis pubis, women should be examined 1 week following initial therapy and retreated with an alternative regimen if live mites are observed.

To avoid reinfection by either pediculosis pubis or scabies, treatment should be prescribed for sexual contacts within the previous 6 weeks and other close household contacts. Those individuals with close physical contact should be treated at the same time as the infected woman whether or not they have symptoms. Clothing and bedding should be decontaminated. Importantly, women and physicians alike should not confuse the 1% cream rinse of permethrin dosage recommended for pubic lice with the permethrin cream 5% being recommended for scabies.

Molluscum Contagiosum

Molluscum contagiosum is a pox virus that causes a chronic localized infection, consisting of flesh-colored, dome-shaped papules with an umbilicated center. The inability to grow the virus in standard tissue culture or in an animal model resulted in limited knowledge about molluscum contagiosum, but now the entire genome has been sequenced. Like many viruses in the pox family, molluscum is spread by direct skin to skin contact. The incubation time is 2 to 7 weeks. In children, molluscum contagiosum may present over the entire body. In adults, it is primarily an asymptomatic disease of the vulvar skin and unlike most sexually transmitted diseases, it is only mildly contagious. However, lesions can be spread by autoinoculation, during contact sports, or by fomites on bath sponges or towels.

Molluscum replicates in cytoplasm of cells. Widespread infection in adults is most closely related to underlying cellular immunodeficiency, such as during an HIV infection. It can also occur in the setting of chemotherapy or corticosteroid administration.

Diagnosis is made by the characteristic appearance of the lesions. The small nodules or domed papules of molluscum contagiosum are usually 1 to 5 mm in diameter (Fig. 22-7). Close inspection reveals that many of the more mature nodules have an umbilicated center. Characteristically, an infected woman will have 1 to 20 solitary lesions randomly distributed over the vulvar skin. A crop of new nodules will persist from several months to years. If the diagnosis cannot be made by simple inspection, the white, waxy material from inside the nodule should be expressed on a microscopic slide. The finding of intracytoplasmic molluscum bodies with Wright or Giemsa stain confirms the diagnosis. The major complication of molluscum contagiosum is bacterial superinfection. The umbilicated papules may resemble furuncles when secondarily infected.

Molluscum contagiosum is usually a self-limiting infection and spontaneously reduces after a few months in immunocompetent individuals. However, treatment of individual papules will decrease sexual transmission and autoinoculation of the virus. Treatment of individual papules is initiated with injection of a local anesthetic with a small subdermal wheal of 1% lidocaine (Xylocaine). The caseous material is then evacuated and the nodule excised with a sharp dermal curette. The base of the papule is subsequently chemically treated with either ferric subsulfate (Monsel solution) or 85% trichloroacetic acid. An alternative method is canthardin, a chemical blistering agent. In one retrospective study, 90% of 300 children had clearance of lesions with an average of two visits. In immunocompromised individuals, treatment is more difficult. In the HIV-infected patient, there have been multiple reports of recalcitrant molluscum lesions resolving only after initiating highly active antiretroviral therapy.

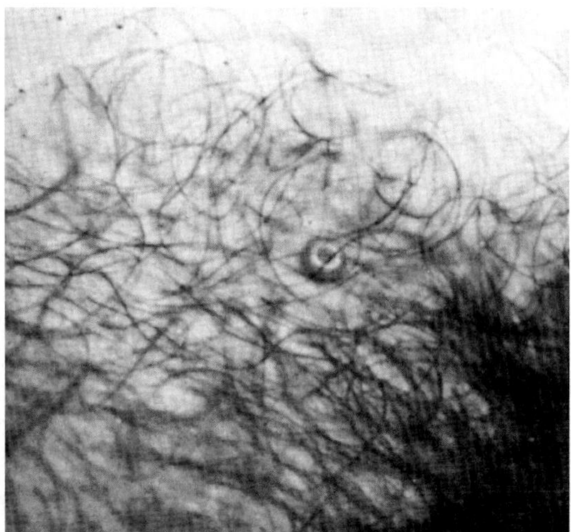

Figure 22-7. Papule of molluscum contagiosum with umbilicated center. (From Brown ST: Molluscum contagiosum. In Holmes KK, Mårdh PA, Sparling PF, et al [eds]: Sexually Transmitted Diseases. New York, McGraw-Hill, 1984.)

Condyloma Acuminatum

Condyloma acuminatum is the most common viral sexually transmitted disease of the vulva, vagina, rectum, and cervix caused by the human papillomavirus (HPV). Synonyms for vulvar condylomata acuminata include genital, venereal, or anogenital warts. In the past few years this disease has reached epidemic levels (Fig. 22-8). It presents as a clinically recognizable macroscopic lesion in 30% of infected women and as an asymptomatic, unrecognized subclinical infection in the remaining 70%. DNA testing demonstrates that the majority of HPV infections are subclinical. Thus the prevalence of the disease depends on the sophistication of the technique used to diagnose subclinical infection, such as cytology, colposcopy, or molecular probes of biopsy material. It is estimated that in the past 20 to 25 years the number of infected individuals has increased approximately 700%. The prevalence of HPV varies widely depending on the population studied. However, it is as high as 50% in sexually active teenagers with multiple partners. The relationship between HPV infection and early lower genital tract intraepithelial neoplasia and invasive squamous cell carcinoma have been the stimuli for expanding research efforts into this complex group of viruses.

More than 70 subtypes of HPV, which differ from one another in their individual genomes, have been identified. At least 25 different subtypes of HPV have been involved in genital infection. Of the most common HPV subtypes, numbers 16 and 18 are high risk to be associated with aneuploid, premalignant, or malignant lesions of the female genital tract. Types 6 and 11 are more commonly associated with benign, euploid lesions (Table 22-3). Women may be infected simultaneously with more than one HPV type. Sexual intercourse is the usual method of transmitting genital HPV infection. Autoinoculation definitely occurs because HPV DNA has been demonstrated on the fingers of women with genital warts suggesting the possibility of this secondary means of inoculation. The virus can be shed from both macroscopic and microscopic lesions. It is highly contagious, with 25% to 65% of sexual partners developing the infection. Oriel discovered that 60% of adults develop the disease following intercourse with a partner who was actively shedding the virus. Studies have demonstrated condoms offer only modest protection against HPV transmission. The average incubation period is 3 months, with a wide range of 1 to 8 months. As with other sexually transmitted diseases, peak incidence occurs between the ages of 15 and 25 years.

Table 22-3 Genital HPV Types

HPV Type	Morphology	Potential for Cancer
6, 11	Genital warts, LSIL, RRP	Low (negligible)
40, 42, 53, 54, 57, 66, 84	LSIL	Low (negligible)
16, 18, 31, 33, 35, 39 45, 51, 52, 56, 58, 59 68, 73, 82	LSIL HSIL Cancer	High
61, 62, 67, 69, 70	?	Uncertain

HSIL, high-grade squamous intraepithelial lesion; LSIL, low-grade squamous intraepithelial lesion; RRP, recurrent respiratory papillomatosis.

In the majority of women, the diagnosis of overt condyloma acuminatum can be made by direct inspection. Condyloma acuminata-type warts tend to occur primarily on moist surfaces. Indications to perform a biopsy include the rare situations when lesions do not respond to standard therapy; the condition

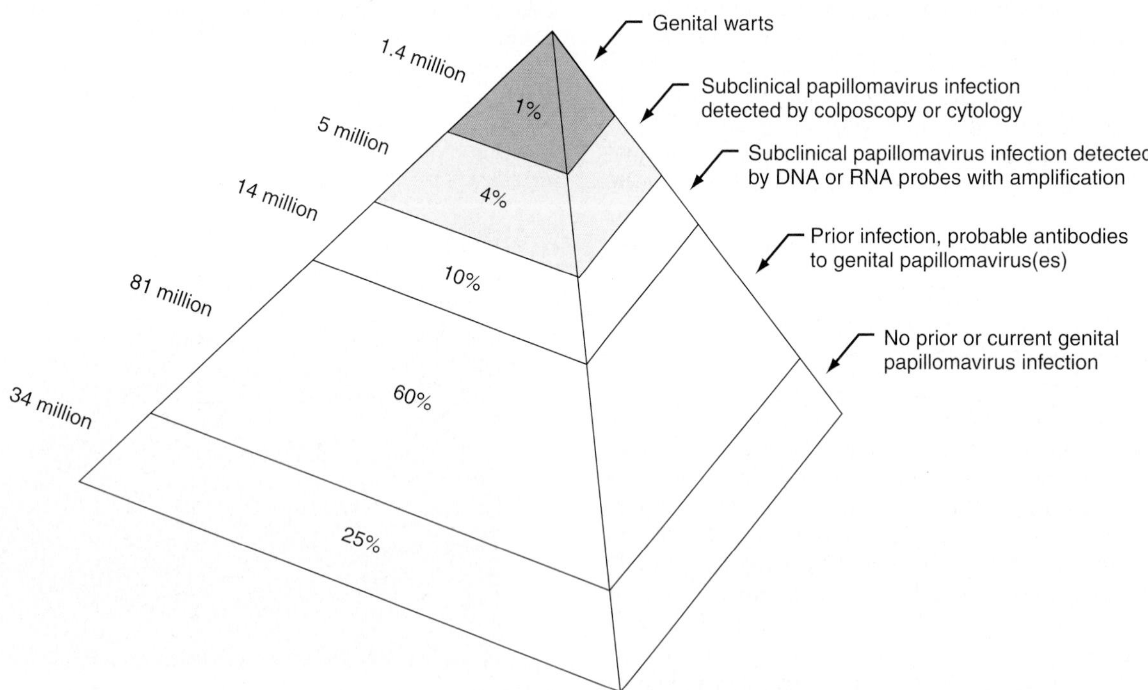

Figure 22-8. Estimated prevalence of genital HPV infection among sexually active men and women 15 to 49 years of age in the United States. (From Koutsky LA, Kiviat NB: Genital human papillomavirus. In Holmes KK, Mårdh PA, Sparling PF, et al [eds]: Sexually Transmitted Diseases. New York, McGraw-Hill, 1984.)

Table 22-4 Anatomic Distribution of Anogenital HPV Infections* in Female Patients

Site	Percentage†
Cervix	70
Vulva	25
Vagina	10
Anus	20

*Including subclinical lesions.
†Total exceeds 100% because of the multicentric distribution of HPV infection.
From Ferenczy A: Epidemiology and clinical pathophysiology of condylomata acuminata. Am J Obstet Gynecol 172:1331, 1995.

accelerates during therapy; the woman is immunocompromised; or when growths are pigmented, indurated, fixed, or ulcerated. Type-specific HPV nucleic acid tests are not indicated, nor are they of benefit in the diagnosis or management of visible genital warts. Pedunculated warts are friable and tend to bleed following minor trauma. Initial infections usually begin in the vestibule and adjacent areas of the labia. However, adjacent, moist epithelium may be involved with condyloma, including the vagina, cervix, urethra, bladder, and rectum (Table 22-4). Initial lesions are pedunculated, soft papules approximately 2 to 3 mm in diameter and 10 to 20 mm long. They may occur as a single papule or in clusters. The infection progresses by means of autoinoculation. As adjacent lesions coalesce, many different presentations may evolve (Fig. 22-9). Lesions vary from pinhead-sized papules to large cauliflower-like masses that may grow to several centimeters in diameter. Uncomplicated condylomata acuminata are usually asymptomatic. Depending on size and location, some warts are symptomatic, producing pain, itching, tendency to bleed when friable, and an odor when secondarily infected. Condylomata in the cervix tend to be flat and sometimes bleed on contact. The presence of condylomata of the cervix, especially subclinical disease, is generally discovered by colposcopic examination. Perianal warts occur in approximately 20% of women with condyloma acuminatum. Subclinical HPV infection of the cervix, vagina, or vulva may be discovered by applying 3% to 5% acetic acid to the epithelium. Often, HPV-infected cells appear shiny white in color, with the area of infection having irregular borders and sometimes satellite lesions. However, application of acetic acid is not a specific test for HPV infection. Thus, in a low-risk population, many false-positives will be encountered if one uses this test for screening. Vaginal condylomata are identified in approximately one of three women with vulvar disease. Common benign skin lesions to consider in the differential diagnosis of condyloma acuminata are micropapillomatosis labialis, seborrheic keratosis, nevi, and other STDs such as condyloma lata and molluscum contagiosum and neoplasms such as giant condyloma or bowenoid papulosis or squamous cell carcinoma.

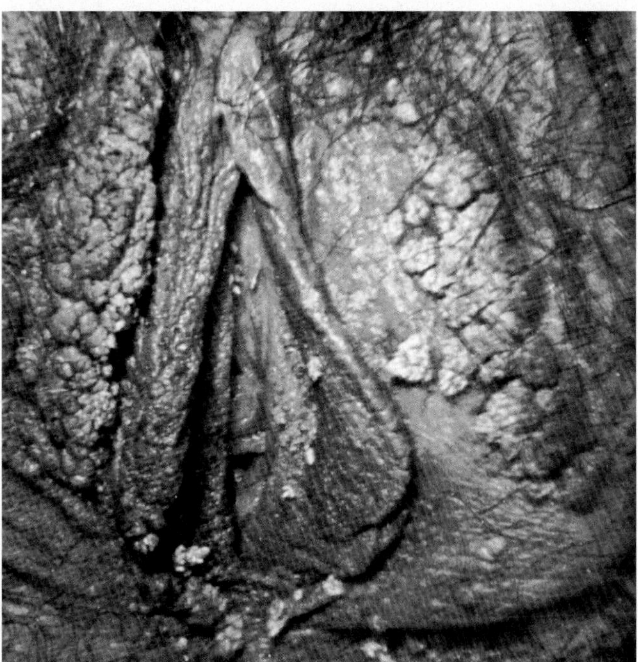

Figure 22-9. Condyloma acuminatum. Often small, younger lesions are present with larger, older lesions. (From Friedrich EG: Vulvar Disease, 2nd ed. Philadelphia, WB Saunders, 1983.)

Several conditions are known to predispose women to infection with HPV and include immunosuppression, diabetes, pregnancy, and local trauma. Often, preexisting vulvovaginitis has provided the moist, excoriated skin on which the HPV colonizes. The vulvovaginitis should be treated as part of the therapeutic plan for condyloma acuminatum.

The management of the individual woman depends on the location, size, and extent of the condyloma and whether the woman is pregnant. Most clinicians attempt to treat the patient until the macroscopic lesions disappear. The most important priority is to remove symptomatic growths. No present therapy of HPV eliminates subclinical infection from the surrounding epithelium. Untreated condylomata usually resolve. However, some remain unchanged or increase in size. There is no evidence that treatment changes infectivity or the natural history of the disease. Serial HPV DNA testing has delineated the natural history of HPV. Almost all low-risk HPV infections and two thirds of high-risk HPV infections are eradicated over a 24-month period. There is a wide range of therapeutic choices, including chemical, cautery, and immunologic therapy. The CDC-recommended treatments for external genital warts are subdivided into patient-applied therapies and provider-administrated therapies (see the following boxes). None of the various treatment regimens is more effective than other acceptable treatments. However, warts located on moist surfaces and in intertriginous areas respond faster to topical treatment than do warts on drier surfaces. Approximately two thirds of women notice moderate burning and pain in the areas that are being treated. Data from randomized clinical trials is presented in Table 22-5. Complications rarely occur unless the treatment is overzealous, which results in ulcerated or infected areas of vulvar skin.

Another chemical alternative treatment is topical 5-fluorouracil/epinephrine/bovine collagen gel. The preparation is injected directly into the base of the wart. This therapy requires frequent visits and the lack of superior efficacy makes it difficult to justify its routine use.

Lesions larger than 2 to 3 cm are best treated by cryotherapy, electrocautery, or laser therapy. It is sometimes best to surgically shave the condyloma and then apply thermal injury to the virus in the base of the lesion. The woman should be advised

Table 22-5 Clearance and Recurrence Rates with Different Treatment Modalities for External Genital Warts

Treatment	CLEARANCE RATES (%) End of Treatment	3 Months or More	Recurrent Rates
Cryotherapy	63–88	63–92	0–39
Electrocautery/electrotherapy	93–94	78–91	24
Interferon			
Intralesional	19–62	36–62	0–33
Systemic	7–51	18–21	0–23
Topical	6–90	33	6
Laser therapy	27–89	39–86	<7–45
LEEP	≤90	—	—
Podophyllin*	32–79	22–73	11–65
Podophyllotoxin (Podofilox)	42–88	34–77	10–91
Surgical/scissor excision	89–93	36	0–29
Trichloroacetic acid	50–81	70	36
5-fluorouracil	10–71	37	10–13

*Studies using more than one treatment strength have been grouped together.
LEEP, loop electrocautery excision procedure.
From Beautner KR, Wiley DJ: Recurrent external genital warts: A literature review. Papillomavirus Report 8:69, 1997. Reprinted with permission. From Maw RD: Treatment of anogenital warts. Dermatol Clin 16:829, 1998.

that changes in skin pigmentation are common following ablative therapy.

To date, effective treatment of condyloma acuminatum with systemic immunotherapy by itself has been disappointing. Interferon, because of its antiviral and antiproliferative properties, was postulated to be an ideal drug to treat HPV infection. Regrettably, interferons, when given parenterally, may result in severe systemic symptoms similar to a viral illness in some women. Interferon treatment of HPV has been accomplished by topical creams and direct injection into the condylomata. Local application exerts antiviral activity by stimulating a focal immune response.

Recurrences usually present within 3 months of successful treatment of the initial treatment. A quadrivalent HPV vaccine is now available against types 16, 18, 6, and 11. In females naïve to HPV virus initial administration of the vaccine followed by repeat inoculation at 2 and 6 months can prevent 90% of genital warts. More vaccines are currently in development (see Chapter 29, Malignant Diseases of the Cervix).

Genital Ulcers

Herpes, granuloma inguinale (donovanosis), lymphogranuloma venereum, chancroid, and syphilis may all present as ulcerations in the genital area. However, their causes, disease courses, and treatments are different. Table 22-6 lists some of their major characteristics. Physicians must always consider the possibility of more than one STD concurrently infecting an individual.

Genital Herpes

Genital herpes is recurrent and incurable and is among the most frequently encountered STDs. It is frequently transmitted by asymptomatic shedding; approximately 80% of the individuals are unaware they are infected. Herpes is highly contagious, with 75% of sexual partners of infected individuals contracting the disease. In a recent study of 5452 asymptomatic adults in private

Treatment of Warts: Patient-Administered

	Podafilox 0.5% Solution or Gel (Condylox)	Imiquimod 5% Cream (Aldera)
Dose	Bid for 3 days, 4 days off up to 4 cycles	Daily and qhs, 3 times/week up to 16 weeks, wash 6–10 min after R_x
Mode of action	Antimitotic	Immune enhancer
Side effects	Mild to moderate pain, local irritation	Mild to moderate local inflammation
Pregnancy	NO	NO

MMWR 55(RR-11), 2006.

Treatment of Warts: Provider-Administered

	Cytotherapy	Podophyllin Resin	Trichloroacetic Acid (TCA)
Dose	Weekly every 1–2 weeks (no cryoprobe in vagina)	Weekly	Weekly, "frosting"
Mode of action	Thermal-induced cytolysis	Antimitotic	Chemical coagulation of proteins
Side effects	Pain, necrosis + blistering	Local irritation	Pain, adjacent damage [use soap, soda]
Pregnancy	OK	NO	OK

MMWR 55(RR-11), 2006.

Table 22-6 Clinical Features of Genital Ulcers

	Syphilis	Herpes	Chancroid	Lymphogranuloma Venereum	Donovanosis
Incubation period	2–4 weeks (1–12 weeks)	2–7 days	1–14 days	3 days–6 weeks	1–4 weeks (up to 6 months)
Primary lesion	Papule	Vesicle	Papule or pustule	Papule, pustule, or vesicle	Papule
Number of lesions	Usually one	Multiple, may coalesce	Usually multiple, may coalesce	Usually one	Variable
Diameter (mm)	5–15	1–2	2–20	2–10	Variable
Edges	Sharply demarcated Elevated, round or oval	Erythematous	Undermined, ragged, irregular	Elevated, round or oval irregular	Elevated, irregular
Depth	Superficial or deep	Superficial	Excavated	Superficial or deep	Elevated
Base	Smooth, nonpurulent	Serous, erythematous	Purulent	Variable	Red and rough ("beefy")
Induration	Firm	None	Soft	Occasionally firm	Firm
Pain	Unusual	Common	Usually very tender	Variable	Uncommon
Lymphadenopathy	Firm, nontender, bilateral	Firm, tender, often bilateral	Tender, may suppurate, usually unilateral	Tender, may suppurate, loculated, usually unilateral	Pseudoadenopathy

From Holmes KK, Mårdh PA, Sparling PF, et al (eds): Sexually Transmitted Diseases, 2nd ed. New York, McGraw-Hill, 1990.

community-based clinics in six geographic regions in the United States the zero prevalence of HSV-2 was 25.5%.

Recent evidence suggests that viral shedding from asymptomatic individuals may occur as frequently as 1 in 5 days. Thus some infectious disease specialists consider herpes a persistent rather than a intermittent disease. It is important that the woman understand the natural history of disease with emphasis on probability of recurrent attacks, the effect of antiviral agents, and the risks of neonatal infection.

Recurrent genital herpes is not a debilitating physical disease, yet it may present an overwhelming psychological burden. To the individual patient there is an immense sense of social isolation and a reluctance to initiate a sexual relationship. This can result in a decrease in self-esteem, depression, and, most important, a feeling of loss of control due to the inability to predict the time of the next recurrence.

There are two distinct types of herpes simplex virus: type 1 (HSV-1) and type 2 (HSV-2). In the past a broad generalization was, HSV-I tends to infect epithelium above the waist, and HSV-2 tends to cause ulceration below the waist. However, depending on the series, HSV-1 may cause lower genital tract infections between 13% and 40% of the time. Currently, HSV-1 is the most commonly acquired genital herpes in women younger than 25. HSV-1 does not protect against HSV-2, but HSV-2 does offer some protection against HSV-1.

The primary infection by herpes is both a local and a systemic disease. The majority of initial genital infections occur in women between the ages of 15 and 35. The incubation period is between 3 and 7 days, with an average of 6 days. Often the patient experiences paresthesias of the vulvar skin before papules and subsequent vesicle formation. Usually there are multiple vesicles that become shallow, superficial ulcers over a large area of the vulva. There is often simultaneous involvement of the vagina and cervix (Fig. 22-10). Patients experience multiple crops of ulcers for 2 to 6 weeks. Often the ulcers coalesce; however, the ulcers heal spontaneously without scarring (Fig. 22-11). Viral shedding may occur for 2 to 3 weeks after vulvar lesions appear. During primary infections, positive cultures for herpesvirus may be obtained from lesions in 80% of women. The majority of symptomatic women have severe vulvar pain, tenderness, and inguinal adenopathy. Nevertheless, subclinical primary herpes infection is common. Regional lymphadenopathy usually develops during primary genital infections.

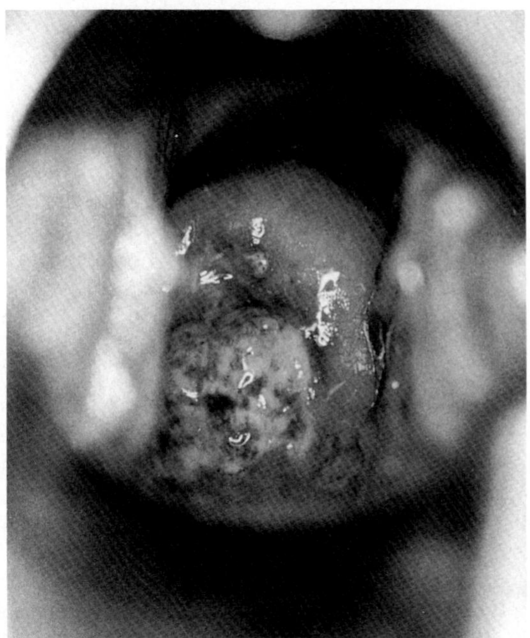

Figure 22-10. Primary herpes involving cervix. Necrotic exophytic mass is seen on posterior lip. This was clinically thought to be invasive carcinoma. Herpes simplex virus culture was positive. Lesion spontaneously disappeared. (From Kaufman RH, Faro S: Herpes genitalis: clinical features and treatment. Clin Obstet Gynecol 28:154, 1985.)

Systemic symptoms, including general malaise and fever, are experienced by 70% of women during the primary infection. Rarely there is central nervous system (CNS) infection, with the reported mortality rate from herpes encephalitis being approximately 50%. Primary infections of the urethra and bladder may result in acute urinary retention, necessitating catheterization. The symptoms of vulvar pain, pruritus, and discharge peak between days 7 and 11 of the primary infection. The average woman experiences severe symptoms for approximately 14 days.

Recurrent genital herpes is a local disease, and the symptoms are much less severe than the primary outbreak. Many women

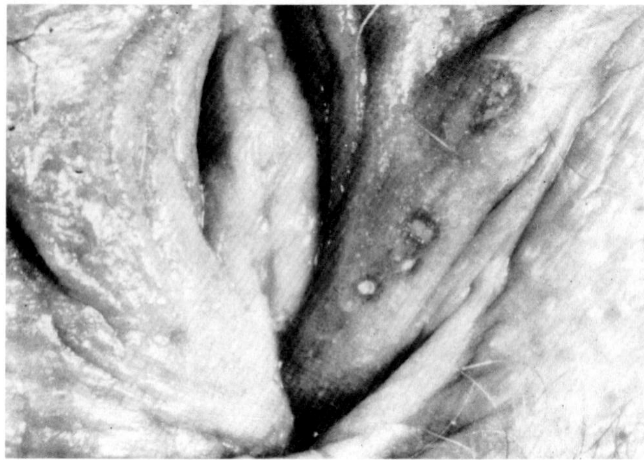

Figure 22-11. Recurrent herpes genitalis. Superficial ulcers are noted following rupture of vesicles. (From Kaufman RH, Faro S: Herpes genitalis: Clinical features and treatment. Clin Obstet Gynecol 28:156, 1985.)

develop asymptomatic recurrences. In 50% of women the first recurrence occurs within 6 months of the initial infection. If a woman's initial genital infection was with HSV-2, she has an approximately 80% chance of having a recurrence within 12 months. Women whose primary HSV-2 infection was severe have recurrences approximately twice as often, with a shorter time to recurrence intervals compared with women with milder initial episodes of the disease. On the average a woman will have four recurrences during the first year. In contrast, if the initial pelvic infection was with HSV-1, there is a 55% chance of a recurrence within 1 year, with the average rate of recurrence slightly less than one episode. There is a general clinical opinion that recurrences are frequently related to the onset of a menstrual period or emotional stress. To generalize, most clinical manifestations of recurrent infection are half as severe as those of primary infections. That is, vulvar involvement is usually unilateral, recurrent attacks last an average of 7 days, and viral shedding occurs for approximately 5 days. The ability to successfully culture herpesvirus from recurrent herpetic ulcers is 40%. A common feature of recurrence is a prodromal phase of sacroneuralgia, vulvar burning, tenderness, and pruritus for a few hours to 5 days before vesicle formation. The probability and frequency of recurrence of herpes is related to the HSV serotype. Extragenital sites of recurrent infection are common. The herpesvirus resides in a latent phase in the dorsal root ganglia of S2, S3, and S4.

The clinical diagnosis of genital herpes is often made by simple clinical inspection. Women come to the physician when they develop symptoms from vulvar ulcers. Herpetic ulcers are painful when touched with a cotton-tipped applicator, whereas the ulcers of syphilis are painless. As stated earlier, viral cultures are useful in confirming the diagnosis in primary episodes when culture sensitivity is 80%, but less useful in recurrent episodes. Most herpesvirus cultures will become positive within 2 to 4 days of inoculation. The most accurate and sensitive technique for identifying herpesvirus is the polymerase chain reaction (PCR) test. Serologic tests are helpful in determining whether a patient has been infected in the past with herpesvirus. Western blot assay for antibodies to herpes is the most specific method for diagnosing recurrent herpes, as well as unrecognized or subclinical infection. However Western blot tests are not widely available and difficult to perform. ELISA and immunoblot tests are available for both HSV-1 and HSV-2. Rapid serologic point-of-care tests are now available for HSV-2 antibodies. Appropriate screening tests for other STDs should be obtained, as they may coexist with herpes.

Treatment of HSV-1 or HSV-2 may be used for three different clinical scenarios:

1. primary episode
2. recurrent episode
3. daily suppression

In primary episodes duration and severity of symptoms is lessened and shedding is shortened with antiviral therapy. Antiviral therapy is recommended for use in all patients with primary episodes.

Episodic therapy for recurrences can shorten duration of outbreak if started within 24 hours of prodromal symptoms or lesion appearance. Due to the necessity of starting antiviral therapy immediately after recognizing symptoms, it is important that the patient with HSV be given a prescription for antiviral therapy to have at home.

Patient-initiated therapy has been found to be superior to therapy ordered by a physician because patients initiate therapy earlier in the course of a recurrence. The antiviral medication should be started as early as possible during the prodrome and definitely within 24 hours of the appearance of lesions. Daily suppressive therapy is recommended when the patient has six or more episodes a year or for psychological distress. It is important for patients to be aware that asymptomatic viral shedding can occur even when on daily suppressive therapy.

In serodiscordant couples a prospective placebo-controlled randomized trial demonstrated daily use of valacyclovir for suppression in the seropositive partner resulted in significantly fewer cases of HSV acquisition in the seronegative partner. Regular use of condoms in serodiscordant couples also decreases transmission, but is not 100% protective. HSV seronegative women are three times as likely to acquire HSV infection from seropositive male partners compared with seronegative males acquiring HSV from infected female partners. A summary of CDC-recommended treatment regimens is presented in the following box.

Acyclovir is a drug with relatively minimal toxicity, and recent reports have documented daily use for as long as 6 years helping to establish the long-term safety of the drug. However, the CDC recommends that acyclovir or other suppressive drug should be discontinued after 12 months of suppressive therapy to determine the subsequent rate of recurrence for each individual woman. Even if herpes is not treated over time, clinical recurrences tend to dramatically decrease in number.

A vaccine would be the logical approach for optimum prevention of herpes. Research is ongoing.

Granuloma Inguinale (Donovanosis)

Granuloma inguinale, also known as donovanosis, is a chronic, ulcerative, bacterial infection of the skin and subcutaneous tissue of the vulva. Rarely the vagina and cervix are involved in advanced, untreated cases. Granuloma inguinale is common in tropical climates such as New Guinea and the Caribbean islands,

Antiviral Treatment for HSV—Nonpregnant Patient

Indication	Valacyclovir	Acyclovir	Famciclovir
First clinical episode	1000 mg bid for 7–10 days	200 mg five times a day or 400 mg tid for 7–10 days	250 mg tid for 7–10 days
Recurrent episodes	1000 mg daily or 500 mg bid for 5 days (or 3 days)	400 mg tid for 5 days or 800 mg bid for 5 days or 800 mg tid for 3 days	125 mg bid for 5 days 1000 mg bid for 1 day
Daily suppressive therapy	500 mg daily (≤8 recurrences per year) or 1000 mg/day or 250 mg bid (>9 recurrences/year)	400 mg bid	250 mg bid

MMWR 55(RR-11), 2006.

but fewer than 20 cases are reported each year in the United States.

This chronic disease is caused by an intracellular gram-negative, nonmotile, encapsulated rod—*Calymmatobacterium granulomatis.* This bacterium shares common antigens with *Klebsiella* and *E. coli.* It is very difficult to culture on standard media but has recently been isolated in cell culture. Serologic tests are nonspecific. This disease can be spread both sexually through close, nonsexual contact. However, it is not highly contagious, and chronic exposure is usually necessary to contract the disease. The incubation period is extremely variable—from 1 to 12 weeks. The mildly contagious disease is found in 1% to 52% of sexual partners of women with the disease. However, it is also found in young children and elderly women, who are not sexually active. Thus some experts hypothesize that the disease may be secondary to autoinoculation following trauma to the infected area.

The initial growth of granuloma inguinale is an asymptomatic nodule. The skin over the nodule ulcerates, and the characteristic lesion is a beefy-red ulcer with fresh granulation tissue. The area around the lesions is highly vascular, thus the ulcers bleed easily when touched. Usually there are multiple nodules and, subsequently, multiple ulcers of the vulva. Adjacent areas of ulceration grow and coalesce and, if untreated, will eventually destroy the normal vulvar architecture. The ulcers are painless unless secondarily infected. Adenopathy is not a prominent feature unless there is a superimposed infection. Vulvar edema, especially of the labia, is a common feature of the disease. If untreated, the chronic form of the disease is characterized by scarring and lymphatic obstruction, which produces marked enlargement of the vulva.

In endemic areas the disease is usually diagnosed by its clinical manifestations. The diagnosis is established by identifying Donovan bodies in smears and specimens taken from the ulcers (Fig. 22-12). Both the deep aspects of the ulcer crater and the fresh edge of an expanding lesion should be sampled. The pathognomonic Donovan bodies are clusters of dark-staining bacteria with a bipolar (safety pin) appearance found in the cytoplasm of large mononuclear cells (Fig. 22-13). Special silver stains highlight the Donovan bodies. However, even a brief period of previous antibiotic therapy may result in an absence of Donovan bodies in women who have granuloma inguinale.

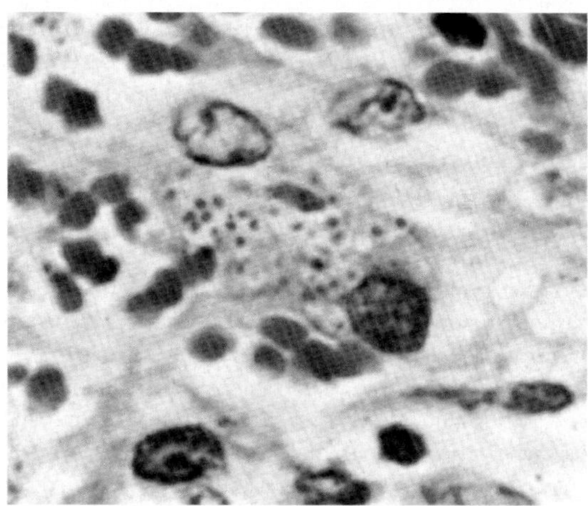

Figure 22-12. Donovanosis. Biopsy specimen shows intracytoplasmic Donovan bodies (H&E stain). (From Hart G: Donovanosis. In Holmes KK, Mårdh PA, Sparling PF, et al [eds]: Sexually Transmitted Diseases. New York, McGraw-Hill, 1984.)

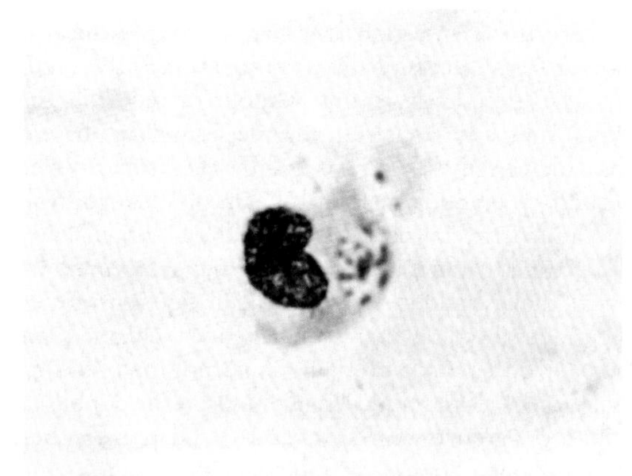

Figure 22-13. Donovanosis. Crust preparation from biopsy specimen shows single cell with many intracytoplasmic Donovan bodies (Giemsa stain). (From Hart G: Donovanosis. In Holmes KK, Mårdh PA, Sparling PF, et al [eds]: Sexually Transmitted Diseases. New York, McGraw-Hill, 1984.)

The differential diagnosis includes lymphogranuloma venereum, vulvar carcinoma, syphilis, chancroid, genital herpes, amebiasis, and other granulomatous diseases.

Granuloma inguinale may be managed by a wide range of oral broad-spectrum antibiotics. The CDC recommends doxycycline 100 mg orally twice a day for a minimum of 3 weeks. Alternative antibiotic regimens are azithromycin 1 g orally per week for 3 weeks, ciprofloxacin 750 mg orally twice a day for a minimum of 3 weeks, or erythromycin base 500 mg or TMP-SMZ one double-strength tablet orally twice a day for a minimum of 3 weeks orally four times a day for a minimum of 3 weeks. Tetracycline is no longer recommended because many strains of the bacteria have developed resistance. The initial response to antibiotic therapy should be apparent within the first 7 days. However, optimal clinical response usually takes 3 to 5 weeks to ensure that the lesions have healed completely. It is best to continue antibiotics until a complete clinical response is noted with healing of the ulcerative lesions. Alternative antibiotic therapy such as an aminoglycoside has been used in refractory cases. Rarely, medical therapy fails and surgical excision is required. Coinfection with another sexually transmitted pathogen is a distinct possibility. Sex partners of women who have granuloma inguinale should be examined if they have had sexual contact during the 60 days preceding the onset of symptoms.

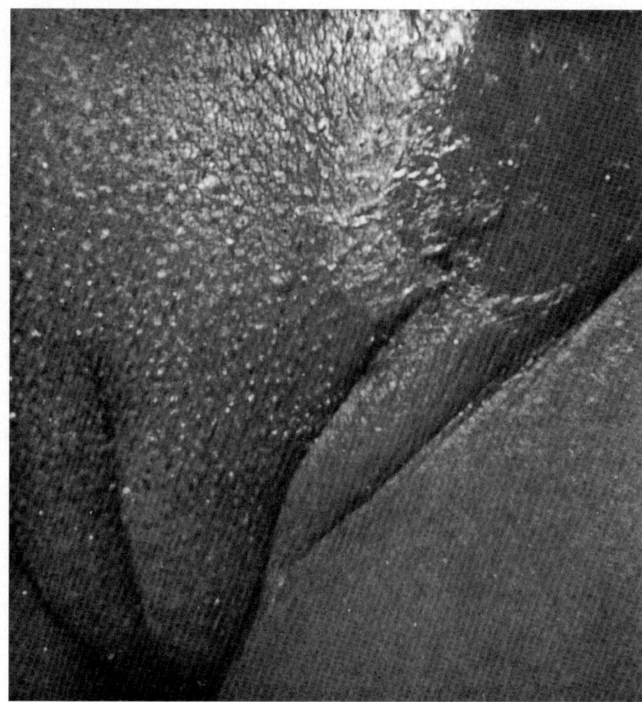

Figure 22-14. Lymphogranuloma venereum bubo with "groove" sign. (From Friedrich EG: Vulvar Disease, 2nd ed. Philadelphia, WB Saunders, 1983.)

Lymphogranuloma Venereum

Lymphogranuloma venereum (LGV) is a chronic infection of lymphatic tissue produced by *Chlamydia trachomatis.* It is found most commonly in the tropics. Cases occur infrequently in the United States, with fewer than 150 new cases being reported each year. The majority of cases are reported to occur in men. In most series the ratio of males to females with the disease is approximately 5:1. The vulva is the most frequent site of infection in women, but the urethra, rectum, and cervix may also be involved. Subclinical infection is common. Studies have demonstrated positive complement fixation tests in more than 50% of prostitutes without demonstrable disease. This STD is produced by serotypes L_1, L_2, and L_3 of *C. trachomatis.* These serotypes are similar to the serotypes that produce trachoma. The incubation period is between 3 and 30 days.

There are three distinct phases of vulvar and perirectal LGV. The primary infection is a shallow, painless ulcer of the vestibule or labia. Occasionally this ulcer is near the urethra or rectum. The ulcer heals rapidly without therapy. The patient usually consults a physician during the secondary phase of the disease, which begins 1 to 4 weeks after the primary infection. The secondary phase is marked by painful adenopathy in the inguinal and perirectal areas. Two thirds of women have unilateral adenopathy, and half have systemic symptoms, including general malaise and fever. When the disease is untreated, the infected nodes become increasingly tender, enlarged, matted together, and adherent to overlying skin, forming bubos (tender lymph nodes). A classic clinical sign of LGV is the double genitocrural fold, or "groove sign" (Fig. 22-14), a depression between groups of inflamed nodes. The groove sign develops in approximately 20% of women with LGV. Within 7 to 15 days the bubo will rupture spontaneously and form multiple draining sinuses and fistulas. These are classic signs of the tertiary phase of the infection. Extensive tissue destruction of the external genitalia and anorectal region may occur during the tertiary phase. This tissue destruction and secondary extensive scarring and fibrosis may result in elephantiasis, multiple fistulas, and stricture formation of the anal canal and rectum.

Diagnosis is established by culture of pus or aspirate from a tender lymph node. With the recent development of monoclonal antibodies for *Chlamydia,* the diagnosis may be confirmed with this technique using fluid aspirated from an infected node. The complement fixation antibody titer is the most frequently used serum method for diagnosis. Antibody titers greater than 1:64 are indicative of active infection. The antibody test will cross-react with other *Chlamydia* infections. However, mucosal *Chlamydia* infections usually are associated with low titers. The differential diagnosis of LGV includes syphilis, chancroid, granuloma inguinale, bacterial lymphadenitis, vulvar carcinoma, genital herpes, and Hodgkin's disease.

The CDC recommends doxycycline 100 mg twice daily for at least 21 days as the preferred treatment. Alternative choices for therapy include azithromycin 1 gm orally once per week for 3 weeks, ciprofloxacin 750 mg orally twice daily for at least 3 weeks, or erythromycin base 500 mg four times daily orally for 21 days. Antibiotic therapy cures the bacterial infection and prevents further tissue destruction. However, fluctuant nodes should be aspirated to prevent sinus formation. Rarely incision and drainage of infected nodes is necessary to alleviate inguinal pain. The late sequelae of the destructive tertiary phase of LGV often require extensive surgical reconstruction. It is important to administer antibiotics during the perioperative period.

Chancroid

Chancroid is a sexually transmitted, acute, ulcerative disease of the vulva. The soft chancre of chancroid is always painful and tender. In comparison, the hard chancre of syphilis is usually asymptomatic. The clinical importance of chancroid is enhanced by recent reports that the genital ulcers of chancroid facilitate the transmission of HIV infection. Chancroid is a common disease in developing countries, but until the early 1980s it was rarely seen in the United States. Recently there has been a substantial decline in reported cases in the United States, with only 30 reported in 2004. However, difficulty in making the diagnosis may cause underreporting. Epidemiologic studies suggest that chancroid tends to occur in clusters and may account for a substantial portion of genital ulcer cases when present.

Chancroid is caused by *Haemophilus ducreyi,* a highly contagious, small, gram-negative rod. *H. ducreyi* is a nonmotile, facultative anaerobe. This bacterium on Gram stain exhibits a classic appearance of streptobacillary chains, or what has been described as an extracellular "school of fish." The incubation period is short—usually 3 to 6 days. Tissue trauma and excoriation of the skin must precede initial infection because *H. ducreyi* is unable to penetrate and invade normal skin.

Women with chancroid who consult a physician have solitary or multiple ulcers, most commonly of the vulvar vestibule and rarely of the vagina or cervix. The initial lesion is a small papule. Within 48 to 72 hours the papule evolves into a pustule and subsequently ulcerates. Multiple papules and ulcers may be in different phases of maturation secondary to autoinoculation. The extremely painful ulcers are shallow with a characteristic ragged edge. The ulcers have a dirty, gray, necrotic, foul-smelling exudate, and there is an absence of induration at the base (the soft chancre). Approximately 50% of women develop acutely tender inguinal adenopathy, a bubo, usually within the first 2 weeks of an untreated infection. In most cases the inguinal adenopathy is unilateral, on the same side of the vulva as the preponderance of infection. Nodes that are fluctuant should be treated by needle aspiration to prevent rupture of the abscess or, if greater than 5 cm in diameter, treated by incision and drainage.

The diagnosis is made by Gram stain and culture of purulent material or by aspiration of tender lymph nodes. The sensitivity of Gram stain for this organism is poor and culture requires special media and growth conditions. No FDA-approved PCR test is available in the United States, but laboratories have developed their own PCR test. Unfortunately, PCR may not be a practical diagnostic tool for most STD clinics. Sometimes the clinical diagnosis is made in a woman with painful vulvar ulcers after the differential diagnosis of the other common STDs that produce vulvar ulcers, including genital herpes, syphilis, lymphogranuloma venereum, and donovanosis has been excluded.

Because of antibiotic resistance to tetracyclines and sulfonamides, the CDC recommends azithromycin 1 g orally in a single dose or ceftriaxone 250 mg intramuscularly in a single dose, or ciprofloxacin 500 mg orally twice for 3 days. All four regimens are effective for treatment of chancroid in HIV-infected women, although such patients may be at higher risk for treatment failures. Large ulcers may require 2 to 3 weeks to heal with clinical resolution of lymphadenopathy slower than that of ulcers. Sexual partners should be treated in a similar fashion. *H. ducreyi* is very sensitive to quinolones, but they are contraindicated in pregnancy.

Successful antibiotic therapy results in both symptomatic and objective improvement within 5 to 7 days of initiating therapy. Following therapy, symptomatic improvement in ulcers occurs within 3 days. Objective improvement occurs within 7 days. Bubos respond at a slower rate than do skin ulcers. Approximately 10% of women whose ulcers initially heal have a recurrence at the same site. Women with HIV infection have an increased rate of failure to the standard treatments for chancroid and therefore often require more prolonged therapy. Approximately 20% of patients with chancroid in large urban areas in the United States are concurrently infected with herpes simplex virus, *Treponema palladium,* or HIV. Often, *H. ducreyi* is resistant to multiple antibiotics. Therefore, susceptibility testing of bacterial isolates should be performed on patients who do not respond to therapy.

Syphilis

Syphilis is a chronic, complex systemic disease produced by the spirochete *Treponema pallidum.* The infection initially involves mucous membranes. Syphilis remains one of the important STDs in the United States. The incidence of primary and secondary syphilis in the United States peaked in 1990. The CDC estimates that 3.2 cases were reported per 100,000 people in the United States in 1998. This is the lowest rate since surveillance began in 1941. However, in 2001 the number of cases of early syphilis reported to the CDC increased for the first time since 1990, and increased 10% from 2003 (6730 cases) to 2004 (7120 cases). The increase is mainly among men who have sex with men. In women, diagnosis of early syphilis declined by 35% between 2000 and 2002. Syphilis remains a devastating disease. Early syphilis is a cofactor in the transmission and acquisition of HIV. Currently 25% of new syphilis cases occur in persons coinfected with HIV. Epidemiologists speculate that only one out of four new cases of syphilis is reported. Even with mandatory screening, congenital syphilis continues to be a public health problem. The mothers experiencing the tragedy of stillbirth or neonatal death from syphilis usually have not received prenatal care. Syphilis should be included in the differential diagnosis of all genital ulcers and cutaneous rashes of unknown origin, and all diagnosed with syphilis should be screened for HIV.

T. pallidum is an anaerobic, elongated, tightly wound spirochete. Because of its extreme thinness, it is difficult to detect by light microscopy. Therefore, the presence of spirochetes is diagnosed by use of specially adapted techniques—dark-field microscopy or direct fluorescent antibody tests (Fig. 22-15). These organisms have the ability to penetrate either skin or mucous membranes. The incubation period is between 10 and 90 days, with the average being 3 weeks. They replicate every 30 to 36 hours, which accounts for the comparatively long incubation period.

Syphilis is a moderately contagious disease. Approximately 3% to 10% of patients contract the disease from a single sexual encounter with an infected partner. Similar studies have documented that 30% of individuals become infected during a 1-month exposure to a sexual partner with primary or secondary syphilis. Patients are contagious during primary, secondary, and probably the first year of latent syphilis. Syphilis can be spread by kissing or touching a person who has an active lesion on the lips, oral cavity, breast or genitals. Case transmission can occur with oral–genital contact.

Diagnosis of syphilis is complicated by the fact that the organism cannot be cultivated in vitro. Hence, serologic tests

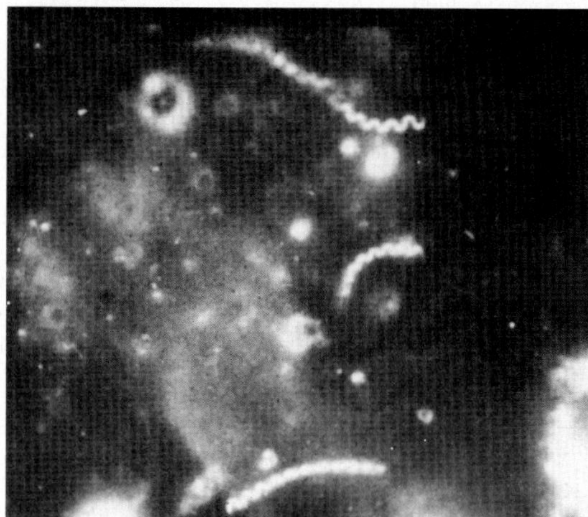

Figure 22-15. Dark-field microscopic appearance of *Treponema pallidum*. (From Larsen SA, McGrew BE, Hunter EF, et al: Syphilis serology and dark field microscopy. In Holmes KK, Mårdh PA, Sparling PF, et al [eds]: Sexually Transmitted Diseases. New York, McGraw-Hill, 1984.)

have been the foundation of screening programs to detect early syphilis. There are two types of serologic tests: the nonspecific, nontreponemal and the specific, antitreponemal antibody tests. The nonspecific tests such as the VDRL (Venereal Disease Research Laboratories) slide test and the RPR (rapid plasma reagin) card test are inexpensive and easy to perform. They are used as screening tests for the disease and also as an index of response to treatment. These tests evaluate the patient's serum for the presence of reagin antibodies as they react with an antigen from beef heart. Quantitative nontreponemal antibody titers usually correlate with the activity of the disease. Approximately 1% of patients have technical or biologic false-positive results with the nonspecific tests. Many conditions produce biologic false-positive results, including a recent febrile illness, pregnancy, immunization, chronic active hepatitis, malaria, sarcoidosis, intravenous drug use, HIV infection, advancing age, acute herpes simplex, and autoimmune diseases such as lupus erythematosus or rheumatoid arthritis. Biologic false-positive serum tests usually are associated with extremely low titers (<1:8). A false-negative result is a possibility, occurring in approximately 1% to 2% of tests. This negative reaction occurs in women in whom there is an excess of anticardiolipin antibody in the serum—termed the *prozone phenomenon.*

If a nonspecific test result is positive, the significance of this result must be confirmed by a specific antitreponemal test. Specific tests are more sensitive; however, occasionally they may produce false-positive results. Most false-positive results occur among women with lupus erythematosus (Table 22-7). The standard for specific tests had been the TPI (*Treponema* immobilization test). It has largely been replaced by the FTA-ABS (fluorescent-labeled *Treponema* antibody absorption) and the MHA-TP (microhemagglutination assay for antibodies to *T. pallidum*). The MHA-TP does not have as high a rate of false-positive results as the FTA-ABS. A woman with a positive reactive treponemal test usually will have this positive reaction for her lifetime regardless of treatment or the activity of the disease.

Table 22-7 Potential Causes of Biologic False-Positive Results in Syphilis Serology

	Acute BFP Reactions	Chronic BFP Reaction
Physiologic	Pregnancy	Advanced age
		Multiple blood transfusions
Infections	Varicella	HIV
	Vaccinia	Tropical spastic paraparesis
	Measles	Leprosy*
	Mumps	Tuberculosis
	Infectious mononucleosis	Malaria*
	Herpes simplex	Lymphogranuloma venereum
	Viral hepatitis	Trypanosomiasis*
	HIV seroconversion illness	Kala-azar*
	Cytomegalovirus	
	Pneumococcal pneumonia	
	Mycoplasma pneumonia	
	Chancroid	
	Lymphogranuloma venereum	
	Psittacosis	
	Bacterial endocarditis	
	Scarlet fever	
	Rickettsial infections	
	Toxoplasmosis	
	Lyme disease	
	Leptospirosis	
	Relapsing fever	
	Rat-bite fever	
Vaccinations	Smallpox	
	Typhoid	
	Yellow fever	
Autoimmune disease		Systemic lupus erythematosus
		Discoid lupus
		Drug-induced lupus
		Autoimmune hemolytic anemia
		Polyarteritis nodosa
		Rheumatoid arthritis
		Sjögren's syndrome
		Hashimoto's thyroiditis
		Mixed connective tissue disease
		Primary biliary cirrhosis
		Chronic liver disease
		Idiopathic thrombocytopenic purpura
Other		Intravenous drug use
		Advanced malignancy
		Hypergammaglobulinemia
		Lymphoproliferative disease

*BFP reaction resolves with resolution of infection.
BFP, biologic false-positive; HIV, human immunodeficiency virus.
Data from Nandwani R, Evans DTP: Are you sure it's syphilis? A review of false positive serology. Int J STD AIDS 1995; 6:241; and Hook EW III, Marra CM: Acquired syphilis in adults. N Engl J Med 1992; 326:1062.

Clinically, syphilis is divided into primary, secondary, and tertiary stages. In primary syphilis, a papule, which is usually painless, appears at the site of inoculation 2 to 3 weeks after exposure. This soon ulcerates to produce the classic finding of primary syphilis, a chancre (Fig. 22-16). The chancre is a painless ulcer, 1 to 2 cm, with a raised indurated margin and a non-exudative base. Most often the chancre is solitary, painless, and found on the vulva, vagina, or cervix. During the first week of clinical disease, the woman develops regional adenopathy that is nontender and firm. An increase in extragenital primary lesions

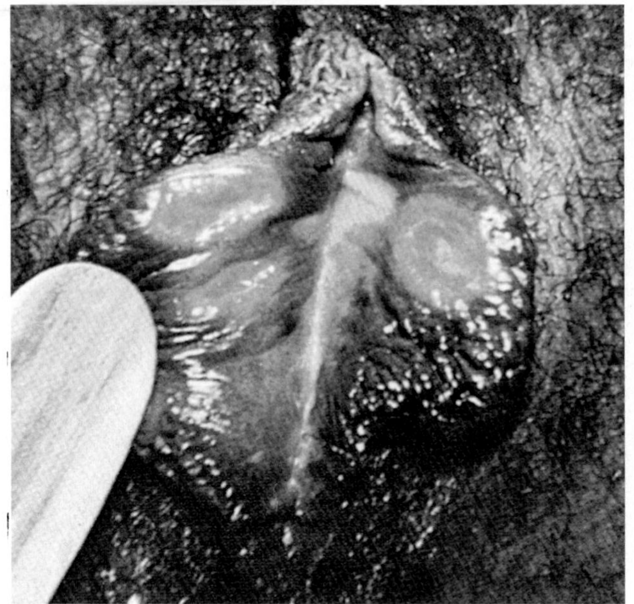

A

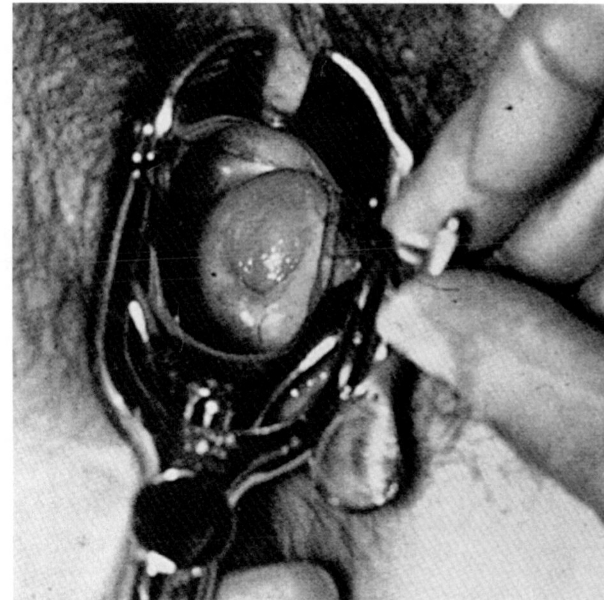

B

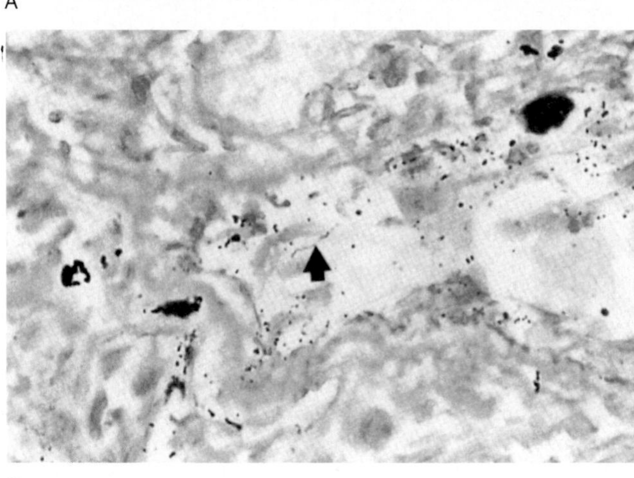

C

Figure 22-16. Primary syphilis. **A** and **B** show primary chancres of syphilis, which began as a papule, erode, and develop into painless ulcers with raised, firm, indurated borders and a clean, smooth base. In **C,** silver staining reveals a spirochete 6–15 μm in length with regularly spaced spiral coils (*arrow*). (**A** and **B**, reprinted from U.S. Public Health Service: Syphilis: A Synopsis. Washington, DC, U.S. Government Printing Office, 1967, pp 47, 50. **C**, from Wong TY, Mihm MC Jr: Images in clinical medicine. Primary syphilis. N Engl J Med 331:1492, 1994. Copyright 1994 Massachusetts Medical Society. All rights reserved.)

has been reported, including lesions of the mouth, anal canal, and nipple of the breast. Approximately 5% of chancres occur in extragenital locations. The painless ulcer heals spontaneously within 2 to 6 weeks without treatment. Hence, many do not seek treatment, a feature that enhances transmission likelihood. Confirmation that the ulcer is primary or secondary syphilis depends on identification of *T. pallidum* by dark-field microscopy from wet smears of the ulcer. Special preparations must be made to obtain suitable smears. It is important to clean and abrade the ulcer with gauze before obtaining the serum for the slides. Syphilis is not frequently diagnosed in the primary stage in women.

Serologic tests for syphilis generally become positive 4 to 6 weeks after exposure—thus 1 to 2 weeks after development of the chancre. At the time of dark-field identification of *T. pallidum* from a primary chancre, approximately 70% of women will have a positive serologic test. If the serologic test result remains negative for 3 months, it is unlikely that the ulcer was syphilis.

Secondary syphilis is the result of hematogenous dissemination of the spirochetes and is a systemic disease. If primary syphilis is untreated, weeks to a few months later approximately 25% of individuals develop a systemic illness that represents secondary syphilis. The stages are not exclusive, with approximately 25% of women still having a primary chancre when the secondary lesions appear. Secondary syphilis develops between 6 weeks and 6 months (with an average of 9 weeks) after the primary chancre. During an attack of secondary syphilis, which if untreated will last 2 to 6 weeks, a multitude of systemic symptoms may occur depending on the major organs involved. The classic rash of secondary syphilis is red macules and papules over the palms of the hands and the soles of the feet (Fig. 22-17). Vulvar lesions include mucous patches and condyloma latum associated with painless lymphadenopathy. The vulvar lesions of condyloma latum are large, raised, flattened, grayish-white areas (Fig. 22-18). On wet surfaces of the vulva, soft papules often coalesce to form ulcers. These ulcers are larger than herpetic ulcers and are not tender unless secondarily infected. A woman

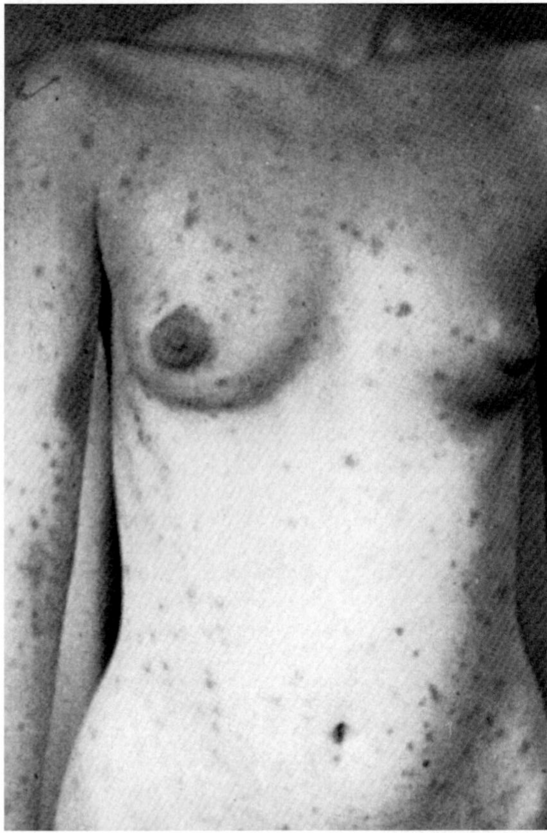

A

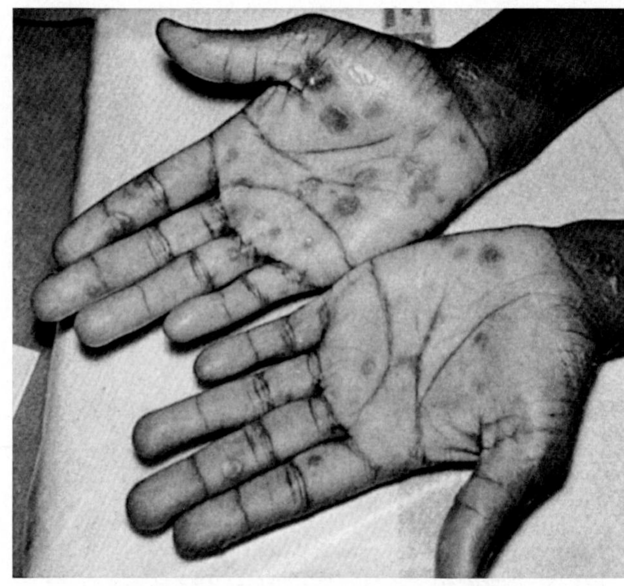

B

Figure 22-17. Rash of secondary syphilis. **A,** Common presentation on the trunk and arms. **B,** Red maculopapular lesions involve palms and soles. (From Kissane JM: Bacterial diseases. In Kissane JM [ed]: Anderson's Pathology. St. Louis, Mosby–Year Book, 1985.)

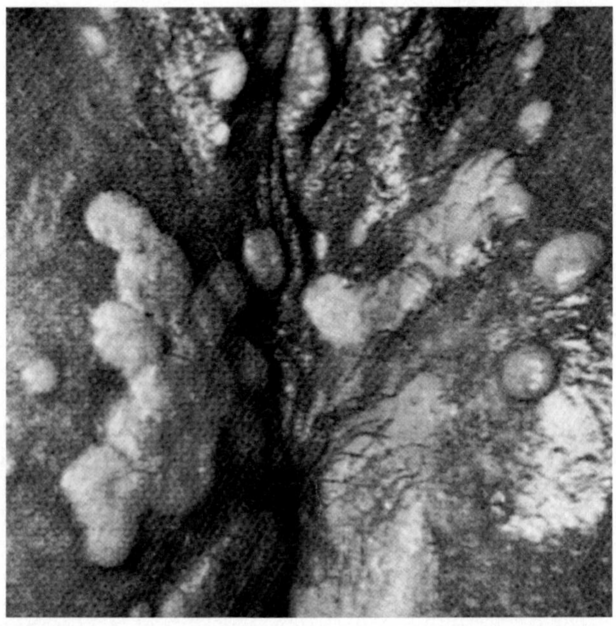

Figure 22-18. Multiple lesions of condylomata lata on vulva and perineum. Dark-field microscopic findings were positive. (From Faro S: Sexually transmitted diseases. In Kaufman RH, Faro S [eds]: Benign Diseases of the Vulva and Vagina, 4th ed. St. Louis, Mosby–Year Book, 1994.)

with syphilis is most infectious during the first 1 to 2 years of her disease with decreasing infectivity thereafter.

The latent stage of syphilis follows the secondary stage and varies in duration from 2 to 20 years. During the latency period, a woman has a positive serology without symptoms or signs of her disease. The majority of women who are diagnosed as having syphilis are discovered by positive blood tests during the latent stage of the disease. Early latent syphilis is an infection of 1 year or less. All other cases are referred to a late latent or latent syphilis of unknown duration. All women who have been sexually active with latent syphilis should have a pelvic exam to discover potential lesions involving the vagina or cervix. Women with latent syphilis should have quantitative nontreponemal serologic tests 6, 12, and 24 months following therapy. During the first 3 to 4 years of the latent phase an individual may experience relapses of secondary syphilis. Women with syphilis in the primary or secondary stages and during the first year of latent syphilis are believed to be infectious.

The tertiary phase of syphilis is devastating in its potentially destructive effects on the central nervous, cardiovascular, and musculoskeletal systems. Tertiary syphilis develops in approximately 33% of patients who are not appropriately treated during the primary, secondary, or latent phases of the disease (Fig. 22-19). The manifestations of late syphilis include optic atrophy, tabes dorsalis, generalized paresis, aortic aneurysm, and gummas of the skin and bones. A gumma is similar to a cold abscess with a necrotic center and the obliteration of small vessels by endarteritis.

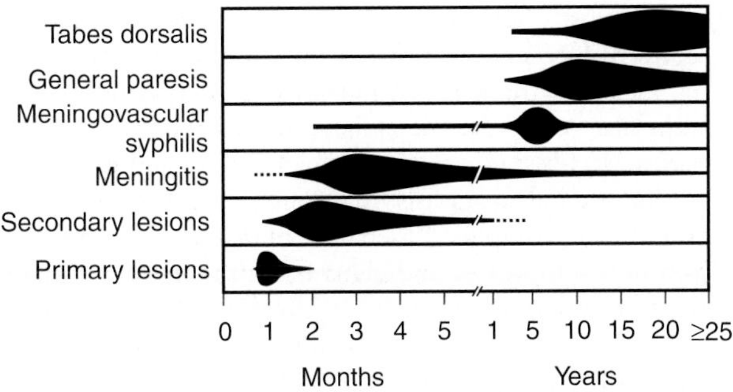

Figure 22-19. Approximate time course of the clinical manifestations of early syphilis and neurosyphilis. Shaded areas corresponding to each syndrome represent the approximate proportion of patients with the syndrome specified and do not indicate the proportion of all patients with syphilis who have that syndrome. (From Hook EW III, Marra CM: Acquired syphilis in adults. N Engl J Med 326:1060, 1992. Copyright 1992 Massachusetts Medical Society. All rights reserved.)

Parenteral penicillin G is the drug of choice for syphilis. *T. pallidum* is exquisitely sensitive to penicillin. However, because of the slow replication time of the spirochete, blood levels must be maintained for 7 to 14 days. The CDC recommends 2.4 million units of benzathine penicillin G intramuscularly in one dose for early syphilis (primary and early latent secondary syphilis). Patients who are allergic to penicillin should receive oral tetracycline 500 mg every 6 hours for 14 days or doxycycline 100 mg orally twice a day for 2 weeks. Standard treatment protocols for syphilis are detailed in the following box. Approximately 60% of women develop an acute febrile reaction associated with flulike symptoms such as headache and myalgia within the first 24 hours after parenteral penicillin therapy for early syphilis. This response is termed the Jarisch-Herxheimer reaction.

All women with early syphilis should be reexamined clinically and serologically at 6 months and 12 months following therapy. With successful therapy in early syphilis, the titer should decline fourfold in 6 months and become negative within 12 months. Women who have a sustained fourfold increase in nontreponemal test titers have failed treatment or have become reinfected. They should be retreated and evaluated for concurrent HIV infection. When women are retreated the recommendation is three weekly injections of benzathine penicillin G 2.4 million units IM. For long-term follow-up the same serologic tests should be ordered. Optimally, the test should be obtained from the same laboratory. The VDRL and RPR are equally valid, but RPR titers tend to be slightly higher than VDRL titers. With successful treatment the VDRL titer will become nonreactive or at most be reactive with a lower titer within 1 year. There is a 1% to 2% chance that the patient will not exhibit a fourfold titer decline, and these cases are considered therapeutic failures. They should be treated once again. Patients with syphilis lasting longer than 1 year should have quantitative VDRL titers for 2 years following therapy because their titers will decline more slowly. A specific test for syphilis, such as the FTA-ABS, remains reactive indefinitely. In summary, all women with a first attack of primary syphilis should have a negative nonspecific serology within 1 year, and women treated for secondary syphilis should have a negative serology within 2 years. If they are not, treatment failure, reinfection, and concurrent HIV infection should be investigated.

Centers for Disease Control Recommended Treatment of Syphilis (2006)

Early Syphilis (primary, secondary, and early latent syphilis of less than 1 year's duration)

Recommended Regimen: benzathine penicillin G, 2.4 million units intramuscularly, one dose

Alternative Regimen (Penicillin-Allergic Nonpregnant Patients): Doxycycline 100 mg orally 2 times a day for 2 weeks

or tetracycline 500 mg orally 4 times a day for 2 weeks

Late Latent Syphilis (of more than 1 year's duration, gummas, and cardiovascular syphilis)

Recommended Regimen: benzathine penicillin G, 7.2 million units total, administered as 3 doses of 2.4 million units intramuscularly at 1-week intervals

Alternative Regimen (penicillin-allergic nonpregnant patients): doxycycline 100 mg orally 2 times a day for 2 weeks if < 1 year; otherwise, for 4 weeks

or tetracycline 500 mg orally 4 times a day for 2 weeks if < 1 year; otherwise, for 4 weeks

Neurosyphilis

Recommended Regimen: aqueous crystalline penicillin G, 18–24 million units daily, administered as 3–4 million units IV every 4 hours, for 10–14 days

Alternative Regimen: Procaine penicillin 2.4 million units IM daily, for 10–14 days plus probenecid 500 mg PO 4 times a day for 10–14 days

Syphilis in Pregnancy

Recommended Regimen: Penicillin regimen appropriate for stage of syphilis. Some experts recommended additional therapy (e.g., a second dose of benzathine penicillin 2.4 million units intramuscularly) 1 week after the initial dose, for those who have primary, secondary, or early latent syphilis.

Alternative Regimen (penicillin allergy): Pregnant women with a history of penicillin allergy should be skin tested and desensitized

Syphilis Among HIV-Infected Patients

Primary and Secondary Syphilis: Recommended benzathine penicillin G 2.4 million units IM. Some experts recommended additional treatments, such as 3 weekly doses of benzathine penicillin G, as in late syphilis. Penicillin-allergic patients should be desensitized and treated with penicillin.

Latent Syphilis (normal CSF examination): Benzathine penicillin G 7.2 million units as 3 weekly doses of 2.4 million units each

From CDC 2006 Guidelines for Treatment of Sexually Transmitted Diseases. MMWR 47:28, 1997.

Syphilis often involves the CNS. The diagnosis is complicated, and there is no established diagnostic test that is a gold standard for neurosyphilis. All women with suspected neurosyphilis should be tested for HIV infection. The diagnosis of neurosyphilis is made on a combination of clinical findings, reactive serologic tests, and abnormalities of cerebrospinal fluid, serology, cell count, or protein. Infection of the CNS by spirochetes may occur during any stage of syphilis. Women should undergo a cerebral spinal fluid examination if they develop neurologic or ophthalmologic signs or symptoms, evidence of active tertiary syphilis, treatment failures, and HIV infection with late latent syphilis or syphilis of an unknown duration. For the treatment for neurosyphilis, the CDC recommends aqueous crystalline penicillin G 18 to 24 million units a day, administered as 3 to 4 million units IV every 4 hours for 10 to 14 days. An alternative regimen is procaine penicillin 2.4 million units IM a day, plus probenecid 500 mg orally four times a day, for 10 to 14 days. The duration of both of these regimens for neurosyphilis are shorter than that of the regimen used for late syphilis in the absence of neurosyphilis. Therefore, some experts administer benzathine penicillin, 2.4 million units IM, after completion of either regimen to provide comparable total duration of therapy.

It is important for all women with syphilis to be tested for HIV infection. Simultaneous syphilis and HIV infection alters the natural history of syphilis, with earlier involvement of the CNS. Women with HIV infection may have a slightly increased rate of treatment failure with currently recommended regimens. Similarly, they may exhibit unusual serologic responses. Most often serologic titers are higher than expected. However, false-negative serologic tests or delayed appearance of seroreactivity has been reported. Nevertheless, the CDC's recommendation for treating early syphilis is the same for women whether or not they are concurrently infected with HIV. Following penicillin treatment for syphilis, women with HIV should be followed with quantitative titers at more frequent intervals, for example 3, 6, 9, 12, and 24 months following therapy.

Sexual partners of women with syphilis in any stage should be evaluated both clinically and serologically. The time intervals used to identify an at-risk sex partner are 3 months plus duration of symptoms for primary syphilis, 3 months plus duration of symptoms for secondary syphilis, and 1 year for early latent syphilis. Individuals who are exposed within the 90 days preceding the diagnosis of primary, secondary, or early latent syphilis in their sexual partners should be treated presumptively because they may be infected even if seronegative.

Vulvar Irritation Caused by Vaginitis

Anatomic distribution of symptoms occasionally creates a semantic misinterpretation of the clinical reality. This is true for vulvar disease. The first symptom of vaginal infection is often vulvar pruritus, and the first sign of vaginal infection may be secondary erythema and edema of the vulvar skin. Sometimes, self-medication for a vaginal infection may produce irritation of the vulva. Women whose chief complaint is vaginal itching or burning may have symptoms because of irritation of the vestibule and adjacent vulvar epithelium. The sensory nerve endings are more numerous in the vulvar skin than in the vagina. The presence of excessive vaginal fluid is not appreciated until the fluid flows from the vagina onto the vulva.

A semantic compromise is to term most vaginal infections as vulvovaginitis. This is especially true with candidiasis. There is a separate clinical entity of primary cutaneous candidiasis, but it is rare and is most often found in women with diabetes mellitus. The skin involvement of primary candidiasis is most prominent on the labia and the genitocrural folds. In this condition, the vulva appears beefy red, the labia are edematous, and the skin of the vulva has fissures and often small vesicles and pustules.

The differential diagnosis for women with symptoms of vulvovaginitis is complex. Discharge, burning, and pruritus are the common symptoms, and signs of vulvar irritation include erythema and excoriation of the vulvar skin. Discharge may be caused by either a cervical or vaginal infection. Vulvar irritation may be produced by primary or secondary infections, a primary skin irritant, or contact dermatitis. Physiologic fluids such as urine and normal cervical secretions and vaginal fluid may cause maceration of the vulvar skin when the epithelium remains constantly moist, such as in the situation produced by tight-fitting synthetic fabric undergarments, especially panty hose.

The clinical symptoms of vulvovaginitis are usually not helpful in establishing the cause. A careful history for contact allergens must be obtained. Sometimes vaginal spermicides, soaps, perfumes, and feminine hygiene sprays will cause skin irritation. The cervical and vaginal secretions should be examined under the microscope for infection. The diagnosis of primary vulvar skin infections should be entertained.

First and foremost in alleviating the symptoms of vulvovaginitis is emphasis on keeping the vulvar skin dry. The patient should be encouraged to wear loose-fitting cotton undergarments. Treatment of vaginal infection is important and will be discussed in the next section.

VAGINITIS

Vaginal discharge is the most common symptom in gynecology. Other symptoms associated with vaginal infection include superficial dyspareunia, dysuria, odor, and vulvar burning and pruritus. The three common infections of the vagina are produced by (1) a fungus (candidiasis), (2) by a protozoon (*Trichomonas*), and (3) a synergistic bacterial infection (bacterial vaginosis). Relative prevalence differs depending on the population studied. However, in a group of middle-class women in the reproductive range, bacterial vaginosis represents approximately 50% of cases, whereas candidiasis and *Trichomonas* infection each constitute approximately 25% of cases. Vaginal discharge resulting from viral infections such as herpes was discussed earlier in the chapter. Vaginitis in prepubertal and postmenopausal women is discussed in chapters dedicated to gynecologic problems in those age groups (Chapters 13, Pediatric and Adolescent Gynecology, and 42, Menopause). Atrophic vaginitis, secondary to low levels of circulating estrogens, predisposes women to secondary infection due to the thin atrophic lining of the vaginal canal.

Accurate diagnosis of vaginitis is critical. HIV acquisition is increased in women with either *Trichomonas vaginitis* or bacterial vaginosis. Hence, timely diagnosis with appropriate treatment is paramount.

The vaginal environment has been described as both a dynamic and a delicate ecosystem. The normal vaginal pH is approximately 4.0 in premenopausal women. The maintenance of an optimum pH balance involves a complex interplay of hormonal, microbiologic, and other unknown factors. In reproductive-age women, estrogen stimulates the glycogen content of vaginal epithelial cells. The glycogen is metabolized to lactic acid and other short-chain organic acids, principally by the lactobacilli but also by other vaginal bacteria and enzymes. *Lactobacillus,* an aerobic gram-positive rod, is found in 62% to 88% of asymptomatic women and is the regulator of normal vaginal flora. Lactobacilli make lactic acid, which maintains the normal vaginal pH of 3.8 to 4.5 and inhibit adherence of bacteria to vaginal epithelial cells. Approximately 60% of vaginal lactobacilli strains make hydrogen peroxide, which inhibits the growth of bacteria and destroys HIV in vitro. Estrogen improves lactobacilli concentration by enhancing vaginal epithelial cell production of glycogen, which breaks down into glucose and acts as a substrate for the bacteria.

One of the most helpful diagnostic aids in the differential diagnosis of vaginitis is to measure vaginal acidity with pH indicator paper. A vaginal pH of greater than 5.0 indicates bacterial vaginosis or *Trichomonas* infection or possibly an atrophic vaginal discharge. A vaginal pH of less than 4.5 represents either a physiologic discharge or a fungal infection. Cervical mucus, vaginal fluids produced during sexual excitement, and semen are all of a neutral or basic pH and may temporarily change the normal acidity. Semen has been found to buffer vaginal acidity for 6 to 8 hours following intercourse. Vaginal pH is slightly higher in postmenopausal women than in premenopausal women.

Normal physiologic vaginal discharge consists of cervical and vaginal epithelial cells, normal bacterial flora, water, electrolytes, and other chemicals. The quantitative concentration of bacterial organisms is 10^8 to 10^9 colonies per milliliter of vaginal fluid. The concentration of anaerobic and aerobic bacteria varies considerably during the menstrual cycle. Qualitatively the number of bacterial species may vary from 17 to 29. Anaerobic bacteria were quantitatively the most prevalent—five times more common than aerobic bacteria.

In addition to lactobacilli other common aerobic bacteria found in the vagina are diphtheroids, streptococci, *Staphylococcus epidermidis,* and *Gardnerella vaginalis.* The most common gram-negative bacillus is *E. coli.* Anaerobic bacteria have been detected in approximately 80% of women, the most prevalent being *Peptococcus, Peptostreptococcus,* and *Bacteroides* species (Table 22-8). *Candida* species and mycoplasmas are also common inhabitants of asymptomatic women. Our knowledge of vaginal flora has relied on classic microbiology. Newer molecular techniques are demonstrating even greater complexity in vaginal flora.

The clinical diagnosis of vaginitis depends on examination of the vaginal secretions under the microscope and measurement of vaginal pH. Nevertheless it is helpful to generalize about the classic characteristics of normal secretions and the three common vaginal infections (Table 22-9).

Table 22-8 Bacterial Vaginal Flora among Asymptomatic Women Without Vaginitis

Organism	Range of Recovery (%)
Facultative Organisms	
Gram-positive rods	
Lactobacilli	50–75
Diphtheroids	40
Gram-positive cocci	
Staphylococcus epidemidis	40–55
Staphylococcus aureus	0–5
Beta-hemolytic streptococci	20
Group D streptococci	35–55
Gram-negative organisms	
Escherichia coli	10–30
Klebsiella sp.	10
Other organisms	2–10
Anaerobic Organisms	
Peptococcus sp.	5–65
Peptostreptococcus spp.	25–35
Bacteroides spp	20–40
Bacteroides fragilis	5–15
Fusobacterium sp.	5–25
Clostridium sp.	5–20
Eubacterium sp.	5–35
Veillonella sp.	10–30

From Eschenbach DA: Vaginal infection. Clin Obstet Gynecol 26:187, 1983.

Table 22-9 Typical Features of Vaginitis

Condition	Symptoms and Signs*	Findings on Examination*	pH	Wet Mount	Comment
Bacterial vaginosis[†]	Increased discharge (white, thin) Increased odor	Thin, whitish gray homogeneous discharge, sometimes frothy	>4.5	Clue cells (>20%) shift in flora Amine odor after adding potassium hydroxide to wet mount	Greatly decreased lactobacilli Greatly increased cocci, bacilli small curved rods
Candidiasis	Increased discharge (white, thick)[‡] Pruritus Dysuria Burning	Thick, curdy discharge Vaginal erythema	<4.5	Hyphae or spores	Can be mixed infection with bacterial vaginosis, *T. vaginalis*, or both, and have higher pH
Trichomoniasis[§]	Increased discharge (yellow, frothy) Increased odor Pruritus Dysuria	Yellow, frothy discharge *with or without* vaginal *or* cervical erythema	>4.5	Motile trichomonads Increased white cells	More symptoms at higher vaginal pH

*Although these features are typical, their sensitivity and specificity are generally inadequate for diagnosis.
†For a diagnosis of bacterial vaginosis, a report of increased discharge has a sensitivity of 50% and a specificity of 49%; odor, a sensitivity of 49% and a specificity of 20%; and a pH above 4.7, a sensitivity of 97% and a specificity of 65%, compared with the use of a Gram stain.
‡Forty percent of patients presenting with symptoms of vaginitis report increased (white) discharge, but this discharge is not related to *Candida albicans* in many studies.
§A report of a yellow discharge has a sensitivity of 42% and a specificity of 80%; a frothy discharge on examination has a sensitivity of 8% and a specificity of 99%.
From Eckert LOD: Clinical practice: Acute vulvovaginitis. N Engl J Med 355:1246, 2006.

Normal vaginal secretions are white, floccular or curdy, and odorless. In a woman with a normal or physiologic discharge it is important to note that the vaginal discharge is present only in the dependent portions of the vagina. Pathologic discharges usually involve the anterior and lateral walls of the vagina. It should be emphasized that vaginal discharge characteristics, especially amount of discharge, is insensitive and nonspecific diagnostic criteria for vaginitis. However, thick white, curdy discharge, when present, is highly associated with fungal infections. Gray-white discharges that are thin and usually profuse suggest a differential diagnosis of *Trichomonas* or bacterial vaginosis as do vaginal discharges that have a foul odor. The odor secondary to necrotic gynecologic tumors of the lower genital tract may be minimized by treating the woman topically for bacterial vaginosis.

Bacterial Vaginosis

Bacterial vaginosis reflects a shift in vaginal flora from lactobacilli-dominant to mixed flora, including genital microplasmas, *G. vaginalis*, and anaerobes, such as peptostreptococci, and *Prevotella* and *Mobiluncus* species. Although *Gardnerella* and anaerobic organisms can be found in women with normal vaginal flora, their concentration increases several-fold in women with bacterial vaginosis concurrent with a marked decrease in lactobacilli.

The origin of bacterial vaginosis remains illusive. No causative agent has been identified. Because of the inability to find a transmissible agent, bacterial vaginosis has not been classified as an STD. However, risk factors for bacterial vaginosis include new or multiple sexual partners. It is also prevalent in women who have sex with women and genotyping has revealed identical bacterial strains between monogamous lesbian partners. Also, bacterial vaginosis is more common in lesbian couples who share sex toys with each other without cleaning the toys between use. Recently, molecular techniques have identified a cluster of noncultivable bacteria related to *Clostridium* in women with bacterial vaginosis. As newer techniques analyzing vaginal flora evolve, it may be possible to determine a causal agent. Currently, bacterial vaginosis is described as a "sexually associated" rather than a true sexually transmitted infection.

Other risk factors include douching as least monthly or within the prior 7 days, and social stressors (e.g., homelessness, threats to personal safety, and insufficient financial resources) have been reported to increase risk. A lack of hydrogen peroxide-producing lactobacilli is also a recognized risk factor for bacterial vaginosis and may explain in part, the higher prevalence of bacterial vaginosis in black women independent of other risk factors. Bacterial vaginosis is the most prevalent cause of symptomatic vaginitis, with a prevalence of approximately 15% to 50%.

Histologically there is an absence of inflammation in biopsies of the vagina, thus the term *vaginosis* rather than vaginitis. Bacterial vaginosis has been associated with upper tract infections, including endometritis, pelvic inflammatory disease, postoperative vaginal cuff cellulitis, and multiple complications of infection during pregnancy, such as preterm rupture of the membranes and endomyometritis, and decreased success with in vitro fertilization and increased pregnancy loss of less than 20 weeks' gestation.

In women with bacterial vaginosis, the most frequent symptom is an unpleasant vaginal odor, which patients describe as "musty" or "fishy" (Table 22-10). The odor is often sensed following intercourse, when the alkaline semen results in a release of aromatic amines.

The vaginal discharge associated with bacterial vaginosis is thin and gray-white. The consistency of the discharge is similar to a thin paste made from flour. Speculum examination reveals that the discharge is mildly adherent to the vaginal walls, in contrast to a physiologic discharge, which is discovered in the most dependent areas of the vagina. The vaginal discharge is frothy in approximately 10% of women, and it is rare to have associated pruritus or vulvar irritation.

Bacterial vaginosis is clinically diagnosed. The classic findings on wet smear are clumps of bacteria and "clue cells," which are vaginal epithelial cells with clusters of bacteria adherent to their external surfaces (Fig. 22-20). Leukocytes are not nearly as frequent as epithelial cells underneath the microscope.

The four criteria for the diagnosis of bacterial vaginosis are (1) a homogeneous vaginal discharge is present; (2) the vaginal discharge has a pH equal to or greater than 4.5; (3) the vaginal discharge has an aminelike odor when mixed with potassium hydroxide; whiff tests; and (4) a wet smear of the vaginal discharge demonstrates clue cells greater in number than 20% of the number of the vaginal epithelial cells. For the clinician three of the four criteria is sufficient for a presumptive diagnosis. Ironically, 50% of women who have three of the four clinical criteria for bacterial vaginosis are asymptomatic. If readily available, a Gram stain of vaginal secretion is an excellent diagnostic method. A colorimetric test that detects proline iminopeptidase has been developed for office use. Enzyme levels in vaginal fluid are elevated in women with bacterial vaginosis.

A positive "test" may be obtained with either bacterial vaginosis or *Trichomonas* infection. It is usually more prominent with bacterial infections because of the amount of anaerobic metabolism. The common aromatic amines are cadaverine and putrescine, both of which result from anaerobic metabolism. It

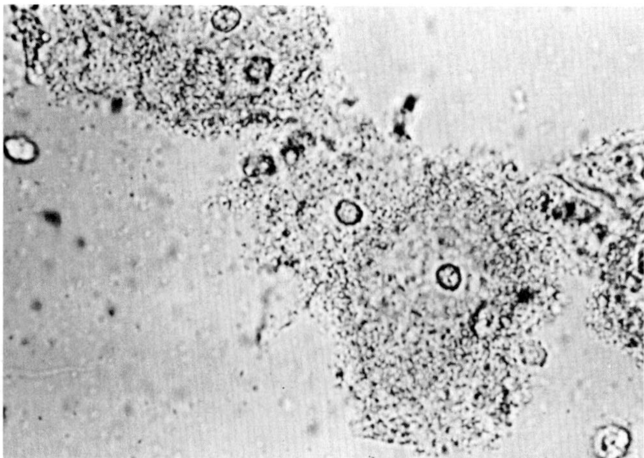

Figure 22-20. Vaginal epithelial cells from woman with bacterial vaginosis. These are typical clue cells, being heavily covered by coccobacilli, with loss of distinct cell margins. (×400.) (From Holmes KK: Lower genital tract infections in women: Cystitis/urethritis, vulvovaginitis, and cervicitis. In Holmes KK, Mårdh PA, Sparling PF, et al [eds]: Sexually Transmitted Diseases. New York, McGraw-Hill, 1984.)

Table 22-10 Diagnostic Tests Available for Vaginitis

Test	Sensitivity (%)	Specificity (%)	Comment
Bacterial Vaginosis			
pH > 4.5	97	64	
Amsel's criteria	92	77	Must meet 3 of 4 clinical criteria (pH > 4.5, thin watery discharge, >20% clue cells, positive "whiff" test), but similar results achieved if 2 of 4 criteria met
Nugent criteria			Gram's stain morphology score (1–10) based on lactobacilli and other morphotypes; a score of 1–3 indicates normal flora, and score of 7–10 bacterial vaginosis; high interobserver reproducibility
Pap smear	49	93	
Point-of-care tests			
QuickVue Advance pH + amines	89	96	Positive if pH >4.7
QuickVue Advance *G. vaginalis**	91	>95	Tests for proline iminopeptidase activity in vaginal fluid; if used when pH >4.5, sensitivity is 95% and specificity is 99%
OSOM BV blue*	90	<95	Tests for vaginal sialidase activity
Candida			
Wet mount			
Overall	50	97	
Growth of 3–4+ on culture	85		*C. albicans* a commensal agent in 15–20% of women
Growth of 1+ on culture	23		
pH ≤ 4.5	Usual		If symptoms present, pH may be elevated if mixed infection with bacterial vaginosis or *T. vaginalis* present
Pap smear	25	72	
Trichomonas Vaginalis			
Wet mount	45–60	95	Increased visibility of microorganisms with a higher burden of infection
Culture	85–90	>95	
pH > 4.5	56	50	
Pap smear	92	61	False positive rate of 8% for standard Pap test and of 4% for liquid-based cytologic test
Point-of-care tests			
OSOM	83	98.8	10 min required to perform tests for *T. vaginalis* antigens

From Eckert LO: Clinical practice: Acute vulvovaginitis. N Engl J Med 355:1248, 2006.

should be stressed that vaginal bacterial culture has no role in the evaluation of bacterial vaginosis.

Because there are no effective means of replacing lactobacilli, the treatment for bacterial vaginosis is to decrease anaerobes with antibiotic therapy and hope the patient will then regenerate her own lactobacilli. Table 22-11 provides treatment alternatives. Cure rates are comparable, and the agent used should depend on patient preference and cost factors. Treatment results in 80% symptomatic and 70% microbiologic cure at 1 month. Single-dose oral therapy of 2 g of metronidazole is no longer recommended due to high failure rates. Currently, Clindesse (clindamycin) is the only single-does therapeutic agent with equivalent efficacy to multiple-dose regimens.

Recurrent bacterial vaginosis (three or more episodes in the previous year) is a common clinical problem. One double-blind, randomized, placebo-controlled trial demonstrated that after 10 days of daily induction therapy with vaginal metronidazole, the twice-weekly use of 0.75% metronidazole gel for 16 weeks maintained a clinical cure in 75% of patients at 16 weeks and 50% by 28 weeks.

Concurrent treatment of the male partner is not recommended at this time. Alternative therapies such as introduction of oral or vaginal *Lactobacillus* are often used to treat symptoms, but studies in women with bacterial vaginosis have not provided evidence of their efficacy.

Trichomonas Vaginal Infection

Trichomonas vaginalis is a unicellular intracellular parasite that is sexually transmitted and inhabits the vagina and lower urinary tract, especially Skene's ducts in the female. It is estimated that there are 5 million new cases of trichomoniasis annually in the United States. The prevalence of the disease remains high despite the availability of effective treatments since the early 1960s. *Trichomonas* vaginal infection is the cause of acute vaginitis in 5% to 50% of cases depending on the population studied and is the most prevalent nonviral, nonchlamydial STD of women.

Many women who harbor *Trichomonas* in their vaginal secretions are free of symptoms. McLellan and coworkers discovered that only one out of two women with positive vaginal cultures had symptoms of a vaginal discharge. In the same study only one out of six women complained of vulvar pruritus. Positive wet smears or cultures for *Trichomonas* are reported in 3% to 10% of asymptomatic gynecology patients, with a much higher percentage being found in women attending a STD clinic. The protozoa is isolated from 30% to 40% of male partners of women with a positive culture and approximately 85% of female partners of a male with a positive culture. *T. vaginalis* infection is a highly contagious STD. Following a single sexual contact, at least two thirds of both male and female sexual

Table 22-11 Recommendations for Acute Vaginitis*

Disease	Drug	Dose	Cost†
Bacterial vaginosis†	Metronidazole (Flagyl)	500 mg orally twice a day for 7 days‡	$
	0.75% Metronidazole gel (Metrogel)	One 5-g application intravaginally daily for 5 days§	$$$
	2% Clindamycin cream (Cleocin vaginal)	One 5-g application intravaginally every night for 7 days	$$$
	2% Extended-release clindamycin cream (Clindesse)	One application intravaginally§,¶	$$
Vulvovaginal candidiasis uncomplicated			
Intravaginal therapy§	Azoles		
	2% Butoconazole cream (Mycelex-3)	5 g per day for 4 days**	$$
	2% Sustained-release butoconazole cream (Gynazole)	One 5-g dose	$$$
	1% Clotrimazole cream (Mycelex-7)	5 g for 7–14 day**	$
	Clotrimazole (Gyne-Lotrimin 3)	Two 100-mg vaginal tablets per day for 3 days	$
		One 500-mg vaginal tablet	$
	2% Miconazole cream	5 g per day for 7 days**	$$
	Miconazole (Monistat-7)	One 100-mg vaginal suppository per day for 7 days**	$$
	Miconazole (Monistat-3)	One 200-mg vaginal suppository per day for 3 days	$$
	Miconazole (Monistat-1)	One 1200 mg vaginal suppository**	
	6.5% Tioconazole oinment (Monistat 1-day)	One 5-g dose**	$
	0.4% Terconazole cream (Terazol 7)	5 g per day for 7 days	$$$
	0.8% Terconazole cream (Terazol 3)	5 g per day for 3 days	$$
	Terconazole vaginal	One 80-mg vaginal suppository per day for 3 days	$$$
	Nystatin vaginal	One 100,000-U vaginal tablet per day for 14 days	$$$
Oral therapy	Fluconazole (Diflucan)	One 150-mg dose orally	$
Vulvovaginal candidiasis, complicated††			
Intravaginal therapy§	Azole	7–14 days	$$
Oral therapy‡‡	Fluconazole (Diflucan)	Two 150-mg doses orally 72 hr apart	$$$
Trichomoniasis	Metronidazole (Flagyl)	One 2-g dose orally	$
		500 mg orally twice daily for 7 days	
	Tinidazole (Tindamax)	One 2-g dose orally§§	$$

*Recommendations are based on the CDC 2006 Guidelines for Treatment of Vaginitis.[37]
†Oral therapy is recommended for pregnant women.
‡Drug may cause gastrointestinal upset in 5 to 10 percent of patients; a disulfuram reaction is possible; alcohol should be avoided for 24 hours after ingestion.
§Vaginal treatments cause local vaginal irritation in 2 to 5 percent of patients.
¶This agent is approved by the Food and Drug Administration but is not listed in the CDC 2006 Guidelines.
**This agent is available over the counter.
††Complicated vulvovaginitis refers to disease in women who are pregnant, women who have uncontrolled diabetes, women who are immunocompromised, or women who have severe symptoms, non–*Candida albicans* candidiasis, or recurrent episodes (four or more per year).
‡‡Oral therapy is not recommended for pregnant women.
§§Drug may cause gastrointestinal upset in 2 to 5 percent of patients; disulfuram reaction is possible; alcohol should be avoided 72 hours after ingestion.
From Eckert LO: Clinical practice: Acute vulvovaginitis. N Engl J Med 355:1250, 2006.

partners become infected. The incubation period for *Trichomonas* infection is 4 to 28 days. *Trichomonas* is a hardy organism and will survive for up to 24 hours on a wet towel and up to 6 hours on a moist surface. However, experimental studies have established that successful vaginal infection depends on the deposition of an inoculum of several thousand organisms. Thus it is unlikely that infection may be related to exposure from infected towels or swimming pools.

Trichomoniasis is caused by the anaerobic, flagellated protozoon, *Trichomonas vaginalis* (Fig. 22-21). Other species of *Trichomonas* reside in the oral pharynx and rectum. These species are site-specific and do not produce disease in the vagina. *T. vaginalis* resides in the paraurethral glands of both the male and female. When a woman is treated with topical medication, reinfection occurs not only from an infected partner but also from the patient's own urethra and Skene's ducts.

T. vaginalis is a unicellular protozoon that is normally fusiform in shape. This organism exists only in the trophozoite form or vegetative cell. It is slightly larger than a white blood cell. Three to five flagella extend from one end of the organism. The flagella provide the active movement of the protozoon, with the direction of motion usually toward the end with the flagella. The *Trichomonas* organism assumes a spherical shape in an acidic environment. Motion is then restricted to waves of the undulating membrane of the protozoon.

Vaginitis from *Trichomonas* is a disease primarily of women in the reproductive years. The normal highly acidic vaginal environment is resistant to *Trichomonas* infection. When lactobacilli predominate in the vaginal fluid, a woman will not develop symptoms. However, menstrual blood, semen, or other vaginal pathogens that alter the vaginal pH to a more basic level favor the growth of *Trichomonas* organisms.

Trichomonas produces a wide variety of patterns of vaginal infection. Women may or may not have symptoms and signs of acute or chronic infection. The primary symptom of *Trichomonas* vaginal infection is profuse vaginal discharge. The volume of discharge associated with symptomatic *Trichomonas* infection is the most abundant of common vaginal infections. Patients often complain that the copious discharge makes them feel "wet." The discharge may be white, gray, yellow, or green. The classic discharge of *Trichomonas* infection has been termed "frothy" (with bubbles) and often has an unpleasant odor. However, a frothy discharge is only noted in 10% to 25% of women with proven *Trichomonas* infection. This discharge is

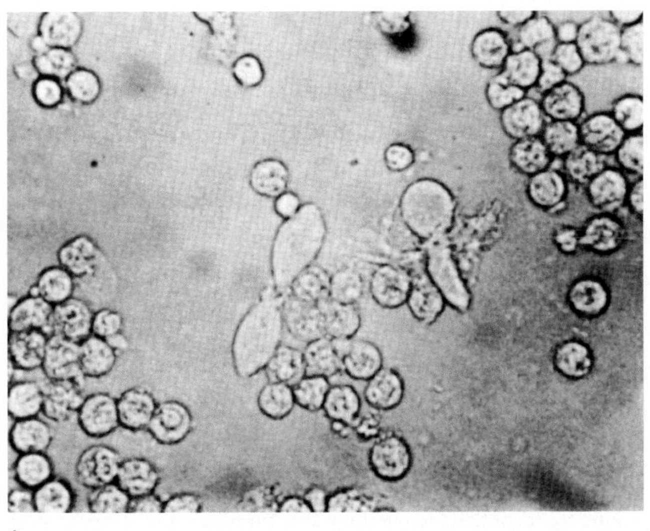

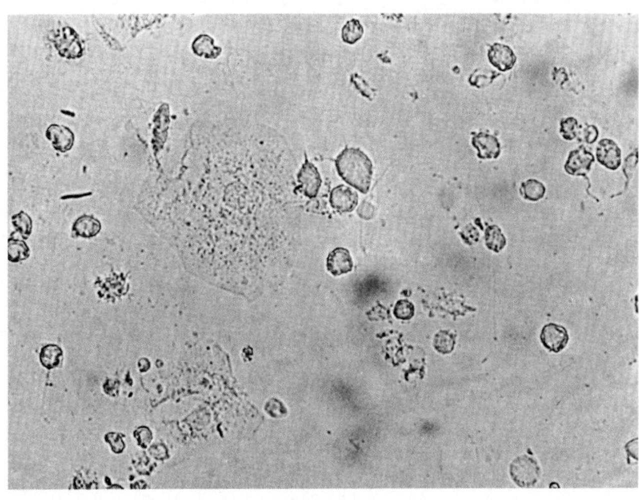

Figure 22-21. **A** and **B,** Trichomonads in wet mount prepared with physiologic saline. (**A** from Faro S: Trichomoniasis. In Kaufman RH, Faro S [eds]: Benign Diseases of the Vulva and Vagina, 4th ed. St. Louis, Mosby-Year Book, 1994. **B** from Friedrich EG: Vulvar Disease, 2nd ed. Philadelphia, WB Saunders, 1983.)

not diagnostic, because it may be seen also with bacterial vaginosis.

Associated with the acute vaginal discharge are erythema and edema of the vulva and vagina. Approximately 50% of symptomatic women detect abnormal vaginal odor and experience vulvar pruritus. The classic sign of a strawberry appearance of the upper vagina and cervix is rare and is noted in less than 10% of women. Approximately 25% of women experience vulvar pruritus. Vulvar skin involvement is limited to the vestibule and labia minora, which helps to distinguish it from the more extensive vulvar involvement of *Candida* vulvovaginitis. Often women with chronic infection have a malodorous discharge as their only complaint. Dysuria is a symptom in approximately one out of five women with symptomatic *Trichomonas* infection. Similar to bacterial vaginosis, *T. vaginalis* is associated with upper genital tract infections, including infections after delivery, surgery, abortion, pelvic inflammatory disease, preterm delivery, infertility, and cervical dysplasia.

The diagnosis of *Trichomonas* vaginal infection is confirmed by examination of vaginal fluid mixed with physiologic saline under the microscope (see Table 22-11). To optimally visualize *Trichomonas* organisms, it is best to use high power and dampen the condenser to produce the greatest contrast. Trichomonads are best discovered in an area of the wet smear with relatively few white blood cells. If the wet smear is fresh and warm, the organisms will exhibit forward motion. If the slide is cold, if the organisms are surrounded by white blood cells, or if the saline is too hypertonic, the *Trichomonas* organisms will assume an ovoid configuration and exhibit minimal motion. The wet smear usually contains a large number of inflammatory cells and many vaginal epithelial cells. The only other vaginitis with an abundance of white blood cells is atrophic vaginitis. The epithelial cells are normal in appearance and have distinct edges. It is postulated that *Trichomonas* excretes a cytotoxic substance that lyses intracellular bridges. This may explain the large number of normal epithelial cells on wet smear seen with severe infection.

The accuracy of diagnosis by wet smear varies widely throughout the literature. If the patient is symptomatic, the sensitivity of a saline wet preparation is 80% to 90%. Therefore a culture for *Trichomonas* is rarely indicated. Attempts to diagnose *T. vaginalis* infection by Papanicolaou smear results in an error rate of at least 50%. There is a large number of both false-positive and false-negative reports. A complementary laboratory test to the wet smear is the measurement of pH of the vaginal fluid with colorimetric paper. The vaginal pH associated with *T. vaginalis* is between 5.0 and 7.0. Vaginal culture for *T. vaginalis* has an 85% to 90% sensitivity and 75% specificity. A point-of-care enzymatic test, OSOM, has 83% sensitivity and 98% specificity and requires only 10 minutes to perform. This test may be particularly useful when a microscope is unavailable.

The major side effects of metronidazole therapy to treat trichomoniasis include nausea, vomiting, a metallic taste, and secondary *Candida* infections. Nausea is the most frequent complication and is experienced by 5% of women. Metronidazole is safe in all trimesters of pregnancy. Patients should be warned that metronidazole inhibits ethanol metabolism. Therefore, they may experience a disulfiram-like reaction if the two drugs are used concurrently. Because tinidazole has a longer half-life, advise patients to abstain from alcohol for 72 hours.

The asymptomatic female who has *Trichomonas* identified in the lower genital urinary tract definitely should be treated. Extended follow-up studies have shown that one out of three asymptomatic females will become symptomatic within 3 months. Furthermore, HIV acquisition is increased in women with *Trichomonas* infection. Obviously, all STDs have common epidemiologic backgrounds, and finding one dictates appropriate studies to rule out colonization or infection with another STD. Frequently, vaginal infections are a mixed infection, with *Trichomonas* and bacterial vaginosis occurring simultaneously in the same individual. Metronidazole gel has been approved for the treatment of bacterial vaginosis, but it is inferior to oral therapy for the treatment of *Trichomonas.*

Women who have a recurrence in most cases have either been reinfected or complied poorly with therapy. The prevalence of low level metronidazole resistance in *T. vaginalis* is 2% to 5%; in case series prolonged treatment with higher doses of metronidazole and tinidazole has been successful. Because *T. vaginalis* is sexually transmitted, treatment of the patient's partner is important and increases cure rates.

Oral nitromidazole therapy is recommended for treatment of *Trichomonas* vaginitis. A single dose (2 g) of metronidazole or tinidazole oral therapy is recommended. Tinidazole is a second-generation nitroimidazole and has a longer half life of 24 hours. A random trial comparing a single dose of metronidazole (2 g) with tinidazole (2 g) showed tinidazole was equivalent or superior to metronidazole, yielding 90% to 95% cure rates. Topical therapy for *Trichomonas* vaginitis is not recommended because it does not eliminate disease reservoirs in Bartholin's and Skene's glands.

Candida Vaginitis

Candida vaginitis (Fig. 22-22) is produced by a ubiquitous, airborne, gram-positive fungus. In most populations greater than 90% of cases are caused by *Candida albicans,* with 5% to 10% of vaginal fungal infections produced by *C. glabrata* or *C. tropicalis. Candida* species are part of the normal flora of approximately 25% of women, being a commensal saprophytic organism on the mucosal surface of the vagina. Its prevalence in the rectum is three to four times greater and in the mouth two times greater than in the vagina. When the ecosystem of the vagina is disturbed, *C. albicans* becomes an opportunistic pathogen. Lactobacilli inhibit the growth of fungi in the vagina. However, when the relative concentration of lactobacilli declines, rapid overgrowth of *Candida* species occurs. Following the traditional regimen of 10 to 14 days of oral broad-spectrum antibiotics, the percentage of women who have vaginal colonization with *Candida* increases threefold.

Vaginitis caused by fungal infection is primarily a disease of the childbearing years. It is estimated that three out of four women will have at least one episode of vulvovaginal candidiasis during their lifetime. The greatest enigma of this condition is the recurrence rate after an apparent cure, varying from 20% to 80%. Approximately 3% to 5% of these women experience recurrent vulvovaginal candidiasis, defined as three or more documented episodes in one year.

C. albicans is responsible for 80% to 95% of vaginal fungal infections. The organisms develop both filamentous (hyphae and pseudohyphae) and ovoid forms, termed *conidia, buds,* or *spores.* In contrast, *C. glabrata* does not produce filamentous forms. Merkus and associates and Montes and Wilborn have reported studies of the pathophysiology of *Candida* infections as viewed with the electron microscope. The filamentous forms of *C. albicans* have the ability to penetrate the mucosal surface and become intertwined with the host cells (Fig. 22-23). This results in secondary hyperemia and limited lysis of tissue near the site of infection.

C. albicans, although normally not pathogenic, may overgrow in the vagina because of a number of well-established host factors that enhance growth of the fungus. Hormonal factors, depressed cell-mediated immunity, and antibiotic use are the three most important. The hormonal changes associated with both pregnancy and menstruation favor growth of the fungus. The prevalence of *Candida* vaginitis increases throughout pregnancy, probably as a result of the high estrogen levels. The literature was initially mixed with respect to the relationship between oral contraceptives and candidiasis. Oriel and colleagues discovered more positive cultures, but fewer symptoms, in women taking oral contraceptives. Presently, with low-dose estrogen oral contraceptives, there is no increase in the incidence of fungal vaginitis. Women tend to report recurrent episodes of vaginitis immediately preceding and immediately following their menstrual periods. Broad-spectrum antibiotics, especially those that destroy lactobacilli (penicillin, tetracycline, cephalosporins), are notorious for precipitating acute episodes of

Figure 22-22. A scanning electron micrograph shows a pure culture of *Candida albicans* (×6030). (From Phillips DM: N Engl J Med 328:1322, 1993. Copyright 1993 Massachusetts Medical Society. All right reserved.)

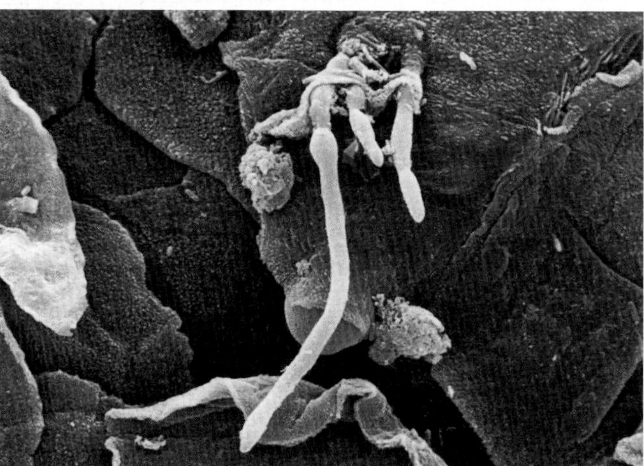

Figure 22-23. Scanning electron microscopy of intraluminal debris of specimen of vaginal wall taken from patient with vaginal candidiasis (×3500). Hyphae of *C. albicans* penetrate epithelial layers of vaginal surface. (From Merkus JM, Bisschop MP, Stolte LA: The proper nature of vaginal candidosis and the problem of recurrence. Obstet Gynecol Surv 40:499, 1985. © Copyright 1985 by Williams & Wilkins.)

C. albicans vaginitis. Women with diabetes mellitus, or even a low renal threshold for sugar, have a higher incidence of vaginal and vulvar candidiasis. Obesity and debilitating disease are other predisposing factors.

Probably the most important host factor is depressed cell-mediated immunity. Women who take exogenous corticosteroids and women with AIDS often experience recurrent *Candida* vulvovaginitis. Altered local immune responses, such as hyper-IgE-mediated response to a small amount of *Candida* antigen, may occur in women with recurrent vulvovaginal candidians. Also, some women with recurrent vulvovaginal candidians have tissue infiltration with polymorphonuclear (PMN) leukocytes. This high density of PMNs correlates with symptomatology but does not result in clearance of *Candida.*

Since fungal vaginitis usually presents as a vulvovaginitis, the predominant symptom is pruritus. Depending on the degree of vulvar skin involvement, pruritus may be accompanied by vulvar burning, external dysuria, and dyspareunia. The vaginal discharge is white or whitish gray, highly viscous, and described as granular or floccular. It does not have an odor. The amount of discharge is highly variable. The vulvar signs include erythema, edema, and excoriation. With extensive skin involvement, pustules may extend beyond the line of erythema. During speculum examination a cottage cheese-type discharge is often visualized with adherent clumps and plaques (thrush patches) attached to the walls of the vagina. These clumps or raised plaques are usually white or yellow. The pH of the vagina associated with this infection is below 4.5. (in contrast to bacterial vaginosis and *Trichomonas* vaginitis, which are associated with elevated pH).

The diagnosis is established by obtaining a wet smear of vaginal secretion and mixing this with 10% to 20% potassium hydroxide (Fig. 22-24). The alkali rapidly lyses both red blood cells and inflammatory cells. It is important always to use a coverslip, because potassium hydroxide will destroy the glass lens of the microscope. Active disease is associated with filamentous forms, mycelia, or pseudohyphae, rather than spores. However, it may be necessary to search the slide and scan many different microscopic fields to identify hyphae or pseudohyphae. The average concentration of organisms is 10^3 to 10^4/mL. Although symptoms can be present at a low colony count, the ability to detect *C. albicans* on a wet mount is 80% when semiquanitative culture growth is 3–4+, and is only 20% when culture growth is −2+. Hence, a negative smear does not exclude *Candida* vulvovaginitis. The diagnosis can be established by culture with either Nickerson or Sabouraud medium. These cultures will become positive in 24 to 72 hours. Vaginal culture for *Candida* is particularly useful when a wet mount is negative for hyphae, but the patients have symptoms and discharge or other signs suggestive of vulvovaginal candidiasis on examination. Fungal culture may also be useful in cases of women who have recently treated themselves with an antifungal agent (up to 90% have a negative culture within 1 week after treatment). A specimen should be cultured from women with recurrent vulvovaginal candidians to ensure it is *C. albicans* because non-albicans *Candida* are often azole-resistant. It should be stressed that obtaining a vaginal culture for bacteria is not useful because the vagina has anaerobes, coliforms and *G. vaginalis* all as part of normal flora. The differential diagnosis includes other common causes of vaginitis such as bacterial vaginosis, *Trichomonas* vaginitis, and atrophic vaginitis. Also, one should consider noninfectious conditions such as allergic reactions, contact dermatitis, chemical irritants, and rare diseases such as lichen planus.

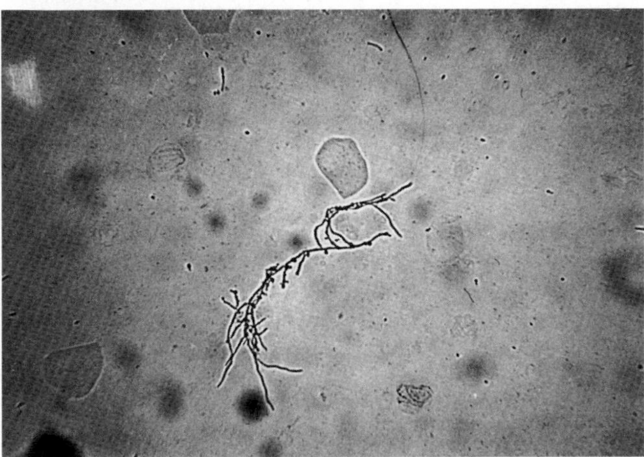

Figure 22-24. Microscopic appearance of vaginal smear in a case of vaginal candidiasis. Potassium hydroxide preparation; yeast cells and pseudomycelia (×320). (From Merkus JM, Bisschop MP, Stolte LA: The proper nature of vaginal candidosis and the problem of recurrence. Obstet Gynecol Surv 40:495, 1985. © Copyright 1985 by Williams & Wilkins.)

The over-the-counter availability of vaginal antifungal therapy makes self-treatment an option for many women. However, it must be recognized that symptoms suggestive of uncomplicated vulvovaginal candidians may reflect an alternative diagnosis. One study of women seen at a clinic for STDs found that self-treatment of the symptoms listed on the package insert of over-the-counter medication of candidians would correctly treat only 28% of patients; 53% had bacterial vaginosis, infection with *T. vaginalis,* gonorrhea, or chlamydia. In another study, involving women purchasing over-the-counter antifungal therapy, only 34% had vulvovaginal candidiasis and no other vaginal infection. If a patient chooses self-treatment, she should be advised to come in for examination if the symptoms are not eliminated with a single course of over-the-counter therapy.

For treatment of vulvovaginal candidiasis, the CDC recommends placing the patient into uncomplicated or complicated category to guide treatment.

Multiple azole vaginal preparations are available for treatment, and a single oral agent, fluconazole, is approved for treatment. In patients with uncomplicated vulvovaginal candidiasis, topical antifungal agents are typically used for 1 to 3 days, or a single oral dose of fluconazole. Patient preference, response to prior therapy, and cost should guide the choice of therapy.

For patients with complicated vaginitis, topical azoles are recommended for 7 to 14 days. In a randomized, placebo-controlled trial involving women with severe vulvovaginal candidiasis, a second dose of fluconazole (150 mg) given 72 hours after the first dose increased the cure rate from 67% to 80%.

In women with recurrent vulvovaginal candidiasis, a randomized, controlled trial demonstrated that after a 10-day course of oral fluconazole (150 mg) every 3 days, 90% of women remained symptom-free during a 6-month suppressive course of weekly fluconazole (150 mg), and symptomatic episodes were reduced by 50% during the subsequent 6 months in these women as compared with placebo for suppression. Women with recurrent vulvovaginitis should receive a vaginal fungal culture to determine species and sensitivities. Infections with *Candida* species other than *C. albicans* are often azole resistant; however, one study of terconazole for non–*C. albicans* fungal vaginitis resulted in a mycologic cure in 56% of patients and a symptomatic cure in 44%. A trial in which women used vaginal boric acid capsules (600 mg in "O" gelatin capsules) for a minimum of 14 days resulted in a symptomatic cure rate of 75% for those with non–*C. albicans* infections. Boric acid inhibits cell wall growth of fungus and may also be used for suppression in women with recurrent vulvovaginal candidiasis. Following 10 days of therapy, one 600-mg capsule intravaginally twice per week for 4 to 6 months decreases symptomatic recurrences. Boric acid is toxic if ingested, so should be stored in a safe manner.

Studies of alternative therapies for vulvovaginal candidiasis (such as oral or vaginal *Lactobacillus,* garlic, or diet alterations such as yogurt ingestion) have not provided evidence of their efficacy.

A summary of diagnostic tools available for determining the cause of vaginitis and a treatment summary are provided in Tables 22-10 and 22-11.

TOXIC SHOCK SYNDROME

Toxic shock syndrome (TSS) is an acute, febrile illness produced by a bacterial exotoxin, with a fulminating downhill course involving dysfunction of multiple organ systems. The cardinal features of the disease are the abrupt onset and the rapidity with which the clinical signs and symptoms may present and progress. It is not unusual for the syndrome to develop from a site of bacterial colonization rather than from an infection. A woman with TSS may develop rapid onset of hypotension associated with multiorgan system failure. TSS was first described in 1978 by Todd as a sometimes fatal sequela of *Staphylococcus aureus* infection in children. In the early 1980s more than 95% of the reported cases of TSS were diagnosed in previously healthy, young (<30 years), menstruating females. *S. aureus* has been isolated from the vagina in more than 90% of these cases.

Between 1979 and 1996, 5296 TSS cases were reported. Menstrual cases account for 74% of total cases, although the proportion has decreased over time (91% from 1979 to 1980, 71% from 1981 to 1986, and 59% from 1986 to 1996). The number of cases of menstrual TSS has declined from 9 out of 100,000 women in 1980 to 1 out of 100,000 women since 1986. The case-fatality rate has also declined and was 1.8% from 1987 to 1996 after a high of 5.5% in 1979 to 1980. Most likely the withdrawal of highly absorbent tampons and polyacrylate rayon containing products from the market partially explains the decrease. However, tampon use remains a risk factor from TSS. Women who develop TSS are more likely to have used higher absorbency tampons, several cycle days of tampons, and kept a single tampon in for a longer period of time.

Presently, approximately 50% of cases of TSS are not related to menses. Nonmenstrual TSS may be a sequela of focal staphylococcal infection of the skin and subcutaneous tissue, often following a surgical procedure. In the past few years it has been recognized that occasionally severe postoperative infections by *Streptococcus pyogenes* produce a similar "streptococcal toxic shocklike syndrome." TSS related to a surgical wound occurs early in the postoperative course, usually within the first 48 hours. The proportion of cases following surgical procedures increased from 14% in 1979 to 1986 to 27% in 1987 to 1996.

There are three requirements for the development of classical TSS: (1) the woman must be colonized or infected with *S. aureus,* (2) the bacteria must produce TSS toxin-1 (TSST-1) or related toxins, and (3) the toxins must have a route of entry into the systemic circulation. The majority of strains of *S. aureus* are unable to produce TSS toxin-1. Interestingly, approximately 85% of adult females have antibodies against TSST-1.

If an individual woman continues to use tampons when the vagina is colonized with *S. aureus,* there is a significant chance of a recurrence. It has been reported that one woman experienced five episodes of the disease. There appears to be no pattern to these recurrent episodes. Interestingly, women with menstrual-related TSS do not respond immunologically to TSST-1 as do women with nonmenstrual-related TSS. It is very rare for a woman with nonmenstrual TSS to have a recurrence.

The signs and symptoms of TSS are produced by the exotoxin named toxin-1. Toxin-1 is a simple protein with a molecular weight of 22,000. It is accepted as the underlying cause of the disease. Thus toxins act as "superantigens." Superantigens are molecules that activate up to 20% of T cells at once, resulting in massive cytokine production. Pathophysiologically, superantigens do not require processing by antigen-presenting cells. The primary effects of toxin-1 are to produce increased vascular permeability and thus profuse leaking of fluid (capillary leak) from the intravascular compartment into the interstitial space and associated profound loss of vasomotor tone, resulting in decreased peripheral resistance.

Studies of the bacteriology of the vagina of normal menstruating females have documented that 5% to 17% of women are colonized with *S. aureus.* Approximately 5% test positive when the culture is obtained at midcycle, and the percentage increases to 10% to 17% during the menses. Rarely are blood cultures positive for *S. aureus* in a woman with TSS. Thus the exotoxin is believed to be absorbed directly from the vagina. It is possible that microulcerations produced by use of tampons facilitate the toxin's entry into the systemic circulation. The risk of nonmenstrual TSS is definitely increased in women who use barrier contraceptives such as the diaphragm, cervical cap, or a sponge containing nonoxynol 9.

Because of the severity of the disease, gynecologists should have a high index of suspicion for TSS in a woman who has an unexplained fever and a rash during or immediately following her menstrual period. The syndrome has a wide range of symptoms. The varying degree of severity of both symptoms and signs depends on the magnitude of involvement of individual organs. Most women experience a prodromal flulike illness for the first 24 hours. Between days 2 and 4 of the menstrual period, the patient experiences an abrupt onset of a high temperature associated with headache, myalgia, sore throat, vomiting, diarrhea, a generalized skin rash, and often hypotension. It is important to consider that not all women with TSS experience the full-blown manifestations of the disease. The rigid criteria developed by the CDC are used for epidemiologic studies. Clinically, many women present with a *forme fruste* of TSS, with low-grade fever and dizziness rather than hypotension.

The most characteristic manifestations of TSS are the skin changes. During the first 48 hours the skin rash appears similar to an intense sunburn. During the next few days the erythema will become more macular and look like a drug-related rash. From days 12 to 15 of the illness, there is a fine, flaky, desquamation of skin over the face and trunk with sloughing of the entire skin thickness of the palms and soles. The vaginal mucosa is hyperemic during the initial phase of the syndrome. During pelvic examination, patients complain of tenderness of the external genitalia and vagina. Myalgia, vomiting, and diarrhea are experienced by more than 90% of women with TSS (see the following box on case definition of toxic shock syndrome). Many abnormal laboratory findings are associated with the disease, and again they reflect the severity of involvement of individual organ systems (see the following box on laboratory abnormalities in early toxic shock syndrome). The differential diagnosis of toxic shock syndrome includes Rocky Mountain spotted fever, streptococcal scarlet fever, and leptospirosis.

The management of a classic case of severe TSS demands an intensive care unit and the skills of an expert in critical care medicine. The first priority is to eliminate the hypotension produced by the exotoxin. Copious amounts of intravenous fluids are given while pressure and volume dynamics are monitored with a pulmonary artery catheter. Mechanical ventilation is required for women who develop adult respiratory distress syndrome.

When the patient is initially admitted to the hospital, it is important to obtain cervical, vaginal, and blood cultures for *S. aureus.* Although there is no controlled series documenting its efficacy, it is prudent to wash out the vagina with saline or dilute iodine solution to diminish the amount of exotoxin that may be absorbed into the systemic circulation.

Women with TSS should be treated with clindamycin 600 mg IV every 8 hours plus nafcillin or oxacillin 2 g IV every 4 hours, and most experts recommend a 1- to 2-week course of therapy with an antistaphyloccocal agent such as clindamycin or dicloxacillin even in the absence of positive *S. aureus* culture. If the diagnosis is questionable, it is best to include the use of an aminoglycoside to obtain coverage for possible gram-negative sepsis. Antibiotic therapy probably has little effect on the course of an individual episode of TSS. However, if the underlying cause of toxic shock syndrome is a skin infection, the infected site should be drained and débrided.

In summary, the treatment of TSS depends on the severity of involvement of individual organ systems. Not all patients develop a temperature of greater than 38.9° C and hypotension. Thus clinicians should be aware of the *forme fruste* manifestations of

Case Definition of Toxic Shock Syndrome

1. Fever (temperature 38.9°C, 102°F)
2. Rash characterized by diffuse macular erythroderma
3. Desquamation occurring 1–2 weeks after onset of illness (in survivors)
4. Hypotension (systolic blood pressure ≤ 90 mm Hg in adults) or orthostatic syncope
5. Involvement of three or more of the following organ systems:
   a. Gastrointestinal (vomiting or diarrhea at onset of illness)
   b. Muscular (myalgia or creatine phosphokinase level twice normal)
   c. Mucous membrane (vaginal, oropharyngeal, or conjunctival hyperemia)
   d. Renal (BUN or creatinine level ≥ twice normal or ≥ 5 WBC/HPF in absence of UTI)
   e. Hepatic (total bilirubin, SGOT, or SGPT twice normal level)
   f. Hematologic (platelets ≤ $100{,}000/mm^3$)
   g. Central nervous system (disorientation or alterations in consciousness without focal neurologic signs when fever and hypotension absent)
   h. Cardiopulmonary (adult respiratory distress syndrome, pulmonary edema, new onset of second- or third-degree heart block, myocarditis)
6. Negative throat and cerebrospinal fluid cultures (a positive blood culture for *staphylococcus aureus* does not exclude a case)
7. Negative serologic tests for Rocky Mountain spotted fever, leptospirosis, rubeola

BUN, blood urea nitrogen; HPF, high-powered field; SGOT, serum glutamic-oxaloacetic transaminase; SGPT, serum glutamic-pyruvic transaminase; UTI, urinary tract infection; WBC, white blood cell count.

From Toxic shock syndrome—United States, 1970–1982. MMWR 31:201, 1982.

Laboratory Abnormalities in Early Toxic Shock Syndrome*

Present in > 85% of patients
Coagulase-positive staphylococci in cervix or vagina
Immature and mature polymorphonuclear cells > 90% of WBCs
Total lymphocyte count < $650/mm^3$
Total serum protein level < 5.6 mg/dL
Serum albumin level < 3.1 g/dL
Serum calcium level < 7.8 mg/dL
Serum creatinine clearance > 1.0 mg/dL
Serum bilirubin value > 1.5 mg/dL
Serum cholesterol level ≤ 120 mg/dL
Prothrombin time > 12 seconds
Present in > 70% of patients
Platelet count < $150{,}000/mm^3$
Pyuria > 5 WBCs/HPF
Proteinuria ≥ 2
(BUN) > 20 mg/dL
Aspartate aminotransferase (formerly SGOT) > 41 U/L

*Results were available for at least 18 patients per category with the following exceptions: cervicovaginal cultures (12 patients), cholesterol level (15 patients), and prothrombin time (14 patients).

BUN, blood urea nitrogen; HPF, high-powered field; SGOT, serum glutamic-oxaloacetic transaminase; WBCs, white blood cells.

From Chesney PJ, Davis JP, Purdy WK, et al: Clinical manifestations of toxic shock syndrome. JAMA 246:746, 1981. Copyright 1981, American Medical Association.

the syndrome. The foundation of treatment of the disease is prompt and aggressive management because of the rapidity with which the disease may progress.

It is possible to decrease the incidence of TSS by a change in use of catamenial products. Women should be encouraged to change tampons every 4 to 6 hours. The intermittent use of external pads is also good preventive medicine. Women will usually accept the recommendation to wear external pads during sleep. The incidence of TSS has decreased dramatically with the removal of superabsorbing tampons from the market. A study by Tierno and Hanna reported that all-cotton tampons are the safest choice to avoid menstrual TSS.

Lastly, there are cases of streptococcal toxic shocklike syndrome that are secondary to life-threatening infections with group A streptococcus *(Streptococcus pyogenes).* Several different exotoxins have been identified and M-type 1 and 3 are the two most common serotypes. In gynecology the majority of these cases involve massive subcutaneous postoperative infections. One of the most distinguishing characteristics of a necrotizing skin infection is the intense localized pain in the involved area. Elderly women and women who are diabetic or immunocompromised are at much greater risk to develop invasive streptococcal infection and streptococcal toxic shocklike syndrome. The mortality rate is approximately 30% when TSS is secondary to group A streptococcal infections.

CERVICITIS

Cervicitis, an inflammatory process in the cervical epithelium and stroma, can be associated with trauma, inflammatory systemic disease, neoplasia, and infection. Although it is clinically important to consider all causes of inflammation, this section will focus on infectious origins.

Cervical infection can be ectocervicitis or endocervicitis. Ectocervicitis can be viral (HSV) or from a severe vaginitis (e.g., "strawberry cervix" associated with *T. vaginalis* infection) or *C. albicans.* The cervix is a potential reservoir for *Neisseria gonorrhoeae, Chlamydia trachomatis,* herpes simplex virus, human papillomavirus, and *Mycoplasma* species. Often the patient is asymptomatic, even though the cervix is colonized with either gonorrheal or chlamydial organisms. The cervix acts as a barrier between the abundant bacterial flora of the vagina and the bacteriologically sterile endometrial cavity and oviducts. Bacterial infection of the endocervix becomes a major reservoir for sexual and perinatal transmission of pathogenic microorganisms. Primary cervical infection may result in secondary ascending infections including pelvic inflammatory disease and perinatal infections of the membranes, amniotic fluid, and parametria. Endocervicitis may be secondary to bacterial infection with either *C. trachomatis* or *N. gonorrhoeae.* Bacterial vaginosis and *M. genitalium* have also been associated with endocervicitis.

The histologic diagnosis of chronic cervicitis is so prevalent that it should be considered the norm for parous women of reproductive age. The histopathology of endocervicitis is characterized by a severe inflammatory reaction in the mucosa and submucosa. The tissues are infiltrated with a large number of PMNs and monocytes, and occasionally there is associated epithelial necrosis. Physiologically, there is a resident population of a small number of leukocytes in the normal cervix. Thus the emphasis is on a severe inflammatory reaction by a large number of PMNs.

Cervical mucus is much more than a simple physical barrier; it exerts a definite bacteriostatic effect. Mucus may also act as a competitive inhibitor with bacteria for receptors on the endocervical epithelial cells. Cervical mucus also contains antibodies and inflammatory cells that are active against various sexually transmitted organisms. This section will focus on mucopurulent cervicitis and techniques to diagnose common cervical infections.

Mucopurulent Cervicitis

The diagnosis of cervicitis continues to rely on symptoms, examination, and microscopic evaluation. Two simple, definitive, objective criteria have been developed to establish mucopurulent cervicitis: gross visualization of yellow mucopurulent material on a white cotton swab (Fig. 22-25) and the presence of 10 or more PMN leukocytes per microscopic field (magnification × 1000) on Gram-stained smears obtained from the endocervix. Alternative clinical criteria that may be adopted are erythema and edema in an area of cervical ectopy or associated with bleeding secondary to endocervical ulceration, or friability when the endocervical smear is obtained. Women may also report increased vaginal discharge and intermenstrual vaginal bleeding. In their original study, the Seattle group discovered that 40% of patients with STDs had mucopurulent cervicitis (24% diagnosed by grossly visualized purulent material and 16% without mucopus but positive Gram stains of cervical mucus). However, the sensitivity, specificity, and positive predictive value of objective criteria have varied markedly in follow-up studies.

The prevalence of mucopurulent cervicitis depends on the population being studied. Approximately 30% to 40% of women attending clinics for STDs and 8% to 10% of women in university student health clinics have the condition. Greater

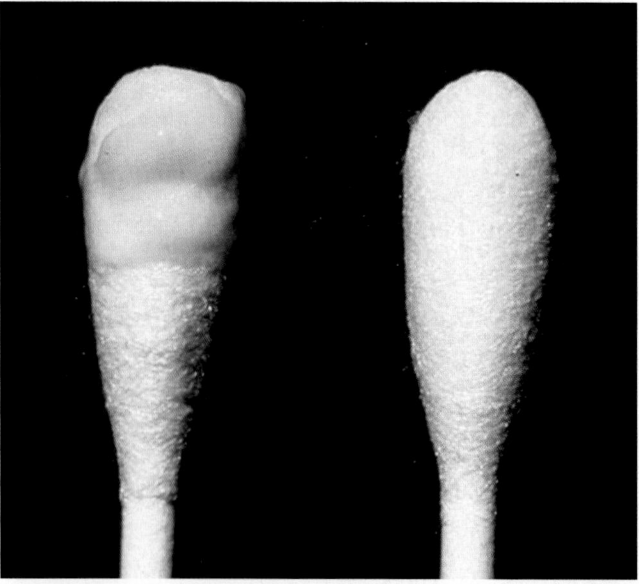

Figure 22-25. Mucopurulent cervicitis demonstrated by cotton swab test.

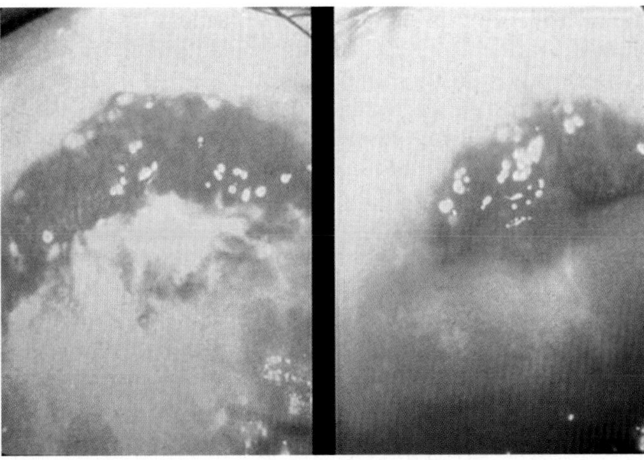

Figure 22-26. Patient with *C. trachomatis* mucopurulent cervicitis with resolution post-treatment.

than 60% of women with this disease are asymptomatic. Symptoms that suggest cervical infection include vaginal discharge, deep dyspareunia, and postcoital bleeding. The physical signs of a cervical infection are a cervix that is hypertrophic and edematous.

C. trachomatis is the cause of cervical infection in many women with mucopurulent cervicitis (Fig. 22-26). Depending on geographic region, gonorrhea is also an important cause of mucopurulent cervicitis. However, the majority of women who have lower reproductive tract infections by *C. trachomatis* or *N. gonorrhoeae* do not have mucopurulent cervicitis. The corollary is that the majority of women who have mucopurulent cervicitis are not infected by *C. trachomatis* or *N. gonorrhoeae.* Mucopurulent cervicitis is present in approximately 40% to 60% of women in whom no cervical pathogen can be identified. Thus this condition often persists following adequate broad-spectrum antibiotic therapy. The presence of active herpes infection is correlated with ulceration of the exocervix but not with mucopus.

When mucopurulent cervicitis is clinically diagnosed, empiric therapy for *C. trachomatis* is recommended in women at increased risk of this common STD (young age ≤ 25 years, new or multiple sex partners, unprotected sex). If the prevalence of *N. gonorrhoeae* is greater than 5%, concurrent therapy for *N. gonorrhoeae* is indicated. Concomitant trichomoniasis should also be treated if detected, as should bacterial vaginosis. If presumptive treatment is deferred, the use of sensitive nucleic acid test for *C. trachomatis* and *N. gonorrhoeae* is needed.

Recommended regimens for presumptive cervicitis therapy include azithromycin 1 g orally in a single dose or doxycycline 100 mg orally twice daily for 7 days. Presumptive gonococcal treatment is indicated if over 5% prevalence in the population assessed. Women treated for chlamydia should be instructed to abstain from sexual intercourse for 7 days after single-dose therapy or until completion of the 7-day regimen.

Recently, *Mycoplasma genitalium,* which is nonculturable, has been associated by DNA testing in women with mucopurulent cervicitis. Bacterial vaginosis has also been associated with mucopurulent cervicitis and the cervicitis resolved with bacterial vaginosis treatment.

The key teaching point is that many women harboring sexually transmitted pathogens in the cervix are asymptomatic.

Detection of Pathogenic Cervical Bacteria

Neisseria Gonorrhoeae

Nucleic acid amplification testing (NAAT) of the urine or cervix is the most sensitive and specific diagnostic tool for identifying gonorrheal infections. Urine tests should be "first void" (either the first void in morning, or at least one hour since last void). This technique allows sensitive detection of DNA particles originating either from either the urethra, or from the endocervix (which fall into the vaginal pool and vestibule). The majority of women who are colonized with *N. gonorrhoeae* are asymptomatic. Therefore, it is important to routinely screen women at high risk for gonorrheal infection. Screening of high-risk individuals is the primary way to control the disease. Gonorrheal NAAT are over 95% sensitive and specific.

It is important to know quinolone resistance patterns in one's geographic region. These changes are based on the increasing trends of the development of antibiotic-resistant *N. gonorrhoeae,* including fluoroquinolones-resistant *N. gonorrhoeae,* and strains with chromosomally mediated resistance to multiple antibiotics, including penicillin and spectinomycin. In 1995 penicillinase-producing strains of *N. gonorrhoeae* caused approximately 13% of gonorrheal infections in the United States. Two other considerations are given high priority when choosing an antibiotic: single-dose efficacy and simultaneously treating coexisting chlamydial infection. *C. trachomatis* has been frequently found to simultaneously colonize women with gonorrhea. The present recommended parenteral regimen is ceftriaxone, 125 mg IM one time. Alternatively, cefixime, cefpodoxime, ciprofloxacin, or ofloxacin may be given in a single oral dose. These regimens have documented cure rates of greater than 95% in uncomplicated anogenital gonorrhea. Ceftriaxone or ofloxacin cure greater than 90% of pharyngeal gonorrhea. For patients who are allergic or intolerant to cephalosporins and quinolones, the number-one alternative is spectinomycin, 2 g IM in a single dose (see the following boxes on treatment regimens for gonorrhea and chlamydial infection). In addition to the antibiotics for gonorrhea,

Recommended Regimens for Treatment of Chlamydial Infection

Recommended Regimens

Azithromycin 1 g PO in a single dose,

or

Doxycycline 100 mg PO bid for 7 days.

Alternative Regimens

Erythromycin base 500 mg PO qid for 7 days,

or

Erythromycin ethylsuccinate 800 mg PO qid for 7 days,

or

Ofloxacin 300 mg PO bid for 7 days.

From CDC 2006 Guidelines for Treatment of Sexually Transmitted Diseases. MMWR 55:11.

Centers for Disease Control Recommended Treatment of Uncomplicated Gonococcal Infections of the Cervix, Urethra, and Rectum in Adults (1997)

Recommended Regimens

Cefixime 400 mg PO in a single dose
or
Cefriaxone 125 mg IM in a single dose
or
Ciprofloxacin 500 mg PO in a single dose,
or
Ofloxacin 400 mg PO in a single dose or levofloxacin 250 mg PO in a single dose
plus
Azithromycin 1 g PO in a single dose,
or
Doxycycline 100 mg PO bid for 7 days
unless *C. trachomatis* is ruled out

Alternative Regimens

1. Spectinomycin 2 g IM in a single dose
2. Injectable cephalosporins such as ceftizoxime 500 mg IM, cefotaxime 500 mg IM, cefoxitin 2 g IM with probenecid 1 g PO, all as a single dose. Cefpodoxime 400 mg PO
3. Other quinolones such as gafifloxin 400 mg PO, lomefloxacin 400 mg PO, or norfloxacin 800 mg PO, all as a single dose

From 2006 CDC treatment guidelines.

the CDC recommends treating with azithromycin 1 g orally in a single dose, or oral doxycycline, 100 mg twice daily for 7 days, or if chlamydia has not been ruled out.

If the woman is asymptomatic, follow-up testing is no longer recommended by the CDC as a test of cure for lower tract infections (uncomplicated gonorrhea). Women with positive cultures for gonorrhea should have a serologic test for syphilis in 4 to 6 weeks, even though patients with incubating syphilis are usually cured by antibiotic combinations of ceftriaxone and tetracycline. Similarly, patients should be offered informed consent and testing for HIV infection.

It is important to remember *N. gonorrhoeae* attaches to columnar epithelium, so a vaginal cuff swab in women with prior hysterectomies is not recommended.

Chlamydia Trachomatis

As with gonorrhea, the gold standard of techniques used to identify *C. trachomatis* infection is NAAT. *C. trachomatis* also attaches to columnar epithelium. Hence, vaginal specimens should not be collected in a women who had a hysterectomy. Because *C. trachomatis* is an obligatory intracellular organism, if a culture is used for diagnosis, it is mandatory to obtain epithelial cells to maximize the percentage of positive cultures. A Dacron, rayon, or calcium alginate swab is placed in the endocervical canal. It is rotated for 15 to 20 seconds to gently abrade the columnar epithelium. The cytobrush, which was developed primarily to enhance sampling of endocervical cells for cytology, has been discovered to be the optimal instrument for appropriate sampling for *Chlamydia* culture as well. Chlamydial antigen detection is insensitive and nonspecific compared with NAAT and is no longer recommended.

C. trachomatis infection is frequently asymptomatic. Chlamydial screening program have been very successful at decreasing the prevalence of the disease. The CDC recommends annual screening of all sexually active women 25 years of age or younger, and screening of older women with risk factors (e.g., those who have a new sex partner or multiple partners).

For all women with either chlamydial or gonorrheal infections, partners should be treated. Patients should be instructed to refer all sex partners of the last 60 days for evaluation and treatment and to avoid sexual intercourse until therapy is completed and they and their partners have resolution of symptoms.

If a patient is unsure if her partner will get treated, delivery of antibiotic therapy (either by prescription or medication) is an option. Recently, studies have demonstrated that patient-delivered partner therapy result in lower rates of chlamydial persistence or recurrence. All women with *C. trachomatis, N. gonorrhoeae* or mucopurulent cervicitis of unknown origin need evaluation to rule out pelvic inflammatory disease.

KEY POINTS

- The three most prevalent primary viral infections of the skin of the vulva are genital herpes, condyloma acuminatum, and molluscum contagiosum.
- Acute bacterial cystitis is characterized by abrupt onset and multiple symptoms, including dysuria, urgency, and frequent voiding. Suprapubic tenderness is a specific sign for acute bacterial cystitis; however, it is not present in the majority of patients.
- The differential diagnosis of dysuria in adult women includes acute cystitis, acute urethritis, or vulvovaginitis.
- The most frequent pathogens involved in uncomplicated lower UTI are *Escherichia coli* (approximately 80%) and *Staphylococcus saprophyticus* (approximately 5% to 15%).
- For the first episode of acute, uncomplicated cystitis the current treatment of choice is 3 days of oral therapy with TMP-SMZ, trimethoprim alone, or one of the quinolones such as ciprofloxacin or norfloxacin.
- More than 90% of recurrences in young women are exogenous reinfection with new isolates arising from local flora.
- A normal Bartholin's gland cannot be palpated. Approximately 2% of adult women develop enlargement of both Bartholin's glands.
- The treatment of choice for a symptomatic Bartholin's cyst or abscess is the development of a fistulous tract from the dilated Bartholin's duct to the vestibule.

KEY POINTS *Continued*

- Excision of Bartholin's duct and gland is indicated for persistent deep infection, multiple recurrences of abscesses, or enlargement of the gland in a woman older than 40. Removal of a Bartholin's gland for recurrent infection should be performed when the infection is quiescent.
- Pediculosis pubis, an infestation by the crab louse *Phthirus pubis,* is characterized by constant itching, predominantly vulvar involvement, and the finding of eggs and lice by visual inspection. It may be treated by topical application of 1% permethrin cream rinse (Nix) or 1% lindane shampoo (Kwell).
- Scabies, an infection by the itch mite *Sarcoptes scabiei,* is characterized by intermittent pruritus, most commonly in the hands, wrists, breasts, vulva, and buttocks. It is diagnosed by a scraping of the papules, vesicles, or burrows in which the mites live and inspection under the microscope. It may be treated by topical application of 5% permethrin cream (Nix) or 1% lindane lotion or 30 g of cream.
- Permethrin is more expensive than lindane, and permethrin has less potential for toxicity in the event of inappropriate use. Seizures have been reported when lindane was applied immediately after a bath or in women with extensive dermatitis. Lindane is not recommended during pregnancy or for lactating women or children younger than 2.
- Molluscum contagiosum in adults is an asymptomatic viral disease primarily of the vulvar skin. It is a common generalized skin disease in adults with immunodeficiency, especially HIV infection.
- Condyloma acuminatum presents as a clinically recognizable macroscopic lesion in 30% of infected women and as a subclinical infection in 70% of women.
- Condyloma acuminatum is an STD spread by skin-to-skin contact. It is caused by the human papillomavirus (HPV). Autoinoculation also occurs. It is a highly contagious disease.
- Vaginal condylomata are identified in approximately one of three women with vulvar disease.
- No present therapy of HPV eliminates subclinical infection from the surrounding epithelium.
- HPV vaccine against types 6 and 11 can prevent 90% of condylomata when administered to HPV-naïve females
- Genital herpes is a recurrent, incurable STD. Approximately 80% of the individuals are unaware they are infected.
- Genital herpes is most frequently transmitted by individuals who are asymptomatic and unaware that they have the infection at the time of transmission.
- From a clinical standpoint the important difference between HSV-1 and HSV-2 is that the frequency of recurrence is four times greater following a primary infection with HSV-2 than with HSV-1.
- The primary infection by herpes is both a local and a systemic disease. The majority of symptomatic women have severe vulvar pain, tenderness, and inguinal adenopathy. However, subclinical primary herpes infection is common.
- Oral medication effective against HSV has been shown to be beneficial in reducing the duration of herpetic ulcerative lesions and in reducing the time that the virus can be isolated from these lesions.
- Patients with frequent episodes of recurrent genital herpes may be successfully treated with prophylactic oral medication. The primary goals of continuous suppressive therapy are to limit the severity and number of occurrences as well as to give the woman a sense of control over her disease. In discordant couples suppressive therapy also decreases acquisition of HSV in the seronegative partner.
- Granuloma inguinale, also known as donovanosis, is a chronic, ulcerative, bacterial infection of the skin and subcutaneous tissue of the vulva.
- Granuloma inguinale may be managed by a wide range of oral broad-spectrum antibiotics.
- Lymphogranuloma venereum (LGV) is an STD produced by serotypes L_1, L_2, and L_3 of *C. trachomatis.*
- The treatment for LGV is oral doxycycline, 100 mg twice a day for 3 weeks. An alternative regimen is erythromycin base 500 mg every 6 hours for 3 weeks.
- Chancroid is a sexually transmitted, acute, ulcerative disease of the vulva. The soft chancre of chancroid is always painful and tender. In comparison, the hard chancre of syphilis is usually asymptomatic.
- Syphilis is a chronic complex systemic disease produced by the spirochete *Treponema pallidum.*
- Early syphilis is a cofactor in the transmission and acquisition of HIV.
- Dark-field microscopy rather than normal light microscopy is used for detection of syphilis because of the extreme thinness of the spirochete *Treponema pallidum.*
- Quantitative nontreponemal antibody titers usually correlate with the activity of syphilis.
- Nonspecific tests for syphilis, the VDRL and RPR, have a 1% false-positive rate. Many conditions produce biologic false-positive results, including a recent febrile illness, pregnancy, immunization, chronic active hepatitis, malaria, sarcoidosis, intravenous drug use, and autoimmune diseases such as lupus erythematosus or rheumatoid arthritis. Therefore, specific tests such as the TPI, FTA-ABS, and MHA-TP must be employed when a positive nonspecific test result is encountered.
- A woman with a positive reactive treponemal test usually will have this positive reaction for her lifetime regardless of treatment or the activity of the disease.
- The characteristic chancre of primary syphilis is a red, round ulcer with firm, well-formed, raised edges, with a nonpurulent clean base and yellow-gray exudate. During the first week of clinical disease, the woman develops regional adenopathy that is nontender and firm.
- A woman with syphilis is most infectious during the first 1 to 2 years of her disease with decreasing infectivity thereafter.
- Tertiary syphilis develops in approximately 33% of patients who are not appropriately treated during the primary, secondary, or latent phases of the disease.

Continued

KEY POINTS *Continued*

- Concurrent HIV infection should be considered in patients with syphilis. It is optimal for all women with syphilis to be tested for HIV infection.
- Sexual partners of women with syphilis in any stage should be evaluated both clinically and serologically.
- In women in the reproductive age range, bacterial vaginosis represents approximately 50% of vaginitis, and candidiasis and *Trichomonas* infection represent approximately 25% each.
- The normal vaginal environment is a dynamic and delicate ecosystem, with a pH of approximately 4.0 in premenopausal women.
- A vaginal pH of greater than 5.0 indicates atrophic vaginitis, bacterial vaginosis, or *Trichomonas* infection, whereas a vaginal pH of less than 4.5 in a symptomatic woman is characteristic of either a physiologic discharge or fungal infection.
- Bacterial vaginosis results when high concentrations of anaerobic bacteria replace the normal H_2O_2-producing *Lactobacillus* species in the vagina. Histologically, there is an absence of inflammation in biopsies of the vagina.
- The classic criteria for the diagnosis of bacterial vaginosis are (1) a homogeneous vaginal discharge is present; (2) the vaginal discharge has a pH equal to or greater than 4.5; (3) the vaginal discharge has an aminelike odor when mixed with potassium hydroxide; and (4) a wet smear of the vaginal discharge demonstrates clue cells greater in number than 20% of the number of the vaginal epithelial cells.
- Ironically, 50% of women who have three of the four clinical criteria for bacterial vaginosis are asymptomatic.
- HIV acquisition is increased in women with bacterial vaginosis and *Trachomatis vaginalis* infection.
- *Trichomonas* vaginal infection is the most prevalent nonviral, nonchlamydial STD of women. *Trichomonas* is the causal factor for approximately one in four episodes of infectious vaginitis.
- *T. vaginalis* infection is a highly contagious STD. Following a single sexual contact, at least two thirds of both male and female sexual partners become infected.
- Dysuria is a symptom in approximately one of five women with symptomatic *Trichomonas* infection.
- The asymptomatic female who has *Trichomonas* identified in the lower female genital urinary tract definitely should be treated. Extended follow-up studies have shown that one in three asymptomatic females will become symptomatic within 3 months.
- *Candida* vaginitis is produced by a ubiquitous, airborne, gram-positive fungus. The vast majority of cases are caused by *Candida albicans,* with 5% to 20% of vaginal fungal infections produced by *C. glabrata* or *C. tropicalis.*
- *Candida* species are part of the normal flora of approximately 25% of women, being a commensal saprophytic organism on the mucosal surface of the vagina. When the ecosystem of the vagina is disturbed, *Candida* becomes an opportunistic pathogen.
- Recurrent vulvovaginal candidiasis is defined as four or more episodes of symptomatic lower tract infection within 12 months.
- Toxic shock syndrome (TSS) is an acute, febrile illness, produced by a bacterial exotoxin with a fulminating downhill course involving dysfunction of multiple organ systems.
- Menstrual associated TSS is decreasing. Severe postoperative infections by *Streptococcus pyogenes* may produce a similar TSS.
- Because of the severity of the disease, gynecologists should have a high index of suspicion for TSS in a woman who has an unexplained fever and a rash during or immediately following her menstrual period.
- The initial rash of TSS over the first 48 hours is similar in appearance to an intense sunburn. Over the next several days it evolves into a macular rash with fine, flaky desquamation over the face and trunk, and sloughing of the entire skin thickness over the palms and soles.
- The differential diagnosis of TSS includes Rocky Mountain spotted fever, streptococcal scarlet fever, and leptospirosis.
- Bacterial infection of the endocervix becomes a major reservoir for sexual and perinatal transmission of pathogenic microorganisms.
- The most common site of *Chlamydia* infection in the female reproductive tract is the columnar cells of the endocervix.
- Symptoms that suggest cervical infection include vaginal discharge, deep dyspareunia, and postcoital bleeding. *Chlamydia trachomatis* is the major infective agent in women with mucopurulent cervicitis.
- The majority of women who have lower reproductive tract infections by *C. trachomatis* or *N. gonorrhoeae* do not have mucopurulent cervicitis. The corollary is the majority of women who have mucopurulent cervicitis are not infected by *C. trachomatis* or *N. gonorrhoeae.*
- Routine dual therapy for gonococcal and chlamydial infections is indicated if the woman has chlamydia and comes from a population in which the prevalence of gonococcal infections is greater than 5%.
- Many women harboring sexually transmitted pathogens in the cervix are asymptomatic.
- Nucleic acid amplification testing is the standard detection method for *C. trachomatis* and *N. gonorrhoeae.* Urine testing requires a first void specimen.
- *N. gonorrhoeae* Gram stain smears are positive for only 50% of women with positive cultures. Culture of a second consecutive endocervical cotton swab will increase detection of *N. gonorrhoeae* by approximately 7% to 10%.
- If the woman is asymptomatic, follow-up cultures are no longer recommended by the CDC as a test of cure for lower tract infections (uncomplicated gonorrhea).

BIBLIOGRAPHY

Key Readings

ACOG Committee on Practice Bulletins: ACOG practice bulletin: Clinical management guidelines for obstetrician-gynecologists, number 72, May 2006: Vaginitis. Obstet Gynecol 107:1195, 2006.

Brunham RC, Paavonen J, Stevens CE, et al: Mucopurulent cervicitis—the ignored counterpart in women of urethritis in men. N Engl J Med 311:1, 1984.

Corey L, Wald A, Patel R, et al; Valacyclovir HSV Transmission Study Group: Once-daily valacyclovir to reduce the risk of transmission of genital herpes. N Engl J Med 350(1):11, 2004.

Eckert LO: Clinical practice: Acute vulvovaginits. N Engl J Med 355:1244, 2006.

Eckert LO, Hawes SE, Stevens CE, et al: Vulvovaginal candidiasis: Clinical manifestations, risk factors, management algorithm. Obstet Gynecol 92: 757, 1998.

Eschenbach DA, Hillier S, Critchlow C, et al: Diagnosis and clinical manifestations of bacterial vaginosis. Am J Obstet Gynecol 158:819, 1988.

Gupta K, Scholes D, Stamm WE: Increasing prevalence of antimicrobial resistance among uropathogens causing acute uncomplicated cystitis in women. JAMA 281:736, 1999.

Hooton TM, Besser R, Foxman B, et al: Acute uncomplicated cystitis in an era of increasing antibiotic resistance: A proposed approach to empirical therapy. Clin Infect Dis 39:75, 2004.

Marrazzo JM, Koutsky LA, Eschenbach DA, et al: Characterization of vaginal flora and bacterial vaginosis in women who have sex with women. J Infect Dis 185:1307, 2002.

Sobel JD, Ferris D, Schwebke J, et al: Suppressive antibacterial therapy with 0.75% metronidazole vaginal gel to prevent recurrent bacterial vaginosis. Am J Obstet Gynecol 194:1283, 2006.

Sobel JD, Wiesenfeld HC, Martens M, et al: Maintenance fluconazole therapy for recurrent vulvovaginal candidiasis. N Engl J Med 351:876, 2004.

Soper D: Trichomoniasis: Under control or undercontrolled? Am J Obstet Gynecol 190: 281, 2004.

Wald A, Zeh J, Selke S, et al: Virologic characteristics of subclinical and symptomatic genital herpes infections. N Engl J Med 333:770, 1995.

Wolner-Hannssen P, Krieger JN, Stevens CE, et al: Clinical manifestations of vaginal trichomoniasis. JAMA 261:571, 1989.

Key References

Abulafia O, Sherer DM: Bartholin gland abscess: Sonographic findings. J Clin Ultrasound 25:47, 1997.

American Medical Association: Genital herpes: A clinician's guide to diagnosis and treatment, part I. Evans RM, Brakl MJ (eds): AMA Continuing Medical Education Program, 1997.

American Medical Association: Genital herpes: A clinician's guide to diagnosis and treatment, part II. Evans RM, Brakl MJ (eds): AMA Continuing Medical Education Program, 1997.

American Medical Association: External genital warts: Diagnosis and treatment. Evans RM, Wiley D (eds): AMA Continuing Medical Education Program, 1997.

Andersen PG, Christensen S, Detlefsen GU, Kern-Hansen P: Treatment of Bartholin's abscess: Marsupialization versus incision, curettage and suture under antibiotic cover. A randomized study with 6 months' follow-up. Acta Obstet Gynecol Scand 71:59, 1992.

Antonelli N, Diehl SJ, Wright JW: A randomized trial of intravaginal nonoxynol 9 versus oral metronidazole in the treatment of vaginal trichomoniasis. Am J Obstet Gynecol 182:1008, 2000.

Armstrong DKB, Maw RD, Dinsmore WW, et al: A randomized, double-blind, parallel group study to compare subcutaneous interferon alpha-2a plus podophyllin with placebo plus podophyllin in the treatment of primary condylomata acuminata. Genitourin Med 70:389, 1994.

Arav-Boger R, Leibovici L, Danon YL: Urinary tract infections with low and high colony counts in young women: Spontaneous remission and single-dose vs multiple-day treatment. Arch Intern Med 154:300, 1994.

Augenbraun M, Feldman J, Chirgwin K, et al: Increased genital shedding of herpes simplex virus Type 2 in HIV-seropositive women. Ann Intern Med 123:845, 1995.

Avorn J, Monane M, Gurqitz JH, et al: Reduction of bacteriuria and pyuria after ingestion of cranberry juice. JAMA 271:751, 1994.

Barbone F, Austin H, Louv WC, Alexander WJ: A follow-up study of methods of contraception, sexual activity, and rates of trichomoniasis, candidiasis, and bacterial vaginosis. Am J Obstet Gynecol 163: 510, 1990.

Barbosa-Cesnik CT, Gerbase A, Heymann D: STD vaccines-an overview. Genitourin Med 73:336, 1997.

Benedetti J, Corey L, Ashley R: Recurrence rates in genital herpes after symptomatic first-episode infection. Ann Intern Med 121:847, 1994.

Beneditti JK, Zeh J, Corey L: Clinical reactivation of genital herpes simplex virus infection decreases in frequency over time. Ann Intern Med 131:14, 1999.

Berkley SF, Hightower AW, Broome CV, Reingold AL: The relationship of tampon characteristics to menstrual toxic shock syndrome. JAMA 258:917, 1987.

Blake DR, Duggan A, Joffe A: Use of spun urine to enhance detection of *Trichomonas vaginalis* in adolescent women. Arch Pediatr Adolesc Med 153:1222, 1999.

Boeke AJP, Dekker JH, Peerbooms PGH: A comparison of yield from cervix versus vagina for culturing *Candida albicans* and *Trichomonas vaginalis.* Genitourin Med 69:41, 1993.

Bonnez W, Elswick RK Jr, Bailey-Farchione A, et al: Efficacy and safety of 0.5% podofilox solution in the treatment and suppression of anogenital warts. Am J Med 96:420, 1994.

Bozbora A, Erbil Y, Berber E, et al: Surgical treatment of granuloma inguinale. Br J Dermatol 138:1079, 1998.

Brook I: Aerobic and anaerobic microbiology of Bartholin's abscess. Surg Gynecol Obstet 169:32, 1989.

Brown ST, Nalley JF, Kraus SJ: Molluscum contagiosum. Sex Transm Dis 8:227, 1981.

Brown TJ, Yen-Moore A, Tyring SK: An overview of sexually transmitted diseases, part I. J Am Acad Dermatol 41:511, 1999.

Brown TJ, Yen-Moore A, Tyring SK: An overview of sexually transmitted diseases, part II. J Am Acad Dermatol 41:661, 1999.

Caruso LJ: Vaginal moniliasis after tetracycline therapy: The effects of amphotericin B. Am J Obstet Gynecol, 90:374, 1964.

Catanzarite VA, Piacquadio KM, Stanco LM, et al: Preventing transmission of AIDS and hepatitis in obstetric-care providers. Contemp OB/GYN 44:39, 1999.

Cavannah DK, Ballas ZK: Pseudoephedrine reaction presenting as recurrent toxic shock syndrome. Ann Intern Med 119:302, 1993.

Centers for Disease Control: 2006 Guidelines for treatment of sexually transmitted diseases. MMWR, Vol. 55, RR-11, 2006.

Chiasson MA, Ellerbrock TV, Bush TJ, et al: Increased prevalence of vulvovaginal condyloma and vulvar intraepithelial neoplasia in women infected with the human immunodeficiency virus. Obstet Gynecol 89:690, 1997.

Chesney PJ: Clinical aspects and spectrum of illness of toxic shock syndrome: Overview. Rev Infect Dis 11:S1, 1989.

Chesney PJ, Davis JP, Purdy WK, et al: Clinical manifestations of toxic shock syndrome. JAMA 246:741, 1981.

Cho JY, Ahn MO, Cha KS: Window operation: An alternative treatment method for Bartholin gland cysts and abscesses. Obstet Gynecol 76:886, 1990.

Chosidow O: Scabies and pediculosis. Lancet 355:819, 2000.

Chouela EN, Abeldaño AM, Pellerano G, et al: Equivalent therapeutic efficacy and safety of Ivermectin and Lindane in the treatment of human scabies. Arch Dermatol 135:651, 1999.

Collier AC, Schwartz MA: Strategies for second-line antiretroviral therapy in adults with HIV infection. Advan Exper Med Biol 458:239, 1999.

Coodley GO, Coodley MK, Thompson AF: Clinical aspects of HIV infection in women. J Gen Intern Med 10:99, 1995.

Condylomata International Collaborative Study Group: Recurrent condylomata acuminata treated with recombinant interferon alfa-2a: A multicenter double-blind placebo-controlled clinical trial. JAMA 265:2684, 1991.

Corey L, Handsfield HH: Genital herpes and public health: Addressing a global problem. JAMA 283:791, 2000.

Corey Leone P: Sex transmitted diseases. N Engl J Med 31(5):311, 2004.

Cox NH: Permethrin treatment in scabies infestation: Importance of the correct formulation. BMJ 320:37, 2000.

Croen KD, Ostrove JM, Dragovic L, Straus SE: Characterization of herpes simplex virus type 2 latency-associated transcription in human sacral ganglia and in cell culture. J Infect Dis 163:23, 1991.

Culhane JF, Rauh V, McCollum KF, et al: Exposure to chronic stress and ethnic differences in rates of bacterial vaginosis among pregnant women. Am J Obstet Gynecol 187:1272, 2002.

del Giudice P: Ivermectin: A new therapeutic weapon in dermatology? Arch Dermatol 135:705, 1999.

Eckert LO, Moore DE, Patton DL, et al: Relationship of vaginal bacteria and inflammation with conception and early pregnancy loss following in-vitro fertilization. Infect Dis Obstet Gynecol 11:11, 2003.

Edwards-Jones V, Foster HA: The effect of topical antimicrobial agents on the production of toxic shock syndrome toxin-1. J Med Microbio 41:408, 1994.

Erbelding EM, Vlahov D, Nelson KE, et al: Syphilis serology in human immunodeficiency virus infection: Evidence for false-negative fluorescent treponemal testing. J Infect Dis 176:1397, 1997.

Eschenbach DA: History and review of bacterial vaginosis. Am J Obstet Gynecol 169:441, 1993.

Eschenbach DA, Hummel D, Gravett MG: Recurrent and persistent vulvovaginal candidiasis: Treatment with ketoconazole. Obstet Gynecol 66:248, 1985.

Faber BM: The diagnosis and treatment of scabies and pubic lice. Prim Care Update Ob/Gyns 3:20, 1996.

Faro S: Systemic vs. topical therapy for the treatment of vulvovaginal candidiasis. Infect Dis Obstet Gynecol 1:202, 1994.

Faro S: A review of famciclovir in the management of genital herpes. Infect Dis Obstet Gynecol 6:38, 1998.

Faro S, Skokos CK: The efficacy and safety of a single dose of Clindesse vaginal cream versus a seven-dose regimen of Cleocin vaginal cream in patients with bacterial vaginosis. Infect Dis Obstet Gynecol 13:155-60, 2005.

Feldman JG, Chirgwin K, Dehovitz JA, Minkoff H: The association of smoking and risk of condyloma acuminatum in women. Obstet Gynecol 89:346, 1997.

Ferenczy A: Epidemiology and clinical pathophysiology of condylomata acuminata. Am J Obstet Gynecol 172:1331, 1995.

Ferris DG, Nyrijesy P, Sobel JD, et al: Over-the-counter antifungal drug misuse associated with patient-diagnoses vulvovaginal candidiasis. Obstet Gynecol 99:419, 2002.

Fidel PL Jr, Barousse M, Espinosa T, et al: An intravaginal live Candida challenge in humans leads to new hypotheses for the immunopathogenesis of vulvovaginal candidiasis. Infect Immun 72:2939, 2004.

Fidel PL Jr, Ginsburg KA, Cutright JL, et al: Vaginal-associated immunity in women with recurrent vulvovaginal candidiasis: Evidence for vaginal Th 1-type responses following intravaginal challenge with Candida antigen. J Infect Dis 176:728, 1997.

Fife KH, Crumpacker SC, Mertz GJ, et al: Recurrence and resistance patterns of herpes simplex virus following cessation of ≥6 years of chronic suppression with acyclovir. J Infect Dis 169:1338, 1994.

Fischbach F, Petersen EE, Weissenbacher ER, et al: Efficacy of clindamycin vaginal cream versus oral metronidazole in the treatment of bacterial vaginosis. Obstet Gynecol 82:405, 1993.

Fong IW, Bannatyne RM, Wong P: Lack of in vitro resistance of *Candida albicans* to ketoconazole, itraconazole and clotrimazole in women treated for recurrent vaginal candidiasis. Genitourin Med 69:44, 1993.

Foxman B: Epidemiology of urinary tract infections: incidence, morbidity, and economic costs, Am J Med 113 Suppl 1A:5S, 2002.

Fredricks DN, Fiedler TL, Marrazzo JM: Molecular identification of bacteria associated with bacterial vaginosis. N Engl Med 353:1899, 2005.

Fu YL, Hu YX, Ling HL, et al: Human papillomaviruses and papillomatosis lesions of the female lower genital tract. Infect Dis Obstet Gynecol 1:235, 1994.

García-Closas M, Herrero R, Bratti C, et al: Epidemiologic determinants of vaginal pH. Am J Obstet Gynecol 180:1060, 1999.

Gardella C, Brown Z, Wald A, et al: Risk factors for herpes simplex virus transmission to pregnant women: A couples study. Am J Obstet Gynecol 193(6): 1891, 2005.

Gaydos CA, Howell MR, Pare B, et al: *Chlamydia trachomatis* infections in female military recruits. N Engl J Med 339:739, 1998.

Giraldo P, von Nowaskonski A, Gomes FAM, et al: Vaginal colonization by *Candida* in asymptomatic women with and without a history of recurrent vulvovaginal candidiasis. Obstet Gynecol 95:413, 2000.

Goldman P: Metronidazole. N Engl J Med 303:1212, 1980.

Goldmeier D, Hay P: A review and update on adult syphilis, with particular reference to its treatment. Int J STD AIDS 4:70, 1993.

Goldschmidt RH, Dong BJ: Treatment of AIDS and HIV-related conditions-1999. JABFP 12:71, 1999.

Gupta K, Hooton TM, Roberts PL, Staff WE: Patient-initiated treatment of uncomplicated recurrent urinary tract infections in young women. Ann Intern Med 135:9, 2001.

Gupta K, Sahm DF, Mayfield D, Stamm WE: Antimicrobial resistance among uropathogens that cause community-acquired urinary tract infections in women: A nationwide analysis. Clin Infect Dis 33:89, 2001.

Gupta R, Wald A, Krantz E, et al: Valacyclovir and acyclovir for suppression of shedding of herpes simplex virus in the genital tract. Infect Dis 15;190(8): 1374, 2004.

Harmanli OH, Cheng GY, Nyirjesy P, et al: Urinary tract infections in women with bacterial vaginosis. Obstet Gynecol 95:710, 2000.

Hart G: Donovanosis. Clin Infect Dis 25:24, 1997.

Hatch KD: Clinical appearance and treatment strategies for human papillomavirus: A gynecologic perspective. Am J Obstet Gynecol 172:1340, 1995.

Hauth JC, Goldenberg RL, Andrews WW, et al: Reduced incidence of preterm delivery with metronidazole and erythromycin in women with bacterial vaginosis. N Engl J Med 333:1732, 1995.

Hawes SE, Hillier SL, Benedetti J, et al: Hydrogen peroxide-producing lactobacilli and acquisition of vaginal infections. J Infect Dis 174:1058, 1996.

Hill GB, Livengood CH III: Bacterial vaginosis-associated microflora and effects of topical intravaginal clindamycin. Am J Obstet Gynecol 171:1198, 1994.

Hillier SL: Diagnostic microbiology of bacterial vaginosis. Am J Obstet Gynecol 169:455, 1993.

Hillier SL, Krohn MA, Klebanoff SJ, Eschenbach DA: The relationship of hydrogen peroxide-producing lactobacilli to bacterial vaginosis and genital microflora in pregnant women. Obstet Gynecol 79:369, 1992.

Hilton E, Isenberg HD, Alperstein P, et al: Ingestion of yogurt containing *Lactobacillus acidophilus* as prophylaxis for candidal vaginitis. Ann Intern Med 116:353, 1992.

Hines JF, Ghrim S, Schlegel R, Jenson AB: Prospects for a vaccine against human papillomavirus. Obstet Gynecol 86:860, 1995.

Hoge CW, Schwartz B, Talkington DF, et al: The changing epidemiology of invasive group A streptococcal infections and the emergence of streptococcal toxic shock-like syndrome: A retrospective population-based study. JAMA 269:384, 1993.

Holmes KK, Mårdh PA, Sparling PF, et al (eds): Sexually Transmitted Diseases, 3rd ed. New York, McGraw-Hill, 1999.

Hook EW III, Marra CM: Acquired syphilis in adults. N Engl J Med 326:1060, 1992.

Hughes VL, Hillier SL: Microbiologic characteristics of Lactobacillus products used for colonization of the vagina. Obstet Gynecol 75:244, 1990.

Hutchison CM, Hook EW III, Shepherd M, et al: Altered clinical presentation of early syphilis in patients with human immunodeficiency virus infection. Ann Intern Med 121:94, 1994.

Jeremias J, Draper D, Ziegert M, et al: Detection of *Trichomonas vaginalis* using the polymerase chain reaction in pregnant and non-pregnant women. Infect Dis Obstet Gynecol 2:16, 1994.

Joesoef MR, Schmid GP: Bacterial vaginosis: Review of treatment options and potential clinical indications for therapy. Clin Infect Dis 20(S1):S72, 1995.

Joesoef MR, Schmid GP, Hillier SL: Bacterial vaginosis: Review of treatment options and potential clinical indications for therapy. Clin Infect Dis 28(S1):S57, 1999.

Joseph AK, Rosen T: Laboratory techniques used in the diagnosis of chancroid, granuloma inguinale, and lymphogranuloma venereum. Dermatol Clin 12:1, 1994.

Kain KC, Schulzer M, Chow AW: Clinical spectrum of nonmenstrual toxic shock syndrome (TSS): Comparison with menstrual TSS by multivariate discriminate analyses. Clin Infect Dis 16:100, 1993.

Kaufman RH, Faro S: Benign Diseases of the Vulva and Vagina, 4th ed. St. Louis, Mosby-Year Book, 1994.

Klebanoff SJ, Coombs RW: Viricidal effect of Lactobacillus acidophilus on human immunodeficiency virus type 1: Possible role in heterosexual transmission. J Exp Med 174: 289, 1991.

Koelle DM, Benedetti J, Langenberg A, Corey L: Asymptomatic reactivation of herpes simplex virus in women after the first episode of genital herpes. Ann Intern Med 116:433, 1992.

Koutsky LA, Stevens CE, Holmes KK, et al: Underdiagnosis of genital herpes by current clinical and viral-isolation procedures. N Engl J Med 326:1533, 1992.

Krebs HB, Helmkamp F: Chronic ulcerations following topical therapy with 5-fluorouracil for vaginal human papillomavirus-associated lesions. Obstet Gynecol 78:205, 1991.

Krieger JN, Jenny C, Verdon M, et al: Clinical manifestations of trichomoniasis in men. Ann Intern Med 118:844, 1993.

Krieger JN, Tam MR, Stevens CE, et al: Diagnosis of trichomoniasis: Comparison of conventional wet-mount examination with cytologic studies, cultures, and monoclonal antibody staining of direct specimens. JAMA 259:1223, 1988.
Langenberg AGM, Corey L, Ashley RL, et al: A prospective study of new infections with herpes simplex virus type 1 and type 2. N Engl J Med 341:1432, 1999.
Larsen B, White S: Antifungal effect of hydrogen peroxide on catalase-producing strains of *Candida* spp. Infect Dis Obstet Gynecol 3:73, 1995.
Lee YH, Rankin JS, Alpert S, et al: Microbiological investigation of Bartholin's gland abscesses and cysts. Am J Obstet Gynecol 129:150, 1977.
Lipsky MS, Waters T, Sharp LK: Impact of vaginal antifungal products on utilization of health care services: Evidence from physician visits. J Am Board Fam Pract 13:178, 2001.
Livengood CH III, McGregor JA, Soper DE, et al: Bacterial vaginosis: Efficacy and safety of intravaginal metronidazole treatment. Am J Obstet Gynecol 170:759, 1994.
Livengood CH III, Soper DE, Sheehan KL, et al: Comparison of once-daily and twice-daily dosing of 0.75% metronidazole gel in the treatment of bacterial vaginosis. Sex Transmit Dis 26:137, 1999.
Louv WC, Austin H, Perlman J, Alexander WJ: Oral contraceptive use and the risk of chlamydial and gonococcal infections. Am J Obstet Gynecol 160:396, 1989.
Lytle CD, Carney PG, Vohra S, et al: Virus leakage through natural membrane condoms. Sex Transm Dis 17:58, 1990.
MacDermott RIJ: Bacterial vaginosis. Br J Obstet Gynaecol 102:92, 1995.
Madico G, Quinn TC, Rompalo A, et al: Diagnosis of *Trichomonas vaginalis* infection by PCR using vaginal swab samples. J Clin Microbiol 36:3205, 1998.
Manders SM: Toxin-mediated streptococcal and staphylococcal disease. J Am Acad Dermatol 39:383, 1998.
Marliére V, Roul S, Labréze C, and Taïeb A: Crusted (Norwegian) scabies induced by use of topical corticosteroids and treated successfully with ivermectin. J Pediatr 135:122, 1999.
Martin DH, DiCarlo RP: Recent changes in the epidemiology of genital ulcer disease in the United States: The crack cocaine connection. Sex Transm Dis 21(S2):S76, 1994.
Martin DH, Mroczkowski TF, Dalu ZA, et al: A controlled trial of a single dose of azithromycin for the treatment of chlamydial urethritis and cervicitis. N Engl J Med 327:921, 1992.
Maskell R: Broadening the concept of urinary tract infection. Br J Urol 76:2, 1995.
Maunder JW: Lice and scabies: myths and reality. Sex Transmit Dis 16:843, 1998.
Maw RD: Treatment of anogenital warts. Dermatol Clin 16:829, 1998.
McCarty JM: Azithromycin (Zithromax). Infect Dis Obstet Gynecol 4:215, 1996.
McLachlin CM: Pathology of human papillomavirus in the female genital tract. Curr Opin Obstet Gynecol 7:24, 1995.
McLellan R, Spence MR, Brackman M, et al: The clinical diagnosis of trichomoniasis. Obstet Gynecol 60:30, 1982.
Meikle SF, Zhang X, Marine WM, et al: *Chlamydia trachomatis* antibody titers and hysterosalpingography in predicting tubal disease in infertility patients. Fertil Steril 62:305, 1994.
Merkus JMWM, Bisschop MPJM, Stolte LAM: The proper nature of vaginal candidosis and the problem of recurrence. Obstet Gynecol Surv 40:493, 1985.
Mertz GJ, Benedetti J, Ashely R, et al: Risk factors for the sexual transmission of genital herpes. Ann Intern Med 116:197, 1992.
Montes LG, Wilborn WH: Fungus-host relationship in candidiasis. Arch Dermatol 121:119, 1985.
Morrow RA, Friedrich D, Meier A, Corey L: Use of "biokit HSV-2 Rapid Assay" to improve the positive predictive value of Focus HerpeSelect HSV-2 ELISA. BMC Infect Dis 14; 5:84, 2005.
Moscicki AB, Shiboski S, Broering J, et al: The natural history of human papillomavirus infection as measured by repeated DNA testing in adolescent and young women. J Pediatr 132:277, 1998.
Mroczkowski TF, Martin DH: Genital ulcer disease. Dermatol Clin 12:753, 1994.
Nahas GT, Goldstein BA, Zhu WY, et al: Comparison of Tzanck smear, viral culture, and DNA diagnostic methods in detection of herpes simplex and varicella-zoster infection. JAMA 268:2541, 1992.
Nandwani R, Evans DTP: Are you sure it's syphilis? A review of false positive serology. Int J STD AIDS, 6:241, 1995.
Neri A, Rabinerson D, Kaplan B: Bacterial vaginosis: Drugs versus alternative treatment. Obstet Gyncol Surv 49:809, 1994.
Nilsen AE, Aasen T, Halsos AM, et al: Efficacy of oral acyclovir in the treatment of initial and recurrent genital herpes. Lancet 2:571, 1982.
Nuovo GJ, Pedemonte BM: Human papillomavirus types and recurrent cervical warts. JAMA 263:1223, 1990.
Nyirjesy P, Seeney SM, Grody MHT, et al: Chronic fungal vaginitis: the value of cultures. Am J Obstet Gynecol 173:820, 1995.
Oriel JD: Natural history of genital warts. Br J Vener Dis 47:1, 1971.
Oriel JD: The increase in molluscum contagiosum. Br Med J 294:74, 1987.
Oriel JD, Partridge BM, Denny MJ, et al: Genital yeast infections. Br Med J 4:761, 1972.
Ortiz-Zepeda C, Hernandez-Perez E, Marroquin-Burgos R: Gross and microscopic features in chancroid: A study in 200 new culture-proven cases in San Salvador. Sex Trans Dis 21:112, 1994.
Patterson BA, Garland SM, Bowden FJ, et al: The diagnosis of *Trichomonas vaginalis*: New advances. Int J STD AIDS 10:68, 1999.
Pearlman MD, Yashar C, Ernst S, Solomon W: An incremental dosing protocol for women with severe vaginal trichomoniasis and adverse reactions to metronidazole. Am J Obstet Gynecol 174:934, 1996.
Peipert JF, Montagno AB, Cooper AS, Sung CJ: Bacterial vaginosis as a risk factor for upper genital tract infection. Am J Obstet Gynecol 177:1184, 1997.
Pfeifer TA, Forsyth PS, Durfee MA, et al: Nonspecific vaginitis: Role of *Haemophilus vaginalis* and treatment with metronidazole. N Engl J Med 298:1429, 1978.
Potter J: Should sexual partners of women with bacterial vaginosis receive treatment? Br J Gen Pract 49:913, 1999.
Priestley CJF, Jones BM, Dhar J, Goodwin L: What is normal vaginal flora? Genitourin Med 73:23: 1997.
Ralph SG, Rutherford AJ, Wilson JD: Influence of bacterial vaginosis on conception and miscarriage in the first trimester: cohort study. BMJ 319:220, 1999.
Raz R, Stamm WE: A controlled trial of intravaginal estriol in postmenopausal women with recurrent urinary tract infections. N Engl J Med 329:753, 1993.
Redondo-Lopez V, Lynch M, Schmitt C, et al: *Torulopsis glabrata* vaginitis: Clinical aspects and susceptibility to antifungal agents. Obstet Gynecol 76:651, 1990.
Reduced incidence of menstrual toxic-shock syndromes: United States 1980–1990. MMWR Morb Mortal Wkly Rep 39:421, 1990.
Reingold AL, Broome CV, Gaventa S, Hightower AW: Risk factors for menstrual toxic shock syndrome: Results of a multistate case-control study. Rev Infect Dis 11 Suppl 1:S35, 1989.
Richart RM, Nuovo GJ: Human papillomavirus DNA in situ hybridization may be used for the quality control of genital tract biopsies. Obstet Gynecol 75:223, 1990.
Rigg D, Miller MM, Metzger WJ: Recurrent allergic vulvovaginitis: Treatment with *Candida albicans* allergen immunotherapy. Am J Obstet Gynecol 162:332, 1990.
Rolfs RT: Treatment of syphilis, 1993. Clin Infect Dis 20(S1):S23, 1995.
Rooney JF, Straus SE, Mannix ML, et al: Oral acyclovir to suppress frequently recurrent herpes labialis: A double-blind, placebo-controlled trial. Ann Intern Med 118:268, 1993.
Rosen DJD, Margolin ML, Menashe Y, Greenspoon JS: Toxic shock syndrome after loop electrosurgical excision procedure. Am J Obstet Gynecol 169:202,1993.
Rosen T, Brown TJ: Genital ulcers: Evaluation and treatment. Sex Transm Dis 16:673, 1998.
Ross RA, Lee MT, Onderdonk AB: Effect of *Candida albicans* infection and clotrimazole treatment on vaginal microflora in vitro. Obstet Gynecol 86:925, 1995.
Royce RA, Jackson TP, Thorp JM Jr, et al: Race/ethnicity, vaginal flora patterns, and pH during pregnancy. Sex Transm Dis 26:96, 1999.
Sacks SL: Famciclovir (FAMVIR). Infect Dis Obstet Gynecol 5:3, 1997.
Sanguineti A, Carmichael K, Campbell K: Fluconazole-resistant *Candida albicans* after long-term suppressive therapy. Arch Intern Med 153:1122, 1993.
Schulte JM, Schmid GP: Recommendations for treatment of chancroid, 1993. Clin Infect Dis 20(S1):S39, 1995.
Schwarcz SK, Zenilman JM, Schnell D, et al: National surveillance of antimicrobial resistance in *Neisseria gonorrhoeae.* JAMA 264:1413, 1990.

Schwartz B, Gaventa S, Broome CV, et al: Nonmenstrual toxic shock syndrome associated with barrier contraceptives: Report of a case-controlled study. Rev Infect Dis 11:S43, 1989.
Schwebke JR: Abnormal vaginal flora as a biological risk factor for acquisition of HIV infection and sexually transmitted diseases. J Infect Dis 192:1315, 2005.
Schwebke JR, Schulien MB, Zajackowski M: Pilot study to evaluate the appropriate management of patients with coexistent bacterial vaginosis and cervicitis. Infect Dis Obstet Gynecol 3:119, 1995.
Shah PN, Kell PD, Barton SE: Gynaecological disorders and human immunodeficiency virus infection. Int J STD AIDS 5:383, 1994.
Sjöberg I, Hakansson S: Endotoxin in vaginal fluid of women with bacterial vaginosis. Obstet Gynecol 77:265, 1991.
Smith KL, Yeager J, Skelton H: Molluscum contagiosum: Its clinical, histopathologic, and immunohistochemical spectrum. Int J Dermatol 38:664, 1999.
Sobel JD: Vaginitis. N Engl J Med 337:1896, 1997.
Sobel JD, Brooker D, Stein GE, et al: Single dose fluconazole compared with conventional clotrimazole topical therapy of *Candida* vaginitis. Am J Obstet Gynecol 172:1263, 1995.
Sobel JD, Chaim W: Treatment of *Torulopsis glabrata* vaginitis: Retrospective review of boric acid therapy. Clin Infect Dis 24:649, 1997.
Sobel JD, Chaim W, Nagappan V, Leaman D: Treatment of vaginitis caused by Candida glabrata: Use of topical boric acid and flucytosine. Am J Obstet Gynecol 189: 1297, 2003.
Sobel JD, Faro S, Force RW, et al: Vulvovaginal candidiasis: Epidemiologic, diagnostic, and therapeutic considerations. Am J Obstet Gynecol 178:203, 1998.
Sobel JD, Kapernick PS, Zervos M, et al: Treatment of complicated candida vaginitis: Comparison of single and sequential doses of fluconazole. Am J Obstet Gynecol 185:363, 2001.
Soper DE: Bacterial vaginosis and trichomoniasis: Epidemiology and management of recurrent disease. Infect Dis Obstet Gynecol 2:242, 1995.
Soper DE: Gynecologic sequelae of bacterial vaginosis. Int J Gynecol Obstet 67:S25, 1999.
Soper DE, Bump RC, Hurt WG: Bacterial vaginosis and trichomoniasis vaginitis are risk factors for cuff cellulites after abdominal hysterectomy. Am J Obstet Gynecol 163:1016, 1990.
Spinillo A, Capuzzo E, Egbe TO, et al: *Torulopsis glabrata* vaginitis. Obstet Gynecol 85:993, 1995.
Spruance SL, Stewart JCB, Rowe NH, et al: Treatment of recurrent herpes simplex labialis with oral acyclovir. J Infect Dis 161:185, 1990.
Staary A, Schuh E, Kerschbaumer M, et al: Performance of transcription-mediated amplification and ligase chain reaction assays for detection of chlamydial infection in urogenital samples obtained by invasive and noninvasive methods. J Clin Microbiol 36:2666, 1998.
Stamm WE: An epidemic of urinary tract infections? N Engl J Med 345, 2001.
Stamm WE, Hooton TM: Management of urinary tract infections in adults. N Engl J Med 329:1328, 1993.
Stamm WE, Wagner KF, Amsel R, et al: Causes of the acute urethral syndrome in women. N Engl J Med 303:409, 1980.
Stanberry LR: Control of STDs-the role of prophylactic vaccines against herpes simplex virus, Sex Transm Dis 74:391, 1998.
Stapleton A, Stamm WE: Prevention of urinary tract infection. Infect Dis Clin North Am 11:719, 1997.
Stern JE, Givan AL, Gonzalez JL, et al: Leukocytes in the cervix: A quantitative evaluation of cervicitis. Obstet Gynecol 91:987, 1998.
St. Louis ME, Wasserheit JN: Elimination of syphilis in the United States. Science 281:353, 1998.
Sumners D, Kelsey M, Chait I: Psychological aspects of lower urinary tract infections in women. BMJ 304:17, 1992.
Sweet RL: The enigmatic cervix. Dermatol Clin 16:739, 1998.
Sweet RL, Gibbs RS: Infectious Diseases of the Female Genital Tract, 3rd ed. Baltimore, Williams & Wilkins, 1995.
Tice AD: Short-course therapy of acute cystitis: A brief review of therapeutic strategies. J Antimicrob Chemother 43(SA):85, 1999.
Tidwell BH, Lushbaugh WB, Laughlin MD, et al: A double-blind placebo-controlled trial of single-dose intravaginal versus single-dose oral metronidazole in the treatment of trichomonal vaginitis. J Infect Dis 170:242, 1994.
Tierno PM, Hanna BA: Propensity of tampons and barrier contraceptives to amplify *Staphylococcus aureus* toxic shock syndrome toxin-1. Infect Dis Obstet Gynecol 2:140, 1994.
Usha V, Nair TVG: A comparative study of oral ivermectin and topical permethrin cream in the treatment of scabies. J Am Acad Dermatol 42:236, 2000.
Van Slyke KK, Michel VP, Rein MF: Treatment of vulvovaginal candidiasis with boric acid powder. Am J Obstet Gynecol 141:145, 1981.
Van Kessel K, Assefi N, Marrazzo J, Eckert L: Common complementary and alternative therapies for yeast vaginitis and bacterial vaginosis: a systematic review. Obstet Gynecol Surv 58: 351, 2003.
Vejtorp M, Bollerup AC, Vejtorp L, et al: Bacterial vaginosis: A double-blind randomized trial of the effect of treatment of the sexual partner. Br J Obstet Gynaecol 95:920, 1988.
Von Krogh G, Hellberg D: Self-treatment using a 0.5% podophyllotoxin cream of external genital condylomata acuminata in women: A placebo-controlled, double-blind study. Sex Transm Dis 19:170, 1992.
Wain AM: Metronidazole vaginal gel 0.75% (MetroGel-Vaginal): a brief review, Infect Dis Obstet Gynecol 6:3, 1998.
Wald A, Langenberg G, Krantz E, et al: The relationship between condom use and herpes simplex virus acquisition. Ann Intern Med 15;143(10):707, 2005.
Wald A, Zeh J, Selke S, et al: Reactivation of genital herpes simplex virus type 2 infection in asymptomatic seropositive persons. N Engl J Med 342:844, 2000.
Wang J: Trichomoniasis. Prim Care Update 7:148, 2000.
Washington AE, Gove S, Schachter J, et al: Oral contraceptives, *Chlamydia trachomatis* infection, and pelvic inflammatory disease. JAMA 253:2246, 1985.
Watts DH, Krohn MA, Hillier SL, Eschenbach DA: Bacterial vaginosis as a risk factor for post-cesarean endometritis. Obstet Gynecol 75:52, 1990.
Waugh MA: Molluscum contagiosum. Dermatol Clin 16:839, 1998.
Williams LA, Klausner JD, Whittington WLH, et al: Elimination and reintroduction of primary and secondary syphilis. Am J Public Health 89:1093, 1999.
Wisenfeld HC, Heine RP, Rideout A, et al: The vaginal introitus: A novel site for *Chlamydia trachomatis* testing in women. Am J Obstet Gynecol 174:1542, 1996.
Witkin SS, Inglis SR, Polaneczky M: Detection of *Chlamydia trachomatis* and *Trichomonas vaginalis* by polymerase chain reaction in introital specimens from pregnant women. Am J Obstet Gynecol 175:165, 1996.
Word B: Office treatment of cyst and abscess of Bartholin's gland duct. South Med J 61:514, 1968.
Workowski KA, Lampe MF, Wong KG, et al: Long-term eradication of *Chlamydia trachomatis* genital infection after antimicrobial therapy: Evidence against persistent infection. JAMA 270:2071, 1993.
Zhang L, Ramratnam B, Tenner-Racz K, et al: Quantifying residual HIV-1 replication in patients receiving combination antiretroviral therapy. N Engl J Med 340:1605, 1999.

Infections of the Upper Genital Tract 23

Endometritis, Acute and Chronic Salpingitis

Linda O. Eckert and Gretchen M. Lentz

KEY TERMS AND DEFINITIONS

Atypical, or Silent, Pelvic Inflammatory Disease. Relatively asymptomatic inflammation of the upper genital tract.

Canaliculus. A small, canallike opening forming a channel for ascension of bacteria from the lower to the upper genital tract.

Commensal Bacteria. An organism that may exist in the genital tract without causing disease.

Fitz-Hugh–Curtis Syndrome. A syndrome of perihepatic inflammation that develops in 5% to 10% of women with acute pelvic inflammatory disease, originating from transperitoneal or vascular dissemination of either *Neisseria gonorrhoeae* or *Chlamydia trachomatis.*

Hydrosalpinx. A collection of watery, sterile fluid in the fallopian tube, secondary to tubal obstruction, an end stage of a pyosalpinx.

Multidrug-Resistant Tuberculosis. Infection from *Mycobacterium tuberculosis* that is resistant to two or more antituberculin drugs, including isoniazid.

Nonoxynol 9. A chemical detergent used in spermicidal preparations that is also bactericidal and viricidal.

Penicillinase-Producing Gonorrhea. Strains of *N. gonorrhoeae* that become resistant to penicillin by acquiring a resistance factor plasmid that enables the gonococcus to produce an enzyme that destroys penicillin.

Pelvic Inflammatory Disease. A nonspecific term that most commonly refers to inflammation caused by infection in the upper genital tract; often used synonymously with the term *acute salpingitis.*

Tuboovarian Complex. A collection of pus within an anatomic space created by adherence of adjacent organs, involving the oviducts, ovaries, and sometimes the intestines.

This chapter considers upper genital tract infections. The primary focus is on acute pelvic inflammatory disease (PID), which is one of the major manifestations of sexually transmitted diseases (STDs). This discussion considers the epidemiology, diagnosis, and treatment of acute PID. The three major sequelae of PID are ectopic pregnancies, chronic pain, and infertility. This chapter will also consider uncommon causes of upper genital tract infection, such as tuberculosis and actinomycosis. For more detail on the infections with *Neisseria gonorrhoeae* and *Chlamydia trachomatis,* the reader is referred to Chapter 22 (Infections of the Lower Genital Tract).

The Centers for Disease Control and Prevention (CDC) regularly revises its treatment protocols for STDs. The recommendations and medications in this edition are based on the 2006 CDC guidelines. Readers are urged to consult any updates in CDC guidelines, since bacterial resistance to antibiotics and epidemiologic concerns may lead to changes in treatment protocols. This information may be accessed online at www.cdc.gov/publications.htm.

ENDOMETRITIS

Nonpuerperal endometritis is infection of the uterine lining. Although endometritis commonly coexists with salpingitis, recently many studies support endometritis as a distinct clinical syndrome. In one large study of 152 women with suspected PID who all underwent laparoscopy and endometrial biopsy, 43 (28%) had neither endometritis nor salpingitis, 26 (17%) had isolated endometritis, and 83 (55%) had acute salpingitis. Those with endometritis alone had distinct risk factors (douching in last 30 days, current IUD in place, and in days 1 to 7 of menstrual cycle). Also, among those women with suspected PID, endometritis was associated with clinical manifestations (cervical motion tenderness, rebound, fever) and infection with *N. gonorrhoeae* and *C. trachomatis* (or both) intermediate in frequency between women with salpingitis and those with neither salpingitis nor endometritis.

The "gold standard" diagnosis of endometritis is based on endometrial biopsy. At least one plasma cell per 120× field of endometrial stroma combined with five or more neutrophils in the superficial endometrial epithelium per 400× field is the histopathologic criteria for endometritis. In severe cases, diffuse lymphocytes and plasma cells in the endometrial stroma or stromal necrosis may be present.

The concept of "subclinical" endometritis has evolved in part, because many women with tubal infertility have no history of clinical symptoms consistent with prior PID. Several large, cross-sectional studies in various geographic regions have studied women without any symptoms or signs of acute salpingitis (no cervical motion or adnexal or uterine tenderness) to further define subclinical endometritis. Most of these studies have been conducted in STD clinics or emergency rooms; endometritis is associated with young age (20 to 22 years old in most studies), abnormal uterine bleeding (menorrhagia or metrorrhagia), menstrual cycle day less than 14, douching in last 30 days, and history of prior PID

Lower genital tract infections with *C. trachomatis, N. gonorrhoeae,* bacterial vaginosis, *M. genitalium,* and *Trichomonas vaginalis* are associated with histologic endometritis with odds ratios of 1.5 to 3.0 depending on the study, as is mucopurulent cervicitis. One study demonstrated that in women with current *N. gonorrhoeae* or *C. trachomatis* infection, endometritis was apparent in 43% of women with a history of prior PID and 23% in women without prior PID. This is suggestive of possible immunologic memory. Some women with endometritis do not have an isolated pathogen.

Because many of the symptoms and signs associated with endometritis are subtle, a clinician needs to have a low threshold for performing an endometrial biopsy to aid in diagnosis. Treatment for endometritis is the same as outpatient salpingitis treatment (Table 23-1). Treatment should last 14 days. Addition of metronidazole should be strongly considered if the patient has bacterial vaginosis.

Antimicrobial therapy for endometritis is effective. One study demonstrated significant reduction in abnormal bleeding, cervicitis, uterine tenderness, and histologic endometritis following treatment with 400 mg orally of cefixime, 1000 mg of azithromycin, and 500 mg orally of metronidazole twice daily for 7 days. Endometritis in human immunodeficiency virus (HIV)-seropositive women has not been well characterized. One series of 42 seropositive women, none of whom had *C. trachomatis* or *N. gonorrhoeae* demonstrated a 38% prevalence of endometritis. Compared with the seropositive women without endometritis, the seropositive women with endometritis did not have increased uterine tenderness, lower CD4+ lymphocytes, or other findings. A small subset of those with endometritis had a repeat endometrial biopsy following antimicrobial therapy, and 50% of the endometritis resolved histologically. The authors concluded that endometritis in HIV-infected women might be related to pathogens that were not evaluated, to prior infection, or to reduced immunity from HIV.

The sequelae of endometritis distinct from salpingitis are difficult to determine. In a series of 614 women in the PID evaluation and clinical health (PEACH) study, women with either endometritis, or upper genital tract infection with *N. gonorrhoeae* or *C. trachomatis* or both were compared with women without endometritis or upper genital tract infection for outcomes of pregnancy, infertility, recurrent PID, and chronic pelvic pain. The women with endometritis or upper genital tract infection had higher age- and race-specific pregnancy rates than the national average after adjusting for age, race, education, PID history, and baseline infertility. In this group with clinically suspected mild PID treated with standard antimicrobial therapy, endometritis or upper genital tract infection was not associated with reproductive morbidity.

Table 23-1 Endometritis Treatment Regimens 2006 CDC Guidelines

Regimen A
Levofloxacin 500 mg PO daily for 14 days or ofloxacin 400 mg PO twice daily for 14 days
with or without
Metronidazole 500 mg PO twice daily for 14 days

Regimen B
Ceftriaxone 250 mg IM in a single dose and
Doxycycline 100 mg PO twice daily for 14 days
with or without
Metromidazole 500 mg PO twice daily for 14 days

PELVIC INFLAMMATORY DISEASE

PID is an infection in the upper genital tract not associated with pregnancy or intraperitoneal pelvic operations. Thus it may include infection of *any or all* of the following anatomic locations: the endometrium (endometritis) (see previous section) the oviducts (salpingitis), the ovary (oophoritis), the uterine wall (myometritis), the uterine serosa and broad ligaments (parametritis), and the pelvic peritoneum. Many authors prefer the term *salpingitis* because infection of the oviducts is the most characteristic and common component of PID. Importantly, most long-term sequelae of PID result from destruction of the tubal architecture by the infection. In most clinical situations the terms acute *salpingitis* and *pelvic inflammatory disease* are used synonymously to describe an acute infection.

The prevalence of STDs and corresponding PID is a major public health concern. However, the incidence of PID in the United States is decreasing. The decline in visit numbers is primarily due to aggressive *Chlamydia* screening and treatment programs nationwide. The estimated number of cases in women 15 to 44 years of age was 189,662 in 2002 and 168,837 in 2003 (national ambulatory medical care survey). The number of hospitalizations for acute PID steadily declined in the 1980s and 1990s and has subsequently remained constant at around 70,000 cases a year. Outpatient visits have also declined, though it is still the most common gynecologic cause for emergency department visits (350,000/year). Presently, it is estimated that the approximately 1 million annual cases of acute PID incurs a total cost of about $1.8 billion per year.

Reduction of the medical impact of acute PID requires aggressive therapy for lower genital tract infection and early diagnosis and treatment of upper genital tract infection. Public health emphasis also must be placed on primary prevention involving attempts to prevent exposure and acquisition of STD. This includes teaching adolescents safe sex practices and promoting the use of condoms and chemical barrier methods. Secondary prevention of PID involves universal screening of women at high risk for chlamydia and gonorrhea; screening for active cervicitis; increasing use of sensitive tests to diagnose lower genital infection; treatment of sexual partners; and education to prevent recurrent infection.

Acute PID results from ascending infection from the bacterial flora of the vagina and cervix in more than 99% of cases. This ascending infection occurs along the mucosal surface, resulting in bacterial colonization and infection of the endometrium and fallopian tubes. The process sometimes extends to the surface of the ovaries and nearby peritoneum and rarely into the adjacent soft tissues, such as the broad ligament and pelvic blood vessels. Acute PID is rare in the woman without menstrual periods, such as the pregnant, premenarcheal, or postmenopausal woman. In less than 1% of cases, acute PID results from transperitoneal spread of infectious material from a perforated appendix or intraabdominal abscess. Hematogenous and lymphatic spread to the tubes or ovaries is another remote possibility. Acute PID is usually a polymicrobial infection that is a mixture of aerobic and anaerobic bacteria clinically appearing as a complex infection. Therapeutic strategies and regimens are broad spectrum, seeking to suppress aerobic and anaerobic organisms. More than 20 species of microorganisms have been cultured from direct aspiration of purulent material from infected tubes. Acute PID is unlike an infection in many other areas of the body, which usually is caused predominantly by one species of microorganism.

Annually, acute PID occurs in 1% to 2% of all young, sexually active women. It is the most common serious infection of women ages 16 to 25. Approximately 85% of infections are spontaneous in sexually active females. The other 15% of infections develop following procedures that break the cervical mucus barrier, allowing the vaginal flora the opportunity to colonize the upper genital tract. These procedures include endometrial biopsy, curettage, intrauterine device (IUD) insertion, hysterosalpingography, and hysteroscopy. For emphasis, PID is extremely rare in women who are either amenorrheic or not sexually active. When PID is found in the postmenopausal woman, associated conditions such as genital malignancies; diabetes; or concurrent intestinal diseases, such as diverticulitis, appendicitis, or carcinoma are usually discovered.

One in four women with acute PID experiences medical sequelae. Conversely, many women with sequelae of the disease, such as infertility related to tubal obstruction, do not have a history of having had the symptoms or signs of an acute infection. Following acute PID, the rate of ectopic pregnancy increases 6- to 10-fold, and the chance of developing chronic pelvic pain increases 4-fold. In the United States each year 26,100 ectopic pregnancies and 90,000 new cases of chronic abdominal pain are directly related to PID. The incidence of infertility following acute PID varies widely (6% to 60%) depending on the severity of the infection, the number of episodes of infection, and the age of the patient. Weström reported that hospitalized patients have an incidence of infertility due to tubal obstruction of 11.4% after one episode of PID, 23.1% after two episodes, and 54.3% after three or more episodes. Women with one episode of acute PID are also more susceptible to developing a subsequent infection. It is difficult to distinguish whether this tendency is related primarily to mucosal damage or to reinfection by a potentially infected mate. Grimes has estimated that 0.29 deaths per 100,000 women ages 15 to 44 are directly related to PID.

The clinical symptoms and signs of acute PID vary considerably and are usually nonspecific. Importantly, some patients may have very little symptomatology, a condition called *silent,* or *asymptomatic, PID* (see Endometritis section).

Ideally, laparoscopy with direct visualization of the internal female organs would not only improve the diagnostic accuracy but also afford the opportunity for direct cultures of purulent material, which might help to establish optimum therapy. However, most women do not undergo this procedure because of the expense.

In summary, the CDC has emphasized that physicians should aggressively treat women if there is any suspicion of the disease, because the sequelae are so devastating and the clinical diagnosis made from symptoms, signs, and laboratory data is often incorrect.

Etiology

Acute PID is usually a polymicrobial infection caused by organisms ascending from the vagina and cervix along the mucosa of the endometrium to infect the mucosa of the oviduct. Two classic sexually transmitted organisms, *N. gonorrhoeae* and *C. trachomatis,* cause acute PID in many cases. These two organisms coexist in the same individual 25% to 50% of the time. Endogenous aerobic and anaerobic bacteria that originated from the normal vaginal flora are cultured from tubal fluid in approximately 50% of cases. In women with bacterial vaginosis (BV) and PID, BV-associated microorganisms have been isolated laparoscopically from the fallopian tubes, demonstrating ascension of these organisms. Direct cultures have proved that tubal infections are usually polymicrobial throughout the active infectious process. Sweet and colleagues discovered an average of seven different species in his series of intraabdominal cultures performed via the laparoscope. However, the type and number of species vary depending on the stage of the disease when the culture is obtained. For example, gonorrheal organisms are frequently cultured during the first 24 to 48 hours of the disease but are often absent later. Similarly, later in the disease process, anaerobic bacteria tend to predominate.

It used to be common practice to divide PID into gonococcal and nongonococcal disease depending on the recovery of *N. gonorrhoeae* from the endocervix. Laparoscopic studies have demonstrated a correlation of no better than 50% between endocervical and tubal cultures. Thus endocervical cultures are a crude index at best of the specific cause of upper genital tract infection.

Because of the virulence of *N. gonorrhoeae* in both in vitro and in vivo studies, its major role in PID is well established. Approximately 15% of women with cervical infection by *N. gonorrhoeae* subsequently develop acute PID. Approximately 50% of women with endocervical cultures positive for *N. gonorrhoeae* at the time of acute PID will have the same organism cultured from the fallopian tubes. If *N. gonorrhoeae* is the only organism cultured from the tubes, a patient will usually respond rapidly to treatment.

The virulence of the strain or colony type of *N. gonorrhoeae* helps to predict the incidence of upper genital tract infection. Transparent colonies of *N. gonorrhoeae* on culture medium attach more readily to epithelial cells and thus produce tubal infection more frequently than opaque-appearing colonies. Immunologic studies have demonstrated that an antibody against the outer membrane protein of the gonococcus develops in approximately 70% of women following severe pelvic infection. The lack of significant antibody titers may help explain why teenagers are more likely to develop upper genital tract disease than women in their late 20s.

There is an extremely wide variation in the recovery rates of *N. gonorrhoeae* depending on the geographic location of the study (Table 23-2). Because these tables are generated from laparoscopic data, and laparoscopy is now infrequently used in the diagnosis of acute salpingitis, more recent data on geographic

Table 23-2 Comparison of *Chlamydia trachomatis* and *Neisseria gonorrhoeae* Cervical Isolation and *N. gonorrhoeae* Tubal Isolation among Women with Acute PID

		CERVICAL INFECTION		TUBAL/PERITONEAL INFECTION*
First Author of Study†	**No. of Patients**	***C. trachomatis***	***N. gonorrhoeae***	***N. gonorrhoeae***
Henry-Suchet	17	6/16 (38%)	0/4	1/4 (25%)
Møller	166	37 (22%)	9 (5%)	
Mårdh	60	23 (38%)	4 (5%)	
Gjønnaess	65	26/56 (46%)	5 (8%)	0/65
Mårdh	63	19/53 (36%)	11 (17%)	1/14 (7%)
Adler	78	4 (5%)	14 (18%)	
Ripa	206	52/156 (33%)	39 (19%)	
Osser	209	52/111 (47%)	41 (20%)	
Paavonen	106	27 (25%)	27 (25%)	
Paavonen	101	32 (32%)	25 (25%)	
Paavonen	228	69 (30%)	60 (26%)	
Eilard	22	6 (27%)	7 (32%)	1/22 (5%)
Bowie	43	22 (51%)	15 (35%)	
Eschenbach	204	20/100 (20%)	90 (44%)	7/54 (13%)
Sweet	39	2 (5%)	18 (46%)	8/35 (23%)
Cunningham	104		56 (54%)	30/104 (29%)
Thompson	30	3 (10%)	24 (80%)	10/30 (33%)
Total	1741	400/1365 (29%)	445/1728 (26%)	58/328 (18%)

*Isolation of *N. gonorrhoeae* from the peritoneum of the total number of woman studied.
†Reference to studies appear in original source.
From Eschenbach DA: Acute pelvic inflammatory disease, vol 1. In Gynecology and Obstetrics, Philadelphia, Harper & Row, 1985, p 8.

variations in tubal isolates of *C. trachomatis* and *N. gonorrhoeae* are not available. However, the prevalence of *N. gonorrhoeae* cervicitis in young women is significantly increased in the South and southeastern regions of the United States. Therefore the proportion of patients with salpingitis from *N. gonorrhoeae* in these regions is likely much higher than in the Pacific Northwest or other geographic regions with low gonorrhea prevalence.

Once the gonococcus ascends to the fallopian tube, it selectively adheres to nonciliated mucus-secreting cells. However, the majority of damage occurs to the ciliated cells, most likely due to an acute complement-mediated inflammatory response with migration of polymorphonuclear leukocytes, vasodilation, and transudation of plasma into the tissues (Figs. 23-1 and 23-2). This robust inflammatory response causes cell death and tissue damage. The process of repair with removal of dead cells and fibroblast presence results in scarring and tubal adhesions.

C. trachomatis is an intracellular, sexually transmitted bacterial pathogen. A report from Edinburgh found a ratio of chlamydial to gonococcal PID diagnosed by laparoscopy of 4:1. However, there is a widespread difference in isolation rates depending on the series and the geographic location (Table 23-3). One of the primary reasons that chlamydial organisms were not recovered in early studies in the United States was the reluctance to perform a biopsy of the fallopian tubes to obtain culture material. Recently, chlamydia has become more prevalent than gonorrhea. From 205 to 40% of sexually active women have

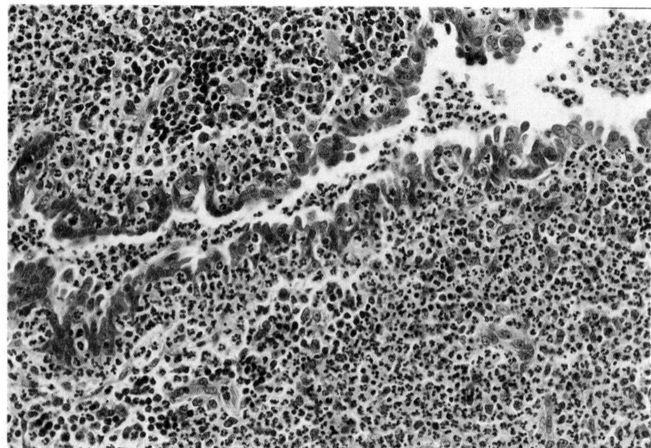

Figure 23-1. Acute salpingitis with a mixture of neutrophils, lymphocytes, and plasma cells in the fallopian tube destroying some of the epithelial lining. (From Voet RL: Color Atlas of Obstetric and Gynecologic Pathology. St. Louis, Mosby, 1997, p 107.)

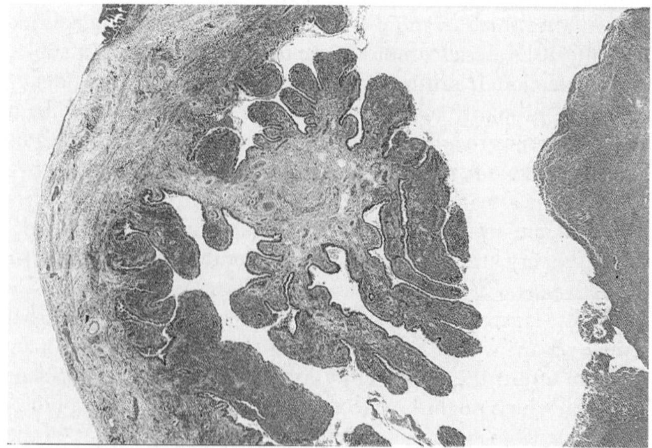

Figure 23-2. Acute salpingitis showing dilatation of the fallopian tube and blunting of the papillary fronds. (From Voet RL: Color Atlas of Obstetric and Gynecologic Pathology. St. Louis, Mosby, 1997, p 102.)

Table 23-3 *Chlamydia trachomatis* in Acute Pelvic Inflammatory Disease

		ISOLATION RATE OF *C. TRACHOMATIS*		
Study (ref)*	**Number of Patients**	**Endocervix (%)**	**Upper Genital and Peritoneal Cavity (%)**	**Fourfold Rise in Serum Antibodies (%)**
Eilard et al	22	6 (27)	2 (9)[†]	5 (23)
Mårdh et al	53	19 (37)	6/20 (30)[†]	
Treharne et al	143			88 (62)[‡]
Paavonen et al	106	27 (26)		19/72 (26)
Paavonen	228	68 (30)		32/167 (19)
Mårdh et al	60	23 (38)		24/60 (40)
Ripa et al	206	52/156 (33)		118 (57)[¶]
Gjønnaess et al	56	26 (46)	5/42 (12)[†]	26/52 (46)
Møller et al	166	37 (22)		34 (21)
Osser and Persson	111	52 (47)		37/72 (51)
Eschenbach et al	100	20 (20)	1/54 (2)[§]	15/74 (20)
Sweet et al	37	2 (5)	0[†]	5/22 (23)
Thompson et al	30	3 (10)	3 (10)**	
Sweet et al	71	10 (14)	17 (24)[††]	
Wasserheit et al	22	10 (45)	8 (36)[††]	
Kiviat et al	55	12 (22)	12 (22)[††]	
Brunham et al	50	7 (14)	4 (8)**	20 (40)
Landers et al	148	41 (28)	32 (22)[††]	
Soper et al	84	13 (15)	1 (1)** 6 (7)[††]	
Kiviat et al	69		16 (23)	

*References appear in the original source.
[†]Fallopian tube.
[‡]Chlamydial IgG ≥ 1:64; 23% had IgM = 1:8.
[¶]Chlamydial IgG ≥ 1:64; fourfold rise in 28/80 (35%).
[§]Culdocentesis.
**Exudate from fallopian tube.
[††]Fallopian tube and/or endometrial cavity
From Sweet RL, Gibbs RS: Infectious Diseases of the Female Genital Tract, 3rd ed. Baltimore, Williams & Wilkins, 1995.

antibodies against *C. trachomatis.* From 10% to 30% of women with acute PID who do not have cultures positive for *Chlamydia* have evidence of acute chlamydial infection by serial antibody titer testing. Overall, *Chlamydia* is involved in at least 40% of women who are hospitalized with PID. Approximately 30% of women with documented acute cervicitis secondary to chlamydia subsequently develop acute PID. Studies have shown upper tract chlamydial infection increases the risk of an ectopic pregnancy from three to six times compared with women without chlamydial infection.

Whereas *N. gonorrhoeae* remains in the fallopian tubes for at most a few days in untreated patients, *Chlamydia* may remain in the fallopian tubes for months after initial colonization of the upper genital tract. It has been detected in tubes of macaques despite adequate antimicrobial therapy and resolution of cervical infection.

Sophisticated polymerase chain reaction (PCR), in situ hybridization, and electron microscopy studies demonstrate persistence of the *C. trachomatis* in the fallopian tubes for years. Whether this represents persistent or recurrent infection of the upper genital tract is unknown.

Cell-mediated immune mechanisms appear to be important in tissue destruction associated with *C. trachomatis* infection. Primary infection appears to be self-limited with mild symptoms and little permanent damage. In animals, repeat genital exposures to *C. trachomatis* can induce a chronic hypersensitivity response to chlamydial antigens. Because chlamydial 57-kDa protein and human 60-kDa heat shock protein have homologous regions, repeat exposures to *Chlamydia,* such as may occur in asymptomatic untreated *C. trachomatis* cervical infection, may lead to an autoimmune circuit causing severe tubal damage even if *C. trachomatis* is no longer present. Immunologically sensitized studies have demonstrated that women with antibodies to chlamydial heat shock protein are more likely to have severe tubal scarring and Fitz-Hugh–Curtis syndrome (adhesions between the liver and diaphragm indicating prior peritonitis) than women who do not mount this antibody response. Recent basic research has demonstrated a genetic modulation of the immune response to *C. trachomatis* infection with an increased risk in women with HLA-1. Preliminary evidence suggests that the specific chlamydial strain also may be an important variable.

The past decade has produced a clinical awareness of a syndrome called *atypical,* or *silent, PID.* This is an asymptomatic, or relatively asymptomatic, inflammation of the upper genital tract often associated with chlamydial infection. The sequelae of repeated asymptomatic chlamydial infections are tubal infertility and ectopic pregnancy. Some investigators believe that atypical PID may be the more common form of upper tract infection, and symptomatic PID may be but the "tip of the iceberg." As many as 40% of women with cervicitis without upper tract symptoms will also have endometritis noted on endometrial biopsy. Studies of women with tubal infertility have noted that many women, though not diagnosed as having had overt PID, have had symptoms of acute pelvic pain (see Endometritis section).

The role of genital mycoplasmas in the etiology of acute PID is unclear. Cervical cultures positive for both *Mycoplasma hominis* and *Ureaplasma urealyticum* may be obtained from the majority of young, sexually active women. The rate of isolation of genital mycoplasmas from the cervix is approximately 75% and similar in populations of women who are sexually active both with and without PID.

Direct tubal cultures demonstrated *M. hominis* in 4% to 17% and *U. urealyticum* in 2% to 20% of women with acute PID. However, serologic studies in women with acute PID have demonstrated that only one woman in four develops a significant rise in antibody titers to these organisms. Experimental inoculation of the cervix of the Grivet monkey demonstrated that the route of spread of mycoplasmas is via the parametria rather than the mucosa. Thus the primary upper genital tract infection is in the parametria and the tissue surrounding the tubes, not in the tubal lumen. This fact may help to explain the low success rate of direct tubal cultures. Histologically, *Mycoplasma* does not appear to produce damage to the tubal mucosa. These organisms are not highly pathogenic. A recent study by Chatwani and coworkers demonstrated that the presence of genital mycoplasmas does not change the clinical presentation and clinical course of acute PID. The investigators found that both *M. hominis* and *U. urealyticum* may colonize or persist in the endometrial cavity after complete recovery from acute PID. In summary, in vitro and in vivo studies suggest that *Mycoplasma* may be a commensal bacterium rather than a pathogen in the oviducts.

However, recently *M. genitalium,* which is nonculturable and identified by PCR, is associated with cervicitis, endometritis, and tubal factor infertility. In one study of 123 women with laparoscopically determined acute salpingitis, *M. genitalium* was detected in 9 (7%), laparoscopically women, including 1 woman with a positive fallopian tube specimen. In a different study, *M. genitalium* was detected in the cervix, endometrium, or both of 58 women with histologically confirmed endometritis.

The endogenous aerobic and anaerobic flora of the vagina frequently ascend to colonize and infect the upper reproductive tract. Direct cultures of purulent material (Fig. 23-3) from the tubal lumen or posterior cul-de-sac have demonstrated a wide range of organisms. The most common aerobic organisms are nonhemolytic *Streptococcus, Escherichia coli,* group B *Streptococcus,* and coagulase-negative *Staphylococcus.* Anaerobic organisms tend to predominate over aerobes, and the most common anaerobic organisms are *Bacteroides* species, *Peptostreptococcus,* and *Peptococcus.* Anaerobic organisms are almost ubiquitous in pelvic abscesses associated with acute PID. Tuboovarian complexes and abscesses are more common in women with concurrent bacterial vaginosis or HIV infection. The finding of concurrent bacterial vaginosis and PID, as well as the association of bacterial vaginosis with endometritis, serve to emphasize the contributory role of these organisms in the pathogenesis of PID. Regardless of the initiating event, the microbiology of PID should be treated as mixed. In addition, BV-associated organisms have been isolated from fallopian tubes of women with salpingitis and in women with endometriosis.

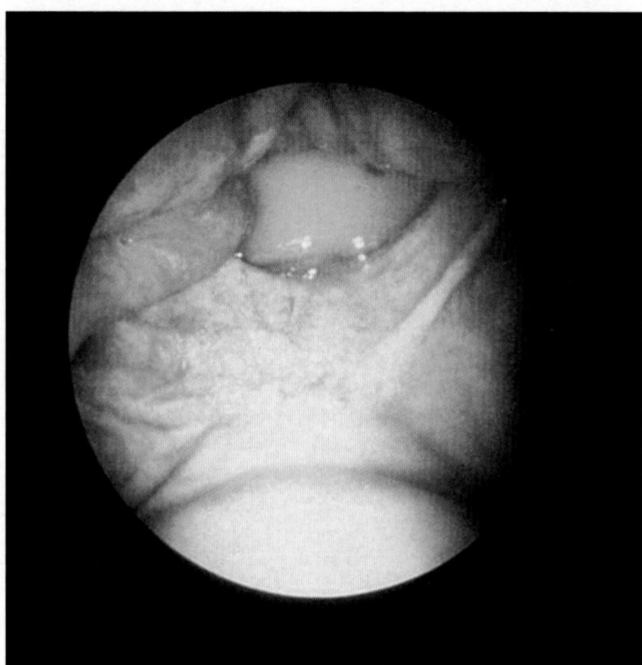

Figure 23-3. Laparoscopic view of the pouch of Douglas with pus from acute PID.

Risk Factors

Risk factors are important considerations in both the clinical management and prevention of upper genital tract infections. In a case-control study among sexually active, inner city adolescents, younger age at first intercourse, older sex partners, involvement with a child protective agency, prior suicide attempt, alcohol use before intercourse, and current *C. trachomatis* infection were all significant risk factors for the development of PID. This study illustrates the multiple risk factors for PID. There is a strong correlation between the incidence of STD and acute PID in any given population. The age distribution of uncomplicated STD is usually the same as that for acute PID.

In epidemiologic studies, age at first intercourse, marital status, and number of sexual partners are all gross indicators of the frequency of exposure to STDs. Having multiple sexual partners increases the chance of acquiring acute PID approximately fivefold. The frequency of intercourse with a monogamous partner is not a risk factor.

The incidence of acute PID decreases with advancing age. Acute PID is a condition of young females, with 75% of cases occurring in women younger than 25 years of age. The risk that a sexually active adolescent female will develop acute PID is 1 in 8. This risk factor decreases to 1 in 80 for women older than age 25. The sexual behaviors of teenagers, including contact with multiple partners and lack of contraception, predispose them to STDs and, correspondingly, acute PID. Younger age also increases the incidence of acute PID. For unknown reasons young women with colonization of the cervix by *Chlamydia* have a higher incidence of upper genital tract infection than older women do. A hypothesis to explain the increased infection rate in teenagers includes the comparative lack of antibody protection and the wider area of cervical columnar epithelium, which allows colonization by *C. trachomatis* and *N. gonorrhoeae.*

Stone and associates have tabulated (Table 23-4) both proven and hypothetical methods of preventing STD and acute PID. Both clinical and laboratory studies have documented that the use of contraceptives changes the relative risk of developing acute PID.

Table 23-4 Methods of Preventing STDs, Mechanisms of Action, and Efficacy

Method	Mechanism	Efficacy in Prevention of STDs
Behavioral		
Monogamy Reducing number of partners Avoiding certain sexual practices Inspecting and questioning partners	Decreases likelihood of exposure to infected persons Decreases likelihood of contact with infectious agents	Not well studied; theoretic efficacy
Barriers		
Condom	Protects partner from direct contact with semen, urethral discharge, or penile lesion Protects wearer from direct contact with partner's mucosal secretions	Effective in vitro barrier to chlamydiae, CMV, and HIV, partial protection HSV Appears to decrease risk of acquiring urethral/cervical GC, PID, and male urethral *Ureaplasma* colonization; partial HPV protection Effect on risk of acquiring NGU not established
Spermicide	Chemically inactivates infectious agents	Nonvaginal use has not been studied Inactivates gonococci, syphilis spirochetes, trichomonads, HSC, ureaplasmas, and HIV in vitro. In vivo studies disappointing. 100 mg gel dose and contraceptive sponge associated with epithelial ulcers and abrasiors
Diaphragm/spermicide	Mechanical barrier covers cervix Used with spermicides	Diaphragm alone has not been studies Appears to decrease risk of acquiring cervical GC and PID
Vaccines	Induce antibody response that renders host immune to disease	Commercially available hepatitis B vaccine is safe and effective Results of clinical trials of gonococcal and herpes simplex vaccines ongoing Gonococcal, HIV, and HSV vaccines research in progress Effective guardravalent HPV vaccine safe and effective
Oral Antibiotics		
Penicillin	Kill infectious agent on or shortly after exposure before infection is established	No studies among women or civilian men
Sulfathioazole		Appears to decrease risk of acquiring GC and hard and soft chancres, but use not recommended
Tetracycline analogues		
Local		
Postcoital urination Postcoital washing	Flushes infectious agents out of urethra and washes infectious agents of genital skin and mucous membrane	Poorly studied
Postcoital antiseptic douching	Inactivates and washes infectious agents out of vagina	Poorly studied. Not recommended. Increases risk of endometritis

CMV, cytomegalovirus; GC, gonorrhea; HIV, human immunodeficiency virus; HPV, human papillomavirus; HSV, herpes simplex virus; NGU, nongonococcal urethritis. PID, pelvic inflammatory disease.
From Stone KM, Grimes DA, Magder LS: Primary prevention of sexually transmitted diseases. A primer for clinicians. JAMA 255:1763, 1986. Copyright 1986, American Medical Association.

Barrier methods (condoms, diaphragms, and spermicidal preparations) are effective both as mechanical obstructive devices and as chemical barriers. Nonoxynol 9, the material ubiquitous in spermicidal preparations, is both bactericidal and viricidal. Laboratory tests have demonstrated that nonoxynol 9 kills *N. gonorrhoeae,* genital *Mycoplasma* species, *Trichomonas vaginalis, Treponema pallidum,* herpes simplex virus, and HIV. However, microbicide trials with nonoxynol 9 have been disappointing. Doses of 100-mg gel, alone or in a contraceptive sponge, are associated with increased epithelial abrasions and ulcers. The porosity of latex in condoms is more than 1000 times smaller than viral particles. Thus routine condom use prevents deposition and transmission of infected organisms from the semen to the endocervix. Many studies have found that women who frequently use a vaginal douche have a threefold to fourfold increased relative risk of PID over women who douche less frequently than once a month.

Oral contraceptive use doubles the risk of cervicitis, but decreases the risk of laparoscopically proven salpingitis fivefold (Table 23-5). This seems contradictory. However, more recent data reveal that the prevalence of minimally symptomatic histologic endometritis is increased in oral contraceptive users. Thus, it appears that when cervical infection is present, women on oral contraceptives have a similar incidence of upper genital tract infection to that of women who do not use oral contraceptives, but the severity of the symptoms and tissue damage is diminished in oral contraceptive users. This may be partially due to thicker cervical mucus produced by the progestin component of oral contraceptives, which inhibits sperm and bacterial penetration. Also, the decrease in duration of menstrual flow accompanying oral contraceptive use theoretically creates a shorter interval for bacterial colonization of the upper tract.

Twenty to thirty years ago, multiple case-controlled studies reported an increased risk of acute PID in women who were

Table 23-5 Comparison of Laparoscopic Findings with Type of Contraceptive Use in 738 Women with Signs and Symptoms Suggestive of Acute Salpingitis

	CONTRACEPTIVE METHOD*		
Lapaoscopic Findings	**Oral Contraceptive (%)**	**Intrauterine Device (%)**	**Reference† (%)**
Salpingitis	171 (59.8)	183 (80.6)	190 (84.4)
Nonsalpingitis	115 (40.2)	44 (19.4)	35 (15.6)

*Relative risk of oral contraceptive use versus reference = 0.27 $\chi^2_1 = 36.9, p < 0.0001$; relative risk of IUD use versus reference = 0.77 (95% confidence interval 0.47 to 1.26, $\chi^2_1 = 1.1, p = 0.28$); and relative risk of oral contraceptive versus IUD use = 0.36 (95% confidence interval 0.24 to 0.54 $\chi^2_1 = 25.7, p < 0.0001$).

†Reference = barrier methods or no contraception.

From Wølner-Hanssen P, Svensson L, Mårdh PA, et al: Laparoscopic findings and contraceptive use in women with signs and symptoms suggestive of acute salpingitis. Obstet Gynecol 66:234, 1985. Reprinted with permission from the American College of Obstetricians and Gynecologists.

using an IUD. There has been just criticism of these early epidemiologic studies for their selection of control groups and the bias of including women with Dalkon shields in their statistics. The increase in risk for PID occurs only at the time of insertion of the IUD and in the first 3 weeks after placement. An analysis from the World Health Organization (WHO) found the rate of PID to be 9.7 per 1000 woman-years for the first 20 days after insertion compared with 1.4 per 1000 woman-years for the next 8 years of follow-up.

Acute salpingitis occurring in a woman with a previous tubal ligation is extremely rare, and when it does occur, the symptoms of the infection are less severe. Phillips and D'Ablaing reported the incidence of acute PID developing in the proximal stump of previously ligated fallopian tubes as 1 in 450 women hospitalized for acute salpingitis.

Epidemiologic studies have documented that previous acute PID is a definite risk factor for future attacks of the disease. Approximately 25% of women with acute PID subsequently develop another acute tubal infection. Ten years ago this reinfection was believed to be "chronic infection" or exacerbations of a "latent" tubal process. Direct cultures have proven that the disease is another primary infection. The microscopic tubal damage produced by the initial upper genital tract infection may facilitate repeat infection. It is possible that prior infection causes an immunological "priming" effect, making upper genital tract infection more likely with repeated cervical exposure (see the previous discussion of *C. trachomatis* pathology). The increased risk may also be related to an untreated male partner. Studies have documented that greater than 80% of male contacts are not treated. Approximately 50% of men with STDs are free of symptoms, and thus they do not seek treatment. Recently, studies have shown that dispensing partner treatment for the affected female to give to her partner decreases *C. trachomatis* reinfection.

Transcervical penetration of the cervical mucus barrier with instrumentation of the uterus is a risk factor, for it may initiate "iatrogenic" acute PID. Approximately 1 million first-trimester abortions are performed each year in the United States. The incidence of upper genital tract infection associated with this procedure is approximately 1 in 200 cases. Recent practice has emphasized the use of prophylactic antibiotics to decrease the incidence of associated acute PID. Women with concurrent bacterial vaginosis have a higher risk for postabortal infection and thus should be treated with oral antibiotics with anaerobic coverage.

A growing area of research involves identification of changes in the virulence of organisms and the host's response to the organisms. Virulence factors of an organism are another risk factor for PID and may explain why some lower tract infections progress to upper tract disease but others do not. The gonococcus possesses different factors that may become activated in certain environments to increase the virulence of the organism. Similarly, other organisms that are usually of low virulence may possess factors that affect their virulence and pathogenicity. Both bacterial virulence factors, such as hemolysin enzymes and proteases, and bacterial defense mechanisms that inhibit host responses may become activated under varying microenvironments. Genetic variation may be another risk factor. Some women may be genetically predisposed to mount a robust inflammatory process that may lead to tubal scarring (such as chlamydial heat shock protein). In a group of Kenyan women with confirmed tubal infertility, two class II alleles were detected less commonly in women seropositive for *C. trachomatis* compared with women seronegative for *Chlamydia,* suggesting these alleles may lead to an immunologically mediated mechanism of protection against *Chlamydia.*

In summary, the primary emphasis in disease prevention is the treatment of sexual partners of women with acute PID. The male partner is frequently asymptomatic and should be treated empirically with antibiotics against both chlamydia and gonorrhea.

Symptoms and Signs

Patients with acute PID present with a wide range of nonspecific clinical symptoms and signs. Thus the diagnosis of acute PID even by experienced clinicians is imprecise. Many women have mild, nonspecific pelvic symptoms that are overlooked by both the woman and her physician. The severity of the clinical presentation of acute PID varies from no discernable symptoms to diffuse peritonitis and a life-threatening illness. Since the diagnosis is usually based on clinical criteria, there is both a high false-positive rate and a high false-negative rate. The differential diagnosis of acute PID includes lower genital tract pelvic infection, ectopic pregnancy, torsion or rupture of an adnexal mass, acute appendicitis, gastroenteritis, and endometriosis.

Laparoscopic studies of women with a clinical diagnosis of acute PID have established the inadequacy of diagnosis by the usual criteria of history and physical and laboratory examination. In these studies approximately 205 to 25% of women had no identifiable intraabdominal or pelvic disease. Another 10% to 15% of patients were found to have other pathologic conditions, such as ectopic pregnancy, acute appendicitis, or torsion of the adnexa. In one of these studies Jacobson reported a series of 814 women in whom laparoscopy was performed because of clinically suspected acute PID. The clinical diagnosis was confirmed at laparoscopy in 532 women (65%). This study also documented the laparoscopic findings in 98 women with a false-positive clinical diagnosis of acute PID and 91 cases of false-negative clinical diagnosis of acute PID (Tables 23-6 and 23-7).

Table 23-6 Laparoscopic Findings in Patients with False Positive Clinical Diagnosis of Acute PID but with Pelvic Disorders Other Than PID

Laparoscopic Finding	Number
Acute appendicitis	24
Endometriosis	16
Corpus luteum bleeding	12
Ectopic pregnancy	11
Pelvic adhesions only	7
Benign ovarian tumor	7
Chronic salpingitis	6
Miscellaneous	15
Total	98

From Jacobson LJ: Differential diagnosis of acute pelvic inflammatory disease. Am J Obstet Gynecol 138: 1006, 1980.

Table 23-7 Preoperative Diagnoses in Patients with False-Negative Clinical Diagnosis of Acute PID Prior to Laparoscopy/Laparotomy

Clinical Diagnosis	Visual Diagnosis: Acute PID (Number)
Ovarian tumor	20
Acute appendicitis	18
Ectopic pregnancy	16
Chronic salpingitis	10
Acute peritonitis	6
Endmetriosis	5
Uterine myoma	5
Uncharacteristic pelvic pain	5
Miscellaneous	6
Total	91

From Jacobson LJ: Differential diagnosis of acute pelvic inflammatory disease. Am J Obstet Gynecol 138: 1006, 1980.

Another interesting finding of laparoscopic studies is the lack of correlation between the number and intensity of symptoms, signs, and degree of abnormality of laboratory values, and the severity of tubal inflammation. Women with *C. trachomatis* infections may exhibit minor symptoms but have a severe inflammatory process visualized by laparoscopic examination. Criteria for establishing the severity of acute PID by laparoscopic examination are listed in Table 23-8.

Historically, the diagnosis of acute PID was not established unless the patient had the triad of fever, elevated erythrocyte sedimentation rate (ESR), and adnexal tenderness or a mass. Only 17% of laparoscopically identified cases have this classic triad. Thus reliance on stringent clinical criteria for establishing the diagnosis of the disease would result in the majority of cases being overlooked and untreated. Obviously, more frequent and liberal use of diagnostic laparoscopy is an important advance in the management of the disease. Laparoscopy allows precise diagnosis and also the opportunity to collect material from the site of the infection for culturing. However, in practice the majority of women with acute PID do not undergo laparoscopy because of the expense of this invasive technique. Endometrial biopsy is more readily available as a diagnostic tool.

Table 23-8 Severity of Disease by Laparoscopic Examination

Severity	Findings
Mild	Erythema, edema, no spontaneous purulent exudates*; tubes freely movable
Moderate	Gross purulent material evident; erythema and edema, more marked; tubes may not be freely movable, and fimbria stoma may not be patent
Severe	Pyosalpinx or inflammatory complex Abscess†

*The tubes may require manipulation to produce purulent exudate.
†The size of any pelvic abscess should be measured.
From Hager WD, Eschenbach DA, Spence MR, et al: Criteria for diagnosis and grading of salpingitis. Obstet Gynecol 61:114, 1983. Reprinted with permission from the American College of Obstetricians and Gynecologists.

Hager and colleagues have established clinical criteria for diagnosing acute PID (Table 23-9). These uniform criteria were adopted by the Infectious Disease Society of Obstetrics and Gynecology. The frequencies of various symptoms, signs, and laboratory data from this series of 414 women are depicted in Tables 23-10 and 23-11. However, more recently the PEACH trial found that for women with endometritis diagnosed on endometrial biopsy, the requirement of all three clinical criteria (lower abdominal tenderness, adnexal tenderness, and cervical motion tenderness) resulted in decreased sensitivity. Hence, the 2006 CDC treatment guidelines state that empiric therapy for PID should be initiated in sexually active young women and other women at risk for STDs with pelvic or lower abdominal pain if cervical motion tenderness or uterine tenderness or adnexal tenderness is present. The CDC diagnostic criteria are summarized in the following box.

Pain in the lower abdomen and pelvis is by far the most frequent symptom of acute PID. In all large series, more than 90% of women present with diffuse bilateral lower abdominal pain. This pain is usually described as constant and dull. On

Table 23-9 Acute Salpingitis: Clinical Criteria for Diagnosis

Criteria	
Abdominal direct tenderness, with or without rebound tenderness Tenderness with motion of cervix and uterus Adnexal tenderness	All 3 necessary for diagnosis
	plus
Gram stain of endocervix—positive for gram-negative intracellular diplococci Temperature (>38° C) Leukocytosis (>10,000) Purulent material (white blood cells present) from peritoneal cavity by culdocentesis or laparoscopy Pelvic abscess or inflammatory complex on bimanual examination or on sonography	1 or more necessary for diagnosis

From Hager WD, Eschenbach DA, Spence MR, et al: Criteria for diagnosis and grading of salpingitis. Obstet Gynecol 61:114, 1983. Reprinted with permission from the American College of Obstetricians and Gynecologists.

Table 23-10 Frequency of Various Symptoms as Reported by Patients in Acute PID and Visually Normal Groups (First-Time PID Patients)

	LAPAROSCOPIC DIAGNOSIS				
	Acute PID (Number = 414)		Normal (Number = 138)		
Symptom	**Number**	**Percent**	**Number**	**Percent**	***P* Value**
Lower abdominal pain	411	99.3	135	97.8	NS
Vaginal discharge	287	69.3	85	61.6	NS
Temperature ≥ 38° C	142	34.4	34	24.6	0.05
Irregular bleeding	165	40.0	54	39.1	NS
Urinary symptoms	82	19.8	29	21.0	NS
Vomiting	43	10.4	13	9.4	NS
Protitis symptoms	30	7.3	4	2.9	NS
Other	33	8.0	8	5.8	NS

From Hadgu A, Weström L, Brooks CA, et al: Predicting acute pelvic inflammatory disease: A multivariate analysis. Am J Obstet Gynecol 155:956, 1986.

Table 23-11 Frequency of Various Objective Findings at Admission in Acute PID and Visually Normal Groups

	LAPAROSCOPIC DIAGNOSIS				
	Acute PID (Number = 414)		Normal (Number = 138)		
Clinical Findings at Admission	**Number**	**Percent**	**Number**	**Percent**	***P* Value**
Bimanual examination					
Marked tenderness	193	95.4	128	92.8	NS
Palpable mass or swelling	198	47.8	36	26.1	0.001
Erythrocyte sedimentation rate > 15 mm/hr	336	81.2	78	56.5	0.001
Abnormal vaginal discharge	337	81.4	80	58.0	0.001
Fever (38° C)	146	35.3	21	15.2	0.001

From Hadgu A, Weström L, Brooks CA, et al: Predicting acute pelvic inflammatory disease: A multivariate analysis. Am J Obstet Gynecol 155:956, 1986.

CDC Guidelines for Diagnosis of Acute PID Clinical Criteria for Initiating Therapy

Minimum Criteria

Empiric treatment of PID should be initiated in sexually active young women and others at risk for STDs if all the following minimum criteria are present and no other causes(s) for the illness can be identified:

- Lower abdominal tenderness or
- Adnexal tenderness or
- Cervical motion tenderness

Routine Criteria for Diagnosing PID

- Oral temperature >38° C
- Abnormal cervical or vaginal discharge (mucopurulent)
- Presence of abundant WBCs on microscopy of vaginal secretions
- Elevated erythrocyte sedimentation rate
- Elevated C-reactive protein
- Laboratory documentation of cervical infection with *N. gonorrhoeae* or *C. trachomatis*

Definitive Criteria for Diagnosing PID

- Histopathologic evidence of endometritis on endometrial biopsy
- Transvaginal sonography or magnetic resonance imaging techniques showing thickened fluid-filled tubes with or without free pelvic or tuboovarian complex
- Laparoscopic abnormalities consistent with PID

Although initial treatment can be made before bacteriologic diagnosis of *C. trachomatis* or *N. gonorrhoeae* infection, such a diagnosis emphasizes the need to treat sex partners.

PID, pelvic inflammatory disease; STD, sexually transmitted disease; WBC, white blood cells.
From Centers for Disease Control and Prevention: 2006 Guidelines for treatment of sexually transmitted disease. MMWR 55:11, 2006

occasion the pain may become cramping, and it is accentuated by motion or sexual activity. Generally the pain is of short duration, usually less than 7 days. If the pain has been present for longer than 3 weeks, it is unlikely that the patient has acute PID. Approximately 75% of patients with acute PID have an associated endocervical infection or a coexistent purulent vaginal discharge. Abnormal uterine bleeding, especially spotting or menorrhagia, is noted in about 40% of patients. Nausea and vomiting are relatively late symptoms in the course of the disease.

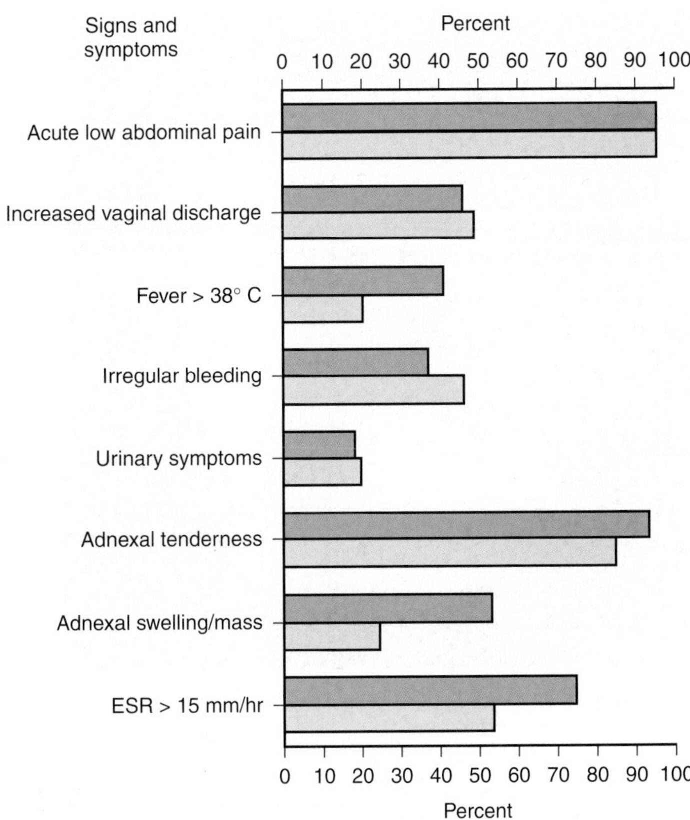

Figure 23-4. Comparison of frequency of symptoms, signs, and laboratory findings between patients with acute pelvic inflammatory disease (PID) *(dark blue)* and suspected PID without pelvic pathology *(light blue bars)* by laparoscopic examination. ESR, erythrocyte sedimentation rate. (From Jacobson LJ: Differential diagnosis of acute pelvic inflammatory disease. Am J Obstet Gynecol 138:1008, 1980.)

When one compares the frequency of individual symptoms and signs between women with laparoscopically proven acute PID and those without the disease, there is no significant difference, with the exception of fever (Fig. 23-4). Acute PID often occurs with minimum symptoms. Most studies have found that approximately 50% of women who are infertile as a result of tubal obstruction do not remember ever having symptoms of acute pelvic infection.

The symptoms of acute pelvic infection secondary to *N. gonorrhoeae* are of rapid onset, and the pelvic pain usually begins a few days after the onset of a menstrual period. Acute pelvic infection caused by *C. trachomatis* alone often may have an indolent course with slow onset, less pain, and less fever.

Five percent to 10% of women with acute PID develop symptoms of perihepatic inflammation—the Fitz-Hugh–Curtis syndrome (Figs. 23-5 and 23-6). The condition is often mistakenly diagnosed as either pneumonia or acute cholecystitis. Persistent symptoms and signs include right upper quadrant pain, pleuritic pain, and tenderness in the right upper quadrant when the liver is palpated. The pain may radiate to the shoulder or into the back. Liver transaminases may be elevated. Fitz-Hugh–Curtis syndrome develops from transperitoneal or vascular dissemination of either the gonococcus or *Chlamydia* organism to produce the perihepatic inflammation. Currently, *Chlamydia* produces the majority of cases. Other organisms, including anaerobic streptococci and coxsackievirus, have also been associated with this syndrome. Laparoscopy may be useful in the diagnosis of this syndrome. The liver capsule will appear inflamed, with classic "violin string" adhesions to the parietal peritoneum beneath the diaphragm. Women with perihepatitis have a higher prevalence of moderate-to-severe pelvic adhesions and a higher prevalence and higher titers of antibodies to the chlamydial heat shock protein 60. Treatment is the same as the treatment for acute salpingitis.

Women with laparoscopically confirmed acute PID are often afebrile. Only one out of three women with acute PID presents with a temperature greater than 38° C. In a study of women

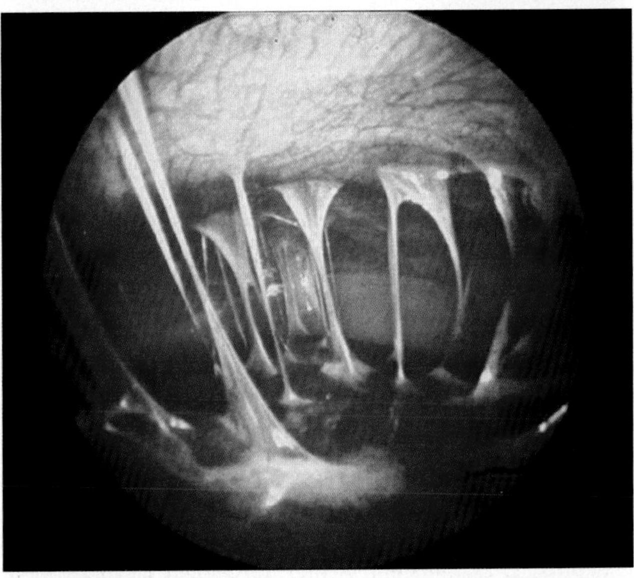

Figure 23-5. Classic "violin strings" sign of Fitz-Hugh–Curtis from PID.

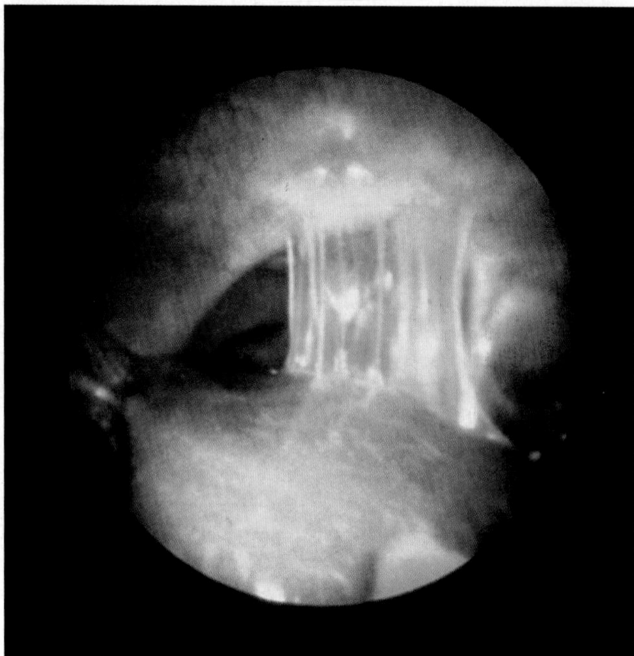

Figure 23-6. Perihepatic adhesions of Fitz-Hugh–Curtis from PID.

with biopsy-proven acute chlamydial salpingitis, only 20% had a fever. Lower abdominal and pelvic tenderness during examination is the hallmark of acute PID. Most women with acute PID have tenderness to direct palpation in the lower abdomen and sometimes may have rebound tenderness. Bilateral tenderness of the parametria and adnexa is usually discovered during pelvic examination. This tenderness is especially noted with movement of the uterus or cervix during the pelvic examination. An ill-defined adnexal fullness is frequently noted. This may represent edema, inflammatory adhesions to either the small or large intestine, or an adnexal complex or abscess. The incidence of true adnexal abscess is approximately 10% in women with acute PID.

Diagnosis

Direct visualization via the laparoscope is the most accurate method of diagnosing acute PID. Laparoscopy also has been indispensable in the clinical research of the disease. In several presentations of acute PID laparoscopy or laparotomy is strongly indicated, such as impending septic shock, acute surgical abdomen, and in a complicated differential diagnosis in a postmenopausal woman. Women who undergo laparoscopy to confirm the diagnosis of acute PID have the additional advantage of concurrent operative procedures such as lysis of adhesions, potential drainage of an abscess, and irrigation of the pelvic cavity. To date, operative laparoscopy during acute infection has not been proven to reduce the prevalence of long-term sequelae. Currently, laparoscopy is used less frequently. More women receive outpatient therapy. Hence, the diagnosis of the majority of episodes of acute PID is made on the basis of clinical history and physical examination. Acute PID should be included in the differential diagnosis of any sexually active young woman with pelvic pain. Laboratory tests may be obtained, but their results lack sufficient sensitivity and specificity to make them an important factor in establishing the diagnosis. Since clinical symptoms and signs are nonspecific for the disease, when the diagnosis is based on clinical criteria, the rates of both false-positives and false-negative are high. Because of the long-term sequelae of the disease, most clinicians maintain a low threshold in entertaining a diagnosis of acute PID, readily accepting that they are treating many women who actually do not have pelvic infection, in order not to omit treating those with early or mild disease. For the CDC guidelines for diagnosis of acute PID, see the previous box.

Leukocytosis is not a reliable indicator of acute PID nor does it correlate with the need for hospitalization or the severity of tubal inflammation. Less than 50% of women with acute PID have a white blood cell count of greater than 10,000 cells per milliliter. For years, ESR was a standard laboratory test for acute PID. This laboratory test is nonspecific. The ESR is elevated (>15 mm/hr) in approximately 75% of women with laparoscopically confirmed acute pelvic infection. However, 53% of women with pelvic pain and visually normal pelvic organs have an elevated ESR. Similarly, the ESR is a crude indicator of severity of disease and is no longer used to guide therapy. Some investigators obtain C-reactive protein levels. We have not found that these levels change clinical management.

Women with acute PID should have a sensitive test for human chorionic gonadotropin to help in the differential diagnosis of ectopic pregnancy. About 3 to 4 of every 100 women who are admitted to a hospital with a diagnosis of acute pelvic infection have an ectopic pregnancy.

Because most cases of upper genital tract infection are preceded by lower genital tract infection, it is important to examine the endocervical mucus for inflammatory cells, and NAAT for both *N. gonorrhoeae* and *C. trachomatis,* and have the laboratory perform a Gram stain. *C. trachomatis* is the most prevalent causative pathogen. Recently, *C. trachomatis* has surpassed *N. gonorrhea* as the most prevalent sexually transmitted bacteria-producing upper tract infection in the developed world. A positive gram-stained smear of the endocervical mucus is nonspecific, and a negative smear does not rule out upper tract infection. A saline prep and pH of vaginal secretions for bacterial vaginosis should also be obtained. Peipert and coworkers has reported that the presence of an increased number of vaginal white blood cells is the most sensitive laboratory indicator of acute PID. However, he concluded that no one diagnostic laboratory test is pathognomonic for upper genital tract infection. Most importantly, combinations of positive tests improved diagnostic specificity and positive predictive value. However, this results in a diminution of sensitivity and negative predictive value (Table 23-12). If the cervical discharge appears normal and no white blood cells are found on the wet prep of vaginal fluid, the diagnosis of PID is unlikely, and alternative causes of pain should be considered.

An endometrial biopsy for evidence of endometritis can be a useful tool. However, because of the time delay between biopsy and the final histopathologic report, this test is primarily used to help confirm a clinical suspicion. It is important to realize that although the majority of women with acute salpingitis have coexisting endometritis, the converse that the majority of women with endometritis have salpingitis has not been established. In

Table 23-12 Diagnostic Test Characteristics of Laboratory Tests for the Diagnosis of Acute Upper Genital Tract Infection

Test	Sensitivity (%)	Specificity (%)	PREVALENCE 30%		PREVALENCE 60%	
			NPV (%)	PPV (%)	NPV (%)	PPV (%)
Entire Cohort (*N* = 120)						
ESR	70	52	80	38	54	69
CRP	71	66	84	47	60	76
WBC	57	88	83	67	58	88
Vaginal WBC	78	39	80	35	54	66
Classical PID (*N* = 70)						
ESR	72	53	82	40	56	70
CRP	76	59	85	44	62	74
WBC	66	80	85	59	61	83
Vaginal WBC	87	38	87	38	66	68
Nonclassical PID (*N* = 50)						
ESR	64	51	77	36	49	66
CRP	58	73	80	48	54	76
WBC	38	97	78	84	51	95
Vaginal WBC	62	41	72	31	42	6

CRP, C-reactive protein; ESR, erythrocyte sedimentation rate; NPV, negative predictive value; PPV, positive predictive value; WBC, white blood cell count.
From Peipert JF, Boardman L, Hogan JW, et al: Laboratory evaluation of acute upper genital tract infection. Obstet Gynecol 87:733, 1996. Reprinted with permission from the American College of Obstetricians and Gynecologists.

one investigation of women with biopsy-proven endometritis, the accuracy of coexistent acute PID confirmed by laparoscopy had a sensitivity of 89% and a specificity of 87%.

The percentage of American women with acute PID who also are infected with HIV has been estimated to be 6% to 22%. Women with acute PID and HIV infection have a higher incidence of adnexal masses. However, the acute pelvic infection responds to antibiotic therapy in a similar fashion to that in women who are not infected with HIV. Because acute PID is usually secondary to an STD, it is ideal to examine, culture, and smear urethral secretions from the male partner. Often this step is not performed for a variety of nonmedical reasons. The CDC continues to emphasize the importance of treating partners of women with STDs.

Ultrasonography is of limited value for patients with mild or moderate PID due to its low sensitivity. However, vaginal ultrasonography is helpful in documenting an adnexal mass and differentiating between a tuboovarian abscess and a tuboovarian complex (Fig. 23-7). Ultrasonography is also a noninvasive diagnostic aid for patients who are so tender during pelvic examination that the physician cannot determine the presence or absence of a pelvic mass. Though ultrasonography is neither specific nor sensitive in distinguishing the cause of a pelvic mass, findings of dilated and fluid-filled tubes, free peritoneal fluid, and adnexal masses may be confirmatory of symptoms and physical signs (Figs. 23-8 to 23-10). Thus vaginal ultrasound does have a high positive predictive value when used in a high-risk population. Magnetic resonance imaging is sensitive, but its expense and limited acute availability in some locations have restricted its role in PID diagnosis.

Laparoscopy is definitely indicated for patients who are not responding to therapy, both to confirm the diagnosis and to obtain cultures of purulent material. Figure 23-11 shows a laparoscopic view of a tuboovarian abscess.

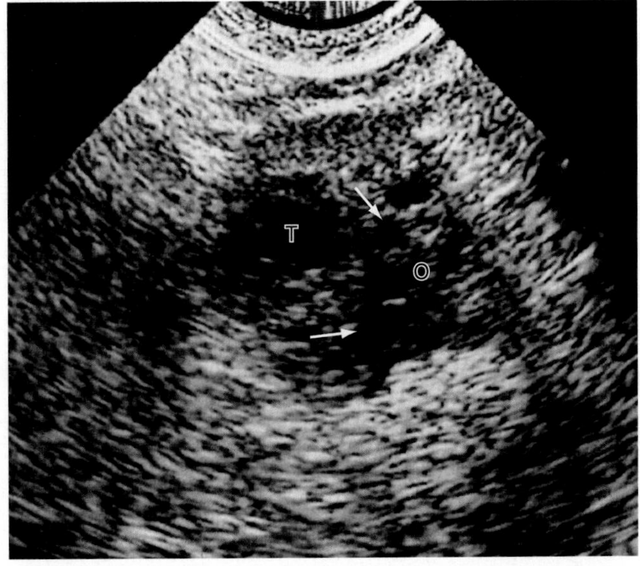

Figure 23-7. Sonogram of a cross-section of an adnexal mass suggestive of tuboovarian complex. The slightly dilated and fluid-filled tube (T) is seen very close to the ovary (O). The ovarian part of the complex can be recognized by the presence of follicles *(arrows)*. Endometrial biopsy showed plasma cell endometritis. (From Cacciatore B, Leminen A, Ingman-Friberg S, et al: Transvaginal sonographic findings in ambulatory patients with suspected pelvic inflammatory disease. Obstet Gynecol 80:912, 1992.)

Management

Treatment of the patient with PID encompasses more than just prescribing the appropriate antimicrobial regimen. Determining the need for hospitalization, patient education, treatment of sexual partners, and careful follow-up are key treatment issues.

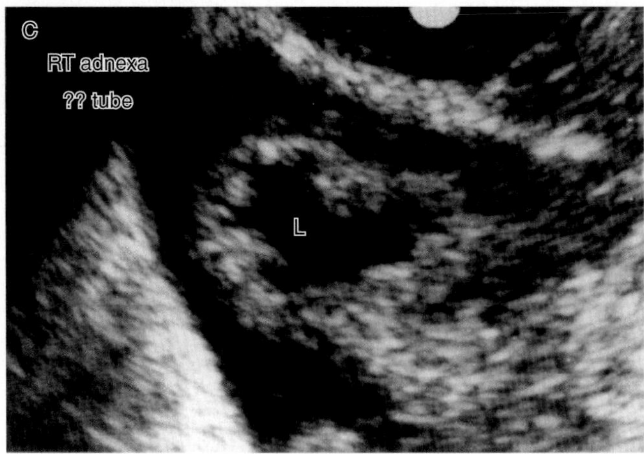

Figure 23-8. Transvaginal sonographic image of acute salpingitis. The central sonolucent fluid in the lumen (L) and the thickened endosalpingeal folds render this the "cogwheel" appearance. (From Timor-Tritsch IE, Lerner JP, Monteagudo A, et al: Transvaginal sonographic markers of tubal inflammatory disease. Ultrasound Obstet Gynecol 12:56, 1998.)

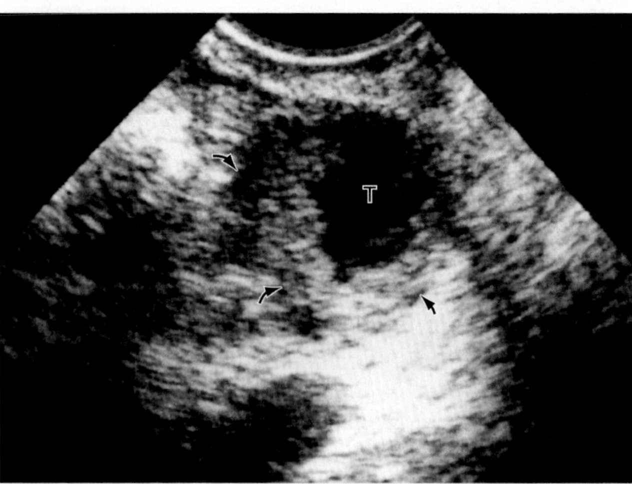

Figure 23-10. Sonographic image of a cross section of a dilated and fluid-filled fallopian tube (T). The wall is thickened and irregular in shape *(arrows)*. Endometrial biopsy showed plasma endometritis. (From Cacciatore B, Leminen A, Ingman-Friberg S, et al: Transvaginal sonographic findings in ambulatory patients with suspected pelvic inflammatory disease. Obstet Gynecol 80:912, 1992.)

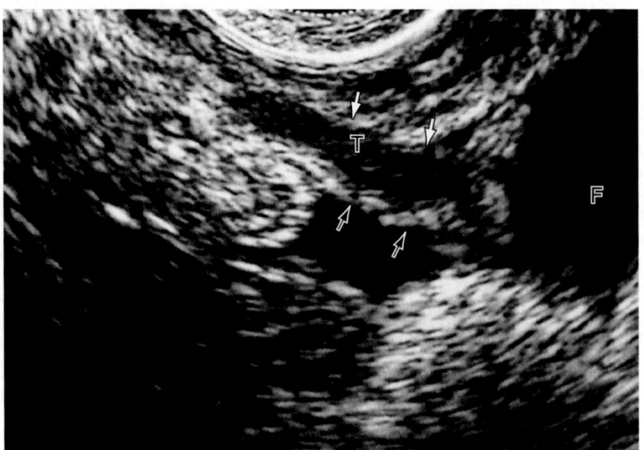

Figure 23-9. Longitudinal section of a slightly dilated and fluid-filled tube (T). Its walls are slightly thickened *(arrows)*. Endometrial biopsy showed plasma cell endometritis. F, free fluid. (From Cacciatore B, Leminen A, Ingman-Friberg S, et al: Transvaginal sonographic findings in ambulatory patients with suspected pelvic inflammatory disease. Obstet Gynecol 80:912, 1992.)

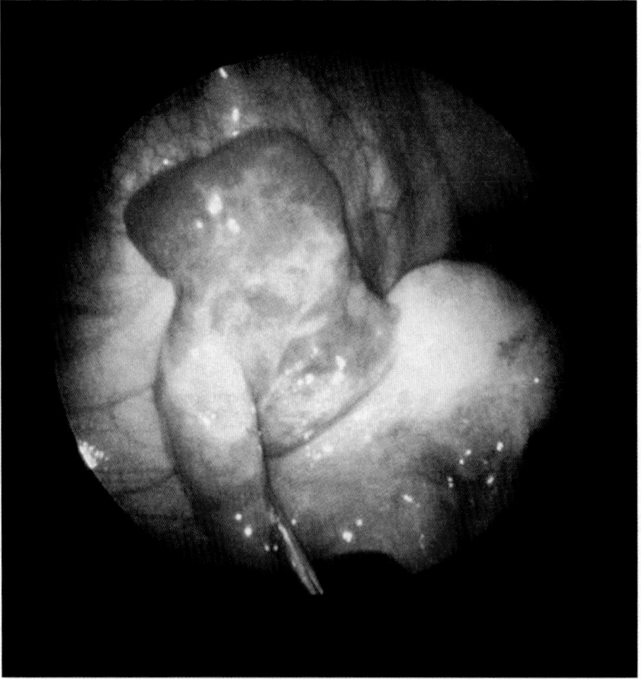

Figure 23-11. Laparoscopic view of acute PID and a tuboovarian abscess.

The two most important goals of the medical therapy of acute PID are the resolution of symptoms and the preservation of tubal function. Antibiotic therapy should be started as soon STD screening has been obtained and the diagnosis is suggested. Early diagnosis and early treatment will help reduce the number of women who suffer from the long-term sequelae of the disease. Women who are not treated in the first 72 hours following the onset of symptoms are three times as likely to develop tubal infertility or ectopic pregnancy as those who are treated early in the disease process. Both animal and human studies have suggested that early antibiotic treatment improves long-term fertility. In the management of acute PID, one should not forget the treatment of the male partner and education for the prevention of the disease, including the use of proper contraceptives, which help to reduce the rate of upper genital tract infection.

Although the choice of antibiotic therapy for most infectious diseases is usually based on cultures and sensitivity of bacteria obtained directly from the site of the infection in PID, direct tubal cultures are not practical. Because most cases of PID are polymicrobial, broad-spectrum antibiotic coverage is indicated. Empirical antibiotic protocols should cover a wide range of

Table 23-13 Microorganisms Isolated from the Fallopian Tubes of Patients with Acute Pelvic Inflammatory Disease

Type of Agent	Organism
Sexually transmitted disease	*Chlamydia trachomatis*
	Neisseria gonorrhoeae
	Mycoplasma hominis
Endogenous agent aerobic or facultative	*Streptococcus* species
	Staphylococcus species
	Haemophilus species
	Escherichia coli
Anaerobic	*Bacteroides* species
	Peptococcus species
	Peptostreptocccus species
	Clostridium species
	Actinomyces species

From Weström L: Introductory address: Treatment of pelvic inflammatory disease in view of etiology and risk factors. Sex Transm Dis 11:439, 1984.

bacteria, including *N. gonorrhoeae, C. trachomatis,* anaerobic rods and cocci, gram-negative aerobic rods, and gram-positive aerobes (Table 23-13). Selection of one antibiotic protocol over another may be influenced by the clinical history. For example, acute PID following an operative procedure is usually caused by endogenous flora of the vagina, whereas acute PID in a 19-year-old college student is likely secondary to *C. trachomatis.*

A failure of outpatient oral therapy may be related to non-compliance, reinfection, or inadequate antibiotic coverage for penicillinase-producing or chromosomally mediated resistant *N. gonorrhoeae* or facultative or anaerobic organisms involved in upper genital tract infection that are resistant to the drug prescribed. It is important to know resistance profiles in your geographic region. Inpatient failure rates for resolution of acute symptoms with intravenous (IV) antibiotics are approximately 5% to 10%.

A variety of oral and parenteral antibiotic regimens have been effective in achieving short-term clinical and microbiologic cures in randomized clinical trials. However, there are a paucity of data comparing the effect of various protocols on the incidence of long-term complications and elimination of bacterial infection in both the endometrium and fallopian tubes. The CDC has published recommendations of outpatient treatment of PID (see the following box). Regimen A is levofloxacin 500 mg PO daily for 14 days with or without metronidazole 500 mg PO twice a day for the same 14 days. Oral levofloxacin is effective as a single agent against both *N. gonorrhoeae* and *C. trachomatis.* Metronidazole is added to this regimen because of the lack of anaerobic coverage with ofloxacin. Regimen B is ceftriaxone 250 mg IM once or cefoxitin 2 g IM plus probenecid 1 g PO in a single dose concurrently once, or another parenteral third-generation cephalosporin such as ceftizoxime or cefotaxime. Regimen B also includes doxycycline 100 mg PO twice a day for 14 days with the cephalosporin. The optimal cephalosporin choice for regimen B is not known. Ceftizoxime has unparalleled coverage against *N. gonorrhoeae;* cefotaxime has better anaerobic coverage. Regimen B is less expensive than regimen A. The clinician should individualize the choice of regimens depending on his or her estimate of the need for anaerobic coverage. Importantly, if the woman has bacterial

Centers for Disease Control Ambulatory Management of Acute PID

Regimen A

Levofloxacin 500 mg PO once daily for 14 days
or
Ofloxacin 400 mg PO once daily for 14 days
with or without
Metronidazole 500 mg PO bid for 14 days

Regimen B

Ceftriaxone 250 mg IM in a single dose
or
Cefoxitin 2 g IM in a single dose and probenecid 1 g PO administered concurrently in a single dose
or
Other parenteral third-generation cephalosporin (e.g., ceftizoxime or cefotaxime)
plus
Doxycycline 100 mg PO bid for 14 days
with or without
Metronidazole 500 mg PO bid for 14 days

From Centers for Disease Control and Prevention: 2006 Guidelines for treatment of sexually transmitted diseases. MMWR 55:11, 2006.

vaginosis, prolonged coverage with metronidazole is preferable. To date there are no data regarding the use of oral cephalosporins for the treatment of PID. Note the dose of ceftriaxone in PID is twice the dose for cervicitis. Completion of all 14 days of therapy, independent of symptom resolution, should be stressed.

Information on alternative oral regimens is limited. Amoxicillin/clavulanic acid plus doxycycline for 14 days was effective in one clinical trial and has broad-spectrum coverage. However, gastrointestinal side effects associated with this regimen may limit its utility.

It is important to reexamine women within 48 to 72 hours of initiating outpatient therapy to evaluate the response of the disease to oral antibiotics. The patient should be hospitalized when the therapeutic response is not optimal. If the disease is responding well, approximately 4 to 6 weeks after therapy the patient should be examined to assess resolution of clinical symptoms and establish post therapy baseline.

In the past, many practitioners preferred to hospitalize nulliparous women for treatment of PID. This is no longer recommended. A multicenter trial of 831 women found no advantage to inpatient treatment of mild-to-moderate PID randomized to inpatient versus outpatient treatment. In over 84 months of follow-up, equivalent number of pregnancies, live births, time to pregnancy, infertility, recurrent PID, chronic pelvic pain, and ectopic pregnancy occurred in both the inpatient and outpatient treatment groups. This was true even in teenagers and women without a previous live birth.

The CDC has established criteria for hospitalization (see following box). These criteria include unsure diagnosis, being too ill to tolerate oral therapy, no improvement with oral therapy, and presence of a tuboovarian abscess or pregnancy.

Indications for Hospitalizing Patients with Acute Pelvic Inflammatory Disease

Surgical emergencies (e.g., appendicitis) cannot be excluded.
The patient is pregnant.
The patient does not respond clinically to oral antimicrobial therapy.
The patient is unable to follow or tolerate an outpatient oral regimen.
The patient has severe illness, nausea and vomiting, or high fever.
The patient has a tuboovarian abscess.

Modified from Centers for Disease Control and Prevention: 2006 Guidelines for treatment of sexually transmitted diseases. MMWR 55:11, 2006.

Acute PID associated with the presence of an IUD is usually more advanced at the time of diagnosis than infection without a foreign body. Both patient and physician delays in diagnosis are not unusual. Often women misinterpret the early signs and symptoms of an infection as being related to the IUD. Pelvic infections with an IUD in place and pelvic infections following operative or diagnostic procedures often are due to anaerobic bacteria. Thus it is best to hospitalize these patients and use IV antibiotics. The IUD should be removed and cultured as soon as appropriate levels of IV antibiotics have been obtained. Concurrent immunodeficiency, especially HIV infection with a low CD4 count is another important criterion for hospitalization. If a therapeutic response or compliance with oral medications has not been optimal or is questionable, or if follow-up in 72 hours is not possible, then the patient should be admitted for IV antibiotic therapy.

The 2006 CDC guidelines for inpatient treatment of acute PID with parenteral therapy are listed in following box. The protocols stress the polymicrobial origin of acute pelvic infection, the increasing importance of *C. trachomatis,* and the emergence of penicillin-resistant *N. gonorrhoeae.* With IV protocols the CDC recommends that IV antibiotics be continued at least 24 hours after substantial improvement in the patient. When the patient has a mass, we add ampicillin to clindamycin and gentamicin. However, for patients without a mass, we switch to oral antibiotics when the symptoms have diminished and the patient has been afebrile for 24 hours. In both regimens doxycycline is continued for a total of 14 days.

Regimen A is a combination of doxycycline and IV cefoxitin. It is excellent for community-acquired infection because it treats both gonorrhea and chlamydial infection. Doxycycline and cefoxitin provide excellent coverage for *N. gonorrhoeae, C. trachomatis,* and also penicillinase-producing *N. gonorrhoeae.* Cefoxitin is an excellent antibiotic against *Peptococcus, Peptostreptococcus,* and *E. coli.* The disadvantage of this combination is that the two drugs are less than ideal for a pelvic abscess or for anaerobic infections. To date cefotetan has been found as effective as cefoxitin. There is no clinically significant difference in bioavailability of doxycycline whether it is given by the oral or IV route. Thus doxycycline should be administered orally whenever possible because of the marked superficial phlebitis produced by IV infusion.

Centers for Disease Control Inpatient Management of Acute PID

Parenteral Regimen A
Cefotetan 2 g IV every 12 hours
OR
Cefoxitin 2 g IV every 6 hours
PLUS
Doxycycline 100 mg PO or IV every 12 hours

Note: Because of pain associated with infusion, doxycycline should be administered orally when possible, even when the patient is hospitalized. Both PO and IV administration of doxycycline provide similar bioavailability.

Parenteral Regimen B
Clindamycin 900 mg IV every 8 hours
PLUS
Gentamicin loading dose IV or IM (2 mg/kg of body weight) followed by a maintenance dose (1.5 mg/kd) every 8 hours. Single daily dosing may be substituted

Alternative Parenteral Regimens
Limited data support the use of other parenteral regimens, but the following three regimens have been investigated in a least one clinical trial, and they have broad-spectrum coverage
Levofloxacin 500 mg IV once daily.
OR
Ofloxacin 400 mg IV every 12 hours
WITH or WITHOUT
Metronidazole 500 mg IV every 8 hours
OR
Ampicillin/Sulbactam 3 g IV every 6 hours
PLUS
Doxycycline 100 mg PO or IV every 12 hours

IV ofloxacin has been investigated as a single agent; however, because of concerns regarding its spectrum, metronidazole may be included in the regimen. Preliminary data suggest that levofloxacin is as effective as ofloxacin and may be submitted; its single daily dosing makes it advantageous.

From Centers for Disease Control and Prevention: 2006 Guidelines for treatment of sexually transmitted diseases. MMWR 55:11, 2006.

Doxycycline should be included in the regimen of follow-up oral therapy. Sweet and associates observed 17 women with PID who initially had endometrial cultures positive for *Chlamydia.* Clinically, 16 of 17 women responded to treatment with cephalosporins alone. However, posttreatment endometrial cultures remained positive for *Chlamydia* in 12 of 13 women. Therefore without tetracycline or erythromycin a patient may appear free of symptoms but may still be harboring *Chlamydia.* Antibiotics active against *C. trachomatis* must be present in effective dosages for at least 7 days for both clinical and microbiologic cures. *C. trachomatis* has a 48- to 72-hour life cycle inside of the mucosal cell. Thus prolonged therapeutic levels of the antichlamydial antibiotic are imperative.

Regimen B is a combination of clindamycin and an aminoglycoside (gentamicin). Regimen B has the advantage of providing excellent coverage for anaerobic infections and facultative gram-negative rods. Therefore it is preferred for patients with an abscess, IUD-related infections, and pelvic infections after a diagnostic or operative procedure. Studies have demonstrated that high IV levels of clindamycin, such as 900 mg every 8 hours, provide activity against 90% of bacterial strains of *Chlamydia.* Most infectious disease experts recommend the use of a single daily dose of gentamicin rather than a dose given every 8 hours. The initial once-daily aminoglycoside dose is based on nomograms that take body weight into consideration. The advantages of a once-daily aminoglycoside program are decreased toxicity, increased efficacy, and a decreased cost. Also, no serum drug levels are needed. Aztreonam, a monobactam, has an antibiotic spectrum similar to that of the aminoglycosides but without renal toxicity. However, it is much more expensive. It may be given in a dose of 2 g IV every 8 hours. Also, a third-generation cephalosporin may be used instead of an aminoglycoside in a patient with renal disease. Parenteral antibiotic therapy may be discontinued when the woman has been afebrile for 24 hours, and oral therapy with doxycycline (100 mg twice daily) should continue to complete 14 days of therapy.

Alternative inpatient regimens include ampicillin/sulbactam plus doxycycline because they have excellent anaerobic coverage and thus would be a good choice for women with a tuboovarian complex. Similarly the combination of ofloxacin with or without metronidazole is reasonable. Levofloxacin with or without metronidazole may be advantageous because it is dosed once a day. The alternative regimens have had less extensive clinical trials.

In summary, no regimen is uniformly effective for all patients. To date there are insufficient clinical data to suggest superiority of one regimen over another, either with respect to initial response or subsequent fertility.

Operative treatment of acute PID has decreased markedly in the past 15 years. Operations are restricted to life-threatening infections, ruptured tuboovarian abscesses, laparoscopic drainage of a pelvic abscess, persistent masses in some older women for whom future childbearing is not a consideration, and removal of a persistent symptomatic mass. Because of the techniques of in vitro fertilization, every effort is made to perform conservative surgery and preserve ovarian and uterine function in women who have not completed their families. Unilateral removal of a tuboovarian complex or an abscess is a frequent conservative operation for acute PID. Similarly, drainage of a cul-de-sac abscess via percutaneous drainage or a culpotomy incision results in preservation of the reproductive organs.

Rigorously defined, an abscess is a collection of pus within a newly created space. In contrast, a tuboovarian complex is a collection of pus within an anatomic space created by adherence of adjacent organs. Abscesses caused by acute PID contain a mixture of anaerobes and facultative or aerobic organisms (Figs. 23-12 and 23-13). The environment of an abscess cavity results in a low level of oxygen tension. Therefore anaerobic organisms predominate and have been cultured from 60% to 100% of reported cases. Basic investigations have discovered that clindamycin penetrates the human neutrophil, and it is possible that this property facilitates the level of clindamycin within the abscess. Clindamycin is also stable in the abscess environment, which is not true of many other antibiotics. Thus a combination of clindamycin and an aminoglycoside is considered the standard for treatment of a tuboovarian abscess. This combination does not treat the enterococcus, and ampicillin should be added if there is suspicion that this organism is involved. Metronidazole alone is an effective alternative to clindamycin for anaerobic infections but does not provide gram-negative coverage. If abscesses do not respond to parenteral broad-spectrum antibiotics, drainage is imperative.

Transvaginal or transabdominal percutaneous aspiration or drainage of pelvic abscesses may be accomplished under ultrasonic or computer tomography guidance. This technique has shown excellent results. In one small randomized trial early transvaginal drainage and intensive antibiotic therapy were compared with intensive antibiotic therapy alone. A favorable short-term outcome occurred in 90% of those who underwent ultrasound-guided transvaginal drainage in contrast to 65% of

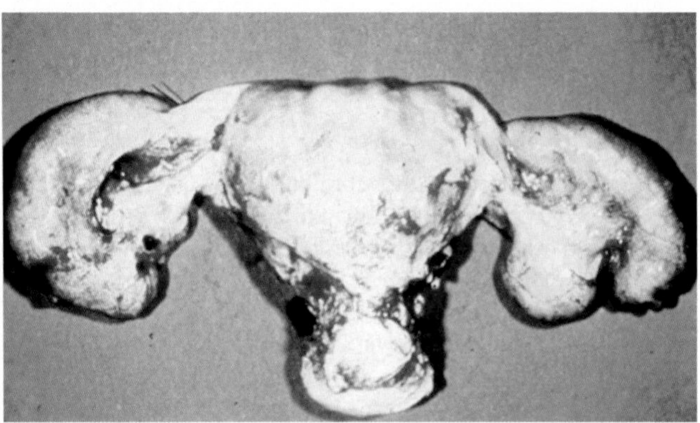

Figure 23-12. Hysterectomy specimen from a 23-year-old patient with bilateral tuboovarian abscesses.

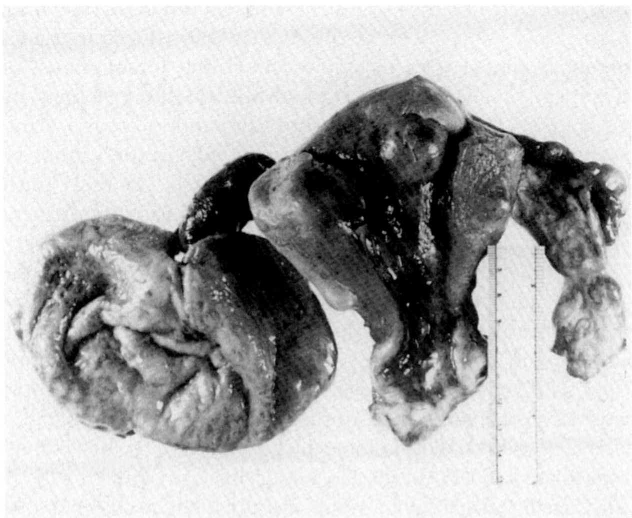

Figure 23-13. Pyosalpinx. Right tube is markedly enlarged and contains 50 mL of creamy pus. Tubal wall is thickened. (From Janovski NA [ed]: Color Atlas of Gross Gynecologic and Obstetric Pathology. New York, McGraw-Hill, 1969, p 131.)

the control group. However, fertility and ectopic pregnancy rates after percutaneous drainage are unknown at this time. Long-term recurrence and sequelae need to be evaluated before this technique is accepted as a therapeutic standard. A strong contraindication to percutaneous aspiration is any suspicion of an infected carcinoma in the differential diagnosis. Laparoscopic aspiration of tuboovarian complexes is another alternative. This procedure has shown good results but does not have greater benefit than percutaneous ultrasound-guided aspiration of abscess cavities. Laparoscopic aspiration obviously carries more operative risks than ultrasound-guided aspiration.

Postmenopausal women with suspected PID should have appropriate imaging studies to rule out other concurrent diseases, especially malignancies. The bacterial etiology in postmenopausal women does not usually include a sexually transmitted microorganism, but rather bacteria from the intestinal tract or normal vaginal flora. The disease process involves tuboovarian complexes and abscesses. Medical treatment should emphasize broad-spectrum antibiotic regimens with adequate anaerobic coverage. Operative intervention in a postmenopausal woman should be considered early in the disease, especially if the condition does not rapidly improve with medical therapy.

Sequelae

Before antibiotic therapy, the mortality rate associated with acute PID was 1%. Grimes has estimated that there is presently one death every other day in the United States directly related to PID. Most of these deaths result from rupture of tuboovarian abscesses. The current mortality rate is 5% to 10% for ruptured tuboovarian abscesses even with modern medical and operative therapy.

Recurrent acute PID is experienced by approximately 25% of women. Younger women become reinfected twice as often as older women. A great challenge to health care providers is to educate women with PID to reduce their chances of a second episode of infection. It is essential and imperative that preventive medicine include treatment and education of the male partner. Selection of contraceptives that will reduce the chance of upper genital tract infections and liberal prescriptions for treatment of lower genital tract disease for these women are also important. Because sequelae to PID, both overt and silent, are related to the number of infections, prevention cannot be overemphasized. Because the majority of PID in the United States is related to STDs, increased attention to partner treatment and education is appropriate.

The morbidity, suffering, and cost of PID arises from the scarring and adhesion formation that accompany healing of damaged tissues after the infection itself is eradicated. These effects result in ectopic pregnancy, chronic pain, and infertility. Approximately 10% to 15% of pregnancies will be ectopic after laparoscopically mild-to-moderate PID, and almost 50% after severe PID. The number of hospitalizations for ectopics peaked around 1989 at 90,000 and declined to 30,000 in 1997. This decline is partially a result of outpatient management of ectopics, but mostly a result of successful chlamydia screening and prevention programs. One case-control study suggested that chlamydia-associated PID alone caused almost one-half of ectopic pregnancies (Table 23-14)

Table 23-14 Summary of the Reproductive Events After Index Laparoscopy in the Total Sample of 1732 Patients and 601 Control Subjects

Category	Patients Number (%)	Control Subjects Number (%)
Total number followed	1732	601
Avoiding pregnancy	370 (21.4)	144 (24.0)
Not pregnant for unknown reasons*	53 (3.1)	6 (1.0)
Attempting pregnancy	1309	451
Pregnant	1100 (80.8)	439 (96.1)
First pregnancy ectopic	100 (9.1)	6 (1.4)
Not pregnant	209 (16.0)	12 (2.7)
Completely examined	162	3
With proved TFI	141	0
With nTFI (other cause of infertility)	21	3
Incompletely examined	47	9

nTFI, nontubular factor infertility. TFI, tubal factor infertility.
*Reporting no use of contraceptive and not consulting for infertility.
From Weström L, Joeseof R, Reynolds G, et al: Pelvic inflammatory disease and fertility. A cohort study of 1,844 women with laparoscopically verified disease and 657 control women with normal laparoscopic results. Sex Transm Dis 19:185, 1992.

Studies have found chronic pain is a common sequela of a symptomatic pelvic infection. In one study the chance that a woman will develop chronic pelvic pain following acute salpingitis was four times greater than the risk for control subjects. Approximately 20% of women with acute pelvic infections subsequently developed chronic pelvic pain, versus approximately 5% among controls without pelvic infection. Other studies have found similar results (Table 23-15). Among women with chronic pelvic pain, approximately two out of three are involuntarily infertile, and a similar percentage have deep dyspareunia. In a study from Oxford of 1355 women with PID and 10,507 controls, chronic abdominal pain developed 10 times more commonly in subjects who had PID (Table 23-16). Chronic pelvic pain may be caused by a hydrosalpinx, a collection of sterile, watery fluid in the fallopian tube. A hydrosalpinx (Fig. 23-14) is the end-stage development of a pyosalpinx. Chronic pain often develops in a woman even though she may have had a normal pelvic examination when examined 4 to 8 weeks following her acute infection. The pain may result from adhesions and the resultant fixation or tethering of organs intended to have freedom of movement during physical activity, coitus, and ovulation (Table 23-17). Women with chronic pelvic pain and a history of acute PID may benefit from laparoscopy to establish the diagnosis and rule out other diseases, such as endometriosis. Often, conservative surgery for this sequela via either laparoscopy or celiotomy is successful.

Acute pelvic infection is one of the major causes of female infertility. Epidemiologic studies estimate that between 4% and 13% of women either are infertile or have an operative procedure secondary to acute PID.

The sequelae of infections vary from a damaged yet patent oviduct, to peritubular and periovarian adhesions that may hinder ovum pickup, to complete tubal obstruction. Tubal obstructions that are secondary to infection are commonly found at the fimbrial end or the cornual region of the oviduct. An alarming factor that has been documented with chlamydial infection is the tubal damage from subacute PID. Patton and colleagues found essentially equally severe tubal damage, adhesion, degeneration of endosalpingeal structures, and cilia dys-

Table 23-15 Frequency and Predictors of Long-Term Sequelae of Acute Pelvic Inflammatory Disease

Sequela	Frequency (Number and %)	Risk Factor	UNIVARIATE ANALYSIS *P*	UNIVARIATE ANALYSIS Relative Risk and 95% Confidence Interval	Multivariate Analysis *P* Value
Involuntary infertility	17/42 (40%)	History of pelvic inflammatory disease	0.05	1.8 (1.0–3.3)	0.05
		Age at time of first sex	0.04	0.39	
		≥2 days of pain before therapy	0.02	2.0 (1.1–3.6)	0.07
Chronic pelvic pain	12/51 (24%)	History of pelvic inflammatory disease	0.03	1.5 (1.0–2.2)	
Pelvic inflammatory disease after index episode	22/51 (43%)	History of pelvic inflammatory disease	0.06	1.7 (0.9–3.1)	0.02
		Mean No. of days of pain before therapy	0.04	—	0.04
		Age at time of first sex	0.0008	—	0.01
Ectopic pregnancy	2/51 (2.4%)	*			

*Risk analysis not performed because of small numbers involved.
From Safrin S Schacter J, Dahrouge D, Sweet RL: Long-term sequelae of acute inflammatory disease. A retrospective cohort study. Am J Obstet Gynccol 166:1300, 1992.

Table 23-16 Standardized (Indirect Standardization) First Event Rates Per 1000 Woman-Years for Specified Outcomes After Admission with Either Acute Pelvic Inflammatory Disease (PID) or a Control Event in Cohorts of Women in the Oxford Record Linkage Study Followed from 1970 to 1985. Number of Women Shown in Parentheses

Outcome Condition	Women with PID *N* = 1200	Women with Control Conditions *N* = 10,507	Relative Risk
Nonspecific abdominal pain	16.7 (155)	1.7 (158)	9.8
Gynaecologic pain	3.6 (38)	0.8 (70)	4.5
Endometriosis	2.2 (18)	0.4 (34)	5.5
Hysterectomy	18.2 (152)	2.3 (204)	7.9
Ectopic pregnancy	1.9 (19)	0.2 (14)	9.5

From Buchan H, Vessey M, Goldacre M, Fairweather J: Morbidity following pelvic inflammatory disease. Br J Obstet Gynaecol 100:558, 1993.

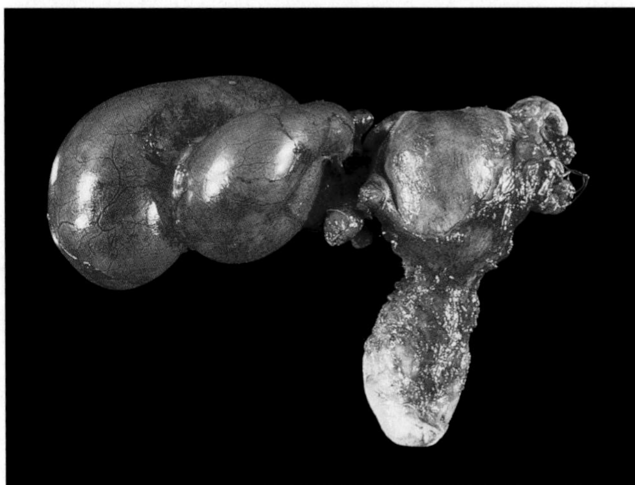

Figure 23-14. Hydrosalpinx with marked dilatation of the fallopian tube and blunting of the fimbriated end. (From Voet RL: Color Atlas of Obstetric and Gynecologic Pathology. St. Louis, Mosby, 1997, p 107.)

function in women with acute chlamydial PID and women with silent chlamydial infection.

Weström followed a large cohort of women with PID in southern Sweden from 1960 through 1984. He discovered that the infertility rate was significantly lower in the younger women than in older women, following a single episode of infection (Table 23-18). The milder the episode of acute PID the less likely a woman was to suffer tubal obstruction and infertility. The infertility rate also increased directly with the number of episodes of acute pelvic infection. These data are not surprising because the prevalence of long-term sequelae is directly proportional to the number and severity of the episodes of acute PID. Lepine and coworkers recently reported additional data from the world's largest and longest prospective cohort study of women with acute PID. The authors found that increasing severity of the initial episode of acute pelvic infection correlates with a longer low-term probability of live birth. The cumulative proportion of women achieving a live birth after 12 years was 90% for women whose initial infection was mild, 82% for women with moderate disease, and 57% for women with severe PID. Subsequent episodes of pelvic infection had a greater effect on women whose initial episode was judged as severe as for those with milder disease.

ACTINOMYCES INFECTION

Actinomyces is a rare cause of upper genital tract infection. *Actinomyces israelii,* the most common species found, is a gram-positive anaerobic bacterium that is difficult to culture. To successfully culture this organism, an anaerobic environment must be maintained for 2 to 3 weeks.

A. israelii is discovered either by histologic examination or culture from women with tuboovarian abscesses. There are many

Table 23-17 Associations between a History of Acute Pelvic Inflammatory Disease and Adnexal Adhesions, Distal Tubal Occlusion, and/or Perihepatic Adhesions

	PELVIC INFLAMMATORY DISEASE				
Laparoscopic Findings	**Yes (*N* = 22)**	**No (*N* = 90)**	**OR**	**95% CI**	***P***
Distal tubal occlusion	4 (18.2%)	7 (7.8%)	2.6	0.7–10.0	0.14
Tubal adhesions	8 (36.4%)	21 (23.3%)	1.9	0.7–5.1	0.16
Ovarian adhesions	9 (40.9%)	21 (23.3%)	2.3	0.9–6.5	0.08
Perihepatic adhesions	3/21 (14.3%)	2/84 (2.4%)	6.8	1.1–43.9	0.05
Any adhesions	11 (50.0%)	25 (27.8%)	2.6	1.0–6.8	0.04

CI, confidence interval; OR, odds ratio.
From Wølner-Hanssen P: Silent pelvic inflammatory disease: Is it overstated? Obstet Gynecol 86:321, 1995.

Table 23-18 Percent and Number of Patients Attempting to Conceive Who Had Tubal Factor Infertility by Age, Number of Acute Pelvic Inflammatory Disease Episodes, and Severity of Pelvic Inflammatory Disease*

	AGE (YEARS)					
	<25		≥25		TOTAL	
Number of Episodes of PID	%	(*n*/*N*)	%	(*n*/*N*)	%	(*n*/*N*)
One	7.7	(59/771)	9.1	(20/220)	8.0	(79/991)
Mild	0.8	(2/241)	0.0	(0/71)	0.6	(2/312)
Moderate	6.4	(23/361)	5.6	(5/89)	6.2	(28/452)
Severe	20.1	(34/169)	25.0	(15/60)	21.4	(49/229)
Two	18.4	(29/158)	25.9	(7/27)	19.5	(36/185)
Three or more	37.7	(23/61)	75.0	(3/4)	40.0	(26/65)
Total	11.2	(111/990)	12.0	(30/251)	11.4	(141/1241)

n, total number of cases followed; *N*, total number of evaluable cases; PID, pelvic inflammatory disease.
*Excluding those with nontubal factor infertility and with incomplete infertility examinations.
From Weström L, Joeseof R, Reynolds G, et al: Pelvic inflammatory disease and fertility. A cohort study of 1,844 women with laparoscopically verified disease and 657 control women with normal laparoscopic results. Sex Transmit Dis 19:185, 1992.

large series of tuboovarian abscesses without a single case of *A. israelii* described. Most cases described have been in women chronically wearing an IUD for an average of 8 years. Usually *A. israelii* is part of a polymicrobial infection, and whether its role is primary or secondary in the infectious process is unknown.

There is a controversy as to the significance of discovering actinomycetes on a Pap smear of women wearing an IUD. The contrasting, relatively high detection rate of actinomycetes observed on Pap smears from IUD users, and extreme rarity of subsequent development of pelvic actinomycosis, leads most experts to conclude that progression to upper tract infection is highly unlikely to be related. The decision to remove the IUD to treat a patient is influenced by the presence or absence of clinical symptoms. Unless there are associated symptoms, such as fever, abdominal pain, or abnormal uterine bleeding, the identification of the organism in any cervical smear should not prompt antibiotic therapy or IUD removal.

Actinomycetes may produce a chronic endometritis with an associated foul-smelling discharge. The clinical infection may be manifest by widespread adhesions, induration, and fibrosis. The diagnosis of *Actinomyces* infection is usually not made until a tuboovarian abscess is examined by the pathologist. Then the classic "sulfur granules" are observed histologically along with gram-positive filaments.

Although much has been written about chronic draining sinuses with *Actinomyces* infection, this complication is unusual in gynecology. However, when this organism is present in a tuboovarian abscess, the patient should receive oral penicillin or doxycycline or fluoroquinolones for 12 weeks following an operative procedure.

TUBERCULOSIS

Tuberculosis of the upper genital tract, primarily chronic salpingitis and chronic endometritis, is a rare disease in the United States. To date most gynecologists will not have encountered a single case. However, pulmonary tuberculosis is steadily increasing in the United States, and it is likely that the incidence of pelvic tuberculosis also will rise. Tuberculosis is a frequent cause of chronic PID and infertility in other parts of the world. Thus it should be suspected in immigrants, especially those from Asia, the Middle East, and Latin America. Though the disease is usually found in premenopausal women, it will occur in postmenopausal women 10% of the time.

Pelvic tuberculosis may be produced by either *Mycobacterium tuberculosis* or *M. bovis.* The primary site of infection for tuberculosis is usually the lung. Early in the course of pulmonary infection the bacteria spread hematogenously, and the infection becomes located in the oviduct. Subsequently the bacilli usually spread to the endometrium and less commonly to the ovaries. However, the oviducts are the primary and predominant site of pelvic tuberculosis. In developing countries without pasteurization of milk, bovine tuberculosis produces primary infections in the human gastrointestinal tract. Subsequent lymphatic or hematogenous dissemination results in pelvic tuberculosis. Autopsy studies published 25 years ago demonstrated that 4% to 12% of women who died of pulmonary tuberculosis concurrently had evidence of upper genital tract infection. In a recent large study from India, 117 women had tubal blockage secondary to tuberculosis. When these women underwent laparoscopy, the findings were 50% simple tubal blockage, 15% tuboovarian masses, and 24% a frozen pelvis.

In general, extrapulmonary tuberculosis may present as either an insidious or as a rapidly progressing disease. The clinical symptoms and signs of pelvic tuberculosis are similar to the chronic sequelae of nontuberculous acute PID. The predominant presentations of this chronic infection are infertility and abnormal uterine bleeding. Mild-to-moderate chronic abdominal and pelvic pain occur in 35% of women with the disease. Advanced cases are often accompanied by ascites. Some women may be asymptomatic. The findings at pelvic examination are normal in approximately 50% of cases. The remaining patients have mild adnexal tenderness and bilateral adnexal masses, with an inability to manipulate the adnexa because of scarring and fixation.

Tuberculous salpingitis may be suspected when a patient is not responding to conventional antibiotic therapy for acute bacterial PID. Results of a tuberculin skin test will be positive. However, approximately one in three women does not have evidence of pulmonary tuberculosis on chest radiographic films. The diagnosis may be established by performing an endometrial biopsy late in the secretory phase of the cycle. A portion of the endometrial biopsy should be sent for culture and animal inoculation, and the remaining portion should be examined histologically. The findings of classic giant cells, granulomas, and caseous necrosis confirm the diagnosis (Fig. 23-15). Approximately two out of three women with tuberculous salpingitis will have concomitant tuberculous endometritis. Pelvic tuberculosis may not be diagnosed until laparotomy or celiotomy, when the characteristic changes may be visualized. The distal ends of the oviduct remain everted, producing a "tobacco pouch" appearance. When the diagnosis has been established, the patient should have a chest radiographic examination, IV pyelogram, serial gastric washings, and urine cultures for tuberculosis. Approximately 10% of women with pelvic tuberculosis have concomitant urinary tract tuberculosis.

The treatment of pelvic tuberculosis is medical. Not uncommonly patients will be admitted to the hospital for initiation of therapy, for observation, and to ensure appropriate compliance. Initial therapy in a patient with newly diagnosed tuberculosis usually will include five drugs because of the emergence of multidrug-resistant organisms. Multidrug-resistant (MDR) tuberculosis is defined as infection from a strain of *M. tuberculous* that is resistant to two or more agents, including isoniazid. The mortality rate in HIV-negative patients who develop MDR infection may be as high as 80%. Often, health care workers become infected during outbreaks of MDR tuberculosis. The CDC has recommended starting a patient on multidrug regimens until the patient's culture results yield specific sensitivity. At that time medications may be decreased to two or three agents. Patients who have infection from MDR strains are usually kept on five drug regimens. Operative therapy for pelvic tuberculosis is reserved for women with persistent pelvic masses, some women with resistant organisms, women older than 40, and women whose endometrial cultures remain positive. Although the major sequelae of pelvic tuberculosis are infertility, occasionally a woman will become pregnant after medical therapy.

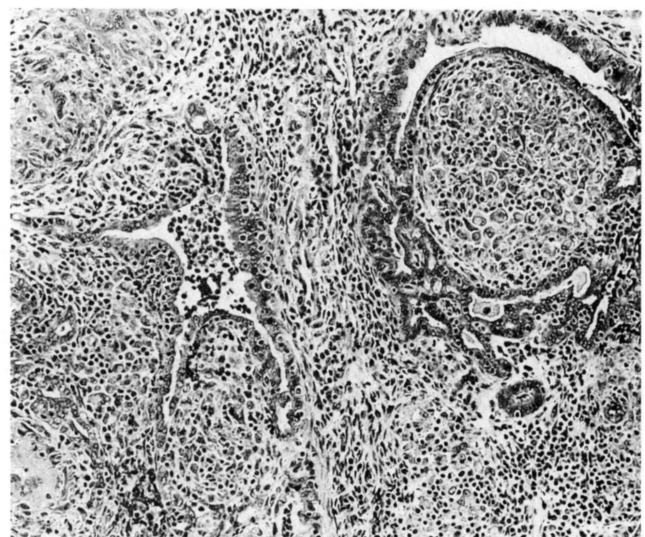

Figure 23-15. Tuberculous salpingitis: Langerhans' giant cell granuloma. (From Gompel C, Silverberg SG (eds): Pathology in Gynecology and Obstetrics, 2nd ed. Philadelphia, JB Lippincott, 1977, p 258.)

KEY POINTS

- The Centers for Disease Control (CDC) regularly revises its treatment protocols for STDs. This information may be accessed online at www.cdc.gov/publications.htm.
- Studies have emphasized that organisms that produce bacterial vaginosis may also produce histologic endometritis even in women without symptoms of upper tract disease.
- The diagnosis of chronic endometritis is established by the finding of plasma cells and neutrophils on endometrial biopsy.
- During days 1 and 2 of the menstrual cycle, it is normal to see scattered polymorphonuclear leukocytes in an endometrial biopsy.
- PID may include infection of *any or all* of the following anatomic locations: the endometrium (endometritis), the oviducts (salpingitis), the ovary (oophoritis), the uterine wall (myometritis), the uterine serosa and broad ligaments (parametritis), and the pelvic peritoneum.

Continued

KEY POINTS *Continued*

- Approximately one in four women with acute PID experiences further medical sequelae, including recurrent acute PID, ectopic pregnancy, and chronic pelvic pain.
- The CDC has emphasized that physicians should aggressively treat women if there is any suspicion of the disease, since sequelae are so devastating and the clinical diagnosis made from symptoms, signs, and laboratory data is often incorrect.
- Acute PID is usually caused by a polymicrobial infection of organisms ascending from the vagina and cervix, traveling along the mucosa of the endometrium to infect the mucosa of the oviduct. The primary bacterial organisms cultured from tubal fluid and mucosa include *Neisseria gonorrhoeae, Chlamydia trachomatis,* and endogenous aerobic and anaerobic bacteria.
- Approximately 20% of women with cervical infection by gonorrhea subsequently develop PID. The virulence of the strain of *N. gonorrhoeae* helps to predict the incidence of upper genital tract infection.
- *C. trachomatis* is the most prevalent organism causing PID. The salpingitis it produces is usually insidious in onset.
- Approximately 30% of women with documented acute cervicitis secondary to chlamydia subsequently develop acute PID.
- Studies of women with tubal infertility have noted that many women, though not diagnosed as having had overt PID, have had symptoms of pelvic pain. Some investigators believe that atypical or silent PID may be the more common form of upper tract infection, and symptomatic PID may be but the "tip of the iceberg."
- Anaerobic organisms are almost ubiquitous in pelvic abscesses associated with acute pelvic inflammatory disease. Tuboovarian complexes and abscesses are more common in women with concurrent bacterial vaginosis or HIV infection.
- There is a strong correlation between the incidence of STD within a population and the incidence of acute PID.
- In epidemiologic studies, age at first intercourse, marital status, and number of sexual partners are all gross indicators of the frequency of exposure to STDs. Having multiple sexual partners increases the chance of acquiring acute PID approximately fivefold.
- Acute PID is a condition of young menstruating women, with 75% of cases occurring in women younger than 25 years of age. The risk for a sexually active adolescent female is 1 in 8. This decreases to 1 in 80 for women older than age 25.
- When PID is found in the postmenopausal woman, genital malignancies, diabetes, or concurrent intestinal disease is usually found.
- The increase in risk for PID occurs primarily at the time of insertion of the IUD and in the first 3 weeks after placement.
- Acute salpingitis occurring in a woman with a previous tubal ligation is rare, and, when it does occur, it presents with less severe symptoms.
- Approximately 20% to 25% of women have no identifiable intraabdominal or pelvic disease by laparoscopy when diagnosed as having acute PID on the basis of history, physical, and laboratory examination.
- Pain in the lower abdomen and pelvis is the most frequent symptom of acute PID, and in all large series more than 90% of women with the diagnosis have some type of abdominal pain.
- Seventy-five percent of patients with acute PID have an associated endocervical infection or a coexistent purulent vaginal discharge.
- Nausea and vomiting are comparatively late symptoms in the course of acute PID.
- From 5% to 10% of women with acute PID develop perihepatic inflammation, Fitz-Hugh–Curtis syndrome.
- Approximately one third of women with acute PID present with a temperature greater than 38° C.
- The incidence of adnexal abscess is approximately 10% in women with acute PID.
- Acute PID should be diagnosed with a minimum of suspicion with the knowledge that overtreatment is preferable to missed diagnosis.
- Acute PID should be included in the differential diagnosis of any sexually active young woman with pelvic pain.
- Because acute PID has a wide range of nonspecific clinical symptoms, there is both a high false-positive rate and a high false-negative rate when the diagnosis is based on clinical findings and laboratory results.
- Less than 50% of women with acute PID have a white blood cell count of greater than 10,000 cells per milliliter.
- Most studies demonstrate that women with acute PID and HIV infection have a higher incidence of adnexal masses. However, the acute pelvic infection responds to antibiotic therapy in a similar fashion as in women who are not infected with HIV.
- Though ultrasonography is neither specific nor sensitive in distinguishing the cause of a pelvic mass, findings of dilated and fluid-filled tubes, free peritoneal fluid, and adnexal masses may be confirmatory of symptoms and physical signs. Vaginal ultrasound does have a high positive predictive value when used in a high-risk population.
- Laparoscopy is the optimum method for accurately diagnosing acute PID.
- Women who are being treated as outpatients for acute PID should be reexamined within 48 to 72 hours of initiation of therapy to evaluate the response of the disease to oral antibiotics.
- Indications for hospitalization for treatment of PID include presence of tuboovarian complex or abscess, pregnancy, concurrent HIV infection, uncertain diagnosis, gastrointestinal symptoms, peritonitis in upper quadrants, history of operative or diagnostic procedures, and inadequate response to outpatient therapy.
- There is no clinically significant difference in bioavailability of doxycycline whether it is given by the oral or IV route.

KEY POINTS *Continued*

Thus doxycycline should be administered orally whenever possible because of the marked superficial phlebitis produced by IV infusion.

- Antibiotics against *C. trachomatis* must be present in effective dosages for at least 7 days for both clinical and microbiologic cures. *C. trachomatis* has a 48- to 72-hour life cycle inside of the mucosal cell. Thus prolonged therapeutic levels of the antichlamydial antibiotic are imperative.
- The advantages of a once daily aminoglycoside program are decreased toxicity, increased efficacy, and a decreased cost.
- Surgical treatment for acute PID is restricted to life-threatening infections, ruptured tuboovarian abscesses, laparoscopic drainage of a pelvic abscess, persistent masses in some older women for whom future childbearing is not a consideration, and removal of a persistent symptomatic mass. Unilateral removal of a tuboovarian complex or abscess is a frequent conservative operation for acute PID for women desiring future childbearing.
- Recurrent acute PID is experienced by approximately 25% of women. The chance that a woman will develop chronic pelvic pain following acute PID is four times greater than is the risk for control subjects.
- Because sequelae of acute PID are related to the number of infections, prevention cannot be overemphasized.
- *Actinomyces* is a rare cause of upper genital tract infection. *Actinomyces israelii* is the most common species found and is a gram-positive anaerobe, which is difficult to culture.
- Pelvic tuberculosis may be produced by either *Mycobacterium tuberculosis* or *M. bovis.* The primary sites of infection are the lung and the gastrointestinal tract.
- The predominant presentations of tuberculous salpingitis are infertility and abnormal uterine bleeding.
- Because of the emergence of multidrug-resistant strains, the CDC has recommended starting a patient on multidrug regimens until the patient's culture results yield specific sensitivity.

BIBLIOGRAPHY

Key Readings

Centers for Disease Control: 2006 Guidelines for treatment of STDs, MMWR Vol 55; No. RR-11, 2006.

Eckert LO, Hawes SE, Wølner-Hanssen PK, et al: Endometritis: The clinical-pathologic syndrome. Am J Obstet Gynecol 186(4):690-5, 2002.

Eschenbach DA, Wölner-Hanssen P, Hawes SE, et al: Acute pelvic inflammatory disease: Associations of clinical and laboratory findings with laparoscopic findings. Obstet Gynecol 89:184, 1997.

Hillier SL, Kiviat NB, Hawes SE, et al: Role of bacterial vaginosis-associated microorganisms in endometritis. Am J Obstet Gynecol 175:435, 1996.

Hillis SD, Owens LM, Marchbanks PA, et al: Recurrent chlamydial infections increase risks of hospitalization for ectopic pregnancy and pelvic inflammatory disease. Am J Obstet Gynecol 176:103, 1997.

Jacobson LJ: Differential diagnosis of acute pelvic inflammatory disease. Am J Obstet Gynecol 138:1006, 1980.

Larsson PG, Platz-Christensen JJ, Thejls H, et al: Incidence of pelvic inflammatory disease after first-trimester legal abortion in women with bacterial vaginosis after treatment with metronidazole: A double-blind randomized study. Am J Obstet Gynecol 166:100, 1992.

Lepine LA, Hillis SD, Marchbanks PA, et al: Severity of pelvic inflammatory disease as a predictor of the probability of live birth. Am J Obstet Gynecol 178:977, 1998.

Lippes J: Pelvic actinomycosis: A review and preliminary look at prevalence. Am J Obstet Gynecol 180:265, 1999.

Weström L: Incidence, prevalence, and trends of acute pelvic inflammatory disease and its consequences in industrialized countries. Am J Obstet Gynecol 138:880, 1980.

Weström L, Joesoef R, Reynolds G, et al: Pelvic inflammatory disease and fertility: A cohort study of 1,844 women with laparoscopically verified disease and 657 control women with normal laparoscopic results. Sex Transmit Dis 19:185, 1992.

Wisenfeld HG, Hillier SL, Krohn MA, et al: Lower genital tract infection and endometritis: Insight into subclinical pelvic inflammatory disease. Obstet Gynecol 100:3, 2002.

Key References

Abbul SB, Muskin EP, Shofer FS: Pelvic inflammatory disease in patients with bilateral tubal ligation. Am J Emerg Med 15:271, 1997.

Aboulghar MA, Mansour RT, Serour GI: Ultrasonographically guided transvaginal aspiration of tuboovarian abscesses and pyosalpinges: An optional treatment for acute pelvic inflammatory disease. Am J Obstet Gynecol 172:1501, 1995.

Ahmad MM: IUDs and actinomyces. IPPF Med Bul 21:3, 1987.

Amin-Hanjani S, Chatwani A: Endometrial cultures in acute pelvic inflammatory disease. Infect Dis Obstet Gynecol 3:56, 1995.

Anthony SJ, Lopez P: Genital amebiasis: Historical perspective on an unusual disease presentation. Urology 54:952, 1999.

Askienazy-Elbhar M, Henry-Suchet J: Persistent "silent" *Chlamydia trachomatis* female genital tract infections. Infec Dis Obstet Gynecol 7:31, 1999.

Baker DA: Re-emergence of tuberculosis. Curr Opin Obstet Gynecol 6:373, 1994.

Bernstien R, Kennedy WR, Waldron J: Acute pelvic inflammatory disease: A clinical follow-up. Int J Fertil 1987; 32:229.

Boardman LA, Peipert JF, Brody JM, et al: Endovaginal sonography for the diagnosis of upper genital tract infection. Obstet Gynecol 90:54, 1997.

Bowie WR: Antibiotics and sexually transmitted diseases. Infect Dis Clin North Am 8:841, 1994.

Buchan H, Vessey M, Goldacre M, Fairweather J: Morbidity following pelvic inflammatory disease. Br J Obstet Gynaecol 100:558, 1993.

Burkman R, Schlesselman S, McCaffrey L, et al. The relationship of genital tract actinomycetes and the development of pelvic inflammatory disease. Am J Obstet Gynecol 143:585, 1982.

Bukusi EA, Cohen CR, Stevens CE, et al: Effects of human immunodeficiency virus 1 infection on microbial origins of pelvic inflammatory disease on efficacy of ambulatory oral therapy. Am J Obstet Gynecol 181:1374, 1999.

Cacciatore B, Leminen A, Ingman-Friberg S, et al: Transvaginal sonographic findings in ambulatory patients with suspected pelvic inflammatory disease. Obstet Gynecol 80:912, 1992.

Cates W, Joesoef MR, Goldman MB: Atypical pelvic inflammatory disease: Can we identify clinical predictors? Am J Obstet Gynecol 169:341, 1993.

Chan Y, Parchment W, Skurnick JH, et al: Epidemiology and clinical outcome of patients hospitalized with pelvic inflammatory disease complicated by tubo-ovarian abscess. Infect Dis Obstet Gynecol 3:135, 1995.

Chatwani A, Amin-Hanjani S: Management of intrauterine device-associated actinomycosis. Infect Dis Obstet Gynecol 1:130, 1993.

Chatwani A, Harmanli OH, Nyirjesy P, Reece EA: Significance of genital mycoplasmas in pelvic inflammatory disease: Innocent bystander. Infec Dis Obstet Gynecol, 4:263, 1996.

Chow JM, Yonekuram L, Richwald GA, et al: The association between *Chlamydia trachomatis* and ectopic pregnancy. JAMA 263:3164, 1990.

Cohen CR, Brunham RC: Pathogenesis of chlamydia induced pelvic inflammatory disease. Sex Transm Infect 75:21, 1999.

Cohen CR, Gichui J, Rukaria R, et al: Immunogenetic correlates for Chlamydia trachomatis-associated tubal infertility. Obstet Gynecol 101(3):438, 2003.

Cohen CR, Manhart LE, Bukusi EA, et al: Association between mycoplasma genitalium and acute endometritis, 359(9308):765, 2002.

Cohen CR, Mugo NR, Astete SG, et al: Detection of Mycoplasma genitalium in women with laparoscopically diagnosed acute salpingitis. Sex Transm Infec 81(6):463, 2005.

Cohen CR, Sinei S, Reilly M, et al: Effects of human immunodeficiency virus type 1 infection upon acute salpingitis: a laparoscopic study. J Infec Dis 178:1352, 1998.

Corsi PJ, Johnson SC, Gonik B, et al: Transvaginal ultrasound-guided aspiration of pelvic abscesses. Infec Dis Obstet Gynecol 7:216, 1999.

Curtis KM, Hillis SD, Kieke BA, et al. Visits to emergency departments for gynecologic disorders in the United States, 1992–1994. Obstet Gynecol 1998; 91:1007.

Dan BB: Sex, lives, and *Chlamydia* rates. JAMA 263:3191, 1990.

Davis JD: Aztreonam. Prim Care Update Ob/Gyns 4:61, 1997.

Devine PA: Extrapelvic manifestations of gonorrhea. Prim Care Update Ob/Gyns 5:233, 1998.

Dieterie S, Rummel C, Bader LW, et al: Presence of the major outer-membrane protein of *Chlamydia trachomatis* in patients with chronic salpingitis and salpingitis isthmica nodosa with tubal occlusion. Fertil Steril 70:774, 1998.

Dodson MG, Faro S: The polymicrobial etiology of acute pelvic inflammatory disease and treatment regimens. Rev Infect Dis 7:S696, 1985.

Eckert LO, Hawes SE, Wolner-Hanssen PK, et al: The antimicrobial treatment of subacute endometritis: A proof of concept study. Am J Obstet Gynecol 190(2):305, 2004.

Eckert LO, Watts DH, Thwin SS, et al: Histologic endometritis in asymptomatic human immunodeficiency virus-infected women: Characterization and effect of antimicrobial therapy. Obstet Gynecol 102(5 Pt 1): 962, 2003.

Farley TMM, Rosenberg MJ, Rowe PJ, et al: Intrauterine devices and pelvic inflammatory disease: An international perspective. Lancet 339:785, 1992.

Faro S, Martens M, Maccato M, et al: Vaginal flora and pelvic inflammatory disease. Am J Obstet Gynecol 169:470, 1993.

Fiorino AS: Intrauterine contraceptive device-associated actinomycotic abscess and actinomyces detection on cervical smear. Obstet Gynecol 87:142, 1996.

Fleenor-Ford A, Hayden MK, Weinstein RA: Vancomycin-resistant enterococci: Implications for surgeons. Surgery 125:121, 1999.

Garland SM, Kelly VN: Role of genital mycoplasmas in bacteremia: Should we be routinely culturing for these organisms? Infec Dis Obstet Gynecol 4:329, 1996.

Gérard HC, Branigan PJ, Balsara GR, et al: Viability of *Chlamydia trachomatis* in fallopian tubes of patients with ectopic pregnancy. Fertil Steril 70:945, 1998.

Gilbert DN, Lee BL, Dworkin RJ, et al: A randomized comparison of the safety and efficacy of once-daily gentamicin or thrice-daily gentamicin in combination with ticarcillin-clavulanate. Am J Med 105:182, 1998.

Grimes DA: Deaths due to sexually transmitted diseases. JAMA 255:1727, 1986.

Hadgu A, Weström L, Brooks CA, et al: Predicting acute pelvic inflammatory disease: A multivariate analysis. Am J Obstet Gynecol 155:954, 1986.

Haeusler G, Tempfer C, Lehner R, et al: Fallopian tissue sampling with a cytobrush during hysteroscopy: A new approach for detecting tubal infection. Fertil Steril 67:580, 1997.

Hager WD, Eschenbach DA, Spence MR, et al: Criteria for diagnosis and grading of salpingitis. Obstet Gynecol 61:113, 1983.

Haggerty CL, Ness RB, Amortegui A, et al: Endometritis does not predict reproductive morbidity after pelvic inflammatory disease. Am J Obstet Gynecol 188(1): 141, 2003.

Hemsell DL, Little BB, Faro S, et al: Comparison of three regimens recommended by the Centers for Disease Control and Prevention for the treatment of women hospitalized with acute pelvic inflammatory disease. Clin Infect Dis 19:720, 1994.

Hoffman IF, Taha TE, Padian NS, et al: Nonoxynol-9 100 mg gel: Multi-site safety study from sub-Saharan Africa. AIDS 5;18(16):2191, 2004.

Irwin KL, Moorman AC, O'Sullivan MJ, et al: Influence of human immunodeficiency virus infection on pelvic inflammatory disease. Obstet Gynecol 95:525, 2000.

Jackson SL, Soper DE: Pelvic inflammatory disease in the postmenopausal woman. Infec Dis Obstet Gynecol 7:248, 1999.

Jacobs RF: Multiple-drug-resistant tuberculosis. Clin Infect Dis 19:1, 1994.

Jamieson DJ, Duerr A, Macasaet MA, et al: Risk factors for a complicated clinical course among women hospitalized with pelvic inflammatory disease. Infec Dis Obstet Gynecol 8:88, 2000.

Jana N, Vasishta K, Saha SC, Ghosh K: Obstetrical outcomes among women with extrapulmonary tuberculosis. N Engl J Med 341:645, 1999.

Janovski NA (ed): Color Atlas of Gross Gynecologic and Obstetric Pathology. New York, McGraw-Hill, 1969.

Jossens MOR, Schachter J, Sweet RL: Risk factors associated with pelvic inflammatory disease of differing microbial etiologies, Obstet Gynecol 83:989, 1994.

Kamwendo F, Forslin L, Bodin L, Danielson D: Programmes to reduce pelvic inflammatory disease—the Swedish experience. Lancet 351:25, 1998.

Kerr-Layton JA, Stamm CA, Peterson LS, McGregor JA: Chronic plasma cell endometritis in hysterectomy specimens of HIV-infected women: a retrospective analysis. Infec Dis Obstet Gynecol 6:186, 1998.

Korn AP, Bolan G, Padian N, et al: Plasma cell endometritis in women with symptomatic bacterial vaginosis. Obstet Gynecol 85:387, 1995.

Korn AP, Hessol N, Padian N, et al: Commonly used diagnostic criteria for pelvic inflammatory disease have poor sensitivity for plasma cell endometritis. Sex Transm Dis 22(6):335, 1995.

Korn AP, Hessol NA, Padian NS, et al: Risk factors for plasma cell endometritis among women with cervical *Neisseria gonorrhoeae,* cervical *Chlamydia trachomatis,* or bacterial vaginosis. Am J Obstet Gynecol 178:987, 1998.

Korn AP, Landers DV, Green JR, et al: Pelvic inflammatory disease in human immunodeficiency virus-infected women. Obstet Gynecol 82:765, 1993.

Landers DV, Wølner-Hanssen P, Paavonen J, et al: Combination antimicrobial therapy in the treatment of acute pelvic inflammatory disease. Am J Obstet Gynecol 164:849, 1991.

Larsen B: Virulence attributes of low-virulence organisms. Infect Dis Obstet Gynecol 2:95, 1994.

Livengood CH III, Hill GB, Addison WA: Pelvic inflammatory disease: findings during inpatient treatment of clinically severe, laparoscopy-documented disease. Am J Obstet Gynecol 166:519, 1992.

Mann SN, Smith JR, Barton SE: Pelvic inflammatory disease. Int J STD AIDS 7:315, 1996.

McCormack WM: Pelvic inflammatory disease. N Engl J Med 330:115, 1994.

McGregor JA, Crombleholme WR, Newton E, et al: Randomized comparison of ampicillin-sulbactam to cefoxitin and doxycycline or clindamycin and gentamicin in the treatment of pelvic inflammatory disease or endometriosis. Obstet Gynecol 83:998, 1994.

McNeeley SG, Hendrix SL, Mazzoni MM, et al: Medically sound, cost-effective treatment for pelvic inflammatory disease and tuboovarian abscess. Am J Obstet Gynecol 178:1272, 1998.

Møller BR, Kristiansen FV, Thorsen P, et al: Sterility of the uterine cavity. Acta Obstet Gynecol Scand 74:216, 1995.

Money DM, Hawes SE, Eschenbach DA, et al: Antibodies to the chlamydial 60 kd heat-shock protein are associated with laparoscopically confirmed perihepatitis. Am J Obstet Gynecol 176:870, 1997.

Monif GRG: Abscesses occurring after acute salpingitis. Contemp OB/GYN 37:55, 1992.

Monif GRG: The great douching debate: to douche or not to douche. Obstet Gynecol 94:630, 1999.

Munday PE: Clinical aspects of pelvic inflammatory disease. Hum Reprod 12 (Suppl):121, 1997.

Ness RB, Hillier SL, Kip KE, Richter HE, Soper DE, Stamm CA, McGregor JA, Bass DC, Rice P, Sweet RL: Douching, pelvic inflammatory disease, and incident gonococcal and chlamydial genital infection in a cohort of high-risk women, Am J Epidemiol 161(2):186-95, 2005.

Ness RB, Keder LM, Soper DE, et al: Oral contraception and recognition of endometritis, Am J Obstet Gynecol 176:580, 1997.

Ness RB, Trautmann G, Richter HE, et al: Effectiveness of treatment strategies of some women with pelvic inflammatory disease: A randomized trial. Obstet Gynecol 106(3) 573, 2005.

Nicolau D, Freeman CD, Belliveau PP, et al: Experience with a once-daily aminoglycoside program administered to 2,184 adult patients. Antimicrob Agent Chemother 39:650, 1995.

Paavonen J: Pelvic inflammatory disease: From diagnosis to prevention. Sex Transmit Dis 16:747, 1998.

Paavonen J, Kiviat N, Brunham RC, et al: Prevalence and manifestations of endometritis among women with cervicitis. Am J Obstet Gynecol 152:280, 1985.

Padian NS, Washington AE: Pelvic inflammatory disease: A brief overview. Ann Epidemiol 4:128, 1994.

Panoskaltsis TA, Moore DA, Haidopoulos DA, McIndoe AG: Tuberculous peritonitis: Part of the differential diagnosis in ovarian cancer. Am J Obstet Gynecol 182:740, 2000.

Parikh FR, Nadkarni SG, Kamat SA, et al: Genital tuberculosis—a major pelvic factor causing infertility in Indian women. Fertil Steril 67:497, 1997.

Patton DL, Moore DE, Spadoni LR, et al: A comparison of the fallopian tube's response to overt and silent salpingitis. Obstet Gynecol 73:622, 1989.

Paukku M, Puolakkainen M, Paavonen T, Paavenen J: Plasma cell endometritis is associated with *Chlamydia trachomatis* infection. Am J Clin Pathol 112:211, 1999.

Pavletic AJ, Wölner-Hanssen P, Paavonen J, et al: Infertility following pelvic inflammatory disease. Infec Dis Obstet Gynecol 7:145, 1999.

Peipert JF, Boardman LA, Sung CJ: Performance of clinical and laparoscopic criteria for the diagnosis of upper genital tract infection. Infec Dis Obstet Gynecol 5:291, 1997.

Peipert JF, Montagno AB, Cooper AS, Sung CJ: Bacterial vaginosis as a risk factor for upper genital tract infection. Am J Obstet Gynecol 177:1184, 1997.

Peipert JF, Ness RB, Soper DE, Bass D: Association of lower genital tract inflammation with objective evidence of endometritis. Infec Dis Obstet Gynecol 8:83, 2000.

Peipert JF, Soper DE: Diagnostic evaluation of pelvic inflammatory disease. Infect Dis Obstet Gynecol 2:38, 1994.

Peipert JF, Sweet RL, Walker CK, et al: Evaluation of ofloxacin in the treatment of laparoscopically documented acute pelvic inflammatory disease (salpingitis). Infec Dis Obstet Gynecol 7:138, 1999.

Perdigon PL: Imaging techniques for diagnosis of serious intraabdominal and pelvic infections. Prim Care Update Ob/Gyns 6:115, 1999.

Perez-Medina T, Huertas MA, Bajo JM: Early ultrasound-guided transvaginal drainage of tubo-ovarian abscesses: A randomized study. Ultrasound Obstet Gynecol 7:435, 1996.

Peterson HB, Galaqid EI, Zenilman JM: Pelvic inflammatory disease: Review of treatment options. Rev Infect Dis 12(S6): S656, 1990.

Phillips AJ, D'Ablaing G: Acute salpingitis subsequent to tubal ligation. Obstet Gynecol 67:55S, 1986.

Reed SD, Landers DV, Sweet RL: Antibiotic treatment of tuboovarian abscess: Comparison of broad-spectrum β-lactam agents versus clindamycin-containing regimens. Am J Obstet Gynecol 164:1556, 1991.

Rein DB, Kassler WJ, Irwin KL, Rabiee L: Direct medical cost of pelvic inflammatory disease and its sequelae: Decreasing, but still substantial. Obstet Gynecol 95:397, 2000.

Richter HE, Holley RL, Andrews WW, et al: The association of interleukin 6 with clinical and laboratory parameters of acute pelvic inflammatory disease. Am J Obstet Gynecol 181:940, 1999.

Rodvold KA, Danziger LH, Quinn JP: Single daily doses of aminoglycosides. Lancet 350:1412, 1997.

Safrin S, Schachter J, Dahrouge D, Sweet RL: Long-term sequelae of acute inflammatory disease: A retrospective cohort study. Am J Obstet Gynecol 166:1300, 1992.

Schaefer G: Female genital tuberculosis. Clin Obstet Gynecol 19:223, 1976.

Scholes D, Daling JR, Stergachis A, et al: Vaginal douching as a risk factor for acute pelvic inflammatory disease. Obstet Gynecol 81:601, 1993.

Sellers J, Mahony J, Goldsmith C, et al: The accuracy of clinical findings and laparoscopy in pelvic inflammatory disease. Am J Obstet Gyneol 164:113, 1991.

Shulman A, Maymon R, Schapiro A, Bahary C: Percutaneous catheter drainage of tubo-ovarian abscesses. Obstet Gynecol 80:555, 1992.

Smith KJ, Ness RB, Roberts MS: Hospitalization for pelvic inflammatory disease: A cost-effectiveness analysis. Sex Transm Dis 2006 Jun 21; [Epub ahead of print].

Soper DE: Pelvic inflammatory disease. Infect Dis Clin North Am 8:821, 1994.

Soper DE: The semantics of pelvic inflammatory disease. Sex Transmit Dis 22:342, 1995.

Soper DE: Pelvic inflammatory disease (PID). Infec Dis Obstet Gynecol 4:62, 1996.

Soper DE, Brockwell NJ, Dalton HP: False-positive cultures of the cul-de-sac associated with culdocentesis in patients undergoing elective laparoscopy. Obstet Gynecol 77:134, 1991.

Soper DE, Brockwell NJ, Dalton HP, Johnson D: Observations concerning the microbial etiology of acute salpingitis. Am J Obstet Gynecol 170:1008, 1994.

Stacey CM, Munday PE, Taylor-Robinson D, et al: A longitudinal study of pelvic inflammatory disease. Br J Obstet Gynaecol 99:994, 1992.

Stamm WE: *Chlamydia trachomatis* infections: Progress and problems. J Infec Dis 179 (Suppl):S380, 1999.

Stevens HA: Clindamycin. Prim Care Update Ob/Gyns 4:251, 1997.

Stone KM, Grimes DA, Magder LS: Primary prevention of sexually transmitted diseases. JAMA 255:2062, 1986.

Sweet RL, Blankfort-Doyle M, Robbie MO, et al: The occurrence of chlamydial and gonococcal salpingitis during the menstrual cycle. JAMA 255:2062, 1986.

Suss AL, Homel P, Hammerschlag M, Bromberg, K. Risk factors for pelvic inflammatory disease in inner-city adolescents. Sex Transm Dis 2000; 27:289.

Teisala K, Heinonen PK, Punnonen R: Laparoscopic diagnosis and treatment of acute pyosalpinx. J Reprod Med 35:19, 1990.

Teisala K, Heinonen PK, Punnonen R: Transvaginal ultrasound in the diagnosis and treatment of tubo-ovarian abscess. Br J Obstet Gynaecol 97:178, 1990.

Telenti A, Iseman M: Drug-resistant tuberculosis: What do we do now? Drugs 59:171, 2000.

Toglia MR, Schaffer JI: Tubo-ovarian abscess formation in users of intrauterine devices remote from insertion: A report of three cases. Infec Dis Obstet Gynecol 4:85, 1996.

Toth A, O'Leary WM, Ledger W: Evidence for microbial transfer by spermatozoa. Obstet Gynecol 59:556, 1982.

Toub DB, Goff BA, Muntz HG: Tuberculous endometritis presenting as postmenopausal bleeding: A case report. J Reprod Med 36:616, 1991.

Walker CK, Kahn JG, Washington AE, et al: Pelvic inflammatory disease: Metaanalysis of antimicrobial regimen efficacy. J Infect Dis 168:969, 1993.

Walker CK, Workowski KA, Washington AE, et al: Anaerobes in pelvic inflammatory disease: Implications for the Centers for Disease Control and Prevention's Guidelines for Sexually Transmitted Diseases. Clin Infec Dis 28 (Suppl):S29, 1999.

Walsh T, Grimes D, Frezieres R, et al: Randomized controlled trial of prophylactic antibiotics before insertion of intrauterine devices. Lancet 351:1005, 1998.

Walters MD, Eddy CA, Gibbs RS et al: Antibodies to *Chlamydia trachomatis* and risk for tubal pregnancy. Am J Obstet Gynecol 159:942, 1988.

Walters MD, Gibbs RS: A randomized comparison of gentamicin-clindamycin and cefoxitin-doxycycline in the treatment of acute pelvic inflammatory disease. Obstet Gynecol 75:867, 1990.

Washington AE, Gove S, Schachter J, et al: Oral contraceptives, *Chlamydia trachomatis* infection, and pelvic inflammatory disease. JAMA 253:2246, 1985.

Washington AE, Katz P: Cost of a payment source for pelvic inflammatory disease. JAMA 266:2565, 1991.

Weström L: Introductory address: Treatment of pelvic inflammatory disease in view of etiology and risk factors. Sex Transm Dis 11:437, 1984.

Weström L: Pelvic inflammatory disease and other sexually transmitted diseases. Curr Opin Obstet Gynecol 1:5, 1989.

Wisenfeld HC, Sweet RL, Ness RB, et al: Comparison of acute and subclinical pelvic inflammatory disease. Sex Transm Dis 32(7):400, 2005.

Wølner-Hanssen P: Silent pelvic inflammatory disease: Is it overstated? Obstet Gynecol 86:321, 1995.

Wølner-Hanssen P, Eschenbach DA, Paavonen J, et al: Association between vaginal douching and acute pelvic inflammatory disease. JAMA 263:1936, 1990.

Wølner-Hanssen P, Svensson L, Mardh PA, et al: Laparoscopic findings and contraceptive use in women with signs and symptoms suggestive of acute salpingitis. Obstet Gynecol 66:233, 1985.

Preoperative Counseling and Management

24

Patient Evaluation, Informed Consent, Infection Prophylaxis, Avoidance of Complications

Vern L. Katz

KEY TERMS AND DEFINITIONS

Antisialagogue. An agent that decreases the production and amount of saliva.

Effective Period of Prophylactic Antibiotics. The first 3 hours of decreased tissue resistance following a surgical insult. Prophylactic antibiotics must be at the site of damaged tissue during this interval.

Informed Consent. An agreement by the patient that she understands the following: the nature and extent of the disease process, the nature and extent of the contemplated operation, the anticipated benefits and results of the surgery including a conservative estimate of successful outcome, the risks and potential complications of the operative procedure, and alternative methods of therapy.

Nosocomial Infection. An infection acquired in a hospital.

Prophylactic Antibiotics. The administration of antibiotics to patients without evidence of infection to prevent postoperative morbidity related to infection.

Thromboprophylaxis. A technique used to prevent thromboembolic disease, usually perioperative heparin or mechanical compression stockings.

Preoperative evaluation is a challenge to the gynecologist, for it involves both the art and the science of clinical medicine. Excellent preparation for the operation facilitates a successful end result. Optimum preparation involves two personality traits: compulsive attention to detailed planning and a deep empathy for the patient. For the gynecologist, preoperative planning can be divided into three basic aspects: obtaining preoperative information, reducing the patient's anxieties and fears, and obtaining informed consent. Francis D. Moore states that the first aphorism of preoperative preparation is to avoid "surprises." This dictum should be applied to protect both the patient and the physician.

The gynecologist, as leader of the surgical team, has an obligation to prepare the patient, her family, and the hospital personnel, including nurses, anesthesiologists, and the operating room team, concerning the anticipated details surrounding the surgical procedure. The majority of gynecologic operations are elective and thus allow sufficient time to prepare. However, even in emergency situations, preoperative preparation should be as detailed as possible because shortcuts during an emergency can result in further compromise to the patient.

For the patient, *there are no small, insignificant, or minor operations.* Almost any operation is a major event in her life. Associated with an elective operation are the anxiety and apprehension of the anticipated surgical procedure coupled with the ambivalence of deciding whether to have the operation. To help her decide, it is important for the physician to outline the natural history of the gynecologic disease so that the patient is able to understand the benefits of surgery. Most women have questions concerning the return of normal body functions and the cosmetic changes produced by the operation; these questions must be answered. Questions concerning the woman's perception of the operation's impact on her sexuality must be discussed. Recent prospective studies have documented that sexual function is most likely to remain the same or improve following gynecologic surgery for benign disease. As always, the physician is an educator. His or her goal should be to outline for the patient the reason and approximate time frame for each preoperative step and procedure. If the patient is ambivalent concerning the need for a surgical procedure, this often may be resolved by suggesting that she seek another professional opinion. Many third-party payer programs insist that patients obtain a second opinion before elective gynecologic operations.

Few events assault human dignity and challenge the emotional defenses as much as the events surrounding an elective operation. The woman is stripped of her clothing, bombarded with questions, and sometimes clipped of her pubic hair, all at a time when she is feeling the most vulnerable because of the impending surgery. It is important for the physician to protect the patient's privacy and human dignity during the preoperative period. The gynecologist must appreciate that the preoperative period is one of great psychological stress for the patient. The time of the anticipated surgical procedure is a catalyst for emotional responses ranging from vulnerability and helplessness to the grief produced by possible anticipated loss of a reproductive organ. The physician–patient relationship is far more than the legally described contractual one. An important aspect of the relationship is the physician's encouragement of the patient to be a partner in the mutual goal of a return to normal function. The understanding and trust built between the patient and physician during the preoperative period will help the patient to build confidence and cope with the stress of the postoperative period.

One of the most important aspects of the preoperative preparation is a discussion with the physician before the procedure. Ideally the physician, the patient, and her family have a private meeting. During this time, it is important for the physician to answer all the patient's questions, as well as those of her family. It is acceptable to answer a question with the statement, "I don't know." Patients admire the honesty this response expresses. The gynecologist must remember that just as he or she studies the patient for both verbal and nonverbal information, so does the patient watch the gynecologist. It is essential for the gynecologist to display gentleness and patience at this time. Sincere interest may be reinforced by eye-to-eye contact and a gentle touch of the hands.

A thorough and detailed history and physical examination, considering the entire patient, not just the pelvis, detect approximately 90% of the facts pertinent to the surgical procedure. Multiple studies have demonstrated that the most significant risk factors for postoperative morbidity are preoperative conditions. Preoperative laboratory screening tests discover fewer than 10% of significant surgical risk factors. It is an established surgical axiom that operative morbidity and mortality are directly proportional to preexisting conditions. Known or unsuspected medical illnesses may affect the operation, anesthesia, and postoperative course and in rare instances may preclude the procedure altogether. Also, it is important to evaluate the influence of gynecologic disease on other organ systems. For example, is a pelvic mass producing obstruction of the ureters?

This chapter outlines the preoperative preparations for gynecologic operations for benign disease. The preparations and plans for surgery extend into the postoperative period in a continuous spectrum. Thus several topics will be started here and continued in Chapter 25 (Postoperative Counseling and Management). Emphasis is placed on obtaining a standard complete history, performing an adequate physical examination, and educating the patient and family (including obtaining informed consent). Special considerations for women with concurrent common medical disease are also included. Two recurrent themes are stressed in the chapter: avoiding surprises during each step in the preoperative period and alleviating the patient's fears and anxiety. This chapter is not intended to be an exhaustive discussion of all medical and surgical conditions that may have some effect on preoperative planning. Rather, the focus is on common preoperative problems encountered in benign gynecologic surgery. Cost containment strategies have placed increasing emphasis on same-day admission for almost all major gynecologic operations regardless of the woman's age. This practice has abruptly changed the timing of many preoperative events. Laboratory tests, electrocardiograms, and radiographic examinations are performed on an outpatient basis before surgery. Even preparation of the large intestine must be performed at home.

Two considerations are helpful to women who must run the preoperative hospital gauntlet. It is very helpful to give the patient a specific list of instructions for the 24 hours prior to surgery. Second, the patient may need a drug that will help relieve anxiety, such as diazepam, lorazepam, or alprazolam to be taken the night before surgery.

PREOPERATIVE HISTORY

A detailed complete history not only obtains information but also helps to relieve the patient's fears and anxieties. When the history is obtained in an unhurried manner, the process is reassuring to the patient. The patient should perceive the gynecologist as a gentle and reassuring clinician rather than as a detective trying to rapidly solve a crime. The extent and depth of the general history may be modified to a minor degree by the age and general health of the woman and the operation contemplated. However, even minor operations may have major complications. Therefore it is best to be overprepared. The possibility of degenerative multiple organ disease necessitates a meticulous review before any surgical procedure in geriatric patients. Even for an emergency operation a detailed history is important.

For elective operations the preoperative history usually is taken on two separate occasions. Studies have documented that patients often omit important medical information, particularly when under stress. Repetitive history taking does provide additional information and helps to decrease the risk of omission of significant historical information. The interview occurs initially in the physician's office several weeks before the operation and is repeated 1 to 7 days before the procedure. The second interval is valuable, for it gives the patient an opportunity to reconsider her decision. Similarly, the physician uses the time to collect necessary information, such as records of previous surgical procedures. An important question to include in the history is whether the patient or anyone in her family has had problems with surgery. This question may provide information about potential medical issues and also alert the surgeon to sources of anxiety for the patient that are better off addressed prior to the procedure. In reviewing the history the second time, often the patient recalls important information that she omitted during the initial history. For example, she may have recently talked to a sister who has a history of excessive bleeding during an operation.

There are two purposes in obtaining a detailed and comprehensive history from the patient. The first is to put the patient at ease; the second is to cover a formalized and extremely thorough set of questions. The two processes demand time and gentle consideration of the patient's anxiety. It is best to let the woman offer her perspective first. Subsequently the physician may direct the questions to a standard format. Obviously the format must be covered in a systematic manner so that essential areas are not omitted. Many gynecologists have the woman complete a standardized historical questionnaire prior to the outpatient appointment.

Although this chapter does not review all the components of a complete history (see Chapter 7, History, Physical Examination, and Preventive Health Care), it is advantageous to group questions under the specific organ systems: pulmonary, cardiovascular, renal, hepatic, metabolic, endocrine, neurologic, hematologic, and immunologic. Several specific questions should be included to fill any holes and to cross-check on the review of symptoms. These questions cover problems with surgery, anesthesia, or bleeding in the patient or her family.

The next general category is drug allergy and current medications. Questions must be constructed so as to include both prescribed and over-the-counter medications as well as herbals and supplements. Approximately 0.5% of the general population and 1.5% of women over the age of 55 are receiving continuous glucocorticoids. Thus a specific question about glucocorticoid therapy for chronic medical problems is essential.

Table 24-1 Herbal Medicine and Other Dietary Supplement-Related Sites on the World Wide Web

Organization	Web Address	Site Information
Center for Food Safety and Applied Nutrition, Food and Drug Administration	http://vm.cfsan.fda.gov/~dms/supplmnt.html	Clinicians should use this site to report adverse events associated with herbal medicines and other dietary supplements. Sections also contain safety, industry, and regulatory information.
National Center for Complementary and Alternative Medicine, National Institutes of Health	http://nccam.nih.gov	This site contains factsheets about alternative therapies, consensus reports, and databases.
Agricultural Research Service, United States Department of Agriculture	http://www.ars-grin.gov/duke	The site contains an extensive phytochemical database with search capabilities.
Quackwatch	http://www.quackwatch.com	Although this site addresses all aspects of health care, there is a considerable amount of information covering complementary and herbal therapies.
National Council Against Health Fraud	http://www.ncahf.org	This site focuses on health fraud with a position paper on over-the-counter herbal remedies.
HerbMed	http://www.herbmed.org	This site contains information on more than 120 herbal medications, with evidence for activity, warnings, preparations, mixtures, and mechanisms of action. There are short summaries of important research publications with MEDLINE links.
ConsumerLab	http://www.consumerlab.com	This site is maintained by a corporation that conducts independent laboratory investigations of dietary supplements and other health products.

From Ang-Lee MK, Moss J, Yuan CS: Herbal medicine and perioperative care. JAMA 286:213, 2001.

It is important to inquire regarding over-the-counter vitamins, nutritional, and herbal supplements. Many of these have the potential to affect surgery through coagulation, healing, and cross-reactivity with other medications. In general herbal treatments should be stopped 7 days prior to surgery. Recommendations regarding commonly used herbs are in Table 24-1.

Many women do not consider aspirin or oral contraceptives as medication; therefore specific questions regarding these substances are needed. General questions regarding smoking, alcohol, exercise tolerance, and recent upper respiratory infections are often grouped together. Specific questions should be directed toward sensitivity to iodine or latex. Latex allergy is directly responsible for 12% of the perioperative anaphylactic reactions in adult patients and for 70% in children. Health care workers are particularly prone to latex allergy.

The woman's contraceptive history, including any recent change, must be known. Over the years there has been no greater embarrassment in the operating room than the realization that a recent contraceptive practice has been abandoned and the patient is pregnant. Included with the contraceptive history are key questions concerning possible exposure to the human immunodeficiency virus (HIV). Also, the physician should estimate the probability of blood transfusion and together with the patient decide whether autologous blood should be donated for possible transfusion. Many women and their families are deeply concerned about the potential risk of acquiring HIV via allogeneic blood. Presently the risk of an HIV-contaminated unit of donated blood passing through screening tests and infecting the woman is approximately one in 1,000,000 units of blood. Using a decision analysis model to assess the cost effectiveness of autologous blood donation, Etchason and colleagues found considerable additional cost ($68 to $4783) per unit of blood. Managed care programs will struggle with this ethical dilemma. Lastly, there is no evidence that blood from directed donors, selected by the patient, is safer than blood from volunteer donors.

PHYSICAL EXAMINATION

The preoperative physical examination should answer three basic questions: Has the primary gynecologic disease process changed since the initial diagnosis? What is the effect of the primary gynecologic disease on other organ systems? What deficiencies in other organ systems may affect the proposed surgery and hospitalization? A pelvic examination performed the day before surgery may demonstrate that a myoma has undergone acute degeneration or an ovarian cyst may have ruptured and "disappeared." Pelvic masses adherent to the large intestine suggest the potential need for mechanical cleansing of the bowel before surgery. A patient with cardiac murmurs secondary to valvular heart disease needs antibiotic prophylaxis against subacute bacterial endocarditis. Often the morbidly obese woman has impairments in the function of the circulatory and respiratory systems. Observations and findings in the physical examination may prompt further laboratory and diagnostic tests.

The most important feature of the preoperative physical is that it should be performed in a thorough and compulsive manner. The gynecologist should use the same sequence every time to help focus attention on the evaluation of each organ system.

The physical examination is best performed in the physician's office. To diminish the patient's anxiety, the physical examination should not be performed in silence. Conversation with the patient may involve further history taking or questions and answers about the proposed operation. Gentle palpation is important. A gentle touch helps to build the trust and confidence that are the foundation of the physician–patient relationship.

Two important axioms should be stressed. First, in emergency situations it is imperative to perform a complete physical examination. This examination should include an evaluation of the blood pressure and pulse in both the recumbent and sitting positions; orthostatic hypotension and tachycardia are crude indexes of a decrease in circulating intravascular volume.

Second, it is important to perform a pelvic and rectal examination the day before the operation and again in the operating room immediately before the surgical incision. Pelvic masses sometimes change in size when the bladder and gastrointestinal tracts are empty. These measures help avoid surprises and may alter the surgical plan.

LABORATORY AND DIAGNOSTIC PROCEDURES

The general purpose of preoperative laboratory procedures is to identify conditions that will alter or aid in perioperative management. Specifically, screening tests are used to find unsuspected, asymptomatic diseases that may affect, alter, or postpone the anticipated surgical procedure. Preoperative laboratory tests also help to establish the extent of known disease that may influence the scheduling of elective surgery. Gynecologists should individualize their preoperative approach to patients and select specific tests for each patient. The downside of multiple routine preoperative testing is that it increases the likelihood of false-positive results, especially if the disease has a low prevalence in the population being tested. A false-positive test has many negative features, including anxiety for the patient, additional testing, financial cost, and often delays scheduling the operation. Sometimes special imaging procedures are used to determine the effects of pelvic disease on other organ systems.

Age-appropriate screening tests should be reviewed with patients prior to elective surgery. For example Pap smears and mammograms should be up to date prior to an elective gynecologic procedure. A workup of a potential breast cancer would take precedence over elective surgery for benign pelvic disease. Screening colonoscopy should be discussed with patients older than 50. However, few women will avail themselves of this test if they are asymptomatic. However, testing the stool for occult blood in women older than age 50 detects bleeding from a colon cancer in approximately 2 of 1000 asymptomatic women.

Presently there is debate over which preoperative laboratory procedures should be standard. Attention has been drawn to the cost–benefit ratio of preoperative screening. Although the cost of each individual test is usually low, the aggregate costs are substantial. Often the cost argument is overcome by the individual gynecologist's concern to practice defensive medicine in the present medicolegal climate. Many preoperative laboratory tests are ordered simply by convention, for years being standard orders in an individual's or hospital's practice.

In a classic study, Kaplan and coworkers retrospectively studied the usefulness of preoperative laboratory procedures. They estimated that 60% of the routinely ordered tests, such as differential cell count, platelet count, and 12-factor automated body chemistry analyses, would not have been performed if tests had been ordered only for an indication discovered by history or physical examination. Most important, only 0.22% of these tests demonstrated an abnormality that might influence perioperative management (Fig. 24-1). The final conclusion in their assessment of 2000 patients undergoing elective operations was

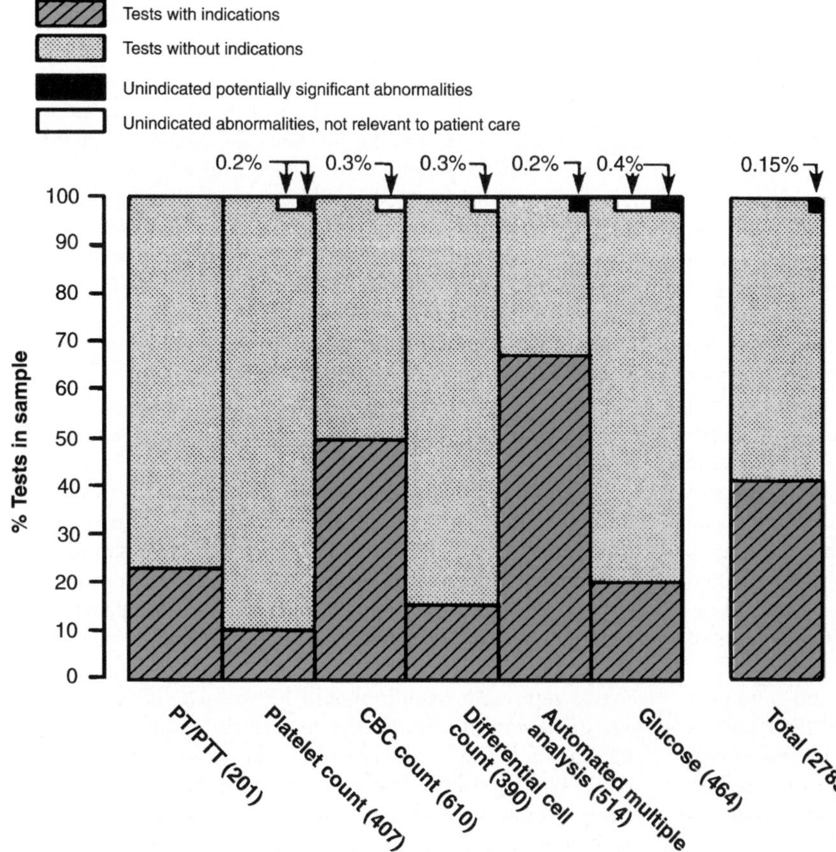

Figure 24-1. Proportions of indicated and unindicated preoperative tests, drawn to scale. Numbers in parentheses represent sample sizes used. PT/PTT, prothrombin time/partial thromboplastin time; CBC, complete blood count. Automated multiple analysis is six factor. (From Kaplan EB, Scheiner LB, Boeckmann AJ, et al: The usefulness of preoperative laboratory screening. JAMA 253:3578, 1985.)

that in the absence of specific indications, routine preoperative laboratory tests do not significantly contribute to patient care and could be eliminated. Many authorities perform no routine preoperative clinic screening test on healthy patients younger than 40.

Two of the most important considerations in the choice of preoperative tests are the age of the patient and the extent of the surgical procedure. Preoperative laboratory procedures should be determined in each patient based on the findings of both a complete history and a physical examination. Women who benefit from preoperative testing have significant risk factors or positive findings discovered during the complete history and physical exam. Most important, abnormal results from any laboratory test should result in some change in perioperative management. Regretfully, unexpected abnormalities in many standard preoperative laboratory tests are frequently overlooked or ignored. Studies have found that between 30% and 60% of unexpected abnormalities detected by preoperative laboratory tests are not actually noted or investigated prior to surgery.

Preoperative complete blood count and urinalysis are required by nearly all hospitals. By far the most important of these for gynecologists is the test for anemia. A woman should not be admitted for elective gynecologic surgery with a low hematocrit level that will necessitate transfusion during the perioperative period, unless a delay in surgery is contraindicated or medical therapy to improve the hematocrit level has been unsuccessful. The results of the urinalysis, white blood cell count, and differential count rarely alter management. Before major gynecologic surgery, with an anticipated potential blood loss of greater than 750 mL, a blood sample should be sent to the blood bank for typing and screening for unusual antibodies. This should replace the expensive routine typing and cross-match. However, it is important that the blood bank have the capability of providing cross-matched blood within a reasonable period of time if serious intraoperative bleeding does occur. Routine preoperative type and screen for uncomplicated abdominal or vaginal hysterectomy is not cost-effective. Also, routine clotting studies are not cost-effective and rarely provide useful clinical information unless indicated by history and physical examination (Table 24-2).

It is beneficial to order limited blood screening tests in women older than age 40 or in women who have positive family histories or questionable past histories of hepatic or renal disease. A preoperative creatinine or blood urea nitrogen (BUN) is especially important if the patient is going to be treated with antibiotics excreted by the kidneys. A test for human chorionic gonadotropin may be appropriate, depending on contraceptive and sexual history. A pregnancy test should almost always be obtained if the patient is a teenager. Menstrual history is at best an imperfect indication of an early pregnancy. Serum electrolytes are ordered in women taking diuretics or for those with a history of renal disease or heart disease. Also, serum electrolytes should be evaluated for patients with vomiting, diarrhea, ileus, bowel obstruction, or any condition that affects water or electrolyte balance.

Table 24-2 Comparison of the Clinical Characteristics of Platelet and Clotting Factor Disorder

	Platelet Disorder	Clotting Factor Disorder
Site of bleeding	Skin	Deep/soft tissue (e.g., muscles, joints)
	Mucous membrane (nasal, oral, vaginal, gastrointestinal, etc.)	
Bleeding after cuts and scratches	Yes	No
Petechiae	Yes	No
Ecchymoses	Small, superficial	Large, deep (often palpable)
Hemarthroses	Rare	Common
Bleeding after surgery	Immediate, usually mild	Delayed (several hours or 1–2 days), then severe

From Clarke-Pearson DL: Obstet Gynecol Forum 6:2, 1992.

The tradition of ordering chest radiographs on all patients has been abandoned. Roizen performed a detailed cost analysis of routine chest X-ray films and determined the practice was not cost-effective unless the patient was over older than age 75 or had known pulmonary or cardiac disease. A history and physical examination are sufficient to screen patients and chest radiographs need be ordered only for patients with positive findings. A meta-analysis of studies of routine preoperative chest radiographs demonstrated that false-positive results leading to invasive procedures and associated morbidity were more frequent than the discovery of new findings leading to a change in management. Currently, chest films should be ordered in women who are 20-pack/year smokers, women with cardiac or pulmonary symptomatology, immigrants who have not had a recent chest film, and women older than 70.

A baseline preoperative electrocardiogram (ECG) has been found to be cost-effective in asymptomatic patients only after age 60 in women without a history of cardiac disease or significant risk factors. It sometimes detects a recent asymptomatic myocardial infarction or serious cardiac arrhythmias. ECG may be indicated in women with a history of smoking and in those with diabetes or renal disease, depending on the severity.

At the conclusion of a complete history, physical examination, and screening laboratory procedures, the gynecologist should determine whether consultation with other specialists is necessary. This decision should be based on the seriousness of the concurrent disease and the complexity of the proposed operation.

PATIENT–FAMILY EDUCATION AND INFORMED CONSENT

One of the primary responsibilities of the gynecologic surgeon is to educate the patient and her family about the anticipated surgical procedure and hospitalization and recovery. Giving this information is both an ethical and legal responsibility. Informed consent is an important principle to ensure that the woman's right to self-determination is respected. The ethical concept of the process of informed consent includes two important components: comprehension and free consent. Most important, in almost all circumstances the patient and her family want to know about the operation. Similar to the history and physical examination, educational discussions should take place on at least two occasions. Throughout the educational process, questions from the patient or family should be welcomed. The patient and family should be informed about the potential use of intravenous fluids, urinary catheters, and monitoring equipment.

Often physicians take these devices for granted, not realizing such equipment may cause anxiety and fears in laypersons not familiar with modern postoperative care.

Educating the patient is a great step in relieving anxiety. If the patient is aware of the sequence of events, the stress of this time becomes more tolerable. It is difficult to overeducate the patient on details of the preoperative area, the operating room, and recovery room routines. Written information, when available, is also helpful. Psychological preparation of the family is equally important, and arrangements should be made for a specific location for a meeting with family members immediately following the operation. An informed family is one of the surgeon's greatest assistants. An uninformed family will often harass the entire health care delivery team.

Few concepts bring more ambivalence and concern to the physician than the doctrine of informed consent. In the present medicolegal climate, the absence of informed consent is cited as a major problem in many lawsuits. Some critics have pointed out that true informed consent would involve sending the patient to medical school and then through several hours of intensive discussion. Some of these issues are discussed further in Chapter 6 (Medical, Legal, and Ethical Issues).

It is important to differentiate between the concepts of consent and informed consent. Consent involves a simple yes-or-no decision, but informed consent is an educational process. If a gynecologist were to operate without consent, he or she would be vulnerable to charges of assault and battery. The right of an adult woman to have final authority to consent to an operation has more than 200 years of legal precedent. The preoperative consent form that is standard in most hospitals simply documents that consent, hopefully informed consent, has been obtained.

To obtain informed consent, the surgeon must explain to the patient in understandable terms the following: the nature and extent of the disease process; the nature and extent of the contemplated operation; the anticipated benefits and results of the surgery, including a conservative estimate of successful outcome; the risks and potential complications of the operative procedure; alternative methods of therapy; and any potential changes in sexual, reproductive, and other functions. The gynecologist should also discuss with the patient what the operation will not accomplish. Many patients expect surgery to magically cure a large constellation of symptoms. Questions from the patient should be encouraged and welcomed. After being educated and considering the information, the patient acquires an understanding of the risks and benefits of the proposed procedures and may make a "fully informed" decision and give informed consent for the operation to be performed.

The possibility of unanticipated pathologic conditions should be discussed with the patient and permission obtained on the written consent form for the most extensive operative procedure that may be necessary. Patients readily accept the necessity of freedom of judgment by the gynecologist during the operation as to the extent of the operative procedure, depending on what is discovered during surgery. For example, permission to remove both fallopian tubes and ovaries along with the uterus should be obtained in the event that extensive adnexal disease is an unanticipated finding.

One of the greatest dilemmas in the doctrine of informed consent is the extent and depth of discussions concerning potential complications of an operation. Attorneys who specialize in defending gynecologists in medical malpractice litigation strongly advise discussing all major complications, including death from surgery and rare, serious complications, such as urinary tract fistulas following hysterectomy. Studies have documented that approximately 70% of patients do not read the consent form before signing it. Ideally, to protect the gynecologist, the final discussion of the informed consent process should be witnessed by a family member and another member of the health delivery team. Highlights of this discussion should be documented by a paragraph written by the gynecologist in the progress notes of the chart.

Regretfully, some patients may become overwhelmed by multiple caregivers' perceived "obligation" to give information. The excessive and conflicting information provided by physicians, nurses, and other caring individuals in the typical tertiary-care hospital may confuse and increase the fears of the woman and her family. Adding to this problem is the abundance of conflicting nonpeer-reviewed information available via the lay press and the Internet. In summary, a caring gynecologist must not only educate the patient, but be prepared to discuss other information that the woman has received.

PREOPERATIVE PREPARATION

Rarely a woman is admitted to the hospital prior to the operation. The preoperative orders should communicate the gynecologist's preoperative preparation for his or her patient. To avoid omissions, it is important to develop a systematic method of writing preoperative orders. The orders should be individualized depending on the previous history and physical examination obtained as an outpatient, the patient's age, and the extent of the proposed surgical procedure. Unusual or infrequent orders should be written in specific detail to avoid confusion by nursing and other hospital personnel. Because of the increasing emphasis on same-day admission to the hospital, most procedures and orders are accomplished on an outpatient basis. Therefore it is important to give the patient a specific list of instructions for the 24 hours before surgery.

The first two or three lines of the order sheet should include the proposed operation, and a list of the patient's diseases. Further orders are subdivided into four broad categories: general measures, medication, laboratory tests, and preventive therapies.

General measures include orders for activity, diet, ordinary medication usage, and vital signs. The patient should have nothing more than sips of water with essential medications for the 2 to 4 hours prior to elective surgery. If the patient's operation is not scheduled until the middle of the afternoon, it is acceptable for the patient to have an early liquid breakfast. Interestingly the extent of preoperative anxiety does not influence gastric fluid volume or acidity.

The second category of orders is for medications. When prophylactic antibiotics are ordered, the time of injection should ensure that significant blood and tissue levels will be present at the time of bacterial contamination during the surgical procedure. An additional subgroup is special medications for specific medical illnesses. It is presumed that the anesthesiologist will write orders for preoperative medication to alleviate anxiety and reduce tracheobronchial secretions.

The third major group of orders involves preoperative laboratory tests. This group includes standard laboratory tests and specifically indicated laboratory tests.

The fourth and last group of orders involves preventive therapies. Thrombophlebitis remains a major complication of gynecologic surgery. Prophylactic subcutaneous heparin or intermittent pneumatic leg compression devices (or both) are indicated in women at moderate and high risk for thromboembolic disease. Patients who have been NPO for a prolonged period or who have lost fluid from cleansing of the gastrointestinal tract should be given intravenous fluids before induction of anesthesia to ensure proper hydration. If removal of hair is necessary for the operation, it should be clipped immediately before the operation.

CONSULTATION WITH THE ANESTHESIOLOGIST

The preoperative interaction between the patient and the anesthesiologist in a preoperative screening clinic is most important. For the patient, both the reassurance of meeting the anesthesiologist and their exchange of information greatly alleviate anxiety. For the anesthesiologist, it is an opportunity to obtain necessary medical information, evaluate the patient, determine the risk of the perioperative period, and write preoperative medication orders. This meeting had traditionally occurred the afternoon or evening before surgery. However, with emphasis on cost containment and greater use of outpatient facilities, and with admission to the hospital the morning of the operation, this meeting frequently occurs in an outpatient clinic several days before surgery. Recently, anesthesiologists have assumed more responsibility for postoperative pain management, primarily using epidural narcotics. This subject should be discussed with the patient. Recovery is more rapid when a patient's concerns are addressed and when she knows what to expect regarding postoperative therapy for pain.

Anesthesiologists classify surgical procedures according to the patient's risk of mortality. In 1961, Dripps first published guidelines to determine the risk of death related to major operative procedures. This physical status scale (Table 24-3) has been adopted by the American Society of Anesthesiologists. With but minor modifications, the anesthetic risk classes are still widely used. An emergency operation doubles the mortality risks for classes 1, 2, and 3; produces a slightly increased risk in class 4; and does not change the risk in class 5. The majority of deaths due to anesthesia are ascribable to human error. The most common serious morbidity associated with elective surgery is cardiovascular complications. Evaluations by anesthesiologists in a preoperative clinic provide information leading to changes in management for more than 15% of healthy patients. In this report, the most common medical conditions of concern that tend to be changed by anesthesia are gastric reflux, insulin-dependent diabetes mellitus, asthma, and anticipated difficulties in intubation.

Table 24-3 Dripps-American Society of Anesthesiologists Classification

Class	Description
1	A normal healthy patient
2	A patient with mild to moderate systemic disease
3	A patient with severe systemic disease with limited activity but not incapacitated
4	A patient with incapacitating, constantly life-threatening systemic disease
5	A moribund patient not expected to survive 24 hours with or without operation

Modified from Anesthesiology 24:111, 1963. From Jewell ER, Persson AV: Preoperative evaluation of the high-risk patient. Surg Clin North Am 65:3, 1985.

A problem frequently encountered by both gynecologists and anesthesiologists is whether to continue or interrupt medications that the patient is taking. If the drug is prescribed for a medical illness, it is best to continue the drug through the perioperative period. The physician must determine whether the drug will adversely affect the course of either the anesthesia or the surgery and whether it will interact with other drugs to be given during the procedure. It is acceptable to have the patient take oral medications the morning of surgery. The 30 to 60 mL of water needed to swallow the oral medication is negligible compared with gastric fluid volumes.

The primary goals of preoperative medication are to relieve anxiety and produce sedation. Many patients desire amnesia. This may not be a reasonable goal for early discharge following the operation. Sedation is easy to accomplish; however, relief of anxiety does not invariably accompany sedation. Narcotics and sedatives should be used with caution in patients with chronic respiratory or liver disease. Recently, a task force of the American Society for Anesthesiologists recommended against the routine prophylactic use of anticholinergics, antihistamines, and histamine-2 (H_2) receptor antagonists to reduce the risks of pulmonary aspiration.

PROPHYLACTIC ANTIBIOTICS

The use of prophylactic antibiotics in gynecologic surgical procedures has become standard practice when a clinically significant risk of postoperative infection exists. Wound infections and pelvic cellulitis, although infrequent, are important causes of postoperative morbidity. Gynecologic operations produce both hypoxic tissue and collections of bloody and serous fluids, both of which are excellent culture media. Rigidly defined, prophylactic antibiotic use involves the administration of antibiotics to women without evidence of pelvic infection to prevent postoperative morbidity related to infection. The major use of prophylactic antibiotics is in operations such as vaginal hysterectomy, following which there is potential for a high incidence of postoperative pelvic cellulitis. The goal of antibiotic therapy is to prevent infection by the endogenous flora of the lower female reproductive tract. Prophylactic antibiotics are given occasionally when the incidence of postoperative infection is low but the results of the surgical procedure would be severely compromised if an infection did occur, such as with reconstructive operations on the fallopian tubes. Approximately 40% of all antibiotics used in hospitals are ordered prophylactically.

The use of prophylactic antibiotics in gynecologic surgery has been the subject of much debate. As in any discussion of preventive medicine, one has to evaluate the benefits, risks, and costs. In general, the use of prophylactic antibiotics results in fewer operative site infections (abdominal wound and pelvic cellulitis), reduced febrile morbidity, and shorter hospital stays. The major risk of allergic or toxic reactions is small, especially with a short course of prophylactic antibiotics. The increased cost of the antibiotics is justified by a lower total cost from a shorter hospitalization. Certainly the economic costs of prolonged hospitalization for even a minor postoperative infection are substantial.

The foundation of our understanding of prophylactic antibiotics is the classic research of John Burke published in 1961. He stressed the fact that maximum antibacterial activity in subcutaneous wounds results from a combination of host resistance and antibiotics. His experimental studies proved that the antibiotic must be present in damaged tissue at the time of contamination with bacteria or shortly thereafter. Burke termed the first 3 hours of decreased tissue resistance following a surgical insult as the *effective period.* He found that there was no protective effect in preventing the development of subcutaneous wound infections if the antibiotics were given later than 3 hours following bacterial contamination.

Subsequent studies have documented two other important facts concerning prophylactic antibiotics in gynecology. First, the goal of prophylactic antibiotics is to reduce the total number of bacteria present in the operative site. It is not necessary to kill all of the bacteria. Second, for prophylaxis to be successful, adequate tissue levels of antibiotics need to be maintained only for the duration of the operation. The normal endogenous vaginal flora has 1×10^8 bacteria per milliliter of vaginal secretions, consisting of a wide spectrum of both aerobic and anaerobic organisms. Thus, theoretically, the choice of a single antibiotic for prophylaxis in gynecology is a most difficult one. Ideally the drug chosen as a prophylactic antibiotic should be nontoxic, inexpensive, and effective against most organisms encountered in the endogenous flora. Multiple reports have documented a linear relationship between the incidence of bacterial vaginosis and the incidence of postoperative pelvic infection. Therefore, a woman should not have an elective hysterectomy if bacterial vaginosis is discovered during the 2 weeks prior to surgery. It is important for the gynecologist to identify women with bacterial vaginosis. Following treatment, the vaginal ecosystem should return to normal prior to the operation.

There is abundant literature supporting the use of prophylactic antibiotics in gynecology. More than 50 studies summarize the data from women who received prophylactic antibiotics for vaginal hysterectomy. The results of these studies show that the incidence of febrile morbidity was reduced from 40% to 15% and the incidence of pelvic infection from 25% to 5%. The results of more than 30 studies of women having abdominal hysterectomies are not as decisive. Some studies demonstrated no significant improvement, whereas positive studies demonstrated less dramatic declines in febrile morbidity, pelvic infection, and wound infection. The average reduction in febrile morbidity was 12%, and the average reduction in operation site infection, 5%. In many studies it is difficult to determine whether the investigators equated postoperative fever with postoperative infection.

No center or expert has demonstrated the specific antibiotic of choice for prophylaxis in gynecology. It is most difficult to compare one prophylactic antibiotic with another. Not only are there differences in methodology between studies but also differences in terminology between definitions of febrile morbidity and documented pelvic infections. However, there are not significant differences in outcome no matter which single broad-spectrum antibiotic is used. Presently, first- or second-generation cephalosporins are the most popular choice for prophylactic antibiotics in gynecology (e.g., a single dose of a cephalosporin, first or second generation, 1 to 2 g intravenously 30 minutes before the operation). A meta-analysis by Tanos and Rojansky suggests a significant reduction in the incidence of infection, but not postoperative fever, with the use of prophylactic cephalosporins by the intravenous rather than the intramuscular route (odds ratio [OR], 0.66, CI, 0.5 to 0.9). Often nursing personnel give prophylactic antibiotics prematurely by optimistically anticipating when the patient will go to the operating room. This practice may result in lower than desirable antibiotic levels during the time of bacterial contamination. Some hospitals have developed standard protocols to ensure that prophylactic antibiotics are given at the appropriate time.

With the wide spectrum of bacteria involved in the constantly changing ecologic system of the vagina, a single antibiotic does not have the spectrum to be bactericidal or bacteriostatic against all the bacteria present. The important feature sought in a prophylactic antibiotic is an ability to reduce the total number of bacteria present in the bacterial inoculum; it does not have to affect all organisms. A reduction in overall number allows the woman's natural defense mechanisms to eradicate the remaining bacteria.

Recent emphasis has focused on an extremely short duration of therapy for prophylactic antibiotics. Comparative studies have documented that single-dose therapy is as effective as 24 hours of antibiotics. No advantage exists to continuing prophylactic antibiotics beyond the immediate operative period. This short duration of administration also reduces cost and complications. The incidence of serious complications, such as drug allergy and resistant bacteria, is directly related to the length of administration of the antibiotic. With prophylactic antibiotics the major concern is the potential threat of increasing bacterial resistance. This results in two problems: more nosocomial infections with resistant organisms and alterations of the normal vaginal flora. If infection does develop following prolonged use of prophylactic antibiotics, one must obtain cultures and select antibiotic coverage different from the antibiotic used for prophylaxis. Other potential complications from prophylactic antibiotics are antibiotic-associated diarrhea or colitis or the more serious pseudomembranous enterocolitis often secondary to *Clostridium difficile* infection. This complication usually follows chronic use of antibiotics, but, rarely, it may occur after a short exposure to antibiotics. Antibiotic therapy any time in the previous 6 weeks may be responsible for precipitating the onset of this disease.

Many factors affect the risk of postoperative infection. The most important include the length of the operation, whether the woman is premenopausal or postmenopausal, obesity, low socioeconomic status, malnutrition, immunosuppression, the use of prophylactic antibiotics, and the operative approach. A randomized clinical trial reported by Greif and coworkers studied supplemental perioperative oxygen in 500 patients undergoing operations involving the large bowel. The authors discovered the administration of supplemental oxygen during the operation and in the first 2 hours of the perioperative period resulted in a 50% reduction in the incidence of wound infection. If this initial report is confirmed by subsequent studies, supplemental oxygen use will become the standard because the cost and risk are not major factors. Keeping a patient warm was also found to reduce perioperative infection in a recent study.

In summary, prophylactic antibiotics are routinely ordered for vaginal or abdominal hysterectomies and gynecologic operations that carry a substantial risk of postoperative infection. The most popular choice is a single dose of a cephalosporin given close enough to surgery such that tissue levels will be adequate when the operation begins. Whatever broad-spectrum antibiotic is selected, the gynecologist must know the pharmacokinetics of the drug. The half-life of the antibiotic is important in selecting the proper timing and route of preoperative administration and the possible necessity of an intraoperative dose for longer operations. The antibiotic selected should be active against the majority of endogenous flora of the vagina. The drug should be present at the time of surgical insult, and it should be used only during the time of the operative procedure. Obviously, prophylactic antibiotics are helpful, but they should not be exchanged or substituted for meticulous surgical technique. Most importantly antibiotic prophylaxis should not be used indiscriminately because of the increasing problem with selection of resistant bacteria.

THROMBOEMBOLIC DISEASE

Thrombophlebitis of either the pelvic or the leg veins is a frequent complication of gynecologic surgery. Studies using sophisticated I^{125} fibrinogen scanning techniques, documented that approximately 15% of women having gynecologic surgery for a benign disease and approximately 22% of women having surgery for malignant disease develop thrombophlebitis (Table 24-4). Many, if not the majority, of these women will be asymptomatic. In one study, almost 40% of patients with deep venous thrombophlebitis (who had no symptoms of pulmonary embolus) had documented evidence of a pulmonary embolus by ventilation perfusion studies of the lung. The two potential serious outcomes associated with thrombosis are pulmonary embolus early in the course of the disease and the chronic complication of postthrombotic venous insufficiency, which may greatly impair the quality of a woman's life. Many aspects of pelvic surgery predispose the woman to develop thrombophlebitis, including venous stasis, surgical injury to the walls of large veins, associated anaerobic infection, and hormonal status. Classically, the three major pathophysiologic changes that facilitate the development of thrombophlebitis and pulmonary embolus are venous injury, circulatory stasis, and hypercoagulable conditions (Virchow's triad).

Table 24-4 Incidence of Venous Thrombosis After Gynecologic Operations with I^{125} Fibrinogen Scanning

Reference*	Number of Patients	Type of Operation	Incidence of Leg Vein Thrombosis
Adolf et al	75	Major	29
Ballard et al	55	Major benign disease	29
Clyton et al	231	Major	16
Endl and Auinger	43	Major	37
Walsh et al	100	Vaginal hysterectomy	7
	117	Abdominal hysterectomy	13
	23	Wertheim's operation	25
	22	Other malignant disease	45

*References are from the original source.

From Bonnar J: Venous thromboembolism and gynecologic surgery. Clin Obstet Gynecol 28:433, 1985.

Approximately 40% of deaths following gynecologic surgery are directly or indirectly related to pulmonary emboli. Although the initial venous injury most often occurs at the time of the operation, approximately 15% of symptomatic emboli do not present until the first week following discharge from the hospital. Because of the significant morbidity and mortality associated with a postoperative pulmonary embolus, every effort should be made to reduce the incidence of thrombophlebitis.

Thromboprophylaxis includes treatments and protocols that are given to a patient to prevent a thrombosis. In order to prescribe the optimum thromboprophylaxis protocol a risk assessment is undertaken of every patient undergoing surgery. The first step is to determine during the history what factors place the patient at increased risk for thromboembolic disease. One category of such factors include a tendency either inherited or acquired to form a thrombosis—a thrombophilia. A history of previous thrombophlebitis or embolus or a family or personal history of hypercoagulability should prompt a laboratory evaluation for a thrombophilia. Unexplained fetal losses particularly in the mid second or third trimester, heart attack at an early age, or stroke in family members are also warning flags for potential thrombophilia. The thrombophilia screen should include assessment of factor V Leiden with an activated protein C resistance or a genetic analysis, prothrombin G20210A mutation, protein C, S, and antithrombin III levels, genotype of the methylenetetrahydrofolate reductase (MTHFR) enzyme for homocysteinemia, and in the case of a personal history, assessment for anticardiolipin antibody and lupus anticoagulant (Fig. 24-2). With a very strong history and a negative thrombophilia workup, consideration is given to a more extensive screen for less common thrombophilias, including plasminogen activator inhibitor levels and factors VIII, IX, XI, and VII. The thrombophilias are discussed at length in Chapter 16 (Spontaneous and Recurrent Abortion).The presence of a thrombophilia places the patient at an increased risk for thrombotic disease during the perioperative period. If there is a potent thrombophilia such as antithrombin III deficiency or high levels of anticardiolipin, then the patient is considered at the highest risk. Women with two thrombophilias are also at the highest risk for thrombosis; for example women who are homozygous for factor V Leiden or who have both the prothrombin mutation and protein C deficiency. A recent review by Donahue and coworkers noted that if thromboprophylaxis was given, than there was no increased risk of a thrombosis from factor V Leiden.

Other risk factors for thrombosis include malignant disease, previous radiation therapy, congestive heart failure, chronic pulmonary disease, nephrotic syndrome, morbid obesity, venous disease, edema of the legs, active pelvic infection, age older than 40, current use of oral contraceptives or hormone replacement therapy up to the time of the operation, and length of immobilization or preoperative hospitalization. Not uncommonly, the clinician is asked to consult of hospitalized patient who is subsequently taken to surgery. Three or more days of limited

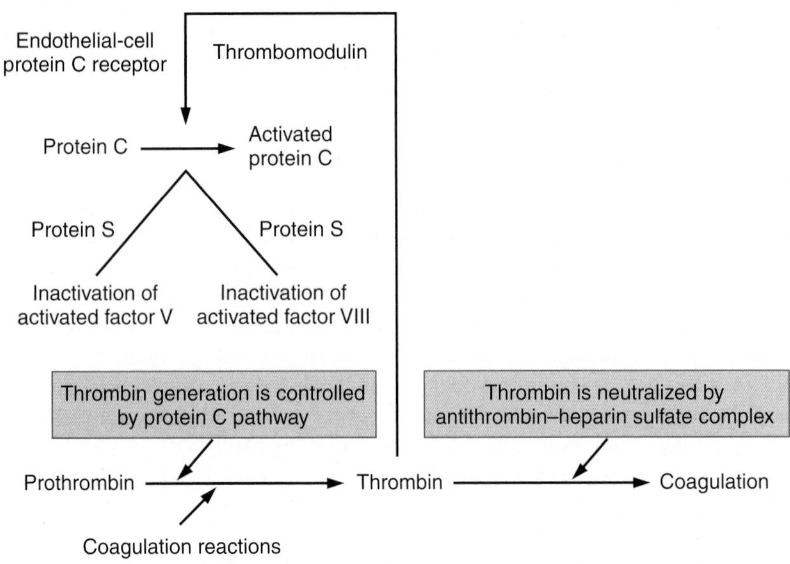

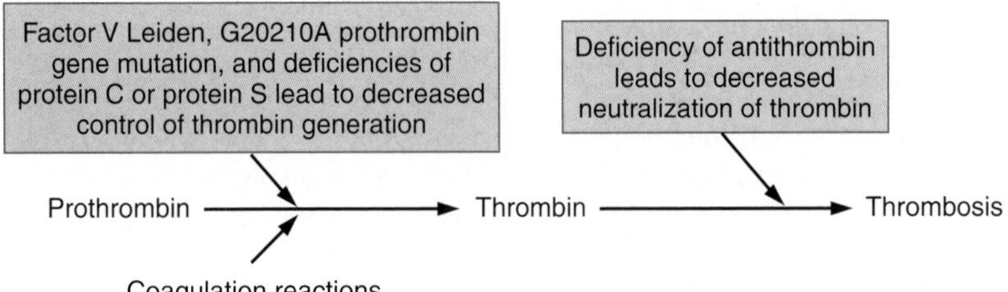

Figure 24-2. Mechanisms in the control of coagulation and inherited thrombophilias. (From Seligsohn U, Lubetsky A: Genetic susceptibility to venous thrombosis. N Engl J Med 344:1223, 2001. Copyright 2001 Massachusetts Medical Society. All rights reserved.)

ambulation confer a greater risk for thromboembolism. The length in time of the procedure is also a risk factor. In general, surgeries greater than 30 minutes put the patient at an increased risk. Laparoscopy is not less of a risk than a laparotomy if the laparoscopy lasts longer than 30 minutes. All of the above factors are evaluated, and the patient is assigned a level of risk: low, moderate, or high risk (Table 24-5). Women in the lowest risk group have less than a 3% risk of thrombosis, women in the moderate group have a 10% to 30% risk of thrombosis, and women in the high-risk groups have a greater than 30% risk of a thrombosis.

Various means are used to prevent thromboembolic disease depending on the level of risk (see the following box). Ideally, the first prophylactic measure to reduce the incidence of embolic disease is to discontinue oral contraceptives or hormone replacement therapy (HRT) 4 weeks before *major* elective operations. The increase in absolute risk from oral contraceptives is small. Thus, pragmatically the risk avoided by stopping oral contraceptives must be weighted against the possible risk of an unwanted pregnancy. The level of risk from HRT is also small. Several large cohort studies have shown no significant increase in incidence of deep vein thrombosis (DVT) in women using hormonal therapies as long as thromboprophylaxis is used. Thus women who are taking HRT or oral contraceptives should receive thromboprophylaxis even if they are younger. Other

Thromboprophylaxis

1. In the low-risk group, provide early mobilization and support stockings.
2. In the moderate-risk group, administer 60 mg enoxaparin or 5000 U dalterparin 6–12 hours after surgery and then give daily as long as patient is hospitalized, or intermittent pneumatic compression stockings intraoperatively and throughout hospitalization.
3. In the high-risk group, intermittent pneumatic compression and low-molecular-weight heparin (LMWH) either 30 mg enoxaparin or equivalent 1/2 dose of other LMWH 1–2 hours before surgery, repeated 12 hours after surgery, and then 60 mg enoxaparin or equivalent per day. Alternatively, heparin may be given as 60 mg enoxaparin or 5000 U dalteparin given 6–12 hours postoperatively and then daily. Note: dosing may be altered in mobidly obese patients or very thin patients.

simple prophylactic measures include elastic stockings, early ambulation, and leg exercises in bed. Support hose should be thigh high so as to avoid venous stasis at the knee. The appearance of the support hose also serves a teaching function to remind women and nursing personnel of the importance of

Table 24-5 Risk Assessment Profile for Thromboembolism in Gynecologic Surgery

Low Risk
Minor surgery (<30 min) with no other risk factors
Major surgery (<30 min) but with age <40 yr and no other risk factors
Age < 40 yr, no other risk factors
Moderate Risk
Minor surgery (<30 min) in patients with a personal or family history or deep vein thrombosis, pulmonary embolism, or thrombophilia
Major surgery (>30 min)
Laparoscopic extended surgery
Obesity (>80 kg)
Moderate to severe varicose veins
Current infection
Immobility before operation (> 3 days)
Major current illness (e.g., cardiovascular disease, cancer, inflammatory bowel disease, nephritic syndrome, malignancies other than gynecologic, chronic pulmonary disease)
Heart failure or recent myocardial infarction
Single thrombophilia other than antithrombin III deficiency, anticardiolipin antibody, or lupus anticoagulant
Recent pregnancy
Hormonal therapy within 4 weeks—including OCP, HRT, or a SERM
Recent surgery or trauma
Long-distance travel within 3 weeks
Intravenous drug use
High Risk
Presence of three moderate risk factors from moderate risk list
Major pelvic or abdominal surgery for gynecologic cancer
Major surgery (>30 min) in patients with personal or family history of previous deep vein thrombosis, pulmonary embolism, or thrombophilia; paralysis or immobilization of lower limbs
Age > 60 yr
Active malignancy
Thrombosis within 1 month
Two thrombophilias, or antithrombin III deficiency, lupus anticoagulant, or anticardiolipin

HRT, hormone replacement therapy; OCP, oral contraceptive pills; SERM, selective estrogen receptor modulator.
Modified from Bonnar J: Can more be done in obstetric and gynecologic practice to reduce morbidity and mortality associated with venous thromboembolism? Am J Obstet Gynecol 180:784, 1999.

ambulation and exercise to prevent venous stasis. The preventive effect from support hose in themselves is quite small; however, the added effects and the risk–benefit ratio is quite large.

The key decision for the prophylaxis of thromboembolic diseases is whether to order prophylactic heparin or pneumatic inflated sleeve devices or a combination of both. A meta-analysis, reviewing more than 70 randomized trials of more than 16,000 general surgery, orthopedic, and urologic patients demonstrated that perioperative subcutaneous heparin prevents approximately two thirds of DVT and 50% of all deaths from pulmonary emboli. The most striking data in this study related the reduction in death directly to pulmonary emboli, with 19 deaths in the patients given perioperative heparin and 55 deaths in the control group. Randomized clinical trials have demonstrated that either pharmacologic agents, such as heparin, or mechanical methods, such as intermittent pneumatic compression of the legs, are equally effective in preventing thrombophlebitis. The complication from heparin prophylaxis is bleeding. Some women are transiently anticoagulated by the heparin, and thus may experience excessive bleeding during or following the operative procedure. This complication is experienced by approximately 2% of women. The risk of bleeding is significantly lower with low-molecular-weight heparins (LMWH). Obese or extremely thin patients should have their dosage of heparin adjusted.

LMWH are superior to standard unfractionated heparin, for they have a longer half-life, almost 100% bioavailability, dose-independent clearance, and thus a more consistent anticoagulation effect from dose to dose. Therefore most studies report significantly fewer hemorrhagic complications with LMWH than with unfractionated heparin. Additionally, the incidence of heparin-induced thrombocytopenia is significantly lower in patients given LMWH than for those receiving unfractionated heparin. There are two major protocols for heparin prophylaxis. One protocol uses a reduced dose prior to the procedure, with 1/2 dose 1 to 2 hours before surgery (i.e., 30 mg enoxaparin or 2500 U. dalteparin). A second dose is then given 12 hours after surgery. A full dose (60 mg. enoxaparin or 5000 U dalteparin) is then given every 24 hours. The second protocol uses a full dose 6 to 12 hours after surgery and every 24 hours thereafter. A meta-analysis of studies summarizing 1600 surgeries for elective hip repair (as high risk as gynecologic procedures) found both perioperative and postoperative LMWH administration to be equally effective. The rates of DVT were 12.4% and 14.4%, respectively. The risks of bleeding were higher in the perioperative protocol groups, 6.3% versus 2.5% for postoperative dosing. The conclusion being that dosing may begin 12 hours after the procedure in most cases, and no less than 6 hours after the procedure. Trials comparing administration 6 and 12 hours postprocedure will help elucidate optimum timing.

The primary alternative to anticoagulation is intermittent pneumatic compression modalities, which include foot pumps, and calf- and thigh-level stockings. Together these devices not only prevent stasis and the endothelial injury that may occur with extreme venous distention but also stimulate the fibrinolytic system. Thus the effect is more than just physical. In one meta-analysis of 11 randomized clinical trials, there was an almost 70% reduction in incidence of DVT in patients using intermittent pneumatic calf compression. One study in trauma patients found full-length compression stockings to be superior to foot pumps. Compression stockings are relatively inexpensive, and their only down side is poorly fitting stockings that produce a tourniquet effect at the knee. They should be used intraoperatively and for the entire hospitalization (since the fibrinolytic effect is maintained only while they are in use). Complications or side effects are extremely rare, but injuries to the common peroneal nerve and compartment syndrome have been reported. Contraindications to the use of pneumatic stockings include known DVT, severe atherosclerotic disease, congestive heart failure, and open wounds on the legs. Both nursing personnel and patients and their families must be educated as to the benefits of the devices or their compliance with this mechanical method is poor. The decision of which method to use is primarily based on the differences in bleeding complications between the two regimens. Maxwell and colleagues randomized 211 gynecologic oncology patients to LMWH or compression stockings. The rates of DVT were similar and quite low in both groups.

In patients who are currently taking oral anticoagulants for thromboprophylaxis because of previous DVT, oral anticoagulants should be stopped 5 days prior to the surgery. Heparin and oral medications should be restarted shortly after surgery. Surgery should be delayed if the previous event was within 3 months. Women who must be operated on within 1 month of a previous DVT should be converted from oral agents to intravenous heparin, and be given perioperative thromboprophylaxis until oral agents can be restarted postoperatively. If the risk for thrombosis is very high, and the surgery cannot be postponed, a temporary vena-cava filter may be placed transcutaneously. These women should have mechanical prophylaxis also. Each patient should have her therapy individualized after assessment of risk.

GASTROINTESTINAL TRACT

Gastrointestinal symptoms are rare in women being evaluated for elective operations for benign gynecologic conditions. However, if the patient has such symptoms, the gynecologist should consider preoperative endoscopy or radiologic studies of the gastrointestinal tract. The effect of nausea, vomiting, or diarrhea on serum electrolytes and also on the nutritional status of the patient needs to be evaluated.

In this era of cost containment, colonoscopy need not be routinely performed on all patients with adnexal masses. These tests do help to establish the differential diagnosis among diverticulitis, carcinoma of the colon, and endometriosis. Colonoscopy may be indicated for benign disease if there is a left-sided adnexal mass in a woman older than age 40, a positive stool guaiac test, or bowel symptoms. Again, the evaluation of each patient must be individualized in an attempt to determine if a primary gynecologic process is pressing on the bowel or directly invading the large intestine.

Proper mechanical cleansing of the gastrointestinal tract is important before every elective gynecologic operation. The patient should not have eaten solid food for 6 to 8 hours before surgery. Clear liquids are emptied from the stomach within minutes; however, fatty foods greatly delay gastric emptying. Obviously, incomplete preparation of the upper gastrointestinal tract increases the risk of aspiration, which is a serious complication of anesthesia and operations. Recent studies have documented the safety of allowing both inpatients and outpatients to ingest clear liquids up until 2 hours before elective surgery.

If there is a suspicion that the operation will necessitate entry into the lumen of the large intestine, both mechanical cleansing and antibiotics to reduce the bacterial count of the colon should be considered. Mechanical cleansing is also desirable in obese patients, and those in whom the intestines will need to be "packed." Colon and rectal surgeons have debated for years about the best methods to accomplish this. Traditionally, mechanical preparation has been accomplished by 3 days of liquid diet, cathartics, and enemas. Almost all gynecologists have modified their mechanical preparation to a single day of an oral gut lavage solution (GoLYTELY or CoLyte) (Table 24-6). The solution is isotonic and contains polyethylene glycol (PEG) in a balanced salt solution. GoLYTELY is ingested at a rate of 1.5 L per hour until diarrheal effluent is clear, usually within 3 to 6 hours. Patients' compliance with GoLYTELY is facilitated if it is chilled. The average woman must ingest 4 L of lavage solution within 4 hours to produce optimal results. Many patients do not accomplish this task in an outpatient setting. Many surgeons prefer oral Fleet's phosphosoda to GoLYTELY. It is better tolerated in most patients. Oliveria and associates recently reported a large randomized trial comparing sodium phosphate and PEG-based oral lavage solutions. The efficacy of the two preparations was similar. However, there was superior subjective patient tolerance to the 90-mL dose of sodium phosphate. Care must be taken in selecting women who receive oral sodium phosphate because it produces hypokalemia and is contraindicated in women with hepatic, renal, or heart disease. In elderly patients, the bowel preparation is often omitted or given as an inpatient with intravenous solutions to prevent dehydration. In summary, the advantages of oral gut lavage are that it is rapid and safe for most patients, with negligible water and sodium absorption or intestinal secretion.

There is a great debate as to the most advantageous method of giving prophylactic antibiotics to prepare the large bowel. The majority of colon and rectal surgeons use a combination of both oral and systemic antibiotics. The alternative choices concerning antibiotic coverage have focused on whether to reduce the high bacterial count inside the bowel lumen (neomycin 1 g and erythromycin base 1 g, each given three times the day before the operation) or to use parenteral prophylactic antibiotics so as to obtain high tissue levels before possible contamination by colon bacteria. Because of concern regarding anaerobic infection, some gynecologists substitute metronidazole (500 mg) for each erythromycin dose. We believe both oral and systemic antibiotic prophylaxis are important and both should be utilized (Table 24-7).

Table 24-6 GoLYTELY Formulation

Components	Concentration
Polyethylene glycol 4000 (PEG)	59.1 g/L
Sodium sulfate (Na_2SO_4)	40 mmol/L
Potassium chloride (KCI)	10 mmol/L
Sodium chloride (NaCI)	25 mmol/L
Sodium bicarbonate ($NaHCO_3$)	20 mmol/L
Distilled water*	
Parabens†	
Final osmolarity	280–300 mOsm/L

*Distilled to a final volume of 1000 mL.
†Methylparabens 0.2 g; prophylparabens 0.1 g.
From Beck DE, Harford FJ, DiPalma JA: Comparison of cleansing methods in preparation for colonic surgery. Dis Colon Rectum 28:492, 1985.

Table 24-7 Mechanical and Antibiotic Preparation of Intestine

Day Before the Operation	Day of the Operation
GoLYTELY orally 1.5 L/hour until effluent is clear	Second-generation cephalosporin 2 g IV 30 minutes before the operation
Neomycin 1 g and erythromycin base 1 g orally at 2, 4, and 10 PM	

URINARY TRACT

The lower urinary tract is in close anatomic proximity to the pelvic organs. Both benign and malignant gynecologic diseases frequently produce anatomic distortion of the urethra, urinary bladder, or ureters. Similarly gynecologic neoplasias may produce partial or complete obstruction of one or both ureters, resulting in hydroureter or hydronephrosis. Preoperative evaluation may include blood chemistry studies such as a BUN or creatinine, imaging studies such as computed tomography (CT) scan, and function studies such as a glomerular filtration rate.

Preoperative imaging may help to diagnose congenital abnormalities of the urinary tract. Congenital urinary anomalies are rare but are more common in women with congenital anomalies of the reproductive tract. The presence of a pelvic kidney is important information in the differential diagnosis of a large, fixed adnexal mass. The presence of a double ureter is another anomaly discovered by preoperative radiologic studies. Preoperative knowledge of a double ureter is advantageous in anatomic identification of structures in the retroperitoneal spaces.

Imaging also helps to confirm the patency of the lower urinary tract. It is important to establish whether the enlargement, inflammation, or displacement of the gynecologic organs has produced distortion, obstruction, and possibly associated chronic infection of the urinary tract. For example, when a uterus is enlarged to the pelvic brim with myomas, hydronephrosis is noted in approximately one third of patients. Common indications for enhanced CT scan with benign gynecologic disease include cervical myomas, lateral projection of uterine myomas, adnexal masses that are fixed and adherent, endometriosis, and large pelvic masses that produce urinary symptoms. Using these conservative indications, approximately 25% of studies will demonstrate an abnormal finding. However, a preoperative intravenous pyelogram (IVP) will not give the gynecologist information that will necessarily reduce the incidence of operative injury to the ureters. During the operation the ureters must be identified along their entire course. The exact incidence of ureteral injury associated with benign surgery is unknown, for many injuries do not produce symptoms.

One serious problem with contrast media that are used for imaging is an allergic reaction triggered by immunoglobulin E antibodies to the radiologic contrast medium. An imaging study of the kidneys using conventional ionic contrast media has an adverse reaction rate of approximately 8%, and life-threatening reactions occur following 1 in every 1000 injections. Pretreating patients with oral corticosteroids, giving methylprednisolone (32 mg) 12 hours and 2 hours before the injection of intravenous contrast material, significantly reduces the incidence of allergic reaction. This treatment is an alternative to using monomeric, nonionic, iodinated compounds as the contrast medium, with a lower incidence of allergic reactions. Studies demonstrate a decrease in severe allergic reactions of fivefold to 30-fold with nonionic compared with ionic contrast media.

Another serious concern in ordering an enhanced imaging study is the possibility of clinically significant nephrotoxicity being caused by the contrast material. Nephropathy has been a common cause of iatrogenic acute renal failure. Women with diabetes, existing renal impairment, chronic hypertension, moderate to severe congestive heart failure, as well as those with reduced effective arterial volume and those receiving drugs that impair renal function are at high risk for contrast nephrotoxicity. A normal serum creatinine level should be verified prior to ordering these scans. For example, 15% of women with diabetic nephropathy will develop renal failure requiring dialysis despite adequate hydration and the use of low-osmolar agents. The pathogenesis of contrast nephrotoxicity is believed to be both direct tubular insult and ischemic injury. Low-osmolar, nonionic contrast media are less nephrotoxic than are high-osmolar, ionic media in high-risk patients. One study of 83 patients with chronic renal insufficiency demonstrated a combination of prophylactic oral administration of the antioxidant acetylcysteine along with hydration was an effective means of preventing further renal damage produced by a nonionic, low-osmolar contrast agent. A recent randomized trial by Aspelin and colleagues using an isoosmolar contrast found a near ninefold reduction in renal toxicity when compared with a low-osmolar contrast medium.

As much as 5% of women have some form of renal disease. Insufficient renal function is a major risk factor in elective operations because of the patient's decreased ability to excrete medications. Women with insufficient renal function do poorly if they develop perioperative infections. Patients with azotemia have a threefold greater risk of adverse drug reactions than women with normal renal function. However, renal insufficiency is very infrequent in an asymptomatic woman younger than age 40, especially compared with the incidence of unsuspected respiratory disease. The frequency of abnormal serum BUN or creatinine levels is directly dependent on the patient's age. Most authorities recommend serum creatinine and BUN levels be obtained in all women with a history of renal disease and in those older than age 45. Baseline and interval tests of renal function in women who are going to be treated with aminoglycosides are necessary and valuable studies. Women with chronic renal disease usually have platelet dysfunction that should be evaluated preoperatively.

Women with chronic renal insufficiency, diabetes, jaundice, and congestive heart failure, as well as the elderly are at high risk of developing acute renal failure during the perioperative period. Prior to surgery, these patients should be evaluated to ensure that they have normal blood volume and osmolar status. These women should be carefully monitored to avoid hypotension and nephrotoxins. Perioperative ketorolac (Toradol) should be avoided in women with elevated serum creatinine levels. Assessment of volume status is particularly important in these women if they have received a mechanical bowel prep. Because women with chronic renal insufficiency have a decreased reserve, small insults to the kidney such as a relative hypovolemia, may push these women into renal failure. A not uncommon scenario occurs when a women with marginal renal function begins to develop a movement of intracellular volume into her third space after surgery. If intravenous hydration is inadequate, the woman will have normal vital signs, but a decreased urine output. The oliguria is a response to the relative hypovolemia. At the same time nonsteroidal antiinflammatory drugs (NSAIDs) may be prescribed. The combination of chronic renal insufficiency with decreased reserve, hypovolemia, and exposure to an NSAID leads to a transient tubular necrosis with a worsening oliguria and azotemia.

RESPIRATORY SYSTEM

Pulmonary complications are the most frequent form of postoperative morbidity experienced by women following gynecologic operative procedures, occurring in more than 1 in every 20 postoperative patients. The goals of the preoperative assessment of the respiratory system are to identify women at risk for developing postoperative pulmonary complications and to prescribe appropriate preoperative therapy to reduce these risks. Common pulmonary complications include bronchospasm, atelectasis, pneumonia, and exacerbation of underlying chronic lung disease. A rare, but most serious problem is respiratory failure with prolonged mechanical ventilation usually seen in women with severely diminished pulmonary reserve. Obviously, predicting and preventing postoperative cardiac problems will dramatically reduce postoperative pulmonary morbidity. Arozullah and coworkers in a study of 161,000 operations was able to derive a model for predicting the likelihood of developing postoperative pneumonia (Table 24-8). Only rarely a patient cannot be anesthetized and well oxygenated intraoperatively. The primary goal should be to avoid postoperative pulmonary complications. Similar to the evaluation of other organ systems, the history and physical examination are the most important parts of the pulmonary evaluation. Pulmonary function tests of lung volumes and flow rates are indicated only to evaluate women with history or physical findings suggestive of restrictive or obstructive pulmonary disease.

Preoperative assessment must determine if the patient has the pulmonary reserve to overcome the normal postoperative decrease in pulmonary function. Women who have compromised preoperative pulmonary function are especially susceptible to develop clinically significant postoperative atelectasis, which occurs following approximately 10% of gynecologic operations. Predisposing factors that increase the incidence of atelectasis include morbid obesity, smoking, pulmonary disease, and advanced age. Increased pain, the supine position, abdominal distention, impaired function of the diaphragm, and sedation also contribute to decreased lung volumes and reduced dynamic measurements of pulmonary function for the postoperative patient. The sequence of events that predispose a woman to postoperative pulmonary complications are depicted in Figure 24-3.

Important questions in the history relate to smoking, recent upper respiratory infection, cough, amount of sputum production, degree of dyspnea, wheezing, and most important, exercise tolerance. In women with known respiratory disease, a complete medication history should be obtained, including antibiotics, bronchodilators, mucolytic agents, and corticosteroids. Some women exhibit suppression of their hypothalamic pituitary axis function if they have received low daily doses of either oral or inhaled corticosteroids. Thus, if low daily doses of either oral or inhalation corticosteroids have been taken during the past year for greater than a 2-week period, the patient should receive parenteral hydrocortisone to cover potential adrenal insufficiency during the perioperative period. The history should also include questions about exposure to industrial air pollution.

If the woman is currently a smoker, the risk of postoperative pulmonary complications increases approximately fourfold. The basic defense mechanisms of the lungs, such as the ciliary action of the epithelial cells that line the respiratory tract, are significantly impaired by smoking. Even young women with "normal lungs" who smoke half a pack of cigarettes a day are at an increased risk. Ideally, women should stop smoking 8 weeks preoperatively. However, abstinence from cigarettes for 2 to 4 weeks preoperatively is a more practical goal. Providing transdermal nicotine replacement is helpful in alleviating the symptoms of acute nicotine withdrawal. Smoking is most detrimental in women with chronic bronchitis or chronic obstructive pulmonary disease (COPD).

Traditionally, anesthesiologists have insisted on at least a 10-day interval between an upper respiratory infection and the date of an elective operation. If the patient has productive sputum, the amount of sputum is estimated, purulent sputum cultured, and appropriate antibiotics given. However, a dramatic change in this practice has affected women without underlying pulmonary disease. Fennelly and Hall state that there is little evidence that anesthesia in adult patients with an upper respiratory tract infection results in respiratory complications.

During the physical examination, special attention should be given to findings of tachypnea, wheezing, rhonchi, rales, decreased breath sounds, and prolonged expiration. Direct observation of exercise tolerance, such as climbing a flight of

Table 24-8 Postoperative Pneumonia Risk Index

Preoperative Risk Factor	Point Value
Type of Surgery	
Abdominal aortic aneurysm repair	15
Thoracic	14
Upper abdominal	10
Neck	8
Neurosurgery	8
Vascular	3
Age	
≥80 yr	17
70–79 yr	13
60–69 yr	9
50–59 yr	4
Functional Status	
Totally dependent	10
Partially dependent	6
Weight loss > 10% in past 6 months	7
History of chronic obstructive pulmonary disease	5
General anesthesia	4
Impaired sensorium	4
History of cerebrovascular accident	4
Blood Urea Nitrogen Level	
<2.86 mmol/L (<8 mg/dL)	4
7.85–10.7 mmol/L (22–30 mg/dL)	2
≥10.7 mmol/L (≥30 mg/dL)	3
Transfusion > 4 units	3
Emergency surgery	3
Steroid use for chronic condition	3
Current smoker within 1 year	3
Alcohol intake > 2 drinks/day in past 2 weeks	2

Class I < 15 pts, probability of pneumonia .24; class II 16–25 pts, 1.20 probability; class III 26–40 pts, probability 4.0: class IV 41–55 pts, probability 9.4; class V >55 pts, probability of pneumonia 15.4.
From Arozullah AMJ, Khuri SF, Henderson WG: Development and validation of a multifactorial risk index for predicting postoperative pneumonia after major noncardiac surgery. Ann Intern Med 135:847, 2001.

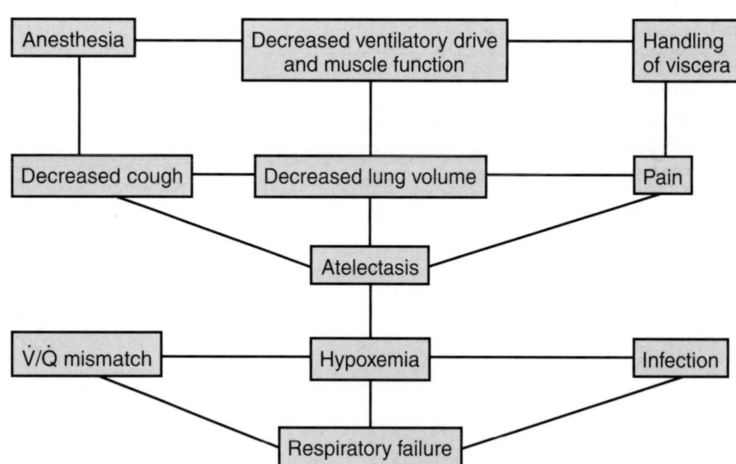

Figure 24-3. The administration of anesthesia and handling of viscera precipitate a series of changes that may lead to postoperative pulmonary complications. V̇/Q, ventilation/perfusion. (From Celli BR: What is the value of preoperative pulmonary function testing? Med Clin North Am 2:309, 1993.)

stairs, is helpful in evaluating the extent of pulmonary reserve. This is a crude index of pulmonary function. Patients with any positive findings on history or physical examination should have a chest radiographic examination, and in selected cases arterial blood gases should be obtained and pulmonary function tests performed. Preoperative pulmonary function tests should be performed on patients with productive sputum (more than 2 ounces per day), age greater than 65 years, 20 pack-years or greater smoking history, morbid obesity, asthma, and COPD. Women with chronic lung disease often have shunting of blood in the lungs and arterial hypoxemia. Thus preoperative arterial blood gases should be measured. When arterial blood gases are evaluated, the oxygen tension should exceed 65 mm Hg, and the carbon dioxide tension should be less than 45 mm Hg. An elevated arterial CO_2 is an important warning sign because the respiratory drive has become refractory to hypercarbia. In a recent study of 272 patients referred for preoperative pulmonary assessment, 8% of whom eventually developed postoperative pulmonary complications. Age greater than 65, 40 pack-year history, and short laryngeal height (<4 cm) were independently associated with pulmonary morbidity. Preoperative hypercarbia and poor forced expiratory volumes and times were related to the independent variables.

Pulmonary function tests help both to assess the pulmonary reserve and to identify the extent to which the dysfunction is reversible. These tests help to identify women at increased risk for pulmonary problems during the postoperative period. Pulmonary function tests that measure lung volumes and flow rates help to distinguish restrictive defects or a decrease in the amount of lung tissue from obstructive defects in which there is a reduction and prolongation of airflow during expiration. The two most common pulmonary function tests used for screening are forced vital capacity (FVC) and forced expiratory volume in 1 second (FEV_1). A woman with a FVC volume of less than 50% of the predicted normal for her age and body size should have more extensive testing for significant lung disease. Similarly, the FEV_1 should be greater than 75% of the predicted normal volume. When pulmonary function tests are lower than predicted, or the history uncovers notable issues, a pulmonology consult should be obtained. Pulmonologists may prescribe bronchodilators, or steroids to maximize pulmonary function in women with obstructive disease. A systematic review by Smith in 2002 found level I evidence for chest physiotherapy, intermittent positive pressure breathing, and epidural anesthesia as three modalities (besides smoking cessation) that reduce postoperative pulmonary morbidity.

Women who are morbidly obese or with symptoms of sleep apnea (or a suspicious history obtained from the patient's spouse or partner) should have a pulmonology consultation. These women may benefit from continuous positive airway pressure (CPAP) devices. Women with sleep apnea should not be placed on low levels of oxygen and narcotics without CPAP, because they have lost their respiratory stimulus from higher levels of CO_2. Thus, if they are given inspired oxygen there will be nothing to stimulate breathing, thereby leading to acidosis. Women with sleep apnea also have a higher incidence of hypertension and cardiac disease secondary to sympathetic nervous system activation during periods of apnea. These women should have an ECG and anesthesia consultation as well.

Over 25 million Americans have asthma. Thus this condition is frequently encountered during the preoperative evaluation. Asthma increases the incidence of perioperative respiratory problems approximately fourfold. Asthmatic women are susceptible to perioperative respiratory complications secondary to bronchial hyperresponsiveness, airflow obstruction, and hypersecretion of mucus. Ideally, an asthmatic patient should have elective surgery when she is free of wheezing and has optimal pulmonary status, as measured by pulmonary function tests (peak flow >80% of the predicted or her personal best value).

Preoperative preparation of patients with asthma or other COPD includes cessation of smoking; instruction in incentive spirometry, the combination of inhaled ipratropium and an inhaled β-adrenergic receptor agonist, chest physiotherapy, and postural drainage; adequate hydration; sometimes high-dose oral corticosteroids; and antibiotics for purulent sputum for several days before the anticipated surgery. Most authorities advise combining multiple therapeutic regimens to try to reduce the risk of postoperative pulmonary complications. Moller and colleagues studied 120 patients randomized to smoking cessation programs versus controls, 6 to 8 weeks prior to their surgery. Eighteen percent of patients in the smoking cessation program developed postoperative pulmonary complications versus 52% of controls, including 5% versus 31% difference in wound infection and 0 versus 10% difference in cardiovascular

Table 24-9 Risk Reduction Strategies

Preoperative
Encourage cessation of cigarette smoking for at least 8 wk
Treat airflow obstruction in patients with chronic obstructive pulmonary disease or asthma
Administer antibiotics and delay surgery if respiratory infection is present
Begin patient education regarding lung-expansion maneuvers
Intraoperative
Limit duration of surgery to less than 3 hr
Use spinal or epidural anesthesia*
Avoid use of pancuronium
Use laparoscopic procedures when possible
Substitute less ambitious procedure for upper abdominal or thoracic surgery when possible
Postoperative
Use deep-breathing exercises or incentive spirometry
Use continuous positive airway pressure
Use epidural analgesia*

*This strategy is recommended, although variable efficacy has been reported in the literature.
Adapted from Smetana GW: Preoperative pulmonary evaluation. N Engl J Med 340:937, 1999. Adapted with permission.

complications, respectively. Ideally, these women should discontinue smoking at least 8 weeks before surgery.

In summary, the major factors in postoperative respiratory morbidity are underlying pulmonary disease, smoking, advanced age, and the associated decrease in functional respiratory capacity normally produced by the events surrounding an operation. Prophylactic lung expansion programs are the foundation of effective plans to decrease the risk of postoperative atelectasis in high-risk individuals. Meta-analysis of studies of either incentive spirometer or deep-breathing exercises find a decrease in relative risk of pulmonary complications by approximately 50%. Effective pain control by epidural analgesia also reduces the risk of pulmonary complications (Table 24-9).

ENDOCRINE SYSTEM

Diabetes Mellitus

The prevalence of diabetes in adult women is approximately 5% in women younger than 65, and the incidence increases rapidly as women get older. The rule of thumb for diabetes management is that elective operations should be scheduled for the diabetic patient only if she is in nutritional balance and under good diabetic control. Associated electrolyte problems must be recognized and corrected before the operation. The stress of an operation and of anesthesia often produces changes in glucose tolerance and insulin resistance. Since pancreatic reserve is a continuum, even women who are not diabetic by standard blood glucose criteria may develop detrimental hyperglycemia secondary to the physiologic stresses of surgery.

During the perioperative period the physiologic stress response involves the release of catecholamines, cortisol, growth hormone, and glucagon, all of which may produce hyperglycemia. The combined effects of these three hormones tend to elevate the blood sugar levels by 20 to 40 mg/dL, physiologically they act with synergism to amplify the proglycemic response at the cellular level. In 2004 the American College of Endocrinology published a position paper, Inpatient Diabetes and Metabolic Control, emphasizing not only the effects of elevated blood glucose levels, but the beneficial effects of adequate insulin (Table 24-10). Insulin decreases lipolysis. Elevated free fatty acids are associated with arrhythmias. Insulin inhibits several inflammatory mediators, in particular the proinflammatory cytokines. Adequate insulin also leads to an increase in nitric oxide levels in the endovasculature, inducing vasodilatation.

The principal postoperative complications in diabetic patients are increased operative site infections, cardiac morbidity, and wound disruptions. The increase in infection rate is believed to be secondary to a decrease in both cellular and humoral responses to bacteria. Women with diabetes have approximately a fivefold increase in incidence of wound infection compared with age-matched controls. The increased incidence of wound disruptions is due to a decreased tensile strength during healing associated with both insulin resistance and elevated blood sugars.

Preoperative evaluation requires meticulous attention to the details of the patient's disease during the history and physical examination. Important questions center on the severity of the diabetes, types of medications, and recent diabetic control, including blood glucose levels. Specific inquiries should be made about the complications of chronic diabetes, especially those affecting the cardiovascular and renal systems. During the physical examination, attention should be directed toward the diagnosis of peripheral neuropathy. Diabetic neuropathy may be the explanation of persistent pain during the perioperative period. Autonomic neuropathy may cause postoperative gastrointestinal or genitourinary dysfunction. Autonomic dysfunction also predisposes the diabetic patient to postural hypotension, cardiac arrhythmias, and cardiac arrest. Preoperative blood studies should include some measurement of recent diabetic control, such as a glycosylated hemoglobin, hemoglobin A1C (HbA_{1C}), and also an electrolyte and renal profiles. An ECG should be obtained regardless of the woman's age. Special

Table 24-10 Mechanisms Causing Adverse Outcomes from Poorly Controlled Diabetes

Hyperglycemia
Dehydration
Academia from keto acids and lactate
Nonenzymatic glycosylation of proteins central to immune function: complement, impaired IgG, inhibited neutrophil activity
Fatigue and muscle wasting from lipolysis and protein catabolism
Increased Circulating Fatty Acids
Increased skeletal muscle breakdown
Cell membrane instability
Decline in myocardial contractility and increased cardiac arrhythmias
Inhibited endothelial function
Insulin Resistance
Increased lipolysis
The presence of insulin inhibits inflammatory factors
Decreased endothelial-derived relaxing factor—nitric oxide
Insulin and glucose inhibit proinflammatory cytokines

Derived from the American College of Endocrinology Position Statement on Inpatient Diabetes and Metabolic Control, 2004.

emphasis should be directed to screening for asymptomatic infection, especially in the urinary tract.

The medical sequelae of diabetes mellitus, such as renal and cardiac insufficiency, peripheral neuropathy, and peripheral vascular disease, are related to both the severity and the chronicity of the disease. The patient's history will help to differentiate mild insulin-dependent diabetes from severe insulin-dependent diabetes. When diabetes is treated with oral agents, consideration should be directed to preoperative dosage. Longer acting sulfonylureas may be discontinued 24 hours before surgery. Short-acting sulfonylureas should be discontinued 12 hours before the operation. Metformin is associated with lactic acidosis in the setting of renal compromise. Many fatalities have occurred in both the peri- and postoperative period. Decreased renal function may occur even in women who have otherwise seemingly normal renal activity. Women who take metformin for treatment of polycystic ovary syndrome should stop their medication 4 days prior to surgery. Women who take metformin for glucose control, should be changed to subcutaneous insulin if necessary 3 to 4 days prior to surgery.

Peri- and postoperative treatment of women with glucose intolerance or overt diabetes is based on tight glucose control, with the general goal of management being to avoid hyperglycemia and hypoglycemia. Regional anesthesia has less of an effect on blood glucose than general anesthesia and, when appropriate, is a better option for diabetic patients. Current evidence compiled over the last 8 years has shown clearly that the closer the blood sugar is maintained toward normal, the greater the improvement in patient outcomes. Populations of patients undergoing surgery for cardiac, vascular, neurosurgical, and bariatric indications, as well as those having general surgery or experiencing trauma and those in intensive care have all been studied. All have been shown to have a decreased incidence of morbidity and mortality with tight glucose regulation compared with control groups, with sliding scales starting at 200 mg/dL or greater. Fasting blood glucose levels greater than 126 mg/dL and random levels greater than 200 mg/dL in general surgery patients were noted to correlate with mortality rates 18 times greater and twice longer lengths of stay compared to patients with tight control, glucose levels less than 120. In a landmark trial by Van Den Berghe and colleagues, 1548 ICU patients were randomized into tight control, glucoses 80 to 110 mg % versus controls where insulin was given for glucose levels above 215 mg %. The mortality rate was 4.6% versus 8% in controls. The increase in mortality was related primarily to sepsis. Tight control was associated with a significant reduction in septicemia by 46%, a reduction in renal failure by 41%, in transfusion by 50%, and in neuropathy by 44%. Importantly, this study evaluated blood glucose levels in all patients, not just diabetics, which emphasizes that the stresses of surgery can produce detrimental hyperglycemia in any patient. The greater the perioperative stress, the greater the insulin resistance. Studies from the Mayo Clinic of 1026 patients showed that the increased morbidity could be directly related to increasing glucose levels, thus threshold glucose levels to start treatment should occur as close to the physiologic range as possible.

The American College of Endocrinology proposed that, based on strong level I evidence, inpatients should have tight insulin control. Preprandial glucoses should be less than 110 mg %, and maximum glucose levels at anytime should not exceed

Table 24-11 Perioperative Insulin Protocol

1. Test patient in preoperative holding area. If patient is on oral medications, and procedure is < 1 hr in duration with anticipated return to regular diet, check glucose regularly. If blood glucose > 180 mg %, begin insulin infusion.
2. If blood glucose < 110 check every 2 hr, IV of D_5W solution should be used.
3. If glucose 110–179, check hourly and begin insulin when glucose surpasses 180 mg %.
4. If glucose is > 200, check every 1/2 hr.
5. If patient is type 1 diabetic, begin insulin infusion in holding area when glucose is > 100 mg %.
6. Begin infusion with solution run through line and on a pump piggy-backed into main line.
7. Sample infusion protocol

Blood Glucose (mg %)	Insulin Bolus (Units)	Insulin Rate (units/hr)
100–120	0	0.5
121–150	0	1
151–180	0	1.5
181–200	1	2
201–220	2	2.5
221–220	3	4
251–280	4	5
281–300	6	6
301–330	8	7

Note: Infusion rates should be adjusted for complexity of surgery, blood loss, emergent nature, patient's degree of control.

180 mg %. ICU patients should have insulin infusions to maintain glucose levels under 110 mg %. For patients with minor surgeries who will be resuming regular oral intake shortly after surgery, glucose levels may be controlled with hourly glucose measurements and subcutaneous insulin. For patients who have mild diabetes and who may resume oral intake, but the gynecologist will have to wait and see, checking hourly glucoses is appropriate. For patients with more complex surgeries, in which oral intake will not be resumed soon, insulin infusions beginning either preoperatively or intraoperatively should be used (Table 24-11). An insulin infusion should be begun when the blood sugar reaches 180 mg %. Patients should have glucose levels checked in the preoperative screening area and then at regular intervals until surgery and recovery are concluded and a steady state is reached. Postoperative glucose management is discussed further in Chapter 25 (Postoperative Counseling and Management).

Continuous intravenous infusion of regular insulin should be mixed in either normal saline with 10 mEq of potassium, or 5% dextrose in 1/2 normal saline (D_5 1/2NS) with 10 mEq of potassium. Lactate induces gluconeogenesis. Thus, one should be cautious in giving large volumes of lactated Ringer's solution as it may produce hyperglycemia. One last caveat: For obvious reasons elective operations on women with diabetes mellitus should be scheduled early in the morning.

THYROID

Patients with thyroid disease should take their regular dose of thyroxine with a sip of water the morning of surgery. If their thyroid has not been checked for several months prior, it is helpful to obtain a thyroid-stimulating hormone (TSH) or a free thyroxine (T_4) during the preoperative evaluation. Additionally, patients with thyroid disease should also have an ECG and their electrolyte levels should be obtained.

Patients with poorly controlled hyperthyroidism may be vulnerable to thyroid storm in response to the stress of surgery. Symptoms of storm may include tachycardia and hyperthermia. Initial treatment is β-blockade, iodine, and antithyroid medications. Patients with poorly controlled hypothyroidism may have hypertension, myocardial dysfunction, and hypoglycemia. Thyroid hormone enhances the cellular response to catecholamines, and patients with hypothyroid disease respond poorly to stresses.

ADRENAL DISEASE

Glucocorticoids are prescribed for a variety of illnesses. Exogenous steroids of the glucocorticoid class will blunt the natural response of the hypothalamic–pituitary–adrenal axis in the necessary response to stress. Steroid use for longer than a 2- to 3-week period within the year prior to surgery necessitates an augmented steroid administration during the perioperative period. Even if the dosing was small (as little as 5 to 7.5 mg of daily prednisone), adrenal insufficiency may occur. Supplemental cortisone should be given as 100 mg every 12 hours for most patients. A minor surgery will only need one dose, major surgeries entail dosing for the surgery and up to 24 hours postoperatively.

CARDIOVASCULAR DISEASE

The greatest single cause of surgical mortality, including postoperative mortality, is cardiovascular disease. It has been estimated that over 1 million postoperative cardiac complications, including fatal myocardial infarctions will occur each year in the United States. Many of these deaths occur with emergency surgeries and are unavoidable. However, for elective procedures it is the responsibility of the gynecologist to assess the risks and if possible take steps to improve the patient's cardiac status or decide if the benefits of the surgery are appropriate for the risks involved.

The goals of cardiovascular assessment are twofold: to determine the risks for women with cardiac symptomatology and to assess levels of risk in women without cardiac disease. Surgery presents a significant challenge to the cardiovascular system. Cardiac output must increase in proportion to the complexity of the operation. Intravascular volume may both increase and at times fall into a hypovolemic or a relative hypovolemic state. Both of these states would be challenges to cardiac and vascular status. One of the greatest challenges comes from the catecholamine surges that accompany an operation and that will produce a rise in myocardial oxygen demand. If the woman has limited reserves, she may not be able to respond adequately to these challenges. The surge in activity of the sympathetic nervous system can sometimes be ameliorated by the use of β-blockers, but at other times may present specific and significant challenges to the gynecologic surgical patient. Additionally, several aspects of surgery and medications, including anesthesia, antidiuretic hormones, and angiotensin, and other hormonal secretions may depress myocardial function.

The American College of Cardiology, in conjunction with the American Heart Association have developed a four-part assessment for evaluating cardiac risk associated with surgery. The first group of risk factors arises from the history, physical examination, laboratory evaluation, and diagnostic tests. The second assessment is the patient's preoperative functional status. The next assessment is the complexity and nature of the anticipated surgery. Fourth is an evaluation of a patient's cardiac disease, which may be low to nonexistent in many women.

For all patients, the assessment of cardiac risk begins with a history and physical. In this step asymptomatic cardiac disease may be uncovered. A history of cardiac symptoms, previous cardiac disease; hypertensive diseases; vascular diseases; comorbidities, including renal disease, hepatic disease, pulmonary disease, and diabetes; a history of hyperlipidemia; obesity; and smoking all need to be taken into account. The physical examination should focus not only on the examination of the heart, but also on lungs and peripheral vasculature including the extremities. Laboratory assessment in many patients should include assessment of renal status, including BUN and creatinine, as well as blood gasses in women with chronic pulmonary disease. An ECG should be obtained in women who are older than 55 years, those with diabetes, those with a previous cardiac history or symptoms, and those with other comorbidities. A routine ECG obtained on postmenopausal women may diagnose asymptomatic myocardial infarction or serious arrhythmias. This may necessitate postponing elective surgery. It is to be noted, though, that an ECG is a fairly nonsensitive test. Two weeks following a documented myocardial infarction, a normal ECG is found in approximately one out of four patients. The potential observation for arrhythmias is valuable at this time. The dangers of an operation in a woman with multiple premature ventricular contractions (PVCs) are most significant if the PVCs are associated with a decrease in left ventricular function. Women with previously uncategorized arrhythmias need to be evaluated by a specialist prior to surgery.

An assessment of the patient's functional capacity is the next step in the preoperative assessment. This assessment uses an evaluation of what the patient can normally do in her day-to-day life (Table 24-12). The question, "can you climb a flight of stairs?" which is the ability to perform an exercise of four metabolic equivalents (METs), is an important separation point. Patients who cannot climb a flight of stairs without difficulty, whose functional capacity is less than 4 METs will usually have more difficulty with surgery. Whereas patients whose functional

Table 24-12 Energy Used for Assessing Functional Capacity Levels

1–3 METS: *Daily household activities*: Eating, dressing using the bathroom without help, walking around the house. Walking on level ground around the block at a slow pace.
4–6 METS: Light housework, climbing a flight of stairs, walking at about 4 mph. Jogging a short distance. Extensive work around the house such as moving furniture or scrubbing floors.
7–10 METS: Tennis, jogging. Moderate recreational activities.
≥10 METS: Strenuous exercises—Running, basketball, skiing, aerobics

METS, metabolic equivalents.

capacity is greater than 4 METs usually do well. Tasks such as dressing oneself and moving about the house are the equivalent of 1 to 2 METs, whereas such activities such as tennis or jogging are closer to 10 METs.

In grading risk, the complexity of the operation may be divided into an associated high, intermediate, or low cardiac risk. High cardiac risk has greater than a 5% risk of cardiac complications, intermediate less than 5%, and low risk less than 1%. Elective major gynecologic procedures usually present an intermediate risk, and endoscopic and minor procedures are usually of low risk; however, extensive gynecologic resections that are lengthy and involve significant fluid shifts pose a high risk. An emergency surgery will increase the risk of cardiovascular complications two- to fivefold over the baseline risk.

When the composite risks are pulled together the risk to the patient can be estimated (Tables 24-13 and 24-14). If the risks of cardiac complications are high or the cardiac history is worrisome, then more intensive evaluation is indicated. Stress or exercise ECG and invasive cardiac angiography may be considered.. The American College of Cardiology in association with the American Hospital Association Guidelines have published an algorithm for assessing risk and guiding clinicians as to further investigations of the patient's cardiac status prior to surgery. If a clinician is unsure about the safety for a patient undergoing surgery, referral is indicated. Additionally, much symptomatology may be ambiguous, such as inability to sleep well at night, atypical chest pain, and questions about functional capacity, which may be due to physical problems other than cardiovascular ones. When such a history is unclear, testing such as exercise stress tests in conjunction with cardiac consultation is indicated.

Table 24-13 American College of Physicians Modified Cardiac Risk Index*

Variable	Points, *n*
Coronary Artery Disease	
Myocardial infarction < 6 months earlier	10
Myocardial infarction > 6 months earlier	5
Canadian Cardiovascular Society Angina Classification†	
Class III	10
Class IV	20
Alveolar Pulmonary Edema	
Within 1 week	10
Ever	5
Suspected critical aortic stenosis	20
High-grade AV block	10
Arrhythmias	
Rhythm other than sinus or sinus plus atrial premature beats on electrocardiogram	5
>5 premature ventricular contractions on electrocardiogram	5
Poor general medical status, defined as any of the following: PO_2 < 60 mm Hg, PCO_2 > 50 mm Hg, K^+ level < 3 mmol/L, blood urea nitrogen level > 50 mmol/L, creatinine level > 260 μmol/L, bedridden, diabetes mellitus	5
Age > 70 years	5
Emergency surgery	10
Low functional capacity	5
Hypertension	5
History of stroke	5

*Class I = 0–15 points; class II = 20–30 points; class III = more than 30 points.
†Canadian Cardiovascular Society classification of angina (2): 0 = asymptomatic; I = angina with strenuous exercise; II = angina with moderate exertion; III = angina with walking 1–2 level blocks or climbing I flight of stairs or less at a normal pace; IV = inability to perform any physical activity without development of angina.
Modified from American College of Physicians: Guidelines for assessing and managing the perioperative risk from coronary artery disease associated with major noncardiac surgery. Ann Intern Med 127:309, 1997.

Table 24-14 Cardiac Risk Classes for Patients Going to Surgery

Risk Class	Point Score	No or Minor Complications (%)	Life-Threatening Complications* (%)	Cardiac Death (%)
I	0–5	99	0.7	0.2
II	6–12	93	5.7	2.7
III	13–25	86	11.7	2.7
IV	>26	22	22.7	56.7

*Myocardial infarction, ventricular tachycardia, pulmonary edema.
Modified from Goldman L, Caldera DL, Southwick FS, et al: Cardiac risk factors and complications in non-cardiac surgery. Medicine 57:357, 1978; from Salem DN, Homans D, McNally JW, et al: Cardiology. In Molitch ME (ed): Management of Medical Problems in Surgical Patients. Philadelphia, FA Davis, 1982, p 76.

If surgery is necessary, but the patient is at an increased risk, several therapies may then be taken to decrease cardiac risk. One of the more commonly used interventions is perioperative β-blockade, which is preferable begun approximately 1 week prior to surgery. Beta-blockade should be titrated to a resting heart rate of approximately 60 beats per minute. In one study the mortality rate was reduced by greater than 55% with the use of β-blockade. It is important to note that mortality rate in this study was decreased for up to 24 months after surgery compared with that for controls. Several studies have looked at the use of β-blockade preoperatively, and there is no consensus as to who should receive preoperative medication. Most physicians feel that any high-risk patient, based on the algorithms explained earlier, should receive perioperative β-blockade. However, some physicians feel that patients at intermediate risk should receive β-blockers as well.

Other mechanisms to decrease cardiac risk include perioperative continuous monitoring for ST-segment changes. The development of ST changes intraoperatively may potentially signify myocardial ischemia. Biochemical markers would then be checked (creatinine, kinase, and MB fraction), which if positive may lead to the need for coronary revascularization. Certainly, all women at high risk should be strongly considered for intensive monitoring. Routine intraoperative transesophageal echocardiography has not been shown to be helpful, nor has prophylactic placement of a pulmonary artery catheter. Other medications, such as angiotensin-converting enzyme (ACE) inhibitors, aspirin, and statins should be continued throughout the perioperative period in women who are at intermediate or high risk for morbidity.

Hypertensive Disease

Women with controlled essential hypertension in the absence of cardiac or renal complications are not at an increased risk for major problems with elective surgery. However, women with poorly controlled hypertension and a diastolic pressure greater than 110 mm Hg should have more intense medical management of their hypertension before elective surgery. No increased risk of cardiovascular complications from surgery occurs in women with uncomplicated mild to moderate hypertension when the diastolic blood pressure is less than 110 mm Hg. If mild or moderate hypertension is complicated by angina, congestive heart failure, abnormal ECG, left ventricular hypertrophy, or renal insufficiency, the surgery should be postponed until the woman is completely evaluated by a cardiologist.

During the induction of anesthesia, there is a potential abrupt rise of blood pressure of 20 to 50 mm Hg. This transient hypertension is experienced during intubation in 6% of normotensive patients and 17% of women with hypertension. Rapid hemodynamic fluctuations are directly related to morbidity in hypertensive women. Major differences between preoperative and intraoperative blood pressures correlate directly with episodes of myocardial ischemia. Perioperative hypotension or hypertension will occur in 20% to 30% of hypertensive women in whom the blood pressure is controlled prior to surgery.

Antihypertensive medication should be continued throughout the perioperative period. The only exception is monoamine oxidase inhibitors, primarily used to treat depression, which should be discontinued for at least 2 weeks before surgery. Discontinuing some antihypertensive agents is potentially harmful. For example, if β-blockers are withdrawn, patients may develop a hypersensitivity to adrenergic stimulation and an exacerbation of ischemic heart disease. Myocardial infarction, ventricular tachycardia, and abrupt cardiac arrest have all been documented in women in whom β-blockers have been abruptly discontinued prior to surgery. Similarly, patients taking clonidine develop abrupt hypertensive rebound if the drug is withdrawn. Diuretic therapy need not be discontinued before surgery. Potential hazards of diuretics include a relative hypovolemia and hypokalemia. Although diuretics often produce hypokalemia, and associated arrhythmias are a concern in women with organic heart disease, they are rarely seen in women without significant heart disease.

Coronary Artery Disease

Medically significant coronary artery disease is a problem of older women. It is unusual for a premenopausal woman to have ischemic heart disease unless she has diabetes, hyperlipidemia, severe hypertension, or a strong family history of coronary disease. Nevertheless, women older than age 50 often have elective gynecologic surgery. Thus considerations of angina and previous myocardial infarctions are essential in planning elective surgery.

Unstable angina of less than 3 months duration is a strong contraindication to an elective operation. Conversely, most women with stable angina without a previous history of myocardial infarction do not have an increased risk of infarction during operations. Regardless of the duration of angina, the patient should be evaluated by a cardiologist prior to elective surgery. When a woman has had a myocardial infarction, it is important to delay an elective operation for approximately 6 months. The excessive mortality rate associated with a noncardiac operative procedure within 3 months of an acute myocardial infarct is 27% to 37%. Following a 6-month interval the chance of a reinfarction is 4% to 6% with elective operations. Randomized controlled studies of preoperative percutaneous transluminal coronary stent placement or coronary angioplasty have not been published. To date, revascularization operations on the heart have not been demonstrated to reduce the short-term likelihood of mortality in patients subsequently undergoing noncardiac surgery within 6 months of an acute myocardial infarction. No advantage exists in delaying surgery longer than 6 months, because the woman's risk remains constant for the rest of her life.

The induction of anesthesia is an especially vulnerable time for myocardial ischemia. Myocardial ischemia occurs when the heart has to increase its rate and respond to an increase in systemic blood pressure. Approximately 60% of postoperative myocardial infarctions are not accompanied by chest pain. The woman develops congestive heart failure, arrhythmia, and, in the elderly woman, confusion. The majority of postoperative myocardial infarcts occur during the first 48 hours following surgery. However, it is not unusual for the heart attack to present on the third or fourth postoperative day. Thus women with coronary artery disease should be closely monitored both hemodynamically and electrocardiographically for at least 3 to 4 days postoperatively.

Valvular Heart Disease

Women with valvular heart disease who are at significant risk during surgery are those with aortic and mitral stenosis. Physiologically, these lesions are similar in that the fixed cardiac output may lead to decompensation secondary to the need for changes in cardiac output during surgical procedures.

The major perioperative consideration in women with valvular heart disease is the use of prophylactic antibiotics to reduce the incidence of subacute bacterial endocarditis developing from a bacteremia associated with the surgical procedure. Even without antibiotic coverage, this is a rare complication. However, because of the substantial morbidity and mortality associated with bacterial endocarditis, antibiotic prophylaxis is the standard of care.

Mitral valve prolapse is presently the leading indication for endocarditis prophylaxis. Mitral valve prolapse is a common finding, being diagnosed in 4% to 8% of women having gynecologic surgery. A report by Fried documented that the prevalence of mitral valve prolapse is considerably lower than previously reported. The prevalence of mitral valve prolapse is highest in young, thin females. The incidence of bacterial endocarditis is threefold to eightfold higher in women with mitral valve prolapse than in the general population. An ad hoc group of the American Heart Association has developed an algorithm to define when prophylaxis is recommended for patients with mitral valve prolapse (Fig. 24-4). Women with a history of mitral valve prolapse should have an echocardiogram after diagnosis to document whether the patient is at risk for endocarditis and thus may need antibiotics.

Women who are in the high-risk category for endocarditis include those with prosthetic cardiac valves, previous endocarditis, complex cyanotic congenital heart disease, and surgically constructed systemic pulmonary shunts or conduits. Women who are in the moderate-risk category include those

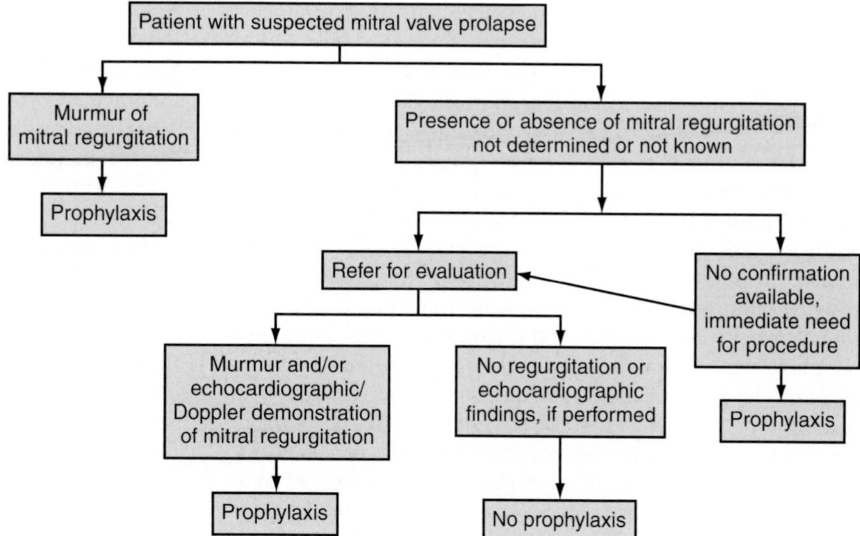

Figure 24-4. Clinical approach to determination of the need for prophylaxis in patients with suspected mitral valve prolapse. (From Dajani AS, Taubert KA, Wilson W, et al: Prevention of bacterial endocarditis. Recommendations by the American Heart Association. JAMA 277:1796, 1997.)

with most other congenital cardiac malformations, acquired valvular dysfunction such as associated with rheumatic heart disease, hypertrophic cardiomyopathy, and mitral valve prolapse with valvular regurgitation or thickened leaflets. Women in both the high-risk and moderate-risk categories definitely should receive antibiotics prophylactically to prevent endocarditis. Women in the negligible-risk category for which endocarditis prophylaxis is not recommended include those with an isolated secundum atrial septal defect; previous coronary artery bypass graft surgery; cardiac pacemakers; and previous surgical repair of atrial septal, ventricular septal, or patent ductus arteriosis. An appropriate antibiotic coverage for moderate-risk women undergoing gynecologic surgery is ampicillin (2 g IV) and for high risk the addition of gentamicin (1.5 mg/kg of body weight not to exceed 120 mg) within 30 minutes of starting the procedure. Depending on the time of expected bacteremia, often the same dosage of both drugs is repeated 6 hours later or amoxicillin 1.0 g orally 6 hours following the parenteral antibiotics. If the woman is allergic to ampicillin, vancomycin (1 g given slowly IV) may be substituted. Vancomycin should be given slowly, over a 2-hour period, to avoid systemic flushing known as *red man syndrome.*

Special consideration should be given to women with valvular heart disease who are receiving chronic oral anticoagulation. It is preferable to discontinue the oral medication 72 hours before surgery. The international normalized ratio (INR) should be less than 1.5 prior to beginning the operation. There has been a recent change in clinical opinion concerning the need for IV heparin in these patients. Kearon and Hirsh postulate that the absolute risk of thromboembolism associated with a few days of perioperative subtherapeutic anticoagulation is generally very low. In contrast, the risk of bleeding associated with perioperative IV heparin is often relatively high. Therefore, they believe that the risk–benefit ratio does not favor the use of perioperative heparin. Oral anticoagulants are usually resumed postoperatively with heparin. Exceptions include patients with caged ball valves and women with recent thromboemboli. These women should be converted to perioperative heparin prior to the procedure.

SURGERY IN THE ELDERLY

Performing surgery in the elderly patient requires careful preoperative preparation. Physical changes of aging affect comorbidities, functional reserve, tissue healing and frailty of tissue, and a delayed return to baseline function after the procedure. The number of elderly patients is increasing. By 2030, one fifth of the American population will be older than 65. The definition of elderly is also increasing, the older the surgeon, the older the definition of elderly. Though risks factors for surgery begin to increase at age 40, and then increase steadily, the general set point for elderly is age 70.

Cardiac morbidity is the single greatest source of morbidity and mortality in the elderly surgical population. Women older than 70 experience a 7% to 10% risk of cardiac morbidity with major surgery. Important physiologic changes that must be accounted for include alterations in the cardiac musculature, with connective tissue and fat replacing myocardial tissue. Rosenthal and Zenilman summarized those changes. Alterations occur in the heart's conduction system, with connective tissue replacing electrical conduction cells. An increased incidence of arrhythmias results. Aging leads to weakening in the valve with dilatation of the valve rings and decreased distensibility, thus impaired functional reserve. A decreased response to sympathetic stimulation leads to poorer diastolic filling, and a reduced compensation to hypovolemic changes. Thus, failure occurs at a lower cardiac threshold. Symptoms of cardiac failure may be less specific in the geriatric population. The first sign may be confusion, which is quite common in the elderly population. Because the elderly patient has less cardiac reserve, anemia is particularly problematic. Preoperative hematocit should be obtained. A study by Wu and coworkers of elderly patients with myocardial infarction, noted that a hematocrit greater than 33% was associated with a significantly increased rate of survival. Similarly hypovolemia must be avoided. Elderly patients who need a bowel prep should be admitted and given IV fluids to maintain normal volume and electrolytes. If there is a less stringent need for mechanical bowel preparation, a Fleet's enema may be sufficient. All women older than 70 are candidates for perioperative β-blockade.

The pulmonary reserve also decreases with advancing age. Chest wall compliance, inspiratory effort, and pulmonary elasticity all decline, leading to a drop in vital capacity. As women age their response to hypoxia decreases. Elderly women are more susceptible to sepsis if they develop pneumonia. The biliary, renal, neurologic, and immune systems all steadily deteriorate with age. All are important components for the necessary response to surgery. Thus, careful preoperative attention to electrolytes, pulmonary reserve, liver function, and preexisting functional capacity are also part of the assessment prior to surgery. Weighing the risks and benefits of the operation must take into account the complication rate, particularly in women with comorbidities. Toglia and Nolan published a series of 54 major gynecologic surgeries in women between the ages of 70 and 85, mean 77. Ten percent of these women developed cardiac complication, including three myocardial infarctions in the perioperative period and two more within a week. Two patients developed significant arrhythmias, one patient had a stroke. Parker and colleagues reported on 62 women between the ages of 80 and 94, mean age 84, who underwent 77 procedures (49 major). These women had a 14% complication rate. Friedman and associates reported on 120 women in their 80s and 90s. Compared to a cohort of women 50 to 79 years of age, length of stay was increased but mortality and major complications were similar.

When obtaining consent from an elderly woman, the American College of Surgery has emphasized several issues. If the patient has a hearing impairment, consent should be obtained in a quiet room with the surgeon speaking slowly. Family members should be present. A discussion of postoperative recovery and any changes in the patient's level of independence need to be discussed. Not all elderly patients judge risks and long-term problems similar to younger women; their perspective is different.

THE MORNING OF THE OPERATION

Preoperative Note

A brief preoperative note helps to serve as a final summary of preoperative preparation. This abbreviated checklist should summarize important findings in the preoperative history, physical examination, and laboratory screening tests. This note is designed to ensure that no step has been forgotten and to summarize in a few words pertinent details for other individuals who subsequently attend the patient. The surgeon should make a brief notation that all the patient's questions have been answered and that both patient and physician are in agreement over the proposed operative procedure.

Hair Removal

Most centers have abandoned the ancient ritual of shaving the abdomen and vulvar areas the day before surgery. Hair removal is not necessary unless dense hair presents a mechanical problem in preoperative washing of the skin. Multiple studies have documented a twofold to threefold increase in infection rate directly related to perioperative shaving. Cruse and Foord studied approximately 63,000 operations over a 10-year period and found a 0.9% incidence of infection when patients were not shaved as opposed to 2.5% when they were shaved. Razors produce macroscopic and microscopic nicks and cuts that allow a protective environment for colonization by skin bacteria. Depilatory agents often produce intense burning if used on the perineum. A systematic review by Kjonniksen and associates concluded that if the hair is mechanically in the way, it should be clipped just before the operation. Patients should be advised not to shave themselves prior to surgery for this reason.

Reassurance

Many women are extremely anxious the morning of their operation, and admission to the hospital the morning of surgery usually intensifies their anxiety. In many hospitals this process offers little emotional support to the individual woman but rather gives her the opinion that she is being "herded" in an impersonal fashion. The physical presence of "her" gynecologist when she enters the operating room provides great reassurance. The kindness of touching the woman's hand or standing by her side as the induction of anesthesia begins is greatly appreciated.

Pelvic Examination

After the patient is asleep or the conduction anesthesia has taken effect, the gynecologic surgeon has two important responsibilities: performing the preoperative pelvic examination and supervising the positioning of the patient. A pelvic examination following catheterization and just before surgical incision should be standard practice, regardless of the type or extent of the proposed gynecologic operation. The relaxation of the abdominal wall produced by anesthesia and the advantage of an empty bladder and lower intestinal tract affords the surgeon the optimum environment for performing a pelvic examination. The findings may change the choice of incision or operative approach. Before draping the patient, the gynecologist should make sure that the patient is properly positioned on the operating room table. This is especially true in obtaining good exposure in the lithotomy position. Pressure points should be avoided to protect against neuromuscular and skin injury, especially over bony prominences.

KEY POINTS

- For the patient, there are no small, insignificant, or minor operations. Almost any operation is a major event in her life.
- The goals of preoperative planning are to obtain appropriate information, reduce the patient's anxieties and fears, and obtain informed consent.
- The first aphorism of preoperative preparation is to avoid "surprises." This dictum should be applied to protect both the patient and the physician.
- Eye-to-eye contact and gentle touching of the hands are appropriate and effective ways to express the physician's sincere interest in caring for the patient.
- An operation without consent makes the gynecologist vulnerable to charges of assault and battery, except in an emergency.
- Highlights of the discussion regarding informed consent should be documented by a paragraph written by the gynecologist in the progress notes of the chart.
- A detailed history and physical examination will detect approximately 90% of the information pertinent to the surgical procedure.
- Surgical morbidity and mortality are directly proportional to the extent of a patient's preexisting medical disease.
- Studies have documented that patients often omit important medical information particularly when under stress. Repetitive history taking does provide additional information and helps to decrease the risk of omission of significant historical information.
- It is important to inquire regarding over-the-counter vitamin, nutritional, and herbal supplements because of the increasing incidence of interactions with drugs.
- Specific questions should be directed toward sensitivity to iodine or latex. Latex allergy is directly responsible for 12% of the perioperative anaphylactic reactions in adult patients and for 70% in children.
- The preoperative physical examination should answer three basic questions: Has the primary gynecologic disease process changed since the initial diagnosis? What is the impact of the primary gynecologic disease on other organ systems? What deficiencies in other organ systems may affect the proposed surgery and hospitalization?
- In emergency situations it is imperative to perform a complete physical examination. This examination should include an evaluation of the blood pressure and pulse in both the recumbent and sitting positions; orthostatic hypotension and tachycardia are crude indices of a decrease in circulating intravascular volume.
- The choice of which preoperative tests to perform should be based on the age of the patient and the extent of the surgical procedure, as well as on details from the history and physical examination.
- Studies have found that between 30% and 60% of unexpected abnormalities detected by preoperative laboratory tests are not actually noted or investigated prior to surgery.
- Routine preoperative type and screen of blood for uncomplicated abdominal or vaginal hysterectomy is not cost-effective.
- A pregnancy test should almost always be obtained if the patient is in her childbearing years.
- Serum electrolyte levels should be evaluated for patients with vomiting, diarrhea, ileus, bowel obstruction, or any condition that affects water or electrolyte balance.
- Routine chest radiographic films are not cost-effective unless the patient is older than 75 or has findings in the history or physical examination suggestive of cardiac or respiratory disease.
- A baseline preoperative ECG is appropriate and cost-effective in women older than 60 and in women with preexisting comorbidities.
- Oral medications that a woman may be taking for a specific condition or illness may be taken the morning before surgery with 30 to 60 mL of water.
- Antibiotic prophylaxis is effective by reducing the number of bacteria present, not by killing all bacteria. To be effective, the antibiotic must be present at the time of tissue injury or shortly thereafter.
- Prophylactic antibiotics are routinely ordered for vaginal or abdominal hysterectomies and gynecologic operations that carry a substantial risk of postoperative infection. The most popular choice is a first-generation cephalosporin. Preferentially the prophylactic antibiotics should be administered intravenously.
- Using sophisticated I^{125} fibrinogen scanning techniques, approximately 15% of women having surgery for a benign disease and approximately 22% of women having surgery for malignant disease develop thrombophlebitis.
- Approximately 40% of deaths following gynecologic surgery are directly or indirectly related to pulmonary emboli.
- The factors that make a woman at high risk for thromboembolic disease include a previous history of thromboembolic disease, a family or personal history of hypercoagulability (thrombophilic state), malignant disease, previous radiation therapy, congestive heart failure, morbid obesity, venous disease, edema of the legs, active pelvic infection, age, current use of oral contraceptives or hormone replacement therapy up to the time of the operation, and length of preoperative hospitalization.
- Patients at high risk for thromboembolic disease should be considered as candidates for both mechanical prophylaxis and prophylactic heparin.
- Colonoscopy need not be performed routinely on all patients with adnexal masses. These tests are indicated in women older than 40 with left-sided masses, women with positive stool guaiac tests, or women with bowel symptoms.
- If there is a possibility that the pelvic pathology may necessitate entry in the lumen of the large intestine, both mechanical cleansing of the bowel and antibiotics to reduce the bacterial count should be considered before surgery.

Continued

KEY POINTS *Continued*

- An imaging study of the kidneys using conventional ionic contrast media has an adverse reaction rate of approximately 8%, and life-threatening reactions occur following 1 in every 1000 injections.
- Nephropathy induced by radiocontrast dye is a common cause of hospital-acquired acute renal failure.
- Pulmonary complications are the most frequent postoperative morbidity experienced by women following gynecologic operative procedures.
- Factors that increase the incidence of atelectasis include morbid obesity, smoking, pulmonary disease, and advanced age.
- Some women exhibit suppression of their hypothalamic pituitary axis function if they have received low daily doses of corticosteroids for a 2-week period within the past year.
- If a woman is currently a smoker, her risk of postoperative pulmonary complications increases approximately fourfold.
- If preoperative arterial blood gases are measured, the oxygen tension should exceed 65 mm Hg, and the carbon dioxide tension should be less than 45 mm Hg.
- Asthma increases the incidence of perioperative respiratory problems approximately fourfold.
- There is a threefold increase in morbidity and a doubling of mortality if surgery is performed on diabetic patients who are in poor glucose control.
- Women with diabetes have approximately a fivefold increase in incidence of wound infection compared with age-matched controls.
- Autonomic neuropathy may cause postoperative gastrointestinal or genitourinary dysfunction. Autonomic dysfunction also predisposes the diabetic patient to postural hypotension, cardiac arrhythmias, and cardiac arrest.
- The perioperative blood glucose levels in diabetic women should be maintained 180 mg/dL. It is preferable to be as close to normoglycemia as possible.
- The use of insulin lispro (Humalog) has facilitated the perioperative management of diabetes. The advantages of this medication are its extremely short onset, peak levels and duration of action, and more predictable subcutaneous absorption.
- Elective operations on diabetic women should be scheduled early in the morning.
- The presence of congestive failure is the single most predictive factor of cardiovascular complications during the perioperative period.
- The cardiovascular risks associated with surgery are increased two- to fivefold during an emergency operation.
- No increased risk of cardiovascular complications from surgery occurs in women with uncomplicated mild to moderate hypertension when the diastolic blood pressure is less than 110 mm Hg.
- The excessive mortality associated with noncardiac surgery within 3 months of an acute myocardial infarction is 27% to 37%.
- The recommended protocol for bacterial endocarditis prophylaxis is ampicillin (2 g intravenously) and gentamicin (1.5 mg/kg of body weight not to exceed 120 mg IV) within 30 minutes of starting the procedure.
- Elderly patients should be given consent in a quiet room with family members present.

BIBLIOGRAPHY

American College of Endocrinology: Position statement on inpatient diabetes and metabolic control. Endocr Pract 10:77, 2004.

American College of Obstetricians and Gynecologists: Ethical dimensions of informed consent. ACOG Committee Opinion 108, 1992.

ACOG Committee on Practice Bulletins: ACOG Practice Bulletin No. 74. Antibiotic prophylaxis for gynecologic procedures. Obstet Gynecol 108:225, 2006.

American Society of Anesthesiologists Practice Guidelines: Practice guidelines for preoperative fasting and the use of pharmacologic agents to reduce the risk of pulmonary aspiration: Application to health patients undergoing elective procedures. Anesthesiology 90:896, 1999.

Ang-Lee MK, Moss J, Yuan CS: Herbal medicines and perioperative care. JAMA 286:208, 2001.

Arozullah AM, Khuri SF, Henderson WG, et al: Development and validation of a multifactorial risk index for predicting postoperative pneumonia after major noncardiac surgery. Ann Intern Med 135:847, 2001.

Aspelin P, Aubry P, Fransson SG, et al: Nephrotoxic effects in high-risk patients undergoing angiography. N Engl J Med 348:491, 2003.

Aspinall ST, Dealler SF: New rapid identification test for *Clostridium difficile.* J Clin Pathol 45:956, 1992.

Barrett BJ: Contrast nephrotoxicity. J Am Soc Nephrol 5:125, 1994.

Bartlett JG: Antibiotic-associated diarrhea. Clin Infect Dis 15:573, 1992.

Bauer KA: Management of thrombophilia. J Thromb Haemost 1:1429, 2003.

Beck DE, Harford FJ, DiPalma JA: Comparison of cleansing methods in preparation for colonic surgery. Dis Colon Rectum 28:491, 1985.

Beck DE, DiPalma JA: A new oral lavage solution vs cathartics and enema method for preoperative colonic cleansing. Arch Surg 126:552, 1991.

Beilman GJ: New strategies to improve outcomes in the surgical intensive care unit. Surg Infect 5:289, 2004.

Bergqvist D, Burmark US, Flordal PA, et al: Low molecular weight heparin started before surgery as prophylaxis against deep vein thrombosis: 2500 versus 5000 XaI units in 2070 patients. Br J Surg 82:496, 1995.

Blom JW, Doggen CJ, Osanto S, et al: Malignancies, prothrombotic mutations, and the risk of venous thrombosis. JAMA 293:715, 2005.

Boersma E, Poldermans D, Bax JJ, et al: Predictors of cardiac events after major vascular surgery: Role of clinical characteristics, dobutamine echocardiography, and β-blocker therapy. JAMA 285:1865, 2001.

Brasch RC: The case strengthens for allergy to contrast media. Radiology 209:35, 1998.

Bratzler DW, Houck PM: Antimicrobial prophylaxis for surgery: An advisory statement from the national surgical infection prevention project. Am J Surg 189:395, 2005.

Burke JF: The effective period of preventive antibiotic action in experimental incisions and dermal lesions. Surgery 50:161, 1961.

Burnand KG, Gaffney PJ, McGuiness CL, et al: The role of monocyte in the generation and dissolution of arterial and venous thrombi. Cardiovas Surg 6:119, 1998.

Burns ER, Lawrence C: Bleeding time: A guide to its diagnostic and clinical utility. Arch Pathol Lab Med 113:1219, 1989.

Capes SE, Hunt D, Malmberg K, et al: Stress hyperglycaemia and increased risk of death after myocardial infarction in patients with and without diabetes: A systematic overview. Lancet 355:773, 2000.

Casadei B, Abuzeid H: Is there a strong rationale for deferring elective surgery in patients with poorly controlled hypertension? J Hypertens 23:19, 2005.

Celli BR: What is the value of preoperative pulmonary function testing? Med Clin North Am 2:309, 1993.

Chalker RB, Celli BR: Special considerations in the elderly patient. Clin Chest Med 14:437, 1993.
Chase JG, Shaw GM, Lin J, et al: Targeted glycemic reduction in critical care using closed-loop control. Diabetes Technol Ther 7:274, 2005.
Choban PS, Flancbaum L: The impact of obesity on surgical outcomes: A review. J Am Coll Surg 185:593, 1997.
Christian SS, Christian JS: The cephalosporin antibiotics. Prim Care Update Ob/Gyns 4:168, 1997.
Clarke-Pearson DL: Prevention of venous thrombosis following gynecologic surgery. J Gynecol Tech 1:11, 1995.
Classen DC, Evans RS, Pestotnik SL, et al: The timing of prophylactic administration of antibiotics and the risk of surgical-wound infection. N Engl J Med 326:281, 1992.
Collins R, Scrimgeour A, Yusuf S, et al: Reduction in fatal pulmonary embolism and venous thrombosis by perioperative administration of subcutaneous heparin. N Engl J Med 318:1162, 1988.
Comerota AJ, Chouhan V, Harada RN, et al: The fibrinolytic effects of intermittent pneumatic compression: Mechanism of enhanced fibrinolysis. Ann Surg 226:306, 1997.
Cooper MS, Stewart PM: Corticosteroid insufficiency in acutely ill patients. N Engl J Med 348:727, 2003.
Cruse PJ, Foord R: A 10-year prospective study of 62,939 wounds,. Surg Clin North Am 60:27, 1980.
Czupryniak L, Strzelczyk J, Pawlowski M, et al: Mild elevation of fasting plasma glucose is a strong risk factor for postoperative complications in gastric bypass patients. Obesity Surg 14:1393, 2004.
Daly E, Vessey MP, Hawkins MM, et al: Risk of venous thromboembolism in users of hormone replacement therapy. Lancet 348:977, 1996.
Davis JD: Prevention, diagnosis, and treatment of venous thromboembolic complications of gynecologic surgery. AJOG 184:759, 2001.
Davis JM, Demling RH, Lewis FR, et al: The Surgical Infection Society's policy on human immunodeficiency virus and hepatitis B and C infection. Arch Surg 127:218, 1992.
Devereux RB, Frary CJ, Kramer-Fox R, et al: Cost-effectiveness of infective endocarditis prophylaxis for mitral valve prolapse with or without a mitral regurgitant murmur. Am J Cardiol 74:1024, 1994.
Devor M, Barrett-Connor E, Renvall M, et al: Estrogen replacement therapy and the risk of venous thrombosis. Am J Med 92:275, 1992.
Dindo D, Muller MK, Weber M, et al: Obesity in general elective surgery. Lancet 361:2032, 2003.
Donahue BS: Factor V Leiden and perioperative risk. Anesth Analg 98:1623, 2004.
Douketis J: Hormone replacement therapy and risk for venous thromboembolism: What's new and how do these findings influence clinical practice? Curr Opin Hematol 12:395, 2005.
Doyle RL: Assessing and modifying the risk of postoperative pulmonary complications. Chest 115:77S, 1999.
Dunn AS, Turpie AG: Perioperative management of patients receiving oral anticoagulants. Arch Intern Med 163:901, 2003.
Eagle KA, Berger PB, Calkins H, et al: ACC/AHA guideline update for perioperative cardiovascular evaluation for noncardiac surgery: Executive summary: A report of the American College of Cardiology/American Heart Association Task Force on Practice Guidelines (Committee to Update the 1996 Guidelines on Perioperative Cardiovascular Evaluation for Noncardiac Surgery). Circulation 105:1257, 2002.
Eason EL, Sampalis JS, Hemmings R, Joseph L: Povidone-iodine gel vaginal antisepsis for abdominal hysterectomy. Am J Obstet Gynecol 176:1011, 1997.
Eiseman B. Surgical decision making and elderly patients. Bull of AM Coll Surg. 81:8, 1996.
Etchason J, Petz L, Keeler E, et al: The cost effectiveness of preoperative autologous blood donations. N Engl J Med 332:719, 1995.
Fennelly ME, Hall GM: Anesthesia and upper respiratory tract infections—a non-existent hazard? Br J Anaesth 64:535, 1990.
Ferguson KJ, Strauss RG, Toy PTCY, et al: Physician recommendation as the key factor in patients' decisions to participate in preoperative autologous blood donation programs. Am J Surg 168:2, 1994.
Ferguson MK: Preoperative assessment of pulmonary risk. Chest 115:58S, 1999.
Fisher QA, Feldman MA, Wilson MD: Pediatric responsibilities for preoperative evaluation. J Pediatr 125:675, 1994.
Fleisher LA: Preoperative evaluation of the patient with hypertension. JAMA 287:2043, 2002.
Fleisher LA, Eagle KM: Lowering cardiac risk in noncardiac surgery. N Engl J Med 345:1677, 2001.
Francis JL: Laboratory investigation of hypercoagulability. Semin Thromb Hemost 24:111, 1998.
Freed LA, Levy D, Levine RA, et al: Prevalence and clinical outcome of mitral-valve prolapse. N Engl J Med 341:1, 1999.
Friedman WH, Gallup DG, Burke JJ 2nd, et al: Outcomes of octogenarians and nonagenarians in elective major gynecologic surgery. Am J Obstet Gynecol 195:547, 2006; discussion 552.
Furnary AP, Gao G, Grunkemeier GL, et al: Continuous insulin infusion reduces mortality in patients with diabetes undergoing coronary bypass grafting. J Thorac Cardiovasc Surg 125:1007, 2003.
Furnary AP, Wu YX, Bookin SO: Effect of hyperglycemia and continuous intravenous insulin infusions on outcomes of cardiac surgical procedures: The Portland diabetic project. Endocrine Practice 10:21, 2004.
Gal TJ: Pulmonary function testing. In Miller RD (ed): Anesthesia, vol 1, 5th ed. Philadelphia, Churchill Livingstone, 2000.
Geerts WH, Heit JA, Clagett GP, et al: Prevention of venous thromboembolism. Chest 119:132S, 2001.
Ginzburg E, Cohn SM, Lopez J, et al: Randomized clinical trial of intermittent pneumatic compression and low molecular weight heparin in trauma,. Br J Surg 90:1338, 2003.
Goldfarb S, Spinler S, Berns JS, Rudnick MR: Low-osmolality contrast media and the risk of contrast-associated nephrotoxicity. Invest Radiol 28(S5):S7, 1993.
Goldman L: Evidence-based perioperative risk reduction. Am J Med 114:763, 2003.
Goldman L, Caldera DL, Nussbaum SR, et al: Multifactorial index of cardiac risk in noncardiac surgical procedures. N Engl J Med 297:845, 1977.
Greif R, Akca O, Horn EP, et al: Supplemental perioperative oxygen to reduce the incidence of surgical-wound infection. N Engl J Med 342:161, 2000.
Guaschino S, De Santo D, De Seta F: New perspectives in antibiotic prophylaxis for obstetric and gynaecological surgery. J Hosp Infect 50:513, 2002.
Haavik PE, Søreide E, Hofstad B, Steen PA: Does preoperative anxiety influence gastric fluid volume and acidity? Anesth Analg 75:91, 1992.
Hamilton GS, Solin P, Naughton MT: Obstructive sleep apnoea and cardiovascular disease. Intern Med J 34:420, 2004.
Handlin DS, Baker T: The effects of smoking on postoperative recovery. Am J Med 93(S1A):32S, 1992.
Hayden SP, Mayer ME, Stoller JK: Postoperative pulmonary complications: risk assessment, prevention, and treatment. Cleve Clin J Med 62:401, 1995.
Hayhurst MD: Preoperative pulmonary function testing. Respir Med 87:161, 1993.
Helström L, Sörbom D, Bäckström T: Influence of partner relationship on sexuality after subtotal hysterectomy. Acta Obstet Gynecol Scand 74:142, 1995.
Hilditch WG, Asbury AJ, Crawford JM: Pre-operative screening: Criteria for referring to anaesthetists. Anesthesia 58:117, 203.
Hirsch IB, Paauw DS: Diabetes management in special situations. Endocrinol Metab Clin North Am 26:631, 1997.
Hirsh J: Advances and contemporary issues in prophylaxis for deep vein thrombosis. Chest 124:347S, 2003.
Holleman DR, Simel DL: Does the clinical examination predict airflow limitation? JAMA 273:313, 1995.
Hollenberg SM: Preoperative cardiac risk assessment. Chest 115:51S, 1999.
Houry S, Georgeac C, Hay JM, et al: A prospective multicenter evaluation of preoperative hemostatic screening tests,. Am J Surg 170:19, 1995.
Hovanessian HC: New-generation anticoagulants: The low molecular weight heparins. Ann Emerg Med 34:768, 1999.
Hurbanek JG, Jaffer AK, Morra N, et al: Postmenopausal hormone replacement and venous thromboembolism following hip and knee arthroplasty. Thromb Haemost 92:337, 2004.
Jick H, Derby LE, Myers MW, et al: Risk of hospital admission for idiopathic venous thromboembolism among users of postmenopausal oestrogens. Lancet 348981, 1996.
Jones T, Isaacson JH: Preoperative screening: what tests are necessary? Cleve Clin J Med 62:374, 1995.
Kallar SK, Everett LL: Potential risks and preventive measures for pulmonary aspiration: New concepts in preoperative fasting guidelines. Anesth Analg 77:171, 1993.
Kaplan EB, Sheiner LB, Boeckmann AJ, et al: The usefulness of preoperative laboratory screening. JAMA 253:3576, 1985.

Karnath BM: Preoperative cardiac risk assessment. Am Fam Physician 66:1889, 2002.

Kearon C, Hirsh J: Management of anticoagulation before and after elective surgery. N Engl J Med 330:1506, 1997.

Khoury W, Klausner JM, Abraham RB, et al: Glucose control by insulin for critically ill surgical patients. J Trauma 57:1132, 2004.

Kjonniksen I, Andersen BM, Sondenaa VG, et al: Preoperative hair removal—A systemic literature review. AORN J 75:928, 2002.

Krämer BK, Kammerl M, Schweda F, Schreiber M: A primer in radiocontrast-induced nephropathy. Nephrol Dial Transplant 14:2830, 1999.

Kreisel D, Savel TG, Silver AL, Cunningham JD: Surgical antibiotic prophylaxis and *Clostridium difficile* toxin positivity. Arch Surg 130:989, 1995.

Krinsley JS: Association between hyperglycemia and increased hospital mortality in a heterogeneous population of critically ill patients. Mayo Clin Proc 78:1471, 2003.

Krinsley JS: Effect of intensive glucose management protocol on the mortality of critically ill patients. Mayo Clin Proc 79:992, 2004.

Kyrle PA, Minar E, Bialonczyk C, et al: The risk of recurrent venous thromboembolism in men and women. N Engl J Med 350:2558, 2004.

Lavelle-Jones C, Byrne DJ, Rice P, Cuschieri A: Factors affecting quality of informed consent. BMJ 306:885, 1993.

Lin L, Song J, Kimber N, et al: The role of bacterial vaginosis in infection after major gynecologic surgery. Infec Dis Obstet Gynecol 7:169, 1999.

Lindenauer PK, Pekow P, Wang K, et al: Perioperative beta-blocker therapy and mortality after major noncardiac surgery. N Engl J Med 353:349, 2005.

Ljungqvist O, Thorell A, Gutniak M, et al: Glucose infusion instead of preoperative fasting reduces postoperative insulin resistance. J Am Coll Surg 178:329, 1994.

Macpherson DS: Preoperative laboratory testing: Should any tests be "routine" before surgery? Med Clin North Am 77:289, 1993.

Madden S, Porter TF: Deep venous thrombosis: prophylaxis in gynecology. Clin Obstet Gynecol 42:895, 1999.

Mangano DT, Layug EL, Wallace A, et al: Effect of Atenolol on mortality and cardiovascular morbidity after noncardiac surgery. N Engl J Med 335:1713, 1996.

Mannino DM, Etzel RA, Flanders WD: Do the medical history and physical examination predict low lung function? Arch Intern Med 153:1892, 1993.

Maxwell GL, Synan I, Dodge R, et al: Pneumatic compression versus low molecular weigh heparin in gynecologic oncology surgery: A randomized trial. Obstet Gynecol 98:989, 2001.

McAlister FA, Khan NA, Straus SE, et al: Accuracy of the preoperative assessment in predicting pulmonary risk after nonthoracic surgery. Am J Respir Crit Care Med 167:741, 2003.

McCray E, Martone WJ, Wise RP, and Culver DH: Risk factors for wound infections after genitourinary reconstructive surgery. Am J Epidemiol 123:1026, 1986.

McIntyre FJ, McCloy R: Shaving patients before operation: a dangerous myth? Ann R Coll Surg Engl 76:3, 1994.

Miriam A, Korula G: A simple glucose insulin regimen for perioperative blood glucose control: the vellore regimen. Anesth Analg 99:598, 2004.

Mittendorf R, Aronson MP, Berry RE, et al: Avoiding serious infections associated with abdominal hysterectomy: A meta-analysis of antibiotic prophylaxis. Am J Obstet Gynecol 169:1119, 1993.

Mizock BA: Alterations in carbohydrate metabolism during stress: a review of the literature. Am J Med 98:75, 1995.

Moghissi E: Hospital management of diabetes: Beyond the sliding scale. Cleveland Clinic J Med 71:801, 2004.

Møller AM, Villebro N, Pedersen T, et al: Effect of preoperative smoking intervention on postoperative complications: a randomized clinical trial. Lancet 359:114, 2002.

Morcos SK, El Nahas AM: Advances in the understanding of the nephrotoxicity of radiocontrast media. Nephron 78:249, 1998.

Morcos SK, Oldroyd S, Haylor J: Contrast media-induced nephrotoxicity: A new insight. Clin Radiol 52:573, 1997.

Moser KM, Fedullo PF, LitteJohn JK, Crawford R: Frequent asymptomatic pulmonary embolism in patients with deep venous thrombosis. JAMA 271:223, 1994.

Mukherjee D, Eagle KA: Perioperative cardiac assessment for noncardiac surgery: Eight steps to the best possible outcome. Circulation 107:2771, 2003.

Murdoch CJ, Murdoch DR, McIntyre P, et al: The pre-operative ECG in day surgery: A habit? Anesthesia 54:907, 1999.

Myers ER, Clarke-Pearson DL, Olt GJ, et al: Preoperative coagulation testing on a gynecologic oncology service. Obstet Gynecol 83:438, 1994.

Narr BJ, Warner ME, Schroeder DS, Warner MA: Outcomes of patients with no laboratory assessment before anesthesia and a surgical procedure. Mayo Clin Proc 72:505, 1997.

Oliveira L, Wexner SD, Daniel N, et al: Mechanical bowel preparation for elective colorectal surgery: A prospective, randomized, surgeon-blinded trial comparing sodium phosphate and polyethylene glycol-based oral lavage solutions. Dis Colon Rectum 40:585, 1997.

Palda VA, Detsky AS: Perioperative assessment and management of risk from coronary artery disease. Ann Intern Med 127:313, 1997.

Parfrey PS, Griffiths SM, Barrett BJ, et al: Contrast material-induced renal failure in patients with diabetes mellitus, renal insufficiency, or both: a prospective controlled study. N Engl J Med 320:143, 1989.

Parker DY, Burke JJ, Gallup DG: Gynecological surgery in octogenarians and nonagenarians. Am J Obstet Gynecol 190:1401, 2004.

Phillips S, Hutchinson S, Davidson T: Preoperative drinking does not affect gastric contents. Br J Anaesth 70:6, 1993.

Platell C, Hall J: What is the role of mechanical bowel preparation in patients undergoing colorectal surgery? Dis Colon Rectum 41:875, 1998.

Polk HC Cheadle WG, Franklin GA: Principles of preoperative preparation. In Townsend CM, Beauchamp RD, Evers MB, et al (eds): Sabiston's Textbook of Surgery, 17th ed. Philadelphia, WB Saunders, 2004.

Poldermans D, Boersma E, Bax JJ, et al: The effect of bisoprolol on perioperative mortality and myocardial infarction in high-risk patients undergoing vascular surgery. N Engl J Med 341:1789, 1999.

Porri F, Lemiere C, Birnbaum J, et al: Prevalence of latex sensitization in subjects attending health screening: Implications for a perioperative screening. Clin Experiment Allergy 27:413, 1996.

Prather CM, Ortiz-Camacho CP: Evaluation and treatment of constipation and fecal impaction in adults. Mayo Clin Proc 73:881, 1998.

Ransom SB, McNeeley SG, Malone JM Jr: A cost-effectiveness evaluation of preoperative type-and-screen testing for vaginal hysterectomy. Am J Obstet Gynecol 175:1201, 1996.

Raskob GE, Hirsh J: Controversies in timing of the first dose of anticoagulant prophylaxis against venous thromboembolism after major orthopedic surgery. Chest 124:379S, 2003.

Robertshaw HJ, McAnulty GR, Hall GM: Strategies for managing the diabetic patient. Best Pract Res Clin Anaesth 18:631, 2004.

Roizen MF: Anesthetic implications of concurrent diseases. In Miller RD (ed): Anesthesia, vol 1, 5th ed. Philadelphia, Churchill Livingstone, 2000.

Roizen MF: Preoperative evaluation of patients with diseases that require special preoperative evaluation and intraoperative management. In Miller RD (ed): Anesthesia, vol 1, 5th ed. Philadelphia, Churchill Livingstone, 2000.

Roizen MF: More preoperative assessment by physicians and less by laboratory tests. N Engl J Med 342:204, 2000.

Roizen MF, Foss JF, Fischer SP: Preoperative evaluation. In Miller RD (ed): Anesthesia, vol 1, 5th ed. Philadelphia, Churchill Livingstone, 2000.

Rosenberg RD, Aird WC: Vascular-bed-specific hemostasis and hypercoagulable states. N Engl J Med 340:1555, 1999.

Rosenthal RA, Zenilman ME: Surgery in the elderly. In Townsend CM, Beauchamp RD, Evers MB, et al (eds): Sabiston's Textbook of Surgery, 17th ed. Philadelphia, WB Saunders, 2004.

Royal College of Obstetricians and Gynaecologists: Hormone replacement therapy and venous thromboembolism. RCOG guideline 19:1, 2004.

Rust OA, Magann EF: Prophylaxis for subacute bacterial endocarditis in obstetrics and gynecology. Prim Care Update Ob/Gyns 1:183, 1994.

Sandham JD, Hull RD, Brant RF, et al: A randomized, controlled trial of the use of pulmonary-artery catheters in high-risk surgical patients. N Engl J Med 348:5, 2003.

Saint S, Bent S, Vittinghoff E, Grady D: Antibiotics in chronic obstructive pulmonary disease exacerbations: A meta-analysis. JAMA 273:957, 1995.

Salem M, Tainsh RE Jr, Bromberg J, et al: Perioperative glucocorticoid coverage: A reassessment 42 years after emergence of a problem. Ann Surg 219:416, 1994.

Saltzman AK, Carter JR, Fowler JM, et al: The utility of preoperative screening colonoscopy in gynecologic oncology. Gynecol Oncol 56:181, 1995.

Schackelford DP, Hoffman MK, Kramer PR Jr, et al: Evaluation of preoperative cardiac risk index values in patients undergoing vaginal surgery. Am J Obstet Gynecol 173:80, 1995.

Schein OD, Katz J, Bass EB, et al: The value of routine preoperative medical testing before cataract surgery. N Engl J Med 342:168, 2000.

Seligsohn U, Lubetsky A: Genetic susceptibility to venous thrombosis. N Engl J Med 344:1222, 2001.
Shackelford DP, Lalikos JF: Estrogen replacement therapy and the surgeon. Am J Surg 179:333, 2000.
Sloand EM, Pitt E, Klein HB: Safety of the blood supply. JAMA 274:1368, 1995.
Smith A: Postoperative pulmonary infections. Clin Evid 8:1428, 2002.
Smith CE, Styn NR, Kalhan S, et al: Intraoperative glucose control in diabetic and nondiabetic patients during cardiac surgery. J Cardiothorac Anesth 19:201, 2005.
Sparrow RA, Hardy JG, Fentem PH: Effect of "antiembolism" compression hosiery on leg blood volume. Br J Surg 82:53, 1995.
Stenchever MA: Too much informed consent? Obstet Gynecol 77:631, 1991.
Strebel N, Prins M, Agnelli G, et al: Preoperative or postoperative start of prophylaxis for venous thromboembolism with low-molecular weight heparin in elective hip surgery? Arch Intern Med 162:1451, 2002.
Strunin L: How long should patients fast before surgery? Time for new guidelines. Br J Anaesth 70:1, 1993.
Sundram CJ: Informed consent for major medical treatment of mentally disabled people. N Engl J Med 318:1368, 1988.
Tanos V, Rojansky N: Prophylactic antibiotics in abdominal hysterectomy. J Am Coll Surg 179:593, 1994.
Tepel M, Van Der Giet M, Schwarzfeld C, et al: Prevention of radiographic-contrast-agent-induced reductions in renal function by acetylcysteine. N Engl J Med 343:180, 2000.
Toglia MR, Nolan TE: Morbidity and mortality rates of elective gynecologic surgery in the elderly woman. Am J Obstet Gynecol 189:1584, 2003.
Tønnesen H: The alcohol patient and surgery. Alcohol Alcohol 34:148, 1999.
Toogood JH: Side effects of inhaled corticosteroids. J Allergy Clin Immunol 102:705, 1998.
Valantas MR, Beck DE, Di Palma JA: Mechanical bowel preparation in the older surgical patient. Curr Surg 61:320, 2004.
Van den Berghe G, Wouters P, Weekers F, et al: Intensive insulin therapy in critically ill patients. N Engl J Med 345:1359, 2001.
Vriesendorp TM, Morélis QJ, DeVries JH, et al: Early post-operative glucose levels are an independent risk factor for infection after peripheral vascular surgery: a retrospective study. Eur J Vasc Endovasc Surg 28:520, 2004.
Watts SA, Gibbs NM: Outpatient management of the chronically anticoagulated patient for elective surgery. Anaesth Intensive Care 31:145, 2003.
Weitz JI: Low-molecular-weight heparins. N Engl J Med, 337:688, 1997.
Wilcox MH, Spencer RC: *Clostridium difficile* infection: Responses, relapses and reinfections. J Hosp Infect 22:85, 1992.
Williams-Russo P, Charlson ME, MacKenzie CR, et al: Predicting postoperative pulmonary complications: is it a real problem? Arch Intern Med 152:1209, 1992.
Wilson AT, Reilly CS: Anesthesia and the obese patient, Int J Obesity 17:427, 1993.
Wu WC, Rathore SS, Wang Y, et al: Blood transfusion in elderly patients with acute myocardial infarction. N Engl J Med 345:1230, 2001.
Zacharoulis D, Kakkar A: Venous thromboembolism in laparoscopic surgery. Curr Opin Pulm Med 9:356, 2003.
Zmora O, Pikarsky AJ, Wexner SD: Bowel preparation for colorectal surgery. Dis Colon Rectum 44:1537, 2001.

Postoperative Counseling and Management 25

Fever, Respiratory, Cardiovascular, Thromboembolic, Urinary Tract, Gastrointestinal, Wound, Operative Site, Neurologic Injury, Psychological Sequelae

Vern L. Katz

KEY TERMS AND DEFINITIONS

Adynamic Ileus. A temporary loss of intestinal peristalsis that may lead to a functional intestinal obstruction.

Antipyretic. A drug or device to lower body temperature.

Atelectasis. Imperfect expansion of the lung.

Biofilm. The adherent layer of bacteria and bacterial by-products that forms around indwelling urinary catheters.

Cuff Cellulitis. One of many terms used for the cellulitis caused by an infection from endogenous bacteria in the serosanguineous fluid that collects in the space immediately above the vaginal apex.

Duplex Ultrasound. A high-resolution ultrasound technique using real time and Doppler, used as a method to diagnose deep venous thrombosis.

Ebb Phase. The first few postoperative days when the physiologic response to surgical stress induces water and sodium retention with increased levels of aldosterone, ADH, and cortisol.

Homans' Sign. Discomfort behind the knee on forced dorsiflexion of the foot; a sign of deep vein thrombophlebitis in the calf.

Impedance Plethysmography. A noninvasive screening method using changes in blood volume, as measured by changes in electrical resistance, for the detection of deep vein thrombosis.

Latzko's Operation. A technique for repair of a vesicovaginal fistula at the vaginal apex that includes partial colpocleisis with denudation of the vaginal mucosa surrounding the fistula and subsequent multilayer closure without entering the bladder.

Lymphocyst. A local collection of lymphatic fluid.

Necrotizing Fasciitis. A virulent, rapidly progressing soft tissue infection that is sometimes fatal and requires prompt surgical débridement.

Phlebography (Venography). Radiography of the venous system, a method of detecting deep vein thrombosis.

Shock. A condition in which circulatory insufficiency prevents adequate vascular perfusion of vital organs.

Ventilation/Perfusion Scan ($\dot{V}/Q$ Scan). A noninvasive imaging technique that may be used to establish or exclude the diagnosis of pulmonary embolus.

Wound Dehiscence. Disruption of any layers of the surgical incision caused by a failure of normal healing. The peritoneum remains intact.

Wound Evisceration. Complete breakdown of the healing process through all levels of the incision, with omentum or bowel presenting through the incision.

The goal of postoperative care is the restoration of a woman's normal physiologic and psychological health. The postoperative period encompasses time from the end of the procedure in the operating room until the patient has resumed her normal routines and lifestyle. Classically, this continuum may be divided into three overlapping phases based on the patient's functional status. The role and concerns of the gynecologist gradually evolve as the patient moves from one phase to another. The first phase, perioperative stabilization, draws the surgeon's attention to the resumption of normal physiologic functions, particularly respiratory, cardiovascular, and neurologic. The older the patient, the more comorbidities she has, and the more complex her procedure, the longer this period lasts. This period encompasses recovery from anesthesia and the stabilization of homeostasis, with resumption of oral intake. Usually the time period is 24 to 48 hours. The second phase, postoperative recovery, usually lasts 1 to 4 days. This phase may occur both in the hospital and at home. During this period, patients will resume regular diet, ambulation, and move from parenteral medications to oral medications for treatment of pain. Most traditional postoperative complications become apparent in this time. The last phase is termed "the return to normalcy," which lasts 1 to 6 weeks. Care during this time occurs primarily in the outpatient setting. During this phase, the patient gradually increases strength and transitions from a sick role back to full and normal activity.

As the patient moves through these phases, both physically and psychologically, her needs will change, and the interaction with staff and her physician also change. She will gradually leave the "patient" role and resume a nondependent role. The communication between physicians, patients, and family varies over the course of recovery. For example, in the immediate postoperative period, the primary psychological task of dealing with pain and nausea is the immediate concern. Whereas late, the return of dignity and dealing with changes in body image will dominate a woman's attention. It is common for the main questions of the first postoperative day to be "When can I get these tubes out?" and "When can I shower?" Information or bad news about surgical findings must be tailored and given honestly but appropriately for the patient's physical and psychological status. In the first phase of recovery, discussion regarding surgical results is usually concrete and simple, as the patient drifts in and out of an awake state. Later in the postoperative recovery, details can be discussed. As the patient enters the third phase of returning to normalcy, the implications, perspectives, and treatments become much more of an issue and are reviewed in detail.

Postoperative complications may occur at any time; however, early recognition and management will often preclude larger problems from developing. Thus, attention to postoperative details cannot be over emphasized. Often the woman and her family judge the competence of the gynecologist by the compassion displayed and attention to detail during this postoperative period. Complications increase the duration of the postoperative stay in the hospital. In a study of women readmitted for postoperative complications, approximately 40% had been discharged earlier than the mean length of stay for the corresponding operative procedure.

General caveats of postoperative management emphasize attention to the particular needs of each patient. Flexibility and individual considerations should take precedence over standard orders, but guidelines can help the physician develop his or her own preferences. Individualization is especially important in the postoperative care of geriatric women. Special nursing attention and minimal doses of narcotics help to prevent confusion and disorientation. Ongoing verbal communications with the nursing staff help eliminate misunderstandings that might result in less than ideal postoperative care.

Surgical stress invokes several physiologic responses meant as the bodies "defenses." Many of these responses may be more problematic than the actual surgery. Peri- and postoperative management strategies are aimed at minimizing or preventing these adverse effects, such as prevention of thromboembolism, or β-blockade in older patients to prevent cardiac complications (Fig. 25-1). Individual patients will respond to the stress differently. For example, some women will respond to the insulin resistance of surgical trauma with severe hyperglycemia, which is detrimental to healing. The clinician must be aware of the physiologic stressors.

This chapter discusses major issues of management during the time period from the end of surgery until the return to normal physiologic and psychological function. Problems and complications arise over the whole spectrum of the postoperative time frame and are interrelated. Thus, the clinician must be aware at all times of a patient's changing status during recovery. For simplicity, the chapter is organized around organ systems and their potential complications. However, very few problems arise in a single organ system.

POSTOPERATIVE FEVER

The exact definition of postoperative febrile morbidity varies greatly among authors. Diurnal fluctuations are characteristic of the normal daily body temperature patterns of humans. A normal temperature is usually 37.2° C in the morning and 37.7° C overall. Most definitions use a temperature greater than 38° C 24 hours after surgery as the indicator of febrile morbidity. It is not unusual for gynecologic patients to have a mild temperature elevation during the first 72 hours of the postoperative period, especially during the late afternoon or evening. Up to 75% of patients develop a temperature greater than 37° C, which is usually not associated with an infectious process. Approximately 25% of women after abdominal hysterectomy and 35% following vaginal hysterectomy exhibit febrile morbidity. In a recent study of 686 women with hysterectomy for benign indications, Peipert and colleagues documented a febrile morbidity rate of 14%.

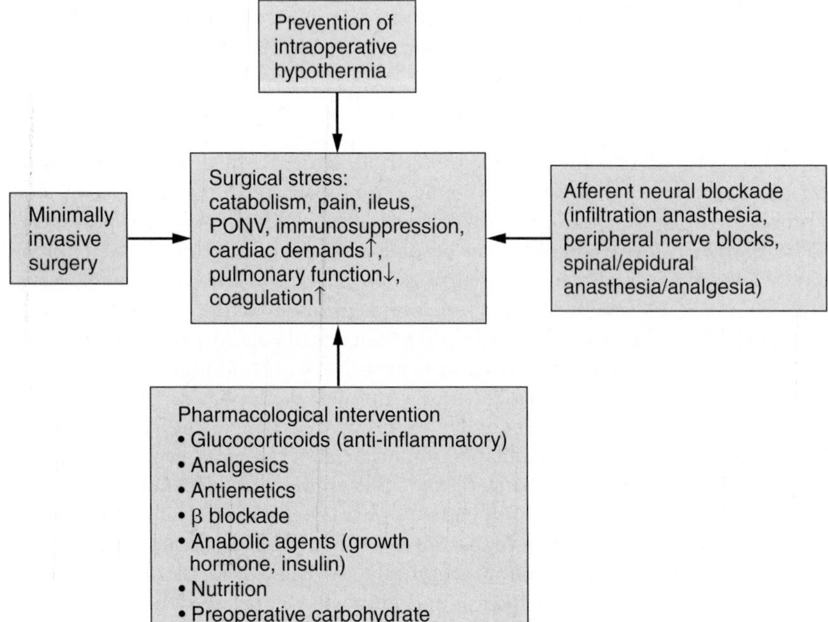

Figure 25-1. Stresses of surgery and interventions to counteract adverse responses. (Adapted from Kehlet H, Dahl JB: Anaesthesia, surgery, and challenges in postoperative recovery. Lancet 362:1922, 2003.)

Table 25-1 Onset of Fever for Various Postoperative Complications

Causes	DAY 1	2	3	4	5	6	1 Week or More
Atelectasis	—	—	→				
Pneumonia			—	—	—	—	→
Wound infection							
Streptococcal or Clostridial	—	→					
Other bacterial					—	—	→
Ovarian abscess							→
Cuff cellulitis				—	—	→	
Phlebitis							
Superficial				—	—	→	
Deep			—	—	—	—	→
Urinary tract infection			—	—	—	—	→
Ureteral or bladder injury							→

Fever is the most common diagnostic problem in the postoperative patient. Common causes of a fever include atelectasis, pneumonia, urinary tract infection (UTI), nonseptic phlebitis, wound infection, and operative site infection. Two intraoperative factors that dramatically increase the risk of postoperative fever are an operative time longer than 2 hours and the necessity for intraoperative transfusion. In Peipert and colleague's study, increased intraoperative blood loss was associated with a 3.5 relative risk (RR) (confidence interval [CI] 1.8–6.8) of developing fever postoperatively.

The physician's primary goal in examining the postoperative febrile patient is to determine whether the fever is caused by an infection. Approximately 20% of postoperative fevers are directly related to infection, and 80% are related to noninfectious causes. Some conditions necessitate active intervention, whereas others are self-limiting. Thus it is imperative not to empirically treat a postoperatively febrile patient with broad-spectrum antibiotics. In addition, it is usually unnecessary to give antipyretics to lower the temperature of an adult. As Duff emphasized, fever is a phylogenic host response to infection in fish, lizards, and in higher mammals, including humans. Fever may be a beneficial response to the host.

Fever is a common postoperative finding, especially a mild temperature elevation during the first 48 to 72 hours following an operation. The pathophysiology of postoperative fever is primarily related to the release of cytokines. The cause of a postoperative fever may be simple and common, such as atelectasis or dehydration, or unusual, such as malignant hyperthermia or septicemia. The temporal relationship of the *onset* of a patient's febrile response to common postoperative complications is depicted in Table 25-1.

Workup for Fever

The initial workup for a postoperative fever should emphasize the most common problems. Medical students memorize the five W's in the differential diagnosis: wind (atelectasis), water (UTI), wound (infection or hematoma), walk (superficial or deep vein phlebitis), and wonder drugs (drug-induced fever).

The proper workup of a postoperative fever, similar to that of any problem in gynecology, involves the three classic steps of history, physical examination, and laboratory evaluations, with major emphasis placed on the physical examination. A chart review and history from the patient may highlight preoperative problems that might cause fever: intraoperative complications, such as aspiration of gastric or oral contents; placement of foreign bodies, such as drains; recent infusion of blood products or drugs; and known allergies. The physical examination emphasizes examination of the lungs for atelectasis and pneumonia; the wound and operative site for infection or hematoma formation; the costovertebral angles for tenderness, which might suggest pyelonephritis; and superficial veins in the arms for superficial phlebitis and deep veins in the legs for deep vein phlebitis.

The findings of the history and especially the physical examination and considerations of cost containment all influence the extent of laboratory tests ordered. Ordering a specific list of laboratory tests is unrewarding. The three most commonly ordered laboratory tests are complete blood count, chest roentgenogram, and urinalysis. A study by Schwandt and coworkers has emphasized that chest radiograph and urine cultures are best ordered only for specific clinical signs not as reflex orders. Other common tests include culture and Gram stains of body fluids, including sputum, urine, and blood. One study of over 300 women who were febrile following hysterectomy did not identify a single positive blood culture. Women with persistent and undiagnosed fevers may need tests of liver function or special imaging studies, such as pelvic ultrasound or computed tomography (CT) to detect problems such as compromised ureters, abscesses, or foreign bodies.

Each major complication will be discussed in detail later in the chapter. However, several specific generalizations concerning the type and characteristics of fever patterns should be emphasized. Fever is a common postoperative finding, occurring in approximately 75% of women. Rarely is the cause of the fever a serious infection. Microatelectasis is thought to be the cause of approximately 90% of fevers occurring in the first 48 hours after operation. Patients who develop fever as a result of an indwelling catheter, such as plastic intravenous (IV) lines or Foley catheters, are afebrile for several days and then experience an abrupt temperature spike. In contrast, wound or pelvic infections, which are usually clinically diagnosed from the fourth to seventh postoperative days, usually are associated with a low-grade fever that begins early in the postoperative period. An empiric trial of IV heparin for 72 hours is often a diagnostic and therapeutic trial for pelvic thrombophlebitis in refractory cases of postoperative fever of unknown origin.

Importantly, infection in the elderly will not always present with classic findings. The amount of temperature elevation may not reflect the severity of the infection. Not uncommonly, the first signs of infection in the elderly will be mental status change. Additionally, the degree of leukocytosis, being blunted or absent, may not reflect infection.

A patient with a drug-induced fever feels better and does not look as ill as her temperature course indicates. The tachycardia associated with the elevated temperature is usually much less than usually anticipated with a similar temperature elevation secondary to inflammation or infection. The presence of eosinophilia suggests a drug-induced fever. However, drug fever is rare and is usually a diagnosis of exclusion. Presumptive evidence of a drug-induced fever is established when the fever disappears after discontinuation of the drug. Scientifically, the diagnosis can only be confirmed by challenging the patient with the medication again after the fever has subsided. Clinically, this latter technique is not pragmatic.

Superficial thrombophlebitis often produces an enigmatic fever. Much of the time there is tenderness at the IV site. Thus it is important to empirically change any IV lines that have been in place for longer than 48 hours. This is particularly true for central venous catheters and epidural catheters, where an infection may not show clinical signs of localized tenderness or erythema. The cause of febrile transfusion reactions is a concern. However, usually the reactions are caused by leukocyte or platelet antibodies. As long as a major blood type incompatibility is not found, treatment may be conservative.

The basic fever workup should be repeated at intervals until the diagnosis is established. The patient should be reexamined and selective laboratory tests reordered. Rare causes of postoperative fever include malignant neoplasms, pulmonary embolus (PE), thyroid storm, and malignant hyperthermia. These diagnoses usually present with other signs and symptoms as well as temperature elevation.

It is important to consider that fever is a potential beneficial physiologic response to the patient. Therefore, unless the adult is markedly symptomatic secondary to the elevated temperature, it is not necessary to order an antipyretic medication. Cellular damage only occurs when the core temperature exceeds 41° C. Active cutaneous cooling does not reduce core temperature and may have undesirable effects such as increasing the metabolic rate and activating the autonomic nervous system.

MANAGEMENT OF A FALLING HEMATOCRIT

Bleeding is one of the most feared postoperative complications because it not only prolongs the hospital stay but also in rare cases may lead to the patient's death. Significant arterial bleeding in the first 24 hours often necessitates reoperation. This complication is discussed along with the management of shock and pelvic hematomas later in the chapter.

Vital signs should be ordered at frequent intervals during the first 24 hours to detect hypovolemia secondary to postoperative bleeding. Most women will have sufficient intravascular volume to compensate (during the early phases of hemorrhage) through the redistribution of blood flow from less vital to more vital organs. Low urine output may be the earliest sign of a decrease in intravascular volume. Thus, following an operation, sizable amounts of unrecognized intraperitoneal or retroperitoneal bleeding sometimes are present without the woman having subjective symptoms or appreciable changes in her vital signs or urine output. Minimum urine output should be 0.5 mL/kg/hr, approximately 20 mL/hr women of medium and larger size should produce more urine, just as petite patients will produce less. A consistent orthostatic decrease in blood pressure of greater than 10 mm Hg may indicate a possible decrease of 20% of the blood volume. Thus a hematocrit may be helpful at two intervals during the postoperative course. We prefer a hematocrit at 24 and 72 hours following the operative procedure. A hematocrit drawn 24 hours following an operation may not truly reflect postoperative blood loss.

The normal physiologic response to the stress of the operation and tissue destruction is a release of increased levels of aldosterone, cortisol, and antidiuretic hormone (ADH). The higher levels of aldosterone produce an increase in both sodium and water retention, whereas increased levels of ADH promote free water retention. This has been called the "ebb phase" of postoperative physiology. It is common for women to have notable lower extremity edema for the first few postoperative days, because they are often given significant amounts of IV fluids. Depending on the type and amount of intraoperative and postoperative IV fluids, the hematocrit on the first postoperative day may be misleading and reflect fluid changes rather than intraoperative or postoperative hemorrhage. The hematocrit from the third postoperative day is a more accurate measurement of postoperative change. If the patient is doing well, the stress hormones decline and water retention stops. The patient will begin to experience a brisk diuresis, sometimes termed the "flow phase," beginning around the third postoperative day. Hematocrits should be obtained in a standard fashion so as to eliminate sampling errors. For example, hematocrit samples drawn from central lines or during blood gas determinations often give false values because of the heparin or saline flush solutions.

After the effects of the operative blood loss are subtracted from the preoperative hematocrit, each further reduction in hematocrit of 3 to 5 points reflects a postoperative hemorrhage of approximately 500 mL. The safe level of postoperative anemia is a controversial issue. Certainly it is not identical to the level needed before an operation. Most young, healthy women without complicating medical illness will tolerate hematocrits of 20% to 22% without transfusion. These patients should be observed for orthostatic changes in their vital signs. Women with cardiac and pulmonary disease, and women over the age of 60 should be transfused to maintain a hematocrit above 30%. The morbidity and mortality associated with a surgical procedure are directly related to the amount of intraoperative and postoperative blood loss and not the corresponding level of preoperative anemia.

RESPIRATORY COMPLICATIONS

Alterations of pulmonary function are an expected physiologic change in women having general anesthesia and operations that open the peritoneal cavity. Of importance, respiratory complications directly cause 25% of deaths in women who die during the first 7 postoperative days. Many respiratory problems are secondary to inadequate ventilation by women as they try to minimize acute pain from the operative incision.

Atelectasis

The term *atelectasis* is derived from two Greek words that mean "imperfect expansion." The severity of atelectasis ranges from lack of expansion of a small group of terminal bronchioles and alveoli to complete collapse of a lung. In most patients, atelectasis is the failure to maintain patency of the small pulmonary airways and alveoli. Microatelectasis is a common occurrence, developing during almost all pelvic operations, and it persists for 24 hours postoperatively in approximately 50% of women. Atelectasis is the most common cause of postoperative temperature elevations. Studies have demonstrated that there is no association between fever and the amount of atelectasis diagnosed radiologically. The incidence of atelectasis depends on the number of predisposing risk factors and the vigor with which the clinical diagnosis is established.

Ninety percent of all postoperative respiratory complications are related to atelectasis. The immediate postoperative period is characterized by a decrease in functional residual capacity and lung compliance (Fig. 25-2). Thus the work of breathing is increased. Microatelectasis is most common where small airways (less than 1 mm in diameter) become blocked by secretions. When small airways remain closed by a combination of mucus plugs and bronchospasm, the gas distal to the obstruction is absorbed. This process results in atelectasis. These changes occur during the first 72 hours following an operation. When atelectasis becomes progressive and involves a large area of lung tissue, there is an associated decrease in oxygen saturation and a decrease in arterial oxygen pressure (Po_2). This is associated with a normal to low arterial carbon dioxide pressure (Pco_2).

Pulmonary and nonpulmonary factors that favor premature airway closure and development of atelectasis are listed in the following box. The supine position decreases the functional residual capacity approximately 20% compared with the erect position. Obesity, smoking, age older than 60 years, prolonged operative time, presence of a nasogastric tube, and coexisting medical conditions, such as cardiac or lung disease and pulmonary infection, all predispose women to atelectasis. In one study, 40% of obese women demonstrated radiologic evidence of atelectasis in their postoperative chest roentgenograms.

Nonpulmonary and Pulmonary Factors That Favor Premature Airway Closure and Atelectasis

Nonpulmonary Factors

- Supine position
- Obesity
- Increased abdominal girth (ileus, pneumoperitoneum)
- Breathing at low lung volumes
  - Bindings around the chest and abdomen
  - Incisional pain
  - Sedative narcotic drugs
  - Prolonged effect of paralyzing drugs
  - Immobility
  - Excessively high concentrations of oxygen for prolonged periods

Pulmonary Factors

- Interstitial edema
- Loss of surfactant with air space instability
- Airway obstruction
  - Inflammatory with swelling of bronchial and interbronchial tissue
  - Constriction of bronchial smooth muscle
  - Retained secretions

From Wellman JJ: Respiratory care in the surgical patient. In Lubin MF, Walker HK, Smith RB (eds): Medical Management of the Surgical Patient. Stoneham, MA, Butterworth, 1982, p 288. Used with permission.

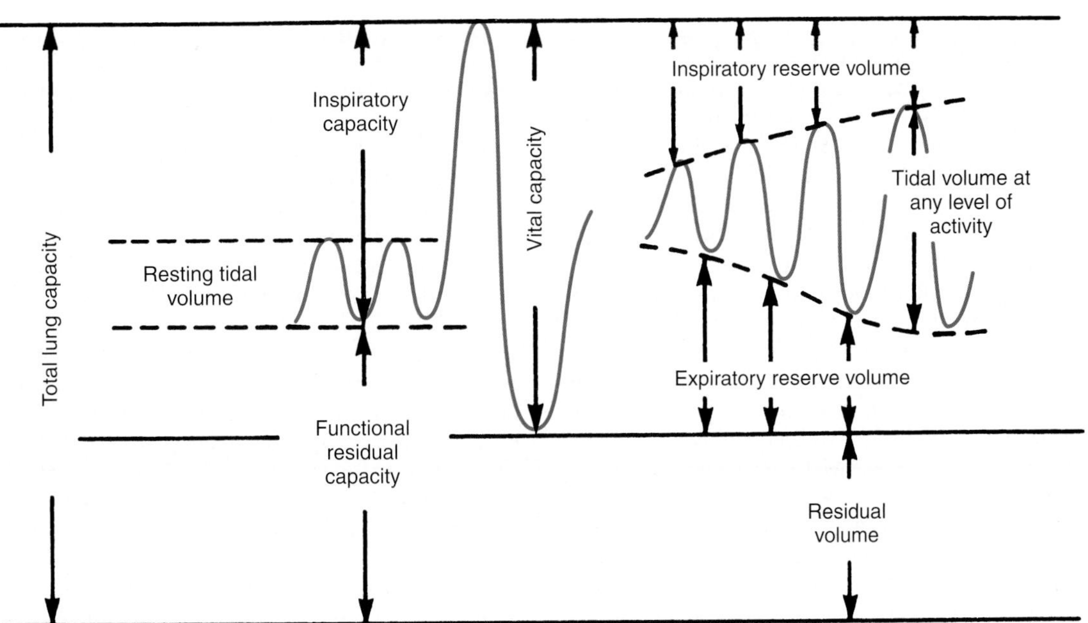

Figure 25-2. Graphic illustration of lung volumes and capacities. (From Wellman JJ: Respiratory care in the surgical patient. In Lubin MF, Walker HD, Smith RB [eds]: Medical Management of the Surgical Patient. Stoneham, MA, Butterworth, 1982, p 285. Used with permission.)

In normal breathing periodic, involuntary, deep inspirations help to expand all areas of the lung. Pain, the supine position, narcotics, and abdominal distention contribute to a pattern of monotonous shallow breathing without spontaneous deep sighs in the postoperative period. Because of the pain of an abdominal incision, chest wall breathing dominates over abdominal breathing. The resultant decrease in the movement of the diaphragm contributes to the development of atelectasis. A further decrease in functional residual capacity, a decrease in surfactant, and a depression of mucociliary transport all contribute to ventilation/perfusion ($\dot{V}/\dot{Q}$) mismatches and reduced $\dot{V}/\dot{Q}$ ratios. The end results are gas trapping, atelectasis, and vascular shunting. In the majority of individuals, microatelectasis is patchy and localized to small areas. However, the severity of atelectasis varies and may involve a complete lung.

Distribution of pulmonary blood flow is influenced by gravity. A greater proportion of pulmonary blood flows to dependent areas of the lungs in the supine patient. This increased blood flow, combined with the atelectasis in dependent areas, results in an increased impairment of oxygenation, as well as a decrease in the elimination of carbon dioxide.

The endotracheal tube may contribute to the development of atelectasis. Even correctly placed endotracheal tubes are associated with destruction of cilia in the respiratory tract epithelium. Women with nasogastric tubes have a higher incidence of atelectasis, more commonly related to a decrease in deep breathing than to aspiration of stomach contents.

Atelectasis may present as the classic triad of fever, tachypnea, and tachycardia developing within the first 72 hours following an operation. On physical examination, tubular breathing, decreased breath sounds, and moist inspiratory rales may be heard. These findings are most prominent over the bases of the lung. If the condition progresses, an increase in productive cough and leukocytosis result. Chest radiographic films may demonstrate a patchy infiltrate with elevations of the diaphragm. There may be a corresponding shift of the trachea and mediastinum when atelectasis involves a large segment of the lung.

Atelectasis usually resolves spontaneously by the third to fifth postoperative day. Nevertheless, major efforts are made to prevent atelectasis, especially in high-risk individuals. The foundations of prevention of atelectasis are the encouragement of uneven ventilation and the production of episodes of prolonged inspiration to increase functional residual capacity. Thus the patient is encouraged to walk, take deep breaths, cough, turn from side to side, and remain semierect rather than supine. Early mobilization and ambulation have been documented to be as effective as chest physical therapy in the prevention of pulmonary complications. Keeping pain relief to a level where the woman will be able to cooperate and not have monotonous shallow breathing is also helpful. The most important aid to prevent and treat atelectasis is a simple bedside incentive spirometry device. Many women need encouragement by the hospital staff to use these devices effectively. The primary risk of atelectasis is progression to pneumonia. Randomized clinical trials and systematic reviews have noted that preventative measures significantly reduce both problematic atelectasis and pneumonia. Thus these simple measures should be ordered for all patients.

In summary, basilar atelectasis is the most common postoperative pulmonary problem experienced by gynecologic patients. If atelectasis does not clear, the woman should be treated with chest physical therapy, intermittent positive pressure breathing, aerosol therapy, or intermittent continuous positive airway pressure by mask. Rarely, bronchoscopy may be indicated to remove large mucus plugs.

Pneumonia

Postoperative pneumonia is commonly associated with atelectasis, because bacterial infections often begin in collapsed areas of the lungs. The infections lead to increased water in the lungs, increased elastic resistance, and decreased lung compliance. In animals the inhalation of infected material does not produce pneumonia without associated atelectasis. In experimental animals the injection of an IV bolus of bacteria was found to cause pneumonia in selectively localized areas of the lung that were obstructed. Predisposing factors to the development of pneumonia include chronic pulmonary disease, heavy cigarette smoking, alcohol abuse, obesity, advanced age, nasogastric tubes, long operative procedures, gram-negative bacterial infections, postoperative peritonitis, and debilitating illnesses.

The symptoms and signs of pneumonia are fever, cough, dyspnea, tachypnea, and purulent sputum. When pain occurs, it may be felt in the back or chest. The classic physical finding of pneumonia is coarse rales over the infected area. The patient usually has a higher temperature and more systemic toxicity than does a woman with atelectasis. Leukocytosis is pronounced in most patients, though it may be delayed or attenuated in the elderly. Chest roentgenograms often demonstrate diffuse, patchy infiltrates of the lung. Radiographic diagnoses are approximately 60% accurate for either bacterial or viral pneumonia in women with laboratory-proven pneumonia. Gram stain of the sputum helps to differentiate between bacterial colonization and infection. In cases of pneumonia the smear contains a large number of inflammatory cells with both intracellular and extracellular bacteria.

The management of pneumonia is similar to the management of atelectasis, with the addition of parenteral antibiotics. The initial choice of parenteral antibiotics is usually based on the Gram stain and subsequently on sputum cultures. Most lung infections result when the contents of the mouth (mucus and bacteria that have a physiologic pH) are inhaled and subsequently produce bacterial pneumonia.

One in 3000 procedures may be complicated by pneumonitis produced by aspiration of gastric fluid (sterile and highly acidic). The aspiration produces a severe chemical pneumonitis. Aspiration and its complications are a cause of approximately 30% of anesthetic mortalities. Women at high risk for aspiration pneumonia include the elderly, obese, and those with a hiatal hernia or emergency surgery associated with a full stomach. The morbidity from aspiration is secondary to particulate matter entering into the lungs. The particulate matter is difficult for the lung defenses to clear. Morbidity also arises from the caustic nature of gastric acid. The combination of these insults leads to a destructive inflammatory response. When aspiration is significant and severe, adult respiratory distress syndrome often develops. Secondary infection usually complicates aspiration pneumonitis, and broad-spectrum antibiotics should be given when this diagnosis is entertained. Preventive measures include early removal of nasogastric suction, antacid ingestion, and H_2 blockers in the perioperative period, as well as careful use of narcotics and sedatives.

SLEEP APNEA

Sleep apnea has become a significant concern as the incidence of obese patients rises. Increased fatty tissue in the neck may produce compression and narrowing of the airway, leading to intermittent apnea while a woman sleeps. In addition, the chronic airway narrowing in obese patients may also lead to hypoventilation. Increased chest wall thickness and adipose tissue in the abdominal wall lead to a decrease in pulmonary compliance. The lowered PO_2 may induce systemic as well as pulmonary hypertension. Patients will also develop a chronically increased PCO_2. Respiratory drive shifts from a CO_2-driven response to a response to low levels of oxygen. When morbidly obese patients are given higher levels of oxygen as well as narcotics they are at increased risk for apnea. These patients develop an increased sensitivity to narcotics that shuts down the respiratory drive. Patients with chronic hypoxia from any cause will often have an increased sensitivity to narcotics, but it is particularly problematic in the obese patient who is dependent on low levels of oxygen for respiratory stimulation. These patients should be given oxygen as needed. However, during the postoperative period when narcotics are given, ongoing pulse oxymetry should be used to keep the oxygen saturation in the 94% range. At saturation levels of 96% to 99% these patients may lose some of their respiratory drive and become hypercarbic and acidotic.

CARDIOVASCULAR PROBLEMS

Hemorrhagic Shock

Shock is defined as a condition in which circulatory insufficiency prevents adequate vascular perfusion of vital organs. Systemic hypotension results in poor tissue perfusion and reduced capillary filling. If this pathophysiologic state is neglected, prolonged hypotension results in oliguria, progressive metabolic acidosis, and multiple organ failure. Shock may be produced by hemorrhage, cardiac failure, sepsis, and anaphylactic reactions. Hypovolemic shock is by far the most common cause of acute circulatory failure in gynecology. Cardiogenic shock and septic shock are rare. Shock from postoperative hemorrhage is most commonly seen in the first few hours following the operation. In the perioperative period, hypovolemia may be secondary to several factors, including preoperative volume deficiency, unreplaced blood loss during surgery, extracellular fluid loss during surgery, inadequate fluid replacement, and, most commonly, continued blood loss following the surgical procedure. Tachycardia is the classic cardiovascular physiologic response to hypotension. Progressive hypovolemia results in diminished urine output. However, relative bradycardia in hypotensive women is also a common hemodynamic response.

The vast majority of perioperative cases of shock are related to hemorrhage secondary to inadequate hemostasis. The development of shock from acute blood loss depends on the rate of bleeding; for example, a slow venous ooze may produce a large amount of blood loss but not produce shock. Rapid loss of 20% of a woman's blood volume produces mild shock, whereas a loss of greater than 40% of blood volume results in severe shock. Actual measurement of intraoperative blood loss is imprecise even with extensive use of suction equipment. Studies have demonstrated that 15% to 45% of surgical blood loss is absorbed on the drapes, laparotomy pads, and other areas. Thus the level of blood in the suction bottle does not accurately represent the true loss from the procedure. Massive blood loss has been defined as hemorrhage that results in replacement of 50% of the circulating blood volume in less than 3 hours.

Hypotension in the immediate postoperative period may be secondary to the residual effects of anesthesia or oversedation. For example, elderly patients often experience prolonged vasodilation secondary to the sympathetic blockade produced by epidural or spinal anesthesia.

The most common cause of postoperative bleeding is either a less than ideal ligature or hemorrhage from a vessel that retracted during the operation. Bleeding may come from an isolated artery or vein or may be more generalized when the bleeding is secondary to a clotting diathesis. The differential diagnosis of postoperative hemorrhagic shock includes conditions such as pneumothorax, PE, massive pulmonary aspiration, myocardial infarction, and acute gastric dilation.

The differential diagnosis of ineffective coagulation includes sepsis, fibrinolysis, diffuse intravascular coagulation, and a previously unrecognized coagulation defect, such as von Willebrand's disease. Inadequate hemostasis sometimes develops from excessive transfusion. The progressive acidosis associated with shock increases hemostatic problems. Hypothermia further complicates hemostasis because it produces platelet dysfunction and coagulopathy secondary to decreased activity of thromboxanes. Thrombocytopenia, impaired platelet function, and a decrease in factors V, VIII, and XI occur with massive transfusions. Coagulopathy begins with the transfusion of greater than 5 units of blood. Hypofibrinogenemia is the first to develop followed by deficiencies of other coagulation factors. Thrombocytopenia is the last recognized defect in the coagulopathy cascade. However, the timing of its development varies from individual to individual. Thus transfusion of platelets should be determined by serial platelet counts (see the following box). Similarly, preset formulas for the transfusion of fresh frozen plasma, such as 2 units of plasma for every 5 units of packed cells, should be replaced by selective transfusion of plasma as needed to match a clotting deficiency.

Tachycardia and decreased urine output are two early signs of hypovolemia caused by hidden internal bleeding. The body's adrenergic response to hemorrhage includes perspiration, tachycardia, and peripheral vasoconstriction. Urine output decreases to less than 0.5 mL/kg/hr (20 to 25 mL/hr) as a result of poor perfusion of the kidneys. With further loss of blood the woman becomes agitated, appears weak, and develops skin pallor with cold and clammy extremities. The systolic blood pressure drops below 80 mm Hg. Again, because of adaptive cardiovascular changes, it takes a rapid loss of approximately one third of the blood volume to produce significant hypotension.

After an operation both occult intraperitoneal and retroperitoneal bleeding often occur without significant local symptoms. Extraperitoneal bleeding may present as bleeding from

Suggested Transfusion Guidelines for Platelets

Recent (within 24 hours) platelet count < 10,000/mm^3 (for prophylaxis)
Recent (within 24 hours) platelet count <50,000/mm^3 with demonstrated microvascular bleeding ("oozing") or a planned surgical/invasive procedure
Demonstrated microvascular bleeding and a precipitous fall in platelet count
Adult patients in the operating room who have had complicated procedures or have required more than 10 units of blood ***and*** have microvascular bleeding. Giving platelets assumes adequate surgical hemotasis has been achieved.
Documented platelet dysfunction (e.g., prolonged bleeding time greater than 15 minutes, abnormal platelet function tests) with petechiae, purpura, microvascular bleeding ("oozing"), or surgical/invasive procedure
Unwarranted indications:
- Empirical use with massive transfusion when patient is not having clinically evident microvascular bleeding ("oozing")
- Prophylaxis in thrombotic thrombocytopenic purpura/hemolytic-uremic syndrome or idiopathic thrombocytopenic purpura
- Extrinsic platelet dysfunction (e.g., renal failure, von Willebrand's disease)

From Rutherford EJ, Skeet DA, Schooler WG: Hematologic principles in surgery. In Townsend CM, Beauchamp RD, Evers BM (eds): Sabiston Textbook of Surgery, 17th ed. Philadelphia, Saunders, 2004, p 128.

the vaginal vault if the vaginal cuff was left open. There may be mild flank or back tenderness with rebound on abdominal palpation. However, abdominal distention, muscle rigidity, and shoulder pain are late signs of intraperitoneal hemorrhage. The diagnosis of clinically significant postoperative bleeding may be confirmed by serial changes in hematocrits or by paracentesis. However, it is important to caution that marked changes in hematocrit and hemoglobin require time to develop. Bimanual examination with the patient under anesthesia may help in the diagnosis of silent retroperitoneal bleeding immediately before reoperation. Imaging studies may demonstrate obliteration of the psoas shadow and deviation of the ureter by a large retroperitoneal hematoma. Preoperative CT may be the most useful imaging modality in this setting.

The goals of management of postoperative shock are to replace, restore, and maintain the effective circulating blood volume and establish normal cellular perfusion and oxygenation (see the following box on Management Priorities in Massive Transfusion). To accomplish this goal, an adequate cardiac output and appropriate peripheral vascular resistance must be maintained. The first priority is to provide adequate ventilation because poor respiratory gas exchange is the most frequent cause of death in these patients. The second, almost simultaneous, priority is rapid fluid replacement with adequate amounts of blood and crystalloid solution (normal saline or

Management Priorities in Massive Transfusion (the Exact Priority Depends on the Circumstances)

Restore circulating blood volume
Maintain oxygenation
Correct coagulopathy
Maintain body temperature
Correct biochemical abnormalities
Prevent pulmonary and other organ dysfunction
Treat underlying cause of haemorrhage

From Donaldson MDJ, Seaman MJ, Park GR: Massive blood transfusion. Br J Anaesth 69:621, 1992.

lactated Ringer's solution). The three-to-one rule suggests a ratio of 3 mL of crystalloid solution for every 1 mL of blood loss. The optimal fluid replacement is a fluid evenly distributed throughout multiple body compartments. Optimal replacement includes packed red blood cells and a balanced electrolyte solution, such as lactated Ringer's solution. In February 1995, the University Hospital Consortium developed guidelines for the use of albumin, nonprotein colloid, and crystalloid solutions. They recommended in hemorrhagic shock that crystalloids should be considered the initial resuscitation fluid of choice; colloids are appropriate for resuscitation in conjunction with crystalloids when blood products are not immediately available. A meta-analysis of patients with hypovolemia found an excess mortality of approximately 6% (1 excess death per 17 treated patients) in those who received albumin instead of or in addition to crystalloid solutions. Guidelines for transfusion of red blood cells are listed in the box on Suggested Transfusion Guidelines for Red Blood Cells.

The goals of fluid replacement are to obtain and maintain a systolic blood pressure that is similar to preoperative readings, maintain urine output greater than 0.5 mL/kg/hr (usually > 30 mL/hr), and maintain a pulmonary wedge pressure between 10 and 15 mm Hg. Table 25-2 lists types of blood components used for replacement therapy. To monitor the rapid replacement of large volumes of IV fluid, a Swan–Ganz catheter is used to determine pulmonary artery pressure, pulmonary wedge pressure, central venous pressure, and cardiac output. These values allow adjustments in the rate of vascular volume replacement. A Foley catheter facilitates measurement of hourly urine outputs. We prefer a pulmonary artery catheter (Swan–Ganz catheter) over a central venous pressure line. However, if one is using a central venous pressure line, it is important to measure the pressure with the patient at a 45-degree angle. Studies have demonstrated that a central venous pressure measurement in the supine position will severely underestimate the volume of intravascular depletion.

The gold standard of imaging studies to detect abdominal and pelvic hemorrhage is a CT scan. An unenhanced CT scan will determine rapidly the precise location of the hemorrhage. During the imaging studies, acute hemorrhage appears as a high attenuation area in contrast to the normal soft tissue. In an emergent situation, the use of a helical scanner allows for an even more rapid acquisition of images.

Table 25-2 Indications for Administration of Various Blood Products

Product	Content	Acceptable Indication	Unacceptable Indication
Red blood cells	Red cells	To increase oxygen-carrying capacity in anemic women For orthostatic hypotension secondary to blood loss	For volume expansion In place of a hematinic To enhance wound healing To improve general well-being
Platelet concentrates	Platelets	To control or prevent bleeding associated with deficiencies in platelet number or function	In patients with immune thrombocytopenic purpura (unless bleeding is life threatening) Prophylactically with massive blood transfusion
Fresh frozen plasma	Plasma, clotting factors	To increase the level of clotting factors in patients with demonstrated deficiency	For volume expansion As a nutritional supplement Prophylactically with massive blood transfusion
Cryoprecipitate	Factors I, V, VIII, XIII, von Willebrand factor, fibronectin	To increase the level of clotting factors in patients with demonstrated deficiency of fibrinogen, factor VIII, factor XIII, fibronectin, or von Willebrand factor	Prophylactically with massive blood transfusion

From ACOG Tech Bull 199:1, 1994.

Suggested Transfusion Guidelines for Red Blood Cells

- Hemoglobin < 8g/dL or acute blood loss in an otherwise healthy patient with signs and symptoms of decreased oxygen delivery with two or more of the following:
  - Estimated or anticipated acute blood loss of > 15% of total blood volume (750 mL in 70-kg male)
  - Diastolic blood pressure < 60 mm Hg
  - Systolic blood pressure drop > 30 mm Hg from baseline
  - Tachycardia (>100 beats/min)
  - Oliguria/anuria
  - Mental status changes
- Hemoglobin < 10 g/dL in patients with known increased risk of coronary artery disease or pulmonary insufficiency who have sustained or are expected to sustain significant blood loss
  - Symptomatic anemia with any of the following:
    - Tachycardia (>100 beats/min)
    - Mental status changes
    - Evidence of myocardial ischemia including angina
    - Shortness of breath or dizziness with mild exertion
    - Orthostatic hypotension
  - Unfounded/questionable indications:
    - To increase wound healing
    - To improve the patient's sense of well-being
    - 7 g/dL < hemoglobin < 10 g/dL (or 21% < hematocrit < 30%) in otherwise stable, asymptomatic patient
    - Mere availability of pre-donated autologous blood without medical indication

From Rutherford EJ, Skeet DA, Schooler WG: Hematologic principles in surgery. In Townsend CM, Beauchamp RD, Evers BM (eds): Sabiston Textbook of Surgery, 17th ed. Philadelphia, Saunders, 2004, p 128.

Returning a patient to the operating room to control hemorrhage is often a difficult decision. However, this decision should not be postponed, and the patient should have an exploratory operation as soon as possible after volume replacement. During this second operation excellent anesthesia, a full selection of surgical instruments, and the value of good assistance cannot be overemphasized. Proper exposure is paramount for the success of this operation. Initially the old clots are removed, and further bleeding is reduced by direct pressure over the pelvic vessels. A systematic search is conducted in an effort to identify the individual vessels that are bleeding. Often the offending artery or vein cannot be identified, or friability of the tissues results in further bleeding.

Bilateral ligation of the anterior divisions of the hypogastric arteries distal to the posterior parietal branch is an effective operation to control persistent postoperative pelvic hemorrhage. This procedure results in a reduction of pulse pressure, which allows a stable clot to form at the site where the pelvic vessels are injured. Classically, two ligatures are placed and tied around each hypogastric artery (Fig. 25-3). The major potential complication of this procedure is injury to the hypogastric vein. If there is generalized oozing, thrombocytopenia, disseminated intravascular coagulation, or factor VIII deficiency should be suspected. If these conditions are excluded, venous oozing from small vessels in the pelvis may be controlled by local

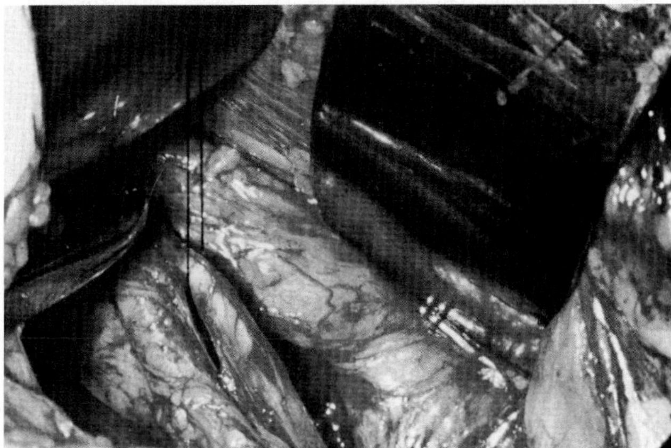

Figure 25-3. Ligation of internal iliac artery. Double loop is being directed toward bifurcation of common iliac artery. (From Breen JL, Gregori CA, Kindzierski JA: Hemorrhage in gynecologic surgery. In Shaefer G, Graber EA [eds]: Complications in Obstetric and Gynecologic Surgery. Hagerstown, MD, Harper & Row, 1981, p 439.)

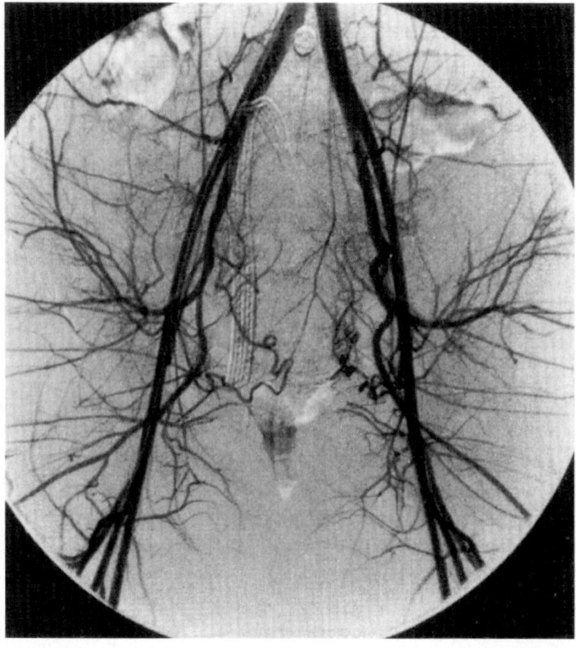
A

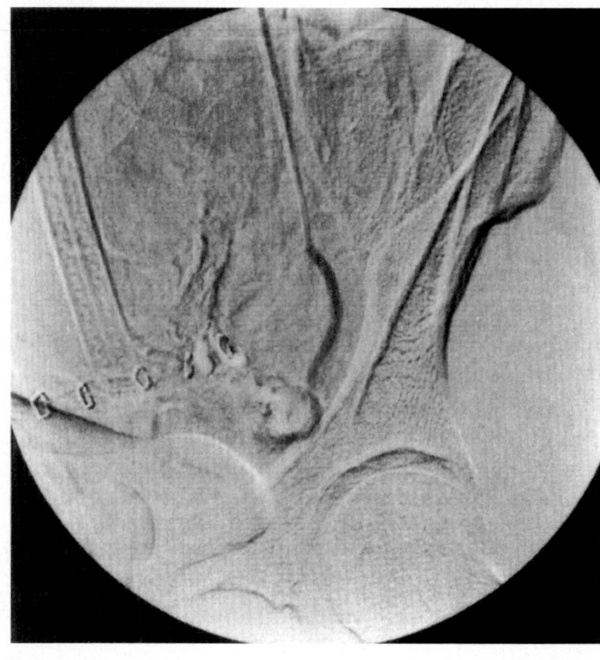
B

Figure 25-4. **A,** Anteroposterior digital subtraction pelvic angiogram in 37-year-old woman with persistent pelvic bleeding after surgical myomectomy for uterine leiomyomas demonstrates contrast pooling (*arrows*) from branches of left uterine artery, consistent with active hemorrhage. **B,** Postembolization left uterine arteriogram shows occluded left uterine artery *(long arrows)* with no evidence of active bleeding. (From Vedantham S, Goodwin SC, McLucas B, Mohr G: Uterine artery embolization: An underused method of controlling pelvic hemorrhage. Am J Obstet Gynecol 176:938, 1997.)

application of microfibrillar collagen compounds (Avitene, Gelfoam, Floseal).

Intraoperative rapid autologous blood transfusion is a technique that is used extensively in cardiovascular and trauma surgery. Regretfully, it is underused or rarely performed by gynecologists. Grimes has described a simple device that can adapt this technique for use in any operating room. The major complication of rapid autologous transfusion is a 10% hemolysis rate. The risks of air embolism or infusion of particulate matter are minimal. Obviously, autologous blood does not contain platelets or clotting factors so that platelets and fresh frozen plasma will have to be given concurrently for severe hemorrhage. Rapid autologous transfusion is contraindicated in advanced pelvic infection or malignancy.

In many situations angiographic embolization instead of exploratory laparotomy is preferable (Fig. 25-4). Introduction of digital road mapping technology has improved the rapid identification of bleeding vessels. Similarly, treatment of recurrent postoperative hemorrhage or hemorrhage late in the postoperative course (7 to 14 days) may be performed with angiographic arterial embolization. Either absorbable gelatin sponges, which produce vascular occlusion for 10 to 30 days, or metal coils with Dacron fibers, which produce permanent occlusion, may be used.

Hematomas

This section will describe the management of wounds or pelvic hematomas that develop slowly and are diagnosed after the first postoperative day. Proper management of postoperative hematomas is one of the most challenging and controversial subjects in operative gynecology. The incidence of hematomas is inversely related to the extent to which meticulous hemostasis is obtained intraoperatively. Women who are given low-dose heparin or chronically take aspirin are at a slightly higher risk of hematoma formation. Hematomas result from intermittent or slow, continuous venous bleeding and are almost always self-limiting. Eventually the pressure of the expanding hematoma will exceed the venous pressure, and a stable clot will form. The extent of the hematoma is determined partially by the potential size of the compartment into which the bleeding occurs. Retroperitoneal or broad ligament hematomas may contain several units of blood. The diagnosis of a wound or pelvic hematoma is usually suspected on the morning of the third postoperative day when the laboratory reports an unexpectedly low hematocrit. The patient may have mild to moderate tenderness over the affected area. By the fifth postoperative day the hematoma liquefies and is easier to outline during bimanual examination. Distinguishing between an uninfected hematoma and a hematoma that has become secondarily infected is difficult before incision and drainage. Both clinical situations produce tenderness and fever secondary to the inflammation surrounding the hematoma. The diagnosis of most retroperitoneal hematomas may be made by physical examination. Most important is a careful rectovaginal examination. Radiologic imaging studies are indicated when the hematoma cannot be palpated.

Hematomas less than 5 cm in diameter may be treated conservatively. Larger hematomas may be drained transcutaneously, either with CT or ultrasound direction as soon as they liquefy. If not treated, most large hematomas will become secondarily infected even when the patient is treated with parenteral antibiotics. Effective drainage of most pelvic and broad ligament hematomas usually can be accomplished vaginally or radiographically. Small subcutaneous hematomas or fascial hematomas usually resolve. However, they are associated with an increased incidence of wound infection.

Any operation is accompanied by the potential risk of an unrecognized retained sponge or laparotomy pad. The exact incidence of this worrisome complication is difficult to establish but is estimated to be between 1 in 1200 and 1 in 1500 laparotomies. Most often the sponge counts at surgery have been correct. When this complication is discovered during the first postoperative week, the patient usually has a tender pelvic mass that is infected. When this mass is discovered after the immediate postoperative course, patients are often asymptomatic or exhibit minimal tenderness. The possibility of a retained foreign body should be considered in the differential diagnosis of pelvic hematomas and abscesses. A retrospective study of retained sponges, by Gawande and associates, noted that retained foreign bodies were more commonly associated with higher body mass index (BMI), emergency surgeries, and an intraoperative change in the type of procedure to be performed.

Thrombophlebitis and Pulmonary Embolus

Surgery is a time of hypercoagulability secondary to the stress response. As such, the surgeon must be aware of the potential complications of thromboembolism throughout the postoperative course. Prophylaxis against deep vein thrombosis (DVT) is discussed in Chapter 24 (Preoperative Counseling and Management). However, prophylaxis needs to be continued throughout the hospital stay and, in certain high-risk cases, even after discharge. For example, patients with both a malignancy, as well as a thrombophilia, or previous DVT and thrombophilia, and those who will have decreased ambulation may benefit from 1 to 3 weeks of low-molecular-weight heparin after leaving the hospital. Studies in patients with hip replacements and with abdominal pelvic malignancies have shown significant reductions (50% to 66%) in the incidence of DVT with prolonged anticoagulation. Currently there is insufficient evidence to make recommendations for prolonged thromboprophylaxis for gynecology patients except in high-risk situations. Without specific guidelines the length of time for thromboprophylaxis should be individualized. Prophylaxis will not prevent all DVTs, thus part of daily rounds includes assessments for this complication.

Superficial Thrombophlebitis

Superficial thrombophlebitis is one of the most frequently occurring postoperative complications and is most commonly associated with IV catheters. Superficial thrombophlebitis is a benign disease. However, it is associated with deep vein thrombophlebitis in approximately 5% of cases. Superficial thrombophlebitis is frequently overlooked or disregarded as a cause of postoperative fever. However, this diagnosis should be suspected whenever an IV line with antibiotics or hypertonic solutions has been used. Superficial tenderness and erythema outline the course of the veins. Women with established superficial varicosities in the lower extremities are especially susceptible because of localized stasis or pressure during the operative procedure and inactivity during the first 24 hours after operation. Patients with superficial thrombophlebitis of the legs also may have concomitant deep venous disease. Thus the finding of superficial thrombophlebitis does not eliminate the necessity to consider DVT as well. Recurrent, superficial phlebitis, in varying anatomic sites, may be a sign of occult malignant disease.

Detailed basic investigations have identified fibrin sheaths surrounding IV catheters in 60% to 100% of patients studied. The exact fate of the several inches of clot and fibrin sheath after the removal of the IV catheter is uncertain. Venography studies have found that these clots and fibrin sheaths do not break up on catheter removal but initially remain in situ. IV catheters are an important source of nosocomial infections. Approximately 30% of all hospital-acquired bacteremias are secondary to IV lines. The most serious complication of IV catheter use is infection of the thrombus, producing suppurative phlebitis or catheter sepsis. The initial infection may occur via the bloodstream or via bacteria from the skin reaching the thrombus along the catheter line. When frank pus is expressed, the treatment of suppurative phlebitis includes excising the infected vein.

The natural history of IV catheter-associated phlebitis was documented by Hershey and colleagues. The classic symptom of phlebitis is inflammation of the subcutaneous tissue along the course of a vein or over the area of merging varicosities. The patient develops a painful, tender, erythematous induration (nodule or core). In the majority of severe cases there is associated fever. In studying 202 episodes of superficial phlebitis, Hershey and colleagues discovered that the disease develops relatively rapidly, giving few symptoms or signs that allow removal of the catheter to prevent the disease (Fig. 25-5). After the process has begun, the inflammation does not consistently terminate with removal of the catheter. In their study, more than 40% of cases occurred 24 hours or more after withdrawal of the IV line. Nevertheless, the duration of phlebitis is prolonged if the catheter is not immediately removed when the diagnosis of superficial phlebitis is made. The authors recommended that all IV catheters be removed and replaced at 48-hour intervals regardless of whether signs or symptoms of superficial phlebitis are present. In addition, the use of an IV team decreased the incidence of catheter-associated phlebitis from 32% to 15% in their series. Strict aseptic techniques should be used during catheter insertion. Catheters inserted into the hand or forearm, through which antibiotics are infused, should be changed at least every 36 hours. Though not all studies have affirmed that recommendation, most authors have suggested all IV lines be changed every 48 to 72 hours. In one study, heparin flushes of IV catheters decreased the risks of phlebitis by 6RR (CI .4–8) over saline flushes in one study. Recent series have documented the association of inherited thrombophilias with superficial phlebitis, increasing the risk by 4- to 13-fold. The more potent the thrombophilia, the higher the risk.

In summary, venous catheters should be removed at the first sign of induration, erythema, or edema. Superficial phlebitis is the leading cause of an enigmatic postoperative fever during the third, fourth, or fifth postoperative day.

The clinical management of mild superficial thrombophlebitis includes rest, elevation, and local heat. Moderate to severe superficial thrombophlebitis may be treated with a nonsteroidal

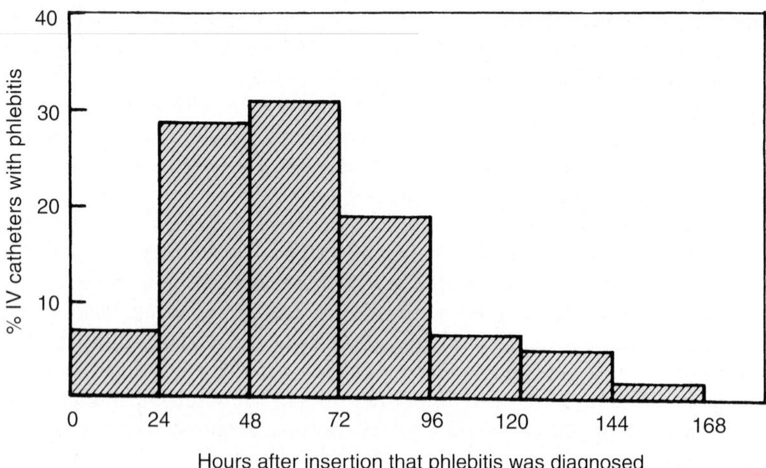

Figure 25-5. Hours after insertion that phlebitis was diagnosed. Time of diagnosis of phlebitis from time of IV catheter insertion. (From Hershey CO, Tomford JW, McLaren CE, et al: The natural history of intravenous catheter-associated phlebitis. Arch Intern Med 144:1374, 1984. © Copyright 1984, American Medical Association.)

antiinflammatory drug (NSAID) such as ibuprofen or low-dose heparin. The rare case of proximal progression of the inflammatory process should be treated with therapeutic doses of IV heparin and antibiotics.

Deep Vein Thrombophlebitis

Thromboembolic complications generally occur early in the postoperative course: 50% within the first 24 hours and 75% within 72 hours. Approximately 15% occur after the seventh postoperative day. Diagnosis of deep vein thrombophlebitis by physical examination is insensitive. Thus imaging studies are essential for establishing the correct diagnosis. Venous thrombosis and PE are the direct causes of approximately 40% of deaths in gynecologic cases. The incidence of fatal pulmonary emboli following gynecologic operations is approximately 0.2%. Because women often die within a few hours of the appearance of initial symptoms, emphasis must be placed on prevention rather than treatment of this complication. PE is not the only major consequence of deep venous thrombophlebitis. Many women develop chronic venous insufficiency or "postphlebitic syndrome" of the legs as a major sequela following thrombophlebitis. The resulting damage to valves of the deep veins produces shunting of blood to superficial veins, chronic edema, pain on exercise, and skin ulceration.

The reported incidence of DVT with gynecologic operations varies from 7% to 45%, with an average of approximately 15%. Walsh and coworkers found the incidence of DVT to be 7% after vaginal hysterectomy, 13% after abdominal hysterectomy for benign disease, 25% after Wertheim hysterectomy, and 45% after extensive gynecologic cancer operations. The incidence of thrombophlebitis is directly dependent on risk factors such as the type and duration of operation, the age of the woman, thrombophilias, history of deep vein thrombophlebitis, peripheral edema, amount of blood lost at operation, restrictions in preoperative ambulation, obesity, immobility, malignancy, sepsis, diabetes, current oral contraceptive or hormone use, and conditions that produce venous stasis, such as ascites and heart failure (Table 25-3). Older and obese women have an increased incidence of thrombophlebitis because of dilation of their deep venous system. There is a two- to fourfold increased risk for venous thrombophlebitis in women taking postmenopausal estrogen therapy. The length of the surgical procedure also has an important influence on the development of thrombophlebitis. If the operation is 1 to 2 hours in duration, approximately 15% of women develop the disease; if the surgery is longer than 3 hours, the risk is greater (Table 25-4).

The process of thrombosis most often begins in the deep veins of the calf. It is estimated that 75% of pulmonary emboli

Table 25-3 Conditions Associated with Increased Risk for Deep Vein Thrombosis

Condition
Advancing age
Obesity
Previous venous thromboembolism
Surgery
Trauma
Active cancer
Acute medical illness (e.g., acute myocardial infarction, heart failure, respiratory failure, infection)
Inflammatory bowel disease
Antiphospholipid syndrome
Dyslipoproteinaemia
Nephrotic syndrome
Paroxysmal nocturnal haemoglobinuria
Myeloproliferative diseases
Behçet's syndrome
Varicose veins
Superficial vein thrombosis
Congenital venous malformation
Long-distance travel
Prolonged bed rest
Immobilisation
Limb paresis
Chronic care facility stay
Pregnancy/puerperium
Oral contraceptives
Hormone replacement therapy
Heparin–induced thrombocytopenia
Other drugs
Chemotherapy
Tamoxifen
Thalidomide
Antipsychotics
Central venous catherer
Vena cava filter
Intravenous drug abuse

From Kyrle PA, Eichinger S: Deep vein thrombosis. Lancet 365:1164, 2005.

Table 25-4 Risk Categories of Thromboembolism in Gynecologic Operations

Risk Category	Low Risk	Medium Risk	High Risk
Age	40 years	40 years	50 years
Contributing factors			
Operation	Uncomplicated or minor	Major abdominal or pelvic	Major, extensive malignant disease
Weight		Moderately obese—75 to 90 kg or > 20% above ideal weight	Morbidly obese— >115 kg or >30% above ideal weight Previous venous thrombosis Varicose veins Cardiac disease Diabetes (insulin dependent)
Calf vein thrombosis	2%	10–35%	30–60%
Iliofemoral vein thrombosis	0.4%	2–8%	5–10%
Fatal pulmonary emboli	0.2%	0.1–0.5%	1%
Recommended prophylaxis	Early ambulation	Low-dose heparin or intermittent pneumatic compression	Low-dose heparin or intermittent pneumatic compression

From Mattingly RF, Thompson JD (eds): Te Linde's Operative Gynecology, 6th ed. Philadelphia, JB Lippincott, 1985, p 106.

originate from a thrombus that began in the leg veins. If one leg is involved, the other leg has thrombophlebitis in approximately 33% of women. Usually the thrombophlebitis remains localized and the clot lyses spontaneously, and the patient is free of symptoms. In approximately 1 in 20 cases the process extends centrally to the veins of the upper leg and pelvis. Involvement of the femoral vein often results in swelling caused by obstruction of this large vein. Pulmonary emboli from calf veins alone are rare, with only 4% to 10% of pulmonary emboli originating from this area. In contrast there is a 50% risk of a PE if thrombophlebitis of the femoral vein is not treated.

In 1854, Virchow described the three key predisposing or precipitating factors in the production of thrombi: an increase in coagulation factors, damage to the vessel wall, and venous stasis. Subsequent studies have documented that all three events occur with gynecologic operations. Blood flow in the iliac vein decreases by approximately 55% during an operation. During an operation there are several normal physiologic changes that produce hypercoagulability, including increases in the following: factors VIII, IX, and X, number of platelets, platelet aggregation and adherence, fibrinogen, and lastly, thromboplastin-like substance from tissue necrosis.

Kakkar described the cascade of events leading to the development of thrombophlebitis. The initial event in the cascade is stasis. Stasis leads to localized anoxia with subsequent generation of thrombi at the anoxic site. This produces changes in the lining of the vessel with exposure of the basement membrane and platelet adhesion and local coagulation. Thus the most important event in thrombophlebitis is the generation of thrombi in the presence of venous stasis. A thrombus may generate in an area of stasis, or it may generate wherever a vessel wall is damaged with resultant exposure of the subendothelial collagen, to which platelets will adhere.

The site of initial formation of the thrombus is most often near the base of a valve cusp in the calf of the leg (Fig. 25-6). The thrombus propagates and grows by repetitive layers of platelet aggregation and deposition of fibrin from fibrinogen. The most recently formed portion of the propagating thrombi are free floating (not attached to the vein) and are most likely to become pulmonary emboli. The body attempts to repair the area of thrombosis through an invasion of fibroblasts from the vein wall to encompass the base of the thrombus. Eventually the thrombus is attached to the vein wall, the area is reepithelialized, organization occurs, and symptoms resolve.

The signs and symptoms of deep vein thrombophlebitis depend directly on the severity and extent of the process. Many localized cases of deep vein thrombophlebitis in the calf are asymptomatic and are only recognized by a screening procedure such as duplex ultrasonography. However, even extensive areas of deep vein thrombophlebitis may be asymptomatic, and the first sign may be the development of a PE. In a woman

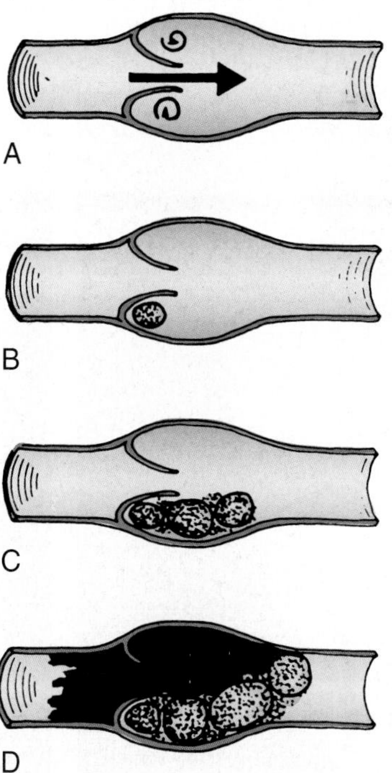

Figure 25-6. Stages in development of thrombus in valve pocket of deep veins of leg. **A,** Stasis in valve pocket results in thrombin generation. **B,** Platelet aggregation and fibrin formation. **C,** Propagation of platelet-fibrin nidus. **D,** Blockage of venous flow with resultant retrograde extension. (From Bloom AL, Thomas DP [eds]: Haemostases and Thrombosis. Edinburgh, Churchill Livingstone, 1981, p 684.)

who is asymptomatic, the pathophysiologic process may not totally obstruct the individual vein and drainage is obtained via associated competent collateral circulation.

Studies using ^{125}I-labeled fibrinogen to screen the legs have documented that approximately one out of two women who develop deep vein thrombophlebitis following gynecologic operation is totally free of symptoms. Among women who develop signs and symptoms, approximately 68% have induration of the calf muscles, 52% have minimum edema, 25% have calf tenderness, and 11% develop a difference of more than 1 cm in diameter of the leg. Homans' sign is present in 10%, and differential pain over the calf with a blood pressure cuff is present in approximately 40%. The clinical diagnosis of iliofemoral thrombosis is much easier, and the patient usually develops severe symptoms due to obstruction of venous return. Usually there is an acute onset of severe pain, swelling, and a sensation that the leg will "burst."

The clinician must have a high degree of suspicion to begin the diagnostic workup for deep vein thrombophlebitis. The clinical symptoms and signs of DVT are nonspecific. A clinical clue is the persistence of a low-grade fever with unexplained tachycardia. The tachycardia is often more rapid than one would expect with a low-grade fever. The finding of a definite difference in leg circumference is supportive evidence of DVT. However, physical examination of the legs produces false-positive findings in approximately 50% of cases. Thus, if the signs and symptoms are suggestive, or the woman is at high risk, the diagnosis should be confirmed by one of the imaging techniques currently available to detect deep vein thrombophlebitis. Interestingly, the more symptomatic the disease, the more adherent the thrombus. Relatively, patients with symptoms are less likely to develop pulmonary emboli.

In the last decade, ascending contrast venography (phlebography) was considered the gold standard (the most accurate method) for detecting deep vein thrombophlebitis (Fig. 25-7). However, duplex ultrasonography, the combination of Doppler and real-time B-mode ultrasound, and color Doppler are the preferred methods for diagnosing deep vein thrombophlebitis. The diagnostic accuracy of venography is estimated to be 95% for peripheral disease and 90% for iliofemoral thrombophlebitis. Contrast venography is superior to duplex ultrasonography for the diagnosis of DVT in asymptomatic women, but is more expensive, painful, and time-consuming.

Duplex ultrasonography has remarkably high sensitivity and specificity in symptomatic women. Real-time ultrasound imaging provides visualization of the larger veins, and sensitive Doppler ultrasound is focused simultaneously on the suspicious vessel. The technology depends on changes in venous flow for a positive diagnosis. A meta-analysis from White and colleagues documented that the sensitivity of duplex ultrasonography in detecting proximal thrombi is 95% (CI 92% to 98%) and the specificity is 99% (CI 98% to 100%).The advantages of this method are that it is noninvasive, easy to use, highly accurate, objective, simple, and reproducible. Color Doppler ultrasonography may improve the diagnostic accuracy in larger veins. The main disadvantage of duplex ultrasonography is its limited accuracy when investigating small vessels in the calf. The inability to compress the deep vein by moderate pressure with the ultrasound probe is the most widely used criterion for the positive diagnosis of DVT.

Lensing and coworkers, in a prospective study of 220 patients, used compressibility of the vein as the sole criterion for diagnosis of DVT. For all patients in their study, including both proximal vein and calf vein thrombosis, the sensitivity was

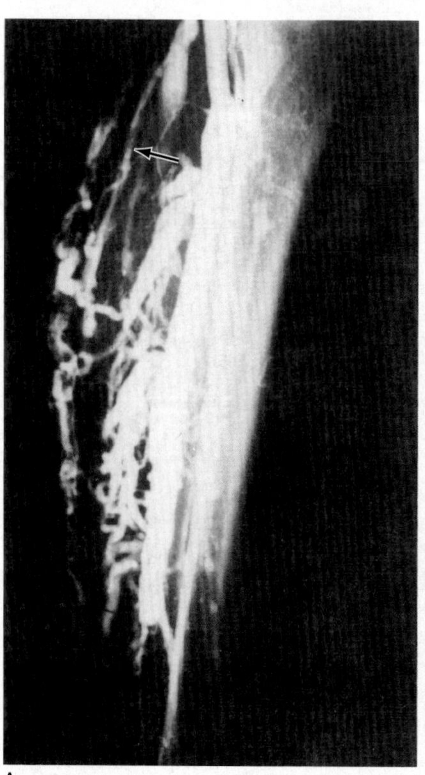

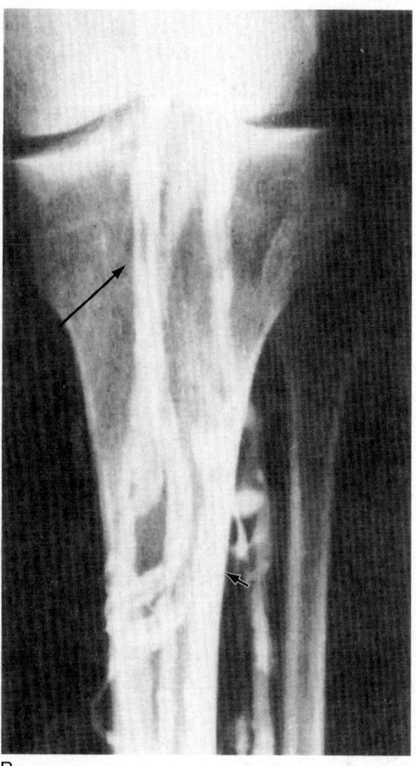

Figure 25-7. **A,** Phlebogram showing small thrombi in veins of calf (*arrow*), which are usually of no clinical significance. **B,** Thrombi in deep vein of calf (*arrow*) showing extension into popliteal vein. (From Bonnar J: Venous thromboembolism and gynecologic surgery. Clin Obstet Gynecol 28:439, 1985.)

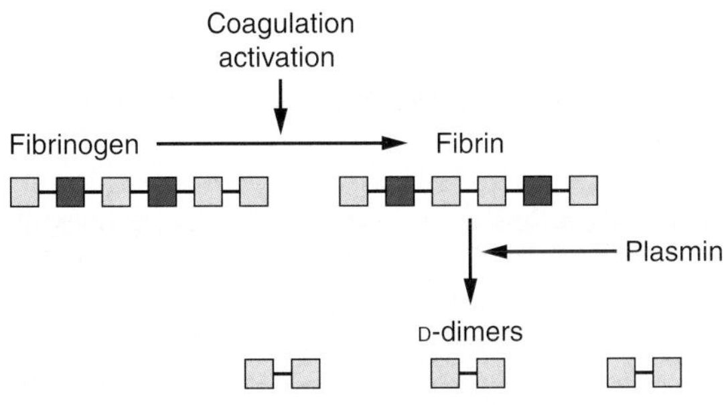

Figure 25-8. D-Dimer production.

91% and the specificity was 99%. Impedance plethysmography, another noninvasive screening method for detecting DVT utilizes a pneumatic cuff applied around the thigh. Changes in blood volume are measured by changes in electrical resistance (impedance). Impedance is reduced with venous thrombi. This method has at least a 15% false-negative rate and a 20% false-positive rate. As with duplex ultrasonography, the accuracy of this method for detecting thrombi of small vessels is limited.

Magnetic resonance angiography (MRA) is noninvasive and is comparable diagnostically to contrast venography and duplex Doppler ultrasonography. The cost of MRA is much greater than contrast or duplex scanning. However, there is the added benefit of soft tissue imaging, which may provide diagnostic information.

At the time of the initial bedside examination, the physician will develop a level of suspicion for DVT based on physical findings and clinical characteristics. If the likelihood is low, and the patient is not perioperative-plasma D-dimer levels may be obtained. D-Dimer is a protein from cross-linked fibrin after it has been degraded by plasmin in the fibrinolytic process (Fig. 25-8). D-Dimer may be elevated due to trauma, surgery, intravascular hemolysis, pregnancy, and other inflammatory states. Thus, in the perioperative setting it is much less helpful. Clinical studies using a relatively low cut-off value for D-dimer with an enzyme-linked immunosorbent assay (ELISA) result in a sensitivity of approximately 99%. When the clinical suspicion is high for a DVT, imaging studies such as ultrasound should be obtained.

The objectives of clinical management of deep vein thrombophlebitis associated with gynecologic operations are early detection and early therapy. In reality antithrombotic therapy is preventive medicine, since the therapeutic agent interrupts progression of the disease (thrombus formation) but does not actively resolve the disease process. Anticoagulation with heparin (unfractionated or low-molecular-weight [LMW]) is the drug of choice for the initial first-line treatment of DVT once the diagnosis is confirmed (Table 25-5). LMW heparin is as effective and is safer than unfractionated heparin. For continuous infusion the initial loading dose is 5000 to 10,000 IU given intravenously, followed by continuous infusion of 1000 to 1500 IU/hour. The dosage of unfractionated IV heparin should be adjusted to prolong an activated partial thromboplastin time (aPTT) to 2.5 times control values. Continuous heparin infusion is preferred over periodic bolus injections because there are fewer hemorrhagic complications (6% vs. 14%). The half-life of heparin on the average is 1 to 2 hours after IV injection. Failure to achieve adequate anticoagulation in the first 24 hours of therapy increases the risk of recurrent venous thromboembolism 15-fold. Heparin should be continued for 5 to 7 days. Oral warfarin (Coumadin), 15 mg daily, should be begun within the first 48 hours of heparin therapy. Following 2 to 3 days of 10 to 15 mg of Coumadin daily, the international normalized ratio (INR) will usually be 1.5 to 2. This therapeutic level the INR of 2 should be maintained by appropriate adjustment of the Coumadin dosage. The biologic half-life of Coumadin is 2 to 3 days. Anticoagulation with Coumadin should be continued for 6 to 9 months for adequate secondary prophylaxis. A meta-analysis from Ost and colleagues evaluated the duration

Table 25-5 Options for the Initial Treatment of Deep-Vein Thrombosis with Anticoagulant Agents

			REPORTED RISKS	
Drug	**Method of Administration**	**Dose***	**Risk of Heparin-Induced Thrombocytopenia†**	**Risk of Major Bleeding**
			no./total no. (%)	
Unfractionated heparin	Intravenous	Loading dose, 5000 U or 80 U/kg of body weight with infusion adjusted to maintain activated partial-thromboplastin time within the therapeutic range†	9/332 (2.7)	35/1853 (1.9)
Low-molecular-weight heparin			0/333 (0)	20/1821 (1.1)
Dalteparin	Subcutaneous	100 U/kg every 12 hr or 200 U/kg daily; maximum, 18,000 U/day		
Enoxaparin	Subcutaneous	1 mg/kg every 12 hr or 1.5 mg/kg daily; maximum, 180 mg/day		
Tinzaparin	Subcutaneous	175 U/kg daily; maximum, 18,000 U/day		
Nadroparin	Subcutaneous	86 U/kg every 12 hr or 171 U/kg daily; maximum, 17,100 U/day		

*Doses vary in patients who are obese or who have renal dysfunction. Monitoring of antifactor Xa levels has been suggested for these patients, with dose adjustment to a target range of 0.6–1.0 U/mL 4 hrs after injection for twice-daily administration or 1.0–2.0 U/mL for once-daily administration. Even though there are few supporting data, most manufactures recommend capping the dose for obese patients at that for a 90-kg patient.

†The therapeutic range of activated partial thromboplastin time corresponds to heparin levels of 0.3–0.7 U/mL, as determined by antifactor Xa assay. High levels of heparin-binding proteins and factor VIII may result in so-called heparin resistance. In patients requiring more than 40,000 U per day to attain a therapeutic activated partial-thromboplastin time, the dosage can be adjusted on the basis of plasma heparin levels.[31]

From Bates SM, Ginsberg JS: Treatment of deep-vein thrombosis. N Engl J Med 351:271, 2004.

Table 25-6 Recommendations for the Duration of Anticoagulant Therapy for Patients with Deep-Vein Thrombosis

Characteristics of Patient*	Risk of Recurrence in the Year after Discontinuation (%)	Duration of Therapy
Major transient risk factor	3	3 mo
Minor risk factor, no thrombophilia	< 10 if risk factor avoided	6 mo
	> 10 if risk factor persistent	Until factor resolves
Idiopathic event; no thrombophilia or low-risk thrombophilia	< 10	6 mo†
Idiopathic event; high-risk thrombophilia	> 10	Indefinite
More than one idiopathic event	> 10	Indefinite
Cancer; other ongoing risk factor	> 10	Indefinite

*Examples of major transient risk factors are major surgery, a major medical illness, and leg casting. Examples of minor transient risk factors are the use of an oral contraceptive and hormone-replacement therapy. Examples of low-risk thrombophilias are heterozygosity for the factor V Leiden and G20210A prothrombin-gene mutations. Examples of high-risk thrombophilia are antithrombin, protein C, and protein S deficiencies; homozygosity for the factor V Leiden or prothrombin gene mutation or heterozygosity for both; and the presence of antiphospholipid antibodies.

†Therapy may be prolonged if the patient prefers to prolong it or if the risk of bleeding is low.

From Bates SM, Ginsberg JS: Treatment of deep-vein thrombosis. N Engl J Med 351:273, 2004.

of anticoagulation following venous thromboembolism. Studies of 3 months of therapy were compared with studies of 6 months or longer. The risks of bleeding (the major complication) were similar between short- and long-term therapy. However, the relative risk of recurrent thromboembolism was 0.21 (CI, 0.14 to 0.31) comparing long-term heparin versus short-term heparin use. Some patients with large DVT, antiphospholipid antibody syndrome, or malignancies may require extended therapy beyond 6 to 9 months due to increased risks of recurrence (Table 25-6).

The primary risk of chronic anticoagulation therapy is the potential for major bleeding complications. Major bleeding occurs in approximately 4% of woman-years of therapy. Thus it is important to carefully follow these women with serial coagulation studies. Approximately 1% of patients on full-dose heparin develop thrombocytopenia (platelet counts less than 100,000). If thrombocytopenia develops, heparin should be discontinued because of the potential risk of paradoxic thrombosis.

LMW heparin, though more expensive than unfractionated heparin, has several advantages, and has effectively replaced unfractionated heparin as the gold standard for treatment of DVT. LMW heparin may be given subcutaneously once or twice daily. It does not require monitoring in women with normal and stable renal function. It induces significantly less heparin-induced thrombocytopenia, and it has a lower risk of inducing bleeding. Because blood levels are more reproducible, there is actually a lower incidence of complications noted in some studies in terms of progression from DVT to pulmonary emboli. Additionally, studies comparing LMW heparin versus unfractionated heparin have shown a greater effect with thrombus regression within the veins themselves.

Testing of levels of LMW heparin is based not on the aPTT, but on the antifactor Xa activity level. Levels are calculated specifically for each LMW heparin. An aPTT of 1.5 times normal corresponds approximately to an antifactor Xa activity level of 0.2. Therapeutic levels are found between 0.4 and 0.8. Bleeding usually occurs when levels of the antifactor Xa activity level rise greater than 1.0 to 1.2. If needed in patients with unstable renal status, levels may be checked approximately 4 hours after dosing.

Rarely patients will not be candidates for anticoagulation. In these patients inferior vena caval filters may be used to protect against pulmonary emboli. Temporary vena caval filters may be placed with fluoroscopic guidance. In some patients with large DVT and other risk factors such as compound thrombophilias and malignancy, consideration may be given to both anticoagulation and filter placement.

Many clinicians will obtain laboratory studies to identify thrombophilic states when a DVT occurs. These tests should be obtained with any idiopathic DVT. However, there is less support for the cost/benefit ratio in obtaining this information for a surgically related DVT. If management decisions including the duration of therapy or the use of estrogens in the future might be changed, then thrombophilia studies should be obtained. Additionally, in a patient with a family history of thrombosis it would be reasonable to obtain these studies.

The recent development and improvement of thrombolytic agents, such as plasminogen activators (streptokinase, urokinase, and recombinant tissue plasminogen activator), has offered an alternative medical therapy to heparin. The efficacy of these drugs in treating acute venous thrombosis has been established. For acute thrombi, IV therapy is prescribed for 72 hours. It is important to underline that gynecologic surgery within the preceding 10 days is a relative contraindication to the use of these agents.

Pulmonary Embolus

The accurate diagnosis of PE is essential for the prevention of morbidity from lack of treatment or from unnecessary anticoagulation therapy. Autopsy studies have documented that pulmonary emboli are undiagnosed clinically in approximately 50% of women who experience this complication. Approximately 10% of women with a PE die within the first hour. The mortality of women with correctly diagnosed and treated pulmonary emboli is 8%, in contrast to approximately 30% if the disease is not treated. Most pulmonary emboli in gynecologic patients originate from thrombi in the pelvic and femoral veins. Predisposing risk factors are found in the majority of women with PE. Anticoagulation therapy is also dangerous, as heparin is one of the leading causes of drug-related deaths in hospitalized patients.

No combination of symptoms or signs is pathognomonic for PE, and many patients are asymptomatic. The signs and symptoms of PE are nonspecific, and similar symptoms are caused by many other forms of cardiorespiratory disease. Common conditions considered in the differential diagnosis of pulmonary embolism include pneumonia, cardiac failure, atelectasis,

Table 25-7 Symptoms and Signs of Pulmonary Embolus

	Patients with Finding (%)
Symptoms	
Predisposing factors*	94
Dyspnea	84
Pleuritic chest pain	74
Apprehension	59
Cough	53
Hemoptysis	30
Syncope	14
Signs	
Tachypnea	92
Rales	58
Accentuation of pulmonic valve closure	53
Tachycardia	44
Cyanosis	20

*Prolonged immobilization, postoperative state, congestive heart failure, carcinomatosis, and so on.
From Blinder RA, Coleman RE: Evaluation of pulmonary embolism. Radiol Clin North Am 23:392, 1985. Data from the Urokinase Pulmonary Embolism Trial—a national cooperative study. Circulation 47 (suppl II):1, 1973.

aspiration, acute respiratory distress syndrome, and sepsis. Although the differential diagnosis is broad in scope, the symptoms should alert the physician to the possibility of a PE, thus allowing a proper diagnostic workup to establish or rule out the disease. A national study of 327 patients with an angiographically proven PE found that chest pain, dyspnea, and apprehension are the most common symptoms. The dyspnea is often of abrupt onset. The classical triad of shortness of breath, chest pain, and hemoptysis is seen in less than 20% of women with proven PE. Tachycardia, tachypnea, rales, and an increase in the second heart sound over the pulmonic area are the most frequently found signs of pulmonary emboli (Table 25-7). Approximately 15% of women with pulmonary emboli have an unexplained low-grade fever associated with a PE. A high fever is rarely associated with a PE but definitely may occur. The clinical manifestations of PE are produced primarily by occlusion of the large branches of the pulmonary arteries by embolic material. Pathophysiologically, associated reflex bronchial constriction and vasoconstriction intensify the symptomatology. More than 50% of clinically recognized pulmonary emboli are multiple. The most frequent location of pulmonary emboli is in the lower lobes of the right lung. Shock and syncope are associated with massive pulmonary emboli.

Although imaging techniques are the gold standard for establishing the diagnosis of pulmonary emboli, several studies have found that clinical assessment is nearly as accurate. Chunilal and associates have referred to the "clinical gestalt," and have noted similar accuracy of diagnosis to imaging. Clinical assessment of signs and symptoms by an experienced clinician may approximate a low, medium, and high probability of PE.

Routine laboratory data, such as electrocardiograms (ECGs), chest radiographs, and blood gas analyses, and assessment of troponin, are important because they may contribute to the overall clinical impression, but individually or collectively they are not diagnostic. Less than 15% of ECGs demonstrate significant changes of right ventricular strain with T wave inversion in V_1 to V_4, with a PE. Diminished pulmonary vascular markings may be a suggestive finding on a chest film, but are fairly nonspecific. In the final analysis, imaging studies are of central importance in confirming the diagnosis of PE. However, the chest radiograph may be helpful in the differential diagnosis by demonstrating other pulmonary complications. The most common findings on chest film examination with a PE are infiltrate, pleural effusion, atelectasis, and enlargement of the heart or descending pulmonary artery, although these findings are nonspecific. The majority of women with pulmonary emboli demonstrate hypoxemia on blood gas determinations, but as with other routine tests, these findings do not occur invariably. The rapid measurement of plasma D-dimer levels may sometimes be useful in screening women with a suspected PE. There is no need to perform pulmonary angiography when the concentration of D-dimer is below the cut-off levels (< 500 ng/mL) *and* the clinical suspicion is low. The negative predictive value is 99% in women with a combination of a low pretest probability of PE and a normal D-dimer. The clinician should appreciate that the units of value for the D-dimer test have widely divergent sensitivities, specificities, and negative predictive values because many different D-dimer tests are used. A negative D-dimer test in women with cancer does not reliably exclude venous thrombosis or PE because the negative predictive value of the test is lower in women with cancer. In the postoperative setting D-dimer is of much less value because it is usually elevated after surgery.

Helical CT has replaced $\dot{V}/Q$ scans as the first step in imaging techniques to establish or exclude the diagnosis of PE (Fig. 25-9). Helical CT, sometimes called spiral CT, uses imaging of the pulmonary vessels. Imaging of the pulmonary vessels is facilitated by the use of IV contrast media. The procedure is minimally invasive and provides a volumetric image of the lung by rotating the detector at a constant rate around the woman. A cost-effective analysis from Doyle and coworkers found that helical CT was the most cost-effective first-line test to diagnose pulmonary embolus. Several algorithms have been published for evaluation of suspected PE, each medical center will establish such an algorithm based on the expertise and imaging equipment available at the institution (Fig. 25-10).

When helical CT, CT angiography, is unavailable, the second choice is the $\dot{V}/Q$, scan. This test is safe and relatively easy to perform. The scan involves the injection of small radiocolloid particles into the circulation. They are trapped in small vessels, and their distribution depends on regional pulmonary blood flow. Ventilation scintigraphy uses radionuclides of technetium aerosol or xenon gas. The combination of lack of symmetry and a mismatch in the ventilation scan is the abnormality that leads to the diagnosis. However, the clinician should not rely too much on the ability of the $\dot{V}/Q$ scan as a single test to diagnose a PE. In patients with a suspected PE, 40% will have a normal scan. A normal result effectively rules out the diagnosis of PE. The multicenter Prospective Investigation of Pulmonary Embolism Diagnosis (PIOPED) found that 4% of patients with normal or near-normal perfusion lung scans subsequently were discovered to have pulmonary emboli. This study emphasized a high sensitivity of 98% but a low specificity of 10% for $\dot{V}/Q$ scans in the diagnosis of PE. The authors pointed out that almost all patients with acute PE had abnormal scans, but so did most patients without emboli.

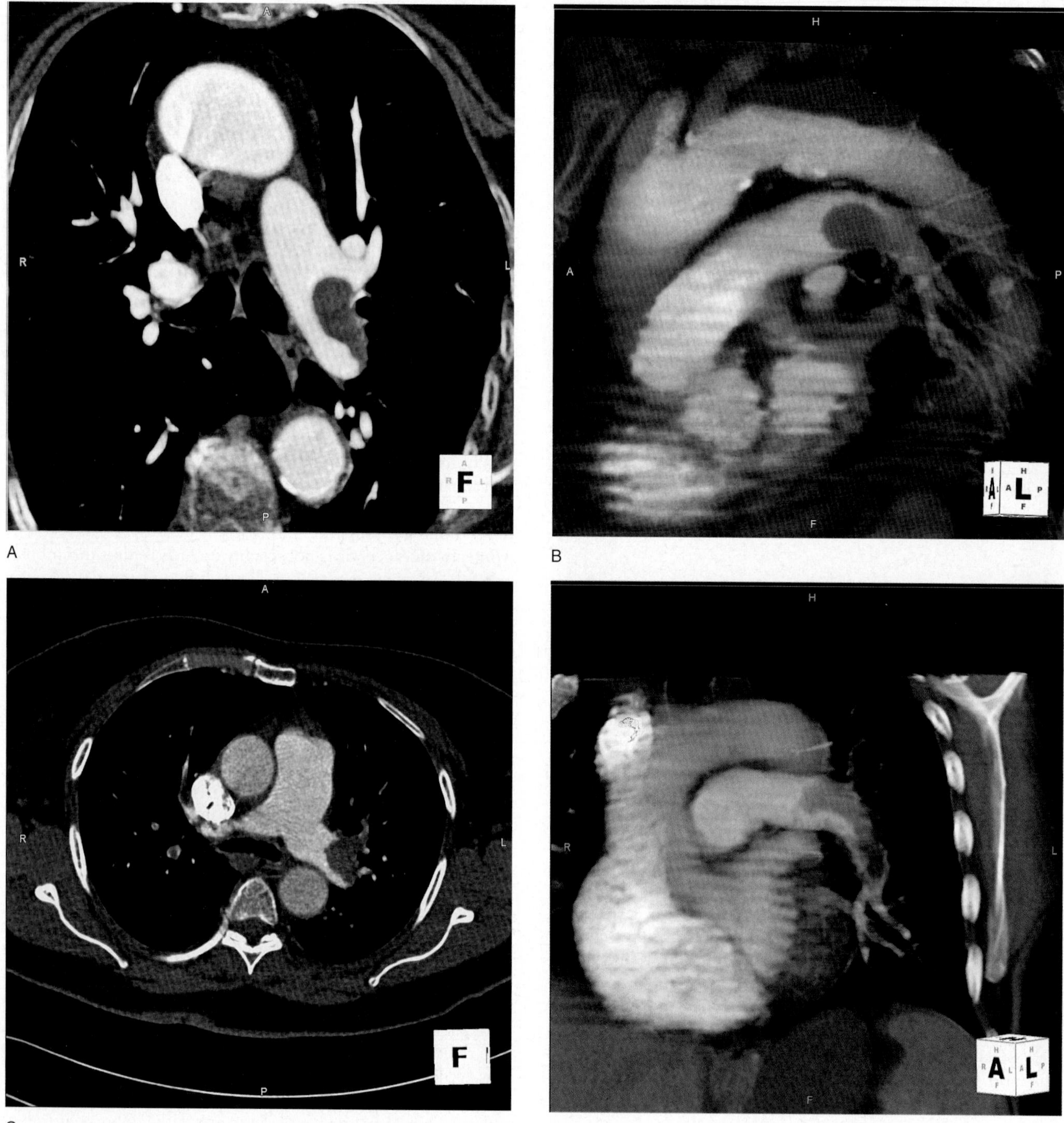

Figure 25-9. Helical CT of pulmonary embolus. The letters on the cube help orient the viewer as the 3-D image is rotated: A, anterior; F, foot; H, head; L, left. (Courtesy of Charles McGlade, MD, Sacred Heart Medical Center, Eugene, OR.)

$\dot{V}/Q$ scans have a high sensitivity but a variable specificity for the diagnosis of PE. For example, other cardiorespiratory diseases such as asthma may result in regional areas of decreased perfusion. If the scan documents multiple segments or lobar perfusion defects with a ventilation mismatch, the probability of pulmonary emboli is greater than 85%. $\dot{V}/Q$ scans with less extensive perfusion abnormalities or matching ventilation defects do not reliably exclude the diagnosis of PE.

Pulmonary angiography is the gold standard (the most definitive test presently available) for detecting pulmonary emboli. This test is not ordered routinely because of the potential morbidity (hypotension and cardiac dysrhythmias) and risk of death associated with its use. Most deaths are directly related to pulmonary hypertension and right ventricular dysfunction. Approximately 5% of patients experience complications from this test, and the mortality is approximately 2 per 1000. The

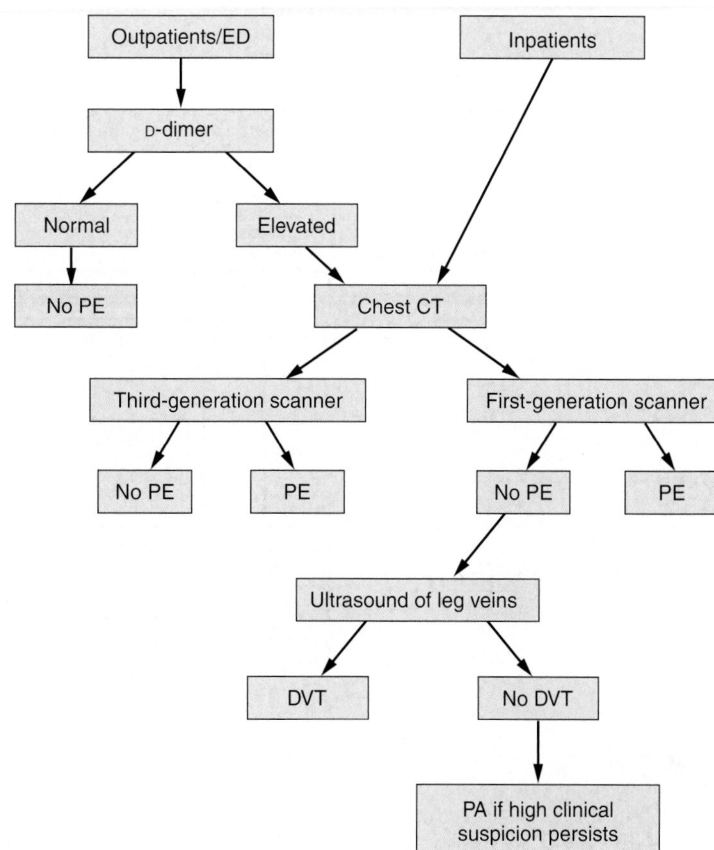

Figure 25-10. Algorithm for diagnostic evaluation of pulmonary embolus. CT, computed tomography; DVT, deep vein thrombosis; ED, emergency department; PA, pulmonary angiogram; PE, pulmonary embolus. (From Goldhaber SZ, Elliott G: Acute pulmonary embolism: Part I: Epidemiology, pathophysiology, and diagnosis. Circulation 108:2728, 2003.)

significance of this imaging technique is unquestioned if one accepts intraluminal filling defects for the definitive diagnosis of PE. A series of 960 patients yielded only two false-positive tests.

The management of the vast majority of pulmonary emboli is with anticoagulation either with IV unfractionated heparin or full-dose LMW heparin, similar to the management of deep vein thrombophlebitis (Fig. 25-11). Prompt and early therapy with heparin provides anticoagulation as well as inhibiting the release of serotonin from platelets. Potentially, this results in a decrease in the associated bronchoconstriction. Some women are candidates for thrombolytic therapy (streptokinase–urokinase). The time window for effective use of thrombolysis has been expanded with initiation of therapy as late as 14 days following the initial symptoms or signs of a PE. Thrombolytic therapy works by transforming plasminogen to plasmin. Use of thrombolytic therapy during the early postoperative period is a subject of great debate because of the increased risk of serious hemorrhage. Goldhaber and associates completed a randomized controlled study comparing urokinase and the new recombinant human tissue-type plasminogen activator. The latter was found to act more rapidly and to be safer than urokinase. Thrombolytic therapy is the method of choice in patients with massive pulmonary emboli (angiographically, greater than 50% obstruction of the pulmonary arterial bed) with associated moderate to severe hemodynamic embarrassment, lobular obstruction, or multiple segmental profusion defects. Random trials of heparin versus thrombolytic therapy have shown that emboli clear more rapidly with initial thrombolytic therapy. The MAPPET-3 trial (Management strategies and prognosis of Pulmonary Embolus-3) found that, in severely affected patients (but not ones in shock), thrombolytic therapy was superior to heparin. However, for all patients, particularly those with small emboli, the increased risks of intracranial bleeding may outweigh the benefits. Recent trials have evaluated thrombolytic therapy with heparin and found the combination superior to heparin alone. A thrombolytic agent is infused intravenously for the first 12 to 24 hours, and heparin therapy is continued for 7 to 10 days. The clinical assumption is that approximately 7 days are needed for the intravascular venous thrombus to become firmly attached to the vein's side wall.

All patients with pulmonary emboli should have warfarin therapy after heparin treatment for 3 to 9 months. The risk of a woman developing a subsequent fatal PE during the 3 months of anticoagulation therapy is approximately 1 in 70 to 1 in 100. Trials from Canada and from Sweden have found better long-term survival with extended anticoagulation, 18 months to 2 years. Some authors feel that if there are additional risk factors such as very potent thrombophilias then indefinite anticoagulation is indicated.

An adjunct for treatment is vena caval filters. The most widely accepted indication for vena cava filters is failure of medical management or a contraindication to heparin therapy. Approximately 35% of vena cava filters are placed for prophylactic indications. A randomized trial reported by Decousos and colleagues compared vena cava filters with LMW or un-

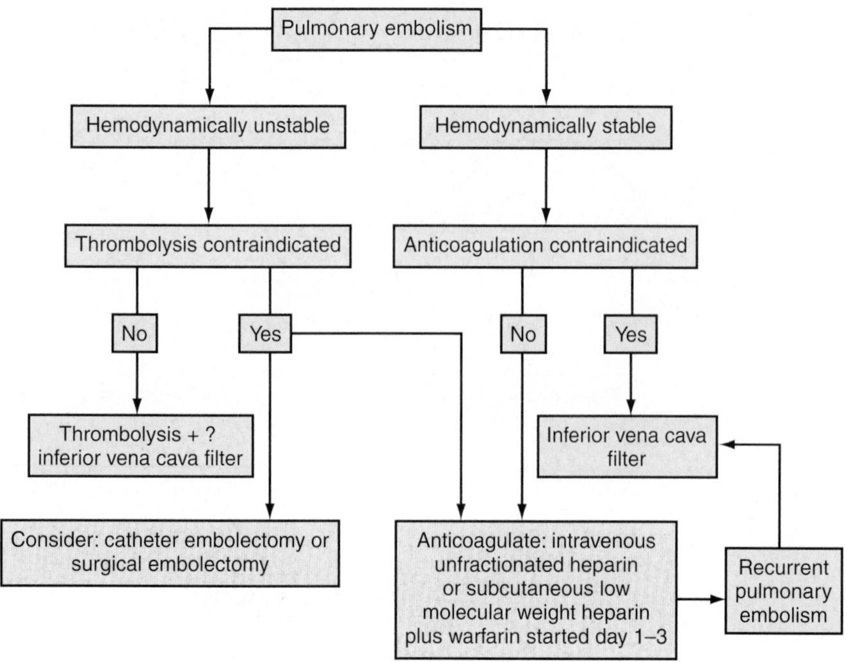

Figure 25-11. Treatment of pulmonary embolism. (From Tai MRM, Atwal AS, Hamilton G: Modern management of pulmonary embolism. Br J Surg 86:853, 1999.)

fractionated heparin. They concluded the initial beneficial effect of vena cava filters for the prevention of PE was counterbalanced by an excess of recurrent DVT without any difference in mortality rates. Treatment of a massive PE in an unstable patient involves a choice of thrombolytic therapy, pulmonary artery embolectomy, transvenous catheter embolectomy, or filter placement in the inferior vena cava.

URINARY TRACT PROBLEMS

Inability to Void

Many women experience an inability to void or an incomplete emptying of the bladder during the postoperative period. The etiology is complex, but the inability to void is more frequent and lasts longer after an operation that involves the urethra or bladder neck. The major pathophysiologic change is the direct trauma and edema produced by the surgical procedure to the perivesical tissues. Other factors that contribute include the potential of overdistention from excessive hydration and dysynchronous contractions from the bladder neck. The differential diagnosis includes anxiety, mechanical interference, obstruction by swelling and edema, neurologic imbalance, and drug-associated detrusor hypotonia.

The woman's initial attempts at voiding should be made in a sitting position. Obviously, privacy is important to minimize performance anxiety. It is best not to remove the Foley catheter until the patient is ambulatory. Most women have difficulty in completely emptying their bladder either on a bedpan or in a semirecumbent position during the first 24 hours after abdominal hysterectomy. Catheter drainage keeps the bladder at rest and avoids acute bladder distention with resulting detrusor dysfunction and possibly retrograde reflux of urine. The age-old tradition of intermittent clamping and releasing of the Foley catheter to regain bladder tone is often counterproductive. We do not believe in this technique. It is not based on sound physiologic principles, and possible overdistention would compound voiding difficulties. There is no evidence to support the outdated practice of gradual emptying of the distended urinary bladder. The optimal management of urinary retention is quick, complete emptying.

Most problems with voiding resolve without medication and with time. If mechanical obstruction is not suspected to be a major factor, intermittent straight catheterization is indicated. This will result in a lower incidence of UTI and a more rapid return to normal function than periodic replacement and removal of a Foley catheter for the evaluation of residual urine volume. Although bacteriuria occurs secondary to intermittent catheterization, development of pyelonephritis is rare unless the patient has concomitant vesicoureteral reflux. Bacteriuria may occur with ever greater incidence with indwelling catheters. Most women prefer self-catheterization. They especially appreciate intermittent self-catheterization because it gives them control over a part of their postoperative care. Routine culture of the urine with removal of a catheter in an asymptomatic patient is not necessary.

Rarely, medications may be given to patients who experience prolonged periods of inability to void. Reflex urethral spasm is common after plastic surgery to repair an enterocele or rectocele. Urethral spasm may be diminished by an α-adrenergic receptor blocking agent, phenoxybenzamine (Dibenzyline), in a dosage of 10 mg every 8 hours. However, hypotension is commonly associated with this drug. Bladder hypotonia may occur as a result of overdistention, prolonged inactivity, or use of medications such as β-blockers. Bladder hypotonia may be treated with bethanechol (Urecholine) in a dosage of 25 to 50 mg every 8 hours. Urecholine effectively produces detrusor contractions. This medication is prescribed rarely in the postoperative setting.

Infection

The most commonly acquired infection in the hospital and the most frequent cause of gram-negative bacteremia in hospitalized patients is catheter-associated UTI. Approximately 40% of nosocomial infections are UTIs, and 60% of these are directly related to an indwelling urethral catheter. One percent of patients with infections from bladder catheters will develop bacteremia. However, patients without catheters may develop overdistention and bladder atony as a result of postoperative pain. Overdistention produces a temporary paralysis of the detrusor activity that may take several days to resolve. The atonic bladder is also prone to UTI. Thus, after a gynecologic operation, the patient is susceptible to UTI either with or without a catheter in place.

The normal uroepithelium inhibits adherence of surface bacteria to the walls of the urethra and bladder. A bladder catheter disrupts this property, and surface bacteria are able to colonize the lower urinary tract. Additionally, bacteria form a sheet or biofilm of microorganisms and bacterial bioproducts that adheres to the catheter. These biofilms protect bacteria from antibiotics. This characteristic of biofilms explains why antibiotic suppression is ineffective for patients with chronic catheterization, and why replacement of a catheter is necessary in the treatment of systemic infection secondary to a colonized urinary tract. The incidence of a positive culture increases dramatically with time. After a Foley catheter has been in place for 36 hours, approximately 20% of women have bacterial colonization, and after 72 hours, more than 75% have positive cultures. If the catheter drains into an open system for longer than 96 hours, 100% develop bacteriuria. Women with an indwelling catheter in place with a closed drainage system develop UTIs at the rate of approximately 5% per 24 hours; this increases to 50% of women after 7 days of continuous catheterization.

Catheter-related UTIs are related to the patient's age. In one study, 30% of women older than 50 developed an infection, compared with 16% of those postoperative women younger than age 50. Diabetes increased the incidence of catheter-related UTIs threefold. The incidence of infection is directly related to the length of time the catheter is in place. The incidence of a positive urine culture after a single in-and-out catheterization is approximately 1%.

Sterile technique used during insertion, strict aseptic catheter care, and maintenance of a closed drainage system are all important steps for reducing the incidence of infection through reduced colonization. Bacteria ascend from the exterior to the bladder either via the lumen of the catheter or around the outside of the catheter. A meta-analysis by Saint and colleagues noted that silver alloy-coated urinary catheters are significantly more effective in preventing UTIs than are silver oxide catheters. The silver alloy-coated catheters are more expensive than standard Foley catheters. However, they reduce nosocomial UTI by approximately 50%. A sterile, closed drainage system is another prophylactic measure to reduce the incidence of UTIs. In one study, strict closed drainage reduced the rate of infection from 80% to 23%. Studies have documented a lower risk of infection with a suprapubic, transabdominal urinary catheter. The latter technique also decreases patient discomfort and permits earlier spontaneous voiding. Systemic prophylactic antibiotics exert a short-term effect, decreasing the initial incidence of infection. However, the negative effect of prophylactic antibiotics is an increased emergence of antibiotic-resistant bacteria. Therefore prophylactic antibiotics are not used to "cover a catheter" except in immunocompromised patients. With catheterization for longer than 3 weeks, all patients have bacterial colonization regardless of the use of prophylactic antibiotics and a closed system.

The symptoms of UTI usually develop 24 to 48 hours after the Foley catheter is removed. Of interest, the signs and symptoms associated with a catheter-acquired lower UTI are not nearly as pronounced or as specific as those associated with cystitis unrelated to catheter use. Patients with lower UTIs usually do not have fever but experience urinary frequency and mild dysuria, which are difficult to distinguish from normal postoperative discomfort. As mentioned previously, elderly women may manifest mental status changes as the first sign of problems. Women with upper UTIs usually have a high fever, chills, and flank pain. If urinary tract symptoms persist after appropriate antibiotic therapy, one should obtain imaging studies to evaluate the possibility of obstruction in the urinary tract. Obstruction of the ureter without associated infection may be asymptomatic or produce only mild flank tenderness. No appreciable change will be noted in urinary output with an isolated unilateral ureteral obstruction.

The diagnosis of UTI is established by urinalysis and urine culture. It is important to identify white blood cells and bacteria with the microscope. However, women with high-volume urine outputs may demonstrate minimal findings on urinalysis but have a positive urine culture. Stark and Maki emphasized that a bacterial concentration of 10^2 organisms per milliliter in a catheterized specimen is significant. In their studies more than 95% of patients with 10^2 colony-forming units per milliliter (cfu/mL) subsequently developed the standard criterion of infection, which is 100,000 cfu/mL for a midstream culture.

We recommend a minimum of 3 days of antibiotic therapy for a woman who has developed cystitis after catheter use. One-day, single-dose antibiotic treatment is not an effective treatment for UTI.

To reduce the incidence of UTI, the Foley catheter should be used judiciously. When possible, use of a suprapubic catheter or intermittent in-and-out catheterization is preferable to continuous drainage with a Foley catheter. If a Foley catheter is used, retrograde flow of urine from the bag to the bladder during ambulation should be avoided. Preventive measures, such as aseptic care of the catheter and a closed, sterile drainage system, are also important. Modern practice is not to treat catheter-associated urinary tract colonization unless the patient becomes febrile (develops infection). If signs and symptoms of infection occur with a Foley in place, the woman should be treated with systemic antibiotic therapy for 10 days. Prophylactic antibiotics are not used unless the patient is immunosuppressed, for they often result in a UTI with a *Proteus* or *Pseudomonas* species rather than the more common *Escherichia coli.*

Urinary Fistula

Vesicovaginal and ureterovaginal fistulas are infrequent yet significant complications of operations for benign gynecologic conditions. In the United States, gynecologic operations are found to be the cause of approximately 75% of urinary tract fistulas. Surprisingly, it is not the difficult cancer operation but rather the simple total abdominal hysterectomy for benign disease, such as myomas or abnormal bleeding, that is the most frequently associated with this complication. Fistulas following gynecologic operations are secondary to abdominal hysterectomy in 75% of cases and to vaginal operations in the remaining 25%. The exact incidence of injury to the ureter associated with gynecologic operations is unknown because many patients do not exhibit symptoms. However, it has been estimated that ureteral injury occurs as frequently as 1 per 200 abdominal hysterectomies. The ratio of injuries to the urinary bladder to ureteral injuries is approximately 5:1.

The classic clinical symptom of a urinary tract fistula is the painless and almost continuous loss of urine, usually from the vagina. On occasion the uncontrolled loss of urine may be related to change in position or posture. When urine loss is intermittent and related to position, one should suspect a ureterovaginal rather than a vesicovaginal fistula. Urinary incontinence may be present within a few hours of the operative procedure. This symptom is secondary to a direct surgical injury to the bladder or ureter that was not appreciated during the operative procedure. The majority of fistulas become symptomatic 8 to 12 days and occasionally as late as 25 to 30 days after the operation. Occlusion of the blood supply from clamping or figure-of-8 sutures produces avascular necrosis and subsequent sloughing of the urogenital tissue. Pelvic examination often reveals a small reddened area of granulation tissue at the site of the fistula. In a review of unilateral ureteral obstruction secondary to gynecologic surgery, Stanhope and coworkers noted a mean increase of only 0.8 mg/dL in serum creatinine. The differential diagnosis of an ureterovaginal fistula includes spontaneous loss of peritoneal fluid or serosanguineous fluid from the retroperitoneal space.

A small fistula may be localized by placing a tampon in the vagina and instilling a dilute solution of methylene blue dye into the urinary bladder. This will also help differentiate between a vesicovaginal fistula and a ureterovaginal fistula. If the blue coloring is discovered on the tampon, then a defect in the bladder should be suspected. If the tampon is not colored, 3 to 5 mL of indigo carmine should be injected intravenously. The subsequent finding of blue coloring on the tampon is presumptive evidence of an ureterovaginal fistula. An IV pyelogram or enhanced CT scan should be obtained in either case to detect obstruction of the ureter and diagnose compound (ureter and bladder) fistulas.

As with most other postoperative complications, preventive medicine is paramount. Optimum operative technique should emphasize the standard axioms in the prevention of urinary tract injury. The patient should have an empty bladder, and the physician should obtain adequate exposure of the site. Sharp dissection should be made along tissue planes with proper traction and countertraction. When operating near the bladder or ureter, bleeding vessels should be ligated individually rather than with random clamping of tissue. If possible, the ureter should not be completely detached from the overlying peritoneum. With extensive dissection of the periureteral tissue, care should be taken to avoid interference with the longitudinal vascular supply of the ureter. In the most difficult cases where anatomic landmarks are obscure, opening of the dome of the bladder and palpation with the index finger and thumb may help to identify the proper surgical plane. The urinary system, especially the bladder, is very "forgiving" if given a short period of rest to recover. If trauma to the bladder is suspected, continuous catheter drainage for 3 to 5 days usually results in spontaneous healing. Selective cystoscopy following complicated or difficult operative procedures when the gynecologist wonders whether the integrity of the lower urinary tract has been compromised should be a strong consideration.

When leakage from the urinary tract is first discovered, the bladder should be drained with a large-bore Foley catheter. Ureteral injuries should be treated with retrograde ureteral catheters. Approximately 20% of bladder injuries and 30% of ureteral injuries heal spontaneously without further operations. Ureteral injuries that occurs secondary to cauterization or coagulation during laparoscopy may present several days to a few weeks after surgery. Symptoms may vary from pain, bloating, ileus, leukocytosis, and urinary ascites. In these cases, splinting of the urinary tract facilitates healing of the defect before epithelialization of the aberrant tract occurs, which would result in a true fistula. Spontaneous healing usually occurs within the first 4 weeks. With a ureteral fistula, follow-up imaging should be ordered at 3, 6, and 12 months to detect delayed ureteral strictures.

Unless the diagnosis is made in the immediate perioperative period, operative repair should usually be delayed 2 to 3 months after the initial injury to obtain optimum results. The workup of a patient before operative repair of a vesicovaginal fistula includes IV pyelography, cystoscopy, and biopsy of the fistula's margins if carcinoma is suspected. Cystoscopy is mandatory and should be performed for two reasons: to establish that edema and inflammation have subsided around the fistulous tract and to establish the relationship of the fistulous tract to the trigone of the bladder, especially the ureteral orifices. Occasionally, repair of a fistula near the ureteral orifice compromises the ureter, and the ureter must be reimplanted into the bladder.

Operative repair of a vesicovaginal fistula is usually accomplished via a multilayered closure performed by the vaginal route. The principles for a successful operation include adequate exposure, dissection and mobilization of each tissue layer; excision of the fistulous tract; closure of each layer without tension on the suture line; and excellent hemostasis with closure of the dead space. Reliable bladder drainage is provided to avoid tension on the suture line for approximately 10 days. Latzko's operation is the simplest means of repairing a fistula at the vaginal apex. This technique of partial colpocleisis involves denudation of the vaginal mucosa surrounding the fistula and subsequent multilayer closure without entering the bladder. The primary disadvantage of the procedure is postoperative shortening of the vagina.

Many ureteral injuries discovered during the immediate postoperative period will heal when treated by percutaneous nephrostomy and ureteral catheters. Ureterovaginal fistulas that do not heal spontaneously are usually repaired 2 to 3 months after the original operation. The surgeon has several choices as to the operative technique. However, most persistent ureterovaginal fistulas involving the lower third of the ureter are repaired by reimplanting the ureter into the bladder.

GASTROINTESTINAL COMPLICATIONS

Postoperative Diet

Most patients may be put on a regular diet as soon as tolerated. The following section discusses nausea and postoperative GI complications. Relevant to postoperative nutrition is glucose control. Part of the physiologic stress response to surgery is a drive for gluconeogenesis. This process is enhanced by a hormonally mediated insulin resistance. The resultant hyperglycemia is advantageous in the teleologic sense of the "fight or flight" response, but is detrimental for wound healing, cardiovascular function, and inflammatory processes. Several studies have correlated clinical outcomes with glucose levels. The American Association of Endocrinology notes an 18-fold increase in hospital mortality in both general medicine and general surgery patients with glucose levels above 200.

Glucose control begins preoperatively, and is discussed in detail in Chapter 24 (Preoperative Counseling and Management). Women who are given insulin infusions during surgery, should have their infusions continued until they are taking regular meals. At this point, they may be given subcutaneous insulin if necessary. Metformin (Glucophage) should not be used in the perioperative setting. In women with a history of insulin resistance, women who are morbidly obese, and those older than 60, glucose levels should be checked at the bedside every 4 to 6 hours during the first postoperative day. If a patient's glucose rises above 180, she should be treated. Target levels are no greater than fasting values under 110 mg%, and a maximum glucose level 180 mg%. Sliding-scale insulin treatments are less effective in the first 24 hours, but are easier than infusions. Sliding-scale regular insulin is most appropriate for women without a previous history of diabetes and without risk factors, and those with short surgeries who will resume normal activity and diet within 24 hours. Infusions are preferable if glucose levels are elevated significantly and early in the postoperative course, and for women with longer surgeries who will not resume regular eating and activity for a few days. Insulin infusions are begun with concomitant infusions of D_5 ½ NS (5% dextrose in half-strength normal saline) with 10 mEq of KCl. The Portland Insulin Protocol allows for tight control of glucose levels and with nursing support can be quite effective (see following box).

When transitioning off of insulin infusions it is reasonable to use the rule of thumb of using 80% of the previous 24-hour total insulin dose. This amount may be divided into split doses of NPH or longer acting glargine. Glargine is associated with less hypoglycemia. Initially, a bolus of fast-acting insulin, lispro, may be added with meals. Bedside glucose is measured every 4 hours.

Portland Continuous Intravenous Insulin Protocol (Version 2001): Target Blood Glucose Level, 100 to 150 mg/dL

1. Start "Portland Protocol" during surgical procedure and continue through 7 AM of the third postoperative day (POD). Patients who are not taking enteral nutrition on POD 3 should remain on this protocol until taking at least 50% of a full liquid or soft American Diabetes Association (ADA) diet.
2. For patients with no previous diagnosis of diabetes mellitus (DM) who present with hyperglycemia: start PDX protocol if blood glucose (BG) level >200 mg/dL. Consult endocrinologist on POD 2 for DM workup and follow-up orders.
3. Start insulin infusion through pump "piggybacked" to maintenance intravenous line, as follows:

		INITIAL INSULIN RATE (U/H) (CIRCLE ONE)	
Blood Glucose (mg/dL)	**Intravenous Insulin Bolus (U)**	**Type 2 DM Preoperatively**	**Type 1 DM Preoperatively**
80–119	0	0.5	1.0
120–179	0	1.0	2.0
180–239	0	2.0	3.5
240–299	4	3.5	5.0
300–359	8	5.0	6.5
≥360	12	6.5	8.0

4. Test blood glucose (BG) level by finger-stick method or arterial line drop sample. The frequency of BG testing should be as follows:
   a. If BG ≥ 200 mg/dL, check BG every 30 minutes.
   b. If BG < 200 mg/dL, check BG every hour.
   c. When titrating vasopressors (such as epinephrine), check BG every 30 minutes.
   d. If BG is 100 to 150 mg/dL with < 15 mg/dL change *and* insulin rate has remained unchanged for 4 hours ("stable infusion rate"), they may test BG every 2 hours.
   e. May stop every-2-hour testing on POD 3 (see items 5 and 8 below).
   f. At night on telemetry unit:

   If BG is 150 to 200 mg/dL, test every 2 hours.
   If BG < 150 mg/dL and stable insulin infusion rate exists, test every 4 hours.

Continued

Portland Continuous Intravenous Insulin Protocol (Version 2001): Target Blood Glucose Level, 100 to 150 mg/dL *Continued*

5. Insulin titration guidelines:

Blood Glucose (mg/dL)	Action
<50	Stop insulin; give 25 mL of 50% dextrose; recheck BG in 30 minutes When BG > 75 mg/dL, restart with rate 50% of previous rate
50–75	Stop insulin; if previous BG > 100 mg/dL, then give 25 mL of 50% dextrose; recheck BG in 30 minutes When BG > 75 mg/dL, restart with rate 50% of previous rate
76–100	If < 10 mg/dL lower than last test, decrease rate by 0.5 U/h If > 10 mg/dL lower than last test, decrease rate by 50% If ≥ last test result, maintain same rate
101–150	Use same rate
151–200	If 20 mg/dL lower than last test, use same rate Otherwise, increase rate by 0.5 U/h
>200	If ≥ 30 mg/dL lower than last test, use same rate If < 30 mg/dL lower than last test (**OR** if higher than last test), increase rate by 1 U/h **AND**—if > 240 mg/dL, give intravenous bolus of regular insulin per "Intravenous insulin bolus" dosage scale (see item 3 above) **Recheck BG in 30 minutes**

If BG > 200 mg/dL and has not decreased after 3 consecutive increases in insulin: give intravenous bolus per item 3 and double the insulin rate

IF BG > 300 mg/dL for 4 consecutive readings: call physician for additional intravenous bolus orders

6. Begin use of 1,800–calorie ADA diabetic diet with any oral intake.
7. Postmeal subcutaneous insulin lispro (Humalog) supplement in addition to insulin infusion when oral intake advances beyond clear liquids:
   a. If patient eats 50% or less of servings on breakfast, lunch, or supper tray, then give 3 U insulin lispro subcutaneously immediately after that meal.
   b. If patient eats more than 50% of serving on breakfast, lunch, or supper tray, then give 6 U of insulin lispro subcutaneously immediately after the meal.
8. On POD 3: Restart preadmission glycemic control medication, unless patient is not tolerating enteral nutrition—then maintain insulin drip per protocol.

Nausea and Gastrointestinal Function

Minor disturbances in gastrointestinal function are a normal consequence of anesthesia, perioperative medications, and surgical manipulation. Most women experience some nausea for approximately 12 hours, pass flatus some time during the first 48 hours, and have a spontaneous bowel movement by the third or fourth postoperative day. Current best practice for women without bowel resections and those younger than age 70 is clear liquids within 6 hours of surgery, and a regular diet with cessation of nausea. Traditionally, patients were to have nothing by mouth until the passage of flatus, and then given a gradual resumption of diet from clear liquid to full liquid to soft to regular diet, *step up diets*. Several studies over the past 10 years have shown that delayed feeding and step-up diets are unnecessary, and in some ways detrimental. Steed and colleagues in a study of major gynecologic surgeries, including oncologic cases, compared restricted oral intake with step-up diets to early full diet and found no adverse effects, as well as a shorter length of stay in the early feeding group. McMillan and coworkers, in a study of major gynecologic surgeries, compared low-residue diet at 6 hours followed by a regular diet with a traditional delayed feeding and step-up after bowel function had returned. These authors found more nausea and emesis in the delayed feeding group, with a shorter length of stay in the early feeding group. Cutillo and associates and Pearl and colleagues found similar results in their studies of gynecologic oncology patients (Table 25-8).

Approximately one third of adult women experience postoperative nausea and vomiting (PONV). Several factors affect the likelihood and severity of postoperative nausea, including preoperative anxiety, decreased threshold for nausea and vomiting, previous history of PONV, duration of surgery, the type and drugs used for anesthesia, obesity, and postoperative pain medications. Certain preventive measures may be used to minimize PONV, including adequate hydration, minimizing use of narcotics and inhalation agents, avoiding nitrous oxide, the choice of regional anesthesia, and avoiding excessive movement

Table 25-8 Gastrointestinal Information

Category	Clear Liquid (*N* = 107)	Regular Diet (*N* = 138)
Morbidity		
Nausea	21 (19.6)	26 (18.8)
Vomiting	10 (9.3)	19 (13.8)
Abdominal distension	10 (9.3)	18 (13.0)
Nasogastric tube use	1 (0.9)	8 (5.8)
Tolerance		
Diet on first attempt	101 (94.4)	121 (87.7)
Regular diet on first attempt	103 (96.3)	
If intolerant, time to tolerance (days)	5.3 ± 1.5	3.6 ± 1.5
Flatus before discharge	55 (51.4)	69 (50.0)
Intervals (days)		
Bowel sounds	1.2 ± 0.5	1.2 ± 0.5
Flatus	2.8 ± 1.4	2.8 ± 1.0
Regular diet*	2.4 ± 2.5	1.1 ± 0.3
Hospital stay	3.6 ± 3.0	3.4 ± 1.7

Data presented as mean ± standard deviation or *N* (%).
*$p < 0.05$; no other significant differences between groups.
From Pearl MI, Frandina M, Mahler L, et al: A randomized controlled trial of a regular diet as the first meal in gynecologic oncology patients undergoing intraabdominal surgery. Obstet Gynecol 100:232, 2002.

in the immediate postoperative period. Many physicians prescribe medications prophylactically for women to prevent PONV (see following box).

A large randomized clinical trial of 5199 patients by Apfel and associates examined several regimens for prophylaxis for PONV. This large multicentered trial documented several important principles for postoperative management. The antiemetic interventions of dexamethasone, the 5-HT_3 antagonist ondansetron as well as droperidol were found to be equally effective for treating nausea. Droperidol is associated with a rare but problematic side effect of prolonged QT intervals and has subsequently led to most pharmacies removing this medication from formularies. Dexamethasone 2.5 to 5 mg should be given at the beginning of surgery to be most effective. The authors noted that treatments work independently and thus have an additive, not synergistic effect. The repeat use of medications for rescue effects are less efficacious if an agent has been given previously. Thus, it is better to reserve use of the more expensive regimen, such as ondansetron, for treatment. Previous studies have found that agents such as metoclopramide are ineffective for prophylaxis. Antiemetics in the phenothiazine class, such as promethazine and prochlorperazine, are effective but have some limitations because of side effects of sedation, dry mouth, and extrapyramidal effects, which may be worse for older women. Apfel and associate's study also looked at risk factors for PONV. The female sex is one of the strongest risk factors for PONV, 3.13 RR (CI 2.33 to 4.20). Thus, all women should be considered for prophylactic measures. Other factors include 1.78 RR (1.35 to 2.95) for patients with hysterectomies, 1.57 RR (1.32 to 1.07) for nonsmokers, and 2.14 (1.75 to 2.61) for use of postoperative opioids.

Ileus

Ileus is an inhibition of the normal propulsive reflexes of the bowel that are regulated by the autonomic nervous system. Adynamic (paralytic) ileus is a normal event defined as an ileus of minor to moderate degree. It may be expected to follow any intraperitoneal or pelvic operation. Brief declines in the motility of the gastrointestinal (GI) tract are normal responses after surgery. The stomach, returns to full motility in 24 to 72 hours after surgery. However some gastric secretions will continually pass into the duodenum. The stomach secretes 500 to 1000 mL of fluid per day. The pancreas secretes an additional liter. The small intestine resumes peristalsis within 6 hours after surgery. The colon resumes full motility in 18 to 48 hours. The incidence and duration of adynamic ileus are less following vaginal hysterectomy than with abdominal hysterectomy and even less following laparoscopic surgery. If adynamic ileus persists longer than 5 days, a diagnosis of mechanical bowel obstruction should be strongly considered.

Adynamic ileus is believed to result from a lack of coordinated motor activity of the intestine, which results in disorganized, propulsive activity. Electrical activity is present, but the pathophysiologic problem is continuous activity of the intrinsic inhibitor neurons in the wall of the small intestine. Usually the process is generalized, but occasionally it may be localized, involving only an isolated loop of small intestine. The cause of prolonged postoperative ileus is a subject of continued debate. Generally, the mechanisms include an increased neurologic inhibition of intestinal motility due to sympathetic nerve activity, as well as an inflammation within the intestinal wall. Bauer and Boeckxstaens describe leukocytic infiltration secondary to cytokine production from manipulation of the bowel during surgery. The inflammation inhibits the appropriate neuromuscular reactions, which then decrease motility. Opioid receptors become stimulated with abdominal surgery, further decreasing motility. Recent experimental trials using selective opioid antagonists have shown promise in decreasing postoperative ileus in gynecologic as well as general surgery patients. To be useful these receptor antagonists must not cross the blood–brain barrier, and when given orally should have little systemic absorption as well. In addition to pharmacologic treatments, other studies have found that preoperative counseling and psychological suggestions will decrease perioperative ileus. Early carbohydrate intake as well as postoperative gum chewing have also improved rates for return of bowel function and decreased rates of postoperative ileus. Importantly, early feeding, as mentioned previously, decreases the incidence of postoperative ileus, most likely through stimulation of intestinal reflexes. Overall, a multifactorial peri- and postoperative approach to postoperative ileus is indicated (Table 25-9).

The classic symptoms of a prolonged ileus include absence of flatus, abdominal distention, and obstipation. Often these symptoms are associated with nausea and effortless vomiting. Bowel sounds may be hypoactive or absent. This condition may be associated with abdominal tenderness, and the abdomen is usually tympanic to percussion. Nausea and vomiting that persist more than 24 hours after surgery are a cause for concern. The difference between small-bowel obstruction and adynamic ileus is a subtle one, because adynamic ileus is normally associated with partial obstruction of the small intestine.

Diagnostic films of the abdomen (supine, erect, and lateral) help to establish the correct diagnosis (Table 25-10). In a woman with adynamic ileus, the intestinal gas is scattered throughout the gastrointestinal tract, including the small intestine and

Sample Adult Post Operative Nausea and Vomiting Order

COMPLETE IN POST-ANESTHESIA CARE UNIT (PACU)

1. Antiemetic(s) given in OR:

Antiemetic	Dose	Time

☐ None

2. Time of arrival in PACU: ____________
   Antiemetic(s) given in PACU:

Antiemetic	Dose	Time
Anzemet		
Compazine		
Haldol		

☐ None

ANTIEMETIC REGIMEN

	Medication	Dose	Time
1	**Dolasetron** (Anzemet)	12.5 mg IV	Over 1 minute
2	**Prochlorperazine** (Compazine)	5 mg IV	5 mg per minute
	If no IV access, may give **Prochlorperazine** (Compazine) 25 mg rectally.		
3	**Halperidol** (Haldol)	1–2 mg IV	Over 1 minute
	■ DO NOT give if patient has Parkinson's		
4	**If there is no response after Halperidol (Haldol), contact the surgeon or ordering physician for further orders.**		
5	If the patient is on IV Morphine via PCA, switch to **Hydromorphone** (Dilaudid), asking the pharmacist for the equivalent dose.		

DISCONTINUE ALL PREVIOUSLY ORDERED MEDICATIONS FOR NAUSEA.
This order supercedes all previous antiemetic orders.

IF < 8 HOURS FROM ARRIVAL IN PACU

1. Check vital signs and if SBP ≤ 25% from baseline or HR > 100, contact physician. (SBP x 0.75. If post-op SBP is less than that, call MD).
2. If the patient has not received any antiemetic, begin with **Dolasetron (Anzemet).**
3. If the patient has already received an antiemetic in OR or PACU, give the next antiemetic listed in Table for Anti-Emetic Regimen.
4. If nausea persist or returns after 20 minutes, use the next antiemetic listed in the table.
5. Continue down the list of antiemetics in 20-minute intervals until nausea is absent or all the antiemetics listed in the table have been administrated.
6. If all medications have been given and nausea persists, contact MD.

IF > 8 HOURS FROM ARRIVAL IN PACU

1. **Dolasetron (Anzemet)** 12.5 mg IV. May repeat every 8 hours prn.
2. If no response in 20 minutes, give **Prochlorperazine (Compazine)** 5 mg IV. May repeat every 8 hours prn. If no IV access, may give **Prochlorperazine (Compazine)** 25 mg rectally. May repeat every 8 hours prn.
3. If patient remains nauseated 20 minutes after above medications, contact physician.
4. Repeat the above sequence (1 and 2) every 8 hours prn.

Courtesy of Sacred Heart Hospital, Eugene, OR.

colon. Air–fluid levels, if present, tend to be at the same level. In some studies, CT has been found to be sensitive and specific in differentiating adynamic ileus from complete obstruction and helpful in differentiating ileus from partial obstruction.

Oral administration of radiocontrast material may be both a therapeutic and diagnostic test. The osmolality of the radiocontrast material is approximately six times greater than that of normal saline. Thus a large amount of fluid enters the small bowel and acts as a direct stimulant of peristalsis. In one study after preliminary abdominal films were obtained, 120 mL of 66% diatrizoate meglumine, 10% diatrizoate sodium (Gastrografin) was administered orally or via nasogastric tube. Passage of liquid stool occurred within a few hours in patients with adynamic ileus. Gastrografin, unlike barium, is nontoxic

Table 25-9 Treatment Options for Postoperative Ileus

Treatment	Potential Mechanism	Comments
Nonpharmacologic Treatment Options		
NG tube	Gastric/small bowel decompression	No evidence NG tubes reduce duration of POI. May increase pulmonary postoperative complications
Early enteral nutrition	Stimulates GI motility by eliciting reflex response and stimulating release of several hormonal factors	Appears safe, well tolerated. Some, but not all, studies suggest decrease in POI
Sham feeding	Cephalic-vagal reflex	Small clinical trials suggest some benefit
Early mobilization	Possible mechanical stimulation	No significant change in duration of POI, but may decrease other postoperative complications
Laparoscopic surgery	Decreased opiate requirements, decreased pain, less abdominal wall trauma	Most studies find decreased duration of POI with laparoscopy
Psychological preoperative preparation	Improves bowel motility through visceral learning	One study found positive benefit in decreasing time to flatus and hospital discharge
Pharmacologic Treatment Options		
Metoclopramide	Dopamine antagonist, cholinergic agent	Majority of RCTs suggest no benefit
Cisapride	Dopamine antagonist, cholinergic agonist, serotonin receptor agonist	Possibly effective, withdrawn from U.S. market due to cardiovascular side effects
Erythromycin	Motilin agonist	2 RCTs suggest no benefit
Opiate antagonists	Block peripheral opiate receptors	One RCT shows ADL8-2698 decreases time to flatus, bowel movement, and hospital discharge, but not currently available outside of clinical trials. Other agents have not been evaluated in POI
Epidural anesthesia	Inhibits sympathetic reflex at cord level, opioid-sparing analgesia	Several RCTs suggest benefit in decreasing POI, most effective when inserted at thoracic level
NSAIDs	Opiate-sparing analgesia, inhibits COX-mediated prostaglandin synthesis	Probable benefit. COX-2 selective medications need further evaluation
Laxatives	Stimulant, prokinetic effects	No RCTs. One nonrandomized, unblinded study suggests possible benefit
Antiadrenergic agents	Blocks sympathetic neural reflex	Little practical benefit in POI drugs often limited by cardiovascular side effects
Cholinergic agents	Acetylcholine modulation	Frequent systemic side effects. Neostigmine has possible benefit
Multimodality therapy	Combination therapy may work via multiple mechanisms	Possible benefit in reducing POI. No RCTs have been reported

COX, cyclooxygenase; NSAIDs, nonsteroidal antiinflammatory drugs; POI, postoperative ileus; RCTs, randomized controlled trials.
From Behm B, Stollman N: Postoperative ileus: Etiologies and interventions. Clin Gastroenterol Hepatol 1:74, 2003.

if it accidentally contaminates the peritoneal cavity during an operation for bowel obstruction. In a different study, Finan and coworkers gave Gastrografin on the third postoperative day to 57 women with ileus. These women were compared with 58 women with ileus who received rectal suppositories. The investigators found no difference in the mean time of return of bowel function between the two groups of women.

Severe adynamic ileus is a self-limiting condition that responds to GI rest, IV fluids, and time. During the period of watchful expectancy, adequate fluid and electrolyte replacement is necessary. Patients experience mild cramping and passage of flatus and regain their appetite with the return of normal peristalsis. If adequate bowel sounds are present, a rectal tube, Fleet's enema, or rectal suppository may facilitate the initial passage of flatus. Some advocate the routine postoperative administration of a wetting agent, such as simethicone (Mylicon), to reduce surface tension of intestinal mucus and liberate entrapped gas. Opinions are mixed as to whether such an agent reduces the incidence or intensity of adynamic ileus. Randomized trials of the prokinetic agents erythromycin and metochlorpropamide

Table 25-10 Differential Radiographic Findings in Ileus and Mechanical Obstruction

Adynamic Ileus	Mechanical Obstruction
Small and large bowel are distended in proportion to each other	In small-bowel obstruction there is dilated small bowel proximal to site of obstruction in colonic obstruction the colon is distended and small-bowel distention is present with incompetent ileocecal valve
Air–fluid levels in small bowel are infrequent; when present, they are at the same levels	Air–fluid levels are common and at different levels in the bowel
Quantitative difference in small-bowel distention	Greater small-bowel distention than with ileus
Small-bowel distention in central part of abdomen with colon in periphery	Small-bowel distention present in central part of abdomen; no peripheral large-bowel distention

From Buchsbaum HJ, Mazer J: The gastrointestinal tract. In Buchsbaum HJ, Walton LA (eds): Strategies in Gynecologic Surgery. New York, Springer-Verlag, 1986, p 100.

Table 25-11 Average Daily Volume and Electrolyte Concentrations of Gastrointestinal Secretions

	Volume (mL/day)	ELECTROLYTE CONCENTRATIONS (mEq/L)		
		Na^+	K^+	Cl^-
Saliva	1000–1500	10–40	10–20	6–30
Gastric juice	2000–2500	60–120	10–20	10–30
Hepatic bile	600–800	130–155	2–12	80–100
Pancreatic juice	700–1000	150–155	5–10	30–50
Duodenal secretions	300–800	90–140	2–10	70–120
Jejunal and ileal secretions	2000–3000	125–140	5–10	100–130
Colonic mucosal secretions	200–500	140–148	5–10	60–90
TOTAL	8000–10,000			

From Buchsbaum HJ, Mazer J: The gastrointestinal tract. In Buchsbaum HJ, Walton LA (eds): Strategies in Gynecologic Surgery. New York, Springer-Verlag, 1986, p 103.

Table 25-12 Composition of Intravenous Solutions

Solutions	Glucose (g/L)	Na^+	Cl^-	HCO_3^-	K^+	Ca^{2+}	Mg^{2+}	HPO_4^-	NH_4^-
		(mEq/L)							
Extracellular fluid	1000	140	102	27	4.2	5	3	0.3	
5% dextrose and water	50								
10% dextrose and water	100								
0.9% sodium chloride (normal saline)		154	154						
0.45% sodium chloride (half-normal saline)		77	77						
0.21% sodium chloride (1/4 normal saline)		34	34						
3% sodium chloride (hypertonic saline)		513	513						
Lactated Ringer's solution		130	109	28*	4	2.7			
0.9% ammonium chloride		168							168

*Present in solution as lactate but is metabolized to bicarbonate.
From Miller TA, Duke JH: Fluid and electrolyte management. In Dudrick SJ, Baue AE, Eiseman B, et al (eds): Manual of Preoperative and Postoperative Care, 3rd ed. Philadelphia, WB Saunders, 1983, p 47.

have shown these agents to be ineffective in relieving ileus. Importantly, prophylactic nasogastric suctioning will not prevent ileus. In many studies, prophylactic nasogastric suctioning is associated with an increased risk of aspiration as well as an increased rate of ileus—the very symptom the treatment is supposed to prevent. However, if a severe ileus does not resolve, then nasogastric suctioning will be necessary. Nasogastric suction prevents progression of the intestinal distention. During periods when nasogastric suctioning is used, special attention should be given to correct replacement of fluid and electrolytes (Tables 25-11 and 25-12). A rare but worrisome complication of prolonged ileus is massive dilation of the cecum. Massive dilatation of the colon related to a pseudoobstruction produced by severe adynamic ileus in the absence of mechanical obstruction is known as Ogilive's syndrome. This condition may be treated medically by evacuating the air with colonoscopy, or, in severe cases, cecostomy may be necessary. An alternative method of treating this condition is IV neostigmine.

Intestinal Obstruction

Adhesions are the most common cause of intestinal obstruction postoperatively. During subsequent operations greater than 90% of women are found to have some adhesions following abdominal laparotomy. In a large retrospective cohort study covering a 10-year period following laparotomy for gynecologic conditions, approximately one in three women had adhesion-related readmissions to the hospital. Less common causes of intestinal obstruction are hernias, mesenteric defects, intussusception, volvulus, and neoplasm. Large raw areas of the pelvis with hypoxic tissue facilitate the attachment of small intestine following pelvic operations. Previous gynecologic operations are the most common cause of small-bowel obstruction in women. The incidence of operation for obstruction of the small intestine after an abdominal hysterectomy is estimated to be approximately 2%. Interestingly, in one series, adhesions involving the pelvic peritoneum were responsible for the intestinal obstruction in 85% of cases, and adhesions to the closure of the anterior abdominal wall accounted for the other 15%. Fortunately the fibrous adhesions that form during the first 2 to 3 weeks after an operation are soft and filmy. Thus intestinal strangulation during the postoperative period is extremely rare. Dense adhesions may develop several months after an operation. The incidence of intestinal obstruction depends on the type of gynecologic operation performed. Approximately 2 women in 1000 develop an obstruction after a benign gynecologic operation, whereas approximately 8% develop intestinal obstruction after radical cancer operations. Intestinal obstruction occurs in the small intestine in approximately 80% of cases and in the colon in the remaining 20%. As mentioned previously, the differential diagnosis between bowel obstruction and ileus is a difficult one (Table 25-13).

The acute symptoms of intestinal obstruction present most commonly between the fifth and seventh postoperative day. The majority of patients have a short period of normal intestinal

Table 25-13 Differential Diagnosis Between Postoperative Ileus and Postoperative Obstruction

Clinical Features	Postoperative Ileus	Postoperative Obstruction
Abdominal pain	Discomfort from distention but not cramping pains	Cramping, progressively severe
Relationship to previous operation	Usually within 48–72 hours of operation	Usually delayed; may be 5–7 days for remote onset
Nausea and vomiting	Present	Present
Distention	Present	Present
Bowel sounds	Absent or hypoactive	Borborygmi with peristaltic rushes and high-pitched tinkles
Fever	Only if related to associated peritonitis	Rarely present unless bowel becomes gangrenous
Abdominal radiograph	Distended loops of small and large bowels; gas usually present in colon	Single or multiple loops of distended bowel, usually small bowel with air–fluid levels
Treatment	Conservative with nasogastric suction, enemas, cholinergic stimulation	Partial: conservative with nasogastric decompression; or Complete: surgical

From Mattingly RF, Thompson JD (eds): Te Linde's Operative Gynecology, 6th ed. Philadelphia, JB Lippincott, 1985, p 102.

function before the onset of symptoms. Women with bowel obstruction appear to have more toxicity and more acute distress than do women with ileus. The abdominal pain is intermittent, colicky, and sharp in nature. Episodes of colicky pain usually last from 1 to 3 minutes. Associated symptoms include vomiting, abdominal distention, and constipation. Bowel sounds are loud, high-pitched, and metallic. Occasionally they may be heard without a stethoscope. Nasogastric drainage is more profuse than in patients with severe adynamic ileus. A patient with a complete small-bowel obstruction may have a bowel movement, eliminating fecal material that already existed in the colon.

Abdominal radiographs demonstrate a stepladder appearance: multiple air–fluid levels throughout the small intestine with an absence of gas in the colon and rectum. Pneumoperitoneum from an exploratory celiotomy usually persists for 7 to 10 days. Thus, in the early postoperative period, free air under the diaphragm is not diagnostic of perforation of a hollow viscus. Obstruction of the colon may be diagnosed by retrograde infusion of contrast material or by flexible endoscopy.

The foundation of early treatment of postoperative intestinal obstruction is decompression of the small intestine and adequate replacement of fluids and electrolytes. Decompression may be accomplished by means of a nasogastric tube or, preferably, a long tube (Miller–Abbott or Cantor tube). Serial monitoring of white blood cell counts with differentials should be performed. Repeat abdominal radiographic examinations at regular intervals are used to assess the degree of intestinal distention. Expectant management is successful in many patients. In an older series by Wolfson and colleagues, less than 40% of 112 patients with small-bowel obstruction due to adhesions required operation. A small series from Gowen also noted a greater than 70% success with long-tube decompression. Conservative therapy was most successful in those patients in whom the long intestinal drainage tube was successfully advanced from the stomach into the small intestine.

The major cause of morbidity and death with bowel obstruction is delay in diagnosis, with resultant strangulation and secondary sepsis. Women who develop strangulation experience a dramatic increase in the intensity of abdominal pain, and the pain becomes continuous. Strangulation of the small bowel is associated with localized peritoneal irritation, increase in temperature, and marked leukocytosis. Bowel obstruction may also lead to translocation of intestinal bacteria across the bowel wall, promoting sepsis. A series by Sagar and coworkers found that the more distal the obstruction, the greater the incidence of anaerobic septicemia.

Fecal impaction is most often seen in elderly patients. It results from loss of peristalsis in the colon, with an impaired perception of rectal fullness. Fecal impaction is a humiliating experience for the woman. She may have either diarrhea around the impaction or obstipation. Treatment involves obtaining partial analgesia with lidocaine jelly and, subsequently, manually fragmenting and extracting the fecal mass.

Rectovaginal Fistula

Rectovaginal fistulas and fecal incontinence secondary to perineal tears are most commonly obstetric complications and are only rarely associated with gynecologic operations. In general, rectovaginal fistulas following hysterectomy or repair of an enterocele are usually located in the upper third of the vagina, whereas those secondary to a posterior colporrhaphy are in the lower third of the vagina. Other causes of rectovaginal fistula are carcinoma, radiation therapy, perirectal abscess, inflammatory bowel disease, lymphogranuloma venereum, and trauma.

The initial signs and symptoms associated with potential fistulous tracts between the rectum and vagina usually present 7 to 14 days after an operation. The first warning may be the rectal passage of several blood clots, indicating that a hematoma has ruptured into the rectum. Distressing symptoms include passage of gas from the vagina and, depending on the size of the opening, the passage of fecal material from the vagina. Associated with these classic symptoms and signs are chronic, foul-smelling vaginal discharge and subsequent dyspareunia. Aside from the physical symptoms of the anatomic defect, fistulas cause severe emotional distress because they affect almost every aspect of the patient's daily life.

The diagnosis is not difficult to establish, and only very small openings present a diagnostic problem. What appears to be granulation tissue in the posterior aspect of the vagina is the dark-red rectal mucosa, which stands out in contrast to the lighter vaginal mucosa. Usually the defect may be successfully defined with a small, malleable metal probe. If this is not successful, a Foley catheter should be placed in the rectum. Methylene blue dye or milk may then be instilled into the rectum with a tampon in the vagina, similar to the procedure establishing the diagnosis of a vesicovaginal fistula.

Table 25-14 Differences Between Antibiotic-Associated Diarrhea from *Clostridium Difficile* and Diarrhea from Other Causes

Characteristic	Diarrhea due to *C. difficile* Infection	Diarrhea from Other Causes
Most commonly implicated antibiotics	Clindamycin, cephalosporins, penicillins	Clindamycin, cephalosporins, or amoxicillin–clavulanate
History	Usually no relevant history of antibiotic intolerance	History of diarrhea with antibiotic therapy common
Clinical features		
Diarrhea	May be florid; evidence of colitis with cramps, fever, and fecal leukocytes common	Usually moderate in severity (i.e., "nuisance diarrhea") without evidence of colitis
Findings on CT or endoscopy	Evidence of colitis (not enteritis) common	Usually normal
Complications	Hypoalbuminemia, anasarca, toxic megacolon, relapses with treatment with metronidazole or vancomycin	Usually none except occasional cases of dehydration
Results of assay for *C. difficile* toxin	Positive	Negative
Epidemiologic pattern	May be epidemic for endemic in hospitals or long-term care facilities	Sporadic
Treatment		
Withdrawal of implicated antibiotic	May resolve but often persists or progresses	Usually resolves
Antiperistaltic agents	Contraindicated	Often useful
Oral metronidazole or vancomycin	Prompt response	Not indicated

CT, computed tomography

From Bartlett JG: Antibiotic associated diarrhea. N Engl J Med 346:335, 2002.

For initial treatment the woman should be obstipated with a low-residue diet and diphenoxylate hydrochloride (Lomotil). Approximately one in four anatomic defects heals spontaneously before epithelialization of the tract. A low-residue diet or hyperalimentation may be helpful in facilitating spontaneous closure of some anatomic defects.

Timing of the operative repair is important. The gynecologist should inspect the area surrounding the fistula to make sure that the tissues are free of edema, induration, and infection. Preoperative evaluation includes visualization of the entire vagina and sigmoidoscopy of the rectal mucosa in an attempt to discover more than one opening. Imaging studies and endoscopy are important diagnostic tools if there is any suspicion of coexistence of Crohn's disease.

The operative technique employed depends on the size and location of the fistula. Standard operative principles include removal of the entire fistulous tract and closure of tissue layers without tension on the suture line. In the repair of large rectovaginal fistulas in the lower part of the vagina, it is usually easier to convert the rectovaginal fistula into a fourth-degree laceration. Diverting colostomy should be used for all radiation-induced fistulas, the majority of fistulas associated with inflammatory bowel disease, and some large postoperative fistulas at the apex of the vagina. The woman may be discharged from the hospital after the first bowel movement. The stool should be kept soft with low-residue diets and stool softeners such as mineral oil for the first 2 weeks after the operation.

Antibiotic-Associated Diarrheas

Patients may develop diarrhea in the postoperative period after exposure to antibiotics. Oral and parenteral antibiotics produce similar rates of diarrhea, with some studies noting that up to a third of patients receiving antibiotics will develop diarrhea. The antibiotic therapy, either for prophylaxis or for treatment, can disrupt the normal intestinal flora. The result is a disturbed breakdown of bile acids and carbohydrates that induce loose stools. Diarrhea may develop secondary to medications other than antibiotics, including oral contrast media, diabetic foods that contain artificial sweeteners, and many cardiac medications. If the patient is afebrile, the diarrhea is mild, and the abdominal examination is unremarkable, then stopping or changing antibiotics and providing supportive care are all that is necessary. If the patient has a temperature greater than 38° C, a leukocytosis, abdominal tenderness, severe abdominal distention, bloody diarrhea, or persistent diarrhea, then evaluation for *Clostridium difficile* infection is indicated (Table 25-14).

Clostridium difficile is a species of spore-forming, gram-positive anaerobic bacteria found normally in 5% of healthy adults. However, after antibiotic treatment and disruption of normal enteric flora, up to 25% of hospitalized adults will become colonized with *C. difficile*. The organism is spread by nosocomial oral–fecal contamination. Persistence of the spores of *C. difficile* and contamination of the environment are primary factors in cross infection. The organism after colonizing the intestine may secrete toxins, which produce a spectrum of clinical disease. Symptoms from the infection are varied and range from a mild diarrhea to colitis to a pseudomembranous colitis that in rare cases may be fatal. Nearly all antibiotics have been associated with the development of *C. difficile* diarrhea (Table 25-15). Second- and third-generation cephalosporins (clindamycin, ampicillin, and amoxicillin) are the antibiotics associated with the highest risk of developing *C. difficile* diarrhea. Symptoms usually appear 5 to 10 days after the initiation of antibiotic therapy. However, they may appear from a few days to a few weeks after antibiotic exposure. Diagnostic tests include culture for the organism; *C. difficile* cell cytotoxin B assay; ELISA kits for the *C. difficile* toxins A and B; stool leukocyte assay, which is nonspecific; colonoscopy for direct evaluation of pseudomembranes; abdominal radiographs; and CT. The test for *C. difficile* cell cytotoxin B in the stool is the gold standard for diagnosis because it is the most sensitive and specific. This test is also relatively inexpensive. The results are usually available within 24 hours.

Discontinuing antibiotic therapy is the only treatment required in approximately one in four women. Use of drugs that slow intestinal transit time such as diphenoxylate atropine

Table 25-15 Antimicrobial Agents That Induce *Clostridium difficile*–Associated Diarrhea and Colitis

Frequent Induction	Infrequent Induction	Rare or No Induction
Ampicillin and amoxicillin	Tetracyclines	Parenteral aminoglycosides
Cephalosporins	Sulfonamides	Bacitracin
Clindamycin	Erythromycin	Metronidazole
	Chloramphenicol	Vancomycin
	Trimethoprim	
	Quinolones	

From Kelly CP, Pothoulakis C, LaMont JT: *Clostridium difficile* colitis. N Engl J Med 330:257, 1994.

(Lomotil) or narcotics are definitely contraindicated because the toxins of *C. difficile* remain in the gastrointestinal tract for a longer period of time. Therapy for the infection is metronidazole given 250 mg by mouth four times a day, or oral vancomycin, 125 mg four times a day. Gastrointestinal symptoms usually improve within the first 72 hours of therapy, and complete resolution of symptoms occurs within 10 days. Host factors are involved in the pathogenesis of the disease; older and more chronically ill patients usually develop more severe symptoms. Patients with ileus may receive high-dose vancomycin through a long tube. Up to 25% of women may develop a recurrence or relapse. Recent studies have confirmed that more than 50% of recurrences of symptoms after initial response to treatment are due to reinfection rather than due to a relapse. Recurrences usually can be successfully treated in the same manner as the initial therapy.

Recent trials have evaluated probiotic agents for the prevention of antibiotic-associated diarrhea as well as for treatment of *C. difficile* disease. Probiotics are live microbes that may act in the intestinal tract to colonize with less problematic organisms. Other actions include the secretion of compounds that may inhibit *C. difficile* or inactivate the toxin. To be most effective, probiotics should be given at the same time as the antibiotic. Several trials in both the United States and Europe have found that the probiotic yeast *Saccharomyces boulardii* significantly decreases the incidence of antibiotic-associated diarrhea. Trials of *Lactobacillus* have not found significant efficacy. Though the complete mechanism of action is theoretical at this point, *S. boulardii* does seem to inactivate the *C. difficile* toxin. The yeast also seems to stimulate IgA production in the intestinal mucosa against *C. difficile* as well.

WOUND COMPLICATIONS

Infection

A major wound infection prolongs the hospital stay approximately 2 to 6 days. In their extensive review of 23,649 operations, Cruse and Foord determined that the incidence of abdominal wound infection varied depending on risk factors; however, for abdominal hysterectomy the incidence was approximately 5%. In a population of women not at high risk, the incidence of infection should be 1% to 2%. Abdominal hysterectomy is classified as a clean-contaminated operative procedure because the bacterial flora of the vagina is in continuity with the operative site during the surgery. The Centers for Disease Control and Prevention has revised their nomenclature describing incisional infection. They subdivide incisional infections into superficial infections that involve only the skin and subcutaneous tissue and deep infections that involve the deep soft tissues including fascia and muscles.

The pathophysiology of wound infection depends on an interaction between the number and virulence of bacterial contamination and the resistance of the patient. Inoculation of bacteria into the wound occurs in the operating room during the surgical procedure. A wide spectrum of common, endogenous bacteria produce wound infections, including most gram-positive cocci and both aerobic and anaerobic rods. Small numbers of bacteria are present in all surgical wounds; however, bacterial growth is facilitated by decreased tissue oxygen and excessive amounts of necrotic tissue. It takes between 100,000 and 1 million bacteria per gram of tissue to produce infection in a surgical wound of the skin and subcutaneous tissue. The incidence of superficial skin infection is directly related to the length of the operative procedure. Each additional hour of surgery results in a doubling of the incidence of superficial skin infections. The primary source of bacterial contamination of an abdominal wound may be exogenous to the patient (such as a break in sterile technique) or endogenous (such as purulent material from a pelvic abscess).

Both local and systemic factors contribute to the level of host resistance and thus to the incidence of wound infections. Local factors are more significant and include the presence of hematomas, necrotic tissue, foreign bodies, dead space, use of cautery, and decreased local tissue perfusion. Systemic factors include obesity, diabetes, liver disease, malnutrition, immunosuppression, defects in the reticuloendothelial system, age, and the duration of preoperative hospitalization. The incidence of postoperative wound infection is increased eightfold when the woman's preoperative weight exceeds 200 pounds. Soper and colleagues noted that the thickness of subcutaneous tissue is the greatest risk factor for wound infection in a series of women undergoing abdominal hysterectomy. If an abdominal incision is more than 4 cm in depth, the risk of a superficial skin infection is increased approximately threefold. Greer and coworkers have described a supraumbilical upper abdominal incision as a method to avoid cutting across a large, thick panniculus for pelvic surgery in the morbidly obese woman. Corticosteroid therapy may suppress the inflammatory phase of the healing process. However, after the first 5 days of wound healing, corticosteroid therapy has no effect on an uninfected wound. Multiple regimens and protocols have been studied to decrease rates of wound infection. Skin warming, to improve circulation, supplemental oxygen, and antibiotics to be given well before incision time, have all been emphasized as techniques for infection prevention.

The first symptom of most wound infections appears between the fifth and the tenth postoperative day. Wound infection may occur as late as several months following surgery, but more than 90% of cases present within the first 2 weeks of the postoperative period. The first sign is usually fever, followed by tachycardia and varying degrees of increased tenderness and pain. As the infection progresses, many wounds develop areas that are either fluctuant or firm, and some develop crepitus. The incision is swollen, erythematous, edematous, and tender.

Occasionally, subcutaneous gas may be seen on radiographic examination. Later in the course of the infection there may be associated spontaneous purulent drainage from the wound.

Fever during the first 24 to 48 hours is usually secondary to atelectasis. However, two rare types of wound infections are so virulent that they produce toxicity within the first 48 hours. Classically, these early infections are those produced by *Clostridium* species and acute β-hemolytic streptococcal infection. Clinically, wound infections secondary to β-hemolytic streptococci appear swollen and red and have an odorless discharge. In contrast, infections secondary to *Clostridium* are boggy and edematous, and the discharge has a sweet odor.

Initial management of any wound infection consists of opening and draining the wound. The wound opens easily following removal of the skin sutures or clips. Purulent material exhibits a wide range of consistency from the thin watery discharge classical of a streptococcal infection to the thick pus associated with staphylococcal subcutaneous infections. Gram stain and both aerobic and anaerobic cultures of the wound should be obtained at this point. These initial cultures are most valuable if the patient does not respond to initial management. In such cases the differential diagnosis would be between infections involving deeper tissue planes and infection for which host resistance has failed even after drainage of the wound.

Once a wound infection has been opened and drained, care is directed toward initial packing of the wound with gauze to effect débridement and periodic irrigation. Rarely are antibiotics needed, unless there is a surrounding cellulitis. If there is a distinct zone of diffuse erythema surrounding a wound infection, the most likely organism is a streptococcal infection, and IV antibiotics are indicated. Systemic antibiotics are always indicated in women with immunosuppression or concomitant diseases with impaired defense mechanisms. Most women with a wound infection will become afebrile within 48 to 72 hours after the wound has been opened and débrided. When the woman becomes afebrile and granulation tissue begins to form, consideration may be given to delayed secondary closure. If the incision is large and débridement has been extensive, closure may be facilitated with the use of vacuum-assisted devices. The wound is cleaned daily and between cleaning, topical negative pressure (TNP) is maintained with the vacuum-assisted device. The vacuum promotes granulation, reduces edema in the subcutaneous tissue, and greatly speeds healing.

Prevention is the foundation of any approach to the management of wound infections. Prevention involves consideration of both local and systemic factors, which if unattended, predispose to infection. Prophylactic antibiotics decrease the incidence of wound infection. These antibiotics are discussed in Chapter 24 (Preoperative Counseling and Management).

If the wound is grossly contaminated, then delayed primary closure on the third or fourth postoperative day may be appropriate. Women who should be considered as candidates for delayed primary closure include those who are immunosuppressed or malnourished, who have far-advanced malignancies, or who are markedly obese. Women having operative procedures that involve a simultaneous abdominal and vaginal approach and those with a surgical opening of unprepared large intestine are also candidates for delayed primary closure. In a small series, Brown and associates reported that the latter technique reduced the incidence of wound infection from 23% in a control group to 2% in the group having delayed closure. When delayed primary closure is planned, sutures may be placed at the time of surgery and secured, but not tied. The incision should be packed loosely with gauze. If the wound is dry and without evidence of infection on postoperative day 3, the edges may be approximated with the preplaced sutures.

Delayed secondary closure may be accomplished in previously infected wounds after several days of drainage and débridement. Delayed secondary closure markedly reduces the time necessary for eventual closure of the skin defect by secondary intention. Patient satisfaction is dramatically increased with delayed secondary closure.

A virulent, rapidly progressing form of soft tissue wound infection is necrotizing fasciitis. Often the diagnosis is not suspected during the early part of the infection because of the relative minor changes in the skin overlying the deeper infection. The early symptoms are local pain with systemic symptoms of tachycardia and fever, which are higher than would be expected with an uncomplicated wound infection. The woman may experience marked tenderness when the infected area is palpated. Conversely, necrotic tissue may become hypoesthetic, or completely numb. An appearance of an area that appears infected but is anesthetic should heighten the suspicion for the diagnosis of necrotizing fasciitis. As the disease progresses, the wound edges usually darken, with crepitance and bullae formation and anesthetic areas develop. Necrotizing fasciitis involves the subcutaneous tissue and superficial fascia. In a series of gynecologic and obstetric patients, Gallup and coworkers found that 35% displayed radiographic evidence of subcutaneous gas.

Obesity and diabetes were common comorbidities in this series. The authors treated many patients with hyperbaric oxygen after débridement. Other authors have also emphasized this management option for necrotizing fasciitis.

The infection rapidly expands in the subcutaneous spaces and often tracks far beyond the superficial margins of the involved skin. If the diagnosis is questionable, a full-thickness core biopsy and frozen section of the tissue should be performed. This condition is a *life-threatening* surgical emergency, and patients should have débridement as soon as possible. It is most important for the gynecologist to have a high degree of suspicion for this condition because even with adequate surgical débridement, the mortality rate is 30% to 50%. This rare but potentially fatal condition necessitates wide débridement of all necrotic tissue, high levels of broad-spectrum antibiotics, and sometimes hyperbaric oxygen. Débridement to freely bleeding tissue helps determine the surgical margin. It is not unusual for the patient to need repetitive débridements. Women with diabetes, malnutrition, immunosuppression, malignancy, obesity, and poor tissue perfusion are most susceptible to this complication.

Dehiscence and Evisceration

Dehiscence is a failure of normal healing and literally means disruption of any of the layers of a surgical incision. The physiologic, biochemical, and structural changes that characterize normal wound healing are complex and, at best, imperfectly understood. However, clinically the most important fact to the clinician is that the strength of the wound increases over

Table 25-16 Qualities of Absorbable Sutures

Name	Material	Configuration	Absorption (days)
Surgical gut (chromic)	Animal collagen	Twisted	Unpredictable (14–80)
Monocryl	Poliglecaprone	Monofilament	Predictable (90)
Coated Vicryl	Polyglactin	Braided	Predictable (80)
Dexon	Polyglycolic acid	Braided	Predictable (90)
PDS	Polydioxanone	Monofilament	Predictable (180)
Maxon	Polyglyconate	Monofilament	Predictable (180)

From Weintraub SL, Weng Y, Hunt JP, O'Leary JP: Principles of perioperative and operative surgery. In Townsend CM, Beauchamp RD, Evers BM, et al (eds): Sabiston Textbook of Surgery, 17th ed. Philadelphia, Saunders, 2004, p 255.

time. The strength of a skin incision increases at a rapid and almost constant rate for the first 4 months and at a much slower rate for the first year. Clinically, dehiscence usually means that the previous incision of the skin, subcutaneous tissue, and fascia has separated, but not the peritoneum. This complication usually occurs during the first 2 postoperative weeks. Often dehiscence is recognized immediately or within the first 24 hours following the removal of skin clips. Evisceration is a complete breakdown of the healing process through all levels of the abdominal incision, with omentum or bowel presenting through the incision.

The incidence of wound dehiscence is approximately 1 in 200 gynecologic operations. The major short-term result of wound dehiscence is the prolongation of hospital stay. Over the long term, dehiscence predisposes to incisional hernias. Wound dehiscence is a rare cause of surgical mortality, especially in debilitated patients. Wound infection is present in approximately 50% of women with wound disruption. As with wound infections, preventive management is the most important therapeutic consideration. The incidence of dehiscence has decreased with the use of longer lasting and stronger sutures. Many clinicians prefer to use PDS, a treated Vicryl, or a permanent suture such as polypropylene (Prolene) for greater strength and prolonged presence in the tissue. The rule of thumb is that the suture should remain strong in the tissue until the tissue can resume its original strength. In patients with the propensity for poor or prolonged healing, such as women with malignancy, diabetes, or immune suppression, the use of permanent suture should be strongly considered. When infection is present, monofilament suture is preferable to a braided or polyfilament suture (Tables 25-16 and 25-17).

The consensus of authorities regarding fascial disruption is that local factors are much more important in the pathophysiology of wound disruption than are systemic factors, although both should be considered in preventive management. Important mechanical factors predisposing to disruption are conditions that increase the tension on the incision line, such as abdominal distention and chronic lung disease, or a technically inadequate closure of the wound. Other factors include obesity, advanced age, malignancy, uremia, liver failure, diabetes, hypoproteinemia, hematoma formation, sepsis, corticosteroids or chemotherapy, prior radiation therapy, and whether the incision is made through an area of a previous incision. Whether an incision is horizontal or vertical has little effect on the incidence of wound disruption. The pathophysiology of fascial dehiscence involves exaggerated collagen lysis in the wound. Clinically the sutures "tear through the fascia" rather than dissolving or becoming "untied." For example, approximating and tying sutures too vigorously, especially with a figure-of-8 suture, may lead to strangulation and necrosis of the tissue and subsequent wound dehiscence. Primary mass closure with a continuous monofilament, delayed-absorbable suture helps to avoid this problem in high-risk patients.

The classic symptom and sign of wound disruption is the spontaneous passage of copious serosanguineous fluid from the abdominal incision. Most often this occurs between the fifth and eighth postoperative days. Patients with uninfected wounds generally have been asymptomatic. Patients who develop wound defects often lack the normal "healing ridge" of tissue that can be palpated in normal healing wounds.

Imperative for prevention of wound dehiscence is proper closure of the incision in a woman at high risk for less than optimum healing. Although there are many regional preferences for the choice of suture and method of closure, the most popular technique is some modification of the Smead–Jones closure with permanent suture (Fig. 15-12). Closure with the Smead–Jones technique results in a dehiscence rate of approximately 1 in 1000 operations. With this technique it is important to place individual sutures at least 1 to 1.5 cm away from the adjacent sutures and include at least 2 cm of fascia on either side of the incision. The alternative technique is a mass closure using a monofilament permanent suture material such as nylon or Prolene. Delayed primary wound closure 3 to 5 days after the operation should be considered if the wound was contaminated during the procedure, such as with rupture of a tuboovarian abscess. Also, delayed closure should be considered for any patient already at high risk for wound complications, such as

Table 25-17 Qualities of Nonabsorbable Sutures

Name	Material	Configuration	Comments
Silk	Silk	Braided	Good handling and knotting characteristics; low durability of tensile strength
Ethilon	Polyamide (nylon)	Monofilament	Tissue reactivity minimal; good tensile strength over time
Dermalon	Polyamide (nylon)	Braided	Less tissue cutting in braided form
Prolene	Polyolefin (polypropylene)	Monofilament	Low reactivity, excellent retained tensile strength
Dacron	Polyester	Braided	Superior strength and durability; poor choice in contaminated field
Tevdek	Polyester (coated with Teflon—heavy)	Braided	Coating minimizes tendency to cut tissue

From Weintraub SL, Weng Y, Hunt JP, O'Leary JP: Principles of perioperative and operative surgery. In Townsend CM, Beauchamp RD, Evers BM, et al (eds): Sabiston Textbook of Surgery, 17th ed. Philadelphia, Saunders, 2004, p 255.

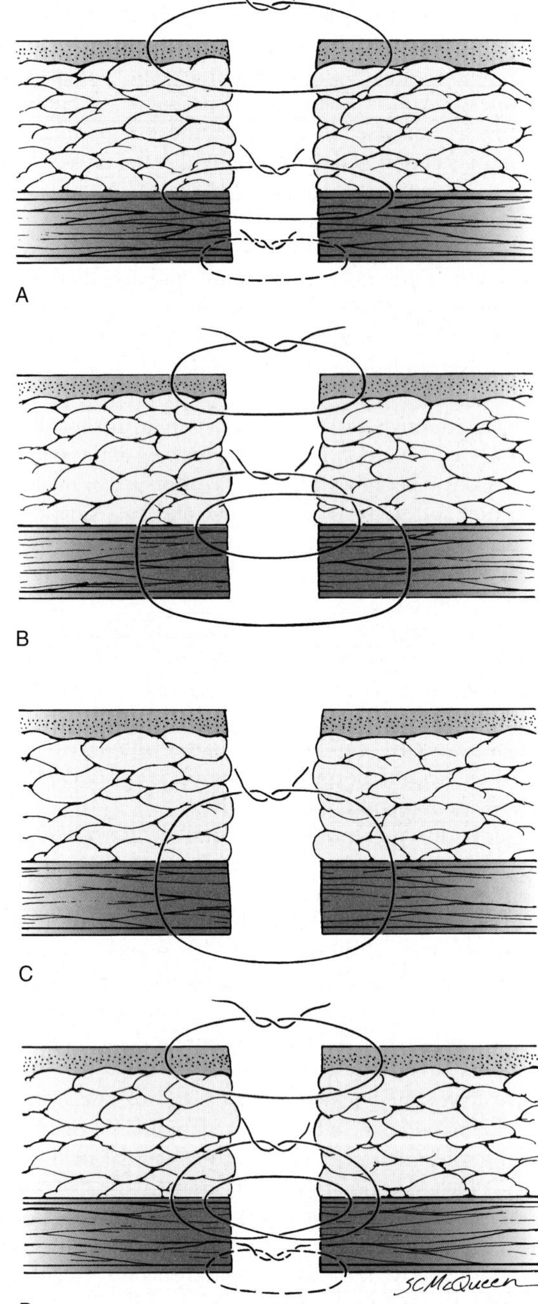

Figure 25-12. Types of abdominal incision closures. **A,** Layered. **B,** Smead–Jones. **C,**Through-and-through. **D,** Far-near. (From Braun TE: Wound dehiscence. In Schaefer G, Graber EA [eds]: Complications in Obstetric and Gynecological Surgery. Hagerstown, MD, Harper & Row, 1981, p 159.)

those who are malnourished, diabetic, markedly obese, or immunosuppressed.

Rarely, the vaginal cuff may rupture, producing dehiscence and vaginal evisceration of abdominal contents. This complication often presents with sudden vaginal bleeding and pain. Croak and colleagues reviewed 12 cases of vaginal evisceration; prior pelvic surgery and postmenopausal surgery for enterocele were common predisposing factors (Table 25-18). If there is no evidence of infection, the vaginal cuff may be closed primarily without opening the abdomen. If secondary issues are present that may inhibit healing (immunosuppression, for example) or if infection is suspected, then an abdominal approach should be considered. Antibiotic treatment with broad-spectrum coverage should be strongly considered. Vaginal evisceration is uncommon, but when it occurs, it is usually several weeks after surgery.

Table 25-18 Predisposing Factors to Evisceration*

Predisposition	Clinical Number/Number with Data Reported (%)
Postmenopausal (age > 51 yr)	9/12 (75)
Prior pelvic surgery	10/12 (83)
Postmenopausal with surgery	9/12 (75)
Enterocele and vaginal vault	10/12 (83)
Posterior enterocele	6/12 (50)
Vaginal cuff defect	4/12 (33)
Coital trauma	1/12 (8)
Spontaneous	7/12 (58)
Trauma	1/12 (8)

*Total numbers reported for each predisposition were limited by availability of data. Some patients had more than one predisposition.
From Croak AJ, Gelshart JB, Kingele CJ, et al: Characteristics of patients with vaginal vault rupture and evisceration. Obstet Gynecol 103:573, 2004.

The treatment of wound disruption is prompt reclosure in the operating room. On the hospital ward, once the diagnosis is recognized, the wound and viscera should be covered with most sterile gauze and broad-spectrum antibiotics begun. Once the patient is anaesthetized, the wound may be completely reopened and evaluated, depending on the size and the depth of the defect. Similar to the management of wound infections, digital examination of the defect is important so that the full extent of the problem will be recognized. With larger defects the wound edges must be débrided and the wound closed with a modified Smead–Jones or mass closure technique.

When a closure of a hernia is indicated during surgery, either as part of the primary surgery or after débridement, two principles are emphasized. The closure should be sterile, with all signs of infection resolved. Secondly, mesh should be used to close the defect. Studies have noted a significantly lower disruption rate with mesh closure than with suture.

OPERATIVE SITE COMPLICATIONS

Pelvic Cellulitis and Abscess

Infections of the contiguous retroperitoneal space immediately above the vaginal apex are common complications following abdominal or vaginal hysterectomy. However, the frequency of this postoperative complication has dramatically decreased in direct relation to the use of prophylactic antibiotics. These soft tissue infections range in severity from localized, minor cellulitis to large pelvic abscesses and have many names, from "cuff cellulitis" to "infected hematoma." Nevertheless, they are similar to soft tissue infections in other parts of the body and are either a cellulitis or an abscess. These infections prolong hospital stay and increase the cost of patient care. The bacterial spectrum that produces these infections includes aerobic and anaerobic bacteria from both exogenous and endogenous sources. Most postoperative pelvic infections are polymicrobial, usually from endogenous vaginal flora, and approximately 60% to 80% involve anaerobic organisms.

The pathophysiology of development of retroperitoneal infection is straightforward. The classic clamp-crush-cut-and-tie technique used in pelvic surgery produces an abundance of hypoxic and anoxic tissue that helps to establish an optimal environment for infection. This environment is further enhanced by the normal retroperitoneal hysterectomy site, producing an average of 40 mL of serosanguineous fluid each day during the first 72 postoperative hours. The endogenous flora of the upper vagina colonize and multiply in this retroperitoneal serosanguineous fluid and in pelvic hematomas after the operation.

The major symptoms of an operative site infection are fever associated with lower quadrant abdominal and pelvic pain. The fever usually becomes prominent between the third and fifth postoperative days. As the infection becomes more severe, the fever becomes spiking in character, the pain intensifies, and the patient develops moderate leukocytosis.

The diagnosis of cuff cellulitis is confirmed by pelvic examination. Pelvic tenderness and induration are prominent during the bimanual examination. A subtle difference exists between normal postoperative pelvic tenderness and induration and the tenderness and induration produced by infection. Postoperative infection is accompanied by an increase in suprapubic pain and lateral parametrial tenderness. Cuff cellulitis sometimes responds to drainage by opening the vaginal cuff. Appropriate cultures of the site are difficult with cellulitis because of vaginal contamination. Persistent cellulites or one encompassing a large area, or a pelvic abscess, necessitate parenteral antibiotic therapy. Often the diagnosis of a retroperitoneal abscess is confirmed when the patient has ongoing fever and pelvic tenderness after 2 to 3 days of parenteral antibiotics for a suspected cuff cellulitis. Eason and associates reported that the volume of pelvic fluid 3 to 5 days postoperatively after a hysterectomy is a nonspecific finding and does not predict febrile morbidity or the need for drainage. They further commented that large or complex fluid collections may be present without adverse clinical consequences. CT-directed biopsy may aid in diagnosis.

Because of their polymicrobial origin, the infections are usually treated with an aminoglycoside (gentamicin) and an antibiotic specific for anaerobic infection (clindamycin). Metronidazole (Flagyl) may be substituted for clindamycin. An alternative therapy is substitution of a third-generation cephalosporin or the monobactam agent aztreonam (Azactam) for the aminoglycoside. Aztreonam has a similar spectrum of antibiotic coverage with much less renal toxicity; however, it is much more expensive. IV antibiotics should be continued until the patient is afebrile for 24 hours. Recent studies have documented that oral antibiotic therapy is unnecessary following successful parenteral therapy. Alternatives to the aminoglycoside/clindamycin regimen include broad-spectrum antibiotics combined with β-lactamase inhibitors such as ampicillin/sulbactam, amoxicillin/clavulanate, piperacillin/tazobactam, or ticarcillin/clavulanate. These drugs have better coverage of Enterobacteriaceae species and *Enterococcus.* Although many pelvic abscesses drain spontaneously, patients should have serial pelvic examinations and endovaginal ultrasound or CT imaging to determine the most appropriate time and modality to effect drainage. Appropriate cultures should be obtained from the center of an abscess cavity when the abscess is operatively incised. If a patient does not become afebrile within 48 hours of adequate drainage of a retroperitoneal abscess, a concomitant complication of pelvic thrombophlebitis should be suspected. If pelvic thrombophlebitis is suspected, a 72-hour trial of IV heparin therapy with concurrent antibiotics should be instituted.

Granulation Tissue

Granulation tissue at the apex of the vaginal vault is a frequent complication following hysterectomy. Small areas of friable, red granulation tissue are seen at the 6-week postoperative pelvic examination in more than 50% of women. Granulation tissue is more common following abdominal than vaginal hysterectomy. Colombo and coworkers found that the incidence of both cuff cellulitis and formation of granulation tissue was no different between women with the vaginal cuff left open and those in whom it was closed after abdominal hysterectomy. Manyonda and colleagues conducted a prospective randomized trial of women with total abdominal hysterectomies, comparing polyglactin (Vicryl) and chromic catgut for closure of the cuff. In this study 32% of the women had developed vault granulation tissue by their 6-week postoperative checkup. Of women who developed granulation tissue, chromic catgut was implicated twice as frequently as polyglactin suture, 68% versus 32%, respectively.

Excessive granulation tissue is the result of an exaggerated healing response of the vascular-rich pelvic tissues. One of the causes is believed to be inversion of the vaginal epithelium between the margins of the edges of the incision at the apex of the vaginal vault.

Some patients are asymptomatic, but many women experience spotting or a bloody discharge after intercourse. A rare patient may have mild pelvic discomfort. On speculum examination the granulation tissue appears as a polypoid projection hanging from the vaginal suture line. The differential diagnosis includes a prolapsed fallopian tube and recurrent carcinoma in a patient with a pelvic malignancy. The polypoid mass is easily avulsed from the vaginal apex. The remaining areas of granulation tissue should be treated with a chemical cautery (silver nitrate or Monsel's solution) or by cryocautery or electrocautery.

Prolapsed Fallopian Tube

Prolapse of the distal end of the fallopian tube is a rare complication of abdominal or vaginal hysterectomy. It is usually discovered during a routine visit during the first few months following the operation. Factors that may predispose a woman to develop prolapse of the fallopian tube include hematoma formation and postoperative pelvic infection.

Many women with this complication are free of symptoms, but others experience a watery discharge, postcoital spotting and pain, or moderate lower abdominal and pelvic pain. Differing from granulation tissue, the fallopian tube is not friable and is firmly attached. Grasping the fallopian tube with an instrument and applying traction produces much more pain than traction on granulation tissue. Treatment is the destruction of the segment of the fallopian tube protruding through the vaginal vault with cryocautery or the laser. Because the fallopian tube is well innervated, any destructive procedure must be performed with anesthesia. The fallopian tube may be removed during a subsequent outpatient procedure with adequate anesthesia. Most clinicians opt for a vaginal approach with ligation of the fallopian tube as high as possible. The stump of the tube is buried retroperitoneally and the vaginal epithelium closed. Some difficult cases must be performed transabdominally via the laparoscope or minilaparotomy. An alternative treatment is coagulation of the segment of fallopian tube protruding through the vaginal apex with cryocautery. Because of the tube's innervation, this must be done with anesthesia. Often the vaginal wall reepithelializes over the area, thereby excluding the tube from any connection with the vaginal cavity.

Lymphocyst

A lymphocyst is a local collection of lymphatic fluid within the retroperitoneal spaces of the pelvis resulting from retrograde drainage of lymph. It is a rare complication, discovered most frequently after pelvic node dissections. In the past this complication occurred in approximately 20% of patients having undergone radical operations. However, with meticulous attention to ligation of distal lymphatic channels and abandonment of the practice of reperitonealization, this complication is reported in less than 5% of such cases. A peritoneal opening or "peritoneal window" allows flow of the lymphatic fluid into the peritoneal cavity with subsequent peritoneal resorption. The incidence is lower in series where palpation alone is used to identify the cysts. If ultrasound examination is used postoperatively to screen for lymphocysts, the incidence is 10-fold greater. Conditions that predispose the patient to formation of a lymphocyst are previous radiation and anticoagulation.

Lymphocysts usually present during the first 6 postoperative weeks. They vary greatly in size and seldom become infected. The cyst usually begins anterior and medial to the iliac vessels. As it expands, it may produce pelvic pain, leg pain, fever, obstruction or angulation of the ureter, pressure symptoms on the bladder, or partial venous obstruction. Small lymphocysts, less than 4 cm in diameter, are usually asymptomatic and regress spontaneously within 8 weeks. Larger cysts may necessitate treatment either by intermittent aspiration or marsupialization performed laparoscopically, or placement of an omental flap.

Ovarian Abscess

Ovarian abscess is a rare but serious postoperative complication. This condition is potentially fatal because of intraperitoneal rupture of the abscess. Ovarian abscesses arise from bacterial colonization of the ovarian cortex without primary involvement of the fallopian tube. This may occur either via disruption of the ovarian capsule by the presence of a recently ruptured corpus luteum or via an operative disruption, such as cystectomy performed during vaginal hysterectomy.

The disease may follow either a slow, indolent course or a rapidly progressive one. Some patients with this complication present during the first postoperative week with high fever and severe pain, which are continuous until rupture occurs. Other patients will be afebrile, but return sometime during the first few months with a persistent low-grade fever and mild pain. Chronologically, most ovarian abscesses appear later in the postoperative course compared with other retroperitoneal abscesses. Ovarian abscesses usually appear 2 to 3 weeks postoperatively, but cases have been reported as late as 3 to 4 months later. Willson and Black, in a classic work describing 28 patients with ovarian abscess, noted that the predominant symptom was abdominal pain associated with persistent tachycardia and high fever. This abscess is found higher in the pelvis than a retroperitoneal abscess at the apex of the vagina.

Initial treatment is medical therapy with IV antibiotics. However, most patients do not respond to medical therapy, and drainage of the abscess becomes a necessity either percutaneously with imaging directed aspiration, or surgically. If surgical drainage is required, the abdominal approach is preferable. This rare problem should be considered in any woman having a gynecologic operation in which the integrity of the ovarian capsule is disrupted either physiologically or operatively.

Postoperative Neuropathy

Postoperative neuropathy is an uncommon but significant and sometimes debilitating problem. A review of gynecologic injuries by Irvin and associates found the three most common causes of neuropathy to be related to self-retaining retractors, overly flexed thighs when women are placed in the dorsal lithotomy position, and by surgical resection.

The femoral nerve is the largest branch of the lumbar plexus and arises from the primary dorsal rami of L2, L3, and L4. It provides motor function to several leg muscles, including the quadriceps, and sensory fibers that innervate the anterior and medial surfaces of the thigh and leg. The vascular supply to the femoral nerve may be compromised during an abdominal or vaginal hysterectomy. The cause of this complication is most commonly related to continuous pressure, usually by a self-retaining retractor producing ischemic necrosis of the nerve. The vascular circulation of the nerve itself is compromised by diminished blood flow in the vasa nervorum. The most common site of nerve compression is 4 to 6 cm above the inguinal ligament where the nerve pierces the psoas muscle.

Factors that contribute to the development of this complication are thinness of the patient, long retractor blades, prolonged operative times, and systemic diseases such as diabetes mellitus, gout, alcoholism, and malnutrition. The classic patient who develops this complication is a short, thin, athletic woman who has a transverse incision in which a self-retaining retractor is used. A similar problem may develop after vaginal operations or laparoscopy in thin women who are placed into exaggerated hip flexion or abduction in the dorsal lithotomy position. Dunnihoo and colleagues reported on 33 cases of femoral neuropathy after vaginal hysterectomy. Femoral neuropathy following vaginal surgery is believed to be secondary to compromise of the nerve by severe angulation of the woman, not secondary to pressure injury from retractors.

Patients with this complication may experience numbness, paresthesias, and difficulty with their gait. Patients may have difficulty lifting the affected knee because of the involvement of the quadriceps. Symptoms may present with a spectrum of severity. Usually the neurologic symptoms develop within the first 24 to 72 hours following an operation. These symptoms are causes of great anxiety to the patient. Because of the inability to lift the leg, climbing stairs is a particular problem. The muscle and sensory function recovers spontaneously over several weeks to several months. The patient should be seen by a physical therapist to facilitate ambulation and prevent muscle atrophy.

To prevent this complication, it is important to palpate the lateral pelvic wall and femoral artery after placement of a self-retaining retractor. With the woman in the lithotomy position, one should check for pulsations in the popliteal or posterior tibial vessels. In a thin patient, placing folded towels between the skin surface and the self-retaining retractor helps to prevent this complication by decreasing the depth of penetration of the lateral retractor blades.

The ilioinguinal and iliohypogastric nerves pass in a transverse and diagonal course through the anterior lower abdominal musculature medial to the inguinal ligament and through the inguinal canal. The nerves supply sensory fibers to the labia, mons pubis, and medial thigh. The nerves may become injured during an operation with a Pfannenstiel incision or during urinary incontinence procedures (Fig. 25-13). Pathophysiologically, the nerve may be transected or entrapped by suture or scar formation. Sharp or burning pain may develop immediately postoperatively or usually within a few days. The pain may radiate to the groin or vulva. Most symptoms will resolve spontaneously. Severe pain may necessitate nerve block or suture removal, or segmented removal of the involved nerve.

When pain does not resolve and becomes chronic, it develops a central nervous system (CNS) component. Thus, many patients with long-standing pain will respond to CNS-directed therapies. Mendell and Sahenk have reviewed sensory neuropathies. Tricyclic antidepressants; selective serotonin-reuptake inhibitor (SSRI) medications; and anticonvulsants such as carbamazepine, gabapentin, and lamotrigine, have been found to be effective adjunctive agents for this complication. Long-term pain in the incision may also be related to small neuromas that may need excision.

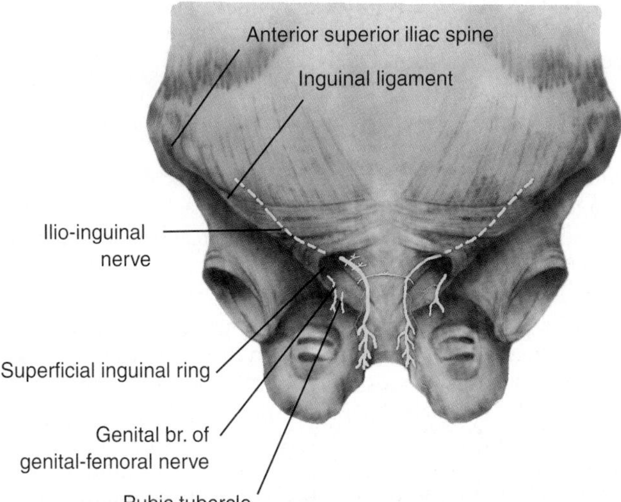

Figure 25-13. Ilioinguinal nerve entrapment during needle suspension for stress incontinence. (From Miyazaki F, Shook G: Ilioinguinal nerve entrapment during needle suspension for stress incontinence. Obstet Gynecol 80:246, 1992.)

ESTROGEN REPLACEMENT

Bilateral salpingo-oophorectomy is sometimes performed on young women for conditions such as pelvic inflammatory disease. National surveys have documented that bilateral salpingo-oophorectomy concomitant with hysterectomy is performed in approximately 25% of premenopausal women. Removal of ovaries in a premenopausal woman reduces the serum estradiol concentrations by approximately 80% and serum testosterone concentrations by approximately 50%. The possible consequences of estrogen deprivation include vasomotor symptoms, urogenital tissue atrophy (atrophic vaginitis, dyspareunia, and urethral syndrome), and osteoporosis. Removal of the ovaries in premenopausal women may lead to clinically significant sexual dysfunction.

Estrogen replacement is indicated in the vast majority of premenopausal women having bilateral oophorectomy. The increase in hypercoagulability produced by the doses of estrogen used for postmenopausal symptoms is negligible. Nevertheless, because of the physiologic hypercoagulability and injury to the intima of vessels associated with the operative procedure, oral estrogen therapy should not be started immediately after the procedure. Theoretically, estradiol given via a cutaneous patch is more acceptable in the immediate postoperative period than oral estrogen because of the difference in effect of the associated relative decrease in the liver's production of clotting factors. An oral tablet of 0.625 mg of conjugated estrogens daily is sufficient to protect from bone demineralization and osteoporosis. A higher dose may be required to alleviate hot flushes. Most women in the perimenopausal age range who undergo oophorectomy will also develop symptomatic hot flushes. In general, women may be given estrogen replacement when they become symptomatic. This may occur within a few days to a week after surgery. Transdermal estrogen produces significantly fewer changes in coagulation factors than oral estrogen. We prescribe a 0.05–0.1 estradiol patch to premenopausal women without risk factors to use estrogen, starting 2 days after surgery. In women older than 40, we await symptoms. The small amount of evidence regarding estrogen replacement in this setting indicates that quality of life improves after hysterectomy, and that sexual function is not adversely affected.

PSYCHOLOGICAL SEQUELAE

Pain Relief

The proper management of pain during the postoperative period should be a primary goal of all gynecologists. Most women experience moderate to severe pain during the first 36 to 48 hours following a gynecologic operation. However, pain and suffering are personal, internal events, the extent and presence of which may best be measured by direct communication with

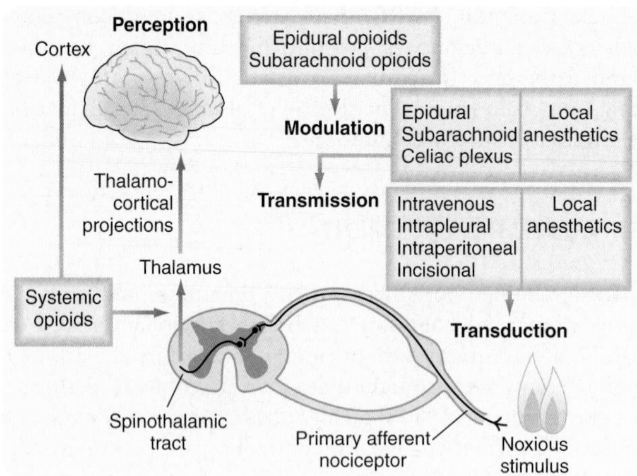

Figure 25-14. Schematic drawing of the pathways for transmission of painful stimuli. (From Sherwood E, Williams CG, Prough DS: Anaesthesiology principles, pain management, and conscious sedation. In Townsend CM, Beauchamp RD, Evers BM, et al [eds]: Sabiston Textbook of Surgery, 17th ed. Philadelphia, Saunders, 2004, p 456.)

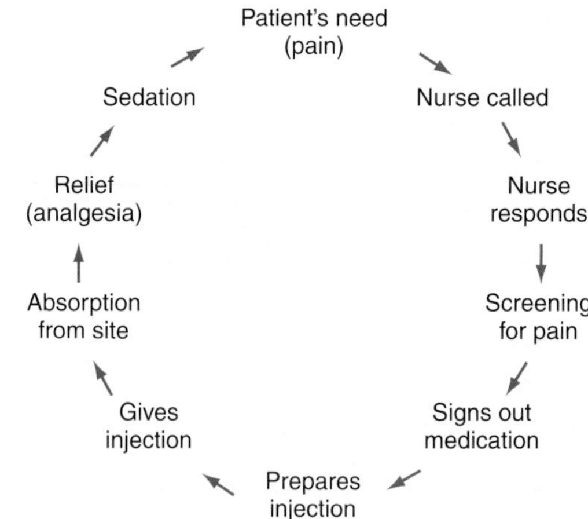

Figure 25-15. Pain cycle. (From White PF: Pain management (special report). Postgrad Med 80:8, 1986.)

the patient. Pain is initiated at the local level through the trauma of the surgery. Systemic and neurologic pathways are then activated (Fig. 25-14). The most effective pain management strategies involve inhibiting the initiation and activation of these broader pain reflexes. Such inhibition is also associated with the fewest side effects.

The current literature documents that pain relief is often treated inadequately in postoperative patients. For many women who undergo gynecologic operations, dosages of analgesics are prescribed that are less than adequate to relieve pain, and many nurses further reduce the amount of medication. The many misconceptions concerning postoperative pain include the dangers of addiction and the fear of respiratory depression. Kuhn and colleagues have emphasized that it is not only physicians and nurses who contribute to ineffective treatment. Patients also contribute by having a lower level of pain relief expectation. These authors believe that pain relief is poor because of inadequate education of patients in what to expect from pain relief. Inadequate pain relief prolongs hospital stay and has adverse psychological consequences. Additionally, several investigators have noted that inadequately treated pain increases secondary morbidities, including atelectasis from decreased mobility, increased inflammatory response, and elevated glucose with higher catecholamines. Studies have shown that epidural anesthesia (presumably by inhibiting the spinal pain reflexes) to have a significantly diminished effect on the immune response in patients undergoing laparotomy. Syndromes of chronic pain are presumed to begin with inadequate pain relief in the postoperative period.

More than two decades ago, White presented a schematic representation of the pain cycle and the potential delays in pain relief with traditional "prn" analgesic regimens (Fig. 25-15). Many studies have confirmed that regular-interval preventive pain relief is superior to conventional "on demand" analgesic medication during the first 36 to 48 hours after the operation. However, there is great variability in absorption. In addition, the therapeutic window (the range of effective blood concentration before undesired side effects occur) is narrow.

In White's study, peak concentrations varied as much as fivefold among the 10 different individuals and the time to reach peak blood level varied as much as sevenfold. Thus patient-controlled analgesic (PCA) systems have become one of the preferred methods of pain relief during the immediate postoperative period (Fig. 25-16). PCA systems dramatically decrease patients' anxiety because they are in control rather than the hospital staff. These systems are both safe and effective as long as there is a lockout period, and they help to minimize individual differences in pharmacokinetics. Modern PCA systems minimize the risk of drug overdose and allow the patient to titrate and therefore maximize analgesic effectiveness. In general, patients use the PCA system for approximately 12 to 36 hours until they are completely tolerating oral feeding. Meta-analysis from Remy and coworkers found that the addition of acetaminophen with an opioid PCA reduces the amount of opioid needed. Sample dosing for PCA is listed in the following box. Women should be given instructions concerning PCA systems to alleviate inherent fears of addiction. Their families need instruction in not pushing the medication for the patient to help alleviate their pain. PCA is less effective in elderly patients who are more affected by confusion and disorientation.

Perioperative injections of opioids intrathecal or epidural effectively relieve postoperative pelvic pain in most situations. Side effects are primarily itching and a small risk of hypotension. Continuous PCA epidurals may also be used. The advantages and disadvantages of patient-controlled analgesia and epidural anesthesia are characterized in Table 25-19.

In addition to narcotics, NSAIDs are valuable as adjunctive agents. NSAIDs are most effective when given as scheduled medications and as early as possible in the postoperative period. Their mechanism of action is the inhibition of prostaglandin production. Through inhibition of prostaglandins, pain is prevented rather than blocked centrally. NSAID have three potential side effects. The first is H_2 blockers or proton pump inhibitors. Renal toxicity may be prevented by using set doses and prescribing only for women with normal renal function with adequate intravascular volume. Third, is inhibition of platelet function with higher doses of NSAID. Some clinicians will wait 1 to 2 hours after surgery before giving these medica-

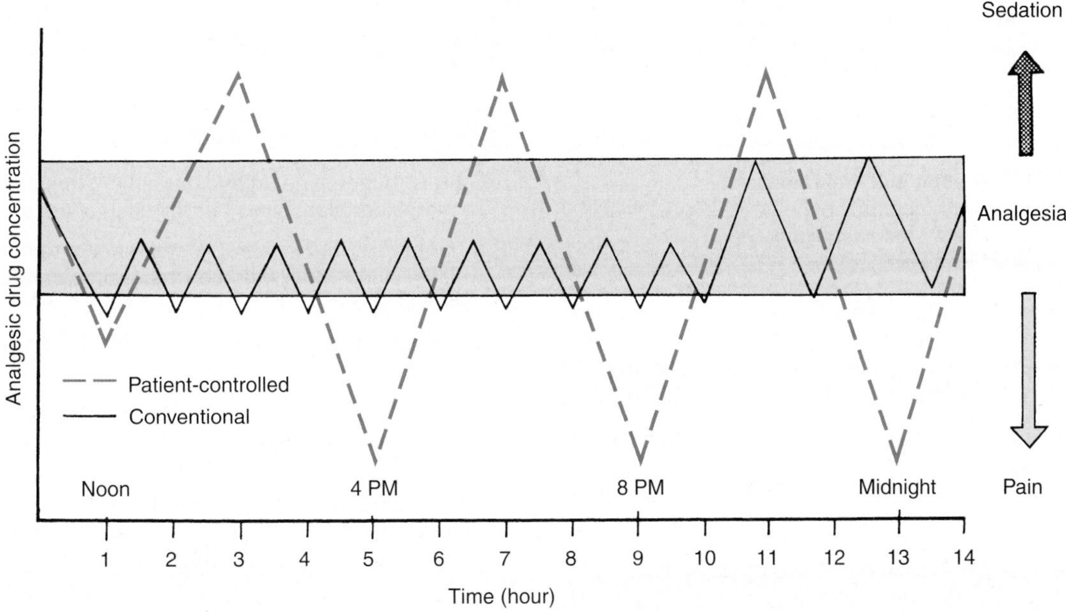

Figure 25-16. Theoretic relationships among dosing interval, analgesic drug concentration, and clinical effects when comparing patient-controlled analgesic (PCA) system *(solid lines)* with conventional intramuscular therapy *(dashed lines)*. (Redrawn from White PF: Semin Anesthesiol 4:255, 1985.)

tions to avoid excessive bleeding. Advantages of prostaglandin synthetase inhibitors are a lack of effect on gastrointestinal motility and a much smaller effect on sensorium than narcotic agents. Commonly used NSAIDs for postoperative pain include ibuprofen, naproxen, and ketorolac (Toradol). Ketorolac may be given as an intramuscular or IV injection during the operative procedure. Intramuscular injections reach peak plasma levels in 40 to 50 minutes, with a half-life of 4 to 6 hours. The dose is an intramuscular loading dose of 30 to 60 mg followed with 15 to 30 mg every 6 hours during the first 24 to 36 hours. More commonly, ketorolac is given intravenously every 4 to 6 hours, 15 to 30 mg. The drug works well when given concomitantly with narcotics. Toradol should not be used for more than 4 consecutive days because of GI side effects. In the elderly, changes in GI function may limit the usefulness of these agents. Stomach colonization with *Helicobacter pylori* increases with increasing age. Eighty percent of women older than 80 are colonized. These bacteria increase sensitivity to gastrointestinal irritation. Prophylactic H_2 blockers or proton pump inhibitors should be considered when administering NSAID to older patients.

Many of the side effects of the NSAIDs are due to cyclo-oxygenase-1 (COX) inhibition. The development of selective COX-2 inhibitors has promise, though warnings regarding cardiovascular side effects have limited their acceptance at this time. Sample protocols for pain orders are listed in the following box.

Many surgeons and anesthesiologists believe that giving analgesics in the perioperative period prior to the patient's sensation of pain (giving them preemptively) leads to better pain control. Many studies have noted that the beneficial effects are significant when infiltration is given prior to the surgical incision. Because much of the pain arises from peritoneal irritation and fascial trauma, incisional infiltration is most effective with minimally invasive procedures such as laparoscopy. Infiltration is most commonly employed with a local anesthetic, lidocaine 1%, or bupivacaine, 0.25%.

Psychosexual Problems and Depression

The time immediately before and after a surgical procedure is a stressful period for all women and their families. Anxiety and fear are normal responses and should be anticipated by health care providers. Any operation on the female reproductive organs

Table 25-19 Advantages and Disadvantages of Epidural Analgesia and Patient-Controlled Analgesia

	Epidural	Patient-Controlled
Advantages	Immediate pain relief May improve colon motility May improve postoperative pulmonary function after lower abdominal and pelvic surgery Less sedating than patient-controlled analgesia	Requires no special nursing or anesthesia support postoperatively Gives the patient "personal control" over administration of pain medication
Disadvantages	Requires a skilled anesthesiologist for correct placement May interfere with ambulation May delay removal of Foley catheter	Patient may experience pain in the recovery room until an adequate serum level of medication is achieved

From Baker VV: Principles of postoperative care. In Baker VV, Deppe G (eds): Management of Perioperative Complications in Gynecology. Philadelphia, WB Saunders, 1997, p 141.

Sample PCA Dosing Guidelines

NOT NPO, NOT POSTOP, PAIN SCORE < 4 to 6

Pain Score	Medication and Treatment
<4	Start with acetaminophen or Darvocet N–100
4–5	Start with Vicodin or Norco
5–6	Start with Percocet

If on ketorolac, discontinue and start ibuprofen

NOT NPO, NOT POSTOP, PAIN SCORE ≥ 6

1. Continue oral meds and supplement with IV push opioids, max 2 doses
2. Discontinue oral meds and start PCA or start IV push opioids

OVERSEDATION

If patient develops a level of sedation score of "4" per Analgesic Sedation/Precaution Scale, or if the respiratory rate ≤ 10 per minute and SaO_2 < 94 on 3 L of O_2:

Start naloxone (Narcan) titration; use oxygen until the patient is fully recovered. Careful titration of the dose of naloxone (Narcan) in cases of mild respiratory depression will reverse the side effects of opioids without reversing analgesia. Hold any further opioid doses until patient awake/alert with SaO_2 > 94, respiratory rate ≥ 10. *Respiratory rate and quality are paramount.*

NPO, POSTOP, or PAIN SCORE ≥ 6

1. Start with morphine unless the patient has a true allergy to morphine: rash, hives, airway edema, anaphylaxis.
2. If the patient has intolerable side effects to morphine, which includes **poor pain control,** switch to hydromorphone.
3. If the patient has a true allergy to morphine, start with fentanyl.
4. If the patient's pain is not controlled with morphine PCA, switch to hydromorphone. If hydromorphone does not control the pain, call the physician.
5. If the patient is on a PCA, **do not** administer oral analgesics for breakthrough pain. Call the physician.
6. If the patient remains alert and oriented after initial IV push dose of opioid, a PCA of that opioid may be initiated. If the patients is mentally or physically incapable of using a PCA and remains painful, continue to administer IV push opioids.
7. Initial PCA settings should be based on the patient's history, age, general condition, and weight. Start at the lowest dose and increase the dose as ordered on the Dosing Regimen for PCA or IV push opioids below before switching to another pain medication.
8. There is no continuous dosing on a PCA while following the Acute Pain Management orders.

Dosing Regimen for PCA or IV push opioids

Maximum hourly total dose includes both IV push per Nurse dose and PCA dose

	IV Push per Nurse			PCA		Hourly Limit
	Nurse Bolus Dose As Needed	Maintenance Dose As Needed	Maximum Hourly Dose	Nurse Bolus Dose	Maintenance Dose	Maximum Dose per Nurse and PCA Doses Combined
MORPHINE						
Pain Score < 6 or Age > 65	1–5 mg every 10 minutes	1–5 mg every 2–3 hours	**15 mg**	1–5 mg	1–2 mg with 6–10 minute lockout	**15 mg**
Pain Score ≥ 6 + Age ≤ 65 + weight > 50 kg	5–10 mg every 10 minutes	5–10 mg every 2–3 hours	**15 mg**	5–10 mg	1–3 mg with 6–10 minute lockout	**15 mg**
HYDROMORPHONE (DILAUDID)						
Pain Score < 6 or Age > 65	0.2–1.0 mg every 10 minutes	0.2–1.0 mg every 2–3 hours	**3 mg**	0.2–1.0 mg	0.2–0.4 mg with 6–10 minute lockout	**3 mg**
Pain Score ≥ 6 + Age ≤ 65 + weight > 50 kg	1–2 mg every 10 minutes	1–2 mg every 2–3 hours	**3 mg**	1–2 mg	0.2–0.6 mg with 6–10 minute lockout	**3 mg**
FENTANYL						
Pain Score < 6 or Age > 65	10–50 µg every 10 minutes	10–50 µg every 1–2 hours	**200 µg**	10–50 µg	10–20 µg with 6–10 minute lockout	**200 µg**
Pain Score ≥ 6 + Age ≤ 65 + weight > 50 kg	50–100 µg every 10 minutes	50–100 µg every 1–2 hours	**200 µg**	50–100 µg	20–30 µg with 6–10 minute lockout	**200 µg**

Notify physician if maximum medication dose is not producing adequate pain relief (i.e. Pain Score > 5)

Courtesy of Sacred Heart Medical Center, Eugene, OR.

second visit at 5 to 6 weeks after the procedure. If vaginal surgery or vaginal pain or pressure is present, then a vaginal examination may be indicated.

The discussion of surgical findings occurs at several points during the postoperative period. Initially patients are drowsy after waking up from anesthesia or IV analgesics. Families may want to know the results prior to the patient hearing them. It is important to clarify preoperatively, with the woman, who in the family can know what information. During the early postoperative period the gynecologist must judge how much information to provide. This should be tailored to what the patient can understand, depending on her level of wakefulness. Honesty at all times is the basic ethical principle; however, if the patient is waking up from anesthesia she obviously will not be able to understand a detailed description of operative findings. The art of medicine is called into play at this point in knowing how much to explain. By the end of the first few days the discussion may move to details of surgical findings as well as treatment options, sequelae, and prognosis if a long-term problem has been found.

KEY POINTS

- Often, the woman and her family judge the competence of the gynecologist by the compassion displayed during the immediate postoperative period.
- Diurnal fluctuations are characteristic of the daily body temperature patterns of humans. A normal temperature is usually 37.2° C in the morning and 37.7° C overall.
- Postoperative febrile morbidity is related to infection in approximately 20% of cases and noninfectious causes in 80% of cases.
- The pathophysiology of postoperative fever is primarily related to the release of cytokines.
- Intraoperative factors that dramatically increase the risk of postoperative fever are an operative time longer than 2 hours and intraoperative transfusion.
- The proper workup of a postoperative fever involves three classic steps of history, physical examination, and laboratory evaluations, with the major emphasis placed on the physical examination.
- The findings of the history and especially the physical examination should guide the extent of the laboratory tests ordered. Ordering a specific list of laboratory tests when a fever occurs is unrewarding.
- Approximately 75% of patients develop a temperature greater than 37° C, which is usually not associated with an infectious process.
- Infection in the elderly will not always present with classic findings. The amount of temperature elevation may not reflect the severity of the infection. Not uncommonly, the first signs of infection in the elderly will be mental status change. Additionally, the degree of leukocytosis may not reflect infection also, being blunted or absent.
- Minimum urine output should be 0.5 mL/kg/hr. The use of 20 mL/hr benchmark for all women is only an approximation, which should be adjusted for a patient's weight.
- Because of the shifts in water balance, the postoperative hematocrit at 72 hours is a more accurate measurement of operative and postoperative blood loss than a hematocrit at 24 hours.
- The normal physiologic response to the stress of an operation and tissue destruction is release of increased levels of antidiuretic hormone and aldosterone, producing both sodium and water retention.
- After subtracting the effects of the operative blood loss from the preoperative hematocrit, a further reduction in hematocrit of 3 to 5 points reflects a postoperative hemorrhage of approximately 500 mL.
- Women older than 60, and those with significant cardiac and pulmonary comorbidity should be transfused if their hematocrit falls below 30%.
- Microatelectasis is a common occurrence developing during almost all pelvic operations, and it is persistent 24 hours postoperatively in approximately 50% of women. Current studies have demonstrated that there is no association between fever and the amount of atelectasis diagnosed radiologically.
- Factors that predispose patients to atelectasis include supine position, obesity, smoking, age older than 60 years, prolonged operative time, presence of nasogastric tube, and coexisting medical conditions such as cardiac disease or pulmonary infection.
- The clinical presentation of fever, tachypnea, and tachycardia within 72 hours of an operation is pathognomonic for atelectasis.
- Early mobilization and ambulation have been documented to be as effective as chest physical therapy in the prevention of pulmonary complications.
- Postoperative pneumonia is commonly associated with atelectasis, with predisposing factors including chronic pulmonary disease, heavy cigarette smoking, alcohol abuse, obesity, older age, nasogastric tubes, long procedures, gram-negative bacterial infections, postoperative peritonitis, and debilitating illnesses.
- Radiographic diagnoses are approximately 60% accurate for either bacterial or viral pneumonia in women with laboratory-proven pneumonia.
- In the perioperative period, hypovolemia may be secondary to several factors, including preoperative volume deficit, unreplaced blood loss during surgery, extracellular fluid loss during surgery, inadequate fluid replacement, and, most commonly, continued blood loss after the surgical procedure.
- Tachycardia is the classic cardiovascular physiologic response of the body to hypotension. However, relative bradycardia in hypotensive women is also a common hemodynamic response.
- Rapid loss of 20% of a woman's blood volume produces mild shock, whereas a loss of greater than 40% of blood volume results in severe shock.

Continued

KEY POINTS *Continued*

- From 15% to 45% of surgical blood loss is absorbed onto drapes, pads, and other areas. Thus blood levels in the suction bottle are inaccurate markers of total operative blood loss.
- Massive blood loss recently has been defined as hemorrhage that results in replacement of 50% of circulating blood volume in less than 3 hours.
- The differential diagnosis of hemorrhagic shock in the postoperative patient includes pneumothorax, pulmonary embolus, massive pulmonary aspiration, myocardial infarction, and acute gastric dilation.
- The goals of management of shock are to replace, restore, and maintain effective circulating blood volume and to establish normal cellular perfusion and oxygenation. To accomplish this goal, an adequate cardiac output and appropriate peripheral vascular resistance must be maintained.
- In hemorrhagic shock crystalloids should be considered the initial resuscitation fluid of choice; colloids are appropriate for resuscitation in conjunction with crystalloids when blood products are not immediately available.
- The gold standard of imaging studies to detect abdominal and pelvic hemorrhage is a CT scan performed without either oral or IV contrast.
- Returning a patient to the operating room to control hemorrhage is often a difficult decision. However, this decision should not be postponed, and the patient should have an exploratory operation as soon as possible after volume replacement.
- The extent of wound or pelvic hematomas is determined by the potential size of the compartment into which the bleeding occurs. Retroperitoneal or broad ligament hematomas may contain several units of blood.
- Superficial thrombophlebitis is frequently overlooked or disregarded as a cause of postoperative fever.
- Recurrent, superficial phlebitis, in varying anatomic sites, may be a sign of occult malignant disease.
- Approximately 30% of all hospital-acquired bacteremias are secondary to IV lines.
- Superficial phlebitis is the leading cause of an enigmatic postoperative fever during the third, fourth, or fifth postoperative day.
- The clinical management of mild superficial thrombophlebitis includes rest, elevation, and local heat. Moderate to severe superficial thrombophlebitis may be treated with nonsteroidal antiinflammatory agents.
- Generally, thromboembolic complications occur early in the postoperative course: 50% within the first 24 hours and 75% within the first 72 hours. Approximately 15% occur after the seventh postoperative day.
- Diagnosis of deep vein thrombophlebitis by physical examination is very insensitive. Thus imaging studies are essential for establishing the correct diagnosis.
- Venous thrombosis and PE are the direct causes of approximately 40% of deaths in gynecologic cases.
- The reported incidence of DVT with gynecologic operations varies from 7% to 45%, with an average of approximately 15%.
- The incidence of thrombophlebitis is directly dependent on the risk factors of type and duration of operation, age of the woman, obesity, immobility, malignancy, sepsis, diabetes, current oral contraceptive use, and conditions producing venous stasis.
- Thrombophlebitis most often begins in the deep veins of the calf. Approximately 75% of pulmonary emboli originate from a thrombus that begins in the leg veins and extends to the femoral veins.
- The three precipitating factors that produce thrombi, as described by Virchow, are an increase in coagulability, damage to the vessel wall, and venous stasis.
- D-Dimer blood assay levels are helpful in excluding the diagnosis of deep vein thrombophlebitis in an individual woman when the clinical result is below the cut-off level.
- Heparin is the drug of choice for the initial treatment of thrombosis or PE once the diagnosis is confirmed.
- Failure to achieve adequate anticoagulation in the first 24 hours of therapy increases the risk of recurrent venous thromboembolism 15-fold.
- The primary risk of chronic anticoagulation therapy is the potential for major bleeding complications. Major bleeding occurs in approximately 4% of woman-years of therapy.
- Autopsy studies have documented that pulmonary emboli are undiagnosed clinically in approximately 50% of women who experience this complication.
- Women with pulmonary emboli have a mortality rate of 30% in untreated cases versus 8% in treated cases.
- Signs and symptoms of pulmonary emboli are nonspecific; however, the most common symptoms are chest pain, dyspnea, apprehension, tachypnea, rales, and an increase in the second heart sound over the pulmonic area.
- Ventilation/perfusion scans are the first line in imaging techniques to rule out the diagnosis of PE. However, pulmonary angiography is the most definitive test in establishing the diagnosis. Five percent of patients experience complications from pulmonary angiography.
- The risk of a woman developing a subsequent fatal PE during the 3 months of anticoagulation therapy is approximately 1 in 70 to 1 in 100.
- The possible causes of postoperative voiding problems include anxiety, mechanical interference, obstruction by swelling and edema, overdistention from hydration, neurologic imbalance, drug-associated detrusor hypotonia, and dysynchronous bladder contractions.
- Intermittent in-and-out catheterization is preferable to continuous drainage with a Foley catheter for women with intermediate-term voiding dysfunction. Women especially appreciate intermittent self-catheterization because it gives them control over a part of their postoperative care.
- The most commonly acquired infection in the hospital and most frequent cause of gram-negative bacteremia in hospitalized patients is catheter-associated UTI.
- Prophylactic antibiotics should not be used with a Foley catheter to cover for the possibility of UTI unless the patient is immunocompromised.

KEY POINTS *Continued*

- In the United States, urinary fistulas following gynecologic operations are secondary to abdominal hysterectomy in 75% of cases and to vaginal procedures in the remaining 25%.
- The ratio of operative injuries to the urinary bladder compared with ureteral injuries is approximately 5:1.
- Although symptoms of urinary incontinence may present within a few hours of the operative procedure, the majority of fistulas usually present 8 to 12 days after operation, occasionally as late as 25 to 30 days after the operation.
- If there is a suspicion that trauma to the bladder has occurred during an operative procedure, continuous catheter drainage for 3 to 5 days usually results in spontaneous healing.
- Approximately 25% of adult women experience postoperative nausea and vomiting.
- An uncomplicated ileus may last 24 to 48 hours in the stomach, only a few hours in the small intestines, and 48 to 72 hours in the colon.
- If adynamic ileus persists for longer than 5 days, a diagnosis of mechanical bowel obstruction should be strongly considered.
- Multiple recent articles report early postoperative oral feeding is safe and efficacious. This practice is preferred by women because it facilitates their recovery and shortens hospital stay.
- The difference between small-bowel obstruction and adynamic ileus is a subtle one, for adynamic ileus is normally associated with partial obstruction of the small intestine.
- Previous gynecologic operations are the most common cause of bowel obstruction in women.
- Pneumoperitoneum from an exploratory celiotomy usually persists for 7 to 10 days. Thus, in the early postoperative period, free air under the diaphragm is not diagnostic of perforation of a hollow viscus.
- After the diagnosis of a defect between the vagina and rectum has been made, the woman should be obstipated with a low-residue diet and diphenoxylate hydrochloride (Lomotil). Approximately one in four anatomic defects heals spontaneously before epithelialization of the tract occurs.
- *Clostridium difficile* is a species of spore-forming, gram-positive anaerobic bacteria found normally in 1% of healthy adults. However, after antibiotic treatment and disruption of normal enteric flora, up to 25% of hospitalized adults will become colonized with *C. difficile.*
- Second- and third-generation cephalosporins, clindamycin, ampicillin, and amoxicillin, are the antibiotics associated with the highest risk of developing *C. difficile* diarrhea.
- The incidence of postoperative wound infection is increased eightfold when the woman's preoperative weight exceeds 200 pounds. The thickness of subcutaneous tissue is the greatest risk factor for wound infection in women undergoing abdominal hysterectomy.
- Symptoms of wound infections occur most commonly between the fifth and tenth postoperative day, with the patient usually exhibiting tachycardia and fever.
- Delayed secondary closure may be accomplished in previously infected wounds after several days of drainage and débridement. Delayed secondary closure markedly reduces the time necessary for eventual closure of the skin defect by secondary intention. Patient satisfaction dramatically increased with delayed secondary closure.
- Necrotizing fasciitis involves the subcutaneous tissue and superficial fascia. It rapidly expands in the subcutaneous spaces. If the diagnosis is questionable, a full-thickness core biopsy and frozen section of the tissue should be performed. This condition is a surgical emergency, and patients should have operative débridement as soon as possible.
- The incidence of wound dehiscence is approximately 1 in 200 gynecologic operations. Wound infection is found in approximately 50% of women with wound disruption.
- The classic symptom and sign of an impending wound disruption is the spontaneous passage of copious serosanguineous fluid from the abdominal incision.
- Most postoperative pelvic infections are polymicrobial, usually from endogenous vaginal flora, and approximately 60% to 80% involve anaerobic organisms.
- The volume of pelvic fluid 3 to 5 days postoperatively after a hysterectomy is a nonspecific finding and does not predict febrile morbidity or the need for drainage.
- If a patient does not become afebrile within 48 hours of adequate drainage of a retroperitoneal abscess, a concomitant complication of pelvic thrombophlebitis should be suspected. If pelvic thrombophlebitis is suspected, a 72-hour trial of IV heparin therapy with concurrent antibiotics should be instituted.
- Granulation tissue at the apex of the vaginal vault is a frequent complication following hysterectomy. Small areas of friable, red granulation tissue are seen at the 6-week postoperative pelvic examination in more than 50% of women.
- Ovarian abscesses arise from bacterial colonization of a disrupted ovarian capsule, usually by the presence of a recently ruptured corpus luteum or by operative disruption during a procedure.
- Ovarian abscesses usually present 2 to 3 weeks postoperatively, but cases have been reported as late as 3 to 4 months.
- Common causes of femoral neuropathy are continuous pressure from self-retaining retractors or exaggerated hip flexion or abduction in the dorsal lithotomy position in thin women.
- Patient-controlled analgesic systems dramatically decrease patients' anxiety because they are in control rather than the hospital staff. These systems are both safe and effective as long as there is a lockout period, and they help to minimize individual differences in pharmacokinetics.
- Any operation on the female reproductive organs stimulates questions and conflicts concerning body image, feminine identity, sexuality, and possibly future childbearing.
- Discharge instructions should be given in both verbal and written forms, and the gynecologist should anticipate the most common questions.

BIBLIOGRAPHY

Acute Respiratory Distress Syndrome Network: Ventilation with lower tidal volumes as compared with traditional tidal volumes for acute lung injury and the acute respiratory distress syndrome. N Engl J Med 342:1301, 2000.

Agnelli G, Becattini C, Kirschstein T: Thrombolysis vs heparin in the treatment of pulmonary embolism. Arch Intern Med 162:2537, 2002.

Ahmed AB, Hobbs GJ, Curran JP: Randomized, placebo-controlled trial of combination antiemetic prophylaxis for day-case gynaecological laparoscopic surgery. Br J Anaesth 85:678, 2000.

Akca O, Doufas AG, Sessler DI: Use of selective opiate receptor inhibitors to prevent postoperative ileus. Minerva Anestesiol 68:162, 2002.

Al-Took S, Platt R, Tulandi T: Adhesion-related small-bowel obstruction after gynecologic operations. Am J Obstet Gynecol 180:313, 1999.

American College of Endocrinology: Position statement on inpatient diabetes and metabolic control. Endocrine Practice 10, 2004.

American College of Obstetricians and Gynecologists: Lower urinary tract operative injuries. ACOG Educ Bull 238:1, 1997.

Apfel CC, Korttila K, Abdalla M, et al: A factorial trial of six interventions for the prevention of postoperative nausea and vomiting. N Engl J Med 350:2441, 2004.

Arcasoy SM, Kreit JW: Thrombolytic therapy of pulmonary embolism: A comprehensive review of current evidence. Chest 115:1695, 1999.

Arozullah AM, Khuri SF, Henderson WG, et al: Development and validation of a multifactorial risk index for predicting postoperative pneumonia after major noncardiac surgery. Ann Intern Med 135:847, 2001.

Asao T, Kuwano H, Nakamura J, et al: Gum chewing enhances early recovery from postoperative ileus after laparoscopic colectomy. J Am Coll Surg 195:30, 2002.

Atkinson TP, Kaliner MA: Anaphylaxis. Med Clin North Am 76:841, 1992.

AuBuchon JP, Birkmeyer JD: Controversies in transfusion medicine: Is autologous blood transfusion worth the cost? Con Transfusion 34:79, 1994.

Baig MK, Wexner SD: Postoperative ileus: A review. Dis Colon Rectum 47:516, 2004.

Baldo BA: Penicillins and cephalosporins as allergens-structural aspects of recognition and cross-reactions. Clin Exp Allergy 29:744, 1999.

Barnes J, Resch KL, Ernst E: Homeopathy for postoperative ileus? A meta-analysis. J Clin Gastroenterol 25:628, 1997.

Barone JG, Cummings KB: Etiology of acute urinary retention following benign anorectal surgery. Am Surg 60:210, 1994.

Bartlett JG: Antibiotic-associated diarrhea. N Engl J Med, 346, 2002.

Bates SM, Ginsberg JS: Treatment of deep-vein thrombosis. N Engl J Med 351:268, 2004.

Bates SM, Kearon C, Crowther M, et al: A diagnostic strategy involving a quantitative latex D-dimer assay reliably excludes deep venous thrombosis. Ann Intern Med, 138:787, 2003.

Batres F, Barclay DL: Sciatic nerve injury during gynecologic procedures using the lithotomy position. Obstet Gynecol 62:92S, 1983.

Bauer AJ, Boeckxstaens GE: Mechanisms of postoperative ileus. Neurogastroenterol Motil 16:54, 2004.

Behm B, Stollman N: Postoperative ileus: Etiologies and interventions. Clin Gastroenterol Hepatol 1:71, 2003.

Beilin B, Shavit Y, Trabekin E, et al: The effects of postoperative pain management on immune response to surgery. Anesth Analg 97:822, 2003.

Belda FJ, Aguilera L, de la Asuncion JG, et al: Supplemental perioperative oxygen and the risk of surgical wound infection. JAMA 294:2035, 2005.

Bergqvist D, Agnelli G, Cohen AT, et al: Duration of prophylaxis against venous thromboembolism with enoxaparin after surgery for cancer. N Engl J Med 346:975, 2002.

Bernardi E, Prandoni P, Lensing AWA, et al: D-dimer testing as an adjunct to ultrasonography in patients with clinically suspected deep vein thrombosis: Prospective cohort study. BMJ 317:1037, 1998.

Birdwell BG, Raskob GE, Whitsett TL, et al: The clinical validity of normal compression ultrasonography in outpatients suspected of having deep venous thrombosis. Ann Intern Med 128:1, 1998.

Bloom SL, Ramin SM, Gilstrap LC: Blood and blood component therapy. Prim Care Update Ob/Gyns 4:200, 1997.

Boardman A: Diagnosis and management of pseudomembranous colitis and *Clostridium difficile*-associated disease. Prim Care Update Ob/Gyns 5:219, 1998.

Bonnar J: Can more be done in obstetric and gynecologic practice to reduce morbidity and mortality associated with venous thromboembolism? Am J Obstet Gynecol 180:784, 1999.

Bounameaux H, Reber-Wasem MA: Superficial thrombophlebitis and deep vein thrombosis: A controversial association. Arch Intern Med 157:1822, 1997.

Breddin HK, Hach-Wunderle V, Nakov R, et al: Effects of a low molecular weight heparin on thrombus regression and recurrent thromboembolism in patients with deep-vein thrombosis. N Engl J Med 344:626, 2001.

Bregenzer T, Conen D, Sakmann P, Widmer AF: Is routine replacement of peripheral intravenous catheters necessary? Arch Intern Med 158:151, 1998.

Broomhead CJ: Physiology of postoperative nausea and vomiting. Br J Hosp Med 53:327, 1995.

Broussard EK, Surawicz CM: Probiotics and prebiotics in clinical practice. Nutr Clin Care 7:104, 2004.

Brown MD, Rowe BH, Reeves MJ, et al: The accuracy of the enzyme-linked immunosorbent assay D-dimer test in the diagnosis of pulmonary embolism: A meta-analysis. Ann Emergency Med 40, 2002.

Bungard TJ, Kale-Pradhan PB: Prokinetic agents for the treatment of postoperative ileus in adults: A review of the literature. Pharmacotherapy 19:416, 1999.

Campbell IA, Fennerty A, Miller AC: British thoracic society guidelines for the management of suspected acute pulmonary embolism. Thorax 58:470, 2003.

Cancio LC, Cohen DJ: Heparin-induced thrombocytopenia and thrombosis. J Am Coll Surg 186:76, 1998.

Caprini JA, Glase CJ, Anderson CB, et al: Laboratory markers in the diagnosis of venous thromboembolism. Circulation 109, 2004.

Carpenter JP, Holland GA, Baum RA, et al: Magnetic resonance venography for the detection of deep vein thrombosis: Comparison with contrast venography and duplex Doppler ultrasonography. J Vasc Surg 18:734, 1993.

Carr JA, Silverman N: The heparin-protamine interaction: A review. J Cardiovasc Surg 40:659, 1999.

Carson JL, Willett LR: Is a hemoglobin of 10 g/dL required for surgery? Med Clin North Am 77:335, 1993.

Carter CJ: The natural history and epidemiology of venous thrombosis. Prog Cardiovasc Dis 36:423, 1994.

Cassar K, Munro A: Surgical treatment of incisional hernia. Br J Surg 89:534, 2002.

Castro CJ, Krammer J, Drake J: Postoperative feeding: A clinical review. Obstet Gynecol Surv 55:571, 2000.

Cataldo PA, Senagore AJ, Kilbride MJ: Ketorolac and patient controlled analgesia in the treatment of postoperative pain. Surg Obstet Gynecol 176:435, 1993.

Caumo W, Schmidt AP, Schneider CN, et al: Risk factors for postoperative anxiety in adults. Anaesthesia 56:720, 2001.

Challis DE, Bennett MJ: Nerve entrapment—an important complication of transverse lower abdominal incisions. Aust N Z J Obstet Gynaecol 34:5, 1994.

Chassany O, Michaux A, Bergmann JF: Drug-induced diarrhoea. Drug Safety 22:53, 2000.

Chumbley GM, Hall GH, Salmon P: Patient-controlled analgesia: an assessment by 200 patients. Anaesthesia 53:216, 1998.

Chunilal JD, Eikelboom JW, Attia J, et al: Does this patient have pulmonary embolism? JAMA 290:2849, 2003.

Clarke-Pearson DL, Synan IS, Dodge R, et al: A randomized trial of low-dose heparin and intermittent pneumatic calf compression for the prevention of deep venous thrombosis after gynecologic oncology surgery. Am J Obstet Gynecol 168:1146, 1993.

Colombo M, Maggioni A, Zanini A, et al: A randomized trial of open versus closed vaginal vault in the prevention of postoperative morbidity after abdominal hysterectomy. Am J Obstet Gynecol 173:1807, 1995.

Correia MI, da Silva RG: The impact of early nutrition on metabolic response and postoperative ileus. Curr Opin Clin Nutr Metab Care 7:577, 2004.

Croak AJ, Gebhart JB, Klingele CJ, et al: Characteristics of patients with vaginal rupture and evisceration. Obstet Gynecol 103:572, 2004.

Cronan JJ: Venous thromboembolic disease: The role of US. Radiology 186:619, 1993.

Cruikshank MK, Levine MN, Hirsch J, et al: A standard heparin homogram for the management of heparin therapy. Arch Intern Med 151:333, 1991.

Cruse PJE, Foord R: A 5-year prospective study of 23,649 surgical wounds. Arch Surg 107:206, 1973.

Cutillo G, Maneschi F, Franchi M, et al: Early feeding compared with nasogastric decompression after major oncologic gynecologic surgery: A randomized study. Obstet Gynecol 93:41, 1999.

Cuzen N, Haque R, Timmis A: Applications of thrombolytic therapy. Intensive Care Med 24:756, 1998.

Dalen JE, Alpert JS: Thrombolytic therapy for pulmonary embolism: Is it effective? Is it safe? When is it indicated? Arch Intern Med 157:2550, 1997.

Darouiche RO, Raad II, Heard SO, et al: A comparison of two antimicrobial-impregnated central venous catheters. N Engl J Med 340:1, 1999.

Dauzat M, Laroche JP, Deklunder G, et al: Diagnosis of acute lower limb deep venous thrombosis with ultrasound: trends and controversies, J Clin Ultrasound 25:343, 1997.

Davis JD: Prevention, diagnosis, and treatment of venous thromboembolic complications of gynecologic surgery. Am J Obstet Gynecol 184, 2001.

Decousus H, Leizorovica A, Parent F, et al: A clinical trial of vena cava filters in the prevention of pulmonary embolism in patients with proximal deep-vein thrombosis. N Engl J Med 338:409, 1998.

DeLancey JOL, Hartman RG: Operations on the abdominal wall. In Sciarra JJ (ed): Gynecology and Obstetrics. Philadelphia, JB Lippincott, 1992.

Demetriades D, Chan LS, Bhasin P, et al: Relative bradycardia in patients with traumatic hypotension. J Trauma Inj Infec Crit Care 45:534, 1998.

DeMoerloose P, Michiels JJ, Bounameaux H: The place of D-Dimer testing in an integrated approach of patients suspected of pulmonary embolism. Semin Thromb Hemost 24:409, 1998.

Di Nisio M, Middeldorp S, Büller HR: Direct thrombin inhibitors. N Engl J Med, 353:1028, 2005.

Dodds C, Allison J: Postoperative cognitive deficit in the elderly surgical patient. Br J Anaesth 81:449, 1998.

Dodson MK, Magann EF, Meeks GR: A randomized comparison of secondary closure and secondary intention in patients with superficial wound dehiscence. Obstet Gynecol 80:321, 1992.

Donaldson MDJ, Seaman MJ, Park GR: Massive blood transfusion. Br J Anaesth 69:621, 1992.

Douketis JD, Kearon C, Bates S, et al: Risk of fatal pulmonary embolism in patients with treated venous thromboembolism. JAMA 279:458, 1998.

Doyle NM, Ramirez MM, Mastrobattista JM, et al: Diagnosis of pulmonary embolism: A cost-effectiveness analysis. Am J Obstet Gynecol 191:1019, 2004.

Ducic I, Moxley M, Al-Attar A: Algorithm for treatment of postoperative incisional groin pain after cesarean delivery or hysterectomy. Obstet Gynecol 108:27, 2006.

Duff GW: Is fever beneficial to the host: a clinical perspective. Yale J Biol Med 59:125, 1986.

Dunn LJ, Van Voorhis LW: Enigmatic fever and pelvic thrombophlebitis. N Engl J Med 276:265, 1967.

Dunnihoo DR, Huddleston HT, North SC: Femoral nerve palsy as a complication of vaginal hysterectomy: Review of the world literature. J Gynecol Surg 10:1, 1994.

Eason E, Aldis A, Seymour RJ: Pelvic fluid collections by sonography and febrile morbidity after abdominal hysterectomy. Obstet Gynecol 90:58, 1997.

Eiseberg E: Post-surgical neuralgia. Pain 111:3, 2004.

Ejlersen E, Andersen HB, Eliasen K, et al: A comparison between preincisional and postincisional lidocaine infiltration and postoperative pain. Anesth Analg 74:495, 1992.

Ellis H, Niran BJ, Thompson JN, et al: Adhesion-related hospital readmissions after abdominal and pelvic surgery: A retrospective cohort study. Lancet 353:1476, 1999.

Engoren M: Lack of association between atelectasis and fever. Chest 107:81, 1995.

Fanning J, Neuhoff RA, Brewer JE, et al: Frequency and yield of postoperative fever evaluation. Infec Dis Obstet Gynecol 6:252, 1998.

Fareed J, Hoppensteadt DA, Bick RL: Management of thrombotic and cardiovascular disorders in the new millennium. Clin Appl Thromb/Hemost 9:101, 2003.

Farrell SA, Kieser K: Sexuality after hysterectomy. Obstet Gynecol 95:1045, 2000.

Fiessinger J-N, Huisman MV, Davidson BL, et al: Ximelagatran vs low-molecular-weight heparin and warfarin for the treatment of deep vein thrombosis. JAMA 293:681, 2005.

Finan MA, Barton DPJ, Fiorica JV, et al: Ileus following gynecologic surgery: Management with water-soluble hyperosmolar radiocontrast material. South Med J 88:539, 1995.

Fleenor-Ford A, Hayden MK, Weinstein RA: Vancomycin-resistant enterococci: Implications for surgeons. Surgery 125:121, 1999.

Fong SY, Pavy TJG, Yeo ST, et al: Assessment of wound infiltration with bupivacaine in women undergoing day-case gynecological laparoscopy. Reg Anesth Pain Med 26:131, 2001.

Francis KR, Lamaute HR, Davis JM, Pizzi WF: Implications of risk factors in necrotizing fasciitis. Am Surg 59:304, 1993.

Fraser JD, Anderson DR: Deep venous thrombosis: recent advances and optimal investigation with US. Radiology 211:9, 1999.

Friera A, Olivera MJ, Suarez C, et al: Clinical validity of negative helical computed tomography for clinical suspicion of pulmonary embolism. Respiration 71:30, 2004.

Frost SD, Brotman DJ, Michota F: Rational use of D-dimer measurement to exclude acute venous thromoembolic disease. Mayo Clin Proc 78:1385, 2003.

Fujii Y, Tanaka H, Somekawa Y: Granisetron, droperidol, and metoclopramide for the treatment of established postoperative nausea and vomiting in women undergoing gynecologic surgery. Am J Obstet Gynecol 182:13, 2000.

Furnary AP, Wu YX, Bookin SO: Effect of hyperglycemia and continuous intravenous insulin infusions on outcomes of cardiac surgical procedures: The Portland diabetic project. Endocr Pract 10:21, 2004.

Gallup DG, Freedman MA, Meguiar RV, et al: Necrotizing fasciitis in gynecologic and obstetric patients: a surgical emergency. Am J Obstet Gynecol 187:305, 2002.

Gallup DG, Nolan TE, Smith RP: Primary mass closure of midline incisions with a continuous polyglyconate monofilament absorbable suture. Obstet Gynecol 76:872, 1990.

Gan TJ, Meyer T, Apfel CC, et al: Consensus guidelines for managing postoperative nausea and vomiting. Anesth Analg 97:62, 2003.

Gandhi GY, Nuttall GA, Abel MD, et al: Intraoperative hyperglycemia and perioperative outcomes in cardiac surgery patients. Mayo Clin Proc 80:862, 2005.

Gawande AA, Studdert DM, Orav EJ, et al: Risk factors for retained instruments and sponges after surgery. N Engl J Med 348:229, 2003.

Ghosh S, Sallam S: Patient satisfaction and postoperative demands on hospital and community services after day surgery. Br J Surg 81:1635, 1994.

Gilmour DT, Dwyer PL, Carey MP: Lower urinary tract injury during gynecologic surgery and its detection by intraoperative cystoscopy. Obstet Gynecol 94:883, 1999.

Ginsberg JS, Wells PS, Kearson C, et al: Sensitivity and specificity in a rapid whole-blood assay for D-dimer in the diagnosis of pulmonary embolism. Ann Intern Med 129:1006, 1998.

Giuntini C, Di Ricco G, Marini C, et al: Epidemiology. Chest 107:S3, 1995.

Goh JTW, Gregora MG, Welch M: Lithotomy position-induced femoral neuropathy. Aust N Z J Obstet Gynaecol 34:596, 1994.

Goldhaber SZ, Elliot CG: Acute pulmonary embolism: part II risk stratification, treatment, and prevention. Circulation 108:2834, 2003.

Goldhaber SZ, Elliott CG: Acute pulmonary embolism: part I epidemiology, pathophysiology, and diagnosis. Circulation 108:2726, 2003.

Goldhaber SZ, Simons GR, Elliott CG, et al: Quantitative plasma D-dimer levels among patients undergoing pulmonary angiography for suspected pulmonary embolism. JAMA 270:2819, 1993.

Gowen GF: Long tube decompression is successful in 90% of patients with adhesive small bowel obstruction. Am J Surgery 185:512, 2003.

Grady D, Sawaya G: Postmenopausal hormone therapy increases risk of deep vein thrombosis and pulmonary embolism. Am J Med 105:41, 1998.

Greer BE, Cain JM, Figge DC, et al: Supraumbilical upper abdominal midline incision for pelvic surgery in the morbidly obese patient. Obstet Gynecol 76:471, 1990.

Grimes DA: A simplified device for intraoperative autotransfusion. Obstet Gynecol 72:947, 1988.

Gunnarsson PS, Sawyer WT, Montague D, et al: Appropriate use of heparin: Empiric vs nomogram-based dosing. Arch Intern Med 155:526, 1995.

Haire WD: Vena cava filters for the prevention of pulmonary embolism. N Engl J Med 338:463, 1998.

Hall JC, Heel KA, Papadimitriou JM, Platell C: The pathobiology of peritonitis. Gastroenterology 114:185, 1998.

Hammond CJ, Hassan TB: Screening for pulmonary embolism with a D-dimer assay: do we still need to assess clinical probability as well? J R Soc Med 98:54, 2005.

Harding GKM, Nicolle LE, Ronald AR, et al: How long should catheter-acquired urinary tract infection in women be treated? A randomized controlled study. Ann Intern Med 114:713, 1991.

Harrison L, McGinnis J, Crowther M, et al: Assessment of outpatient treatment of deep-vein thrombosis with low-molecular-weight heparin. Arch Intern Med 158:2001, 1998.

Hemsell DL: Post-hysterectomy cuff and pelvic cellulitis. Contemp Obstet Gynecol 32:39, 1990.

Hemsell DL: Infection after hysterectomy. Infec Dis Obstet Gynecol 5:52, 1997.

Hendrix SL, Schimp V, Martin J, et al: The legendary superior strength of the Pfannenstiel incision: A myth? Am J Obstet Gynecol 182:1446, 2000.

Hershey CO, Tomford JW, McLaren CE, et al: The natural history of intravenous catheter-associated phlebitis. Arch Intern Med 144:1373, 1984.

Hirsh J, Raschke R, Warkentin TE, et al: Heparin: Mechanism of action, pharmacokinetics, dosing considerations, monitoring, efficacy, and safety. Chest 108:S258, 1995.

Hohler A, Katz VL, Dotters DJ, Rogers RG: *Clostridium difficile* infection in obstetric and gynecologic patients. SMJ 90:889, 1997.

Horowitz E, Dekel A, Yogev Y, et al: Urine culture at removal of indwelling catheter after elective gynecologic surgery: Is it necessary? Acta Obstet Gynecol Scand 83:1003, 2004.

Hull RD, Raskob GE, Pineo GF, Brant RF: The low-probability lung scan: a need for change in nomenclature. Arch Intern Med 155:1845, 1995.

Hull RD, Raskob GE, Pineo GF, et al: A comparison of subcutaneous low-molecular-weight heparin with warfarin sodium for prophylaxis against deep-vein thrombosis after hip or knee implantation. N Engl J Med 329:1370, 1993.

Hull RD, Raskob GE, Pineo GF, et al: Subcutaneous low-molecular-weight heparin compared with continuous intravenous heparin in the treatment of proximal-vein thrombosis. N Engl J Med 326:975, 1992.

Irvin W, Andersen W, Taylor P, et al: Minimizing the risk of neurologic injury in gynecologic surgery. Obstet Gynecol 103:374, 2004.

Jacobs DG, Sing RF: The role of vena caval filters in the management of venous thromboembolism. Southeastern Surgical Congress, annual meeting, 2003.

Johnson S, Samore MH, Farrow KA, et al: Epidemics of diarrhea caused by a clindamycin-resistant strain of *Clostridium difficile* in four hospitals. N Engl J Med 341:1645, 1999.

Jones EM, MacGowan AP: Back to basics in management of *Clostridium difficile* infections. Lancet 352:505, 1998.

Joshi GP, Ogunnaike BO: Consequences of inadequate postoperative pain relief and chronic persistent postoperative pain. Anesthesiology Clin North Am 23:21, 2005.

Kakkar VV: Pathophysiologic characteristics of venous thrombosis. Am J Surg 150:1, 1985.

Kakkar VV, Cohen AT, Edmonson RA, et al: Low molecular weight versus standard heparin for prevention of venous thromboembolism after major abdominal surgery. Lancet 341:259, 1993.

Kanne JP, Lalani TA: Role of comuted tomography and magnetic resonance imaging for deep venous thrombosis and pulmonary embolism. Circulation 109:I-15, 2004.

Katz DS, Lane MJ, Mindelzun RE: Unenhanced CT of abdominal and pelvic hemorrhage. Semin Ultrasound CT MR 20:94, 1999.

Katz DS, Leung AN: Radiology of pneumonia. Clin Chest Med 20:549, 1999.

Ke RW, Portera SG, Bagous W, et al: A randomized, double-blinded trial of preemptive analgesia in laparoscopy. Obstet Gynecol 92:972, 1998.

Kearon C: Duration of venous thromboembolism prophylaxis after surgery. Chest 124:386S, 2003.

Kehlet H, Dahl JB: The value of multimodal or balanced analgesia in postoperative pain treatment. Anesth Analg 77:1048, 1993.

Kehlet H, Dahl JB: Anaesthesia, surgery, and challenges in postoperative recovery. The Lancet 362:1921, 2003.

Kelly CP, Pothoulakis C, LaMont JT: *Clostridium difficile* colitis. N Engl J Med 330:257, 1994.

Killewich LA, Sandager GP, Nguyen AH, et al: Venous hemodynamics during impulse foot pumping. J Vasc Surg 22:598, 1995.

Koltun WA, Bloomer MM, Tilberg AF, et al: Awake epidural anesthesia is associated with improved natural killer cell cytotoxicity in the perioperative period. Anesth Analg 82:492, 1996.

Konstantinides S, Geibel A, Heusel G, et al: Heparin plus alteplase compared with heparin alone in patients with submassive pulmonary embolism. N Engl J Med 347:1143, 2002.

Kraus K, Fanning J: Prospective trial of early feeding and bowel stimulation after radical hysterectomy. Am J Obstet Gynecol 182:996, 2000.

Krebs HB: Intestinal injury in gynecologic surgery: a ten-year experience. Am J Obstet Gynecol 155:509, 1986.

Krinsley JS: Effect of an intensive glucose management protocol on the mortality of critically ill patients. Mayo Clin Proc 79:992, 2004.

Kuhn S, Cooke K, Collins M, et al: Perceptions of pain relief after surgery. BMJ 300:1687, 1990.

Kuno K, Menzin A, Kauder HH, et al: Prophylactic ureteral catheterization in gynecologic surgery. Urology 52:1004, 1998.

Kyne L, Warny M, Qamar A, Kelly CP: Asymptomatic carriage of *Clostridium difficile* and serum levels of IgG antibody against toxin A. N Engl J Med 342:390, 2000.

Kyrle PA, Eichinger S: Deep vein thrombosis. The Lancet 365:1163, 2005.

Kyrle PA, Minar E, Hirschl M, et al: High plasma levels of factor VIII and the risk of recurrent venous thromboembolism. N Engl J Med 343:457, 2000.

Lam KW, Pun TC, Wong KS: Efficacy of preemptive analgesia for wound pain after laparoscopic operations in infertile women: A randomized, double-blind and placebo control study. BJOG 111:340, 2004.

Landefeld CS, Beyth RJ: Anticoagulant-related bleeding: clinical epidemiology, prediction, and prevention. Am J Med 95:315, 1993.

Leith S, Wheatley RG, Jackson IJB, et al: Extradural infusion analgesia for postoperative pain relief. Br J Anaesth 73:552, 1994.

Leizorovicz A, Simonneau G, Decousus H, Boissel JP: Comparison of efficacy and safety of low molecular weight heparins and unfractionated heparin in initial treatment of deep venous thrombosis: A meta-analysis. BMJ 309:299, 1994.

Lenhardt R, Negishi C, Sessler DI, et al: The effects of physical treatment on induced fever in humans. Am J Med 106:550, 1999.

Lensing AW, Prandoni P, Brandjes D, et al: Detection of deep-vein thrombosis by real-time B-mode ultrasonography. N Engl J Med 320:342, 1989.

Linkins LA, Bates SM Ginsberg JS, et al: Use of different D-dimer levels to exclude venous thromboembolism depending on clinical pretest probability. J Thromb Haemost 2:1256, 2004.

Liu S, Carpenter RL, Neal JM: Epidural anesthesia and analgesia: Their role in postoperative outcome. Anesthesiology 82:1474, 1995.

Lopes AD, Hall JR, Monaghan JM: Drainage following radical hysterectomy and pelvic lymphadenectomy: Dogma or need? Obstet Gynecol 86:960, 1995.

Luijenoijk RW, Hop WCJ, van den Tol P, et al: A comparison of suture repair with mesh repair for incisional hernia. N Engl J Med 343:392, 2000.

Lundberg GD: Practice parameter for the use of fresh-frozen plasma, cryoprecipitate, and platelets. JAMA 271:777, 1994.

MacFarland LV: Epidemiology, risk factors and treatments for antibiotic-associated diarrhea. Dig Dis 16:292, 1998.

Macintyre PE: Intravenous patient-controlled analgesia: one size does not fit all. Anesthesiology Clin N Am 23:109, 2005.

Mackowiak PA, Wasserman SS, Levine MM: A critical appraisal of 98.6° F, the upper limit of the normal body temperature, and other legacies of Carl Reinhold August Wunderlich. JAMA 268:1578, 1992.

Macmillan SLM, Kammerer-Doak D, Rogers RG, et al: Early feeding and the incidence of gastrointestinal symptoms after major gynecologic surgery. Obstet Gynecol 96:604, 2000.

Madan M, Alexander DJ, McMahon MJ: Influence of catheter type on occurrence of thrombophlebitis during peripheral intravenous nutrition. Lancet 339:101, 1992.

Majeski J, Majeski E: Necrotizing fasciitis: Improved survival with early recognition by tissue biopsy and aggressive surgical treatment. SMJ 90:1065, 1997.

Malins AF, Field JM, Nesling PM, Cooper GM: Nausea and vomiting after gynaecological laparoscopy: comparison of premedication with oral ondansetron, metoclopramide and placebo. Br J Anaesth 72:231, 1994.

Manganelli D, Palla A, Donnamaria V, Giuntini C: Clinical features of pulmonary embolism: doubts and certainties. Chest 107:S25, 1995.

Mann MC, Votto J, Kambe J, McNamee MJ: Management of the severely anemic patient who refuses transfusion: lessons learned during the care of a Jehovah's Witness. Ann Intern Med 117:1042, 1992.

Mann WJ, Arato M, Patsner B, et al: Ureteral injuries in an obstetrics and gynecology training program: Etiology and management. Obstet Gynecol 72:82, 1988.

Manyonda IT, Welch CR, McWhinney NA, et al: The influence of suture material on vaginal vault granulations following abdominal hysterectomy. Br J Obstet Gynaecol 97:608, 1990.

Marcantonio ER, Goldman L, Orav EJ, et al: The association of intraoperative factors with the development of postoperative delirium. Am J Med 105:380, 1998.

Marik PE: Aspiration pneumonitis and aspiration pneumonia. N Engl J Med, 344:665, 2001.

Martinelli I, Cattaneo M, Taioli E, et al: Genetic risk factors for superficial vein thrombosis. Thromb Haemost 82:1215, 1999.

McClean KL, Sheehan GJ, Harding GKM: Intraabdominal infection: A review. Clin Infect Dis 19:100, 1994.

McIntosh DG, Rayburn WF: Patient-controlled analgesia in obstetrics and gynecology. Obstet Gynecol 78:1129, 1991.

McKenzie R, Kovac A, O'Connor T, et al: Comparison of ondansetron versus placebo to prevent postoperative nausea and vomiting in women undergoing ambulatory gynecologic surgery. Anesthesiology 78:21, 1993.

Meeks GR, Waller GA, Meydrech EF, Flautt H Jr: Unscheduled hospital admission following ambulatory gynecologic surgery. Obstet Gynecol 80:446, 1992.

Melling AC, Ali B, Scott EM, et al: Effects of preoperative warming on the incidence of wound infection after clean surgery: A randomized controlled trial. The Lancet 358:876, 2001.

Mendell JR, Sahenk Z: Painful sensory neuropathy. N Engl J Med 348:1243, 2003.

Mermel LA: Prevention of intravascular catheter-related infections. Ann Intern Med 132:391, 2000.

Meyer MA, Lalich RA, Meyer MM, Widener J: Outpatient vaginal hysterectomy in a community hospital. Wis Med J 93:422, 1994.

Miyazaki F, Shook G: Ilioinguinal nerve entrapment during needle suspension for stress incontinence. Obstet Gynecol 80:246, 1992.

Mizock BA: Alterations in carbohydrate metabolism during stress: A review of the literature. Am J Med 98:75, 1995.

Moser KM, Fedullo PF, LitteJohn JK, Crawford R: Frequent asymptomatic pulmonary embolism in patients with deep vein thrombosis. JAMA 271:223, 1994.

Moss GS, Gould SA: Plasma expanders: An update. Am J Surg 155:425, 1988.

Murry BE: Vancomycin-resistant enterococcal infections. N Engl J Med 342:710, 2000.

Nelson R, Tse B, Edwards S: Systematic review of prophylactic nasogastric decompression after abdominal operations. B J Surg 92:673, 2005.

Neu HC: Emerging trends in antimicrobial resistance in surgical infections: A review. Eur J Surg S573:7, 1994.

Nyman MA, Schwenk NM, Silverstein MD: Management of urinary retention: Rapid versus gradual decompression and risk of complications. Mayo Clin Proc 72:951, 1997.

Oger E, Alhene-Gelas M, Lacut K, et al: Differential effects of oral and transdermal estrogen/progesterone regimens on sensitivity to activated protein C among postmenopausal women a randomized trial. Arterioscler Thromb Vasc Biol 23:1671, 2003.

Ost D, Tepper J, Mihara H, et al: Duration of anticoagulation following venous thromboembolism a meta-analysis. JAMA 294:706, 2005.

Page GG: The immune-suppressive effects of pain. In Machelska H, Stein C: Immune Mechanisms of Pain and Analgesia. New York, Kluwer Academic/ Plenum, 2003.

Palla A, Giuntini C: Diagnosis of pulmonary embolism: Have we reached our goal? Respiration 71:22, 2004.

Palla S, Petruzzelli S, Donnamaria V, Giuntini C: The role of suspicion in the diagnosis of pulmonary embolism. Chest 107:S21, 1995.

Patsner B: Closed-suction drainage versus no drainage following radical abdominal hysterectomy with pelvic lymphadenectomy for stage 1B cervical cancer. Gynecol Oncol 57:232, 1995.

Pearl ML, Frandina M, Mahler L, et al: A randomized controlled trial of a regular diet as the first meal in gynecologic oncology patients undergoing intraabdominal surgery. Obstet Gynecol 100:230, 2002.

Pearl ML, Valea VA, Fischer M, et al: A randomized controlled trial of early postoperative feeding in gynecologic oncology patients undergoing intra-abdominal surgery. Obstet Gynecol 92:94, 1998.

Peipert JF, Weitzen S, Cruickshank C, et al: Risk factors for febrile morbidity after hysterectomy. Obstet Gynecol 103:86, 2004.

Perrier A: Noninvasive diagnosis of pulmonary embolism. Hosp Pract 15:47, 1998.

Petty TL: The acute respiratory distress syndrome-historic perspective. Chest 105:S44, 1994.

PIOPED investigators: Value of the ventilation/perfusion scan in acute pulmonary embolism: Results of the Prospective Investigation of Pulmonary Embolism Diagnosis. JAMA 263:2753, 1990.

Ponec RJ, Saunders MD, Kimmey MB: Neostigmine for the treatment of acute colonic pseudo-obstruction. N Engl J Med 341:137, 1999.

Prandoni P, Lensing AWA, Büller HR, et al: Comparison of subcutaneous low-molecular-weight heparin with intravenous standard heparin in proximal deep-vein thrombosis. Lancet 339:441, 1992.

Ramin SM, Ramin KD, Hemsell DL: Fallopian tube prolapse after hysterectomy. SMJ 92:963, 1999.

Rathbun SW, Raskob GE, Whitsett TL: Sensitivity and specificity of helical computed tomography in the diagnosis of pulmonary embolism: a systematic review. Ann Intern Med 132:227, 2000.

Remy C, Marret E, Bonnet F: Effects of acetaminophen on morphine side-effects and consumption after major surgery meta-analysis of randomized controlled trials. B J Anaesth 94:505, 2005.

Ripley DL: Necrotizing fasciitis. Prim Care Update Ob/Gyn 7:142, 2000.

Robertson PL, Goergen SK, Waugh JR, Fabiny PJ: Colour-assisted compression ultrasound in the diagnosis of calf deep venous thrombosis. Med J Aust 163:515, 1995.

Russell JA: Management of sepsis. N Engl J Med 355:16, 2006.

Sabiston DC Jr (ed): Textbook of Surgery, 14th ed. Philadelphia, WB Saunders, 1991.

Sagar PM, Sedman P, May J, et al: Intestinal obstruction promotes gut translocation of bacteria. Dis Colon Rectum 38:640, 1995.

Saint S, Elmore JG, Sullivan SD, et al: The efficacy of silver alloy-coated urinary catheters in preventing urinary tract infection: A meta-analysis. Am J Med 105:236, 1998.

Saleh A, Fox G, Felemban A, et al: Effects of local bupivacaine instillation on pain after laparoscopy. J Am Assoc Gynecol Laparosc 8:203, 2001.

Scarabin PY, Oger E, Plu-Bureau G, et al: Differential association of oral and transdermal oestrogen-replacement therapy with venous thromboembolism risk. Lancet 362:428, 2003.

Schulman S: Care of patients receiving long-term anticoagulant therapy. N Engl J Med 349:675, 2003.

Schulman S, Rhedin AS, Lindmarker P, et al: A comparison of six weeks with six months of oral anticoagulant therapy after a first episode of venous thromboembolism. N Engl J Med 322:1661, 1995.

Schwandt A, Andrews SJ, Fanning J: Prospective analysis of a fever evaluation algorithm after major gynecologic surgery. Am J Obstet Gynecol 184:1066, 2001.

Sessler DI, Akca O: Nonpharmacological prevention of surgical wound infections. Healthc Epidemiol 35:1397, 2002.

Shifren JL, Braunstein GD, Simon JA, et al: Transdermal testosterone treatment in women with impaired sexual function after oophorectomy. N Engl J Med 343:682, 2000.

Simonneau G, Sors H, Charbonnier B, et al: A comparison of low-molecular-weight heparin with unfractionated heparin for acute pulmonary embolism. N Engl J Med 337:663, 1997.

Smith A: Postoperative pulmonary infections. Clin Evid 8:1428, 2002.

Smith AJ, Nissan A, Lanouette NM, et al: Prokinetic effect of erythromycin after colorectal surgery: Randomized, placebo-controlled, double-blind study. Dis Colon Rectum 43:333, 2000.

Soper DE, Bump RC, Hurt WG: Wound infection after abdominal hysterectomy: Effect of the depth of subcutaneous tissue. Am J Obstet Gynecol 173:465, 1995.

Spirt MJ: Antibiotics in inflammatory bowel disease: New choices for an old disease. Am J Gastroenterol 89:974, 1994.

Standards Care Committee of British Thoracic Society: Suspected acute pulmonary embolism: A practical approach. Thorax 52:S2, 1997.

Stanhope CR, Wilson TO, Utz WJ, et al: Suture entrapment and secondary ureteral obstruction. Am J Obstet Gynecol 164:1513, 1991.

Stark RP, Maki DG: Bacteriuria in the catheterized patient. N Engl J Med 311:560, 1984.

Steed HL, Capstick V, Flood C, et al: A randomized controlled trial of early versus "traditional" postoperative oral intake after major abdominal gynecologic surgery. Am J Obstet Gynecol 186:861, 2002.

Stein PD, Afzal A, Henry JW, Villareal CG: Fever in acute pulmonary embolism. Chest 117:39, 2000.

Stein PD, Hull RD, Pineo G: Strategy that includes serial noninvasive leg tests for diagnosis of thromboembolic disease in patients with suspected acute pulmonary embolism based on data from PIOPED. Arch Intern Med 155:2101, 1995.

Stephenson H, Dotters DJ, Katz V, Droegemueller W: Necrotizing fasciitis of the vulva. Am J Obstet Gynecol 166:1324, 1992.
Strickler B, Blanco J, Fox HE: The gynecologic contribution to intestinal obstruction in females. J Am Coll Surg 178:617, 1994.
Suzuki M, Ohwada M, Sato I: Pelvic lymphocysts following retroperitoneal lymphadenectomy: Retroperitoneal partial "no-closure" for ovarian and endometrial cancers. J Surg Oncol 68:149, 1998.
Swan MC, Banwell PE: The open abdomen: aetiology, classification and current management strategies. J Wound Care 14, 2005.
Swisher ED, Kahleifeh B, Polh JF: Blood cultures in febrile patients after hysterectomy: Cost-effectiveness. J Reprod Med 42:547, 1997.
Symmonds RE: Ureteral injuries associated with gynecologic surgery: prevention and management. Clin Obstet Gynecol 19:623, 1976.
Tagalakis V, Kahn SR, Libman M, et al: The epidemiology of peripheral vein infusion thrombophlebitis: A critical review. Am J Med 113:146, 2002.
Taguchi A, Sharma N, Saleem RM, et al: Selective postoperative inhibition of gastrointestinal opioid receptors. N Engl J Med 345:935, 2001.
Tai NRM, Atwal AS, Hamilton G: Modern management of pulmonary embolism. Br J Surg 86:853, 1999.
Tarkington MA, Dejter SW Jr, Bresette JF: Early surgical management of extensive gynecologic ureteral injuries. Surg Gynecol Obstet 173:17, 1991.
Thakar R, Clarkson P: Bladder, bowel and sexual function after hysterectomy for benign conditions. Br J Obstet Gynaecol 104:983, 1997.
Thomas JH: Pathogenesis, diagnosis, and treatment of thrombosis. Am J Surg 160:547, 1990.
Tønnesen H, Kehlet H: Preoperative alcoholism and postoperative morbidity. Br J Surg 83:869, 1999.
Tønnesen E, Wahlgreen C: Influence of extradural and general anaesthesia on natural killer cell activity and lymphocyte subpopulations in patients undergoing hysterectomy. Br J Anaesth 60:500, 1988.
Traill ZC, Gleeson FV: Venous thromboembolic disease. Br J Radiol 71:129, 1998.
Van Strijen MJL, de Monye W, Schiereck J, et al: Single-detector helical computed tomography as the primary diagnostic test in suspected pulmonary embolism: A multicenter clinical management study of 510 patients. Ann Intern Med 138:307, 2003.
Vedantham S, Goodwin SC, McLucas B, Mohr G: Uterine artery embolization: An underused method of controlling pelvic hemorrhage. Am J Obstet Gynecol 176:938, 1997.
Verma A, Mittal S, Kumar S: Primary ovarian abscess. Int J Gynecol Obstet 68:263, 2000.
von Gruenigen VE, Coleman RL, King MR, Miller DS: Abdominal compartment syndrome in gynecologic surgery. Obstet Gynecol 994:830, 1999.
Wallace D, Hernandez W, Schlaerth JB, et al: Prevention of abdominal wound disruption utilizing the Smead-Jones closure technique. Obstet Gynecol 56:226, 1980.
Walsh JJ, Bomar J, Wright FW: A study of pulmonary embolism and deep leg vein thrombosis after major gynaecological surgery using labelled fibrinogen-phlebography and lung scanning. J Obstet Gynaecol Br Comm 81:311, 1974.
Walters MD, Dombroski RA, Davidson SA, et al: Reclosure of disrupted abdominal incisions. Obstet Gynecol 76:597, 1990.
Ware LB, Matthay MA: The acute respiratory distress syndrome. N Engl J Med 342:1334, 2000.
Warkentin TE, Levine MN, Hirsh J, et al: Heparin-induced thrombocytopenia in patients treated with low-molecular-weight heparin or unfractionated heparin. N Engl J Med 332:1330, 1995.
Watkins DT, Robertson CL: Water-soluble radiocontrast material in the treatment of postoperative ileus. Am J Obstet 152:450, 1985.
Wells PS, Ginsberg JS, Anderson DR, et al: Use of a clinical model for safe management of patients with suspected pulmonary embolism. Ann Intern Med 129:997, 1998.
Wells PS, Hirsh J, Anderson DR, et al: Accuracy of clinical assessment of deep-vein thrombosis. Lancet 345:1326, 1995.
Wells PS, Owen C, Doucette S: Does this patient have deep vein thrombosis? JAMA 295:199, 2006.
Wetchler SJ, Dunn LJ: Ovarian abscess. Obstet Gynecol Surv 40:476, 1985.
Wheeler AP, Bernard GR: Treating patients with severe sepsis. N Engl J Med 340:207, 1999.
White PF: Pain management (special report). Postgrad Med 80:7, 1986.
White PF: Prevention of postoperative nausea and vomiting—A multimodal solution to a persistent problem. N Engl J Med 350:3511, 2004.
White RH, McGahan JP, Daschbach MM, Hartling RP: Diagnosis of deep-vein thrombosis using duplex ultrasound. Ann Intern Med 1989 111:297, 1989.
Willson JR, Black JR: Ovarian abscess. Am J Obstet Gynecol 90:34, 1964.
Wolfson PJ, Bauer JJ, Gelernt IM, et al: Use of the long tube in the management of patients with small-intestinal obstruction due to adhesions. Arch Surg 120:1001, 1985.
Wong HY, Carpenter RL, Kopacz DJ, et al: A randomized, double-blind evaluation of ketorolac tromethamine for postoperative analgesia in ambulatory surgery patients. Anesthesiology 78:6, 1993.
Writing Group for the Christopher Study Investigators: Effectiveness of managing suspected pulmonary embolism using an algorithm combining clinical probability, D-dimer testing, and computed tomography. JAMA 295:172, 2006.
Wu WC, Raathore SS, Wang Y, et al: Blood transfusion in elderly patients with acute myocardial infarction. N Engl J Med 345:1230, 2001.

PART IV

GYNECOLOGIC ONCOLOGY

Principles of Radiation Therapy and Chemotherapy in Gynecologic Cancer 26

Basic Principles, Uses, and Complications

Charles Kunos and Steven E. Waggoner

KEY TERMS AND DEFINITIONS

Alkylating Agent. Antineoplastic agents that covalently bind (alkylate) with DNA to inhibit growth of dividing cells.

Alpha Particle. A type of particulate radiation that is the same as a helium nucleus.

Antimetabolites. Antineoplastic agents resembling natural purines or pyrimidines and can interfere with cell metabolism.

Antitumor Antibiotic. Antineoplastic agents derived from bacterial or fungal cultures.

Atomic Mass Number (A). The number of protons plus neutrons within an atom's nucleus.

Atomic Number (Z). The number of protons within an atom's nucleus.

Brachytherapy. A form of radiation therapy in which a radiation source is placed close to a tumor. The source may be in the form of wires implanted into the tumor (interstitial) or placed adjacent to a tumor, including the vagina, cervical canal, and endometrial cavity (intracavitary).

Centigray (cGy). One hundredth of a gray; a measure of radiation absorbed dose equal to 1 rad.

Complete Response. Total disappearance of all clinical, radiographic, and biochemical evidence of cancer, normally for at least 1 month.

Curie (Ci). A measure of radioisotopes disintegration equivalent to 3.7×10^{10} disintegrations per second.

Depth Dose. The specific dose of irradiation absorbed at a given distance beneath the surface.

Electron Volt (eV). A unit of electromagnetic energy equal to 1.6×10^{-19} joules. MeV = 1 million eV; keV = 1000 eV.

Erythropoietin. A protein produced by the kidneys that stimulates red blood cell production. Now synthesized and often administered to patients receiving chemotherapy.

Fractionation. Dividing a prescribed dose of radiation into smaller doses administered over time to reduce damage to normal tissues.

Gamma Rays. Electromagnetic radiation derived from the nucleus of decaying radioactive isotopes.

Granulocyte-Cell-Stimulating Factor. A cytokine growth factor that stimulates neutrophil production from the bone marrow.

Gray (Gy). A measure of absorbed radiation dose by tissue. 1 Gy = 1 J/kg (100 rads).

Growth Fraction. The proportion of tumor cells undergoing cellular division at a given time point.

Isodose Curve. A curve connecting points that receive equivalent radiation doses derived from one or more sources of radiation.

Linear Accelerator. A machine that accelerates electrons under vacuum using microwaves to a high energy to produce photon or electron treatment beams.

Linear Energy Transfer (LET). The amount of energy transferred by ionizing radiation per unit of distance traveled.

Log Cell Kill. The proportion of cells killed by treatment: 90% equals a 1-log cell kill; 99% equals a 2-log cell kill.

Partial Response. The tumor burden (usually estimated by summation of the longest diameter of one or more target lesions) is reduced by at least 30% during treatment, for a duration of at least 1 month.

Percent Depth Dose. The specific dose of irradiation absorbed at a given depth beneath the surface.

Photons. A form of electromagnetic radiation whose energy is proportional to their frequency and inversely proportional to their wavelength.

Planck's Constant. A physical constant describing the unit size of light (i.e., a photon), $h = 6.626 \times 10^{-34}$ joules/second.

Progression. Increase in size (normally > 20% increase in the sum of the longest

Continued

KEY TERMS AND DEFINITIONS—*continued*

diameter of target lesions) or number of tumors.

Radiation. The emission and propagation of energy through space or a material by particulate matter or electromagnetic waves (photons).

Radioprotector. A chemical that lessens the adverse radiobiologic effects of ionizing radiation.

Radiosensitivity. The susceptibility of a biologic system to the radiobiologic effects of ionizing radiation.

Radiosensitizer. A chemical that promotes the radiobiologic effects of ionizing radiation.

RECIST (Response Evaluation Criteria in Solid Tumors) Criteria. A formal process for measuring tumor target lesions and assessing response to treatment.

Source-to-Surface Distance (SSD). The distance from the external radiation source to the skin of the patient.

Stable Disease. Small changes in tumor volume that do not qualify as response or progression.

Targeted Therapy. Use of compounds targeted against the epidermal growth factor receptor (EGFR) tyrosine kinase cell proliferation pathway or the angiogenesis signaling pathway. These agents are not directed against the genetic and/or mitotic apparatus of dividing cells.

Taxane. Antineoplastic agents originally extracted from the bark of the Western yew tree (*Taxes baccata*) and now synthesized.

Teletherapy. A form of radiation therapy with the placement of the radioactive source at a distance from the patient (external beam radiotherapy).

Vinca Alkaloids. Antineoplastic agents derived from periwinkle plant (*Vinca rosea*) extracts.

X-ray. Extranuclear electromagnetic radiation formed by accelerated electrons in a vacuum striking a high Z target.

In this chapter, the general principles of radiation therapy and chemotherapy are discussed with the intent of describing the underlying concepts and principles of therapy that pertain to the treatment of gynecologic malignancies. The rationale and logistics of individual cancer treatments are detailed separately in other chapters specifically dedicated to each gynecologic malignancy.

Included with the basic concepts of radiation physics are atomic and nuclear structure, particles, and nomenclature, radiation production, interactions of radiation with bodily tissues, the biologic effects of radiation on cells, and the factors that modify these effects. Common radiation sources and their properties are illustrated as they relate to the treatment of specific gynecologic malignancies. Basic principles of normal tissue tolerance and the complication risks of radiation therapy as they relate to gynecologic malignancies are also presented.

Cell growth, division, and metabolism are modified both by cancer-related changes in gene expression and protein regulation and by chemotherapeutic alteration of cellular metabolism. Treating physicians must recognize the various classes of chemotherapeutic agents, their actions in gynecologic malignancies, and their treatment-related toxicities. General approaches are to be followed in administering chemotherapy, specifically including the monitoring of patients receiving these agents. These are reviewed in this chapter.

RADIATION THERAPY

Radiation Therapy Principles

Radiation therapy is the safe clinical application of radiation for the local treatment of abnormally proliferating benign or malignant tumors. The principles of radiation physics and radiobiology underlying treatment are discussed, but several key therapeutic goals deserve mentioning first. The dose response of tumor cells after radiation treatment follows a sigmoid curve, with increasingly effective tumor cell kill or arrest of division associated with increasing dose (Fig. 26-1). A similar treatment response exists for normal tissues, and the ability of radiation therapy to control malignancy depends on the greater tolerance of normal tissues to radiation exposure and a diminished capacity of cancer cells to recover from radiation-induced damage. Thus, if one were to treat up to the total radiation dose that causes

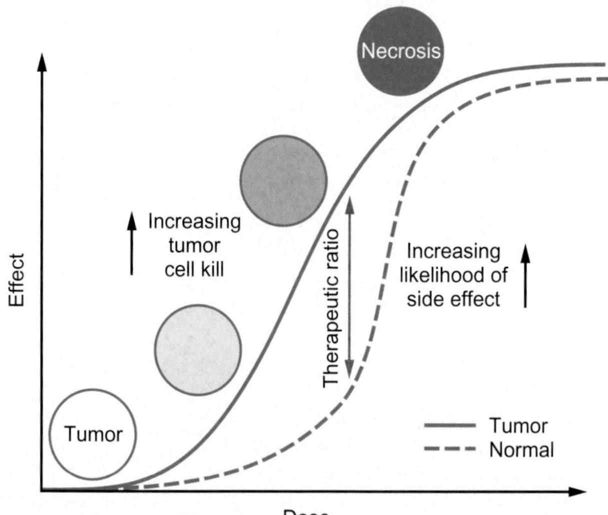

Figure 26-1. Therapeutic ratio. The concept of the therapeutic ratio for radiation therapy that compares the radiation dose–response curves for tumor control and normal tissue side effect rate. Optimally, the tumor control curve lies to the left of the normal tissue curve. For every incremental increase in total dose needed to control tumor, there is a corresponding increase in the likelihood of normal tissue side effects from treatment. The magnitude of the difference between effective tumor cell kill and the likelihood of treatment-related side effects corresponds to the therapeutic ratio (*gray arrow*). Improved tumor-directed, image-guided radiotherapy planning, use of radiation sensitizers, and use of chemotherapeutic agents (which push the tumor control curve to the left) or the use of radioprotectors (which push the normal tissue curve to the right) can widen the therapeutic ratio.

no normal tissue damage, only a small proportion of a tumor would be controlled by radiation-induced damage. Conversely, if one were to treat to a total dose that could eradicate almost the entire tumor, irreparable damage to normal tissue would often occur. This would lead to an unacceptable series of complications or even patient death after radiation treatment. The therapeutic goal of radiation therapy is to balance attempts at maximum local tumor control while minimizing adverse symptoms of treatment and normal tissue damage. Basic radiation therapy principles are detailed throughout the chapter, but briefly include the following:

- *Fractional cell kill:* Each radiation dose kills a constant fraction of the tumor cell population. Tumor cell kill follows a linear-quadratic relationship with the potential for cell-mediated repair of radiation-induced damage between radiation dose fractions.
- *Radiation dose rate:* Large radiation doses per fraction produce the greatest number of tumor cell kills; these same large radiation doses also produce the greatest damage burden on normal tissues leading to early and late adverse complications.
- *Radiation resistance:* Although all tumor cells are sensitive to the effects of radiation, select malignant tumor cells show reduced radiosensitivity, resulting in slow tumor regression or renewed tumor repopulation during or after radiation treatment. Radiation resistance is associated with (1) enhanced cell-mediated repair of radiation-induced damage, (2) active concentration of chemical radioprotectors, or (3) cellular hypoxia or nutritional deficiency.
- *Cell-cycle dependency of cell kill:* Actively proliferating tumor cells are most often killed by radiation therapy. Ionizing radiation imparts its greatest cell-kill effect during the mitotic phase (M phase) and to a lesser extent during the late Gap1 phase and early DNA synthesis phase (G_1/S). Radiation has little effect during the late synthetic phase (S phase). Before each phase of the cell cycle, genomic integrity is monitored, and, if found intact, a cell then progresses through the next phase. If, however, genomic damage is detected, a cell arrests the cell cycle so that the damage may be repaired. If the normal monitors of genomic integrity are faulty, as in the case of most cancers, then a cell traverses the cell cycle with radiation-induced damage leading to mitotic cell death or loss of critical genomic information vital to future cell survival.

With these basic fundamental principles of radiation therapy discussed, it is important to examine in depth the effects of electromagnetic radiation on biologic systems as it pertains to the treatment of gynecologic malignancies.

Basic Radiation Physics

Matter is made up of subatomic particles that are bound together by energy to form atoms. The simplest representation of the atom consists of a central core of one or more positively charged protons (+1, 933 MeV) and zero or more uncharged neutrons (±0, 933 MeV) surrounded by a cloud of negatively charged orbital electrons (−1, 0.511 MeV). As described by Bowland, four fundamental forces hold these subatomic particles together and include the strong force (10^1 N), electromagnetic or coulomb force (10^{-2} N), weak force (10^{-13} N), and gravitational force (10^{-42} N). The strong nuclear force acts over a short range (10^{-14} m), keeping an atom's protons from repelling one another because of similar electrostatic charge. The coulomb force of attraction binds orbital electrons to the nucleus such that the closer an electron is to the nucleus, the higher the binding energy an electron has. As described later, the strength of the binding energy of orbital electrons relates to the interaction of radiation on matter and its subsequent biologic effects. The chemical identity of an atom relates to its number of protons, and this number identifies the atom's atomic number (Z). Neutron number (N) varies among atoms and increases as the atomic number increases to stabilize the nucleus. An atom's atomic mass number (A) is approximately the sum of the proton number and the neutron number (A = Z + N). Radionuclides are represented by the following notation: ^{A}X.

When an atom is neutral, it has no electric charge, meaning the number of protons equals the number of electrons. If incident energy is transferred to an atom, an ionization event can occur whereby the atom acquires a positive or negative charge. When charge is acquired, an atom is said to be ionized. Removal of an orbital electron results in an atom with a positive charge, and the energy required to strip an electron off an atom must exceed the binding energy of that particular electron. Addition of an orbital electron results in an atom with a negative charge. This can occur when an electron passes close enough to an atom to experience a strong attractive force from the nucleus. Atoms can also undergo excitation, a process whereby an incident particle's energy is not sufficient to eject an atom's orbital electron but rather raises one or more electrons to a higher orbital energy state. It is through these types of interactions in atoms that radiation therapy elicits biologic consequences within tissues.

Radiation itself can be defined as the emission and propagation of energy through space or a physical medium. Radiation can be particulate, meaning that units of matter with discrete mass and momentum propagate energy (for example, alpha particles, protons, neutrons, electrons) or can be electromagnetic (photons), meaning energy travels in oscillating electric and magnetic fields that have no mass and no charge and that have a velocity of the speed of light ($c = 3.8 \times 10^8$ m/s). Both particulate radiation and electromagnetic radiation can ionize atoms, events occurring randomly throughout the medium.

In the treatment of gynecologic malignancies, the most common source of radiation is electromagnetic (photon) radiation. Photons are generally referred to as either x-rays (extranuclear or from the atom) or gamma rays (from the nucleus) based on their origin. Important properties of photons include its wavelength (λ), frequency (ν), speed $c = (\lambda\nu)$, and energy $E = (h\nu)$, where h is Planck's constant. A photon's energy (E) is proportional to its frequency; that is, higher energies are transmitted at a higher frequency. Because the frequency of a photon is inversely proportional to the wavelength, electromagnetic radiation with shorter wavelengths has a higher frequency and thus a higher energy. As described by Kahn in his textbook on the physics of radiaton therapy, the energy that is produced is measured in electron volts; 1 eV = 1.6×10^{-19} J, and it takes approximately 34 eV to generate one ion pair in water. The photons used to treat gynecologic malignancies can be generated either externally at a distance from the patient's tumor (teletherapy) or internally close to the patient's tumor (brachytherapy). Teletherapy x-ray radiotherapy units can deliver a range of photon energies from

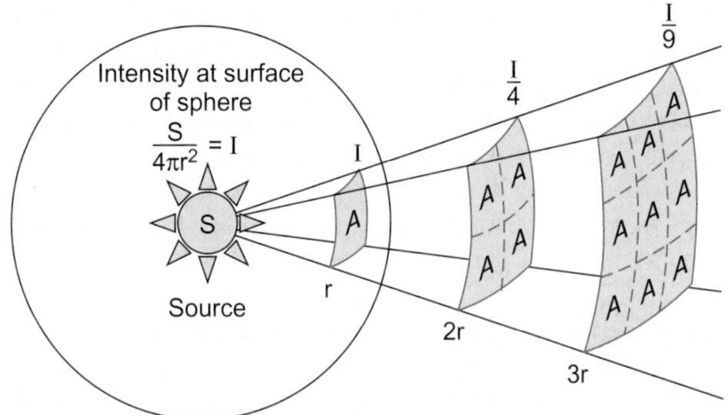

Figure 26-2. Inverse square law. Radiation intensity decreases with the square of the distance away from a point source of radiation. The intensity (I) of radiation at any given radius (r) is the source strength (S) divided by the area (A) of the sphere. For example, the energy intensity three times as far from a point source is spread over nine times the area, hence one ninth the intensity.

50,000 eV (50 keV) to more than 30 MeV, depending on their radiation source or linear accelerator design. Nuclear decay of radioactive isotopes generates the gamma ray photons used in brachytherapy, and such decay or disintegration was measured historically in curies. One Ci is defined as 3.7×10^{10} disintegrations per second, which is equivalent to the rate of disintegration of 1 g of radium. The modern standard unit for activity is the becquerel (Bq), which is one disintegration per second or 2.7×10^{-11} Ci.

Regardless of the source of electromagnetic or photon radiation, the transmitted energy diverges as the distance it travels from the source increases. This divergence causes a decrease in energy, and the relationship is described by the inverse square law. The inverse square law states that the energy dose of radiation per unit area decreases proportionately to the square of the distance from the site to the source ($1/r^2$). For example, the dose of radiation 3 cm from a point source is only one ninth of the value of the dose at 1 cm (Fig. 26-2).

Therapeutic Radiation Production

In general, two techniques are utilized in radiation therapy treatment: teletherapy (external) and brachytherapy (internal). Teletherapy in the form of external beam radiation treatment produces ionizing radiation through radioactive decay of unstable radionuclides such as cobalt (^{60}Co) or, more commonly, through acceleration of electrons. In a typical ^{60}Co teletherapy unit, the shielded ^{60}Co source resides in a treatment head mounted to a gantry that has 360-degree rotation around a patient. Collimators consisting of interleaved bars or custom-made blocks of high Z materials can shape the treatment beam to conform the dose to the target volume. With the decay of each ^{60}Co atom, two gamma ray photons are emitted at 1.17 and 1.33 MeV (1.25 MeV average). Over a specified time limit of exposure, these gamma ray photons deliver a specific radiation dose. Absorbed radiation dose is measured in gray (Gy = 1 J/kg). Typical dose rates are 3 Gy/min at 80 cm from the source. The ^{60}Co source decays with a half-life of 5.263 years, and thus the source must be replaced every 5 to 7 years.

In a typical linear accelerator teletherapy unit, electrons are "boiled" off a filament and accelerated under vacuum along an accelerating wave guide using alternating microwave fields. These accelerated electrons can be used to treat the patients themselves or can hit a high Z material transmission target to produce photons of various energies by a interaction known as *bremsstrahlung* or "braking radiation." Currently, most treatment machines generate photon energies of 4 to 20 MeV and similar to ^{60}Co teletherapy units have 360-degree gantry rotation around a patient. Typical linear accelerator dose rates are 3 Gy/min at 100 cm from the source. It is important to realize key differences between these two types of treatment machines: (1) a ^{60}Co unit is always "on" when the source is not shielded because radioactive decay always occurs, whereas a linear accelerator is "on" only when energized because there is no radionuclide source; (2) the photon spectra are different in that ^{60}Co has a discrete average monoenergetic energy, whereas linear accelerators produce photons of variable energies and an average energy of one third the maximum generated energy; and (3) ^{60}Co produces treatment beams using only gamma ray photons, whereas a linear accelerator produces treatment beams of either electrons or x-ray photons depending on its treatment mode.

Alternative forms of teletherapy treatment are available, but are uncommonly used to treat gynecologic malignancies. Teletherapy radiation dose can be delivered using alpha particles (helium nucleus), neutrons, or protons. Alpha particles produce a large number of ionizations over a short distance, but have limited use as a mode of therapy because of their short range in tissue. Neutrons are highly penetrating into tissue because of their lack of charge and cause high-energy collisions with atomic nuclei, principally of hydrogen, to produce recoil protons that then lose energy in surrounding tissues by ionization. Accelerated protons, as positively charged particles, used as therapy deposit radiation dose sparingly along their path until near the end of their range where peak dose is delivered, the so-called Bragg peak. Both neutron and proton therapies are used currently to treat cancer, but are not used routinely in the treatment of gynecologic malignancies.

To produce a consequential radiobiologic effect in tissues or tumor, incident photons or other forms of radiation must interact with matter. Kahn notes that there are five possible electromagnetic (photon) interactions with matter:

1. *Coherent scattering* (<10 keV) occurs when an incident photon scatters off an atom's outer orbital electron without losing energy. This produces no radiobiologic effect.
2. *Photoelectric effect* (10 to 60 keV) occurs when an incident photon interacts with an inner orbital electron and the photon's energy is completely absorbed by that electron. If enough energy is transferred to the orbital electron to exceed the binding energy of the inner orbital electron, it is ejected, leaving a vacancy that an outer orbital electron fills. When an outer orbital electron fills the vacancy, a characteristic x-ray is produced with energy equal to the difference in binding energy between the two electron orbitals. The probability of a photoelectric effect event happening is proportional to Z^3/E^3. Diagnostic radiographic or computed tomography images that are acquired at relatively low photon energies have high tissue–bone contrast detail because the Z^3/E^3 ratio is maximized.

3. *Compton effect* (60 keV to 10 MeV)-occurs when an incident photon (Eγ) loses some or all of its energy to an outer orbital electron. The photon, if it remains, is scattered at some angle away from the atom. An electron that has acquired energy exceeding its binding energy (E_{BE}) leaves the atom with sufficient kinetic energy ($E_{KE} = E\gamma - E_{BE}$) to penetrate tissue and produce molecular damage through downstream ionizations. For simplicity, at common therapeutic photon energies (4 to 18 MeV), the Compton effect is biologically most important in that incident photons interact predominantly with cellular water. Human and mammalian tissues are principally composed of water (~90%) and functional biomolecules such as proteins and DNA (Fig. 26-3). Incident photons ionize water to produce an ion radical (H_2O^+) and a free electron (e^-). The ion radical is highly reactive (10^{-10} second half-life) and can interact with another molecule of water to form a hydroxyl radical (·OH). Hydroxyl radicals are also highly reactive (10^{-9} second half-life) and can break chemical bonds in target molecules such as proteins and DNA (·R). Breaks in the chemical bonds of DNA can lead to DNA base damage, DNA cross-links, DNA single-stranded breaks, and DNA double-stranded breaks. As discussed later, DNA strand breaks can result in loss of vital genomic material during subsequent cell divisions, potentially leading to mitotic death of the damaged cell. In this way, therapeutic radiation leads to significant radiobiologic effects by functionally modifying cellular proteins and damaging DNA.
4. *Pair production* (>10 MeV) occurs when an incident photon has an energy greater than 1.022 MeV. This threshold is required because the photon disappears to form an electron–positron pair, each particle having an energy of 0.511 MeV. Once formed, free electrons slow by nuclear attraction and are quickly stopped in tissue. However, the formed positron is highly reactive and short-lived in that it annihilates with surrounding electrons to create two photons of 0.511 MeV, each traveling 180 degrees apart from one another. Positron emission tomography scanners build images based on coincident detection of photons formed by this process.
5. *Photodisintegration* (>10 MeV) occurs when an energetic photon penetrates the nucleus of an atom and dislodges a neutron. Emitted neutrons cannot ionize tissue themselves because they have no charge, but rather collide with surrounding atomic nuclei to produce recoil, positively charged protons that elicit radiobiologic effects through subsequent ionizations.

Radiation Biology

Munro has shown that nuclear DNA is unquestionably one essential target of therapeutic radiation. In his textbook on radiobiology, Hall reported that one third of radiation-induced DNA damage is from the direct interaction of incident photons ionizing atoms within DNA itself. Two thirds of radiation-induced DNA damage is a consequence of the indirect damage done by freely diffusing hydroxyl radicals (·OH). Recently, however, Hall and Hei have described a bystander effect whereby lethal damage to cellular proteins, organelles, or the cell membrane in an irradiated cell can lead to neighboring cell death in cells that would not have died on their own. The bystander effect suggests that damage to cellular proteins or organelles in one cell may also result in cell lethality. Note that not all radiation damage is lethal to the cell; some damage to DNA can undergo repair, namely, sublethal DNA damage repair. Sublethal DNA damage repair occurs both in normal cells and malignant cells, but much less so in malignant cells because malignant cells often have abnormal DNA repair mechanisms. A variety of complex and redundant repair mechanisms have been identified including base excision repair and nucleotide excision repair for damage to the DNA base and deoxyribose backbone, homologous recombination repair for DNA single-strand breaks, and nonhomologous end-joining repair for DNA double-strand breaks. As the time interval between radiation doses lengthens, cell survival increases due to the prompt repair of radiation-induced damage. The repair process is usually complete within 1 to 2 hours, although this period may be longer in some slowly

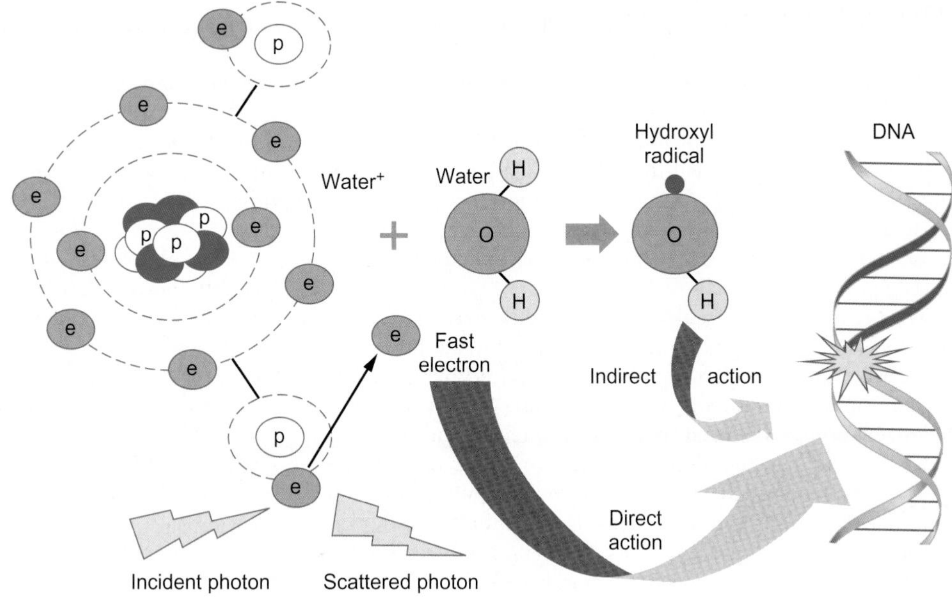

Figure 26-3. Compton effect. Cells are composed of biomolecules dissolved in an aqueous (~90% water by weight) solution. Incident photons (p) randomly ionize (*left*) cellular water to produce an ion radical (water$^+$) and a free fast electron (e^-) that can damage biomolecules such as DNA. The water ion radical interacts with another molecule of water to form a hydroxyl radical (OH). Most often (~66%), formed hydroxyl radicals diffuse throughout the cell, breaking chemical bonds in target molecules such as proteins and DNA (R, *right*). Breaks in the chemical bonds of DNA can lead to DNA base damage, DNA cross-links, DNA single-strand breaks, and DNA double-strand breaks contributing to the loss of vital genomic material during subsequent cell divisions and possibly mitotic death of the damaged cell.

renewing cellular tissues. Before discussing the consequences of DNA damage, it is important to understand key factors that can modify the rate at which DNA damage accumulates.

Intracellular molecular oxygen importantly modifies radiation-induced DNA damage as it "fixes" damage done by free hydroxyl radicals. Palcic and Skarsgard have reported that molecular oxygen, when present during or within microseconds of photon-induced ionization events, reacts with the altered chemical bonds of ionized molecules (·R) to produce organic peroxides (RO_2), a nonreparable form of the target molecule. Molecules "fixed" in this manner are permanently altered and may function abnormally. Thus, tumor and tissue oxygenation have practical implications in radiation therapy insofar as rapidly proliferating gynecologic malignancies may have poor blood supplies, which decreases tumor cell oxygenation, particularly at the center of large tumors. Tumor tissue hypoxia leads to radiation resistance as reflected by increased cell survival after radiation treatment. Laboratory experiments have shown that the radiation dose necessary to kill the same proportion of hypoxic cells as compared to aerated approaches 3:1. This ratio is commonly referred to the *oxygen enhancement ratio*. For oxygen to have its maximal effect, dissolved oxygen concentration in tumor must be approximately 3 mm Hg (venous blood is 30–40 mm Hg), according to Hall. In the treatment of gynecologic malignancies, Dunst and coworkers have found that cervical cancer patients undergoing radiation therapy with serum hemoglobin greater than 10 mg/dL have improved tumor oxygenation, resulting in superior local control and superior clinical outcomes compared with patients whose hemoglobin is less than 10 mg/dL. Also, hypoxic cell sensitizers such as the nitroimidazoles, as studied by Adams and colleagues, and the bioreductive drug tirapazamine, as reported by Goldberg and coworkers, improve radiosensitivity of hypoxic cells within tumors. The potential benefit of these agents in the treatment of gynecologic cancers is being explored in clinical trials.

The rate at which energy is lost per unit path length of medium or LET also imparts an effect on the accumulation of radiation-induced DNA damage. For photons, energy loss is infrequent along its path length, typical of low LET radiations. Sparsely ionizing, low LET radiations produce one or more sublethal events and thus necessitate multiple "hits" to kill the cell. Heavy particulate radiation resulting from alpha particles or protons is densely ionizing as energy is deposited more diffusely along its path length. This is typical of high LET radiation. Because the probability of producing a lethal event in a cell is much higher with high LET radiation, cell death in this case is independent of tumor oxygenation. For this reason, research efforts have been directed toward the development of heavy particle generators that overcome the limitation of poor oxygenation of cancer cells.

Within the cell, molecules that have sulfhydryl moieties at one end and a strong base such as an amine at the other end are capable of scavenging free radicals produced by radiation-induced ionization events. These molecules can also donate hydrogen atoms to ionized molecules before molecular oxygen can "fix" the damage done by radiation-induced hydroxyl radicals. As reported by Utley and associates, amifostine is a nonreactive phosphorothioate that (1) accumulates readily in normal tissues by active transport to be metabolized into an active compound to scavenge free radicals and (2) accumulates slowly in tumors by passive diffusion with limited or no conversion to the active compound. It is reasonable to conclude that the presence of a radioprotector such as amifostine would decrease radiation-induced DNA damage and limit normal tissue radiation-related side effects. Clinical trials are investigating the radioprotective effect of amifostine in gynecologic malignancies, but, at present, amifostine has shown the most promise as a chemoprotectant and has been approved to reduce the renal toxicity associated with repeated administration of cisplatin chemotherapy in women with advanced ovarian cancer.

What constitutes cell death in the traditional sense (cessation of cellular respiration and vital function) is not the same in radiation biology. Death in radiation biology is the loss of reproductive integrity or the inability to maintain uninterrupted cellular proliferation with high fidelity. Thus, radiation "kills" without actual physical disappearance of malignant cells (although body macrophages often remove the dead cells causing tumors to shrink in size). Malignant cells may remain a part of a tumor, but have discontinued cellular metabolism and proliferation. Most cells when exposed to radiation die a mitotic death, meaning that cells die at the next or a subsequent cell division with all progeny also dying. Inflammation can accompany mitotic cell death, potentially resulting in local adverse side effects. Jonathan and associates noted that alternative forms of loss in reproductive capacity due to radiation include terminal differentiation, senescence, or apoptosis. In apoptosis, cells undergo a complex process of programmed cellular involution and phagocytosis by neighboring cells. There is no inflammatory response resulting from apoptosis. One remarkable example of apoptosis is the formation of the spaces between the digits of the hand during human fetal development.

Returning to radiation-induced DNA damage, electromagnetic radiation (x-ray or gamma) deposits energy within cells, which may damage DNA directly or indirectly through hydroxyl radicals (·OH). In relative terms, more than 1000 DNA-base-damaging events, 1000 DNA single-stranded breaks, and 40 DNA double-stranded breaks occur with each typical radiation dose fraction. Although base and DNA single-stranded breaks need to be repaired so that mutations are not propagated, DNA double-stranded breaks are believed to be the most crucial radiobiologic effect of radiation therapy. There is an increased statistical probability that a cell will be unable to repair a DNA double-stranded break resulting in the loss of genetic material at cell division. Also, attempts by cells to repair the DNA double-stranded breaks often result in bizarre chromosome arrangements that interfere with normal division of the cell. Through either loss of critical genes or impaired cell division, cell death ensues.

Cell death following radiation therapy is modeled by a linear-quadratic relationship (Fig. 26-4). The initial slope of the cell survival curve is shallow and curvilinear, whereas the terminal slope is more linear. In the low-dose region of the survival curve typical of daily-dose fractions used in radiation therapy, the fraction of cells surviving is high due to the repair of single-event sublethal damage (such as multiple base damage or DNA single-stranded breaks). In the high-dose region of the survival curve, the fraction of cells surviving is low due to multiple event damage in the form of DNA double-stranded breaks or accumulation of too many sublethal events that can be repaired before the next cell division. Capacity to repair sublethal damage

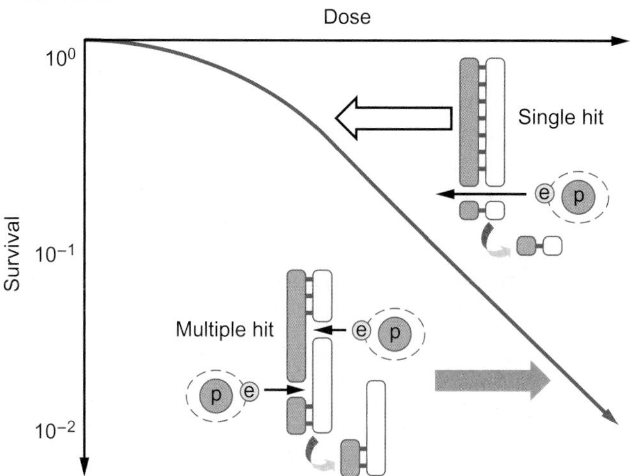

Figure 26-4. Cell survival curves. A radiation survival curve plots cell survival on a logarithmic scale against radiation dose on a linear scale. Survival represents the number of cells retaining reproductive capacity to form approximately 50 cell colonies (i.e., approximately five to six cell divisions) after a specified radiation dose. The initial slope is shallow, forming a "shoulder" in the low-dose region (1 to 3 Gy per fraction) due to repair of sublethal damage. Occasionally, a single hit will produce a DNA double-strand break, resulting in the loss of genetic material (*open arrow*). In the high-dose region (>3 Gy per fraction), the slope steepens due to multiple damaging events leading to DNA double-strand breaks. If not repaired, significant vital genetic material may be lost at a subsequent cell division and the cell may die. e, electron; p, photon.

depends on radiation quality (LET), tissue oxygenation, and cell-cycle time.

As shown in Figure 26-5 and as described by Deshpande and associates and by Pawlik and Keyomarsi, there are four highly regulated phases of the cell cycle. After completing mitosis, cells enter a gap phase (G_1) variable in time span in which the cell performs protein synthesis and other functional metabolic and biologic processes. Under the influence of complex, finely regulated intercellular and intracellular signaling, cells then enter the DNA replication phase (S phase) in which the cell must exactly replicate its DNA to produce an identical set of chromosomes. Entry into the S phase is controlled by sequentially activated, highly regulated cyclin-dependent kinases (CDKs) responsible for differentially recruiting and amplifying specific gene products necessary for DNA replication. Moreover, there are corresponding cell-cycle inhibitory proteins (CDKIs) that negatively regulate cell-cycle progression. After DNA replication, the cell enters a second gap phase (G_2), in part to ensure high DNA replication fidelity in the newly formed chromosomes. At the completion of the G_2 phase, cells undergo mitosis whereby two identical daughter cells are produced.

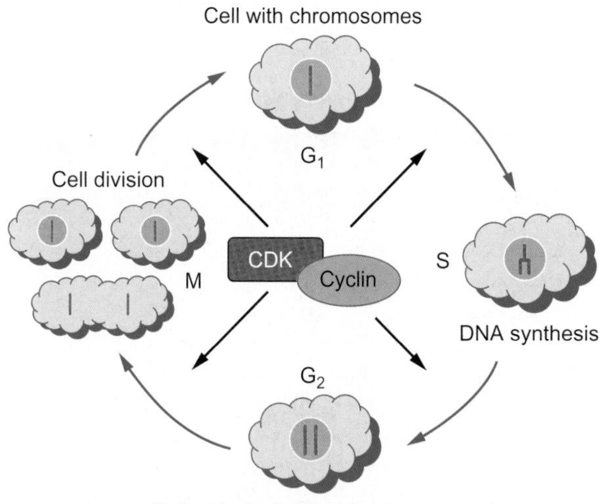

Figure 26-5. Phases of the cell. After mitosis (M), there is an interval of variable duration during which there is RNA and protein synthesis and a diploid DNA content (G_1 [Gap1]). The cell may also enter a prolonged or resting phase (G_0) and then reenter the cycle during DNA synthesis, the S phase, in which DNA is duplicated. During the G_2 (Gap2) phase, there again is protein and RNA synthesis. During the M phase, the cell divides into two cells, each of which receives diploid DNA content. CDK, cyclin-dependent kinase.

To maintain genetic integrity through the cell cycle, the cell has multiple checkpoints through which it must pass, notably at the G_1/S and G_2/M transitions, as described by Pawlik and Keyomarsi. The G_1/S checkpoint prevents replication of damaged DNA, as in the case of radiation therapy. Malumbres and Barbacid have reported that proteins critical to the G_1/S checkpoint include p53, p21, and the retinoblastoma protein (Rb), all of which modulate the activity of CDKs responsible for the transition to S phase. Briefly, Rb lacks phosphorylated subunits in its active form, binding to the E2F transcription factors and preventing E2F translocation to the nucleus to recruit genes needed for S phase. Sequential phosphorylation of RB by CDK 4/6-cyclin D and CDK2-cyclin E complexes releases the E2F transcription factors. Radiation-induced DNA damage results in the accumulation of the G_1 checkpoint regulatory protein p53, which in turn activates the CDKI p21. p21 inhibits phosphorylation of RB, delaying the G_1/S transition. The G_2/M checkpoint prevents segregation of aberrant chromosomes at mitosis. Two molecularly distinct checkpoints have been identified: one that is regulated by the ataxia-telangiectasia mutated gene product (ATM) and one that is ATM independent. ATM has multiple phosphorylation products that modulate CDKs at the G_2/M transition (Chk1 and Chk2) as well as p53 expression through modification of its degradation pathway. Indeed, according to Xu and associates, phosphorylation of the Chk1 and Chk2 inhibits the cdc2 protein kinase, blocking cells at the G_2/M transition. ATM's essential role in DNA damage recognition is highlighted by the extreme radiosensitivity of patients with mutated ATM. Malignant cells that often have mutated cell-cycle checkpoint proteins have an impaired ability to repair damage done to nuclear DNA, and thus accumulate lethal DNA-damaging events that lead to cell kill in a few cell cycles.

Cells show different radiosensitivities during the cell cycle. M-phase cells are particularly radiosensitive because the DNA is packaged tightly into chromosomes such that ionization events have a high likelihood of causing lethal DNA double-stranded breaks. S-phase cells are particularly radioresistant because enzymes responsible for ensuring high-fidelity DNA replication are relatively overexpressed and recognize altered DNA bases or inappropriate strand breaks. Cells in the G_1 or G_2 phase of the cell cycle are relatively radiosensitive compared with S phase. Chemotherapies that inhibit cell-cycle dependent pathways or impede DNA repair enhance the radiobiologic effect of radiation.

Radiation Treatment: Brachytherapy and Teletherapy Therapy

In general, two techniques are used in radiation treatment: brachytherapy (internal) and teletherapy (external). Brachytherapy involves the placement of radioactive sources within an existing body cavity (e.g., the vagina) in close proximity to the tumor. In the treatment of gynecologic malignant tumors, radioactive sources can be placed either within hollow needles that are implanted directly into the tissue to be irradiated (interstitial implant) or within a hollow cylinder or inserted in tandem into the vagina or through the cervical os, respectively. For the treatment of cervical cancer, two vaginal ovoids, one on each side of the tandem, are positioned in the vaginal fornices (intracavitary therapy). In clinical practice, interstitial or intracavitary brachytherapy needles or applicators without radioactive sources are placed first in the operating room with a patient under anesthesia. After post-anesthesia patient recovery, the position of the needles or applicators is confirmed by radiographic imaging. These radiographic images help guide radiotherapy planning. Radioactive sources are "afterloaded" some time later to reduce radiation exposure to medical personnel treating the patient. The most widely used intracavitary applicator is the Fletcher-Suit applicator, which is useful for treatment of a cervical tumor or a tumor located near the cervix (Fig. 26-6). For both interstitial and intracavitary brachytherapy, radiation dose delivery to the tumor and surrounding tissues follows the inverse square law as modified by source and tissue photon attenuation and scattering.

Several radioisotopes with various photon energies and half-lives are used in gynecologic brachytherapy. Although uncommon, radioisotopes with a short half-life (such as ^{198}Au [gold]) may be placed within the patient and left permanently. Those radioisotopes with a long half-life (^{137}Cs [cesium]) are placed temporarily within interstitial or intracavitary needles or applicators and are removed after a prescribed radiation dose has been administered. Historically, brachytherapy for most gynecologic malignancies consisted of temporary low-dose rate (40 to 70 cGy/hr) sources in place for 1 to 3 days. Low-dose rate requires the patient to be in a shielded hospital room with medical personnel supervision, under bed rest with prolonged analgesia and prophylactic anticoagulation, and limited family contact during radiation dose administration. Recently, high-dose rate, catheter-based brachytherapy has become popular because the procedure can be performed in 1 day on an outpatient basis. High-dose rate uses a thin wire tipped with iridium (^{192}Ir) to deliver radiation dose at rates exceeding 200 cGy/min. Unlike low-dose rate, high-dose rate is performed in a shielded treatment room requiring patient immobilization for a short period and minimal patient analgesia and anesthesia. Table 26-1 indicates the half-lives of some of the isotopes commonly used in treating gynecologic cancers. It is also important that a uniform

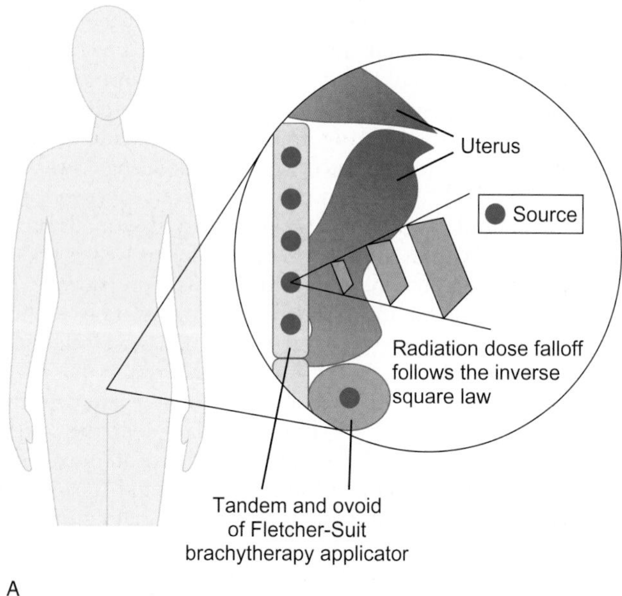

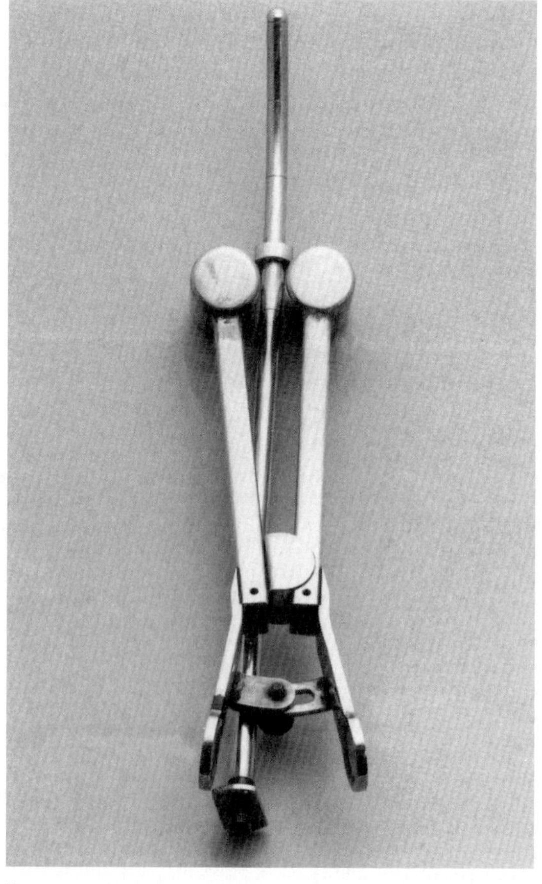

Figure 26-6. Brachytherapy. For the treatment of gynecologic malignancies, brachytherapy usually consists of placement of radiation sources (*dark circles*) in close proximity to the tumor. This can be accomplished by intracavitary placement of hollow applicators such as the Fletcher-Suit device (*pictured*) placed within the uterine cavity and vaginal vault or by interstitial placement of hollow needles through the tissues themselves. Radiation dose decreases as the square of the distance away from the radiation source.

Table 26-1 Half-Lives of Commonly Used Radioisotopes for Gynecologic Malignancies

Radionuclide	Half-life
Gold (^{198}Au)	2.7 days
Phosphorus (^{32}P)	14.3 days
Iridium (^{192}Ir)	73.8 days
Cobalt (^{60}Co)	5.26 years
Cesium (^{137}Cs)	30 years
Radium (^{226}Ra)	1620 years

distribution of radiation be achieved in the adjacent tissues to avoid "hot spots," which can damage normal tissue, as well as "cold spots," which can lead to reduced dose delivery to the tumor.

Teletherapy in the form of external beam radiotherapy means that the source of radiation is at a distance from the patient, sometimes located at a distance 5 to 10 times greater than the depth of the tumor being irradiated. This distance is referred to as the SSD and is used to calculate dose using the inverse square law. When using a SSD patient treatment setup, the SSD is used along with tumor depth, radiation beam energy, depth of the point of maximum dose, and output parameters for a given treatment field size to determine daily radiation dose. Alternatively, with the use of different angles and ports of treatment, the concept of source axis distance has been introduced; it denotes the distance from the radiation source to the central axis of machine rotation. The patient is positioned so that this axis passes through the center of the tumor, and treatment ports are arranged around this axis to optimize tumor dose. When using a source axis distance patient treatment setup, daily radiation dose is calculated using machine output and beam attenuation at the depth for a given treatment field size.

Conventional external beam radiation is delivered with beams of uniform intensity. Advances in computer-guided planning and treatment have made the use of beams of varying intensity more commonplace. This approach of planned dose intensification allows the high-dose region to be conformed precisely to the shape of the planned treatment volume, and this technique is called intensity-modulated radiotherapy. Recent advances in radiotherapy delivery systems have allowed linear accelerators to be coupled with helical computed tomography scanners. Image-guided radiation therapy using this type of device is called helical tomotherapy. In conventional therapy and both intensity-modulated radiotherapy and helical tomotherapy, beams from the external radiation source can be sculpted using high electron-dense material collimators. Collimators limit scatter radiation and block portions of the treatment beam from delivering intolerant radiation dose to critical tissues (Fig. 26-7). In general, the higher the energy source of the radiation is, the deeper the beam can penetrate into tissue. Thus, high-energy radiation has its predominant effect in deeper tissues and spares the surface or the skin of radiation effect.

An isodose curve is a line that connects points in the tissue that receive equivalent doses of irradiation. Figure 26-7 contrasts the isodose curves for 6- and 22-MeV machines. For the 6-MeV machine, the maximum dose is near the surface with a more rapid falloff in the deeper tissues. For the 22 MeV machine, the maximum dose is deep to surface, sparing the effects of radiation on the overlying skin.

In addition to the energy of the beam, the energy of radiation absorbed at various depths is affected by the size of the field being treated. Larger fields contain more scattered radiation, which leads to a greater dose at a given depth. Figure 26-7 demonstrates the effect of increasing the size of the field with increasing dose at a given depth for three different types of energy sources.

Thus, the radiation dose delivered to the tumor is affected by the energy of the source, the depth of the tumor beneath the surface, and the size of the field undergoing irradiation. With external therapy, usually 160 to 200 cGy/day is given five times per week. Recently, there has been experimental work evaluating hyperfractionation, which involves smaller multiple doses given more frequently (for example, 120 cGy three times per day or 160 cGy two times per day with 6 hours between doses to allow sublethal damage repair in normal tissues). Hyperthermia, or the use of high temperature heat to denature cellular proteins, has also been explored to enhance the therapeutic effectiveness of radiation because malignant cells are particularly vulnerable to heat-induced killing during the S-phase portion of the cell cycle. It appears to offer the most promise for tumors localized in an area that can effectively and safely tolerate increased temperatures (42° to 43° C).

Tissue Tolerance and Radiation Complications

Adverse radiation effects are commonly divided into two broad categories, early and late, which demonstrate markedly different patterns of response to radiation dose fractionation. It is important for the treating physician to understand critical tissues and organ systems at risk of radiation damage. Table 26-2 presents the *approximate* tolerance of tissues to radiation therapy.

Early or acute effects manifest as the result of death in a large population of cells and can occur within days to weeks after the start of radiation therapy. For early effects, the total dose of radiation and, to a lesser extent, the dose per fraction determine the severity of the side effect. Radiation acutely affects tissues undergoing rapid cell division to replace lost normal functioning cells. Examples of where this is most pronounced include the skin, the intestinal mucosa, the mucosa of the vagina and bladder, and the hematopoietic system in which precursor stem cells are renewing functional mature cells. The radiation dose given in multiple small fractions reduces the untoward adverse effects of cell damage on normal tissue and allows normal healing to occur between treatment fractions through sublethal DNA damage repair (the shallow, curvilinear portion of the cell survival curve). During treatment of gynecologic malignancies, most adverse early treatment-related toxicities can be managed with medications. It is preferred practice that radiation treatment not be interrupted for treatment-related toxicities due to radiation-induced tumor accelerated repopulation. Only rarely does a treatment program need to be temporarily discontinued for treatment-related toxicities.

Late effects occur after a delay of months or years after radiation therapy. Late effects are often the product of parenchymal connective tissue cell loss and vascular damage. Late effects may be seen in slowly renewing tissues such as lung, kidney, heart,

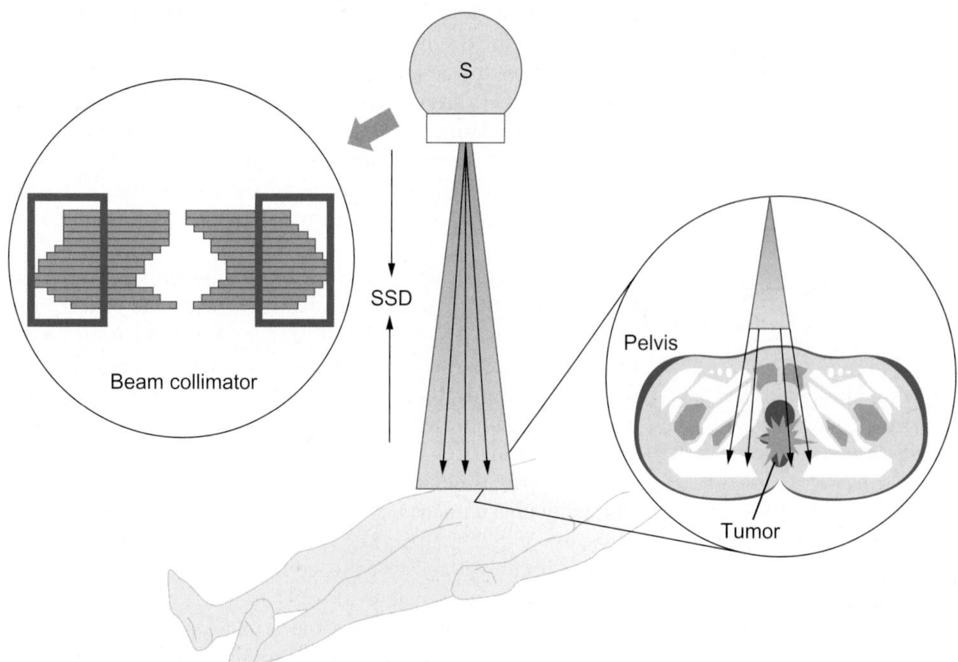

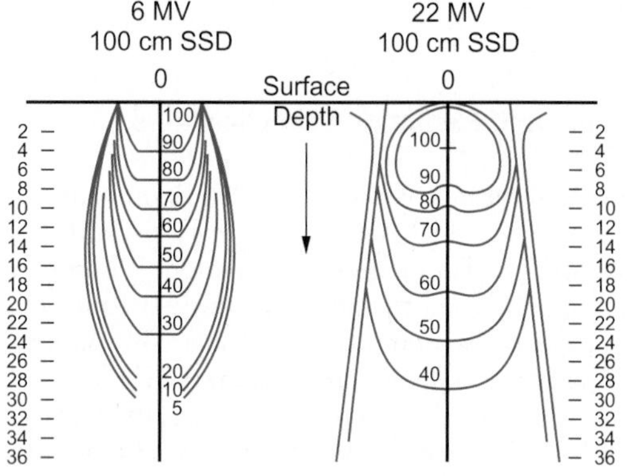

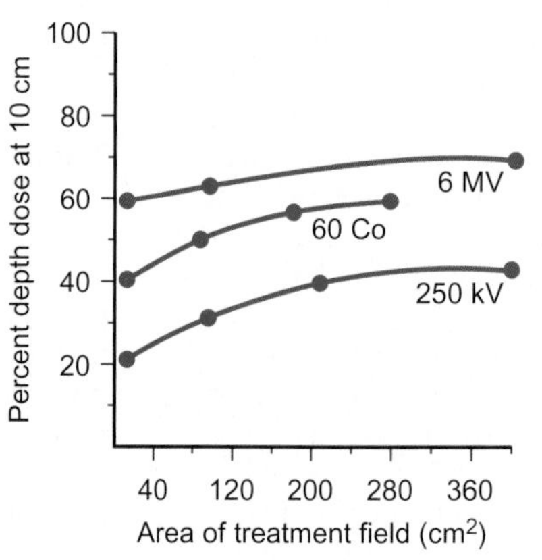

Figure 26-7. Teletherapy. Conventional external beam radiotherapy is the delivery of radiation dose to tissues at a distance (source-to-surface distance [SSD]) away from the radiation source (S). As the beam emerges from the treatment machine, the beam diverges and can be shaped by high Z material leaflets of a beam collimator (*top*) or custom blocks. As the treatment beam "hits" the patient, photon interactions occur producing ionization events (*inset*). Energy deposition within tissue creates isodose curves. Isodose curves and depth-dose distributions for 6 and 22 MV photons are shown (*bottom left*). Note that the higher energy machine delivers radiation to a greater depth for same surface dose, resulting in skin sparing. As treatment field size varies, the dose delivered at a specified depth varies (*bottom right*).

and liver and in the central nervous system. In the treatment of gynecologic malignancies, late adverse effects include tissue necrosis and fibrosis as well as fistula formation and ulceration. In contrast to early effects, late effects depend primarily on dose per fraction. Fractionated radiation therapy using a daily radiation dose of 160 to 200 cGy minimizes the risk of late effects. Second cancers (mostly sarcomas) induced after radiation are rare (1:500 to 1000 cases) and do not usually appear until 15 to 20 years after radiation exposure. Arai and associates noted an excess of rectal cancer, bladder cancer, and leukemia among patients with carcinoma of the cervix treated by radiation in comparison with those treated by surgery.

Table 26-2 Normal Tissue Tolerance to Radiation Therapy

Tissue	Tolerance (Gy)
Kidney	20–23 Gy
Liver	25–35 Gy
Small bowel	45–50 Gy
Rectum	60–70 Gy
Bladder	60–70 Gy
Vaginal mucosa	70–75 Gy
Cervix	>120 Gy

The skin overlying the tumor being treated visibly manifests the effects of radiation-induced normal tissue damage. Skin effects are manifest by reddening of the skin and loss of hair where the radiation treatment beam enters the body. Erythema may progress to dry or moist skin breakdown or desquamation due to loss of the actively proliferating basal layer of the epidermis that renews the overlying epithelium. This is less common now than in prior years because higher energy radiation beams that spare surface dose are used. However, during the treatment of vulvar malignancies, the skin surface and superficial groin nodes are the radiotherapeutic target, and thus desquamation is more commonly observed. Medical management consisting of non-metal-containing creams and emollients during therapy reduces discomfort and allows healing within 2 to 4 weeks after completion of radiation therapy. Late skin fibrosis may produce a rough leathery texture to the skin in the irradiated field. Chiao and Lee, as well as Gothard and coworkers, have reported on the use of pentoxifylline and vitamin E to promote healing of late subcutaneous and deep tissue fibrosis after radiation.

In the treatment of gynecologic malignancies, the other sites at risk of radiation-induced normal tissue damage are the bladder, rectum, and large and small bowel. The bladder epithelium consists of a basal layer of small diploid cells covered by large transitional cells. Radiation damage to the diploid cells results in slow renewal of the overlying transitional cells that are periodically sloughed off during urination. Radiation cystitis manifested as dysuria and urinary frequency results in bladder irritation. Treatment with analgesics such as pyridium can alleviate symptoms. Hematuria may also occur. Therapy with sclerosing solutions or fulguration through a cystoscope may be necessary. McIntyre and colleagues noted that ureteral stricture after radiation for stage I carcinoma of the cervix was 1% at 5 years and 2.5% at 20 years, a rare but important complication. In rare instances, urinary diversion may be required. Bladder fibrosis and reduced bladder capacity are late effects of pelvic radiation therapy.

In the intestine, the renewing stem cells are found at the bottom of the crypts of Lieberkuhn. Within 2 to 4 days after the start of radiation, these cells can become depleted, leading to atrophy of intestinal mucosa. Damage to the bowel usually occurs in the form of inflammation (sigmoiditis or enteritis), which commonly results in increased bowel motility or diarrhea but also may be rarely associated with severe bleeding and cramping pain. Less severe cases can often be controlled with a low-roughage diet and antispasmodic medications. Although uncommon, severe cases may require bowel resection or permanent bowel diversion through a colostomy. Covens and coworkers noted that those who required operation for radiation damage to the bowel had an approximately 25% risk of dying in 2 years, with ileal damage being the most risky. Those with complications not requiring surgery frequently have decreased vitamin B_{12} and bile acid absorption. Late bowel toxicities include radiation proctitis due to small vessel vascular damage in the epithelium, which may progress to intermittent rectal bleeding. Bowel stenosis or obstructions resulting from fibrosis and adhesion formation may occur, especially in those patients who have had previous pelvic or abdominal surgery. Occasionally, enteric fistulas can develop, and bowel perforation may occur. In the latter case, surgical therapy is required, usually to bypass the affected area of the intestine. As a rule, extensive dissection of irradiated tissue is avoided. Montana and Fowler showed that the risks of proctitis and cystitis are dose-related. For example, they found severe proctitis and cystitis at doses of 6750 and 6900 cGy, respectively, whereas such complications were not observed in patients whose median dose was 6500 and 6300 cGy.

A lowering of circulating lymphocytes, granulocytes, platelets, and red blood cells can be seen with pelvic radiation therapy for gynecologic malignancies. The stem cells of the bone marrow in an adult reside in the axial skeleton (vertebrae, ribs, and pelvis). Usual external beam radiation therapy treatment fields for gynecologic malignancies encompass the sacrum and lower vertebrae and pelvis and thereby reduce precursor stem cells for circulating blood cells. This is an important consideration if the patient is to receive concurrent radiosensitizing chemotherapy or subsequent cytotoxic chemotherapy. Growth factor support with synthetic erythropoietin and/or granulocyte colony-stimulating factors is often required for patients receiving multiagent chemotherapy following treatment with pelvic radiation therapy.

Last, fistulas between the vagina and bladder or between the vagina and rectum may develop when there has been extensive radiation damage to the intervening tissues. This usually takes place during therapy for large carcinomas of the cervix (see Chapter 29). As a rule, such complications will occur 6 months to 2 years after treatment, although they may occur many years after primary therapy. Diverting surgery or resection of the fistulas is often needed to correct these serious complications.

CHEMOTHERAPY

Although many patients with cancer present initially with a clinically appreciable mass or tumor, only a minority of patients have localized disease, curable with local treatment alone. More often, the cancer has spread to regional lymph nodes or disseminated to other organs even though these sites may not be clinically appreciated. Thus, numerous compounds have been tested and used to treat human cancers. Li and colleagues demonstrated the first successful effort in gynecologic cancer using the antimetabolite methotrexate that could cause permanent remission of metastatic trophoblastic disease. A number of general principles have been developed during the study of chemotherapeutic agents that provide guidelines for their recommended use and administration.

Chemotherapy Principles and Guidelines

Some of the concepts used in antibiotic therapy for infections have been applied to the chemotherapeutic approach to cancer management. However, major differences exist. Infections are frequently caused by a single agent or even multiple types of bacteria with specific growth patterns and sensitivities to antibiotics. Although it is believed that a cancer can originate from a single cell, clinically evident disease is composed of a heterogeneous population of cells with different cell-cycle durations, varying growth fractions, and diverse expression of genes and proteins responsible for cell proliferation and metastasis. Larger tumors are more likely to contain cells capable of acquiring resistance to a single cytotoxic chemotherapeutic agent. Basic principles for cancer chemotherapy arose from experiments in murine tumor models, notably mice leukemias, conducted by Skipperand colleagues at the Southern Research Institute. These principles include the following:

- *Fractional cell kill:* Each dose of chemotherapy kills a constant fraction of the tumor cell population. Tumor cell kill correlates usually in a linear relationship with the pharmacokinetic parameter of area under the drug concentration curve (AUC).
- *Dose intensity:* High chemotherapy doses interspersed with short rest periods produce greatest tumor cell kill in rapidly proliferating malignancies.
- *Drug resistance:* Single-agent chemotherapy administration selectively isolates drug-resistant tumor cells, leading to an

outgrowth of hardy, resistant malignant cells. Chemotherapy drug resistance has been associated with (1) cell-mediated modification of drug targets, (2) active drug transport out of the cell, and (3) alteration of drug activation or targeting.

- *Cell cycle dependency of cell kill:* Actively proliferating tumor cells are most often killed by chemotherapy agents; drugs inhibiting DNA processing act during the S phase and those impairing cell division act during the M phase. If the normal monitors of genomic integrity are intact, then a cell may suspend the cell cycle to repair any detected damage. If, however, these monitors are abnormal, a cell may continue progression through the cell cycle, which may lead to unrecoverable cell-cycle arrest or irreparable damage to critical genes vital for future cell survival. Malignant cancer cells often demonstrate abnormal monitors of genomic integrity, in part permitting their rapid proliferation but also increasing their sensitivity to chemotherapies.

Approaches to Treatment

The dose of an anticancer chemotherapy agent is usually calculated as a function of body surface area (square meters), which provides a better measure of potential toxicity than body weight. This is in part because of the observation that body surface area more closely reflects cardiac output and blood flow than just body weight alone. Chemotherapeutic agents have varying toxicities, which is considered in the next section. A major problem with most agents is bone marrow toxicity, requiring careful monitoring of mature and stem cell turnover within the hematopoietic system. Most gynecologic chemotherapy agents are administered intravenously in cycles varying from weekly to 3- or 4-week intervals between each cycle. If mature white blood cells (i.e., absolute neutrophil count) and platelets have not recovered adequately by the time the next cycle of chemotherapy is due to be administered, the subsequent dose of the agent or agents is usually reduced or the time interval between treatments extended until recovery is documented. In case of persistent marrow toxicity, growth factor support is often useful in allowing chemotherapy treatments to continue.

An additional consideration in toxicity of chemotherapeutic agents relates to hepatic metabolism and/or renal excretion. It may be necessary to modify the dose of the drug administered when either renal or hepatic function is compromised. For example, doxorubicin (Adriamycin) and vincristine are metabolized in the liver, and dose reductions must be made if the drug is administered to a patient with hepatic dysfunction; methotrexate and cisplatin effects are increased in patients with renal damage, necessitating dose reduction in these patients; cisplatin not only has its effects intensified in patients with renal damage but also is toxic to the kidney, requiring particular caution if it is administered to individuals with compromised renal function or patients receiving therapy with other renal toxic medications. Methotrexate and cisplatin are also bound to albumin, and this binding is decreased in patients taking sulfonamides or salicylates, both of which increase the toxicity and effects of the chemotherapy. In general, low serum albumin leads to an increase in free circulating chemotherapeutic agent, one reason malnourished patients have heightened toxicity to chemotherapy.

Various chemotherapeutic agents can be differentially toxic to other organ systems of the body, including the gastrointestinal, nervous, pulmonary, and reproductive systems. Loss of ovarian function and fertility is often an important consideration in selecting adjuvant treatments for younger women, and chemotherapy-induced toxicity of the ovary deserves mention here. The impact of chemotherapy on the ovary is principally a function of cumulative dose and patient age. Chemotherapy-induced gonadal toxicity results from ovarian stromal fibrosis, loss of follicles, and impaired granulosa cell and follicular cell development, as reported by Bines and coworkers, Warne and associates, Gradishar and Schilsky, and Ataya and Moghissi. Warne and coworkers, as well as Wallace and colleagues, noted that alkylating agents and platinum analogues confer the greatest risk of ovarian dysfunction whereas Sutton and associates reported that anthracyclines are less toxic to the ovary. As a consequence, cessation of menstrual function occurs commonly in premenopausal women receiving chemotherapy, but in most cases it returns in a few months following completion of therapy. Subsequent successful pregnancies do occur with no evidence at present of an increased risk of congenital anomalies in those who have had chemotherapy. Certainly, the physician must be aware of the individual adverse affects when administering these agents, including those on ovarian function when ovarian cell lines are not the chemotherapeutic target. The goal of treatment is to provide as high a dose of the chemotherapeutic agent as possible to produce maximum chemotherapeutic effectiveness without causing unacceptable toxicity or side effects.

There are four ways in which chemotherapy is generally used: (1) as an induction treatment for advanced disease (neoadjuvant therapy) in which additional treatment following chemotherapy is planned, (2) as an adjunct to radiation therapy, (3) as primary treatment for cancer, and (4) by direct instillation into specific regions of the body (e.g., intraperitoneal chemotherapy).

In assessment of the effect of chemotherapeutic agents, a number of definitions are used to describe the response of the tumor being treated. Clinical response should be assessed on an individual basis, with tumors in some patients monitored by physical examination and in some patients through imaging, typically with computed tomography or magnetic resonance imaging. Other means of assessing response to therapy include serial assessment of specific tumor markers (i.e., CA 125 for ovarian cancer and β-human chorionic gonadotropin for gestational trophoblastic disease) or identification of changes in hypermetabolic foci through positron emission tomography. In 2000, an international committee endorsed a technique for measuring tumors on computed tomography and magnetic resonance imaging that is easy and highly reproducible. This is known as RECIST (Response Evaluation Criteria in Solid Tumors) and is applicable for subjects with at least one measurable target lesion. The greatest diameters of all target lesions are summed, and changes in this sum during treatment are used to assign response (Table 26-3).

Evaluation of New Agents

In the development of new drugs, serial evaluations are necessary to assess the effectiveness of the drug as well as to ascertain its toxicity. A number of trials are necessary to move a new agent

Table 26-3 RECIST (Response Evaluation Criteria in Solid Tumors) Criteria to Assess Clinical Response to Therapy

- CR (complete response) = disappearance of all target lesions
- PR (partial response) = 30% decrease in the sum of the greatest diameters of target lesions
- PD (progressive disease) = 20% increase in the sum of the greatest diameters of target lesions
- SD (stable disease) = small changes that do not meet above criteria

from the point of evaluation to allow it to be used in regular medical practice. Such phase trials are defined as follows:

Phase I trial: A phase I trial tests new drugs at various doses to evaluate toxicity and to determine tolerance to the drug. At the various doses tested, some therapeutic effects may be observed, although this is not the primary aim of the trial.

Phase II trial: A phase II trial tests the therapeutic effectiveness and extent of the toxicity of the drug at doses expected to be effective against a specific tumor type.

Phase III trial: A phase III trial compares new treatment therapies against treatment currently in use. For instance, this trial design assesses whether a new drug therapy is superior, equivalent, or inferior to the chemotherapy currently used.

A standard method frequently used to measure a patient's general functional condition before enrollment in clinical chemotherapy trials of new agents is the Karnofsky Performance Status (Table 26-4). In general, patients are poor candidates from clinical trials if their Karnofsky Performance Status score is 50 or less. Cooperative research groups, such as the Gynecologic Oncology Group, have modified the Karnofsky Performance Status scoring system to reflect a five-point graded classification (see Table 26-4).

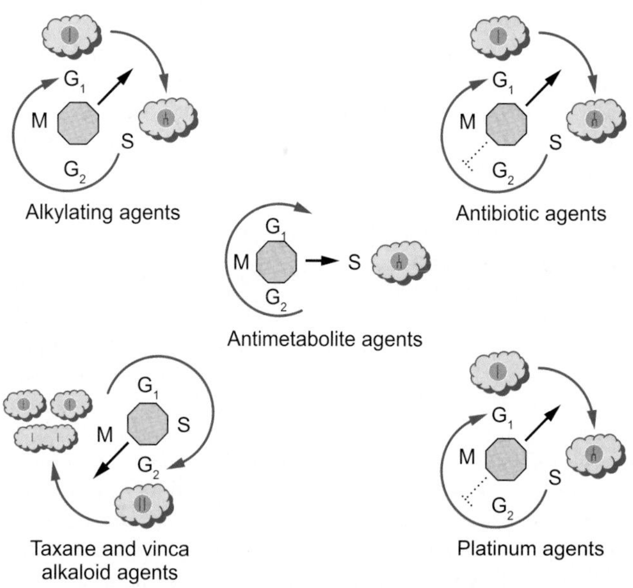

Figure 26-8. Chemotherapy cell-cycle activity. Chemotherapy agents demonstrate variable antitumor cytotoxic and radiosensitizing activities depending on their mechanism of action during the cell cycle. Alkylating agents facilitate transfer of alkyl groups to DNA, disrupting the G_1/S transition (*top left*). Agents derived from bacteria deregulate normal DNA and RNA processing, slowing progression through the G_1/S and G_2/M transitions (*top right*). Antimetabolites result in faulty base insertion into replicated DNA or specifically inhibit rate-limiting enzymes such as ribonucleotide reductase that are needed to produce deoxyribonucleotides for DNA replication during the S phase (*center*). Taxane and vinca alkaloid agents alter the mitotic spindle during mitosis, preventing cell division (*bottom left*). Platinum agents show activity throughout the cell and cycle form DNA structural adducts limiting progression at various cell-cycle checkpoints. Chemotherapeutic agents themselves are cytotoxic, but also increase tumor cell sensitivity to ionizing radiation during critical periods of the cell cycle in which radiation has maximal effect. The safe combination of these various classes of chemotherapies and radiation is an area of active clinical research.

Chemotherapeutic Agents Commonly Used in Gynecologic Cancer

A large number of chemotherapeutic drugs have been used in the therapy of gynecologic cancers (Fig. 26-8). In general, these agents can be classified into platinum compounds, taxanes, antitumor antibiotics, antimetabolites, alkylating agents, vinca (plant) alkaloids, camptothecans, and hormones. Examples of agents currently used alone or in combination for the treatment of gynecologic cancer are discussed.

Table 26-4 Assessment of Performance Status

Score	Karnofsky Performance Status	Grade	Gynecologic Oncology Group Performance Status Scale
100	Normal, no complaints; no evidence of disease	0	Fully active, able to carry on all predisease performance without restriction
90	Able to carry on normal activity; minor signs or symptoms of disease		
80	Normal activity with effort; some signs or symptoms of disease	1	Restricted in physically strenuous activity but ambulatory and able to carry out work of a light or sedentary nature, e.g., light housework, office work
70	Cares for self but unable to carry on normal activity or do active work		
60	Requires occasional assistance but is able to care for most personal needs	2	Ambulatory and capable of all self-care but unable to carry out any work activities; Up and approximately ≥50% of waking hours
50	Requires considerable assistance and frequent medical care		
40	Disabled; requires special care and assistance	3	Capable of only limited self-care, confined to bed or chair >50% of waking hours
30	Severely disabled; hospitalization indicated, although death not imminent		
20	Very sick; hospitalization necessary; active support treatment necessary	4	Completely disabled; cannot carry on any self-care; totally confined to bed or chair
10	Moribund; fatal process progressing rapidly		
0	Dead	5	Dead

Platinum Agents

Cisplatin and carboplatin are two of the most active and widely used chemotherapy agents in the treatment of gynecologic malignancies. As noted by Wang and Lippard, these synthetic compounds are used in the primary treatment of ovarian, tubal, peritoneal, endometrial, cervical, and vulvar cancers as well as some cases of metastatic gestational trophoblastic disease.

Lawrence and coworkers note that cisplatin (cis-diamminedichloroplatinum [CDDP]) binds to DNA causing intrastrand, interstrand, and protein adducts and thereby interferes with DNA processing and replication synthesis. Although its cell-cycle specificity has not been clearly defined, cisplatin's radiosensitizing mechanisms include formation of toxic intermediates in the presence of radiation-induced free radicals, as reported by Lawrence and associates; radiation-induced increased cellular platinum uptake, as noted by Yang and coworkers; inhibition of radiation-induced DNA repair, as described by Amorino and colleagues; and cell-cycle arrest at the G_2/M transition, according to Wang and Lippard. For the treatment of most gynecologic malignancies, cisplatin is given by an intravenous or an intraperitoneal infusion. Because cisplatin is nephrotoxic, copious hydration and mannitol infusion usually accompanies cisplatin administration to prevent renal tubular necrosis because the drug is excreted in the urine in its active form. Cisplatin also induces myelosuppression and high-frequency ototoxicity. Audiograms may be obtained before and during treatment to assess ototoxicity. Cisplatin induces severe peripheral neuropathy, which may improve somewhat after cessation of therapy but tends to be long lasting. Metabolic changes including hypomagnesemia and hypokalemia occur, and seizures have been reported in severe cases. Severe nausea with vomiting accompanies administration of the drug, so antiemetic medications are given before cisplatin infusion.

Carboplatin is an analogue of cisplatin, and a study conducted by Ozols and colleagues reported that it has activity in ovarian epithelial carcinoma comparable with that of cisplatin. Its mechanism of action and antitumor activity throughout the cell cycle are similar to that of cisplatin, yet carboplatin is less potent in producing DNA interstrand cross-links compared with cisplatin. Of recent clinical interest, Yang and coworkers found that the cellular uptake of carboplatin increases after ionizing radiation treatment with a concomitant increase in drug–DNA binding. Carboplatin is relatively nontoxic to the kidneys but appears more prone to cause leukopenia, thrombocytopenia, and anemia (nadir at 15 to 20 days). Rare toxicities include rash, alopecia, hepatotoxicity, neurotoxicity, and ototoxicity. Dose is usually based on the AUC. A typical outpatient dose range is an AUC = 5 to 7 mg/mL calculated using the formula: dose (mg) = AUC × (creatinine clearance + 25).

Taxanes

Paclitaxel (Taxol) and its synthetic analogue docetaxel (Taxotere) are derived from the bark of the Western yew tree (*Taxus baccata*). Both chemotherapeutic agents promote microtubule assembly and inhibit depolymerization of tubulin during mitosis. By arresting cell division through a functional block of the M phase, paclitaxel and docetaxel are potent chemotherapeutic agents with activity in most solid tumors. Administration of these drugs can be accompanied by severe hypersensitivity reactions and hypotension. Thus, premedication with antihistamines and steroids are recommended to minimize hypersensitivity reactions. Neutropenia is the major toxic side effect, but sensory peripheral neuropathy is also a serious problem. Bradycardia and severe cardiac problems have been reported with the administration of paclitaxel, but they are rare. A rare complication has been the report of bowel perforation in a few individuals while on paclitaxel therapy, as noted by Rose and Piver. In addition to its use in the treatment of ovarian cancer, paclitaxel and/or docetaxel are being used in the treatment of other cervical cancer, endometrial cancer, and uterine sarcomas.

Antitumor Antibiotics

Antitumor antibiotics are derived from products of bacterial or fungal cultures. The chemotherapeutic agents used most commonly in gynecologic malignancies are actinomycin D (Dactinomycin), doxorubicin (Adriamycin), and bleomycin (Blenoxane).

Actinomycin D is derived from the bacteria *Streptomyces parvulus* and is used primarily in the treatment of gestational trophoblastic disease. This drug lodges between adjacent purine–pyrimidine (guanine–cytosine) base pairs blocking DNA-dependent ribosomal RNA synthesis by RNA polymerase. Actinomycin D is maximally effective in G_1 phase of the cell cycle, but data suggest that this drug may act throughout the entire cell cycle. Because bound actinomycin D dissociates slowly from DNA, cells actively progressing through the cell cycle are stopped from doing so at the G_1/S checkpoint for genomic integrity leading to cell death. If radiation is delivered in the presence of the drug, treated cells show a radiosensitizing effect. The drug causes severe myelosuppression, often leading to leukopenia and thrombocytopenia (nadir 7 to 10 days). Toxicity to the gastrointestinal mucosa is associated with emesis within 20 hours, stomatitis, and nonbloody diarrhea. Reversible alopecia may also occur. Dermatitis resulting from "radiation recall" has been noted, meaning skin erythema and inflammation arise in skin areas previously irradiated.

Doxorubicin (Adriamycin) and its newer liposomal formulation (Doxil) are anthracyclines derived from the bacteria *Streptomyces peucetius* var. *caesius*. Within the cell nucleus, doxorubicin wedges between stacked nucleotide pairs in the DNA helix and, because of its bulk, inhibits binding of enzymes needed for DNA-directed RNA and DNA transcription as well as DNA replication. Doxorubicin therefore has maximal activity in the G_1 and S phases of the cell cycle. A second mechanism of action noted for doxorubicin includes inhibition of topoisomerase II in the G_2 phase of the cell cycle. Topoisomerase II assists in the coiling and supercoiling of DNA prior to mitosis by facilitating enzymatic DNA double-strand breaks. Doxorubicin has been shown to stabilize the double-stranded break generated by topoisomerase II, thereby promoting loss of genetic material during mitotic division. Doxorubicin must be administered carefully by intravenous injection because extravasation leads to soft-tissue and skin necrosis and ulceration. Doxorubicin is metabolized by the liver, and doses must be reduced in patients with compromised hepatic function. Myelosuppression occurs regularly with therapeutic doses. Complete but reversible alopecia is a side effect (Table 26-5). Because the drug binds to cardiac myocytes, doxorubicin predisposes to congestive heart failure. Therefore, cardiac function is assessed routinely before administration and cumulative doses are kept to less than 550 mg/m^2.

Table 26-5 Side Effects of Drugs Often Used or Being Tested in Gynecologic Oncology

	Bone Marrow	Phlebitis Sclerosant	Neurologic	Skin	Pulmonary	Renal	Hepatic	Cardiac	Endocrine	Bladder	Gut Mucositis	Allergic	Alopecia	Metabolic	Nausea Vomiting
Antimetabolites															
Methotrexate	+++		+	+	+	+	++				+++		+		+
5-Fluorouracil	+++		+	+							++		+		+
Gemcitabine	++		+	+			+				+		+		+
Alkylating Agents															
Cyclophosphamide	+++			+			+	+	+	++	++		++	+	++
Ifosfamide	++		++							++			++		+
Antitumor Antibiotics															
Actinomycin D	+++	+	+	+							++		++	+	++
Doxorubicin	+++	++	+					++			++		++		++
Bleomycin	+		++	+++	+++		+					+			++
Vinca Alkaloids															
Vinblastine	+++	+					+						+		
Vincristine	+	+	+++				+						+	+	
Etoposide (VP-16)	+++										+		++		+
Taxanes															
Paclitaxel	+++	+	++	+				+			+	++	++		+
Docetaxel	+++	+	++	+				+			+	++	++		+
Platins															
Cisplatin	+		+			+++									++
Carboplatin	++		+			+					+				+
Growth Factor Inhibitors															
Cetuximab	+			++	+	+					+	+			++
Transtuzumab	+		+	+	+	+		++			+			+	+
Bevacizumab	+			++		+		++			++				+

+++, dose limiting; ++, common; +, rare.
Modified from Tattersall MHN: Pharmacology and selection of cytotoxic drugs. In Coppleson M (ed): Gynecologic Oncology, 2nd ed. Edinburgh, Churchill Livingstone, 1992, p 180.

Adriamycin has been encapsulated with liposomes (Doxil) that form a synthetic lipid-like membrane around the doxorubicin molecule. The half-life of this compound is longer than that of its parent compound, and there is some evidence that the agent is taken up preferentially by tumor cells. Cardiomyopathy is less common with liposome-encapsulated Adriamycin, but skin toxicity, notably palmar planter dysesthesia, is more common.

Bleomycin is derived from the bacteria *Streptomyces verticillis* and, when complexed with ferrous iron, is a potent oxidase, producing single-stranded DNA breaks by hydroxyl radical formation. Bleomycin may be administered intravenously, intramuscularly, or subcutaneously. It is excreted via the kidney, and some dose reduction is made if renal function is compromised. The drug does *not* produce significant myelosuppression, in contrast to most of the other cytotoxic agents. It is, however, highly toxic to the lungs in that pneumonitis and pulmonary fibrosis occurs in 10% of patients. Thus, particular care must be used in persons with compromised lung function. To prevent this complication, cumulative doses of less than 400 mg are given. If pneumonitis develops as evident by symptoms of low-grade fever and nonproductive cough, treatment is a tapered course of oral corticosteroid therapy. Bleomycin is also toxic to skin and can produce erythema, peeling, and pigmentation. It has been used as part of combination therapy with particular effectiveness against ovarian germ cell tumors and has been tried for a variety of other gynecologic malignancies, particularly carcinoma of the cervix.

Antimetabolites

Antimetabolites interfere with cell metabolism by competing with naturally occurring purines or pyrimidines, whose chemical structure they resemble. In this way they interfere or prevent vital biochemical reactions.

5-Fluorouracil (5-FU) is a fluorinated pyrimidine analogue resembling the DNA nucleoside thymine and different from the RNA nucleoside uracil by a fluorinated carbon in the fifth position in the nucleoside ring, as described by Grem. Conversion of 5-FU into fluorodeoxyuridine monophosphate blocks DNA synthesis by covalently binding to thymidylate synthase. This inhibits the formation of de novo thymidylate, a necessary precursor of thymidine triphosphate that is essential for DNA synthesis and cell division. Conversion of 5-FU into fluorouridine triphosphate results in the erroneous incorporation of fluorouridine triphosphate into RNA. This incorporation interferes with RNA processing and protein synthesis. By these actions, 5-FU perturbs normal progression through the G_1/S transition, bringing about impaired cell division due to altered nucleotide pools and DNA repair. As such, 5-FU is a potent radiosensitizer. One advantage of the drug is that 5-FU can be administered as a bolus or continuous intravenous infusion or orally as a prodrug that is metabolized to 5-FU (capecitabine [Xeloda]). 5-FU suppresses the bone marrow, although less so than many other cytotoxic agents used in gynecologic cancer treatment. Stomatitis, diarrhea, alopecia, nail changes, dermatitis, acute cerebellar syndrome, cardiac toxicity, hyperpigmentation over the vein used for infusion, and hand–foot syndrome have been reported. The drug is normally used in conjunction with cisplatin as a radiation sensitizer in the treatment of advanced cervical and vulvar cancer.

Methotrexate is a folic acid analogue that binds tightly to dihydrofolate reductase, which plays a critical role in intracellular folate metabolism. This prevents metabolic transfer of one carbon unit within the cell and thereby arrests DNA, RNA, and protein synthesis. Cells show sensitivity to this drug predominantly in the S phase portion of the cell cycle. The effects of methotrexate can be overcome by the administration of folinic acid (citrovorum factor) 24 hours after methotrexate, which replenishes the tetrahydrofolate. Some chemotherapy protocols have used very high doses of methotrexate to treat the tumor, followed by citrovorum rescue to avoid severe toxic side effects (see Table 26-5). Methotrexate is administered intravenously, intramuscularly, or orally using a variety of dose regimens. It is excreted in the urine and dose adjustments must be made if there is decreased renal function. Methotrexate results in severe myelosuppression (nadir 6 to 13 days). Stomatitis, nausea, and emesis are reported. Hepatotoxicity resulting in liver enzyme elevation may be seen within 12 hours after high-dose treatment. Therapeutic serum methotrexate levels are evident long after treatment in patients with ascites or pleural effusion because these act as a reservoir for the drug. The predominant use of the drug in the treatment of gynecologic malignancies has been the effective treatment of trophoblastic disease.

Gemcitabine, a synthetic deoxycytidine nucleoside analogue, targets ribonucleotide reductase (RR), the rate-limiting enzyme in deoxyribonucleotide metabolism during the S phase, as described by Cory. Mammalian cells use the RR enzyme to transform ribonucleotides into deoxyribonucleotides needed for DNA replication. Elford and coworkers have found a correlation between tumor growth rate and the specific activity of RR. As such, inhibitors of RR may decrease the rate of tumor cell replication and tumor growth in vivo. Kuo and Kinsella reported that ionizing radiation can induce a demonstrable increase in RR protein and enzyme activity in cancers, such as human cervical carcinoma cells, leading to increased capacity to repair DNA damage. This lowers the radiobiologic effect of ionizing radiation. As a nucleoside analogue, gemcitabine is incorporated as a fraudulent base pair in DNA; as a diphosphate, it inhibits the regulatory subunit of the RR enzyme, which leads to depletion of deoxyribonucleotide pools needed for DNA synthesis in the S phase of the cell cycle. Both mechanisms contribute to gemcitabine's cytotoxic and radiosensitizing properties. Reported treatment toxicities include myelosuppression (20%), transient elevation of liver enzymes, nausea, vomiting, flulike symptoms, and fatigue. Gemcitabine is used in the treatment of recurrent ovarian cancer and uterine sarcomas.

Alkylating Agents

Alkylating agents are chemical compounds that facilitate the replacement of hydrogen for an alkyl group, potentially disrupting normal function of the altered molecule. As chemotherapeutic agents, alkylating agents interact directly with DNA by transferring positively charged alkyl groups to negatively charged chemical groups intrinsic to the DNA molecule. Examples of this class include cyclophosphamide and ifosfamide. In general, the effectiveness of these agents appears similar, but there are some variations in toxicity. The alkylating agents as a drug class affect rapidly dividing cells and are particularly toxic to the bone marrow, leading to severe myelosuppression.

Cyclophosphamide and its structural analogue ifosfamide are bifunctional cyclic phosphamide esters of nitrogen mustard. Both drugs interact with the N7 position of guanine within the DNA helix to form cross-link bridges between the same strand of DNA (intrastrand), opposite strands of DNA (interstrand), and between DNA and cellular proteins. By forming intrastrand and interstrand DNA bridges, cyclophosphamide and ifosfamide impair the functional binding of enzymes used to process and replicate DNA, disrupting the G_1/S phase traverse of the cell cycle. These drugs are inactivated in the liver and exclusively excreted by the kidney. Their urinary metabolite acrolein may accumulate within the urinary system causing severe urothelial damage that may result in hemorrhagic cystitis within 24 hours or weeks later after administration. Prophylactic hydration (3 L/day) to increase dilute urinary output and administration of 2-mercaptoethane sulfonate (Mesna), a compound that binds to acrolein and prevents urotoxicity, can be used to prevent this complication. Administration of these agents also leads to leukopenia (nadir 8 to 14 days) and thrombocytopenia (nadir 18 to 21 days), alopecia, nausea and emesis, and amenorrhea. Therapy with alkylating agents has been associated with the subsequent risk of developing acute leukemia. This risk may range from 2% to 10% and appears to be related to dose of and duration of alkylating agent treatment. They may be administered intravenously or orally but are only rarely used in the primary treatment of gynecologic malignancies.

Antimicrotubular (Antimitotic) Drugs

A number of cytotoxic drugs have been isolated from plant extracts. Most of the antimitotics are plant alkaloids. These include naturally occurring vinca alkaloids, such as vincristine, vinblastine, and the semisynthetic analogues. The vinca alkaloids bind to the β-tubulin subunits of the mitotic spindles, blocking polymerization of the microtubules in mitosis.

Vinca (Plant) Alkaloids

For gynecologic malignancies, the most often used vinca alkaloids include vinblastine, vincristine, and VP-16 (etoposide). Vinblastine and vincristine are derived from the periwinkle plant (*Vinca rosea*). Both drugs act in a cell-cycle-dependent manner, blocking the assembly of tubulin and causing toxic destruction of the mitotic spindle, which arrests cellular mitosis. Vinorelbine is a semisynthetic vinca alkaloid derived from vinblastine and is a radiation-sensitizing agent. VP-16 (etoposide) is an epipodophyllotoxin derived from the root of the May apple or mandrake plant. VP-16 stabilizes DNA strand breaks made by topoisomerase II during coiling and supercoiling of DNA during mitosis. By affecting the late G_2 and M phases of the cell cycle, these drugs are potent cytotoxins and increase cell radiosensitivity by slowing the G_2/M transition in which radiation effects are maximal. Vincristine is severely neurotoxic and can produce numbness, motor weakness, and constipation as a result of its autonomic effects. There is little myelosuppression. Vinblastine is myelotoxic, and this tends to be a dose-limiting factor. However, vinblastine and vinorelbine are less neurotoxic than vincristine. VP-16 is myelotoxic, leading to depression of leukocytes and platelets. VP-16 induces anorexia, nausea and emesis, stomatitis, and severe hypotension if infused in less than 30 minutes. Uncommon toxicities include cardiotoxicity, bronchospasm, and somnolence. These drugs are used to treat ovarian germ cell tumors, cervical cancer (vinorelbine) and trophoblastic disease.

Topoisomerase Inhibitors

As mentioned, topoisomerases are DNA enzymes that control the topology of DNA double-helix cellular functions during transcription and replication of genetic material. There are two classes of topoisomerases: I and II. Drugs that prevent these functions are referred to as inhibitors. Topotecan, a topoisomerase I inhibitor, is used in the treatment of cervical cancer and epithelial ovarian cancer.

Topotecan is a semisynthetic analogue of camptothecin, a chemical derived from the *Camptotheca accuminata* tree native to China. This drug stabilizes single-strand breaks made by topoisomerase I, an enzyme that relaxes DNA structural tension by facilitating single-strand breaks and subsequent religation. Topotecan has the greatest activity during the G_1/S phases of the cell cycle. Toxicities include bone marrow suppression, nausea and vomiting, alopecia, mucositis, and diarrhea.

Growth Factor Receptor Targeting and Hormone Therapy

In the past 5 years, there has been a substantial increase in the number of targeted chemotherapeutics directed against specific growth factor receptors. Both normal and malignant cells show a growth response to specific endocrine, paracrine, and autocrine chemical stimuli activating cell surface growth factor receptors. Both the EGF family and vascular endothelial growth factor (VEGF) family of receptors have been targeted for cytotoxic and radiosensitizing agents in studies by Sartor and by Siemann and Shi. The EGF family of receptors comprises four transmembrane receptor kinases: HER2, HER3, HER4, and EGFR. Clinical studies have confirmed that EGFR and HER2 overexpression results in relative radioresistance among cancers, and therefore drugs that target these receptors may promote radiosensitization as has been shown among cancers of the head and neck by Bonner and coworkers and of the breast by Rao and associates. The chimeric antibodies against EGFR (cetuximab, Erbitux) and HER2 (trastuzumab, Herceptin) are being investigated in clinical trials of gynecologic malignancies.

VEGF-receptor-targeted therapies have emerged as clinically efficacious antiangiogenic and tumor-vasculature-stabilizing agents. It is known that tumor cells grow rapidly, often outpacing new blood vessel proliferation needed to ensure reliable oxygen and nutrient supply. Drugs such as bevacizumab (Avastin) that inhibit new blood vessel proliferation limit successful growth of proliferation malignant cells. Furthermore, Hicklin and Ellis have suggested that VEGF target therapies render small vessels hyperpermeable to circulating macromolecules, promoting steady tumor cell oxygenation (and thereby enhancing radiation sensitivity) and limiting intermittent tumor hypoxia from the random opening and closing of small vessels (which adversely confers radioresistance). Clinical activity in the treatment of recurrent ovarian cancer by such researchers as Monk and others has prompted study of more extensive study of VEGF target therapies as part of the primary therapy of advanced ovarian cancer.

Hormone therapy has been effectively developed in the treatment of breast cancer. Estrogen and progesterone receptors have been clearly identified in endometrial carcinomas and have been recently found in other types of gynecologic cancers, particularly ovarian epithelial carcinomas. Progestins such as megestrol (Megace), depo-medroxyprogesterone (Depo-Provera), and 17-OH progesterone caproate (Delalutin), as well as antiestrogens such as tamoxifen and raloxifene, have been used in the treatment of endometrial carcinomas and seem to have their best effects against well-differentiated tumors.

KEY POINTS

- Electromagnetic radiation is a form of energy that has no mass or charge and travels at the speed of light.
- Inverse square law states that the energy measured from a radiation source is inversely proportional to the square of the distance from the radiation source.
- Each delivered radiation dose kills a constant fraction of tumor cells irradiated. Oxygen can render radiation-induced DNA damage permanent.
- The effect of photon radiation (low LET) on tissues is altered by tissue oxygenation, whereas neutron (high LET) radiation is independent of oxygenation.
- The cell replication cycle consists of M (mitosis), G_1 (Gap1 = RNA and protein synthesis), S (DNA synthesis), and G_2 (Gap2 = RNA and protein synthesis). When the cell is not in the replication cycle, it is in the G_0 phase.
- The dose of radiation delivered to a tumor depends on the energy of the source, the size of the treatment field, and the depth of the tumor beneath the surface. Increasing the dose increases the depth of maximum dose beneath the skin surface.
- Radiation acts on cells primarily in the M phase, making rapidly proliferating cells the most radiosensitive.
- Normal tissues repair the radiobiologic effects of radiation more effectively than tumor tissue.
- Radiation side effects most commonly involve erythema of the skin without desquamation and mild fatigue.
- Uncommon side effects include lowering of the circulating blood cells, dysuria and urinary frequency, diarrhea, bowel injury, and fistula formation.
- Multiple chemotherapeutic agents have been used alone to kill cancer cells and have been used to sensitize cells to radiation. Often, chemoradiation improves clinical outcomes, particularly with squamous cell cancers.
- Cytotoxic chemotherapeutic agents act on various phases of the cell cycle, primarily affecting rapidly proliferating cells, and at a given dose destroy a constant fraction of tumor cells.
- The major classes of cytotoxic chemotherapeutic agents used in gynecologic oncology are alkylating agents, antitumor antibiotics, antimetabolites, vinca (plant) alkaloids, topoisomerase inhibitors, and specially synthesized compounds.
- Topoisomerase inhibitors such as topotecan and CPT 11 are drugs that stabilize DNA breaks during uncoiling.
- Most chemotherapeutic drugs are severely myelosuppressive, with the exception of bleomycin and vincristine.
- Vincristine and cisplatin cause severe peripheral neurotoxicity.
- Bleomycin is associated with severe pulmonary toxicity.
- Doxorubicin is associated with severe cardiomyopathy.
- Cisplatin is nephrotoxic and myelosuppressive. Its analogue carboplatin is also excreted by the kidney but is not nephrotoxic.
- Paclitaxel (Taxol) and docetaxel (Taxotere) are powerful antineoplastic agents that disrupt the function of microtubules. These drugs are effective particularly in cases of ovarian cancer. They can cause severe infusion reactions, neutropenia, and neurotoxicity.
- New chemotherapies targeting growth factor receptors are under clinical study for cytotoxic and radiosensitizing applications.
- Alopecia can occur with any chemotherapy, but it is total and severe with doxorubicin, actinomycin, and paclitaxel. Hair growth resumes after cessation of treatment.
- Growth factors or granulocyte colony-stimulating factor are used to limit the hematologic toxicity of chemotherapy.

BIBLIOGRAPHY

Adams GE, Stratford IJ, Bremner JC, et al: Nitroheterocyclic compounds as radiation sensitizers and bioreductive drugs. Radiother Oncol 20(suppl 1):85–91, 1991.

Amorino GP, Freeman ML, Carbone DP, et al: Radiopotentiation by the oral platinum agent, JM216: role of repair inhibition. Int J Radiat Oncol Biol Phys 44:399–405, 1999.

Arai T, Nakano T, Fukuhisa K, et al: Second cancer after radiation therapy for cancer of the uterine cervix. Cancer 67:398–405, 1991.

Ataya K, Moghissi K: Chemotherapy-induced premature ovarian failure: mechanisms and prevention. Steroids 54:607–626, 1989.

Bines J, Oleske DM, Cobleigh MA: Ovarian function in premenopausal women treated with adjuvant chemotherapy for breast cancer. J Clin Oncol 14:1718–1729, 1996.

Bonner JA, Trigo J, Humblet Y, et al: Phase 3 trial of radiation therapy plus cetuximab versus radiation therapy alone in locally advanced squamous cell carcinomas of the head and neck [abstract]. Proc ASCO 2004;5507.

Bowland JD: Radiation oncology physics. In Gunderson LL, Tepper JE (eds): Clinical Radiation Oncology. New York, Churchill Livingstone, 2000, pp 64–118.

Chiao TB, Lee AJ: Role of pentoxifylline and vitamin E in attenuation of radiation-induced fibrosis. Ann Pharmacother 39:516–522, 2005.

Cory JG: Role of ribonucleotide reductase in cell division. In Cory JC, Cory AM (eds): International Encyclopedia of Pharmacology and Therapeutics—Inhibitors of Ribonucleotide Diphosphate Reductase Activity, Vol 128. New York, Pergamon Press, 1989, pp 1–16.

Covens A, Thomas G, DePetrillo A, et al: The prognostic importance of site and type of radiation-induced bowel injury in patients requiring surgical management. Gynecol Oncol 43:270–274, 1991.

Deshpande A, Sicinski P, Hinds PW: Cyclins and CDKS in development and cancer: a perspective. Oncogene 24:2909–2915, 2005.

Dunst J, Kuhnt T, Strauss HG, et al: Anemia in cervical cancers: impact on survival, patterns of relapse, and association with hypoxia and angiogenesis. Int J Radiat Oncol Biol Phys 56:778–787, 2003.

Elford HL, Freese M, Passamani E, et al: Ribonucleotide reductase and cell proliferation. I. Variations of ribonucleotide reductase activity with tumor growth rate in a series of rat hepatomas. J Biol Chem 245:5228–5233, 1970.

Goldberg Z, Evans J, Birrell G, et al: An investigation of the molecular basis for the synergistic interaction of tirapazamine and cisplatin. Int J Radiat Oncol Biol Phys 49:175–182, 2001.

Gothard L, Cornes P, Brooker S, et al: Phase II study of vitamin E and pentoxifylline in patients with late side effects of pelvic radiotherapy. Radiother Oncol 75:334–341, 2005.

Gradishar WJ, Schilsky RL: Ovarian function following radiation and chemotherapy for cancer. Semin Oncol 16:425–436, 1989.

Grem J: 5-Fluoropyrimidines. In Chabner BA, Longo D (eds): Cancer Chemotherapy and Biotherapy Principles and Practice, 2nd ed. Philadelphia, Lippincott–Raven, 1996, pp 149–212.

Hall EJ: Radiobiology for the Radiologist, 5th ed. Philadelphia, Lippincott Williams & Wilkins, 2000.

Hall EJ, Hei TK: Genomic instability and bystander effects induced by high-LET radiation. Oncogene. 22:7034–7042, 2003.

Hicklin DJ, Ellis LM: Role of the vascular endothelial growth factor pathway in tumor growth and angiogenesis. J Clin Oncol 23:1011–1027, 2005.

Jonathan EC, Bernhard EJ, McKenna WG: How does radiation kill cells? Curr Opin Chem Biol 3:77–83, 1999.

Kahn FM: The Physics of Radiation Therapy, 3rd ed. Philadelphia, Lippincott Williams & Wilkins, 2003.

Kuo ML, Kinsella TJ: Expression of ribonucleotide reductase after ionizing radiation in human cervical carcinoma cells. Cancer Res 58:2245–2252, 1998.

Lawrence TS, Blackstock AW, McGinn C: The mechanism of action of radiosensitization of conventional chemotherapeutic agents. Semin Radiat Oncol 13:13–21, 2003.

Li MC, Hertz R, Spencer DB: Effect of methotrexate therapy upon choriocarcinoma and chorioadenoma. Proc Soc Exp Biol Med 93:361–366, 1956.

Malumbres M, Barbacid M: To cycle or not to cycle: a critical decision in cancer. Nat Rev Cancer 1:222–231, 2001.

McIntyre JF, Eifel PJ, Levenback C, et al: Ureteral stricture as a late complication of radiotherapy for stage IB carcinoma of the uterine cervix. Cancer 75:836–843, 1995.

Monk BJ, Han E, Josephs-Cowan CA, et al: Salvage bevacizumab (rhuMAB VEGF)-based therapy after multiple prior cytotoxic regimens in advanced refractory epithelial ovarian cancer. Gynecol Oncol 102:140–144, 2006.

Montana GS, Fowler WC: Carcinoma of the cervix: analysis of bladder and rectal radiation dose and complications. Int J Radiat Oncol Biol Phys 16:95–100, 1989.

Munro TR: The relative radiosensitivity of the nucleus and cytoplasm of the Chinese hamster fibroblasts. Radiat Res 42:451–470, 1970.

Ozols RF, Bundy BN, Greer BE, et al: Phase III trial of carboplatin and paclitaxel compared with cisplatin and paclitaxel in patients with optimally resected stage III ovarian cancer: a Gynecologic Oncology Group study. J Clin Oncol 21:3194–3200, 2003.

Palcic B, Skarsgard LD: Reduced oxygen enhancement ratio at low doses of ionizing radiation. Radiat Res 100:328–329, 1984.

Pawlik TM, Keyomarsi K: Role of cell cycle in mediating sensitivity to radiotherapy. Int J Radiat Oncol Biol Phys 59:928–942, 2004.

Rao GS, Murray S, Ethier SP: Radiosensitization of human breast cancer cells by a novel ErbB family receptor tyrosine kinase inhibitor. Int J Radiat Oncol Biol Phys 48:1519–1528, 2000.

Rose PG, Piver MS: Intestinal perforation secondary to paclitaxel. Gynecol Oncol 57:270–272, 1995.

Sartor CI: Epidermal growth factor family receptors and inhibitors: radiation response modulators. Semin Radiat Oncol 13:22–30, 2003.

Siemann DW, Shi W: Targeting the tumor blood vessel network to enhance the efficacy of radiation therapy. Semin Radiat Oncol 13:53–61, 2003.

Skipper HE: The effects of chemotherapy on the kinetics of leukemic cell behavior. Cancer Res 25:1544–1550, 1965.

Skipper HE: Dose intensity versus total dose of chemotherapy: an experimental basis. Import Adv Oncol 43–64, 1990.

Sutton R, Buzdar AU, Hortobagyi GN: Pregnancy and offspring after adjuvant chemotherapy in breast cancer patients. Cancer 65:847–850, 1990.

Utley JF, Marlowe C, Waddell WJ: Distribution of 35S-labeled WR-2721 in normal and malignant tissues of the mouse. Radiat Res 68:284–291, 1976.

Wallace WH, Shalet SM, Crowne EC, et al: Gonadal dysfunction due to cis-platinum. Med Pediatr Oncol 17:409–413, 1989.

Wang D, Lippard SJ: Cellular processing of platinum anticancer drugs. Nat Rev Drug Disc. 4:307–320, 2005.

Warne GL, Fairley KF, Hobbs JB, et al: Cyclophosphamide-induced ovarian failure. N Engl J Med 289:1159–1162, 1973.

Xu B, Kim S-T, Lim D-S, et al: Two molecularly distinct G(2)/M checkpoints are induced by ionizing irradiation. Mol Cell Biol 22:1049–1059, 2002.

Yang LX, Douple EB, Wang HJ: Irradiation enhances cellular uptake of carboplatin. Int J Radiat Oncol Biol Phys 33:641–646, 1995.

Yang LX, Douple E, Wang HJ: Irradiation-enhanced binding of carboplatin to DNA. Int J Radiat Biol 68:609–614, 1995.

Immunology and Molecular Oncology in Gynecologic Cancer 27

Immunologic Response, Cytokines, Tumor Cell Killing, and Immunotherapy

S. Diane Yamada and Steven E. Waggoner

KEY TERMS AND DEFINITIONS

Active Immunity. A form of adaptive immunity that is the result of exposure to a foreign antigen and activation of lymphocytes.

Adaptive Immunity. Also known as specific immunity. The use of extracts derived from sensitized lymphocytes to transfer "immunologic memory" and induce an antitumor response.

Adenovirus. An RNA virus that can be used as a vector in gene therapy.

Allele. The form of DNA sequences in a gene on a given chromosomal locus. If the genes are identical, the individual is homozygous. Different genes result in heterozygosity. One allele is inherited from the mother and the other from the father.

Amplification. Increase in the number of copies of a DNA sequence in a cell.

Angiogenesis. The formation of new blood vessels. A process in neoplasia whereby malignant cells release substances that eventually lead to the activation and production of endothelial cells and the establishment of new capillary blood supply to a growing tumor.

Antibody. Produced by B lymphocytes. Also known as an immunoglobulin. Binds antigen with high specificity to result in neutralization of antigen, activation of complement, or leukocyte-dependent destruction of antigen.

Antigen. A molecule that can bind an antibody or T-cell receptor (TCR).

Antigen-Presenting Cell (APC). A cell, often a macrophage or dendritic cell, that digests the antigen involved in cellular immunity and then displays the foreign antigen as peptide fragments on its surface in conjunction with major histocompatibility complex (MHC) molecules to activate T cells. APCs also express molecules to specifically activate T cells.

Apoptosis. The process of programmed cell death leading to degradation of DNA, fragmentation of the cell, and phagocytosis by macrophages.

B Lymphocyte. A central mediator of the humoral immune response. B lymphocytes produce antibodies in response to an antigenic stimulus. They differentiate into plasma cells, which secrete antibody.

BRCA1, BRCA2. Breast cancer and ovarian susceptibility genes. Thought to function primarily as DNA repair genes. Mutation of *BRCA1* or *BRCA2* confers a high lifetime risk of breast or ovarian cancer.

Cellular Immunity. A form of adaptive immunity in which lymphoid cells, usually CD4+ T cells, activate macrophages or CD8+ cells and directly kill infected cells.

Cluster of Differentiation (CD). Cell surface markers on the surface of T cells that recognize antibodies and allow for characterization of specific T-cell subunits.

Colony-Stimulating Factors. Cytokines that promote the production of specific progenitor cells within the bone marrow such as red blood cells, granulocytes, and lymphocytes.

Complement. A component of the immune system consisting of serum and cell surface proteins activated by antigen–antibody complexes (the classic pathway) or microbial surfaces (alternative pathway) to generate an inflammatory response and cytotoxicity.

Cytokines. Modulators of the immune and inflammatory system that act as communicators between members of the immune system.

Cytotoxic T Lymphocytes. CD8+-expressing cells that kill cells expressing peptides in conjunction with MHC class I molecules.

Epitope. The portion of an antigen to which an antibody binds, e.g., the portion of an antigen that binds an MHC molecule that is recognized by a TCR.

Fab. The variable portion of the immunoglobulin molecule that binds to the antigen.

Fc. The "constant" region of the immunoglobulin molecule that is responsible for biologic activity. It allows for antibody binding to a phagocyte.

Helper T Cells. A T-cell lymphocyte subset that is usually CD4+. Their main effector function is to activate macrophages in cell-mediated immunity and stimulate B-cell immunoglobulin production in humoral immunity.

Humoral Immunity. A type of adaptive immunity mediated by antibody production from B lymphocytes.

Immunoglobulin. Synonymous with antibody. Five basic types are recognized (IgG, IgM, IgA, IgD, IgE).

Interferon (IFN). A cytokine produced by lymphocytes or fibroblasts in response to viral infection. There are three types: alpha, beta, and gamma. IFN-γ is produced by T cells and natural killer (NK) cells and activates macrophages.

Interleukin (IL). A class of cytokines secreted by monocytes, lymphocytes, and macrophages. They are numerically designated.

Continued

KEY TERMS AND DEFINITIONS *Continued*

Lymphokine. See Cytokine.

Macrophage. A cell derived from monocytes that can act as an APC, phagocytotic cell, or a producer of cytokines.

Major Histocompatibility Complex. A cluster of genes coded for on chromosome 6 that include HLA antigens. The gene complex is found in nearly all nucleated cells of the body and codes for the peptide-binding molecules recognized by T lymphocytes. The MHC molecules include class I and II MHC molecules. Class I molecules bind peptides derived from cytosolic proteins and are recognized by CD8+ cells. Class II molecules bind peptides endocytosed by APCs and are recognized by CD4+ T cells.

Mutation. An alteration of normal genetic composition that leads to a change in the DNA sequence that is perpetuated in subsequent cell divisions.

Natural Killer (NK) Cell. A type of lymphocyte that produces IFN-γ and functions in the innate immune system to directly kill cells.

Oncogene. A class of genes that can be mutated, overexpressed, or amplified and is associated with the development of malignant growth.

Opsonization. A process whereby opsonins, IgG, or complement fragments are attached to the cell surface of marked cells to target them for phagocytosis.

Overexpression. Increase in the amount of protein product produced by a gene.

Passive Immunity. The transfer of specific antibodies or lymphocytes from one individual who has responded to and is immune to an antigen to another individual to try to enhance the immune response.

Plasma cell. Terminally differentiated B lymphocyte that secretes antibody.

Proto-oncogene. A normal gene component in cells that plays a role in physiologic growth and development. When abnormally activated, they become oncogenes.

Retrovirus. An RNA tumor virus that, when integrated into certain animal cells, leads to oncogene development. It has an RNA genome and can propagate by reverse transcription of its RNA into DNA.

Suppressor T Cell. A differentiated T-cell lymphocyte that functions to suppress B-cell production and T-cell cytotoxicity.

T Lymphocytes. Lymphocytes that exhibit cell surface antigenicity via the TCR and mediate cellular immunity within the adaptive immune system. Subsets include CD4+ T helper cells and CD8+ cytotoxic T lymphocytes.

T-Cell Receptor (TCR). An antigen receptor present on CD4+ and CD8+ T cells that recognizes peptides complexed with MHC molecules on APCs.

Transfection. The transfer of DNA sequences (genetic material) into a cell.

Translocation. The transfer or exchange of genetic material between two nonhomologous chromosomes.

Transcription. Process by which messenger RNA is synthesized from a DNA template in the nucleus, then enters the cytoplasm, and serves as a template for protein synthesis.

Tumor Necrosis Factor (TNF). A cytokine that mediates endotoxic shock and is capable of inhibiting tumor cell growth. It is produced by activated mononuclear phagocytes and recruits neutrophils and monocytes to sites of infection.

Tumor-Specific Antigen. Antigen expression restricted to tumor cells and not normal cells. They can act as targets for immunotherapy.

Tumor Suppressor Gene. A normal genetic component of the cell that controls cell growth and proliferation. Mutations in the gene can lead to malignancy.

This chapter summarizes general principles of tumor immunology, which is followed by a description of molecular genetics, signaling pathways, and regulation of angiogenesis as they apply to gynecologic tumors. These are rapidly expanding fields, and it is not possible in this chapter to explore them in great detail. However, in the following sections, some basic immunologic mechanisms are reviewed and the possible application of this information to gynecologic tumor therapy is explored. This is followed by a summary of the molecular and genetic changes associated with malignant cellular growth and a consideration of the application of this knowledge to cancer therapy.

THE IMMUNOLOGIC RESPONSE

The immune system has adapted to fight off foreign intruders such as bacteria and viruses, but it also plays a role in the surveillance and control of cancer cell growth. The immune system is divided into that part that is *innate*, present at birth, and that part that is *adaptive,* as a response to infection. Components of the innate immune system include physical barriers such as epithelial surfaces, macrophages, NK cells, and dendritic cells. Dendritic cells and macrophages are phagocytic cells that act as APCs. Macrophages also play an important role in the production of cytokines, which act as growth factors for other immune cells. Other members of the innate immune system include components of the complement system and cytokines that regulate these cells. The major components of the adaptive immune system are the T lymphocytes (T cells) and the B lymphocytes (B cells). Two types of adaptive immune response exist: *cell-mediated immunity* and *humoral immunity.* Although cell-mediated immunity is mediated by T lymphocytes, humoral immunity is mediated by antibodies and B lymphocytes.

Innate Immunity

In contrast to the adaptive immune system that can recognize a variety of foreign substances including tumor antigens, the innate immune system can only recognize microbial substances. The main effector cells of the innate immune system include neutrophils, macrophages, and NK cells. Neutrophils and macrophages are recruited to sites of infection and inflammation where they phagocytose and destroy microbes. Receptors on the surface of these effectors, such as the *Toll-like receptors* recognize bacterial lipopolysaccharides among other bacterial specific surface molecules to stimulate the production of cytokines that can recruit additional phagocytic cells to the site of infection. NK cells are a subset of the lymphocyte population and can directly kill infected cells. They recognize cells that lack MHC class I molecules such as bacteria. Recently, Moretta and coworkers reported that NK cells are cytotoxic to tumor cells likely due to a similar lack of surface MHC class I molecules. NK cells produce IFN-γ, which activates phagocytic macrophages.

The *complement system* is also an important component of the innate immune system. This is a complicated system that consists of a large group of interacting plasma proteins. Activation by binding to antigen-complexed antibody molecules activates the *classic pathway*, whereas the *alternative pathway* is activated by recognition of microbial surface structures in the absence of antibody. Activation of these pathways converges in cleavage of C3 protein into a larger C3b fragment that is deposited on the microbial surface leading to complement activation and C3a, which acts as a chemoattractant for neutrophils. Complexing of downstream complement proteins C6, C7, C8, and C9 produces a membrane pore in tagged cells that ultimately results in cell lysis. Unfortunately, tumor cells seem to be resistant to complement-dependent cytotoxicity. The innate immune system is intimately linked to the adaptive immune system by cells such as activated macrophages that enhance T-cell activation and complement fragments that can activate B cells and antibody production.

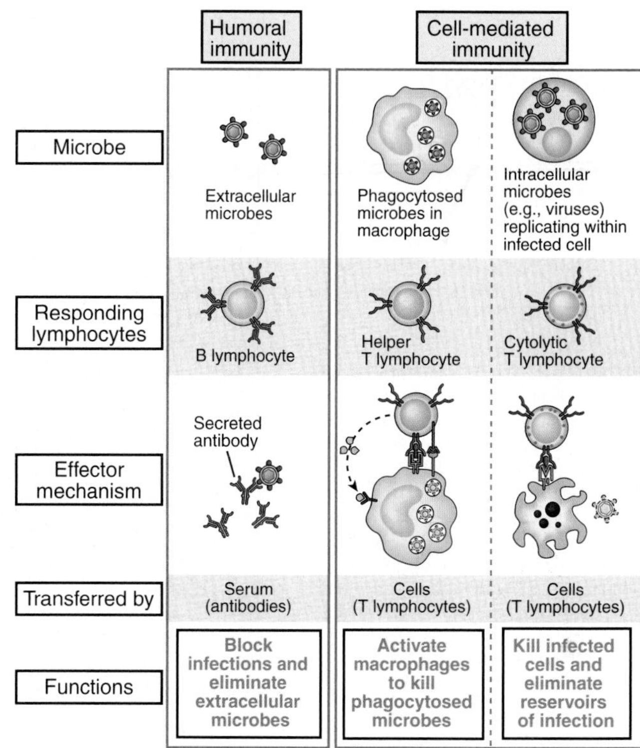

Figure 27-1. Differences in adaptive immunity. In cell-mediated immunity, helper T lymphocytes activate macrophages or dendritic cells that kill phagocytosed molecules or cytotoxic T lymphocytes that kill infected cells. In humoral immunity, B lymphocytes eradicate microbes by secreting antibodies. (From Abbas AK, Lichtman AH: Cellular and Molecular Immunology, 5th ed. Philadelphia, Elsevier, 2005, p 8.)

Adaptive Immunity

Cellular Immunity: T Cells

Cell-mediated immunity (Fig. 27-1) occurs in response to antigens. APCs such as macrophages or dendritic cells process the antigen in the context of different MHC molecules or HLA molecules. The T cells recognize cell surface–associated antigens in the context of two classes of MHC molecules, class I and II. Specific reactivity of a T-cell clone depends on antigen presentation by an APC followed by recognition by a TCR. Unfortunately, not all cancers express class I or II MHC antigens, and, as such, this can be a mechanism of evading the cellular immune response. The T cells themselves originate in the bone marrow and differentiate in the thymus. They are found circulating in the blood or are harbored in the lymph nodes, spleen, or Peyer's patches in the intestine.

T cells are characterized by their cell surface lymphocyte markers, which are termed CD groups. T cells, in general, have the CD 2 surface marker, whereas CD 3 is linked to the TCR. Th (helper/inducer) cells have a CD 4 surface marker, whereas Ts (suppressor/cytotoxic) cells have CD 8 surface markers. The CD 4 surface markers are on T cells that recognize antigens presented with HLA (MHC) class II molecules (Th cell), and the CD 8 surface markers are on T cells that recognize antigens presented with HLA (MHC) class I (suppressor/cytotoxic) molecules (Fig. 27-2). In both of these situations, the CD 2 surface marker is present, and interactions between the TCR and antigen–HLA complex are stabilized by the CD 3 surface marker.

Within the class of CD4+ helper T cells, there are two helper T cell subsets: Th1 and Th2 cells. Th1 cells produce IFN-α and IL-12, cytokines that induce recruitment of macrophages and CD8+ cells. Activated CD8+ cells directly lyse infected cells harboring the antigen determinant or signal B cells to produce antibodies. The latter is mediated through the production of cytokines. Th2 cells produce IL-4, which induces an antibody or humoral response from B cells. Recently, Zhang and colleagues reported that the presence of tumor-infiltrating T cells in ovarian cancer sites has been associated with a significant improvement in progression-free and overall patient survival.

Humoral Immunity: B Cells and Immunoglobulins

In humans, B cells are derived from hematopoietic stem cells and aggregate in lymph nodes, the spleen, or the GI tract. Antibodies are synthesized from B lymphocytes in response to activated CD8+ cells or Th2 cells. In turn, the B lymphocytes differentiate into plasma cells that secrete large quantities of antibody (immunoglobulin) in response to the antigenic stimulant. In contrast to the immune response initiated by T cells where the antigen must be processed, B cells recognize antigens in an unprocessed state. Each B cell is programmed to secrete a specific type of antibody, and it is estimated that more than 10^7 different antibodies are capable of being produced in response to the presence of foreign antigens. All antibodies have the same basic structural characteristics but exhibit extensive variability in the portion of the structure that specifically binds antigen.

Figure 27-2. The antigen is processed by the antigen-presenting cell and broken into smaller fragments. These fragments and major histocompatability complex (MHC) or HLA molecules (class I or II) then interact with the receptor on the surface of the T cell (T-cell receptor) to activate either CD4+ T cells or CD8+ T cells (cytotoxic T lymphocytes). CTL, cytotoxic T lymphocyte; ER, endoplasmic reticulum; TAP, transporter associated with antigen processing. (From Abbas AK, Lichtman AH: Cellular and Molecular Immunology. Philadelphia, Elsevier, 2005, 5th ed, p 91.)

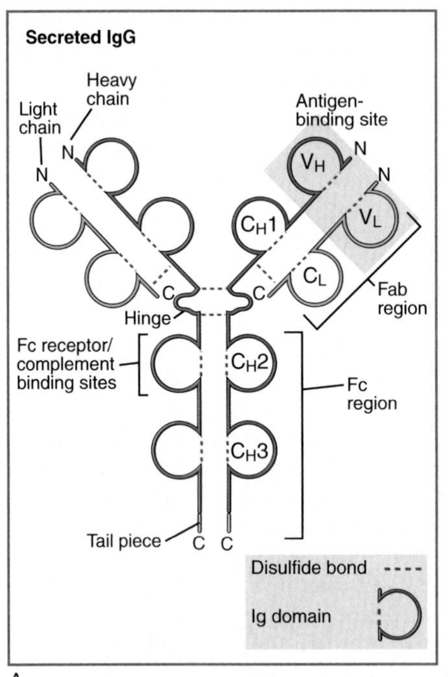

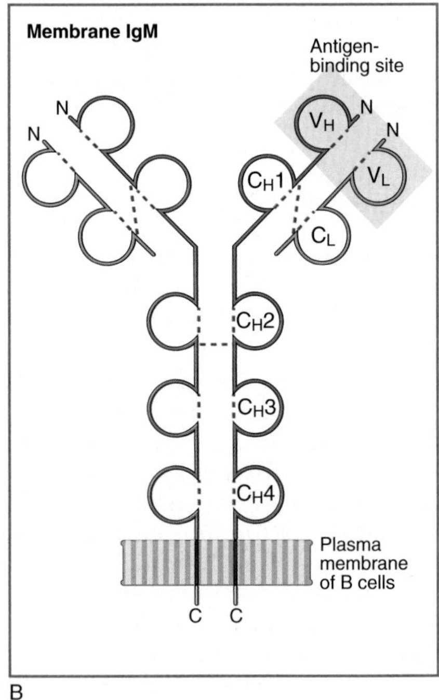

Figure 27-3. Structure of immunoglobulins. Antigen binding sites are formed by the apposition of a variable light chain (V_L) and variable heavy chain (V_H). The N terminal contains the variable regions (Fab) that bind antigen. The C terminal contains the constant region (Fc) that facilitates effector functions such as activation of complement pathways or binding to phagocytic cells. C_H, heavy chain C region; C_L, light chain C region. (From Abbas AK, Lichtman AH: Cellular and Molecular Immunology. Philadelphia, Elsevier, 2005, 5th ed, p 48.)

The basic immunoglobulin structure consists of two identical heavy chains and two identical light chains. Each pair is connected by a disulfide bond. Both heavy and light chains have a variable region (V) at the amino terminal and a constant region (C) at the carboxy terminal (Fig. 27-3). The V region participates in antigen recognition and confers specificity, and the C region mediates effector function by allowing the antibody to bind to a phagocyte. Five types of related immunoglobulin molecules are recognized (IgG, IgM, IgA, IgD, IgE [see the following box]) that serve different effector functions. IgM and IgD production occurs early in the antibody response. The membrane-bound form of IgM and IgD binds antigen and activates naive B cells leading to B-cell proliferation and *clonal selection*. IgM is also involved in activation of the classic pathway of the complement system. IgG production occurs later in the antibody response and is of higher specificity for particular antigens. IgG is responsible

Classes of Immunoglobulins

IgG, the major class of immunoglobulin, comprises approximately 70% of total serum immunoglobulin and is the predominant form of antibody. Only IgG crosses the placenta and is important for the transfer of passive immunity to the newborn.

IgA comprises approximately 20% of total serum immunoglobulin. It is found in saliva, milk colostrums, and genitourinary secretions.

IgM represents approximately 10% of total serum immunoglobulin. It is the predominant antibody produced early in the humoral immune responses and is the most efficient in activating complement.

IgD accounts for less than 1% of total serum immunoglobulin and is found on the surface of B cells. The precise role of IgD is not understood but presumably it plays a role in B-lymphocyte activation.

IgE is associated with hypersensitivity and also infection with parasites.

for neonatal immunity in the transfer of maternal antibodies across the placenta and gut. Its main effector functions include opsonization of antigen for phagocytosis by macrophages and neutrophils as well as activation of the classic pathway of the complement system. NK cells and other leukocytes can bind to IgG- and IgE-coated cells to facilitate antibody-dependent cytotoxicity. Finally, IgA is responsible for mucosal immunity, whereas IgE mediates hypersensitivity reactions.

CYTOKINES

Cytokines, proteins secreted by immune cells, mediate other immune cell functions. During the activation phase of the immune response system, cytokines stimulate the growth and differentiation of lymphocytes, whereas in the effector phase of the immune response, they activate other effector cells to help eliminate antigens and microbes. The major classes of cytokines include those that regulate innate immunity, those that regulate adaptive immunity, and, finally, those that stimulate hematopoiesis.

Cytokines That Mediate Innate Immunity

Tumor Necrosis Factor

TNF mediates the acute inflammatory response to bacterial infections and microbes. It is secreted principally by macrophages, T cells, NK cells, and mast cells. TNF is produced in response to lipopolysaccharide production by bacteria. IFN-γ, which is produced by T cells and NK cells, can augment TNF production by macrophages. The primary action of TNF is to recruit neutrophils and monocytes to sites of infection to facilitate eradication of bacteria. One complication of sepsis, largely as a result of TNF production, is septic shock, which results in intravascular collapse and disseminated intravascular coagulation (DIC).

Interleukins

ILs are potent cytokines that are produced by some leukocytes to affect other leukocytes. They are designated numerically. IL-1 is released in response to cell damage by macrophages, endothelial cells, and some epithelial cells. Many of its actions are similar to those of TNF. However, it lacks the ability to produce the septic shock symptoms that TNF can. Other important ILs include IL-12, IL-10, IL-6, IL-15, and IL-18. All are produced by macrophages. IL-12 plays a key role in the transition between cell-mediated immunity and adaptive immunity. IL-12 stimulates NK cells and T cells to produce IFN-γ, which activates macrophages to kill phagocytosed foreign substances including microbes. It also increases cytolytic activity by stimulating CD8+ cells. The other ILs stimulate NK- and T-cell activation and proliferation as well as IFN-γ synthesis. IFNs protect against viral infection; increase expression of class I MHC molecules, which increases cytotoxic T lymphocyte–mediated cytotoxicity; and stimulate production of Th cells. Marth and colleagues have found that high levels of IFN-γ expression in ovarian cancer specimens are associated with longer survival in patients.

Cytokines That Mediate Adaptive Immunity

IL-2, IL-4, IL-5, and IL-13 are all involved in regulation of adaptive immunity in addition to IFN-γ and transforming growth factor β. After T cells recognize antigen, the T cells produce IL-2, which leads to clonal expansion of activated T cells and additional production of cytokines such as IFN-γ and IL-4. IL-2 also affects B cells by acting as a growth factor and stimulus for antibody synthesis. IL-4 plays a key role in stimulating IgE production from B cells and, most importantly, stimulates the development of Th2 cells from naive T cells. IFN-γ, as mentioned previously, can stimulate class I and II MHC production in addition to stimulating Th1 differentiation, activating neutrophils, and promoting cytolytic activity of NK cells. Transforming growth factor β, on the other hand, inhibits proliferation and differentiation of T cells.

Cytokines That Mediate Hematopoiesis

Colony-Stimulating Factors

IL-3 is a multilineage colony-stimulating factor that allows for differentiation of cells into all known cell types. Granulocyte colony–stimulating factor, a cytokine, is produced by macrophages, fibroblasts, and endothelial cells. It promotes mobilization of neutrophils from the bone marrow. Granulocyte–macrophage colony-stimulating factor is produced by T cells, macrophages, endothelial cells, and fibroblasts. It stimulates maturation of bone marrow cells into dendritic cells and monocytes. Both granulocyte colony–stimulating factor and granulocyte–macrophage colony-stimulating factor are used in patients undergoing chemotherapy and bone marrow transplant.

TUMOR-CELL KILLING AND IMMUNOTHERAPY

Immunotherapy has been developed to recognize and destroy tumor cells. Three major classes of immunotherapy exist:

immune modulation, passive therapy, and active therapy. Immune modulation relies on nonspecific means such as the administration of IL-2, IFNs, or bacille Calmette–Guérin to elicit an immune response. Passive therapy transfers components of the acquired immune system to the recipient with cancer. Examples include the use of monoclonal antibodies directed toward tumor-specific antigens. Active therapy makes use of the patient's own immune system to elicit a response. Vaccines making use of peptides, proteins, DNA, or RNA would fall into this category.

Immune modulation has been used in ovarian cancer in the form of adjuvant IFN treatment after surgery and as consolidation therapy after surgery and standard chemotherapy. One randomized prospective trial in patients with advanced-stage ovarian cancer randomized patients to cisplatin and cyclophosphamide chemotherapy versus the same regimen with intraperitoneal IFN-γ. The study of Windbichler and coworkers showed an improvement in both progression-free survival and 3-year survival in the IFN arm with manageable toxicity. In contrast, prospective studies reported by Alberts and coworkers and by Hal and associates showed that using IFN-α as consolidation therapy after surgery and standard chemotherapy did not improve progression-free or overall survival, but these studies were hampered by patient numbers insufficient to detect a difference in outcome.

Tumor cells are known to have specific tumor-associated antigens or receptors on their surface that may distinguish them from normal cells. One example of successful passive therapy is the use of monoclonal antibodies directed toward overexpressed growth factor receptors such as Her-2/*neu* (*erb*-B2) or epidermal growth factor receptor (EGFR). In studies reported by Vogel and coworkers and by Slamon, Leyland-Jones, and associates, the humanized monoclonal antibody trastuzumab (Herceptin) has been used very successfully in metastatic breast cancer where 20% to 30% of patient tumors overexpress Her-2/*neu*. In contrast, in a study by Bookman and associates of ovarian cancer, treatment with trastuzumab has met with limited success because only 10% of patients overexpress Her-2/*neu*. Bevacizumab (Avastin), a monoclonal antibody directed against vascular endothelial growth factor (VEGF), is currently approved by the U.S. Food and Drug Administration for frontline treatment with chemotherapy for metastatic colorectal cancer and has undergone phase II testing in ovarian cancer, with encouraging results reported by Burger and coworkers.

One promising immunotherapy that has come out recently has been the human papillomavirus (HPV) vaccine for the prevention of cervical dysplasia and cervical cancer. Koutsky and colleagues reported on the use of an HPV 16 virus–like particle vaccine in 2392 women who were negative for HPV 16 DNA and antibodies at enrollment. There was a significant reduction in the number of women with persistent HPV 16 infection in the vaccine group: 0 per 100 woman-years at risk versus 3.8 per 100 woman-years at risk in the placebo group ($P < .001$). There were no cases of cervical dysplasia in the vaccine group as opposed to nine in the placebo group. A study conducted by Villa and coworkers showed that use of a quadrivalent vaccine against HPV types 6, 11, 16, and 18 decreases the incidence of persistent infection or dysplasia by 90% ($P < .0001$). The use of HPV vaccine therapy is efficacious and will have tremendous implications for the prevention of cervical cancer.

MOLECULAR ONCOLOGY

A cancer may arise as a result of acquired mutations or through inheritance of a mutated gene followed by acquisition of an acquired mutation in the other allele. The former is known as a sporadic cancer, and the latter is known as a hereditary cancer. Genetic alterations occur in three major categories of genes: oncogenes, tumor suppressor genes, and DNA mismatch repair genes. Knowledge of how these genes function is a rapidly expanding field and well beyond the scope of this text, but a general overview is provided.

The term *oncogene* has been applied to one set of genes that, when altered, is associated with the development of a malignant cell. Most studies describing oncogenes have been done in animals such as chickens, mice, and rats. Many of the oncogenes described in the literature probably do not play a role in human disease. Functionally, oncogenes are involved in cell proliferation, signal transduction, and transcriptional alteration. Mechanisms of alteration in oncogene function include gene amplification (increase in numbers of copies of genes in the cell), translocation, or overexpression. The term *overexpression* refers to excessive and abnormal protein production.

Oncogenes

Several classes of oncogenes exist including the peptide growth factors, cytoplasmic factors, and nuclear factors. Representative examples are described in the following sections (Table 27-1).

Peptide Growth Factors

Epidermal Growth Factor Receptor Family. The family of *erb*-B receptors has been reviewed recently by Britten and includes the EGFR (*erb*-B1), Her-2 (*erb*-B2), *erb*-B3, and *erb*-B4. All *erb*-B receptors share the same structure including

Table 27-1 Classes of Genes Involved in Growth Stimulatory Pathways

Peptide Growth Factors	**Corresponding Receptors**
Epidermal growth factor (EGF) and transforming growth factor (TGF) α	EGF receptor (*erb*-B1) *erb*-B2 (Her-2/*Neu*), *erb*-B3, *erb*-B4
Heregulin	
Insulin-like growth factors (IGF-I, IGF-II)	IGF-I and II receptors
Platelet-derived growth factor (PDGF)	PDGF receptor
Fibroblast growth factors (FGFs)	FGF receptors
Macrophage colony–stimulating factor (M-CSF)	M-CSF receptor (*FMS*)
Cytoplasmic Factors	**Examples**
Nonreceptor tyrosine kinases	ABL, SRC
G proteins	K-Ras, H-Ras
Serine-threonine kinases	AKT2
Nuclear Factors	**Examples**
Transcription factors	MYC, JUN, FOS
Cell-cycle progression factors	Cyclins, E2F

From Boyd J, Berchuck A: Oncogenes and tumor suppressor genes. In Hoskins WJ, Young RC, Markman M, et al (eds): Principles and Practice of Gynecologic Oncology. Philadelphia, Lippincott Williams & Wilkins, 2005, p 103.

an extracellular domain that binds ligand, a transmembrane domain, and an intracellular tyrosine kinase domain. EGFR, *erb*-B3, and *erb*-B4 can bind their respective receptors and dimerize with one another. Her-2 does not have an identifiable ligand and dimerizes with the other receptors in response to ligand binding. A cascade of phosphorylation events then occurs that ultimately results in cellular processes such as cell growth, proliferation, and differentiation. Although the *erb*-B receptors share activation of some signaling pathways, there are certain pathways that are activated preferentially by specific receptors. For instance, activation of the *erb*-B3 receptor preferentially activates the phosphatidylinositol 3′ kinase pathway discussed later. A number of different mechanisms exist that are associated with malignant transformation. Activating mutations have been found in the tyrosine kinase domain of EGFR in lung cancer by Lynch and colleagues and by Paez and associates. This finding has led to the development of a number of EGFR inhibitors that include monoclonal antibodies directed at the ligand binding domain and tyrosine kinase inhibitors directed at the catalytic domain. Gene amplification is also a well-characterized mechanism of EGFR family alteration. Slamon, Godolphin, and coworkers have reported that Her-2/*neu* amplification, for instance, is found in 20% to 30% of breast cancers and 10% of ovarian cancers. According to a study by Vogel and coworkers, trastuzumab, a humanized monoclonal antibody to HER-2/*neu*, produces a response rate of 34% in women with HER-2/*neu*–positive breast cancer as measured by fluorescent in situ hybridization. In addition to combining trastuzumab with chemotherapeutic agents such as carboplatin, ongoing studies are also looking at combining trastuzumab with EGFR tyrosine kinase inhibitors in the hope that multiple downstream signaling pathways necessary for cancer cell proliferation will be blocked.

Vascular Endothelial Growth Factor and Angiogenesis. The process of angiogenesis involves the development of new vasculature to bring nutrients and necessary substrates to tumors. One key modulator of this process is VEGF and its receptors, as reviewed by Ferrara and associates. Tumors frequently express growth factors such as epidermal growth factor, transforming growth factors α and β and platelet-derived growth factor that up-regulate VEGF. VEGF, in turn, acts as a potent mitogen for endothelial cells. Strategies to target VEGF have included the use of a humanized monoclonal antibody (bevacizumab) directed against VEGF. Currently, this treatment is approved by the U.S. Food and Drug Administration for use in colorectal cancer where, in a study reported by Hurwitz and coworkers, it yielded a 30% increase in median survival in conjunction with chemotherapy when compared with chemotherapy alone. Bevacizumab has also shown promise in phase II studies as a single agent in ovarian cancer and will undergo phase III testing as frontline therapy in newly diagnosed, advanced stage ovarian cancer patients in conjunction with standard paclitaxel and carboplatin chemotherapy.

Cytoplasmic Factors

Phosphatidylinositol 3′ Kinase Pathway. As described by Hennessy and associates, the phosphatidylinositol 3′ kinases (PI3Ks) are lipid kinases that control second messengers governing cellular proliferation, survival, motility, and morphology. With growth factor stimulation, p110α, the catalytic subunit of PI3K, phosphorylates a series of proteins, among them AKT, a serine threonine kinase with multiple isoforms. AKT activates several downstream targets, one of which is mTOR (mammalian target of rapamycin), a regulator of cellular proliferation and translation. PTEN (phosphatase and tensin homologue) is the regulatory counterpart to PI3K and a tumor suppressor gene. It dephosphorylates proteins phosphorylated by PI3K. Aberrant PI3K signaling in cancer has been attributed to alterations in a number of members of this pathway. Mutations in p110α were first described in 2004 by Samuels and associates and may lead to gain of function activity. Levine and colleagues have found that the *PIK3CA* gene, which encodes for the p110α catalytic subunit of PI3K, has missense somatic mutations in 12% of ovarian cancers and 18% of breast cancers. Other mechanisms of PI3K signaling dysfunction include loss of PTEN function by mutation or transcriptional down-regulation or gain of AKT function by amplification, overexpression, or increased phosphorylation, as reported by Bellacosa and coworkers. Somatic mutations in PTEN have been described in endometrial and ovarian cancers, whereas AKT2 amplification has been identified in breast and ovarian cancers. As reported by Adjei and Hidalfo, current drugs under study that target this pathway include PI3K and AKT inhibitors as well as mTOR inhibitors such as rapamycin and the rapamycin analogue CCI-779.

Another class of cytoplasmic factors that is involved in growth stimulation is the G protein class of *RAS* genes. Adjei has reported that the protein products of the *RAS* genes regulate a number of processes including cellular differentiation and cytoskeletal organization. This class of genes plays a central role in the regulatory pathway that controls signal transduction from the cell surface to the nucleus. The Ras proteins localize to the inner surface of the cell membrane and, in response to activation of cell surface receptor tyrosine kinases, activate pathways such as the mitogen-activated protein kinase signaling pathway, which, in turn, activates the production of nuclear transcription factors such as c-myc, c-jun, and c-fos. In turn, as described by Neves and colleagues and by Adjei and Hidalgo, these transcription factors modulate a number of proliferation genes. According to a review article by Bos, oncogenic Ras proteins have been found in 30% of human cancers. Current therapeutic approaches that target the oncogenic Ras signaling pathway include the use of antisense oligonucleotides, producing viruses to specifically kill Ras-transformed cells, and inhibition of downstream Ras effector pathways.

Tumor Suppressor Genes

Tumor suppressor genes restrain cellular proliferation. In this capacity, they serve vital functions in normal cell regulation. The retinoblastoma gene (*Rb*) was the first tumor suppressor gene to be characterized and is described in a 1986 study by Friend and colleagues. Baretk and coworkers have shown that *Rb* encodes a nuclear protein that regulates G1 phase cell cycle arrest. In the inherited form of retinoblastoma, two gene copies are inherited. Affected individuals inherit one defective copy of the *Rb* gene, but because there is a normal intact copy, a malignancy does not develop until the second copy of the gene is inactivated, presumably as a result of mutation. Thus, there is a "two-hit" theory of action of the tumor suppressor gene, with the first "hit" being present in the inherited abnormal gene and the second "hit" the consequence of somatic mutations that occur later, manifesting in cancer.

The most widely known tumor suppressor gene in gynecologic oncology is the *p53* gene, which is located on the short arm of human chromosome 17, as described by Finlay and associates. *p53* functions as a transcription factor and regulator of the cell cycle and apoptosis. One key function of normal *p53* is to bind to transcriptional regulatory elements in DNA. As gatekeeper of the genome, in response to DNA damage, *p53* activates genes regulating apoptosis (*Bax, Fas, bcl-2*). Hollstein and coworkers have shown that the most common mutations in *p53* are missense mutations within exons 5 to 8. The resultant mutant proteins can no longer bind to DNA yet can complex with and inactivate any normal *p53* in the cell. Cells expressing mutant *p53* do not undergo cell cycle arrest at the typical G1-S checkpoint before DNA replication nor do they undergo apoptosis.

Tumor suppressor genes play an active role in the modulation of gynecologic malignancy. For instance, the role of *Rb* and *p53* in cervical carcinogenesis attributable to high-risk HPV types has recently been elucidated. The E6 oncoprotein of HPV types 16 and 18 has been shown by Werness and colleagues and by Scheffner and associates to bind to *p53* and target it for degradation. The E7 oncoprotein of HPV type 16 associates with the *Rb* gene product in infected cells to up-regulate proliferation.

Although *p53* mutations are one of the most common in human cancer, attempts to target and modulate this tumor suppressor pathway have met with disappointing results. Use of an adenovirus to replace defective *p53* in recurrent ovarian cancer has not resulted in any clinically significant benefit to patients in two studies published by Buller and associates in 2002.

BRCA1 and BRCA2

Approximately 5% to 10% of breast and ovarian cancers have a hereditary basis, as shown in studies published by Rosen and colleagues and by Risch and coworkers. According to Frank and colleagues, the vast majority are attributable to the inheritance of mutations in *BRCA1* and *BRCA2*. In 1990, Hall and associates performed genetic studies that linked familial breast cancer risk to chromosome 17q21. In 1994, *BRCA1*, located on chromosome 17, was identified by positional cloning done by Miki and associates. Because only 45% of familial breast cancers could be linked to *BRCA1*, Wooster and coworkers searched for a second breast cancer susceptibility gene, now known as *BRCA2*, which was localized to chromosome 13q12.3 and reported their findings in 1994 and 1995. The pattern of inheritance is autosomal dominant in nearly all families studied. Approximately 0.5% to 0.6% of U.S. women are carriers of an altered *BRCA1* or *BRCA2* gene; however, certain groups such as Ashkenazi Jewish women are at particularly high risk with more than 1% carrying a mutated gene. It is estimated that for carriers of *BRCA1* mutations, breast cancer will develop by age 70 in 36% to 85% of women and ovarian cancer in 40% to 60%. Cass, Holscheider, and colleagues have reported that development of fallopian tube carcinoma is also a part of the BRCA phenotype. An analysis conducted by Antoniou concluded that the lifetime risk of development of ovarian cancer with *BRCA2* is far lower, approximately 10%. Inheritance of mutated *BRCA2*, however, is associated with other cancers including male breast cancer and pancreatic, urinary tract, and biliary tract cancers. Unfortunately, the women who develop these hereditary forms of cancer develop breast and ovarian cancers at a younger age than is typically seen with sporadic cancers. Personal characteristics associated with an increased likelihood of a *BRCA1* or *BRCA2* mutation include breast cancer diagnosed at an early age (younger than age 50), bilateral breast cancer, and/or a history of both breast and ovarian cancers. Family history characteristics associated with an increased likelihood of carrying a BRCA1 or BRCA2 mutation include multiple cases of breast cancer in the family, both breast and ovarian cancers in the family, male breast cancer, and one or more family members with two primary cancers.

Sowter and Ashworth reviewed *BRCA1* and *BRCA2* as tumor suppressor genes that encode for large proteins, 1863 amino acids and 3418 amino acids, respectively. Inheritance of a mutated allele followed by inactivation of the normal allele allows for tumorigenesis. Both *BRCA1* and *BRCA2* code for proteins that play a role in repair of DNA strand breaks. There are more than 200 mutations that have been identified in *BRCA1*; the vast majority of these mutations result in truncated proteins. *BRCA1* has been found by Scully and coworkers to colocalize in vivo and associate in vitro with RAD51, a protein known to repair double-stranded DNA breaks. In addition to interacting directly with RAD51, *BRCA2* has also been identified as a *FANCD1* gene, a member of the Fanconi anemia complex of proteins. Cells with deficient *BRCA1* or *BRCA2* are incapable of repairing DNA strand breaks, which results in genetic instability. Why mutations in *BRCA1* particularly predispose to breast and ovarian cancers is unclear. *BRCA1* has been shown by Ma and associates to interact with the estrogen receptor α directly, implicating it as a regulator of preventing estrogen-independent proliferation. *BRCA2* contains a region known as the ovarian cancer cluster region (nucleotides 4075–6503 in exon 11) where mutations in this region have been reported by Thompson and the Breast Cancer Linkage Consortium to be associated with increased ovarian cancer and decreased breast cancer risk. For *BRCA1*, Gayther and coworkers have reported that mutations in the C terminal end, required for DNA repair and transcriptional activation, predispose to breast cancer, whereas mutations in the N terminal end are associated with development of ovarian cancer. The outcome of patients with *BRCA1* or *BRCA2* mutations who develop ovarian cancer has been somewhat controversial. Recent studies by Boyd and colleagues, Ben David and associates, and Cass, Baldwin, and coworkers have demonstrated that these women survive longer than their sporadic cancer counterparts. It has been suggested by Bhattacharyya and colleagues that this longer survival may be the result of improved response to platinum-based chemotherapy due to inability to repair chemotherapy-induced DNA damage.

DNA Mismatch Repair Genes

The role of the DNA mismatch repair gene system is to recognize and fix errors in the DNA helix resulting from incorrect pairings of nucleotides. In addition, the system repairs single-stranded DNA loops that occur in the helix when an extra nucleotide has been inserted or deleted in one of the DNA strands. During the repair process, Markowitz suggests, the system digests the individual bases and resynthesizes the correct sequences. The most common germline mutations in DNA mismatch repair genes are acquired in an autosomal-dominant fashion and occur on chromosomes 2 and 3 in the genes *MSH2*, *MLH1*, *MSH6*, and *PMS2*, according to a study reported by Fishel and coworkers. More than 400 mutations in the mismatch repair genes have been identified; Peltomaki reports that the majority (50%) occur in *MLH1*, 40% in *MSH2*, 10% in *MSH6*, and less than 5% in *PMS2*. Patients who acquire these mutations develop chromosomal aberrations and an accumulation of abnormal cells resulting in hereditary nonpolyposis colon cancer syndrome. In this syndrome, patients inherit a mutated DNA mismatch repair gene followed by subsequent loss of the wild-type allele. The clinical criteria for diagnosis of this syndrome are known as the Amsterdam criteria and consist of three individuals diagnosed with colon cancer. As described by Vasen and colleagues, the three individuals must represent two different generations, one member must be a first-degree relative of the other two, and one of the three individuals must have developed colon cancer before the age of 50. The colon cancers are frequently found in the proximal, as opposed to the distal, colon. In addition to colorectal cancer, cancers of the ovary and endometrium, GI tract, upper urologic tract, and sebaceous glands (Muir–Torre syndrome) are also frequently found. Endometrial cancer is the second most common cancer found in this cohort of patients. The lifetime risk of developing ovarian cancer in patients with hereditary nonpolyposis colon cancer is 5% to 10%, whereas the risk of developing endometrial cancer is 40% to 60%.

KEY POINTS

- The immune system consists of the innate and adaptive immune systems. The innate system is present at birth and consists of natural barriers, NK cells, macrophages, and the complement system. The adaptive immune system adapts to infection or foreign invasion and consists of the T cells and B cells.
- The cellular immune response occurs as a result of T lymphocytes reacting via a surface TCR that processes antigens presented to it by an APC in conjunction with HLA (MHC) molecules.
- T-cell activation can result in activation of helper/inducer (Th) cells, cytotoxic/suppressor (Ts) cells, or cytokine production.
- Helper/inducer (Th) cells recruit macrophages and cytotoxic/suppressor cells.
- Cytotoxic T cells have the ability to lyse infected cells or signal B cells to produce antibody.
- Humoral immunity results from antigen stimulation of a B lymphocyte, which differentiates into a plasma cell and secretes antibody (immunoglobulin).
- There are five types of immunoglobulins (IgG, IgM, IgD, IgA, and IgE). The immunoglobulin molecule consists of a fixed region (Fc), which carries the biologic activity, and a variable region (Fab), which reacts to a specific antigen.
- The complement cascade provides a basis for the inflammatory response and can also mediate cytotoxicity.
- T cells are characterized by cell surface markers, which are termed clusters of differentiation (CD), and are numbered CD1 to CD80.
- Cytokines (lymphokines) are regulatory substances of the immune system produced as a result of T-cell activation, cell damage by a virus, or other cells, such as macrophages and monocytes, involved in the immune response.
- IFNs are a group of cytokines produced in response to viral infections. They also have antiproliferative effects and can enhance the antitumor immune response as well as interact with other cytokines and chemotherapeutic agents.
- Colony-stimulating factors are a group of cytokines that can stimulate various parts of the bone marrow and can help to overcome the suppressive effects of chemotherapy.
- Immune modulation is a nonspecific form of immunotherapy that consists of administration of IL-2, IFNs, or bacille Calmette–Guérin to elicit an immune response.
- Passive therapy transfers components of the acquired immune system to the recipient with cancer, e.g., monoclonal antibodies directed toward tumor-specific antigens.
- Active immunotherapy uses a patient's own immune system for protection against infection, e.g., vaccines.
- There are three types of genes associated with malignant development: oncogenes, tumor suppressor genes, and DNA mismatch repair genes.
- Proto-oncogenes are protein sequences of oncogenes that occur in normal cells and regulate physiologic growth and development. When activated, they can lead to malignant change.
- Malignant change is seen with point mutations, chromosomal aberration, gene amplification (increase in number of copies), or chromosomal translocation.
- Overexpression is excessive protein production in the cytoplasm, a result of gene alterations that can lead to abnormal cell growth.
- *Ras* oncogenes are part of a group of signal transducer oncogenes that relay messages from the membrane to the cell interior. They are activated generally by point mutations.
- Growth factor genes include C-*erb*-B2 (Her-2/*neu*), which can be overexpressed and act as a tumor-specific target for monoclonal antibody therapy.
- Nuclear oncogenes include *myc* and *fos* and can activate other genes as well as stimulate DNA replication.
- Tumor suppressor genes restrain cell growth. They have two copies, and, in general, alteration of both copies leads to a mutant expression, which allows malignant growth to occur.
- *Rb* (retinoblastoma) and *p53* are two widely studied tumor suppressor genes.

Continued

KEY POINTS *Continued*

- Mutant *p53* prevents normal *p53* from interacting with DNA, which prevents cellular growth inhibition.
- *BRCA1* and *BRCA2* mutations confer a high lifetime risk of breast and/or ovarian cancer. Mutation screening may be appropriate for women with family histories suggesting a hereditary predisposition to breast or ovarian cancer.
- DNA mismatch repair genes act by recognizing and fixing errors in the DNA helix resulting from incorrect pairings of nucleotides. They prevent accumulation of genetically damaged material in the cell.
- Angiogenesis is the formation of new capillary blood vessels that can bring nutrients and necessary substrates to tumors.

REFERENCES

Adjei AA: Blocking oncogenic Ras signaling for cancer therapy. J Natl Cancer Inst 193:1062–1074, 2001.

Adjei AA, Hidalgo M: Intracellular signal transduction pathway proteins as targets for cancer therapy. J Clin Oncol 23:5386–5403, 2005.

Alberts DS, Hannigan EV, Liu PY, et al: Randomized trial of adjuvant intraperitoneal alpha-interferon in stage III ovarian cancer patients who have no evidence of disease after primary surgery and chemotherapy: An intergroup study. Gynecol Oncol 100:133–138, 2006.

Antoniou A, Pharaoh PD, Narod S, et al: Average risks of breast and ovarian cancer associated with *BRCA1* or *BRCA2* mutations detected in case series unselected for family history: A combined analysis of 22 studies. Am J Hum Genet 72:1117–1130, 2003.

Baretk J, Bartkova J, Lukas J: The retinoblastoma protein pathway in cell cycle control and cancer. Exp Cell Res 237:1–6, 1997.

Bellacosa A, de Feo D, Godwin AK, et al: Molecular alterations of the AKT2 oncogene in ovarian and breast carcinomas. Int J Cancer 64:280–285, 1995.

Ben David Y, Chetrit A, Hirsch-Yechezkel G, et al: Effect of *BRCA* mutations on the length of survival in epithelial ovarian tumors. J Clin Oncol 20:463–466, 2002.

Bhattacharyya A, Ear US, Koler BH, et al: The breast cancer susceptibility gene *BRCA1* is required for subnuclear assembly of RAD51 and survival following treatment with the DNA crosslinking agent cisplatin. J Biol Chem 275:23899–23903, 2000.

Bos JL: Ras oncogenes in human cancer. A review. Cancer Res 49:4682–4689, 1989.

Boyd J, Sonoda Y, Federici MG, et al: Clinicopathologic features of *BRCA*-linked and sporadic ovarian cancer. JAMA 283:2260–2265, 2000.

Britten CD: Targeting ErbB receptor signaling: A pan-ErbB approach to cancer. Mol Cancer Ther 3:1335–1342, 2004.

Buller RE, Runnebaum IB, Karlan BY, et al: A phase I/II trial of rAd/p53 (SCH 58500) gene replacement in recurrent ovarian cancer. Cancer Gene Ther 9:553–566, 2002.

Buller RE, Shalin MS, Horowitz JH, et al: Long term follow up of patients with recurrent ovarian cancer after Ad *p53* gene replacement with SCH 58500. Cancer Gene Ther 9:567–572, 2002.

Burger RA, Sill M, Monk BJ, et al: Phase II trial of bevacizumab in persistent or recurrent epithelial ovarian cancer (EOC) pr primary peritoneal cancer (PPC): A Gynecologic Oncology Group study. ASCO Proc Abstract 5009, 2005.

Cass I, Baldwin RL, Varkey T, et al: Improved survival in women with BRCA-associated ovarian carcinoma. Cancer 97:2187–2195, 2003.

Cass I, Holschneider C, Datta N, et al: BRCA-mutation-associated fallopian tube carcinoma. A distinct clinical phenotype? Obstet Gynecol 106:1327–1334, 2005.

Chang DZ, Sabatini PJ, Divgi CR, et al: Immunotherapy of gynecologic malignancies. In Hoskins WJ, Young RC, Markman M, et al (eds): Principles and Practice of Gynecologic Oncology. Philadelphia, Lippincott Williams & Wilkins, 2005.

Ferrara N, Gerber HP, LeCouter J: The biology of VEGF and its receptors. Nat Med 9:669–676, 2003.

Finlay CA, Hinds PW, Levine AJ: The p53 proto-oncogene can act as a suppressor of transformation. Cell 57:1083–1093, 1989.

Fishel R, Lescoe MK, Rao MRS, et al: The human mutator gene homolog MSH2 and its association with hereditary nonpolyposis colon cancer. Cell 75:1027, 1993.

Frank TS, Mankley SA, Olopade OI, et al: Sequence analysis of *BRCA1* and *BRCA2*: Correlation of mutations with family history and ovarian cancer risk. J Clin Oncol 16:2417, 1998.

Friend SH, Bernards R, Rogelj S, et al: A human DNA segment with properties of the gene that predisposes to retinoblastoma and osteosarcoma. Nature 323:643–646, 1986.

Gayther SA, Warren W, Mazoyer S, et al: Germline mutations of the *BRCA1* gene in breast and ovarian cancer families provide evidence for a genotype-phenotype correlation. Nat Genet 11:428–433, 1995.

Hal GD, Brown JM, Coleman RE, et al: Maintenance treatment with interferon for advanced ovarian cancer: Results of the Northern and Yorkshire Gynaecology Group randomized phase III study. Br J Cancer 91:621–626, 2004.

Hall JM, Lee MK, Newman B, et al: Linkage of early-onset familial breast cancer to chromosome 17q21. Science 250:184–189, 1990.

Hennessy BT, Smith DL, Ram PT, et al: Exploiting the PI3K/AKT pathway for cancer drug discovery. Nat Rev 4:988–1004, 2005.

Hollstein M, Sidransky D, Vogelstein B, et al: p53 mutations in human cancers. Science 253:49–53, 1991.

Hurwitz H, Fehrenbacher L, Novotny W, et al: Bevacizumab plus irinotecan, fluorouracil, and leucovorin for metastatic colorectal cancer. N Engl J Med 350:2335–2342, 2004.

Koutsky LA, Ault KA, Wheeler CM, et al: A controlled trial of a human papillomavirus type 16 vaccine. N Engl J Med 347:1645–1651, 2002.

Levine DA, Bogomolniy F, Yee CJ, et al: Frequent mutations of the PIK3CA gene in ovarian and breast cancers. Clin Cancer Res 11:2875–2878, 2005.

Lynch TJ, Bell DW, Sordella R, et al: Activating mutations in the epidermal growth factor receptor underlying responsiveness of non-small cell lung cancer to gefitinib. N Engl J Med 350:2129–2139, 2004.

Ma YM, Tomita Y, Fan S, et al: Structural determinants of the *BRCA1*: Estrogen receptor interaction. Oncogene 24:1831–1846, 2005.

Markowitz S: DNA repair defects inactivate tumor suppressor genes and induce hereditary and sporadic colon cancers. J Clin Oncol 21S:75S–80S, 2000.

Marth C, Fiegl H, Zeime AG, et al: Interferon-γ expression is an independent prognostic factor in ovarian cancer. Am J Obstet Gynecol 191:1598–1605, 2004.

Miki Y, Swensen J, Shattuck-Eidens D, et al: A strong candidate for the breast and ovarian cancer susceptibility gene *BRCA1*. Science 266:66–71, 1994.

Moretta L, Bottino C, Pende D, et al: Human natural killer cells: Molecular mechanisms controlling NK cell activation and tumor cell lysis. Immunology Lett 100:7–13, 2005.

Olayioye MA, Neve RM, Lane HA, Hynes NE: The ErbB signaling network: Receptor heterodimerization in development and cancer. EMBO J 19:3159–3167, 2000.

Neves SR, Ram PT, Iyengar R: G protein pathways. Science 296:1636–1639, 2002.

Peltomaki P: Role of DNA mismatch repair defects in the pathogenesis of human cancer. J Clin Oncol 21:1174–1179, 2003.

Paez JG, Janne PA, Lee JC, et al: EGFR mutations in lung cancer: Correlation with clinical response to gefitinib therapy. Science 304:1497–1500, 2004.

Risch HA, McLaughlin JR, Cole DE, et al: Prevalence and penetrance of germline *BRCA1* and *BRCA2* mutations in a population series of 649 women with ovarian cancer. Am J Hum Genet 68:700–710, 2001.

Rosen EM, Fan S, Pestell RG, Goldberg ID: *BRCA1* gene in breast cancer. J Cell Physiol 196:19–41, 2003.

Samuels Y, Wang Z, Bardelli A, et al: High frequency of mutations of the PIK3CA gene in human cancers. Science 334:504, 2004.

Scheffner M, Werness BA, Huibregtse JM, et al: The E6 oncoprotein encoded by human papillomavirus types 16 and 18 promotes the degradation of p53. Cell 63:1129–1136, 1990.

Scully R, Chen J, Plug A, et al: Association of BRCA1 with Rad51 in mitotic and meiotic cells. Cell 88:265–275, 1997.

Slamon DJ, Godolphin W, Jones LA, et al: Studies of the HER-2/neu proto-oncogene in human breast and ovarian cancer. Science 244:707–712, 1989.

Slamon DJ, Leyland-Jones B, Shak S, et al: Use of chemotherapy plus a monoclonal antibody against HER2 for metastatic breast cancer that overexpresses HER2. N Engl J Med 344:783–792, 2001.

Sowter HM, Ashworth A: *BRCA1* and *BRCA2* as ovarian cancer susceptibility genes. Carcinogenesis 26:1651–1656, 2005.

Thompson D, Easton DF, the Breast Cancer Linkage Consortium: Variation in risks, by mutation position, in BRCA2 mutation carriers. Am J Hum Genet 68:410–419, 2001.

Vasen H, Mecklin J, Khan P, et al: The International Collaborative Group on Hereditary Non-Polyposis Colorectal Cancer (ICG-HNPCC). Dis Colon Rectum 34:424–425, 1991.

Villa LL, Costa RL, Petta CA, et al: Prophylactic quadrivalent human papillomavirus (types 6, 11, 16, and 18) L1 virus-like particle vaccine in young women: A randomized double-blind placebo-controlled multicentre phase II efficacy trial. Lancet Oncol 6:271–278, 2005.

Vogel CL, Cobleigh MA, Tripathy D, et al: Efficacy and safety of trastuzumab as a single agent in first-line treatment of HER2 overexpressing breast cancer. J Clin Oncol 20:719–726, 2002.

Werness B, Levine A, Howley P: Association of human papillomavirus types 16 and 18 E6 proteins with p53. Science 248:76–79, 1990.

Windbichler GH, Hausmaninger H, Stummvoll W, et al: Interferon-gamma in the first line therapy of ovarian cancer: A randomized phase III trial. Br J Cancer 82:1138–1144, 2000.

Wooster R, Bignell G, Lancaster J, et al: Identification of the breast cancer susceptibility gene BRCA2. Nature 378:789–792, 1995.

Wooster R, Neuhausen SL, Mangion J, et al: Localization of a breast cancer susceptibility gene. *BRCA2*, to chromosome 13q12-13. Science 265:2088–2090, 1994.

Zhang L, Conejo-Garcia JR, Katsaros D, et al: Intratumoral T cells, recurrence, and survival in epithelial ovarian cancer. N Engl J Med 348:203–213, 2003.

Intraepithelial Neoplasia of the Lower Genital Tract (Cervix, Vulva) 28

Etiology, Screening, Diagnostic Techniques, Management

Kenneth L. Noller

KEY TERMS AND DEFINITIONS

Atypical Squamous Cells (ASC). Bethesda System term used to indicate that abnormal squamous cells are present that do not fulfill all the criteria for a diagnosis of a squamous intraepithelial lesion. It is commonly abbreviated as ASC. Two subtypes are recognized: ASC of undetermined significance (ASC-US) and ASC, cannot exclude a higher grade lesion (ACS-H).

Atypical Glandular Cells (AGC). A Bethesda System term used to indicate that there are abnormal glandular cells present that do not fulfill all the criteria for a diagnosis of an adenocarcinoma in situ or adenocarcinoma. The term can often be further qualified if the cells of origin can be identified.

The Bethesda System (TBS). A system of terminology for the reporting of cervical cytology test results that is used by virtually all cytology laboratories in the United States as well as in many other countries. It was last revised in 2002.

Carcinoma In Situ. An older term, now mostly abandoned, to represent full epithelial thickness neoplastic changes. It has been replaced by the term cervical intraepithelial neoplasia 3.

Cervical Intraepithelial Neoplasia (CIN). A premalignant change in the cervical epithelium. The cells have altered nuclei that have at least some features of a neoplastic process. CIN is graded in three steps. CIN 1 is of little or no clinical consequence as it is usually a result of a transient human papillomavirus infection only. In the past, CIN 1 was referred to as mild dysplasia. If the cellular changes are more extensive and include one half to two thirds of the thickness of the epithelium, it is referred to as CIN 2. Full-thickness cellular changes are referred to as CIN 3. CIN 3 includes those changes previously referred to as severe dysplasia and carcinoma in situ.

Colposcope (Colposcopy). A low-power, binocular microscope that is mounted on a stand. It is focused approximately 30 cm from the objective lens. It is used to view the uterine cervix after a speculum has been introduced into the vagina. It is the diagnostic method of choice for the evaluation of most Pap test abnormalities.

Conization. Removal of the central cervix for the purpose of diagnosis or treatment of cervical neoplasia. It may be performed either with a scalpel (cold knife cone) or by a loop electroexcision procedure.

Cryocautery. An office method for the destruction of areas of CIN. Although its success rate is similar to that of a loop electroexcision procedure, it is used less frequently than in the past. One limitation is that no tissue sample is obtained.

Dysplasia. An outdated term for the changes now called CIN.

Endocervical Sampling. This refers to obtaining a sample from the endocervix to determine whether CIN is present. The sample can be collected with an endocervical brush (cytology) or an endocervical curette (histology).

High-Grade Squamous Intraepithelial Lesion (HSIL). This is a term used in TBS to report cellular changes that are consistent with a histologic report of CIN 2 or CIN 3. It is slowly replacing the CIN terminology for histology specimens.

Human Papillomavirus (HPV). This is a group of more than 100 types of DNA-containing viruses known to infect humans. More than 15 types may be found in the genital area. Cervical cancer virtually always contains HPV DNA. The vast majority of all sexually active individuals are infected with the virus at some time. In most cases, the infection is self-limited. Recently, vaccines have been developed that prevent HPV infection with the more common HPV types.

Loop Electroexcision Procedure (LEEP). This is the most commonly used procedure for the removal of areas of CIN. It is an office procedure in which a thin electric wire loop is used to excise squamous intraepithelial lesions.

Low-Grade Squamous Intraepithelial Lesion (LSIL). This is a term used in TBS to report cellular changes that are consistent with a histologic report of CIN 1. In most cases, it indicates that an active HPV infection is present.

Metaplasia. The process by which an area of glandular epithelium is replaced by squamous epithelium. It is a normal process and its presence on a biopsy specimen is considered normal.

Mosaic. A colposcopic term used to describe a tissue pattern that is often associated with neoplasia.

Pap Test (Pap Smear). The concept that cancer could be diagnosed by the examination of cells was conceived by Dr. Papanicolaou, and the test retains his name. Originally, a sample of cells was scraped from the uterine cervix, spread on a glass slide, and fixed in alcohol. Samples are now most often placed in a vial of transport medium, and the actual slide is prepared in the laboratory. The Pap test is the most effective cancer screening procedure ever developed. In countries where most adult women are screened regularly, the incidence of invasive cervical cancer is reduced by approximately 70%.

Continued

KEY TERMS AND DEFINITIONS *Continued*

Punctation. A colposcopic term used to describe a tissue pattern that is often associated with neoplasia.

Satisfactory Colposcopy. A colposcopic examination in which the entire transformation zone can be seen. All other examinations are termed unsatisfactory.

Transformation Zone. This is the area between the border of squamous epithelium and glandular epithelium in the central cervix. Almost all significant squamous neoplasia originates in this area.

Carcinoma of the cervix is one of the most common malignancies in women. According to a 2002 ACOG Practice Bulletin, it is estimated to be the second or third most common cause of cancer death in women worldwide, despite the fact that a screening test, the Pap smear, is available that has been demonstrated to reduce the incidence of the disease by at least 70%. Unfortunately, many developing countries lack the ability to carry out widespread Pap screening.

The epidemiology of cervical cancer has been studied for more than a century. This work paved the way for the discovery that an infection with the HPV is a necessary, but insufficient cause of the disease (Bosch and coworkers). The recent introduction of a vaccine that protects against the most prevalent cancer-associated types of HPV infection has the potential to reduce the occurrence of this cancer dramatically (Mao and associates).

Cervical neoplasia is also increased in women who are immunosuppressed whether through infection (e.g., HIV), medications (e.g., chemotherapy), or genetics, according to a 2003 study by Schuman and coworkers. Smoking also increases a woman's risk of developing significant CIN, probably by altering the local immune response of the cervix.

HISTORY, EPIDEMIOLOGY, AND INFECTION

It is likely that carcinoma of the cervix has been a major cause of cancer death for centuries, although histologic confirmation has only been available more recently. In Paris in the 19th century, cervical cancer was reported to be the most common malignancy in women.

In the early part of the 20th century, epidemiologic studies demonstrated that the cancer was closely linked to sexual activity. Early age at first intercourse and multiple sexual partners were the most consistent risk factors. This suggested that there might be an infectious agent passed through sexual activity that is the "cause" of cervical carcinoma. Although some studies found associations with herpes simplex virus infections, *Chlamydia* infections, and gonorrhea, all these were ultimately discarded. It was only when it became possible to identify HPV infection that the true "cause" of cervical cancer was discovered.

The papillomaviruses are found in virtually all mammalian species and are generally species-specific. They are double-stranded DNA viruses that replicate within epithelial cells, as described in a 2005 ACOG Practice Bulletin. The group that infects humans (HPV) includes more than 100 types. Within these types there is further grouping such that the types that commonly are found on one anatomic part of the body are not the same as found on other parts. For example, plantar warts on the feet are not caused by the same HPV types as warts on the hands. In several locations, infection with HPV is associated with a clinically evident lesion, the wart. Unfortunately, this has led to HPV being labeled as the "wart virus" despite the fact that many infections, indeed most in the genital tract, do not form warts.

Approximately 40 types of HPV are known to infect the genital tract of both men and women. Of these, at least 12 are associated with cancer. The other types are either associated with genital warts or unimportant infections with no clinical symptoms. Because it is not possible to grow the virus in the laboratory, it has taken many years and much indirect evidence to determine that an infection with one of the cancer-associated types is a necessary precursor to squamous cell carcinoma and most of the cases of adenocarcinoma of the uterine cervix. However, the virus is an "incomplete" cause as the vast majority of genital HPV infections do not result in cancer.

Epidemiologic evidence is conclusive that the virus can be passed from one individual to another through sexual activity. However, HPV DNA can be found on clothing and other surfaces and thus fomite transmission might be possible, although, according to Winer and colleagues, it is unlikely. It will not be possible to determine whether such material is infective until a method of culturing HPV is developed.

Studies of college students and other groups performed by Wheeler and colleagues in 1996 and Moscicki and associates in 1998 have confirmed that most men and women acquire a genital HPV infection within a few years of the onset of sexual activity. The most common type identified in the general U.S. population is type 16, which is also the type most highly associated with cancer. Studies by Ho and associates in 1995 and 1998 tested participants for evidence of the virus at regular intervals several months apart, and most of the detected infections cleared within a few months, although some persisted for as long as 36 months. Recently, it has been found that many infections last only a few weeks, suggesting that the previous studies underestimated the cumulative incidence of the disease. Many investigators now believe that in sexually active individuals, infection with HPV at some time is almost universal.

Despite nearly uniform infection with HPV, the vast majority of women do not develop cervical cancer (Koutsky and colleagues). That is, of the millions and millions of women who are infected with HPV, only a few will ever develop cervical cancer, even if they are never screened and/or treated for preinvasive lesions. Longitudinal studies have now confirmed this fact (Fig. 28-1). The search for a predictive measure that will distinguish between those women who are infected and will clear the disease and those in whom the infection will persist and lead eventually to carcinoma has been frustrating. Although it is clear

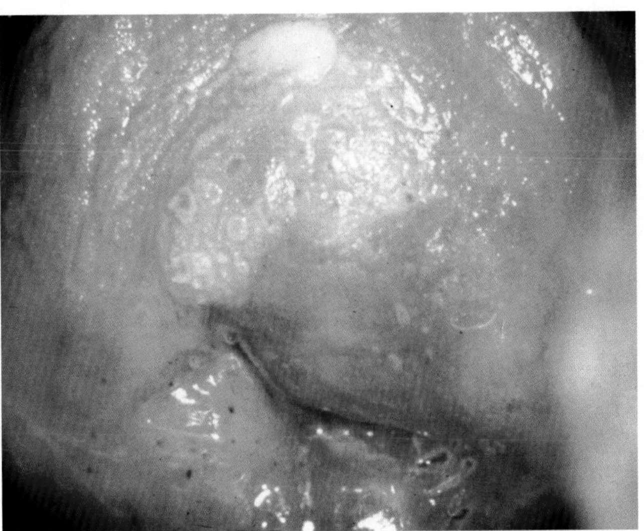

Figure 28-1. Colpophotograph of a cervix with an active human papillomavirus infection. The patient had a cytology sample reported as low-grade squamous intraepithelial lesion. She was followed without treatment, and the lesions regressed over the next year.

that those women who have a compromised immune system from any cause (genetic, iatrogenic, or infectious) have a greater risk of developing a persistent HPV infection, there is as yet no way to predict which healthy women will be unable to clear the disease spontaneously (Aldieh and associates). The only other independent risk factor that has been identified is smoking.

A cancer-associated HPV type causes neoplastic cellular changes when its DNA becomes integrated into the host cell genome. When this happens, certain repressor areas of the viral genome are lost. Consistently, the loss of these control mechanisms allows for the expression of the viral E6 and E7 genes. As described by Munger and colleagues, the production of oncoproteins results in the inactivation of the p53 and retinblastoma tumor repressors). These changes theoretically lead to cell immortalization and rapid cell proliferation. However, in most cases, the transformed cells are managed by the individual's immune system, and the infection/intraepithelial neoplasia is defeated. In some women, for reasons that are still not clear, the transformed cells begin to replicate, and if the lesion is not treated, after a period of several years, a cancer can develop.

Testing for the presence of HPV DNA is useful in a few specific clinical settings, and these are described in the sections on cytology screening and management of abnormal cytology reports.

Recently, vaccines that protect against the acquisition of HPV types 16 and 18, the two most common cancer-associated HPV types, have become available commercially. Studies, in particular one by Mao and colleagues, have confirmed that they protect against the development of significant preinvasive neoplasia and that the protection remains effective for at least 3.5 years. These vaccines have the potential to prevent approximately 70% of all cases of squamous cancer of the cervix. However, to be most effective, they must be given before exposure, that is, at the onset of sexual activity (Noller and associates, 1987). Ideally, all girls (and boys, although the studies showing efficacy in males have not yet been completed) would receive the series of three injections around age 11 and 12. It is not yet known whether vaccination protection is lifelong or whether a booster dose will be needed later. The vaccine is derived from "virus-like particles" that do not contain any of the viral DNA.

Because the vaccines currently available do not provide protection against all cancer-associated HPV types, screening with the Pap test will need to be continued indefinitely. Indeed, it is possible that suppression of types 16 and 18 will provide an opportunity for other carcinogenic types to become more prevalent. Newer vaccines that have the potential to protect against a greater number of the common cancer-associated types are in development.

CERVICAL CYTOLOGY TESTING (THE PAP TEST)

Cervical cytology testing became available in many developed countries in the 1950s after the studies of Dr. Papanicolaou had shown that by examining a cellular sample scraped from the uterine cervix and properly prepared and stained, the presence of cancer and its precursors could be identified. The 1941 monograph by Drs. Papanicolaou and Traut remains one of the sentinel breakthroughs in the history of preventive medicine. Their work led to the demonstration that when cancer precursors were identified, local therapy prevented the development of cancer. Despite the fact that Pap testing has a low sensitivity (many false-negatives), in virtually all countries that use it, the incidence of cervical cancer has been reduced by approximately 70%, according to Fahey and Nanda and their coworkers. The success of the technique relies on the facts that it takes many years for invasive cancer to develop following an HPV infection and that most women are tested repeatedly. Indeed, most women who develop invasive cervical cancer in the United States have either never been tested or have not been tested for many years.

The technique requires that the cervix be visualized after placement of a speculum into the vagina. The portio of the cervix is then scraped using either a "broom" or the combination of a plastic spatula and an endocervical brush (Figs. 28-2 and 28-3) (Martin-Hirsch and coworkers, Lancet, 1999). Noller and colleagues' 2003 survey of the Fellows of the American College of Obstetricians and Gynecologists showed great uniformity the use of Pap testing. This survey was conducted before the new cytology guidelines, discussed later, had become widely accepted.

Originally, the clinician would place the collected sample on a glass slide and fix it with alcohol. In recent years, that method has been replaced almost entirely by a "liquid-based" approach. The sample is now placed in a liquid medium for transport to the laboratory where the slide is prepared. This technique is slightly more sensitive for the detection of CIN, but its greatest value is that the medium can be used for HPV DNA testing and for the detection of some sexually transmitted diseases (Hutchinson and colleagues).

ACOG has recommended Pap testing for all women within 3 years of the onset of sexual activity or at age 21 (ACOG Practice Bulletin Number 45, 2003; ACOG Committee Opinion Number 330, 2006). Invasive cervical cancer is virtually never found in women younger than the age of 21 as the disease takes many years to develop after an initial HPV infection.

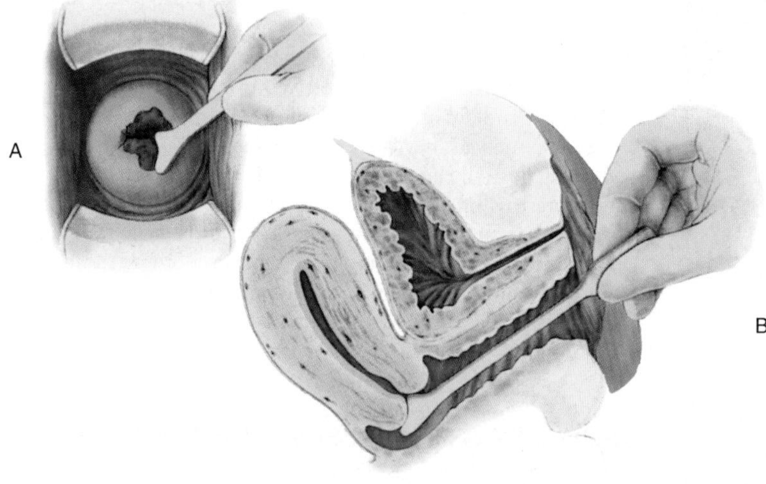

Figure 28-2. A plastic spatula is often used to obtain a specimen from the exocervix. It must be used with an instrument that samples the endocervix. **A,** Cervix as seen through a speculum, with the spatula being used to obtain a cell sample. **B,** Longitudinal view at the same point in the procedure.

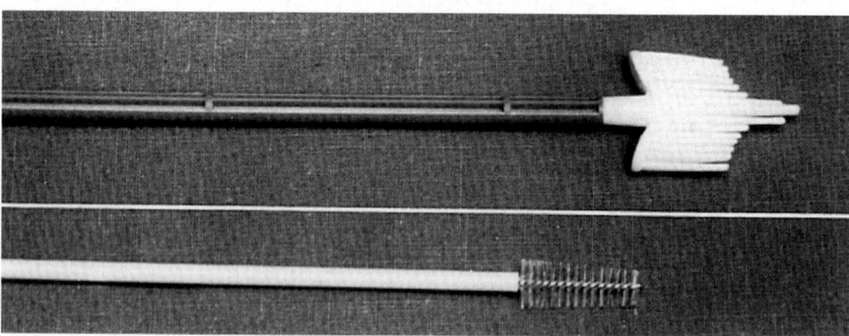

Figure 28-3. Both of these instruments can be used to obtain a cytologic sample from the endocervix. Cervical broom (Unimar) (*top*). Cytobrush (Medscand) (*bottom*).

Nonsexually active women should be tested at age 21 as there is some evidence that HPV infections might occur from fomite transmission. In addition, childhood sexual abuse might also transmit HPV.

The frequency of Pap testing has always been controversial. Although annual testing was the norm for many years, there has never been a study conducted to determine the optimum frequency. Currently, most organizations that make recommendations suggest annual testing until age 30. After age 30, if there has been no evidence of HSIL and the most recent previous tests have been negative, the interval can be extended to every 2 or 3 years. Perhaps the most effective testing after age 30 is the use of the combination of the Pap test and HPV DNA, per studies by Bellinson and Schiffman and their associates. If both of these tests are negative, the risk of HSIL during the next 3 years is extremely small. (This is the only U.S. Food and Drug Administration–sanctioned use of HPV DNA testing as a screening procedure.) Annual testing with cytology alone is acceptable, although not necessary for most women.

Of course, the combination of two tests for screening will occasionally result in disparate results, i.e., when one test is positive and the other is negative. A group of experts in this area met under the leadership of the National Cancer Institute to develop interim guidelines for patient management in these situations. Results were published by Wright and colleagues in 2004. In general, if one test is positive and one negative, the clinician can either perform colposcopy or repeat both tests in 6 to 12 months. Eventually, data will emerge to support or modify these opinions.

In the past, according to the ACOG Practice Bulletin 45, most women were advised to continue to have Pap testing after hysterectomy, despite the fact that vaginal carcinoma is exceedingly rare. Indeed, Pearce and colleagues showed that most abnormal Pap tests after hysterectomy result in false-positives. Therefore, the current recommendation is that women cease to have Pap testing after a total hysterectomy, i.e., the cervix has been removed completely. The only exceptions are women who have a history of an HSIL, are immunocompromised, or were exposed in utero to diethylstilbestrol.

Testing may also be discontinued in women who have no history of HSIL, have no new sexual partner, and have reached an advanced age, according to a study by Sawaya and associates. Unfortunately, the various organizations do not agree on the age at which testing can be stopped, but the age range of 65 to 70 is most commonly cited.

Several investigators have examined the cost benefit of various cytology methods, intervals, and techniques. In most cases, according to studies by Brown and Garber and Kim and coworkers, following the current guidelines is the most efficient method both to care for a patient and to maximize the expense of screening.

Cervical Cytology Reporting:The Bethesda System

In 1988, the National Cancer Institute convened a conference to develop a uniform terminology for the reporting of Pap test reports. It has been modified twice, the most recent modification

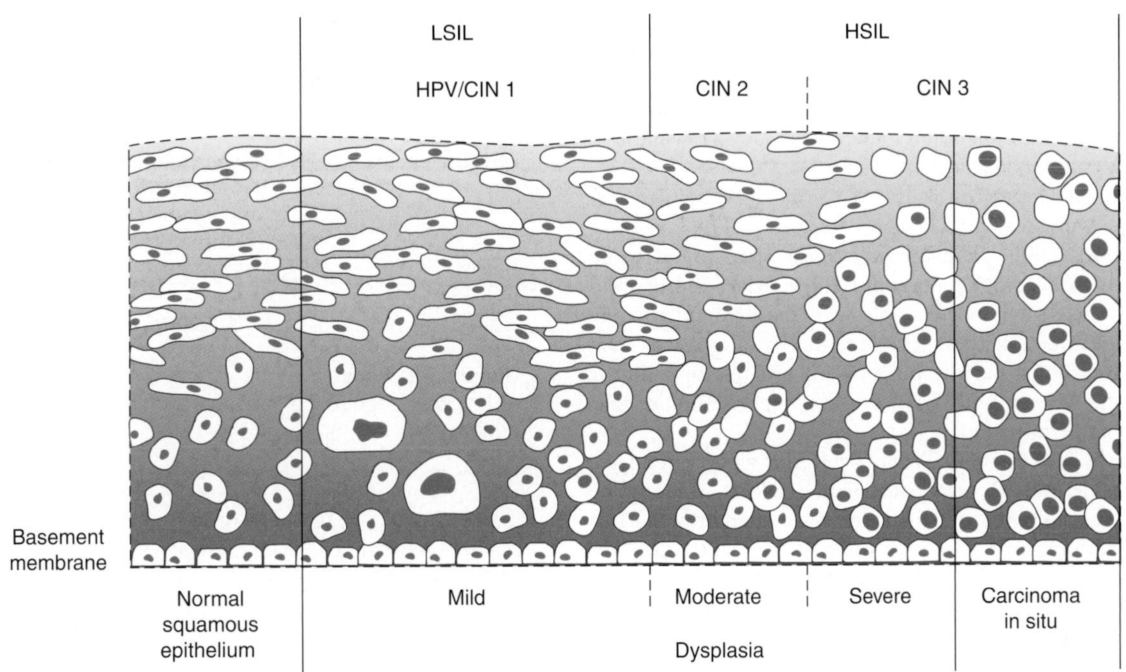

Figure 28-4. Diagram of cervical epithelium showing various terminologies used to characterize progressive degrees of cervical neoplasia. CIN, cervical intraepithelial neoplasia; HSIL, high-grade squamous intraepithelial lesion; HPV, human papillomavirus; LSIL, low-grade squamous intraepithelial lesion.

occurring in 2001 (Broder). The box shows the currently used classification. Virtually all laboratories in the United States (and many countries throughout the world) use this terminology. The management of patients with various abnormal reports is outlined here. ACOG Practice Bulletin Number 66 and a summary article by Noller in 2005 are sources for more information on this topic. Unfortunately, this cytology nomenclature is often confused with the terms used to describe histologic diagnoses. Figure 28-4 shows how TBS, CIN, and dysplasia categories correspond to tissue changes.

The first part of any TBS report states whether the sample was satisfactory or unsatisfactory. Reasons for an unsatisfactory report include such things as lack of a label, loss of transport medium, scant cellularity, and contamination by foreign material. Few samples are reported as unsatisfactory if a liquid-based technique is used.

The report next indicates whether the cellular material was normal. If other than normal, the abnormalities are further divided into squamous and glandular. The cytologist may also comment on the presence of evidence of infections such as yeast and changes consistent with a diagnosis of bacterial vaginosis.

Squamous abnormalities are found in approximately 5% to 6% of all cytology samples. The most common is ASC-US. This indicates that there are cells on the slide that show some of the features associated with squamous lesions, but either there are very few of these cells present or the changes are not consistent with a more precise report. In most laboratories, ASC-US changes are reported in 3% to 5% of all samples.

ASC-US reports require a management plan. Kinney and associates have demonstrated that although an ASC-US report is usually not indicative of HSIL, because ASC-US reports are common, the absolute number of women with HSIL and ASC-US is high. The National Cancer Institute sponsored a prospective, randomized study, the ASCUS LSIL Transmission Study (ALTS), to determine the most efficacious method of further evaluation of women with this report. One third of the women had immediate colposcopy, one third had repeat cytology in 4 to 6 months, and one third had HPV DNA testing, followed by colposcopy if the test was positive for high-risk HPV types. Although the HPV DNA arm performed slightly better than the others, all three approaches were found to be acceptable (Solomon and coworkers).

The Bethesda System for Reporting Cervical Cytology

- Adequacy of sample
  - Satisfactory
  - Unsatisfactory
- Squamous cell abnormalities
  - Atypical squamous cells (ASC)
    - ASC of undetermined significance
    - ASC, cannot exclude high-grade lesion
  - Low-grade squamous intraepithelial lesion
  - High-grade squamous intraepithelial lesion
  - Squamous cell carcinoma
- Glandular cell abnormalities
  - Atypical glandular cells, specify site of origin, if possible
  - Atypical glandular cells, favor neoplastic
  - Adenocarcinoma in situ
  - Adenocarcinoma
- Other cancers (e.g., lymphoma, metastatic, sarcoma)

The second abnormality is ASC-H. This report indicates that there are cells present that are worrisome for a significant lesion, but are few in number. All women with this report should be evaluated with a colposcopic examination as there is a high likelihood that a significant lesion is present, as reported by Sherman and associates in 1999.

LSIL is the next category. In the ALTS trial, it was shown that most of the women with this report were HPV DNA positive (ALTS Report, 2000). This report is most often found to be consistent with histology reports of CIN 1, HPV, and/or mild dysplasia. Indeed, it is not possible with the light microscope to determine which of these lesions represents a transient viral infection and which has the potential to progress to a higher grade lesion. Women with LSIL cytology reports should have a colposcopic examination.

HSIL is the next category. Women with this report often have a CIN 2 or 3 lesion, and, very occasionally, cancer. All should be evaluated with colposcopy. This is the most straightforward of all the categories in TBS (Sherman and associates, 2001). In fact, there is such good correlation between an HSIL cytology report and the finding of CIN 2 or 3 by colposcopy, if the two techniques do not agree, an excisional procedure is recommended to determine the actual nature of the lesion.

If solid evidence of carcinoma is present in the cytology specimen, it will be reported as such. In countries where cytology screening has been in place for many years, this is a rare finding. Other malignancies can also rarely be identified on cytology, e.g., lymphoma, sarcoma, metastatic cancer.

As discussed in Zweitig and colleagues' study, about 3 times in 1000, a cytology sample will contain abnormal glandular cells. Sometimes these can be classified by the site of origin (e.g., endometrium, ovary), but often cannot. The classification of these glandular lesions is long and complicated (see Box), but the all are managed similarly. All these women should have colposcopy, and if no lesion is identified, additional tests are needed. Conization of the cervix, scalpel excision is preferred to LEEP in this instance, should be performed unless there are other explanations for the abnormal glandular cells. For example, in pregnancy and with certain cervical infections such as *Chlamydia*, abnormal glandular cells are occasionally seen. If colposcopy is negative, these women can be followed until after the condition is resolved. However, if the abnormal glandular cells persist, conization is necessary. If the woman is older than age 35, an endometrial biopsy should be performed. When atypical glandular cells are present, there is approximately a 7% to 10% risk of an invasive cancer being present, making this a very worrisome report.

The first step in the management of women with the various abnormal cytology reports is shown in the following box. Because colposcopy is the predominant method of evaluation of women with abnormal reports, the technique is discussed in detail below.

First Step in the Evaluation of a Woman with an Abnormal Cervical Cytology Report

Squamous lesions

ASC-US	HPV DNA testing for HR types Repeat Pap in 6 months Colposcopy (all three options acceptable)
ASC-H	Colposcopy
LSIL	Colposcopy
HSIL	Colposcopy

Glandular lesions

All reports require colposcopy and further evaluation if negative

ASC-H, atypical squamous cells, cannot exclude a higher grade lesion; ASC-US, atypical squamous cells of undetermined significance; HR, high risk; HSIL, high-grade intraepithelial lesion; HPV DNA, human papillomavirus DNA; LSIL, low-grade squamous intraepithelial lesion.

Natural History of Cervical Intraepithelial Neoplasia

CIN is "graded" as 1, 2, or 3 depending on the percentage of the thickness of the epithelium that demonstrates cells with nuclear atypia. There is now general agreement that the histologic changes known as CIN 1, mild dysplasia, or HPV all result from infection with HPV (Fig. 28-5). In the vast majority of cases, these lesions disappear spontaneously, often within weeks to months, although, according to Moscicki and associates, it may take up to 36 months in some cases. For reasons that have not as yet been discovered, in a few women, these infections persist and the virus becomes integrated into the host genome, allowing for the development of malignant transformation. Fortunately, this process is slow and requires several years from first infection to the development of cancer.

When the process of cell transformation involves one half to two thirds of the thickness of the epithelium, it is designated CIN 2 (Fig. 28-6). The process still remains reversible at this stage with approximately half disappearing spontaneously without treatment.

When the neoplastic process involves the full or nearly full thickness of the epithelium, it is designated CIN 3 (Fig. 28-7). This term encompasses what was once called severe dysplasia and carcinoma in situ. Studies demonstrated that histopathologists could not differentiate between these categories in a consistent manner. Because CIN 3 is believed to be the precursor to invasive cancer, treatment is recommended (see later). However, even CIN 3 changes spontaneously disappear approximately one third of the time.

Fortunately, it takes several to many years for CIN to progress to invasive cancer (Kiviat). Treatment at any time during the intraepithelial stage will halt further progression. There is even an early stage of invasive cancer that is sometimes called microinvasive carcinoma. These lesions are not visible to the naked eye, but may be identified by colposcopic examination (Fig. 28-8). Management of theses lesions is covered in Chapter 29.

EVALUATION OF ABNORMAL CYTOLOGY: COLPOSCOPY

As discussed previously, the technique of colposcopy is almost always the first step in the evaluation of women with abnormal

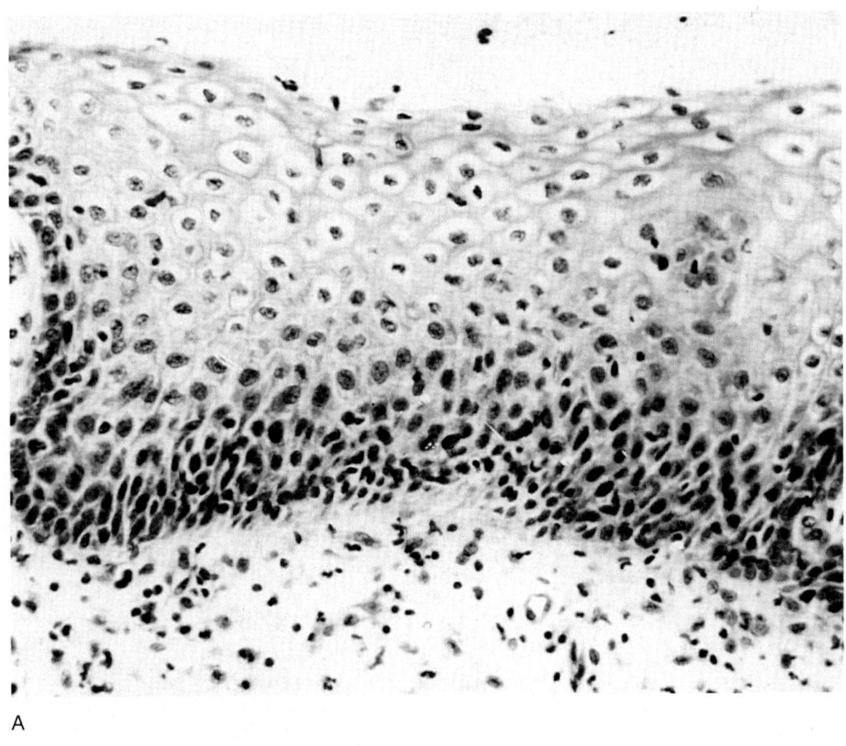

A

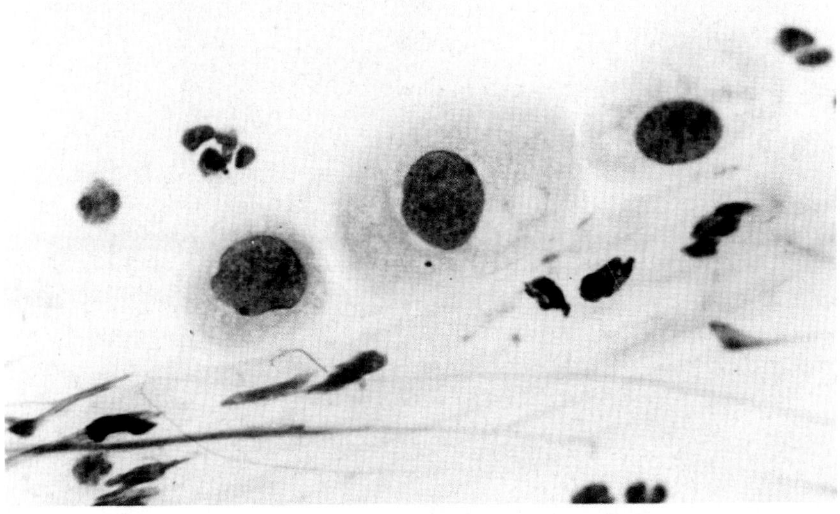

B

Figure 28-5. **A,** Cervical intraepithelial neoplasia 1 (mild dysplasia). Atypical cells are present in the lower one third of the epithelium. (H&E stain, ×250.) **B,** Low-grade squamous intraepithelial lesion cytology. These cells show an altered nuclear-to-cytoplasmic ratio with enlargement and have granular chromatin. (Pap stain, ×800.)

cytology results. The only exception is the category of ASC-US in which there are three equally appropriate first steps in the evaluation: repeat cytology in 6 months, HPV DNA testing, and colposcopy. If the repeat cytology specimen is positive or if the HPV DNA test is positive, the patient needs a colposcopic examination. Thus, for most abnormal reports, colposcopy is the first step in management (ACOG Bulletin #65, September 2005).

The colposcope is a low-power binocular microscope that is mounted on a stand with a powerful light source that is focused 30 cm beyond the front objective. Its useful magnification is from approximately 3× to 15×. The instrument is placed just outside the vagina after a speculum has been inserted and the cervix brought into view. After any obscuring mucus is removed with a swab, the cervix is carefully examined for the presence of lesions. In most cases, none will be visible. Diluted acetic acid, 3% to 5%, is then applied to the cervix, and after approximately 30 seconds, the cervix is again examined. Although the exact mechanism of action has never been determined, the acetic acid causes areas of increased nuclear density to be seen. With experience, a colposcopist can distinguish those tissue patterns that are associated with CIN from normal epithelium.

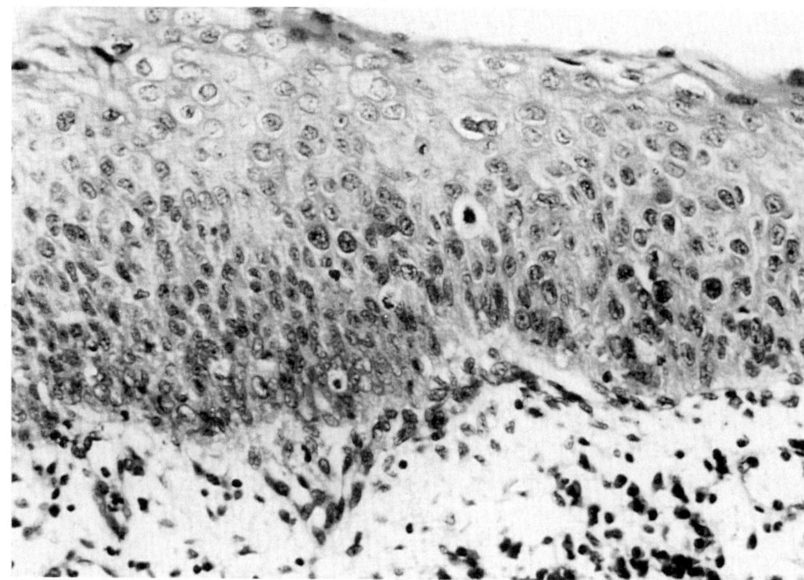

Figure 28-6. Cervical intraepithelial neoplasia 2 (moderate dysplasia). The atypical cells extend approximately halfway to through the epithelium. (H&E, ×300.)

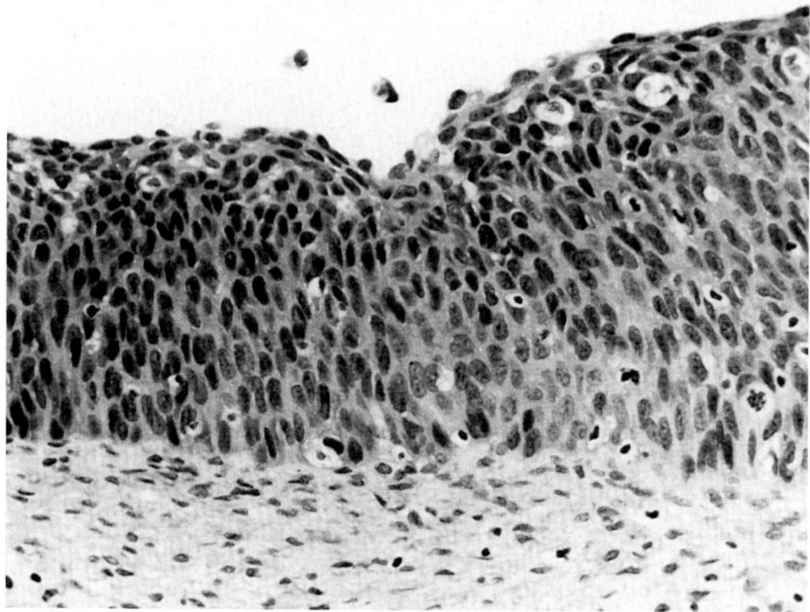

A

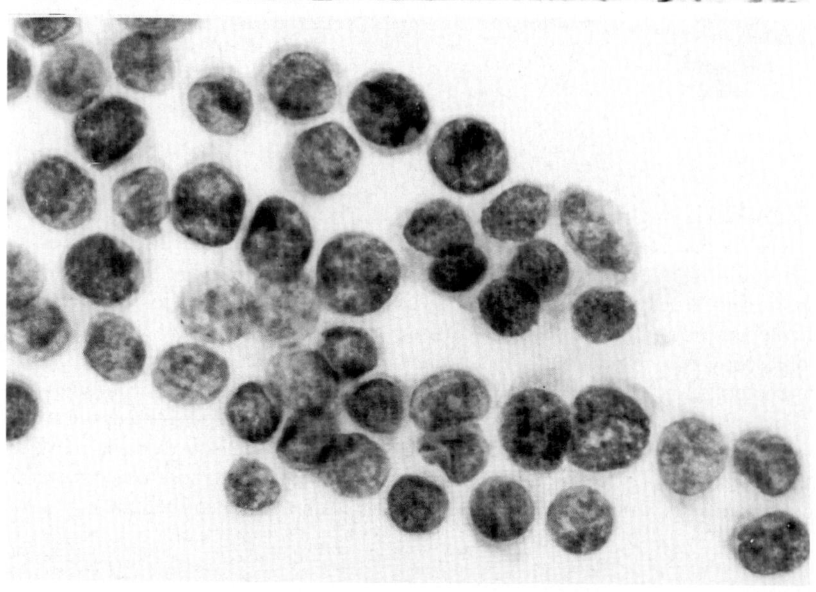

B

Figure 28-7. A, Cervical intraepithelial neoplasia 3 (severe dysplasia/carcinoma in situ). There is a lack of squamous maturation throughout the thickness of the epithelium. Virtually all the cells have enlarged nuclei with granular chromatin. Note that the basement membrane is intact showing that this process is confined to the epithelial layer only. **B,** High-grade squamous intraepithelial lesion. These cells exhibit large nuclei with granular chromatin. Very little cytoplasm can be seen. (Pap stain, ×800.)

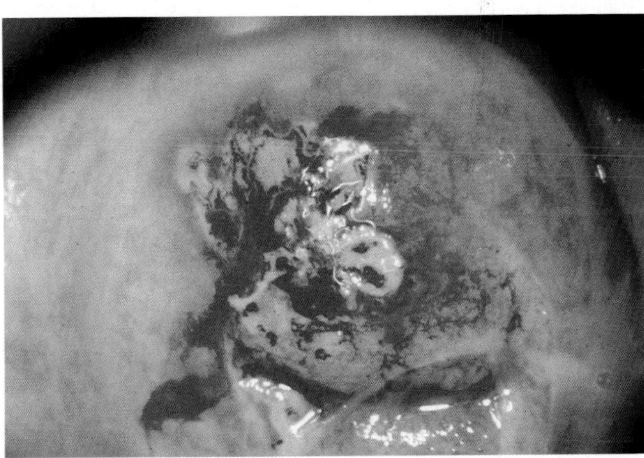

Figure 28-8. Colpophotograph of a microinvasive carcinoma of the anterior lip of the cervix at 6× magnification. Abnormal vessels can be seen, and one of these is bleeding due to the application of acetic acid.

A good colposcopist becomes facile in the recognition of tissue patterns, much as a pathologist relies on that ability to make histologic diagnoses. Although published several decades ago, there are no better descriptions and illustrations of the technique and findings of colposcopy than in the textbooks of Coppleson and colleagues and Kolstad and Stafl.

The colposcopist must also determine whether the transformation zone (TZ) can be seen in its entirety (Fig. 28-9). The TZ is the area that lies between normal columnar epithelium and mature squamous epithelium. The TZ is important because the vast majority of cases of squamous neoplasia of the cervix begin in this anatomic area, probably because it is an area of rapid cell turnover. Virtually all women are born with an area of columnar epithelium on the portio (face) of the cervix. When the vagina becomes very acidic at the time of menarche, this single columnar cell layer is gradually replaced by squamous epithelium through the process of squamous metaplasia. Squamous epithelium is much more resistant to the low pH of the mature vagina.

It is important to be able to assess the entire TZ. If some portions extend into the endocervical canal beyond visibility, the examiner will not be able to determine whether there is more significant disease above. In these cases, the lesion should not be treated with ablative methods (see later), but rather by one of the techniques that provides a tissue sample for histologic examination. If the entire TZ is visible, and the patient has not previously been treated for CIN, any of the common methods of treatment of CIN can be employed. However, if there is any finding that suggests that the lesion might extend into the canal or if it is not possible to see the TZ, it is wise to evaluate the endocervix with either a cytologic specimen from the canal or an endocervical curettage.

If a lesion is seen, one or more biopsy specimens should be taken to confirm the diagnosis (Fig. 28-10). Because the cervix has few if any pain fibers that respond to a cutting action, the samples can be taken with minimal or no pain. However, it is

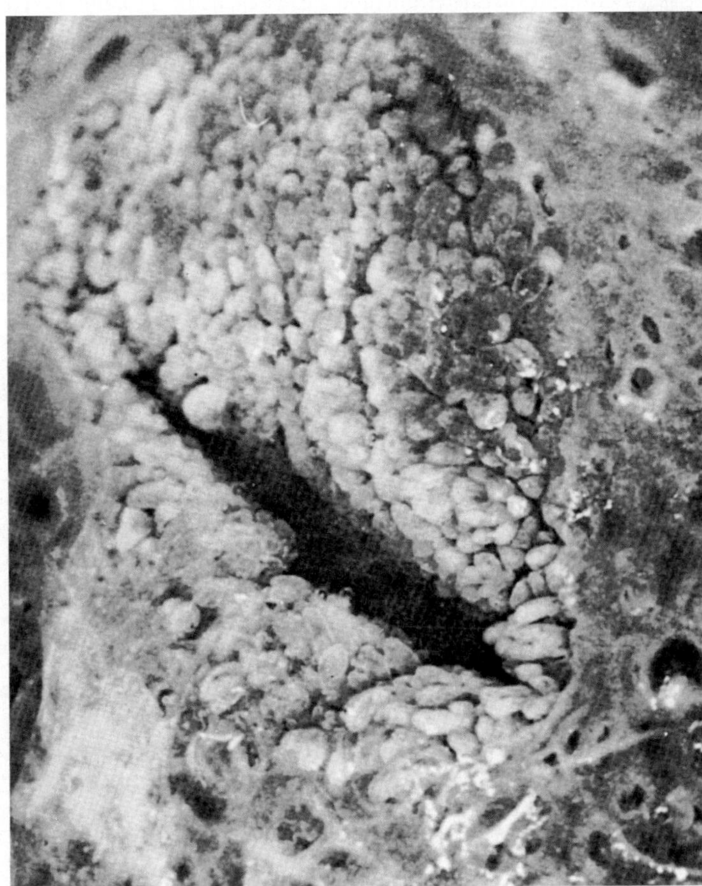

Figure 28-9. Normal cervix as seen through a colposcope at approximately 6× magnification. The central grapelike structures are covered with columnar epithelium. The tissue outside this area represents squamous metaplasia. There are multiple "gland" openings in this area, indicating that columnar epithelium is being replaced by squamous epithelium. This area between the columnar and squamous epithelia is known as the transformation zone. (From Coppleson M, Pixley E, Reid B: Colposcopy—A Scientific and Practical Approach to the Cervix in Health and Disease. Springfield, IL, Charles C Thomas, 1971.)

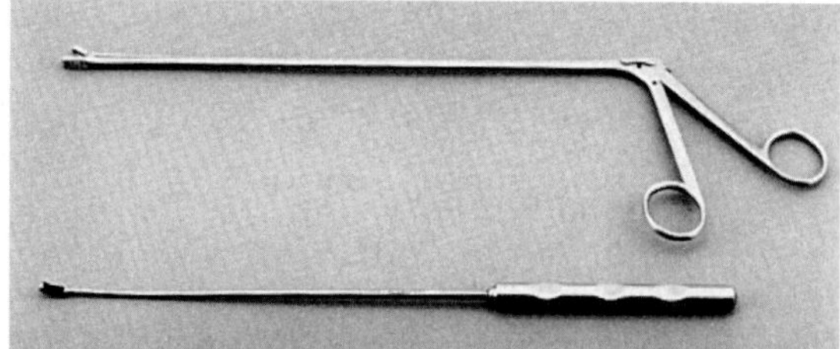

Figure 28-10. Cervical biopsy instruments. Punch biopsy (*top*). Endocervical curette (*bottom*).

important to maintain a sharp cutting edge on the biopsy instruments as the cervix has pain fibers that respond to stretch. If bleeding occurs, the base of the biopsy site can be touched with Monsel's solution or a silver nitrate stick. Cervical biopsy specimens are very small, usually only approximately 4 × 5 mm. Therefore, no restrictions are needed. The sites heal within a few days (Fig. 28-11). The exception is if a biopsy is performed during pregnancy. In that case, the patient should be advised to place nothing in the vagina for 3 weeks.

Colposcopy during pregnancy is difficult. The cervix becomes larger, the vaginal side walls tend to obstruct the view of the cervix, the blood supply to the cervix is increased, and decidual changes in the epithelium can be confused with CIN. Nonetheless, colposcopy plays a key role in a pregnant woman with an abnormal Pap test (Wright and coworkers). Invasive cancer must be ruled out, and that determination can be made by a careful colposcopic examination of the cervix. If there is no evidence of invasion, further evaluation can be postponed until after delivery. Biopsies during pregnancy can be performed safely in the physician's office. However, the examiner must be ready to respond with prolonged local pressure and, on rare occasions, with suture ligation should brisk bleeding occur.

The only indication for an excisional procedure in pregnancy is the possible presence of invasive disease. In those cases, a conization procedure under anesthesia is recommended.

If CIN was identified during pregnancy, a follow-up colposcopic examination should be scheduled postpartum. However, it should not be attempted until at least 6 weeks have passed. Many times the lesion will have disappeared, even if it was CIN 3.

TREATMENT

There has been a great change in the approach to treatment of CIN lesions over the past 30 years. Now that it is known that the vast majority of the lesions disappear spontaneously, treatment is indicated for only those lesions that have demonstrated a potential for further progression.

Cervical Intraepithelial Neoplasia 1

Treatment of CIN 1 is no longer the preferred method of management of these lesions at any age. Exceptions should be made on a patient-by-patient basis and only if the lesion has persisted for at least 12 months. Treatment of CIN 1 in women younger than age 21 is not recommended, even if the lesion persists. Virtually all CIN 1 is a manifestation of a transient HPV infection, and these resolve with the development of anti-HPV antibodies. Although many lesions regress within months, resolution may take up to 36 months. Because the lesion is so far removed from cancer, it should not be regarded as a serious finding. Although patients with CIN 1 require follow-up to ensure that the lesion regresses, clinicians should not present the finding in a way that alarms the patient.

Some small fraction of CIN 1 lesions progress to CIN 2 or 3, but, at present, it is not possible to determine which have that potential. However, because the treatment of CIN 2 and 3 is easy and office-based, there is no penalty for waiting to determine whether spontaneous resolution of a CIN 1 lesion will occur. In addition, all the treatments are associated with a risk of long-term complications such as cervical stenosis and premature delivery, according to Kyrgiou and associates (Fig. 28-12).

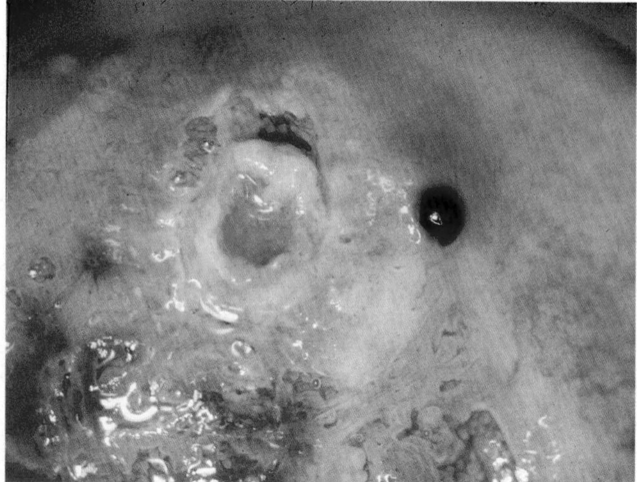

Figure 28-11. Colpophotograph (approximately ×12) of a cervical biopsy site 72 hours after the procedure. The eschar is already beginning to separate from the cervix.

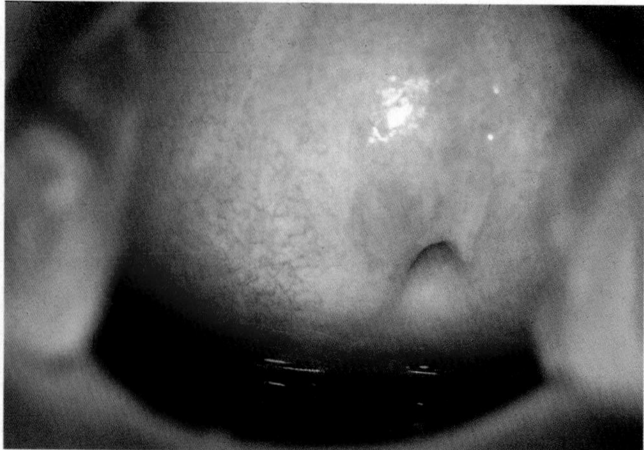

Figure 28-12. Mild cervical stenosis following cryocautery for cervical intraepithelial neoplasia 2. The colposcopic examination is unsatisfactory because the transformation zone cannot be seen (colpophotograph approximately ×6).

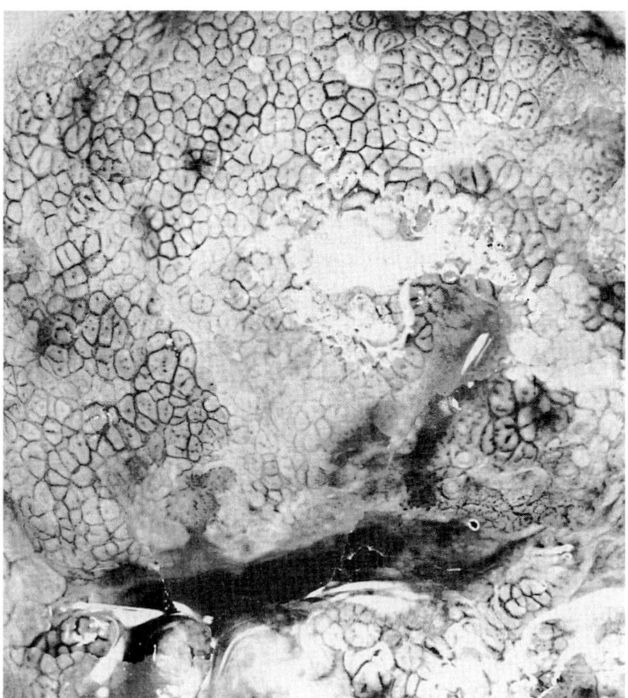

Figure 28-13. Extensive cervical intraepithelial neoplasia 3 (CIN 3) lesion covering most of the epithelium visible in this colpophotograph. The predominant feature is a mosaic pattern. There is "umbilication" of many of the tiles with a punctuate vessel, a common feature of CIN 3. Although this large lesion needs to be examined carefully for evidence of atypical vessels, a hallmark of invasive cancer, none are seen in this view. (Colpophotograph ×8.) (From Kolstad P, Stafl A: Atlas of Colposcopy. Baltimore, University Park Press, 1972.)

Cervical Intraepithelial Neoplasia 2

The majority of CIN 2 lesions also regress spontaneously. For many years, virtually all CIN 2 lesions were treated. It slowly became more common not to treat women younger than age 21. As the transient nature of these lesions has become more evident, many clinicians now follow patients beyond age 21, particularly if they are not through with childbearing. If a lesion progresses to CIN 3, it should be treated.

Cervical Intraepithelial Neoplasia 3

Although some of these lesions regress, most either persist or, in some cases, progress to invasive cancer (Fig. 28-13). Therefore, according to ACOG Practice Bulletin 66, they should be treated. If the involved area is removed in its entirety, the disease is cured. Several methods have similar treatment success, and these are discussed.

Women who have had one CIN 3 lesion are slightly more likely to develop another lesion in the future. Therefore, long-term follow-up is necessary.

Treatment Methods

The goal of treatment of CIN is to remove the lesion, and any technique that accomplishes that goal can be used. Currently, most treatment is office-based. Indeed, it is hard to justify the expense and increased risk of treatment under general anesthesia, except in rare cases with specific indications.

Treatment can be accomplished either by ablation (cryotherapy, thermoablation, CO_2 laser ablation) or excision (LEEP [also known as LLETZ], cold knife conization, CO_2 laser conization). All these methods have first-treatment success rates of approximately 95%, and the choice of method depends on the availability of equipment and the experience and expertise of the clinician (Martin-Hirsch and colleagues, Cochrane Database, 1999) Hysterectomy is *not* recommended for treatment of CIN, even if cervical biopsy specimens have been reported as showing "carcinoma in situ." As early as 1976, Kolstad and Klem demonstrated that hysterectomy for carcinoma in situ was no better than an excisional cone. In addition, hysterectomy carries risks that are much more common and serious than office-based therapy of CIN 3.

When a first treatment fails, it is because of incomplete excision of the entire lesion. Involved tissue can be left behind either in the endocervix or on the exocervix. The latter does not represent a difficult treatment problem as colposcopy can easily identify the area and office excision is both easy and curative.

When the endocervical margin of an excised specimen is positive for CIN, the patient should be followed with endocervical evaluation and colposcopy in 3 to 4 months. Many of these women will not have persistent disease, according to Lopes and colleagues, probably because very little of the lesion remained and the normal healing process destroyed the remainder. However, when there is evidence that CIN remains in the endocervical canal 4 to 6 months after the procedure, repeated excision of the canal is indicated. An endocervical margin that is positive is not an indication for hysterectomy or immediate repeat excision.

Ablative Methods

Cryotherapy

This outpatient method was the most commonly used treatment for CIN lesions in the 1970s and 1980s, but has largely been supplanted by LEEP. If patients are carefully selected, the success rate is approximately 95%. Larger CIN lesions have higher failure rates, most likely because the whole lesion is not covered by the cryoprobe. It is not appropriate to use cryotherapy if the lesion extends into the endocervix.

The procedure is simple. After colposcopy and sampling has shown that the lesion is confined to the exocervix, a probe is selected that will cover the entire lesion (Fig. 28-14). In most systems, N_2O is used as the refrigerant. The probe is applied to the cervix and the system is activated. The cervix will freeze quickly, but the probe must remain in place until the ice ball that forms extends to at least 5 mm beyond the edge of the instrument. In most cases, this takes 3 to 4 minutes. The refrigerant is then turned off, and the probe allowed to thaw and separate from the cervix. Several studies have suggested that repeating the freeze–thaw cycle a second time results in a higher success rate, whereas others have shown equal success with a single freeze.

Most patients experience almost no discomfort during the procedure, although some complain of menstrual-type cramping. Because the tissue that was destroyed remains on the cervix,

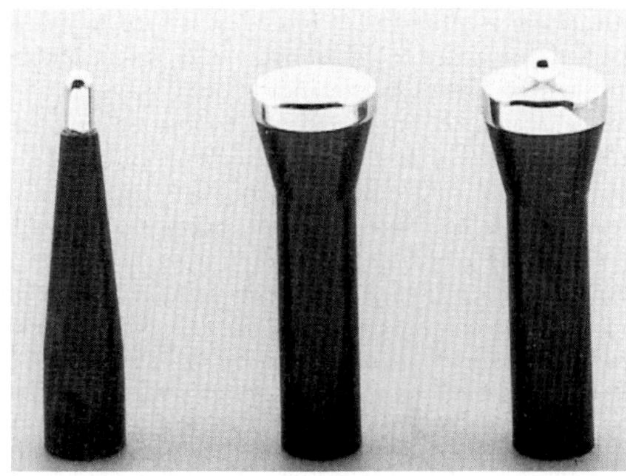

Figure 28-14. Three varieties of cryotherapy probes.

within a few hours to a day, the patient will begin to experience vaginal discharge. As the tissue sloughs, the amount of discharge increases, and malodor is common. It may take as long as 3 weeks for the discharge to stop. The patient should be cautioned to place nothing in the vagina for at least 3 weeks after the procedure to avoid causing dislodgment of the escar.

The first follow-up should occur in approximately 4 to 6 months and include cytology and colposcopy. The cytology sample should include the endocervix.

Short-term complications from the procedure include the nuisance of the discharge and occasionally bleeding. Long-term complications include cervical stenosis and a small increase in preterm labor. Unfortunately, the instrument was sometimes used by inexperienced individuals, and cases of invasive cancer following treatment were reported. In almost every case, an appropriate evaluation had not been performed before treatment.

Thermoablation

This technique is almost never used in the United States at present. Various loops, needles, and paddles were used to destroy CIN lesions. Although the success rate was as high as other techniques, it often required general anesthesia and perhaps resulted in more cervical stenosis than other methods.

CO_2 Laser Ablation

This technique became available to clinicians in the 1980s. When a focused CO_2 laser beam is directed at the cervical epithelium, the laser energy is absorbed by the water in the cells. The water turns to steam and the cell wall disrupts, killing the cell. The cell protein is largely "exploded" in a plume of smoke that is drawn out of the vagina by suction. Because very little dead tissue is left after the procedure, there is no prolonged vaginal discharge as there is with cryotherapy. The success rate is similar to other techniques.

The technique became popular both because the area of tissue destruction could be minimized and there was no prolonged discharge as with cryotherapy. In addition, because the instrument is attached to a colposcope, usually those who used the technique were very familiar with CIN. Additional training is required as treatment success depends on the correct choice of laser energy delivered (calculated as a "power density") and proper depth and extent of treatment.

For several years, CO_2 laser ablation was the method of choice for treatment of CIN. It can be performed in the office with no anesthesia. (I have personally treated several hundred patients in the office with this technique.) However, the equipment is very expensive. When LEEP became available, laser treatment began to wane. Currently, it is used almost exclusively in those cases in which there the lesion extends far out onto the exocervix. In these cases, CO_2 laser can be effective with less tissue destruction than other methods.

Excisional Methods

Loop Electrosurgical Excision (LEEP)

This procedure is currently the most common method for the treatment of CIN 2 and 3. It involves the removal of the TZ of the cervix under local anesthesia and can be performed safely and without discomfort in the office.

Typically, 3 or 4 mL lidocaine with epinephrine is injected into the cervix in a circumferential manner, making five to eight injections at the distal edge of the resection margin. The lidocaine is injected just under the epithelium rather than deep into the cervix. One to 2 minutes should be allowed for the epinephrine to cause vasoconstriction. A wire loop attached to a cautery machine that can provide a cutting current is then used to remove the tissue. Various sizes of loops are available (Fig. 28-15). If there is any bleeding, the edge of the defect can be cauterized with a ball electrode attached to the current generator. In most cases, there is less than 5 mL of blood loss. There is no reason to perform curettage of the endocervical canal above the resected margin as the management of the patient is the same whether the sample is positive or negative, and curettage can cause additional scarring.

The LEEP specimen is sent to the laboratory for histologic evaluation. In most cases, the whole lesion will have been excised and the margins of the specimen will be free of CIN. If either margin is positive for CIN, a colposcopic examination should be performed with the first follow-up cytology in 4 to 6 months. If the exocervical margin was positive, that area should be evaluated carefully. If a small bit of the original lesion was left behind, treatment is usually very easy.

If the endocervical margin showed signs of CIN, there is no urgency to perform a repeat procedure. Many of these women will have no residual disease at the time of follow-up. In all cases, the endocervix should be evaluated either by cytology or endocervical curettage. Only if persistent CIN is demonstrated in the canal should a repeat LEEP be performed. A positive endocervical margin or evidence of persistent disease in the canal is *not* an indication for hysterectomy. Indeed, hysterectomy is almost never indicated for the treatment of CIN. Only if CIN 3 persists despite multiple treatment attempts should it be considered, and evaluation by an expert colposcopist is strongly recommended.

Cold Knife Conization

This term is used to describe removal of the CIN lesion with a scalpel (the cold knife). Before colposcopy was widely used in the evaluation of women with abnormal Pap tests, cold knife conization was the standard diagnostic procedure. Under general anesthesia, the cervix would be stained with an iodine-containing

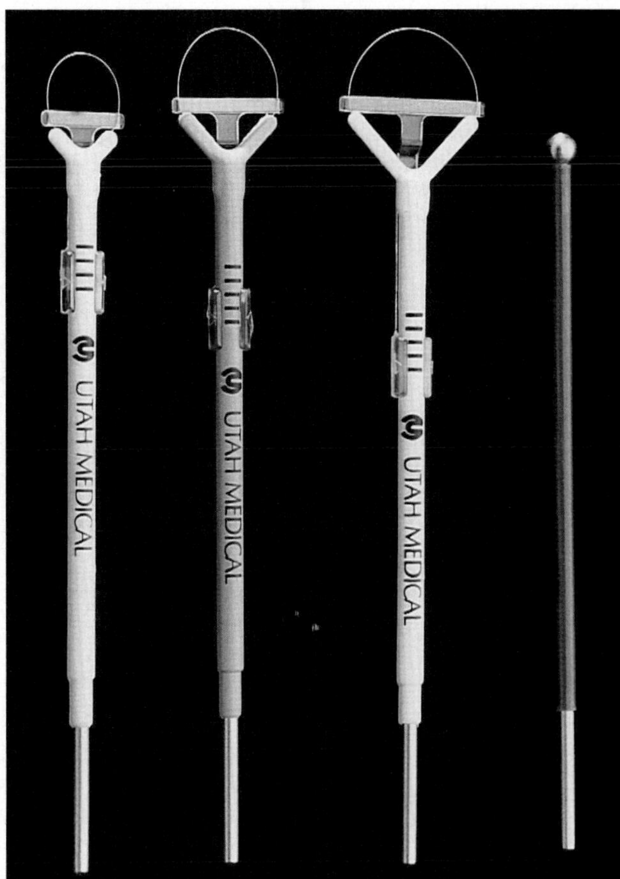

Figure 28-15. Examples of electrodes (Utah Medical Corp., Midvale, UT) used for a loop electroexcision procedure. The width of the excised tissue specimens can range from 1.0 to 2.0 cm, and the specimen depth can be adjusted by sliding the guard attached to the electrode shaft. Following excision, the base of the cervix is often gently cauterized with a ball electrode. (Courtesy Steven E. Waggoner, MD, The University of Chicago.)

solution, and all the epithelium that did not stain would be removed. The knife would be angled toward the endocervical canal, thus removing a cone-shaped piece of tissue that could be evaluated by a pathologist. Often, extensive suturing of the defect bed would be performed.

With the advent of colposcopy and office-based therapy, cold knife conization is used less and less often. For the evaluation of squamous lesions, it offers no advantage over LEEP, which does not require the use of general anesthesia. Its sole unique indication at present is in the diagnostic evaluation of patients with glandular lesions in which the absence of the thermal artifact introduced at the endocervical margin by LEEP is problematic. In addition, some clinicians still use the technique when a LEEP has failed, although there are few data to support this approach.

The technique has evolved over time. Because colposcopy should always be performed before cold knife conization, the exocervical extent of the lesion will be known. There is no reason to excise more tissue than necessary, so the excision should be tailored to the lesion. In many cases, a small cylinder of tissue can be removed instead of the larger "cone." In most cases, bleeding can be controlled with application of Monsel's solution (ferrous subsulfate) to the defect, especially if a vasoconstrictive solution is injected into the cervix before the excision. Sutures are only rarely necessary. If a bleeding site is encountered, a simple or figure-of-eight ligature of the bleeder suffices. There is no indication for the Sturmdorf sutures often used in the past. This technique rolled the exocervical epithelium into the canal, making subsequent evaluation virtually impossible. In addition, it is not necessary to control bleeding.

Follow-up

All the treatment methods described have a first-time success rate of approximately 95% (Martin-Hirsch and colleagues, Cochrane Database, 1999). According to ACOG Practice Bulletin Number 66, because women who have been treated for CIN 2 and 3 have a somewhat higher risk of developing a new lesion, they should be followed closely. A first Pap test should be taken 4 to 6 months after the treatment and repeated at that interval until three negative cytology results have been reported. At that time, the woman can be returned to annual screening examinations.

If a Pap test is reported as showing a squamous abnormality, colposcopy should be performed. The examination should include an evaluation of the endocervix, either with cytology or endocervical curettage. If a lesion is seen on the distal exocervix, it most likely represents an edge that was not included in the initial treatment. However, if a lesion is either seen to be involving the endocervical canal or if the endocervical specimen is positive, an excisional procedure that includes the endocervix should be performed.

VAGINAL INTRAEPITHELIAL NEOPLASIA

The least common malignancy of the lower female genital tract is vaginal cancer. The lesions are virtually all squamous carcinomas, and it it believed that most are preceded by an intraepithelial lesion (Audet-Lapointe and coworkers, Cardosi and colleagues). However, cancer is so rare that it is no longer advised to screen for the malignancy in women who have had a total hysterectomy unless they have a history of CIN 2 or 3. In fact, because the majority of abnormal vaginal cytology specimens are falsely positive, women who have undergone hysterectomy should be actively discouraged from having cytology samples taken. The exceptions, according to Kalogirou and colleagues, are women who have been treated for HSIL, women exposed in utero to diethylstilbestrol, and women who are immunocompromised.

VULVAR INTRAEPITHELIAL NEOPLASIA

Vulvar cancer occurs primarily in postmenopausal women who have had an untreated preinvasive lesion for many years. Unfortunately, cytologic screening of the vulva is not useful as it is unreliable. Most cases are identified either through a patient complaint of a "sore" or an area that "itches." Some asymptomatic cases are identified when a clinician performs a vulvar examination and identifies an abnormal-appearing area.

Natural History

The natural history of vulvar intraepithelial neoplasia (VIN) lesions is not as well worked out as for CIN lesions. Although it is believed that most cases of invasive squamous cancer of the vulva go through an intraepithelial stage similar to cervical lesions, is not known for certain (van Seters and colleagues). It is known that many invasive squamous cancers of the vulva contain HPV DNA, but the percentage of positive cases is lower than those of the cervix where it is almost 100%. When vulvar cancer occurs in a reproductive-age woman (a rather rare event), HPV DNA can almost always be identified. In postmenopausal women, the percentage of cancers with HPV DNA is small.

Vulvar histology is much less helpful than cervical histology. For example, it is known that a fraction of CIN 3 lesions will progress to cancer if not treated. However, a much larger fraction of VIN 3 lesions disappear spontaneously, particularly when they occur in women younger than age 35. Currently, VIN 1 lesions are not treated, as are fewer and fewer VIN 2 lesions.

Invasive vulvar cancer is probably preceded by VIN 3 in the majority of cases. However, many VIN 3 lesions never progress, especially when they occur in women younger than age 35. In that age group, VIN 3 most often represents HPV infection. Because there is no way to distinguish between those that will and will not regress, treatment of VIN 3 is still recommended at all ages.

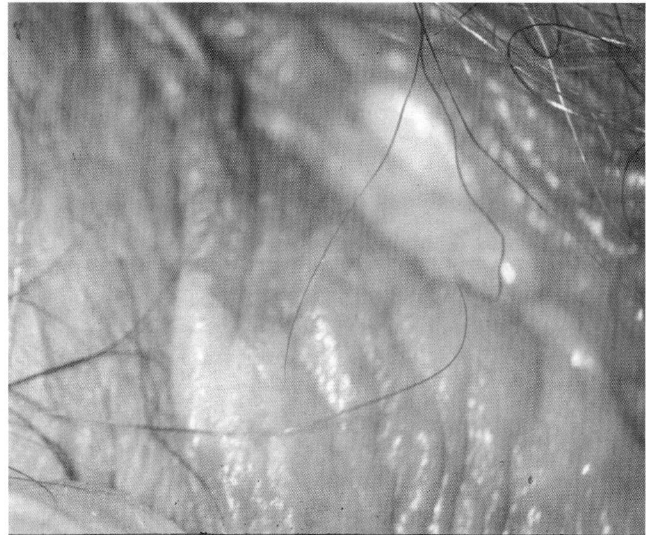

Figure 28-16. Vulvar intraepithelial neoplasia (VIN) 3 lesion as seen through a colposcope after the application of acetic acid. A second lesion is out of focus, but can be seen in the background. VIN is often multifocal.

Treatment of VIN

Before a decision to treat is made, following Wright and Chapman, it is important to have histologic confirmation of the lesion, both to be certain that it is truly VIN 3 and also to rule out invasion (Fig. 28-16). For some reason, many clinicians are reluctant to perform vulvar biopsies in the office. These can be done with a minimal of discomfort by using a very small (30 gauge) needle and lidocaine.

If a decision is made to treat a VIN lesion, there are several different techniques that can be used. The goal is to destroy the lesion, and any method that removes the epithelium can accomplish that goal. Unlike the cervix, there are no crypts (commonly called glands) in the vulvar epithelium, so excisions can be very superficial.

In the past, excision with a scalpel was used almost universally to treat VIN. Fortunately, many of these lesions are small and require only a small excision, especially in younger women. Because of the multiple folds of skin on the vulva, it is almost always possible to close the incision primarily. If lesions recur, a relatively common event, there may not be sufficient skin remaining for primary closure without relaxing incisions. It is not necessary to remove more than the lesion. In the past, "skinning vulvectomy" in which all the skin of the vulva was removed and a skin graft placed on the defect, was commonly used to treat vulvar carcinoma in situ (VIN 3). That procedure is no longer indicated, as simple excision of the individual lesion(s) has a similar cure rate.

The CO_2 laser can be used to ablate areas of VIN. It is especially useful in the area surrounding the clitoris where it is appropriate to remove the minimum amount of tissue consistent with removal of the entire lesion. However, the skill of the operator is important with this technique as the ablation should not be carried through the dermis. The raw edges, actually burns, left after laser surgery are much more painful than excision and primary closure.

Cryosurgery has been used, but there is poor control of the depth of the tissue destruction and healing is slow and painful. LEEP is used by some. There is better control of depth with LEEP than with cryosurgery, but it is still rarely used.

A novel approach in young women with VIN 3 lesions, particularly in the clitoral area, is the application of imiquimod. Although no large studies have been reported, small case series have shown a good rate of clearance for those who can tolerate the irritation that always accompanies its use. Long-term data are also not available.

KEY POINTS

- The Pap test is the most effective cancer screening procedure ever developed.
- When it is used widely, it decreases the incidence of cervical cancer by approximately 70%.
- TBS terminology is used for the reporting of cervical cytology specimens.
- Cervical cancer is caused by HPV.
- Virtually all HPV infections regress spontaneously.

KEY POINTS *Continued*

- Smoking increases the likelihood that an HPV infection will persist or progress.
- A vaccine is available that prevents HPV infection if given before exposure to the HPV types in the vaccine.
- In some cases, an HPV infection can lead to a precancer of the cervix called CIN. CIN is graded as 1, 2, or 3 depending on the percentage of the epithelial thickness that is involved in the process.
- CIN 1 should be observed rather than treated as it usually regresses spontaneously.
- Treatment of CIN 2 and 3 can be performed in the office with any one of several techniques.
- CIN 2 and 3 occur more commonly in women who are immunocompromised.
- An HPV DNA test can be used to triage women with ASC-US cytology reports. It can also be combined with cervical cytology for screening for CIN in women older than age 30.
- The colposcope is used to evaluate women with abnormal Pat tests.
- The LEEP procedure is the most common method used to treat CIN 2 and 3.
- Cervical stenosis, infertility, and premature birth are increased slightly in women who have been treated for CIN, regardless of the treatment method used.

BIBLIOGRAPHY

ACOG Practice Bulletin Number 45: Cervical cytology screening. Obstet Gynecol 102:417–427, 2003.

ACOG Practice Bulletin Number 61: Human papillomavirus. Obstet Gynecol 105:905–918, 2005.

ACOG Committee Opinion Number 330: Evaluation and management of abnormal cervical cytology and histology in the adolescent. Obstet Gynecol 107:963–968, 2006.

ACOG Practice Bulletin Number 66: Management of abnormal cervical cytology and histology. Obstet Gynecol 106:645–664, 2005.

ACOG Practice Bulletin Number 35. Diagnosis and treatment of cervical carcinomas. Obstet Gynecol 99:855–867, 2002.

Aldieh L, Klein RS, Burk R, et al: Prevalence, incidence and type-specific persistence of human papillomavirus in human immunodeficiency virus (HIV)-positive and HIV-negative women. J Infect Dis 184:682–690, 2001.

Audet-Lapointe P, Body G, Vauclair R, et al: Vaginal intraepithelial neoplasia. Gynecol Oncol 35:232–239, 1990.

Bellinson J, Qiao YL, Pretorius RG, et al: Shanxi province cervical cancer screening study: A cross-sectional comparative trial of multiple techniques to detect cervical neoplasia. Gynecol Oncol 83:439–444, 2001.

Bosch FX, Manos MM, Munoz N, et al: International Biological Study on Cervical Cancer (IBSCC) Study Group. Prevalence of human papillomavirus in cervical cancer: A Worldwide perspective. J Natl Cancer Inst 87:796–802, 1995.

Broder S: Rapid Communication—the Bethesda System for reporting cervical/vaginal cytologic diagnoses—report of the 1991 Bethesda Workshop. JAMA 267:1892, 1992.

Brown AD, Garber AM: Cost effectiveness of 3 methods to enhance the sensitivity of Papanicolaou testing. JAMA 281:347–353, 1999.

Cardosi RJ, Bomalaski JJ, Hoffman MS: Diagnosis and management of vulvar and vaginal intraepithelial neoplasia. Obstet Gynecol Clin North Am 28:685–702, 2001.

Coppleson M, Pixley E, Reid B: Colposcopy—A Scientific and Practical Approach to the Cervix in Health and Disease. Springfield, IL, Charles C Thomas, 1971.

Fahey MT, Irwig L, Macaskill P: Meta-analysis of Pap test accuracy. Am J Epidemiol 141:680–689, 1995.

Ho GYF, Bierman R, Beardsley L, et al: Natural history of cervicovaginal papillomavirus infection in young women. N Engl J Med 338:423–428, 1998.

Ho GYF, Burk RD, Klein S, et al: Persistent genital human papillomavirus infection as a risk factor for persistent cervical dysplasia. J Natl Cancer Inst 87:1365–1371, 1995.

Human papillomavirus testing for triage of women with cytologic evidence of low-grade squamous intraepithelial lesions: Baseline date from a randomized trial. The atypical squamous cells of undetermined significance/low-grade squamous intraepithelial lesions triage study (ALTS) group. J Natl Cancer Inst 92:397–402, 2000.

Hutchinson ML, Zahniser DJ, Sherman ME, et al: Utility of liquid-based cytology for cervical carcinoma screening: Results of a population-based study conducted in a region of Costa Rica with a high incidence of cervical carcinoma. Cancer 87:48–55, 1999.

Kalogirou A, Antoniou G, Karakitsos P, et al: Vaginal intraepithelial neoplasia (VAIN) following hysterectomy in patients treated for carcinoma in situ of the cervix. Eur J Gynaecol Oncol 18:188–191, 1997.

Kim JJ, Wright TC, Goldie SJ: Cost-effectiveness of alternative triage strategies for atypical squamous cells of undetermined significance. JAMA 287:2382–2390, 2002.

Kinney WK, Manos MM, Hurley LB, Ransley JE: Where's the high-grade cervical neoplasia? The importance of minimally abnormal Papanicolaou diagnoses. Obstet Gynecol 91:973–976, 1998.

Kiviat N: Natural history of cervical neoplasia: Overview and update. Am J Obstet Gynecol 175:1099–1104, 1996.

Kolstad P, Klem V: Long-term follow-up of 1121 cases of carcinoma in situ. Obstet Gynecol 48:125, 1976.

Kolstad P, Stafl A: Atlas of Colposcopy. Baltimore, University Press, 1972.

Koutsky LA, Galloway DA, Holmes KK: Epidemiology of genital human papillomavirus infection. Epidemiol Rev 10:122–163, 1988.

Kyrgiou M, Koliopoulos G, Martin-Hirsch P, et al: Obstetric outcomes after conservative treatment for intraepithelial or early invasive cervical lesions: Systematic review and meta-analysis. Lancet 367:489–498, 2006.

Lopes A, Morgan P, Murdoch J, et al: The case of conservative management of "incomplete excision" of CIN after laser conization. Gynecol Oncol 49:247–249, 1993.

Manos MM, Kinney WK, Hurley LB, et al: Identifying women with cervical neoplasia: Using human papillomavirus DNA testing for equivocal Papanicolaou results. JAMA 281:1605–1610, 1999.

Mao C, Koutsky LA, Ault KA, et al: Efficacy of human papillomavirus-16 vaccine to prevent cervical intraepithelial neoplasia: A randomized controlled trial. Obstet Gynecol 107:18–27, 2006.

Martin-Hirsch P, Lilford R, Jarvis G, Kitchner HC: Efficacy of cervical-smear collection devices: A systematic review and meta-analysis. Lancet 354:1763–1770, 1999.

Martin-Hirsch PL, Paraskevaidis E, Kitchener H: Surgery for cervical intraepithelial neoplasia. Cochrane Database Syst Rev 3(CD001318), 1999.

Moscicki AB, Shiboski S, Broering J, et al: The natural history of human papillomavirus infection as measured by repeated DNA testing in adolescent and young women. J Pediatr 132:277–284, 1998.

Moscicki AB, Shiboski S, Hills NK, et al: Regression of low-grade squamous intra-epithelial lesions in young women. Lancet 364:1642–1644, 1678–1683, 2004.

Munger K, Baldwin A, Kirsten M, et al: Mechanisms of human papillomavirus-induced oncogenes. J Virol 78:11451–11460, 2004.

Nanda K, McCrory DC, Myers ER et al: Accuracy of the Papanicolaou test in screening for and follow-up of cervical cytologic abnormalities: A systemic review. Ann Intern Med 132:810–819, 2000.

Noller KL: Cervical cytology screening and evaluation. Obstet Gynecol 106:391–397, 2005.

Noller KL, Bettes B, Zinberg S, Schulkin J: Cervical cytology screening practices among obstetrician-gynecologists. Obstet Gynecol 102:259–265, 2003.

Noller KL, O'Brien PC, Melton LJ 3rd, et al: Coital risk factors for cervical cancer. Sexual activity among white middle class women. Am J Clin Oncol 10:222–226, 1987.

Papanicolaou GN, Traut HF: The diagnostic value of vaginal smears in carcinoma of the uterus. Am J Obstet Gynecol 42:193–206, 1941.

Pearce KF, Haefner HK, Sarwar SF, Nolan TE: Cytopathological findings on vaginal Papanicolaou smears after hysterectomy for benign gynecologic disease. N Engl J Med 335:1559–1562, 1996.

Sawaya GF, Grady D, Kerlikowske K, et al. The positive predictive value of cervical smears in previously screened postmenopausal women: The Heart and Estrogen/Progestin Replacement Study (HERS). Ann Intern Med 133:942–950, 2000.

Schiffman M, Herrero R, Hildesheim A, et al: HPV DNA testing in cervical cancer screening: Results from women in a high-risk province of Costa Rica. JAMA 283:87–93, 2000.

Schuman P, Ohmit SE, Klein RS, et al: Longitudinal study of cervical squamous intraepithelial lesions in human immunodeficiency virus (HIV)-seropositive and at-risk HIV-seronegative women. J Infect Dis 188:28–36, 2003.

Sherman ME, Solomon D, Schiffman M, ASCUS LSIL Triage Study Group: Qualification of ASCUS. A comparison of equivocal LSIL and equivocal HSIL cervical cytology in the ASCUS LSIL Triage Study. Am J Clin Pathol 116:386–394, 2001.

Sherman ME, Tabbara SO, Scott DR, et al: "ASCUS rule out HSIL": Cytologic features, histologic correlates and human papillomavirus detection. Mod Pathol 12:335–343, 1999.

Solomon D, Schiffman M, Tarone R, ALTS Study Group: Comparison of three management strategies for patients with atypical squamous cells of undetermined significance: Baseline results from a randomized trial. J Natl Cancer Inst 93:293–299, 2001.

USPHA/IDSA guidelines for the prevention of opportunistic infections in persons infected with human immunodeficiency virus. MMWR Recomm Rep 48:1–59, 1999.

van Seters M, van Beurden M, de Crain AJ: Is the assumed history of vulvar intraepithelial neoplasia III based on enough evidence? A systematic review of 3322 published patients. Gynecol Oncol 97:645–651, 2005.

Wheeler CM, Greer CI, Becker TM, et al: Short-term fluctuations in the detection of cervical human papillomavirus DNA. Obstet Gynecol 88:261–268, 1996.

Winer RL, Lee SK, Hughes DE, et al: Genital human papillomavirus infection: Incidence and risk factors in a cohort of female university students. Am J Epidemiol 157:218–226, 2003.

Wright VC, Chapman WB: Colposcopy of intraepithelial neoplasia of the vulva and adjacent sites. Obstet Gynecol Clin North Am 20:231–255, 1993.

Wright TC Jr, Cox JT, Massad LS, et al: American Society for Colposcopy and Cervical Pathology. 2001 consensus guidelines for the management of women with cervical intraepithelial neoplasia. Am J Obstet Gynecol 189:295–304, 2003.

Wright TC, Cox JT, Massad LS, et al: 2001 consensus guidelines for the management of women with cervical cytological abnormalities. JAMA 287:2120–2129, 2002.

Wright TC Jr, Cox JT, Massad LS, et al: ASCCP-Sponsored Consensus Conference. 2001 Consensus Guidelines for the management of women with cervical cytological abnormalities. JAMA 287:2120–2129, 2002.

Wright TC Jr, Schiffman M, Soloman D, et al: Interim guidance for the use of human papillomavirus DNA testing as an adjunct to cervical cytology for screening. Obstet Gynecol 103:304–309, 2004.

Zweitig S, Noller K, Reale F, et al: Neoplasia associated with atypical glandular cells of undetermined significance on cervical cytology. Gynecol Oncol 65:314–318, 1997.

Malignant Diseases of the Cervix

29

Microinvasive and Invasive Carcinoma: Diagnosis and Management

Anuja Jhingran and Charles Levenback

KEY TERMS AND DEFINITIONS

Adenoma Malignum. A virulent adenocarcinoma of the cervix that histologically consists of glands that appear well differentiated (minimal deviation adenocarcinoma).

Barrel-Shaped Cervix. A cervix containing a large carcinoma, generally of endocervical origin, that has replaced much of the cervix, causing its diameter to widen (usually > 4 cm).

Brachytherapy. A form of radiation therapy in which the source is placed close to the tumor. The application may be in the form of needles implanted into the tumor (interstitial therapy) or into the vagina or cervical canal (internal therapy). For cervical tumors, an intracervical tandem and vaginal ovoids (colpostats) are usually used.

Endophytic. A term used to describe a tumor that begins in the endocervical canal.

Exophytic. A term used to describe a cervical tumor that grows on the outside surface primarily of the cervix (portio).

Extrafascial Hysterectomy. An operation that develops the pubocervical fascia to allow total removal of the cervix and uterus (class I hysterectomy).

Fletcher-Suit Applicator. A system that delivers brachytherapy to cervical carcinomas by use of a tandem in the cervical canal and ovoids (colpostats) in the vagina.

Glassy Cell Carcinoma. A virulent adenosquamous carcinoma that occurs in the cervix and metastasizes early in the course of the disease.

Microinvasive Carcinoma. A small (stage IA) carcinoma detected by microscopic examination with little or no risk of spread to regional lymph nodes (see text for detailed discussion).

Modified Radical Hysterectomy. An operation that removes the uterus and cervix and some paracervical tissues but does not dissect the ureters distal to the uterine artery (class II hysterectomy).

Pelvic Exenteration. An extensive pelvic operation usually employed to treat a central pelvic recurrence of cervical carcinoma after radiation. A total exenteration involves removal of the bladder, uterus, cervix, and rectum. An anterior exenteration spares the rectum, whereas a posterior exenteration spares the bladder.

Persistent Tumor. The identification of invasive disease at the site of primary therapy less than 6 months after therapy.

Point A. A term used in radiation therapy of carcinoma of the cervix to identify a point 2 cm above the external os of the cervix and 2 cm lateral to the cervical canal.

Point B. A term used in the radiation treatment of carcinoma of the cervix to identify a point 3 cm lateral to point A or 5 cm from the cervical canal.

Radical Hysterectomy. An operation that removes the uterus, upper third of the vagina, cervix, and paracervical-parametrial tissues. The pelvic ureters are dissected to the uterovesical junction. It is usually combined with a pelvic lymph node dissection (class III hysterectomy).

Recurrent Tumor. The identification of invasive disease 6 months or more after therapy.

Summary of Stages of Carcinoma.

Stage I: Tumor confined to the cervix

Stage IA: Microinvasion (preclinical)

Stage IB: All other cases confined to the cervix

Stage IIA: Tumor spread to the upper two thirds of the vagina

Stage IIB: Tumor spread to paracervical tissue but not to the pelvic walls

Stage IIIA: Tumor spread to the lower third of the vagina

Stage IIIB: Tumor spread to the pelvic wall or obstruction of either ureter by tumor

Stage IV: Tumor spread to the mucosa of the bladder or rectum or outside the pelvis.

Teletherapy. A form of radiation with placement of the radioactive source at a distance from the patient (external therapy). It is usually used to treat the pelvis and occasionally the paraaortic nodes in patients with cervical carcinoma.

Verrucous Carcinoma. A wart-appearing, well-differentiated squamous malignancy that rarely metastasizes.

Malignancies of the cervix are almost always carcinomas, and a summary of the more common histologic types are shown in the following box. Approximately 80% to 85% of these tumors are squamous cell carcinomas and from 15% to 20% are adenocarcinomas. The incidence of adenocarcinomas has increased in most developing countries, particularly among younger women.

Carcinoma of the cervix is closely associated with early and frequent sexual contact and cervical viral infection, particularly human papillomavirus (HPV), as detailed in Chapter 28 (Intraepithelial Neoplasia of the Lower Genital Tract). According to the American Cancer Society, the frequency of cervical cancer has been steadily decreasing, in part because of the effect of

Summary of Major Categories of Cervical Carcinoma

Squamous Cell Carcinomas
- Large cell (keratinizing or nonkeratinizing)
- Small cell
- Verrucous

Adenocarcinomas
- Typical (endocervical)
- Endometrioid
- Clear cell
- Adenoid cystic (basaloid cylindroma)
- Adenoma malignum (minimal deviation adenocarcinoma)

Mixed Carcinomas
- Adenosquamous
- Glassy cell

widespread screening for premalignant cervical changes by cervical cytology (Pap smear). Approximately 9710 new cases of cervical cancer will be diagnosed in the United States in 2006, making it the third most frequent malignancy of the lower female genital tract after endometrial and ovarian carcinomas. Approximately 3700 deaths annually result from cervical cancer, which is less than the approximately 15,310 for ovarian cancer. The incidence of cervical carcinoma in the United States is higher among the Hispanic/Latin population (15%) compared with whites (8.7) and African Americans (11.1). However, the mortality rate from cervical cancer is the highest among African Americans compared with other races. This is partially because African Americans tend to have their cancers diagnosed at a late stage. Invasive cervical cancers are diagnosed at a localized stage in 56% of white women and 48% of African American women. This chapter details the various types of cervical carcinomas and consider their natural history, methods of diagnosis and evaluation, and the details of therapy. Primary sarcomas and melanomas of the cervix are extremely rare and are not considered separately (Fig. 29-1).

HISTOLOGIC TYPES

Varieties of squamous cell carcinoma of the cervix are illustrated in Figure 29-2. An early form, microinvasive carcinoma, is considered separately in the next section. Most squamous cell carcinomas of the cervix are reported to be of the large cell, nonkeratinizing type, but many are keratinized, and squamous pearls may be seen. The degree of differentiation of tumors is usually designated by three grades: G1, well differentiated; G2, intermediate; and G3, undifferentiated. However, there is no consensus on the value of tumor grade as a major prognostic factor for squamous cell carcinoma of the cervix.

A rare variety of squamous cell carcinoma is the so-called verrucous carcinoma, which is morphologically similar to those found in the vulva (see Chapter 32). These warty tumors appear as large, bulbous masses (Fig. 29-3). They rarely metastasize but unfortunately may be admixed with the more virulent, typical squamous cell carcinomas, in which case metastatic spread is more likely.

Adenocarcinomas may have a number of histologic varieties. As noted by Brinton and colleagues, adenocarcinomas do not appear to be affected by the usual sexual factors associated with squamous carcinomas. However, HPV DNA, oral contraceptive use, and lack of cervical cytologic screening heightened the risk of developing these tumors. The typical variant often contains intracytoplasmic mucin and is related to the mucinous cells of the endocervix (endocervical pattern) (Fig. 29-4). However, on occasion, the cells contain little or no mucin, and then the tumor may resemble an endometrial carcinoma (endometrioid pattern). It may be difficult histologically to ascertain whether these carcinomas arise in the cervix or endometrium. Endocervical tumors more frequently stain positive for carcinoembryonic antigen than do endometrial tumors, and this

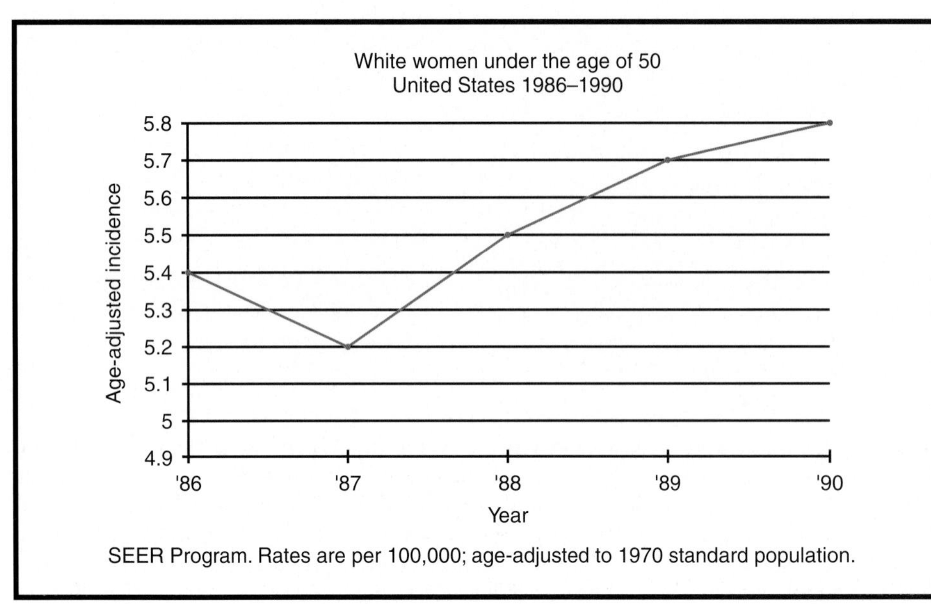

Figure 29-1. Incidence rates of invasive carcinoma. (From Ries LAG, Harkins D, Krapcho M, et al [eds]: SEER Cancer Statistics Review. Washington, DC, U.S. Department of Health and Human Services, 1973–1991, 136–144, 1994.)

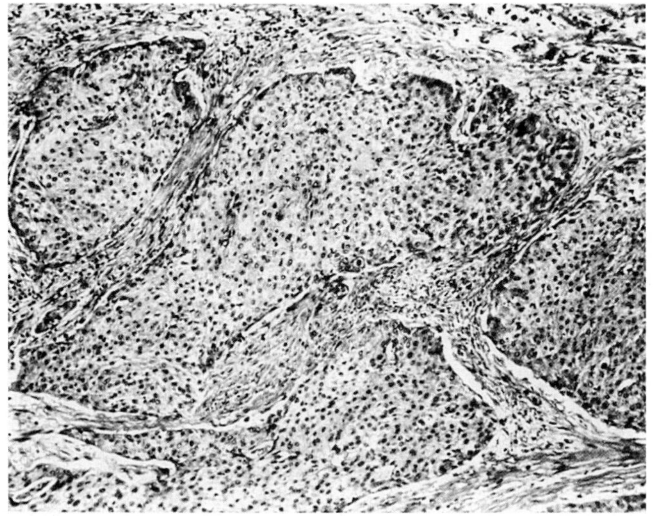

A

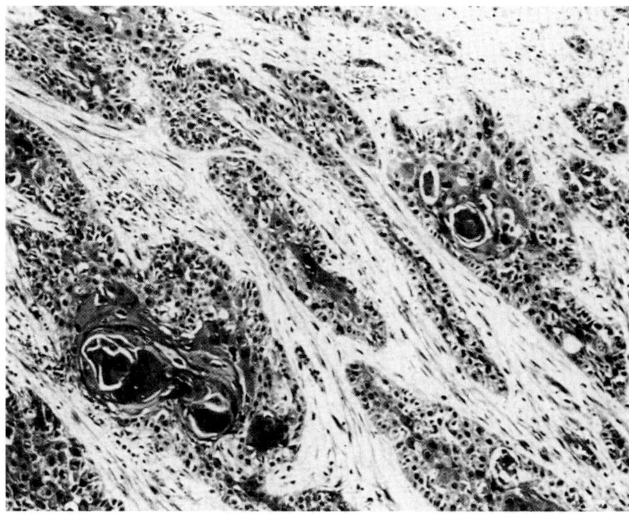

B

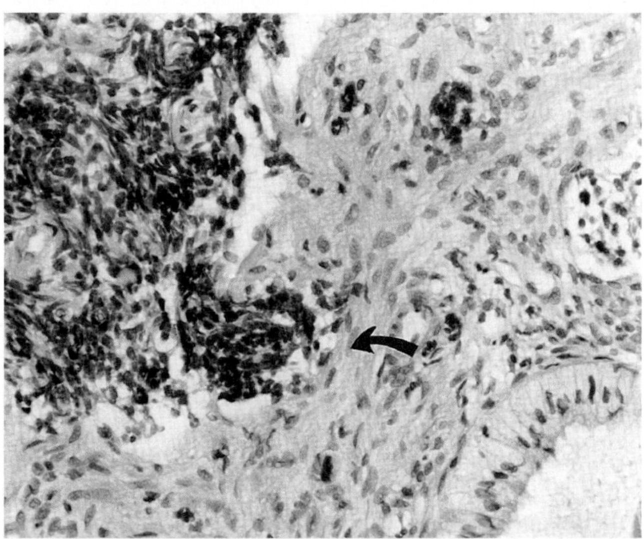

C

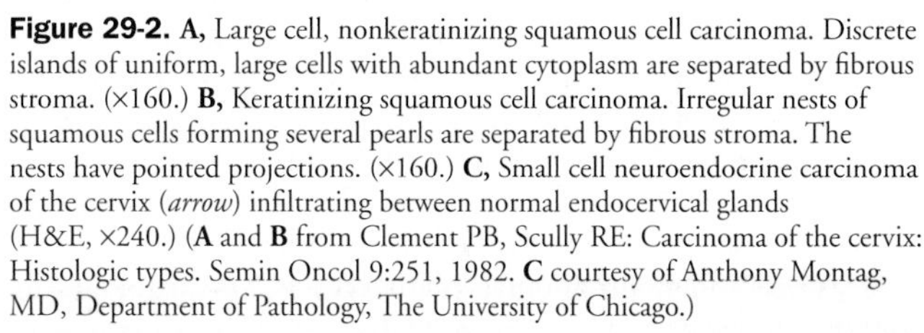

Figure 29-2. **A,** Large cell, nonkeratinizing squamous cell carcinoma. Discrete islands of uniform, large cells with abundant cytoplasm are separated by fibrous stroma. (×160.) **B,** Keratinizing squamous cell carcinoma. Irregular nests of squamous cells forming several pearls are separated by fibrous stroma. The nests have pointed projections. (×160.) **C,** Small cell neuroendocrine carcinoma of the cervix (*arrow*) infiltrating between normal endocervical glands (H&E, ×240.) (**A** and **B** from Clement PB, Scully RE: Carcinoma of the cervix: Histologic types. Semin Oncol 9:251, 1982. **C** courtesy of Anthony Montag, MD, Department of Pathology, The University of Chicago.)

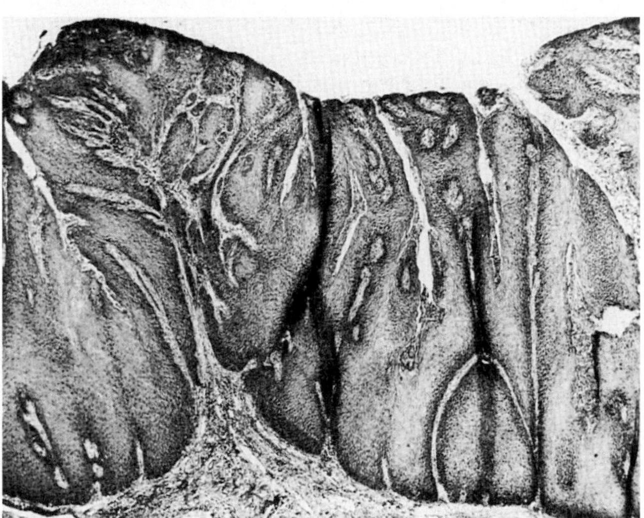

Figure 29-3. Verrucous carcinoma. Downgrowns of papillae have broad bases. Tumor cells are well differentiated. (×34.) (From Clement PB, Scully RE: Carcinoma of the cervix: Histologic types. Semin Oncol 9:251, 1982.)

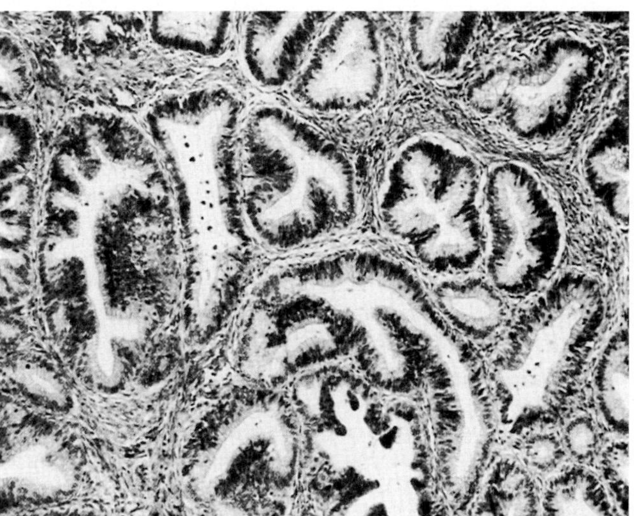

Figure 29-4. Typical adenocarcinoma. Irregular glands are lined by stratified mucin-containing epithelium. Mitotic figures are numerous. (×160.) (From Clement PB, Scully RE: Carcinoma of the cervix: Histologic types. Semin Oncol 9:251, 1982.)

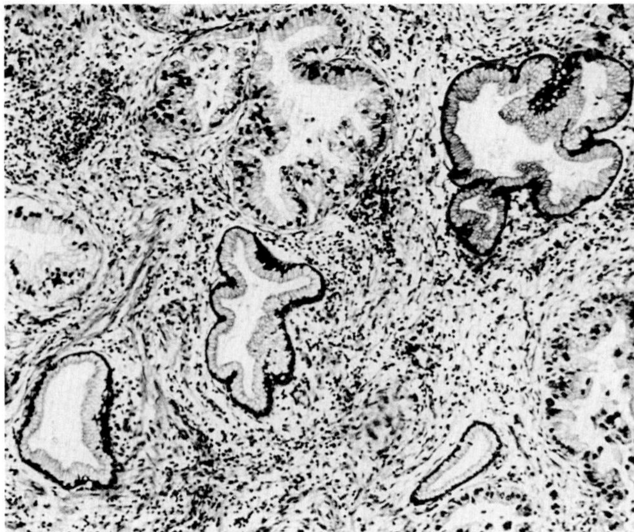

Figure 29-5. Adenoma malignum. Glands are mostly well differentiated, appearing normal except for their irregular shapes. A few obviously malignant glands are also present. (×160.) (From Clement PB, Scully RE: Carcinoma of the cervix: Histologic types. Semin Oncol 9:251, 1982.)

histochemical observation has been used to try to distinguish the tumors microscopically by an immunoperoxidase reaction.

A rare but important virulent variety of adenocarcinoma is the adenoma malignum. These microscopically innocuous-appearing tumors consist of well-differentiated mucinous glands (Fig. 29-5) that vary in size and shape and infiltrate the stroma. Despite their bland histologic appearance, they tend to be deeply invasive and metastasize early. The term *minimal deviation adenocarcinoma* is applied to these tumors. According to McGowan and associates, patients with Peutz-Jeghers syndrome are at increased risk of the development of these tumors.

Clear cell adenocarcinomas of the cervix are histologically identical to those of the ovary (see Chapter 33) and vagina (see Chapter 31). They are uncommon in the cervix and can also be associated with intrauterine diethylstilbestrol exposure (see Chapter 15), although they also often develop spontaneously in the absence of diethylstilbestrol exposure.

Adenoid cystic carcinomas are rare. Berchuk and Mullin summarized 88 cases reported in the literature. These tumors are aggressive and may resemble cylindromas of salivary gland or breast origin and histologically may resemble basal cell carcinomas of the skin (adenoid basal, or basaloid, carcinomas). Most patients with these tumors are older than age 60 years. The basaloid variety appears to be less aggressive. King and coworkers reported four unusual cases in women younger than age 40. One patient was noted to survive more than 5 years.

Adenosquamous carcinomas, as the name implies, consist of both squamous carcinoma and adenocarcinoma elements in varying proportions (Fig. 29-6). They occur frequently in pregnant women. A particularly virulent variety is termed *glassy cell carcinoma* (Fig. 29-7). This is an undifferentiated tumor consisting of large cells containing cytoplasm with a ground-glass appearance. Glassy cell carcinomas tend to metastasize early to lymph nodes as well as to distant sites and usually have a fatal outcome.

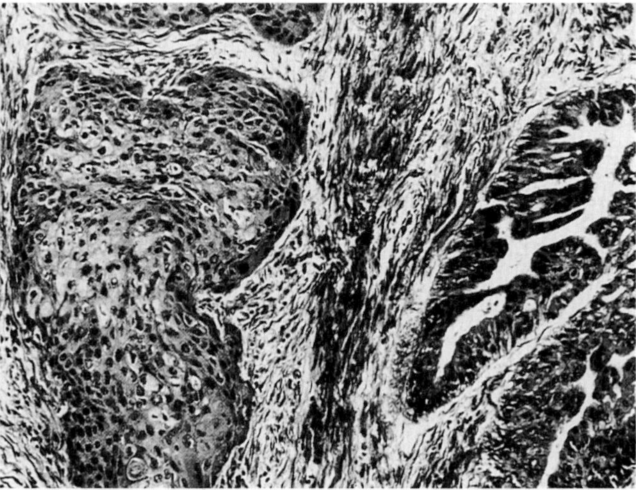

Figure 29-6. Well-differentiated adenosquamous carcinoma. Glandular structure lies adjacent to nest of nonkeratinizing, large squamous cells. (×400.) (From Clement PB, Scully RE: Carcinoma of the cervix: Histologic types. Semin Oncol 9:251, 1982.)

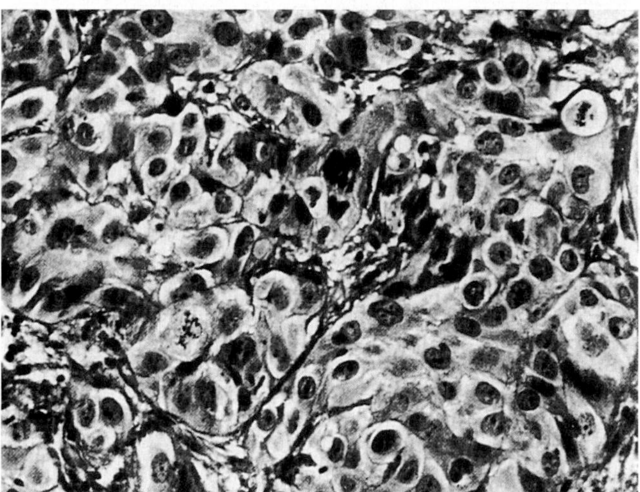

Figure 29-7. Glassy cell carcinoma. Cells have sharp borders, ground-glass-type cytoplasm, and nuclei containing prominent nucleoli. (×1000.) (From Clement PB, Scully RE: Carcinoma of the cervix: Histologic types. Semin Oncol 9:251, 1982.)

Small cell carcinoma of the cervix is rare, compromising less than 5% of all carcinomas of the cervix. Women with small cell carcinoma are likely to be 10 years younger than those with squamous cell carcinoma. The cells are small anaplastic cells with scan cytoplasm. They behave very aggressively and frequently associated with widespread metastasis to multiple sites, including bone, liver, skin, and brain. Efforts to treat these cancers with approaches typically used for small cell carcinoma of the lung have had mixed results.

Another variant that is not in the World Health Organization classification is non-small cell neuroendocrine tumors. The tumors contain intermediate to large cells, high-grade nuclei, and eosinophilic cytoplasmic granules of the type seen in neuroendocrine cells. Reported survival rates for patients with these aggressive carcinomas are similar to those patients with small cell tumors and optimal therapy has yet to be established.

MICROINVASIVE CARCINOMA OF THE CERVIX

Microinvasive carcinoma of the cervix is part of the spectrum of cervical neoplasia between intraepithelial carcinoma (Chapter 28) and frankly invasive carcinoma. These are tiny lesions that have begun to invade the cervical stroma (Fig. 29-8), but can often be treated by less extensive measures than those required for larger invasive cancers. In the International Federation of Gynecology and Obstetrics (FIGO) staging classification, these preclinical carcinomas are designated as stage IA.

A major problem in gynecologic oncology is that there is no uniform agreement on the appropriate definition of microinvasive carcinoma. The ideal definition is one that would have widespread clinicopathologic applicability and describe an early invasive lesion that has little or no risk of spread beyond the cervix, such as to regional pelvic lymph nodes. It is important to consider some of the definitions that have been used to describe this entity and also to consider the results of therapy that have been obtained. The important factors are the depth of stromal invasion, the presence or absence of vascular or lymphatic space involvement (capillary-like spaces), the presence or absence of tumor confluence, and the lateral extent (width) of the lesion.

FIGO (1994) defines a stage IA lesion as a preclinical cervical carcinoma and divides microinvasion into two categories: stages IA1 and IA2. Stage IA1 is minimal stromal invasion that most authorities believe can be treated as a carcinoma in situ. Stage IA1 is a microinvasive tumor whose dimensions are less than 3 mm depth of invasion and 7 mm width. It is not clear whether this definition provides reliable criteria for lack of risk of tumor spread to regional nodes. Stage IA2 is microscopic tumor that is 3 to 5 mm in depth and less than 7 mm in width (Table 29-1). Kolstad summarized 411 patients with stage IA2, 245 of whom

Table 29-1 Clinical Stages of Carcinoma of the Cervix Uteri (International Federation of Gynecology and Obstetrics, Revised 1994)

Stage	Characteristics
I	Carcinoma is strictly confined to the cervix (extension to the corpus should be disregarded)
IA	Invasive cancer identified only microscopically. All gross lesions, even with superficial invasion, are stage IB cancers. Invasion is limited to measured stromal invasion with a maximum depth of 5 mm and no wider than 7 mm*
IA1	Measured invasion of stroma no greater than 3 mm in depth and no wider than 7 mm
IA2	Measured invasion of stroma greater than 3 mm and no greater than 5 mm in depth and no wider than 7 mm
IB	Clinical lesions confined to the cervix or preclinical lesions greater than IA
IB1	Clinical lesions no greater than 4 cm in size
IB2	Clinical lesions greater than 4 cm in size
II	Carcinoma extends beyond the cervix but has not extended to the pelvic wall; it involves the vagina, but not as far as the lower third
IIA	No obvious parametrial involvement
IIB	Obvious parametrial involvement
III	Carcinoma has extended to the pelvic wall; on rectal examination, there is no cancer-free space between the tumor and pelvic wall; the tumor involves the lower third of the vagina; all cases with hydronephrosis or a nonfunctioning kidney should be included unless they are known to be due to another cause
IIIA	No extension to the pelvic wall, but involvement of the lower third of the vagina
IIIB	Extension to the pelvic wall or hydronephrosis or a nonfunctioning kidney due to tumor
IV	Carcinoma has extended beyond the true pelvis or has clinically involved the mucosa of bladder or rectum
IVA	Spread of growth to adjacent pelvic organs
IVB	Spread to distant organs

*The depth of invasion should not be more than 5 mm taken from the base of the epithelium, either surface or glandular, from which it originates. Vascular space involvement, either venous or lymphatic, should not alter the staging.

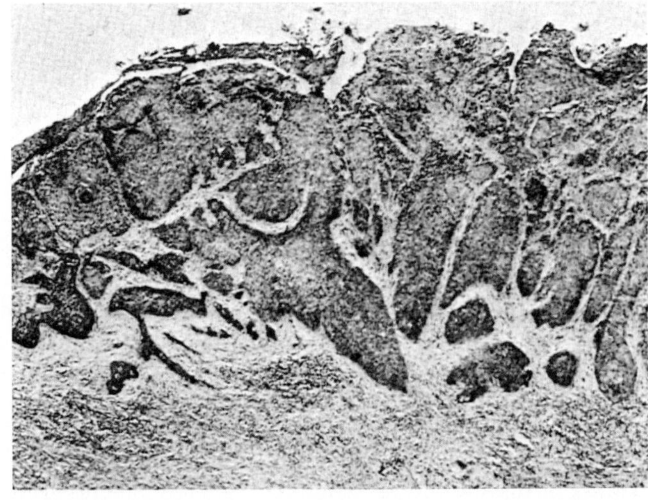
A

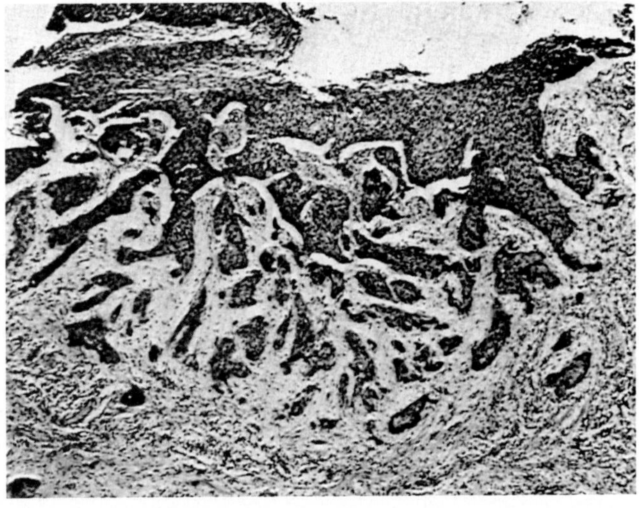
B

Figure 29-8. A, Tumor with only 0.5 mm of invasion. (×40.) **B,** Example of so-called spray pattern with multiple invasive nodules in stroma. Invasion is only 1 mm. (×50.) (From Creasman WT, Fetter BF, Clarke-Pearson DL, et al: Management of stage IA carcinoma of the cervix. Am J Obstet Gynecol 153:164, 1985.)

were treated with hysterectomy and 166 with more radical therapy. Two patients had node metastases, and four died. The poor outcome occurred primarily in those with vascular space involvement. Kolstad recommends conservative therapy if the margins of the cone are clearly negative and there is no lymphatic or vascular space involvement.

The Society of Gynecologic Oncologists in 1974 described microinvasive carcinoma of the cervix as "a lesion in which the neoplastic epithelium invades the stroma in one or more places to a depth of 3 mm or less below the basement membrane of the epithelium and in which lymphatic or vascular involvement is not demonstrated." Currently available studies indicate that almost all lesions meeting the latter definition will not have spread beyond the cervix, but the definition, although widely used, does not provide sufficient precision for many clinical situations. As pointed out by Burghardt and colleagues, these 0- to 3-mm cases include very early cases of early stromal invasion. For these tumors, a small band of eosinophilic neoplastic tissue invades overlying carcinoma in situ (Fig. 29-9). These cases are virtually 100% curable, and if they are removed from the analysis of the 0- to 3-mm invasive category, the stages IA1 and IA2 appear to have a similar prognosis (see therapy discussion later).

A further refinement has been reported by investigators from Western Europe, who used a meticulous and time-consuming three-dimensional microscopic study to calculate the *volume* of neoplastic tissue. Using a 50-mm^2 two-dimensional criterion, Lohe and associates reported no positive nodes in 134 cases studied in numerous centers in Western Europe. This two-dimensional definition has the advantage of considering both the depth of invasion and the width of tumor and provides a general guide that is used by many pathologists for determination of microinvasive disease. The current stage IA1 definition allows for an area of 21 mm^2 and 35 mm^2 for IA2.

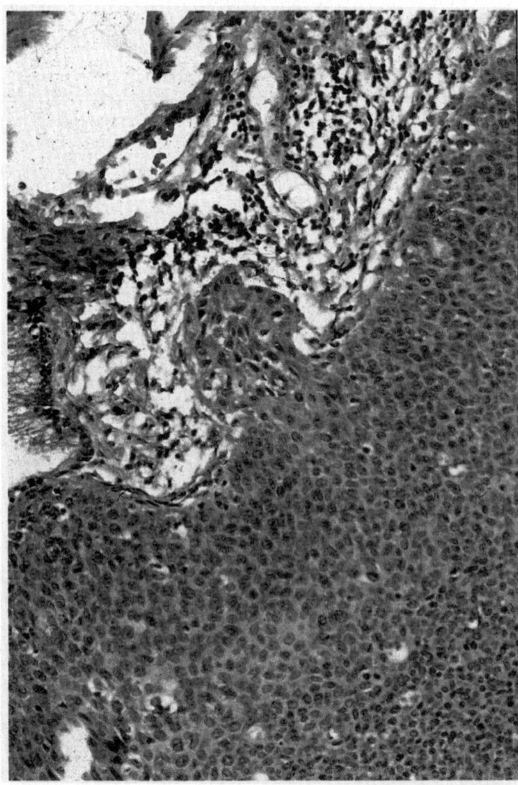

Figure 29-9. Photomicrograph showing early stromal invasion. (Courtesy of Anthony Montag, MD, Department of Pathology, The University of Chicago.)

These area measurements provide the general guidelines, but there are other factors to consider when undertaking conservative treatment for suspected microinvasive tumors. First, the diagnosis of microinvasive tumor cannot be made based on a biopsy specimen alone and a cervical conization must be performed. Second, if the margin of the cervical cone specimen contains neoplastic epithelium, the risk of invasive tumor in the remaining uterus is increased. Third, endocervical tumors have an increased risk of being associated with invasion, and this may occur when the exocervix is covered with normal squamous epithelium. Östor and Rome evaluated 200 patients from Australia with microinvasive tumors, 91 of which invaded less than 5 mm and were less than 7 mm in width. Four of the latter recurred in the vagina, and one patient has died. Twenty-three patients had conization as the sole treatment. None of these have recurred, but none had more than 3 mm of invasion. Morris and coworkers studied 14 patients treated by conization and followed for a mean of 26.5 months. All had lesions with less than 3 mm of invasion without capillary-lymphatic space involvement. One patient had a hysterectomy that showed mild dysplasia in the specimen. The remaining 13 were free of disease at the time of the report. A study of 51 patients with 3 to 5 mm invasion by Creasman and colleagues indicated that if the tumor had these dimensions, subsequent radical hysterectomy and node dissection showed no cases of lymph node metastases. Impressively, no patients died of cancer at 5 years and none recurred despite the fact that one fourth of the cases showed vascular invasion. Thus, truly negative margins that existed in these cases are an excellent prognostic sign despite the fact that these cases belong to stage IA2.

In considering the therapy of microinvasive carcinoma of the cervix, the clinician must weigh the risk that an invasive lesion may be mistakenly treated by conservative means. If an early invasive carcinoma is present, it can usually be successfully treated by means of a radical or modified radical hysterectomy (see later discussion). The risk of death or serious morbidity from such operation is probably approximately 1%, and the risk of error or misdiagnosis of a lesion should be comparably small.

At present, a patient suspected of having microinvasive carcinoma of the cervix should first have conization of the cervix. If the lesion is less than 21 to 35 mm^2, the patient can often be treated by conservative means, which is usually a simple hysterectomy, particularly if invasion from the basement membrane is less than 3 mm. If the lesion is less than 21 mm^2 and there is only infrequent capillary-like space involvement, such conservative treatment is usually adequate. Conization may be used as sole therapy in carefully selected cases in which the cone margins are free of tumor and accurate measurements of the tumor dimensions are available. The presence of capillary-like space involvement does not preclude conservative therapy, but the risk of invasive disease or future recurrence increases with capillary-like space involvement and larger lesions. Conservative therapy should not be attempted if the conization margins are involved with neoplasia. It is usually wise to do an endocervical curettage after the conization to be sure neoplastic epithelium is not higher in the canal. All patients must be followed with periodic physical and cytologic (Pap smear) examinations because recurrences may develop late and have been noted more than 15 years after primary therapy. The 5-year survival rate following appropriately chosen therapy of microinvasive carcinoma of the cervix should approach 100%.

CARCINOMA OF THE CERVIX

Clinical Considerations

Patients with carcinoma of the cervix characteristically present with abnormal bleeding or brownish discharge, frequently noted following douching or intercourse and also occurring spontaneously between menstrual periods. The patients often have a history of not having had a cytologic (Pap) smear for many years. Other symptoms, such as back pain, loss of appetite, and weight loss, are late manifestations and occur when there is extensive spread of cervical carcinoma. The patients tend to be in their 40s to 60s, with a median age of 52 years noted worldwide by Pecorelli and associates. Preinvasive intraepithelial carcinoma of the cervix (see Chapter 28, Intraepithelial Neoplasia of the Lower Genital Tract [Cervix, Vulva]) occurs primarily in women in their 20s and 30s and has become more common among those in their 20s, leading to a gradual increase in the incidence of invasive carcinoma in younger patients.

The diagnosis is established by biopsy of the tumor; a specimen can be easily obtained at office examination. A Kevorkian, Eppendorf, Tishler, or similar punch biopsy instrument is convenient to use. Occasionally it is necessary to biopsy nodularity or induration in the vagina near the cervix to ascertain the limit of tumor spread and to define a correct tumor stage. If the patient's cytologic smear is suggestive of invasive carcinoma with no gross lesion visible and endocervical curettage does not demonstrate carcinoma or if an adequate biopsy specimen to establish carcinoma cannot be obtained, then cervical conization should be performed.

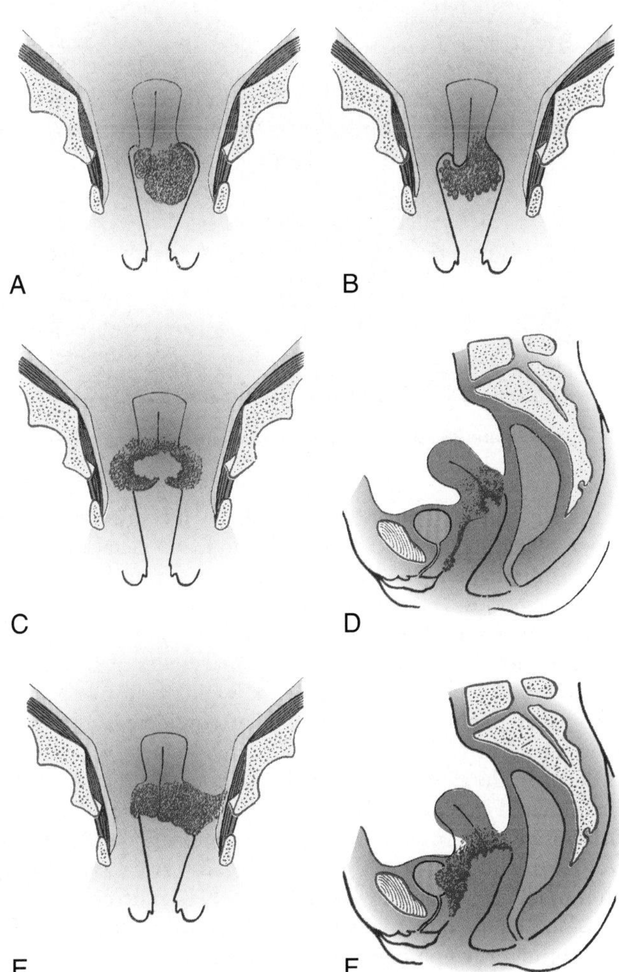

Figure 29-10. Staging of cervical carcinoma. **A,** Stage IB: nodular cervix. **B,** Stage IIA: carcinoma extending into left vault. **C,** Stage IIB: parametrium involved on both sides, but carcinoma has not invaded pelvic wall; endocervical crater. **D,** Stage IIIA: submucosal involvement of anterior vaginal wall and small, papillomatous nodule in its lower third. **E,** Stage IIIB: parametrium involved on both sides; at left, carcinoma has invaded pelvic wall. **F,** Stage IVA: involvement of bladder. (From Pettersson F, Bjorkholm E: Staging and reporting of cervical carcinoma. Semin Oncol 9:289, 1982.)

Staging

The staging of carcinoma of the cervix depends primarily on the pelvic examination, and the designation may be modified by general physical examination, by chest radiographic examination, by intravenous pyelography (IVP), or computed tomography (CT) and is not changed based on operative findings. Table 29-1 shows the definition of the four stages of cervical carcinoma according to FIGO (revised in 1994), and the various types of tumor distribution that may be observed in the various stages are illustrated in Figure 29-10.

Natural History and Spread

Carcinoma of the cervix is initially a locally infiltrating cancer that spreads from the cervix to the vagina and paracervical and parametrial areas. Grossly, the tumors may be ulcerated (Fig. 29-11), similar to carcinomas occurring elsewhere in the female genital tract, and may have an exophytic growth pattern or cauliflower-like appearance extruding from the cervix, usually producing abnormal bleeding and staining. Alternatively, they may be endophytic, in which case they are asymptomatic, particularly in the early stage of development, and tend to be deeply invasive when diagnosed. These usually start initially from an endocervical location and often fill the cervix and lower uterine segment, resulting in a barrel-shaped cervix. The latter tumors tend to metastasize to regional pelvic nodes, and because of the tendency of late diagnosis, they are often more advanced than the exophytic variety. The primary path for distant spread is through lymphatics to the regional pelvic nodes. Blood-borne metastases from cervical carcinomas do occur, but they are less frequent and usually are seen late in the course of the disease.

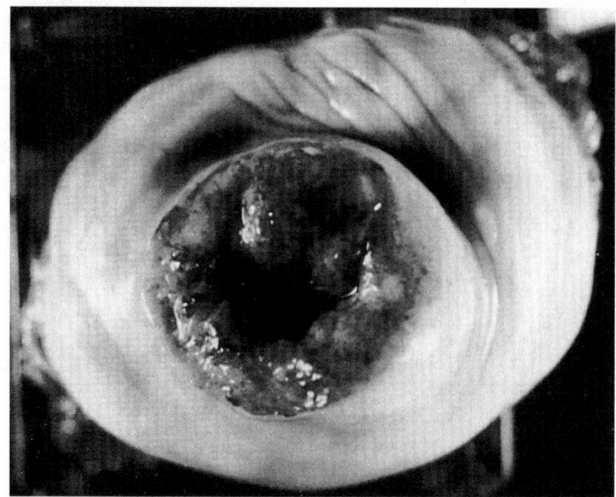

Figure 29-11. Carcinoma of cervix (gross specimen).

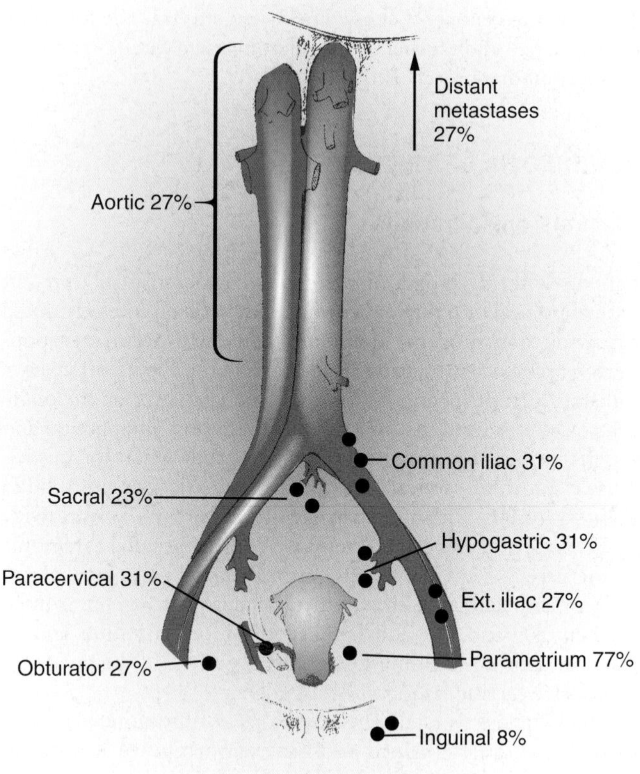

Figure 29-12. Frequency of lymph node metastases in cervical carcinoma. Incidence of node group involvement in 26 nontreated cases of cervical carcinoma. (From Henriksen E: The lymphatic spread of carcinoma of the cervix and of the body of the uterus. Am J Obstet Gynecol 58:924, 1949.)

Initially, cervical carcinoma spreads to the primary pelvic nodes, which include the pericervical node, presacralthe hypogastric (internal iliac) and external iliac nodes, and the nodes in the obturator fossa near the vessels and nerve. From this primary group, tumor spread proceeds secondarily to the common iliac and paraaortic nodes. Rarely the inguinal nodes are involved; however, if the lower one third of the vagina is involved, then the median inguinal nodes should be considered a primary node. The distribution of lymph node involvement was studied in detail in 26 cases of untreated carcinoma of the cervix by Henriksen (Fig. 29-12). A series studying the incidence and distribution pattern of retroperitoneal lymph node metastases in 208 patients with stage IB, IIA, and IIB cervical carcinomas who underwent radical hysterectomy and systemic pelvic node dissection reported that 53 patients (25%) had node metastasis. The obturator lymph nodes were the most frequently involved, with a rate of 19% (39 of 208), and the authors proposed them as sentinel nodes for cervical cancers. An important distal node that becomes involved after the paraaortic group is the left scalene node, that is, the left supraclavicular node. A clinical correlation is that biopsy of this node is frequently performed in the assessment of advanced cervical carcinoma to clarify whether the tumor has spread outside the abdomen. In addition to nodal spread, hematogenous spread of cervical carcinoma occurs primarily to the lung, liver, and, less frequently, bone (see "Recurrence").

Prognostic Factors

FIGO stage is the most important determinant of prognosis for carcinoma of the cervix (Table 29-2); however, there are other factors including tumor characteristics and patient characteristics that are prognostic and are not including in the FIGO staging system. One of the most important predictors is tumor size for both local recurrence and death for patients treated with either surgery or radiation therapy. In fact, the FIGO staging classification for stage I disease was recently modified to include tumor diameter (i.e., ≤4 cm, stage IB1; >4 cm, stage IB2). Another very important prognostic factor is involvement of lymph nodes, which also is not part of the clinical stage system. In several surgical series, after a radical hysterectomy, patients with positive pelvic lymph nodes had a 35% to 40% lower 5-year survival rate than patients with negative nodes. Patients with positive paraaortic nodes have a survival rate that is approximately half that of patients with similar-stage disease and negative paraaortic nodes. With extended-field radiation

Table 29-2 Carcinoma of the Uterine Cervix: Distribution by Stage and 5-Year Survival Rates for Patients Treated in 1990–1992 (N = 11,945)

Stage	Patient (*n*)	5-Year Survival
Ia	902	95.01%
Ib	4657	80.1%
II	3364	64.2%
III	2530	38.31%
IV	492	14%

Modified from Pecorelli S, Creasman WT, Pettersson F, et al: FIGO annual report on the results of treatment in gynaecological cancer, Vol. 23. Milan, Italy, International Federation of Gynecology and Obstetrics. J Epidemiol Biostat 3, 1998.

therapy, patients with positive paraaortic nodes have approximately a 40% to 50% 5-year survival rate. There is a strong correlation between positive nodes and positive lymph-vascular space invasion (LVSI) in the tumor specimen in patients with cervical carcinoma. However, LVSI may be an independent predictor of prognosis as shown in a number of larger surgical series.

In patients who have had a radical hysterectomy, histologic evidence of extracervical spread (≥10 mm), deep stromal invasion (>70% invasion), and LVSI are associated with a poorer prognosis. In fact, a randomized trial from the Gynecologic Oncology Group (GOG) compared observation versus adjuvant radiation therapy in patients after radical hysterectomy with combination of two of the factors mentioned previously, and patients who received radiation therapy had a better local control as well as improved overall survival. Involvement of the parametrium in the hysterectomy specimen has been correlated with higher rates of lymph node involvement, local recurrence, and death from cancer. Uterine body involvement is associated with an increased rate of distant metastases in patients treated with radiation or surgery.

Patients with adenocarcinomas of the cervix have a poorer prognosis than patients with squamous cell carcinomas of the cervix. Investigators have found among patients treated surgically, patients with adenocarcinomas had high relapse rates compared with rates in patients with squamous cell carcinomas. In an analysis of 1767 patients treated with radiation for FIGO stage IB disease, Eifel and colleagues found that independent of age, tumor size, and tumor morphology, patients with adenocarcinomas had the same pelvic control rate but twice as high a rate of distant metastasis as patients with squamous cell carcinomas of the cervix. Although the prognostic significance of histologic grade for squamous carcinomas has been disputed, there is a clear correlation between the degree of differentiation and clinical behavior of adenocarcinomas.

Recently, there has been a great interest in molecular markers regarding prognosis and treatment in carcinoma of the cervix. The most studied marker to date is the serum squamous cell carcinoma antigen. Studies have shown that pretreatment levels of this antigen correlate well with stage of disease, tumor histology, grade, type of tumor (exophytic versus infiltrative), microscopic depth of invasion, and risk of lymph node metastases in patients with early-stage disease. However, the most important properties of this antigen may be its ability to predict clinical outcome as well as a marker for monitoring the course of disease and response to treatment in patients with cervical cancer. Several investigators have reported significantly lower survival rates in patients with very elevated values compared with patients with normal baseline levels, independent of stage. For detection of tumor recurrence, serial squamous cell carcinoma antigen testing has been proven to be more specific than sensitive, with specificities ranging from 90% to 100% and sensitivities ranging from 60% to 90%. Further investigation is need in these areas. Some investigators have a higher rate of recurrence in patients with HPV-positive nodes (although negative for malignancies) and poor prognosis with presence of HPV mRNA in the peripheral blood of cervical cancer patients. Other markers under investigation include epidermal growth factor receptor, cyclooxygenase-2, DNA ploidy, tumor vascularity, and S-phase fraction.

MANAGEMENT

Pretherapy Evaluation

Once the patient has been diagnosed as having an invasive carcinoma, pretreatment evaluation is conducted to determine the extent of disease, to arrive at an accurate clinical staging, and to plan the program of therapy. The usual evaluation consists of a thorough history and physical examination, routine blood studies, an intravenous pyelogram or a CT scan, and chest radiograph. Demonstration of an obstructed ureter or nonfunctioning kidney caused by tumor automatically assigns the case at least to stage III (see Table 29-1). A barium enema test or flexible sigmoidoscopy as well as a cystoscopy is sometimes performed, in the case of large tumors, or for those who will be receiving radiation treatment.

The CT and magnetic resonance imaging (MRI) is more expensive than IVP, but has the advantage of being able to provide greater information concerning tumor spread to lymph nodes, particularly in cases of higher stage disease. CT, MRI, and IVP provide approximately equivalent information for most cases of stages I and IIA, but CT or MRI allows detection of enlarged pelvic and paraaortic nodes that were suspicious for involvement of tumor. However, CT is not particularly useful to detect the parametrial extent of cervical carcinoma, which is evaluated more reliably by pelvic examination. MRI has also been used to evaluate local spread, but the test is not used routinely. The suggestion of tumor in retroperitoneal nodes by CT does not affect stage, which relies primarily on clinical examination and the status of the ureters.

The best radiographic imaging technique for detecting lymph node metastases is unclear. CT and MRI are good for identifying enlarged nodes; however, the accuracy of these techniques in the detection of positive nodes is compromised by their failure to detect small metastases, and many enlarged nodes are due not to metastases but to inflammation associated with advanced disease. The accuracy of MRI in the detection of lymph node metastases (72% to 93%) is similar to that of CT, but is better than CT and physical examination in the evaluation of tumor location, tumor size, depth of stromal invasion, vaginal extension, and parametrial extension of cervical cancer. However, with regard to detecting lymph node metastases or other distant disease, positron emission tomography (PET) shows promise. Several studies from a single institution show the fluorodeoxyglucose PET detects abnormal lymph nodes more often than does CT and that the findings on PET are a better predictor of survival than are those on CT or MRI in patients with carcinoma of the cervix. Multiinstitutional studies are needed to confirm the superiority of PET scans.

Low-Stage (IB–IIA) Disease

Radical hysterectomy and radiation therapy are equally effective as treatments for low-stage disease, and comparable survival statistics have been reported for stage IB and early stage IIA (i.e., minimal spread to the vagina). Numerous studies have been conducted to try to ascertain which tumors will respond preferentially either to radiation or to surgery, but no reliable method of predicting which modality is optimal for a given tumor has been developed. Five-year survival rates from some centers of approximately 80% to 90% have been reported for stage IB and 70% to 80% for stage IIA with either radiation or radical hysterectomy; these statistics are somewhat better than most recently published, collated worldwide percentages (see Table 29-2).

Both modalities have advantages and disadvantages. Surgery allows preservation of ovarian function and completion of therapy in one hospitalization and causes less vaginal radiation fibrosis and compromise of sexual function. It also permits a thorough exploration of the abdomen. Chambers and colleagues reported on 38 patients whose ovaries were transposed laterally and superiorly. This procedure often preserves ovarian function in patients who are subsequently radiated, but ovarian cyst development can be a troublesome postoperative problem. The best results are obtained when operation is performed on small tumors, particularly those that are exophytic. Short-term complications such as infection, thromboembolic disease, and rarely fistula formation may occur, but there are few long-term complications (see later discussion). Short-term serious complications will occur in 1% to 2% of cases. Patients selected for radical hysterectomy are usually younger and in general in better health and thus are better able to tolerate a major surgical procedure. Patients who have had salpingitis or inflammatory bowel disease or who have unexplained pelvic masses are also treated by surgery because of the increased risk of complications with radiation. Radiation therapy is also effective to treat low-stage carcinomas of the cervix. Attempts have been made to combine full radiation treatment with radical hysterectomy, but this leads to frequent severe complications, including lack of healing and fistula formation.

Operative Therapy: Radical Hysterectomy, Pelvic Node Dissection

Radical hysterectomy and bilateral pelvic lymphadenectomy are effective for treatment of many stage IB and some early stage IIA cancers. It is important that the operation remove the same volume of tissues that receive cancerocidal doses of radiation in cases for which radiation is the sole therapy. The amount of tissue removed, particularly in the paracervical and parametrial areas near the ureter, depends on the extent and location of the tumor. Piver and colleagues defined five classes to describe the extent of the operation. Class I guarantees the removal of the entire cervix and uterus. The ureter is not disturbed from its bed. In many instances, this is described as an extrafascial hysterectomy, the type used after preoperative radiation for treatment of a barrel-shaped cervix (see later discussion). A class II operation (Fig. 29-13) removes more paracervical tissue than class I, but the ureters are retracted laterally yet are not dissected from their attachments distal to the uterine artery, and the uterosacral ligaments are ligated approximately halfway between the uterus and rectum. The operation is usually performed with pelvic lymphadenectomy and is often termed a *modified radical hysterectomy.* The operation is useful to treat small microscopic carcinomas of the cervix. Magrina and colleagues used modified radical hysterectomy primarily for tumors smaller than 2 cm (median 1.1 cm) with 5-year survival of 96%. This procedure may occasionally be used to treat small, central cervical recurrences of carcinoma that are diagnosed following radiation therapy of the primary tumor. For a class III operation, the uterine artery is ligated at its origin from the anterior division of the hypogastric artery, and the uterosacrals are ligated deep in the pelvis near the rectum (see Figure 29-12). This operation

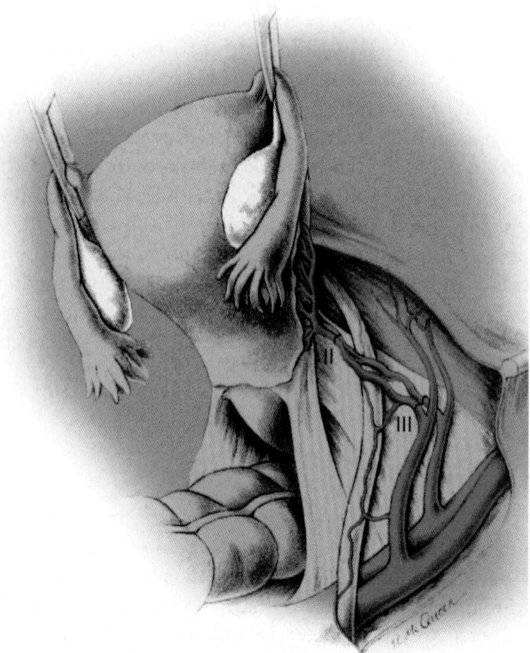

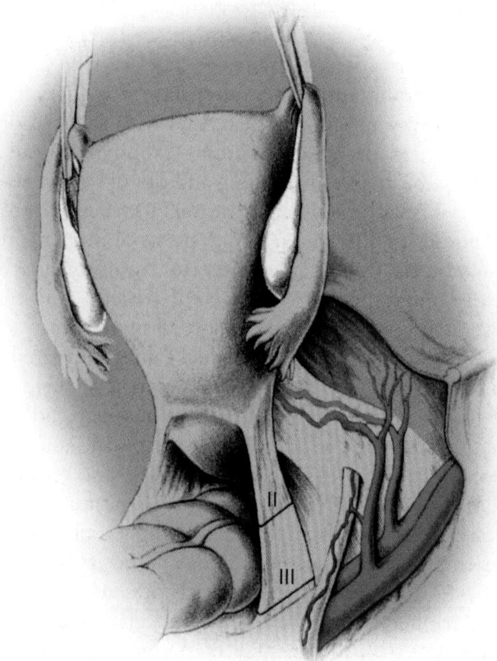

Figure 29-13. Class I and II radical hysterectomy with points of dissection shown (see text).

is usually termed a *radical hysterectomy* (Meigs-Wertheim hysterectomy) and is performed for stage IB and rarely for stage IIA carcinomas of the cervix.

Class IV and V operations are infrequently performed. The former involves a complete dissection of the ureter from its bed and sacrifice of the superior vesical artery. A class V operation involves resection of the distal ureter or bladder or both with reimplantation of the ureter into the bladder (ureteroneocystotomy). Both operations are designed to remove small, central recurrent disease and would be attempted to avoid an anterior exenteration (see following discussion). Extensive data are not available, but the latter two procedures appear to have high complication rates.

Preoperative preparation for a patient who is to undergo radical hysterectomy includes the same basic considerations for anyone undergoing a major operative procedure. Graduated-compression, below-the-knee leg stockings are used to reduce the risk of thromboembolism. Prophylactic antibiotics are also frequently prescribed (see Chapter 24). During the course of the operation, care is taken not to grasp the ureters with instruments such as forceps to avoid damaging the periureteral capillary blood supply.

An important complication of pelvic lymphadenectomy is lymphocyst formation. Most gynecologic oncologists have abandoned the use of closed suction drains in radical hysterectomy patients and leave the pelvic peritoneum open to allow lymph fluid to drain internally in the peritoneal cavity.

Ovarian function may be preserved in younger patients if there is little likelihood of postoperative radiation. If intraoperative findings suggest that radiotherapy will be given postoperatively, the ovaries may be transposed superior and lateral to preserve their function. This technique has some liabilities including early loss of ovarian function and abdominal pain from ovarian cysts.

In stage I cases treated by radical hysterectomy and node dissection, the results obtained are related primarily to the status of the pelvic nodes, as well as the surgical resection margins around the primary tumor (ideally more than 1 cm). If the pelvic nodes are free of tumor, the 5-year survival rate can be expected to exceed 90%, whereas if the nodes are found to contain tumor, the 5-year survival rate drops to 45%–50%. Lerner and coworkers reported a 5-year survival rate (life table technique) of 93.4% for 108 patients using class III hysterectomy for stage IB carcinomas of the cervix. All but five of these tumors were less than 5 cm in diameter. Six patients experienced prolonged bladder dysfunction after operation. Only one postoperative ureterovaginal fistula developed, and there were no postoperative deaths, indicating that excellent results can be obtained with surgery, particularly if the patients are carefully selected. If the patient is found to have extensive spread of gross disease to pelvic nodes, the studies of Potter and coworkers suggest that it is preferable to cease the operation and complete radiation therapy to improve pelvic control of tumor. However, Hacker and associates reported an estimated 5-year survival of 80% for 34 patients whose tumor-positive pelvic or paraaortic nodes were resected and the areas subsequently radiated. In a recent GOG study, Sedlis and coworkers evaluated disease-free survival for patients treated with radical hysterectomy who have negative lymph nodes and surgical margins but with intermediate risk factors including more than one third stromal invasion, capillary lymphatic space involvement, adenocarcinoma, and large tumor diameter by randomizing patients to pelvic radiotherapy or observation. Survival was improved in those who received postoperative pelvic radiation; however, there were radiation complications including bowel obstruction and death.

Numerous studies have been published evaluating low-dose preoperative radiation followed by radical hysterectomy and pelvic node dissection. The technique has been particularly widely used in Western Europe, and Einhorn and colleagues evaluated the Swedish experience comparing complete treatment with full radiation therapy alone or preoperative partial radiation (two intracavitary radiums) and radical hysterectomy for patients under age 41 with stage IB or IIA carcinoma of the cervix. A significant ($P < 0.004$) improvement was noted in stage IB for the combined-therapy group as compared with radiation alone (5-year survival rate: 96% versus 81%). No significant difference was noted in stage IIA. Calais and associates used combined therapy for tumors less than 4 cm in diameter in 70 patients and reported a 10-year survival of 96%, an excellent result. However, definitive trials have not proven the superiority of this technique.

Fertility-Sparing Surgery for Patients with Cervical Cancer. Until recently, stage Ib cervical cancer was considered incompatible with fertility preservation; however, this assumption has been proven incorrect. Radical trachelectomy, either vaginal or abdominal, can be performed with adequate safety and with acceptable pregnancy rates. In the 1980s, Dr. Daniel Dargent developed a combined laparoscopic and vaginal approach for patients with 2 cm or smaller stage Ib1 cervical cancers. The pelvic lymphadenectomy was performed laparoscopically and then a radical vaginal trachelectomy was performed. Plante and colleagues have reported more than 300 cases treated with this approach with a relapse rate of less than 10% and less than 5% mortality due to cancer. Approximately one third of patients can be expected to conceive and almost three fourths of them will carry the fetus more than 37 weeks.

The vaginal approach is difficult for most gynecologic oncologists in North America to master because most are not trained in radical vaginal surgery during fellowship and many do not have the required laparoscopy skills. Recently, abdominal radical trachelectomy is being performed with increasing frequency. There are no series with long-term results available at present; however, results similar to those of radical vaginal trachelectomy are anticipated.

Laparoscopic Surgery for Cervical Cancer. Laparoscopic approaches to the surgical management of cervical cancer are very attractive for several reasons. First, the tumor itself can be removed through the vagina, avoiding the need for an abdominal incision to remove the tumor. The pelvic and paraortic lymph nodes can be removed through laparoscopic ports. Most laparoscopists will not attempt to remove grossly involved lymph nodes through laparoscopic ports due to concern about port site metastases as described by Ramirez and associates. Noninvasive imaging should be performed before surgery to try to exclude patients with gross adenopathy from laparoscopic procedures.

According to a report by Occelli and colleagues, laparoscopy is associated with a reduction of surgical adhesions, especially to the anterior abdominal wall and lymphadenectomy sites compared with laparotomy. Laparoscopy is also associated with less postoperative pain and shorter length of hospital stay.

These factors make this approach especially attractive for surgical staging of patients with advanced cervical cancer who are not candidates for radical hysterectomy. Vasilev and associates, Sonoda and associates, and Schaerth and associates have described a laparoscopic retroperitoneal lymphadenectomy with high success rates when performing a complete lymphadenectomy from the common iliac vessels to the renal vessels, keeping the dissection out of the pelvic radiation field.

Diffusion of innovative laparoscopic approaches is slowed by the lack of laparoscopic surgical skills among many practicing gynecologic oncologists, a relatively slow learning curve, and the decreasing numbers of cases in North America owing to the success of screening and detection programs. The introduction of HPV vaccines will likely continue to reduce the numbers of invasive cervix cancer patients immunized populations. Fortunately, advanced laparoscopic surgery is being taught in most fellowship training programs and improvements in training with simulators should shorten the learning curve for gynecologic oncologist.

Sentinel Lymph Nodes. Sentinel lymph node biopsy has been incorporated into the standard management of several solid tumors, notably breast cancer and cutaneous melanoma. This technique identifies the first site of nodal metastases in a regional lymph node basin. Levenback and coworkers showed that, if the sentinel node is free of disease, the chance that the remaining regional lymph nodes are also disease free is over 95%. In breast and melanoma patients, regional lymphadenectomy is not performed in sentinel-lymph-node-negative patients. This technique has been applied to many other disease sites including cervical cancer by Levenback and colleagues (2002) and Plante and colleagues (2003). Sentinel lymph node biopsy can be performed laparoscopically, an especially attractive feature, allowing it to be combined with laparoscopic radical hysterectomy. Pelvic lymphadenectomy remains the standard for patients with cervical cancer; however, use of sentinel lymph node biopsy will likely increase.

Complications

Following radical hysterectomy, many patients experience long-term complications. Montz and colleagues noted a 5% frequency of small bowel obstruction, which increased to 20% if radiation was used postoperatively. Fistulas from the urinary tract, particularly ureterovaginal fistulas, have been reported to occur in approximately 1% of cases. The low rate appears to result from administration of antibiotics, the prevention of retroperitoneal serosanguineous collections, and avoidance of direct manipulation of the ureter to avoid injury to the periureteral blood supply. Some therapists do not reperitonealize the pelvis, which causes drainage directly to the peritoneal cavity, in which case, suction catheters are not usually used.

Many patients suffer postoperative bladder dysfunction. In part, this appears to be due to disruption of the sympathetic nerve supply to the bladder. However, the dysfunction may be temporary. Low and associates noted an increase in bladder pressure with a decrease in urethral pressure following radical hysterectomy. There was reduced bladder compliance with detrusor instability. The bladder can develop hypotonicity, and overdistention can then become a problem. If overdistention of the bladder and infection are avoided, progressive improvement of bladder function usually occurs. Forney correlated the degree of bladder dysfunction after radical hysterectomy with the extent of resection of the cardinal ligament. Those who had a complete resection of cardinal ligaments could void satisfactorily in an average of 51 days compared with 20 days for those with only partial resection of the ligaments. All the patients experienced a decrease in bladder sensation. In a few patients, the decrease in bladder sensation can be permanent. For patients in whom it is temporary, recovery usually occurs after continuous drainage of the bladder with an indwelling catheter. Westby and Asmussen observed that by 1 year after surgery, a slight decrease in urethral pressure persists but that the decrease is not as great as that noted immediately after the operation. After 1 year, the postoperative changes and bladder function usually recover. In a 1999 study from Sweden, Bergmark and associates noted compromised sexual activity, decreased lubrication, and shortened vagina in women treated for cervical cancer both by surgery and/or radiation.

Outcomes after Surgical Treatment. Reported 5-year survival rates for women with stage IB cervical cancer treated with radical hysterectomy and pelvic lymphadenectomy are approximately 80% to 90%. Patients with positive or close margins or positive lymph nodes are at the highest risk of recurrence and poor outcome. In large prospective studies, 3-year disease-specific survival rates of 85.6% in patients with negative nodes and 50% to 74% in patients with positive nodes were reported. A recent randomized study showed that postoperative chemoradiation improved survival in patients with positive lymph nodes and positive surgical margins.

Radiation Treatment

The majority of patients with carcinoma of the cervix are treated by radiation. The principles of external megavoltage treatment (teletherapy) and local implants (brachytherapy) are reviewed in Chapter 26. External beam radiation is administered in fractions, usually 180 cGy/day 5 days per week to destroy the tumor without causing permanent damage to normal tissues. This delivers uniform doses to the entire pelvis, including the regional pelvic nodes. The local implant delivers its highest energy locally to the cervix and surface of the vagina and paravaginal and paracervical tissues. The radiation from the implant diminishes according to the inverse square law, and the uterus and cervix serve as a receptacle for arranging and holding the intracavitary applicator stem (tandem) and accompanying vaginal applicators (ovoids) in a fixed and optimal position for delivering the desired radiation dosimetry (Fletcher-Suit applicator, see Fig. 29-14). Current low-dose rate treatment delivers approximately 40 cGy/hr to point A with shielding in the ovoids both anteriorly and posteriorly to protect the bladder and rectum. The tandem and ovoids are inserted with the patient anesthetized, and a pack is placed in the vagina to stabilize the apparatus and increase the distance from the mucosa of the bladder and rectum. After the position of the applicator has been confirmed to be satisfactory by radiographs, the radioactive sources, such as cesium 137, are inserted (afterloading technique). Other types of applicators are available, but the principle of delivering intense radiation to the cervix and paracervical areas is the same. The goal is to increase the total dose of radiation to the maximum allowable to achieve tumor control without introducing a major risk of complications and injury to adjacent normal tissue. The specific protocols followed in various treatment centers differ, and individualization for specific patients is often needed depending on the stage and size of the cervical tumor as well as the patient's local anatomy. In general, external therapy is given first both to treat the regional pelvic nodes and to shrink the central tumor mass, which then is more amenable for a local implant. In some patients, external therapy can lead to excessive shrinkage of the vaginal apex, making safe, effective implantation of local radiation sources difficult. This can be a problem, particularly in older or postmenopausal patients. Occasionally in those patients, the implant is done first, especially for smaller stage I tumors. Rotmensch and associates also used intraoperative ultrasonography to provide optimal implant positioning in these difficult patients. In some instances, the central pelvis is shielded during external radiation therapy to allow for subsequent higher doses from the implant. Occasionally, interstitial therapy in the form of needles implanted into the area of the tumor is needed to achieve effective local tumor control. Recently, high-dose rate brachytherapy given on an outpatient basis has been introduced. Multiple randomized and nonrandomized studies have suggested that survival rates and complications rates with high-dose rate brachytherapy are similar to those with traditional low-dose rate treatment. At least two studies from the United States have shown similar results with high- and low-dose rate treatment in early-stage disease; however, in stage IIIB disease, the survival rate was lower with high-dose rate than with low-dose rate therapy. In calculating the doses of radiation, two reference points, A and B, are used (Fig. 29-14). Point A is 2 cm above the external os and 2 cm lateral to the cervical canal. Point B is 5 cm lateral to the cervical canal and 3 cm lateral to point A, which places point B in the vicinity of the lateral pelvic wall. The total dose administered depends on tumor stage, but, in general, at the pelvic wall, it is in the range of 50 to 65 Gy, with the higher doses used for high-stage disease. At point A, it varies but approximately 80 Gy is given for small IB1 lesions, and doses higher than 85 Gy for larger lesions. The normal cervix is particularly resistant to radiation and can tolerate doses as high as 200 to 250 Gy over 2 months, whereas the adjacent bladder and in particular the rectum are much more sensitive, and their exposure in general should be limited at the point of maximal radiation to 80 Gy to the bladder and 70 Gy to the rectum, with overall average doses in the range of 65 to 70 Gy. The small bowel can be damaged at doses above 45 to 50 Gy, especially if adhesions limit intestinal mobility and a large volume is treated.

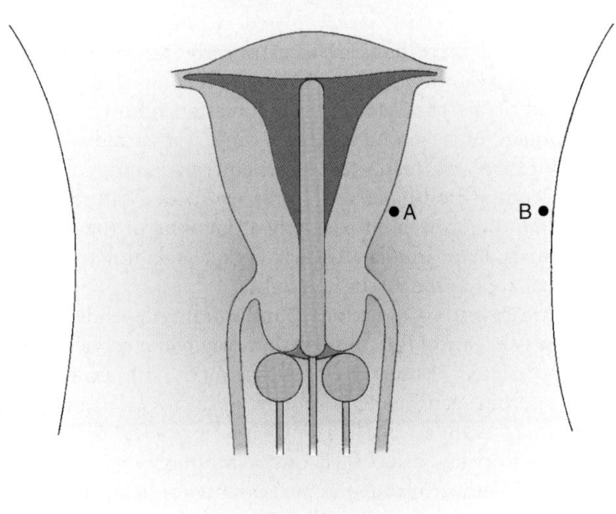

Figure 29-14. Points *A* and *B* with central stem (tandem) and two ovoids in place.

The sum of external radiation therapy (Gy/10) plus the implant dose (mg hr/1000) equals approximately 10. At many treatment centers, this sum varies from 9.0 to 10.0, and, in general, as the sum increases, the risk of complications from radiation therapy increases (see following discussion). In addition, as the volume of tissue that receives high doses of radiation increases, the risk of complications also increases. Therapeutic results with radiation therapy in the past have been generally similar to those with surgery for low-stage disease, and representative values are shown in Table 29-2.

Outcomes. Radical radiation therapy achieves excellent survival and pelvic disease control rates in patients with stage IB–IIA cervical cancer. Eifel and colleagues reported 5-year disease-specific survival of 90%, 86%, and 67% in patients with stage IB tumors with cervical diameters of less than 4 cm, 4.0 to 4.9 cm, and greater than 5 cm, respectively. In 1961, there was report that suggested that adjuvant hysterectomy improved local control in patients with stage IB disease with tumors greater than 6 cm; however, several studies since then have shown no improvement in local control but an increase in toxicity. One of these studies is a large GOG study in which patients were randomized to a trial of radiation with or without extrafascial hysterectomy, and preliminary results showed no difference in survival or local control, but a higher complication rate. Mendenhall and colleagues reported an 18% rate of major complication at 6 years for patients who underwent adjuvant hysterectomy, compared with 7% for patients who received radiation therapy alone. Therefore, there is no clear evidence that adjuvant hysterectomy improves outcome in patients with early stage disease and large tumor size. The 5-year survival for patients with IIA disease is very similar to that of IB disease. For patients with more advanced disease, 5-year survival rates of 65% to 75%, 35% to 50%, and 15% to 20% have been reported for stage IIB, IIIB, and IV tumors, respectively. The addition of chemotherapy has further improved local control and survival for stage IB2 and higher and is discussed in the next section.

CHEMORADIATION

In 1999, prospective randomized trials involving concurrent cisplatin-containing chemotherapy to standard radiotherapy have shown such improved survival that the trials were preliminarily halted in order to release the results, which changed clinical practice.

Rose and colleagues treated patients with advanced squamous cell, adenosquamous, or adenocarcinoma of the cervix (stages IIB, III, and/or IVA) in a recent GOG study. The patients received external radiation therapy (40.8 to 51.0 Gy) followed by one or two brachytherapy implants. Total doses to point B were 55 Gy for stage IIB cases and 60 Gy for stages III and IVA. The patients were randomized to receive one of three concomitant chemotherapy regimens (hydroxyurea; cisplatin, 5-fluorouracil, and hydroxyurea; or cisplatin alone). The best results were obtained with the cisplatin-containing regimens with the least complications that with weekly cisplatin (40 mg/m^2) alone. Progression-free survival at 24 months was an impressive 67% for this very high-risk group of patients.

In a further collaborative trial, Keys and associates studied 369 women with bulky stage Ib carcinoma (>4 cm) in diameter. They were randomized to receive radiation alone or with concomitant weekly cisplatin (40 mg/m^2). Total dose to point B was 55 Gy. Patients with radiographic evidence of hydronephrosis or lymphadenopathy were excluded. Adjuvant extrafascial hysterectomy was performed in 3 to 6 weeks after conclusion of the chemoradiation treatments. Acute severe toxicity, especially hematologic but also GI, was noted. However, the therapeutic results were markedly better in the chemoradiation group with a 3-year 83% disease-free survival compared with 74% in the radiation group alone (P = .008). Recurrences and death were higher in the radiation-alone group.

At the same time, the Radiation Therapy Oncology Group also conducted a trial comparing paraaortic/pelvic radiation therapy to concurrent chemotherapy and pelvic radiation in patients with stage IB–IVA tumors and also found a significant improvement in outcome for all stage disease with concurrent chemotherapy compared with radiation therapy alone. Another trial looked at concurrent chemotherapy with radiation therapy in patients who had a radical hysterectomy for cervical cancer and were found to have pelvic lymph node metastases, positive margins, or parametrial involvement. In this trial, patients who received chemoradiation had a better disease-free survival rate than patients who received radiation therapy alone.

Only one large randomized trial has failed to demonstrate a significant advantage from concurrent cisplatin-based chemotherapy in cervical cancer patients. This trial was done in Canada and was the smallest of six trials looking at concurrent cisplatin and radiation therapy. Taken together, the randomized trials provide strong evidence that the addition of concurrent cisplatin-containing chemotherapy to pelvic radiotherapy benefits patients with locally advanced cervical cancer as well as some select patients with early stage cervical cancer. In a recent meta-analysis of 18 trials with concurrent chemotherapy and radiation (4580 patients) in patients with cervical cancer, concomitant chemotherapy and radiotherapy improved overall and progression-free survival and reduced local and distant recurrence.

Paraaortic Nodes

Numerous small series of patients having documented paraaortic node involvement have demonstrated that some patients have a long-term disease-free survival duration. Patients having microscopic involvement have a better survival duration than those having gross involvement; however, even patients with gross involvement have a 15% to 20% survival rate with aggressive management. Laparoscopy and laparotomy using the extraperitoneal approach allow the removal of positive nodes and sampling of other paraaortic nodes, which may enhance control with radiation therapy and help design the treatment field.

Patients with paraaortic lymph node involvement can be treated effectively with extended-field radiation. The superior boundary of the extended field is usually placed at the T12 vertebra body to cover the paraaortic nodes. Patients are treated with a combination of external beam radiation therapy and brachytherapy. The 5-year survival rates range from 25% to 50%. One of these trials of biopsy-proven paraaortic node metastases, Varia and associates treated 96 patients with extended-field radiation and concomitant 5-fluorouracil and cisplatin weeks 1 and 5. The trial showed that chemoradiation was feasible in this group, and a progressive-free survival at 3 years of 33% was obtained. In a recent Radiation Therapy Oncology Group study, patients with positive paraaortic nodes were treated with concurrent weekly cisplatin and extended-field radiation therapy, and in the phase I part of the study, toxicity was high; the study currently is accruing to the phase II portion in which patients are also receiving aminofostine with the treatment to see whether it decreases the toxicity. At present, the standard treatment in most places for patients with positive paraaortic nodes is extended-field radiation therapy with concurrent weekly cisplatin.

Radiation Complications

Complications following radiation therapy are related to dose, volume treated, and sensitivity of the various tissues receiving radiation. The patient's habitus and presence of diseases that affect circulation, such as diabetes and high blood pressure, increase the risk, as does previous intraabdominal operation. Acute minor complications, such as diarrhea and nausea, subside after radiation therapy is completed. Complications usually arise in 1 to 2 years, but can occur as early as 6 months or as late as many years after radiation therapy is completed. Scarring of normal tissues can lead to severe radiation fibrosis. The rare development of a second primary cancer after radiation for cervical cancer was reported by Kleinerman and colleagues from 13 population-based European registries. With 30 years of survival, there was approximately a doubling of the risk of a new primary in an irradiated pelvic organ, including ovary and bladder, as well as the vagina and vulva.

The treatment of radiation complications depends on the symptoms and site of the complication. Vaginal or cervical ulcerations occasionally occur, and local treatment with topical antibiotics and estrogen creams is usually satisfactory. Postradiation cystitis may manifest itself as urinary frequency or dysuria. After infection has been ruled out, symptomatic treatment is undertaken with drugs such as antispasmodics or urinary analgesics (e.g., phenazopyridine [Pyridium], 100 mg three times daily), and these are prescribed until the symptoms clear. Occasionally hemorrhagic cystitis develops, and this may require hospitalization for continuous bladder irrigation or instillation of agents to control bleeding, such as silver nitrate or sometimes fulguration of the bleeding points. In cases of hematuria, recurrent tumor should first be ruled out. Periureteral fibrosis can lead to ureteral obstruction and loss of kidney function. McIntyre and coworkers studied 1784 patients with stage IB carcinomas who were treated by radiation therapy and found 29 cases of ureteral stenoses, which increased from a frequency of 1% at 5 years to 2.5% at 20 years. Although tumor recurrence was the most common cause of early ureteral obstruction, radiation fibrosis can be a rare but occasionally fatal late complication.

Bowel complications tend to be more frequent than urinary complications. Proctosigmoiditis can lead to diarrhea, severe pain on defecation, or GI bleeding. Conservative therapy with stool softeners and a low-roughage diet may suffice; occasionally, local corticosteroids (Cortisone enema) are of assistance. Fistulas or rectal ulcerations are occasionally seen in the area adjacent to the tip of the cervix, which is also the area maximally radiated during the local vaginocervical implant. If a fistula develops or in cases of ulceration or severe bleeding and pain, a diverting colostomy is required. Serious small bowel complications may occur, leading to obstruction, fistula formation, or necrosis. The use of parenteral nutrition and intravenous hyperalimentation has provided an excellent mechanism to help deal with these problems. Follow-up studies by Klee and coworkers show bladder and bowel symptoms tend to be chronic in some patients, but long-term fatigue was also reported. In most patients, it regressed in a few months.

The rate of complications also is related to the frequency of cure, especially for high-stage disease. Montana and Fowler noted a 19.5% complication rate in the therapy of 251 patients with stage II disease, and the risk of complications increased with radiation dose. For example, patients with complications had a mean dose of 7877 cGy to point A compared with 7593 cGy for those without complications. In a follow-up study, the risk of proctitis was also related to increasing doses of external beam treatment. The balancing of the risk of complication with increasing radiation dose to improve cure rates was further demonstrated by Orton and Wolf-Rosenblum, who studied patients with stages IIB and III carcinoma of the cervix. Higher doses had been used in women who survived 5 years, and their complication rate was 21% compared with only 6% for those who did not survive 5 years. Compromise of sexual function due to inelastic vagina and decreased utilization was noted in the studies of Bergmark and coworkers. In a randomized trial of experimental psychoeducational intervention involving regular vaginal dilation, Robinson and colleagues noted reduced fear of sexual activity post-treatment in the experimental group.

Cervical Stump Tumors

Some patients undergo supracervical hysterectomy for nonmalignant disease. Carcinomas that subsequently develop in the cervical stump pose special problems because of the shortness of the cervical canal and absence of the uterus, both of which curtail the effective use of brachytherapy, especially insertion of an intracervical tandem. There is also the risk that bowel adhesions to the apex of the vagina and cervix will increase the chances of radiation complications, and a pretherapy barium study of the small and large bowel may be helpful to identify loops that adhere to the cervical apex. For patients with small stage IB tumors, an operative approach similar to radical hysterectomy can be considered. However, most patients are treated with radiation. External treatment is emphasized because of the difficulty of an optimal intracavitary implant. A transvaginal cone may also be used to supplement external pelvic therapy. Effective treatment of cervical stump carcinoma can be achieved, and an overall 5-year survival rate of 45% in 173 patients was reported by Wolff and coworkers, and 60% for 70 patients was reported by Kovalic and associates Stage for stage, the survival rates are comparable to those achieved for invasive carcinoma of the cervix, but because of the previous supracervical hysterectomy, there is an increased risk of complications. Chemoradiation studies of these tumors are not currently available, but based on data already presented, radiation combined with weekly cisplatin appears to be optimal.

Carcinoma of the Cervix Inadvertently Removed at Simple Hysterectomy

Unfortunately, the situation occasionally arises in which a patient undergoes simple total hysterectomy and an invasive carcinoma of the cervix is found after operation. Patients with unsuspected invasive cervical carcinoma detected after simple hysterectomy have been classified in five groups according to the amount of disease and presentation: (1) microinvasive cancer, (2) tumor confined to the cervix with negative surgical margins, (3) positive surgical margins but no gross residual tumor, (4) gross residual tumor by clinical examination documented by biopsy, and (5) patients referred for treatment more than 6 months after hysterectomy (usually for recurrent disease). The treatment plan is based on the amount of residual disease. Sometimes the surgeon can subsequently perform a radical operation, removing the tissues that would normally be removed at radical hysterectomy, including the regional pelvic nodes. Such an approach has been used particularly in younger patients, particularly those with small tumors. A 5-year survival of 89% for 18 patients was reported by Chapman and colleagues. However, most of the time, the patient is treated with some sort of radiation therapy. Patients with minimal or no known residual disease at most require brachytherapy to the vaginal apex; patients with gross disease at the specimen margin require full-intensity therapy. Patients with minimal or no gross residual disease (groups 1 to 3) have excellent 5-year survival rates (59% to 79%), whereas rates for patients with gross residual disease (groups 4 and 5) are poorer (in the range of only 41%). Chemoradiation is unproven in this setting, but may have value, especially in patients with gross or recurrent disease.

Carcinoma of the Cervix in Pregnancy

Rarely, an invasive carcinoma of the cervix is discovered in a pregnant patient. Within each stage, survival statistics are similar in pregnant and nonpregnant women. A concern has been that the delivery of a fetus through a cervix replaced by carcinoma might worsen the prognosis due to tumor dissemination, but there is no clear evidence to indicate that tumor dissemination is caused by the birth process. However, tumor recurrence in episiotomy sites following vaginal delivery has been reported by

Cliby and associates. The major risk to the patient of delivery through a cervix containing invasive carcinoma is the risk of hemorrhage as a result of tearing of the tumor during cervical dilation and delivery.

A problem arising in pregnancy is whether a patient with an abnormal cytologic smear has intraepithelial neoplasia or invasive cancer. In general, if the cytologic and histologic findings of colposcopically directed biopsies are comparable and suggest intraepithelial neoplasia or carcinoma in situ, the patient is observed and delivered, with final evaluation and therapy completed approximately 6 weeks after delivery. Even if there is a question of microinvasion, a patient so diagnosed in the last trimester of pregnancy is usually followed and evaluated further after delivery. Cervical conization during pregnancy can lead to severe complications, particularly hemorrhage and also loss of the fetus. If it is necessary to perform a conization or preferably a wedge resection of the cervix during pregnancy, it is probably best to perform this during the second trimester, when the risks of fetal loss and hemorrhage are minimal. For patients in whom invasive cancer is diagnosed, a therapeutic plan must be developed to deliver appropriate care, with regard also for the outcome of the pregnancy.

The therapy of carcinoma during pregnancy is influenced by the stage of the disease, the time in pregnancy the cancer is diagnosed, and the beliefs and desires of the patient in terms of initiating therapy that can terminate the pregnancy as opposed to postponing the therapy until fetal viability is achieved. If carcinoma is diagnosed in the first trimester or early in the second trimester (before 20 weeks), treatment may be undertaken immediately because of the concern that a delay could lead to tumor progression or spread. However, Duggan and colleagues had delays of 2 to 7 months in eight pregnant patients with stage I disease and demonstrated no adverse effects from the delay. If the patient has resectable tumor (stage IB or early IIA), then effective treatment consists of radical hysterectomy and node dissection (class III). This procedure can usually be carried out without difficulty on a pregnant woman. Increased uterine motility and edema of the pelvic tissue planes help to simplify the procedure for the experienced surgeon, but pregnancy does increase the risk of blood loss. For higher stage tumors, therapy is begun with external beam radiation (teletherapy), and usually in 4 to 6 weeks, this leads to spontaneous abortion. The dose of external therapy prescribed varies depending on the stage of the tumor, but approximately 40 to 50 Gy is given. Although the results of a published series are not available, it would appear preferable to augment the radiation with weekly cisplatin because the pregnancy in this instance would be terminated. Following abortion, the uterus involutes, and an implant (brachytherapy) is placed. If the pregnancy does not spontaneously abort, dilation and curettage, prostaglandin-assisted delivery, or, rarely, hysterotomy may be necessary to empty the uterus before brachytherapy. Alternatively, if the initial tumor was small and has completely regressed, an extrafascial hysterectomy or modified radical hysterectomy may be performed.

For patients beyond the 20th week of gestation, therapy is often delayed until fetal viability. The health and maturity of the fetus are determined by appropriate ultrasound studies and amniotic fluid analysis to ensure fetal lung maturity. Delivery is usually accomplished by cesarean section, and after this, therapy is completed by surgery or radiation with the usual considerations of tumor stage and size. Overall, treatment results in pregnant patients are similar to those in nonpregnant patients, stage for stage, as recently confirmed by van der Vange and coworkers. The reader should be aware that many published studies dealing with carcinoma of the cervix in pregnancy include cases treated as long as 1 year postpartum, which assumes the carcinoma was present during pregnancy. Hacker and associates summarized the results of 1249 cases reported in various series in the literature. Overall, a 5-year survival rate of 49.2% was recorded for pregnant patients compared with 51% for nonpregnant patients treated during the same period. Their statistics included not only patients treated during pregnancy but also those treated up to 6 months after delivery, and the postpartum group had the poorest survival statistics. Survival was most closely related to stage, as expected, and persons diagnosed during the first trimester had a better prognosis than those diagnosed during the third trimester.

RECURRENCES

Approximately one third of patients treated for cancer of the cervix will experience tumor recurrence, which is defined as the reappearance of tumor 6 months or more after therapy. Metastases can occur anywhere, but most are in the pelvis (centrally in the vagina or cervix or laterally near the pelvic walls) or less frequently distally in the periaortic nodes, lung, liver, or bone. It should be noted that liver, lung, and distal bone metastases outside the pelvis likely result from hematogenous tumor spread.

The symptoms caused by recurrence depend on the site and extent of metastatic disease. Vaginal discharge and abnormal bleeding are often symptoms of an early central pelvic recurrence. Malaise, loss of appetite, and general symptoms associated with widespread metastatic disease are late manifestations of recurrence. Lateral pelvic recurrences often have a retroperitoneal component, which can lead to sciatic nerve irritation and cause severe pain around the distribution of the sciatic nerve in back of the leg as well as loss of muscle strength causing the patient to walk with a limp. Unilateral leg edema frequently accompanies such metastases, or leg swelling may occur from fibrosis of lymphatics following surgery or radiation. In addition, tumor recurrence can also cause ureteral obstruction, leading to unilateral or bilateral compromise of kidney function. Low back pain frequently occurs.

Patients treated for carcinoma of the cervix are examined according to the same schedule as patients with other malignancies: every 3 months the first 2 years, every 6 months from years 3 to 5, and yearly thereafter. More frequent examinations are done if abnormal symptoms or signs develop. Examination consists of vaginal and cervical cytology (Pap smear) as well as complete physical and pelvic examinations. Generally, chest radiographs are obtained annually, and IVP or abdominal pelvic CT is also performed annually, particularly during the first 2 years after treatment when the majority of recurrences will develop. Renal function tests may be indicated because ureteral fibrosis can occur more than 5 years after the completion of radiation therapy. A blood test for squamous cell carcinoma antigen has been studied as a modality to follow patients who have detectable levels of the antigen in their blood. Holloway and colleagues noted elevated levels in 72 of 153 patients (53%) and found the test useful for following patients who initially had elevated levels. Once recurrent disease is suspected, verification is usually obtained by biopsy of an accessible mass or CT-directed thin-needle aspiration, depending on the location of the tumor recurrence.

Pelvic Recurrences

Approximately half of the recurrences will develop in the pelvis. In addition to clinical assessment and CT, a vaginal ultrasound scan is often useful to document pelvic recurrence. Recurrences of adenocarcinoma are less frequent in the pelvis and are more likely to be at distant sites, such as the lung or supraclavicular areas. For patients who were initially treated by surgery, radiation is usually prescribed for pelvic recurrences, and approximately 50-Gy whole pelvic irradiation is given. Supplemental interstitial or intracavitary radiation is also prescribed, depending on the size and location of recurrence in the pelvis. As described previously, chemoradiation is preferably used. Patients who have isolated central recurrences without pelvic wall fixation or regional metastasis can be cured in as many as 60% to 70% of cases. The prognosis is much poorer when the pelvic wall is involved (usually 10% to 20% of patients survive 5 years after radiation therapy). For patients who were initially treated with radiation who have developed a localized pelvic recurrence, surgical eradication of the tumor should be considered because further effective radiation is not possible and limited surgical resection of the pelvic recurrence may not lead to a cure but will often cause severe complications of wound healing and intestinal and urinary fistulas. However, in rare, carefully selected patients initially treated with primary radiation therapy, radical hysterectomy may be a feasible alternative to exenterative surgery. Coleman and colleagues reported on 50 patients who underwent a radical hysterectomy for persistent or recurrent disease and found 5- and 10-year survival rates of 72% and 60%, respectively, with complications rates of 64% of severe complication and 42% permanent complications. The authors conclude that a radical hysterectomy was an alternative to exenteration in patients with small, centrally recurrent cervical cancer but that it should be used only in carefully selected patients. If neither surgery nor radiation is a feasible alternative, palliative chemotherapy is considered.

Pelvic Exenteration

Exenterative therapy for central pelvic tumor recurrence is an extensive operative procedure used only if the preoperative evaluation suggests that the patient's condition can be cured by this procedure. Exenteration is not performed for palliation. Three types of operation may be used. Anterior pelvic exenteration is the removal of the bladder, uterus, cervix, and part or all of the vagina. Posterior pelvic exenteration is the removal of the anus and rectum and resection of the uterus, cervix, and all or part of the vagina. Total exenteration is combined anteroposterior exenteration to remove all the pelvic contents. Shepherd and associates noted that patients older than age 69, those who had a recurrence within 3 years, or those who had persistent disease or positive resection margins had a poorer prognosis for the procedure.

Before an exenterative operation is undertaken, the patient is thoroughly evaluated for any evidence of disease spread outside the pelvis, and if there is any evidence of disease spread, the procedure is not performed. At operation, abdominal exploration is carried out to be sure the tumor is resectable. Biopsy specimens of any enlarged lymph nodes or suspicious areas outside the pelvis are taken, and frozen-section studies are performed, including evaluation of the operative margins. Usually total exenteration is performed. The recent introduction of a continent urinary pouch has contributed to patient comfort; the operation is well described by Penalver and coworkers. Generally, the urinary stoma is located in the abdomen on the right side and the intestinal stoma on the left side. However, three of 39 patients (7%) died of operative complications. The use of intestinal stapling devices sometimes allows preservation of the rectal sphincter and anal function and avoids a permanent colostomy. Long-term complications are usually ureteral stricture and/or difficulty catheterizing the intestinal reservoir.

Severe postoperative and intraoperative complications can occur with this extensive procedure, and perioperative mortalities as high as 10% to 20% have been reported in the past. Infection and bowel obstruction are the major risks. However, current surgical techniques of preoperative bowel preparation, use of antibiotics, careful intraoperative fluid and volume monitoring, and the use of parenteral nutrition have reduced the immediate postoperative mortality to less than 5%. The use of a peritoneal graft or an omental flap, created from the right or left side of the omentum and placed in the pelvis to protect the denuded pelvic floor, can help to avoid bowel obstruction and reduce postoperative morbidity, as noted by Miller and coworkers. Occasionally, gracilis myocutaneous grafts are used both to create a new vagina and to bring a new blood supply to the previously irradiated pelvis, which aids in wound healing. Morley and colleagues reported a 5-year survival rate of 61% in 100 patients ages 21 to 74 years. No patients with positive nodes in the operative specimen survived.

Nonpelvic Recurrences

Recurrences outside of the pelvis can be treated with radiation, surgery, or chemotherapy. Localized recurrences in areas not previously irradiated are occasionally treated by means of radiation. Resection of the metastasis is rarely done, and it is usually restricted to a localized lesion that occurs 3 to 4 years after primary therapy on the assumption that such a solitary metastasis can be effectively treated with local resection. However, in general, distant metastases are usually manifestations of systemic disease and are not cured with local therapy.

Chemotherapy

Patients with advanced, recurrent, or persistent cervical cancer are the most difficult to treat, and for this patient population, chemotherapy offers the best hope. Many studies, including some by Bonomi and associates and McGuire and associates, have attempted to identify active agents in this patient population, and most of the studies have established cisplatin as the most active agent. Several phase II studies have evaluated novel single agents or the combination of cisplatin with other agents including mitolactol, ifosfamide, gemcitabine, topotecan, paclitaxel, and vinorelbine, all showing promising results. This has led to several phase III studies evaluation chemotherapy in patients with recurrent, advanced, or persistent cervical cancer.

The GOG has published results from four randomized phase III trials (protocols 110, 149, 169, and 179) trying to find the optimal platinum doublet to treat women with metastatic disease. The first of these trials to be published was GOG protocol 110. This trial compared single-agent cisplatin with cisplatin/mitolactol and cisplatin/ifosfamide. Despite the fact that overall response rates were 17.8% in the cisplatin-only arm, 21.1% in the cisplatin/mitolactol, and 31.1% in the cisplatin/ifosfamide arm ($P = .004$), there was no significant difference in overall survival and greater toxicity with the cisplatin/ifosfamide regimen. GOG protocol 149 demonstrated that the addition of bleomycin did not enhance the activity of the cisplatin/ifosfamide doublet, and GOG protocol 169 showed that the addition of paclitaxel to cisplatin or increasing the dose of cisplatin only improved response rate and prolonged progression-free survival but not overall survival.

The only trial that has been positive is GOG protocol 179. In this trial, patients were randomized to single-agent cisplatin versus cisplatin and topotecan. There was a 2.9-month improvement in median survival in patients receiving the combination of cisplatin/topotecan versus cisplatin alone with no increase in toxicity, making this the new standard regimen in the setting of stage IVB or recurrent cervical cancer. In the ongoing phase III trial, GOG protocol 204 is comparing cisplatin/paclitaxel with cisplatin/topotecan, cisplatin/gemcitabine, and cisplatin/vinorelbine in patients with advanced, recurrent, or persistent disease in an attempt to find the optimal platinum doublet. Despite all these efforts, survival rates are poor and newer agents are needed to move from palliation to cure.

Sarcomas

Very rare sarcomas of the cervix have been reported. Brand and colleagues summarized 21 cases of sarcoma botryoides with encouraging results using multiagent chemotherapy followed by operation. A report by Daya and Scully suggests that patients with these tumors may have a better prognosis than those with tumors of similar histology arising in the vagina.

KEY POINTS

- Carcinomas of the cervix are predominantly squamous cell carcinomas (85% to 90%), and approximately 10% to 15% are adenocarcinomas.
- Squamous cell carcinomas appear to have a viral and venereal association, particularly with HPV. In the United States, squamous cell carcinoma is more frequent in blacks than in whites.
- Cervical carcinoma is the third most frequent malignancy of the lower female genital tract, after endometrial and ovarian cancer, and the second most frequent cause of death, after ovarian cancer.
- The definitive diagnosis of microinvasive carcinoma is established only by means of cervical conization, not biopsy. The margins of the cone should be free of neoplastic epithelium before conservative therapy is undertaken
- Microinvasive carcinoma of the cervix can be effectively treated by total hysterectomy, with a 5-year survival rate of almost 100%, but recurrent neoplasia can develop after 5 years. However, a precise and reliable definition of microinvasion is controversial.
- Prognosis in squamous cell cancer of the cervix is related to tumor stage and lesion volume (size), depth of invasion, and spread to lymph nodes. Older patients tend to have a worse prognosis, and HPV-positive younger patients have a better prognosis.
- The prognosis of adenocarcinoma of the cervix is related to tumor stage, size, grade, and depth of invasion. Large adenocarcinomas tend to be poorly differentiated.
- Metastases to regional pelvic nodes in stage I squamous carcinomas correlate with lesion size, depth of invasion, presence of capillary lymphatic space involvement, and correlate inversely with patient age.
- Cervical carcinomas are locally invasive tumors that spread primarily to the pelvic tissues and then to the pelvic and paraaortic lymph nodes. Less frequently, hematogenous spread to the liver, lung, and bone occurs.
- The risk of the spread of cervical carcinoma to pelvic nodes is approximately 15% for stage I, 29% for stage II, and 47% for stage III. For the paraaortic nodes, percentages are 6% for stage I, 19% for stage II, and 33% for stage III.
- Stage IB carcinomas of the cervix may be treated equally effectively by radical hysterectomy and pelvic node dissection or radiation. The 5-year survival rate is approximately 80%. If lymph nodes are free of tumor, the 5-year survival rate is approximately 90%, and if the nodes contain metastatic tumor, the rate is 50%. Improved overall survival rates have been reported for patients with tumors less than 4 cm in diameter treated by preliminary brachytherapy followed by radical hysterectomy.
- During radical hysterectomy, the ureter should never be grasped with surgical instruments to avoid damaging the periureteral blood supply.
- Surgery is often used for treating stage IB and early stage IIA carcinomas of the cervix, particularly for smaller tumors and for younger patients to preserve their ovarian function. Surgery produces less scarring and vaginal fibrosis than does irradiation and is preferred for women with a pelvic mass, pelvic infection, or history of conditions such as inflammatory bowel disease, which increase the risk for radiation complications.

KEY POINTS *Continued*

- High-stage tumors are treated by chemoradiation. Current programs usually use cisplatin 40 mg/m^2 weekly during external treatment and with brachytherapy.
- Urinary fistulas follow radical hysterectomy in approximately 1% of cases.
- Most cancers of the cervix are treated by radiation therapy (teletherapy and brachytherapy). Radiation doses vary with tumor size and stage but approximate 50 to 65 Gy at point B and 85 Gy at point A. Current practice is to combine radiation with simultaneous chemotherapy to optimize the results.
- Improved cure rates of cervical cancers are obtained with increased doses, which also lead to an increased frequency of complications. Large increments in dose may increase complications without increasing cure rates.
- Complications following radiation are related to dose and volume of tissue treated and include radiation inflammation of the bladder or bowel, which may lead to pain, bleeding, or, infrequently, fistula formation. The normal cervix is resistant to radiation, and the dose can be as high as 200 to 250 Gy over 2 months. The bladder and rectum can be injured at average doses in the range of 65 to 75 Gy. Overall, the rate of moderate to severe radiation complications for treatment of all stages is approximately 10%.
- Radiation complications of the intestine are more frequent than bladder complications. Bowel complications tend to occur within the first 2 years after treatment, whereas bladder complications can occur up to 20 years after treatment.
- Worldwide 5-year survival rates reported for patients with carcinomas of the cervix are as follows: stage Ia, 95%; stage Ib, 80%; stage II, 70%; stage III, 50%; and stage IV, 20% with radiation therapy alone.
- Pregnancy does not adversely affect the survival rate for women with carcinoma of the cervix, stage for stage.
- Approximately one third of patients treated for cervical carcinoma develop tumor recurrence, and approximately half of these recurrences are located in the pelvis and most occur within 2 years.
- Patients whose recurrences occur more than 3 years after primary therapy have a better prognosis than those with earlier recurrence.
- Pelvic exenteration in carefully selected patients with central pelvic recurrence can lead to a 5-year survival rate of 50% or better.
- Chemotherapy of recurrent squamous cell carcinoma of the cervix does not produce long-term cures, but response rates of approximately 50% (partial and complete) have been obtained with multiple-agent regimens that contain cisplatin.
- Leg pain following the distribution of the sciatic nerve or unilateral leg swelling is often an indication of pelvic recurrence of carcinoma of the cervix.

BIBLIOGRAPHY

Abell MR, Ramirez JA: Sarcomas and carcinosarcomas of the uterine cervix. Cancer 31:1176, 1973.

Alvarez RD, Soong S-J, Kinney WK, et al: Identification of prognostic factors and risk groups in patients found to have nodal metastasis at the time of radical hysterectomy for early-stage squamous cell carcinoma of the cervix. Gynecol Oncol 35:130, 1989.

Andras EJ, Fletcher G, Rutledge F: Radiotherapy of carcinoma of the cervix following simple hysterectomy. Am J Obstet Gynecol 115:647–655, 1973.

Angioli R, Estape R, Cantuaria G, et al: Urinary complications of Miami pouch: Trend of conservative management. Am J Obstet Gynecol 179:343, 1998.

Anton-Culver H, Bloss JD, Bringman D, et al: Comparison of adenocarcinoma and squamous cell carcinoma of the uterine cervix: A population-based epidemiologic study. Am J Obstet Gynecol 166:1507, 1992.

Balderson K, Tewari K, Gregory WT, et al: Neuroendocrine small cell uterine cervix cancer in pregnancy: Long-term survival following combined therapy. Gynecol Oncol 71:128, 1998.

Berchuk A, Mullin TJ: Cervical adenoid cystic carcinoma associated with ascites. Gynecol Oncol 22:201, 1985.

Berek JS, Hacker NF, Fu YS, et al: Adenocarcinoma of the uterine cervix: Histologic variables associated with lymph node metastasis and spread. Obstet Gynecol 65:46, 1985.

Bergmark K, Avall-Lundqvist E, Dickman PW, et al: Vaginal changes and sexuality in women with a history of cervical cancer. N Engl J Med 340:1383, 1999.

Berman ML, Keys H, Creasman W: Survival and patterns of recurrence in cervical cancer metastatic to periaortic lymph nodes. Gynecol Oncol 19:8, 1984.

Bloss JD, DiSaiia PJ, Mannel RS, et al: Radiation myelitis: A complication of concurrent cisplatin and 5-fluorouracil chemotherapy with extended field radiotherapy for carcinoma of the uterine cervix. Gynecol Oncol 43:305, 1991.

Bloss JD, Blessing J, Behrens R, et al: Randomized phase III trial of cisplatin and ifosfamide with or without bleomycin in squamous carcinoma of the cervix: A Gynecology Oncology Group study. J Clin Oncol 20:1832–1837, 2002.

Bosch FX, Manos MM, Munoz N, et al: Prevalence of human papillomavirus in cervical cancer: A worldwide perspective. J Natl Cancer Inst 87:796, 1995.

Brand E, Berek JS, Hacker N: Controversies in the management of cervical adenocarcinoma. Obstet Gynecol 71:261, 1988.

Brand E, Berek JS, Nieberg RK, Hacker NF: Rhabdomyosarcoma of the uterine cervix. Cancer 60:1552, 1987.

Brinton LA, Herrero R, Reeves WC, et al: Risk factors for cervical cancer by histology. Gynecol Oncol 51:301, 1993.

Bonomi P, Blessing J, Stehman F, et al: Randomized trial of three cisplatin dose schedules in squamous cell carcinoma of the cervix: A Gynecologic Oncology Group study. J Clin Oncol 3:1079–1085, 1985.

Burghardt E, Ostor A, Fox H: The new FIGO definition of cervical cancer stage IA: A critique [editorial]. Gynecol Oncol 65:1, 1997.

Calais G, Le Floch O, Chauvet B, et al: Carcinoma of the uterine cervix stage Ib and early stage II: Prognostic value of the histological tumor regression after initial brachytherapy. Int J Radiat Oncol Biol Phys 17:1231, 1989.

Chambers SK, Chambers JT, Kier R, et al: Sequelae of lateral ovarian transposition in irradiated cervical cancer patients. Int J Radiat Oncol Biol Phys 20:1305, 1991.

Chapman JA, Mannel RS, Disala PJ, et al: Surgical treatment of unexpected invasive cervical cancer found at total hysterectomy. Obstet Gynecol 80:931, 1992.

Clark BG, Souhami L, Roman TN, et al: Rectal complications in patients with carcinoma of the cervix treated with concomitant cisplatin and external beam irradiation with high dose rate brachytherapy: A dosimetric analysis. Int J Radiat Oncol Biol Phys 28:1243, 1994.

Clement PB, Scully RE: Carcinoma of the cervix: Histologic types. Semin Oncol 9:251, 1982.

Cliby WA, Dodson MK, Podratz KC: Cervical cancer complicated by pregnancy: Episiotomy site recurrences following vaginal delivery. Obstet Gynecol 84:179, 1994.

Coleman RL, Keeney ED, Freedman RA, et al: Radical hysterectomy after radiotherapy for recurrent carcinoma of the uterine cervix. Gynecol Oncol 1994;55:29–35.

Covens A, Kirby J, Shaw P, et al: Prognostic factors for relapse and pelvic lymph node metastases in early stage I adenocarcinoma of the cervix. Gynecol Oncol 74:423, 1999.

Covens A, Shaw P, Murphy J, et al: Is radical trachelectomy a safe alternative to radical hysterectomy for patients with stage IA-B carcinoma of the cervix? Cancer 86:2273, 1999.

Crane CH, Schneider BF: Occult carcinoma discovered after simple hysterectomy treated with postoperative radiotherapy. Int J Radiat Oncol Biol 43:1049, 1999.

Creasman WT: New gynecologic cancer staging. Gynecol Oncol 58:157, 1995.

Creasman WT, Zaino RJ, Major FJ, et al: Early invasive carcinoma of the cervix (3 to 5 mm invasion): Risk factors and prognosis. Am J Obstet Gynecol 178:62, 1998.

Cunningham MJ, Dunton CJ, Corn B, et al. Extended-field radiation therapy in early-stage cervical carcinoma: Survival and complications. Gynecol Oncol 1991;43:51–54.

Dargent D, Ansquer Y, Mathevet P: Technical development and results of left extraperitoneal laparoscopic paraaortic lymphadenectomy for cervical cancer. Gynecol Oncol 77:87–92, 2000.

Dattoli MJ, Gretz HF III, Beller U, et al: Analysis of multiple prognostic factors in patients with stage Ib cervical cancer: Age as a major determinant. Int J Radiat Oncol Biol Phys 17:41, 1989.

Davidson SE, Symonds RP, Lamont D, Watson ER: Does adenocarcinoma of uterine cervix have a worse prognosis than squamous carcinoma when treated by radiotherapy? Gynecol Oncol 33:23, 1989.

Daya DA, Scully RE: Sarcoma botryoides of the uterine cervix in young women: A clinicopathological study of 13 cases, Gynecol Oncol 29:290, 1988.

Delgado G, Bundy BN, Fowler WC, et al: A prospective surgical pathological study of stage I squamous carcinoma of the cervix: A gynecologic oncology group study. Gynecol Oncol 35:314, 1989.

Delgado G, Bundy B, Zaino R, et al: Prospective surgical-pathologic study of disease-free interval in patients with stage IB squamous cell carcinoma of the cervix: A Gynecologic Oncology Group study. Gynecol Oncol 38:352, 1990.

Duggan B, Muderspach LI, Roman LD, et al: Cervical cancer in pregnancy: Reporting on planned delay in therapy. Obstet Gynecol 82:598, 1993.

Eifel PJ, Morris M, Wharton JT, Oswald MJ: The influence of tumor size and morphology on the outcome of patients with FIGO stage IB squamous cell carcinoma of the uterine cervix. Int J Radiat Oncol Biol Phys 29:9, 1994.

Einhorn N, Patek E, Sjöberg B: Outcome of different treatment modalities in cervix carcinoma Stage IB and IIA. Observations in a well-defined Swedish population. Cancer 55(5):949–955, 1985.

Forney JP: The effect of radical hysterectomy on bladder physiology. Am J Obstet Gynecol 138:374, 1980.

Fuller AF, Elliott N, Kosloff C, et al: Determinants of increased risk for recurrence in patients undergoing radical hysterectomy for stage IB and IIA carcinoma of the cervix. Gynecol Oncol 1989;33:34–39.

Green JA, Kirwan JM, Tierney JF, et al: Survival and recurrence after concomitant chemotherapy and radiotherapy for cancer of the uterine cervix: A systematic review and meta-analysis. Lancet 358:781–786, 2001.

Greenlee RT, Murray T, Bolen S, Wingo PA: Cancer statistics, 2000. CA Cancer J Clin 50:7, 2000.

Greer BE, Koh W, Stelzer KJ, et al: Expanded pelvic radiotherapy fields for treatment of local-regionally advanced carcinoma of the cervix. Am J Obstet Gynecol 174:1141, 1996.

Grigsby PW: Rectal complications in patients with carcinoma of the cervix: The concept of a rectal reference dose, Int J Radiat Oncol Biol Phys 28:1271, 1994.

Grigsby PW, Siegel BA, Dehdashti F: Lymph node staging by positron emission tomography in patients with carcinoma of the cervix. J Clin Oncol 19:3745–3749, 2001.

Grogan M, Thomas GM, Melamed I, et al: The importance of hemoglobin levels during radiotherapy for carcinoma of the cervix. Cancer 86:1528, 1999.

Hacker NF, Wain GV, Nicklin JL: Resection of bulky positive lymph nodes in patients with cervical carcinoma. Int Gynecol Cancer 5(4):250–256, 1995.

Henriksen E: The lymphatic spread of carcinoma of the cervix and of the body of the uterus. Am J Obstet Gynecol 58:924, 1949.

Holloway RW, To A, Moradi M, et al: Monitoring the course of cervical carcinoma with the squamous cell carcinoma serum radioimmunoassay. Obstet Gynecol 74:944, 1989.

Hong JH, Tsai CS, Chang JT, et al. The prognostic significance of pre- and posttreatment SCC levels in patients with squamous cell carcinoma of the cervix treated by radiotherapy. Int J Radiat Oncol Biol Phys 41:823–830, 1998.

Hoskins PJ, Wong F, Swenerton KD, et al: Small cell carcinoma of the cervix treated with concurrent radiotherapy, cisplatin, and etoposide. Gynecol Oncol 56:218, 1995.

Inoue T, Okumura M: Prognostic significance of parametrial extension in patients with cervical carcinoma stages IB, IIA, and IIB. A study of 628 cases treated by radical hysterectomy and lymphadenectomy with or without postoperative irradiation. Cancer 54:1714–1719, 1984.

Inoue T, Morita K: Long-term observation of patients treated by postoperative extended-field irradiation for nodal metastases from cervical carcinoma stages IB, IIA, and IIB. Gynecol Oncol 58:4, 1995.

Inoue T, Morita K: The prognostic significance of number of positive nodes in cervical carcinoma stages Ib, IIa, and IIb, Cancer 65:1923, 1990.

Kamura T, Tsukamoto N, Tsuruchi N, et al. Multivariate analysis of the histopathologic prognostic factors of cervical cancer in patients undergoing radical hysterectomy. Cancer 69:181–186, 1992.

Kaspar HG, Dinh TV, Doherty MG, et al: Clinical implication of tumor volume measurement in stage I adenocarcinoma of the cervix. Obstet Gynecol 81:296, 1993.

Keys H, Bundy B, Stehman F, et al. Adjuvant hysterectomy after radiation therapy reduces detection of local recurrence in "bulky" stage IB cervical cancer without improving survival: Results of a prospective randomized GOG trial. Cancer J Sci Am 3:117, 1997.

Keys HM, Bundy BN, Stehman FB, et al: Cisplatin, radiation, and adjuvant hysterectomy compared with radiation and adjuvant hysterectomy for bulky stage IB cervical carcinoma. N Engl J Med 340:1154, 1999.

King LA, Talledo OE, Gallup DG, et al: Adenoid cystic carcinoma of the cervix in women under age 40. Gynecol Oncol 32:26, 1989.

Kinney WK, Alvarez RD, Reid GC, et al: Value of adjuvant whole-pelvis irradiation after Wertheim hysterectomy for early-stage squamous carcinoma of the cervix with pelvic nodal metastasis: a matched-control study. Gynecol Oncol 34:258, 1989.

Klee M, Thranov I, Machin D: The patients' perspective on physical symptoms after radiotherapy for cervical cancer. Gynecol Oncol 76:14, 2000.

Kleinerman RA, Boice JD, Storm HH, et al: Second primary cancer after treatment for cervical cancer. Cancer 76:442, 1995.

Kobayashi Y, Yoshinouchi M, Tianqi G, et al: Presence of human papilloma virus DNA in pelvic lymph nodes can predict unexpected recurrence of cervical cancer in patients with histologically negative lymph nodes. Clin Cancer Res 1998;4:979–983.

Kolstad P: Follow-up study of 232 patients with stage Ia1 and 411 patients with stage Ia2 squamous cell carcinoma of the cervix (microinvasive carcinoma). Gynecol Oncol 33:265, 1989.

Komaki R, Mattingly RF, Hoffman RG, et al: Irradiation of para-aortic lymph node metastases from carcinoma of the cervix or endometrium: Preliminary results. Radiology 147:245–248, 1983.

Kovalic JJ, Grigsby PW, Perez CA, et al: Cervical stump carcinoma. Int J Radiat Oncol Biol Phys 20:933, 1991.

Kristensen GB, Abeler VM, Risberg B, et al: Tumor size, depth of invasion, and grading of the invasive tumor front are the main prognostic factors in early squamous cell cervical carcinoma. Gynecol Oncol 74:245–251, 1999.

Lagasse LD, Creasman WT, Shingleton HM: Results and complications of operative staging in cervical cancer: Experience of the Gynecologic Oncology Group. Gynecol Oncol 9:90, 1980.

Larsen NS: Invasive cancer rising in young white females. J Natl Cancer Inst 86:6, 1994.

Levenback C, Coleman R, van der Zee AGJ (eds): Clinical Lymphatic Mapping in Gynecologic Cancers. London, Martin Dunitz Ltd., 2004.

Levenback C, Coleman RL, Burke TW, et al: Lymphatic mapping and sentinel node identification in patients with cervix cancer undergoing radical hysterectomy and pelvic lymphadenectomy. J Clin Oncol 20:688–693, 2002.

Lewandowski GS, Copeland LJ: A potential role for intensive chemotherapy in the treatment of small cell neuroendocrine tumors of the cervix. Gynecol Oncol 48:127, 1993.

Liang C-C, Tseng C-J, Soong Y-K: The usefulness of cystoscopy in the staging of cervical cancer. Gynecol Oncol 76:200, 2000.

Lohe KJ, Burghardt E, Hillemanns HG, et al: Early squamous cell carcinoma of the uterine cervix. II. Clinical results of a cooperative study in the management of 419 patients with early stromal invasion and microcarcinoma. Gynecol Oncol 6:31, 1978.

Long HJ 3rd, Bundy B, Grendys EC, et al: Randomized phase III trial of cisplatin with or without topotecan in carcinoma of the uterine cervix. A Gynecologic Oncology Group study. J Clin Oncol 23:4626–4633, 2005.

Low JA, Mauger GM, Carmichael JA: The effect of Wertheim hysterectomy on bladder and urethral function. Am J Obstet Gynecol 139:826, 1981.

Magrina JF, Goodrich MA, Lidner TK, et al: Modified radical hysterectomy in the treatment of early squamous cervical cancer. Gynecol Oncol 72:183, 1999.

McGowan L, Young RH, Scully RE: Peutz-Jeghers syndrome with "adenoma malignum" of the cervix. Gynecol Oncol 10:125, 1980.

McGuire W III, Arseneau J, Blessing J, et al: A randomized comparative trial of carboplatin and iproplatin in advanced squamous carcinoma of the uterine cervix: A Gynecologic Oncology Group study. J Clin Oncol 7:1462–1468, 1989.

McIntyre JF, Eifel PJ, Levenback C, et al: Ureteral stricture as a late complication of radiotherapy for stage Ib carcinoma of the uterine cervix. Cancer 75:836, 1995.

McKelvey JL, Goodlin RR: Adenoma malignum of the cervix: A cancer of deceptively innocent histological pattern. Cancer 16:549, 1963.

Mendenhall WM, McCarty PJ, Morgan LS, et al: Stage IB-IIa-B carcinoma of the intact uterine cervix greater than or equal to 6 cm in diameter: Is adjuvant extrafascial hysterectomy beneficial? Int J Radiat Oncol Biol Phys 21:899–904, 1991.

Miller B, Morris M, Gershenson DM, et al: Intestinal fistulae formation following pelvic exenteration: A review of the University of Texas MD Anderson Cancer Center experience, 1957–1990. Gynecol Oncol 56:207, 1995.

Monk BJ, Cha DS, Walker JL, et al: Extent of disease as an indication for pelvic radiation following radical hysterectomy and bilateral pelvic lymph node dissection in the treatment of stage Ib and IIa cervical carcinoma. Gynecol Oncol 54:4, 1994.

Montana GS, Fowler WC: Carcinoma of the cervix: Analysis of bladder and rectal radiation dose and complications. Int J Radiat Oncol Biol Phys 16:95, 1989.

Montz FJ, Holschneider CH, Solh S, et al: Small bowel obstruction following radical hysterectomy: Risk factors, incidence, and operative findings. Gynecol Oncol 53:114, 1994.

Moore D, Blessing J, McQuellon R, et al: Phase III study of cisplatin with or without paclitaxel in stage IVB, recurrent or persistent squamous cell carcinoma of the cervix: A Gynecologic Oncology Group study. J Clin Oncol 22:3113–3119, 2004.

Morley GW, Hopkins MP, Lindenauer SM, Roberts JA: Pelvic exenteration, University of Michigan: 100 patients at 5 years. Obstet Gynecol 74:934, 1989.

Morris M, Eifel P, Lu J, et al: Pelvic radiation with concurrent chemotherapy compared with pelvic and para-aortic radiation for high risk cervical cancer. N Engl J Med 340:1137, 1999.

Morris M, Gershenson DM, Eifel P, et al: Treatment of small cell carcinoma of the cervix with cisplatin, doxorubicin, and etoposide. Gynecol Oncol 47:62, 1992.

Morris M, Mitchell MF, Silva EG, et al: Cervical conization as definitive therapy for early invasive squamous carcinoma of the cervix. Gynecol Oncol 51:193, 1993.

Mundt AJ, Connel PP, Campbell T, et al: Race and clinical outcome in patients with carcinoma of the uterine cervix treated with radiation therapy. Gynecol Oncol 71:151, 1998.

Nash JD, Burke TW, Woodward JE, et al: Diagnosis of recurrent gynecologic malignancy with fine-needle aspiration cytology. Obstet Gynecol 71:333, 1988.

Noguchi H, Shiozawa I, Kitahara T, et al: Uterine body invasion of carcinoma of the uterine cervix as seen from surgical specimens. Gynecol Oncol 30:173–182, 1988.

Occelli B, Narducci F, Lanvin D, et al: De novo adhesions with extraperitoneal endosurgical para-aortic lymphadenectomy versus transperitoneal laparoscopic para-aortic lymphadenectomy: A randomized experimental study. Am J Obstet Gynecol 183:529–533, 2000.

Omura G, Blessing J, Vaccarello L, et al: Randomized trial of cisplatin versus cisplatin plus mitolactol versus cisplatin plus ifosfamide in advanced squamous carcinoma of the cervix: A Gynecologic Oncology Group study. J Clin Oncol 15:165–171, 1997.

Orton CG, Wolf-Rosenblum S: Dose dependence of complication rates in cervix cancer radiotherapy. Int J Radiat Oncol Biol Phys 12:37, 1986.

Östor AG: Studies on 200 cases of early squamous cell carcinoma of the cervix. Int J Gynecol Pathol 12:193, 1993.

Östor AG: Early invasive adenocarcinoma of the uterine cervix. Int J Gynecol Pathol 19:29, 2000.

Östor AG, Rome RM: Micro-invasive squamous cell carcinoma of the cervix: A clinico-pathologic study of 200 cases with long-term follow-up. Int J Gynecol Cancer 4:257, 1994.

Pearcey R, Brundage M, Drouin P, et al: Phase III trial comparing radical radiotherapy with and without cisplatin chemotherapy in patients with advanced squamous cell cancer of the cervix. J Clin Oncol 20:966–972, 2002.

Pecorelli S, Creasman WT, Pettersson F, et al: FIGO annual report on the results of treatment in gynaecological cancer, vol. 23. Milan, Italy, International Federation of Gynecology and Obstetrics. J Epidemiol Biostat 3, 1998.

Penalver MA, Bejany DE, Averette HE, et al: Continent urinary diversion in gynecologic oncology. Gynecol Oncol 34:274, 1989.

Penalver M, Donato D, Sevin B, et al: Complications of the ileocolonic continent urinary reservoir (Miami Pouch). Gynecol Oncol 52:360, 1994.

Peters WAI, Liu PY, Barrett R, et al: Cisplatin, 5-fluorouracil plus radiation therapy are superior to radiation therapy as adjunctive therapy in high-risk, early-stage carcinoma of the cervix after radical hysterectomy and pelvic lymphadenectomy. Report of a Phase III Intergroup Study. Gynecol Oncol 72:443, 1999.

Piver MS, Rutledge F, Smith JR: Five classes of extended hysterectomy for women with cervical cancer. Obstet Gynecol 44:265, 1974.

Plante M, Renaud M-C, et al: Vaginal radical trachelectomy: An oncologically safe fertility-preserving surgery. An updated series of 72 cases and review of the literature. Gynecol Oncol 94:614–623, 2004.

Plante M, Renaud MC, Roy M: Radical vaginal trachelectomy: A fertility-preserving option for young women with early stage cervical cancer. Gynecol Oncol 99(3 Suppl 1):S143–S146, 2005.

Plante M, Renaud MC, Tetu B, et al: Laparoscopic sentinel node mapping in early-stage cervical cancer. Gynecol Oncol 91:494–503, 1993.

Plentl AA, Friedman EA: Lymphatic System of the Female Genitalia. Philadelphia, WB Saunders, 1971.

Potter ME, Alvarez RD, Shingleton HM, et al: Early invasive cervical cancer with pelvic lymph node involvement: To complete or not to complete radical hysterectomy? Gynecol Oncol 37:78, 1990.

Ramirez PT, Frumovitz M, Wolf JK, Levenback C: Laparoscopic port-site metastases in patients with gynecological malignancies. Int J Gynecol Cancer 14:1070–1077, 2004.

Reich O, Tamussino K, Lahousen M, et al: Clear cell carcinoma of the uterine cervix: Pathology and prognosis in surgically treated stage IB-IIB disease in women not exposed in utero to diethylstilbestrol. Gynecol Oncol 76:331, 2000.

Riou G, Barrois M, Le MG, et al: C-myc proto-oncogene expression and prognosis in early carcinoma of the uterine cervix. Lancet 1(8536): 761–763, 1987.

Robinson JW, Faris PD, Scott CB: Psychoeducational group increases vaginal dilation for younger women and reduces sexual fears for women of all ages with gynecologic carcinoma treated with radiotherapy. Int J Radiat Oncol Biol Phys 44:497, 1999.

Roman LD, Morris M, Mitchell MF, et al: Prognostic factors for patients undergoing simple hysterectomy in the presence of invasive cancer of the cervix. Gynecol Oncol 50:179–184, 1993.

Rose PG, Blessing JA, Gershenson DM, McGehee R: Paclitaxel and cisplatin as first-line therapy in recurrent or advanced squamous cell carcinoma of the cervix: A gynecologic Oncology Group Study. J Clin Oncol 17:2676, 1999.

Rose PG, Bundy BN, Watkins EB, et al: Concurrent cisplatin-based radiotherapy and chemotherapy for locally advanced cervical cancer. N Engl J Med 340:1144, 1999.

Rotman M, Pajak TF, Choi K, et al: Prophylactic extended-field irradiation of para-aortic lymph nodes in stages IIb and bulky Ib and IIa cervical carcinoma. JAMA 274:387, 1995.

Rotmensch J, Rosenshein NB, Woodruff JD: Cervical sarcoma: A review. Obstet Gynecol Surv 38:456, 1983.

Rotmensch J, Waggoner SE, Quiet C: Ultrasound guidance for placement of difficult intracavitary implants. Gynecol Oncol 54:159, 1994.

Runowicz CD, Wadler S, Rodriguez-Rodriguez L, et al: Concomitant cisplatin and radiotherapy in locally advanced cervical carcinoma. Gynecol Oncol 34:395, 1989.

Rutledge FN, Mitchell MR, Munsell M, et al: Youth as a prognostic factor in carcinoma of the cervix: A match analysis. Gynecol Oncol 44:123–130, 1992.

Sagal S, Kuzumaki N, Hisada T, et al: Ras oncogene expression and prognosis of invasive squamous cell carcinoma of the uterine cervix. Cancer 63:1577, 1989.

Sardi J, Sananes C, Giaroli A, et al: Results of a prospective randomized trial with neoadjuvant chemotherapy in stage Ib bulky, squamous carcinoma of the cervix. Gynecol Oncol 49:156, 1993.

Sarkaria JN, Petereit DG, Stitt JA, et al: A comparison of the efficacy and complication rates of low dose-rate versus high dose-rate brachytherapy in the treatment of uterine cervical carcinoma. Int J Radiat Oncol Biol Phys 30:75, 1994.

Schlaerth JB, Spirtos NM, Carson LF, et al: Laparoscopic retroperitoneal lymphadenectomy followed by immediate laparotomy in women with cervical cancer: A Gynecologic Oncology Group study. Gynecol Oncol 85:81–88, 2002.

Sedlis A, Bundy BN, Rotman MZ, et al: A randomized trial of pelvic radiation therapy versus no further therapy in selected patients with stage IB carcinoma of the cervix after radical hysterectomy and pelvic lymphadenectomy: A Gynecologic Oncology Group study. Gynecol Oncol 73:177, 1999.

Shepherd JH, Ngan HYS, Neven P, et al: Multivariate analysis of factors affecting survival in pelvic exenteration. Int J Gynecol Cancer 4:361, 1994.

Shepherd JH: Staging announcement FIGO staging of gynecologic cancers: Cervical and vulva. Int J Gynecol Cancer 5:319, 1995.

Soisson AP, Soper JT, Clarke-Pearson DL, et al: Adjuvant radiotherapy following radical hysterectomy for patients with stage Ib and IIa cervical cancer. Gynecol Oncol 37:390, 1990.

Sonoda Y, Leblanc E, Querleu D, et al: Prospective evaluation of surgical staging of advanced cervical cancer via a laparoscopic extraperitoneal approach. Gynecol Oncol 91:326–331, 2003.

Sorosky JI, Squatrito R, Ndubisi BU, et al: Stage 1 squamous cell cervical carcinoma in pregnancy: Planned delay in therapy awaiting fetal maturity. Gynecol Oncol 59:207, 1995.

Spirtos NM, Schlaerth JB, Kimball RE, et al: Laparoscopic radical hysterectomy (type III) with aortic and pelvic lymphadenectomy. Am J Obstet Gynecol 174:1763, 1996.

Stock RG, Chen ASJ, Flickinger JC, et al: Node-positive cervical cancer: Impact of pelvic irradiation and patterns of failure. Int J Radiat Oncol Biol Phys 31:31, 1995.

U.S. Department of Health and Human Services. Ries ALG, Miller BA, Hankey BF, et al: SEER Cancer Statistics Review, 1973–1991, 136–144, 1994.

van der Vange N, Weverling GJ, Ketting BW, et al: The prognosis of cervical cancer associated with pregnancy: A matched cohort study. Obstet Gynecol 85:1022, 1995.

van Nagell JR, Maruyama Y, Donaldson ES, et al: Phase II clinical trial using californium 252 fast neutron brachytherapy, external pelvic radiation and extrafascial hysterectomy in the treatment of bulky, barrel-shaped stage Ib cervical cancer. Cancer 57:1918, 1986.

van Nagell JR, Powell DE, Gallion HH, et al: Small cell carcinoma of the uterine cervix. Cancer 62:1586, 1988.

Varia MA, Bundy BN, Deppe G, et al: Cervical carcinoma metastatic to para-aortic nodes: Extended field radiation therapy with concomitant 5-fluorouracil and cisplatin chemotherapy: A Gynecologic Oncology Group study. Int J Radiat Oncol Biol Phys 42:1015, 1998.

Vasilev SA, Vora N, Lee Y: Laparoscopically assisted transperineal interstitial brachytherapy with omental flap for locally recurrent endometrial cancer. J Laparoendosc Surg 5:393–397, 1995.

Vigliotti AP, Wen B, Hussey DH, et al: Extended field irradiation for carcinoma of the uterine cervix with positive periaortic nodes. Int J Radiat Oncol Biol Phys 23:501, 1992.

Westby M, Asmussen M: Anatomical and functional changes in the lower urinary tract after radical hysterectomy with lymph node dissection as studied by dynamic urethrocystography in simultaneous urethrocystometrics. Gynecol Oncol 21:261, 1985.

Wolff JP, Lacour J, Chassagne D, et al: Cancer of the cervical stump: A study of 173 patients. Obstet Gynecol 39:10, 1972.

Neoplastic Diseases of the Vulva

30

Lichen Sclerosus, Intraepithelial Neoplasia, Paget's Disease, Carcinoma

Michael Frumovitz and Diane C. Bodurka

KEY TERMS AND DEFINITIONS

Carcinoma In Situ. Premalignant epithelial change throughout the full thickness of the vulvar epithelium. It is also comparable with vulvar intraepithelial neoplasia (VIN) III.

Keyes Punch. An instrument used to biopsy the vulva.

Lichen Sclerosus. A vulvar abnormality usually characterized by thinning of the epithelium with a loss of subcutaneous adnexal structures, hyalinization of the superficial dermis, and lymphocytic infiltrates below the zone of dermal homogenization.

Clark's Level. A system (I to V) used to define the depth or level to which a malignant melanoma invades the epithelium.

Microinvasive Vulvar Carcinoma. A term used to describe a superficially invasive carcinoma of the vulva that is not expected to be associated with lymph node metastasis. The lesion is less than 2 cm in diameter; the invasion is less than 1 mm into the stroma (stage IA).

Paget's Disease of the Vulva. A pruritic, usually erythematous, lesion microscopically containing large cells similar to Paget cells seen in the breast. The squamous epithelium is studded with large cells containing clear cytoplasm and pleomorphic nuclei with prominent nucleoli.

Radical Vulvectomy. An operation that removes the entire vulva, including subcutaneous and fatty tissue, the labia minora and majora, perineal skin, and clitoris, to treat cancer.

Skinning Vulvectomy. An operation that removes the skin of the vulva, including the labia majora and minora, the clitoris, and perineal skin.

Surgical Staging of Vulvar Cancer.
Stage I: Less than 2 cm in diameter and confined to the vulva and/or perineum

Stage II: More than 2 cm in diameter and confined to the vulva and/or perineum

Stage III: Extends to the anus and/or lower urethra, and/or unilateral regional node metastasis

Stage IV: Spreads to the bladder or rectum or pelvic bone or upper urethra or nonvulvar sites, or bilateral regional node metastases

TNM System. A system used to describe the extent of tumor (T), node status (N), and presence of metastatic disease (M).

Verrucous Carcinoma. An uncommon well-differentiated squamous carcinoma with a gross wartlike appearance that is curable with a local excision.

Vulvar Atypia. A mild, moderate, or severe neoplastic or dysplastic change in the vulvar squamous epithelium. It may also be termed *vulvar intraepithelial neoplasia* (VIN I, II, or III).

Cancer of the vulva accounts for approximately 5% of malignancies of the lower female genital tract, ranking it fourth in frequency after cancers of the endometrium, ovary, and cervix.

Well-defined predisposing factors for the development of vulvar carcinoma have not been identified. In general, premalignant and malignant changes frequently arise at multifocal points on the vulva. Occasionally, invasive carcinoma arises from areas of carcinoma in situ, similar to the mechanism in cervical squamous cell carcinoma (see Chapter 29, Malignant Diseases of the Cervix). However, many cases of squamous cell carcinoma of the vulva appear to develop in the absence of premalignant changes in the vulvar epithelium. Human papillomavirus (HPV) has been noted in many young patients with carcinoma of the vulva. Other factors, such as granulomatous disease of the vulva, diabetes, hypertension, smoking, and obesity, have all been suggested as etiologic factors, but current data do not provide consistent evidence regarding their association with vulvar carcinoma. Carcinoma of the vulva occurs with increasing frequency in those who have been treated for squamous cell carcinoma of the cervix or vagina, presumably as a result of the increased risk of carcinogenesis in the squamous epithelium of the lower genital tract in these patients. It appears that HPV DNA is involved in the development of a subset of vulvar carcinomas that tend to occur in younger patients, as noted by Crum and associates. Monk and colleagues demonstrated that not only were the HPV DNA–associated carcinomas found in younger patients, but also the HPV-negative patients appear to have a poor prognosis with tumors that were more likely to recur and lead to patient death. As demonstrated by Hording and coworkers, HPV-positive tumors tend to have a warty or basaloid appearance whereas HPV-negative tumors tend to be keratinized. The former tend to be associated with premalignant vulvar changes (vulvar intraepithelial neoplasia).

Most vulvar malignancies are squamous cell carcinomas. Although this is a disease of older women, Franklin and Rutledge noted that 15% of cancers of the vulva in their series occurred in women younger than the age of 40. The incidence of squamous cell carcinoma of the vulva increases progressively with age.

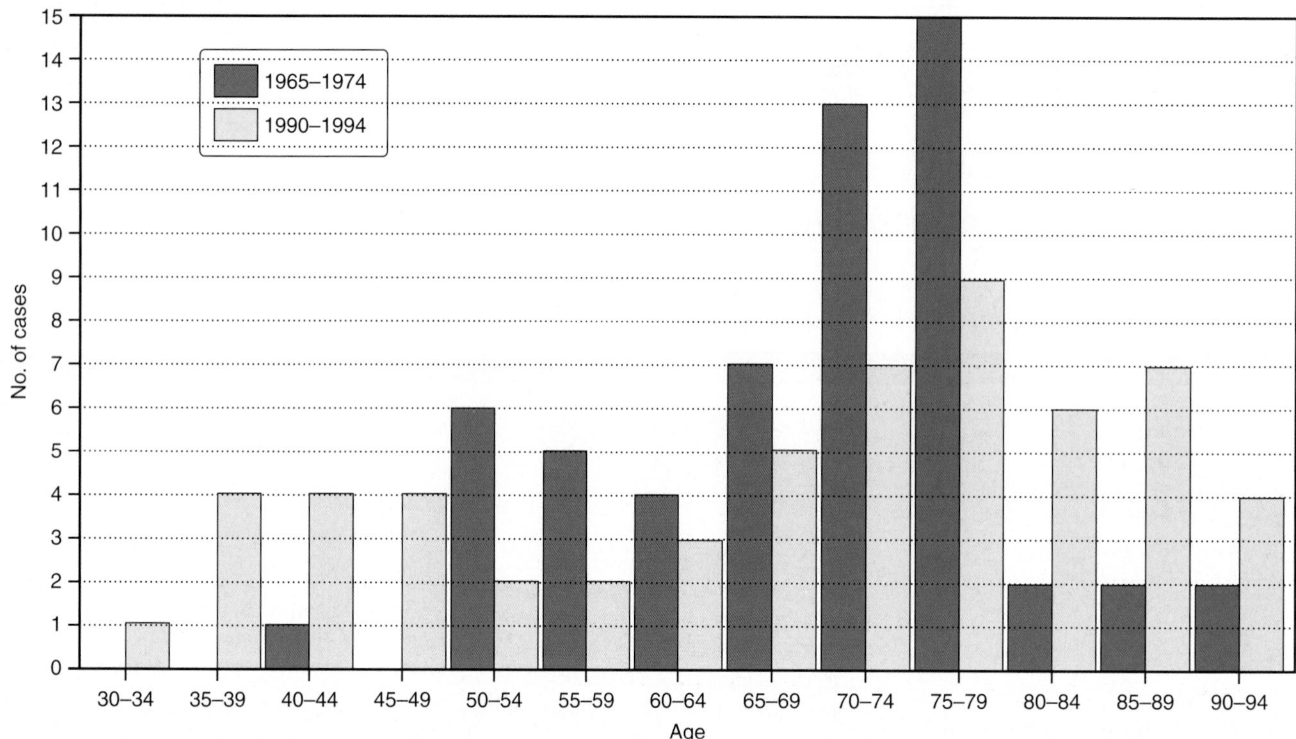

Figure 30-1. Age incidence curve for carcinoma of vulva in women from two different decades. (From Jones RW, Baranyai J, Stables S: Trends in squamous cell carcinoma of the vulva: The influence of vulvar intraepithelial neoplasia. Obstet Gynecol 90:448, 1997.)

Although more than half of patients with carcinoma of the vulva are older than 60 years of age at the time of diagnosis, Jones and colleagues have shown an increasing trend of squamous cell carcinomas of the vulva in women younger than 50 (Fig. 30-1). Although most patients with carcinoma of the vulva are older than 60, those with carcinoma in situ of the vulva are usually 10 to 15 years younger, that is, 40 to 55 years of age. In recent years, premalignant changes of the vulva are being seen with increasing frequency among younger patients, often in their 20s and 30s, possibly as a result of an increasing rate of multiple sexual contacts and increased exposure to venereal infections, particularly HPV, in this population. Carter and colleagues reported a link between immunosuppression and invasive squamous cell carcinoma of the vulva in women younger than 40. Similar to cervical cancer, HPV-related infections would presumably progress through dysplasia to invasive cancer in these immune-compromised women. This chapter reviews the clinical and pathologic aspects of premalignant vulvar lesions and vulvar atypias. This is followed by consideration of the diagnosis, natural history, and management of invasive cancers of the vulva, which includes not only the squamous cell carcinomas but also the rarer melanomas and sarcomas.

VULVAR ATYPIAS

Specific Conditions

Vulvar Atypias: Intraepithelial Neoplasia

Lichen sclerosus (Fig. 30-2) is a change in the vulvar skin that often appears whitish. Microscopically, the epithelium becomes markedly thinned with a loss or blunting of the rete ridges. In some cases, there is also a thickening or hyperkeratosis of the surface layers (Fig. 30-3). Inflammation is usually present. Hart and associates studied 107 patients with lichen sclerosus, and only one followed for 12 years eventually developed vulvar carcinoma. Five patients had vulvar carcinoma at the time that lichen sclerosus was diagnosed. Twelve other patients subsequently developed malignancies at other sites, such as the cervix, colon, breast, ovary, and endometrium. Patients with lichen

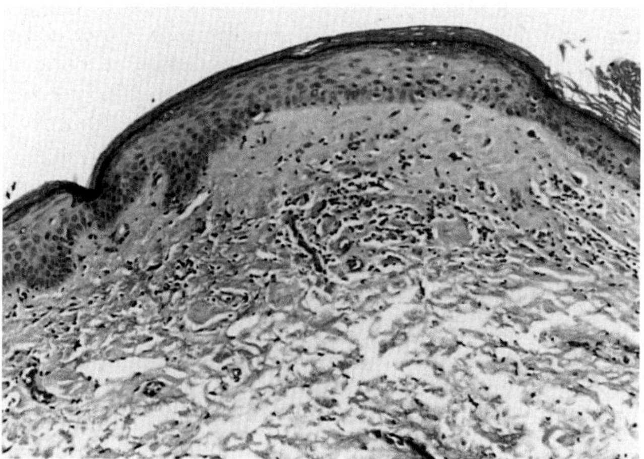

Figure 30-2. Lichen sclerosus et atrophicus. Homogeneous collagen in the papillary dermis is accompanied by a scattered lymphocytic infiltrate and atrophy of the epithelium. (H&E, ×80.) (Courtesy of Anthony Montag, MD, Department of Pathology, The University of Chicago.)

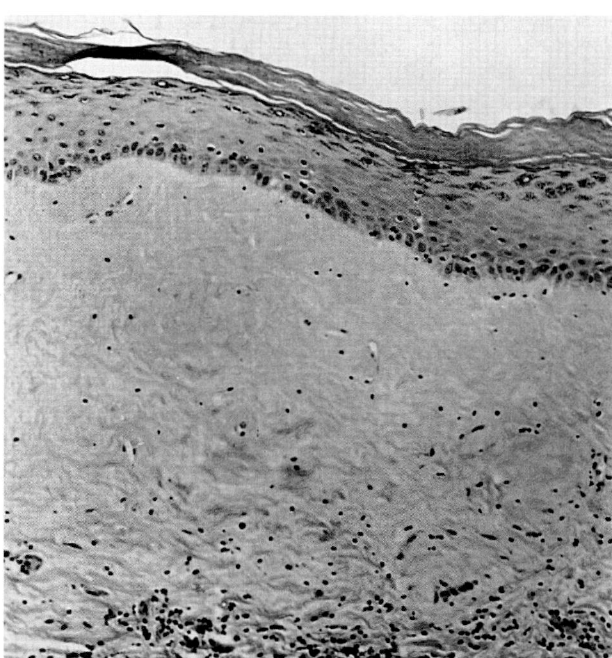

Figure 30-3. Lichen sclerosus. Hyperkeratosis is occasionally present. (From Friedrich EG, Wilkinson EJ: The vulva. In Blaustein A [ed]: Pathology of the Female Genital Tract. New York, Springer-Verlag, 1982.)

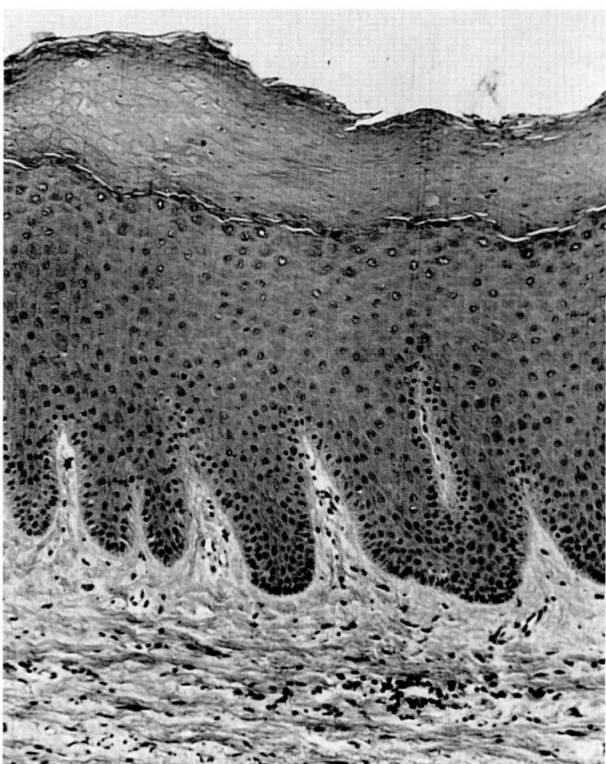

Figure 30-4. Squamous hyperplasia (formerly hyperplastic dystrophy), benign. Hyperkeratosis, acanthosis, and mild inflammation are present. (From Friedrich EG, Wilkinson EJ: The vulva. In Blaustein A [ed]: Pathology of the Female Genital Tract. New York, Springer-Verlag, 1982.)

sclerosus in the past were thought not to be at increased risk for the development of vulvar carcinoma. A study by Carlson and colleagues supports a small premalignant potential of lichen sclerosus. Their study and a literature review showed a risk of lichen sclerosus and squamous cell carcinoma was 4.5% with an average of 4 years latency between symptomatic lichen sclerosus and squamous cell carcinoma. The tumors that developed tended to be clitoral in location.

Squamous hyperplasia (formerly hyperplastic dystrophy) involves elongation and widening of the rete ridges, which may be confluent (Fig. 30-4). There may also be hyperkeratotic surface layers, and the tissue grossly often is whitish or reddish.

Atypical changes may appear in the vulvar epithelium. These changes are usually marked by a loss of maturation process usually seen in squamous epithelium as well as an increase in mitotic activity and in the nuclear-cytoplasmic ratio (Fig. 30-5). Mild dysplasia (atypia) is diagnosed if these changes involve the lower third of the epithelium; moderate dysplasia (atypia) if half to two thirds of the epithelium is involved; and severe dysplasia (atypia) if more than two thirds of the epithelium is affected. Carcinoma in situ involves the full thickness of the epithelium. The term *VIN I* is used for mild atypia, *VIN II* for moderate atypia, and *VIN III* for severe atypia, as well as carcinoma in situ. It is sometimes difficult to distinguish between squamous hyperplasia and intraepithelial neoplasia. Crum has suggested that VIN usually contains nuclei that are fourfold or greater different in size, whereas differences in the size of nuclei in condyloma or nonneoplastic epithelia are threefold or less. Furthermore, abnormal mitoses are usually observed in VIN.

Carcinoma In Situ (Vulvar Intraepithelial Neoplasia III)

Carcinoma in situ is diagnosed if the full thickness of the epithelium is abnormal (Fig. 30-6*A*). Occasionally, the process may histologically resemble carcinoma in situ of the cervix, and in many lesions, there are multinucleated cells, abnormal mitoses, an increased density in cells, and an increase in the nuclear-to-cytoplasmic ratio.

Paget's Disease

Paget's disease is a rare intraepithelial disorder that occurs in the vulvar skin and histologically resembles Paget's disease in the breast. Paget cells are large pale cells (Fig. 30-7). The cells often occur in nests and infiltrate upward through the epithelium. Frequently, histologic abnormalities of the apocrine glands of the skin may be noted in these lesions. There is an increased association of Paget's disease of the vulva with underlying invasive adenocarcinoma of the vulva, vagina, and anus as well as distant sites including the bladder, cervix, colon, stomach, and breast. Paget's disease of the vulva tends to spread, often in an occult fashion, and recurrences are frequent after treatment.

Diagnosis

Clinical Presentation

Atypias of the vulva present with a variety of symptoms and signs. Irritation or itching is common, although some patients

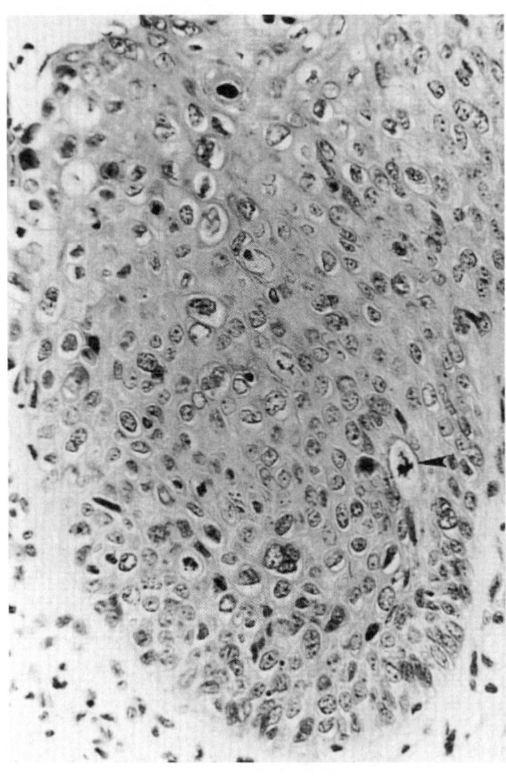

A

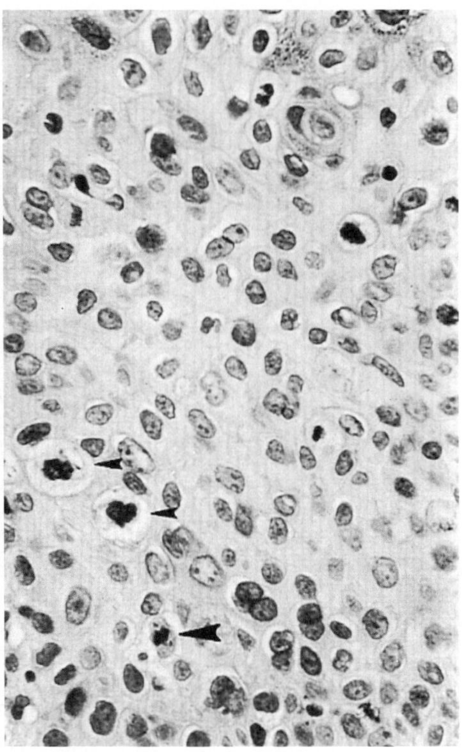

B

Figure 30-5. **A,** Vulvar intraepithelial neoplasia from which human papillomavirus type 16 was isolated. Characteristic features displayed here include abnormal mitoses (a two-group metaphase is denoted by the *arrowhead*), a full-thickness population of abnormal cells, and abnormal differentiation. Superficial cells contain perinuclear halos, which in contrast to condylomata are small and concentric. **B,** The higher power photomicrograph of vulvar intraepithelial neoplasia illustrates the marked variability in nuclear size and staining with both enlarged nuclei and multinucleated cells. Coarsely clumped mitoses (*small arrowheads*) and a three-group metaphase (*large arrowhead*) are present. (From Crum CP: Pathology of the Vulva and Vagina. New York, Churchill Livingstone, 1987.)

do not report these symptoms. The vulva often has a whitish change due to a thickened keratin layer. In the past, the term *leukoplakia* was used. This term has been discarded in part because abnormal lesions of the vulva require biopsy to establish a correct diagnosis. When lichen sclerosus is present, there is usually a diffuse whitish change to the vulvar skin (Fig. 30-8). The vulvar skin often appears thin, and there may be scarring and contracture. In addition, fissuring of the skin is often present, accompanied by excoriation secondary to itching. Areas of squamous hyperplasias (formerly called hyperplastic dystrophy without atypia) also appear as whitish lesions in general, but the tissues of the vulva usually appear thickened and the process tends to be more focal or multifocal than diffuse (Fig. 30-9).

Abnormal areas of vulvar atypia or VIN may also appear as white, red, or pigmented areas on the vulva. However, the clinical appearance of VIN is variable. Friedrich and colleagues estimate that approximately one third of patients with carcinoma in situ will present with pigmented lesions, emphasizing the importance of a biopsy to establish the diagnosis. The lesions tend to be discrete and multifocal and occur more frequently in those who have had squamous cell neoplasia of the cervix. In addition, reddish nodules may also be foci of Paget's disease as well as carcinoma in situ. Paget's disease often has a reddish, eczematoid appearance. It should be reemphasized that these conditions cannot be accurately diagnosed from their clinical appearance, and biopsies are needed.

Diagnostic Methods

In general, cytologic evaluation (Pap smear) of the vulva has not proven helpful, in part because the vulvar skin is thick and keratinized and does not shed cells as readily as the epithelium of the vagina and cervix. However, in some cases, particularly if there is ulceration of the vulva, a cytologic smear can be helpful diagnostically (see Fig. 32-6*B*). A tongue depressor moistened with normal saline or tap water is scraped over the surface portion of the vulva to be sampled, and the specimen is placed on a glass slide and then fixed.

The toluidine blue test (1% toluidine blue applied for 1 minute followed by 1% acetic acid) with biopsy of the retained blue staining areas has generally been discarded because it appears to be so nonspecific.

Colposcopy of the vulva is difficult because the characteristic changes in vascular appearance and tissue patterns that are seen in the cervix are not present (see Chapter 28, Intraepithelial Neoplasia of the Lower Genital Tract [Cervix, Vulva]). Nevertheless, the magnification of the colposcope may be used to help follow patients with VIN as well as to identify the discrete whitish or pigmented areas that warrant biopsy. The colposcope is not used for routine vulvar examination but is primarily used for those who are being evaluated or followed for vulvar atypia or VIN. However, the addition of 3% acetic acid highlights whitish areas for biopsy.

Biopsy of the vulva can be conveniently accomplished with a Keyes dermal punch (Fig. 30-10). Usually, a 3- to 5-mm diameter punch is used. Each area in which a biopsy sample is to be obtained is usually infiltrated with local anesthesia using a fine 25-gauge needle. The punch is then rotated and downward pressure applied so that a disk of tissue is circumscribed. When the entire thickness of the skin has been incised, the specimen is elevated with forceps and then removed with a sharp

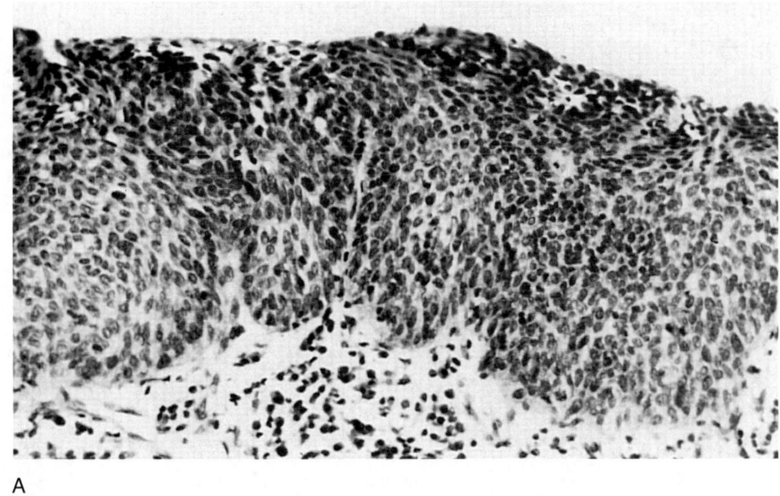

A

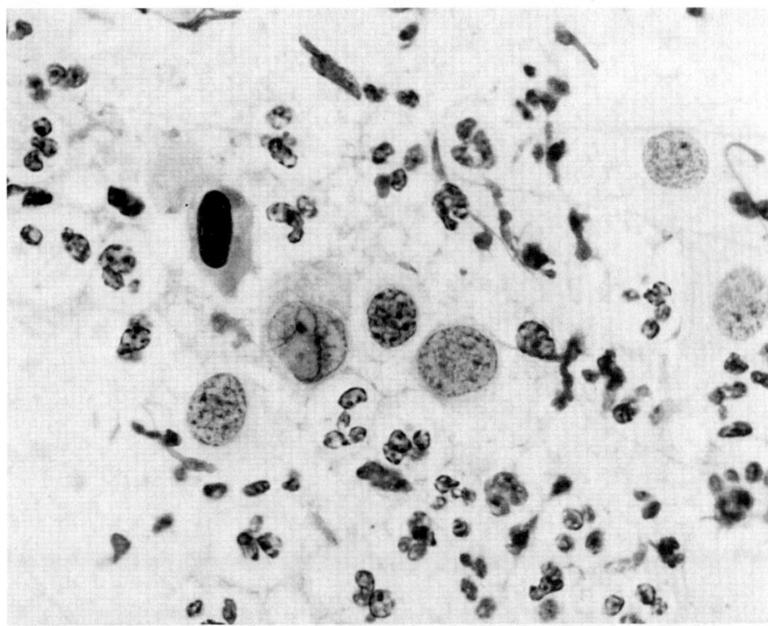

B

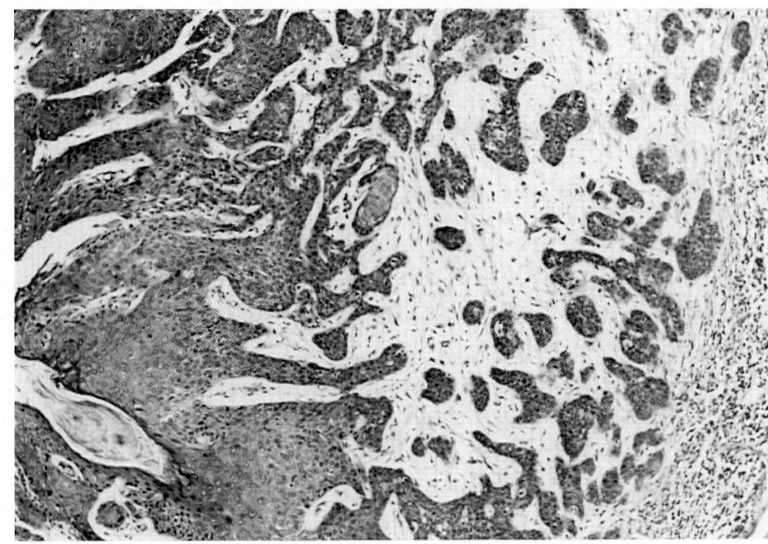

C

Figure 30-6. A, Carcinoma in situ: histology. Full thickness of epithelium is replaced by hyperchromatic cells with poorly defined cellular borders. (×80.) **B,** Carcinoma in situ: cytology. Cells derived from carcinoma in situ of vulva may exhibit varying sizes and shapes as depicted in this photomicrograph. Note variation in nuclear pattern from one nucleus to another. Degenerated polymorphonuclear leukocytes are present in background. (×800.) **C,** Invasive squamous carcinoma: histology. Tumor nests and cords infiltrate stroma. The squamous nature of tumor is more apparent on surface (*left*), where cells have abundant dense cytoplasm. Keratin is also seen. (×80.)

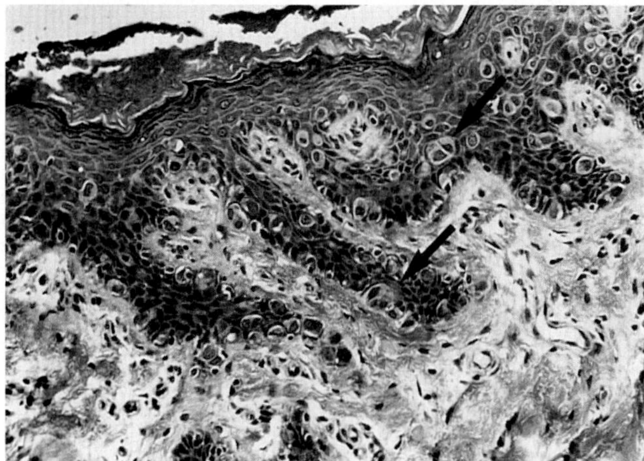

Figure 30-7. Vulvar epidermis with Paget's disease. Malignant cells (*arrows*) are seen infiltrating the epidermis and spreading along the dermal-epidermal junction. (H&E, ×160.) (Courtesy of Anthony Montag, MD, Department of Pathology, The University of Chicago.)

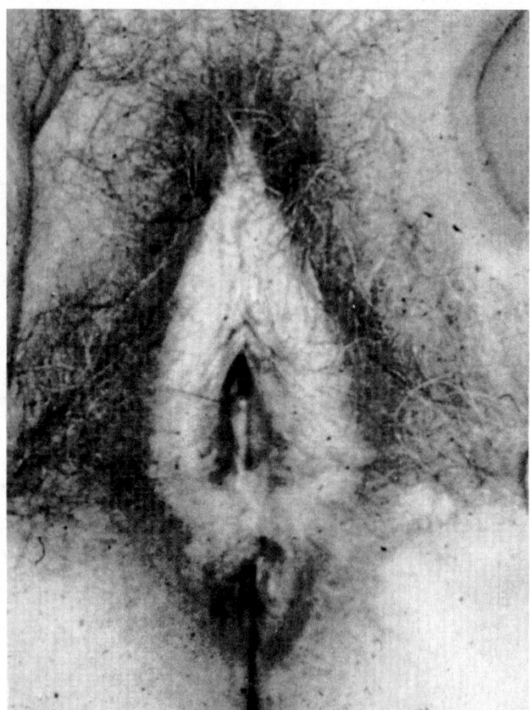

Figure 30-8. Vulva: lichen sclerosus. Tissue of labia minora and perineum has white, brittle "cigarette paper" appearance. (From Kaufman RH, Gardner HL, Merrill JA: Diseases of the vulva and vagina. In Romney SL, Gray MJ, Little AB, et al [eds]: Gynecology and Obstetrics. New York, McGraw-Hill, 1980.)

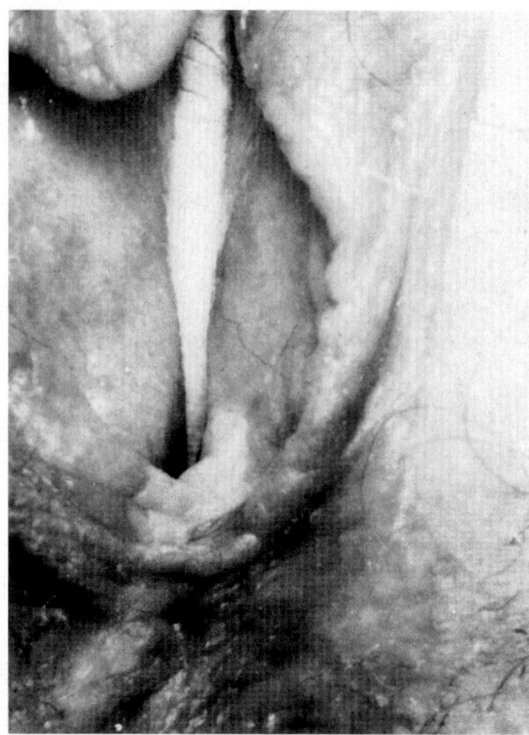

Figure 30-9. Vulva: hyperplastic dystrophy. Sharply demarcated, raised, white area is noted at lower tip of white pointer. (From Kaufman RH, Gardner HL, Merrill JA: Diseases of the vulva and vagina. In Romney SL, Gray MJ, Little AB, et al [eds]: Gynecology and Obstetrics. New York, McGraw-Hill, 1980.)

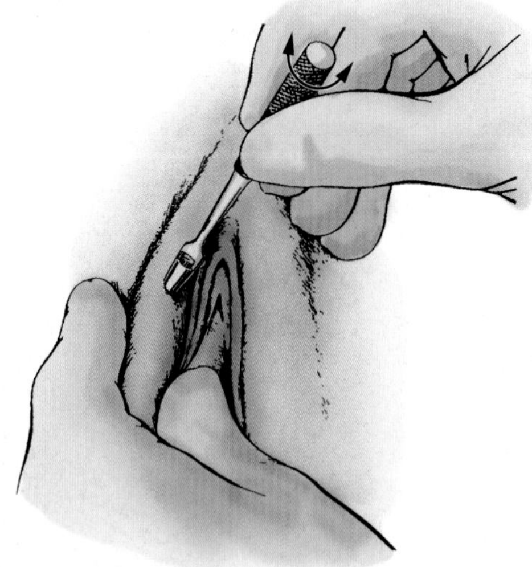

Figure 30-10. Diagnostic Keyes punch biopsy. (From Friedrich EG: Vulvar Disease, 2nd ed. Philadelphia, WB Saunders, 1983.)

scissors. Occasionally, a larger biopsy is needed, in which case a larger field is anesthetized and a small scalpel or cervical punch biopsy (see Fig. 28-14) is used to obtain the specimen. Usually little bleeding is encountered, and it can generally be controlled by applying silver nitrate or ferrous subsulfate (Monsel's solution). Depending on the size of the atypical area and the variety of atypical-appearing areas, one or multiple biopsies may be needed.

Management

Vulvar Atypias

Most vulvar atypias have pruritus as the major symptom, so the relief of itching is often the main concern of the patient. Once the correct diagnosis has been established by biopsy, appropriate therapy can be undertaken. Most whitish lesions will be benign, as lichen sclerosus is the most common condition encountered.

Topical testosterone can be used for atrophic conditions of the vulva, particularly lichen sclerosus. An effective preparation is 2% testosterone propionate in petrolatum, which is used twice daily. Once daily is often sufficient maintenance after the first week. Side effects, such as clitoral hypertrophy and increased hair growth, can occur. If there are undesirable side effects with testosterone, then local progesterone cream is sometimes tried, with variable success. Those who have a beneficial response to testosterone should be continued on the medication indefinitely. Often testosterone cream twice weekly is a sufficient maintenance dose. Another option for the treatment of lichen sclerosus is 0.05% clobetasol propionate ointment. This can be used twice weekly for 2 weeks and then used to retreat as necessary. Although lichen sclerosus can be associated with the development of squamous cell carcinoma, some believe that use of a potent steroid cream has a protective effect from malignant evolution.

The control of local irritation of the vulva is discussed in Chapter 18 (Benign Gynecologic Lesions). In addition to local measures to diminish irritation (cotton underclothes, avoidance of strong soaps and detergents, and avoidance of synthetic undergarments), topical fluorinated corticosteroids are helpful to control itching. Frequently used preparations are 0.025% or 0.1% triamcinolone acetonide (Aristocort, Kenalog), fluorocinolone acetonide (Synalar), or 0.01% or 0.1% betamethasone valerate. These are usually applied twice daily to control the itching, which is often relieved in 1 to 2 weeks. Unfortunately, the prolonged use of fluorinated topical steroids can lead to vulvar atrophy and contraction. Thus, once the symptoms of itching are controlled, the dose of topical corticosteroids is tapered off, or if long-term therapy is needed, a nonfluorinated compound such as 1.0% hydrocortisone is used to avoid vulvar contraction. Occasionally, 1% hydrocortisone is sufficient for initial therapy. In some cases, the corticosteroids are not successful, and numerous types of topical therapy need to be tried to control symptoms. Gentle soaps are helpful. Burow's solution (5% solution of aluminum acetate) is frequently used as a wet dressing to help control irritation and itching. Three percent Doak tar in petrolatum (USP) or in 1% hydrocortisone ointment is useful for severe cases.

In some patients with lichen sclerosus, severe contracture of the vulva, particularly in the area of the posterior fourchette, will occur with concomitant scarring and tenderness. Intercourse may then become painful in these patients. Woodruff and coworkers have described a useful surgical technique to treat these vaginal outlet disorders by plastic repair of the perineum. The contractured and fissured area in the posterior fourchette is excised, which results in an elliptical defect. This defect is then closed by undermining the distal 3 to 4 cm of the posterior vaginal mucosa and suturing the freed mucosa to the perineal skin (Fig. 30-11).

Vulvar Intraepithelial Neoplasia

Once the diagnosis of VIN has been established by biopsy, therapy is performed to eradicate the area containing the neoplasia. The clinician must be aware that the progress of vulvar atypia (mild dysplasia [VIN I]) to moderate dysplasia (VIN II) to severe dysplasia and carcinoma in situ (VIN III) and then to invasive carcinoma is not as well documented for vulvar neoplasia as it is for squamous cell neoplasia of the cervix. Moreover, vulvar neoplasia is frequently multifocal, requiring treatment of several areas. An additional complication is that some cases originally diagnosed as intraepithelial neoplasia have been reported to regress spontaneously.

In 1972, Friedrich reported Bowenoid atypia (histologically similar to carcinoma in situ) in a pregnant patient who regressed spontaneously postpartum. Others also reported spontaneous regression of this lesion. These spontaneously regressing lesions tend to be discrete elevations in young women. Some may be explained by studies of the nuclear DNA content of vulvar atypias that suggest not all lesions with this designation are premalignant. Fu and colleagues noted that only four of eight cases of vulvar atypia had an aneuploid (neoplastic) distribution. A polyploid distribution was noted in four of the cases, which is consistent with a benign process, whereas aneuploidy is consistent with intraepithelial neoplasia.

Although VIN is being diagnosed more commonly in younger women, the risk of progression to invasive cancer is higher for those who are older and for those who are immunosuppressed, such as transplant recipients. Chafe and associates studied 69 patients with a diagnosis of VIN treated by surgical excision. Unsuspected invasion was found in 13 patients. The median age was 36 years for those without invasive carcinoma, whereas the median age was 58 years ($p = 0.003$) for those with invasion found in the excision specimen, emphasizing the increased risk of invasion in the older patients. Furthermore, the risk of invasion was higher in those who had raised lesions with irregular surface patterns. Thus, patients who were older and those with irregular raised lesions had the greatest risk of unrecognized invasive carcinoma. A study by Modesitt and colleagues of 73 women with a mean age of 45 years found an invasive carcinoma in 22% of VIN III excision specimens. Not surprisingly, the risk of recurrence was almost 50% if the margins were positive and only 17% if they were negative. A frequency of 20% invasive disease in 78 patients was also reported by Husseinzadeh and Recinto. Twelve of the 16 malignancies occurred in patients older than age 40 years. The risk of progression from intraepithelial disease to invasive carcinoma appears to be less for vulvar cases than for cervical disease (see Chapter 28, Intraepithelial Neoplasia of the Lower Genital Tract [Cervix, Vulva]).

Current evidence suggests that the potential of VIN to develop into invasive cancer is low. Buscema and coworkers followed 102 patients with vulvar carcinoma in situ for 1 to 15 years without treatment, and four patients developed invasive disease, two of whom were immunosuppressed. Unfortunately, current techniques do not allow precise prediction of which lesions of VIN are at the greatest risk of progression to invasive disease. A recent population-based study from Norway confirms an increasing frequency of VIN III that nearly tripled in frequency in that country from the mid-1970s to 1988–1991. However, during the same period, the age-adjusted frequency of invasive vulvar carcinomas remained virtually constant. Iversen and Tretli further noted an estimated conversion rate of VIN III to invasive carcinoma of approximately 3.4% for these in situ lesions. Jones

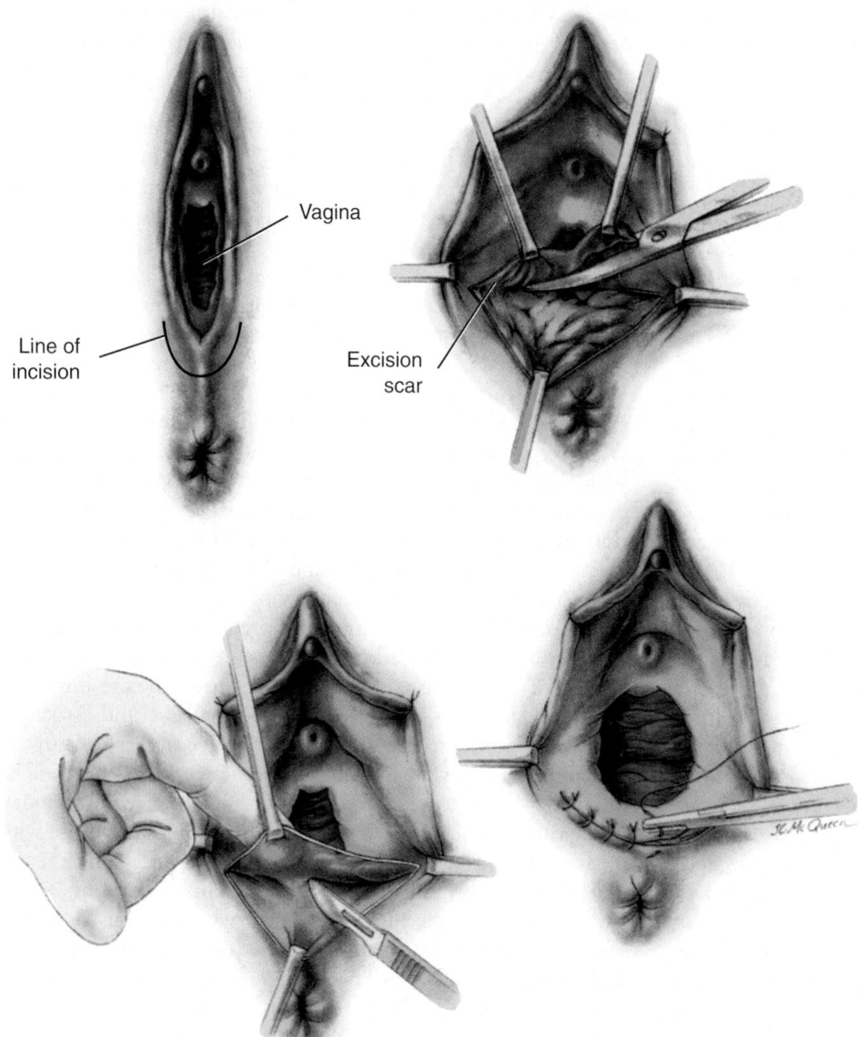

Figure 30-11. Surgical correction of perineal scars. (From Woodruff JD, Julian CJ: Surgery of the vulva. In Ridley JH [ed]: Gynecologic Surgery: Errors, Safeguards, Salvage. Baltimore, Williams & Wilkins, 1974.)

and coworkers recently noted spontaneous regression of VIN II–III pigmented lesions in young women younger than age 30 years.

Currently, HPV types 6 and 11 are generally recognized as being found most frequently in benign vulvar warts, whereas primarily HPV types 16, 18, 31, 33, and 35 are more frequently associated with intraepithelial neoplasia or invasive carcinoma (see Chapter 28, Intraepithelial Neoplasia of the Lower Genital Tract [Cervix, Vulva]). The Centers for Disease Control and Prevention estimate that 80% of women aged 50 will have acquired a genital HPV infection at some point in their life. Beutner and associates, on behalf of the American Medical Association, predicted that as many as 1 million new cases of perineal warts will occur annually in the United States. An additional complication is that HPV type 16 infection is not always accompanied by histologic evidence of VIN. Moreover, HPV types 6, 11, and 16 can be recovered from a single site, including those that show only condyloma as well as those that show carcinoma. Thus, a unique role for HPV types in VIN has not been elucidated. With the current state of our knowledge, therapy should be based on histologic findings and not on the presence or absence of HPV infection or specific HPV types. Studies by Buscema and associates suggest that HPV type 16 is frequently found in vulvar neoplasia, and, as noted previously, HPV 16 has been frequently associated with some vulvar carcinomas.

Therapy

The problem of the management of vulvar HPV infection is particularly complicated because it is extremely prevalent and the risk of progression from HPV infection to VIN is small. Planner and Hobbs evaluated 148 women with cytologic evidence of vulvar HPV infection and found that two thirds of them had pruritus and dyspareunia. Results of the biopsy revealed that 11 of the 148 women had VIN. Follow-up showed spontaneous regression of HPV infection in 56 patients, whereas VIN III developed in two and invasive cancer eventually developed in one. It appears that the best approach is to restrict therapy to individuals with clinically bothersome symptoms such as warts or to eradicate lesions with VIN, particularly VIN II and III. Cytologic or histologic evidence of an asymptomatic HPV infection, such as koilocytosis, is not an indication for therapy. Riva and colleagues treated lower genital tract HPV infection with laser to include the cervix, vagina, and vulva. Twenty-five patients had proven subclinical HPV infection, and the male partners were also evaluated and treated. All 25 patients suffered severe pain, and many required hospitalization. At 3 months after therapy, 24 of the 25 had evidence again of subclinical HPV infection and 22 had persistent histologic evidence of koilocytosis, indicating the futility of trying to eradicate HPV infection by this method.

Many lesions of intraepithelial neoplasia of the vulva tend to be posterior, predominantly in the perineal area. Surgical removal has been effectively used, but the type of operation has changed in recent years. In the past, simple vulvectomy was widely practiced to treat carcinoma in situ of the vulva, but this disfiguring operation is now infrequently used, particularly because the disease is occurring in younger women. To improve the cosmetic result and sexual function, Rutledge and Sinclair introduced the method of "skinning vulvectomy." This removes the superficial vulvar skin, preserving the clitoris, and replaces the removed skin with a split-thickness vulvar graft. In many cases, however, such extensive surgery is not needed. Often the abnormal area of the vulva can be removed only with wide local excision. Sixty-two of the patients in the series reported by Buscema and coworkers were treated with local excision; 68% showed no recurrence. For comparison, in 28 patients treated by vulvectomy, 70% showed no recurrence. The risk of recurrence is higher if neoplastic epithelium is found at the resection margin. Friedrich noted a 10% risk of recurrence if the surgical margins were free of disease compared with a 50% risk if the surgical margins were involved with neoplasia. However, because recurrence may develop even if the resection margins are negative, long-term follow-up is mandatory.

The carbon dioxide laser has been used to treat VIN, usually to a depth of 1 to 3 mm, with deeper depth being used for areas that contain hair. This results in eradication of the abnormal vulvar tissue and healing without scarring. Most patients require a single treatment, but some patients require more, particularly those with large or multiple lesions. Usually, patients can be treated on an outpatient basis with local, general, or regional anesthesia. The laser is particularly useful for younger patients. It is essential to be certain that the patient does not have invasive disease before using the laser, and therefore a biopsy of any suspicious lesions should be performed before laser ablation. The therapist should be experienced in the diagnosis and treatment of vulvar disease before using laser ablation. Older patients or those with raised lesions should be treated by surgical excision. Treatment is usually carried out to a depth of 3 to 4 mm, and healing is usually complete within 2 to 3 weeks. Leuchter and associates treated 142 patients with carcinoma in situ of the vulva. Of the 42 treated by laser, 17% had recurrence; four (25%) of the 16 treated with vulvectomy and 15 (33%) of 45 treated by local excision also had recurrence. In view of the risk of unsuspected carcinoma in older patients, as noted by the studies of Chafe and colleagues, those older than the age of 45 and those with raised or irregular lesions should have an excision performed and have the entire tissue submitted for histologic evaluation. Posterior lesions near the anus require particular attention because often the anal canal is involved, and this abnormal tissue also needs to be removed.

5-Fluorouracil (5-FU) cream has been tried to treat carcinoma in situ of the vulva, but it causes severe burning and is generally not used. More recently, investigators have explored using 5% imiquimod cream as primary treatment for VIN III with promising results. Using an escalating dose regimen of 5% imiquimod cream, Le and colleagues reported complete response in 53% of assessable patients with VIN II/III and another 29% undergoing partial response. Median time to response was 7 weeks, and the treatment was well tolerated with minimal burning and itching at the application site.

Paget's Disease of the Vulva

Paget's disease is generally seen in postmenopausal women and typically appears grossly as a diffuse erythematous eczematoid lesion that has usually been present for a prolonged time. Itching is a common problem. The disease is primarily seen in whites, and the average age of the patient is approximately 65 years. The major importance of Paget's disease of the vulva is the frequent association with other invasive carcinomas. Squamous cell carcinoma of the vulva or cervix or an adenocarcinoma of the sweat glands of the vulva or Bartholin's gland carcinoma may be present. Cases of adenocarcinoma of the GI tract and breast accompanying Paget's disease have also been reported. Once a diagnosis of Paget's disease of the vulva is made, it is important for the gynecologist to rule out the presence of breast and GI malignancy. In a review by Lee and associates, a total of 75 cases of Paget's disease of the vulva were identified, and an underlying invasive carcinoma of the adnexal structures of the skin was reported in only 16 (22%) and a carcinoma in situ in 7 (9%). Twenty-two of the patients (29%) had cancer at distant sites, including adenocarcinoma of the rectum, carcinoma of the breast, carcinoma of the urethra, basal cell carcinoma of the skin, and carcinoma of the cervix.

If no local or distant primary malignancy is uncovered, a wide excision of the affected area can be performed. It is important to remove the full thickness of the skin to the subcutaneous fat to be certain that all the skin adnexal structures are excised, as they may have a subclinical malignancy. Bergen and colleagues evaluated 14 patients with Paget's disease of the vulva treated by surgery, usually vulvectomy, skinning vulvectomy with graft, or hemivulvectomy. With a median follow-up of 50 months, all patients were free of disease, although two with positive margins and one with negative margins required treatment for recurrence. Fishman and coworkers studied 14 patients treated by various surgical procedures for Paget's disease. Either frozen section or gross visual inspection was used to judge the operative margins. In this series, visual estimation was as useful as frozen section insofar as the error rate for judging margins by the final pathology report was approximately 35%. In addition, two of five patients with positive margins had a recurrence after the initial operation compared with three of nine with negative margins. This small series, therefore, suggests that gross visual inspection may be as useful as frozen section when judging the extent of surgical operation. Other small series evaluating Mohs micrographic surgery for treating vulvar extramammary disease have failed to significantly reduce recurrence. A conservative approach involving removal of gross Paget's disease with approximately a 1-cm margin appears to be most appropriate, with the understanding that re-excision may be required for recurrence in the future. The full thickness of the vulvar skin to the adipose layer should be removed.

Even if resection margins are free of Paget's disease at the time of surgical excision, local recurrence remains a risk. Women who have been treated for Paget's disease of the vulva should have as part of their routine follow-up an annual examination of the breast, cytologic evaluation of the cervix and vulva, and screening for GI disease at least by testing for occult blood in the stool. Progression of Paget's disease of the vulva to invasive adenocarcinoma has been rarely reported.

MALIGNANT CONDITIONS

Squamous Cell Carcinoma

Squamous cell carcinomas comprise approximately 90% of primary vulvar malignancies, but a variety of other vulvar cancers are encountered; the primary ones are listed in the following box. Melanomas account for approximately 4% to 5% and the other types for the remainder.

Morphology and Staging

Grossly, vulvar carcinomas usually appear as raised, flat, ulcerated, plaquelike, or polypoid masses on the vulva (Fig. 30-12*A*). Biopsy sample of the lesion reveals the characteristic histologic appearance of squamous cell carcinoma (see Fig. 30-6*C*).

Four clinical stages are defined for carcinoma of the vulva according to the International Federation of Gynecology and Obstetrics (FIGO), similar to the system used for other gynecologic malignancies. In addition, many centers use the TNM (tumor, nodes, metastases) classification: T denotes the size and extent of the tumor, N the clinical status of the nodes, and M the presence or absence of metastatic disease.

In the clinical staging system, lymph node status was assessed clinically and incorporated into the stage. Enlarged or clinically suspicious lymph nodes were assigned a higher stage regardless of disease status documented at surgery. Clinically negative nodes were assigned an earlier stage, which was upheld even if they were found to harbor metastasis after surgical removal and pathologic examination. Therefore, in 1988, the FIGO staging was modified to a surgical staging system to more accurately reflect lymph node status. In addition, a location on the perineum is no longer assigned to stage III. This system with the modifications introduced in 1994 for stages IA and IB is shown in the following box.

Classification of Vulvar Atypias

Squamous cell hyperplasia (formerly hyperplastic dystrophy)
Lichen sclerosus
Intraepithelial neoplasia
VIN I: Mild dysplasia
VIN II: Moderate dysplasia
VIN III: Severe dysplasia-carcinoma in situ
Others
- Paget's disease
- Melanoma in situ (level 1)

VIN, vulva intraepithelial neoplasia

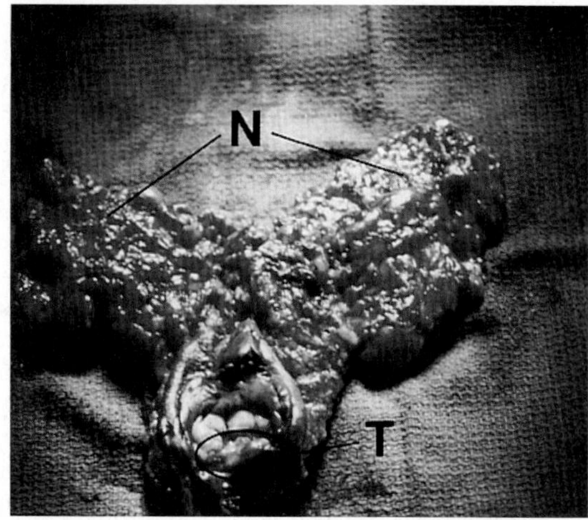

A

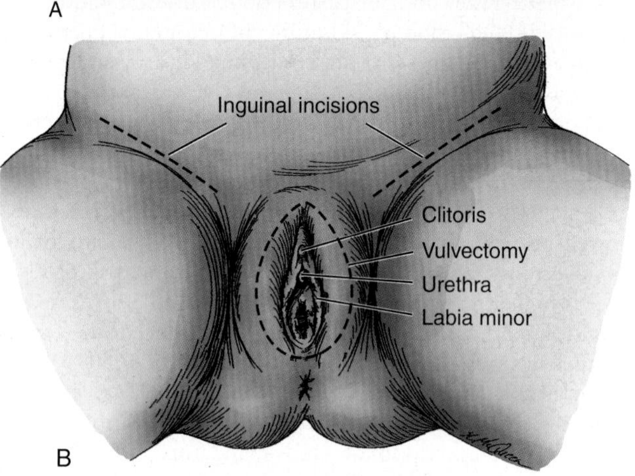

B

Figure 30-12. **A,** Radical vulvectomy specimen. **B,** Vulvectomy with operative incision lines shown. Note groin incisions.

Natural History, Spread, and Prognostic Factors

The vulvar area is rich in lymphatics with numerous cross connections. The main lymphatic pathways are illustrated in Figure 30-13. Tumors located in the middle of either labium tend to drain initially to the ipsilateral femoral-inguinal nodes, whereas perineal tumors can spread to either the left or the right side. Tumors in the clitoral or urethral areas can also spread to either side. From the inguinal-femoral nodes, the lymphatic spread of tumor is cephalad to the deep pelvic iliac and obturator nodes. Although there has been concern in the past that tumors in the clitoral-urethral area would spread directly to the deep pelvic nodes, this rarely, if ever, occurs. The characteristics of lymph drainage of the vulva were evaluated by Iverson and Aas, who injected technetium 99m colloid subcutaneously into the anterior and posterior labia majora, anterior and posterior labia minora, clitoral area, and perineum. They then measured the radioactivity in the pelvic lymph nodes, which were surgically removed 5 hours later. More than 98% of the radioactivity was found in the ipsilateral node and less than 2% on the contralateral side. The anterior labial injections resulted in

TNM and Staging Classifications of Carcinoma of the Vulva

TNM

T:	Primary tumor
Tis:	Preinvasive carcinoma (carcinoma in situ)
T1:	Tumor confined to the vulva and/or perineum, 2 cm or less in diameter
T2:	Tumor confined to the vulva and/or perineum, more than 2 cm in diameter
T3:	Tumor of any size with adjacent spread to the urethra, vagina, anus, or all of these
T4:	Tumor of any size infiltrating the bladder mucosa or the rectal mucosa or both, including the upper part of the urethral mucosa or fixed to the anus
N:	Regional lymph nodes
N0:	No nodes palpable
N1:	Unilateral regional lymph node metastases
N2:	Bilateral regional lymph node metastases
M:	Distant metastases
M0:	No clinical metastases
M1:	Distant metastases (including pelvic lymph node metastases)

Staging (FIGO) Modified 1994

Stage	TNM	Description
Stage 0	Tis:	Carcinoma in situ; intraepithelial carcinoma
Stage I	T1 N0 M0:	Tumor confined to the vulva and/or perineum, 2 cm or less in greatest dimension, no nodal metastases
IA		Invasion 1 mm or less
IB		Invasion more than 1 mm
Stage II	T2 N0 M0:	Tumor confined to the vulva and/or perineum, more than 2 cm in greatest dimension, no nodal metastases
Stage III	T3 N0 M0:	Tumor of any size with the following:
	T3 N1 M0 (1):	Adjacent spread to the lower urethra, vagina, anus, and/or the following:
	T1 N1 M0 (2)	
	T2 N1 M0 (1):	Unilateral regional lymph node metastases
Stage IVA	T1 N2 M0:	Tumor invades any of the following:
	T2 N2 M0	
	T3 N2 M0	
	T4 Any N M0:	Upper urethra, bladder mucosa, rectal mucosa, pelvic bone, and/or bilateral regional node metastases
Stage IVB	any T, any N, M1:	Any distant metastases, including pelvic lymph nodes

Modified from Shepherd JH: Staging announcement: FIGO staging of gynecologic cancers: Cervix and vulva. Int J Gynecol Cancer 5:319, 1995.
FIGO, International Federation of Gynecology and Obstetrics; TNM, Tumor—Nodes—Metastases.

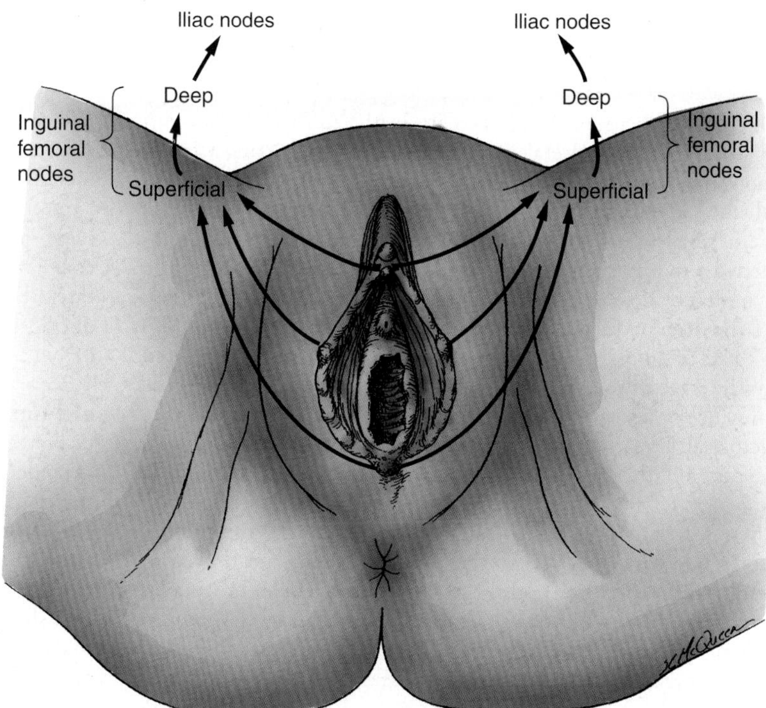

Figure 30-13. Vulva lymph drainage. General schematic representation of major drainage channels of vulva.

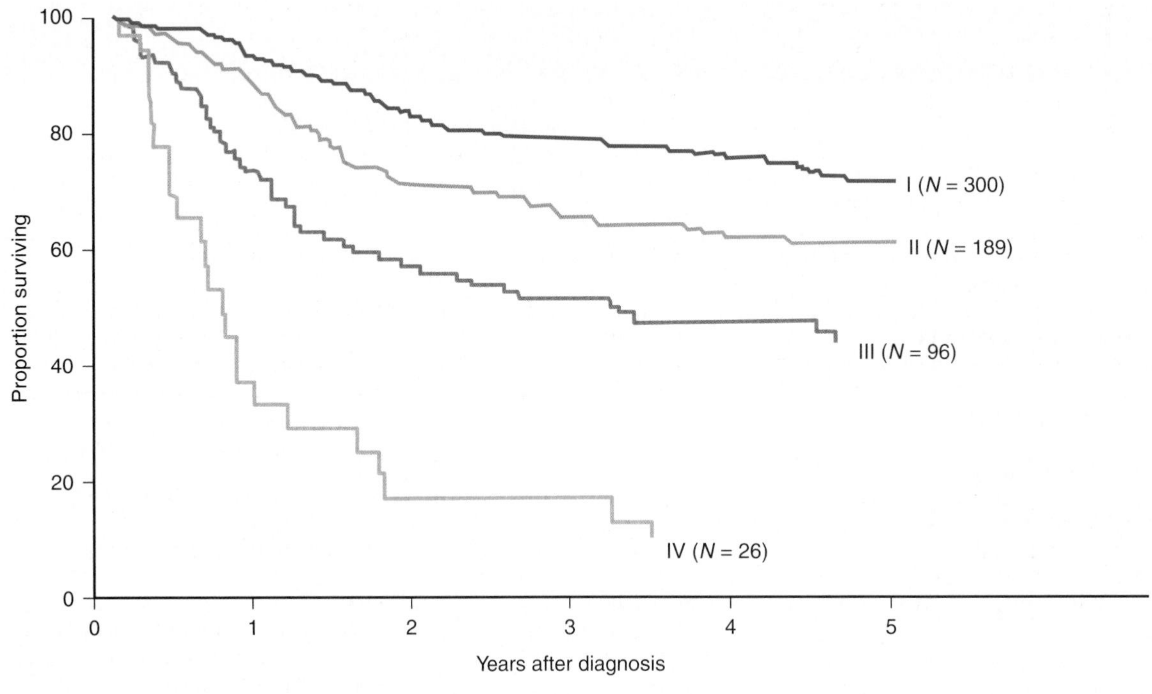

Strata	Patients (N)	Mean age (years)	Overall survival at 1 year	2 year	3 year	4 year	5 year	Hazards ratio[a] (95% Confidence intervals)
I	300	64.7	92.3%	82.3%	78.7%	75.7%	71.4%	Reference
II	189	67.4	86.5%	71.0%	65.8%	62.2%	61.3%	1.94 (1.36–2.75)
III	96	69.4	72.0%	57.2%	51.3%	47.5%	43.8%	3.84 (2.55–5.78)
IV	26	72.8	33.3%	16.7%	16.7%	8.3%	8.3%	12.2 (7.08–21.2)

[a]Hazards ratio and 95% confidence intervals obtained from a Cox model adjusted for country

Figure 30-14. Carcinoma of the vulva: Patients treated in 1990–1992. Survival by International Federation of Gynecology and Obstetrics stage (epidermoid invasive cancer only) (N = 611). [a]Hazards ratio and 95% confidence intervals obtained from a Cox model adjusted for country. (From Pecorelli S, Creasman WT, Pettersson F, et al: FIGO annual report on the results of treatment in gynaecological cancer, vol. 23. Milano, Italy. Epidemiol Biostat 1998.)

92% concentration of radioactivity in the ipsilateral side with 8% on the contralateral side. The clitoral and perineal injections developed a bilateral nodal distribution of radioactivity in all the patients. It is of interest that two thirds of the patients with labial injections had a small amount of detectable radioactivity in the contralateral nodes. Thus, anastomoses of the lymphatics do exist, but a direct connection from the clitoris to the deep nodes was not demonstrated.

The prognosis of a patient with vulvar carcinoma is related to the stage of the disease (Fig. 30-14), lesion size, as well as the presence or absence of cancer in regional nodes. The worldwide actuarial 5-year survival results from the 25th FIGO Annual Report on the Results of Treatment of Gynaecologic Cancer are stage I, 76.9%; stage II, 54.8%; stage III, 30.8%; and stage IV, 8.3%. The presence of carcinoma in regional lymph nodes correlates with the size of the primary lesion, the degree of tumor differentiation, and the extent of involvement of vascular spaces by tumor. Tumor size is usually estimated by the greatest tumor diameter; for example, smaller than 2 cm or larger than 2 cm separates stage I from stage II disease.

The status of the regional lymph nodes is the most important factor prognostically and therapeutically. Numerous studies, including a multicenter collaborative investigation from the Gynecologic Oncology Group (GOG), indicate that tumor stage, location on the vulva, microscopic differentiation, presence or absence of vascular space involvement, and tumor thickness are all important prognostic factors. In a GOG study of 588 patients reported by Homesley and colleagues, the risk of lymph node metastases was related to lesion size (19% for < 2 cm and 42% > 2 cm). Additional independent predictors of positive nodes were (1) tumor grade; (2) suspicious, fixed, or ulcerated lymph nodes; (3) lymphvascular space involvement; (4) older age of the patient; and (5) tumor thickness. Table 30-1 summarizes these factors.

Lymphvascular space invasion also appears to be a factor in vulvar tumors as it is in cervical carcinoma (see Chapter 28, Intraepithelial Neoplasia of the Lower Genital Tract [Cervix, Vulva]). In a small study of 22 patients, Rowley and associates noted no metastases in 20 patients without lymphvascular space invasion and in two of two patients with lymphvascular space invasion.

Table 30-1 Factors Related to Positive Inguinal Nodes (588 Cases)

GOG Grade	% Positive Nodes	Tumor Thickness (mm)	% Positive Nodes	Age (yr)	% Positive Nodes	LVSI	% Positive Nodes
1	2.8	≤1	2.6	<55	25.2	+	75
2	15.1	2	8.9	55–64	25.4	–	27
3	41.2	3	18.6	65–74	36.4		
4	59.7	4	30.9	>75	46		
		≥5	43				

GOG, Gynecologic Oncology Group. LVSI, lymphvascular space invasion.
Modified from Homesley H, Bundy BN, Sedlis A, et al: Prognostic factors for groin node metastasis in squamous cell carcinoma of the vulva (a Gynecologic Oncology Group study). Gynecol Oncol 49:279, 1993.

Stage IA: Carcinoma of the Vulva (Early or Microinvasive Carcinoma)

Definition and Clinicopathologic Relationships

The term *microinvasive carcinoma of the vulva* typically refers to lesion considered to be stage IA definition, that is, smaller than 2 cm with less than 1 mm invasion and is used to identify early tumors unlikely to spread to regional nodes. However, varying clinicopathologic results are reported when this definition is used.

Part of the confusion is due to different reference points from which the depth of invasion is measured, that is, from the surface or basement membrane. Dvoretsky and colleagues carefully analyzed the microscopic aspects of 36 cases of superficial vulvar carcinoma. Tumor penetration into the stroma was measured from the surface of the squamous epithelium (neoplastic thickness) (Fig. 30-15*A*) and also from the tip of the adjacent epithelial ridge (stromal invasion) (see Fig. 30-15*B*). Six of the 36 cases had spread to regional nodes, and all had invaded more than 3 mm from the surface. Kneale and associates have pointed out that although there is almost no risk of metastases to regional nodes in stage IA lesions, late recurrence of these tumors can develop years after primary therapy, and in a literature review, 8 instances of recurrence were reported in 88 cases of superficial vulvar carcinoma. All tumors were less than 2 cm diameter and invaded less than 1 mm into the stroma measured from the adjacent rete peg, which would approximately correspond to 3 mm measured from the surface because the vulvar epithelium is approximately 2 mm thick.

The presence of carcinoma in situ in the primary lesion decreases the risk of node involvement in these cases. Ross and Ehrman noted only one of 35 cases with adjacent carcinoma in situ had nodal metastases, and this tumor penetrated the

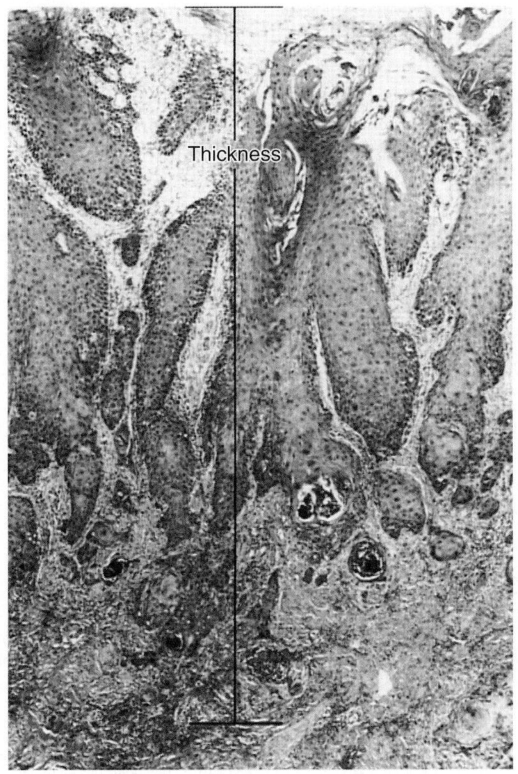

A

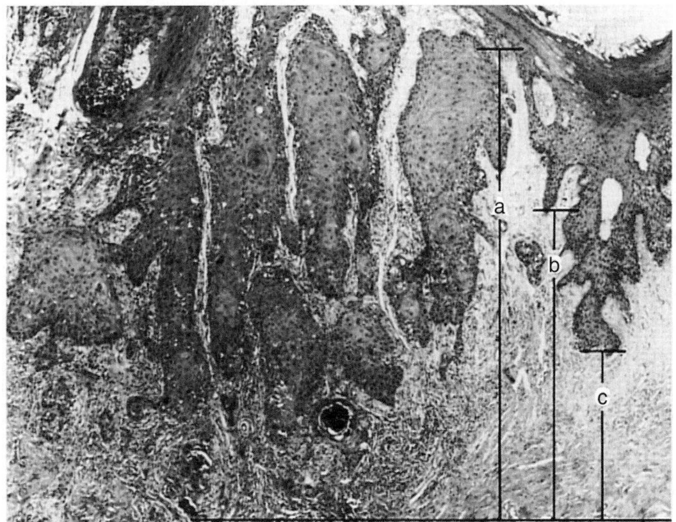

B

Figure 30-15. A, Measurement of neoplastic thickness in squamous cell carcinoma. (×35.) **B,** Superficially invasive squamous cell carcinoma. Reference point used to measure depth of stromal invasion is demonstrated by line *b.* Note striking variation in measurement of stromal invasion, depending on which reference point is chosen (line *a, b,* or *c*). (×35.) (From Dvoretsky PM, Bonfiglio TA, Helkamp BF, et al: The pathology of superficially invasive thin vulva squamous cell carcinoma. Int J Gynecol Pathol 3:331, 1984.)

stroma 1.7 mm. In contrast, 5 of 27 cases of superficial stage I cases (2.1 to 5.0 mm penetration) without adjacent carcinoma in situ had positive nodes. Thus, spread to regional lymph nodes in stage IA carcinoma of the vulva is unlikely, particularly if the tumor is well differentiated (grade 1), invades less than 3 mm measured from the surface or has a depth of invasion measured from the adjacent rete pegs of less than 1 mm, and is without vascular space involvement. The presence of carcinoma in situ is a favorable factor. Less well-differentiated tumors or those with vascular involvement or confluence and with greater depths of invasion have an increased risk of lymph node involvement by cancer.

Management

Based on available evidence, it would appear prudent that most patients with stage IA carcinoma of the vulva by the criteria previously described should be treated at least with a wide excision to give a margin of 1 to 2 cm. Depending on the location of the tumor, a hemivulvectomy may be needed. The lymph node dissection may be omitted or deferred, depending on the final pathologic evaluation of the tumor in the surgical specimen. For younger patients, especially with tumors that involve either the labia or the perineum at a distance from the clitoris, an operation that spares the clitoris should be used. Even if the criteria for stage IA is rigorously applied, a rare nodal metastasis may occur, as reported by Van der Velden and associates. However, a recent report by Magrina and coworkers on 40 patients with T1 lesions (less than 2 cm in diameter) and less than 1 mm invasion could be effectively treated with wide excision. No nodal metastases were noted in this small group, and excision appeared to be as effective as a more radical operation in preventing recurrent disease.

Invasive Carcinoma of the Vulva

Figure 30-12*A* shows a typical carcinoma of the vulva, which usually appears as a polyploid mass. The patient frequently reports a "sore" that has not healed. The patient may also report bleeding, but this does not usually occur early in the course of the disease. Unfortunately, the delay in diagnosis is common because older patients frequently fail to seek prompt medical attention, and often when they do, a biopsy is not initially performed. For example, some patients have their symptoms of irritation or itching treated with various medications to eradicate the symptoms. It is vital that a biopsy sample be taken of any vulvar lesion before undertaking therapy, as was emphasized earlier. A biopsy of a tumor like that shown in Figure 30-12*A* can easily be obtained on an outpatient basis using local anesthesia and biopsy forceps such as a Kevorkian punch as illustrated in Chapter 28, Intraepithelial Neoplasia of the Lower Genital Tract (Cervix, Vulva).

Effective therapy of clinical stage I or II and early stage III vulvar carcinoma can be accomplished with a wide radical excision and inguinal-femoral node dissection. Lesions located more than 2 cm from the midline typically need only an ipsilateral inguinal-femoral lymphadenectomy, whereas midline lesions necessitate bilateral groin dissections. Because the deep pelvic nodes are virtually never involved unless the inguinal nodes are also involved, only the inguinal-femoral nodes are removed at the time of the primary operation and the deep pelvic nodes subsequently treated with external radiation if the superficial nodes are involved with tumor. The inguinal-femoral node dissection is performed through separate inguinal incisions followed by the vulvectomy portion. Figure 30-12*A* shows the type of specimen that can be obtained through separate groin incisions. The operative incisions are shown in Figure 30-12*B*. It appears that an adequate surgical dissection with decreased wound complications can be accomplished by this technique. It is advisable to use suction drainage in the inguinal area until all drainage is complete, which usually takes 7 to 10 days, and drains are frequently also used in the vulvar area. It is important that an adequate margin, usually 1 to 2 cm, be obtained around the primary tumor at the time of surgery. Grimshaw and colleagues reported on 100 cases operated on through separate incisions and noted superb results with a corrected 5-year survival rate in stage I of 96.7% and stage II of 85%. Similar excellent results for separate skin incisions were reported by Farias-Eisner and associates on 74 patients with 5-year survival rates of 97% and 90% for stages I and II, respectively. Tumor recurrence has occurred rarely in the skin bridge over the symphysis when separate groin incisions are used, without an en-bloc dissection of the vulva and intervening lymph tissue. Magrina and coworkers noted comparable survival rates with fewer complications in those undergoing modified radical vulvectomy with inguinal incisions done separately.

In treating clinical stage I and stage II tumors of the vulva, the results of histologic evaluation of the inguinal-femoral nodes are important. Many therapists initially treat the superficial nodes above the cribriform fascia (Fig. 30-16). If these nodes are negative, the deep nodes are spared. The procedure can usually be accomplished with preservation of the saphenous vein, which was traditionally sacrificed. These modifications reduce the risk of leg edema. If the lymph nodes, particularly the upper femoral group, are involved with tumor, the deep pelvic nodes require treatment. Homesley and coworkers reported improved survival for those who received radiation (4500 to 5000 rad) to the deep pelvic nodes in comparison with those who had a pelvic node dissection.

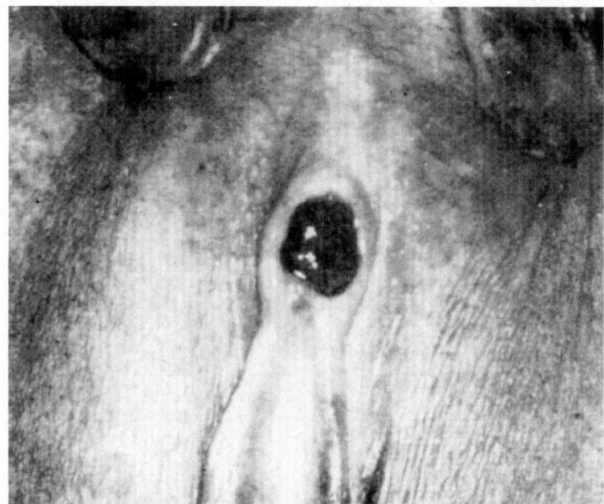

Figure 30-16. Nodular melanoma arising directly from glans clitoris. (Courtesy of J. McL. Morris, MD, deceased, Yale University School of Medicine, New Haven, CT.)

The results of therapy in clinical stage I and II disease relate not only to the stage of the disease but also to the status of the regional pelvic nodes. If the nodes do not contain metastatic tumor and the patient can be successfully treated by radical vulvectomy and bilateral node dissection, 5-year survival rates of approximately 95% are reported. Iversen and associates in a series of 424 patients noted lymph node metastasis in 10.5% of clinical stage I cases, 30% of clinical stage II, 66% of clinical stage III, and 100% of clinical stage IV. The number of positive nodes in the radical vulvectomy specimen correlates with the size of the primary tumor and also with the patient's survival. Andrews and coworkers noted in a study of T1 and T2 tumors that only unilateral inguinal node metastases occurred, and, furthermore, the deep nodes were involved only if the superficial nodes were positive. However, there is a small (2% to 3%) risk of contralateral node involvement of the larger T2 lesions. In a study of 113 patients, Hacker and colleagues noted an actuarial 5-year survival rate of 96% for those with negative nodes, but there was a progressive decrease in the survival rate to 94% for those having one positive node, 80% for two positive nodes, and 12% for three or more positive nodes. In various cases that have been studied, the deep pelvic nodes do not contain tumor unless the upper inguinal-femoral nodes contain metastatic disease. The number of nodes involved and the size of the metastasis are both important. Hoffman and coworkers noted that 14 of 15 patients with inguinal lymph node metastasis measuring less than 36 mm^2 survived free of disease 5 years compared with 12 of 29 whose lymph node metastases measured more than 100 mm^2. These results should be taken into consideration when planning additional therapy for patients with positive nodes.

If tumor spread to the regional inguinal-femoral nodes is identified, further treatment should be considered. If only one node is microscopically involved with tumor and the patient has undergone a complete lymph node dissection of the groin, usually no further therapy is needed, particularly if only a small volume is present. However, if one node is microscopically positive and the patient underwent a superficial inguinal-femoral lymph node dissection, many clinicians would be uncomfortable not treating the groin with adjuvant radiation therapy. If three or more nodes are involved, pelvic radiation as outlined is usually prescribed. For patients with only two nodes involved, the decision for further therapy will depend on the location of the nodes, the extent of groin dissection performed, and the size of the metastatic deposit of tumor, although most therapists would opt for radiotherapy in such cases.

Advanced Vulvar Tumors

Large tumors of the vulva, particularly those that encroach on the anal-rectal area or the urethra, may require more extensive treatment than radical vulvectomy to achieve effective tumor control. In such instances, it may be necessary to remove the anus or urethra as part of a primary operative procedure, in which case, diversion of the urinary or fecal stream is required (see discussion of exenterative surgery for carcinoma of the cervix in Chapter 29, Malignant Diseases of the Cervix).

For tumors that encroach on the urethra or anus, making procurement of negative margins improbable, multidisciplinary organ-sparing approaches may be used in an effort to reduce the morbidity of exenterative procedures. A useful therapeutic approach has been to treat large vulvar tumors with external radiation and then after the tumor has been reduced in size, remove the residual tumor surgically, usually by radical vulvectomy. External radiation is used to deliver approximately 4000 cGy to the tumor and 4500 cGy to the pelvis and inguinal nodes. The operation is usually performed approximately 5 weeks after the completion of radiation therapy. Although a large series of patients has not been treated by this technique, a sufficient number has been treated to demonstrate that marked tumor regression does occur. The primary cancer can be eradicated by an operation that does not require diversion of the urine or feces. Boronow and associates initially summarized the treatment of 26 patients with primary carcinoma of the vaginal vulvar area with this technique and noted a 5-year survival rate of 80%. Rotmensch and colleagues reported on 16 patients, 13 stage III and three stage IV, and achieved an overall 5-year survival rate of 45% with this technique, somewhat better than might be expected with stage III–IV (see Fig. 30-14). Recurrences are more likely if the resection margins were within 1 cm of the tumor. The introduction of chemotherapy with radiation appears to offer therapeutic advantage. Koh and coworkers studied 20 patients with stage III to IV disease and three with recurrence, using 5-FU with radiation. In addition, some patients also received cisplatin with concurrent radiotherapy. Actuarial 3- and 5-year survival rates in this small group were 59% and 49%, respectively. Similar results with 5-FU and radiation, occasionally with the addition of cisplatin, in 25 patients were also reported by Russell and coworkers. Moore and colleagues reported on a phase II GOG study and noted the need for a less extensive operation when chemotherapy with cisplatin and 5-FU were combined with preoperative radiation. Multiple chemoradiation programs are available, but a convenient outpatient regimen consists of weekly IV cisplatin with radiation usually to 4500 cGy. Other complications reported include stenosis of the introitus, urethral stenosis, and rectovaginal fistula, but this technique is an effective alternative to primary exenteration for large vulvar vaginal carcinomas and is preferred in most treatment centers, although success with exenteration can occasionally be achieved, as noted by Miller and associates.

Radiation Therapy and Recurrences

In a few instances, the medical condition of the patient precludes surgery, and radiation therapy may be employed as the sole treatment. However, the vulvar skin is prone to radiation dermatitis fibrosis and ulceration, making irradiation, as the sole form of therapy, a less desirable treatment. Therefore, irradiation is seldom used as the sole treatment of carcinoma of the vulva. To manage recurrences, reoperation is often tried. Piura and colleagues analyzed 73 patients whose disease recurred only on the vulva. Salvage was achieved with wide radical local excision, which appeared to be successful in 30 of the patients in whom the recurrence was only on the vulva.

As may be expected, the risk of recurring carcinoma rises as the stage of the disease increases. In an analysis of 224 patients with vulvar carcinoma, Podratz and associates noted a recurrence rate of 14% in stage I and 71% in stage IV. Local vulvar recurrences were the most common and occurred in 40 of

74 cases of recurrence (54%). The remaining recurrences were in the groin, pelvis, or distant sites. Radiation therapy or additional operations for local vulvar recurrences usually provide effective control and 5-year survival rates of approximately 50%. The risk of recurrence of the disease in the vulva requires careful attention to the surgical resection margins at the time of initial operation.

Combined chemotherapy and radiation has been used for primary treatment of late-stage advanced vulvar tumors as previously described. It has also been applied to recurrences, especially those near the anus and/or urethra. Radiation alone may also be used for vulvar recurrences, as reported by Perez and coworkers, although chemoradiation would appear to be a more effective choice.

Treatment of patients with disseminated disease requires chemotherapy, but, unfortunately, no chemotherapeutic regimen has been very successful in this disease. Squamous cell carcinomas of the female genital tract have generally not been responsive to cytotoxic chemotherapy, and the protocols followed are similar to those described for recurrent squamous cell carcinomas of the cervix (see Chapter 29, Malignant Diseases of the Cervix).

Quality of Life and Vulvar Carcinoma

Limited data have been published regarding quality of life in patients with vulvar cancer. Body image disturbance is significant and may account for decreased or absent sexual activity in women who have undergone vulvectomy. Interestingly, Green and colleagues noted that the extent of surgery or type of vulvectomy performed did not correlate well with degree of sexual dysfunction. The authors demonstrated a significant need to address sexual problems with all women undergoing any type of vulvectomy. The newly developed Functional Assessment of Cancer Therapy–Vulvar (FACT-V) is a valid and reliable instrument to assess quality of life in women with vulvar cancer. Perhaps this tool will be used to help assess quality of life and also to facilitate vital communication about quality-of-life issues in women with this disease.

Lymphatic Mapping and Sentinel Lymph Node Biopsy

As discussed, regional lymph node dissections are routinely performed in the surgical treatment of vulvar cancer as the status of regional lymph nodes is essential for therapeutic planning and overall prognosis. More than 80% of women with clinical stage I and II disease, however, will have no metastatic disease found in the lymph nodes, therefore making an extensive lymphadenectomy unnecessary while increasing postoperative morbidities such as lymphedema and lymphocyst formation. Lymphatic mapping and sentinel lymph node biopsy, as currently used in the treatment of patients with melanoma and breast cancer, are appealing techniques for patients with vulvar cancer. The sentinel node(s) are those nodes that directly drain the primary tumor and are thought to predict the metastatic status of the upper echelon or nonsentinel nodes in the groin. If the sentinel node is negative, in theory, all the other groin nodes would be negative too and surgeons could abandon full groin dissections, thereby greatly reducing the associated morbidities of lymphocyst, lymphedema, and wound separation. Frumovitz and colleagues recently reviewed the combined data on 279 patients with vulvar cancer who had undergone lymphatic mapping and sentinel lymph node identification. They found the overall sensitivity of the sentinel node for detecting metastatic disease in patients with vulvar cancer to be 97.7%, and the false-negative rate for the procedure to be 2.3%. The overall negative predictive value was 99.3%. Although these numbers are promising, at this time, lymphatic mapping and sentinel lymph node biopsy are considered experimental, with the standard of care remaining full inguinal-femoral node dissection.

Other Vulvar Malignancies

Bartholin's Gland Carcinoma

Bartholin's gland carcinomas are adenocarcinomas that comprise approximately 1% to 2% of vulvar carcinomas. An enlargement of Bartholin's gland in a postmenopausal woman should raise suspicion for this malignancy. These tumors are treated similarly to primary squamous cell carcinoma of the vulva, and radical vulvectomy with bilateral inguinal-femoral lymphadenectomy is the treatment of choice. If the regional lymph nodes are free of tumor, the prognosis is good. Rosenberg and associates reported five cases of adenoid cystic carcinoma of Bartholin's gland, a variant of invasive adenocarcinoma, treated by surgery (usually hemivulvectomy) and postoperative radiation therapy. Four of the five patients were living and free of disease 28 to 57 months after treatment.

Basal Cell Carcinoma

Basal cell carcinoma can arise in the vulva as it can arise in the skin elsewhere in the body. It is rare and comprises approximately 2% of vulvar carcinomas. Therapy consists of wide local excision of the lesion, which is generally ulcerated. If the surgical resection margins are free of tumor, the disease is cured.

Verrucous Carcinoma

Verrucous carcinomas of the vulva are also rare. They are a special variant of squamous cell cancer with distinctive histologic features. Clinically, they appear as a large condylomatous mass on the vulva. Histologically, they consist of mature squamous cells and extensive keratinization with nests that invade the underlying vulvar tissue. It is often necessary to perform multiple biopsies of the condylomatous lesion to establish a diagnosis of malignancy. Radiation therapy is ineffective and can worsen the prognosis by causing anaplastic change in the tumor and is therefore contraindicated. The treatment of an authentic verrucous carcinoma is wide excision.

In 24 cases of verrucous carcinoma, Japaze and coworkers noted no lymph node metastases. Some of the primary tumors were as large as 10 cm in diameter. Recurrences developed in nine of the patients, five of whom had previous radiation therapy. Wide local excision is effective therapy. Depending on the size and location of the tumor, simple vulvectomy may be needed, but a radical vulvectomy or inguinal node dissection is not indicated. The 17 cases treated surgically and reported by Japaze and coworkers had a 5-year survival rate of 94%. As noted by Crowther and associates, it is important to take a large biopsy specimen to establish the diagnosis. This is particularly important when dealing with a malignant-appearing tumor from a biopsy specimen that has been reported as benign. This can lead to incorrect therapy for condyloma acuminatum. Conversely, too shallow a biopsy may fail to show areas of squamous cell carcinoma that can coexist with verrucous carcinoma. However, in the presence of areas of squamous cell carcinoma, local excision is inadequate therapy. Verrucous tumors with squamous cell carcinoma elements can metastasize to regional nodes, and such tumors should not be treated as true verrucous carcinomas.

Melanoma

Melanoma is the most frequent nonsquamous cell malignancy of the vulva. It comprises approximately 5% of primary cancers of this area. As is true elsewhere in the body, melanomas arise from junctional or compound nevi. Pigmented lesions of the vulva are usually junctional nevi, and all such lesions should be removed by excision.

Patients with malignant melanoma of the vulva vary widely in age from the late teens to women in their 80s. The average age is approximately 50 years. Clinically, melanomas appear as brown, black, or blue-black masses on the vulva. The lesion can be flat or ulcerated. Occasionally, it is nodular, and small, darkly pigmented areas (satellite nodules) may surround the primary lesion. Some melanomas may be without pigment and can grossly resemble squamous cell carcinoma of the vulva. Most melanomas of the vulva occur on the labia minora or the clitoris (see Fig. 30-16).

Vulvar melanomas, if staged, use the same FIGO classification used for squamous carcinomas (see following box). However, staging is not as useful a prognostic indicator as is the depth of invasion. A system for vulvar melanoma analogous to that used by Clark for cutaneous melanomas has been adopted. Five levels (I–V) have been defined based on the Clark classification. Figure 30-17 shows the depth of invasion for each level of superficial spreading melanoma and nodular melanoma, the two most common varieties of melanomas that occur on the vulva. Superficial spreading melanoma is more common and fortunately has a better prognosis, with a 5-year survival rate of 71% reported in the series by Podratz and associates. The 5-year survival for nodular melanoma, which is more invasive, was only 38%. The level of invasion correlates with survival, which varies from 100% for level II, to 83% for level IV, to 28% for level V.

Tumor thickness is also useful to evaluate the tumor. Breslow reported that overall prognosis is excellent, and spread to regional node is not likely for melanomas whose thickness measured from the surface epithelium to the deepest point of penetration is less than 0.76 mm. Most of these lesions would correspond to level I or II penetration by the modified Clark system. Stefanon and coworkers, in a study of 28 patients, noted no lymph node metastasis if melanoma thickness was less than 3 mm and the 5-year survival rate in this group was 50% compared with 25% for those whose melanomas were more than 3 mm thick. In a comprehensive long-term study of 219 Swedish females, Ragnarsson-Olding and coworkers noted that tumor thickness and ulceration were prognostic factors. In addition, gross amelanosis and advanced age worsened the prognosis. The authors further noted that amelanotic tumors were seen in approximately one fourth of the patients and that overall the vulvar melanomas were approximately 2.5 times more frequent than cutaneous melanomas. A preexisting nevus was not necessary and de novo melanoma development does

Primary Vulvar Malignancies

- Squamous cell carcinoma
- Adenocarcinoma (including Bartholin's gland)
- Verrucous carcinoma
- Basal cell carcinoma
- Melanoma
- Sarcoma

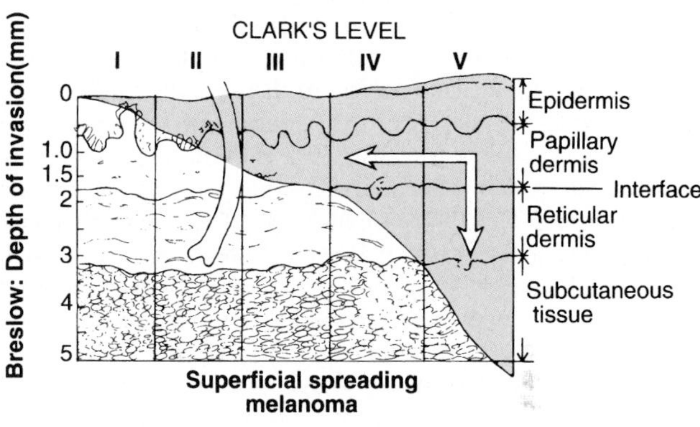

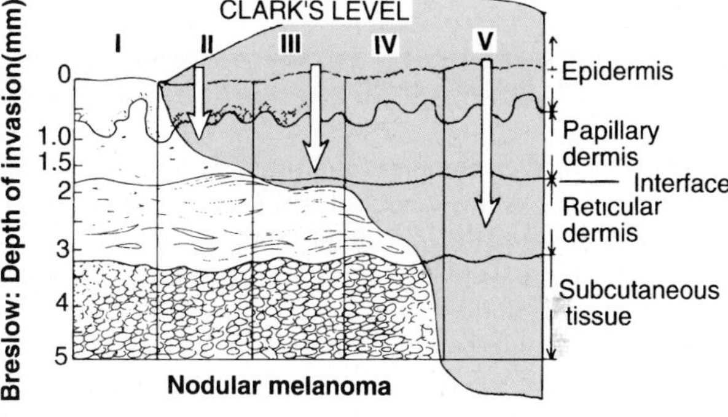

Figure 30-17. Level of invasion for superficial spreading melanoma and nodular melanoma. (From Podratz KC, Gaffey TA, Symmonds RE, et al: Melanoma of the vulva: An update. Gynecol Oncol 16:153, 1983.)

appear to occur on the vulva, particularly in the glabrous (hairless) skin.

The standard therapy for vulvar melanoma is a wide excision of the primary tumor. Because the tumors are rare, a large clinical experience is not available. It was believed that melanoma of the vulva could metastasize to pelvic nodes, bypassing the inguinal femoral nodes; current evidence indicates that there is no pelvic node involvement without previous inguinal node involvement. A further therapeutic consideration is that patients with melanoma whose pelvic nodes are involved with tumor usually do not survive the disease.

Excision margins have been extensively studied for cutaneous melanomas. Veronesi and colleagues found that cutaneous melanomas less than 2 mm thick could be adequately treated with a 1-cm margin, which was as effective as a 3-cm margin for these thin lesions. Although comparable data do not exist for vulvar melanomas, the data from cutaneous melanomas suggest that a 1-cm margin could be used for very thin vulvar melanomas. In a report of 36 melanoma cases, Rose and associates noted that wide excision was as effective as radical vulvectomy. They noted that the prognosis was improved in younger patients, presumably because most of them had superficial spreading (good prognosis) rather than nodular (poor prognosis) melanomas. Although firm recommendations from available data are not possible, a reasonable approach would be to excise a melanoma with a 2-cm margin without node dissection for tumors that are less than 0.76 mm thick. An excision with a 2- to 3-cm margin combined with node dissection would be carried out for more advanced melanomas.

For lesions that correspond to Clark's level 1 or 2, that is, less than 0.76 mm thick, a wide local excision results in 5-year survival rates in the vicinity of 100%. The prognosis is poor for patients with melanomas more than 3 mm thick. If the regional nodes are negative, the survival rate is greater than 60%, but decreases to less than 30% if the regional nodes are involved with tumor. Most series of malignant melanoma report overall survival rates of approximately 50%. Although metastases of melanoma to regional inguinal nodes are usually fatal, isolated prolonged survivals have been observed, as was reported by Trimble and colleagues and also by Tasseron and associates, who noted in a series of 30 patients that 6 had positive nodes and 2 survived for more than 5 years.

Distant metastases are frequently noted, and no effective program of chemotherapy has been described. Regressions (but not cures) have been reported with various multiagent cytotoxic programs. Current efforts are devoted to developing an effective program of bioimmunotherapy.

Sarcoma

Sarcomas of the vulva are extremely rare, accounting for less than 3% of vulvar cancers. Leiomyosarcomas are the most common histologic subtype found followed by liposarcomas, neurofibrosarcomas, angiosarcomas, and epithelioid sarcomas. To date, the largest series of vulvar sarcomas in the literature are 12 cases reported by DiSaia and associates. In their series, they found surgical removal of the primary tumor to be the treatment of choice. Chemotherapeutic considerations are the same as those for sarcomas of other sites in the female genital tract.

Granular Cell Myoblastomas

Granular cell myoblastoma is also an extremely rare tumor that is almost invariably benign but does morphologically show pleomorphism. Local excision is generally sufficient therapy. The tumor appears as a solitary, firm, nontender, slowly growing nodule in the subcutaneous tissue of the vulva.

KEY POINTS

- Squamous cell carcinomas comprise 90% of primary vulvar malignancies. More than half the patients are older than 60 years of age at the time of diagnosis.
- Cancer of the vulva accounts for approximately 4% of malignancies of the lower female genital tract and is less frequent than uterine, ovarian, and cervical cancers.
- Paget's disease generally occurs in postmenopausal women and is usually treated by wide excision. Invasive carcinomas at other sites should be ruled out.
- Prolonged use of fluorinated corticosteroids to treat itching accompanying vulvar dystrophy can lead to vulvar contraction.
- Topical testosterone is often beneficial to treat lichen sclerosus but is absorbed systemically and occasionally can produce masculinizing symptoms.
- Recent studies indicate symptomatic lichen sclerosus is a premalignant condition preceding carcinoma by a mean of 4.0 years. The tumors that do develop tend to be clitoral in location and are in patients older than age 40 years.
- HPV vulvar infection is common. Intraepithelial neoplasia occurs much less frequently.
- HPV-positive tumors tend to occur in younger patients, and these tumors tend to have a better prognosis than HPV-negative tumors.
- A clear progression of dysplasia–carcinoma in situ (VIN I, II, and III) to invasive carcinoma in the vulva has not been clearly established. VIN may spontaneously regress. VIN III has an approximate 3.4% risk of progression to invasive carcinoma.
- Intraepithelial neoplasia of the vulva is usually treated by local excision. Laser therapy of the atypical area may be used in younger patients who do not have raised lesions.
- Vulvar carcinomas less than 2 cm in diameter and with a depth of invasion less than 1 mm (3-mm thickness) rarely metastasize to regional nodes.
- Unilateral vulvar tumors (>2 cm from midline) usually metastasize to ipsilateral inguinal-femoral nodes only.
- Prognosis in vulvar cancer is primarily related to lesion size, lymph node status, and stage.
- The risk of lymph node groin metastases is related to tumor differentiation, lesion thickness, lymphvascular space involvement, patient age, and tumor size.
- The deep pelvic nodes do not become involved with metastatic vulvar cancer unless the inguinal-femoral nodes are affected.
- The 5-year survival rate of vulvar carcinoma with negative nodes is more than 95%. With one positive node, the 5-year survival is approximately the same, that is, 94%; with two nodes, it decreases to 80%; with three or more, to 12%.
- The worldwide 5-year survival rate for carcinoma of the vulva by stage is I, 71.4%; II, 61.3%; III, 43.8%; and IV, 8.3%.
- Advanced vulvar tumors encroaching on the urethra and/or anus may be treated by preliminary radiation followed by wide radical excision rather than exenteration. Enhanced results have also been reported with the combined use of chemotherapy and radiation.
- Verrucous carcinomas are a variant of squamous cancer that do not metastasize to regional nodes. Radiation therapy is

KEY POINTS *Continued*

contraindicated, and local surgical excision is the treatment of choice.

- Melanomas comprise 5% of vulvar cancers and are the most frequent nonsquamous cell malignancies.
- The overall 5-year survival of patients with vulvar melanoma is approximately 50%.
- Superficial spreading melanomas tend to occur in younger patients and have a better prognosis than nodular melanomas.
- Prognosis of vulvar melanoma is related to tumor invasion (Clark's level) and to tumor thickness.
- Basal cell carcinoma of the vulva is treated by wide local excision.

BIBLIOGRAPHY

Andrews SJ, Williams BT, DePriest PD, et al: Therapeutic implications of lymph nodal spread in lateral T_1 and T_2 squamous cell carcinoma of the vulva. Gynecol Oncol 55:41, 1994.

Baehrendtz H, Einhorn N, Pettersson F, Silfersward C: Paget's disease of the vulva: The Radiumhemmet series 1975–1990. Int J Gynecol Cancer 4:1, 1994.

Beller U, Maisonneuve P, Benedet JL, et al: Carcinoma of the vulva. Int J Gynaecol Obstet 83:7, 2003.

Bergen S, DiSaia PJ, Liao SY, et al: Conservative management of extramammary Paget's disease of the vulva. Gynecol Oncol 33:151, 1989.

Berman ML, Soper JT, Creasman WT, et al: Conservative surgical management in superficially invasive stage I vulvar carcinoma. Gynecol Oncol 35:352, 1989.

Beutner KR, Reitano MV, Richwald GA, et al: External genital warts: Report of the American Medical Association consensus conference. Clin Infect Dis 27:796, 1998.

Boronow RC, Hickman BT, Reagan MT, et al: Combined therapy as an alternative to exenteration for locally advanced vulvovaginal cancer. Am J Clin Oncol 10:1711, 1987.

Breslow A: Thickness, cross-sectional areas, and depth of invasion in the prognosis of cutaneous melanoma. Ann Surg 172:908, 1970.

Buscema J, Woodruff JD, Parmley TH, et al: Carcinoma in situ of the vulva. Obstet Gynecol 55:225, 1980.

Carlson JA, Ambros R, Malfetano J, et al: Vulvar lichen sclerosus and squamous cell carcinoma: A cohort, case control, and investigational study with historical perspective; implications for chronic inflammation and sclerosus in the development of neoplasia. Hum Pathol 29:932, 1998.

Carter J, Carlson J, Fowler J, et al: Invasive vulvar tumors in young women—a disease of the immunosuppressed? Gynecol Oncol 51:307, 1993.

Chafe W, Richards A, Morgan L, Wilkinson E: Unrecognized invasive carcinoma in vulvar intraepithelial neoplasia (VIN). Gynecol Oncol 31:154, 1988.

Chamorro T: Cancer of the vulva and vagina. Semin Oncol Nurs 6:198, 1990.

Christopherson W, Buchsbaum HJ, Vort R, et al: Radical vulvectomy and bilateral groin lymphadenectomy utilizing separate groin incisions: Report of a case with recurrence in the intervening skin bridge. Gynecol Oncol 21:247, 1985.

Creasman WT: New gynecologic cancer staging. Gynecol Oncol 58:157, 1995.

Crowther ME, Lowe DG, Shepherd JH: Verrucous carcinoma of the female genital tract. A review. Obstet Gynecol Surv 43:263, 1988.

Crum CP: Vulvar intraepithelial neoplasia: histology and associated viral changes. In Wilkinson EJ (ed): Pathology of the Vulva and Vagina. New York, Churchill Livingstone, 1987.

Curtin JP, Rubey SR, Jones WB, et al: Paget's disease of the vulva. Gynecol Oncol 39:374, 1990.

DiSaia PJ, Rutledge F, Smith JP: Sarcoma of the vulva-report of 12 patients. Obstet Gynecol 38:180, 1971.

Dvoretsky PM, Bonfiglio TA, Helkamp BF, et al: The pathology of superficially invasive thin vulva squamous cell carcinoma. Int J Gynecol Pathol 3:331, 1984.

Farias-Eisner R, Cirisano FD, Grouse D, et al: Conservative and individualized surgery for early squamous carcinoma of the vulva: the treatment of choice for stage I and II (T_{1-2} N_{0-1} M_0) disease. Gynecol Oncol 53:55, 1994.

Fishman DA, Chambers SK, Schwartz PE, et al: Extramammary Paget's disease of the vulva. Gynecol Oncol 56:266, 1995.

Franklin EW 3rd, Rutledge FD: Epidemiology of epidermoid carcinoma of the vulva. Obstet Gynecol 39:165, 1972.

Friedrich EG Jr: Reversible vulvar atypia: a case report. Obstet Gynecol 39:173, 1972.

Friedrich EG, Wilkinson EJ, Fu YS: Carcinoma in situ of the vulva: a continuing challenge. Am J Obstet Gynecol 136:830, 1980.

Frumovitz M, Ramirez PT, Levenback CL: Lymphatic mapping and sentinel node detection in gynecologic malignancies of the lower genital tract. Curr Oncol Rep 7:435, 2005.

Fu YS, Reagan JW, Townsend DE, et al: Nuclear DNA study of vulvar intraepithetial and invasive squamous neoplasms. Obstet Gynecol 57:643, 1981.

Green MS, Naumann RW, Elliot M, et al: Sexual dysfunction following vulvectomy. Gynecol Oncol 77:73, 2000.

Grimshaw RN, Murdoch JB, Monaghan JM: Radical vulvectomy and bilateral inguinal-femoral lymphadenectomy through separate incisions: Experience with 100 cases. Int J Gynecol Cancer 3:18, 1993.

Hacker NF, Berek JS, Lagasse LD, et al: Management of regional lymph nodes and their prognostic influence in vulvar cancer. Obstet Gynecol 61:408, 1983.

Hart WR, Norris HJ, Helwig ED: Relation of lichen sclerosus et atrophicus of the vulva to development of carcinoma. Obstet Gynecol 45:369, 1975.

Hoffman JS, Kumar NB, Morley GW: Prognostic significance of groin lymph node metastases of squamous carcinoma of the vulva. Obstet Gynecol 66:402, 1985.

Homesley HD, Bundy BN, Sedlis A, Adcock L: A randomized study of radiation therapy versus pelvic node resection for patients with invasive squamous cell carcinoma of the vulva having positive groin nodes (a Gynecologic Oncology Group study). Obstet Gynecol 68:733, 1986.

Homesley HD, Bundy BN, Sedlis A, et al: Assessment of current International Federation of Gynecology and Obstetrics staging of vulvar carcinoma relative to prognostic factors for survival (a Gynecologic Oncology Group study). Am J Obstet Gynecol 164:997, 1991.

Homesley HD, Bundy BN, Sedlis A, et al: Prognostic factors for groin node metastasis in squamous cell carcinoma of the vulva (a Gynecologic Oncology Group study). Gynecol Oncol 49:279, 1993.

Hording U, Junge J, Daugaard S, et al: Vulvar squamous cell carcinoma and papillomaviruses: Indications for two different etiologies. Gynecol Oncol 52:241, 1994.

Husseinzadeh N, Recinto C: Frequency of invasive cancer in surgically excised vulvar lesions with intraepithelial neoplasia (VIN 3). Gynecol Oncol 73:119, 1999.

Iversen T, Aas M: Lymph drainage from the vulva. Gynecol Oncol 16:179, 1983.

Iversen T, Abler V, Aalder J: Individual treatment of stage I carcinoma of the vulva. Obstet Gynecol 57:85, 1981.

Iversen T, Elders JG, Christensen A, et al: Squamous cell carcinoma of the vulva: Review of 424 patients, 1957–1974. Gynecol Oncol 9:271, 1980.

Iversen T, Tretli S: Intraepithelial and invasive squamous cell neoplasia of the vulva: Trends in incidence, recurrence, and survival rate in Norway. Obstet Gynecol 91:969, 1998.

Janda M, Obermair A, Cella D, et al: The functional assessment of cancer-vulvar: Reliability and validity. Gynecol Oncol 97:568, 2005.

Japaze H, Dinh TV, Woodruff JD: Verrucous carcinoma of the vulva: Study of 24 cases. Obstet Gynecol 60:462, 1982.

Jemal A, Siegel R, Ward E, et al: Cancer statistics, 2006. CA Cancer J Clin 56:106, 2006.

Jones RW, Baranyai J, Stables S: Trends in squamous cell carcinoma of the vulva: The influence of vulvar intraepithelial neoplasia. Obstet Gynecol 90:448, 1997.

Jones RW, Rowan DM: Spontaneous regression of vulvar intraepithelial neoplasia 2-3. Obstet Gynecol 96:470, 2000.

Kaufman RH: Distinguished professor series. Intraepithelial neoplasia of the vulva. Gynecol Oncol 56:8, 1995.

Kim YJ, Kim JW, Koh BK: Successful treatment of vulvar Bowen's disease with topical imiquimod 5% cream. Int J Dermatol 45:151, 2006.

Koh WJ, Wallace HJ, Greer BE, et al: Combined radiotherapy and chemotherapy in the management of local-regionally advanced vulvar cancer. Int J Radiat Oncol Biol Phys 26:809, 1993.

Le T, Hicks W, Menard C, et al: Preliminary results of 5% imiquimod cream in the primary treatment of vulva intraepithelial neoplasia grade 2/3. Am J Obstet Gynecol 194:377, 2006.

Leuchter RS, Hacker NF, Voet RL, et al: Primary carcinoma of the Bartholin gland: A report of 14 cases and review of the literature. Obstet Gynecol 60:361, 1982.

Lieb SM, Gallousis S, Freedman H: Granular cell myoblastoma of the vulva. Gynecol Oncol 8:12, 1979.

Magrina JF, Gonzalez-Bosquet J, Weaver AL, et al: Primary squamous cell cancer of the vulva: Radical versus modified radical vulvar surgery. Gynecol Oncol 71:116, 1998.

Magrina JF, Gonzalez-Bosquet J, Weaver AL, et al: Squamous cell carcinoma of the vulva stage IA: Long-term results. Gynecol Oncol 76:24, 2000.

Marchitelli C, Secco G, Perrotta M, et al: Treatment of bowenoid and basaloid vulvar intraepithelial neoplasia 2/3 with imiquimod 5% cream. J Reprod Med 49:876, 2004.

Messing MJ, Gallug DG: Carcinoma of the vulva in young women. Obstet Gynecol 86:51, 1995.

Miller B, Morris M, Levenback C, et al: Pelvic exenteration for primary and recurrent vulvar cancer. Gynecol Oncol 58:202, 1995.

Modesitt SC, Waters AB, Walton L, et al: Vulvar intraepithelial neoplasia III: Occult cancer and the impact of margin status on recurrence. Obstet Gynecol 92:962, 1998.

Monk BJ, Burger RA, Lin F, et al: Prognostic significance of human papillomavirus DNA in vulvar carcinoma. Obstet Gynecol 85:709, 1995.

Pecorelli S, Creasman WT, Pettersson F, et al: FIGO annual report on the results of treatment in gynaecological cancer, vol 23. Milano, Italy. Epidemiol Biostat 1998.

Perez CA, Grigsby PW, Galakatos A, et al: Radiation therapy in management of carcinoma of the vulva with emphasis on conservation therapy. Cancer 71:3707, 1993.

Piura B, Masotina A, Murdoch J, et al: Recurrent squamous cell carcinoma of the vulva: A study of 73 cases. Gynecol Oncol 48:189, 1993.

Planner RS, Hobbs JB: Intraepithelial and invasive neoplasia of the vulva in association with human papillomavirus infection. J Reprod Med 33:503, 1988.

Podratz KC, Gaffey TA, Symmonds RE, et al: Melanoma of the vulva: An update. Gynecol Oncol 16:153, 1983.

Ragnarsson-Olding BK, Kanter-Lewensohn LR, Lagerlof B, et al: Malignant melanoma of the vulva in a nationwide, 25-year study of 219 Swedish females. Clinical observations and histopathologic features. Cancer 86:1273, 1999.

Ragnarsson-Olding BK, Nilsson BR, Kanter-Lewensohn LR, et al: Malignant melanoma of the vulva in a nationwide, 25-year study of 219 Swedish females. Predictors of survival. Cancer 86:1285, 1999.

Renaud-Vilmer C, Cavelier-Balloy B, Porcher R, Dubretret L: Vulvar lichen sclerosus: Effect of long-term topical application of a potent steroid on the course of the disease. Arch Dermatol 140:709, 2004.

Riva JM, Sedlacek TV, Cunnane MF, Mangan CE: Extended carbon dioxide laser vaporization in the treatment of subclinical papillomavirus infection of the lower genital tract. Obstet Gynecol 73:25, 1989.

Rose PG, Piver S, Tsukada Y, et al: Conservative therapy for melanoma of the vulva. Am J Obstet Gynecol 159:57, 1988.

Rosenberg P, Simonsen E, Risberg B: Adenoid cystic carcinoma of Bartholin's gland: A report of 5 new cases treated with surgery and radiotherapy. Gynecol Oncol 34:145, 1989.

Ross MJ, Ehrmann RL: Histologic prognosticators in stage I squamous cell carcinoma of the vulva. Obstet Gynecol 70:774, 1987.

Rotmensch J, Rubin SJ, Sutton HG, et al: Preoperative radiotherapy followed by radical vulvectomy with inguinal lymphadenectomy for advanced vulvar cancer. Gynecol Oncol 36:181, 1990.

Russell AH, Mesic JB, Scudder SA, et al: Synchronous radiation and cytotoxic chemotherapy for locally advanced or recurrent squamous cancer of the vulva. Gynecol Oncol 47:14, 1992.

Rutledge F, Sinclair M: Treatment of intraepithelial carcinoma of the vulva by skin excision and graft. Am J Obstet Gynecol 102:807, 1968.

Sedlis A, Homesley H, Bundy BN, et al: Positive groin lymph nodes in superficial squamous vulvar cancer. Am J Obstet Gynecol 156:1159, 1987.

Shepherd JH: Staging announcement: FIGO staging of gynecologic cancers: Cervix and vulva. Int J Gynecol Cancer 5:319, 1995.

Siller BS: Vulvar cancer: A case-control study of triple incision vs. en bloc radical vulvectomy and inguinal lymphadenectomy. Gynecol Oncol 57:335, 1995.

Skinner MS, Sternberg WH, Ichinose H, et al: Spontaneous regression of bowenoid atypia of the vulva. Obstet Gynecol 42:40, 1973.

Stefanon B, Clemente C, Lupi G, et al: Malignant melanoma of the vulva: A clinicopathologic study of 28 cases. Cervix IFGT 5:223, 1987.

Stehman FB, Bundy BN: Sites of failure and times to failure in carcinoma of the vulva treated conservatively: A Gynecologic Oncology Group report. Am J Obstet Gynecol 174:1128, 1996.

Tasseron EWK, Van der Esch EP, Hart AAM, et al: A clinicopathological study of 30 melanomas of the vulva. Gynecol Oncol 46:170, 1992.

Thomas G, Dembo A, DePetrillo A: Concurrent radiation and chemotherapy in vulvar carcinoma. Gynecol Oncol 34:263, 1989.

Trimble EL, Lewis JL, Williams LL, et al: Management of vulvar melanomas. Gynecol Oncol 45:254, 1992.

Van der Velden J, Kooyman CD, Van Lindert ACM, Heintz APM: A stage Ia vulvar carcinoma with an inguinal lymph node recurrence after local excision: A case report and literature review. Int J Gynecol Cancer 2:157, 1992.

Veronesi V, Cascinelli N, Adams J, et al: Thin stage I primary cutaneous malignant melanomas: Comparison of excision with margins of 1 or 3 cm. N Engl J Med 318:1159, 1988.

Woodruff JD, Genadry R, Poliakoff S: Treatment of dyspareunia and vaginal outlet distortions by perineoplasty. Obstet Gynecol 57:750, 1981.

Malignant Diseases of the Vagina 31

Intraepithelial Neoplasia, Carcinoma, Sarcoma

Deborah Jean Dotters and Vern L. Katz

KEY TERMS AND DEFINITIONS

Clear-Cell Adenocarcinoma. A vaginal or cervical malignancy occurring primarily after 14 years of age, often associated with prenatal exposure to diethylstilbestrol (DES).

Endodermal Sinus Tumor. A rare adenocarcinoma of the vagina occurring in infants younger than 2 years of age.

Field Defect. The propensity of squamous epithelium of the lower genital tract (cervix, vagina, and vulva) to undergo premalignant change due to infection with the human papillomavirus (HPV).

Pelvic Exenteration. An extensive pelvic operation usually employed to treat a central pelvic recurrence of cervical or vaginal carcinoma after radiation. A total exenteration involves removal of the bladder, uterus, cervix, and rectum. An anterior exenteration spares the rectum, whereas a posterior exenteration spares the bladder.

Pseudosarcoma Botryoides. A benign tumor occurring in the vagina of infants and pregnant women that has a polyploid shape. Microscopically it may be confused with sarcoma botryoides.

Sarcoma Botryoides (Embryonal Rhabdomyosarcoma). A rare, often fatal, malignancy of the vagina that occurs in infants and children.

Vaginal Tumor Stage. A clinical classification describing the extent of spread of vaginal carcinoma.

Stage I: Limited to vaginal wall
Stage II: Extends to subvaginal tissue
Stage III: Reaches the pelvic sidewall
Stage IV: Extends beyond the true pelvis or into mucosa of the bladder or rectum

Vaginal Intraepithelial Neoplasia (VAIN) 1. VAIN of the least severe type (comparable to mild dysplasia), occupying the lower one third of the epithelium. Also termed *low-grade squamous intraepithelial lesion.*

VAIN-2. VAIN of intermediate severity (comparable to moderate dysplasia), occupying the lower two thirds of the epithelium.

VAIN-3. VAIN of the most severe type (comparable to severe dysplasia and carcinoma in situ), replacing the full thickness of the epithelium. VAIN-2 and VAIN-3 are also combined into high-grade squamous intraepithelial lesion.

This chapter focuses on premalignant and malignant diseases of the vagina. Premalignant changes in the vagina occur less frequently than comparable lesions in the cervix and vulva. However, the histologic appearance of intraepithelial neoplasia of the vagina is similar to that described for the cervix (see Chapter 28). These changes are also similarly designated as dysplasia (mild, moderate, or severe) and carcinoma in situ. The term *VAIN* (vaginal, *VA;* intraepithelial, *I;* neoplasia, *N*) has been used to describe these histologic changes; the comparable categories are VAIN-1 (mild dysplasia), VAIN-2 (moderate dysplasia), and VAIN-3 (severe dysplasia to carcinoma in situ). VAIN-1 is classified as a low-grade squamous intraepithelial lesion, whereas VAIN-2 and VAIN-3 are grouped as high-grade squamous intraepithelial lesions. The cytologic and histologic features of these changes are illustrated in Figure 31-1.

VAIN occurs more commonly in patients previously treated for cervical intraepithelial neoplasia. The frequency of vaginal premalignancy in these patients is approximately 1% to 3%. Similarly, there is an increased risk of VAIN in those previously treated for squamous cell neoplasia of the vulva. The tendency to develop premalignant changes in the lower genital tract has been termed a *field defect* and denotes the increased risk of squamous cell neoplasia arising anywhere in the lower genital tract in such individuals. The vast majority of VAIN is related to infection with HPV. Additional risk factors include HIV infection, cigarette smoking, previous radiation therapy of the genital tract, and immunosuppressive therapy.

Primary cancer of the vagina is rare and constitutes less than 2% of gynecologic malignancies. Most vaginal malignancies are metastatic, primarily from the cervix and endometrium. Less commonly, ovarian and rectosigmoid carcinomas, as well as choriocarcinoma, metastasize to the vagina. The most common histologic type of primary vaginal cancer is squamous cell carcinoma, which is usually seen in women older than 60. Other types of carcinoma, including melanoma and adenocarcinomas, occur less commonly. Malignant transformation of endometriosis has been described in the vagina and rectovaginal septum. Clear-cell adenocarcinoma, historically associated with young women exposed in utero to DES, may also occur in unexposed women. Primary vaginal sarcomas are rare and are primarily a disease of children. Table 31-1 summarizes the major primary malignancies of the vagina arranged according to the age at occurrence.

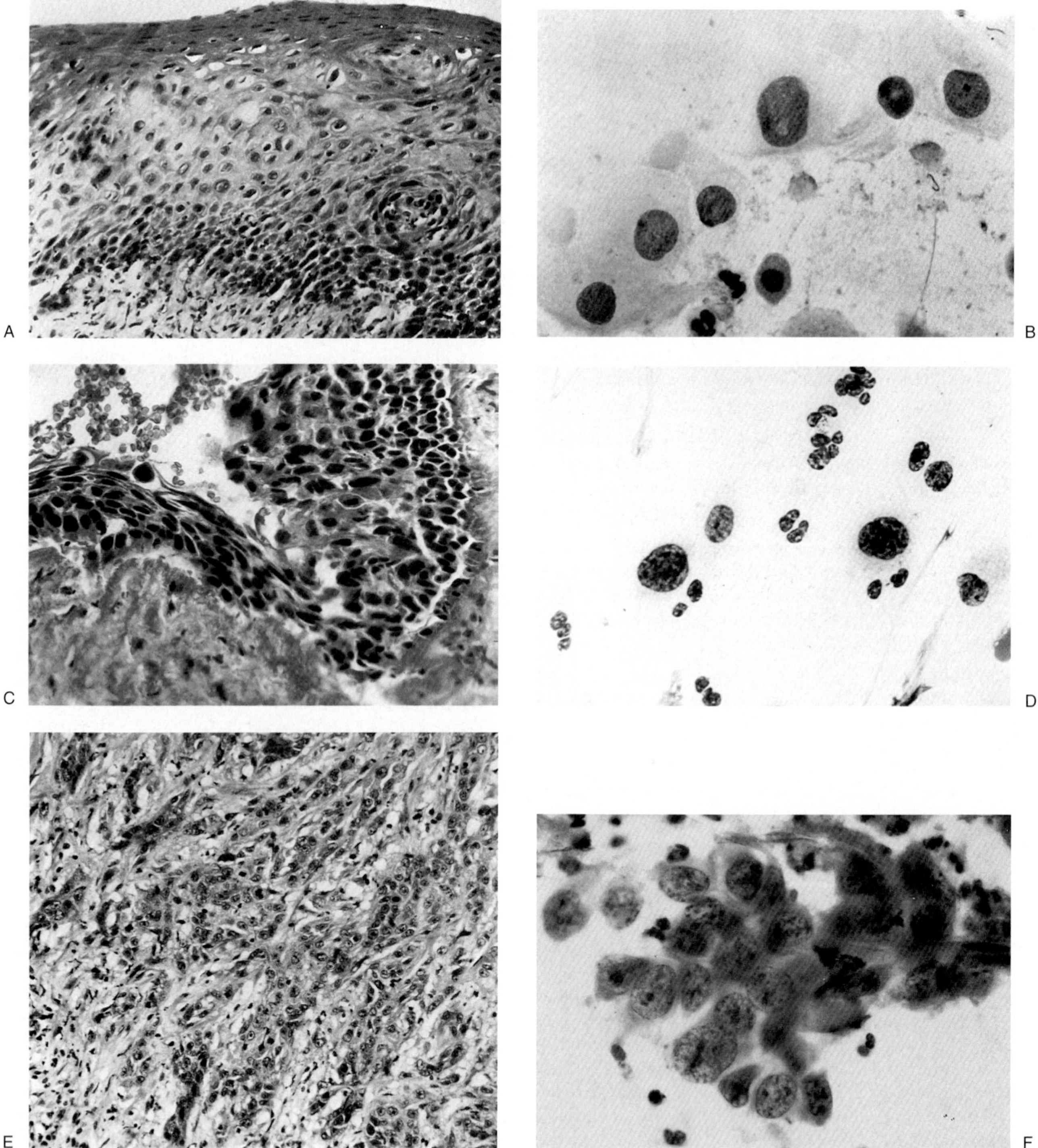

Figure 31-1. **A,** Section of a vagina showing dysplasia. Epithelium appears thickened and shows abnormal maturation. Immature, hyperchromatic cells occupy the lower two to four layers. The middle and upper thirds of mucosa show evidence of cytoplasmic differentiation with well-defined cellular borders. Nuclei in these areas are enlarged and pleomorphic. Parakeratosis is apparent on the surface. Because immature cells are confined to the lower third of the mucosa, dysplasia is classified as mild. (H&E stain, ×250.) **B,** Cytologic specimen showing mild dysplasia. Note the sheet of dysplastic cells. Cells show well-defined cytoplasmic borders. Nuclei are enlarged, and the nuclear contour is smooth. Chromatin is uniformly, finely granular. Focal condensations of chromatin (chromocenters) are present in some nuclei. Nucleoli are not present. (Pap stain, ×1000.) **C,** Section showing severe dysplasia to carcinoma in situ. Entire epithelial thickness is occupied by hyperchromatic, dysplastic cells. Marked nuclear variation and mitoses are seen. Because of occasional cells with squamous differentiation (spindle-shaped cells, cells with well-defined cytoplasmic borders) in superficial layers, this lesion is sometimes classified as severe dysplasia. In carcinoma in situ, immature cells replace the full thickness, and there is no evidence of squamous differentiation on the surface. (H&E stain, ×400.) **D,** Cytologic specimen showing carcinoma in situ. Several isolated immature cells with a high nuclei-to-cytoplasm ratio and poorly defined cytoplasmic borders can be seen. Chromatin is coarsely granular, and no nucleoli are present. In the background are several polymorphonuclear leukocytes and strings of mucus. (Pap stain, ×1000.) **E,** Section showing invasive squamous carcinoma. Cords and sheets of poorly differentiated tumor cells infiltrate the stroma. Nuclei are pleomorphic, and nucleoli are distinct. The mitotic rate is high. Squamous differentiation (keratin pearl formation, single-cell keratinization) was present in other areas of tumor. (H&E stain, ×200.) **F,** Cytologic specimen showing invasive squamous cell carcinoma. Note aggregate of tumor cells. Cellular boundaries are poorly defined, and nuclear orientation is lacking. Chromatin is irregularly distributed and has areas of clumping and clearing. Note nucleoli in some cells, which were absent in cells of patients with dysplasia and carcinoma in situ (Pap stain, ×800).

Table 31-1 Common Primary Vaginal Cancers

Tumor Type	Predominant Age (years)	Clinical Correlations
Endodermal sinus tumor (adenocarcinoma)	<2	Extremely rare, α-fetoprotein secretion, often fatal, multimodality therapy
Sarcoma botryoides	<8	Aggressive malignancy, multimodality therapy
Clear-cell adenocarcinoma	>14	Associated with intrauterine exposure to diethylstilbestrol
Melanoma	>50	Very rare, poor survival
Squamous cell carcinoma	>50	Most common primary vaginal cancer

PREMALIGNANT DISEASE OF THE VAGINA

Detection and Diagnosis

Because premalignant disease of the vagina is generally asymptomatic, detection depends primarily on cytologic screening (see Fig. 31-1*B* and *D*). Most commonly, the changes will be observed in patients who have undergone previous therapy for intraepithelial disease of the cervix. This fact underscores the importance of continued examinations and Pap smears for women even after hysterectomy for dysplastic conditions. VAIN usually occurs in the upper one half of the vagina or along the vaginal cuff suture line. Once an abnormal smear from vaginal epithelium is identified, a biopsy is required for histologic identification (see Fig. 31-1*A* and *C*). A colposcopic examination is usually performed to identify the areas requiring biopsy. As in the case of cervical neoplasia, a repeat Pap smear is often taken before the colposcopic examination. Vaginal colposcopic techniques are similar to those described for the cervix. A large speculum is used to aid in visualizing the entire vaginal wall. Although the abnormal colposcopic findings resemble those of the cervix (see Chapter 28), full visualization of the entire vaginal wall is often difficult and time consuming. A useful adjunct to colposcopy for identifying an area in which to perform a biopsy is to stain the vaginal epithelium with Lugol's solution and to take a biopsy sample from the nonstaining areas. The vaginal epithelium must be adequately estrogenized so that sufficient epithelial glycogen is present for the normal tissue to stain dark brown. The more rapidly dividing dysplastic epithelium uses up its glycogen and thus does not pick up the iodine stain. Vaginal estrogen cream used for 1 to 2 weeks before examination is helpful in evaluating postmenopausal women and those with atrophic vaginitis who present with cytologic atypia. The estrogen cream will not only increase epithelial glycogen, but also helps mature the squamous epithelium, reducing the number of parabasal cells at the surface. Parabasal cells, with their large nuclei, are a common cause of false-positive Pap tests in this age group.

A biopsy is performed with small instruments, such as the Kevorkian or Eppendorf punch biopsy forceps (Fig. 31-2) or similar instruments also used for the cervix. Occasionally, it is necessary to use a fine instrument, such as a nerve hook, to provide traction on the vaginal epithelium to obtain a biopsy sample. Most patients experience some discomfort during the biopsy. Local anesthesia is often helpful, although injection of the anesthetic may be as uncomfortable as the biopsy itself. Vaginal neoplasia is often multifocal. Although the process is most often located in the vaginal apex, it can occur anywhere along the vaginal tube, necessitating examination of the vagina in its entirety.

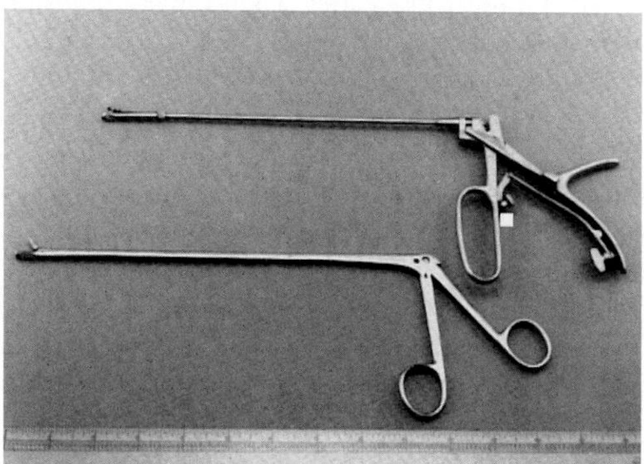

Figure 31-2. Eppendorf (*upper*) and Kevorkian (*lower*) punch biopsy instruments.

Management

There is limited information on the natural history of VAIN. The risk of progression to invasive cancer is thought to be low, around 9%. Those at highest risk of progression are women with high-risk strains of HPV, those with VAIN-3, cigarette smokers, and immunocompromised women. Significantly, Aho and colleagues found that 28% of women undergoing evaluation for VAIN-3 had an underlying invasive carcinoma. This has led many authors to recommend surgical excision rather than destructive procedures for the treatment of VAIN-3.

The principles of managing VAIN are to rule out and prevent invasive disease and to preserve vaginal function. As is true for cervical dysplasia, biopsy-proven VAIN-1, particularly those lesions associated with low-risk strains of HPV, can be observed, provided the patient is compliant with follow-up. VAIN-2 and VAIN-3 are generally treated. Treatment options include topical 5-fluorouracil (5-FU) cream, CO_2 laser vaporization, and wide local excision. The choice of treatment depends largely on the number of lesions, their location, and the level of concern for possible invasion. Radiation therapy, although used in the past, often leads to scarring and fibrosis and is generally not recommended for treatment of noninvasive disease. Because of the proximity of the bladder and rectum, cryotherapy is usually not used.

The main advantage of the CO_2 laser is that it vaporizes the abnormal tissue without shortening or narrowing the vagina, preserving vaginal function. Criteria for CO_2 laser vaporization include a lesion that is discreet and easily visible, and invasive cancer has been ruled out. The beam is directed colposcopically. Iodine staining of the vagina can help outline those areas requiring therapy. Treatment is occasionally performed on an outpatient basis with a local anesthetic and an analgesic. More frequently, general or regional anesthesia is required. The intensity of therapy is regulated by adjusting the wattage of the laser, most commonly 15 to 20 W carried to a depth of 1.5 to 2 mm. Care must be taken not to apply the laser too deeply because of the proximity of the bladder and bowel, particularly in elderly women whose vaginal epithelium may be quite thin. The patient will experience a discharge for 1 to 2 weeks after therapy. Healing usually requires a few weeks. The success rates of laser in treating VAIN vary in the literature, but generally are in the range of 60% to 85%. Regular follow-up every 4 months, including a Pap smear and colposcopy, is required during the first year and usually 6 to 12 months thereafter. The primary disadvantages of laser treatment are the lack of a pathologic specimen for evaluation of the adequacy of margins and to ascertain the absence of invasion, and the procedure can be quite tedious and difficult due to the many folds and crevices at the vaginal apex. It is often difficult to obtain a uniform depth of destruction in these areas.

Topical chemotherapy, 5% 5-FU cream, has the advantage of self-administration and coverage of the entire area at risk (all the vaginal epithelium). It is most often used for widespread, multifocal lesions of HPV-associated VAIN-1 or VAIN-2. One half of a vaginal applicator (approximately 5 g) is inserted into the vagina at bedtime for 7 days. Because the cream is irritating, some protective ointment such as zinc oxide should be applied to the vulva. If excess leakage occurs, less than half of an applicator should be used. In addition, the treatment should be discontinued before 7 days if the patient notes excessive irritation. A cycle of therapy should be repeated in 3 to 4 weeks if intraepithelial neoplasia persists. In some cases, the application of 5-FU is continued for 10 to 14 days, in which case the nontherapy interval is increased to 2 or 3 months. Lesions with a thickened white crust (hyperkeratosis) appear to be less sensitive to this treatment. In contrast, postmenopausal women tolerate only small doses of 5-FU, presumably because of the relative thinness of the vaginal epithelium. In one study, one third of an applicator of 5% 5-FU was used weekly for 10 weeks. It was noted that 17 of 20 patients with vaginal condyloma were free of disease at 3 months. Three patients received a second cycle, and 16 of 18 were free of disease at 10 to 20 months. Success rates of 80% to 90% for patients with VAIN after multiple treatment cycles have been reported. The disadvantage of topical therapy with 5-FU cream is that patients must be highly motivated to complete therapy. 5-FU causes exfoliation and erosion of the vaginal mucosa and can be extremely painful. Only a small percentage of patients are able to complete a full course. Thus, use of topical therapy is quite limited.

Wide local excision (upper vaginectomy) is the treatment of choice for VAIN-3, especially for lesions occurring at the cuff of a hysterectomy. Excision offers the advantage of a surgical specimen to rule out invasion and to ascertain margin adequacy. Excision also has a high success rate (84%). Upper vaginectomy can result in vaginal shortening, which can be ameliorated by the use of topical estrogen cream and a vaginal dilator (or frequent intercourse) once healing is complete.

MALIGNANT DISEASE OF THE VAGINA

Symptoms and Diagnosis

Primary vaginal cancers usually occur as squamous cell carcinomas in women older than age 60. To be considered a primary vaginal tumor, the malignancy must arise in the vagina and not involve the external os of the cervix superiorly or the vulva inferiorly. Otherwise the tumor is classified as cervical or vulvar. This is also an important therapeutic consideration, insofar as the same management techniques apply to small tumors of the upper one third of the vagina and cervical carcinomas. Tumors of the lower one third of the vagina are treated similarly to vulvar cancers (see Chapter 32). Table 31-2 lists the staging criteria for vaginal cancers according to the International Federation of Gynecology and Obstetrics, which are illustrated in Figure 31-3.

Table 31-2 International Federation of Gynecology and Obstetrics Staging Classification for Vaginal Cancer

Stage	Characteristics
0	Carcinoma in situ
I	Carcinoma limited to vaginal wall
II	Carcinoma involves subvaginal tissue but has not extended to pelvic wall
III	Carcinoma extends to pelvic wall
IV	Carcinoma extends beyond true pelvis or involves mucosa of bladder or rectum (bullous edema as such does not assign a patient to stage IV)

Delay in the diagnosis of these cancers frequently occurs, in part because of their rarity and because of a lack of recognition that the abnormal symptoms may be due to a malignancy. The most common symptom of vaginal cancer is abnormal bleeding or discharge. Pain is usually a symptom of an advanced tumor. Urinary frequency is also reported occasionally, particularly in the case of anterior wall tumors, whereas constipation or tenesmus may be reported when the tumors involve the posterior vaginal wall. In general, the longer the delay in diagnosis is, the worse the prognosis and the more difficult the therapy. Vaginal cancer is usually diagnosed by direct biopsy of the tumor mass (see Fig. 31-1*E*). Abnormal cytologic findings (see Fig. 31-1*F*) may prompt a thorough pelvic examination that will lead to diagnosis of vaginal cancer. It is important during the course of the pelvic examination to inspect and palpate the entire vaginal tube and to rotate the speculum carefully to visualize the entire vagina because often a small tumor may occupy the anterior or posterior vaginal wall.

Tumors of Adult Vagina

Squamous Cell Carcinoma

Squamous cell carcinoma is the most common of the vaginal malignancies and accounts for 90% of primary vaginal cancers. Although reported in women in their 30s, the disease occurs primarily in those older than age 60, and 20% are older than the age of 80. Most squamous cell carcinomas occur in the upper third of the vagina, but primary tumors in the middle third and lower third may occur. Grossly, the tumor appears as a fungating, polypoid, or ulcerating mass, often accompanied by a foul smell and discharge related to a secondary infection. Microscopically (see Fig. 31-1*E*), the tumor demonstrates the classic findings of an invasive squamous cell carcinoma infiltrating the vaginal epithelium.

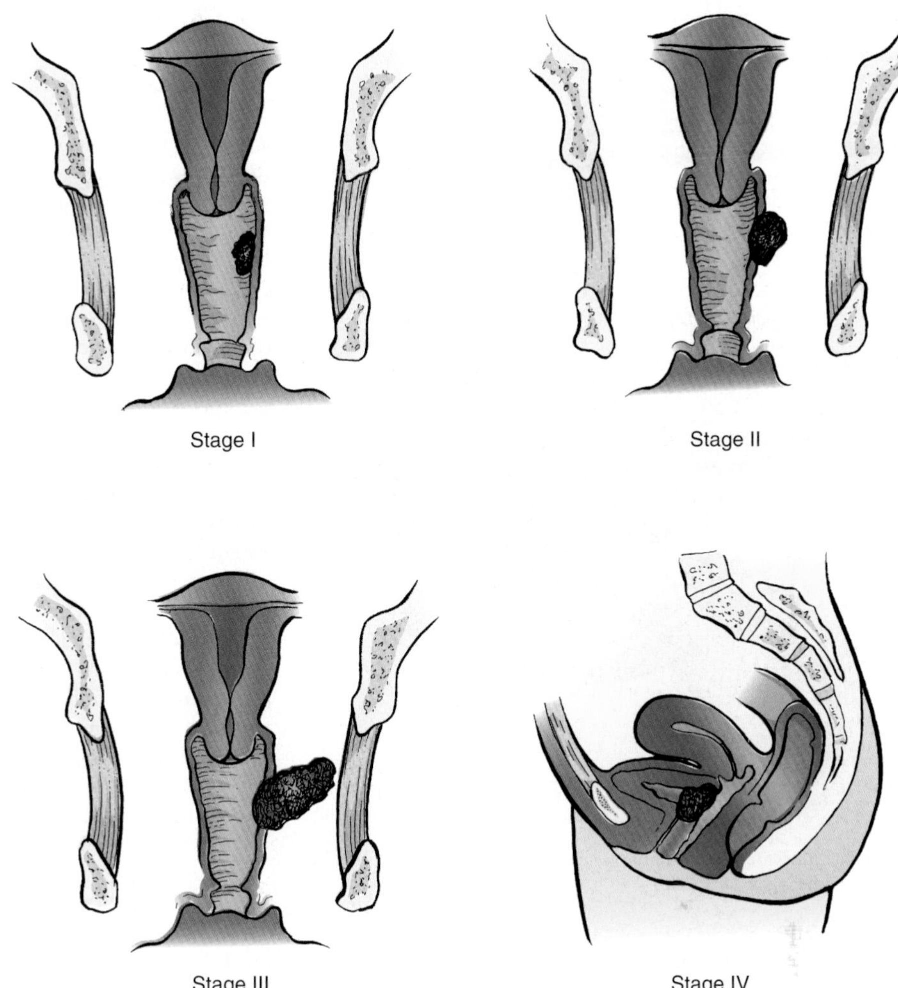

Figure 31-3. Staging of vaginal cancer.

Treatment of these tumors is based on the size, stage, and location. Therapy is limited by the proximity of the bladder anteriorly and the rectum posteriorly. It is also influenced by the location of the tumor in the vagina, which determines the area of lymphatic spread (Fig. 31-4).

The lymphatics of the vagina envelop the mucosa and anastomose with lymphatic vessels in the muscularis. Those of the middle to upper vagina communicate superiorly with the lymphatics of the cervix and drain into the pelvic nodes of the obturator and internal and external iliac chains. In contrast, the lymphatics of the distal third of the vagina drain to both the inguinal nodes and the pelvic nodes, similar to the drainage of the vulva. The posterior wall lymphatics anastomose with the rectal lymphatic system and then to the nodes that drain the rectum, such as the inferior gluteal, sacral, and rectal nodes.

Management. Once the diagnosis of vaginal malignancy is established, a thorough bimanual and visual examination, documenting the size and location of the tumor, and assessment of spread to adjacent structures (submucosa, vaginal sidewall, bladder, and rectum) should be done to determine the clinical stage. Cystoscopy and/or proctoscopy may be helpful, depending on clinical concern, to rule out bladder or rectal invasion. Distant spread may be evaluated with a computed tomography scan of the abdomen, pelvis, and chest. Grigsby has demonstrated that positron emission tomography scanning is the most sensitive and specific imaging test to detect lymph node involvement in cervical cancer and recommends this modality to assess patients with vaginal cancer before embarking on a plan of therapy.

Similar to patients with cervical carcinoma, early stage vaginal carcinoma, without lymph node involvement (stage I or II), may be treated with either surgery or radiation. Young patients with early-stage disease and upper vaginal lesions may be treated with radical upper vaginectomy, parametrectomy, and pelvic lymphadenectomy. Radiation therapy is the most frequently used mode of treatment and can be used for both early and advanced disease. Radiation is the most common therapy because the majority of patients with vaginal carcinoma are elderly with a poorer surgical risk, and radiation is highly effective. Pelvic exenteration can be used primarily to treat advanced disease in the absence of lymph node metastasis, but is usually reserved for patients with localized recurrence after radiation. Cisplatin-based concurrent chemotherapy with irradiation is being used in increasing frequency for squamous carcinomas of the vagina because of the well-documented improvements in outcome for patients with squamous lesions of the cervix treated in this fashion. Although to date, there are no randomized, prospective trials proving its effectiveness in this disease, the numerous similarities in pathophysiology between squamous lesions of

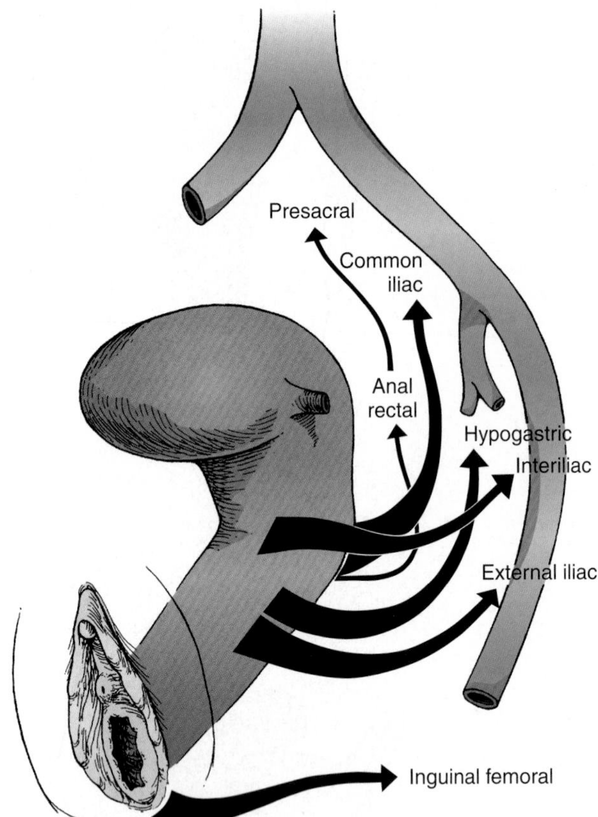

Figure 31-4. Lymphatic drainage of the vagina. Predominant pathways from various parts of the vagina are shown.

the cervix and vagina would lead to the logical conclusion that concurrent radiation/chemotherapy will have increased efficacy over radiation alone in the treatment of vaginal carcinoma.

Stage I vaginal carcinoma may be treated with brachytherapy alone, without external beam therapy. Grigsby recommends vaginal brachytherapy using vaginal cylinders, in one or two applications, delivering a dose of 65 to 80 Gy to the entire length of the vagina. For more advanced lesions, a combination of external beam and brachytherapy is used. External radiation therapy with megavoltage equipment is initially used to shrink the tumor. The size and extent of the radiation field will be determined by the presence or absence of nodal disease, as determined by the pretreatment positron emission tomography or computed tomography scan. The whole pelvis is generally treated to a dose of approximately 5040 cGY. This is followed by a local cesium or radium implant placed interstitially with needles or by intracavitary radiation using a vaginal cylinder or tandem and ovoids, if the cervix is still present. The brachytherapy will bring the total dose to between 7000 and 8500 cGy. Prognosis appears to improve if the interval from the end of external therapy to the initiation of brachytherapy is less than 28 days.

DiSaia and coworkers reported using a fixed perineal template (Syed/Neblett applicator) to achieve reproducible isodose delivery to a large vaginal tumor volume. For lesions of the upper vagina after hysterectomy, a laparotomy or laparoscopy may be done to remove any bowel loops from the vaginal apex. Omentum may be used to provide additional separation of the bowel from the vaginal apex. Paley and associates reported using a retropubic approach in a small series of six patients to achieve direct visualization of needle placement. The treatment is individualized depending on tumor size and stage. For larger lesions, the dose of the external component of radiation therapy is increased, with a concomitant reduction in the local vaginal component of treatment of the primary tumor. Usually a total tumor dose of approximately 7500 cGy is administered. Implants cannot be used in some patients with stage III or IV carcinoma; in such cases, only external therapy can be used, and a central "boost" is given after an initial 5000-cGy whole-pelvic treatment. Severe complications have been noted if the vaginal dose exceeds 9800 cGy. Kucera and Vavra, in a series of 434 patients treated with irradiation, noted results were best for low-stage tumors, those in the upper one third of the vagina, and when the tumor was well differentiated. Kirkbride and colleagues reported that stage, tumor size, and tumor grade were prognostic and that the tumor dose must reach at least 7000 cGy, consistent with other studies. Treatment time is also important, and it is preferable as noted by Lee and colleagues to complete the radiation within 9 weeks.

Survival. Overall 5-year survival rates for patients with primary carcinoma of the vagina have been reported to be approximately 45%. Stage of tumor is the most important predictor of prognosis. In one series of 89 patients treated with surgery and/or irradiation, the 5-year survival rate for stage I was 82% and 53% for stage II. The use of concomitant chemotherapy with radiation can be expected to produce improved survival rates.

Clear-Cell Adenocarcinoma

Clear-cell adenocarcinomas in young women have been seen more frequently since 1970 as a result of the association of many of these cancers with intrauterine exposure to DES. Therapeutic considerations are similar to those for squamous cell carcinoma, taking into account the young age of the patients undergoing therapy. Cervical clear-cell adenocarcinomas are treated like primary cervical carcinomas. The results of therapy for both vaginal and cervical clear-cell adenocarcinoma in young women are discussed together in this section. These tumors are also staged according to the International Federation of Gynecology and Obstetrics classification (see Table 31-2). The majority (80%) have been diagnosed as stage I or II. The overall results of therapy, based on the stage of the tumor at the time of treatment, are shown in Table 31-3. As can be seen, the

Table 31-3 5- and 10-Year Survival Rates for 588 Patients with Clear-Cell Adenocarcinoma of the Vagina and Cervix

Stage	5-Year Survival (%)	10-Year Survival (%)
Stage I	91	85
Stage IIA	80	67
Stage IIB	56	47
Stage II (vagina)	82	67
Stage III	37	25
Stage IV	0	0

Modified from unpublished Registry Data, The University of Chicago.

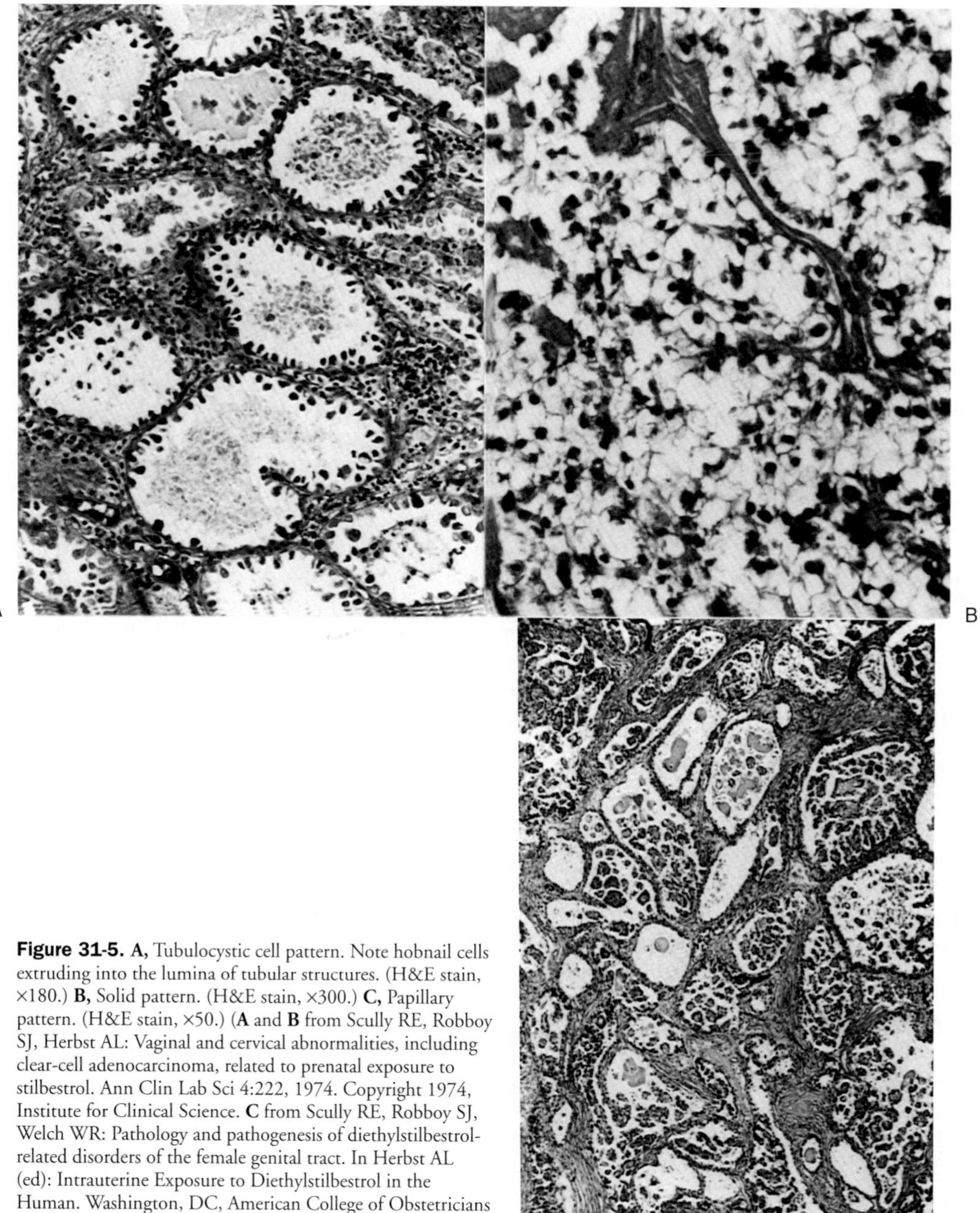

Figure 31-5. **A,** Tubulocystic cell pattern. Note hobnail cells extruding into the lumina of tubular structures. (H&E stain, ×180.) **B,** Solid pattern. (H&E stain, ×300.) **C,** Papillary pattern. (H&E stain, ×50.) (**A** and **B** from Scully RE, Robboy SJ, Herbst AL: Vaginal and cervical abnormalities, including clear-cell adenocarcinoma, related to prenatal exposure to stilbestrol. Ann Clin Lab Sci 4:222, 1974. Copyright 1974, Institute for Clinical Science. **C** from Scully RE, Robboy SJ, Welch WR: Pathology and pathogenesis of diethylstilbestrol-related disorders of the female genital tract. In Herbst AL (ed): Intrauterine Exposure to Diethylstilbestrol in the Human. Washington, DC, American College of Obstetricians and Gynecologists, 1978.)

survival rate is related directly to the stage of the tumor, similar to other gynecologic malignancies at these sites.

In general, surgery is the primary treatment modality because of the young age of the patients. For stage I and early stage II tumors, radical hysterectomy with partial or complete vaginectomy, pelvic lymphadenectomy, and replacement of the vagina with split-thickness skin grafts have been the most common approach. In most cases, ovarian function is preserved. In addition, efforts have been made to preserve fertility in patients who have small tumors of the vagina by the use of local irradiation of the primary tumor and immediate adjacent tissues to spare the ovaries. Because metastases to regional pelvic nodes can occur even with small stage I tumors, retroperitoneal lymph node dissections are usually performed before local therapy.

Usually local excision of the tumor has been performed before irradiation to facilitate local application. Senekjian and associates in 1987 noted that the survival of patients with small vaginal tumors treated by local excision and then local irradiation is comparable with that obtained with conventional extensive therapy. The best candidates are those with tumors less than 2 cm in diameter, a predominant tubulocystic pattern (Fig. 31-5*A*), and depth of invasion less than 3 mm. After wide local excision, the pelvic nodes are sampled to rule out tumor spread. If these are negative, local irradiation can then be given. Pregnancies have occurred in patients so treated. Larger tumors, however, are treated with full pelvic irradiation, in addition to an intracavitary implant. In a few instances, exenterative surgery has been successfully performed. This procedure is preferably applied to central recurrences after primary irradiation. Local vaginal excision as the sole therapy is not usually adequate for small tumors because the tumor frequently recurs.

Three predominant histologic patterns are found in patients with clear-cell adenocarcinoma (Fig. 31-5). In addition, a number of prognostic factors have been identified. The older patients (older than 19 years of age) have been found to have a more favorable prognosis in comparison to younger patients (younger than 15 years of age). This difference is associated with a more favorable outcome for those with the tubulocystic pattern of clear-cell adenocarcinoma, which is the most frequent histologic pattern found in older patients. In addition, smaller tumor diameter and superficial depth of invasion correlate with improved patient survival. Waggoner and coworkers showed that patients with clear-cell adenocarcinoma and a positive maternal DES history did better than those with a negative maternal DES history. If the regional pelvic nodes are free of tumor, the prognosis is also more favorable. It is more likely that the regional pelvic lymph nodes will be free of tumor if other factors are favorable.

Clear-cell adenocarcinomas can spread locally as well as by lymphatics and blood vessels. Metastases to regional pelvic nodes are found in approximately one sixth of stage I cases. The spread to regional pelvic nodes becomes more frequent in higher stage tumors. Depending on the location of the tumor recurrence, therapy has consisted of additional radical surgery or extensive radiation in localized pelvic disease and systemic chemotherapy in cases of metastatic disease. Unfortunately, no single agent or combination of chemotherapeutic agents has currently emerged as an effective therapy. Prolonged follow-up is necessary for these patients because recurrences have been reported as long as 20 years after primary therapy, particularly in the lungs and supraclavicular areas. Data from the Registry on Hormonal Transplacental Carcinogenesis indicate that ovarian preservation with concomitant estrogen stimulation does not adversely affect survival in clear-cell adenocarcinoma

Malignant Melanoma

Vaginal melanomas are rare and highly malignant. Only approximately 2% to 3% of primary vaginal cancers are melanomas. The most common presenting symptoms are vaginal discharge, bleeding, and a palpable mass. Vaginal melanomas appear as darkly pigmented, irregular areas and may be flat, polyoid, or nodular. The average age of affected women is 57 years. Vaginal melanomas tend to metastasize early, via the bloodstream and lymphatics, to the iliac and/or inguinal nodes, lungs, liver, brain, and bones. Patients with vaginal melanoma have a worse prognosis than those with vulvar melanoma, in part probably due to delay in diagnosis in comparison with vulvar carcinomas and in part due to their mucosal location, which seems to predispose to earlier metastasis.

Treatment usually consists of surgery with wide excision of the vagina and dissection of the regional nodes (pelvic or inguinal-femoral, or both), depending on the location of the lesion. Improved outcomes have been associated with the removal of all gross disease. Therapy is usually tailored to the extent of disease. Surgery, radiation, chemotherapy, and immunotherapy have all been described, but no single or combination treatment is uniformly successful.

Both local and distant recurrences are common, and the disease is usually fatal. Even with local control, distant failure is common in patients with melanoma. The overall 5-year survival rate is 8.4%, with an overall median survival of 20 months. Prognostic indicators include tumor size, mitotic index, and Breslow tumor thickness. Improved survival has been noted for patients whose tumors had fewer than six mitoses per 10 high-power fields. Van Nostrand and associates reported a 2-year survival for three of four patients with tumors less than 10 cm^2, that is, approximately 3.0 cm in diameter. However, Neven and coworkers noted that among nine patients, all those with melanomas more than 2 mm thick either died or had a recurrence regardless of therapy, emphasizing the importance of tumor thickness in melanoma prognosis.

Vaginal Adenocarcinomas Arising in Endometriosis

The malignant transformation of extraovarian endometriosis is rare, but is being reported with increasing frequency. Why the disease is being noted more frequently is not known. The rectovaginal septum is the most common extragonadal location. When these tumors occur in the vagina or rectovaginal septum, the typical clinical presentation is pain, vaginal bleeding, and/or a vaginal mass in a patient who has previously undergone extirpative surgery for endometriosis. Risk factors include unopposed estrogen and tamoxifen use. Common histologic types of malignancy include endometrioid adenocarcinoma as the most common, followed by sarcomas (25%), and other tumors of müllerian differentiation. Treatment usually includes surgery plus radiation or chemotherapy. Leiserowitz and colleagues reported a relatively favorable prognosis for women with endometriosis-related malignancies, with 70% alive at a mean follow-up of 31 months.

Vaginal Tumors of Infants and Children

Endodermal Sinus Tumor (Yolk-Sac Tumor)

This type of adenocarcinoma is a rare germ-cell tumor that usually occurs in the ovary. The tumor secretes α-fetoprotein, which provides a useful tumor marker to monitor patients treated for these neoplasms. Approximately 20 cases of this unusual malignancy originating in the vagina of infants, predominantly those younger than 2 years of age, have been reported. The tumor is aggressive, and most patients have died. Young and Scully reported six patients who were free of disease 2 to 9 years after surgery or irradiation or both, with vincristine, actinomycin D, and cyclophosphamide (VAC) chemotherapy. Copeland and colleagues reported similar good results with combination chemotherapy and excision. Collins and associates noted tumor regression in a 5-month-old patient after VAC therapy alone.

Sarcoma Botryoides (Embryonal Rhabdomyosarcoma)

This rare sarcoma is usually diagnosed in the vagina of a young female. Rarely does it occur in a young child older than 8 years of age, although cases in adolescents have been reported. The most common symptom is abnormal vaginal bleeding, with an occasional mass at the introitus (Fig. 31-6). The tumor grossly will resemble a cluster of grapes forming multiple polypoid masses.

The tumors are believed to begin in the subepithelial layers of the vagina and expand rapidly to fill the vagina. These

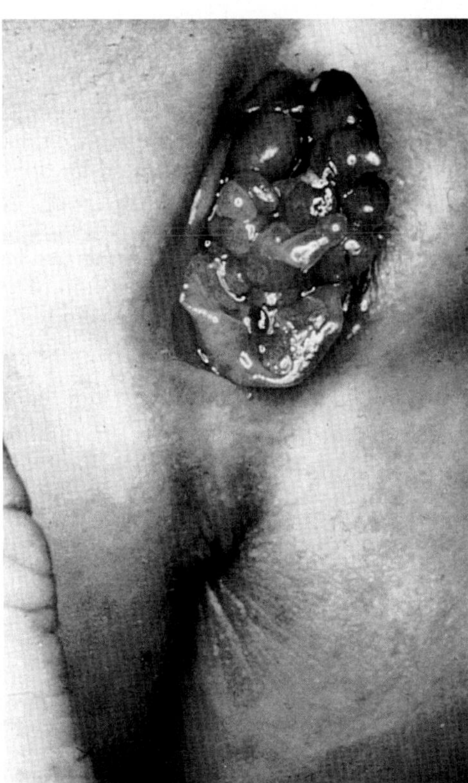

Figure 31-6. Sarcoma botryoides protruding through the vaginal introitus. (From Herbst AL: Cancer of the vagina. In Gusberg SB, Frick HC (eds): Gynecologic Cancer, 5th ed. Baltimore, Williams & Wilkins, 1978. Copyright 1978 by Williams & Wilkins Co.)

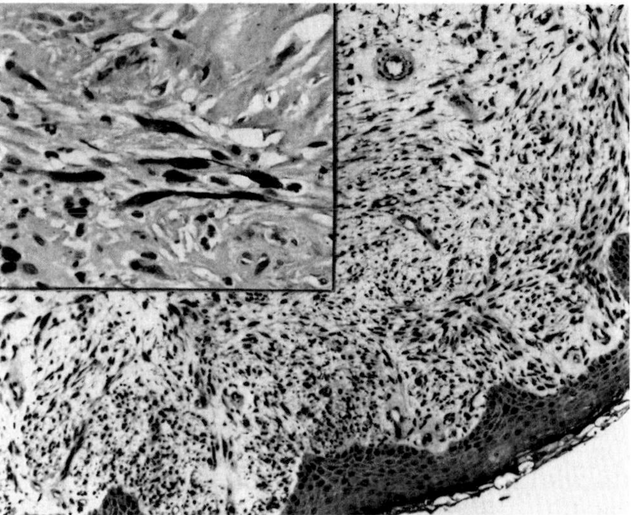

Figure 31-7. Vaginal mucosa with sarcoma botryoides showing condensation of malignant cells under the epithelium (H&E, ×100). *Insert:* Immunohistochemical stain for desmin illustrating strap cells. (×240.) (Courtesy of A. Montag, MD, University of Chicago.)

sarcomas often are multicentric. Histologically, they have a loose myxomatous stroma with malignant pleomorphic cells and occasional eosinophilic rhabdomyoblasts that often contain characteristic cross-striations (strap cells) (Fig. 31-7).

These virulent tumors have been treated in the past by radical surgery, such as pelvic exenteration. However, effective control with less radical surgery has been achieved with a multimodality approach consisting of multiagent chemotherapy (VAC), usually combined with surgery. Radiation therapy has also been used. Hays and associates reported 21 patients with vaginal rhabdomyosarcomas who received chemotherapy. Seven relapsed, five of whom had residual disease after incomplete resection. One had disseminated disease. In 17 patients who received chemotherapy for 8 to 48 weeks, a delayed excision could be performed. Long-term survival data for a large number of patients are not available, but such a combined approach appears to result in effective treatment with less mutilating surgery. A multimodality approach including chemotherapy was used by Flamant and coworkers in 17 females with rhabdomyosarcoma of the vagina or vulva. At the time of their report, 15 appeared cured and 11 of 12 pubescent females have had menses, whereas 2 have successfully conceived and delivered healthy children. This was emphasized in a report from the Intergroup Rhabdomyosarcoma Study by Maurer and colleagues. They found VAC to be effective for disease confined to the vagina without nodal spread. Therapy was effective without irradiation for disease that was locally resected, suggesting that, for these patients, chemotherapy plus surgery can be effective therapy.

Pseudosarcoma Botryoides

A rare, benign vaginal polyp that resembles sarcoma botryoides is found in the vagina of infants and pregnant women. Although large atypical cells may be present microscopically, strap cells are absent. Grossly, these polyps do not resemble the grapelike appearance of sarcoma botryoides. They are called *pseudosarcoma* botryoides. Treatment by local excision is effective.

KEY POINTS

- Predisposing factors associated with the development of vaginal intraepithelial neoplasia include infection with HPV, previous radiation therapy to the vagina, immunosuppressive therapy, and HIV infection.
- The tendency of intraepithelial squamous neoplasia to develop anywhere in the lower female genital tract is termed *field defect* and describes the increased risk of premalignant changes occurring in the cervix, vagina, or vulva.
- Most cases of VAIN occur in the upper one third of the vagina.
- VAIN can be treated by excision, laser, or 5-FU. Excision is often used for VAIN-3, and if the apex is involved, particularly after hysterectomy, laser treatment is generally used for discreet lesions once invasion has been ruled out, and 5-FU cream is used to treat diffuse, multicentric, low-grade disease.

Continued

KEY POINTS *Continued*

- The most common primary vaginal malignancy is squamous cell carcinoma (90%).
- Most cancers occurring in the vagina are metastatic.
- Vaginal cancers constitute less than 2% of gynecologic malignancies.
- Tumors of the upper vagina have a lymphatic drainage to the pelvis similar to cervical tumors, whereas those of the lower one third of the vagina go to the pelvic nodes and also the inguinal nodes similar to vulvar tumors.
- Radical surgery may be used to treat low-stage tumors primarily of the upper vagina in younger patients.
- Radiation therapy is the most frequently used modality for treatment of squamous cell carcinoma of the vagina. Ideally, at least 7000 to 7500 cGy is administered in less than 9 weeks. Concurrent chemoradiation should strongly be considered.
- The overall 5-year survival rate of patients treated for squamous cell carcinoma of the vagina is approximately 45%.
- Clear-cell adenocarcinoma is often associated with prenatal DES exposure and has an improved prognosis if the patient is older than age 19 years and has a predominant tubulocystic tumor pattern and low-stage disease. Those with a positive DES maternal history have a better prognosis.
- Local therapy for small, stage I clear-cell adenocarcinomas of the vagina is best considered if the tumor is less than 2 cm in diameter, invades less than 3 mm, and is predominantly of the tubulocystic histologic type. Pelvic nodes should be sampled and be free of tumor.
- The overall 5-year survival rate of patients treated for clear-cell adenocarcinoma is approximately 80%, in part due to the high proportion of low-stage cases.
- Vaginal melanomas are usually fatal. They occur primarily in patients older than age 50 years.
- Endometrioid adenocarcinomas of the vagina may occur through the malignant transformation of endometriosis, often associated with the use of unopposed estrogen or tamoxifen.
- Endodermal sinus tumors occur in children younger than age 2 years. They secrete α-fetoprotein and are usually treated by multiagent chemotherapy followed by surgical excision.
- Sarcoma botryoides occurs primarily in children younger than age 8 years. It is treated by a multimodality approach using multiagent chemotherapy with surgical removal and occasionally irradiation.

BIBLIOGRAPHY

Aho M, Vesterinen E, Meyer B, et al: Natural history of vaginal intraepithelial neoplasia. Cancer 68:195, 1991.

Andersen WA, Sabio H, Durso N, et al: Endodermal sinus tumor of the vagina. Cancer 56:1025, 1985.

Audet-Lapointe P, Body G, Vauclair R, et al: Vaginal intraepithelial neoplasia. Gynecol Oncol 36:232, 1990.

Buchanan DJ, Schlaerth J, Kurosaki T: Primary vaginal melanoma: Thirteen-year disease-free survival after wide local excision and review of recent literature. Am J Obstet Gynecol 178:1177, 1998.

Cardois RJ, Bomalaski JJ, Hoffman MS: Diagnosis and management of vulvar and vaginal intraepithelial neoplasia. Obstet Gynecol Clin 28:1, 2001.

Coleman RL: Primary vaginal melanoma: A rare and problematic clinical entity. Ann Surg Oncol 11:4, 2003.

Collins HS, Burke TW, Heller PB, et al: Endodermal sinus tumor of the infant vagina treated exclusively by chemotherapy. Obstet Gynecol 73:507, 1989.

Copeland LJ, Gershenson DM, Saul PB, et al: Sarcoma botryoides of the female genital tract. Obstet Gynecol 66:262, 1985.

Creasman WT, Phillips JL, Menck HR: The National Cancer Database report on cancer of the vagina. Cancer 83:1033, 1998.

Davis KP, Stanhope CR, Garton GR, et al: Invasive vaginal carcinoma: Analysis of early-stage disease. Gynecol Oncol 42:131, 1991.

Diakomanolis E, Stefanidis K, Rodolakis A, et al: Vaginal intraepithelial neoplasia: Report of 102 cases. Eur J Gynaecol Oncol 23:457, 2002.

DiSaia PJ, Syed AMN, Puthawala AA: Malignant neoplasia of the upper vagina. Endocr Hypertherm Oncol 6:251, 1990.

Elliott GB, Reynolds HA, Fidler HK: Pseudosarcoma botryoides of cervix and vagina in pregnancy. J Obstet Gynaecol Br Comm 74:728, 1967.

Flamant F, Gerbaulet A, Nihoul-Fekete C, et al: Long-term sequelae of conservative treatment by surgery, brachytherapy, and chemotherapy for vulval and vaginal rhabdomyosarcoma in children. J Clin Oncol 8:1847, 1990.

Gokaslan H, Sismanoglu A, Pekin T, et al: Primary malignant melanoma of the vagina: A case report and review of the current treatment options. Eur J Obstet Gynaecol 121:243, 2005.

Grigsby PW: Vaginal cancer. Curr Treat Options Oncol 3:125, 2002.

Gupta D, Malpica A, Deavers MT, Silva EG: Vaginal melanoma. Am J Surg Pathol 26:1450, 2002.

Herbst AL, Anderson D: Recent advances in clear cell adenocarcinoma of the vagina and cervix secondary to intrauterine exposure to DES. Semin Surg Oncol 6:343, 1990.

Herbst AL, Ulfelder H, Poskanzer DC: Adenocarcinoma of the vagina. N Engl J Med 284:878, 1971.

Indermaur MD, Martino MA, Fiorica JV, et al: Upper vaginectomy for the treatment of vaginal intraepithelial neoplasia. Am J Obstet Gynecol 193:575, 2005.

Kirkbride P, Fyles A, Rawlings GA, et al: Carcinoma of the vagina—experience at the Princess Margaret Hospital (1974–1989). Gynecol Oncol 56:435, 1995.

Kucera H, Vavra N: Radiation management of primary carcinoma of the vagina: Clinical and histopathological variables associated with survival. Gynecol Oncol 40:12, 1991.

Lee WR, Marcus RB, Sombeck MD, et al: Radiotherapy alone for carcinoma of the vagina: The importance of overall treatment time. Int J Radiat Oncol Biol Phys 29:983, 1994.

Leiserowitz GS, Gumbs JL, Oi R, et al: Endometriosis-related malignancies. Int J Gynecol Cancer 13:466, 2003.

Liu L, Davidson S, Singh M: Mullerian adenosarcoma of the vagina arising in persistent endometriosis: Report of a case and review of the literature. Gynecol Oncol 90:486, 2003.

Miettinen M, Wahlstrom T, Vesterinen E, et al: Vaginal polyps with pseudosarcomatous features: A clinicopathologic study of seven cases. Cancer 51:1148, 1983.

Miner TJ, Delgado R, Zeisler J, et al: Primary vaginal melanoma: A critical analysis of therapy. Ann Surg Oncol 11:34, 2004.

Neven P, Shepherd TH, Masotina A, et al: Malignant melanoma of the vulva and vagina. Int J Gynecol Cancer 4:383, 1994

Paley PJ, Koh W-J, Stelzer KJ, et al: A new technique for performing Syed template interstitial implants for anterior vaginal tumors using an open retropubic approach. Gynecol Oncol 73:121, 1998.

Pecorelli S, Creasman WT, Pettersson F, et al: FIGO annual report on the results of treatment in gynaecological cancer. vol 23, Milano, Italy. Epidemiol Biostat, 1998.

Petrilli ES, Townsend DE, Morrow CP, et al: Vaginal intraepithelial neoplasm: Biologic aspects and treatment with topical 5-fluorouracil and the carbon dioxide laser. Am J Obstet Gynecol 38:321, 1980.

Pingley S, Shrivastava SK, Sarin R, et al: Primary carcinoma of the vagina: Tata Memorial Hospital experience. Int J Radiat Oncol Biol Phys 46:101, 2000.

Piver MS, Rose PG: Long-term follow-up and complications of infants with vulvovaginal embryonal rhabdomyosarcoma treated with surgery, radiation therapy, and chemotherapy, Obstet Gynecol 71:435, 1988.

Senekjian EK, Frey KW, Anderson D, Herbst AL: Local therapy in stage I clear cell adenocarcinoma of the vagina. Cancer 60:1319, 1987.

Senekjian EK, Frey KW, Herbst AL: Pelvic exenteration in clear cell adenocarcinoma of the vagina and cervix. Gynecol Oncol 34:413, 1989.

Senekjian EK, Frey KW, Stone C, Herbst AL: An evaluation of stage II vaginal clear cell adenocarcinoma according to substages. Gynecol Oncol 31:56, 1988.

Sulak P, Barnhill D, Heller P, et al: Nonsquamous cancer of the vagina. Gynecol Oncol 29:309, 1988.

Ulrich U, Rhiem K, Kaminski M, et al: Parametrial and rectovaginal adenocarcinoma arising from endometriosis. Int J Gynecol Cancer 15:1206, 2005.

Van Nostrand KM, Lucci JA III, Schell M, et al: Primary vaginal melanoma: Improved survival with radical pelvic surgery. Gynecol Oncol 55:234, 1994.

Waggoner SE, Mittendorf R, Biney N, et al: Influence of in utero diethylstilbestrol exposure on the prognosis and biologic behavior of vaginal clear cell adenocarcinoma. Gynecol Oncol 55:238, 1994.

Young RH, Scully RE: Endodermal sinus tumor of the vagina: A report of nine cases and review of the literature. Gynecol Oncol 18:380, 1984.

Yazbeck C, Poncelet C, Chosidow D, Maldelenat P: Primary adenocarcinoma arising from endometriosis of the rectovaginal septum: A case report. Int J Gynecol Cancer 15:1203, 2005.

Neoplastic Diseases of the Uterus 32

Endometrial Hyperplasia, Endometrial Carcinoma, Sarcoma: Diagnosis and Management

Karen Lu and Brian M. Slomovitz

KEY TERMS AND DEFINITIONS

Carcinosarcoma. A term used to describe uterine cancers that contain adenocarcinoma and sarcoma components; also termed *malignant mixed müllerian tumor.* Depending on the appearance of the sarcomatous elements, it is designated as homologous or heterologous (malignant mixed müllerian tumor):

Heterologous Uterine Sarcoma. A sarcoma consisting of mesenchymal elements foreign to the uterus, that is, chondrosarcoma, osteosarcoma, liposarcoma, and rhabdomyosarcoma.

Homologous Uterine Sarcoma. A sarcoma consisting of mesenchymal elements normally found in the uterus, i.e., leiomyosarcoma and endometrial stromal sarcoma (ESS).

Clear-Cell Carcinoma. A virulent form of endometrial carcinoma that histologically is similar to clear-cell adenocarcinomas that arise in the ovary, cervix, and vagina.

Endometrial Carcinoma Grade. A pathologic classification that describes the degree of differentiation of endometrial carcinoma: G1, well differentiated; G2, intermediate; G3, poorly differentiated.

Endometrial Carcinoma Stage. A classification that describes the extent of spread of endometrial carcinoma:

Stage I: Tumor confined to the uterine corpus.

Stage II: Tumor involving the corpus and cervix.

Stage III: Tumor spreading outside the uterus but confined in the pelvis; tumor involving the pelvic or paraaortic lymph nodes.

Stage IV: Tumor spreading outside the pelvis or into the mucosa of the bladder or rectum.

Endometrial Hyperplasia. A general term that encompasses a variety of proliferative endometrial patterns. Unless there is cellular atypia, the hyperplasias are not generally considered to have marked malignant potential:

Simple Hyperplasia. A type of endometrial hyperplasia consisting of a proliferation of glands, some of which are dilated, and with abundant stroma. In the absence of cytologic atypia, the potential for malignant transformation is approximately 1%.

Complex Hyperplasia Without Atypia. A type of endometrial hyperplasia in which the glands are irregular in shape and often close together and there is no cytologic atypia. If untreated, approximately 3% will progress to carcinoma.

Complex Atypical Hyperplasia. A variant of endometrial hyperplasia that is premalignant. The glands are often severely crowded and have abnormal outpouchings, and there is an abnormal appearance to the epithelial cells of the glands (cytologic atypia). If untreated, approximately 29% will progress to carcinoma.

Leiomyosarcoma. A smooth muscle malignancy with more than five mitoses per 10 high-power fields (hpf), bizarre cells with nuclear atypia, and necrosis.

Malignant Mixed Müllerian Tumor. See Carcinosarcoma.

Uterine Papillary Serous Carcinoma. A virulent form of endometrial carcinoma that histologically resembles papillary serous adenocarcinoma of the ovary.

Endometrial carcinoma is the most common malignancy of the lower female genital tract in the United States. Approximately 41,000 new cases develop in the United States each year, according to recent figures (2006) from the American Cancer Society. This is approximately 1.3 times the frequency of ovarian cancer and approximately twice the number of new cases of cervical cancer. However, 8000 deaths occurred annually from uterine cancer, slightly more than for cervical cancer and much less than the approximately 14,000 for ovarian cancer. Overall, approximately 3 women in 100 in the United States will develop this disease during their lives.

This chapter reviews the clinical and pathologic features of endometrial hyperplasias and carcinomas. The factors that contribute to the development of these diseases and the appropriate methods of management are discussed. Sarcomas of the uterus and their clinical behavior and therapy are also presented.

EPIDEMIOLOGY

Adenocarcinoma of the endometrium affects women primarily in the perimenopausal and postmenopausal years and is most frequently diagnosed in those between the ages of 50 and 65. However, these cancers can also develop in young women during their reproductive years. Approximately 5% of the cases are diagnosed in women younger than 40 and approximately 10% to 15% in women younger than age 50. Figure 32-1 plots a typical age–incidence curve for cancers of the endometrium

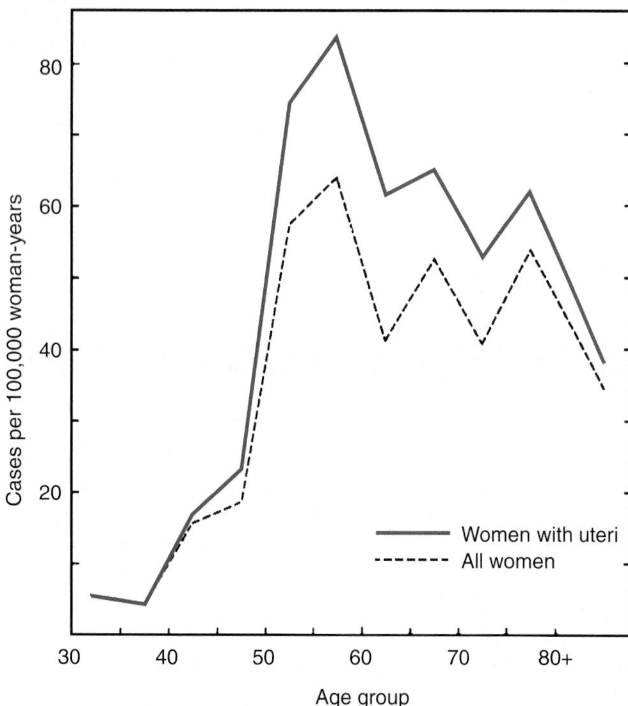

Figure 32-1. Incidence curve for carcinoma of the endometrium by age. (From Elwood JM, Cole P, Rothman KJ, Kaplan SD: Epidemiology of endometrial cancer. J Natl Cancer Inst 59:1055, 1977.)

according to age. The curve rises sharply after age 45 and peaks between 55 and 60; then there is a gradual decrease.

Complex atypical hyperplasia results from increased estrogenic stimulation of the endometrium and is a precursor to endometrioid endometrial cancer. Some endometrial cancers develop without previous hyperplasia. These nonestrogen-related carcinomas tend to be poorly differentiated of serous histology and aggressive (see later discussion).

Multiple factors increase the risk of developing endometrial carcinoma (and hyperplasia) (see the following box). Obesity is a strong risk factor for endometrial cancer. Women who are obese (body mass index >30) have a two- to threefold increased risk. The association is believed to be due to increased circulating estrogen levels that result from conversion of androstenedione to estrone in the adipose tissue and decreased sex hormone-binding globulin. Although more historical than clinically relevant, unopposed estrogen stimulation is strongly associated with endometrial cancer, increasing the risk four to eight times for a woman using estrogen alone for menopausal replacement therapy. The risk increases with higher doses of estrogen (>0.625 mg conjugated estrogens), and more prolonged use but can be markedly reduced with the use of progestin (see Chapter 42, Menopause). Similarly, combination (progestin-containing) oral contraceptives decrease the risk. As noted by Grimes and Economy, combination oral contraceptives protect against endometrial cancer, with most studies showing a relative risk reduction to approximately 0.5. The protection begins after 1 year of use and lasts approximately 15 years after discontinuation. Other conditions leading to long-term estrogen stimulation of the endometrium, including the polycystic ovary syndrome (Stein-Leventhal syndrome) and the much more rare feminizing ovarian tumors, are also associated with increased risk of endometrial carcinoma.

Endometrial Carcinoma Risk Factors

Increases the Risk
Unopposed estrogen stimulation
Unopposed menopausal estrogen (4–8×) replacement therapy
Menopause after 52 years (2.4×)
Obesity (2–5×)
Nulliparity (2–3×)
Diabetes (2.8×)
Feminizing ovarian tumors
Polycystic ovarian syndrome
Tamoxifen therapy for breast cancer

Diminishes the Risk
Ovulation
Progestin therapy
Combination oral contraceptives
Menopause before 49 years
Normal weight
Multiparity

Patients who receive the selective estrogen receptor modulator (SERM) tamoxifen are also at increased risk of developing endometrial carcinoma. In the National Surgical Adjuvant Bowel and Breast B-14 trial examining tamoxifen as adjuvant therapy in women with breast cancer, risk of endometrial cancer was elevated 7.5-fold. This may be an overestimate as the risk of endometrial cancer in the control group was lower than expected. In the National Surgical Adjuvant Bowel and Breast P-1 trial examining tamoxifen as a chemopreventive agent, risk of endometrial cancer was elevated 2.5-fold. Risk increased with duration of use. The majority of endometrial cancers that developed in tamoxifen users were endometrioid histology and low grade and stage. However, high-grade endometrial cancers and sarcomas have also been reported in women taking tamoxifen. Screening strategies including transvaginal ultrasonography and office endometrial sampling have been studied in this cohort. There is a high false-positive rate with transvaginal ultrasonography because tamoxifen causes subendometrial cyst formation, which makes the endometrial stripe appear abnormally thick. Barakat and colleagues performed endometrial pipelle sampling on a large cohort of women taking tamoxifen. They found very few cancers and concluded that women do not benefit from endometrial screening. Rather women should be counseled that tamoxifen increases the risk of endometrial cancer, and all women on tamoxifen who have irregular vaginal bleeding (if premenopausal) or any vaginal bleeding (if postmenopausal) should undergo endometrial sampling or dilatation and curettage (D&C).

Various other factors increase the risk of endometrial cancer. Nulliparity is associated with a twofold increased risk in endometrial cancer. Diabetes increases the risk by 2.8-fold and has been found to be an independent risk factor. Hypertension is often related to obesity and diabetes and is not considered an independent risk factor. Regarding racial factors, the incidence of endometrial cancer among white women is approximately twice the rate in black women. Studies of Hill and coworkers demonstrated that black women tend to develop a much higher percentage of poorly differentiated tumors. The National Cancer Database report by Partridge and colleagues confirms that patients who are black and have a low income do present at an advanced stage and have a poor survival compared with non-Hispanic whites. The difference in survival between blacks and non-Hispanic whites do not appear to be solely based on access to care issues, and there are likely to be biologic differences that account for the disparity in survival.

Lynch syndrome, or hereditary nonpolyposis colorectal cancer syndrome, is an autosomal dominant hereditary cancer susceptibility syndrome caused by a germline defect in a DNA mismatch repair gene (MLH1, MSH2, or MSH6). Women with Lynch syndrome have a 40% to 60% lifetime risk for developing endometrial cancer, a 40% to 60% lifetime risk of developing colon cancer, and a 12% lifetime risk of developing ovarian cancer. This contrasts sharply with the general population risk of 3% for endometrial cancer, 5% for colon cancer, and 1.7% risk of ovarian cancer. Endometrial cancers in Lynch syndrome can be of any histology and grade, and Broaddus and Lu reported that although most were early stage, approximately one fourth were high grade, high stage, or poor histology. Given that there are few longitudinal cohort studies, screening recommendations for gynecologic cancers are based on expert opinion and include annual endometrial biopsy and transvaginal ultrasound to evaluate the ovaries. Colonoscopy every 1 to 2 years has been shown to decrease mortality from colon cancer in Lynch syndrome. Schmeler reported on the efficacy of prophylactic hysterectomy and salpingo-oophorectomy to decrease endometrial and ovarian cancer risk, and women with Lynch syndrome should be offered this option after childbearing is complete. Lynch syndrome is likely to account for approximately 5% of all endometrial cancers. Women with endometrial cancer and a family history of colon, endometrial, or ovarian cancer should be referred for genetic evaluation and colonoscopy.

In the past several years, investigators have begun to define the molecular alterations present in endometrial cancer. PTEN mutations are frequently seen in endometrioid endometrial cancer and have also been seen in complex endometrial hyperplasia. Microsatellite instability occurs in approximately 25% to 30% of all endometrial cancers and is the result of either germline mutations in DNA mismatch repair proteins (MLH1, MSH2, or MSH6) or more frequently from the somatic methylation of the MLH1 promoter. In contrast to endometrioid endometrial cancers, uterine papillary serous carcinomas have a high frequency of p53 mutations. HER-2/neu amplification is seen in 10% to 20% of uterine papillary serous carcinomas and is likely associated with advanced stage and poor prognosis of this histology. Future studies will continue to elucidate our understanding of the molecular alterations of endometrial cancer.

ENDOMETRIAL HYPERPLASIA

The normal morphologic changes that occur in the endometrium during the menstrual cycle are reviewed in Chapter 4, Reproductive Endocrinology. Endometrial hyperplasia is believed to result from an excess of estrogen or an excess of estrogen relative to progestin, such as occurs with anovulation.

Table 32-1 Classifications of Endometrial Hyperplasias

World Health Organization
Simple hyperplasia
Complex hyperplasia
Atypical simple hyperplasia
Atypical complex hyperplasia

Kurman and Norris introduced terminology that has been adopted by the World Health Organization to describe endometrial hyperplasias and their premalignant potential. There are two important separate categories: atypical hyperplasia and hyperplasia without atypia. In these categories, two types are recognized: simple hyperplasia and complex hyperplasia (Table 32-1).

Simple Hyperplasia

This term defines an endometrium with dilated glands that may contain some outpouching and abundant endometrial stroma (Fig. 32-2). The term *cystic hyperplasia* has been used to describe dilation of the endometrial glands, which often occurs in a hyperplastic endometrium in a menopausal or postmenopausal woman (cystic atrophy). It is considered to be weakly premalignant.

Complex Hyperplasia (without Atypia)

In this condition, glands are crowded with very little endometrial stroma and a very complex gland pattern and outpouching formations (Fig. 32-3). In traditional terminology,

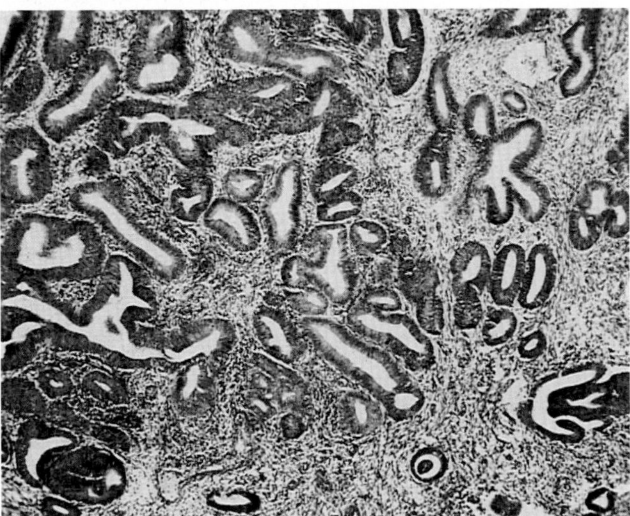

Figure 32-2. Benign simple hyperplasia. (From Kurman RJ, Kaminski PF, Norris HJ: Behavior of endometrial hyperplasia: A long-term study of "untreated" hyperplasias in 170 patients. Cancer 56:403, 1985.)

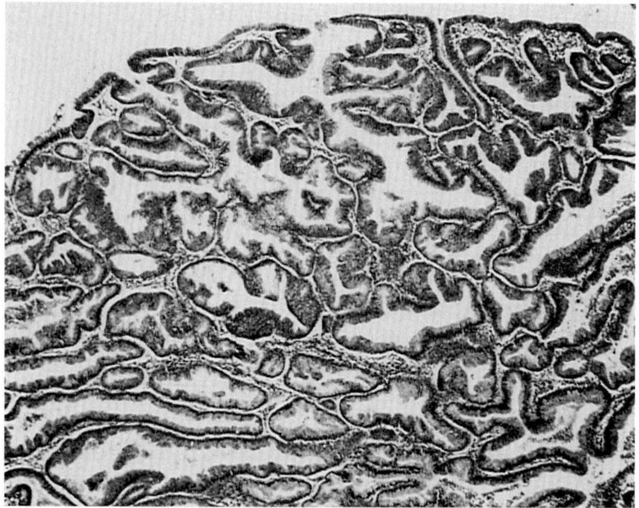

Figure 32-3. Complex hyperplasia characterized by crowded back-to-back glands with complex outlines. (From Kurman RJ, Kaminski PF, Norris HJ: Behavior of endometrial hyperplasia: A long-term study of "untreated" hyperplasias in 170 patients. Cancer 56:403, 1985.)

this is a variant of adenomatous hyperplasia with moderate to severe degrees of architectural atypia but with no cytologic atypia. These hyperplasias have a low premalignant potential.

Complex Atypical Hyperplasia

This term refers to hyperplasias that contain glands with cytologic atypia and are considered premalignant. There is an increase in the nuclear/cytoplasmic ratio with irregularity in the size and shape of the nuclei (Fig. 32-4). Cytologic atypia occurs primarily with complex hyperplasia, and simple hyperplasia with atypia is rarely seen. Complex atypical hyperplasia has the greatest malignant potential.

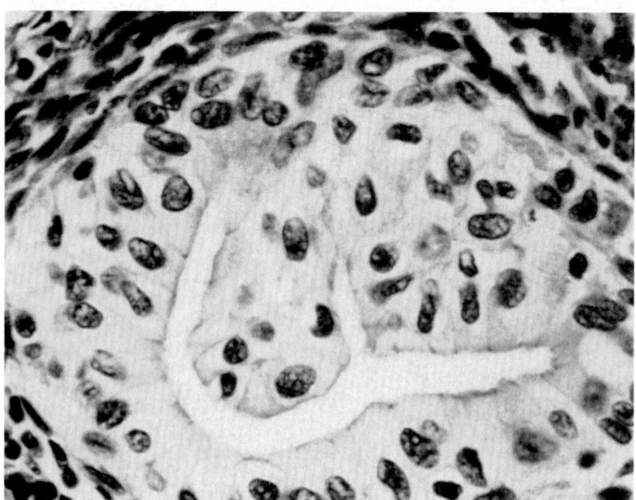

Figure 32-4. Severely atypical hyperplasia (complex) of the endometrium with marked irregularity of nuclei. (×720.) (From Welch WR, Scully RE: Hum Pathol 8:503, 1977. Reprinted with permission from WB Saunders Co.)

A recent study from the Gynecologic Oncology Group has shed light on the difficulty of making the diagnosis of complex atypical hyperplasia. In this large prospective study, one third of cases with a diagnosis of complex atypical hyperplasia were reproduced when evaluated by a gynecologic pathologist that was part of the study. However, one third of the cases were deemed to be "less than" complex atypical hyperplasia by the study pathologists and one third were "greater than" complex atypical hyperplasia, that is, they were considered endometrial cancers. The clinician benefits by directly consulting with the pathologist interpreting the endometrial histologic picture. The fact that demarcations between various diagnostic categories are not sharply defined and reproducible makes this communication important.

Natural History

The rate at which endometrial hyperplasia progresses to endometrial carcinoma has not been accurately determined. Studies addressing this area have been retrospective, based on samples obtained from D&C specimens at a single institution, and therefore are not necessarily generalizable. Kurman and associates studied 170 patients with endometrial hyperplasia diagnosed by D&C at least 1 year before hysterectomy. Table 32-2 shows the results of their study. Overall, complex atypical hyperplasias had the highest risk of progression to carcinoma. Simple hyperplasia had a 1% rate of progression to cancer, complex hyperplasia without atypia had a 3% rate of progression to cancer, and complex atypical hyperplasia had a 29% rate of progression to cancer. In addition to concern about progression to cancer, a recent Gynecologic Oncology Group (GOG) study showed that 40% of women with complex atypical hyperplasia had endometrial cancer in their hysterectomy specimen. This high rate of cancer suggests that complex atypical hyperplasia may frequently be present with low-grade endometrial cancer and that endometrial sampling, whether by D&C or by office endometrial pipelle, may not identify an endometrial cancer when admixed with a complex atypical hyperplasia. Clearly, there is a spectrum of histology that makes a definitive diagnosis of complex atypical hyperplasia difficult, and the clinician must be aware of this fact when planning management strategies.

Diagnosis and Endometrial Sampling

Abnormal vaginal bleeding is the most frequent symptom of endometrial hyperplasia. In younger patients, hyperplasia may develop during anovulatory cycles and may even be detected after prolonged periods of oligomenorrhea or amenorrhea. It can occur at any time during the reproductive years but is most common with abnormal bleeding in the perimenopausal period. Premenopausal women with irregular vaginal bleeding and postmenopausal women with any vaginal bleeding should be evaluated with an office endometrial sampling or a D&C. The office sampling instruments, such as a thin plastic pipelle, are introduced through the cervical os into the endometrial cavity and can provide very accurate information (see Chapter 10, Rape, Incest, and Domestic Violence). Many patients tolerate

Table 32-2 Endometrial Hyperplasia Follow-up

Type	Number	Age	(Mean)	Regressed*	PROGRESSED TO CARCINOMA No. of Cases	PROGRESSED TO CARCINOMA Mean (Years)	Follow-up (Years)
Simple hyperplasia[†]	93	17–71	(42)	74 (80%)	1	11	1–26.7 10 pregnancies
Complex hyperplasia[‡]	29	20–67	(39)	23 (79%)	1	8.3	2–26 3 pregnancies
Atypical hyperplasia	48	20–70	(40)	28 (58%)	11	4.1	1–25 3 pregnancies
Atypical simple hyperplasia	13			9	1		
Atypical complex hyperplasia	35			20	10		

*A total of 34 patients with simple hyperplasia, 7 with complex hyperplasia and 15 with atypical hyperplasia, had no further therapy
[†]Benign proliferation of the glands.
[‡]Greater crowding of glands, no cytologic atypia present.
Adapted from Kurman RJ, Kaminski PF, Norris HJ: Cancer 56:403, 1985; and Kurman RJ, Norris HJ: Endometrial hyperplasia and related cellular changes. In Blaustein's Pathology of the Female Genital Tract, 4th ed. New York, Springer-Verlag, 1994.

office endometrial sampling without an analgesic agent, but paracervical block can be an effective anesthetic aid, particularly in nulliparous women. Some patients benefit from an oral nonsteroidal antiinflammatory drug taken approximately 30 minutes before biopsy.

Transvaginal ultrasonongraphy has been evaluated as an adjunct for the diagnosis of endometrial hyperplasia and cancer. These studies have been studied in different populations, including asymptomatic postmenopausal women, women taking tamoxifen, and women presenting with postmenopausal bleeding. Langer and associates, in a study of 448 asymptomatic postmenopausal women, found a threshold of 5-mm endometrial thickness had only a 9% predictive value for detecting endometrial abnormalities. Its greater use was eliminating the diagnosis of neoplasia for those with thickness less than 5 mm (negative predictive value of 99%). These findings were confirmed in a literature review by Smith-Bindman and colleagues, who found that 96% of women with carcinoma had an abnormal ultrasound scan (endometrial thickness > 5 mm). Conversely, 8% of postmenopausal women with an abnormal scan had no histologic abnormality, and the percentage grew to 23% for those on hormone replacement therapy. However, both of these studies were conducted in postmenopausal asymptomatic women.

Cecchini and coworkers biopsied 108 postmenopausal patients on long-term tamoxifen with endometrial thickness greater than 6 mm. One case of hyperplasia and one of carcinoma were found, and most patients had atrophic endometrium. The authors concluded that the false-positive rate of transvaginal ultrasonography in this population was too high to warrant its use as a screening modality, and they recommended using irregular vaginal bleeding as an indication for endometrial sampling. Similarly, Love and associates found that endometrial thickness is not necessarily a useful guide for biopsy in tamoxifen. In the study by Barakat and colleagues (see earlier discussion), routine screening with transvaginal ultrasonography was not of value, and they concluded that sampling should be done if the patient experiences bleeding.

In postmenopausal women with any vaginal bleeding, Gull and colleagues found that an endometrial stripe of less than 4 mm had a 100% negative predictive value. A finding of endometrial thickness less than 4 mm is a reasonable predictor of lack of endometrial pathology, even in a postmenopausal patient with bleeding. However, persistent vaginal bleeding should lead to endometrial sampling regardless of the ultrasound findings.

Endometrial ablation is sometimes undertaken to control severe uterine bleeding (see Chapter 37, Abnormal Uterine Bleeding). However, thorough evaluation of the endometrium should be performed before ablation in order to rule out an underlying endometrial hyperplasia or cancer.

Management

The therapy employed for endometrial hyperplasia depends on the degree of atypicality of the hyperplasia and the patient's age. For women with simple hyperplasia or complex hyperplasia without atypia, the risk of developing endometrial cancer is low, 1% and 3%, respectively. A diagnostic D&C can also be therapeutic, and progestins or combination oral contraceptive agents will likely be effective.

For complex atypical hyperplasia, the risk of developing endometrial cancer may be 29%, and as stated previously, a concurrent endometrial cancer may be present. Women who desire preservation of childbearing function are treated with high-dose progestin therapy, usually megestrol acetate 40 mg tid to qid. The patient should have long-term follow-up and periodic sampling, the first at 3 months and at least every 6 months thereafter (Fig. 32-5*A*). In these patients, the risk factors that led to the development of complex atypical hyperplasia are likely to remain. Therefore, once the complex atypical hyperplasia is cleared, consideration should be given to periodic progestin treatment or oral contraception until the patient chooses to attempt pregnancy.

Studies have shown that younger patients with chronic anovulation and hyperplasia who desire children may also be treated by induction of ovulation with clomiphene citrate (Clomid) (see Chapter 41, Infertility), especially if the hyperplasia is mildly atypical. Weight reduction for very obese patients is also advised.

For older patients with complex atypical hyperplasia, the risk of carcinoma may be increased. For example, Kurman and associates studied the uteri of patients after curettage had been performed, and atypical hyperplasia was found in the curettings. In their study, 11% of those younger than age 35,

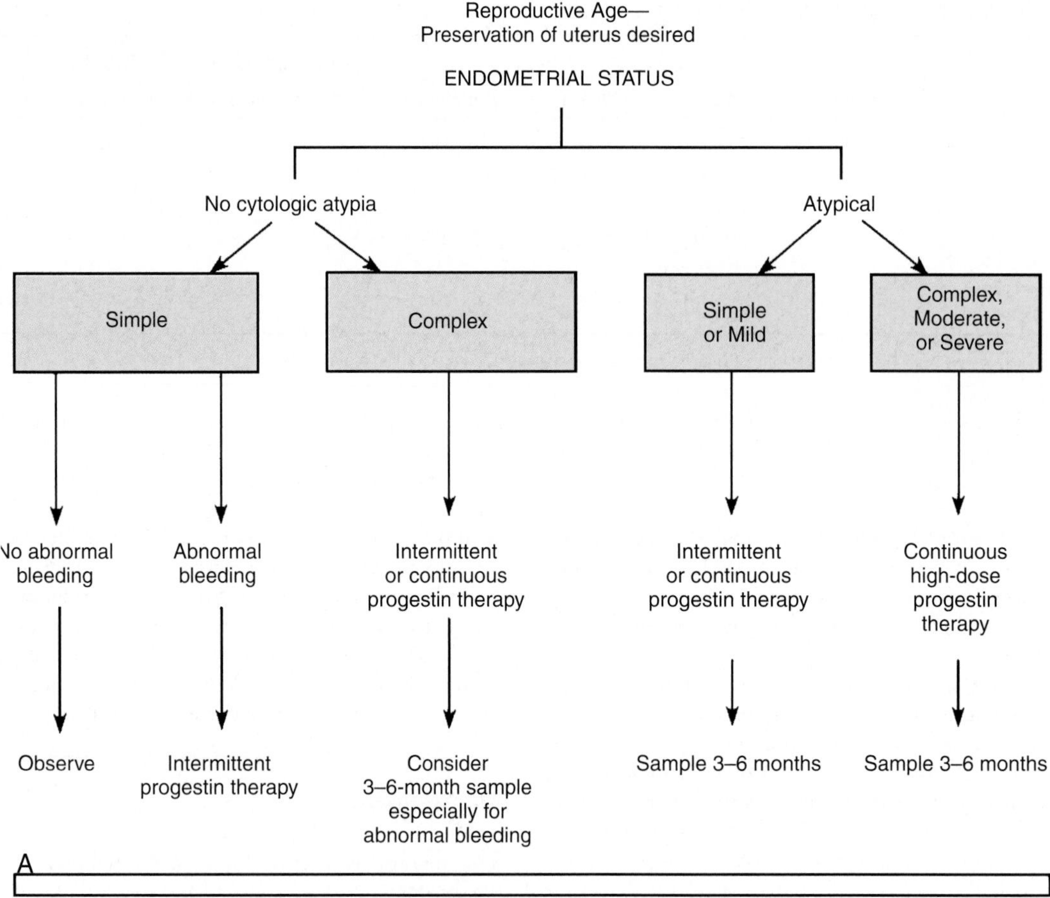

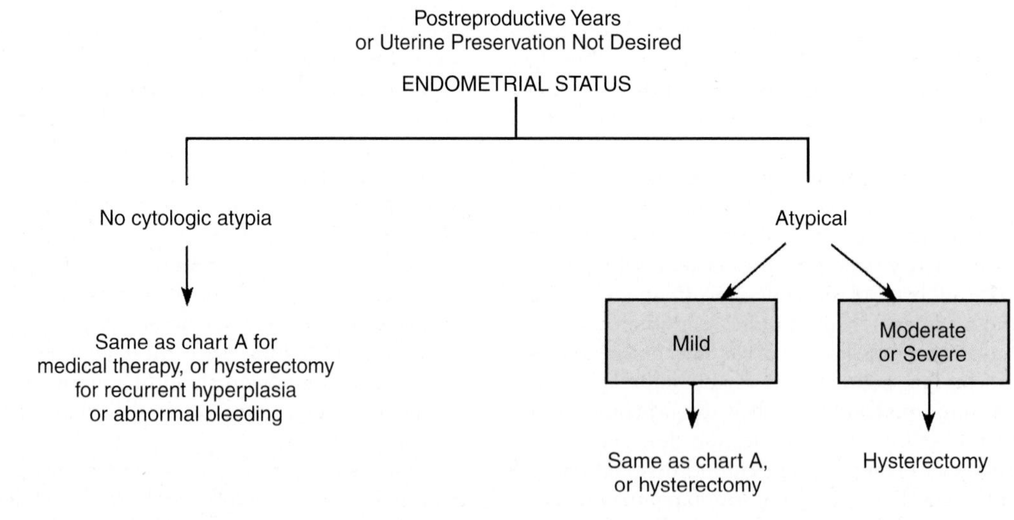

Figure 32-5. Schematic diagram of endometrial hyperplasia management for reproductive (**A**) and postreproductive (**B**) patients.

12% of those 36 to 54, and 28% of those older than age 55 with atypical hyperplasia were found to have carcinoma in their uterus. Thus, older patients with moderate or severe atypical hyperplasia generally require hysterectomy. In addition, those who fail progestin therapy and especially those with severe cytologic atypia should also be considered for hysterectomy (see Fig. 32-5*B*). If hysterectomy is not medically advisable, long-term high-dose progestin therapy can be used (megestrol acetate 40 to –160 mg/day or its equivalent depending on the endometrial response). Periodic sampling of the endometrium is also performed. Figure 32-5 displays a flow chart as a guide to the management of endometrial hyperplasia. It is important to emphasize that the diagnoses are not precisely defined, and these proliferative disorders are a continuum from mild abnormalities to malignant change.

ENDOMETRIAL CARCINOMA

Symptoms, Signs, and Diagnosis

Postmenopausal bleeding and abnormal premenopausal and perimenopausal bleeding are the primary symptoms of endometrial carcinoma.

The diagnosis of endometrial carcinoma is established by histologic examination of the endometrium. Initial diagnosis can frequently be made on an outpatient basis, with an endometrial biopsy. If endometrial carcinoma is found, endocervical curettage may be performed to rule out invasion of the endocervix. A routine cytologic examination (Pap smear) from the exocervix, which screens for cervical neoplasia, detects endometrial carcinoma in only approximately 50% of the cases.

If adequate outpatient evaluation cannot be obtained or if the diagnosis or cause of the abnormal bleeding is not clear from the tissue obtained, a fractional D&C, usually with hysteroscopy, should be performed. The endocervix is first sampled to rule out cervical involvement by endometrial cancer, hysteroscopy is done to visualize the endometrial cavity, and then a complete uterine curettage is performed.

Histologic Types

The various types are listed in the following box.

Figure 32-6 illustrates typical adenocarcinomas of the endometrium and demonstrates varying degrees of differentiation (G1, well differentiated; G2, intermediate differentiation; G3, poorly differentiated). Grading is determined by the percentage of solid components are found in the tumor: grade 1 has less than 6% solid components, grade 2 has 6% to 50% solid components, and grade 3 has more than 50% solid components.

Squamous epithelium commonly coexists with the glandular elements of endometrial carcinoma. Previously, the term *adenoacanthoma* was used to describe a well-differentiated tumor and *adenosquamous carcinoma* to describe a poorly differentiated carcinoma with squamous elements. More recently, the term *adenocarcinoma with squamous elements* has been used with a description of the degree of differentiation of both the glandular and squamous components. Zaino and colleagues, in a GOG study of 456 cases with squamous elements, showed that prognosis was related to the grade of the glandular component and the degree of myometrial invasion. They suggested the term *adenocarcinoma with squamous differentiation*, and this has been generally adopted.

Uterine papillary serous carcinomas are a highly virulent and uncommon histologic subtype of endometrial carcinomas (5%–10%). These tumors histologically resemble papillary serous carcinomas of the ovary (Fig. 32-7). Slomovitz and associates evaluated 129 patients with uterine papillary serous carcinoma (UPSC) and found a high rate of extrauterine disease even in cases without myometrial invasion. They recommend a thorough operative staging (see next section) in all cases of these tumors because of the high risk of extrauterine disease even in cases admixed with other histologic types (endometrial and/or clear-cell).

Clear-cell carcinomas of the endometrium are less common (<5%). Histologically, they resemble clear-cell adenocarcinomas of the ovary, cervix, and vagina. Clear-cell tumors tend to develop in postmenopausal women and carry a prognosis much worse than typical endometrial adenocarcinomas. Survival rates of 39% to 55% have been reported, much less than the 65% or better usually recorded for endometrial carcinoma. Abeler and Kjorstad reviewed 97 cases and noted the best prognosis (90%) for those without myometrial invasion. Patients whose tumors had vascular invasion experienced a 15% 5-year survival. Carcangiu and Chambers reviewed 29 cases and found 5-year survival rates for stages I and II of 72% and 59%, respectively.

Endometrial Primary Adenocarcinomas

Typical endometrioid adenocarcinoma
Adenocarcinoma with squamous elements*
Clear cell carcinoma
Serous carcinoma
Secretory carcinoma
Mucinous carcinoma
Squamous carcinoma

*Previously termed *adenoacanthoma* or *adenosquamous carcinoma.*

Staging

In 1988, a surgical staging classification was introduced (Table 32-3) that relies on an operative evaluation with particular emphasis on myometrial invasion in stage I. Figure 32-8 displays the various stages of endometrial carcinoma based on the varying degrees of uterine involvement according to the new International Federation of Gynecology and Obstetrics (FIGO) system.

Table 32-3 Corpus Cancer Staging (Adopted 1988)

Stages	Characteristic
IA G123	Tumor limited to endometrium
IB G123	Invasion to less than half of the myometrium
IC G123	Invasion to more than half of the myometrium
IIA G123	Endocervical glandular involvement only
IIB G123	Cervical stromal invasion
IIIA G123	Tumor invades serosa and/or adnexae and/or positive peritoneal cytology
IIIB G123	Vaginal metastases
IIIC G123	Metastases to pelvic and/or paraaortic lymph nodes
IVA G123	Tumor invasion of bladder and/or bowel mucosa
IVB	Distant metastases including intraabdominal and/or inguinal lymph node

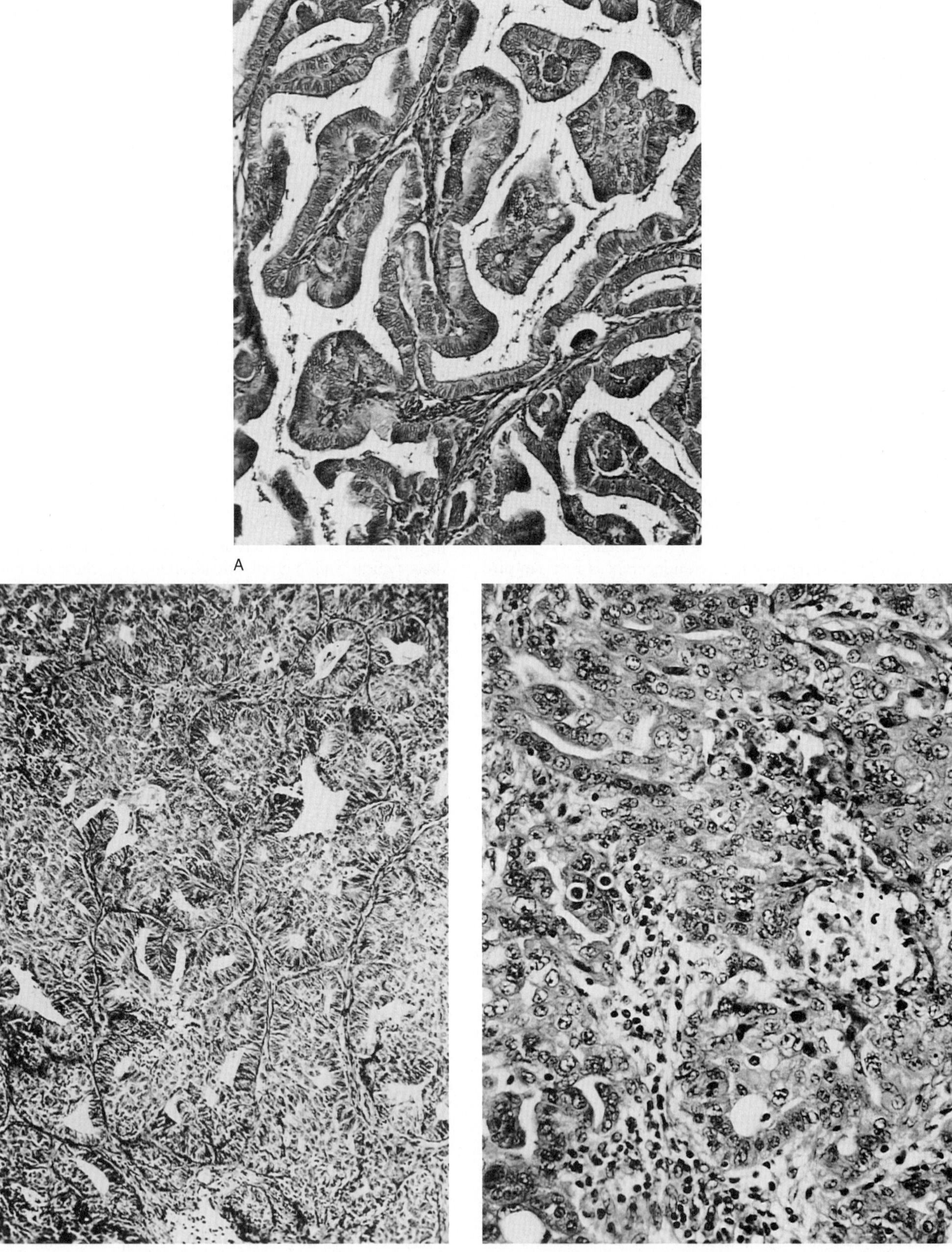

Figure 32-6. **A,** Well-differentiated adenocarcinoma of the endometrium. The glands are confluent. (×130.) **B,** Moderately differentiated adenocarcinoma of the endometrium. The glands are more solid, but some lumens remain. (×100.) **C,** Poorly differentiated adenocarcinoma of the endometrium. The epithelium shows solid proliferation with only a rare lumen. (×100.) (From Kurman RJ, Norris HJ: Endometrial neoplasia: Hyperplasia and carcinoma. In Blaustein A [ed]: Pathology of the Female Genital Tract, 2nd ed. New York, Springer-Verlag, 1982.)

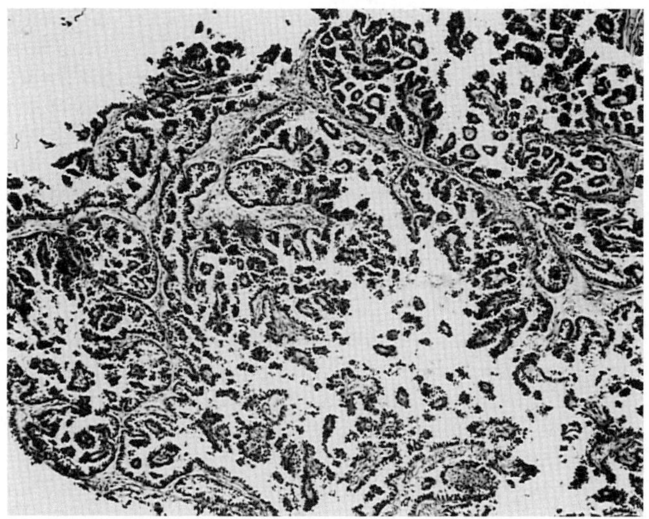

Figure 32-7. Serous carcinoma characterized by a complex papillary architecture resembling serous carcinoma of the ovary. (From Kurman RJ: Blaustein's Pathology of the Female Genital Tract, 3rd ed. New York, Springer-Verlag, 1987.)

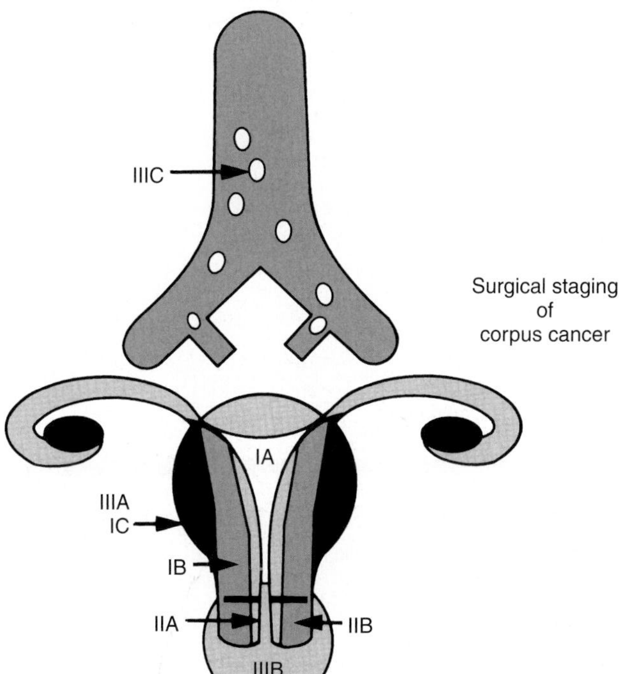

Figure 32-8. Schematic for surgical staging for endometrial carcinoma according to 1988 International Federation of Gynecology and Oncology definitions (see Table 30-4). (Courtesy of Dr. James Orr, Watson Clinic, Lakeland, FL.)

Prognostic Factors

Many variables affect the behavior of endometrial adenocarcinomas. These variables can be conveniently divided into clinical and pathologic factors. The clinical determinants are patient age at diagnosis, race, and clinical tumor stage. The pathologic determinants are tumor grade, histologic type, uterine size, depth of myometrial invasion, microscopic involvement of vascular spaces in the uterus by tumor, and spread of tumor outside the uterus to the retroperitoneal lymph nodes, peritoneal cavity, or uterine adnexa.

Clinical Factors

Older patients have tumors of a higher stage and grade than younger patients. White patients have a higher survival rate than black patients, a finding partially explained by higher stage and higher grade tumors among black women. In addition, black women are more likely to develop UPSC. The 10-year survival of 136 black patients in the series of Aziz and coworkers was 40% compared with 72% for 135 white patients.

Pathologic Factors

Tumor stage is a well-recognized prognostic factor for endometrial carcinoma (Table 32-4), and the results reflect a combination of clinical and operative staging because the latter was introduced in 1988, which was the midpoint of the reporting period. Fortunately, most cases are diagnosed in stage I, which provides a favorable prognosis.

The histologic grade of the tumor is a major determinant of prognosis. Endometrial carcinomas are divided into three grades: grade 1, well differentiated; grade 2, intermediate differentiation; and grade 3, poorly differentiated. Figure 32-9 shows the survival of 895 patients studied by the GOG that relates endometrial carcinoma survival to tumor grade and demonstrates the worsening of prognosis with advancing grade.

The histologic type of the endometrial carcinoma (Fig. 32-10) is also related to prognosis, with the best prognosis associated with typical adenocarcinomas, as well as better differentiated tumors with or without squamous elements, and secretory carcinomas. Approximately 80% of all endometrial carcinomas fall into the favorable category. Poor prognostic histologic types are papillary serous carcinomas, clear-cell carcinomas, and poorly differentiated carcinomas with or without squamous elements, as previously noted.

The degree of myometrial invasion correlates with the risk of tumor spread outside the uterus, but the higher grade and higher stage tumors in general have the deepest myometrial penetration (Fig. 32-11). The importance of tumor grade and myometrial invasion is also illustrated by a study of their relationship to their spread to the retroperitoneal pelvic and paraaortic lymph nodes. Studies of 142 patients by Schink and colleagues indicate that tumor size is also prognostic. Only

Table 32-4 Carcinoma of the Corpus Uteri: Patients Treated in 1990–1992: Survival by FIGO Surgical Stage, $N = 5562$

Stage	5-Year Survival Rate
IA	90.9%
IB	88.2%
IC	81.0%
II	71.6%
III	51.4%
IV	8.9%

Modified from Pecorelli S, Creasman WT, Pettersson F, et al: FIGO annual report on the results of treatment in gynaecological cancer. Vol 23. Milano, Italy. J Epidemiol Biostat 1998.

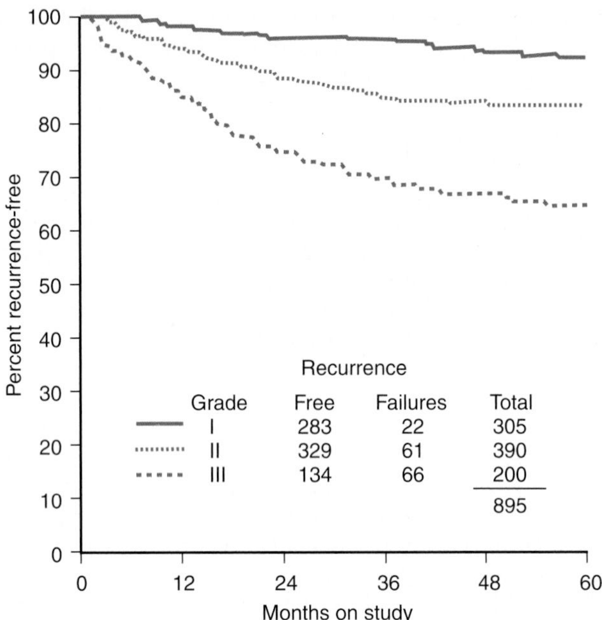

Figure 32-9. Recurrence-free interval by histologic grade. (Redrawn from Morrow CP, Bundy BN, Kurman RJ, et al: Relationship between surgical-pathologic risk factors and outcome in clinical stage I and II carcinoma of the endometrium: A Gynecologic Oncology Group study. Gynecol Oncol 40:55, 1991.)

4% of those with tumors 2 cm or less in size had lymph node metastases. The rate increased to 15% for those with tumors greater than 2 cm to 35% when the entire endometrial cavity was involved. Table 32-5 summarizes the clinical and pathologic factors affecting outcome in early stage tumors.

Peritoneal cytology has been studied as a prognostic factor, and the results are conflicting. In a study of 567 surgical stage I cases, Turner and associates found that positive peritoneal cytology was an independent prognostic factor. In contrast, Grimshaw and coworkers evaluated 322 clinical stage I cases and found that positive peritoneal cytology was an adverse prognostic factor, but they did not find it to be an independent risk factor when other variables were considered. More recently, Kadar and associates and Lurain and colleagues noted that positive peritoneal cytology was associated primarily with adverse features such as extrauterine disease and that therapy (see following discussion) for positive peritoneal cytology as an isolated finding did not appear to improve survival.

Patterns of Spread of Endometrial Carcinoma. Plentl and Friedman noted four major channels of lymphatic drainage from the uterus that serve as sites for extrauterine spread of tumor: (1) a small lymphatic branch along the round ligament that runs to the inguinal femoral nodes, (2) branches from the tubal and (3) ovarian pedicles (infundibulopelvic ligaments), which are large lymphatics that drain into the paraaortic nodes,

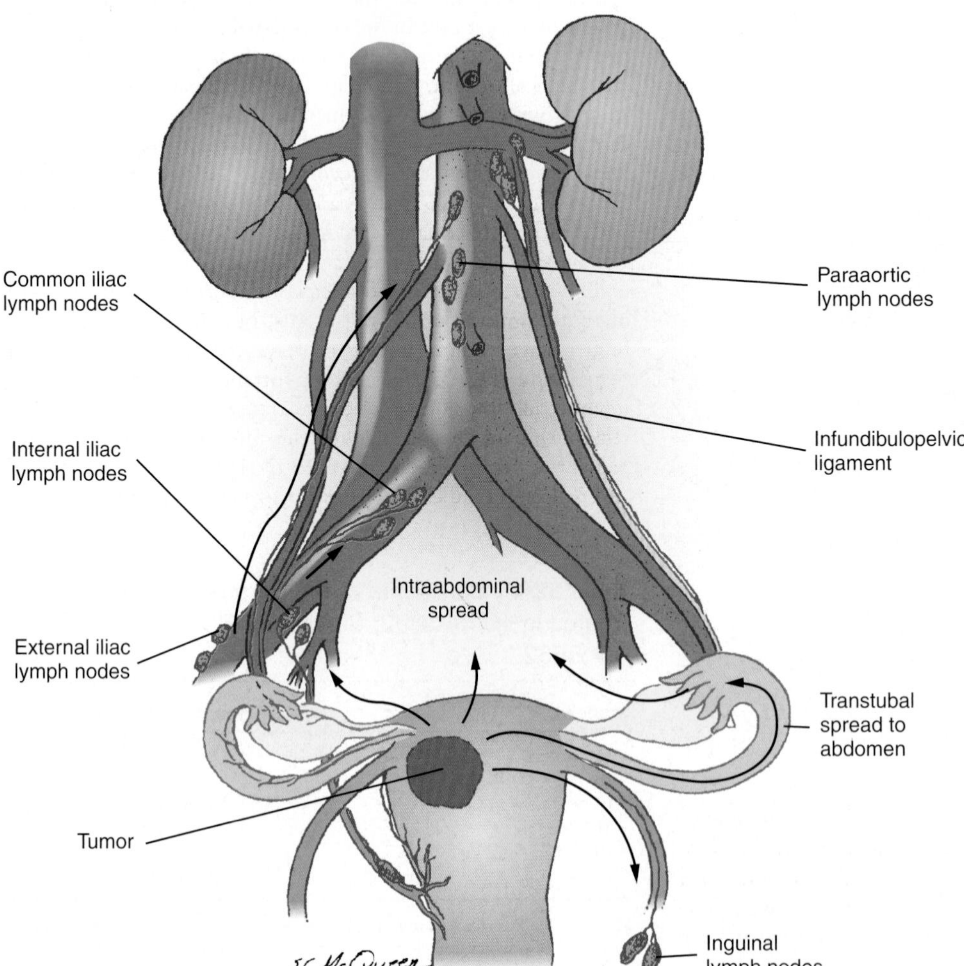

Figure 32-10. Spread of endometrial carcinoma. The major pathways of tumor spread are illustrated (see text).

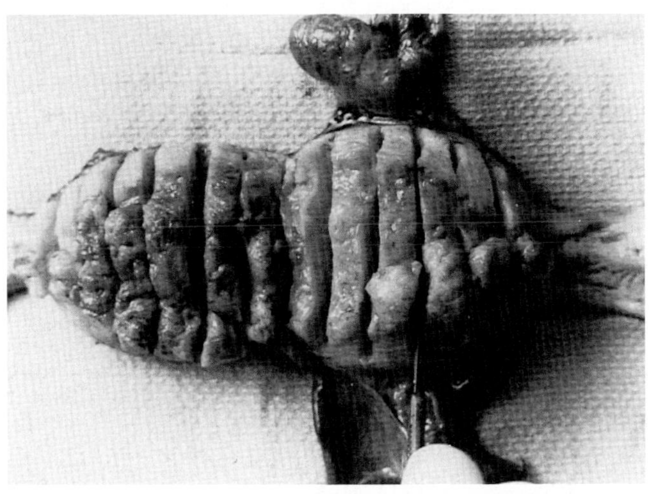

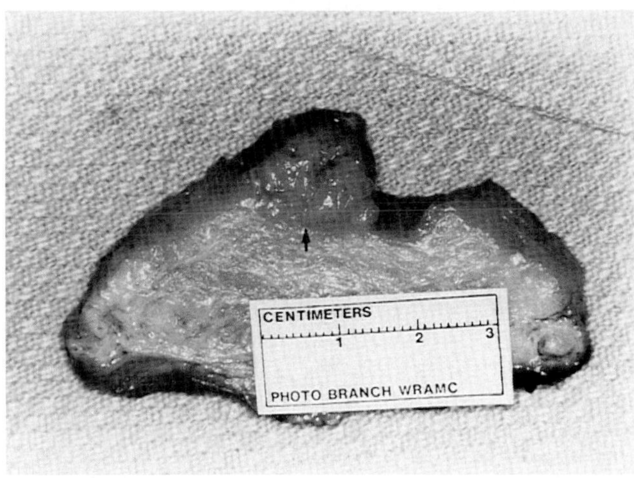

A B

Figure 32-11. **A,** Technique for intraoperative assessment of the depth of myometrial invasion. **B,** Cross section of uterine wall demonstrating superficial myometrial invasion. *Arrow* shows the tumor–myometrial junction. (From Doering DL, Barnhill DR, Weiser EB, et al: Intraoperative evaluation of depth of myometrial invasion in stage I endometrial adenocarcinoma. Obstet Gynecol 74:930, 1989.)

and (4) the broad ligament lymphatics that drain directly to the pelvic nodes. The pelvic and paraaortic node drainage sites (2, 3, and 4) are the most important clinically. In addition, direct peritoneal spread of tumor can occur through the uterine wall or via the lumen of the fallopian tube. Clinically, therefore, the clinician must assess the retroperitoneal nodes, the peritoneal cavity, and the uterine adnexa for the spread of endometrial carcinoma (see Fig. 32-10).

Extensive studies by the GOG have elucidated both the frequency of lymph node metastases in endometrial carcinoma and the pathologic factors that modify this risk in stage I disease. Tumor grade, size of the uterus, and degree of myometrial invasion were studied. Table 32-6 illustrates the frequency of lymph node metastases according to uterine size and tumor grade. There are differences in the proportion of positive nodes between stages IB and IA (pre-1988 staging) cases as well as

Table 32-5 Surgical Stage I and II Tumors: The Proportional Hazards Modeling of Relative Survival Time

Variable	Regression Coefficient	Relative Risk	Significance Test* (*P* value)
Endometrioid			
Grade 1	—	1.0	—
Grade 2	0.28	1.3	2.7 (0.1)
Grade 3	0.56	1.8	
Endometrioid with squamous differentiation			0.1 (0.7)
Grade 1	0.20	1.2	
Grade 2	−0.01	1.0	0.3 (0.6)
Grade 3	0.22	0.8	
Villoglandular			2.2 (0.1)
Grade 1	−4.91	0.01	
Grade 2	−0.59	0.5	10.4 (0.001)
Grade 3	3.73	41.9	
Myometrial invasion			
Endometrium only	—	1.0	
Superficial	0.39	0.5	
Middle	1.20	3.3	19.6 (0.0002)
Deep	1.53	4.6	
Age	0.17	—	
Age^2	−0.000837	—	20.7 (0.0001)
45 (arbitrary reference)	—	1.0	
55	0.85	2.3	
65	1.52	4.6	
75	2.03	7.6	
Vascular space involvement	0.32	1.4	1.2 (0.3)

*Wald χ^2 test.
P value for grading is for overall grade within cell type.
Modified from Zaino RJ, Kurman RJ, Diana KL, Morrow CP: Pathologic models to predict outcome for women with endometrial adenocarcinoma. Cancer 77:1115, 1996.

Table 32-6 Grade, Depth of Myometrial Invasion, and Node Metastasis—Stage I

Depth of Invasion	PELVIC G1 $n = 180$	G2 $n = 288$	G3 $n = 153$
Endometrium only (n = 86)	0 (0%)	1 (3%)	0 (0%)
Inner (n = 281)	3 (3%)	7 (5%)	5 (9%)
Middle (n = 115)	0 (0%)	6 (9%)	1 (4%)
Deep (n = 139)	2 (11%)	11 (19%)	23 (34%)
Depth of Invasion	**AORTIC G1 $n = 180$**	**G2 $n = 288$**	**G3 $n = 153$**
Endometrium only (n = 86)	0 (0%)	1 (3%)	0 (0%)
Inner (n = 281)	1 (1%)	5 (4%)	2 (4%)
Middle (n = 115)	1 (5%)	0 (0%)	0 (0%)
Deep (n = 139)	1 (6%)	8 (14%)	15 (23%)

G, grade.
Adapted from Creasman WT, Morrow CP, Bundy BN, et al: Surgical pathologic spread patterns of endometrial cancer. Cancer 60:2035, 1987.

tumor grade. Table 32-7 shows the effects of tumor grade and depth of myometrial invasion. The frequency of nodal involvement becomes much greater with higher grade tumors and with greater depth of myometrial invasion. The risk of lymph node involvement appears to be negligible for endometrial carcinoma involving only the endometrium. With invasion of the inner third of the myometrium, there is negligible risk of node involvement for grade 1 and 2 cases. If the outer third of the myometrium is involved, the risk of nodal metastases is greatly increased. These data emphasize the importance of myometrial invasion and tumor spread, providing the basis for the FIGO Operative Staging System. Table 32-8 summarizes the risk of nodal metastases based on the GOG studies published by Creasman and colleagues. In a more recent GOG study cited previously, Morrow and coworkers noted that for patients without metastases at operation, the greatest risk of future recurrence was grade 3 histology. Furthermore, among 48 patients with histologically documented aortic node metastases, 47 were found to have positive pelvic nodes, adnexal metastases, or tumor invasion to the outer one third of the myometrium, emphasizing the poor prognostic aspects of these three findings.

Steroid Hormone Receptors. Steroid hormones affect the growth of target cells by binding with steroid receptors in the cell. The receptor steroid complex then interacts with DNA in the cell nucleus, stimulating the synthesis of messenger RNA, which acts in the cytoplasm to stimulate protein synthesis.

The steroid receptor level in endometrial carcinoma is lower than in normal endometrium. The highest levels of estrogen and progesterone receptors in tumors have been found in the well-differentiated (grade 1) tumors and the lowest in grade 3 tumors. Despite extensive research in this area, receptor status in endometrial carcinoma does not appear to have the same clinically relevant role as it does in cases of breast carcinoma.

Table 32-7 FIGO Staging and Nodal Metastasis

Staging	METASTASIS Pelvic	Aortic
IA G1 (n = 101)	2 (2%)	0 (0%)
G2 (n = 169)	13 (8%)	6 (4%)
G3 (n = 76)	8 (11%)	5 (7%)
IB G1 (n = 79)	3 (4%)	3 (4%)
G2 (n = 119)	12 (10%)	8 (7%)
G3 (n = 77)	20 (26%)	12 (16%)

FIGO, International Federation of Gynecology and Oncology; G, grade.
From Creasman WT, Morrow CP, Bundy BN, et al: Surgical pathologic spread patterns of endometrial cancer. Cancer 60:2035, 1987. Reprinted with permission.

Table 32-8 Risk Factors for Nodal Metastases—Stage I

Factor	Pelvic	Aortic
Low risk Grade 1 Endometrium only No intraperitoneal spread	0/44 (0%)	0/44 (0%)
Moderate risk Grade 2 or 3 Invasion to middle third	15/268 (6%)	6/268 (2%)
High risk Invasion to outer third	21/116 (18)	17/118 (15%)

Adapted from Creasman WT, Morrow CP, Bundy BN, et al: Surgical pathologic spread patterns of endometrial cancer. Cancer 60:2035, 1987.

Evaluation

In addition to the usual routine preoperative evaluation, the patient should have a chest radiographic examination, intravenous pyelogram, and/or a chest and abdominal pelvic computed tomography scan. However, a study by Connor and associates noted that preoperative computed tomography scan had only a 50% positive predictive value for nodal disease. Furthermore, postoperative computed tomography monitoring did not appear to improve survival. The measurement of cancer antigen 125 (CA 125), usually used in cases of ovarian carcinoma, may occasionally be useful. If elevated preoperatively, it usually indicates extrauterine disease. It may be a particularly useful marker for those with serous carcinoma of the endometrium.

Management

Stage I

Surgery is the primary treatment modality to treat patients with endometrial carcinoma, except in those patients with significant medical comorbidities. Complete surgical staging includes hysterectomy, bilateral salpingo-oophorectomy, pelvic cytology (washings), and pelvic and paraaortic lymph nodes. According to Orr and Chamberlin, the exceptions include young, premenopausal women with grade 1 endometrial adenocarcinoma associated with endometrial hyperplasia and women with significant medical comorbidities.

Surgical staging allows accurate surgical and histologic assessment of (1) tumor spread in the uterus, (2) degree of penetration into the myometrium, and (3) extrauterine spread to retroperitoneal nodes, adnexa, and/or the peritoneal cavity. This is the approach used for cases that are staged according to the 1988 FIGO system (see Table 32-3).

The use of laparoscopy in the treatment of early stage endometrial cancer has gained popularity over the past several years. This approach combines either a laparoscopy-assisted vaginal hysterectomy or a total laparoscopic hysterectomy with a laparoscopic lymphadenectomy. If this approach is used, it is still important to do a thorough inspection of the peritoneal cavity, peritoneal washings, and appropriate staging biopsies. The GOG recently concluded a phase III randomized trial of surgical staging for endometrial carcinoma comparing the laparoscopic approach to the more traditional abdominal approach. In addition, laparoscopic node dissection can be used particularly for patients who are incompletely staged at the time of initial operation.

For patients with significant medical comorbidities, radiation therapy alone can be used. However, radiation as the sole method of therapy yields inferior results, as Bickenbach and colleagues noted, with an 87% 5-year survival rate for patients with stage I carcinoma treated by surgery alone, in comparison with a 69% survival rate for those treated with radiation therapy alone. For those who cannot tolerate surgery or external beam therapy, treatment by intracavitary radiation alone (Heyman's capsules, see Fig. 32-12) offers some benefit. Lehoczky and associates reported on 170 elderly patients treated with brachytherapy alone with uncorrected 5-year survival rates for stages IA and IB of 46% and 30%, respectively.

Occasionally, morbidly obese patients are encountered for whom an abdominal operation is very risky. Sood and coworkers noted that for stage I patients with preoperative CA 125 less than 20 U/mL, the risk of extrauterine disease was only 3%, making vaginal hysterectomy a therapeutic option. Dotters reported CA 125 more than 35 U/mL usually predicted extrauterine disease, although approximately one third of patients needing full operative staging were not identified by an elevated CA 125 for grade 1 or 2 cases, whereas for grade 3, the sensitivity increased to 88%. However, a few false-positive cases were noted, making the results a useful guide but not sufficiently precise to be the sole criterion for performing lymphadenectomy.

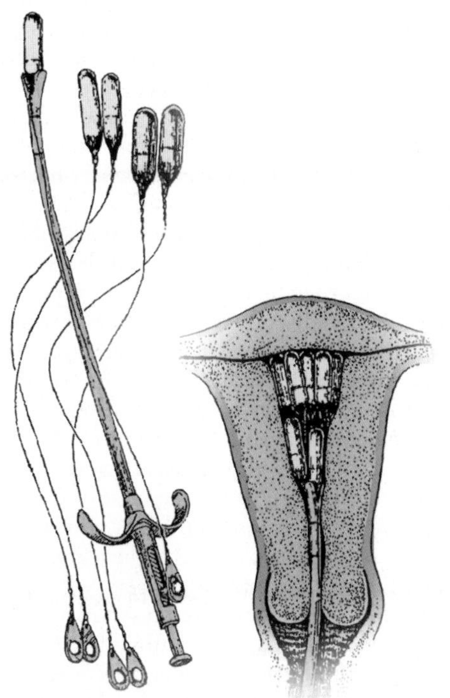

Figure 32-12. Heyman's capsules used to pack and distend the endometrial cavity. (From Wheeless CR: Atlas of Pelvic Surgery. Philadelphia, Lea & Febiger, 1981.)

Stage I, Grade 1. The risk of spread of grade 1 tumor to pelvic nodes is extremely small (see Table 32-7). Operatively, the abdomen is explored, peritoneal cytology is obtained, and an extrafascial total abdominal hysterectomy with bilateral salpingo-oophorectomy is performed.

In patients with stage I, grade 1 tumors, postoperative radiation (vaginal brachytherapy and/or external beam irradiation) may be considered if there is deep myometrial invasion to the outer one third or if there is any invasion and the surgical staging was limited. Postoperative irradiation delivered to the vaginal cuff provides a surface dose to the vagina of approximately 5000 to 6000 cGy (50 to 60 Gy)

Stage I, Grades 2 and 3. Regardless of the surgeon's preference for the extent of surgical staging, all patients with grade 2 or 3 lesions should undergo complete surgical staging. Mariani and coworkers reported improved survival in patients at high risk of nodal disease who underwent paraaortic lymphadenectomy in compared with those who did not have this procedure (Fig. 32-13).

Use of postoperative irradiation depends on the pathologic findings. For grade 2 tumors that invade the myometrium to the middle third or beyond or for grade 3 tumors that invade the myometrium, full pelvic irradiation is may be given in view of the risk of pelvic recurrence. However, if the pelvic nodes are free of tumor, no radiation or local vaginal irradiation alone may be sufficient.

Radiation Therapy Considerations. Three phase III randomized trials evaluated the use of adjuvant radiotherapy in patients with high-risk stage I endometrial cancer (see Table 32-9). In a Norwegian study comparing brachytherapy versus brachytherapy and pelvic radiation, local recurrences were decreased in the group of patients receiving pelvic radiation. In the PORTEC trial from The Netherlands, Creutzberg and colleagues reported on 714 patients with stage I disease. Patients received full pelvic radiotherapy or observation. While locoregional control was better in the treatment arm, there was no difference in overall survival. In a GOG trial, Keys and associates randomized almost 400 patients between whole pelvic radiation and observation. Similar to the PORTEC trial, there was a decrease of local recurrences in the radiation arm with no difference in survival. Current and future trials will evaluate vaginal brachytherapy and chemotherapy as better options to prevent recurrences in patients with intermediate-risk disease.

Stage II

Three therapeutic options have been employed for the treatment of stage II carcinoma of the endometrium that also involves the endocervix: (1) primary operation (radical hysterectomy and pelvic node dissection), (2) primary radiation (intrauterine and vaginal implant and external irradiation) followed by an operation (extrafascial hysterectomy), and (3) simple hysterectomy followed by external beam irradiation.

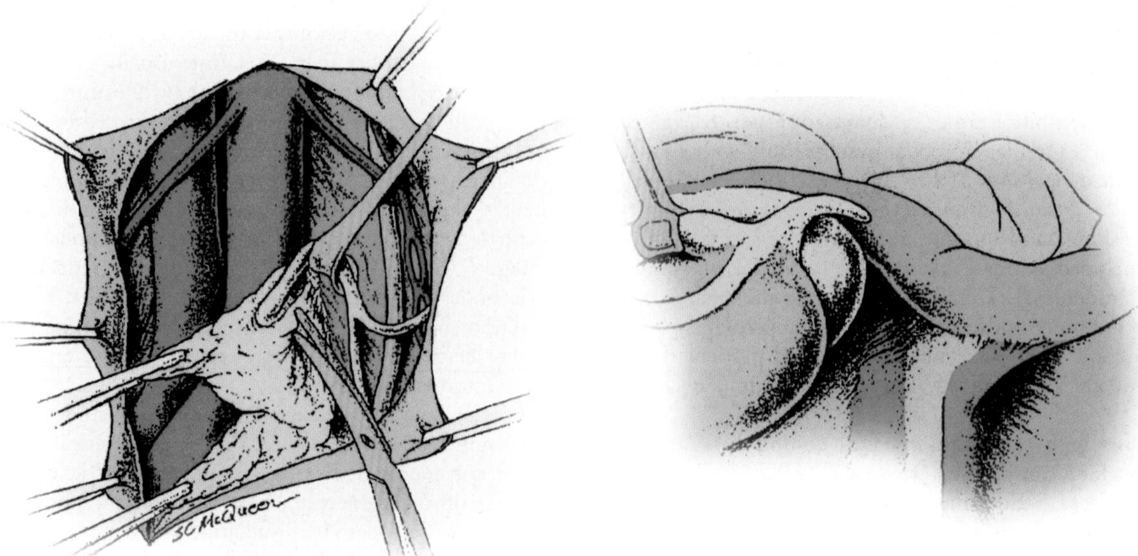

Figure 32-13. Removal of lymph node tissue. The technique of removal of retroperitoneal paraaortic nodes is demonstrated with the important anatomic landmarks.

Radical hysterectomy and pelvic node dissection have been used as effective therapy and have resulted in a 75% 5-year survival rate for the 26 patients treated by Homesley and colleagues and 65% for the 20 patients reported by Wallin and associates.

Most patients with stage II carcinoma of the endometrium are treated with a combination of radiation and extrafascial hysterectomy. A widely used protocol includes external radiation (45 Gy) and a single brachytherapy implant usually followed in 4 to 6 weeks by extrafascial total abdominal hysterectomy, bilateral salpingo-oophorectomy, and paraaortic node sampling. Podczaski and coworkers noted that those with gross cervical tumor had a poor prognosis and were likely to have extrauterine disease at operation. For patients with cervical involvement on biopsy but no gross tumor, Trimble and Jones found radiation treatment by a single implant alone followed by a hysterectomy to be effective, and they added external therapy depending on the nodal findings and myometrial invasion. Andersen reported on 54 patients with stage II tumors and found a 70.6% survival rate in patients treated by abdominal hysterectomy followed by radiation.

Comparable outcomes have recently been reported using high-dose-rate brachytherapy approaches in stage I–II patients unable to undergo surgery. Nguygen and coworkers reported a 3-year disease-free survival rate of 85% in 36 stage I patients treated with definitive radiation therapy. Nineteen patients were considered inoperable due to morbid obesity, and the remainder had significant medical problems precluding anesthesia. All patients were treated as outpatients with five weekly brachytherapy applications performed under conscious sedation. At a median follow-up of 32 months, the 3-year actuarial uterine-control rate was 88%.

Adjuvant Systemic Therapy for Early Stage Endometrioid Endometrial Cancer. In addition to radiation therapy, adjuvant therapeutic options for patients with endometrial cancer and high-risk features include hormonal agents and cytotoxic chemotherapy. Although the addition of postoperative radiation to high-risk patients does reduce the local recurrence rate, distant metastasis continues to be problematic. In approximately 25% of patients with low-stage, grade 3 lesions, the disease will recur at a distant site. In addition, 20% of clinical stage II patients and at least 30% of patients who present with extrauterine disease recur at distant sites even after patients have received adjuvant pelvic radiation.

Several studies have been performed evaluating the use of progestins as an adjuvant therapy for patients with endometrial carcinoma. In trials that have recruited more than 2500 patients, no difference in survival was demonstrated. A meta-analysis of randomized trials of progestins as an adjuvant therapy for patients with early stage endometrial cancer failed to demonstrate any decrease in endometrial-cancer-related deaths. These earlier trials, however, were limited by including patients with low-risk prognostic features or by including only stage I patients. Recently, a large prospective, randomized trial evaluated adjuvant progestin therapy in patients who were at high risk of recurrence. The study enrolled 1012 patients with grade 3 tumors, tumors with high-risk histologic subtypes, or tumors with more than one third myometrial invasion. There was a significant decrease in recurrences among the progestin-treated patients. There was, however, no difference in survival. The 5-year survival rate in the progestin-treated arm was 75% and 72% in the control arm. The use of progestins in the adjuvant treatment of endometrial cancer is currently not standard.

Similar to progestins, there is no benefit from tamoxifen as an adjuvant therapy after primary surgery.

No studies have demonstrated a survival advantage of chemotherapy given in the adjuvant setting. In a GOG study of high-risk patients who received postoperative whole pelvic irradiation alone or with doxorubicin, there was no statistical difference in survival rates or progression-free interval rates. In a phase II study, Burke and colleagues documented an excellent disease-free survival in high-risk patients without extrauterine disease who received six cycles of cisplatin, doxorubicin, and cyclophosphamide. In those patients with disease limited to the uterus, the 3-year survival rate was 82%. In patients with disease outside of the uterus, the 3-year survival rate was 46%.

Stage I or II Uterine Papillary Serous Carcinoma

Over the past few years, several academic centers have tried to determine the best treatment for patients with early stage UPSC. Even with minimal uterine disease limited to the uterus, patients with UPSC often have metastatic disease. In a retrospective, multi-institutional study, Huh and associates reported on 60 patients with stage I UPSC who underwent comprehensive surgical staging. The investigators found that recurrence rates were lower than previously reported and inferred that complete staging may provide a potential benefit. In their study, none of the seven patients who received chemotherapy had a recurrence. In a multi-institutional retrospective study of early-stage UPSC, Dietrich and colleagues found that the combination of carboplatin and paclitaxel in the adjuvant setting was effective in improving survival and limiting recurrences. Further investigation is necessary.

Combined chemotherapy and radiation therapy may play a role in the management of patients with early stage disease. Turner and associates reported the application of vaginal irradiation at a high-dose rate in combination with chemotherapy in surgical stage I patients. The 5-year survival rate was 94%, which is higher than that of most other studies for patients with stage I disease.

Management of Stage III/IV or Recurrent Endometrial Cancer

Because of the hematogenous and lymphatic spread of endometrial cancer, patients with recurrent or advanced disease often present with tumor outside of the pelvis. Systemic therapy, therefore, plays an important role in the management of these patients. Both hormonal and cytotoxic agents have activity in patients with advanced or recurrent endometrial cancer. In addition, there continues to be a role of radiation therapy to obtain local control or to treat disease in the pelvis.

In stage III carcinoma, the disease has spread outside the uterus but remains confined to the pelvis with the exception of stage IIIc, which involves the retroperitoneal nodes. These tumors do not involve the mucosa of the rectum or bladder. They account for approximately 7% of all endometrial carcinomas and occur in patients who are older than those with lower stage tumors and often medically less able to undergo an operation.

Patients with stage IIIA disease include those with disease spread to the adnexa, serosa, and/or positive cytology. Those patients with nonendometrioid histology or spread to the serosa or adnexa require adjuvant therapy (either radiation, chemotherapy, or both). Studies by Slomovitz and colleagues and Mariani and associates have found that patients with stage IIIA disease by positive cytology alone do well without adjuvant therapy.

Approximately 3% of endometrial carcinomas are at stage IV, and many of these patients have tumor metastases outside the pelvis. If possible, optimal surgical debulking has been associated with a prolonged survival. Bristow and coworkers reported that the amount of residual disease after cytoreductive surgery, age, and performance status appear to be important determinants of survival in patients with stage IVB endometrial carcinoma.

Since 10% of recurrences will occur more than 5 years after initial diagnosis, patients with adenocarcinoma of the endometrium need prolonged follow-up. In the series of Aalders and associates involving 379 patients, half of the recurrences were in the pelvis and vagina; the most frequent sites of nonpelvic metastases were the lung (17%), upper portion of the abdomen (10%), and bone (6%). Radiation was the primary treatment of localized recurrent disease in patients who had an operation alone as the initial treatment, but operative excision of resectable nodules was also done when feasible. The 5-year survival rate for those patients who received progestins with other forms of treatment for grade 1 and 2 recurrences was 26% compared with 14% for those who did not. For undifferentiated tumors, the comparable survival rate was 9%.

Radiotherapy can be useful to salvage patients with pelvic recurrence who had only operation for primary therapy. Ackerman and coworkers treated 21 patients with pelvic relapse and found radiation achieved pelvic control of disease in 14 (67%). The best results were with recurrences in the vaginal mucosa. Similarly, Sears and colleagues treated 45 patients with vaginal recurrence of endometrial cancer with radiation and achieved a 44% 5-year survival rate. As noted previously, Carey and associates salvaged 15 of 17 patients with vaginal recurrence initially treated by operation alone.

Systemic treatment options for patients with advanced or recurrent disease may vary depending on the histologic subtype of endometrial cancer.

Chemotherapy for Advanced and Recurrent Endometrioid Endometrial Cancer

Several chemotherapeutic agents or combinations of agents have demonstrated activity in patients with endometrioid endometrial cancer. Combination therapy is more effective than single-agent therapy in treating this disease. The challenge has been to combine agents to maximize efficacy while attempting to limit toxicity.

Doxorubicin was one of the first drugs identified with good activity against endometrial cancer. Single-agent doxorubicin has a response rate of approximately 25% with a median duration of response of less than 1 year. Single-agent cisplatin also has demonstrated response rates between 20% and 42% when used as a first-line agent. The duration of response was again very short (3 to 5 months). In several phase II studies, adding cisplatin to doxorubicin resulted in response rates between 45% and 60%. In a GOG randomized phase III study, cisplatin and doxorubicin in combination had a higher response rate compared with single-agent doxorubicin (45% vs. 27%). There was no difference in overall survival. The EORTC performed a similar trial comparing the same two regimens. Again, the combination arm had a higher response rate than the doxorubicin-alone treatment group. In this study, there was a modest survival advantage in those patients who received the combination regimen. The median overall survival in cisplatin- and doxorubicin-treated patients was 9 months compared with 7 months in the patients who received doxorubicin alone ($p = 0.065$).

More recently, phase II studies of paclitaxel found significant activity in chemonaive patients with recurrent endometrial cancer with a response rate of 36%. In patients who failed previous chemotherapy, paclitaxel also demonstrated activity with a response rate up to 43%. The antitumor effect of single-agent paclitaxel led to the incorporation of paclitaxel into combination therapy regimens. In a phase II study, the combination of cisplatin and paclitaxel demonstrated a 67% response rate. In a phase III study, the GOG found similar activity between the combination of cisplatin and doxorubicin versus doxorubicin and paclitaxel. Following this study, the GOG performed a phase III trial evaluating doxorubicin and cisplatin compared with doxorubicin, cisplatin, and paclitaxel (TAP) with granulocyte-colony-stimulating factor. The TAP regimen yielded a superior response rate (57% vs. 34%, $p < 0.001$), longer progression-free survival (8.3 vs. 5.3 months, $p < 0.001$), and longer overall survival (15.3 vs. 12.3 months, $p = 0.037$). The results of this study set the TAP regimen as the standard of care for the first-line treatment of advanced or recurrent endometrial cancer.

In an attempt to decrease the toxicity related to cisplatin therapy, carboplatin has been investigated. Single-agent carboplatin demonstrates modest activity in chemonaive patients with little or no activity in patients pretreated with chemotherapy. In a phase II study, the combination of paclitaxel and carboplatin was evaluated in patients with advanced and recurrent disease. In patients with advanced endometrioid endometrial cancer, there was a 78% response rate to this combination. The median failure-free survival time was 23 months and the 3-year overall survival rate was 62%. In patients with recurrent disease, the response rate was 56% and the median failure-free interval was 6 months.

The combination of carboplatin and paclitaxel has a more favorable toxicity profile than cisplatin and paclitaxel. For this reason, many community physicians have preferred this combination in the setting of advanced or recurrent endometrial cancer rather than the TAP regimen. The GOG is currently accruing to a phase III randomized study to evaluate TAP compared with carboplatin and paclitaxel to address this question.

In a phase III randomized trial, the GOG recently reported that the combination of doxorubicin and cisplatin demonstrated improved progression free and overall survival compared with whole abdominal irradiation in patients with advanced disease.

Despite higher response rates, more effective cytotoxic agents with longer durations of response are needed. The alkylating agent ifosfamide demonstrated a response rate of 24% in chemonaive patients and a 0% to 15% response rate in patients pretreated with platinum agents. 5-Fluorouracil has demonstrated activity both as a single agent and in combination with melphalan in the phase II setting. Oral etoposide has been shown to have some activity against chemonaive patients with a tolerable toxicity profile, but this was not seen in patients who had received previous chemotherapy.

Prognosis is very poor for patients who fail first-line chemotherapy. The response rates for second- and third-line agents are often less than 10% and the overall survival is less than 9 months. Paclitaxel may have better activity than other agents in this setting. In patients who have failed previous chemotherapy, paclitaxel has response rates up to 43%. In particular, in a cohort of patients who were refractory to platinum, paclitaxel was shown to have a 22% response rate. Preliminary data suggest that retreatment with a platinum/paclitaxel-based regimen may be effective in patients who previously responded to these agents.

Hormone Therapy

Progestins for Advanced or Recurrent Disease

For the past 50 years, progestational agents have been valuable in the armamentarium against endometrial cancer, particularly in patients with recurrent disease. Progestins are generally well tolerated. Side effects are usually minor and include weight gain, edema, thrombophlebitis, headache, and occasional hypertension. In patients with medical comorbidities, use of hormonal agents may be preferable to cytotoxic chemotherapy. Initial clinical trials in patients with advanced or recurrent endometrial cancer demonstrated response rates of 30% to 50%. Larger studies with more specific response criteria demonstrate more modest response rates, usually between 11% and 24%. Podratz and colleagues treated 155 patients with advanced or recurrent endometrial cancer with progestational agents. The objective response rate was 11%. Overall, survival after initiation of hormone therapy was 40% at 1 year, 19% at 2 years, and 8% at 5 years. In a GOG phase II study, patients who had no previous exposure to chemotherapy or hormonal agents were treated with megesterol acetate (800 mg/day). The overall response rate was 24%. The progression-free survival and overall survival were 2.5 months and 7.6 months, respectively.

Current recommendations for progestin therapy include oral medroxyprogesterone acetate (Provera), intramuscular medroxyprogesterone acetate (Depo-Provera), and megesterol acetate (Megace). Although there are no randomized studies that have directly compared different formulations of progestins, response rates are similar. In addition, although a dose-response effect of progestin therapy has been reported in breast cancer, there is no evidence of this effect in patients with endometrial cancer. In a randomized trial of oral medroxyprogesterone acetate, patients receiving the low-dose regimen (200 mg/day) had a higher response to therapy than those receiving the high-dose regimen (1000 mg/day).

There are a number of tumor characteristics that increase the likelihood of response to hormone therapy. These include low-grade tumors, the presence of steroid hormone receptors (i.e., progesterone-receptor [PR] and estrogen-receptor [ER]-positive), and a longer disease-free interval. The GOG demonstrated a response rate of 8% in women whose tumors were PR-negative and 37% for women whose tumors were PR-positive. In addition, there was a 7% response rate in women with ER-negative tumors compared with a 26% response rate in women with ER-positive tumors. Patients with poorly differentiated tumors or hormone-receptor-negative tumors have significantly lower response rates to progestin therapy.

Because of the low-toxicity profile and modest efficacy, progestins should be considered in patients with recurrent endometrial cancer. In particular, all patients not eligible for clinical trials with well-differentiated hormone-receptor-positive recurrent or advanced disease can be given a trial of progestin therapy. If the patient has an objective response, the progestin may be continued indefinitely until there is disease progression.

Selective Estrogen Receptor Modulators and Aromatase Inhibitors. SERMs with antiestrogenic effects in the uterus have been used to treat women with recurrent endometrial cancer. First-generation SERMs such as tamoxifen have mixed estrogenic agonist and antagonist activity. Early response rates for tamoxifen in advanced or recurrent endometrial cancer were between 20% and 36%. However, in a GOG phase II study of tamoxifen given at a dose of 20 mg twice daily, only 10% of patients demonstrated an objective response. Grade 1 and 2 tumors are more likely to respond to tamoxifen than grade 3 tumors.

Short-term administration of tamoxifen can cause an increase in the progesterone receptor levels in postmenopausal women with endometrial cancer. Studies with alternating tamoxifen and progestins have been performed to determine whether this upregulation increases the response to progestin therapy. Phase II trials of tamoxifen plus alternating cycles of progestin demonstrated a 27% to 33% response rate. The Eastern Cooperative Oncology Group found no difference in response rates between patients treated with progestin alone and those treated with progestin in combination with tamoxifen.

Second- and third-generation SERMs, such as raloxifene and arzoxifene, have more selective estrogen antagonism in the uterus. The third-generation agent arzoxifene has enhanced bioavailability and potent estrogen antagonist activity in the uterus. Arzoxifene is 30 to 100 times more potent than raloxifene in antagonizing the effects of estrogen in the uterus. In a phase II GOG study, the response rate in patients with advanced or recurrent endometrial cancer was 31% (9/29) with one complete response and eight partial responses. All patients in this study had tumors that were either ER- or PR-positive or were low grade. These findings suggest that SERMS are an effective alternative to progestins.

Anastrozole, an oral nonsteroidal aromatase inhibitor, is approved by the U.S. Food and Drug Administration for postmenopausal women with progressive breast cancer following tamoxifen therapy. Aromatase is elevated in the stroma of endometrial cancer. In a phase II trial by the GOG, anastrozole was found to have minimal activity (9% response rate) in an unselected population of patients with advanced or recurrent endometrial cancer. More than 25% of the patients in this study had nonendometrioid histologic subtypes, and only 22% of the patients had ER- and PR-positive tumors or demonstrated a response to previous therapy. In the subset of women with FIGO grade 1 and 2 tumors with endometrioid histology, the response rate was 30%.

Chemotherapy for Advanced and Recurrent Uterine Papillary Serous Carcinoma

The majority of information available for patients with UPSC is from retrospective, nonrandomized case series. In addition, response rates to therapy often come from subset analysis of studies of all types of advanced or recurrent endometrial cancer, including phase III GOG studies. Levenback and associates reported 20 patients with recurrent or advanced UPSC treated with cyclophosphamide, doxorubicin, and cisplatin. Fifty-eight percent of the patients were alive without disease after 24 months. However, this regimen was highly toxic. Price and coworkers also evaluated cyclophosphamide, doxorubicin, and cisplatin in 19 patients with advanced disease and 11 patients with recurrent disease. Of the patients treated in the adjuvant setting for advanced disease, 58% were alive without evidence of disease with a median follow-up of 24 months. In the patients with recurrent disease, the response rate was 27%. In addition, all the patients developed treatment-related toxicities. Most of these toxicities were hematologic. One treatment-related death was due to cardiotoxicity.

Recently, more favorable results using paclitaxel with and without carboplatin have been demonstrated. In a phase II study evaluating carboplatin and paclitaxel, the response rate was 60% in 20 patients with high-stage UPSC. The failure-free survival time was 18 months and the 3-year overall survival rate was 39%. Two of four patients with recurrent UPSC demonstrated a response to carboplatin and paclitaxel. Zanotti and colleagues evaluated 24 patients with measurable disease (either progressive disease after initial surgery or recurrent disease). There was an 89% response rate in patients treated after initial surgery, and a 64% response rate for patients with recurrent disease. At the University of Texas M. D. Anderson Cancer Center, single-agent paclitaxel demonstrated a 77% response rate in patients with recurrent disease. Despite this activity, the duration of response in these studies is less than 1 year. Other agents are under investigation for the treatment of UPSC.

SARCOMAS

Sarcomas comprise less than 5% of uterine malignancies and are much less frequent than endometrial carcinomas, particularly in Western countries. Numerous terms have been used to describe the many histologic types. One useful classification is based on determination of the resemblance of the sarcomatous elements to mesenchymal tissue normally found in the uterus (homologous sarcomas) in contrast to tissues foreign to the uterus (heterologous sarcomas). Homologous types include leiomyosarcomas, ESSs, and rarely angiosarcomas. Heterologous types include rhabdomyosarcomas, chondrosarcomas, osteosarcomas, and liposarcomas. These sarcomas may exist exclusively or may be admixed with epithelial adenocarcinoma, in which case the term *carcinosarcoma* (malignant mixed müllerian tumor) is applied. The following box shows a morphologic classification for uterine sarcomas. A study by Zelmanowicz and colleagues suggests risk factors for these tumors are similar to those of endometrial carcinoma, that is, estrogens and obesity increase the risk and oral contraceptive use decreases the risk. No uniformly defined staging criteria exist for these tumors, and the most widely used definitions are similar to those for endometrial carcinoma, that is, stage I, confined to the corpus; stage II, corpus and cervix involved; stage III, spread outside the uterus but confined to the pelvis; and stage IV, spread outside the true pelvis or into the mucosa of the bladder or rectum. Similar to endometrial adenocarcinoma, operative stage is the most important predictor of survival.

Leiomyosarcoma

Leiomyosarcomas represent 1% to 2% of uterine malignancies and approximately one third of uterine sarcomas (Fig. 32-14).

Modified Classification of Uterine Sarcomas

I. Pure sarcoma
  A. Homologous
    1. Smooth muscle tumors
      a. Leiomyosarcoma
      b. Leiomyoblastoma
      c. Metastasizing tumors with benign histologic appearance
        i. Intravenous leiomyomatosis
        ii. Metastasizing uterine leiomyoma
        iii. Leiomyomatosis peritonealis disseminata
    2. Endometrial stromal sarcomas
      a. Low grade: endolymphatic stromal myosis
      b. High grade: endometrial stromal sarcoma
  B. Heterologous
    1. Rhabdomyosarcoma
    2. Chondrosarcoma
    3. Osteosarcoma
    4. Liposarcoma
  C. Other sarcomas
II. Carcinosarcoma—malignant mixed müllerian tumors
  A. Homologous (carcinosarcoma): carcinoma + homologous sarcoma
  B. Heterologous: carcinoma + heterologous sarcoma
III. Müllerian adenosarcoma
IV. Lymphoma

Modified from Clemet P, Scully RE: Pathology of uterine sarcomas. In Coppleson M (ed): Gynecologic Oncology. New York, Churchill Livingstone, 1981. p 591. Reprinted by permission.

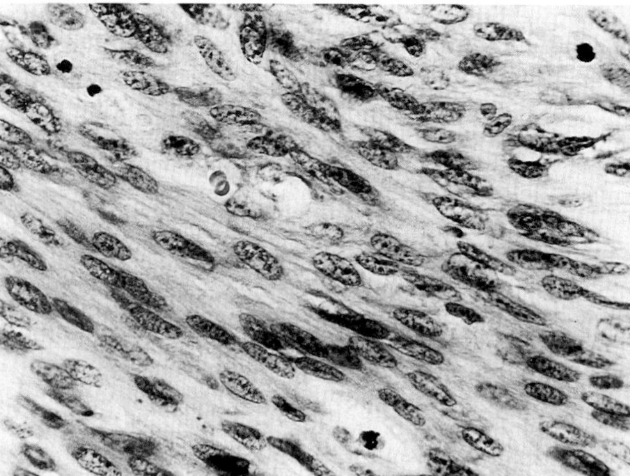

Figure 32-14. Leiomyosarcoma. Nuclear hyperchromatism and mitotic figures are present. (×660.) (From Clement PB, Scully RE: Pathology of uterine sarcomas. In Coppleson M [ed]: Gynecologic Oncology. Edinburgh, Churchill Livingstone, 1981. Reprinted by permission.)

Although the exact cause is unknown, leiomyosarcomas are not thought to arise from benign leiomyomas. Leibsohn and coworkers noted that among 1423 patients who had hysterectomies for presumed leiomyomas with a uterine size comparable with a 12-week pregnancy or larger, the risk of sarcoma increased with age, from 0.4% for those in their 30s to 1.4% for those in their 50s. The determination of malignancy is made in part by ascertaining the number of mitoses in 10 hpf as well as the presence of cytologic atypia, abnormal mitotic figures, and nuclear pleomorphism (see Fig. 32-14). Vascular invasion and extrauterine spread of tumor are associated with worse prognoses. A finding of more than five mitoses per 10 hpf with cytologic atypia leads to a diagnosis of leiomyosarcoma; when there are four or fewer mitoses per 10 hpf, the tumors usually have a more benign clinical course. The prognosis worsens for tumors with more than 10 mitoses per 10 hpf. The presence of bizarre cells may not necessarily establish the diagnosis because they can occasionally be seen in benign leiomyomas and in patients receiving progestational agents. Furthermore, it is important to note that an increase in mitotic count in leiomyomas occurs in pregnancy as well as during oral contraceptive use. This can occasionally cause confusion in the histologic diagnosis.

Usually, the patient has an enlarged pelvic mass, occasionally accompanied by pain or vaginal bleeding. Leiomyosarcomas are suspected if the uterus undergoes rapid enlargement, particularly in patients in the perimenopausal or postmenopausal age group.

Approximately 85% of women diagnosed with a leiomyosarcoma have clinical stage I or II disease (i.e., disease that is limited to the uterus and cervix). Primary treatment includes total hysterectomy, bilateral salpingo-oophorectomy, and staging. Despite the low incidence of high-stage disease, approximately 50% of patients will have a recurrence within 2 years. The recurrence in most of these patients is outside the pelvis.

The GOG evaluated the role of adjuvant radiation therapy in patients (N = 48) with clinical stage I and II disease (Table 32-9). There was no difference in the progression-free interval, abso-lute 2-year survival rate, or site of first recurrence between patients who received pelvic radiation (N = 11) and those that did not (N = 37). This is not surprising because most recurrences were outside the pelvis (83%). There was recurrence in 48% of the patients, and most of these patients had a recurrence within 17 months of diagnosis. In the adjuvant chemotherapy trial by the GOG, patients treated with Adriamycin had a recurrence less frequently than those in the observation arm (44% vs. 61%). This difference was not statistically significant.

Table 32-9 Summary of Randomized Trials of Adjuvant Radiotherapy in Stage I Endometrial Carcinoma

Trial	Surgery	Randomization	Locoregional recurrences	Survival
Norwegian 1968–1974	TAH-BSO	Brachytherapy vs brachy and pelvic RT	7% vs 2% at 5 years, $P < 0.01$	89% vs 91% at 5 years, P = NS
PORTEC	TAH-BSO	Obs vs pelvic RT	14% vs 4% at 5 years, $P < 0.001$	85% vs 81% at 5 years, $P = 0.31$
GOG	TAH-BSO, nodes	Obs vs pelvic RT	12% vs 3% at 2 years, $P < 0.01$	86% vs 92% at 4 years, $P = 0.56$

Unfortunately, there is limited information regarding treatment of advanced or recurrent leiomyosarcoma. Hannigan and colleagues used vincristine, actinomycin D, and cyclophosphamide (Cytoxan) (VAC protocol; see Chapter 31, Malignant Diseases of the Vagina) and noted a 13% complete response rate and 16% partial response rate in 74 patients with advanced metastatic uterine sarcomas. A large collaborative trial was conducted by the GOG and reported by Omura and associates. The best responses were obtained for patients with lung metastases who received doxorubicin and DTIC. Current evidence suggests that a multidrug program offers the greatest potential for inducing remission of uterine sarcomas. Cisplatin, Adriamycin, paclitaxel (Taxol), ifosfamide, and VP 16 all appear to have some effectiveness. Most recently, gemcitabine and docetaxel have been evaluated in a phase II study for patients with recurrent leiomyosarcoma. In this study, 34 patients with leiomyosarcoma were treated. Overall response rate was 53%; however, the duration of response was only 5.6 months.

Endometrial Stromal Sarcoma

Overall, stromal tumors comprise approximately 10% of uterine sarcomas. Their behavior correlates primarily with mitotic rate. Although these tumors were once divided into low grade and high grade, more recently all ESSs are considered low grade. If high-grade elements are present, these tumors would be classified as undifferentiated high-grade sarcomas. Undifferentiated sarcomas have a greater degree of anaplasia and lack the branching vasculature characteristic of ESSs.

ESSs have a peak incidence in the fifth decade of life. There is no association with previous radiation nor are risk factors of endometrial carcinoma associated with the development of ESS. Histologically, ESS most resembles proliferative endometrial stroma.

Prognosis depends on the extent of disease and ability to remove all of the tumor at the time of surgery. In general, ESSs are indolent, slowly progressing tumors.

Recurrent disease may be diagnosed as many as 30 years after diagnosis. ESS tends to recur locally in the pelvis or peritoneal cavity and frequently spreads to the lungs. In treating metastatic disease, it should be remembered that these tumors contain estrogen and progestin steroid hormone receptors and are sensitive to hormone therapy. Complete resolution has been reported with megestrol acetate (Megace), medroxyprogesterone (Provera), letrozole (Femara), tamoxifen, and 17α-hydroxyprogesterone caproate (Delalutin).

Radiation has also been used to treat recurrences of these tumors, especially in the pelvis, with resolution of all residual tumors, but extensive experience with radiation therapy is not available. Systemic chemotherapy with cytotoxic agents has not been reported generally to be effective, although good responses to doxorubicin (Adriamycin) have been reported.

Undifferentiated Sarcomas

These high-grade tumors behave aggressively and have a poor prognosis. These tumors must be evaluated carefully as they are often confused with other large cell undifferentiated tumors (lymphoma, leukemia, high-grade endometrial cancer, carcinosarcoma).

Microscopically, more than 10 mitoses per 10 hpf are present, and frequently 20 or more mitoses per 10 hpf are present. Some series have reported 100% fatalities, although Vongtama and coworkers reported survival of more than 60% for 24 patients with stage I and one patient with stage II disease.

Recurrences are common in the pelvis, lung, and abdomen. If there has not been previous radiation treatment and the recurrence is confined to the pelvis, usually pelvic irradiation is prescribed. If there is disseminated disease, multiple-agent chemotherapy is used.

Carcinosarcoma (Malignant Mixed Müllerian Tumors)

As shown in the box on p. 830, these tumors consist of carcinomatous and sarcomatous elements native to the uterus that may resemble the endometrial stroma of smooth muscle (homologous) or of sarcomatous tissues foreign to the uterus (heterologous). Spanos and colleagues reviewed 188 patients with mixed mesodermal tumor and found both the prognosis and the pattern of survival similar for both homologous and heterologous tumors. The study of George and coworkers showed that patients with these tumors had a markedly worse prognosis than patients with high-grade endometrial carcinomas. Unlike patients with endometrial stromal sarcoma or leiomyosarcoma, those with carcinosarcoma tend to be older and primarily postmenopausal, usually beyond the age of 62 years. Previous pelvic irradiation has been identified as an occasional predisposing factor and was experienced by 17 of the 136 patients reviewed by Norris and Taylor. The heterologous and homologous tumors occur with approximately equivalent frequency. These tumors spread into the myometrium and then to the pelvis, to the abdomen including the peritoneum, and frequently to the lungs and pleura, a pattern similar to the spread of endometrial carcinoma.

A common symptom is postmenopausal bleeding, often accompanied by a large uterus. Occasionally, the diagnosis is made in tissue removed with D&C, and the tumor may appear to be a polypoid excrescence from the cervix; diagnosis may be made also by vaginal ultrasound examination.

As is true for other sarcomas, the primary treatment is surgical removal of the uterus. The extent of the tumor and the depth of myometrial invasion are important prognostic factors. Those with deep myometrial invasion are more likely to have spread to pelvic or paraaortic nodes, as in endometrial carcinomas. Patients with tumors confined to the uterus and little or no myometrial spread have the best prognosis. Total abdominal hysterectomy and bilateral salpingo-oophorectomy are completed with stage I tumors; more extensive procedures are occasionally attempted for stage II tumors as well as for those with early extrauterine spread. Nielsen and coworkers reported a 5-year survival rate of 58% for these when the disease was confined to the uterus.

In a phase I/II study of ifosfamide and cisplatin as adjuvant therapy in patients with high-stage carcinosarcoma, the GOG found this combination to be tolerable. Progression-free and overall survival rates at 2 years were 69% and 82%, respectively. This study lacked appropriate controls so the impact of this regimen on improving survival could not be evaluated.

For patients with advanced or recurrent disease, the GOG evaluated ifosfamide versus ifosfamide and cisplatin in a phase

III randomized study. The response rate to the combination therapy was superior (54% vs. 36%); however, the toxicity was significantly higher. In addition, no significant difference in overall survival was seen.

Müllerian Adenosarcoma

Müllerian adenosarcoma is a rare low-grade malignancy composed of both a sarcomatous stroma (homologous) and a proliferation of benign glandular elements that are intimately associated. It occurs predominantly in women older than 60 years. Ten cases were described initially by Clement and Scully. Total abdominal hysterectomy with bilateral salpingo-oophorectomy is the treatment of choice, but Kaku and colleagues reported on the GOG experience and found a few cases behave aggressively and these authors recommend a staging laparotomy for apparent stage I and II cases. In a retrospective study at the M. D. Anderson Cancer Center, 41 patients with adenosarcoma were evaluated. In this study, 38% of patients had recurrent disease (median time to recurrence 12 months). Adjuvant therapy did not affect the clinical course in patients with no measurable disease after surgery. Mitotic index and sarcomatous overgrowth were related to prognosis. In patients with advanced-stage disease or recurrent disease, there was a moderate rate of response to platinum-based chemotherapy and chemosensitizing radiation. Sixty percent of patients with recurrent disease had a complete response to treatment.

Lymphoma

On rare occasions, the uterus can be the original site for lymphoma, or, more commonly, involvement of the uterus may be the initial presentation of disseminated lymphoma. Approximately 40 cases of primary lymphoma of the uterus have been reported. They are usually treated by radiation after hysterectomy.

KEY POINTS

- Endometrial carcinoma is the most common malignancy of the female genital tract. In the United States, the lifetime risk of endometrial cancer is 3%.
- Most women who develop endometrial cancer are between 50 and 65 years of age.
- Women with Lynch syndrome (hereditary nonpolyposis colorectal cancer syndrome) have a 40% to 60% lifetime risk of endometrial cancer, which is similar to their lifetime risk of colon cancer.
- Chronic unopposed estrogen stimulation of the endometrium leads to endometrial hyperplasia and in some cases adenocarcinoma. Other important predisposing factors include obesity, nulliparity, late menopause, and diabetes.
- The risk of a woman developing endometrial carcinoma is increased three times if her body mass index is greater than 30.
- Tamoxifen use increases the risk of endometrial neoplasia two- to threefold.
- The primary symptom of endometrial carcinoma is postmenopausal bleeding. Women with abnormal bleeding should undergo an endometrial sampling to rule out endometrial pathology.
- Cytologic atypia in endometrial hyperplasia is the most important factor in determining malignant potential.
- Simple hyperplasia will develop into endometrial cancer in 1% of patients, whereas complex hyperplasia will develop into cancer in 29% of patients.
- Recent studies have found that there is a 40% concurrent rate of endometrial cancer in patients with a preoperative diagnosis of complex atypical hyperplasia.
- Prognosis in endometrial carcinoma is related to tumor grade, tumor stage, histologic type, and degree of myometrial invasion.
- Older patients with atypical hyperplasia are at increased risk of malignant progression compared with younger patients.
- Computed tomography scans may miss as many as 50% of patients with nodal disease.
- A key determinant of the risk of nodal spread of endometrial carcinoma is depth of myometrial invasion, which is often related to tumor grade.
- Well-differentiated (grade 1) endometrial carcinomas usually express steroid hormone receptors, whereas poorly differentiated (grade 3) tumors usually do not express receptors.
- Uterine papillary serous carcinoma is an aggressive histologic subtype associated with metastatic disease even in the absence of myometrial invasion.
- Ninety percent of recurrences of adenocarcinoma of the endometrium occur within 5 years.
- Overall survival rates for patients with adenocarcinoma of the endometrium by stage are as follows: stage I, 86%; stage II, 66%; stage III, 44%; stage IV, 16% (overall 72.7% 5-year survival rate combining clinical and operative staging systems).
- Histologic variants of endometrial carcinoma with a poor prognosis include uterine papillary serous carcinoma and clear-cell carcinoma.
- Patients with uterine papillary serous or clear-cell carcinoma of the endometrium should have a full staging laparotomy similar to that for ovarian carcinoma.
- The most frequent sites of distant metastasis of adenocarcinoma of the endometrium are the lung, retroperitoneal nodes, and abdomen.
- Primary treatment of endometrial cancer includes hysterectomy, bilateral salpingo-oophorectomy, pelvic cytology, bilateral pelvic and paraaortic lymphadenectomy, and resection of all disease. The exceptions include young perimenopausal women with stage I and grade 1 endometrial carcinoma associated with endometrial hyperplasia, and women with increased risk of mortality secondary to medical comorbidities.

KEY POINTS *Continued*

- Postoperative adjuvant radiation has not been shown to improve overall survival.
- Patients with high stage or recurrent disease should be treated in a multimodality approach including chemotherapy, radiation, and/or hormone therapy.
- Uterine sarcomas comprise less than 5% of uterine malignancies.
- Uterine sarcomas are treated primarily by operation including removal of the uterus, tubes, and ovaries.
- Endometrial stromal sarcomas are low-grade sarcomas with an indolent course.
- Multiagent chemotherapeutic regimens are usually prescribed for metastatic sarcomas; complete responses are rare and usually temporary.

BIBLIOGRAPHY

Aalders J, Abeler V, Kolstad P, Onsrud M: Postoperative external irradiation and prognostic parameters in stage I endometrial carcinoma: Clinical and histopathologic study of 540 patients. Obstet Gynecol 56:419–427, 1980.

Aalders JG, Abeler V, Kolstad P: Clinical (stage III) as compared to subclinical intrapelvic extrauterine tumor spread in endometrial carcinoma: A clinical and histopathological study of 175 patients. Gynecol Oncol 17:64, 1984.

Aalders JG, Abeler V, Kolstad P: Stage IV endometrial carcinoma: A clinical and histopathological study of 83 patients. Gynecol Oncol 17:75, 1984.

Aalders JG, Abelar V, Kolstad P: Recurrent adenocarcinoma of the endometrium: A clinical and histopathological study of 379 patients. Gynecol Oncol 17:85, 1984.

Aapro MS, Van Wijk FH, Bolis G, et al: Doxorubicin versus doxorubicin and cisplatin in endometrial carcinoma: Definitive results of a randomised study (55872) by the EORTC Gynaecological Cancer Group. Ann Oncol 14:441–448, 2003.

Abeler VM, Kjorstad KE: Clear cell carcinoma of the endometrium: A histopathological and clinical study of 97 cases. Gynecol Oncol 40:207, 1991.

Ackerman I, Malone S, Thomas G, et al: Endometrial carcinoma: Relative effectiveness of adjuvant irradiation vs therapy reserved for relapse. Gynecol Oncol 60:177, 1996.

ACOG Practice Bulletin: Management of endometrial cancer. Obstet Gynecol 65:413, 2005.

Ahmad K, Kim YH, Deppe G, et al: Radiation therapy in stage II carcinoma of the endometrium. Cancer 63:854, 1989.

Andersen ES: Stage II endometrial carcinoma: Prognostic factors and the results of treatment. Gynecol Oncol 38:220, 1990.

Aquino-Parsons C, Lim P, Wong F, et al: Papillary serous and clear cell carcinoma limited to endometrial curettings in FIGO stage 1a and 1b endometrial adenocarcinoma: Treatment implications. Gynecol Oncol 71:83, 1998.

Aziz H, Rotman M, Hussain F, et al: Poor survival of black patients in carcinoma of the endometrium. Int J Radiat Oncol Biol Phys 27:293, 1993.

Ball HG, Blessing JA, Lentz SS, Mutch DG: A phase II trial of paclitaxel in patients with advanced or recurrent adenocarcinoma of the endometrium: A Gynecologic Oncology Group study. Gynecol Oncol 62:278–281, 1996.

Barakat RR, Wong G, Curtain JP, et al: Tamoxifen use in breast cancer patients who subsequently develop corpus cancer is not associated with a higher incidence of adverse histologic features. Gynecol Oncol 55:164, 1994.

Barrett RJ, Blessing JA, Homesley HD, et al: Circadian-timed combination doxorubicin-cisplatin chemotherapy for advanced endometrial carcinoma. A phase II study of the Gynecologic Oncology Group. Am J Clin Oncol 16:494–496, 1993.

Barter JF, Smith EB, Szpak CA, et al: Leiomyosarcoma of the uterus: Clinicopathologic study of 21 cases. Gynecol Oncol 21:220, 1985.

Berchuck A, Anspach C, Evans A, et al: Postsurgical surveillance of patients with FIGO stage I/II endometrial carcinoma. Gynecol Oncol 59:20, 1995.

Berchuck A, Boyd J: Molecular basis of endometrial cancer. Cancer 76:2034, 1995.

Berchuck A, Rodriguez G, Kinney RB, et al: Overexpression of HER-2/*neu* in endometrial cancer is associated with advanced stage disease. Am J Obstet Gynecol 164:15, 1991.

Berchuck A, Rubin SC, Hoskins WJ, et al: Treatment of uterine leiomyosarcoma. Obstet Gynecol 71:845, 1988.

Bernstein L, Deapen D, Cerhan JR, et al: Tamoxifen therapy for breast cancer and endometrial cancer risk. J Natl Cancer Inst 91:1654, 1999.

Braly PS: Flow cytometry as a prognostic factor in endometrial cancer: What does it add? Gynecol Oncol 58:145, 1995.

Brinton LA, Berman ML, Mortel R, et al: Reproductive, menstrual, and medical risk factors for endometrial cancer: Results from a case-control study. Am J Obstet Gynecol 167:1317–1325, 1992.

Bristow RE, Zerbe MJ, Rosenshein NB, et al: Stage IVB endometrial cancer: The role of cytoreductive surgery and determinants of survival. Gynecol Oncol 78:85–91, 2000.

Broaddus RR, Lu KH: Women with HNPCC: A target population for the chemoprevention of gynecologic cancers. Front Biosci 11:207–280, 2006.

Bruckman JE, Bloomer WD, Marck A, et al: Stage III adenocarcinoma of the endometrium: Two prognostic groups. Gynecol Oncol 9:12, 1980.

Burke TW, Gershenson DM, Morris M, et al: Postoperative adjuvant cisplatin, doxorubicin, and cyclophosphamide (PAC) chemotherapy in women with high-risk endometrial carcinoma. Gynecol Oncol 55:47–50, 1994.

Burke TW, Munkarah A, Kavanagh JJ, et al: Treatment of advanced or recurrent endometrial carcinoma with single-agent carboplatin. Gynecol Oncol 51:397–400, 1993.

Calais G, Descamps P, Vitu L, et al: Lymphadenectomy in the management of endometrial carcinoma stage I and II. Retrospective study of 155 cases. Clin Oncol (R Coll Radiol) 2:318–323, 1990.

Carbone PP, Carter SK: Endometrial cancer: Approach to development of effective chemotherapy. Gynecol Oncol 2:348–353, 1974.

Carcangiu ML, Chambers JT: Early pathologic stage clear cell carcinoma and uterine papillary serous carcinoma of the endometrium: Comparison of clinicopathologic features and survival. Int J Gynecol Pathol 14:30, 1995.

Carey MS, O'Connell GJ, Johanson CR, et al: Good outcome associated with a standardized treatment protocol using selective postoperative radiation in patients with clinical stage I adenocarcinoma of the endometrium. Gynecol Oncol 57:138, 1995.

Carlson JA Jr, Allegra JC, Day TG Jr, Wittliff JL: Tamoxifen and endometrial carcinoma: Alterations in estrogen and progesterone receptors in untreated patients and combination hormonal therapy in advanced neoplasia. Am J Obstet Gynecol 149:149–153, 1984.

Caudell JJ, Deavers MT, Slomovitz BM, et al: Imatinib mesylate (Gleevec)-targeted kinases are expressed in uterine sarcomas. Appl Immunohistochem Mol Morphol 13:267–270, 2005.

Cecchini S, Ciatto S, Bonardi R, et al: Screening by ultrasonography for endometrial carcinoma in postmenopausal breast cancer patients under adjuvant tamoxifen, Gynecol Oncol 60:409, 1996.

Chambers JT, Rutherford TJ, Schwartz PE, Carcangiu SK: A pilot study of topotecan for the treatment of serous endometrial cancer. Proc Am Soc Clin Oncol 872, 2001.

Childers JM, Spirtos NM, Brainard P, et al: Laparoscopic staging of the patient with incompletely staged early adenocarcinoma of the endometrium. Obstet Gynecol 83:597, 1994.

Cirisano FD, Robboy SJ, Dodge RK, et al: Epidemiology and surgicopathologic findings of papillary serous and clear cell endometrial cancers when compared to endometrioid carcinoma. Gynecol Oncol 74:385, 1999.

Clement PB, Scully RE: Müllerian adenosarcoma of the uterus. Cancer 34:1138, 1974.

Clement PB, Scully RE: Pathology of uterine sarcomas. In Coppleson M (ed): Gynecologic Oncology, 2nd ed. Edinburgh, Churchill Livingstone, 1992.

Cohen CJ, Deppe G, Bruckner HW: Treatment of advanced adenocarcinoma of the endometrium with melphalan, 5-fluorouracil, and medroxyprogesterone acetate: A preliminary study. Obstet Gynecol 1977;50:415–417.

Connelly PJ, Alberhasky RC, Christopherson WM: Carcinoma of the endometrium. III. Analysis of 865 cases of adenocarcinoma and adenoacanthoma. Obstet Gynecol 59:569, 1982.

Connor JP, Andrews JI, Anderson B, Buller RE: Computed tomography in endometrial carcinoma. Obstet Gynecol 95:692, 2000.

Cook LS, Weiss NS, Schwartz SM, et al: Population-based study of tamoxifen therapy and subsequent ovarian, endometrial, and breast cancers. J Natl Cancer Inst 87:1359, 1995.

Cornelison TL, Baker TR, Piver MS, Driscoll DL: Cisplatin, Adriamycin, etoposide, megestrol acetate versus melphalan, 5-fluorouracil, medroxyprogesterone acetate in the treatment of endometrial carcinoma. Gynecol Oncol 59:243–248, 1995.

COSA-NZ-UK Endometrial Cancer Study Groups: Adjuvant medroxyprogesterone acetate in high-risk endometrial cancer. Int J Gynecol Cancer 8:387, 1998.

Cramer DW, Cutler SJ, Christine B: Trends in the incidence of endometrial cancer in the United States. Gynecol Oncol 2:130, 1974.

Creasman WT: New gynecologic cancer staging. Obstet Gynecol 75:287, 1990.

Creasman WT: Estrogen replacement therapy: Is previously treated cancer a contraindication? Obstet Gynecol 77:308, 1991.

Creasman WT, DeGeest K, DiSaia PJ, et al: Significance of true surgical pathologic staging: A Gynecologic Oncology Group Study. Am J Obstet Gynecol 181:31, 1999.

Creasman WT, Henderson D, Hinshaw W, et al: Estrogen replacement therapy in the patient treated for endometrial cancer. Obstet Gynecol 67:326, 1986.

Creasman WT, Morrow CP, Bundy BN, et al: Surgical pathologic spread patterns of endometrial cancer. Cancer 60:2035, 1987.

Creutzberg CL, van Putten WLJ, Kiper PCM, et al: Surgery and postoperative radiotherapy versus surgery alone for patients with stage-1 endometrial carcinoma: Multicentre randomised trial. Lancet 355:1404, 2000.

Currie JL, Blessing JA, Muss HB, et al: Combination chemotherapy with hydroxyurea, dacarbazine (DTIC), and etoposide in the treatment of uterine leiomyosarcoma: A Gynecologic Oncology Group study. Gynecol Oncol 61:27, 1996.

Dietrich CS 3rd, Modesitt SC, DePriest PD, et al: The efficacy of adjuvant platinum-based chemotherapy in Stage I uterine papillary serous carcinoma (UPSC). Gynecol Oncol 299:557–563, 2005.

Dimopoulos MA, Papadimitriou CA, Georgoulias V, et al: Paclitaxel and cisplatin in advanced or recurrent carcinoma of the endometrium: Long-term results of a phase II multicenter study. Gynecol Oncol 78:52–57, 2000.

Dotters DJ: Preoperative CA 125 in endometrial cancer: Is it useful? Obstet Gynecol 182:1328, 2000.

DuBeshter B: Endometrial cancer: Predictive value of cervical cytology [editorial]. Gynecol Oncol 72:271, 1999.

Dunton CJ, Pfeifer SM, Braitman LE, et al: Treatment of advanced and recurrent endometrial cancer with cisplatin, doxorubicin, and cyclophosphamide. Gynecol Oncol 41:113–116, 1991.

Edmonson JH, Krook JE, Hilton JF, et al: Randomized phase II studies of cisplatin and a combination of cyclophosphamide-doxorubicin-cisplatin (CAP) in patients with progestin-refractory advanced endometrial carcinoma. Gynecol Oncol 28:20–24, 1987.

Eifel PJ, Ross J, Hendrickson M, et al: Adenocarcinoma of the endometrium: Analysis of 256 cases with disease limited to the uterine corpus: Treatment comparison. Cancer 52:1026, 1983.

Fleming GF, Brunetto V, Mundt AJ, et al: Randomized trial of doxorubicin (DOX) plus cisplatin (CIS) versus DOX plus CIS plus paclitaxel (TAX) in patients with advanced or recurrent endometrial carcinoma: A Gynecologic Oncology Group (GOG) study. J Clin Oncol 22:2159–2166, 2004.

Fleming GF, Brunetto V, Bentley R, et al: Randomized trial of doxorubicin (Dox) plus cisplatin (Cis) versus Dox plus paclitaxel (Tax) plus granulocyte colony-stimulating factor (G-CSF) in patients with advanced or recurrent endometrial cancer: A report on Gynecologic Oncology Group (GOG) protocol. Ann Oncol 15:1173–1178, 2004.

Fornander T, Cedermark B, Mattsson A, et al: Adjuvant tamoxifen in early breast cancer: Occurrence of new primary cancers. Lancet 1:17, 1989.

Franchi M, Ghezzi F, Donadello N, et al: Endometrial thickness in tamoxifen-treated patients: An independent predictor of endometrial disease. Obstet Gynecol 93:1004, 1999.

Fukuda K, Mori M, Uchiyama M, et al: Preoperative cervical cytology in endometrial carcinoma and its clinicopathologic relevance. Gynecol Oncol 72:273, 1999.

Gallion HH, van Nagell JR, Powell DF, et al: Stage I serous papillary carcinoma of the endometrium. Cancer 63:2224, 1989.

Geisler JP, Geisler HE, Melton ME, Wiemann MC: What staging surgery should be performed on patients with uterine papillary serous carcinoma? Gynecol Oncol 74:465, 1999.

George E, Lillemoe TJ, Twiggs LB, et al: Malignant mixed müllerian tumor versus high-grade endometrial carcinoma and aggressive variants of endometrial carcinoma: A comparative analysis of survival. Int J Gynecol Pathol 14:39, 1995.

Gitsch G, Friedlander ML, Wain GV, et al: Uterine papillary serous carcinoma: A clinical study. Cancer 75:2239, 1995.

Goff BA, Kato D, Schmidt RA, et al: Uterine papillary serous carcinoma: Patterns of metastatic spread. Gynecol Oncol 54:264, 1994.

Goldschmidt R, Katz Z, Blickstein I, et al: The accuracy of endometrial pipelle sampling with and without sonographic measurement of endometrial thickness. Obstet Gynecol 82:727, 1993.

Goodman A, Zukerberg LR, Rice LW, et al: Squamous cell carcinoma of the endometrium: A report of eight cases and a review of the literature. Gynecol Oncol 61:54, 1996.

Granberg S, Wikland M, Karlsson B, et al: Endometrial thickness as measured by endovaginal ultrasonography for identifying endometrial abnormality. Am J Obstet Gynecol 164:47, 1991.

Green JB 3rd, Green S, Alberts DS, et al: Carboplatin therapy in advanced endometrial cancer. Obstet Gynecol 75:696–700, 1990.

Greven KM, Curran WJ, Whittington R, et al: Analysis of failure patterns in stage III endometrial carcinoma and therapeutic implications. Int J Radiat Oncol Biol Phys 17:35, 1989.

Greven KM, Lanciano RM, Corn B, et al: Pathologic stage III endometrial carcinoma. Prognostic factors and patterns of recurrence. Cancer 71:3697–3702, 1993.

Greven KM, Randall M, Fanning J, et al: Patterns of failure in patients with stage I, grade 3 carcinoma of the endometrium. Int J Radiat Oncol Biol Phys 19:529–534, 1990.

Grice J, Ek M, Greer B, et al: Uterine papillary serous carcinoma: Evaluation of long-term survival in surgically staged patients. Gynecol Oncol 69:69, 1998.

Grigsby PW, Perez CA, Camel HM, et al: Stage II carcinoma of the endometrium: Results of therapy and prognostic factors. Int J Radiat Oncol Biol Phys 11:1915–1923, 1985.

Grigsby PW, Perez CA, Kuske RR, et al: Results of therapy, analysis of failures, and prognostic factors for clinical and pathologic stage III adenocarcinoma of the endometrium. Gynecol Oncol 27:44–57, 1987.

Grimes DA, Economy KE: Primary prevention of gynecologic cancers. Am J Obstet Gynecol 172:227, 1995.

Grimshaw RN, Tupper WC, Fraser RC, et al: Prognostic value of peritoneal cytology in endometrial carcinoma. Gynecol Oncol 36:97, 1990.

Gull B, Carlsson SA, Karlsson B, et al: Transvaginal ultrasonography of the endometrium in women with postmenopausal bleeding: Is it always necessary to perform an endometrial biopsy? Am J Obstet Gynecol 182:509, 2000.

Hall J, Higgins R, Naumann R, Groblewski M: Phase II study of topotecan and cisplatinum stages III and IV or for recurrent endometrial cancer. Proc Am Soc Clin Oncol 1622, 2000.

Hannigan EV, Freedman RS, Elder KW, Rutledge FN: Treatment of advanced uterine sarcoma with vincristine, actinomycin, and cyclophosphamide. Gynecol Oncol 15:224–229, 1983.

Hensley ML, Maki R, Venkatraman E, et al: Gemcitabine and docetaxel in patients with unresectable leiomyosarcoma: Results of a phase II trial. J Clin Oncol 20:2824–2831, 2002.

Hill HA, Coates RJ, Austin H, et al: Racial differences in tumor grade among women with endometrial cancer. Gynecol Oncol 56:154, 1995.

Hoffman MS, Roberts WS, Cavanagh D, et al: Treatment of recurrent and metastatic endometrial cancer and cisplatin, doxorubicin, cyclophosphamide, and megestrol acetate. Gynecol Oncol 35:75, 1989.

Homesley HD, Boronow RC, Lewis JL: Stage II endometrial adenocarcinoma. Obstet Gynecol 49:604, 1977.

Horton J, Begg CB, Arseneault J, et al: Comparison of Adriamycin with cyclophosphamide in patients with advanced endometrial cancer. Cancer Treat Rep 62:159–161, 1978.

Hoskins PJ, Swenerton KD, Pike JA, et al: Paclitaxel and carboplatin, alone or with irradiation, in advanced or recurrent endometrial cancer: A phase II study. J Clin Oncol 19:4048–4053, 2001.

Huh W, Powell M, Leath CA 3rd, et al: Uterine papillary serous carcinoma: comparisons of outcomes in surgical Stage I patients with and without adjuvant therapy. Gynecol Oncol 91:470–475, 2003.

Kadar N, Homesley HD, Malfetano JH: Positive peritoneal cytology is an adverse factor in endometrial carcinoma only if there is other evidence of extrauterine disease. Gynecol Oncol 46:145, 1992.

Kaku T, Silverberg SG, Major FJ, et al: Adenosarcoma of the uterus: A Gynecologic Oncology Group clinicopathologic study of 31 cases. Int J Gynecol Pathol 11:75, 1992.

Kato DT, Ferry JA, Goodman A, et al: Uterine papillary serous carcinoma (UPSC): A clinicopathologic study of 30 cases. Gynecol Oncol 59:384, 1995.

Kauppila A: Progestin therapy of endometrial, breast and ovarian carcinoma. A review of clinical observations. Acta Obstet Gynecol Scand 63:541–450, 1984.

Kelley RM, Baker WH: Progestational agents in the treatment of carcinoma of the endometrium. N Engl J Med 264:216–222, 1961.

Kendall BS, Ronnett BM, Isacson C, et al: Reproducibility of the diagnosis of endometrial hyperplasia, atypical hyperplasia, and well-differentiated carcinoma. Am J Surg Pathol 22:1012, 1998.

Kennedy AS, DeMars LR, Flannagan LM, et al: Primary squamous cell carcinoma of the endometrium: A first report of adjuvant chemoradiation. Gynecol Oncol 59:117, 1995.

Keys HM, Roberts JA, Brunetto VL, et al: A phase III trial of surgery with or without adjunctive external pelvic radiation therapy in intermediate risk endometrial adenocarcinoma: A Gynecologic Oncology Group study. Gynecol Oncol 92:744–751, 2004.

Koss LG, Schreiber K, Oberlander SG, et al: Detection of endometrial carcinoma and hyperplasia in asymptomatic women. Obstet Gynecol 64:1, 1984.

Kurjak A, Kupesic S, Shalan H, et al: Uterine sarcoma: A report of 10 cases studied by transvaginal color and pulsed Doppler sonography. Gynecol Oncol 59:342, 1995.

Kurjak A, Shalan H, Sosic A, et al: Endometrial carcinoma in postmenopausal women: Evaluation by transvaginal color Doppler ultrasonography. Am J Obstet Gynecol 169:1597, 1993.

Kurman RJ, Kaminski PF, Norris HJ: Behavior of endometrial hyperplasia: A long-term study of "untreated" hyperplasias in 170 patients. Cancer 56:403, 1985.

Kurman RJ, Norris HJ: Endometrial hyperplasia and related cellular changes. In Blaustein's Pathology of the Female Genital Tract, 4th ed. New York, Springer-Verlag, 1994.

Kurman RJ, Scully RE: Clear cell carcinoma of the endometrium. Cancer 37:872, 1976.

Lanciano RM, Greven KM: Adjuvant treatment for endometrial cancer: Who needs it? [editorial]. Gynecol Oncol 57:135, 1995.

Langer RD, Pierce JJ, O'Hanlan KA, et al: Transvaginal ultrasonography compared with endometrial biopsy for the detection of endometrial disease. N Engl J Med 337:1792, 1997.

Lee RB, Burke TW, Park RC: Estrogen replacement therapy following treatment for stage I endometrial carcinoma. Gynecol Oncol 36:189, 1990.

Leibsohn S, Mishell DR, d'Ablaing G, Schlaerth JB: Leiomyosarcomas in a series of hysterectomies performed for presumed uterine leiomyomata. Am J Obstet Gynecol 162:968, 1990.

Lentz SS, Brady MF, Major FJ, et al: High-dose megestrol acetate in advanced or recurrent endometrial carcinoma: A Gynecologic Oncology Group Study. J Clin Oncol 14:357–361, 1996.

Levenback C, Burke TW, Silva E, et al: Uterine papillary serous carcinoma (UPSC) treated with cisplatin, doxorubicin, and cyclophosphamide (PAC). Gynecol Oncol 46:317–321, 1992.

Lewis GC Jr, Slack NH, Mortel R, Bross ID: Adjuvant progestogen therapy in the primary definitive treatment of endometrial cancer. Gynecol Oncol 2:368–376, 1974.

Lincoln S, Blessing JA, Lee RB, Rocereto TF: Activity of paclitaxel as second-line chemotherapy in endometrial carcinoma: A Gynecologic Oncology Group study. Gynecol Oncol 88:277–281, 2003.

Lissoni A, Zanetta G, Losa G, et al: Phase II study of paclitaxel as salvage treatment in advanced endometrial cancer. Ann Oncol 7:861–863, 1996.

Long HJ, Pfeifle DM, Wieand HS, et al: Phase II evaluation of carboplatin in advanced endometrial carcinoma. J Natl Cancer Inst 80:276–278, 1988.

Love CDB, Muir BB, Scrimgeour JB, et al: Investigation of endometrial abnormalities in asymptomatic women treated with tamoxifen and an evaluation of the role of endometrial screening. J Clin Oncol 17:2050, 1999.

Lurain JR, Piver MS: Uterine sarcomas: Clinical features and management. In Coppleson M (ed): Gynecologic Oncology, 2nd ed. Edinburgh, Churchill Livingstone, 1992, p 827.

Mackillop WJ, Pringle JF: Stage III endometrial carcinoma. A review of 90 cases. Cancer 56:519–2523, 1985.

MacMahon B: Risk factors for endometrial cancer. Gynecol Oncol 2:122, 1974.

Magriples U, Naftolin F, Schwartz PE, et al: High-grade endometrial carcinoma in tamoxifen-treated breast cancer patients. J Clin Oncol 11:485, 1993.

Malfetano JH: Tamoxifen-associated endometrial carcinoma in postmenopausal breast cancer patients. Gynecol Oncol 39:82, 1990.

Mariani A, Sebo TJ, Katzmann JA, et al: Pretreatment assessment of prognostic indicators in endometrial cancer. Am J Obstet Gynecol 182:1535, 2000.

Mariani A, Webb MJ, Galli L, Podratz KC: Potential therapeutic role of para-aortic lymphadenectomy in node-positive endometrial cancer. Gynecol Oncol 76:348, 2000.

Mariani A, Webb MJ, Keeney GL, et al: Assessment of prognostic factors in stage IIIA endometrial cancer. Gynecol Oncol 86:38–44, 2002.

Markman M, Fowler J: Activity of weekly paclitaxel in patients with advanced endometrial cancer previously treated with both a platinum agent and paclitaxel. Gynecol Oncol 92:180–182, 2004.

Markman M, Kennedy A, Webster K, et al: Persistent chemosensitivity to platinum and/or paclitaxel in metastatic endometrial cancer. Gynecol Oncol 73:422–423, 1999.

McMeekin DS, Gordon A, Fowler J, et al: A phase II trial of arzoxifene, a selective estrogen response modulator, in patients with recurrent or advanced endometrial cancer. Gynecol Oncol 90:64–69, 2003.

Melhem MF, Tobon H: Mucinous adenocarcinoma of the endometrium: A clinico-pathological review of 18 cases. Int J Gynecol Pathol 6:347, 1987.

Mignotte H, Lasset C, Bonadana V, et al: Iatrogenic risks of endometrial carcinoma after treatment for breast cancer in large French case-control study. Int J Cancer 76:325, 1998.

Miller B, Umpierre S, Tornas C, Burke T: Histologic characterization of uterine papillary serous adenocarcinoma. Gynecol Oncol 56:425, 1995.

Miller DS, Blessing JA, Lentz SS, Waggoner SE: A phase II trial of topotecan in patients with advanced, persistent, or recurrent endometrial carcinoma: A Gynecologic Oncology Group study. Gynecol Oncol 87:247–251, 2002.

Moore TD, Phillips PH, Nerenstone SR, Cheson BD: Systemic treatment of advanced and recurrent endometrial carcinoma: Current status and future directions. J Clin Oncol 9:1071–1088, 1992.

Moore DH, Fowler WC, Walton LA, Droegemueller W: Morbidity of lymph node sampling in cancers of the uterine corpus and cervix. Obstet Gynecol 74:180, 1989.

Morrow CP, Bundy BN, Homesley HD, et al: Doxorubicin as an adjuvant following surgery and radiation therapy in patients with high-risk endometrial carcinoma, stage I and occult stage II: A Gynecologic Oncology Group study. Gynecol Oncol 36:166–171, 1990.

Morrow CP, Bundy BN, Kurman RJ, et al: Relationship between surgical-pathological risk factors and outcome in clinical stage I and II carcinoma of the endometrium: A Gynecologic Oncology Group study. Gynecol Oncol 40:55, 1991.

Mortel R, Levy C, Wolff JP, et al: Female sex steroid receptors in postmenopausal endometrial carcinoma and biochemical response to an antiestrogen. Cancer Res 41:1140–1147, 1981.

Muss HB, Case LD, Capizzi RL, et al: High- versus standard-dose megestrol acetate in women with advanced breast cancer: A phase III trial of the Piedmont Oncology Association. J Clin Oncol 8:1797–1805, 1990.

Nielsen SN, Podratz KC, Scheithauer BW, O'Brien PC: Clinicopathologic analysis of uterine malignant mixed müllerian tumors. Gynecol Oncol 34:372, 1989.

Norris HJ, Taylor HB: Mesenchymal tumors of the uterus. I. A clinical and pathologic study of 53 endometrial stromal tumors. Cancer 19:755, 1966.

Omodei U, Ferrazzia E, Ruggeri C, et al: Endometrial thickness and histological abnormalities in women on hormonal replacement therapy: A transvaginal ultrasound/hysteroscopic study. Ultrasound Obstet Gynecol 15:317, 2000.

Omura GA, Blessing JA, Major FJ, et al: A randomized clinical trial of adjuvant Adriamycin in uterine sarcomas: A Gynecologic Oncology Group study. J Clin Oncol 3:1240, 1985.

Omura GA, Major FJ, Blessing JA, et al: A randomized study of Adriamycin with and without dimethyl-triazeno-imidazole-carboxamide in advanced uterine sarcomas. Cancer 52:626, 1983.

Onsrud M, Kolstad P, Normann T: Postoperative external pelvic irradiation in carcinoma of the corpus, stage I: A controlled clinical trial. Gynecol Oncol 4:222, 1976.

Pandya KJ, Yeap BY, Weiner LM, et al: Megestrol and tamoxifen in patients with advanced endometrial cancer: An Eastern Cooperative Oncology Group Study (E4882). Am J Clin Oncol 24:43–46, 2001.

Parker SL, Tong T, Bolden S, Wingo PA: Cancer statistics, 1996. CA Cancer J Clin 46:5, 1996.

Partridge EE, Shingleton HM,Menck HR: The National Cancer Data Base report on endometrial cancer. J Surg Oncol 61:111, 1996.

Pasmantier MW, Coleman M, Silver RT, et al: Treatment of advanced endometrial carcinoma with doxorubicin and cisplatin: Effects on both untreated and previously treated patients. Cancer Treat Rep 69:539–542, 1985.

Patsner B, Mann WJ, Cohen H, Loesch M: Predictive value of preoperative serum CA-125 levels in clinically localized and advanced endometrial carcinoma. Am J Obstet Gynecol 158:399, 1988.

Pawinski A, Tumolo S, Hoesel G, et al: Cyclophosphamide or ifosfamide in patients with advanced and/or recurrent endometrial carcinoma: A randomized phase II study of the EORTC Gynecological Cancer Cooperative Group. Eur J Obstet Gynecol Reprod Biol 86:179–183, 1999.

Pecorelli S, Creasman WT, Pettersson F, et al: FIGO annual report on the results of treatment in gynaecological cancer. Vol. 23. Milano, Italy. J Epidemiol Biostat 1998, pp 75–102.

Perez-Medina T, Bajo J, Folgueira G, et al: Atypical endometrial hyperplasia treatment with progestogens and gonadotropin-releasing hormone analogues: Long-term follow-up. Gynecol Oncol 73:299, 1999.

Petereit DG, Tannehill SP, Grosen EA, et al: Outpatient vaginal cuff brachytherapy for endometrial cancer. Int J Gynecol Cancer 9:456, 1999.

Peters WA, Rivkin SE, Smith MR, Tesh DE: Cisplatin and Adriamycin combination chemotherapy for uterine stromal sarcomas and mixed mesodermal tumors. Gynecol Oncol 34:323, 1989.

Pisani AL, Barbuto DA, Chen D, et al: Her-2/*neu,* p53, and DNA analyses as prognosticators for survival in endometrial carcinoma. Obstet Gynecol 85:729, 1995.

Piver MS, Barlow JJ, Lurain JR, Blumenson LE: Medroxyprogesterone acetate (Depo-Provera) vs. hydroxyprogesterone caproate (Delalutin) in women with metastatic endometrial adenocarcinoma. Cancer 45:268–272, 1980.

Piver MS, Rutledge FN, Copeland L, et al: Uterine endolymphatic stromal myosis: A collaborative study. Obstet Gynecol 64:173, 1984.

Piver MS, Lele SB, Patsner B, Emrich LJ: Melphalan, 5-fluorouracil, and medroxyprogesterone acetate in metastatic endometrial carcinoma. Obstet Gynecol 67:261–264, 1986.

Plentl AA, Friedman EA: Lymphatic System of the Female Genitalia. Philadelphia, WB Saunders, 1971.

Pliskow S, Penalver M, Averette H: Stage III and stage IV endometrial carcinoma: A review of 41 cases. Gynecol Oncol 38:210, 1990.

Podczaski ES, Kaminski P, Manetta A, et al: Stage II endometrial carcinoma treated with external-beam radiotherapy, intracavitary application of cesium, and surgery. Gynecol Oncol 35:251, 1989.

Podratz KC, O'Brien PC, Malkasian GD Jr, et al: Effects of progestational agents in treatment of endometrial carcinoma. Obstet Gynecol 66:106–110, 1985.

Poplin EA, Liu PY, Delmore JE, et al: Phase II trial of oral etoposide in recurrent or refractory endometrial adenocarcinoma: A Southwest Oncology Group study. Gynecol Oncol 74:432–435, 1999.

Press MF, Scully RE: Endometrial "sarcomas" complicating ovarian thecoma, polycystic ovarian disease and estrogen therapy. Gynecol Oncol 21:135, 1985.

Preyer O, Obermair A, Formann E, et al: The impact of positive peritoneal washings and serosal and adnexal involvement on survival in patients with stage IIIA uterine cancer. Gynecol Oncol 86:269–273, 2002.

Price FV, Chambers SK, Carcangiu ML, et al: Intravenous cisplatin, doxorubicin, and cyclophosphamide in the treatment of uterine papillary serous carcinoma (UPSC). Gynecol Oncol 51:383–389, 1993.

Quinn MA, Campbell JJ: Tamoxifen therapy in advanced/recurrent endometrial carcinoma. Gynecol Oncol 32:1–3, 1989.

Quinn MA, Cauchi M, Fortune D: Endometrial carcinoma: Steroid receptors and response to medroxyprogesterone acetate. Gynecol Oncol 21:314–319, 1985.

Ramondetta L, Burke TW, Levenback C, et al: Treatment of uterine papillary serous carcinoma with paclitaxel. Gynecol Oncol 82:156–161, 2001.

Randall ME, Filiaci VL, Muss H, et al: Randomized phase III trial of whole-abdominal irradiation versus doxorubicin and cisplatin chemotherapy in advanced endometrial carcinoma: A Gynecologic Oncology Group Study. J Clin Oncol 24:36–44, 2006.

Reisinger SA, Asbury R, Liao SY, Homesley HD: A phase I study of weekly cisplatin and whole abdominal radiation for the treatment of stage III and IV endometrial carcinoma: A Gynecologic Oncology Group pilot study. Gynecol Oncol 63:399–303, 1996.

Rendina GM, Donadio C, Fabri M, et al: Tamoxifen and medroxyprogesterone therapy for advanced endometrial carcinoma. Eur J Obstet Gynecol Reprod Biol 17:285–291, 1984.

Rose PG, Blessing JA, Lewandowski GS, et al: A phase II trial of prolonged oral etoposide (VP-16) as second-line therapy for advanced and recurrent endometrial carcinoma: A Gynecologic Oncology Group study. Gynecol Oncol 63:101–104, 1996.

Rose PG, Brunetto VL, Van Le L, et al: A phase II trial of anastrozole in advanced recurrent or persistent endometrial carcinoma: A Gynecologic Oncology Group study. Gynecol Oncol 78:212–216, 2000.

Rose PG, Sommers RM, Reale FR, et al: Serial serum CA 125 measurements for evaluation of recurrence in patients with endometrial carcinoma. Obstet Gynecol 84:12, 1994.

Rutqvist LE, Johansson H, Signomklao T, et al: Adjuvant tamoxifen therapy for early stage breast cancer and second primary malignancies. J Natl Cancer Inst 87:645, 1995.

Sagae S, Udagawa Y, Susumu N, et al: Randomized phase III trial of whole pelvic radiotherapy vs cisplatin-based chemotherapy in patients with intermediate risk endometrial carcinoma. J Clin Oncol (2005 ASCO Annual Meeting Proceedings) 23(Suppl):5002, 2005.

Sarcoma Meta-Analysis Collaboration: Adjuvant chemotherapy for localised resectable soft-tissue sarcoma of adults: Meta-analysis of individual data. Lancet 350:1647, 1997.

Sato M, Turner CH, Wang T, et al: LY353381.HCl: A novel raloxifene analog with improved SERM potency and efficacy in vivo. J Pharmacol Exp Ther 287:1–7, 1998.

Schink JC, Rademaker AW, Miller DS, et al: Tumor size in endometrial cancer. Cancer 67:2791, 1991.

Schmeler KM, Lynch HT, Chen LM, et al: Prophylactic surgery to reduce the risk of gynecologic cancers in the Lynch syndrome. N Engl J Med 354:261–269, 2006.

Sears JD, Greven KM, Hoen HM, et al: Prognostic factors and treatment outcome for patients with locally recurrent endometrial cancer. Cancer 74:1303, 1994.

Seski JC, Edwards CL, Herson J, Rutledge FN: Cisplatin chemotherapy for disseminated endometrial cancer. Obstet Gynecol 59:225–228, 1982.

Slomovitz BM, Burke TW, Oh JC, et al: Clinical and pathologic characteristics of uterine papillary serous carcinoma: A single institution review of 129 cases. Gynecol Oncol 91:463–469, 2003.

Slomovitz BM, Broaddus RR, Schmandt R, et al: Expression of imatinib mesylate-targeted kinases in endometrial carcinoma. Gynecol Oncol 95:12–16, 2004.

Slomovitz BM, Ramondetta LM, Lee CM, et a l: Heterogeneity of stage IIIA endometrial carcinomas: Implications for adjuvant therapy. Int J Gynecol Cancer 15:310–316, 2005.

Smith-Bindman R, Kerlikowske K, Feldstein VA, et al: Endovaginal ultrasound to exclude endometrial cancer and other endometrial abnormalities. JAMA 280:1510, 1998.

Sonoda Y, Zerbe M, Barakat RR, et al: High incidence of positive peritoneal cytology in low-risk endometrial cancer treated by laparoscopically assisted vaginal hysterectomy (LAVH). SGO Abstracts 19, 2000.

Sood AK, Buller RE, Burger RA, et al: Value of preoperative CA 125 level in the management of uterine cancer and prediction of clinical outcome. Obstet Gynecol 90:441, 1997.

Sood BM, Timmins PF, Gorla GR, et al: Concomitant cisplatin and extended field radiation therapy in patients with cervical and endometrial cancer. Int J Gynecol Cancer 12:459–464, 2002.

Spanos WJ Jr, Wharton JT, Gomez L, et al: Malignant mixed Mullerian tumors of the uterus. Cancer 53:311–316, 1984.

Sutton G, Brunetto VL, Kilgore L, et al: A phase III trial of ifosfamide with or without cisplatin in carcinosarcoma of the uterus: A Gynecologic Oncology Group Study. Gynecol Oncol 79:147–153, 2000.

Sutton G, Kauderer J, Carson LF, et al: Adjuvant ifosfamide and cisplatin in patients with completely resected stage I or II carcinosarcomas (mixed

mesodermal tumors) of the uterus: A Gynecologic Oncology Group study. Gynecol Oncol 96:630–634, 2005.
Sutton GP, Blessing JA, DeMars LR, et al: A phase II Gynecologic Oncology Group trial of ifosfamide and mesna in advanced or recurrent adenocarcinoma of the endometrium. Gynecol Oncol 63:15–27, 1996.
Thatcher SS, Woodruff JD: Uterine stromatosis: A report of 33 cases. Obstet Gynecol 59:428, 1982.
Thigpen JT, Blessing J, DiSaia P: Oral medroxyprogesterone acetate in advanced or recurrent endometrial carcinoma: Results of therapy and correlation with estrogen and progesterone levels. The gynecology oncology experience. In Banlieu EE, Slacobelli S, McGuire WL (eds): Endocrinology of Malignancy. Park Ridge, NJ, Parthenon, 1986, p 446.
Thigpen JT, Blessing J, Homesley H, et al: Phase III trial of doxorubicin +/– cisplatin in advanced or recurrent endometrial carcinoma: A Gynecologic Oncology Group (GOG) study. Proc Am Soc Clin Oncol 12:261, 1993.
Thigpen JT, Blessing JA, DiSaia PJ, et al: A randomized comparison of doxorubicin alone versus doxorubicin plus cyclophosphamide in the management of advanced or recurrent endometrial carcinoma: A Gynecologic Oncology Group study. J Clin Oncol 12:1408–1414, 1994.
Thigpen JT, Blessing JA, Homesley H, et al: Phase II trial of cisplatin as first-line chemotherapy in patients with advanced or recurrent endometrial carcinoma: A Gynecologic Oncology Group Study. Gynecol Oncol 33:68–70, 1989.
Thigpen JT, Brady MF, Alvarez RD, et al: Oral medroxyprogesterone acetate in the treatment of advance or recurrence endometrial carcinoma: A dose-response study by the Gynecology Oncology Group. J Clin Oncol 17:1736, 1999.
Thigpen T, Brady MF, Homesley HD, et al: Tamoxifen in the treatment of advanced or recurrent endometrial carcinoma: A Gynecologic Oncology Group study. J Clin Oncol 19:364–367, 2001.
Thigpen JT, Buchsbaum HJ, Mangan C, Blessing JA: Phase II trial of Adriamycin in the treatment of advanced or recurrent endometrial carcinoma: A Gynecologic Oncology Group study. Cancer Treat Rep 63:21–27, 1979.
Thoms WM, Eifel PJ, Smith TL, et al: Bulky endocervical carcinoma: A 23-year experience. Int J Radiat Oncol Biol Phys 23:491, 1992.
Tiltman AJ: Mucinous carcinoma of the endometrium. Obstet Gynecol 55:244, 1980.
Trimble CL, Kauderer J, Zaino R, et al: Concurrent endometrial carcinoma in women with a biopsy diagnosis of atypical endometrial hyperplasia. A Gynecologic Oncology Group study. Cancer 106:812–819, 2006.
Trimble EL, Jones HW 3rd: Management of stage II endometrial adenocarcinoma. Obstet Gynecol 71(3 Pt 1):323–326, 1988.
Trope C, Johnsson JE, Simonsen E, et al: Treatment of recurrent endometrial adenocarcinoma with a combination of doxorubicin and cisplatin. Am J Obstet Gynecol 149:379–381, 1984.
Turbow MM, Ballon SC, Sikic BI, Koretz MM: Cisplatin, doxorubicin, and cyclophosphamide chemotherapy for advanced endometrial carcinoma. Cancer Treat Rep 69:465–467, 1985.
Turner BC, Knisely JP, Kacinski BM, et al: Effective treatment of stage I uterine papillary serous carcinoma with high dose-rate vaginal apex radiation (192Ir) and chemotherapy. Int J Radiat Oncol Biol Phys 40:77–84, 1998.
Turner DA, Gershenson DM, Atkinson N, et al: The prognostic significance of peritoneal cytology for stage I endometrial cancer. Obstet Gynecol 74:775, 1989.
Valle RF, Baggish MS: Endometrial carcinoma after endometrial ablation: High-risk factors predicting its occurrence. Am J Obstet Gynecol 179:569, 1998.
van Wijk FH, Lhomme C, Bolis G, et al: Phase II study of carboplatin in patients with advanced or recurrent endometrial carcinoma. A trial of the EORTC Gynaecological Cancer Group. Eur J Cancer 39:78–85, 2003.
Vergote I, Kjorstad K, Abeler V, et al: A randomized trial of adjuvant progestogen in early endometrial cancer. Cancer 64:1011, 1989.
Verschraegen CF, Vasuratna A, Edwards C, et al: Clinicopathologic analysis of mullerian adenosarcoma: The M. D. Anderson Cancer Center experience. Oncol Rep 5:939–944, 1998.
von Minckwitz G, Loibl S, Brunnert K, et al: Adjuvant endocrine treatment with medroxyprogesterone acetate or tamoxifen in stage I and II endometrial cancer—a multicentre, open, controlled, prospectively randomised trial. Eur J Cancer 38:2265–2271, 2002.
Wadler S, Levy DE, Lincoln ST, et al: Topotecan is an active agent in the first-line treatment of metastatic or recurrent endometrial carcinoma: Eastern Cooperative Oncology Group Study E3E93. J Clin Oncol 21:2110–2114, 2003.
Wallin TE, Malkasian GD Jr, Gaffey TA, et al: Stage II cancer of the endometrium: A pathologic and clinical study. Gynecol Oncol 18:1–17, 1984.
Watanabe K, Sasano H, Harada N, et al: Aromatase in human endometrial carcinoma and hyperplasia. Immunohistochemical, in situ hybridization, and biochemical studies. Am J Pathol 146:491–500, 1995.
Whitney CW, Brunetto VL, Zaino RJ, et al: Phase II study of medroxy-progesterone acetate plus tamoxifen in advanced endometrial carcinoma: A Gynecologic Oncology Group study. Gynecol Oncol 92:4–9, 2004.
Wilson TO, Podratz KC, Gaffey TA, et al: Evaluation of unfavorable histologic subtypes in endometrial adenocarcinoma. Am J Obstet Gynecol 162:418, 1990.
Wolfson AH, Wolfson DJ, Sittler SY, et al: A multivariate analysis of clinicopathologic factors for predicting outcome in uterine sarcomas. Gynecol Oncol 52:56, 1994.
Woo HL, Swenerton KD, Hoskins PJ: Taxol is active in platinum-resistant endometrial adenocarcinoma. Am J Clin Oncol 19:290–291, 1996.
Yamada SD, Burger RA, Brewster WR, et al: Pathologic variables and adjuvant therapy as predictors of recurrence and survival for patients with surgically evaluated carcinosarcoma of the uterus. Cancer 88:2782, 2000.
Zaino RJ, Kurman RJ, Diana KL, Morrow CP: Pathologic models to predict outcome for women with endometrial adenocarcinoma. Cancer 77:1115, 1996.
Zaino RJ, Kurman R, Herbold D, et al: The significance of squamous differentiation in endometrial carcinoma: Data from a Gynecologic Oncology Group study. Cancer 68:2293, 1991.
Zanotti KM, Belinson JL, Kennedy AW, et al: The use of paclitaxel and platinum-based chemotherapy in uterine papillary serous carcinoma. Gynecol Oncol 74:272–277, 1999.
Zelmanowicz A, Hildescheim A, Sherman ME, et al: Evidence for a common etiology for endometrial carcinomas and malignant mixed mullerian tumors. Gynecol Oncol 69:253, 1998.
Zerbe MJ, Zhang J, Bristow RE, et al: Retrograde seeding of malignant cells during hysteroscopy in endometrial cancer. SGO Abstracts 20, 2000.

Neoplastic Diseases of the Ovary

33

Screening, Benign and Malignant Epithelial and Germ Cell Neoplasms, Sex-Cord Stromal Tumors

Robert L. Coleman and David M. Gershenson

KEY TERMS AND DEFINITIONS

Adenofibroma. An epithelial tumor that consists of glandular elements and large amounts of ovarian stromal (fibroblast) elements.

Adenoma. A benign ovarian epithelial tumor consisting of glandular (adenomatous) elements.

α-Fetoprotein. A secretory product from endodermal sinus tumors that can be measured in serum and serves as a specific tumor marker.

Borderline Tumors. A term used to describe an epithelial carcinoma of low malignant potential (grade 0). The malignant cells do not invade the stroma.

Brenner Tumor. An epithelial neoplasm that consists of cells resembling urothelium and so-called Walthard nests of the ovary. These are mixed with ovarian stroma.

CA 125. A dominant antibody-based biomarker recognizing the OC-125 surface epithelial antigen. It is expressed most often in nonmucinous epithelial ovarian, peritoneal, and fallopian tube cancers.

Carcinoid. A rare type of teratoma that histologically resembles the carcinoid tumors that arise in the gastrointestinal tract.

Clear-Cell Tumor (Mesonephroma). An ovarian neoplasm that consists of clear cells (containing glycogen) or "hobnail" cells. Histologically, they resemble clear-cell tumors that arise in the endocervix, endometrium, and vagina.

Cyst. A descriptive term added as a prefix to the designation of epithelial tumors to indicate the presence of cystlike spaces, for example, cystadenoma.

Cytoreductive Surgery. The practice of reducing the bulk of malignant tissue and removing, if possible, all gross disease.

Dermoid. A benign cystic germ cell tumor (cystic teratoma) that may contain elements of all three germ cell layers. It is the most common ovarian neoplasm in those younger than 30 years of age.

Dysgerminoma. The most common of ovarian malignant germ cell tumors. It consists of primitive germ cells.

Endodermal Sinus Tumor. A malignant germ cell tumor. It recapitulates extraembryonic tissue and may resemble the yolk sac of the rodent placenta.

Endometrioid Tumor. An ovarian epithelial tumor whose cells resemble those of uterine endometrial adenocarcinoma.

Epithelial Stromal Tumors. The most common type of ovarian neoplasms. They are derived from the surface (coelomic) epithelium and ovarian stroma and were previously termed *common epithelial tumors.* The most common cell types are serous, mucinous, and endometrioid.

Fibroma. The most common benign ovarian solid tumor. It is composed of stromal cells (fibroblasts) and in some cases is associated with benign ascites and hydrothorax (Meigs' syndrome).

FIGO. International Federation of Gynecology and Obstetrics; organization that designates criteria for tumor stage.

Germ Cell Tumor. The second most common type of ovarian neoplasm after epithelial tumors. Germ cell tumors contain cells that recapitulate embryonic tissues (ectoderm, mesoderm, or endoderm) or extraembryonic elements.

Gonadoblastoma. A rare tumor that arises in abnormal (dysgenetic) gonads and consists of sex cord–stromal elements and germ cells.

Granulosa-Thecal Cell Tumor. A sex cord–stromal tumor that often secretes estrogens and consists of granulosa cells (sex cord) and ovarian stromal cells (thecal cells or fibroblasts).

Immature Teratoma. A teratoma with malignant (immature) embryonic elements (ectoderm, mesoderm, or endoderm).

Interval Cytoreduction. A surgical debulking procedure performed in the middle of planned primary therapy.

Krukenberg's Tumor. A tumor metastatic to the ovary, usually bilateral, consisting of signet ring cells that usually originate from the gastrointestinal tract, most frequently the stomach, and then from the large intestine.

Mucinous Tumor. An ovarian epithelial tumor whose cells contain mucin and resemble those of the endocervix.

Neoadjuvant Chemotherapy. This is the practice of delivering primary chemotherapy to patients with advanced disease before a planned surgical debulking.

Ovarian Neoplasm. An ovarian tumor that is not physiologic and will not regress with time. It may be benign or malignant.

Papillary. A descriptive term added to the designation of epithelial tumors if papillary-like projections are present, for example, papillary cystadenocarcinoma.

Papillary Serous Carcinoma of the Ovary. A variant of carcinoma leading to widespread peritoneal carcinomatosis. Microscopically, the architecture is papillary. A tumor of similar histology may arise from the peritoneum directly, in which case, it is termed *primary peritoneal carcinoma.*

Primary Peritoneal Carcinoma. A malignant process predominantly involving

Continued

KEY TERMS AND DEFINITIONS *Continued*

the peritoneum and histologically resembling serous carcinoma. The ovaries are usually of normal size with surface metastatic deposits (up to 5 mm).

Pseudomyxoma Peritonei. Intraperitoneal spread of mucin-secreting cells that originate from ovarian mucinous cystadenoma or cystadenocarcinoma or frequently from the appendix that may lead to recurrent abdominal masses and bowel obstruction.

Secondary Cytoreduction. A surgical debulking procedure after a course of therapy that usually includes primary surgical resection and chemotherapy. It is most accurately used to describe surgical resection for recurrent disease.

Second-Look Operation. A procedure with extensive biopsy sampling and cytologic sampling of the peritoneal cavity, as well as evaluation of the retroperitoneal nodes. It is usually performed after chemotherapy in a patient who is clinically in complete remission.

Serous Tumor. An ovarian epithelial tumor whose cells resemble those of the fallopian tube.

Sertoli-Leydig Cell Tumor. A rare sex cord–stromal tumor with male elements. It often causes virilization.

Sex Cord–Stromal Tumors. A class of ovarian tumors in which the constituents of the ovary or testes are recapitulated.

Small Cell Carcinoma. A highly virulent, usually fatal ovarian malignancy occurring in young women, often accompanied by hypercalcemia.

Stages of Ovarian Cancer (FIGO).

Stage I: Growth limited to the ovaries.

Stage IA: Growth limited to one ovary; no ascites. No tumor on the external surface; capsule intact.

Stage IB: Growth limited to both ovaries; no ascites. No tumor on the external surfaces; capsules intact.

Stage IC: Tumor either stage IA or IB but with tumor on the surface of one or both ovaries; or with capsule ruptured; or with ascites present containing malignant cells or with positive peritoneal washings.

Stage II: Growth involving one or both ovaries with pelvic extension.

Stage IIA: Extension and/or metastases to the uterus and/or tubes.

Stage IIB: Extension to other pelvic tissues.

Stage IIC: Tumor either stage IIA or IIB but with tumor on the surface of one or both ovaries; or with capsule(s) ruptured; or with ascites present containing malignant cells or with positive peritoneal washings.

Stage III: Tumor involving one or both ovaries with peritoneal implants outside the pelvis and/or positive retroperitoneal or inguinal nodes. Superficial liver metastasis equals stage III. Tumor is limited to the true pelvis but with histologically verified malignant extensions to small bowel or omentum.

Stage IIIA: Tumor grossly limited to the true pelvis with negative nodes but with histologically confirmed microscopic seeding of abdominal peritoneal surfaces.

Stage IIIB: Tumor of one or both ovaries with histologically confirmed implants of abdominal peritoneal surfaces, none exceeding 2 cm in diameter. Nodes negative.

Stage IIIC: Abdominal implants more than 2 cm in diameter and/or positive retroperitoneal or inguinal nodes.

Stage IV: Growth involving one or both ovaries with distant metastasis. If pleural effusion is present, there must be positive cytologic test results to allot a case to stage IV. Parenchymal liver metastasis equals stage IV.

Struma Ovarii. A specialized ovarian teratoma that consists of thyroid tissue as a major or exclusive component. It may rarely produce sufficient thyroid hormone to induce hyperthyroidism.

Teratoma. An ovarian germ cell tumor that recapitulates any one or all tissues of the ectoderm, mesoderm, or endoderm. The tissues can be benign (mature) or malignant (immature).

Thecoma. A benign ovarian stromal tumor consisting of thecal cells.

Ovarian cancer is the second most common malignancy of the lower part of the female genital tract, occurring less frequently than cancers of the endometrium but more frequently than cancers of the cervix. However, it is the most frequent cause of death from gynecologic neoplasms in the United States. Cancer Statistics 2006 reports that approximately 20,810 new cases of ovarian cancer will be diagnosed yearly in the United States, and there will be 15,310 deaths. A major contributing factor to the high death rate from the relatively few cases stems from the frequent detection of the disease after metastatic spread when symptoms direct clinical investigation or raise clinical concern. Surprisingly, most women diagnosed with ovarian cancer do report symptoms for months before diagnosis. As detailed later, only severity and duration of symptoms differentially reflect cancer patients from noncancer patients. The incidence of ovarian cancer (Fig. 33-1) increases with age, becoming most marked beyond 50 years, with a gradual increase continuing to age 70 years followed by a decrease for those older than age 80. Moreover, Yancik and associates noted that those older than 65 were more likely to have their cancers diagnosed at an advanced stage, leading to a worse prognosis and poorer survival compared with those younger than age 65 years.

Despite numerous epidemiologic investigations, a clear-cut cause of ovarian cancer has not been defined. A number of theories have been advanced. It is thought that these malignancies are related to frequent ovulation, and therefore women who ovulate regularly appear to be at higher risk. Included are those with a late menopause, a history of nulliparity, or late childbearing. Conversely, women who have had several pregnancies or who have used oral contraceptives appear to have some protection against ovarian cancer. Casagrande and colleagues related the development of ovarian cancer to "ovulatory age," that is, the number of years during which the patient has ovulated. This number would be reduced by pregnancy, breast-feeding, or oral contraceptive use. Schildkraut and associates correlated overexpression of mutant p53 protein in ovarian

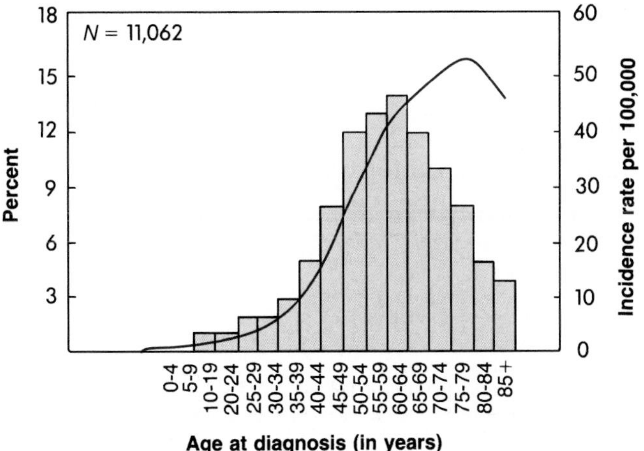

Figure 33-1. Ovarian cancer incidence rates by age, 1973 to 1982. (From Yancik R, Ries LG, Yates JW: An analysis of surveillance, epidemiology, and end results program data. Am J Obstet Gynecol 154:639, 1986.)

cancers with reproductive histories and found that overexpression was more likely in those who had high ovulatory cycle histories. In addition, talcum powder used on the perineum has been postulated to increase the risk, but, as noted by Cramer and coworkers, it is a weak association. The use of oral contraceptives decreases the risk by approximately 50% after 5 years of use (approximately 10% to 12% per year). The protection increases with duration of use to 10 years and appears to last for approximately 15 years after discontinuation of use. Schlesselman calculated a decrease of 369 ovarian cancer cases per 100,000 women for 8 years of use. Given that the approximate occurrence of ovarian cancer cases in this group would be expected to be 1400, such a decrease approximates 25%. Breast-feeding, pregnancy, tubal ligation, and, to a lesser extent, hysterectomy with ovarian preservation also lower the risk of ovarian cancer. It has been suggested that ovulation-inducing drugs such as Clomid increase the risk of ovarian cancer, as noted by Whittemore and colleagues. Rossing and coworkers reported an increase in risk from a population-based study that suggested that the risk was associated with prolonged use of clomiphene insofar as no association was noted with less than 1 year of use. The study was significant but had wide 95% confidence limits, and only 11 cancer cases occurred in the clomiphene group among 3837 women studied in the infertility clinic. However, Venn and associates from Australia did not demonstrate an increase in ovarian cancer for those using fertility drugs for in vitro fertilization. Mahdavi and colleagues assembled a review of cohort and case-control studies evaluating the relationship of fertility agents to ovarian cancer. In this report, little evidence supports the hypothesis that ovulation induction substantially increases cancer risk. However, three reports specifically evaluating the association of these agents and the development of borderline tumor or low malignant potential tumors suggest that a relationship may exist. The frequent presence of hormone receptors in these lesions as well as the hyperestrogenic microenvironment may support this observation. Cramer and coworkers found women with ovarian cancer to have a diet high in animal fat in compared with control subjects, and studies of Risch and associates suggest that saturated fat increases the risk of ovarian

Table 33-1 Putative Associations of Increasing and Decreasing Risks of Ovarian Epithelial Carcinoma

Increases	Decreases
Age	Breast-feeding
Diet	Oral contraceptives
Family history	Pregnancy
Industrialized country	Tubal ligation and hysterectomy with ovarian conservation
Infertility	
Nulliparity	
Ovulation	
Ovulatory drugs	
Talc?	

From Herbst AL: The epidemiology of ovarian carcinoma and the current status of tumor markers to detect disease. Am J Obstet Gynecol 170:1099, 1994.

cancer whereas vegetable fiber may reduce it. Table 33-1 shows the various factors that alter the risk of ovarian cancer. The familial or inherited aspects of the disease are considered subsequently.

There are geographic and racial differences in the distribution of ovarian cancers. These cancers occur most frequently in industrialized and affluent countries such as the United States and Western Europe and less frequently in Asia and Africa. The disease is more frequent among white than black women. Finally, patients with ovarian carcinoma have an increased risk of developing breast and endometrial cancer. The major factors, however, appear to be related to the frequency of ovulation and residence in an industrialized country.

FAMILIAL OVARIAN CANCER

In a case-control study, Hartge and colleagues showed that a familial history of breast cancer and a personal history of breast cancer were ovarian cancer risk factors. Lynch and associates have reported on families with these hereditary ovarian cancers and noted that they tend to occur at a younger age than in the general population. It appears that germline mutations of the *BRCA* tumor suppressor gene on chromosome 17q are responsible for a large proportion of hereditary cancers (see later discussion). However, these are a small proportion of all ovarian carcinomas. Risk alteration in these patients through oral contraceptive use is of uncertain impact. Narod and coworkers suggested that it might be possible to reduce incident risk by their administration. However, Modan and colleagues conducted a case-control study of Jewish women in whom *BRCA* founder mutational analysis was done and evaluated the risk of cancer development based by parity and oral contraceptive use. They were able to establish a protective effect by oral contraceptive use in the cohort, but subanalysis by carrier status demonstrated no effect in those harboring a *BRCA* founder mutation (odds ratio = 1.07, 95% confidence interval: 0.63–1.83). Further study is needed.

Hereditary ovarian cancers are uncommon, accounting for approximately 10% to 15% of all incident cases. However, identification of affected or unaffected women with significant familial risk is important given their accelerated risk of ovarian and other cancers. In addition, these patients are frequently diagnosed at a younger age (median, 50 years), and unaffected individuals are able to consider prophylactic procedures that can affect their lifetime risk. The term *familial ovarian cancer* denotes an inherited trait that predisposes to ovarian cancer development. It has been widely studied and two definitions are important: A first-degree relative is a mother, sister, or daughter of an affected individual; a second-degree relative is a maternal or paternal aunt or grandmother. As noted in the review by Kerlikowske and colleagues, previous studies suggest an increase from approximately 1.5% to 5% in the lifetime risk of ovarian cancer with one first-degree relative; with two or more, the risk reaches approximately 7%. Unfortunately, many of the studies showing statistical significance were based on self-reporting of family history rather than documentation by medical records. Thus, the increase in risk may well be less.

Most ovarian cancers develop sporadically. For the woman with a familial history of ovarian cancer (not the dominant genetic hereditary type), periodic surveillance with transvaginal ultrasonography 6 months after the age of 35 has been suggested (see ultrasonography discussion later in this chapter). Unfortunately, such a strategy has not been shown to be worthwhile or cost effective in disease prevention and may on occasion lead to additional tests or unnecessary procedures when a questionable ultrasound result is obtained (see subsequent discussion on ultrasound screening and natural history of ovarian cancer). The use of prophylactic oophorectomy in patients whose mothers had ovarian cancer has been a controversial topic. Kerlikowske and colleagues and Herbst provided reasons against the widespread use of such a practice. However, the use of prophylactic oophorectomy to reduce the risk of ovarian or peritoneal cancer in mutation carriers may have validity. Finch and associates studied 1828 women enrolled in an international registry over an 11-year period ending in 2003. In this cohort, 575 (30%) had undergone oophorectomy before enrollment, 490 (27%) underwent the procedure after study entry, and 783 (43%) did not undergo the procedure. After a median follow-up of 3.5 years, 50 incident cases were identified: 18 in women undergoing oophorectomy and 32 in women with intact ovaries. The protective effect was 80% (hazard ratio [HR] = 0.2, 95% CI: 0.02–0.58, p = .003). It is reasonable that patients with a significant family history in whom an operation such as hysterectomy is required, removal of both ovaries at the time of operation is appropriate. Likewise, mutation carriers who have finished childbearing may reduce their subsequent cancer risk by salpingo-oophorectomy. The recommendation for hysterectomy at this time is controversial but advocated by some to ensure complete removal of the fallopian tube (cornual segment). The patient must be aware that peritoneal carcinomatosis, a process resembling serous carcinoma of the ovary, can rarely develop despite the removal of both ovaries.

The following describes the classification and histology of the major ovarian neoplasms. Pertinent microscopic findings, clinical behavior, and appropriate therapy are presented.

CLASSIFICATION OF OVARIAN NEOPLASMS

The most widely used classification of ovarian neoplasms is that of the World Health Organization. This classification, along with frequency of occurrence of the primary ovarian neoplasms, is shown in Table 33-2.

Table 33-2 Frequency of Ovarian Neoplasms (World Health Organization Classification)

Class	Approximate Frequency (%)
Epithelial stromal (common epithelial) tumors	65
Germ cell tumors	20–25
Sex cord–stromal tumors	6
Lipid (lipoid) cell tumors	<0.1
Gonadoblastoma	<0.1
Soft-tissue tumors (not specific to ovary)	
Unclassified tumors	
Secondary (metastatic) tumors	
Tumor-like conditions (not true neoplasm)	

The epithelial stromal (common epithelial) tumors are the most frequent ovarian neoplasms. They are believed to arise from the surface (coelomic) epithelium. Germ cell tumors are the second most frequent and are the most common among young women. Histologically, they may be composed of extraembryonic elements or may have features that resemble any or all of the three embryonic layers (ectoderm, mesoderm, or endoderm). Germ cell tumors are the main cause of ovarian malignancy in young women, particularly those in their teens and early 20s. Sex cord–stromal tumors are the third most frequent and contain elements that recapitulate the constituents of the ovary or testis. These tumors may secrete sex steroid hormones or may be hormonally inactive. Lipid (lipoid) cell tumors are extremely rare and histologically resemble the adrenal gland. Gonadoblastomas consist of germ cells and sex cord–stromal elements. They occur in individuals with dysgenetic gonads, particularly when a Y chromosome is present. All these ovarian neoplasms are discussed later in this chapter.

Soft tissue tumors not specific to the ovary, such as hemangioma or lipoma, are extremely rare and are categorized according to the criteria for soft tissue tumors arising elsewhere in the body. Unclassified tumors, as the name implies, cannot be placed in any of the preceding categories. One example is small cell carcinoma, which is a highly virulent cancer affecting primarily young women (see discussion later in chapter). Metastatic tumors to the ovary may arise elsewhere in the reproductive tract or from distant sites such as the bowel or stomach (Krukenberg's tumors). Tumor-like conditions refer to enlargements of the ovary, such as extensive edema, pregnancy luteoma, endometriomas, and follicular or luteal cysts, none of which are true neoplasms. With the exceptions of metastatic tumors and small cell carcinoma of the ovary, none of these are considered further in this chapter.

EPITHELIAL OVARIAN NEOPLASMS

According to Scully, two thirds of ovarian neoplasms are epithelial tumors; malignant epithelial tumors account for approximately 85% of ovarian cancers, probably arising from inclusion cysts lined with surface (coelomic) epithelium within the adjacent ovarian stroma. Table 33-3 summarizes the five cell types that most commonly comprise epithelial ovarian tumors, indicating their relative frequency.

Table 33-3 Epithelial Ovarian Tumor Cell Types

	APPROXIMATE FREQUENCY (%)	
	All Ovarian Neoplasms	**Ovarian Cancers**
Serous	20–50	35–40
Mucinous	15–25	6–10
Endometrioid	5	15–25
Clear cell (mesonephroid)	<5	5
Brenner	2–3	Rare

Modified from Scully RE: Tumors of the ovary and maldeveloped gonads. In Atlas of Tumor Pathology, fascicle 16, series 2. Washington, DC, Armed Forces Institute of Pathology, 1979.

Epithelial tumors can be categorized as benign (adenoma), malignant (adenocarcinoma), or of an intermediate form, known as *borderline malignant adenocarcinoma* or *tumors of low malignant potential.* The term *papillary* or the prefix *cyst* (as in cystadenoma) is used when the tumor has, respectively, papillae or cystic structures. The suffix *fibroma* (as in adenofibroma) is added when the ovarian stroma predominates, with the exception of a Brenner tumor, which normally contains a large amount of ovarian stroma.

Well-differentiated serous tumors (Fig. 33-2*A* and *B*) consist of ciliated epithelial cells that resemble those of the fallopian tube. Serous tumors (Fig. 33-2*C*) are the most frequent ovarian epithelial tumors. The malignant forms account for 40% or more of ovarian cancers; the benign forms (serous cystadenomas) occur primarily during the reproductive years; the borderline tumors occur in women 30 to 50 years of age; the carcinomas typically occur in women older than 40 years of age. Molecular investigation of genetic changes associated with well-differentiated serous tumors support the recent consideration of classifying serous ovarian cancers into low- or high-grade cancer.

Two histologically similar variants of serous tumors occur. One is an aggressive tumor with small ovaries that are usually less than 4 to 5 cm in diameter, with extensive disease on the ovarian surface and metastatic disease in the abdomen. The process is termed *serous surface papillary carcinoma of the ovary.* The other type presents in a clinically similar fashion as a primary peritoneal serous adenocarcinoma. It is often difficult histologically to distinguish these entities.

Mucinous tumors (Fig. 33-3*A* and *B*) consist of epithelial cells filled with mucin; most are benign. These cells resemble cells of the endocervix or may mimic intestinal cells, which can pose a problem in the differential diagnosis of tumors that appear to originate from the ovary or intestine. Benign mucinous tumors are found primarily during the reproductive years, and mucinous

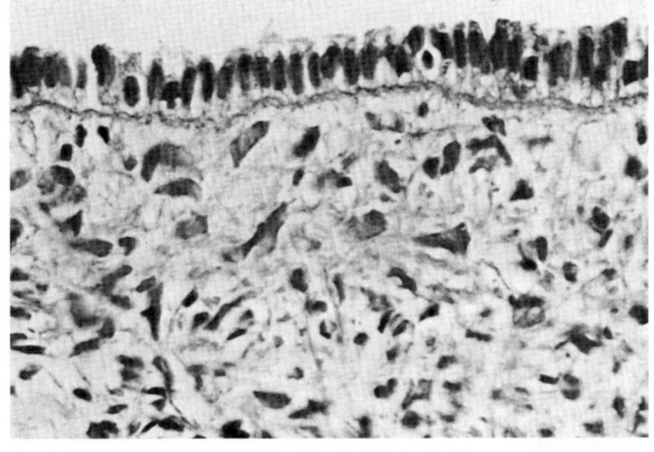

A

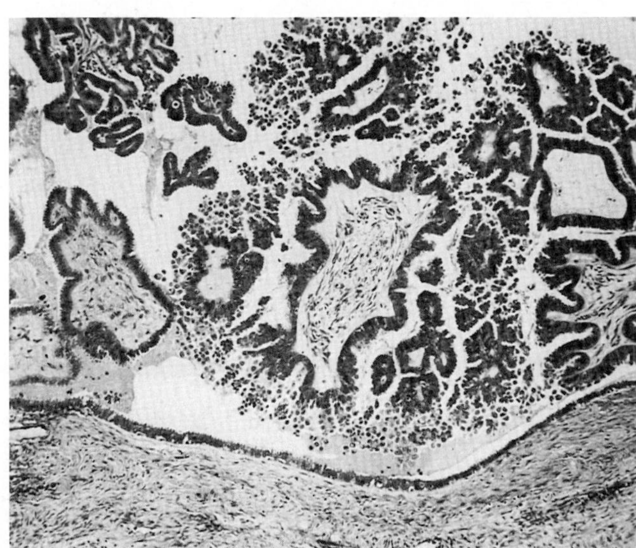

B

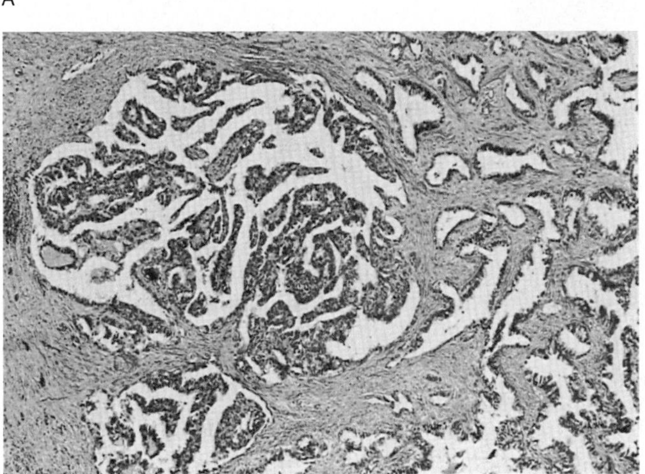

C

Figure 33-2. A, Ciliated epithelium of a well-differentiated serous tumor. (×800.) **B,** Serous papillary cystadenoma of borderline malignancy. The epithelium resembles that of the fallopian tube, and a well-developed papillary pattern is present. (×80.) **C,** Serous papillary adenocarcinoma. (×50.) The neoplastic epithelium invades the stroma. (**A** and **C** from Serov SF, Scully RE, Sobin LH: Histologic Typing of Ovarian Tumors. Geneva, World Health Organization, 1973. **B,** Courtesy of Dr. R. E. Scully.)

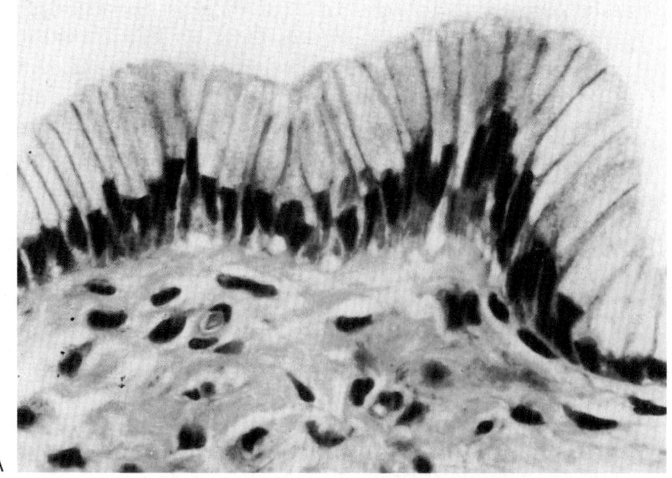

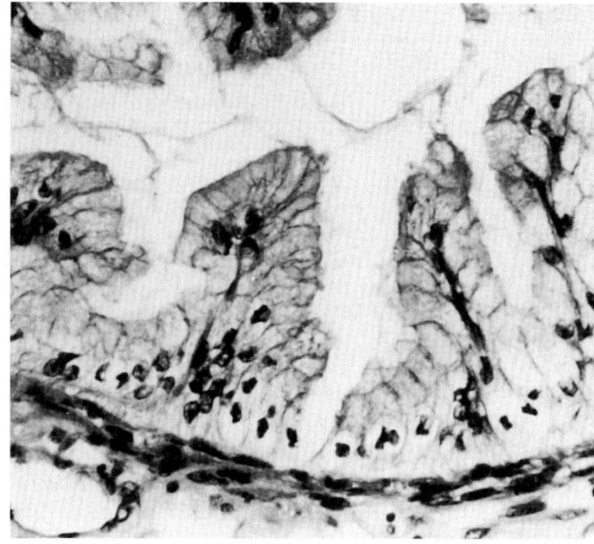

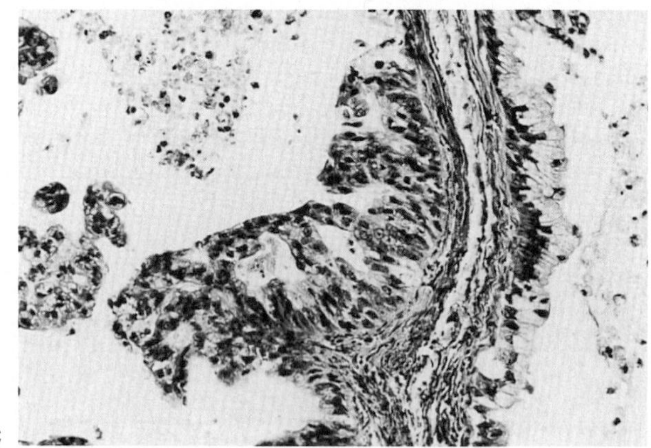

Figure 33-3. **A,** Mucinous cystadenoma. (×800.) **B,** Mucinous borderline tumor. Epithelium resembles that of the endocervix. **C,** Mucinous carcinoma. (×120.) Incomplete stratification of cells and atypicality is present. (**A** and **C** from Serov SF, Scully RE, Sobin LH: Histologic Typing of Ovarian Tumors, Geneva, World Health Organization, 1973. **B**, Courtesy of Dr. R. E. Scully.)

carcinomas (see Fig. 33-3*C*) usually occur among those in the 30- to 60-year age range. Overall they can account for approximately one fourth of ovarian tumors and as many as 10% of ovarian cancers.

Endometrioid tumors (Fig. 33-4), as the name implies, consist of epithelial cells resembling those of the endometrium. In the ovary, these neoplasms are less frequent (approximately 5%) than either the serous or mucinous tumors, but the malignant variety accounts for approximately 20% of ovarian carcinomas. Endometrioid carcinomas usually occur in women in their 40s and 50s. They may be seen in conjunction with endometriosis and ovarian endometriomas, although an origin from endo-

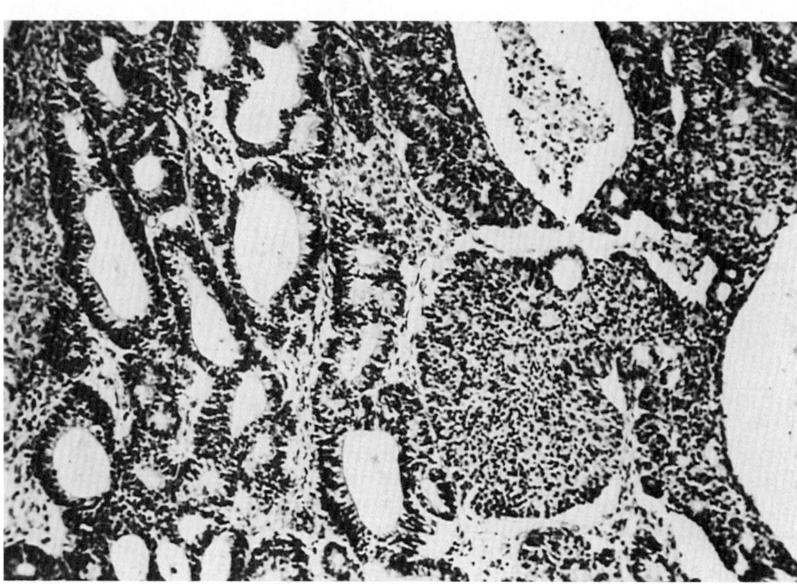

Figure 33-4. Endometrioid carcinoma. Tubular glands are lined by stratified endometrium. (×80.) (From Meadowbrook Staff J 1:148, 1968. Courtesy of Dr. R. E. Scully.)

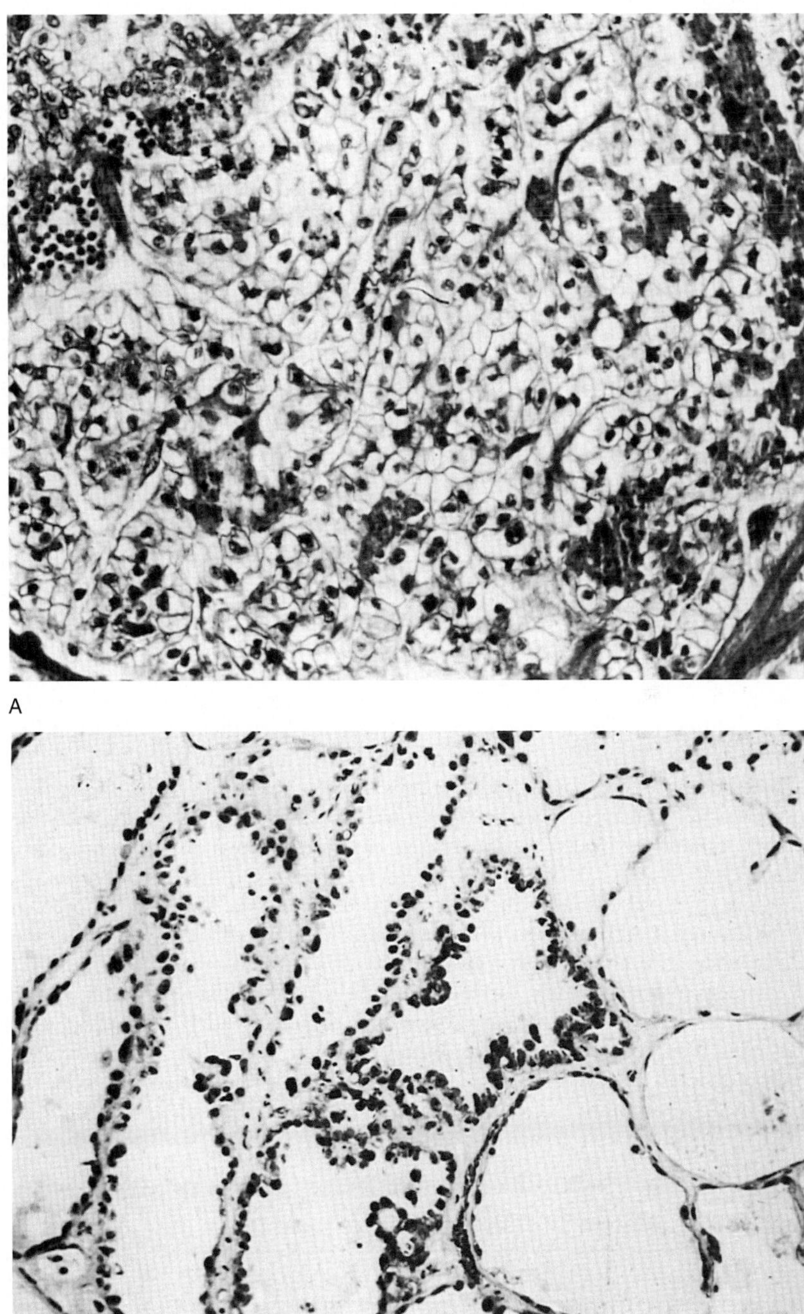

Figure 33-5. **A,** Clear-cell adenocarcinoma. (×200.) Solid pattern of abundant polyhedral tumor cells containing abundant clear cytoplasm is present. **B,** Clear-cell adenocarcinoma. (×200.) *Left:* Hobnail cells with scant cytoplasm: protruding nuclei line shows tubules. *Right:* Cysts lined by flattened tumor cells. (**A**, from Barlow JF, Scully RE: "Mesonephroma" of ovary. Tumor of Mullerian nature related to the endometrioid carcinoma. Cancer 20:1405, 1967. **B**, from Meadowbrook Staff J 1:148, 1968. Courtesy of Dr. R. E. Scully.)

metriosis is rarely demonstrated. Most endometrioid carcinomas arise directly from the surface epithelium of the ovary, as do the other epithelial tumors.

Clear-cell (mesonephroid) tumors contain cells with abundant glycogen (Fig. 33-5*A*) and so-called hobnail cells (see Fig. 33-5*B*), in which the nuclei of the cells protrude into the glandular lumen. Tumors with identical histologic features are found in the endometrium, cervix, and vagina, the latter two often associated with intrauterine diethylstilbestrol exposure. Clear-cell ovarian tumors are not related to diethylstilbestrol exposure and comprise approximately 5% of ovarian cancers. They occur primarily in women 40 to 70 years of age and are highly aggressive.

The major cell types of ovarian epithelial tumors recapitulate the müllerian-duct-derived epithelium of the female reproductive system (serous-endosalpinx, mucinous-endocervix, endometrioid-endometrium). This differentiation occurs even though the ovary is not derived directly from the müllerian ducts (see Chapter 2, Reproductive Genetics). The clear-cell tumors also mimic this müllerian tendency, frequently being admixed with endometrioid carcinomas, as well as with ovarian endometriomas.

Brenner tumors (Fig. 33-6) consist of cells that resemble the transitional epithelium of the bladder and Walthard nests of the ovary. There is abundant stroma. These tumors constitute only 2% to 3% of all ovarian tumors.

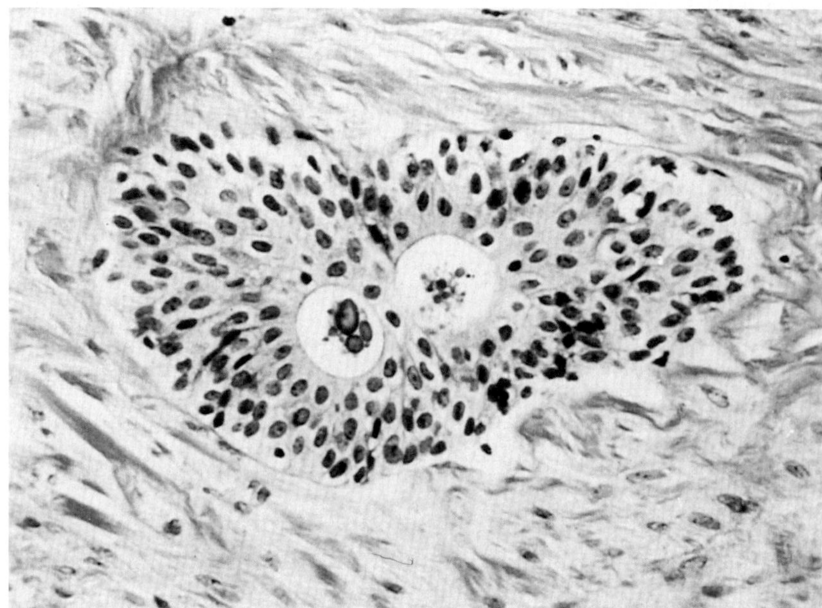

Figure 33-6. Brenner tumor. (×350.) Note nest of transition-like epithelium containing spaces with eosinophilic material. (From Atlas of Tumor Pathology, fascicle 16, series 2. Washington, DC, Armed Forces Institute of Pathology, 1979.)

In addition to the cell types shown in Table 33-3, epithelial tumors may be classified as undifferentiated if the tumor consists of poorly differentiated epithelial cells not characteristic of any particular cell type. They may be considered unclassifiable if they cannot be placed in any of the categories shown in Table 33-3.

Many epithelial ovarian tumors can be bilateral, and the risk of bilaterality is an important consideration in therapy, particularly when an ovarian tumor is discovered in a young woman of reproductive age. Widely varying percentages have been reported for bilaterality in ovarian tumors, and the most widely quoted are summarized in Table 33-4. Malignant epithelial tumors tend to involve both ovaries more frequently than do benign epithelial tumors. Serous tumors also tend to be bilateral more frequently than do mucinous tumors.

Table 33-4 Bilaterality of Ovarian Tumors

Type of Tumor	Occurrence (%)
Epithelial Tumors	
Serous cystadenoma	10
Serous cystadenocarcinoma	33–66
Mucinous cystadenoma	5
Mucinous cystadenocarcinoma	10–20
Endometrioid carcinoma	13–30
Benign Brenner tumor	6
Germ Cell Tumors	
Benign cystic teratoma (dermoid)	12
Immature teratoma (malignant)	2–5
Dysgerminoma	5–10
Other malignant germ cell tumors	Rare
Sex Cord–Stromal Tumors	
Thecoma	Rare
Sertoli–Leydig cell tumor	Rare
Granulosa-theca cell tumor	Rare

Benign Epithelial Ovarian Tumors: The Adnexal Mass

As noted in Chapter 7 (History, Physical Examination, and Preventive Health Care), enlargement of the ovary beyond 5 cm is considered abnormal. However, age and menstrual status must also be considered before the appropriate course of action is chosen. A 5- to 8-cm ovarian mass in a woman with regular menses, even if she is in her 40s, is frequently a functioning ovarian cyst, such as a follicular or corpus luteum cyst. It will usually regress spontaneously during a subsequent menstrual cycle. Enlargements of this type in young patients in their 20s or early 30s do not automatically require immediate operative intervention and can be observed for two menstrual cycles. A potential exception would be a mass in a patient who is taking oral contraceptives. Because the principle mechanism of contraception is anovulation, the index of suspicion for neoplastic growth should be raised. However, contemporary oral contraceptives have lower sex steroids and may permit follicular development. Careful observation or immediate evaluation as noted above is warranted. Shushan and colleagues reported ovarian cysts detected by ultrasonography in pre- and postmenopausal women taking tamoxifen for breast cancer. Unilocular 5- to 8-cm cysts are likely to be functional (see Chapter 18, Benign Gynecologic Lesions), whereas multilocular or partially solid tumors are more likely to be neoplastic. After the age of 40, the risk of malignancy rises. The ovary shrinks during menopause and normally is approximately 1.5 to 2.0 cm in size. A transvaginal ultrasound scan can reliably detect an ovary greater than 1.0 cm in diameter. Higgins and associates estimated the upper limit of the volume of a postmenopausal ovary was approximately 8 cm^3 in compared with 18 cm^3 for the premenopausal ovary. Ten of their patients who exceeded these criteria and had solid or complex echo patterns had neoplastic tumors, and one carcinoma was discovered. An ultrasound examination, preferably with a vaginal probe, helps to differentiate these adnexal masses (see following discussion).

Occasionally, it is discovered that the adnexal mass is paraovarian. In a study of 168 paraovarian tumors, Stein and coworkers noted that only three (2%) were malignant. The three cysts all had solid components, and the cysts were 8 to 12 cm size in patients 19 to 48 years of age.

Adnexal Mass and Ovarian Cancer

CA 125 (cancer antigen 125) was described by Bast and colleagues in the 1980s. It is expressed by approximately 80% of ovarian epithelial carcinomas but less frequently by mucinous tumors. The marker is increased in endometrial and tubal carcinoma, in addition to ovarian carcinoma, and in other malignancies, including those originating in the lung, breast, and pancreas. A level higher than 35 U/mL is generally considered increased. The following box lists some of the benign conditions for which CA 125 also has frequently been found to be increased. As can be seen, many of these are frequently found in women of childbearing age. This lack of specificity must be remembered when one is interpreting increased CA 125 values in younger women with adnexal masses or when screening is being considered (see following discussion). In addition (R.C. Bast, personal communication), there are rare individuals who have no disease but are found to have levels of CA 125 as high as 200 to 300 U/mL, as a consequence of developing idiopathic antibodies to mouse IgG.

One must also be cautious in the interpretation of an increased CA 125 level, particularly in a premenopausal patient with an adnexal mass. The specificity appears to be better for increased values in the postmenopausal patient. In a study of 182 patients, Vasilev and coworkers noted that the CA 125 level was increased in 22% of cases of benign masses, but for postmenopausal patients, an increased level usually indicated malignancy, as was also shown in the CA 125 vaginal ultrasound study of 290 postmenopausal patients by Maggino and colleagues.

Use of Ultrasound Screening and Cancer Antigen 125 in the Evaluation of the Adnexal Mass

Ultrasound has helped to define criteria to allow conservative follow-up and the risk of malignancy of some adnexal masses. Goldstein and associates studied 42 postmenopausal patients whose ultrasound scans showed unilocular cysts less than 5 cm in diameter. Twenty-eight were explored, and none had malignancy. Fourteen were followed for as long as 6 years with no change in ultrasound appearance. Finkler and colleagues noted that the addition of a CA 125 serum assay to their ultrasound criteria in postmenopausal women increased the accuracy of preoperative evaluation. In a clinical pathologic study to define ultrasound criteria of malignancy, Granberg and coworkers studied the ovarian tumors in 1017 women. Of 296 with unilocular cysts, only one was malignant and had visible papillary formations on the cyst wall; 60% of these women were older than age 40. In contrast, malignancy rates were 8% (20 of 229) for multilocular cysts, 65% (147 of 201) for multilocular solid tumors, and 39% (31 of 80) for solid ovarian masses. In a follow-up study of 180 women, the authors noted that 45 of 45 unilocular cysts were benign. In an ultrasound study of cystic ovarian masses in women older than age 50 years, Bailey and coworkers noted that unilocular cysts smaller than 10 cm in diameter are rarely malignant, whereas complex cysts or those with solid areas are at high risk of malignancy.

Several scoring systems have been proposed to try to determine the risk of an ovarian mass being malignant. They usually include the following: (1) Is the finding a simple (unilocular) or complex (multicystic/multilocular with solid components) cyst? (2) Are there papillary projections? (3) Are the cystic walls and/or septa regular and smooth? (4) What is the echogenicity (tissue characterization)? These components help to refine the likelihood of malignancy. Shalev and coworkers combined transvaginal ultrasonography and normal CA 125 values in 55 postmenopausal women with simple cystic or septate cystic ovarian masses, and all 55 had benign disease. Although this is a small study, it suggests the potential of applying stringent ultrasound criteria with CA 125 evaluation of ovarian masses in postmenopausal women.

Others have advocated using transvaginal pulsed Doppler color-enhanced flow studies to differentiate benign from malignant masses. The resistance index, which measures resistance to flow in the vessels, has been employed and presumably is low in the presence of neovascularization that is seen with malignant tumors. The vessels of neoangiogenesis are abnormal in their distribution with disorganized branching and a loss of the muscularis layer, all of which contribute to the decreased resistance to flow. A resistance of 0.40 or less was found useful by Kurjak and coworkers in a study of 254 women. In contrast, Bromley and colleagues, in a study of 33 postmenopausal women, used a cutoff of 0.6, which did not greatly add to their specificities, and these authors rely on morphologic criteria (i.e., solid elements, papillary projections) to diagnose malignancy.

Valentin and associates evaluated the characteristics of 1066 adnexal masses of which 266 were malignant (55 borderline ovarian tumors, 144 primary invasive epithelial cancers, 25 nonepithelial ovarian cancers, and 42 metastatic cancers). A scoring system was used as well as information from color Doppler studies. They reported that borderline and stage I ovarian cancers shared similar morphology but had different characteristics from more advanced-stage tumors. They were larger, contained more papillary projections, and more often were multilocular without solid components but were less often purely solid and less likely to be associated with ascites. Significant variation was noted, however. Similarly, Twickler and colleagues described a scoring model to create an ovarian tumor index for women with adnexal disease. Of 244 women with follow-up, 214 had nonmalignant findings and 30 had cancer. In addition to age, transvaginal ultrasound variables, including ovarian volume, the Sassone morphology scale, and Doppler determination of angle-corrected systole, diastole, and time-averaged velocity, were evaluated. An ovarian tumor index was created from discriminant

Benign Conditions in Which CA-125 Has Been Found to Be Elevated

- Endometriosis
- Peritoneal inflammation, including pelvic inflammatory disease
- Leiomyoma
- Pregnancy
- Hemorrhagic ovarian cysts
- Liver disease

variables (both continuous and weighted) correctly classifying the two cohorts. The area under the receiver operator characteristic curve (AUC) was highly significant (AUC = 0.91). Unfortunately, scoring systems such as these, developed from data produced by highly skilled and proficient sonographers, are difficult to generalize and, although promising, are highly operator dependent.

It should be noted that there is a difference in using ultrasonography to screen for ovarian cancer as opposed to using different modalities of ultrasonography to characterize an ovarian mass as benign or malignant. For example, the addition of color Doppler sonography, which measures blood flow and direction of flow, and power Doppler sonography, which can detect slow flow in small vessels, can add useful information. These permit visualization of flow location (peripheral or central or within a septum). Most malignant tumors have a central flow (75% to 100%) compared with only 5% to 40% of benign ovarian tumors. Schelling and colleagues studied transvaginal B-mode and color Doppler sonography for the diagnosis of malignancy in 257 adnexal masses with unclear malignant status. They achieved 92% sensitivity and 94% specificity. The recent development of three-dimensional (3-D) ultrasonography may allow more accurate volume assessments. In addition, color Doppler with 3-D ultrasonography may permit better detection of vessel irregularity, coiling, and branching. A future possibility is the use of contrast media to quantify and permit earlier detection of abnormal angiogenesis as noted by Abramowicz. Contrast-enhanced (microbubble) power three-dimensional Doppler sonography is beginning to be investigated to evaluate the efficacy of antiangiogenic biologic in serial scanning.

Ovarian Cancer Screening

Although ovarian cancer is characterized by advanced-stage disease at diagnosis and high mortality, early-stage disease is often curable. The greatest impact on these statistics, other than prevention, would be screening to identify early-stage disease. Three modalities, used either individually or in combination, have been the common theme of this effort, physical examination, biomarkers (such as CA 125), proteomics/genomics (experimental) and sonography. For a disease to be amenable to screening, it should be sufficiently severe (high mortality) and have a natural history from latency to overt disease that is well characterized, and there should be successful outcome if early disease is treated. The screening modality should have high positive and negative predictive value and high sensitivity and specificity and be acceptable to the population, cost effective, and widely available to the population. The screening population should be identifiable, and for those in whom early disease is identified, effective therapy should be available. Although ovarian cancer satisfies many of these mandates, it is rare in the general population and not readily characterized by an identifiable precursor, thus producing a high bar for any modality.

Of the three most commonly used modalities, the least sensitive and specific is physical examination. It is estimated that just one early ovarian cancer will be identified in 10,000 physical examinations. Although the easiest to implement, poor sensitivity limits this intervention as an effective strategy.

Biomarkers such as CA 125 are of great interest as they are easy to obtain and serial evaluation can be tracked. CA 125 has been used most consistently since being discovered as a reliable biomarker of epithelial nonmucinous ovarian cancer. Early large population-based studies highlighted the limitation of this as a sole strategy for ovarian cancer screening. Einhorn and associates screened 5550 women and reported in 1992 that just two stage I cancers in 175 women with elevated CA 125 values were identified. As noted previously, a differential effect would be expected between pre- and postmenopausal women. Using the modality in women with a pelvic mass (in whom prevalence is increased) has substantial effects on test characteristics but overlooks the obvious need for cancer identification before gross ovarian enlargement. This has led to the development of combined evaluation (sonography) described here.

Ultrasonography as an isolated modality has also been advocated for screening. Although more expensive and less amenable to population screening, the modality has become increasingly accurate in identifying early changes within the ovary as outlined previously. Campbell and coworkers screened 5479 patients and obtained 338 abnormal scans. Five early-stage ovarian cancers were identified. The positive predictive value was just 1.5%. Similarly, van Nagell screened 1300 patients and obtained 33 abnormal scans. Two early-stage ovarian cancers were identified. As with single-modality testing, sonography is too insensitive to be widely used for screening.

Population-based ovarian cancer screening programs have been difficult to recommend and implement because poor sensitivity and positive predictive value characteristics accompany expensive and inefficient testing methodology and triage algorithms. Menon and colleagues approached this problem by evaluating a new prospectively based algorithm among a population-based screening program currently under way in the United Kingdom. The population cohort used to evaluate the new screening strategy comprised 13,582 menopausal women 50 years of age or older with at least one ovary, of whom 6532 completed a first screen; the remainder served as controls. The screening strategy was a staged process in which each CA 125 sample drawn underwent a calculation for risk of ovarian cancer. The calculation is based on the woman's age and CA 125 value relative to her personal baseline. In this trial, an estimated risk of less than one in 2000 was considered normal, whereas a risk of greater than one in 500 was considered increased; those in between were considered intermediate and required repeat testing. Those not considered normal were referred for a second stage of screening that incorporated a transvaginal ultrasound scan and repeat CA 125 testing. A transvaginal ultrasound scan was considered normal, abnormal, or equivocal based on ovarian volume and morphology. From the combination of CA 125 risk estimation and transvaginal ultrasound scan, a follow-up recommendation was made that could be a gynecologic oncology referral, repeat CA 125 testing, and/or transvaginal ultrasound scan or annual screening. Among the screened group, nearly 80% continued with annual screening; 91 (1.4%) were considered at increased risk. Among the intermediate group, repeat testing was normal in 92%, leaving 188 (2.9% of initial population) who were to undergo second-stage evaluation. Of the 144 who stayed in the program, 95 were returned to annual screening based on CA 125 and transvaginal ultrasound scan findings; 6 were found to have nongynecologic malignancies; 43 were referred to a gynecologic oncologist, of whom 27 were returned to annual screening; and 16 women underwent surgery. From this group, 5 ovarian cancers were identified (4 malignant epithelial and 1 borderline); 11 remaining women had benign ovarian neoplasms. Compared with the authors' previous algorithm based on flat CA 125 values (normal = 30 U/mL), the new process referred less than half to secondary screening. They concluded that the new algorithm increases screening precision. Its effect on cost and survivorship are to be determined when accrual of 200,000 women to the trial is completed.

Successful prediction of cancer in the general public is limited by low prevalence of disease. Creasman and DiSaia estimated that if a vaginal ultrasound scan and CA 125 testing were performed annually on all women older than the age of 45 in the United States, the cost would exceed $10 billion per year.

One strategy to improve the predictive index is to address a population in which prevalence is increased. A number of studies have been undertaken using transvaginal ultrasonography to screen for ovarian malignancy in higher-risk women. Bourne and colleagues screened 775 women who had at least one first- (677) or second-degree (98) relative with ovarian cancer. Overall, 43 women were referred for surgery with abnormal-appearing ovaries and 39 underwent surgery, with three stage IA ovarian carcinomas discovered (3.9 of 1000 screened); one of these was a borderline tumor. One screened patient was found to have peritoneal carcinomatosis 11 months after a normal screening study. The remainder had nonmalignant findings. DePriest and associates screened 6470 asymptomatic postmenopausal women and defined abnormality as an ovary with a volume greater than 10 cm^3 and/or papillary projections in a cystic ovarian tumor. Ninety patients who had persistent findings by repeat ultrasound scan at 4 to 6 weeks had an operation, with the finding of five early (stage IA; see subsequent discussion) and one advanced (stage IIIB) carcinomas. There were 37 serous cystadenomas and 20 assorted benign ovarian conditions. One patient with a normal scan was found to have peritoneal carcinomatosis 11 months later. These investigators noted that normal ovarian volume in a postmenopausal woman is less than 10 cm^3, and in a premenopausal woman, it is as much as 20 cm^3, as reported by Pavlik and colleagues.

Clinicopathologic studies of Bell and Scully, as well as ultrasound screening trials by Crayford and colleagues, provide an explanation for the lack of success with ultrasound screening in detecting low-stage ovarian carcinomas. Bell and Scully proposed the term *early de novo carcinoma* to explain their findings of 14 carefully studied cases. None of these patients had clinical evidence of ovarian carcinoma at the time of operation. All cases had microscopic foci of carcinoma in their ovaries, and three cases were detected only years postoperatively when the patients were discovered to have widespread carcinoma consistent with what was found in their ovaries on retrospective study. Crayford and colleagues screened 5479 self-referred asymptomatic women by vaginal ultrasonography and removed all persistent ovarian cysts in an attempt to reduce the frequency of ovarian cancer. Eighty-eight patients had cysts removed. Twelve years after the conclusion of the study, a slight nonsignificant increase in ovarian cancer deaths for this group was found. Therefore, it appears that the majority of ovarian carcinomas (particularly serous) arise from a tiny cancer of the surface of the ovary, from which it can spread rapidly before the ovary enlarges. Some ovarian tumors such as endometrioid carcinoma may have their origin in endometriosis. These carcinomas, as well as mucinous, tend to be detected more frequently in lower stages. Therefore, they appear more likely to have a cystic rather than a de novo origin. These observations strongly suggest that current strategies to use vaginal ultrasound screening to detect early ovarian carcinoma will have only limited success, as noted by Herbst.

Nonmalignant Neoplasms

Most nonmalignant epithelial ovarian tumors are asymptomatic unilateral adnexal masses that can be treated by oophorectomy or occasionally cystectomy (see "Benign Cystic Teratomas [Dermoids]"). In the past, some have recommended bisecting the opposite ovary to rule out bilaterality in the case of benign epithelial ovarian tumors (see Table 33-4), but in view of the risk of adhesions and infertility as well as the availability of vaginal ultrasonography, this is no longer done. In a woman beyond her reproductive years, especially in the presence of a serous cystadenoma, which tends to be bilateral, hysterectomy and bilateral salpingo-oophorectomy are usually performed.

Mucinous tumors can become particularly large and reach sizes of 30 cm or more. Possible complications of mucinous cystadenoma are perforation and rupture, which can lead to the deposit and growth of mucin-secreting epithelium in the peritoneal cavity (pseudomyxoma peritonei, discussed later with borderline mucinous tumors).

Adenofibromas consist of fibrous and epithelial elements. The epithelial component may be serous, mucinous, clear-cell, or endometrioid, the architectural subtypes of these benign ovarian tumors. Their appearance will depend on the predominant histologic features: epithelial or fibrous. These tumors are also managed by simple excision. Endometriomas are considered in Chapter 19 (Endometriosis).

Brenner tumors (see Fig. 33-6) are rare and often incidental findings when oophorectomy is performed for an indication other than ovarian enlargement. Most often, these tumors occur in women in their 40s and 50s, but both younger and older patients have been found to have them. Brenner tumors are almost always benign and can usually be managed by oophorectomy. When the ovary is palpably enlarged, approximately 5% of Brenner tumors will prove to be malignant. These tumors often occur in perimenopausal and postmenopausal women, in which case, hysterectomy and bilateral salpingo-oophorectomy are indicated. Unfortunately, malignant Brenner tumors appear to have a poor prognosis despite this operative therapy, and an effective program of chemotherapy has not been developed.

The differential diagnosis for and approach to an adnexal mass in female patients of various ages are discussed in Chapter 7 (History, Physical Examination, and Preventive Health Care). Ovarian enlargement in the premenarchal female is usually the result of a germ cell tumor, which may be malignant but is usually benign (see later discussion of germ cell tumors). During the reproductive years, ovarian neoplasms are usually benign. For the woman in her 20s or 30s, most ovarian enlargements can be approached surgically through a lower abdominal transverse (Pfannenstiel) incision or by laparoscope, unless there is a likelihood of malignancy, such as a solid tumor or one with papillae viewed on ultrasound examination. However, the risk of laparoscopic excision was emphasized in a report by Maiman and colleagues. They conducted a national survey and discovered 42 cases of ovarian malignancy in women who had laparoscopic aspiration and/or excision of an adnexal mass that subsequently proved to be malignant. More recently, Lehner and associates and Leminen and Lehtovirta reported early spread of malignancy after laparoscopic removal of ovarian masses that were found postoperatively to be malignant. In these cases, as well as in women older than age 40 or those with a large mass extending out of the pelvis and into the abdomen, a vertical incision is indicated. The tumor should be removed intact, and if malignancy is present, as is more likely in older patients, a thorough surgical evaluation is indicated (outlined in "Epithelial Carcinomas").

A frozen section should be obtained if gross examination of the ovarian tumor is at all suspicious for malignancy. For women of reproductive age desiring fertility, if the diagnosis of malignancy is suspected but uncertain even after a frozen section is obtained, the operation should be terminated after removal of the ovarian tumor. A second procedure can be performed if malignancy is confirmed after detailed histologic study of the permanent sections. This is preferable to risking an unnecessary hysterectomy or bilateral salpingo-oophorectomy in a patient who desires to preserve childbearing function. Patients in whom childbearing is not desired should undergo careful counseling to describe the potential need for a staging procedure in case a documented or suspected malignancy is identified from frozen section.

Epithelial Carcinomas

Diagnosis, Staging, Spread, and Preoperative Evaluation

Ovarian carcinomas are usually diagnosed by detection of an adnexal mass on pelvic or abdominal examination. Occasionally, the diagnosis is made from radiographic survey executed for evaluation of nonspecific gastrointestinal symptoms. Unfortunately, the diagnosis is frequently made only after the disease has spread beyond the ovary, as noted in the previous section describing the de novo origin of these tumors. Scully estimates that the risk of malignancy in a primary ovarian tumor increases to approximately 33% in a woman older than the age of 45, whereas it is less than 1 in 15 for women who are 20 to 45 years of age. In general, more than half of ovarian carcinomas occur in women older than the age of 50. In a hospital-based study of ovarian neoplasms in 861 women, Koonings and associates noted that the risk of malignancy was 13% in premenopausal women but rose to 45% in postmenopausal women. In their study, benign ovarian neoplasms were most common among those 20 to 29 years of age.

More than 90% of women diagnosed with ovarian cancer report symptoms before diagnosis. Unfortunately, these symptoms are vague and not specific for early-stage disease or even ovarian cancer. Goff and colleagues conducted a prospective survey of women seeking medical care. The case patients were those about to undergo surgery for a known or suspected pelvic or ovarian mass; the controls were women presenting to one of two primary care clinics, in which approximately two thirds were being seen for a specific problem. The voluntary questionnaire instrument administered to both cohorts asked the respondents to score the severity, frequency, and duration of 20 symptoms generally reported by ovarian cancer patients. In both groups, recurring symptoms were common and nonspecific. Symptomatology in control patients was related to the purpose of their visit (general checkup vs. specific complaint), their underlying disease comorbidities, and their menopausal status. Not surprisingly, women with the final diagnosis of ovarian cancer generally reported numerically more symptoms and of greater severity but of shorter duration of onset compared with either the clinic controls or patients with benign ovarian tumors. Ovarian cancer patients were also statistically more likely to report increased abdominal size, bloating, urinary urgency, and pelvic pain. Because the combination of increased abdominal size, bloating, and urinary urgency was reported five times more often and of greater severity in cancer patients than in controls, the authors recommended further clinical investigation when identified. Cervix cytologic testing can detect ovarian carcinoma cells because of their transmigration through the tubes, uterus, and cervix into the vagina. However, an ovarian carcinoma is rarely initially detected from cytologic smears. The diagnosis is established by histologic examination of tumor tissue removed at operation. Occasionally, the initial diagnosis is suggested by malignant cells found in ascitic fluid obtained at paracentesis.

The staging of ovarian cancer (Table 33-5) is designed according to the criteria of the International Federation of Gynecology and Obstetrics and is based on the results of operative exploration.

Before surgical exploration for suspected ovarian carcinoma, the patient has the preoperative workup usual for a major abdominal operation (see Chapter 24, Preoperative Counseling and Management). Additional diagnostic studies may include a computed tomography (CT) scan of the abdomen to search for retroperitoneal node enlargement or parenchymal liver masses. Occasionally, a barium enema or colonoscopy is performed to

Table 33-5 Staging of Ovarian Carcinomas (International Federation of Gynecology and Obstetrics) Modified 1985

Stage	Characteristics
I	Growth limited to the ovaries.
IA	Growth limited to one ovary; no ascites present containing malignant cells. No tumor on the external surface; capsule intact.
IB	Growth limited to both ovaries; no ascites present containing malignant cells. No tumor on the external surfaces; capsules intact.
IC	Tumor either stage IA or IB but with tumor on surface of one or both ovaries; or with capsule ruptured; or with ascites present containing malignant cells; or with positive peritoneal washings.
II	Growth involving one or both ovaries with pelvic extension.
IIA	Extension and/or metastases to the uterus and/or tubes.
IIB	Extension to other pelvic tissues.
IIC	Tumor either stage IIA or IIB, but with tumor on surface of one or both ovaries; or with capsule(s) ruptured; or with ascites present containing malignant cells; or with positive peritoneal washings.
III	Tumor involving one or both ovaries with peritoneal implants outside the pelvis and/or positive retroperitoneal or inguinal nodes. Superficial liver metastasis equals stage III. Tumor is limited to the true pelvis but with histologically proven malignant extension to small bowel or omentum.
IIIA	Tumor grossly limited to the rule pelvis with negative nodes but with histologically confirmed microscopic seeding of abdominal peritoneal surfaces.
IIIB	Tumor of one or both ovaries with histologically confirmed implants of abdominal peritoneal surfaces, none exceeding 2 cm in diameter. Nodes are negative.
IIIC	Abdominal implants greater than 2 cm in diameter and/or positive retroperitoneal or inguinal nodes.
IV	Growth involving one or both ovaries with distant metastases. If pleural effusion is present, there must be positive cytology to allot a case to stage IV.
IVA	Parenchymal liver metastasis equals stage IV.

evaluate pelvic and/or gastrointestinal symptoms. Consideration of gastrointestinal pathology is of importance for the potential of a primary colon carcinoma, which may present initially as an adnexal mass in the older patient. Approximately 4% of colon cancers will have metastatic involvement of the ovary at diagnosis. A serum carcinoembryonic antigen may be useful in this setting and is recommended as part of the preoperative evaluation of a pelvic mass. An endoscopic or gastrointestinal radiographic examination is performed if there is evidence of gastrointestinal bleeding or the suggestion of any gastrointestinal pathology. A CA 125 sample is obtained and if increased at the time of operation, it is useful for following the progress of the patient during and after treatment and for demonstrating the response to therapy or detecting tumor progression. Buller and associates studied the regression slope for CA 125 during chemotherapy and found the slope of the regression curve to be predictive of therapeutic outcome. Other investigators have shown that patients whose CA 125 values decrease from increased to normal rapidly while undergoing primary chemotherapy have an improved prognosis over those whose values decrease more slowly. Markman evaluated the survival impact of CA 125 values reaching 50% of pretreatment baseline at 8 weeks after surgery and cisplatin-based chemotherapy. Survival was 21 months for those achieving this decrease versus just 10 months for those not achieving a 50% decrease. Clearly this imperfect marker has prognostic significance in many situations. Serum inhibin has been reported to be elevated in mucinous carcinomas and may serve as a marker, according to the studies of Henley and associates. Frias and coworkers reported pretreatment levels of inhibin A to be a prognostic factor for survival in postmenopausal women with ovarian cancer.

Preoperatively, a program to cleanse the bowel is instituted in case intestinal resection is required. One widely used program uses 4 L of GoLYTELY given over 3 to 4 hours the evening before surgery. Neomycin sulfate 1 g, with 1 g erythromycin base, may be given three times (3 PM, 7 PM, and 11 PM) on the day before surgery or IV broad-spectrum antibiotics prophylactically just before the operation. Alternatively, magnesium citrate (16 oz) with oral Dulcolax tablets may be used. It is preferable to initiate bowel preparation early preoperatively so that liquid stool is evacuated before night sleep. Mechanical cleansing of the bowel is of some controversy though.

Venous thromboembolism prophylaxis is of particular importance in patients with ovarian cancer as large tumor burden is associated with venous stasis and prolonged operation times. Treatment with variable compression leg support stockings and heparin (fractionated and unfractionated) appears to reduce the risk of thromboembolism in gynecologic oncology patients undergoing surgical tumor extirpation.

Ovarian carcinomas infiltrate the peritoneal surfaces of both the parietal and intestinal areas, as well as the undersurface of the diaphragm, particularly on the right side (Fig. 33-7). This is particularly important because tumors that appear at operation to be confined to the ovary may have small areas of diaphragmatic involvement as the sole site of extraovarian spread. As noted earlier, most ovarian carcinomas, particularly the serous type, appear to arise from microscopic ovarian sites and do not become clinically evident until there is widespread metastatic disease. Lymphatic dissemination is also a prominent part of disease spread (Fig. 33-8), and it is particularly important to note that the paraaortic nodes are at risk through lymphatics that run parallel to the ovarian vessels. Knapp and Friedman

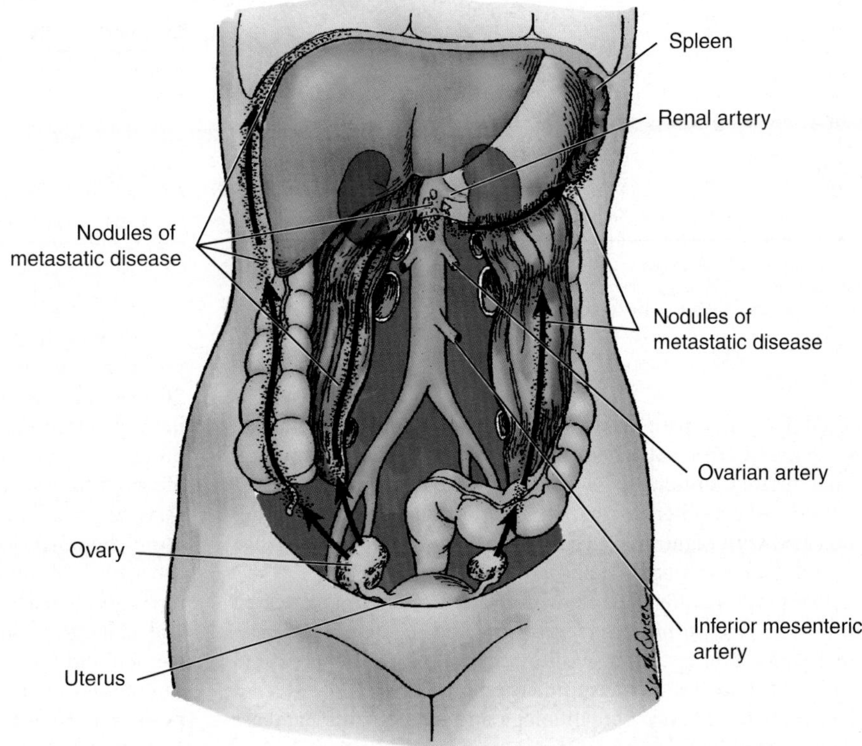

Figure 33-7. Peritoneal spread of ovarian cancer. Portions of omentum, small intestine, and transverse colon have been resected. (From Knapp RC, Berkowitz RS, Leavitt T Jr: Natural history and detection of ovarian cancer. In Gynecology and Obstetrics, Vol 4. Philadelphia, JB Lippincott, 1986.)

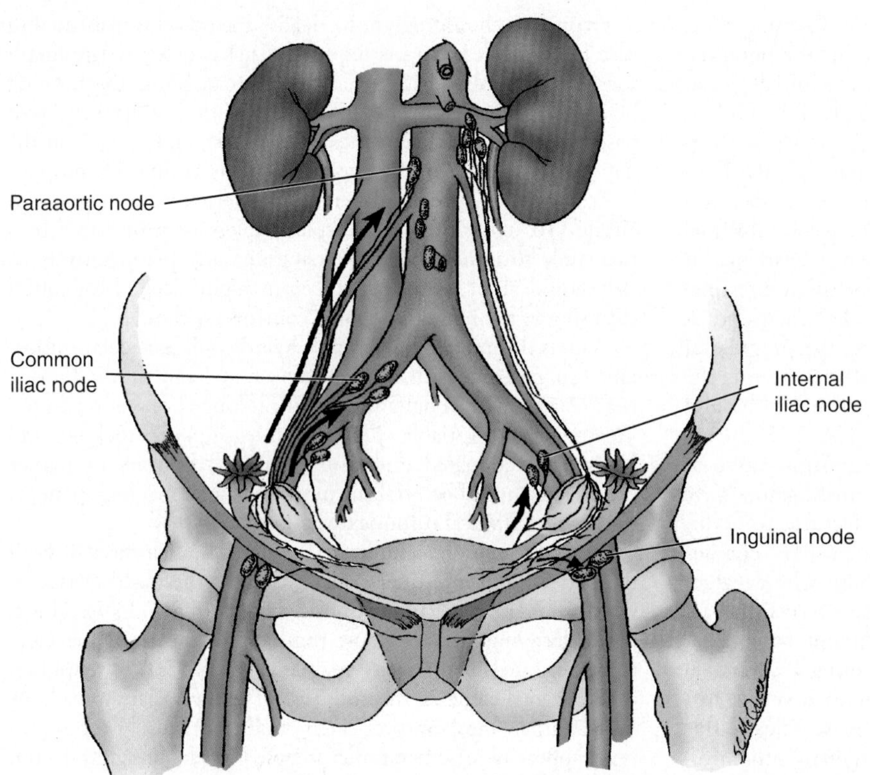

Figure 33-8. Lymph nodes draining ovaries. Primary routes of spread to the pelvic and paraaortic nodes are illustrated. (Redrawn from Musumeci R, Banfi A, Bolis G, et al: Lymphangiography in patients with ovarian epithelial cancer: An evaluation of 289 consecutive cases. Cancer 40:1444, 1977.)

Table 33-6 Carcinoma of the Ovary: Survival by FIGO Stage for Patients Treated 1990–92

Stage	Number	5-Year Survival (%)
IA	342	86.9
IB	49	71.3
IC	352	79.2
IIA	64	66.6
IIB	92	55.1
IIC	136	57.0
IIIA	129	41.1
IIIB	137	24.9
IIIC	1193	23.4
IV	360	11.1

FIGO, International Federation of Gynecology and Obstetrics.
Modified from Pecorelli S, Creasman WT, Pettersson F, et al: FIGO annual report on the results of treatment in gynaecological cancer, Vol 23. Milano, Italy. J Epidemiol Biostat, 1998.

Table 33-7 Summary of Primary Endpoints in the Three Largest Randomized Phase III Studies

	ALBERTS ET AL (1996) *N* = 546		MARKMAN ET AL (2001) *N* = 462		ARMSTRONG ET AL (2006) *N* = 415	
Outcome	**IV**	**IP**	**IV**	**IP**	**IV**	**IP**
Pathologic CR	36%	47%			41%	57%
P value	—					
PFS	—	—	22 mos	28 mos	18 mos	24 mos
P value	—		.01		.05	
OS	41 mo	49 mo	52 mo	63 mo	50 mo	66 mo
P value	.02		.05		.03	

CR, Complete response; OS, overall survival; PFS, progressive-free survival.

noted that, of 26 patients with ovarian cancer apparently limited to the ovary, 19% had paraaortic involvement, and all had poorly differentiated tumors. In a study of 180 patients, Burghardt and coworkers observed that the proportion of positive nodes increased with higher stage tumors: 24% in stage I, 50% in stage II, and 73.5% in stages III and IV.

The prognosis for patients with ovarian carcinoma is related to tumor stage, tumor grade, cell type, and the amount of residual tumor after resection. Worldwide results for patients treated from 1990 to 1992 are summarized in Table 33-6. Recent data from the Survey Epidemiology and End Results database are presented in Table 33-7.

Cell type has been reported to be an important factor in prognosis, as shown in Figure 33-9, which summarizes the 20-year survival rate of a group of patients. The most common invasive epithelial cancers, serous carcinomas, have the worst prognosis; prognosis may be better for mucinous and endometrioid tumors. A variant of papillary serous carcinoma termed *transitional cell carcinoma* is thought by some to be a rare but more chemosensitive tumor. However, this has not been established in multiinstitutional studies. Endometrioid carcinoma is rarely associated with endometriosis, and according to McMeekin and colleagues, such cases more commonly occur in younger women and have a better prognosis than typical endometrioid carcinomas of the ovary. Clear-cell cancers have a worse prognosis, but Kennedy and associates noted that mitotic activity and tumor stage were important prognostic features of this

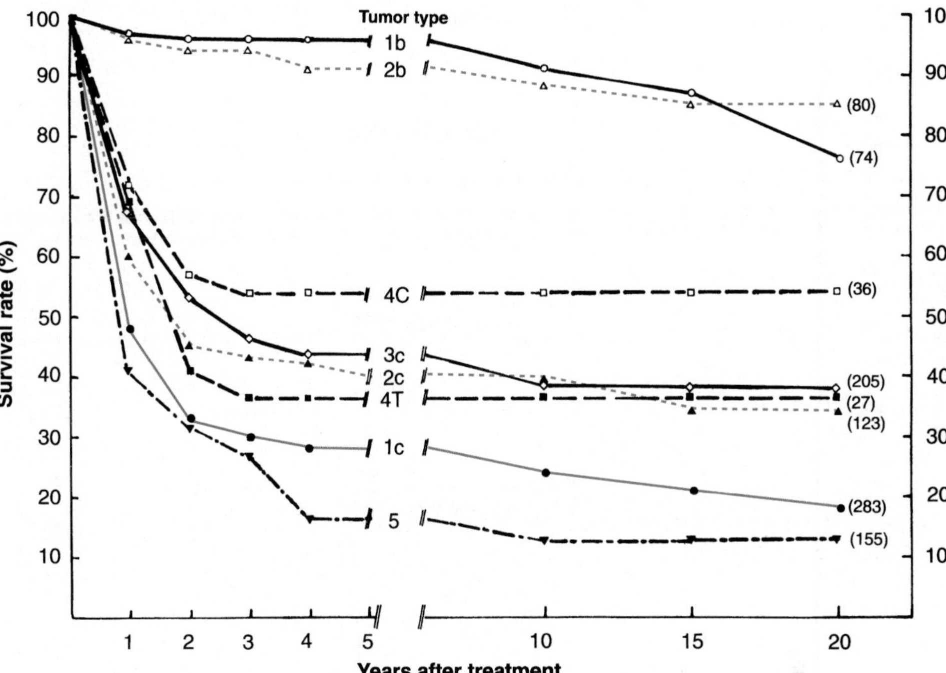

Figure 33-9. Survival rates for 983 patients with all stages of ovarian cancer by histologic type. *1b*, Serous, low malignant potential (74 cases). *2b*, Mucinous, low malignant potential (80 cases), *1c*, Serous carcinoma (283 cases). *2c*, Mucinous carcinoma (123 cases). *3c*, Endometrioid carcinoma (205 cases). *4c*, Clear cell (36 cases). *4T*, Tubulocystic pattern of clear cell (27 cases). *5*, Undifferentiated (155 cases). (Redrawn from Aure JC, Hoeg K, Kolstad P: Clinical and histologic studies of ovarian carcinoma. Long-term follow-up of 990 cases. Obstet Gynecol 37:1, 1971. Reprinted with permission from The American College of Obstetricians and Gynecologists.)

tumor in their series. Tubulocystic pattern did not appear to affect prognosis, as was suggested by the earlier studies of Aure and colleagues, depicted in Figure 33-9. Nonetheless, these are aggressive tumors with a propensity for recurrence even in stage I. In a follow-up analysis, Kennedy and associates noted a survival probability of only 50% for stages I–II, which was similar to that of high-grade epithelial cancers of comparable stage. It should be noted that both stage and grade affect these observations. Serous tumors tend to be more poorly differentiated and discovered at a higher stage than are mucinous tumors.

In some cases, patients are found to have small ovaries (<4 cm in diameter) and widespread papillary serous carcinoma in the abdomen. In such cases, the term *serous surface papillary carcinoma of the ovary* is applied. Fromm and coworkers reported on 74 patients and found survival improved if the patients were treated postoperatively with combination chemotherapy (see later discussion for therapy of advanced-stage carcinoma of the ovary). Another variety of serous carcinoma is primary peritoneal carcinoma. In these cases, the ovaries may be of normal size with surface metastatic tumor deposits. There is widespread intraabdominal spread of carcinoma of serous histology. These cases can be associated with *BRCA1* and *BRCA2* mutations, as shown by the studies of Karlan and colleagues

The cloning of the *BRCA1* gene has advanced our knowledge of the molecular genetics of ovarian cancer, but the role of this gene that resides on chromosome 17q21 is not clear. It appears to be a tumor suppressor gene that is highly expressed in ovarian borderline carcinoma. Mutations in *BRCA1* are strongly associated with increased risk of breast and ovarian cancer and a similar increase in risk occurs with mutations in *BRCA2* (Table 33-8). These mutations are seen in approximately 2% to 2.5% of Ashkenazi Jewish women, who appear to be an appropriate target group for testing whether breast cancer is diagnosed before age 50 in the patient or a close relative according to the analysis of Warner and associates. Prophylactic oophorectomy reduces the risk of ovarian cancer in those with a mutation, but does not eliminate the problem because of the potential for primary peritoneal carcinoma. The study of Rebbeck and colleagues of *BRCA1* mutation carriers suggests prophylactic oophorectomy may also reduce the subsequent risk of breast cancer. Boyd and coworkers reported that, stage for stage, the hereditary ovarian cancer group may have a better prognosis than the spontaneously occurring tumors. Lu and associates noted a high proportion of microscopic carcinomas in apparently normal ovaries removed from patients with *BRCA* mutations, an observation consistent with the de novo origin of serous and poorly differentiated carcinomas.

In addition to stage, the grade of the tumor is a major determinant of patient prognosis. Figure 33-10 demonstrates the survival of 442 patients with ovarian carcinoma by grade, with a markedly worse prognosis for poorly differentiated tumors (grade 3). The relationship between grade and survival also exists when the results are examined separately for each stage of disease. Grade 0 (borderline) tumors have the best prognosis (see Fig. 33-9).

Table 33-8 Carcinoma of the Ovary: Survival by SEER Registration for Patients Treated 1995–2001

Category	5-Year Survival (%)
Localized	94
Regional	69
Distant	9
All stages	45

SEER, Surveillance Epidemiology and End Results.
From Jemal A, Siegel R, Ward E, et al: Cancer statistics, 2006. CA Cancer J Clin 56:106, 2006.

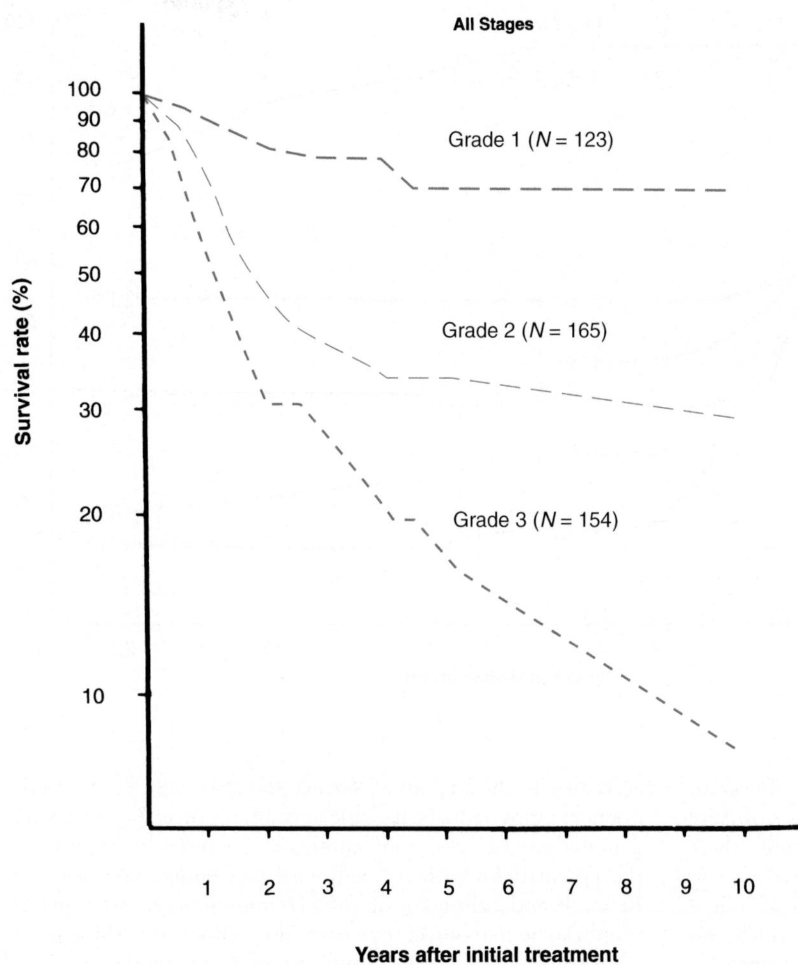

Figure 33-10. Survival rates for patients with ovarian cancer by tumor grade. Survival curves for the complete series according to the histologic degree of differentiation. All differences between curves are highly significant. (From Sorbe B, Frankendal B, Veress B: Importance of histologic grading in the prognosis of epithelial ovarian carcinoma. Obstet Gynecol 59:576, 1982. Reprinted with permission from the American College of Obstetricians and Gynecologists.)

The development of gene expression profiling has enabled a more precise evaluation of clinical behavior in some tumors. Bonome and coworkers studied the gene expression of low malignant potential (LMP) serous neoplasms and invasive low-grade and high-grade serous tumors. A distinct and separate clustering was observed between LMP tumors and high-grade cancers. Low-grade tumors generally clustered with LMP neoplasms. High-grade tumors differentially expressed genes linked to cell proliferation, chromosomal instability, and epigenetic silencing. Based on these findings, high-grade epithelial cancers appear to have a distinct profile relative to LMP neoplasms. Low-grade serous tumors are remarkably similar to LMP serous neoplasms, highlighting their different natural history. These observations have ushered in the consideration of reclassifying invasive malignant cancers into two categories: low-grade and high-grade.

Studies of flow cytometry indicate that the ploidy of the tumor is also prognostic with aneuploidy being a negative prognostic factor. Klemi and colleagues noted an independent prognostic association with the DNA index and S-phase fraction. A better prognosis was observed if the proportion of S-phase cells was less than 11% or if the DNA index (the relative DNA content of aneuploid cells compared with diploid) was less than 1.3. Genetic studies by Slamon and coworkers have shown that the HER-2/*neu* oncogene is found to be amplified in ovarian and breast cancers. As noted in a review by Berchuck and associates, the overexpression of HER-2/*neu* was suspected to occur in approximately 30% of epithelial ovarian cancers and appears associated with a worse prognosis. However, a recent Gynecologic Oncology Group (GOG) study of trastuzumab (a monoclonal antibody to the extracellular domain of HER-2) in patients with recurrent ovarian cancer suggested the incident overexpression by fluorescence in situ hybridization is much lower. In this study, 837 samples were screened for immunohistochemistry overexpression (2+ or 3+) or fluorescence in situ hybridization positivity. Only 95 patients (11.4%) met criteria for therapy. The prospective trial likely more accurately represents the incidence of this factor in ovarian cancer. The p53 tumor suppressor gene is mutated in approximately half of ovarian epithelial cancers studied, whereas the C-*myc* oncogene is overexpressed more commonly in serous cases and the K-*ras* oncogene has been identified more frequently in borderline ovarian cancers. The molecular genetic events surrounding ovarian carcinoma development and biologic behavior are incompletely understood.

The size of residual nodules and the presence or absence of tumor after surgery has been shown to be related to the survival of patients treated for ovarian carcinoma. Aure and colleagues, in their classic studies, noted a 5-year survival rate of more than 30% for stage III tumors that were completely resected compared with 10% when resection was incomplete. Frequently used categories are microscopic (present on biopsy, but not grossly), less than 1.0 cm, or greater than 1.0 cm. The impact of cytoreduction for advanced stage disease is discussed next.

Management

Borderline Ovarian Tumors (Ovarian Carcinomas of Low Malignant Potential). Approximately 20% of ovarian epithelial cancers are tumors of LMP and usually have an excellent prognosis regardless of stage. Most studies have been confined to borderline tumors of the serous (see Fig. 33-2*B*) and mucinous (see Fig. 33-3*B*) varieties, which are the most common histologies; however, other epithelial types (see Table 33-3) can occur. The cells of these epithelial tumors do not invade the stroma of the ovary. It is extremely important that the ovarian tumor be thoroughly sampled by the pathologist to be certain that a borderline tumor is not mixed with invasive elements. Numerous studies have confirmed that borderline tumors have a slower growth rate than do invasive ovarian carcinomas, manifested by prolonged survival (see Fig. 33-9).

Because these tumors tend to occur in young women during the reproductive years, it is desirable to ascertain the safety of conservative therapy for patients with borderline stage 1A tumors (confined to one ovary). Leake and colleagues reported on 200 patients with borderline serous tumors. With a median follow-up of 11.2 years, the 5-year survival rate for *all* stages was 97% and 89% for 20 years.

Recurrences in stages I and II were rare and despite recurrences, the 20-year survival rate in stage III was approximately 40%. Patients with stage I disease can be treated by unilateral adnexectomy and if the opposite ovary is normal, a biopsied need not be performed. Lim-Tan and associates reported on 33 cases of stage I serous borderline tumors initially treated by cystectomy. Only 3 of 33 patients undergoing cystectomy had recurrence or persistence, and these three patients had positive resection margins and/or multiple cysts present in the ovary, emphasizing the effectiveness of conservative operation. However, for most stage IA cases, unilateral adnexectomy is performed, and if the opposite ovary looks normal, no biopsy or wedge resection is done.

Mucinous borderline tumors also are associated with an excellent prognosis. Hart and Norris reviewed 97 patients with stage I tumors who were 9 to 70 years of age with a median of 35 years. More than 10% of the tumors were discovered during pregnancy or in the immediate postpartum period. Follow-up data were available on 87 of the patients, and there were only three tumor-related deaths during the 5- to 10-year follow-up. The actuarial survival was 98% at 5 years and 96% at 10 years. This was also noted by Bostwick and colleagues, who reported on 109 borderline tumors, 33 of which were mucinous, and all of which were stage I, contributing to the good prognosis.

Borderline mucinous tumors have also been associated with widespread growth of mucin-producing cells in the peritoneum (pseudomyxoma peritonei). The result may be the accumulation of large amounts of mucinous material, which is sometimes associated with recurrent bouts of bowel obstruction. Studies by Young and coworkers suggest that pseudomyxoma peritonei usually arise in the appendix. The review of Ronnett and coworkers supports a primary appendicial origin for these tumors, and therefore appendectomy is indicated in these cases. Those associated with appendicial adenoma have a better prognosis than those associated with appendicial carcinoma, and the same is true of ovarian tumors, as noted by Wertheim and associates. The disease tends to recur and to require repeated laparotomy to relieve bowel obstruction. Chemotherapy and mucolytic agents have been tried but are usually not successful. However, Jones and Homesley reported a single case with a complete remission following eight courses of cyclophosphamide (Cytoxan) 500 mg/m^2, doxorubicin (Adriamycin) 50 mg/m^2, and cisplatin 50 mg/m^2.

Conservative therapy of borderline ovarian tumors with preservation of childbearing function may be carried out by unilateral oophorectomy if the following criteria are met: the tumor is confirmed to be at stage IA, extensive histologic sampling of the tumor confirms it to be a borderline tumor, the contralateral ovary appears normal, biopsy specimens of areas of omental or peritoneal nodularity are negative, and results of peritoneal cytologic tests are negative for tumor cells. Retroperitoneal nodes are rarely involved and are not routinely sampled. No recurrences were noted in 156 stage I patients in a GOG study treated by operation alone, as reported by Barnhill and colleagues.

For borderline tumors beyond stage I, both radiation therapy and chemotherapy have been prescribed to attempt to improve survival. However, as noted in Figure 33-9, the 5-year survival rate of patients with all stages of borderline tumors is high (>90%) after resection alone. Operative removal of all gross disease remains the most important factor in primary treatment, with extensive biopsy of any peritoneal or omental implants. As emphasized by Prat, peritoneal implants should be meticulously sampled to determine whether they are noninvasive or invasive. Noninvasive implants occur more frequently than invasive implant and are generally associated with a better survival. Bell and associates studied peritoneal implants (Figs. 33-11 and 33-12) in 56 patients with 368 person-years of follow-up. Patients with benign implants (i.e., endometriosis or endosalpingosis (benign tubal-appearing epithelium) were eliminated because they require no therapy. Three adverse histologic features were identified in the implants: invasiveness, cytologic atypia, and mitotic count. Gross residual disease after primary operation was also a factor. A group of 27 patients without adverse features had a 100% survival. The risk of death was least (4%) for those whose invasive implants were confined to the pelvis, but increased to 20% for stage III cases. Additional therapy should be reserved for those with implants with adverse features, primarily invasiveness and cytologic atypia. Although somewhat controversial in concept, a variant of borderline ovarian tumor frequently associated with invasive implants is the micropapillary serous borderline ovarian tumor. There is no consensus as to whether the implant characteristics define this pathology or are a result of a tumor that essentially is acting as a precursor to invasive disease. Mooney and coworkers noted spontaneous regression of invasive implants postpartum in patients whose borderline tumors were diagnosed during pregnancy. Gershenson and Silva recommend six cycles of chemotherapy (see later discussion) for patients with invasive implants. Histologic examination of the implants may provide a basis to choose patients who might potentially benefit from therapy. However, definite evidence of a survival benefit by treating these cases is lacking. Based on current evidence, surgical removal offers the best treatment for borderline tumors. Other features

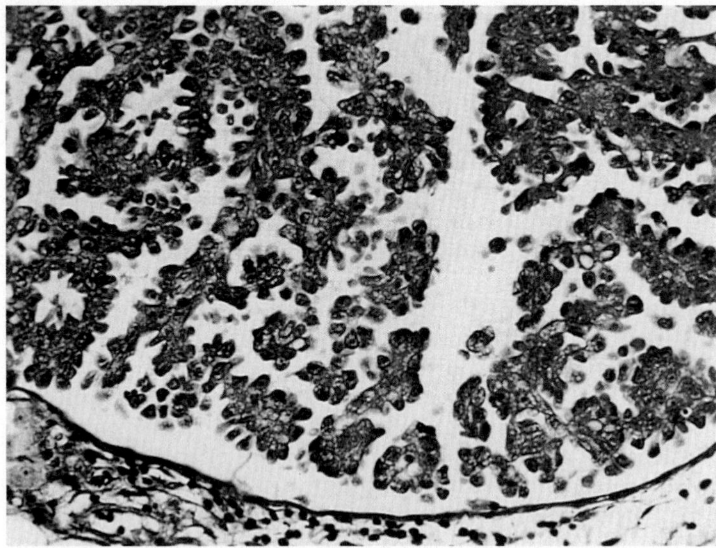

Figure 33-11. Noninvasive implant of epithelial type. Branching papillae and detached clusters of polygonal cells showing moderate cytologic atypicality are present. (H&E, ×313.) (From Bell DA, Weinstock MA, Scully RE: Peritoneal implants of ovarian serous borderline tumors. Histologic features and prognosis. Cancer 62:2212, 1988.)

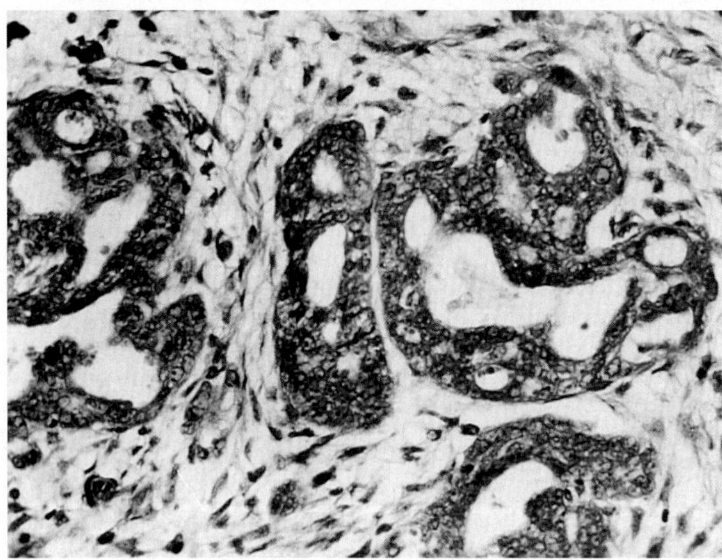

Figure 33-12. Invasive implant. Glands with an irregular contour lined by severely atypical epithelial cells with extensive intraglandular bridging are present (H&E, ×313). (From Bell DA, Weinstock MA, Scully RE: Peritoneal implants of ovarian serous borderline tumors: Histologic features and prognosis. Cancer 62:2212, 1988.)

described with borderline ovarian tumors are nodal metastasis, which occurs in approximately 20% to 25% of cases, and microinvasive ovarian features. The former appears to be unrelated to outcome; however, there is no consensus as to whether the presence of microinvasion or the depth of microinvasion is prognostic. This remains an area of investigation.

Invasive Epithelial Carcinomas. The primary treatment of ovarian epithelial carcinoma is removal of all resectable gross disease. The patient's abdomen is explored through a vertical incision. If ascitic fluid is present, it is sent for cytologic evaluation; if ascites is not present, 200 to 400 mL of normal saline solution is used to obtain cytologic samples from the peritoneum by irrigating at least the pelvis, upper abdomen, and right and left paracolic gutters before any resection is done. The diaphragm can be cytologically sampled by scraping the undersurface with a sterile tongue depressor and the sample placed on a glass slide and sprayed with a fixative. Biopsy or, preferably, excision of any suspicious nodules is performed. A total abdominal hysterectomy, bilateral salpingo-oophorectomy, and appendectomy as well as infracolic omentectomy are performed if technically possible. When there is no gross disease outside the pelvis, paraaortic and pelvic lymph node sampling is recommended, with care taken to remove enlarged nodes. Although the impact of systematic lymphadenectomy has been addressed in one randomized clinical trial by Benedetti-Panici and associates without significant effect, it is reasonable to explore these areas as inspection by palpation is notoriously inaccurate. Current evidence suggests that if all gross disease can be resected, duration of patient survival is enhanced. Although randomized clinical trials have not been performed to document this effect, a recent meta-analysis of 6885 patients gathered from 81 cohorts suggested a linear relationship between the degree of cytoreduction and overall survival. In this report, Bristow and colleagues noted that for each 10% increase in cytoreduction, a 5.5% increase in survival was observed. The surgical procedures required to achieve maximal cytoreduction may be extensive and involve splenectomy, diaphragmatic stripping/resection, and posterior exenteration. It may occasionally be necessary to resect bowel to relieve impending obstruction or to remove a tumor nodule and thereby eliminate all gross disease from the peritoneal cavity. Heintz and coworkers noted prognosis was improved for younger patients (younger than 50 years of age), those with good initial performance status (Karnofsky > 80, see Table 26-4), as well as those whose disease could be cytoreduced to less than 1.5 cm. Adverse factors were large metastases before initial operation, ascites, and peritoneal carcinomatosis. In a small collaborative GOG study, Hoskins and colleagues found that those who started with large-volume disease did worse than those who initially had small-volume disease and no survival advantage could be demonstrated for the debulking operation in the large-volume disease group. Chi and associates noted that those with advanced disease and a preoperative CA 125 level of more than 500 U/mL had less than a 20% chance of an optimal surgical debulking (see later).

One exception to the required removal of the uterus and opposite ovary occurs in the case of well-differentiated (grade 1) ovarian tumors confined to one ovary (stage IA). DiSaia and coworkers outlined criteria for preserving childbearing function in a young woman with stage IA, grade 1 ovarian epithelial carcinoma, as follows:

1. Tumor confined to one ovary
2. Tumor well differentiated (grade 1) with no invasion of capsule, lymphatics, or mesovarium
3. Peritoneal washings negative
4. Omental biopsy specimen negative
5. Young woman of childbearing years with strong desire to preserve reproductive function

These criteria can be applied to all types of epithelial ovarian tumors but are more likely to be satisfied in the case of mucinous tumors, which are more frequently well differentiated and unilateral than serous carcinomas. Wedge resection of a normal-appearing contralateral ovary is unlikely to uncover an occult tumor. It is reasonable to follow the patient closely for any evidence of future ovarian enlargement with vaginal ultrasonography in these cases.

Low-Stage Ovarian Carcinomas. ***Stage I.*** Surgical exploration is performed. It is important to emphasize that careful assessment of the subdiaphragmatic areas and inspection of the entire peritoneum and the retroperitoneal paraaortic and pelvic nodes are important, particularly in view of the risk of diaphragmatic and nodal spread in higher-grade tumors that initially appear to be at stage I, particularly those on frozen section that appear to be less well differentiated than grade 1. In addition, the omentum, uterus, tubes, and contralateral ovary are removed. Frequently, nodal evaluation is performed during the staging procedure. For women undergoing a conservative approach, limited unilateral sampling of the nodal tissue is considered.

Rupture of ovary. Occasionally during removal, a stage I ovarian carcinoma is inadvertently ruptured (stage IC, Table 33-6). There are conflicting opinions as to the potential adverse effects on patient prognosis. In an analysis of 394 patients, Sjövall and associates found that rupture during surgery did not affect survival, whereas there was marked reduction in survival in that study among those whose ovarian rupture occurred *before* the operation. In general, the spilled fluid and all residual tumor should be removed promptly from the operative field after a rupture (see later discussion). Presumably higher grade and larger tumors are most prone to rupture.

A study by Dembo and colleagues of 519 stage I patients found that adverse factors were grade of tumor, dense pelvic adherence (no invasion but adhesion), or more than 250 mL of ascites. Patients without these features had a 98% 5-year survival rate. It appears that patients with stage I grade 3 tumors should have postoperative therapy, but data are unclear for stage I grade 2 patients.

Stage II. Stage II ovarian cancer is initially treated by removal of all gross disease, including the uterus, tubes, and ovaries, and an omentectomy (infracolic) is performed. The pelvic and paraaortic nodes are sampled.

Postoperative management for stages I–II. Recommendations for postoperative or adjuvant therapy generally have evolved around identification of patients in whom a sufficient risk of recurrence is observed. The precision to make this assessment is low and currently based on morphologic features such as grade, histology, and presence of rupture and residuum. Historically, several modalities have been evaluated alone and in combination by prospective studies of unselected patients including chemotherapy, radiation therapy, IP radiocolloids, and immunotherapy. Guthrie and colleagues evaluated 656 patients treated for epithelial ovarian carcinomas that had been totally excised. Most carcinomas were stage I or II, and patients were randomly assigned to receive postoperative treatment of radiation therapy alone, chemotherapy alone, radiation therapy and chemotherapy, or no postoperative therapy. Follow-up was for at least 2 years. Approximately 20% of the tumors were borderline malignancies, and the rest were invasive carcinomas. Perhaps surprisingly, the lowest frequency of death or recurrence was noted in the group receiving no postoperative therapy (2%), whereas in the other groups, the death or recurrence incidence was 14% to 17%. Thus, this study showed no benefit for adjuvant therapy and highlights the need for careful case selection and pathologic review. In addition, because survivorship of low-stage cancer is better, long-term follow-up is necessary to tease out the merits of intervention. Two large multicenter trials have been conducted and were combined for analytical purposes to address this issue. The International Collaborative Ovarian Neoplasm 1 (ICON1) and Adjuvant ChemoTherapy in Ovarian Neoplasm (ACTION) trials compared platinum-based chemotherapy with observation in patients after surgery with early-stage ovarian cancer. The two trials differed somewhat in patient eligibility with ICON1 enrolling postoperative predominantly stage I and II patients with limited staging and ACTION enrolling postoperative stage IA and IB grade 2 and 3, stage IC–IIA, all grades, and clear cell patients. Overall, 925 patients were collectively enrolled (477 in ICON1 and 448 in ACTION) and followed for a median 4 years. The overall survival rate at 5 years was 82% in the chemotherapy arm and 74% in the observation arm (HR = 0.67, 95% CI: 0.5–0.9, p = .001). Recurrence-free survival at 5 years was also significantly higher in the chemotherapy arm compared with observation (HR = 0.64, 95% CI: 0.5–0.82). In selected patients, platinum-based therapy appears to improve survival and lower recurrence at 5 years over observation.

Radioactive colloids have also been used postoperatively in patients with stage I and II disease or with no gross residual tumor after surgery. ^{32}P, a primary beta emitter, has been used most commonly. A standard infusion of 15 mCi of ^{32}P in 500 mL of saline solution is injected intraperitoneally and distributed widely throughout the peritoneal cavity. Radioactive gold (^{198}Au) had also been used in the past but because of gamma ray emission (see Chapter 26, Principles of Radiation Therapy and Chemotherapy in Gynecologic Cancer), it is associated with more posttherapy complications and is not used.

Young and associates conducted two randomized studies for adjuvant therapy of patients with stage I disease. The first showed that those with stage IA grades 1 and 2 had 5-year survival rates of greater than 90% and did not benefit from adjuvant alkylating agent chemotherapy. The second study showed comparable results both for adjuvant ^{32}P and platinum-based therapy for a higher risk cohort including stage I grade 3 as well as completely resected stage II cases. The assessable cohort included 229 randomized patients. The cumulative incidence of recurrence at 10 years was 29% lower for those receiving chemotherapy compared with ^{32}P (28% vs. 35%, p = .15) but was not statistically significant. The recurrence risk in this cohort of patients was substantial; all stage I, 27% and stage II, 44%. Inadequate distribution and small bowel perforation are cited as reasons that ^{32}P is less desirable as adjuvant therapy. Piver and coworkers reported 93% 5-year survival for stage IC or stage I grade 3 patients who received multiagent chemotherapy containing cisplatinum. Vergote and colleagues analyzed 313 patients treated with ^{32}P either after the primary operation or the second-look (see discussion later in chapter) operation. Bowel complications occurred in 22 (7%), and 13 required operations. Bolis and colleagues reported two randomized trials comparing ^{32}P and chemotherapy with cisplatinum at 50 mg/m^2 for six cycles. Stages IA and IB grades 2 to 3 and stages IC showed significantly reduced relapse rates in the cisplatinum arms. Unfortunately, a survival advantage was not demonstrated, and those who had a recurrence after receiving chemotherapy did worse than those who received ^{32}P. Currently, when indicated, the most frequently used modality is chemotherapy, although the ideal regimen and number of courses need are still debated. Bell and coworkers reported the results of a GOG randomized study comparing three and six cycles of adjuvant paclitaxel and carboplatin for women with stage IA and IB grade 3, all stage IC, clear cell, and completely resected stage II epithelial ovarian cancer. The study was powered for a 50% or greater decrease in recurrence for six cycles of therapy. A total of 457 patients were recruited of whom 344 are alive a median 6.8 years since entry. The overall treatment effect is a non-significant 24% reduction in recurrence for the six-cycle arm (HR = 0.76, 95% CI: 0.51–1.13, p = 0.18). The improved impact on estimated recurrence at 5 years was 5%, and there was no difference in overall survival between the arms. Approximately one third of patients in both arms had stage II disease. Forest plot analysis by stage does not demonstrate any alteration in the study's conclusions in this cohort. Although no difference was observed in this trial, many investigators have questioned the pretreatment statistical goals and continue to recommend six cycles of therapy in patients with early-stage disease requiring treatment. It should be noted the carboplatin dose used in this trial was AUC 7.5. Although the optimal treatment is still not known, clearly high-risk early-stage patients benefit from therapy. An ongoing trial is evaluating the benefit maintenance therapy in this category of patients.

Postoperative Therapy for Advanced Epithelial Carcinomas (Stages III and IV). For historical interest, early adjuvant therapy attempts in advanced disease included single-agent and combination chemotherapy regimens based on the alkylating agents. A limited number of responses were observed and treatment frequently continued for 1 to 3 years. With the discovery of cisplatin (and carboplatin subsequently), several randomized trials were conducted comparing platinum and platinum combinations with nonplatinum regimens. These pivotal trials secured platinum as the agent of choice in primary adjuvant therapy, which continues to this day. In addition, several clinical trials established that little additional benefit to treatment was observed beyond four cycles of therapy. Most recently, the discovery of the taxanes has documented the importance this agent, as described below. By convention, six to eight cycles of combination platinum- and taxane-based therapy are now recommended as adjuvant therapy for most patients with advanced disease.

The pivotal trial establishing the importance of paclitaxel in primary ovarian cancer management was reported by McGuire and colleagues on behalf of the GOG. They conducted a randomized trial comparing cisplatinum 75 mg/m^2 with either cyclophosphamide 750 mg/m^2 or paclitaxel 135 mg/m^2 over 24 hours and demonstrated a survival advantage in the paclitaxel arm. All patients had residual disease of more than 1 cm after the primary operation. Response rates were improved with paclitaxel relative to control in patients with measurable disease (73% vs. 60%). The median progression-free survival (PFS) was 18 months in the paclitaxel arm compared with 13 months in the platinum arm ($p < 0.001$). Overall survival was similarly improved (38 months vs. 24 months, HR = 0.6, 95% CI: 0.5–0.8, $p < 0.001$). The results of this study have been confirmed in similar randomized clinical trials conducted worldwide, and the taxane/platinum combination has generally been considered the recommended first-line therapy for ovarian cancer. The platinum analogue carboplatin was found to be less renal toxic and neurotoxic and easily administered without prehydration, thus shortening the time of infusion. After several randomized clinical studies demonstrating the equivalence of this agent to cisplatin in ovarian cancer, carboplatin was substituted for cisplatin in taxane-based regimens. In addition, paclitaxel infused over 3 hours was found to be likely equivalent to paclitaxel infused over 24 hours and, in combination with carboplatin, enabled the combination to be given an outpatient basis. Phase III studies by Ozols and Neijt and associates showed that paclitaxel and carboplatin is a feasible outpatient regimen with less toxicity than paclitaxel-cisplatin and associated with equivalent survival. It should be noted that carboplatin is quantitatively excreted by the kidney, and its effective serum concentration can be calculated from a formula based on the patient's glomerular filtration rate. This can be determined in a number of ways but is generally estimated by calculating one's creatinine clearance. The Calvert formula is most commonly used and gives a total dose by the formula: carboplatin total dose = desired AUC × (GFR +25), where AUC is the area of the elimination concentration curve and GFR is the estimated glomerular filtration rate. AUC-based dosing is preferred for carboplatin because the AUC most accurately reflects observed dose-specific toxicity and is more reliable across patients than dosing based on body mass index. A usual dose for carboplatin is calculated for AUC values of 5.0 to 7.5. Both paclitaxel and platinum compounds are neurotoxic, as noted by Warner, and this is often the dose-limiting toxicity. The taxane docetaxel was found to be potentially less neurotoxic than paclitaxel. Vasey and colleagues reported a large phase III study comparing docetaxel and carboplatin with paclitaxel and carboplatin in patients with stage IC–IV ovarian cancer. Nearly identical survival parameters were observed between the two agents. The docetaxel arm was significantly less neurotoxic; however, it was associated with more myelosuppression. Neurotoxicity, as evaluated on several objective measures, returned to parity several months after treatment. Granulocyte colony-stimulating factor is occasionally needed to reduce the duration of significant neutropenia in these programs. A commonly used program is paclitaxel 175 mg/m^2 over 3 hours or docetaxel 75 mg/m^2 over 1 hour and carboplatin (AUC = 5–6) given in a 1-hour infusion every 3 weeks. Premedication is required for both taxanes to combat hypersensitivity reactions, which have been attributed to both the taxane itself and the carrier vehicle required to make these agents water soluble. In addition, steroid administration is necessary after treatment for docetaxel to combat fluid retention/effusion, a complication that may occur in as many as 25% of patients without prophylaxis.

Alterations in Frontline Treatment Strategies. Although the preferred sequence in primary advanced ovarian cancer management is surgery followed by chemotherapy, several authors have attempted to take advantage of the disease's intrinsic chemosensitivity to improve outcomes in patients with extensive disease. Two avenues have been pursued: neoadjuvant chemotherapy, in which, following biopsy or limited surgery, chemotherapy is administered for a reduced number of cycles (usually three to four) and an operation is planned for removal of the primary tumor (if present) and residual metastases, and interval cytoreduction, when an unsuccessful maximal attempt at cytoreduction is followed by a reduced number of chemotherapy cycles (usually three to four) followed by a second cytoreduction attempt. Both strategies are followed by three to four cycles of chemotherapy after surgery. This latter strategy has been evaluated in randomized clinical trials with conflicting results; the former is currently undergoing randomized evaluation.

Neoadjuvant Chemotherapy. Neoadjuvant chemotherapy is practiced as an alternative for patients thought to have substantial operative risk or preoperative disease distribution that could preclude optimal cytoreduction. Several authors have pointed out the potential benefits to this strategy including the opportunity to allow for an improvement in performance status, decreasing operative morbidity through less extensive surgery, and increasing the opportunity to achieve an optimal result. Each of these goals has been demonstrated in series of small, single-institution retrospective and prospective studies. For instance, in a series of 85 women treated with either neoadjuvant chemotherapy ($N = 57$) or primary cytoreduction ($n = 28$), Morice and associates reported a significant decrease in major morbidity, defined as morbidity requiring a second operation (7% vs. 36%, $p = 0.01$). Survival in this trial was similar between the cohorts, although with wide confidence limits. Schwartz reported on 59 women undergoing neoadjuvant chemotherapy and compared their surgical morbidity with 206 patients treated in the same time period by standard approach. They found patients in the former group to have shorter intensive care unit stay and postoperative hospital stay compared with conventional patients. Both groups received platinum-based chemotherapy. Because patients in these small trials are selected for the modality based on presenting disease volumes or medical status, it has been difficult to determine whether there is a detriment to survival by this approach. Clearly, patients too infirm to be operated on gain from this approach because if they have chemoresistant disease, surgery would have little value and would likely hasten an adverse outcome. Conversely, patients able to undergo the procedure could have a poorer outcome because there could be further expansion of a large population of resistant clones by delaying cytoreductive disease. Loizzi and colleagues reported a case-control study of neoadjuvant chemotherapy in 60 patients (30 each group). Patients were matched 1:1 based on date of diagnosis, histology, and stage. These investigators document that although the neoadjuvant cohort was older and representing a poorer performance status, these patients underwent optimal cytoreduction at a favorable rate (76% vs. 60%) and following platinum-based chemotherapy had similar progression-free and overall survival compared with the control cohort. A critical question to be answered in this methodology is one of biology, which can only be addressed in a prospective clinical study of potentially operable patients. Fortunately, such a study is ongoing.

Interval Cytoreduction. In distinction to neoadjuvant therapy presented previously, interval cytoreduction refers to a secondary attempt at maximal surgery after surgery and adjuvant chemotherapy. Lawton and associates administered three cycles of platinum-based multiagent chemotherapy to 31 incompletely resected ovarian cancer patients. They concluded that such therapy improved the likelihood of subsequent successful resection and subsequent effectiveness of chemotherapy. Two randomized clinical trials followed subsequently to evaluate this hypothesis. In a collaborative effort, Van der Burg and colleagues studied 319 randomized patients with residual nodules larger than 1 cm after primary operation. They gave three cycles of platinum-based chemotherapy and then randomized the patients to a second operation or no operation followed by additional chemotherapy. Only 9% of patients progressed before randomization. Progression-free survival and overall survival were both significantly improved by the performance of interval surgery (18 vs. 13 months, $p = 0.013$, and 26 vs. 20 months, $p = 0.012$). In contrast, on behalf of the GOG, Rose and associates presented a similarly designed trial of 425 randomized patients who received paclitaxel and cisplatin before and after randomization. They reported that only 5% of patients progressed before randomization, and there was no difference in outcome between the cohorts (10.5 vs. 10.8 months, $p = 0.54$; and 32 vs. 33 months, $p = 0.92$). Numerous differences have been described between the two trials, but a principle factor is believed to be the intent of the primary surgical approach; approximately one third of patients in the van der Burg and coworkers trial underwent essentially documentation of disease rather than a complete attempt at surgical cytoreduction before chemotherapy. Currently, this approach is infrequently practiced for those patients who undergo a maximal but incomplete resection at initial surgical evaluation.

Evaluation of Chemotherapy Results

Chemotherapy is usually administered every 3 weeks. The patient is monitored with careful physical examination; blood tests to measure hematologic, liver, and kidney functions; and radiographic studies, such as chest radiographic examinations, ultrasound tests, or (usually) CT scans of the abdomen and the pelvis. Granulocyte colony-stimulating factor is added as needed to combat neutropenia. Mild neutropenia after chemotherapy can be managed expectantly, but for the patient who develops severe neutropenia with fever and an absolute neutrophil count of less than 500 cells/μL, antibiotics are prescribed to prevent septic complications.

If tumor is suspected on CT scan, fine-needle biopsy can frequently document the presence of persistent or recurrent disease. A negative CT scan, however, does not guarantee complete clinical response. Goldhirsch and coworkers noted that 5 of 26 patients with tumor nodules larger than 1 cm had negative CT scans, and the examination was most effective (80%) for detecting metastasis in retroperitoneal nodes. In 1989, Reuter and colleagues reported improved results of 8% false negatives using newer equipment with CT slices at 10- to 15-mm intervals. Patsner reported that 24 of 60 patients with negative CT scans had positive second-look operations, calling into question the value of this imaging study. Vaginal ultrasonography is particularly useful to assess the pelvis. CA 125 levels are used to monitor the course of the patient with carcinoma. As noted previously, Buller and associates calculated that CA 125 level followed an exponential regression curve in successfully treated patients. This provides the possibility of mathematically estimating early in treatment the patient's response to chemotherapy. Bridgewater and coworkers reported that a greater than 50% decrease in CA 125 was a good sign of clinical response.

Second-Look Procedures

Some gynecologic oncologists perform a laparoscopy before a second-look laparotomy. If a second-look laparotomy is performed, it is important to extensively sample the peritoneal surfaces and lymph nodes. Particular attention is paid to areas that contained residual disease at the conclusion of the initial surgical procedure.

There are conflicting opinions regarding the value and indications of a second-look procedure in the therapy of ovarian cancer, and these are mostly done by major centers as part of large-scale protocol studies. Many patients with a negative second-look operation eventually develop recurrent disease. Early studies of a second-look laparotomy showed approximately half (range, 25% to 75%) of the patients thought clinically and radiographically to be free of disease actually had persistent disease at a second-look operation. Walton and coworkers showed that patients who initially have stage I or II disease rarely have positive second-look procedures, and they recommend that the operation not be done for those with low-stage tumors, a result confirmed by Sonnendecker. Favorable factors for a negative second-look operation are low tumor grade, no residual disease after primary operation, young age (younger than 55 years), and rapid regression to normal of increased CA 125 values during chemotherapy.

Maintenance Therapy. Unfortunately, many patients develop recurrent disease, even after a negative second-look operation. Rubin and colleagues noted a high (45%) rate of recurrence in patients with a negative second-look laparotomy. Those initially with higher stage and higher grade tumors are more likely to recur after a negative second-look operation. However, those who were disease-free at 5 years were likely to remain disease-free at subsequent follow-up. Nonetheless, this high recurrence risk has prompted several authors to consider additional treatment at the identification of a complete response to primary treatment. This is often referred to as *maintenance* or *consolidation therapy*, although the former term is favored given that the decision for treatment is based on the effect of primary therapy. Several randomized and nonrandomized clinical trials have been conducted in this arena including hormones, vitamins, radiation therapy, chemotherapy, radioimmunoconjugates, immunotherapy, vaccines, gene therapy, biologic therapy, complementary medicines, and holistic approaches. Unfortunately, all have been negative in regard to improving overall survival. However, one randomized study did show an improvement in PFS. Markman and colleagues studied whether 3 or 12 additional months of paclitaxel could influence time until progression in women who had achieved a complete clinical remission after primary treatment. The trial was designed to accrue 450 patients; however, at a planned interim analysis (after 277 patients were randomized), a statistically significant benefit for the longer treatment was demonstrated, which closed the trial to further accrual. The initial report demonstrated a 7-month improvement in median PFS (28 months vs. 21 months, $p = 0.0035$); a later report with long follow-up confirmed these earlier results (median PFS: 21 months vs. 14 months, $p = 0.006$). No effect on survival was demonstrated however. More work in this area is under way.

Intraperitoneal Therapy. One promising, but relatively old strategy being investigated is IP administration of chemotherapy. Ovarian cancer appears to be "IP friendly" because the distribution of disease is largely confined to this space, the pharmacokinetics of drug delivery are favorable, and the tumor is considered chemosensitive. Early experience with IP administration of chemotherapy documented that it could be used to control ascites. Pharmacologic studies in the 1970s and 1980s demonstrated favorable profiles of high relative direct drug exposure (high C_{max} and area under the dose-response curve [AUC]) for a number of agents subsequently identified to be important for ovarian cancer treatment. In this regard, both platinum (cisplatin and carboplatin) and taxanes (paclitaxel and docetaxel) have been shown to have superior pharmacokinetic profiles when delivered into the peritoneum directly compared with IV administration. Contemporary administration is done principally via an implantable vascular access device placed during surgery or via minilaparotomy subsequently (Fig. 33-13). A sizable number of phase I and II clinical studies have been performed in the past 35 years to document safety of the strategy and to suggest efficacy. This has led to the performance and reporting of eight randomized clinical studies formally evaluating the efficacy of IP-based chemotherapy to intravenous-based chemotherapy in patients with advanced-stage ovarian cancer. A recent meta-analysis of these studies has been published and concludes the route of administration "has the potential to improve cure rates from ovarian cancer." Similarly, the National Cancer Institute issued a clinical announcement accompanying the publication of a large GOG study stating that the IV and IP regimen "conveys a significant survival benefit among women with optimally debulked epithelial ovarian cancer, compared to intravenous administration alone." In this latter study, patients with stage III epithelial ovarian cancer rendered optimal (defined as postsurgical disease residual of $\leq$ 1 cm) were eligible for

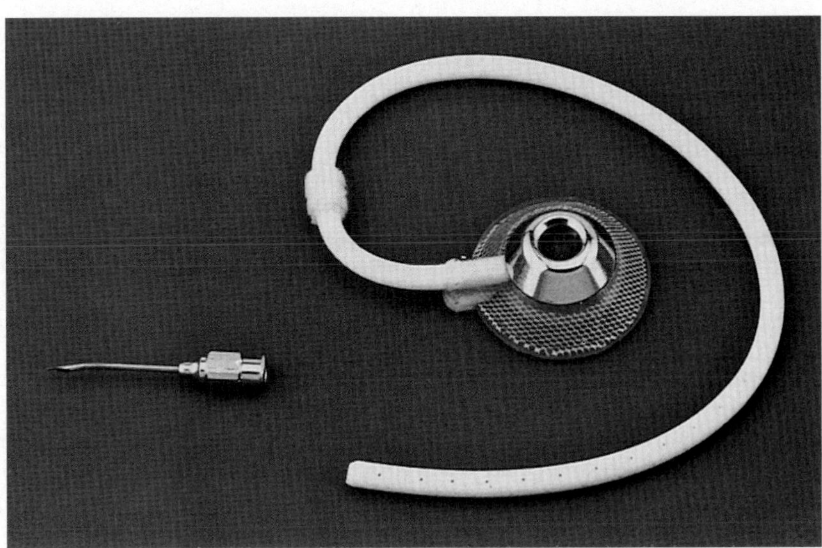

Figure 33-13. Peritoneal catheter with access port for infusion of drugs. (Port-A-Cath, Pharmacia Deltec, Inc.)

randomization to either standard IV cisplatin and paclitaxel (24-hour infusion) or IV paclitaxel (135 mg/m^2 on day 1), IP cisplatin (100 mg/m^2 on day 2), and IP paclitaxel (60 mg/m^2 on day 8). This was the first phase III study to include IP paclitaxel in primary ovarian cancer therapy. Both cohorts were to undergo repeat cycles every 21 days for six total infusions. The primary endpoints were PFS and overall survival, and reassessment operations, if planned, were indicated at randomization. This study was also the first to formally evaluate the impact of treatment on health-related quality of life. Assessment was made at baseline, after the third cycle, after treatment completion, and 12 months after treatment completion. Overall, 415 eligible patients comprised the study population. Both PFS and OS were significantly improved in the intent-to-treat IP cohort (HR_{PFS} = 0.80, 95% CI: 0.64–1.00 and HR_{Death} = 0.75, 95% CI: 0.58–0.97, respectively). The recorded median overall survival of 65.6 months is among the longest ever observed in an adjuvant therapy phase III ovarian cancer study. The results are even more impressive given that the majority (58%) of randomized IP patients did not complete all six cycles of their assigned therapy via IP administration. This was largely due to significant differences in both hematologic and nonhematologic toxicities associated with the IP regimen. Leukopenia and thrombocytopenia were significantly more common in the IP arm, as were pain (11-fold increase), fatigue (fourfold increase), metabolic (fourfold increase), renal (threefold increase), fever (2.5-fold increase), infection (2.5-fold increase), neurologic (twofold increase), and gastrointestinal (twofold increase) events among others. In addition, nearly one in five (40 of 205 patients) randomized IP patients experienced a catheter failure necessitating treatment discontinuation. A detailed assessment of IP catheter complications in this trial has been published. A clear profile for catheter malfunction risk was not identified, although timing and accompanying surgical procedures were closely scrutinized. In a reflection of these observed adverse events, health-related quality of life assessments were significantly lower throughout the trial but returned to parity 12 months after therapy. The authors concluded the IP regimen provided superior survival efficacy and was associated with significant, but manageable toxicity. They encouraged use of IP therapy in clinical practice. Unfortunately, toxicity concerns and a number of unanswered fundamental questions regarding efficacy such as optimal agent, schedule, future trial designs, and the impact of alternative agents such as biologic therapies (vascular endothelial growth factor and epidermal growth factor targeting) have limited the general acceptance of this strategy in the clinical community. Clinical investigation is ongoing.

Recurrent Ovarian Cancer Management. Unfortunately, as many as 70% of patients who present with advanced staged disease, will exhibit recurrent or persistent disease after primary treatment. These patients may have prolonged survival despite developing recurrence; however, they are rarely cured. Because this treatment is generally considered palliative and must balance efficacy with toxicity. The choice of therapy is largely empirical, and the treatment plan usually involves several agents in sequence depending on treatment history, observed and expected toxicity, and performance status. Surgery, chemotherapy, immunotherapy, radiation therapy, biotherapy and hormone therapy are options, alone and in combination, in this cohort of patients, and it is not uncommon for a patient to undergo five or more different chemotherapy regimens including cycles of retreatment with one or more agents. This characteristic is reflective of the increasing number of agents available for use, the short duration of response, and the general health of those receiving therapy.

Although there are few specific treatment guidelines as to how recurrence should be approached, initial consideration is most often guided by the interval of time until recurrence is identified. Patients are categorized as potentially platinum-sensitive, -resistant, or -refractory based on the length of time from the completion of primary therapy until recurrence is identified. By convention, patients exhibiting a treatment-free interval of 6 months or longer are considered as having potentially platinum-sensitive disease. Those who achieved a complete response and were identified with recurrence under this benchmark are considered platinum-resistant and those who did not achieve a complete response or had disease progression during frontline therapy are considered platinum-refractory. In reality, the probability for subsequent chemotherapy response likely represents a continuum based on this interval of time. However, clinically, the arbitrary division is used frequently to make treatment decisions.

Platinum-Refractory Disease. Patients who fall into this designation have very difficult disease to treat as objective response to most all agents available is low and the duration of any individual therapy is short. The choice of therapy depends on patient wishes and comorbidities. Because expectations for response to standard agents are low, these women are good candidates for investigative clinical studies in which new agents with alternative mechanisms of action or targets are being evaluated. Under these expectations, some patients may opt to continue active treatment, whereas others may choose supportive care.

Platinum-Resistant Disease. Patients demonstrating an abbreviated initial response to frontline therapy represent cohorts who are unlikely to respond well to platinum retreatment. That is not to imply that some of these patients would not respond to retreatment with a platinum compound, just that the probability of response would be no greater than with any other agent and potentially lower. A current recommendation for most of these patients is to consider an alternative nonplatinum agent for the first treatment of recurrence. Table 33-9 lists the potential agents for treating these patients, their respective response rates, and significant common toxicities. Patients achieving stable disease or better are usually treated until the agent no longer demonstrates a clinical benefit or toxicity precludes further infusion.

Platinum-Sensitive Disease. Patients in whom disease recurrence is identified more than 6 months after frontline treatment completion are considered potentially platinum-sensitive. These patients are good candidates for retreatment with platinum or a platinum-based combination regimen. In many instances, this combination is similar to that received in frontline treatment: paclitaxel and carboplatin. However, other two-drug and three-drug combinations have been investigated. A limited number of phase III studies have been conducted in this setting; currently, only one has demonstrated an overall survival advantage for use of a taxane- and platinum-based regimen. The ICON4-AGO-OVAR 2.2 study randomized 802 women with recurrent ovarian cancer to either paclitaxel and platinum or a nontaxane platinum regimen. Objective response was 66% in the taxane arm compared with 54% in the conventional arm (p = 0.06). PFS was significantly improved (12 months vs. 9 months, HR = 0.76, 95% CI: 0.66–0.89) as was overall survival (29 months vs. 24 months, HR = 0.82, 95% CI: 0.69–0.97). Approximately 75% of women in both groups had a treatment-free interval of at least 12 months and 64% were taxane-naïve at randomization. These are important factors when considering the study's conclusions. One additional phase III trial has been completed demonstrating a PFS advantage for the combination of gemcitabine and carboplatin compared with single-agent carboplatin in platinum-sensitive patients. This study predominantly conducted by the AGO (Arbeitsgemeinschaft Gynakologische Onkologie), randomized 356 women to either single-agent carboplatin or the combination. Patients were stratified by the duration of their treatment-free interval from completion of primary therapy (6 to 12 months vs. >12 months). PFS was 8.6 months in the combination compared with 5.8 months with single-agent carboplatin (p = 0.0038). Overall survival was nearly identical however (18.0 months vs. 17.3 months, p = 0.73) and underpowered to evaluate this endpoint. Currently gemcitabine is approved for use in combination with carboplatin based on these data.

Secondary Cytoreduction. Because patients with long treatment-free intervals have disease that is considered potentially chemotherapy-sensitive, investigators have evaluated the role of surgery in this setting as well. Although there is some inconsistency in the definition of secondary cytoreduction procedures, the specific intent in this setting is resection of disease at recurrence with the intent of debulking. No randomized trials have been conducted to identify a clinical benefit in this setting. However, several prospective and retrospective reports have suggested only patients with extended treatment-free intervals and those who achieve a complete resection (no visible residual) benefit from the procedure. Tay and associates conducted a multivariate analysis for survival on 46 women undergoing secondary cytoreduction for disease recurrence. They identified that only time to recurrence of 24 months or greater and resection to no visible residual as independent predictors of survival. The optimal resection rate in this study was 41%. Eisenkop and coworkers conducted a prospective study of 106 patients identified with recurrence 6 months or longer from primary treatment. In this study, 82% of the patients were rendered free of visible tumor. In their multivariate analysis, four variables were found to be independent predictors of survival: disease-free interval, residual disease after secondary surgery, administration of chemotherapy before secondary surgery, and size of recurrent tumor. They concluded that complete resection can be obtained in the majority of selected patients and should be considered before administration of second-line chemo-

Table 33-9 Clinical Efficacy of Cytotoxic Agents in Platinum-Resistant and -Sensitive Ovarian Cancer

Agent	Platinum-Resistant Response Rate (%)	Platinum-Sensitive Response Rate (%)	Principle Toxicity
PLD	14–20	28	PPE, mucositis
Topotecan	14–18	33	Myelosuppression
Hexamethylmelamine	10–18	27	Nausea/vomiting
Gemcitabine	16		Myelosuppression
Etoposide	27	35	Myelosuppression, leukemia
Ifosfamide	12		Hemorrhagic cystitis, CNS
Tamoxifen	10–15	10–15	Hot flashes/thromboembolic
Docetaxel	22–25	38	Myelosuppression
Paclitaxel	12–33	20–41	Myelosuppression
Vinorelbine	21	29	Myelosuppression

CNS, central nervous system neurotoxicity; PLD, pegylated liposomal doxorubicin; PPE, palmar-plantar erythrodysthesia.

therapy. In this light, preoperative criteria for exploration include limited disease, lack of carcinomatosis or disease likely not resectable, and absent ascites. A randomized trial is planned to specifically address the role of surgery in platinum-sensitive patients.

Targeted Therapy. The processes that govern cell transformation and immortalization, tumor growth, and metastases for ovarian cancer are complex and not uniform. Nonetheless, several critical targets have been identified that appear to be differentially expressed in tumors cells relative to normal cells. New agents that "target" disruption or inhibition of these specific processes are being developed and incorporated into the care of ovarian cancer patients. Currently, the most developed of these are agents that disrupt the signals to engender new vessel growth and development or angiogenesis. This process appears critical for a tumor to continue its growth beyond 8 mm^3. A number of cytokines have been described which tip the balance to sustained angiogenesis, but the most potent is vascular endothelial growth factor or VEGF. Prognostically, VEGF expression has been documented in all stages of ovarian cancer and has been correlated with impaired survival. VEGF overexpression has also been directly associated with ascites formation. This clinical feature is the result VEGF-induced endothelial hyperpermeability. The compound furthest in development for the treatment for ovarian cancer is bevacizumab, which is undergoing investigation in primary and recurrent ovarian cancer. However, a number of agents targeting VEGF, its receptors, the epidermal growth factor receptor family, glutathione S-transferase as well as various cellular signaling pathways are also under investigation. In addition, new cytotoxics with alternative mechanisms of action such as the tubulin poisons and an agent that binds the minor groove of DNA are under phase III investigation.

Clearly, the spectrum of treatment likely available to women with this disease in the future will require some rational parameters for their use. In this manner, detailed tumor profiling will likely help customize treatment on an individual basis.

Complications and Alternative Considerations

Malignant Effusions. Patients with ovarian cancer frequently develop ascites or hydrothorax or both, requiring repeated drainage by paracentesis or thoracentesis. Occasionally, sclerosing solutions are used in the thoracic cavity to prevent reaccumulation of fluid, with resultant adherence of the pleural surfaces. A number of strategies have been studied in prospective trials. Most efficacious for problematic pleural effusion is either pleurodesis with a sclerotic agent (talc slurry or antibiotic), decortication, or placement of an infusion catheter that can be operated by the patient. A systematic review has been conducted by Tan and coworkers. Symptomatic ascites can also be problematic because few sclerodesis or surgical decortication-type procedures are available for long-term care. These patients typically undergo frequent percutaneous aspirations, which, over time, become self-limiting as a result of adhesions and tumor progression. It is also not uncommon for patients to develop implants of tumor in the subcutaneous tissues after aspiration. Numnum and associates have reported some success using bevacizumab as an adjuvant for this problem.

Immunotherapy. Immunotherapy agents, such as *Corynebacterium parvum* and bacille Calmette–Guérin, have been administered to try to augment the immunologic response and promote tumor resistance in the host. These agents have also been used in combination with cytotoxic chemotherapy, and preliminary improved results have been reported. IP immunotherapy approaches have been evaluated with such agents as interferon, lymphokine-activated killer cells, interleukin-2, and tumor necrosis factor. Berek and coworkers conducted a phase I–II trial of IP cisplatinum (60 mg/m^2) and interferon-α (25×10^6 IV) given every 4 weeks. Among 18 patients, there were three complete and four partial responses. Unfortunately, a randomized trial comparing interferon-α with no further treatment in women achieving complete response after primary chemotherapy showed no benefit. A frontline study of adding interferon-γ to paclitaxel and carboplatin was recently completed with results pending.

The use of monoclonal antibodies as a form of site-directed therapy has been investigated. Epenetos and colleagues have used tumor-associated antigens linked to ^{131}I to treat recurrent ovarian carcinoma. After IP administration to 24 patients, responses were noted primarily in those with small-volume disease, with some responses evaluated by follow-up laparoscopy lasting as long as 3 years. Canevari and associates noted responses in three of 26 patients treated with autologous T lymphocytes targeted with a bispecific monoclonal antibody. Berek and coworkers reported a phase III study of oregovomab in women achieving a complete clinical response after primary therapy. This novel, murine-derived immunotherapeutic agent targets the CA 125 antigen. In a placebo-controlled, randomized trial, 145 women underwent infusion. The time to relapse was 13.3 months in the treatment arm and 10.3 months in the placebo arm ($p = .71$). Although no benefit was observed, an exploratory analysis identified a subgroup in whom this therapy may have a better opportunity for efficacy.

Gene Therapy. The therapeutic impact of gene therapy in ovarian cancer has yet to reach maturity. Although the IP nature of this disease makes it well suited for this approach, various gene- or virus-based gene therapy programs have yielded mixed results at best. Several therapeutic models have been used in early investigation including replacement of a tumor suppressor gene (such as *BRCA* and *P53*), suicide gene therapy, and inhibition of growth factor suppressors and regulators. As noted by Berchuck and Bast, there are a number of hurdles to developing this type of therapy to clinical usefulness. However, intensive investigation is under way in a few centers to develop efficient and efficacious therapeutic programs.

Chemotherapy Sensitivity Assays. A chemotherapy sensitivity and resistance assay is a laboratory algorithm wherein a sample of human tumor is subjected, under experimental conditions, to various chemotherapeutic agents and concentrations to assess response (tumor survival). Two broad categories of assay intent separate the available technologies: those that evaluate the inhibition of cell growth and those that address chemotherapy-associated cell death. Although these intents appear similar, they are very different in their laboratory protocol and may produce vastly disparate results. In most cases, several agents alone and in combination are evaluated. Theoretically, the most active agent or combination could be picked (sensitivity assay) or eliminated (resistance assay) from an empirical program, offering a more precise decision tool. The hypothesis is that differential selection will improve patient outcome. Although the concept is simplistic and rational, the effects of chemotherapy response and patient survival are complex and sometime counterintuitive. It is frequently commented that a limited sample of tissue obtained from either the primary or a metastatic site, at primary diagnosis or in recurrence and after previous chemotherapy or radiation exposure would not necessarily be representative of active disease at any one time. However, Tewari and colleagues reviewing 119 synchronous and 334 metachronous ovarian primary, metastatic, and recurrent samples demonstrated remarkable consistency in the tumor's drug resistance profile. However, efficacy requires clinical correlation. Loizzi and coworkers reported a case-control study on 100 recurrent ovarian cancer patients treated either by assay or empirical therapy. Overall response (65% vs. 35%, $p = 0.02$), PFS (15 months vs. 7 months, $p = 0.0002$), and overall survival (38 months vs. 21 months, $p = 0.005$) were all improved using the assay. Similarly, however, inherent selection bias and treatment overlap necessitate validation by a randomized clinical trial. In 2004, the American Society of Clinical Oncology issued a statement based on the extensive review of the world's reported literature and concluded that this technology needs further investigation before widespread adoption. This represents one area of active area of research.

Radiation Therapy. As presented previously in early-stage disease, radiation has been used for curative intent in women with early-stage cancer with some success. Treatment planning involves a field that treats the entire abdomen as well as higher doses to the pelvis. Long-term efficacy must be balanced against uncommon toxicities of therapy, which include gastrointestinal stricture and fistulas and compromise of the bone marrow should chemotherapy be needed subsequently. The modality has also been used to treat recurrent disease. Cmelak and Kapp treated 41 patients with platinum refractory ovarian cancer who had undergone secondary cytoreduction. They treated the whole abdomen with 28 Gy and a pelvic boost to 48 Gy. For 28 patients with residual disease less than 1.5 cm, the 5-year survival rate was 53%, which is better than would be expected with chemotherapy. However, no large-scale trial data are available for this technique and because of the risk of complications and the lack of extensive data regarding its effectiveness, whole abdominal radiation has generally not been used in these cases. However, localized radiation can be of utility in selected patients with isolated recurrences or persistent disease after chemotherapy or to manage localized symptomatic disease, such as bone metastases. The discovery of intensity modulated radiation therapy has widened the therapeutic index by reducing toxicity to surrounding unaffected tissues.

Summary. Therapy for epithelial ovarian carcinoma is based on removal of all gross disease and sampling of areas at high risk of spread in the peritoneal cavity and retroperitoneal nodes. Postoperative therapy is employed depending on the stage and grade of the primary tumor. For accurately staged cases, postoperative ^{32}P may be used in low-stage tumors, such as stage IC carcinomas in which there is a risk of IP tumor seeding but no residual disease. Multiagent platinum- and taxane-based chemotherapy is frequently employed as adjunctive treatment for poorly differentiated tumors, such as stage I grade 3, or for stage II cases without residual tumor.

For high-stage tumors and for patients with residual disease after initial operation, multiple-agent chemotherapy, usually paclitaxel and carboplatin, is used. It is accompanied by multiple short- and long-term toxic side effects, but results in initial response rates in stage III cases may exceed 90%. Five-year survival rates decrease to 30% or less. Long-term randomized trials and the development of new agents will be needed to improve rates of salvage and to optimize therapy for epithelial ovarian carcinomas. Currently, second-line chemotherapy offers remission to some patients, but the best response rates are achieved with initial chemotherapy.

SMALL CELL CARCINOMA

Dickerson and colleagues described a new and virulent type of ovarian malignancy that occurs in young women, usually between the ages of 15 and 30 years. Because of its histologic appearance, it has been designated a small cell carcinoma. The tumor is often but not always accompanied by hypercalcemia as noted by Young and associates in an analysis of 150 cases. Most patients have died, although a few stage I survivors have been reported, some of whom have been treated with adjuvant multiagent chemotherapy. Reed reported a patient with stage IC disease treated with cisplatinum, etoposide, and bleomycin who survived 5 years. Benrubi and coworkers treated a patient with stage II small cell carcinoma with debulking and multiagent chemotherapy followed by radiation, and the patient was disease-free for 4 years at the time of the report. Other isolated stage I 5-year survivals have been reported with multiagent chemotherapy programs augmented with subsequent pelvic radiation. However, for advanced-stage disease and even in most stage I cases, the course of the tumor has been fatal. Harrison and associates reported the findings of the combined experience of the Gynecological Cancer Intergroup, which included 17 patients with small cell carcinoma of the ovary, hypercalcemic type. All patients were initially treated with surgery and platinum-based chemotherapy. Seven also received adjuvant radiotherapy with either pelvic and paraaortic radiotherapy or pelvic and whole abdominal radiotherapy. For 10 stage I patients, 6 received adjuvant radiotherapy, and 5 were alive and disease-free at the time of the report. All but one of the seven patients with stage III or unknown stage had died.

MALIGNANT MIXED MÜLLERIAN TUMORS (CARCINOSARCOMAS)

These are extremely rare ovarian malignancies that histologically resemble comparable tumors in the uterus. Treatment involves operation for cytoreduction, as noted by Muntz and coworkers, with added therapy usually in the form of multiagent chemotherapy. Stage is prognostic, and those with advanced stages usually do not survive.

As noted by Hellstrom and colleagues, approximately 500 of these rare tumors have been reported. In their series of 36 such cases over 20 years, the median survival was 16.6 months with a 5-year actuarial survival rate of only 18%. Low-stage tumors and those treated with multiagent chemotherapy (cytoxan, Adriamycin, cisplatin) had an improved survival. Although there remains some question about the efficacy of postoperative platinum-based chemotherapy for treatment of these tumors, as noted by Bicher and associates, this approach continues to be the standard. The most commonly employed regimens include the combination of cisplatin plus ifosfamide and the combination of paclitaxel and carboplatin.

GERM CELL TUMORS

These tumors are derived from the germ cells of the ovary. As a group, they are the second most frequent of ovarian neoplasms and account for approximately 20% to 25% of all ovarian tumors. The classification of germ cell tumors according to the World Health Organization designation is shown in the following box.

WHO Classification of Germ Cell Tumors

- Dysgerminoma
  - Endodermal sinus tumor
  - Embryonal carcinoma
  - Polyembryoma
  - Choriocarcinoma
  - Teratomas
  - Immature
  - Mature
    - Solid
    - Cystic
- Dermoid cyst (mature cystic teratoma)
- Dermoid cyst with malignant transformation
  - Monodermal and highly specialized
    - Struma ovarii
    - Carcinoid
    - Struma ovarii and carcinoid
    - Others
  - Mixed forms

The most frequent germ cell tumor is the benign cystic teratoma (dermoid); overall, only 2% to 3% of germ cell tumors are malignant. Among the malignant germ cell tumors, the most frequent is the dysgerminoma, which accounts for approximately 45% of malignant germ cell tumors. Next in frequency are immature teratomas and then endodermal sinus tumors. In female patients younger than age 30, germ cell tumors are the most frequent ovarian neoplasm, and approximately one third of the germ cell tumors encountered in those younger than age 21 are malignant.

The histogenesis of germ cell tumors has been extensively studied and summarized by Talerman. Figure 33-14 shows the theory of the histogenesis of these tumors; they originate from the primitive germ cell and then gradually differentiate to mimic the developmental tissues of embryonic origin (ectoderm, mesoderm, or endoderm) and the extraembryonic tissues (yolk sac and trophoblast). Germ cell tumors that originate in the ovary have homologous counterparts in the testes, that is, dysgerminoma and seminoma. Germ cell tumors are usually unilateral, with the exception of teratomas and dysgerminomas (see Table 33-4). The morphologic and clinical aspects of each of the various types of germ cell tumors are considered separately.

Teratomas

Teratomas consist of tissues that recapitulate the three layers of the developing embryo (ectoderm, mesoderm, and endoderm). One or more of the layers may be represented, and the tissues can be mature (benign) or immature (malignant). Chromosomal studies indicate that teratomas appear to arise from a single germ and have an XX karyotype. In the older literature, terms such as *malignant teratoma* and *teratocarcinoma* were used to denote the malignant variety of these tumors, but these terms have been replaced by the nomenclature shown in the box at left.

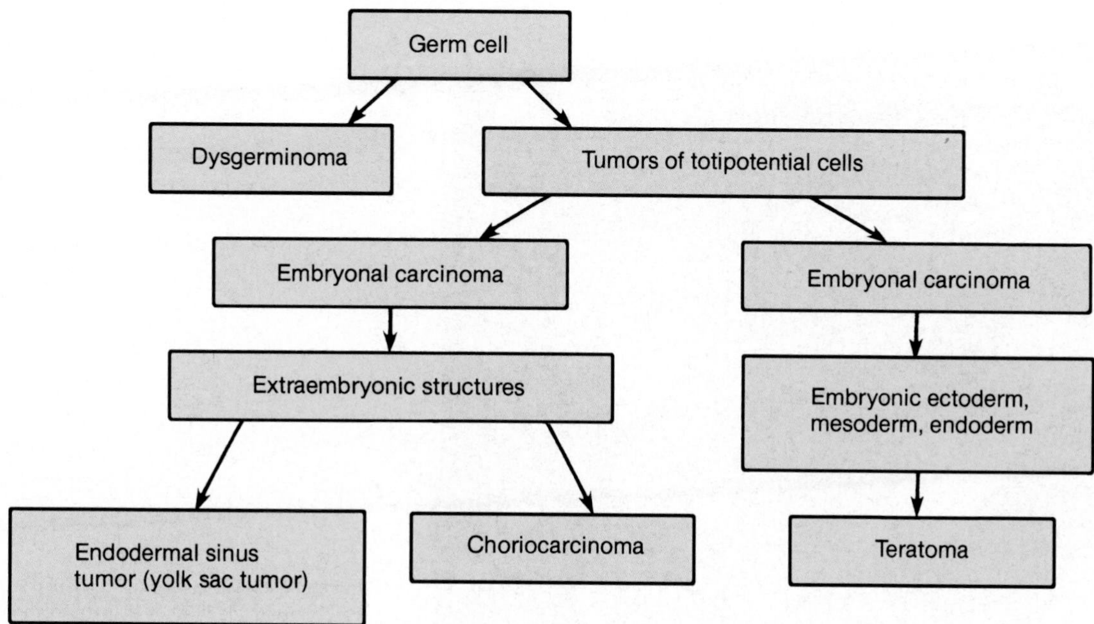

Figure 33-14. Histogenesis of germ cell tumors. (Modified from Talerman A: Germ cell tumors of the ovary. In Blaustein A [ed]: Pathology of the Female Genital Tract. New York, Springer-Verlag, 1982.)

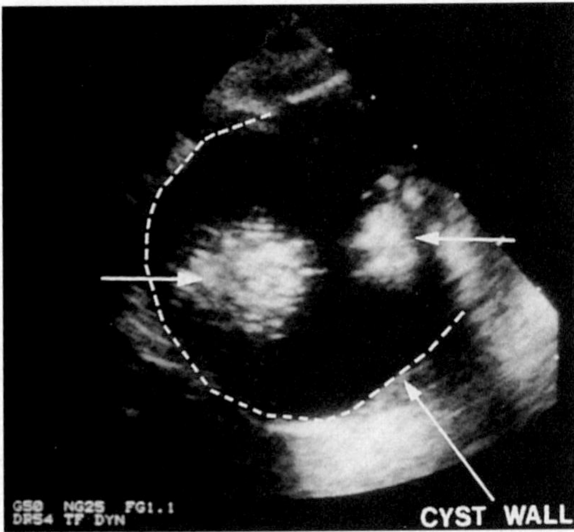

Figure 33-15. Transvaginal ultrasound image of an ovarian dermoid cyst. The *arrows* indicate balls of hair. (Courtesy of Dr. Zubie Sheikh, Department of Obstetrics and Gynecology, The University of Chicago.)

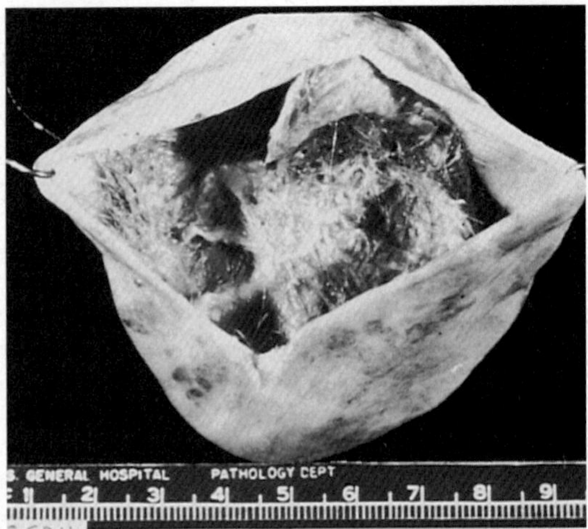

Figure 33-16. Gross specimen of a dermoid cyst that was filled with sebaceous material and hair. (Courtesy of Dr. R. E. Scully.)

Benign Cystic Teratomas (Dermoids)

Benign cystic teratomas are the most common germ cell tumors and account for 25% of all ovarian neoplasms. They primarily occur during the reproductive years but may occur in postmenopausal women and in children. The risk of malignant transformation (see later discussion) is markedly increased if these tumors are found in postmenopausal women. One of the interesting facets of teratomas is their ability to produce adult tissue, including skin, bone, teeth, hair, and dermal tissue. The presence of calcified bone or teeth allows the tumor to be diagnosed preoperatively with ultrasonography or radiography (Fig. 33-15).

Dermoids are usually unilateral, but 10% to 15% are bilateral. The outside wall of the tumor tends to be smooth with a yellowish appearance caused by the sebaceous fatty material that fills the tumor. Hair is also a prominent feature once the cyst is opened (Fig. 33-16). Usually the tumors are asymptomatic, but they can cause severe pain if there is torsion or if the sebaceous material perforates the cyst wall, leading to a reactive peritonitis. This rare complication is severe and can occur during pregnancy. Microscopically, a number of adult tissues are seen (Fig. 33-17).

Treatment of the reproductive-age female patient or of the child consists of either cystectomy or unilateral oophorectomy. In most cases, it should be possible to remove only the cyst and preserve normal ovarian tissue. The technique at open laparotomy is demonstrated in Figure 33-18. The opposite ovary should be inspected. If it is grossly normal, nothing further needs

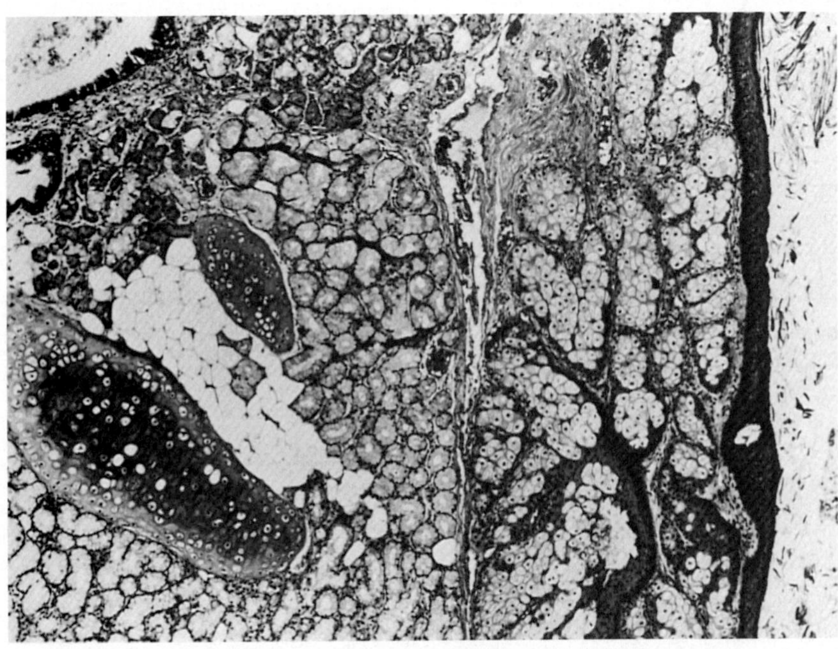

Figure 33-17. Photomicrograph of dermoid. Cartilage is shown *(right)* lined by epidermis and accompanying appendages *(left)*. (×50.) (From Serov SF, Scully RE, Sobin LH: Histologic Typing of Ovarian Tumors. Geneva, World Health Organization, 1973.)

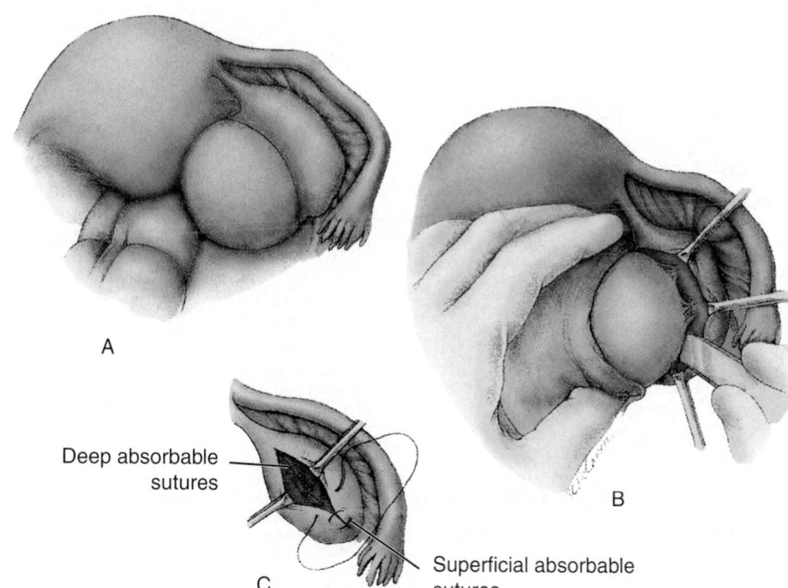

Figure 33-18. Shelling out of teratoma. **A,** Scalpel incision in ovary at intersection of dermoid and normal ovary. **B,** Dermoid being separated. Note how upper part peels away. **C,** Reconstruction of normal ovary.

to be done. Some therapists remove the mass laparoscopically, but rupture can result in local chemical peritonitis unless all irritating substances are completely removed with saline lavage. Current treatment involves preservation of the contralateral ovary without any biopsy if it grossly appears normal. In women beyond childbearing years, therapy for a dermoid usually consists of removal of the uterus, both tubes, and the ovaries.

Occasionally, teratomas may be solid and may consist only of adult tissues, leading to the diagnosis of solid, mature teratoma. These benign germ cell tumors are rare.

A cystic teratoma can undergo malignant degeneration, usually after menopause. Generally, it occurs in the squamous epithelial elements of the dermoid, producing a squamous cell carcinoma. It is a rare complication, estimated to occur in less than 2% of these tumors. If the malignant tissue has spread beyond the confines of the ovary, the prognosis is poor. In such case, additional therapy for squamous cell carcinoma with radiation therapy or chemotherapy or both is used.

Immature Teratomas

Immature teratomas are malignant and account for as many as 20% of the malignant ovarian tumors found in women younger than the age of 20 but less than 1% of all ovarian cancers. They do not occur in women after menopause. They consist of immature embryonic structures that can be admixed with mature elements. Approximately one third of immature teratomas express serum α-fetoprotein.

The prognosis for patients with immature teratomas is related to the stage (FIGO) and grade of the tumor. The grade of the tumor is based on the degree of immaturity of the various tissues. Grade 3 tumors consist of the most immature tissues and often have a high proportion of immature neuroepithelium. Figure 33-19 shows the survival of patients with immature teratomas by stage and grade before the advent of modern chemotherapy. Kurman and Norris reported that patients with stage IA immature teratoma had a 10-year actuarial survival rate of 70% after unilateral salpingo-oophorectomy; this rate is comparable with that recorded after bilateral salpingo-oophorectomy.

Dysgerminomas

Dysgerminomas are the most common type of malignant germ cell tumors. They consist of primitive germ cells with stroma infiltrated by lymphocytes (Fig. 33-20). They are analogous to seminoma in the male testis and comprise approximately 1% of ovarian malignancies. Dysgerminomas occur primarily in women younger than the age of 30. The tumor can be discovered during pregnancy. Some arise in dysgenetic gonads (see later discussion of gonadoblastomas). Unlike other malignant germ cell tumors, dysgerminomas are bilateral in approximately 10% of cases (see Table 33-4). Approximately 15% of dysgerminomas produce human chorionic gonadotropin related to areas of syncytiotrophoblast tissue.

Endodermal Sinus Tumors (Yolk Sac Tumors)

The endodermal sinus tumor, or yolk sac tumor, which comprises 10% of malignant germ cell tumors, in part resembles the yolk sac of the rodent placenta, thus recapitulating extraembryonic tissues (see Fig. 33-14). One typical histologic pattern is shown in Figure 33-21. The tumor secretes α-fetoprotein, which is a specific marker that is useful in identifying and following these tumors clinically. These rapidly growing tumors occur in females between 13 months and 45 years of age. A median age of 19 years at diagnosis was noted by Kurman and Norris. The yolk sac tumor is the prototype for α-fetoprotein production.

Choriocarcinomas

Nongestational choriocarcinoma is a highly malignant rare germ cell tumor resembling extraembryonic tissues. Like gestational choriocarcinoma (see Chapter 35, Gestational Trophoblastic Disease), it consists of malignant cytotrophoblasts and syncytiotrophoblasts; human chorionic gonadotropin is a useful tumor marker. This tumor develops mostly in women younger than the age of 20, primarily in the ovary. The disease was usually fatal

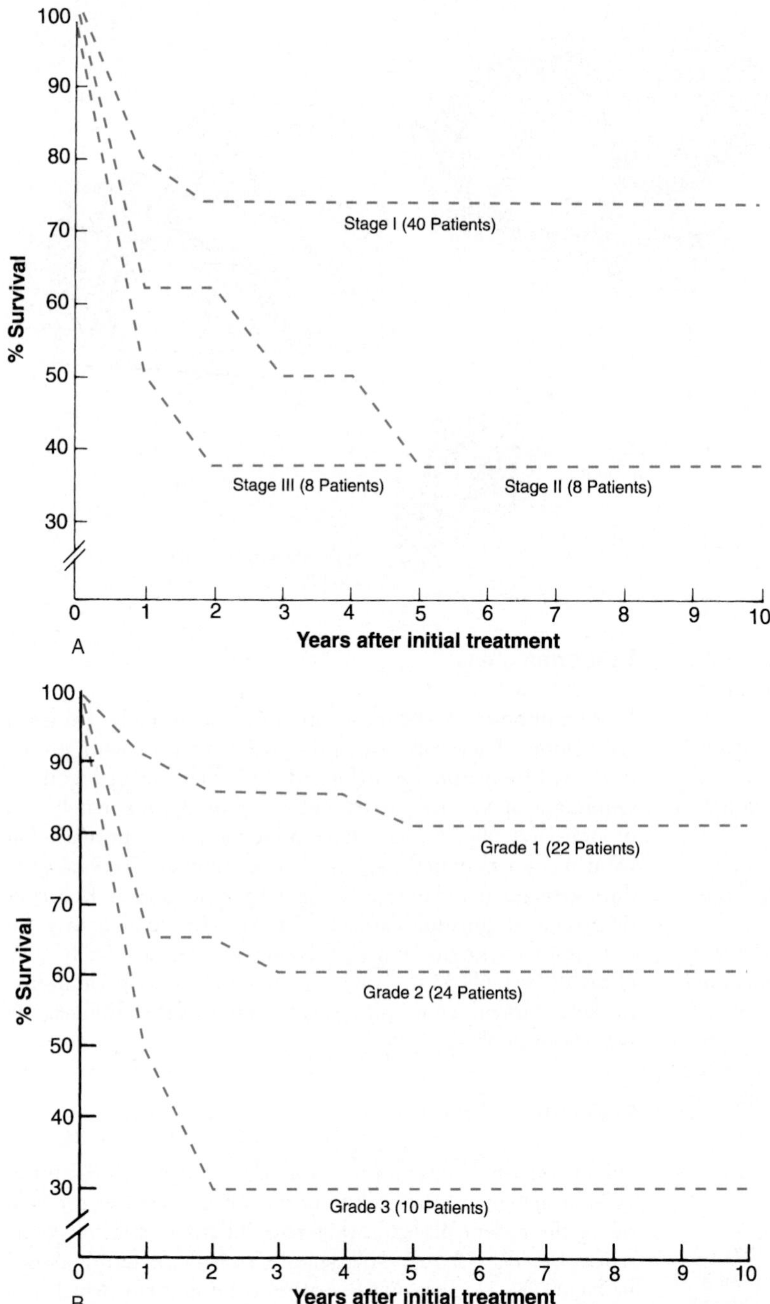

Figure 33-19. A, Actuarial survival of 56 patients with malignant teratoma by neoplasm stage. **B,** By neoplasm grade. (From Norris HJ, Zirkin JH, Benson WL: Immature (malignant) teratoma of the ovary: A clinical and pathologic study of 58 cases. Cancer 37:2359, 1976.)

in the past and does not appear to respond to single-agent chemotherapy, such as methotrexate or actinomycin D, with the same frequency as gestational trophoblastic disease. This lack of response may be due in part to the occurrence of these tumors in combination with other malignant germ cell tumors (mixed germ cell tumor), and, occasionally, the other germ cell elements may not be histologically recognized.

Embryonal Carcinomas

An embryonal carcinoma is a rare malignant germ cell tumor composed of primitive embryonal cells. It occurs in young females between the ages of 4 and 28 years. Kurman and Norris summarized 15 cases. Trophoblastic elements may be present, and both human chorionic gonadotropin and α-fetoprotein have been reported to be present.

Polyembryomas

Polyembryomas are exceedingly rare tumors that are usually found in the testes. They can occur in the ovary and consist of embryonal bodies that resemble early embryos. Trophoblastic elements with human chorionic gonadotropin and placental lactogen secretion have been reported.

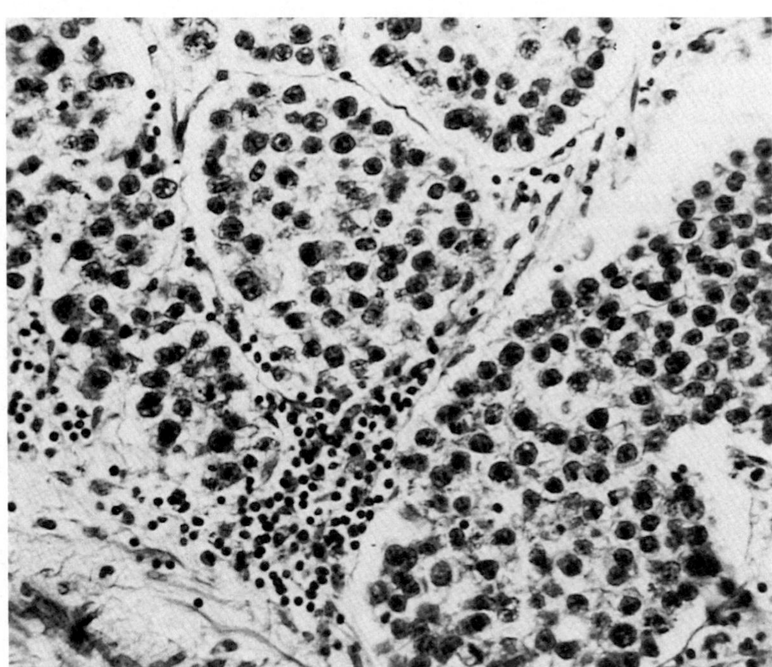

Figure 33-20. Dysgerminoma. (×300.) Dysgerminoma cells are demonstrated as well as infiltration of stroma by lymphocytes. (From Scully RE: Germ cell tumors of the ovary and fallopian tube. In Meigs JV, Sturgis SH [eds]: Progress in Gynecology, Vol 4. New York, Grune & Stratton, 1963.)

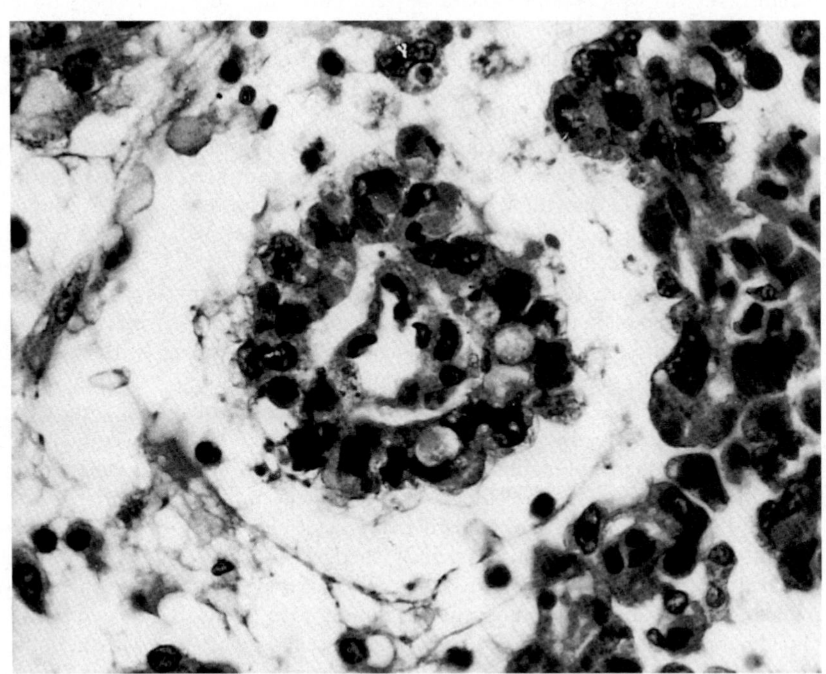

Figure 33-21. Schiller–Duvall body associated with numerous hyaline droplets in an endodermal sinus tumor. (×350.) (From Kurman RJ, Norris HJ: Malignant germ cells of the ovary. Hum Pathol 8:551, 1977. Reprinted with permission from WB Saunders, Philadelphia, 1977.)

Mixed Germ Cell Tumors

Mixed germ cell tumors are combinations of any of the previously described germ cell tumors of the ovary. They can be bilateral if dysgerminoma elements are involved; otherwise, they are unilateral.

Contemporary Treatment of Malignant Germ Cell Tumors

Contemporary management results in cure rates approaching 100% for patients with stage I malignant germ cell tumors and more than 75% for patients with advanced-stage (stage III and IV) disease. Because most patients are young and most of these tumors are unilateral, fertility-sparing surgery consisting of unilateral salpingo-oophorectomy with preservation of the contralateral ovary and the uterus is appropriate. After unilateral adnexal excision, frozen-section examination should be performed to preliminarily confirm the diagnosis. Once a malignant ovarian germ cell tumor is documented, routine biopsy of a normal contralateral ovary should be avoided because such an intervention could lead to future infertility related to peritoneal adhesions or ovarian failure. If bilateral ovarian masses are encountered at surgery, a unilateral salpingo-oophorectomy of the more suspicious side is appropriate. If the opposite ovary contains tumor or is dysgenetic, then bilateral salpingo-oophorectomy is generally indicated. Although not proven to be entirely safe, in the case of bilateral ovarian dysgerminomas in nondysgenetic ovaries, unilateral salpingo-oophorectomy and contralateral ovarian cystectomy may be considered in an effort to preserve fertility. Conversely, if a contralateral ovary contains a mature cystic teratoma (which is much more likely because it is present in 10% to 15% of cases), ovarian cystectomy is indicated.

If the tumor appears to be grossly confined to the ovary, in general, comprehensive surgical staging is recommended, with cytologic washings, omentectomy, peritoneal biopsies, and bilateral pelvic and paraaortic lymphadenectomy. If obvious extra-ovarian metastases are present, then the guiding principle is maximum cytoreductive surgery.

For most patients with malignant ovarian germ cell tumors, postoperative chemotherapy is indicated. Notable exceptions include patients with stage IA pure dysgerminoma and patients with stage IA, grade 1 immature teratoma; these patients have a high cure rate with surgery alone. The VAC regimen (vincristine 1.5 mg/m^2 given intravenously weekly for 12 weeks and actinomycin D 0.5 mg with cyclophosphamide [Cytoxan] 5 to 7 mg/kg/day given intravenously daily for 5 days every 4 weeks) was the first effective combination chemotherapy regimen for patients with malignant germ cell tumors. VAC was the most widely used regimen during the 1970s and early 1980s and produced a relatively high proportion of cures in stage I disease (82%), but in patients with metastatic disease, the cure rate was less than 50%. During the VAC era, conversion of an immature teratoma to a mature teratoma under the influence of chemotherapy, so-called retroconversion, was observed.

By the late 1970s, based on the experience in testicular cancer, the combination of vinblastine, bleomycin, and cisplatin (VBP) was beginning to be used for malignant ovarian germ cell tumors, with superior outcomes compared with those achieved with the VAC regimen, particularly for patients with advanced-stage disease. By the mid-1980s, the VBP regimen was replaced by the combination of bleomycin, etoposide, and cisplatin (BEP) because of the latter's superior toxicity profile. The BEP regimen remains the standard today. Generally, most patients require three to four cycles of therapy. In 1990, Gershenson and coworkers reported that 25 of 26 patients treated with BEP for malignant germ cell tumors were in sustained remission. Subsequently, Williams and associates, reporting the GOG experience, noted that 89 of 93 patients (96%) with completely resected stage I, II, or III disease remained continuously disease-free.

Special note should be made regarding dysgerminoma. Historically, for patients with metastatic dysgerminoma, the traditional postoperative treatment was radiotherapy. Although dysgerminoma is exquisitely radiosensitive and survival rates with such treatment were excellent, most patients suffered loss of fertility. With the advent of successful combination chemotherapy, such as BEP, chemotherapy has almost exclusively supplanted radiotherapy, with a high rate of fertility preservation.

Although second-look surgery was part of standard management for patients with malignant germ cell tumors until the mid-1980s, reports from the University of Texas M. D. Anderson Cancer Center and the GOG called into question the value of this procedure. Gershenson and colleagues reported their experience with second-look surgery, with negative findings in 52 of 53 patients; only 1 of the 52 negative patients relapsed and died of tumor. Subsequently, the GOG experience confirmed that the value of second-look surgery in patients with completely resected malignant germ cell tumors and incompletely resected malignant germ cell tumors not containing an immature teratoma element was negligible; for patients with incompletely resected malignant germ cell tumors with an immature teratoma element, however, second-look surgery appeared to have some impact. Of course, advances in imaging technology may further minimize the need for second-look surgery, even in the latter group.

Over the past few years, there has been a trend toward surveillance with careful follow-up after surgery as an alternative to chemotherapy in selected patients. Bonazzi and associates treated 32 patients with operation alone for stage I–II grade 1–2 tumors. All patients with grade 3 tumors or stage III tumors or those with tumor recurrence received cisplatin, etoposide, and bleomycin. Most patients underwent fertility-sparing surgery. Ten received chemotherapy. All patients were free of disease with a median follow-up of 47 months, and five had delivered healthy infants. A recent Pediatric Oncology Group Study reported by Cushing and associates indicated that patients younger than age 15 with a pure immature teratoma could be followed without chemotherapy; however, more than 90% of the tumors in their series were grade 1 or 2. In addition, a study by Billmire and coworkers found that survival in 131 girls with malignant ovarian germ cell tumors was unaffected by less than comprehensive surgical staging.

The Children's Oncology Group is currently conducting a clinical trial in the pediatric population that the GOG is planning to join. This trial includes surveillance of the low-risk cohort, consisting of all patients with apparent stage I disease with close follow-up of serum markers and initiation of chemotherapy only if relapse occurs. In the intermediate-risk cohort, patients with stage II–IV disease receive a modified BEP regimen over 3 days instead of the standard 5-day regimen.

There is no standard surveillance for patients with malignant ovarian germ cell tumors after completion of primary therapy. For patients who have completed standard surgery plus chemotherapy, we generally recommend serum tumor markers monthly for up to 2 years and then gradually less frequently. Patients treated with fertility-sparing surgery should be closely followed with periodic transvaginal ultrasound and/or CT evaluations. Office visits with physical examination are generally recommended every 3 months for the first 2 years and gradually less frequently thereafter.

With the success of cure in a high proportion of young patients with malignant ovarian germ cell tumors has come an increasing focus on the late effects of therapy, particularly fertility preservation. In a report of 40 patients, Gershenson and coworkers noted that 27 had normal menses after multiagent chemotherapy for germ cell tumors, and 11 of 16 patients who attempted pregnancy were successful in bearing 22 children. Most of these patients received nonplatinum-based chemotherapy. Peccatori and colleagues reported on 139 patients with malignant germ cell tumors, 108 of whom had fertility-sparing operations. Multiagent platinum-containing chemotherapy was used with a 96% survival rate with a mean follow-up of 55 months. In a GOG study, Williams and associates reported on 93 patients treated adjuvantly with cisplatinum, etoposide, and bleomycin for three cycles. Ninety-one of 93 patients were free of disease 4 to 90 months after treatment, although leukemia developed in one patient and lymphoma in a second patient. Brewer and coworkers reported on 26 patients treated with BEP, with 25 alive and disease-free with median follow-up of 89 months. They reported 71% resumed normal menstrual function and six patients conceived. Three additional large studies from Australia, Italy, and the United States (Yale University) have provided further support for the concept of preservation of fertility in the majority of patients treated with fertility-sparing surgery and chemotherapy.

There are now several nonrandomized studies suggesting that gonadotropin-releasing hormone agonist prophylaxis may be worthwhile to preserve ovarian function in young patients receiving chemotherapy. Blumenfeld and coworkers administered gonadotropin-releasing hormone agonist during chemotherapy for nongynecologic tumors to women of reproductive age, and 15 of 16 surviving patients (93.7%) resumed menses and ovulation. However, randomized trials are needed to validate this approach.

Specialized Germ Cell Tumors—Struma Ovarii and Carcinoids

Specialized ovarian germ cell tumors are rare; two types are commonly recognized (see box on p. 865): the struma ovarii and carcinoids. Struma ovarii are dermoids with thyroid tissue exclusively or as a major component. The thyroid tissue can be functional, leading to clinical hyperthyroidism. Most of these tumors are benign, but malignant changes are possible. Metastatic disease, if present, has been reported to be effectively treated with iodine 131, as in the case of primary thyroid carcinoma.

Carcinoids are ovarian teratomas that histologically resemble similar tumors in the gastrointestinal tract. Carcinoids are rare and are unilateral in the ovary. In approximately 30% of cases, a true carcinoid syndrome will develop, and 5-hydroxyindoleacetic acid can be detected and used to monitor the tumor postoperatively. These tumors occur primarily in older women and tend to grow slowly; the prognosis after hysterectomy and bilateral salpingo-oophorectomy is excellent. For a young woman desiring preservation of childbearing function, a stage IA carcinoid can be treated by unilateral salpingo-oophorectomy.

GONADOBLASTOMAS (GERM CELL SEX CORD–STROMAL TUMORS)

The term *gonadoblastoma* was introduced by Scully in 1953 to describe a tumor that consists of germ cell and sex cord–stromal elements. Approximately 100 cases have been reported. The germ cells usually resemble dysgerminoma, whereas the sex cord–stromal elements may consist of immature granulosa and Sertoli cells. Leydig cells and luteinized cells may be present. The tumor usually occurs in patients with abnormal (dysgenetic) gonads. Most patients have a female phenotype but may be virilized. These patients have a Y chromosome detected in their karyotype, and patients with gonadal dysgenesis and a Y chromosome are at risk of the development of gonadoblastoma or malignant germ cell tumors, predominantly dysgerminoma, which may occur in an individual as young as 6 months of age. Removal of these gonads is indicated when they are discovered. Both gonads should be removed, and if the presence of pure gonadoblastoma is confirmed, the prognosis is excellent because these tumors have not been reported to metastasize.

SEX CORD–STROMAL TUMORS

The sex cord–stromal tumors are derived from the sex cords of the ovary and the specialized stroma of the developing gonad. The elements can have a male or female differentiation, and some of these tumors are hormonally active. The group accounts for approximately 6% of ovarian neoplasms and the majority of hormonally functioning ovarian tumors. For the female derivatives, the sex cord component is the granulosa cell, and the stromal component is the theca cell or fibroblast. For the male counterpart, the similar components are the Sertoli cell and the Leydig cell. Granulosa-theca cell tumors and Sertoli–Leydig cell tumors tend to behave as low-grade malignancies. Their clinical and morphologic aspects considered separately.

Granulosa—Theca Cell Tumors

Granulosa cell tumors consist primarily of granulosa cells and a varying proportion of theca cells or fibroblasts or both. One characteristic microscopic pattern is shown in Figure 33-22, which demonstrates the so-called Call Exner bodies, eosinophilic bodies surrounded by granulosa cells. Functional granulosa cell tumors are primarily estrogenic. Approximately 5% occur before puberty, and they can be one of the causes of precocious puberty, but the tumors have been described in women of all ages. In postmenopausal women, these tumors can produce increased levels of blood estrogens, uterine bleeding, and occasionally endometrial carcinoma. It is estimated that approximately 5% of the granulosa cell tumors in adults are associated with endometrial carcinoma. In menstruating women, the functional granulosa cell tumor can produce abnormal menstrual patterns, menorrhagia, and even amenorrhea.

These tumors can become large and may present as a ruptured mass, leading to laparotomy for an acute abdomen with hemoperitoneum. Because of the low-grade malignant character of these tumors, recurrences are frequently more than 5 years after primary therapy. In general, prognosis does not correlate with the histologic pattern of the tumor. A total of 90% of granulosa cell tumors present as stage I. Advanced clinical stage, the presence of tumor rupture, a large primary tumor (>15 cm), and a high mitotic rate have been associated with a poorer prognosis. Overall 10-year survival rates of 90% have been reported. Studies by Klemi and colleagues and others suggest that most granulosa cell tumors have a diploid pattern and a low (<60%) S-phase fraction when analyzed by flow cytometry. Those with an aneuploid pattern had a worse prognosis in the study of Klemi and colleagues. However, it is important to recognize that granulosa cell tumors can be confused histologically

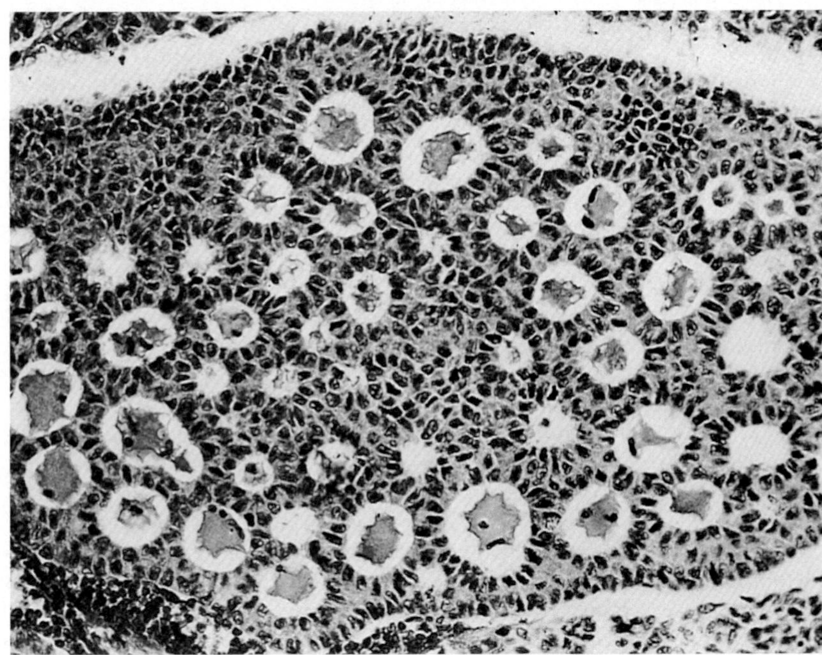

Figure 33-22. Granulosa cell tumor. (×460.) (From Scully RE, Morris J: Functioning ovarian tumors. In Meigs JV, Sturgis SH [eds]: Progress in Gynecology, Vol 3. New York, Grune & Stratton, 1957.)

with poorly differentiated adenocarcinomas, and the latter would also have an aneuploid pattern as well as a poor prognosis. A variant found predominantly in females younger than 20 years of age is known as juvenile granulosa cell tumor. It was described by Young and associates and has an excellent prognosis, particularly if the tumor is confined to one ovary.

The primary therapeutic approach is the surgical removal of the tumor. Because these tumors are rarely bilateral (<5%), young patients with stage IA tumors can be treated by unilateral adnexectomy. Lack and coworkers reported 10 cases of granulosa cell tumors in premenarchal female patients, all of whom were treated by unilateral salpingo-oophorectomy. Two tumors were ruptured. All 10 of the patients were alive with no evidence of disease 2 to 33 years after therapy. Evans and colleagues did note a higher recurrence rate among women who were treated by unilateral salpingo-oophorectomy for stage IA cases compared with those treated with bilateral salpingo-oophorectomy. This finding has led to the recommendation that women of reproductive age treated for granulosa cell tumor by unilateral salpingo-oophorectomy have close follow-up. The removal of the contralateral ovary is considered after reproductive function is completed or if there is evidence of ovarian enlargement. For women who have completed childbearing, abdominal hysterectomy and bilateral salpingo-oophorectomy are recommended. Regardless of management of the pelvic organs, if a granulosa cell tumor is diagnosed on frozen-section examination, comprehensive surgical staging is recommended. Whether complete pelvic and paraaortic lymphadenectomy is indicated remains unresolved; there is some information that the incidence of lymph node metastases associated with this tumor type is low.

Tumor markers may be helpful in monitoring the clinical course of granulosa cell tumors. Studies by Lappohn and associates suggest that the peptide hormone inhibin is secreted by some granulosa cell tumors and serum measurements could serve as a tumor marker. In addition, serum CA 125, serum estradiol, or serum testosterone may occasionally serve as markers that should be followed serially.

Historically, radiotherapy, the VAC regimen (see previously), or the combination of cisplatin, doxorubicin, and cyclophosphamide have been used for treatment of metastatic granulosa cell tumors, but none of these options are currently recommended for general application. Many questions remain regarding recommendations for postoperative treatment. For patients with stage IA granulosa cell tumors, surgery alone is recommended. The recommendation for those with stage IC disease remains controversial, but consideration can be given to adjuvant therapy based on the probable increased risk of relapse. Postoperative therapy is recommended for all patients with stage II–IV disease as well as for those patients with recurrent tumor.

Because of the rarity of granulosa cell tumors, no standard regimen exists. The GOG has reported the largest series of women treated with the BEP regimen. Homesley and coworkers reported on 57 eligible patients; 41 had recurrent disease and 16 had primary metastatic disease. Forty-eight of the patients had granulosa cell tumors. Overall, 11 of 16 primary disease patients and 21 of 41 recurrent-disease patients remained progression-free at a median follow-up of 3 years. However, toxicity was fairly severe, with two bleomycin-related deaths reported.

More recently, Brown and colleagues reported the M. D. Anderson Cancer Center experience with taxane-based chemotherapy. They reported 44 patients with sex cord–stromal tumors of the ovary treated for either primary metastatic or recurrent disease. The response rate for 30 patients treated with a taxane + platinum for recurrent, measurable disease was 42%. Thus, the combination of paclitaxel and carboplatin is also an option for these patients.

Hormone therapy may also be considered for patients with metastatic granulosa cell tumors. Responses of these tumors to medroxyprogesterone acetate and to gonadotropin-releasing hormone antagonists have been reported. Fishman and associates

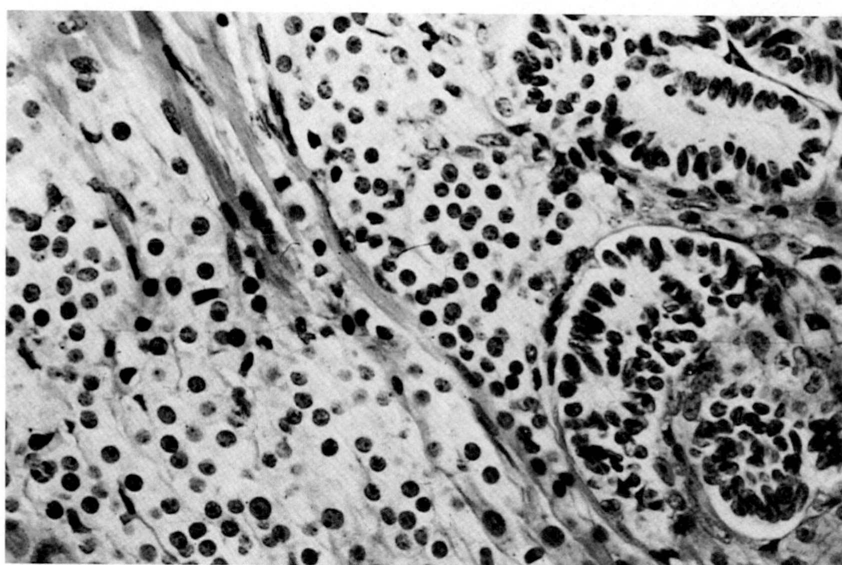

Figure 33-23. Sertoli–Leydig cell tumor. Tubules of Sertoli cells (*right*) and Leydig cells (*left*) are shown. (×250.) (Courtesy of Dr. R. E. Scully.)

treated six patients with recurrent or persistent granulosa cell tumors with leuprolide acetate; of five patients with assessable disease, two had partial responses and three had stable disease.

Thecomas and Fibromas

Thecomas are benign tumors that consist entirely of stroma (theca) cells. They occur in women predominantly in the perimenopausal and menopausal years. These tumors can be associated with estrogen production but not as frequently as are granulosa cell tumors. Removal of the tumor alone is adequate treatment in women in the reproductive years. For older women, total abdominal hysterectomy and bilateral salpingo-oophorectomy are performed. Rarely, thecomas have been reported to be malignant, and these are most likely fibrosarcomas. A closely related tumor is the fibroma, which is the most common benign solid ovarian tumor and accounts for 4% of all ovarian tumors. Like the thecoma, it can occur at any age but is more common in older women; it does not secrete hormones. These tumors contain spindle cells, and the tumors can grow to a large size. They are benign, and excision is adequate treatment. These tumors are associated with ascites in approximately 40% of cases if the tumor exceeds 10 cm, according to Samanth and Black. They can also be responsible for hydrothorax with a benign ascites (Meigs' syndrome), which regresses following tumor removal.

Sertoli–Leydig Cell Tumors (Androblastomas)

Sertoli–Leydig cell tumors are very rare. Sertoli (sex cord) and Leydig (stromal) cells are present in varying amounts, and the tumor may consist almost entirely of either Sertoli or Leydig cells (Fig. 33-23). These tumors tend to occur in young women of reproductive age and frequently are the cause of masculinization and hirsutism. The symptoms of virilization usually regress after tumor removal, but temporal hair recession and a deeper voice tend to remain. Rarely, they have been reported also to have estrogenic activity, leading to the same symptoms and signs as those of granulosa cell tumors. The tumors tend to behave as low-grade malignancies, and the 5-year survival rate is reported to vary from 70% to 90%. Poorly differentiated types tend to have a poor prognosis, as do higher stage tumors. Young and Scully reviewed 207 cases. Seventy-five percent were 30 years of age or younger, and less than 10% were older than 50 years old. One third had evidence of androgen excess. Both ovaries were involved in only three cases. The well-differentiated tumors behaved clinically as benign tumors, whereas recurrence or extrauterine spread was noted occasionally in women with intermediate differentiation (11%) and frequently in those with poor differentiation (59%). Of 164 patients available for follow-up, 18% had metastasis or recurrence.

Treatment of metastatic Sertoli–Leydig cell tumors is similar to that for granulosa cell tumors. In addition, because the prognosis for patients with stage I poorly differentiated Sertoli–Leydig cell tumors is so poor, consideration should be give for adjuvant treatment. However, it should be emphasized that there are no therapeutic data in this setting, and if treatment is recommended, the optimal regimen remains unclear. The BEP regimen or the combination of paclitaxel and carboplatin might be considered in such patients.

Gynandroblastomas

Gynandroblastomas are rare sex cord–stromal tumors consisting of both female and male cell types.

Sex Cord Tumors with Annular Tubules

Sex cord tumors with annular tubules are unusual. As suggested by the name, there is a prominent tubular pattern. Features of both Sertoli and granulosa cell tumors are present. Seventy-four cases were reviewed by Young and associates, and 27 were

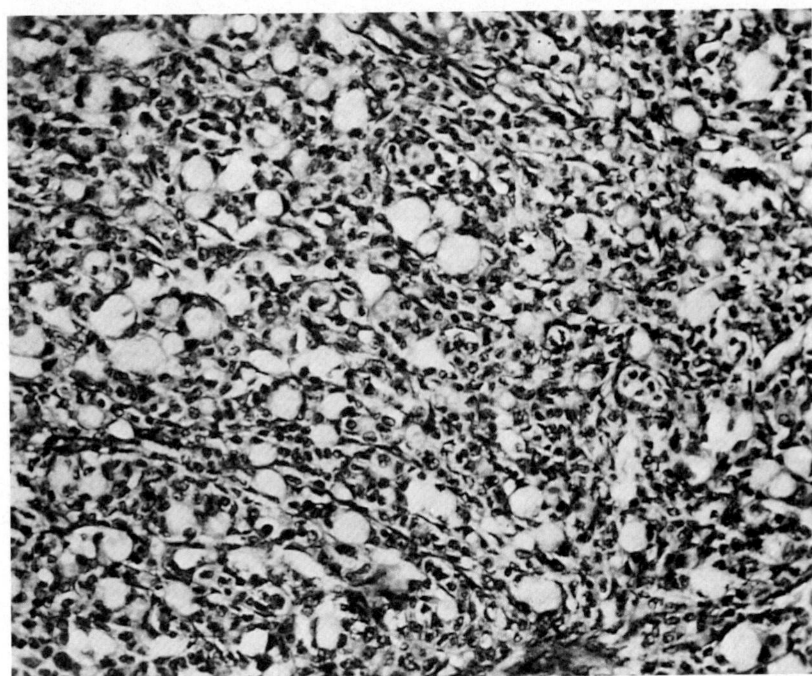

Figure 33-24. Krukenberg's tumor. (×256.) Mucin-filled signet-ring cells are present. (Courtesy of Dr. R. E. Scully.)

associated with mucocutaneous pigmentation and gastrointestinal tract polyposis (Peutz–Jeghers syndrome). The tumors may have estrogenic manifestations. Those associated with Peutz–Jeghers syndrome are benign, and those not associated with this syndrome can be malignant. It is of interest that 4 of the 74 cases reported by Young and associates were associated with a virulent form of cervical adenocarcinoma (adenoma malignum).

Leydig Cell and Hilus Cell Tumors

Leydig cell and hilus cell tumors are rare and are composed of Leydig cells or cells of the ovarian hilus. Their cytoplasm contains hyaline bodies known as *crystalloids of Reinke.* They usually cause virilization and are benign. They tend to be small (<6 cm) and develop primarily in perimenopausal women.

LIPID (LIPOID) TUMORS

Lipid tumors are infrequently occurring ovarian tumors composed of large cells that resemble Leydig cells, luteinized cells, or cells that arise in the adrenal cortex. Approximately 100 tumors have been reported. These tumors usually cause virilization but have also been associated with excess cortisol production. There is not enough experience with them to delineate an effective form of treatment. However, metastases of lipid cell tumors have been reported.

METASTATIC OVARIAN TUMORS

Tumors from distant primary sites can metastasize to the ovary. Frequently, metastases are from primary tumors that originate elsewhere in the female reproductive tract, particularly from the endometrium and fallopian tube. Distant sites of origin occur most frequently from the breast and gastrointestinal tract. Metastatic tumors from the gastrointestinal tract to the ovary can be associated with sex hormone production, which usually leads to estrogenic manifestations. One special type of metastatic ovarian tumor is known as Krukenberg's tumor, which histologically consists of nests of mucin-filled signet-ring cells in a cellular stroma (Fig. 33-24). The most common gastrointestinal tract origin for these tumors is the stomach, and the next frequent is the large intestine. However, breast metastases to the ovary can on occasion give the same histologic picture. A few cases of Krukenberg's tumors have been described with no apparent distant primary malignancy, suggesting the rare possibility of a primary ovarian tumor with the histologic features of a Krukenberg's tumor. A primary gastrointestinal tract malignancy should be considered in older women with an adnexal mass, particularly if it is bilateral and solid. Pretherapy evaluation to rule out a gastrointestinal tract or breast primary tumor is indicated. The tumor should be removed when discovered, and the primary site should be treated. The prognosis is poor, and it is rare for a patient to survive for 5 or more years after treatment.

KEY POINTS

- Ovarian cancer is the leading cause of death from gynecologic cancer, but it occurs less frequently than endometrial cancers.
- Ovarian cancers of women older than age 50 are diagnosed at a more advanced stage, leading to a worse prognosis than for younger women.
- The risk of ovarian cancer is decreased by oral contraceptive use. Tubal ligation and hysterectomy also appear to decrease the risk.
- Most ovarian carcinomas are diagnosed in stage III or IV.
- Ovarian cancer risk rises from approximately 1.4% in general to 5% to 7%, with one to two first- or second-degree relatives with ovarian cancer.
- Patients with ovarian cancer are at increased risk of developing breast cancer and endometrial cancer. It is important that the follow-up of ovarian cancer patients include monitoring for breast cancer.
- Epithelial tumors are the most frequent ovarian neoplasm. They account for two thirds of all ovarian neoplasms and 85% of ovarian cancers.
- The major ovarian epithelial tumor cell types recapitulate müllerian-type epithelium (serous-endosalpinx, mucinous-endocervix, and endometrioid-endometrium).
- Serous ovarian neoplasms are the most common type of epithelial tumors. Serous adenocarcinomas tend to be high grade, are the most virulent, and have the worst prognosis of epithelial adenocarcinomas. They are bilateral in 33% to 66% of cases.
- A cystic adnexal mass less than 8 cm in diameter in a menstruating female is most frequently functional.
- The normal postmenopausal ovary is approximately 1.5 to 2 cm in diameter.
- The risk of an ovarian tumor being malignant is approximately 33% in a woman older than age 45, whereas it is less than 1 in 15 for those 20 to 45 years of age. More than half of ovarian cancers occur in women older than the age of 50.
- There are three types of ovarian tumors with a serous histology: traditional serous adenocarcinoma, surface papillary tumors (ovary < 4 cm), and primary peritoneal carcinomas (serous carcinoma metastatic to the ovary with normal ovarian size).
- Most ovarian carcinomas start from small microscopic foci and spread throughout the peritoneum before becoming clinically evident (de novo origin), particularly serous and poorly differentiated tumors.
- Ovarian carcinomas having a cystic origin are primary mucinous or endometrioid, and these are more likely to be discovered at a low stage.
- A vaginal ultrasound finding of a unilocular cyst of 5 cm or less in a perimenopausal woman can usually be followed without surgical intervention.
- Vaginal ultrasonography may detect early ovarian carcinoma but has not been proven to be a cost-effective screening technique.
- The primary distribution spread of epithelial carcinoma is transcoelomic to the visceral and parietal peritoneum and diaphragm and to the retroperitoneal nodes.
- The risk of retroperitoneal node spread of epithelial carcinoma in apparent stage I cases is greatest for poorly differentiated tumors, for which the risk can reach 10% to 20%. The risk of retroperitoneal node spread increases in higher stage cases.
- The prognosis of a patient with ovarian epithelial carcinoma is related primarily to tumor stage and tumor grade as well as to the amount of residual tumor remaining after primary resection.
- The 5-year survival rate for patients with borderline epithelial ovarian carcinoma (grade 0) is close to 100% for stage I cases and more than 90% for all stages.
- The overall 5-year survival rate for patients with stage I ovarian carcinoma is 65%. For stage I grade 1, the survival rate is reported to be more than 80%.
- Optimal surgical debulking (<1 cm residual nodules) appears to confer a survival advantage in cases of stage III–IV ovarian carcinoma.
- Interval cytoreduction has little additional effect on overall survival if a maximal attempt is made at primary surgery.
- Neoadjuvant chemotherapy can reduce surgical morbidity; however, its efficacy has not been subjected to formal investigation.
- Intraperitoneal chemotherapy appears to benefit patients with optimal cytoreduction over conventional IV chemotherapy, albeit with greater toxicity.
- CT for patients with ovarian cancer can be approximately 80% to 90% effective for detecting tumor in retroperitoneal nodes, but is much less successful in detecting intra-abdominal disease.
- The ovarian CA 125 is useful in helping to monitor patients with ovarian carcinoma. Reaction to the antigen is positive in approximately 80% of cases.
- A rapid decrease in CA 125 values after treatment indicates a more favorable prognosis.
- The initial response rate of ovarian epithelial carcinomas multiple-agent chemotherapy is more than 90%, but the proportion of patients who survive decreases to approximately 30% in 5 years. Initial treatment is usually with platinum and taxane agents.
- Approximately half of patients thought initially to be clinically free of disease are found at second-look laparotomy to have gross or microscopic tumor.
- The 5-year survival rate after negative second-look operation is approximately 50%.
- Recurrent ovarian cancer is very difficult to cure.
- Factors determining response to recurrent chemotherapy regimens include time to treatment progression, distribution and volume of disease, and performance status.
- Combination chemotherapy for platinum-sensitive recurrent disease improves response rates with a less clear effect on survival.

Continued

KEY POINTS *Continued*

- Secondary cytoreduction appears to benefit patients with limited recurrent disease who undergo complete tumor removal. The benefit may be most realized before chemotherapy for recurrence.
- Germ cell tumors are the second most common type of ovarian neoplasms and account for approximately 20% to 25% of all ovarian tumors.
- In young women under age 30, the most frequent ovarian neoplasm is a germ cell tumor, and approximately one third of these germ cell tumors are malignant in those younger than age 21.
- The most common germ cell tumor is the benign cystic teratoma (dermoid). It is bilateral in 10%–15% of the cases. Approximately 30% are calcified.
- For women younger than age 30, the most common ovarian neoplasm is the dermoid.
- Malignant germ cell tumors are usually unilateral except dysgerminomas, which are bilateral in approximately 10% of the cases.
- Dysgerminomas are the most common malignant germ cell tumors and account for 1% to 2% of ovarian cancers.
- The prognosis for a patient with immature teratoma is related to tumor grade and tumor stage. These tumors are the second most common type of malignant germ cell tumor.
- The 5-year survival rate of stage IA pure dysgerminoma treated by unilateral salpingo-oophorectomy is more than 90%.
- Pure dysgerminomas are radiocurable. However, multiagent chemotherapy, particularly with etoposide and platinum with or without bleomycin, will frequently result in complete remission. About two thirds of cases present as stage IA.
- Most patients with malignant ovarian germ cell tumors can be treated successfully with fertility-sparing surgery followed by BEP chemotherapy. Patients who clearly do not require postoperative chemotherapy include those with stage IA dysgerminoma and stage IA grade 1 immature teratoma. However, there is a trend toward the study of surveillance rather than chemotherapy for patients with stage I tumors of any histologic subtype.
- Multiple-agent chemotherapy has improved the survival in patients with malignant germ cell tumors, preserving childbearing function in most cases. Standard chemotherapy consists of the BEP regimen.
- Gonadoblastomas are sex cord–stromal germ cell tumors that arise in dysgenetic gonads in patients with a Y chromosome and are cured by removal.
- Granulosa cell tumors and Sertoli–Leydig tumors usually behave as low-grade malignancies, but there may be late recurrences.
- For patients with primary metastatic or recurrent sex cord–stromal tumors of the ovary, platinum-based chemotherapy is the treatment of choice. Commonly employed regimens include BEP and paclitaxel/carboplatin.
- Some metastatic granulosa cell tumors may respond to hormone therapy, such as leuprolide acetate.
- Fibroma is the most common benign solid ovarian tumor.
- The most frequent sites of origin of tumors metastatic to the ovary are the lower reproductive tract, gastrointestinal tract, and breast.

BIBLIOGRAPHY

Abramowicz JS: Ultrasound contrast media and their use in obstetrics and gynecology. Ultrasound Med Biol 23:1287, 1997.

A'Hern RP, Gore ME: Impact of doxorubicin on survival in advanced ovarian cancer. J Clin Oncol 13:726, 1995.

Alberts DS, Liu PY, Hannigan EV, et al: Intraperitoneal cisplatin plus intravenous cyclophosphamide versus intravenous cisplatin plus intravenous cyclophosphamide for stage III ovarian cancer. N Engl J Med 335:1950–1955, 1996.

Altaras MM, Aviram R, Cohen I, et al: Primary peritoneal papillary serous adenocarcinoma: Clinical and management aspects. Gynecol Oncol 40:230, 1991.

Armstrong DK, Bundy B, Wenzel L, et al: Intraperitoneal cisplatin and paclitaxel in ovarian cancer. N Engl J Med 354:34–43, 2006.

Aure JC, Hoeg K, Kolstad P: The clinical and histologic studies of ovarian carcinoma: Long-term follow-up of 990 cases. Obstet Gynecol 37:1, 1971.

Bailey CL, Ueland FR, Land GL, et al: The malignant potential of small cystic ovarian tumors in women over 50 years of age. Gynecol Oncol 69:3, 1998.

Barakat RR, Almadrones L, Venkatramman ES, et al: A phase II trial of intraperitoneal cisplatin and estoposide as consolidation therapy in patients with stage II-IV epithelial ovarian cancer following negative surgical assessment. Gynecol Oncol 69:17, 1998.

Bast RC, Feene M, Lazarus H, et al: Reactivity of a monoclonal antibody with human ovarian carcinoma. J Clin Invest 68:1331, 1981.

Behbakht K, Randall TC, Benjamin I, et al: Clinical characteristics of clear cell carcinoma of the ovary. Gynecol Oncol 70:255, 1998.

Bell DA, Scully RE: Early de novo ovarian carcinoma. Cancer 73:1859, 1994.

Bell DA, Weinstock MA, Scully RE: Peritoneal implants of ovarian serous borderline tumors: Histologic features and prognosis. Cancer 62:2212, 1988.

Bell J, Brady MF, Young MC, et al: Randomized phase III trial of three versus six cycles of adjuvant carboplatin and paclitaxel in early stage epithelial ovarian carcinoma: A Gynecologic Oncology Group study. Gynecol Oncol 102:432–439, 2006.

Ben-Baruch G, Siven E, Moran O, et al: Primary peritoneal serous papillary carcinoma: A study of 25 cases and comparison with stage III-IV ovarian papillary serous carcinoma. Gynecol Oncol 60:393, 1996.

Benrubi GI, Pitel P, Lammert N: Small cell carcinoma of the ovary with hypercalcemia responsive to sequencing chemotherapy. South Med J 86:247, 1993.

Berchuck A, Bast RC: P53-based gene therapy of ovarian cancer: magic bullet? Gynecol Oncol 59:169, 1995.

Berchuck A, Elbendary A, Havrilesky L, et al: Pathogenesis of ovarian cancers. J Soc Gynecol Invest 1:181, 1994.

Berek JS, Knapp RC, Malkasian GD, et al: CA-125 serum levels correlated with second-look operations among ovarian cancer patients. Obstet Gynecol 67:685, 1986.

Berek JS, Taylor PT, Gordon A, et al: Randomized, placebo-controlled study of oregovomab for consolidation of clinical remission in patients with advanced ovarian cancer. J Clin Oncol 22:3507–3516, 2004.

Bicher A, Levenback C, Silva EG, et al: Ovarian malignant mullerian tumors treated with platinum-based chemotherapy. Obstet Gynecol 85:735, 1995.

Billmire D, Vinocur C, Rescoria F, et al: Outcome and staging evaluation in malignant germ cell tumors of the ovary in children and adolescents: An intergroup study. J Pediatr Surg 39:424, 2004.

Bjorkholm E, Silfversward C: Prognostic factors in granulosa cell tumor. Gynecol Oncol 11:261, 1981.
Blumfeld Z, Aviv I, Linn S, et al: Prevention of irreversible chemotherapy-induced ovarian damage in young women with lymphoma by a gonadotrophin-releasing hormone agonist in parallel to chemotherapy. Hum Reprod 11:1620, 1996.
Bolis G, Colombo N, Pecorelli S, et al: Adjuvant treatment for early epithelial ovarian cancer: Results of two randomised clinical trials comparing cisplatin to no further treatment or chromic phosphate (32P). Ann Oncol 6:887, 1995.
Bonazzi C, Peccatori F, Colombo N, et al: Pure ovarian immature teratoma, a unique and curable disease: 10 years' experience of 32 prospectively treated patients. Obstet Gynecol 84:598, 1994.
Bonome T, Lee JY, Park DC, et al: Expression profiling of serous low malignant potential, low-grade, and high-grade tumors of the ovary. Cancer Res 65:10602–10612, 2005.
Bostwick DG, Tazelaar HD, Ballon SC, et al: Ovarian epithelial tumors of borderline malignancy: Clinical and pathologic study of 109 cases. Cancer 58:2052, 1986.
Bourne TH, Whitehead MI, Campbell S, et al: Ultrasound screening for familial ovarian cancer. Gynecol Oncol 43:92, 1991.
Boyd J, Sonoda Y, Frederici MG, et al: Clinicopathologic features of BRCA-linked and sporadic ovarian cancer. JAMA 283:2260, 2000.
Braly PS, Berek JS, Blessing JA, et al: Intraperitoneal administration of cisplatin and 5-fluorouracil in residual ovarian cancer: A phase II Gynecologic Oncology Group trial. Gynecol Oncol 56:164, 1995.
Brewer M, Gershenson DM, Herzog CE, et al: Outcome and reproductive function after chemotherapy for ovarian dysgerminoma. J Clin Oncol 17:2670, 1999.
Bridgewater JA, Nelstrop AE, Rustin GJS, et al: Comparison of standard and CA-125 response criteria in patients with epithelial ovarian cancer treated with platinum and paclitaxel. J Clin Oncol 17:501, 1999.
Bristow RE, Montz FJ, Lagasse LD, et al: Survival impact of surgical cytoreduction in stage IV epithelial ovarian cancer. Gynecol Oncol 72:278, 1999.
Bristow RE, Tomacruz RS, Armstrong DK, et al: Survival effect of maximal cytoreductive surgery for advanced ovarian carcinoma during the platinum era: A meta-analysis. J Clin Oncol 20:1248–1259, 2002.
Brown J, Shvartsman HS, Deavers MT, et al: The activity of taxanes in the treatment of sex cord-stromal ovarian tumors. J Clin Oncol 22:351, 2004.
Buller RE: BRCA1: What do we know? What do we think we know? What do we really need to know? [editorial]. Gynecol Oncol 76:291, 2000.
Buller RE, Berman ML, Bloss JD, et al: CA-125 regression: A model for epithelial ovarian cancer response. Am J Obstet Gynecol 165:360, 1991.
Buller RE, Vasilev S, DiSaia PJ: CA 125 kinetics: A cost effective clinical tool to evaluate clinical trial outcomes in the 1990s. Am J Obstet Gynecol 174:1241, 1996.
Burghardt E, Girardi F, Lahousen M, et al: Patterns of pelvic and paraaortic lymph node involvement in ovarian cancer. Gynecol Oncol 40:103, 1991.
Campbell S, Bhan V, Royston P, et al: Transabdominal ultrasound screening for early ovarian cancer. BMJ 299:1363–1367, 1989.
Canevari S, Stoter G, Arienti F, et al: Regression of advanced ovarian carcinoma by intraperitoneal treatment with autologous T lymphocytes retargeted by bispecific monoclonal antibody. J Natl Cancer Inst 87:1463, 1995.
Casagrande JT, Louie EW, Pike MC, et al: "Incessant ovulation" and ovarian cancer. Lancet 2:170, 1979.
Chadha S, Cornelisse CJ, Schaberg A: Flow cytometry DNA ploidy analysis of ovarian granulosa cell tumor. Gynecol Oncol 36:240, 1990.
Chi DS, Venkatraman ES, Masson V, Hoskins WJ: Ability of preoperative serum CA-125 to predict optimal primary tumor cytoreduction in stage III epithelial ovarian carcinoma. Gynecol Oncol 77:237, 2000.
Childers JM, Lang J, Surwit EA, Hatch KD: Laparoscopic surgical staging of ovarian cancer. Gynecol Oncol 59:25, 1995.
Cmelak AJ, Kapp DS: Long-term survival with whole abdominal irradiation in platinum-refractory persistent or recurrent ovarian cancer. Gynecol Oncol 65:453, 1997.
Colditz GA, Hankinson SE, Hunter DJ, et al: The use of estrogens and progestins and the risk of breast cancer in postmenopausal women. N Engl J Med 332:1589, 1995.
Columbo N, Sessa C, Landoni F, et al: Cisplatin, vinblastine and bleomycin, combination chemotherapy in metastatic granulosa cell tumor of the ovary. Obstet Gynecol 67:265, 1986.
Cooper BC, Ritchie JM, Broghammer CL, et al: Preoperative serum vascular endothelial growth factor levels: Significance in ovarian cancer. Clin Cancer Res 8:3193–3197, 2002.
Cramer DW, Liberman EF, Titus-Ersntoff L, et al: Genital talc exposure and risk of ovarian cancer. Int J Cancer 81:351, 1999.
Cramer DW, Welch WR, Hutchinson GB, et al: Dietary animal fat in relation to ovarian cancer risk. Obstet Gynecol 63:833, 1984.
Crayford TJB, Campbell S, Bourne TH, et al: Benign ovarian cysts and ovarian cancer: A cohort study with implications for screening. Lancet 355:1060, 2000.
Creasman WT: New gynecologic cancer staging. Obstet Gynecol 75:287, 1990.
Creasman WT, DiSaia PJ: Screening in ovarian cancer. Am J Obstet Gynecol 165:7, 1991.
Creasman WT, Soper JT: Assessment of the contemporary management of germ cell malignancies of the ovary. Am J Obstet Gynecol 153:828, 1985.
Cushing B, Giller R, Ablin A, et al: Surgical resection alone is effective treatment for ovarian immature teratoma in children and adolescents: A report of the Pediatric Oncology Group and the Children's Cancer Group. Am J Obstet Gynecol 181:353, 1999.
Dembo AJ, Bush RS, Beale FA, et al: Ovarian carcinoma: Improved survival following abdominopelvic irradiation in patients with a completed pelvic operation. Am J Obstet Gynecol 134:793, 1979.
Dembo AJ, Davy M, Stenwig AE, et al: Prognostic factors in patients with stage I epithelial ovarian cancer. Obstet Gynecol 75:263, 1990.
DePriest PD, Gallion HH, Pavlik EJ, et al: Transvaginal sonography as a screening method for the detection of early ovarian cancer. Gynecol Oncol 65:408, 1997.
Dickersin GR, Kline IW, Scully RE: Small cell carcinoma of the ovary with hypercalcemia: A report of 11 cases. Cancer 49:188, 1982.
DiSaia PJ, Saltz A, Kagan AR, et al: Chemotherapeutic retroconversion of immature teratoma of the ovary. Obstet Gynecol 49:347, 1977.
Einhorn LH, Donahue J: Cis-diaminedichloroplatinum, vinblastine, and bleomycin combination chemotherapy in disseminated testicular cancer. Ann Intern Med 87:87, 1977.
Einhorn N, Sjovall K, Knapp RC, et al: Prospective evaluation of serum CA 125 levels for early detection of ovarian cancer. Obstet Gynecol 80:14–18, 1992.
Eisenkop SM, Friedman RL, Spirtos NM: The role of secondary cytoreductive surgery in the treatment of patients with recurrent epithelial ovarian carcinoma. Cancer 88:144–153, 2000.
Epenetos AA, Munro AJ, Stewart S, et al: Antibody guided irradiation of advanced ovarian cancer with intraperitoneally administered radiolabeled monoclonal antibodies. J Clin Oncol 5:1890, 1987.
Evans AT, Gaffey TA, Malkasian GD: Clinical pathologic review of 118 granulosa and 82 theca cell tumors. Obstet Gynecol 55:231, 1980.
Finch A, Beiner M, Lubinski J, et al: Salpingo-oophorectomy and the risk of ovarian, fallopian tube, and peritoneal cancers in women with a BRCA1 or BRCA2 mutation. JAMA 296:185–192, 2006.
Finkler NJ, Benacerraf B, Lavin PT, et al: Comparison of serum CA-125, clinical impression, and ultrasound in the preoperative evaluation of ovarian masses. Obstet Gynecol 72:659, 1988.
Fishman A, Kudelka AP, Tresukosol D, et al: Leuprolide acetate for treating refractory or persistent ovarian granulosa cell tumor. J Reprod Med 41:393, 1997.
Ford D, Easton DF, Bishop DT, et al: Risks of cancer in BRCA1-mutation carriers. Lancet 343:692, 1994.
Fox H: Primary neoplasia of the female peritoneum. Histopathology 23:103, 1993.
Frasci G, Conforti S, Zullo F, et al: A risk model for ovarian carcinoma patients using CA 125. Cancer 77:1122, 1996.
Frias AE, Li H, Keeney GL, et al: Preoperative serum level of inhibin A is an independent prognostic factor for the survival of postmenopausal women with epithelial ovarian carcinoma. Cancer 85:465, 1999.
Fromm GL, Gershenson DM, Silva EG: Papillary serous carcinoma of the peritoneum. Obstet Gynecol 75:89, 1990.
Gershenson DM: Menstrual and reproductive function after treatment with combination chemotherapy for malignant ovarian germ cell tumors. J Clin Oncol 6:270, 1988.
Gershenson DM: The obsolescence of second-look laparotomy in the management of malignant ovarian germ cell tumors [letter to the editor]. Gynecol Oncol 52:283, 1994.
Gershenson DM, Copeland LJ, Del Junco G, et al: Second-look laparotomy in the management of malignant germ cell tumors of the ovary. Obstet Gynecol 67:789, 1986.

Gershenson DM, Copeland LJ, Kavanagh JJ, et al: Treatment of malignant non-dysgerminomatous germ cell tumors of the ovary with vincristine, actinomycin-D, and cyclophosphamide. Cancer 56:2756, 1985.

Gershenson DM, Copeland LJ, Kavanagh JJ, et al: Treatment of metastatic stromal tumors of the ovary with cisplatin, doxorubicin, and cyclophosphamide. Obstet Gynecol 70:765, 1987.

Gershenson DM, Del Junco G, Herson J, et al: Endodermal sinus tumor of the ovary: The MD Anderson experience. Obstet Gynecol 61:194, 1983.

Gershenson DM, Del Junco G, Silva EG, et al: Immature teratoma of the ovary. Obstet Gynecol 68:624, 1986.

Gershenson DM, Morris M, Cangir A, et al: Treatment of malignant germ cell tumors of the ovary with bleomycin, etoposide, and cisplatin (BEP). J Clin Oncol 8:715, 1990.

Gershenson DM, Silva EG: Metastatic serous ovarian tumors of low malignant potential. Cancer 65:578, 1990.

Gershenson DM, Silva EG, Levy L, et al: Ovarian serous tumors with invasive peritoneal implants. Cancer 82:1096, 1998.

Gershenson DM, Silva EG, Mitchell MF, et al: Transitional cell carcinoma of the ovary: A matched control study of advanced-stage patients treated with cisplatin-based chemotherapy. Am J Obstet Gynecol 168:1178, 1993.

Gershenson DM, Silva EG, Tortolero-Luna G, et al: Serous borderline tumors of the ovary with noninvasive peritoneal implants. Cancer 83:2157, 1998.

Gloeckler LA, Hankey BF, Edwards BK (eds): Cancer statistics review 1973–87. Prepared by the Surveillance Program, Division of Cancer Prevention and Control, National Cancer Institute, Bethesda, MD, 1992. Available from U.S. Department of Health and Human Services, National Institutes of Health (NIH), National Cancer Institute, PB90-2789.

Goff BA, Mandel LS, Melancon CH, Muntz HG: Frequency of symptoms of ovarian cancer in women presenting to primary care clinics. JAMA 291:2705–2712, 2004.

Goldhirsch A, Greiner R, Dreher E, et al: Treatment of advanced ovarian cancer with surgery, chemotherapy, and consolidation of response by whole-abdominal radiotherapy. Cancer 62:40, 1988.

Goldhirsch A, Triller JF, Greiner R, et al: Computed tomography prior to second-look operation in advanced ovarian cancer. Obstet Gynecol 62:630, 1983.

Goldstein SR, Subramanyam B, Snyder JR, et al: The postmenopausal cystic adnexal mass: The potential role of ultrasound in conservative management. Obstet Gynecol 73(1):8–10, 1989.

Greenlee RT, Murray T, Bolden S, et al: Cancer Statistics, 2000. CA Cancer J Clin 50:7, 2000.

Grimes DA, Economy KE: Primary prevention of gynecologic cancers. Am J Obstet Gynecol 172:227, 1995.

Gross TP, Schlesselman JJ: The estimated effect of oral contraceptive use on the cumulative risk of epithelial ovarian cancer. Obstet Gynecol 83:419, 1994.

Guthrie D, Davy MLJ, Philips PR: A study of 656 patients with "early" ovarian cancer. Gynecol Oncol 17:363, 1984.

Hacker NF: Systematic pelvic and paraaortic lymphadenectomy for advanced ovarian cancer: Therapeutic advance or surgical folly? Gynecol Oncol 56:325, 1995.

Hankinson SE, Colditz GA, Hunter DJ, et al: A quantitative assessment of oral contraceptive use and risk of ovarian cancer. Obstet Gynecol 80:708, 1992.

Hankinson SE, Hunter DJ, Colditz GA, et al: Tubal ligation, hysterectomy, and risk of ovarian cancer: a prospective study. JAMA 270:2813, 1993.

Harrison ML, Hoskins P, du Bois A, et al: Small cell of the ovary, hypercalcemic type-analysis of combined experience and recommendation for management. A GCIG study. Gynecol Oncol 100:233, 2006.

Hart WR, Norris HJ: Borderline and malignant mucinous tumors of the ovary: Histologic criteria and clinical behavior. Cancer 31:1031, 1973.

Hartge P, Schiffman MH, Hoover R, et al: A case-control study of epithelial ovarian cancer. Am J Obstet Gynecol 161:10, 1989.

Healy DL, Burger HG, Mamers P, et al: Elevated serum inhibin concentrations in postmenopausal women with ovarian tumors. N Engl J Med 329:1539, 1993.

Heintz AP, Van Oosterom AT, Trimbos JB, et al: The treatment of advanced ovarian carcinoma (I): Clinical variables associated with prognosis. Gynecol Oncol 30:347–358, 1988.

Hellstrom A-C, Tegerstedt G, Silfversward C, Pettersson F: Malignant mixed mullerian tumors of the ovary: Histopathologic and clinical review of 36 cases. Int J Gynecol Cancer 9:312, 1999.

Herbst AL: The epidemiology of ovarian carcinoma and the current status of tumor markers to detect disease. Am J Obstet Gynecol 170:1099, 1994.

Herbst AL: Letter to the editor: Efficacy of transvaginal sonographic screening in asymptomatic women at risk for ovarian cancer. Gynecol Oncol 80:421, 2001.

Higgins RV, van Nagell JR, Donaldson ES, et al: Transvaginal sonography as a screening method for ovarian cancer. Gynecol Oncol 34:402, 1989.

Hoerl HD, Hart WR: Primary ovarian mucinous cystadenocarcinomas. Am J Surg Pathol 22:1449, 1998.

Homesley HD, Bundy BN, Hurteau JA, et al: Bleomycin, etoposide, and cisplatin combination therapy of ovarian granulosa cell tumors and other stromal malignancies: A Gynecologic Oncology Group Study. Gynecol Oncol 72:131, 1999.

Hoskins WJ, Bundy BN, Thigpen JT, Omura GA: The influence of cytoreductive surgery on recurrence-free interval and survival in small-volume stage III epithelial ovarian cancer: A Gynecologic Oncology Group study. Gynecol Oncol 47:159, 1992.

Hunter VJ, Daly L, Helms M, et al: The prognostic significance of CA-125 half-life in patients with ovarian cancer who have received primary chemotherapy after surgical cytoreduction. Am J Obstet Gynecol 163:1164, 1990.

Ignoffo RJ: Overview of bevacizumab: A new cancer therapeutic strategy targeting vascular endothelial growth factor. Am J Health Syst Pharm 61(21 Suppl 5):S21–S26, 2004.

Iversen O-E, Skaarland E: Ploidy assessment of benign and malignant ovarian tumors by flow cytometry. Cancer 60:82, 1987.

Jaaback K, Johnson N: Intraperitoneal chemotherapy for the initial management of primary epithelial ovarian cancer. Cochrane Database Syst Rev 1:CD005340, 2006.

Jacobs A, Deppe G, Cohen CJ: Combination chemotherapy of ovarian granulosa cell tumor with cis-platinum and doxorubicin. Gynecol Oncol 14:294, 1982.

Jacobs I, Lancaster J: The molecular genetics of sporadic and familial epithelial ovarian cancer. Int J Gynecol Cancer 6:337, 1996.

Jemal A, Siegel R, Ward E, et al: Cancer statistics, 2006. CA Cancer J Clin 56:106–130, 2006.

Jones HW III, Homesley HD: Successful treatment of pseudo-myxoma peritonei of ovarian origin with cis-platinum, doxorubicin, and cyclophosphamide. Gynecol Oncol 22:257, 1985.

Julian CG, Barrett JM, Richardson RC, et al: Bleomycin, vinblastine, and cis-platinum in the treatment of advanced endodermal sinus tumors. Obstet Gynecol 56:396, 1980.

Kaldor JM, Day NE, Pettersson F, et al: Leukemia following chemotherapy for ovarian cancer. N Engl J Med 322:1, 1990.

Kamiya N, Mizuno K, Kawai M, et al: Simultaneous measurement of CA 125, CA 19-9, tissue polypeptide antigen, and immunosuppressive acidic protein to predict recurrence of ovarian cancer. Obstet Gynecol 76:417, 1990.

Karlan BY, Baldwin RL, Lopez-Luevanos E, et al: Peritoneal serous papillary carcinoma, a phenotypic variant of familial ovarian cancer: Implications for ovarian cancer screening. Am J Obstet Gynecol 180:917, 1999.

Kennedy AW, Biscotti CV, Hart WR, et al: Histologic correlates of progression-free interval and survival in ovarian clear cell adenocarcinoma. Gynecol Oncol 50:334, 1993.

Kennedy AW, Markman M, Biscotti CV, et al: Survival probability in ovarian clear cell adenocarcinoma. Gynecol Oncol 74:108, 1999.

Kerlikowske K, Brown JS, Grady DG: Should women with familial ovarian cancer undergo prophylactic oophorectomy? Obstet Gynecol 80:700, 1992.

Kim DS, Park MI: Maternal and fetal survival following surgery and chemotherapy of endodermal sinus tumor of the ovary during pregnancy: A case report. Obstet Gynecol 73:503, 1989.

Kirmani S, Lucas WE, Kim S, et al: A phase II trial of intraperitoneal cisplatin and etoposide as salvage treatment for minimal residual ovarian carcinoma. J Clin Oncol 9:649, 1991.

Klemi PJ, Joensuu H, Salmi T: Prognostic value of flow cytometric DNA content analysis in granulosa cell tumor of the ovary. Cancer 65:1189, 1990.

Knapp RC, Friedman EA: Aortic lymph node metastases in early ovarian cancer. Am J Obstet Gynecol 119:1013–1017, 1975.

Koonings PP, Campbell K, Mishell DR, Grimes DA: Relative frequency of primary ovarian neoplasms: A 10-year review. Obstet Gynecol 74:921, 1989.

Kurjak A, Kupesic S, Breye B, et al: The assessment of ovarian tumor angiogenesis: What does three-dimensional power Doppler add? Ultrasound Obstet Gynecol 12:136, 1998.

Kurman RJ, Norris HJ: Embryonal carcinoma of the ovary: A clinical pathogenic entity distinct from endodermal sinus tumor resembling embryonal carcinoma of the adult testes. Cancer 38:2420, 1976.

Kurman RJ, Norris HJ: Malignant germ cell tumors of the ovary. Hum Pathol 8:551, 1977.

Lack EE, Perez-Atayde AR, Murthy ASK, et al: Granulosa theca cell tumors in premenarcheal girls: A clinical and pathologic study of 10 cases. Cancer 48:1846, 1981.

Lappohn RE, Burger HG, Bouma J, et al: Inhibin as a marker for granulosa-cell tumors. N Engl J Med 321:790, 1989.

Lawton FG, Hilton C, Mould JJ, et al: Short-duration (three cycles) cisplatin combination chemotherapy with alkylating agent consolidation in advanced epithelial ovarian cancer. Gynecol Oncol 40:225–229, 1991.

Leake JF, Currie JL, Rosenshein NB, Woodruff D: Long-term follow-up of serous ovarian tumors of low malignant potential. Gynecol Oncol 47:150, 1992.

Lehner R, Wenzl R, Heinzl H, et al: Influence of delayed staging laparotomy after laparoscopic removal of ovarian masses later found malignant. Obstet Gynecol 92:967, 1998.

Leminen A, Lehtovirta P: Spread of ovarian cancer after laparoscopic surgery: Report of eight cases. Gynecol Oncol 75:387, 1999.

Lenhard RE Jr: Cancer statistics: A measure of progress. CA Cancer J Clin 46:3, 1996.

Lim-Tan SK, Cajigas HE, Scully RE: Ovarian cystectomy for serous borderline tumors: A follow-up of 35 cases. Obstet Gynecol 72:775, 1988.

Linder D, McCaw BK, Hecht F: Pathogenetic origin of benign ovarian teratomas. N Engl J Med 292:63, 1975.

Loizzi V, Chan JK, Osann K, et al: Survival outcomes in patients with recurrent ovarian cancer who were treated with chemoresistance assay-guided chemotherapy. Am J Obstet Gynecol 189:1301–1307, 2003.

Loizzi V, Cormio G, Resta L, et al: Neoadjuvant chemotherapy in advanced ovarian cancer: A case-control study. Int J Gynecol Cancer 15:217–223, 2005.

Low JJH, Perrin LC, Crandon AJ, et al: Conservative surgery to preserve ovarian function in patients with malignant ovarian germ cell tumors. Cancer 89:391, 2000.

Lu KH, Garber JE, Cramer DW, et al: Occult ovarian tumors in women with BRCA1 or BRCA2 mutations undergoing prophylactic oophorectomy. J Clin Oncol 18:2728, 2000.

Lund B, Williamson P: Prognostic factors for outcome of and survival after second-look laparotomy in patients with advanced ovarian carcinoma. Obstet Gynecol 76:617, 1990.

Lynch HT, Watson P, Bewtra C, et al: Hereditary ovarian cancer: Heterogeneity in age at diagnosis. Cancer 67:1460, 1991.

Maggino T, Gadducci A, D'Addario V, et al: Prospective multicenter study on CA 125 in postmenopausal pelvic masses. Gynecol Oncol 54:117, 1994.

Mahdavi A, Pejovic T, Nezhat F: Induction of ovulation and ovarian cancer: A critical review of the literature. Fertil Steril 85:819–826, 2006.

Maiman M, Seltzer V, Boyce J: Laparoscopic excision of ovarian neoplasms subsequently found to be malignant. Obstet Gynecol 77:563, 1991.

Malfetano JH: The appendix and its metastatic potential in epithelial ovarian cancer. Obstet Gynecol 69:396, 1987.

Markman M: CA-125: An evolving role in the management of ovarian cancer. J Clin Oncol 14:1411, 1996.

Markman M, Berek JS, Blessing JA, et al: Characteristics of patients with small-volume residual ovarian cancer unresponsive to cisplatin-based IP chemotherapy: Lessons learned from a Gynecologic Oncology Group phase II trial of ip cisplatin and recombinant α-interferon, Gynecol Oncol 45:3, 1992.

Markman M, Bundy BN, Alberts DS, et al: Phase III trial of standard-dose intravenous cisplatin plus paclitaxel versus moderately high-dose carboplatin followed by intravenous paclitaxel and intraperitoneal cisplatin in small-volume stage III ovarian carcinoma: An intergroup study of the Gynecologic Oncology Group, Southwestern Oncology Group, and Eastern Cooperative Oncology Group. J Clin Oncol 19:1001–1007, 2001.

Markman M, Lewis JL Jr, Saigo P, et al: Impact of age on survival of patients with ovarian cancer. Gynecol Oncol 49:236, 1993.

Markman M, Liu PY, Rothenberg ML, et al: Pretreatment CA-125 and risk of relapse in advanced ovarian cancer. J Clin Oncol 24:1454–1458, 2006.

Markman M, Liu PY, Wilczynski S, et al: Phase III randomized trial of 12 versus 3 months of maintenance paclitaxel in patients with advanced ovarian cancer after complete response to platinum and paclitaxel-based chemotherapy: A Southwest Oncology Group and Gynecologic Oncology Group trial. J Clin Oncol 21:2460–2465, 2006.

McGuire WP, Hoskins W, Brady MF, et al: Cyclophosphamide and cisplatin compared with paclitaxel and cisplatin in patients with stage III and stage IV ovarian cancer. N Engl J Med 334:1, 1996.

McMeekin DS, Burger RA, Manetta A, et al: Endometrioid adenocarcinoma of the ovary and its relationship to endometriosis. Gynecol Oncol 59:81, 1995.

Menczer J, Ben-Baruch G, Modan M, Brenner H: Intraperitoneal cisplatin chemotherapy versus abdominopelvic irradiation in ovarian carcinoma patients after second-look laparotomy. Cancer 63:1509, 1989.

Menczer M, Modan M, Brenner J, et al: Abdominal pelvic irradiation for stage II-IV ovarian carcinoma patients with limited or no residual disease at second-look laparotomy after completion of cis-platinum-based combination chemotherapy. Gynecol Oncol 24:149, 1986.

Menon U, Skates SJ, Lewis S, et al: Prospective study using the risk of ovarian cancer algorithm to screen for ovarian cancer. J Clin Oncol 23:7919–7926, 2005.

Mishell DR: Contraception. N Engl J Med 320:777, 1989.

Modan B, Hartge P, Hirsh-Yechezkel G, et al: Parity, oral contraceptives, and the risk of ovarian cancer among carriers and noncarriers of a *BRCA1* or *BRCA2* mutation. N Engl J Med 345:235–240, 2001.

Mooney J, Silva E, Tornos C, et al: Unusual features of serous neoplasms of low malignant potential during pregnancy. Gynecol Oncol 65:830, 1997.

Morgan RJ, Braly P, Leong L, et al: Phase II trial of combination intraperitoneal cisplatin and 5-fluorouracil in previously treated patients with advanced ovarian cancer: Long-term follow-up. Gynecol Oncol 77:433, 2000.

Morice P, Dubernard G, Rey A, et al: Results of interval debulking surgery compared with primary debulking surgery in advanced stage ovarian cancer. J Am Coll Surg 197:955–963, 2003.

Mulhollan TJ, Silva EG, Tornos C, et al: Ovarian involvement by serous surface papillary carcinoma. Int J Gynecol Pathol 13:120, 1994.

Munkarah A, Gershenson DM, Levenback C, et al: Salvage surgery for chemorefractory ovarian germ cell tumors. Gynecol Oncol 55:217, 1994.

Muntz HG, Jones MA, Godd BA, et al: Malignant mixed müllerian tumors of the ovary. Cancer 76:1209, 1995.

Narod SA, Risch H, Moslehi R, et al: Oral contraceptives and the risk of hereditary ovarian cancer. N Engl J Med 339:424, 1998.

Neijt JP, Engelholm SA, Tuxen MK, et al: Exploratory phase III study of paclitaxel and cisplatin versus paclitaxel and carboplatin in advanced ovarian cancer. J Clin Oncol 18:3084, 2000.

Nichols CR, Tricot G, Williams SD, et al: Dose-intensive chemotherapy in refractory germ cell cancer: A phase I/II trial of high-dose carboplatin and etoposide with autologous bone marrow transplant. J Clin Oncol 7:932, 1989.

Norris HJ, Zirkin HJ, Benson WL: Immature (malignant) teratoma of the ovary: A clinical and pathologic study of 58 cases. Cancer 37:2359, 1976.

Numnum TM, Rocconi RP, Whitworth J, Barnes MN: The use of bevacizumab to palliate symptomatic ascites in patients with refractory ovarian carcinoma. Gynecol Oncol 102:425–428, 2006.

Ozols RF: Intraperitoneal therapy in ovarian cancer: Time's up. J Clin Oncol 9:197, 1991.

Ozols RF, Bundy BN, Greer BE, et al: Phase III trial of carboplatin and paclitaxel compared with cisplatin and paclitaxel in patients with optimally resected stage III ovarian cancer: A Gynecologic Oncology Group study. J Clin Oncol 21:3194–3200, 2003.

Panici PB, Maggioni A, Hacker N, et al: Systematic aortic and pelvic lymphadenectomy versus resection of bulky nodes only in optimally debulked advanced ovarian cancer: A randomized clinical trial. J Natl Cancer Inst 97:560–566, 2005.

Parmar MK, Ledermann JA, Colombo N, et al: Paclitaxel plus platinum-based chemotherapy versus conventional platinum-based chemotherapy in women with relapsed ovarian cancer: The ICON4/AGO-OVAR-2.2 trial. Lancet 361:2099–2106, 2003.

Patsner B: Is there a role for CT scanning to monitor therapy of optimally debulked patients with advanced ovarian epithelial cancer? Int J Gynecol Cancer 4:19, 1994.

Pavlik EJ, DePriest PD, Gallion HH, et al: Ovarian volume related to age. Gynecol Oncol 77:410, 2000.

Peccatori F, Bonazzi C, Chiari S, et al: Surgical management of malignant ovarian germ-cell tumors: 10 years' experience of 129 patients. Obstet Gynecol 86:367, 1995.

Pecorelli S, Creasman WT, Pettersson F, et al: FIGO annual report on the results of treatment in gynaecological cancer, vol 23, Milano, Italy. J Epidemiol Biostat 1998.

Pfisterer J, Vergote I, Du Bois A, et al: Combination therapy with gemcitabine and carboplatin in recurrent ovarian cancer. Int J Gynecol Cancer 15(Suppl 1):36–41, 2005.

Piver MS, Malfetano J, Baker TR, Hempling RE: Five-year survival for stage Ic or stage I grade 3 epithelial ovarian cancer treated with cisplatin-based chemotherapy. Gynecol Oncol 46:35, 1992.

Prat J: Ovarian tumors of borderline malignancy (tumors of low malignant potential): A critical appraisal. Adv Anat Pathol 6:247, 1999.

Pujade-Lauraine E, Guastalla JP, Colombo N, et al: Intraperitoneal recombinant interferon gamma in ovarian cancer patients with residual disease at second-look laparotomy. J Clin Oncol 14:343, 1996.

Randall ME, Barrett RJ, Spirtos NM, et al: Chemotherapy, early surgical reassessment and hyperfractionated abdominal radiotherapy in stage III ovarian cancer: Results of a Gynecologic Oncology Group study. Int J Radiat Oncol Biol Phys 34:139, 1996.

Rebbeck TR, Levin AM, Eisen A, et al: Breast cancer risk after bilateral prophylactic oophorectomy in BRCA1 mutation carriers. J Natl Cancer Inst 91:1475, 1999.

Reed WC: Small cell carcinoma of the ovary with hypercalcemia: Report of a case of survival without recurrence 5 years after surgery and chemotherapy. Gynecol Oncol 56:452, 1995.

Reimer RR, Hoover R, Fraumeini JF, et al: Acute leukemia after alkylating-agent therapy of ovarian cancer. N Engl J Med 297:177, 1977.

Risch HA, Jain M, Marrett LD, et al: Dietary fat intake and risk of epithelial ovarian cancer. J Natl Cancer Inst 86:1409, 1994.

Robey SS, Silva EG, Gershenson DM, et al: Transitional cell carcinoma in high-grade high-stage ovarian carcinoma. Cancer 63:839, 1989.

Ronnett BM, Kurman RJ, Zahn CM, et al: Pseudomyxoma peritonei in women: A clinicopathologic analysis of 30 cases with emphasis on site of origin, prognosis, and relationship to ovarian mucinous tumors of low malignant potential. Hum Pathol 26:509, 1990.

Rose PG, Nerenstone S, Brady MF, et al: Secondary surgical cytoreduction for advanced ovarian carcinoma. N Engl J Med 351:2489–2497, 2004.

Rossing MA, Daling JR, Weiss NS, et al: Ovarian tumors in a cohort of infertile women. N Engl J Med 331:771, 1994.

Rota SM, Zanetta G, Ieda N, et al: Clinical relevance of retroperitoneal involvement from epithelial ovarian tumors of borderline malignancy. Int J Gynecol Cancer 9:477, 1999.

Rubin SC, Randall TC, Armstrong KA, et al: Ten-year follow-up of ovarian cancer patients after second-look laparotomy with negative findings. Obstet Gynecol 93:21, 1999.

Rustin G, Nelstrop AE, McClean P, et al: Defining response of ovarian carcinoma to initial chemotherapy according to serum CA-125. J Clin Oncol 14:1545, 1996.

Samanth KK, Black WC: Benign ovarian stromal tumors associated with free peritoneal fluid. Am J Obstet Gynecol 197:538, 1970.

Santoso JT, Tang D, Lane SB, et al: Adenovirus-based p53 gene therapy in ovarian cancer. Gynecol Oncol 59:171, 1995.

Schelling M, Braun M, Kuhn W, et al: Combined transvaginal B-mode and color Doppler sonography for differential diagnosis of ovarian tumors: results of a multivariate logistic regression analysis. Gynecol Oncol 77:78, 2000.

Schildkraut JM, Bastos E, Berchuck A: Relationship between lifetime ovulatory cycles and overexpression of mutant p53 in epithelial ovarian cancer. J Natl Cancer Inst 89:932, 1997.

Schlesselman JJ: Net effect of oral contraceptive use on the risk of cancer in women in the United States. Obstet Gynecol 85:793, 1995.

Schneider J, Erasun F, Hervas JL, et al: Normal pregnancy and delivery 2 years after adjuvant chemotherapy for grade III immature ovarian teratoma. Gynecol Oncol 29:245, 1988.

Schwartz PE, Rutherford TJ, et al: Neoadjuvant chemotherapy for advanced ovarian cancer: Long-term survival. Gynecol Oncol 72:93–99, 1999.

Schwartz PE, Smith JP: Treatment of ovarian stromal tumors. Am J Obstet Gynecol 125:402, 1976.

Scully RE: Gonadoblastoma: A gonadal tumor related to dysgerminoma (seminoma) and capable of sex hormone production. Cancer 6:455, 1953.

Scully RE: Sex cord-stromal tumors. In Blaustein A (ed): Pathology of the Female Genital Tract, 4th ed. New York, Springer-Verlag, 1994.

Scully RE: Influence of origin of ovarian cancer on efficacy of screening [commentary]. Lancet 355:1028, 2000.

Scully RE, Young RH, Clement PB: Tumors of the ovary, maldeveloped gonads, fallopian tube, and broad ligament. In Atlas of Tumor Pathology, fascicle 23, series 3, Washington, DC, Armed Forces Institute of Pathology, 1998.

Serov SF, Scully RE, Sobin LH: Histological Typing of Ovarian Tumors. Geneva, World Health Organization, 1973.

Sevinc A, Buyukberber S, Sari R, et al: Elevated serum CA-125 levels in hemodialysis patients with peritoneal, pleural, or pericardial fluids. Gynecol Oncol 77:254, 2000.

Shakfeh AM, Woodruff JD: Primary ovarian sarcomas: Report of 46 cases and review of literature. Obstet Gynecol Surv 42:331, 1987.

Shalev E, Eliyahu S, Peleg D, Tsabari A: Laparoscopic management of adnexal cystic masses in postmenopausal women. Obstet Gynecol 83:594, 1994.

Sharp F, Blackett AD, Leake RE, Berek JS: Conclusions and recommendations from the Helene Harris Memorial Trust Fund Biennial International Forum on ovarian cancer, May 4–7, 1995, Glasgow, UK. Int J Gynecol Cancer 5:449, 1995.

Shushan A, Peretz T, Uziely B, et al: Ovarian cysts in premenopausal and postmenopausal tamoxifen-treated women with breast cancer. Am J Obstet Gynecol 174:141, 1996.

Sjövall K, Nilsson B, Einhorn N: Different types of rupture of the tumor capsule and the impact on survival in early ovarian carcinoma. Int J Gynecol Cancer 4:333, 1994.

Slamon DJ, Godolophin W, Jones LA, et al: Studies of the HER-2/neu protooncogene in human breast and ovarian cancer. Science 244:707, 1989.

Sonnendecker EW: Is routine second-look laparotomy for ovarian cancer justified? Gynecol Oncol 31:249–255, 1988.

Sorbe B, Frankendal B, Veress B: Importance of histologic grading in the prognosis of epithelial cancer. Obstet Gynecol 59:576, 1982.

Stein AL, Koonings PP, Schlaerth JB, et al: Relative frequency of malignant paraovarian tumors: Should paraovarian tumors be aspirated? Obstet Gynecol 75:1029, 1990.

Swanson SA, Norris HJ, Kelsten ML, Wheeler JE: DNA content of juvenile granulosa tumors determined by flow cytometry. Int J Gynecol Pathol 9:101, 1990.

Talerman A: Germ cell tumors of the ovary. In Blaustein A (ed): Pathology of the Female Genital Tract, 4th ed. New York, Springer-Verlag, 1994.

Tan C, Sedrakyan A, Browne J, et al: The evidence on the effectiveness of management for malignant pleural effusion: A systematic review. Eur J Cardiothorac Surg 29:829–838, 2006.

Tangir J, Zelterman D, Ma W, et al: Reproductive function after conservative surgery and chemotherapy for malignant germ cell tumors of the ovary. Obstet Gynecol 101:251, 2003.

Tay EH, Grant PT, Gebski V, Hacker NF: Secondary cytoreductive surgery for recurrent epithelial ovarian cancer. Obstet Gynecol 99:1008–1013, 2002.

Tewari KS, Mehta RS, Burger RA, et al: Conservation of in vitro drug resistance patterns in epithelial ovarian carcinoma. Gynecol Oncol 98:360–368, 2005.

Thigpen JT, Blessing JA, Ball H, et al: Phase II trial of paclitaxel in patients with progressive ovarian carcinoma after platinum-based chemotherapy: A Gynecologic Oncology Group study. J Clin Oncol 12:1748, 1994.

Travis LB, Holowaty EJ, Bergfelt K, et al: Risk of leukemia after platinum-based chemotherapy for ovarian cancer. N Engl J Med 340:351, 1999.

Tresukosol D, Kudelka AP, Edwards CL, et al: Recurrent ovarian granulosa cell tumor: A case report of a dramatic response to taxol. Int J Gynecol Cancer 5:156, 1995.

Trimbos JB, Parmar M, Vergote I, et al: International Collaborative Ovarian Neoplasm Trial 1 and Adjuvant Chemotherapy in Ovarian Neoplasm Trial: Two parallel randomized phase III trials of adjuvant chemotherapy in patients with early-stage ovarian carcinoma. J Natl Cancer Inst 95:105–112, 2003.

Troche V, Hernandez E: Neoplasia arising in dysgenetic gonads. Obstet Gynecol Surv 41:74, 1986.

Trope C, Kaern J, Vergote IB, et al: Are borderline tumors of the ovary overtreated both surgically and systemically? A review of four prospective randomized trials including 253 patients with borderline tumors. Gynecol Oncol 51:236, 1993.

Twickler DM, Forte TB, Santos Ramos R, et al: The Ovarian Tumor Index predicts risk for malignancy. Cancer 86:2280–2290, 1999.

Vaccarello L, Rubin SC, Vlamis V, et al: Cytoreductive surgery in ovarian carcinoma patients with a documented previously complete surgical response. Gynecol Oncol 57:61, 1995.

Valentin L, Ameye L, Testa A, et al: Ultrasound characteristics of different types of adnexal malignancies. Gynecol Oncol 102:41–48, 2006.
van der Burg MEL, van Lent M, Buyse M, et al: The effect of debulking surgery after induction chemotherapy on the prognosis in advanced epithelial ovarian cancer. N Engl J Med 332:629, 1995.
Van Nagell JR Jr, DePriest PD, Puls LE, et al: Ovarian cancer screening in asymptomatic postmenopausal women by transvaginal sonography. Cancer 68:458–462, 1991.
Vasey PA, Jayson GC, Gordon A, et al: Phase III randomized trial of docetaxel-carboplatin versus paclitaxel-carboplatin as first-line chemotherapy for ovarian carcinoma. J Natl Cancer Inst 96:1682–1691, 2004.
Venesmaa P: Epithelial ovarian cancer: Impact of surgery and chemotherapy on survival during 1977–1990. Obstet Gynecol 84:8, 1994.
Venn A, Watson L, Bruinsma F, et al: Risk of cancer after use of fertility drugs with in-vitro fertilisation. Lancet 354(9190):1586–1590, 1990.
Vergote I, De Wever I, Tjalma W, et al: Neoadjuvant chemotherapy or primary debulking surgery in advanced ovarian carcinoma: A retrospective analysis of 285 patients. Gynecol Oncol 71:431, 1998.
Vergote IB, Winderen M, De Vos LN, Trope CG: Intraperitoneal radioactive phosphorus therapy in ovarian cancer. Cancer 71:2250, 1993.
Von Hoff DD, Kronmal R, Salmon SE, et al: A Southwest Oncology Group study for the use of a human tumor cloning assay for predicting response in patients with ovarian cancer. Cancer 67:20, 1991.
Walker JL, Armstrong DK, Huang HQ, et al: Intraperitoneal catheter outcomes in a phase III trial of intravenous versus intraperitoneal chemotherapy in optimal stage III ovarian and primary peritoneal cancer: A Gynecologic Oncology Group study. Gynecol Oncol 100:27–32, 2006.
Warner E: Neurotoxicity of cisplatin and taxol. Int J Gynecol Cancer 5:161, 1995.
Warner E, Foulkes W, Goodwin P, et al: Prevalence and penetrance of *BRCA1* and *BRCA2* gene mutations in unselected Ashkenazi Jewish women with breast cancer. J Natl Cancer Inst 91:1241, 1999.
Wertheim I, Fleischhacker D, McLachlin CM, et al: Pseudomyxoma peritonei: A review of 23 cases. Obstet Gynecol 84:17, 1994.
Westhoff C, Randall MC: Ovarian cancer screening: Potential effect on mortality. Am J Obstet Gynecol 165:502, 1991.
Whittemore AS, Harris R, Itnyre J, et al: Characteristics relating to ovarian cancer risk: Collaborative analysis of 12 U.S. case-control studies. Am J Epidemiol 136:1184, 1992.
Wick MR, Mills SE, Dehner LP, et al: Serous papillary carcinomas arising from the peritoneum and ovaries. Int J Gynecol Pathol 8:179, 1989.
Willemse PHB, Aalders JG, Bouma J, et al: Long-term survival after vinblastine, bleomycin, and cisplatin treatment in patients with germ cell tumors of the ovary: An update. Gynecol Oncol 28:268, 1987.
Willemse PHB, Oosterhuis JW, Aalders JG, et al: Malignant struma ovarii by ovariectomy, thyroidectomy, and ^{131}I administration. Cancer 60:182, 1987.
Williams S, Blessing JA, Liao SY, et al: Adjuvant therapy of ovarian germ cell tumors with cisplatin, etoposide, and bleomycin: A trial of the Gynecologic Oncology Group. J Clin Oncol 12:701, 1994.
Williams SD, Blessing JA, DiSaia PJ, et al: Second-look laparotomy in ovarian germ cell tumors: The Gynecologic Oncology Group experience. Gynecol Oncol 52:287, 1994.
Williams SD, Blessing JA, Hatch KD, Homesley HD: Chemotherapy of advanced dysgerminoma: Trials of the Gynecologic Oncology Group. J Clin Oncol 9:1950, 1991.
Wingo PA, Tong T, Bolden S: Cancer statistics, 1995. CA Cancer J Clin 45:8, 1995.
Wu PC, Huang RL, Lang JH, et al: Treatment of malignant ovarian germ cell tumors with preservation of fertility: A report of 28 cases. Gynecol Oncol 40:2, 1991.
Yancik R, Ries LG, Yates JW: An analysis of surveillance, epidemiology, and end results program data. Am J Obstet Gynecol 154:639, 1986.
Young RC, Walton LA, Ellenberg SS, et al: Adjuvant therapy in stage I and stage II epithelial ovarian cancer: Results of two prospective randomized trials. N Engl J Med 332:1021, 1990.
Young RH, Dickersin GR, Scully RE: Juvenile granulosa cell tumor of the ovary. Am J Surg Pathol 8:575, 1984.
Young RH, Gilks CB, Scully RE: Mucinous tumors of the appendix associated with mucinous tumors of the ovary and pseudomyxoma peritonei. Am J Surg Pathol 15:415, 1991.
Young RH, Olivia E, Scully RE: Small cell carcinoma of the ovary, hypercalcemia type. Am J Surg Pathol 18:1102, 1994.
Young RH, Scully RE: Ovarian Sertoli-Leydig cell tumors: A clinicopathological analysis of 207 cases. Am J Surg Pathol 9:543, 1985.
Young RH, Welch WR, Dickersin GR, et al: Ovarian sex cord tumor with annular tubules. Cancer 50:1384, 1982.
Zambetti M, Escobedo A, Pilotti S, De Palo G: Cis-platinum/vinblastine/bleomycin combination chemotherapy in advanced or recurrent granulosa cell tumors of the ovary. Gynecol Oncol 36:317, 1990.
Zanetta G, Bonazzi C, Cantu MG, et al: Survival and reproductive function after treatment of malignant germ cell ovarian tumors. J Clin Oncol 19:1015, 2001.

Neoplastic Diseases of the Fallopian Tubes

34

Screening, Benign and Malignant Epithelial and Germ Cell Neoplasms, Sex-Cord Stromal Tumors

Deborah Jean Dotters and Vern L. Katz

KEY TERMS AND DEFINITIONS

Hydrops Tubae Profluens. A symptom complex of intermittent, watery, or serosanguinous vaginal discharge; crampy pain; and an adnexal mass that may disappear after the pain is noted. This complex occasionally occurs in patients with tubal carcinoma, but most patients do not have this complex.

Primary Tubal Carcinoma. An adenocarcinoma usually of papillary serous variety arising within the lumen of the oviduct. A transition from nonneoplastic to malignant tubal epithelium must be demonstrated to confirm the diagnosis.

Tubal Carcinoma Staging Summary. **Stage 1:** Confined to the tubes

Stage 2: Spread to the ovaries, uterus, or other pelvic tissues

Stage 3: Intraperitoneal spread or involvement of retroperitoneal nodes

Stage 4: Metastases to liver parenchyma, outside the peritoneum, or malignant pleural effusion

Primary cancers of the fallopian tube are among the rarest of gynecologic malignancies, comprising only 0.3% of gynecologic cancers. Almost all are adenocarcinomas of papillary serous histology, arising from the tubal epithelium. The approximate incidence in the United States is 3.6 cases per million women per year. Carcinomas metastatic to the fallopian tube occur much more commonly, usually arising from the ovary, uterus, or GI tract. This chapter reviews current information, with particular emphasis on diagnosis, natural history, and management.

ETIOLOGY AND AGE DISTRIBUTION

The etiology of fallopian tube carcinoma is unclear. Large reviews have found an association with tuberculous salpingitis, chronic pelvic inflammatory disease, infertility, low parity, and tubal endometriosis. Rosen et al. found a decreased risk associated with oral contraceptive use and pregnancy, similar to that seen in ovarian cancer. More recently, several reports have documented an increase in fallopian tube cancers in families with germline mutations in the *BRCA1* and *BRCA2* genes. Retrospective studies have shown that 17% of women with tubal carcinoma harbor germline *BRCA* mutations. Additionally, occult carcinomas and foci of epithelial dysplasias have been found in the tubes of asymptomatic *BRCA*-positive women undergoing risk-reducing bilateral salpingo-oophorectomy. This suggests that the *BRCA1*/*BRCA2* mutations have a role in fallopian tube tumorigenesis. Overexpression of P53 has been described in patients with fallopian tube carcinoma as well as in adjacent, dysplastic fallopian tube epithelium. Overexpression of Her2-*neu* and *c-myc* has also been described.

The mean age of women with fallopian tube carcinoma ranges from 54 to 65 years, with a wide range (Fig. 34-1). In a review of 105 cases, Alvarado-Cabrero and colleagues noted a range of 26 to 85 years, with an average of 58.5 years. A recent study by Cass and associates compared *BRCA*-associated fallopian tube cancers with sporadic cases and found the *BRCA*-associated cases to occur at a somewhat younger age than the sporadic cases (57 vs. 65 years), similar to what is seen in *BRCA*-associated ovarian cancers.

DIAGNOSIS

These tumors are often asymptomatic, and the diagnosis is frequently not made until the patient has undergone surgical

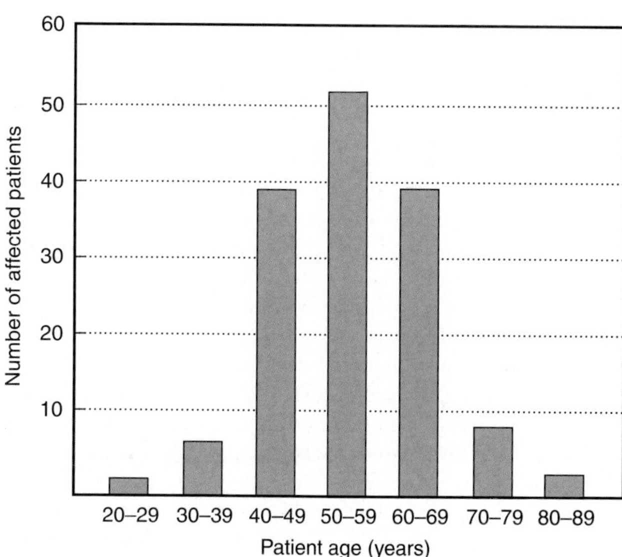

Figure 34-1. Histogram illustrating age distribution of patients with tubal carcinomas. (From Podczaski E, Herbst AL: Cancer of the vagina and fallopian tube. In Knapp RC, Berkowitz RS (eds): Gynecologic Oncology. New York, Macmillan, 1983.)

exploration. The symptoms and spread pattern of fallopian tube carcinoma are largely related to the degree of obstruction of the distal tube. If the fimbriated end of the tube is obstructed, by either tumor or previous injury or infection, the by-products of tumor growth, such as blood and increased serous fluid, distend the tube and are discharged intermittently through the vagina. If the distal portion of the fallopian tube is patent, the malignancy spreads more easily out the distal end of the tube, resulting in tumor seeding of the peritoneal cavity, ascites, and omental caking. Intraperitoneal spread may also occur as the tumor grows through the muscular wall of the tube.

The most commonly reported signs and symptoms of fallopian tube cancer are abnormal vaginal bleeding (47.5%), a palpable adnexal mass (61%), crampy lower abdominal pain (39%), and watery discharge (20%). Latzko's triad of intermittent serosanguinous discharge, colicky pain, and a mass is considered pathognomonic of fallopian tube cancer, but only occurs in about 15% of patients. Hydrops tubae profluens is the term used to describe the expulsion of watery fluid from the vagina by contraction of a distended tube blocked at the distal end.

Abnormal cervical cytology is occasionally present in women with fallopian tube carcinoma, with a reported range of 10% to 40%. A woman with a Pap smear showing adenocarcinoma or atypical glandular cells (AGUS) in whom endocervical and endometrial carcinoma have been ruled out should be evaluated with a CA 125 and endovaginal ultrasound scan to rule out ovarian and/or tubal malignancy. Classic ultrasound findings are that of a fluid-filled, tubular or ovoid mass with internal papillations, mural nodules, or septations, separate from the uterus and ovaries. Ascites may be present. Duplex sonography may show low impedance flow. CA 125 is elevated in more than 85% of women with fallopian tube carcinoma and is useful in monitoring response to treatment or evaluating someone in whom the disease is suspected. It is not recommended as a screening test. In a patient with fallopian tube cancer, the level of CA 125 is an independent prognostic factor in both disease-free and overall survival.

PATHOLOGY

On gross examination, the fallopian tube containing primary adenocarcinoma often appears dilated and may resemble a hydrosalpinx. When the tube is opened, an infiltrating tumor is visible (Figs. 34-2 and 34-3). Sometimes it is difficult to be certain that the tumor is of tubal origin, and confusion with metastatic carcinoma, particularly from the ovary, can be a diagnostic problem. Hu et al. created a set of criteria in 1950 to allow the diagnosis of fallopian tube carcinoma, modified by Sedlis in 1978, and are useful currently (See the following box).

Figures 34-4 and 34-5 demonstrate a primary fallopian tube carcinoma showing a papillary-alveolar pattern. More than 90% of fallopian tube carcinomas are papillary serous adenocarcinomas, which appear and behave like ovarian serous carcinomas. Less commonly, endometrioid or clear cell adenocarcinomas may occur and, rarely, sarcomas, carcinosarcomas, germ cell tumors, or gestational trophoblastic tumors. Fallopian tube carcinomas can arise in either tube with equal frequency and occasionally may be bilateral.

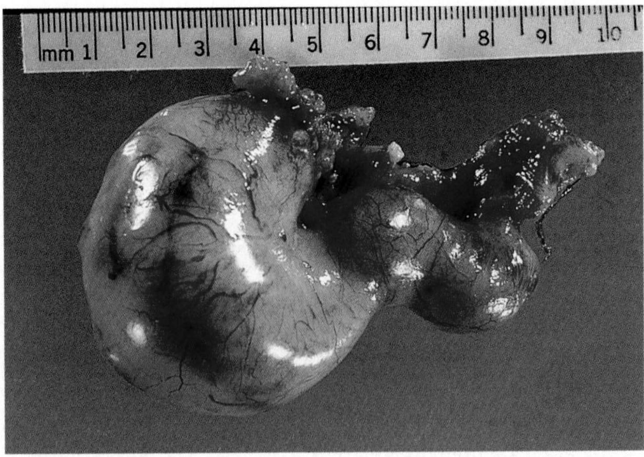

Figure 34-2. Adenocarcinoma of the fallopian tube revealing a dilated fallopian tube with an obstructed fimbriated end. (From Voet RL: Color Atlas of Obstetric and Gynecologic Pathology. St. Louis, Mosby-Wolfe, 1997, fig. 5.29.)

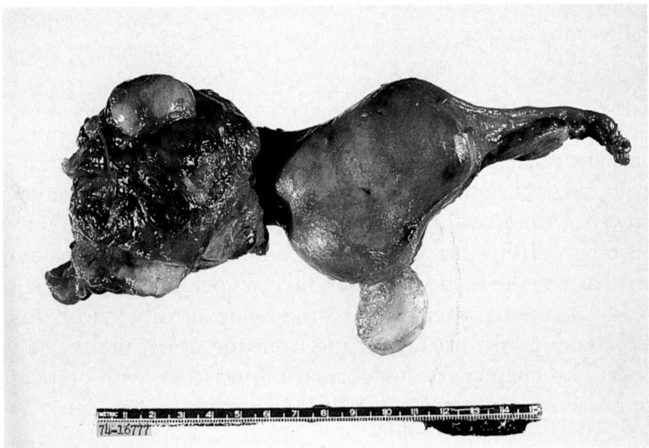

Figure 34-3. Adenocarcinoma of the fallopian tube. (From Anderson MC, Robboy SJ, Russell P: The fallopian tube. In Robboy SJ, Anderson MC, Russell P (eds): Pathology of the Female Reproductive Tract. Edinburgh, Churchill Livingstone, 2002, fig. 16.57.)

Diagnostic Criteria for Fallopian Tube Carcinaoma

1. The main tumor lies in the tube and arises from the endosalpinx.
2. The histologic pattern reproduces the epithelium of tubal mucosa (papillary).
3. Transition can be demonstrated between the malignant and nonmalignant tubal epithelium.
4. The ovaries and uterus must be normal or contain less tumor than the fallopian tube.

STAGING AND NATURAL HISTORY

Fallopian tube carcinoma is surgically staged. The pattern of spread, surgical approach, and staging are very similar to that of epithelial ovarian carcinoma (Table 34-1).

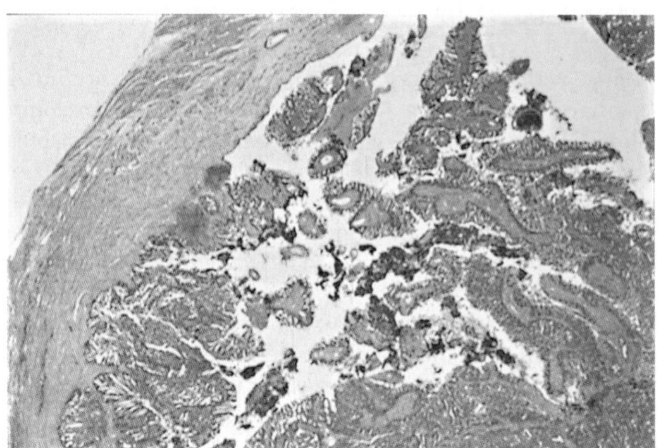

Figure 34-4. Microscopic appearance adenocarcinoma of fallopian tube confined to the endosalpinx with minimal invasion into the muscular wall. (From Voet RL: Color Atlas of Obstetric and Gynecologic Pathology. St. Louis, Mosby-Wolfe, 1997, fig. 5.31.)

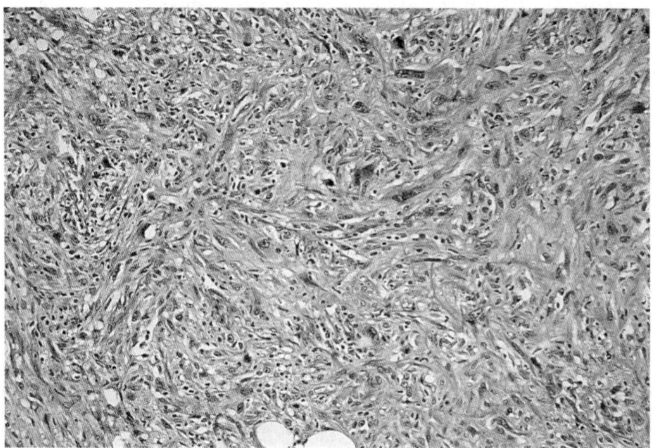

Figure 34-5. Poorly differentiated tubal carcinoma. (From Anderson MC, Robboy SJ, Russell P: The fallopian tube. In Robboy SJ, Anderson MC, Russell P (eds): Pathology of the Female Reproductive Tract. Edinburgh, Churchill Livingstone, 2002, fig. 16.63.)

Table 34-1 FIGO Staging System for Tubal Carcinoma

Stage	Characteristics
0	Carcinoma in situ (limited to tubal mucosa)
I	Growth limited to the fallopian tube
IA	Growth is limited to one tube with extension into the submucosa and/or muscularis, but not penetrating the serosal surface; no ascites
IB	Growth is limited to both tubes with extension into the submucosa and/or muscularis, but not penetrating the serosal surface; no ascites
IC	Tumor either stage IA or IB, but with tumor extension through or onto the tubal serosa or with ascites present containing malignant cells or with positive peritoneal washings.
II	Growth involving one or both fallopian tubes with pelvic extension
IIA	Extension and/or metastasis to the uterus and/or ovaries
IIB	Extension to other pelvic tissues
IIC	Tumor either stage IIA or IIB and with ascites present containing malignant cells or with positive peritoneal washings
III	Tumor involves one or both fallopian tubes with peritoneal implants outside the pelvis and/or positive retroperitoneal or inguinal nodes. Superficial liver metastasis equals stage III. Tumor appears limited to the true pelvis, but with histologically proven malignant extension to the small bowel or omentum
IIIA	Tumor is grossly limited to the true pelvis with negative nodes, but with histologically confirmed microscopic seeding of abdominal peritoneal surfaces
IIIB	Tumor involving one or both tubes with histologically confirmed implants of abdominal peritoneal surfaces, none exceeding 2 cm in diameter, lymph nodes are negative
IIIC	Abdominal implants greater than 2 cm in diameter and/or positive retroperitoneal or inguinal nodes
IV	Growth involving one or both fallopian tubes with distant metastases. If pleural effusion is present, there must be positive cytology to be stage IV. Parenchymal liver metastases equals stage IV.

Note: Staging for fallopian tube is by the surgical-pathologic system. Surgical findings designating stage are determined before tumor debulkin.

The carcinoma is initially confined to the lumen of the tube, but may penetrate through the muscularis to the serosa or out the fimbriated end of the tube. The carcinoma may then spread intraperitoneally to involve the parietal peritoneum, surface of the bowel, and omentum. The peritoneum is the most frequent site of metastatic spread. Lymphatic spread also occurs to both pelvic and paraaortic nodes with approximately equal frequency. Tamimi and Figge noted metastases to the paraaortic nodes in 5 of 15 patients, and these nodes were the only site of metastatic disease in two patients. Others have noted an incidence of greater than 30% of nodal metastasis in patients whose disease was clinically grossly confined to the fallopian tube. Thus, the retroperitoneal nodes must be considered as sites of common spread, and thorough surgical staging with pelvic and paraaortic node dissection is important, especially in patients with apparent stage I disease.

Prognosis in tubal carcinoma is most strongly related to the extent, or stage, of the disease. The grade of tumor and presence of vascular invasion also affect prognosis. Peters et al. noted that in stage I, the depth of invasion of the tubal wall is of prognostic significance. In advanced stages, the amount of residual tumor after debulking surgery is strongly correlated with survival, as in ovarian cancer. Gadducci noted a 55% 5-year survival rate in optimally debulked, advanced-stage patients (<1 cm residual disease) compared to a 21% 5-year survival in patients who were left with a larger residual tumor burden after debulking surgery. Fallopian tube cancer patients have a better prognosis, stage for stage, than their counterparts with ovarian cancer. In 2002, Kosary and colleagues published the following 5-year survival rates in a large, population-based study of more than 350 women with fallopian tube carcinoma: stage I, 95%; stage II, 76%; stage III, 69%; and stage IV, 45%.

MANAGEMENT

The surgical management of fallopian tube carcinoma is similar to that of ovarian cancer. Once the diagnosis is established, the goals of surgery are to remove as much tumor as is possible (optimal debulking, with residual disease < 1 cm) and to determine the stage of the tumor so that the need for postoperative adjuvant therapy can be determined and prognostic information can be shared with the patient and her family. This generally includes a total abdominal hysterectomy and bilateral salpingo-oophorectomy; collection of four-quadrant cytology (collecting peritoneal washings from the pelvis, right and left paracolic gutters, and diaphragm area above the right lobe of the liver); omentectomy; pelvic and paraaortic node dissection; and removal of as much visible tumor as possible. The importance of a thorough pelvic and paraaortic node dissection cannot be overemphasized because of the propensity for lymphatic spread of this tumor.

Patients with stage Ia or Ib fallopian tube carcinoma with no ascites, no intraoperative rupture, grade 1 tumor, no deep invasion into the muscular wall who have undergone comprehensive surgical staging do not require adjuvant therapy. Platinum-based systemic chemotherapy is usually recommended for all other patients with fallopian tube carcinoma. For advanced disease, combination chemotherapeutic regimens similar to those used in ovarian cancer are often used, such as carboplatin-paclitaxel. Radiation therapy has little, if any, role. The installation of intraperitoneal radiocolloids such as P32 has not been shown to be of value in preventing recurrences in early-stage disease. Because of the tendency for fallopian tube cancer to spread throughout the abdominal cavity, external beam radiation therapy cannot be administered in therapeutic doses without causing excessive side effects, minimizing its usefulness.

Measurement of serum CA 125 is generally used to follow patients with fallopian tube carcinoma during and after treatment. An elevation of the CA 125 level is usually the first sign of a clinical recurrence and precedes detection by symptoms or radiographic findings by an average of about 3 months.

MANAGEMENT OF *BRCA*-POSITIVE WOMEN

Women with a germline mutation in the *BRCA1* or *BRCA2* gene have as much as a 120-fold increased risk of developing fallopian tube carcinoma compared with the general population. Of all women with fallopian tube cancer, 16% to 17% have been shown to be positive for this mutation. In addition, *BRCA*-positive women undergoing risk-reducing salpingo-oophorectomy have been shown to have an increase in dysplastic lesions of the fallopian tube as well as occult carcinomas (2% to 10% of cases). The fimbria seems to be the preferred site of abnormalities of the fallopian tube in this group of women. Therefore, the following recommendations with respect to *BRCA*-positive women undergoing risk-reducing surgery (prophylactic salpingo-oophorectomy) seem prudent:

1. The entire tube, or as much as is possible, should be removed along with the ovary. Most authors do not think that a hysterectomy is necessary to remove the intramural portion of the tube, as these lesions are primarily distal.
2. Peritoneal fluid should be obtained for cytology.
3. The pathologist should be notified of the patient's high-risk status and the entire fallopian tube and ovary should be carefully sectioned with serial 2-mm sections or according to the SEE-FIM protocol (sectioning and extensively examining the fimbriated end of the fallopian tube) as described by Lee and colleagues.
4. The entire peritoneal cavity should be evaluated (laparoscopically or via laparotomy, depending on the operation being used) to look for seeding, studding, or other signs of carcinomatosis.

KEY POINTS

- Primary tubal carcinoma is the rarest gynecologic malignancy (0.3% 1.1%).
- Ninety percent of tubal cancers are metastatic, mostly from the ovary, uterus, or GI tract.
- The average age of patients with tubal carcinoma is 58 years.
- Predisposing factors for primary tubal carcinoma appear to be infertility, nulliparity or low parity, pelvic infection, and a family history of ovarian cancer. Women harboring germline mutations of *BRCA1* or *BRCA2* seem to be at especially high risk.
- The most common histologic subtype of fallopian tube carcinoma is papillary serous (90%).
- The triad of abnormal bleeding, adnexal mass, and watery discharge in a postmenopausal woman is suggestive of fallopian tube cancer, although few patients actually present with all three.
- The diagnosis of fallopian tube carcinoma should be considered for anyone with cervical cytology positive for adenocarcinoma or AGUS in whom the diagnosis of endometrial and endocervical cancers has been ruled out. It should also be considered for any woman with postmenopausal bleeding in whom a hysteroscopy or D & C fails to reveal a cause. Ultrasonography and CA 125 are useful diagnostic aids in this setting.
- Ultrasound findings suggestive of fallopian tube carcinoma include a fluid-filled, ovoid or sausage-shaped pelvic mass, with internal mural nodules or solid papillary projections, separate from the uterus and ovaries. Ascites may be present.
- The most common route of spread of fallopian tube carcinoma is to the peritoneal cavity and the retroperitoneal lymph nodes.
- Prognosis in tubal carcinoma is most strongly related to the stage of disease and the amount of residual tumor left after the initial debulking procedure.
- Platinum-based combination chemotherapy is the mainstay of adjuvant treatment for fallopian tube cancers beyond stages Ia and Ib.
- Thorough surgical staging and aggressive debulking surgery are the most important surgical principles for a successful outcome.
- When performing risk-reducing surgery (prophylactic bilateral salpingo-oophorectomy) in high-risk women, the entire fallopian tube should be removed along with the ovaries, peritoneal washings should be obtained for cytologic evaluation, and the entire tubes and ovaries should be serially sectioned by the pathologist at 2-mm intervals.

BIBLIOGRAPHY

Ajithkumar TV, Minimole AL, Manju MJ, Ashokkumar OS: Primary fallopian tube carcinoma. Obstet Gynecol Surv 60:247, 2005.

Agoff SN, Mendelin JE, Grieco VS, Garcia RL: Unexpected gynecologic neoplasms in patients with proven or suspected *BRCA-1* or *2* mutations. Am J Surg Pathol 26:171, 2002.

Alvarado-Cabrero I, Young RH, Vamvakas EC, et al: Carcinoma of the fallopian tube: A clinicopathologic study of 105 cases with observations on staging and prognostic factors. Gynecol Oncol 72:367, 1999.

Asmussen M, Kaern J, Kjoerstad K, et al: Primary adenocarcinoma localized to the fallopian tubes: Report on 33 cases. Gynecol Oncol 30:183, 1988.

Baekelandt M, Kock M, Wesling F, Gerris J: Primary adenocarcinoma of the fallopian tube: Review of the literature. Int J Gynecol Cancer 3:65, 1993.

Barakat R, Rubin SC, Saigo PE, et al: Second-look laparotomy in carcinoma of the fallopian tube. Obstet Gynecol 82:748, 1993.

Barakat RR, Rubin SC, Saigo PE, et al: Cisplatin-based combination chemotherapy in carcinoma of the fallopian tube. Gynecol Oncol 42:156, 1991.

Carcangiu ML, Radice P, Manoukian S, et al: Atypical epithelial proliferation in fallopian tubes in prophylactic salpingo-oophorectomy specimens from BRCA1 and BRCA2 germline mutation carriers. Int J Gynecol Pathol 23:35, 2003.

Cass I, Holschneider C, Datta N, et al: BRCA-mutation associated fallopian tube carcinoma. Obstet Gynecol 106:1327, 2005.

Clayton NL, Jaaback KS, Hirshowitz L: Primary fallopian tube carcinoma—the experience of a UK cancer centre and a review of the literature. J Obstet Gynecol 25:694, 2005.

Colgan TJ, Murphy J, Cole DE, et al: Occult carcinoma in prophylactic oophorectomy specimens. Am J Surg Pathol 25:1283, 2001.

Daya D, Young RH, Scully RE: Endometrioid carcinoma of the fallopian tube resembling an adnexal tumor of probable wolffian origin: A report of six cases. Int J Gynecol Pathol 11:122, 1992.

Gadducci A: Current management of fallopian tube carcinoma. Curr Opin Obstet Gynecol 14:27, 2002.

Hefler LA, Rosen AC, Graf AH, et al: The clinical value of serum concentrations of cancer antigen 125 in patients with primary fallopian tube carcinoma. Cancer 89:1555, 2000.

Hellström AC, Silfversward C, Nillson B, Petterson F: Carcinoma of the fallopian tube: A clinical and histopathologic review. The Radiumhemmet series. Int J Gynecol Cancer 4:395, 1994.

Hirai Y, Kaku S, Teshima H, et al: Clinical study of primary carcinoma of the fallopian tube: Experience with 15 cases. Gynecol Oncol 34:20, 1989.

Hu CY, Taymor ML, Hertig AT: Primary carcinoma of the fallopian tube. Am J Obstet Gynecol 59:58, 1950.

Lacy MQ, Hartmann CL, Kenney GL, et al: c-erbB-2 and p53 expression in fallopian tube carcinoma. Cancer 75:2891, 1995.

Lee Y, Medeiros F, Kindelberger D, et al: Advances in the recognition of tubal intraepithelial carcinoma. Adv Anat Pathol 13:1, 2006.

Levine DA, Argenta PA, Yee CJ, et al: Fallopian tube and primary peritoneal carcinomas associated with *BRCA* mutations. J Clin Oncol 21:4222, 2003.

Medeiros F, Muto MG, Lee Y, et al: The tubal fimbria is a preferred site for early adenocarcinoma in women with familial ovarian cancer syndrome. Am J Surg Pathol 30:230, 2006.

Morris M, Gershenson DM, Burke TW, et al: Treatment of fallopian tube carcinoma with cisplatin, doxorubicin, and cyclophosphamide. Obstet Gynecol 76:1020, 1990.

Peters WA, Andersen WA, Hopkins MP, et al: Prognostic features of carcinoma of the fallopian tube. Obstet Gynecol 71:757, 1988.

Podczaski E, Herbst AL: Cancer of the vagina and fallopian tube. In Knapp RC, Berkowitz RS (eds): Gynecologic Oncology, 2nd ed. New York, Macmillan, 1990.

Podratz KC, Podczaski ES, Gaffey TA, et al: Primary carcinoma of the fallopian tube. Am J Obstet Gynecol 154:1319, 1986.

Puls LE, Davey DD, DePriest D, et al: Immunohistochemical staining for CA-125 in fallopian tube carcinomas. Gynecol Oncol 48:360, 1993.

Rose PG, Piver MS, Tsukada Y: Fallopian tube cancer: The Roswell Park experience. Cancer 66:2661, 1990.

Rosen B, Aziz S, Narod S, et al: Hereditary and reproductive influences on fallopian tube carcinoma (abstract). Gynecol Oncol 76:231, 2000.

Sedlis A: Carcinoma of the fallopian tube. Surg Clin North Am 58:121, 1978.

Tamini HK, Figge DC: Adenocarcinoma of the uterine tube: Potential for lymph node metastases. Am J Obstet Gynecol 141:132, 1981.

Tresukosol D, Kudelka AP, Edwards CL, et al: Primary fallopian tube adenocarcinoma: Clinical complete response after salvage treatment with high-dose paclitaxel. Gynecol Oncol 58:258, 1995.

Wu JP, Tanner WS, Fardal PM: Malignant mixed müllerian tumor of the uterine tube. Obstet Gynecol 41:707, 1981.

Zweemer RP, van Diest PJ, Verheijen RHM, et al: Molecular evidence linking primary cancer of the fallopian tube to *BRCA1* mutations, Gynecol Oncol 76:45, 2000.

Gestational Trophoblastic Disease 35

Hydatidiform Mole, Nonmetastatic and Metastatic Gestational Trophoblastic Tumor: Diagnosis and Management

John J. Kavanagh and David M. Gershenson

KEY TERMS AND DEFINITIONS

Androgenesis. Impregnation of an inactive egg by a paternal haploid sperm that duplicates its chromosomes to provide a diploid complement. This results in a complete mole.

Choriocarcinoma. A morphologic term applied to a highly malignant type of trophoblastic neoplasia in which both the cytotrophoblast and syncytiotrophoblast grow in a malignant fashion.

Complete Mole. A molar pregnancy with swelling of all placental villi. Fetal tissues are absent.

Gestational Trophoblastic Disease (GTD). Disease that results from the abnormal proliferation of trophoblast associated with pregnancy. The disease is considered persistent or recurrent if it remains active or returns after therapeutic intervention.

Hydatidiform Mole. A placental abnormality involving swollen placental villi and trophoblastic hyperplasia with loss of fetal blood vessels. There are two types: partial and complete.

Invasive Mole. A variant of hydatidiform mole in which the hydropic villi invade the myometrium or blood vessels. It may spread to extrauterine sites.

Partial Mole. A molar pregnancy with some normal and some swollen villi plus fetal, cord, and/or amniotic membrane elements.

Placental-Site Trophoblastic Tumor. A rare type of GTD arising in the uterus that secretes human placental lactogen and human chorionic gonadotrophin (HCG).

Gestational trophoblastic disease (GTD) refers to the spectrum of abnormalities of the trophoblast associated with pregnancy. These neoplasias have been known for hundreds of years, and they specifically secrete HCG. The availability of extremely sensitive and specific assays to measure HCG allows prediction of the clinical status of the disease as well as monitoring of treatment. The initial use of methotrexate in 1956 by Li and associates to successfully treat malignant trophoblastic disease completely altered the prognosis of patients with these tumors and represented a milestone in the cure of human tumors by chemotherapeutic agents.

This chapter presents the current classification of GTDs and the factors that appear to be associated with their development. The methods of diagnosis, therapy, and follow-up of these patients are reviewed.

CHARACTERISTICS

Trophoblastic tissue normally shares certain characteristics with malignancies, such as the ability to divide rapidly, to invade locally, and occasionally to metastasize to distant sites such as the lung, yet these activities usually cease at the end of pregnancy, and the trophoblasts disappear. However, in GTD, abnormal growth and development continue beyond the end of pregnancy.

Hydatidiform Mole

A hydatidiform mole has three morphologic characteristics: (1) a mass of vesicles (distended villi) that appear as large, grapelike dilations (Fig. 35-1); (2) a loss of fetal blood vessels, which are either diminished or absent from the villi; and (3) hyperplasia of the syncytiotrophoblast and cytotrophoblast.

The terms *complete mole* and *partial mole* have been used to describe the variations of molar pregnancies. With a complete mole, all placental villi are swollen, and the fetus, cord, and amniotic membranes are absent. With partial molar pregnancy, only some chorionic villi are swollen, and fetal tissues are present, such as amniotic membrane, cord, or even rarely a full-term fetus. The fetus is usually chromosomally abnormal. With a partial mole, the trophoblastic hyperplasia is limited to the syncytiotrophoblast.

The genetics of molar pregnancy has been extensively studied. In normal pregnancy, half the chromosomes of the conceptus are paternal and the other half are maternal, resulting in a diploid content. In complete mole, only paternal chromosomes are believed to be present; there are 46 chromosomes and nearly always 46,XX, although a few moles with 46,XY karyotype have been reported. The development of complete mole appears to result from the fertilization of an "empty egg," one with an absent or inactive nucleus. The haploid paternal set of chromosomes from the sperm impregnate the inactive egg. These

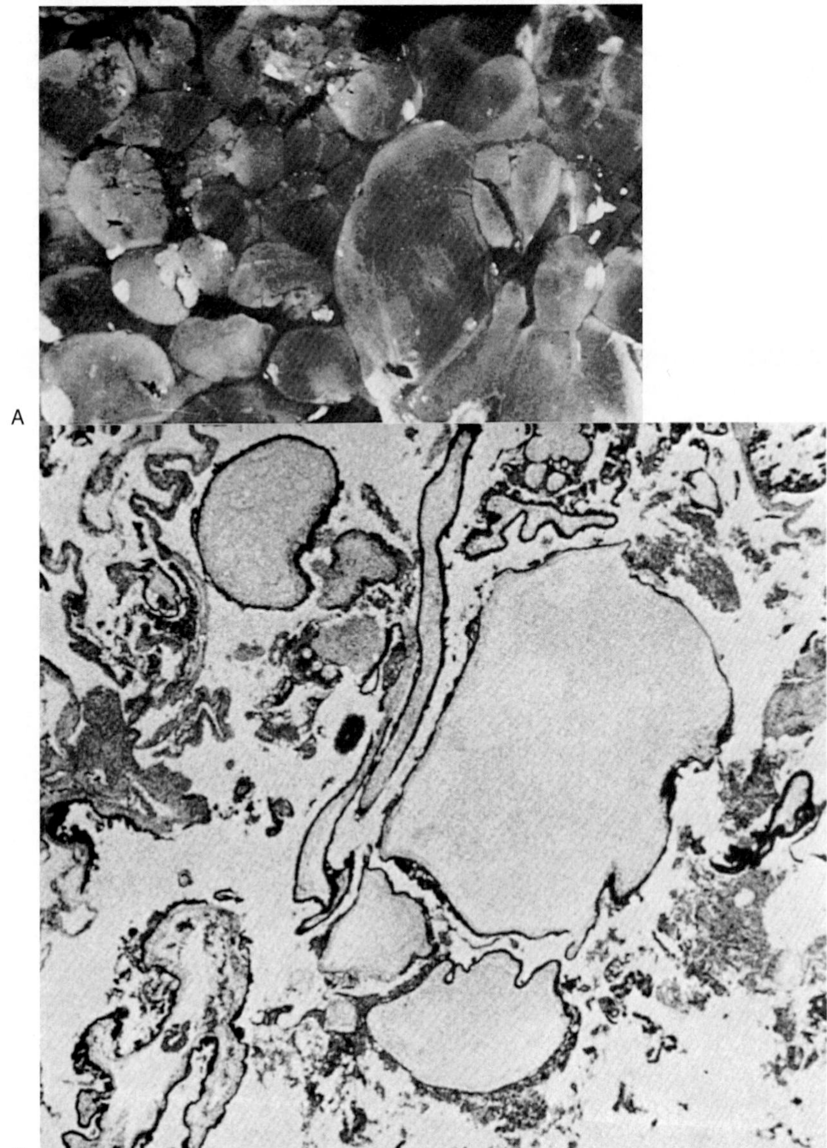

Figure 35-1. **A,** Hydatidiform mole. A few vesicles approach 1 cm in diameter. The background is formed by smaller vesicles. **B,** Hydatidiform mole aborted by suction curettage. A large intact vesicle is near the center. Many vesicles, however, have been ruptured and have collapsed. (From Bigelow B: Gestational trophoblast disease. In Blaustein A [ed]: Pathology of the Female Genital Tract, 2nd ed. New York, Springer-Verlag, 1982.)

paternal chromosomes then duplicate to give the diploid number, a process known as androgenesis, the development of an embryo due only to chromosomes from an X-bearing sperm (Fig. 35-2). In the rare case of complete mole with an XY chromosomal content, the empty egg appears to be fertilized by two haploid sperm, one X and one Y.

Incomplete, or partial, moles are usually triploid and have 69 chromosomes of both maternal and paternal origin. The most common mechanism for the origin of partial mole (Fig. 35-3) is a haploid egg being fertilized by two sperm, resulting in three sets of chromosomes. Alternatively, triploidy could result when an abnormal diploid sperm fertilizes the haploid egg. It is also possible for an abnormal diploid egg to be fertilized by a haploid sperm, but this latter mechanism usually results in an abnormal conceptus with congenital abnormalities rather than a partial mole. Partial mole is often difficult to diagnose and may present as a missed abortion in the second trimester. Although these fetuses are usually abnormal, Watson et al. noted that some partial moles have occurred with phenotypically normal fetuses. In such cases, the uterus is small for dates. As noted by Lage and associates, a few partial moles are diploid, and these very rare cases may be less sensitive to chemotherapy than triploid moles if subsequent GTD develops.

Partial moles are rarely associated with the subsequent development of GTD. Bagshawe and colleagues reported that neoplasia requiring chemotherapy occurs in approximately one in 200 cases of partial mole compared with one in 12 with complete mole. However, Rice and coworkers noted 16 of 240 partial moles (6.6%) had malignant sequelae, all of which responded to chemotherapy. Goldstein and colleagues summarized a number of published reports that indicated that GTD followed partial mole in 39 of 1125 (3.5%) cases. Despite rare subsequent malignancy, patients with partial moles need the same follow-up as those with complete moles.

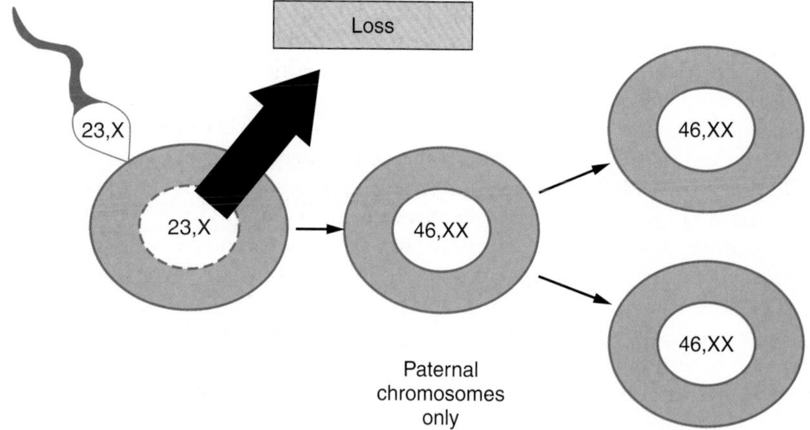

Figure 35-2. Paternal chromosomal origin of a complete classic mode (46,XX). *Left to right:* Entry of normal sperm with haploid set of 23,X into egg whose 23,X haploid set is lost; egg is taken over by paternal chromosomes, which duplicate (without cell's division) to reach requisite complement of 46. Observe that virtually the same result can be obtained through a fertilization by two sperm gaining entry into an empty egg" (dispermy). (From Szulman AE, Surti UL: The syndromes of partial and complete molar gestation. Clin Obstet Gynecol 27:172, 1984.)

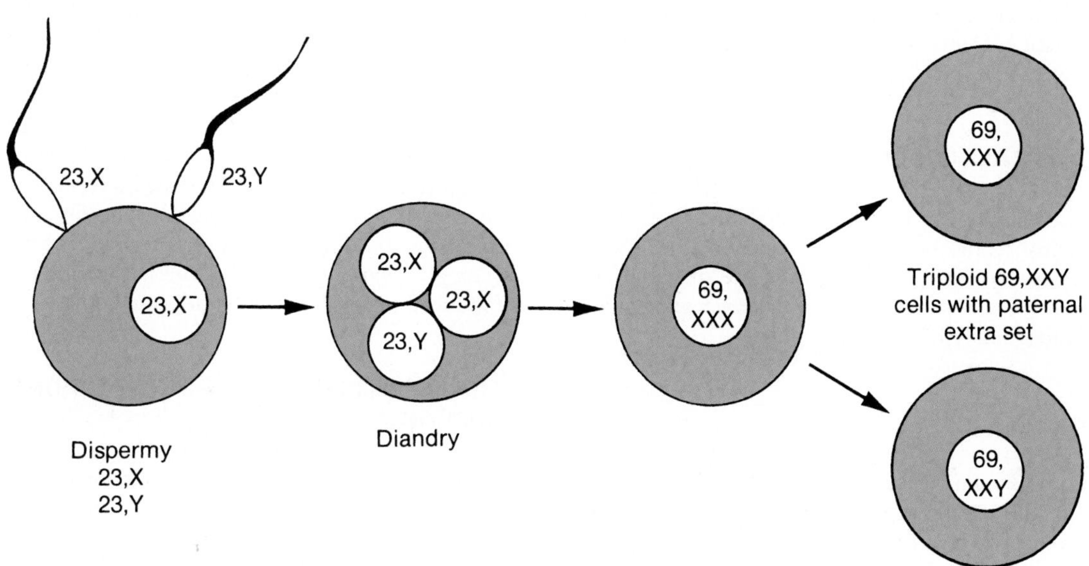

Figure 35-3. Triploid chromosomal origin of partial mole (69,XXY-dispermy). Fertilization of an egg equipped with a normal 23,X complement by two independently produced sperm (dispermy) to give total of 69 chromosomes. Observe that triploidy can also result through fertilization by sperm carrying father's total complement of 46,XY. (From Szulman AE, Surti UL: The syndromes of partial and complete molar gestation. Clin Obstet Gynecol 27:172, 1984.)

Choriocarcinoma

Choriocarcinomas are malignancies that occur after or in association with pregnancy, although the same histologic tumor can develop without pregnancy as a primary neoplasm in the ovaries. The prognosis for primary gonadal choriocarcinomas, which also occur in testes, is worse than for those associated with gestation.

The diagnosis is made histologically, and the term is applied to the finding of malignant cytotrophoblast and syncytiotrophoblast. Chorionic villi are absent. These tumors tend to be hemorrhagic and necrotic. The latter is common because these tumors frequently outgrow their blood supply. Metastases are common.

Most, but not all, gestational choriocarcinomas develop after molar pregnancies. Trophoblastic tissue normally regresses within 2 to 3 weeks after delivery, including cells that may have spread to the lung. The normal processes leading to this regression are unknown, but the finding of trophoblastic cells in the uterus more than 3 weeks after delivery should lead one to consider the possibility of choriocarcinoma.

It is important to recognize that persistent or metastatic GTD has several histologic patterns. The level of HCG determines tumor activity and guides therapeutic intervention.

Placental-Site Trophoblastic Tumor

The term placental-site trophoblastic tumor (trophoblastic pseudotumor) was introduced by Young and Scully to describe a rare tumor that consists of excessive groups of mononucleate and multinucleate trophoblastic cells at the implantation site accompanied by an inflammatory cell reaction. Immunohistochemical studies have shown that the cells of these tumors tend to stain more for human placental lactogen than for HCG, and both HCG and human placental lactogen should be monitored. The tumor can lead to hemorrhage and uterine perforation. It tends to be locally invasive, and most patients do not develop metastases. Hysterectomy is the treatment of choice. Baergen and associates reported 55 of their own patients, and an additional 180 cases from a literature review. In the results of the combined studies, there were 186 treated with hysterectomy. Ninety-four also received chemotherapy. In the combined patient population, there was an 80% to 86% survival rate at 48 months.

Chemotherapy is usually administered for metastatic disease when it occurs, but is less effective with these tumors than with other gestational trophoblastic tumors, which is another reason for prompt operative treatment. EMA/CO (etoposide, high-dose methotrexate with citrovorin (folinic acid) rescue, actinomycin D, cyclophosphamide, and vincristine [Oncovin]) has been reported on by Ajithkumar and colleagues for the treatment of metastatic placental-site trophoblastic tumor, achieving a response rate of 71% and a complete response rate of 38%.

EPIDEMIOLOGY AND INCIDENCE

Extensive investigation has been performed to ascertain the factors that enhance the occurrence of trophoblastic disease. The major areas that have been evaluated are maternal age, history of fetal wastage or hydatidiform mole, geographic and racial distribution, and ABO blood groupings.

Hydatidiform Mole

There is wide variation in the reported incidence of hydatidiform mole. The rates are usually expressed in terms of molar gestations per numbers of pregnancies. Studies by Berkowitz and associates and Eifel and associates showed that in the United States, the rate is estimated to be approximately one in 1500 to 2000 pregnancies and in one in 600 therapeutic abortions. According to the study by Eifel and colleagues, the rates from Southeast Asia are 5 to 15 times higher with much larger variations, and rates up to 13 per 1000 have been reported by Altieri and colleagues. The high rates reported in some studies result from hospital-based rather than population-based statistics. As already noted, hydatidiform mole develops because of abnormal fertilization.

Maternal age is an extremely important risk factor. The lowest rates are among women in their 20s and 30s, with a great increase in those older than age 40, after which the risk progressively increases with age. There is also an increase in risk among those younger than age 20, but the magnitude is not nearly as great as it is among older women. An additional risk factor is a history of hydatidiform mole, which increases the risk of subsequent mole by 20 to 40 times. Previous recurrent spontaneous abortion is also a risk factor.

The increased frequency among those of lower socioeconomic status as well as in underdeveloped areas, particularly in Southeast Asia, has led to the suggestion that poor nutrition is a factor in the development of this disease. However, evidence is conflicting, and as noted by Grimes, a dietary cause for hydatidiform mole has not been supported. A report by Palmer and associates suggests a slight increase in risk of GTD (but not hydatidiform mole) with oral contraceptive use, particularly if conception occurs while using oral contraceptives.

The risk appears to vary with race and ethnic origin. In Southeast Asia, the rates are double for Eurasians compared with those of Chinese, Malaysian, or Indian origin. Studies from the United States across racial groups by Hayashi and colleagues, Gul and Yilmazturk, and Matsuura and colleagues have produced inconsistent results. These studies have shown that black women have a higher, lower, or similar incidence to that in white women. Mexicans and Filipinos appear to have elevated rates compared with Japanese and Chinese.

Choriocarcinoma

Choriocarcinoma occurs in approximately 3% to 5% of those who have previously had a complete mole. However, Secki and colleagues recently reported choriocarcinoma after partial mole. In Western countries, choriocarcinomas are reported at rates between 0.014 and 0.2 per 1000 pregnancies. The rate in the United States is approximately one per 20,000 pregnancies. Rare choriocarcinomas have developed after normal pregnancy (one per 40,000 term pregnancies). The disease also follows incomplete abortion and ectopic pregnancy. The risk factors for complete mole, particularly maternal age and pregnancy loss, are indirectly associated with choriocarcinoma.

CLINICAL CLASSIFICATION OF GESTATIONAL TROPHOBLASTIC DISEASE

The histologic terminology used to describe GTD may be confusing because the previous terms were based on the morphologic appearance of the abnormal tissue. With the use of sensitive and specific assays for HCG, clinical terminology is more useful in describing GTD. This offers an effective way of analyzing the treatment and the biologic behavior of these abnormal trophoblastic conditions. The serum level of HCG is the major guide to therapy.

CLINICAL ASPECTS OF GESTATIONAL TROPHOBLASTIC DISEASE

Hydatidiform Mole

Symptoms and Signs

The most common presenting symptom is abnormal bleeding in a patient who has experienced delayed menses and seems to be pregnant. Abnormal bleeding is present in almost all patients, and associated symptoms often mimic an incomplete or threatened abortion. Occasionally, the patient notices a bloody gelatinous tissue that has been passed from the uterus. The uterus is frequently large for dates; Curry et al. noted this change in approximately half of their patients with molar pregnancy. However, as many as one fourth of the patients may have a uterus small for dates. Sequelae appear to be more common among those with an enlarged uterus. In approximately 20% of the patients, an additional physical finding is enlargement of the ovaries (theca-lutein cysts), which is associated with a higher frequency of future sequelae (approximately 50%) compared with less than 15% for those without ovarian enlargement. The development of these theca-lutein cysts is believed to be secondary to the luteinizing-hormone-like effect of excessive HCG stimulation. However, in a study of 102 patients with theca-lutein cysts, Montz and colleagues noted that cyst growth did not correlate with changes in HCG concentrations and that some persisted after HCG disappeared from the circulation. Three of the cysts ruptured; the remaining spontaneously regressed.

Nausea and vomiting are common complaints, as is true in normal pregnancy, and hyperemesis gravidarum has been reported. Additionally, preeclamptic toxemia may occur in as many as one fourth of the patients, although its frequency has been reported to be less in many series.

Insofar as molar pregnancies are frequently diagnosed in the latter part of the first trimester of pregnancy, GTD should be considered in any patient with signs of toxemia during this time or during the early part of the second trimester. In addition, laboratory manifestations of hyperthyroidism have been reported, but clinical manifestations of hyperthyroidism are rare. The changes are in part due to the production of thyrotrophin-like hormone by the abnormal trophoblastic tissue, although a weak thyroid-stimulating hormone action for HCG has also been hypothesized. These changes are reversible and usually abate after treatment of trophoblastic disease. The signs and symptoms of hydatidiform moles are summarized here.

Clinically, the behaviors of partial and complete moles differ. Complete mole is the more common and also has a more serious prognosis, with increased risk of the subsequent development of a GTD. Partial moles usually present as an incomplete or missed abortion. Serum HCG levels tend to be lower in partial moles. The differences in complete and partial moles are summarized in Table 35-1 and the box below.

Symptoms and Signs of Hydatidiform Mole

Abnormal bleeding in early pregnancy
Lower abdominal pain
Toxemia before 24 weeks of gestation
Hyperemesis gravidarum
Hyperthyroidism (rare)
Uterus large for dates (50%)
Enlargement of ovaries (20%)
Absent fetal heart tones and fetal parts
Expulsion of swollen villi

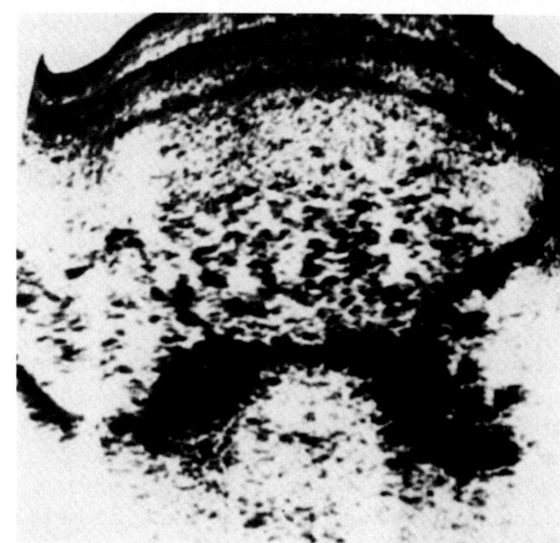

Figure 35-4. Ultrasound scan of uterus demonstrating snowstorm appearance of hydatidiform mole.

Diagnosis

In a patient suspected of having a molar pregnancy, the most valuable diagnostic tool is an ultrasound scan. The examination usually reveals the absence of a fetus (in the case of a complete mole) and characteristic swollen villi that produce a snowstorm-like pattern or multicystic appearance (Fig. 35-4). The examination may also demonstrate ovarian enlargement secondary to the development of a theca-lutein cyst. If a fetal sac is detected, the possibility of a partial mole still exists. However, beyond the seventh week, a fetal heartbeat should be detected by ultrasonography; its absence may suggest a missed abortion. If hydropic villi are present, it is possible that a blood clot in the uterus has been mistaken for a fetal sac. If there is doubt concerning the presence of fetal tissue and the existence of a partial mole, follow-up ultrasonographic examinations are indicated.

Table 35-1 Features of Complete and Partial Hydatidiform Moles

Feature	Complete Moles	Partial Moles
Fetal or embryonic tissue	Absent	Present
Hydatidiform swelling of chronic villi	Diffuse	Focal
Trophoblastic hyperplasia	Diffuse	Focal
Trophoblastic stormal inclusions	Absent	Present
Genetic parentage	Paternal	Bipaternal
Karyotype	46XX; 46XY	69XXY; 69XYY
Persistent human chorionic gonadotropin	20% of cases	0.5% of cases

From Eifel PJ, Gershenson DM, Kavanagh JJ, Silva EG: Gynecologic Cancer (M.D. Anderson Cancer Center Series, Buzdar AU, Freedman RS, eds). New York, Springer, 2006, p 230.

The measurement of HCG is an integral part of the diagnosis and evaluation of the patient suspected of having GTD. Immunoassays allow the measurement of extremely small amounts of HCG in blood and urine. The levels in normal pregnancy reach a peak at approximately 10 to 14 weeks and rarely exceed levels of 100,000 mIU/mL. They can be higher in twin gestation, are frequently elevated in GTD, and may appear elevated in patients whose dates are not accurate. With molar pregnancy, it is possible that the initial level of HCG may not be elevated. A single determination is not diagnostic and will not necessarily differentiate normal pregnancy, multiple pregnancy, and GTD. However, a level in excess of 100,000 mIU/mL suggests GTD. The HCG levels tend to be elevated above normal pregnancy values in a complete mole, whereas a partial mole tends to produce lower levels.

Management

Once the diagnosis of molar pregnancy is made, the uterus should be evacuated. Medical problems, such as anemia due to blood loss, pregnancy-induced hypertension, pulmonary insufficiency, congestive heart failure, and hyperthyroidism, should be evaluated and, when necessary, corrected. Hyperemesis gravidarum may develop, necessitating antiemetic and intravenous fluid therapy. Occasionally, disseminated intravascular coagulation occurs, leading to a consumptive coagulopathy that requires correction as well as prompt uterine evacuation. Pre-evacuation radiographic chest examination is performed to rule out the spread of GTD to the lungs and also for comparison in future follow-up. Unless a viable fetus is found, the pregnancy should be promptly terminated. If hyperthyroidism is present, it should be treated before surgical removal of the molar tissue. Theca-lutein cysts usually regress spontaneously and do not require surgical intervention unless an acute episode (e.g., rupture) occurs. In general, they regress spontaneously in approximately 2 months.

Pulmonary insufficiency may also occur following evacuation of a molar pregnancy. Acute dyspnea and cyanosis may develop, usually within 4 hours of evacuation. As noted by Cotton et al., this risk is greatest in patients whose uterus is more than 16 weeks' gestation in size. Trophoblastic embolization and fluid overload with blood volume expansion contribute to cardiac decompensation and pulmonary edema. If there are signs of pulmonary distress, arterial Po_2 should be monitored. In severely compromised patients, ventilatory assistance, monitoring of pulmonary arterial pressure, and management in an intensive care unit may be needed. Respiratory failure can occur.

Goldstein et al. have advocated the use of prophylactic cytotoxic chemotherapy to prevent the neoplastic sequelae of molar pregnancy. However, this practice has not gained widespread acceptance because giving chemotherapy at the time of evacuation of the mole exposes the patient to toxic drugs, even though most patients with hydatidiform mole do not require further treatment. Approximately 80% of the patients require only uterine evacuation as definitive therapy. If persistent GTD develops, which is a risk for the remaining 20%, chemotherapy can then be used. Chemotherapy in young females does increase the risk of ovarian failure and menopause. Byrne and associates studied 1067 females treated with chemotherapy before age 19 and noted a markedly increased risk of menopause for these women once they reached their 20s.

The most effective and widely used method of emptying the uterus of a molar pregnancy is suction curettage. In many instances, the molar pregnancy will have already begun to abort, and suction can complete the process. The level of HCG is determined before evacuation. Intravenous uterotonic agents are used during the evacuation and immediately postoperatively to aid in uterine contraction and to help reduce blood loss, unless the uterus is only minimally enlarged. However, it is not advisable to use uterotonic drugs before evacuation of the molar pregnancy because of the risk of disseminating abnormal trophoblastic cells. If possible, a large suction curette (12 mm) should be used to aid in evacuation. The operator should begin the evacuation in the lower part of the uterus near the cervix and gradually extend it toward the fundus. After evacuation by suction curettage is complete, a gentle sharp curettage may be performed to ensure completion of the procedure. Intravenous uterotonic agents should be continued post-evacuation to ensure uterine contraction.

Follow-up

After evacuation of the uterus, the patient should be carefully monitored for the potential development of persistent intrauterine or metastatic GTD. The key is the serial determination of β-HCG in the patient's serum. The HCG levels following evacuation of a hydatidiform mole should regress to normal usually within 3 months.

Evaluation of the patient treated for a molar pregnancy should include the data summarized (see the following box), which allows identification of those at higher risk of persistent GTD. The risk of persistence is increased in those with a large uterus, high HCG level, lutein cysts, and a history of molar pregnancy and toxemia as well as in older exposed patients, particularly individuals older than 40. The risk of adverse sequelae is less in the absence of these factors and also when fetal tissue is present (partial mole).

To follow the course of the disease after evacuation of a molar pregnancy, the physician must carefully monitor the HCG levels. Following evacuation of hydatidiform mole, a normal range is usually reached by the 12th week. However, in some instances, the level returns to normal after a longer interval. Weekly HCGs are measured until the level reaches normal values on three consecutive measurements. The patient must not become pregnant, and usually oral contraceptives are prescribed. There has been a controversial suggestion in the literature that birth control pills might increase the risk of GTD, but data from Deicas and colleagues suggest that birth control pills are safe and effective in this situation. A study by Deicas and associates indicates that oral contraceptives actually offer a therapeutic advantage with fewer patients developing GTD who used birth control pills (see box).

After molar evacuation, a pelvic examination is performed within approximately 2 weeks and then repeated as clinically indicated until the uterus and ovaries have returned to normal

Baseline Data for Patient with Molar Pregnancy

Human chorionic gonadotropin serum level (pre-evacuation)
Chest radiograph*
Age
Uterus size
Presence or absence of ovarian theca-lutein cysts
Presence or absence of fetal tissue
History of molar pregnancy
Assessment for medical complications
- Anemia
- Toxemia
- Hyperemesis
- Hyperthyroidism
- Pulmonary compromise

*If chest radiograph is abnormal, full metastatic evaluation should be completed after uterine evacuation.

size. Theca-lutein cysts characteristically resolve within 2 months, but Montz and associates showed they may last as long as 4 months. However, patients with the high-risk factors listed earlier are approximately 10 times more likely to develop the sequelae of neoplasia in comparison to those without these factors. Once the HCG reaches undetectable levels, it is preferable to monitor them monthly for 6 to 12 months, after which the patient may be advised that she can safely attempt another pregnancy. For partial moles, 6 months of follow-up is probably sufficient. However, the isolated recurrence of trophoblastic disease 16 months after complete molar evacuation in a patient on oral contraceptives has been reported.

An increase in HCG (a doubling over a 2-week period) or a plateau in HCG (failure to decrease by at least 10% per week) indicates the presence of persistent GTD. Chemotherapy, after risk assessment, is usually started (Fig. 35-5). As noted by Kohorn, a higher plateau of HCG values is an indication for chemotherapy. He suggests that a level of 10^5 or greater over two values requires treatment, whereas at 10^4 to 10^5, three values are appropriate over 2 weeks, with a range up to a month of follow-up for values that appear to plateau at less than 100 mIU/mL. A general rule suggested by Berkowitz et al. is a level greater than 20,000 mIU/mL more than 4 months post-mole evacuation is an indication for initiation of chemotherapy. The finding of a

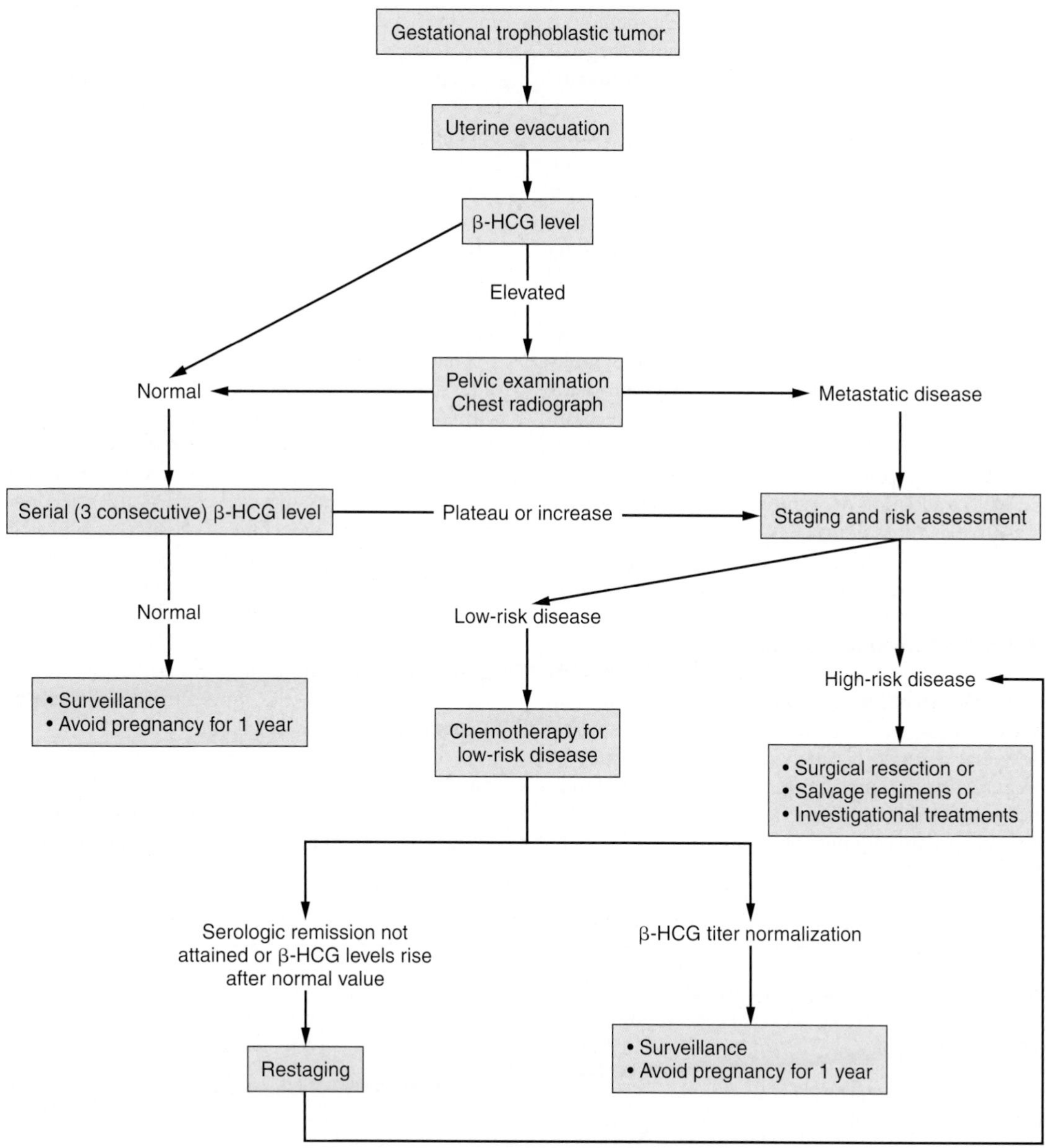

Figure 35-5. Treatment algorithm. Diagnostic and therapeutic to gestational trophoblastic disease as practiced at the University of Texas M.D. Anderson Cancer Center. HCG, human chorionic gonadotropin. (Modified from Kudela AP, Freedman RS, Kavanagh JJ: Gestational trophoblastic tumors. In Pazdur R, Coia LR, Hoskins WJ, Wagman LD: Cancer Management: A Multidisciplinary Approach, 7th ed. New York, The Oncology Group, 2003, p 230. From Eifel PJ, Gershenson DM, Kavanagh JJ, Silva EG: Gynecologic Cancer (M.D. Anderson Cancer Center Series, Buzdar AU, Freedman RS, eds). New York, Springer, 2006, p 235.)

placental-site trophoblastic tumor would be an indication for hysterectomy if the disease were confined to the uterus.

Gestational Trophoblastic Disease: Persistent and Metastatic

Incidence and Diagnosis

As has been noted by Cohn and Herzog, persistent GTD develops after approximately 15% to 20% of complete hydatidiform moles. Conversely, approximately half the cases of persistent GTD arise after molar pregnancy, whereas one fourth occur after normal pregnancy and one fourth after abortion or ectopic pregnancy. Therefore, patients who continue to have abnormal bleeding after any pregnancy should have an HCG assay. Once persistent GTD is diagnosed, chemotherapy is initiated unless complications, such as uterine hemorrhage or perforation, arise that require hysterectomy. The type of therapy is defined by the risk factor analysis.

First, a thorough evaluation must be done, including a complete physical examination, measurement of HCG level, and diagnostic tests to rule out metastatic disease. These patients may have symptoms of metastatic disease, such as hemoptysis (due to pulmonary lesions), or neurologic complaints (secondary to brain metastases). The physical examination should include pelvic and neurologic evaluations.

Because of the fatal ramifications of brain and liver metastases, these areas are usually assessed with a computed tomography (CT) scan or magnet resonance image (MRI). Asymptomatic patients with a normal chest X-ray are unlikely to have brain or other visceral metastasis. Because 97% to 100% of patients with CNS metastasis have concomitant pulmonary disease, one may forgo the CNS evaluation in asymptomatic patients with a normal chest x-ray. For those whose CNS evaluation is needed, a computed tomography or magnetic resonance imaging scan of the brain to exclude brain metastasis should be performed, according to Athanassiou and colleagues. In cerebral involvement, the level of HCG is often elevated in the cerebrospinal fluid (CSF). Bagshawe and Harland reported that the plasma/CSF HCG ratio tends to be less than 60 in the presence of brain metastases. However, as reported by Bagshawe and associates and Ng and Wong, a single plasma/CSF HCG ratio may be misleading because of very rapid changes in plasma HCG levels, which may not be promptly reflected in the CSF, which makes it less accurate compared with imaging. Therefore, MRI may be the preferred way to evaluate the brain, as it can capture even small lesions on the posterior fossa.

A pelvic ultrasound examination allows reasonable definition of the uterus and adnexae. A more complete examination of the anatomy requires a CT scan of pelvis and abdomen. Ha and coworkers reported that an MRI evaluation may be preferred for evaluation of local invasion of the uterus. The most frequent site of metastatic GTD are the lungs (80% to 90% of cases), and less frequently the liver, brain, ovary, and vagina are involved. Chest CT will be more sensitive in detecting chest metastases than a chest radiograph. In addition, metastatic disease can occur at any anatomic site; however, bone and lymph node involvement is rare. The kidney and GI tract are rarely involved, usually presenting as gross hematuria or a bowel perforation, respectively. These may occur soon after therapy. Tests of renal and liver functions should also be performed in addition to a hematologic profile.

Depending on the location and extension of the disease, levels of HCG, and history of chemotherapy and pregnancy, it is possible to categorize the patient as having low-risk or high-risk GTD. The World Health Organization and The International Federation of Gynecology and Obstetrics have jointly agreed on a new staging system that includes both staging and risk categorization, as shown on Table 35-2. The ABO blood groups as a risk factor for GTD were excluded from the newest FIGO classification because, according to Kohorn and colleagues, their significance has not been confirmed.

There are several reports of therapeutic outcomes using the older staging systems. Gordon and colleagues noted that patients with a score of 8 or higher required multiagent chemotherapy. In 1989, Bagshawe et al. summarized results on 487 patients. In this report, a score of 5 or less was considered low risk, and 347 of 348 patients survived. In a multivariate analysis, Soper et al. noted that the clinical classification provided the best method of identifying patient prognosis and the indication for single or multiagent initial chemotherapy. Newer classifications have eliminated the middle risk category. Patients with low risk receive single agents; those with high risk receive multiple agents. It is important to emphasize that regardless of the classification system, the most important factor for following the patient is the level of HCG.

Management

Low-Risk Gestational Trophoblastic Disease. There are several published reports of first-line treatment of low-risk GTD.

Table 35-2 The Scoring System for the International Federation of Gynecology and Obstetrics (FIGO) 2000

FIGO Score	0	1	2	4
Age	≤39	>39		
Antecedent pregnancy	Hydatidiform mole	Abortion	Term pregnancy	
Interval from index pregnancy (months)	<4	4–6	7–2	>12
Pretreatment β-human chorionic gonadotropin (mIU/mL)	<1000	1000–10,000	>10,000–100,000	>100,000
Largest tumor size including uterus (cm)	3–4	5		
Site of metastases	Lung	Spleen, kidney	GI tract	Brain, liver
Number of metastases identified	0	1–4	5–8	>8
Previous failed chemotherapy			Single drug	Two or more drugs

Score value: ≤6 = low risk; ≥7 = high risk.
Modified from Kohorn EI: The new FIGO 2000 staging and risk factor scoring system for gestational trophoblastic disease: Description and critical assessment. Int J Gynecol Cancer 11:73–77, 2001; and Ngan HY: The practicability of FIGO 2000 staging for gestational trophoblastic disease. Int J Gynecol Cancer 14:202–205, 2004.

A commonly used and safe one is methotrexate, 1 to 1.5 mg/kg intramuscularly or intravenously on days 1, 3, 5, and 7, followed by citrovorum factor rescue (leucovorin), 0.1 to 0.15 mg/kg intramuscularly on days 2, 4, 6, and 8, inducing remission in approximately 90% of patients. Studies by Berkowitz and colleagues and Gleeson and colleagues have shown that there is little toxicity and this treatment has the advantages of being easy to administer intramuscularly and includes self-administration and no risk of extravasation injury. Other schedules and drugs include methotrexate, 0.4 mg/kg body weight (maximum, 25 mg) intravenously or intramuscularly daily for 5 days every 2 weeks; actinomycin D, 10 to 12 μg/kg intravenously daily for 5 days every 2 weeks.

Pulse actinomycin D, 1.25 mg/m^2 intravenously once every 2 weeks, has also been used. Petrilli et al. reported on single-dose actinomycin D for 31 patients in a cooperative Gynecologic Oncology Group study. Twenty-nine (94%) achieved remission after a median of four courses of therapy. Another alternative was reported by Homesley et al., who summarized a Gynecologic Oncology Group study of 63 patients with nonmetastatic GTD. Fifty-one responded completely to weekly intramuscular methotrexate, initially 30 mg/m^2 and increased as tolerated 5 mg/m^2 per week to 50 mg/m^2. However, 11 patients failed and subsequently required 5-day actinomycin D therapy. Some experts consider this an unacceptable failure rate.

The 5-day actinomycin D and methotrexate courses have been found to be equally effective. Toxicities differ according to the agent used and metabolic condition of the patient. High-dose methotrexate with citrovorum rescue has not been proven to be more effective than the other single agents given alone. Some investigators have alternated the 5-day actinomycin D and methotrexate courses in the belief that this results in reduced toxicity and more rapid resolution of the disease. VP-16 (etoposide) has also been effectively used as single-agent therapy of 100 mg/m^2 given for 5 days repeated approximately every 2 weeks. The single-dose weekly methotrexate regimen at 30 mg/m^2 intramuscularly or actinomycin D 1.25 mg/m^2 every 2 weeks may provide a cost-effective advantage in terms of outpatient therapy. As noted by Homesley, however, weekly methotrexate has less GI toxicity. Oral etoposide is expensive and causes total alopecia, with GI and hematologic toxicity.

There are no randomized trials that compare one regimen to the other. As Ng and Wong demonstrated, the choice of protocol in any center is often one of familiarity. Patients who fail to respond to one single agent are usually switched to the other single agent. Patients who fail to respond to both single agents receive the combination chemotherapy used for high-risk patients.

Patients are treated until a normal HCG level has been obtained; then one to two additional courses of chemotherapy are usually given. Although recurrence rates of approximately 5% may be expected after therapy, recurrence more than 6 to 12 months after treatment is extremely unusual. Weekly serum HCG determinations are made until three negative HCG levels are obtained. Then monthly levels are taken for at least 6 to 12 months, after which pregnancy may be attempted. Even with recurrence, chemotherapy can be expected to cure 100% of patients with low-risk nonmetastatic trophoblastic disease.

High-Risk Gestational Trophoblastic Disease. The treatment of high-risk GTD requires multiagent chemotherapy.

Table 35-3 Chemotherapy Regimens for Intermediate- and High-Risk Gestational Trophoblastic Disease

Drug Regimen	Administration
EMA-CO (Preferred regimen)	
Course I (EMA)*	
Day 1	
Etoposide	100 mg/m^2 IV over 30 min
Methotrexate	100 mg/m^2 IV bolus
Methotrexate	200 mg/m^2 IV as 12-hr continuous infusion
Dactinomycin	0.5 mg IV bolus
Day 2	
Etoposide	100 mg/m^2 IV over 320 min
Folinic acid	15 mg IV/IM/PO every 6 hr for four doses
Dactinomycin	0.5 mg IV bolus
Course II (CO)	
Day 8	
Cyclophosphamide	600 mg/m^2 IV over 30 min
Vincristine	1 mg/m^2 (up to 2 mg) IV bolus

*Cytokine support may be used.
Modified from Kantarjian HM, Wolf RA, Koller CA: M.D. Anderson Manual of Medical Oncology. New York, McGraw-Hill, 2006.

As discussed in Cohn's 2000 study, the standard treatment is EMA/CO (Table 35-3).

In a study of 36 high-risk patients, Bolis and colleagues noted EMA/CO to be effective, including a 64% response rate when used as second-line therapy, which was higher than methotrexate dactinomycin cyclophosphamide (MAC) or other multiagent protocols. Schink and colleagues reported a complete response in 10 of 12 patients when used as primary therapy for high-risk disease. EMA/CO is widely used for high-risk GTD. Using this protocol in 272 high-risk patients (including 121 with previous chemotherapy), Bower and coworkers reported 213 (78%) complete responses, with 112 subsequent live births and five secondary malignancies. The use of granulocyte colony-stimulating factor can reduce neutropenic toxicity. Recently, platinum and etoposide have been reported for the treatment of high-risk disease. Soper et al. reported six of seven chemorefractory GTD patients had a complete response but with serious side effects, including grade IV neutropenia and severe renal toxicity. Newlands et al. reported a multiagent regimen of etoposide/platinum alternating weekly with EMA to treat EMA/CO failures and rare metastatic placental site trophoblastic tumors, which are usually resistant to chemotherapy. Thirty of 34 patients with gestational trophoblastic tumors and four of eight with placental site trophoblastic tumors survived. Surgery was used in some cases. This appears to be an effective regimen with frequent severe toxicity, especially hematologic. Generally, patients are treated with two cycles of chemotherapy after achieving remission. However, patients in whom remission has been difficult to achieve may benefit from longer therapy.

If brain metastases are diagnosed, one option is to treat with radiation therapy in a dose greater than 22 Gy. However, in the absence of control of systemic disease, the recurrence rates of GTD are high despite high doses of radiation. The long-term effects of high-dose radiation therapy to the brain are not known, as discussed in Schechter and associates' study. According to Rustin and colleagues' study, another option is to treat with chemotherapy regimens containing high-dose methotrexate.

A third option would be surgical resection if it presents as one single lesion, and Ghaemmaghami and associates demonstrated that combinations of these approaches are a valid treatment strategy.

Treatment of Chemotherapy Failures

As mentioned previously, low-risk patients failing one agent may be treated with another single agent chemotherapy, i.e., methotrexate failures may be treated with actinomycin D. Occasionally, they may need EMA/CO treatment, bearing in mind the small risk of secondary leukemia with that regimen.

As many as 20% of patients with high-risk GTD who attain a negative HCG level have a recurrence. In comparison, the recurrence rate for those with low-risk GTD is 5%, whereas those with nonmetastatic GTD have recurrence rates of 1% to 2%.

EMA/CO failures are very problematic patients. Lurain's 2005 study described the strategy for cure: a balance of surgical resection of chemotherapy-resistant sites, including the uterus, and cisplatin-based regimens, such as EMA/etoposide and cisplatin (substituting etoposide and cisplatin for cyclophosphamide and vincristine in the EMA/CO protocol), BEP (cisplatin, etoposide, and bleomycin), VIP (etoposide, ifosfamide, cisplatin), and ICE (ifosfamide, carboplatin, etoposide) (Lurain, 2005) Rustin and colleagues and Bower discussed use of both modalities either singly or together. High-dose salvage therapy has resulted in remission. Giacalone and associates used high-dose chemotherapy with autologous bone marrow transplantation in a refractory patient who is still disease free 3 years after treatment.

Follow-up

After a negative HCG level is achieved for three cycles in patients with high-risk GTD, HCG measurements are repeated every 2 weeks for 3 months and then monthly for 1 year. Some physicians continue the measurement of HCG levels every 6 months for as long as 5 years because of the slight risk of late recurrence of the disease. Radiographic examinations are repeated as clinically indicated. Central nervous system lesions are imaged more regularly. The HCG level is the crucial element in following the patient. Approximately 1 year of a normal HCG is appropriate in a high-risk patient. The patient may then again attempt pregnancy. Six-month follow-up may be appropriate in a low-risk patient.

Post-treatment Issues

According to Rustin and colleagues and Bower, there is an increased percentage of secondary malignancies including solid tumors (absolute risk of approximately 3%) and particularly secondary leukemia. The neurologic impact of whole-brain radiation is not known.

Fertility after Treatment for Gestational Trophoblastic Disease

There is concern, particularly among patients who have been treated for GTD, that a subsequent pregnancy will lead to repeat GTD or recrudescence of the disease. There is a slight increased risk of repeat molar pregnancy; however, normal pregnancy usually results. Alterieri and associates' study proved that it is not a familial disease (Altieri et al., 2004). Data from Rustin and associates indicate no increased frequency of congenital anomalies among infants whose mothers received chemotherapy. Goldstein and coworkers reported that 67.4% of 929 individuals treated at various centers for GTD subsequently had a normal term delivery, whereas only 1.4% experienced a recurrent molar pregnancy. Green et al. reported that those treated with chemotherapy for a variety of tumors are not at increased risk of having offspring with congenital anomalies. However, the patients receiving actinomycin D had the greatest frequency of congenital anomalies, suggesting that further study is indicated for this drug. If pregnancy occurs following GTD, it is important to perform an ultrasound examination early to identify a gestational sac in the uterus as well as a fetal heart, which should be evident by the seventh week of pregnancy. HCG levels should be obtained after delivery to rule out any recurrence of GTD. Products of conception or placentas should be examined histopathologically.

KEY POINTS

- Persistent abnormal bleeding following normal pregnancy, abortion, or ectopic pregnancy should lead to a consideration of the diagnosis of GTD. The finding of pulmonary nodules on chest radiograph after normal pregnancy suggests GTD. The HCG is elevated in these situations.
- A young woman with an unknown primary neoplasm or poorly explained hyperthyroidism should have her serum HCG tested.
- Approximately half the cases of GTD follow molar pregnancy, one fourth follow normal pregnancy, and one fourth follow abortion or ectopic pregnancy.
- The major risk factors for molar pregnancy include maternal age (older than 40 and younger than 20 years) and a history of molar pregnancy. There appears to be an increased frequency of these diseases in Southeast Asia and Mexico.
- The risk of hydatidiform mole is approximately 0.75 to 1.0 per 1000 pregnancies in the United States.
- The risk of developing a second molar pregnancy after a primary mole is approximately 20 to 40 times greater than the initial risk.
- The monitoring of trophoblastic disease and its follow-up is accomplished by the measurement of β-HCG.
- Complete moles are of paternal origin, are diploid, and carry a 20% risk of GTD sequelae.
- Partial moles are of maternal and paternal origin, are triploid, and rarely are followed by GTD, but require the same follow-up for potential malignant sequelae as a complete mole.
- The diagnosis of a molar pregnancy can be established with ultrasonography and may coexist with a normal pregnancy.

KEY POINTS *Continued*

- Hydatidiform moles are effectively and safely evacuated from the uterus using suction curettage.
- Medical complications of hydatidiform mole include anemia, toxemia, hyperthyroidism, hyperemesis gravidarum, cardiac failure, and rarely pulmonary insufficiency.
- Patients are classified into low- or high-risk categories. Low-risk categories receive single agent chemotherapy, usually methotrexate. High-risk patients receive combination chemotherapy, usually EMA/CO.
- Low-risk patients have a cure rate of greater than 90%.
- Patients with high-risk metastatic GTD are successfully treated with chemotherapy in more than 70% of the cases.
- Patients treated for GTD should not become pregnant for approximately 6 to 12 months after treatment to allow accurate assessment of HCG levels.
- Fertility rates and pregnancy outcomes are similar in patients treated for GTD compared with the general population.
- Patients treated with EMA/CO regimens have an increased rate of second malignancies, particularly hematologic.

ACKNOWLEDGMENT

The authors would like to thank Vanessa Fabriccio, Regina G. Richard, Nakarin Sirisabya, Atthapon Jaishuen, and Hong Zheng for corrections and assistance in preparing this chapter.

BIBLIOGRAPHY

Acaia B, Parazzini F, La Vecchia C, et al: Increased frequency of complete hydatidiform mole in women with repeated abortion. Gynecol Oncol 31:310, 1988.

Ajithkumar TV, Abraham EK, Rejnishkumar R, Minimole AL: Placental site trophoblastic tumor. Obstet Gynecol Survey 58:484–488, 2003.

Altieri A, Franceschi S, Ferlay J, et al: Epidemiology and aetiology of gestational trophoblastic disease. Lancet 4:670–678, 2003.

Athanassiou A, Begent RHL, Newlands ES, et al: Central nervous system metastases of choriocarcinoma: Twenty-three years' experience at Charing Cross Hospital. Cancer 52: 1728-1735, 1983.

Atrash HK, Hogue CJR, Grimes DA: Epidemiology of hydatidiform mole during early gestation. Am J Obstet Gynecol 154:906, 1986.

Baergen RN, Rutgers JL, Young RH, et al: Placental site trophoblastic tumor: A study of 55 cases and review of the literature emphasizing factors of prognostic significance. Gynecol Oncol 100:511–520, 2006.

Bagshawe KD: Treatment of high-risk choriocarcinoma. J Reprod Med 29:813, 1984.

Bagshawe KD, Harland S: Immunodiagnosis and monitoring of gonadotrophin-producing metastases in the central nervous system. Cancer 38:112, 1976.

Bagshawe KD, Lawler SD, Paradinas FJ, et al: Gestational trophoblastic tumours following initial diagnosis of partial hydatidiform mole. Lancet 335:1074, 1990.

Bagshawe KD, Rawlings G, Pike MC, et al: The ABO blood groups in trophoblastic neoplasia. Lancet 1:553, 1971.

Bakri Y, Berkowitz RS, Goldstein DP, et al: Brain metastases of gestational trophoblastic tumor. J Reprod Med 39:179, 1994.

Bandy LC, Clarke-Pearson DL, and Hammond C: Malignant potential of gestational trophoblastic disease at the extreme ages of reproductive life. Obstet Gynecol 64:395, 1984.

Berkowitz RS, Bernstein MR, Laborde O, Goldstein DP: Subsequent pregnancy experience in patients with gestational trophoblastic disease: New England Trophoblastic Disease Center, 1965–1992. J Reprod Med 39:228, 1994.

Berkowitz RS, Goldstein DP: Gestational Trophoblastic Diseases: Principals and Practice of Gynecologic Oncology, 3rd ed. Philadelphia, Lippincott Williams & Wilkins, 2000, pp 1117–1137.

Berkowitz RS, Goldstein DP, Bernstein MR: Ten years' experience with methotrexate and folinic acid as primary therapy for gestational trophoblastic disease. Gynecol Oncol 23:111–118, 1986.

Berkowitz RS, Goldstein DP, DuBeshter B, et al: Management of complete molar pregnancy. J Reprod Med 32:634, 1987.

Bigelow B: Gestational trophoblast disease. In Blaustein A (ed): Pathology of the Female Genital Tract, 2nd ed. New York, Springer-Verlag, 1982.

Bolis G, Bonazzi C, Landoni F, et al: EMA/CO regimen in high-risk gestational trophoblastic tumor (GTT). Gynecol Oncol 31:439, 1988.

Bower M, Newlands ES, Holden D, et al: EMA/CO for high-risk gestational trophoblastic tumors: Results from a cohort of 272 patients. J Clin Oncol 15:2636, 1997.

Buckley JD: The epidemiology of molar pregnancy and choriocarcinoma. Clin Obstet Gynecol 27:153, 1984.

Byrne J, Fears TR, Gail MH, et al: Early menopause in long-term survivors of cancer during adolescence. Am J Obstet Gynecol 166:788, 1992.

Chang Y-L, Chang T-C, Hsueh S, et al: Prognostic factors and treatment for placental site trophoblastic tumor-report of 3 cases and analysis of 88 cases. Gynecol Oncol 73:216, 1999.

Cohn DE, Herzog TJ: Gestational trophoblastic diseases: New standards for therapy. Curr Opin Oncol 12:492–496, 2000.

Cotton DB, Bernstein SG, Read SA, et al: Hemodynamic observations in evacuation of molar pregnancy. Am J Obstet Gynecol 138:6, 1980.

Curry SL, Blessing J, DiSaia P, et al: A prospective randomized comparison of methotrexate, dactinomycin, and chlorambucil versus methotrexate, dactinomycin, cyclophosphamide, doxorubicin, melphalan, hydroxyurea, and vincristine in "poor prognosis" metastatic gestational trophoblastic disease: A Gynecologic Oncology Group study. Obstet Gynecol 73:357, 1989.

Deicas RE, Miller DS, Rademaker AW, et al: The role of contraception in the development of postmolar gestational trophoblastic disease. Obstet Gynecol 78:221, 1991.

Dessau R, Rustin GJS, Paradinas FJ, et al: Surgery and chemotherapy in the management of placental site tumor. Gynecol Oncol 39:56, 1990.

Eifel PJ, Gershenson DM, Kavanagh JK, Silva EG: Gynecologic Cancer (M.D. Anderson Cancer Care Series). New York, Springer, 2006, pp 226–243.

Elmer DB, Granai CO, Ball HG, Curry SL: Persistence of gestational trophoblastic disease for longer than 1 year following evacuation of hydatidiform mole. Obstet Gynecol 81:888, 1993.

Gamer EI, Garrett A, Goldstein DP, Berkowitz RS. Significance of chest computed tomography findings in the evaluation and treatment of persistent gestational trophoblastic neoplasia. J Reprod Med 49:411, 2004.

Ghaemmaghami F, Behtash N, Memarpour N, et al: Evaluation and management of brain metastatic patients with high-risk gestational trophoblastic tumors. Int J Gynecol Cancer 14:966–971, 2004.

Giacalone PL, Benos P, Donnadio D, Laffargue F: High-dose chemotherapy with autologous bone marrow transplantation for refractory metastatic gestational trophoblastic disease. Gynecol Oncol 58:383, 1995.

Gleeson NC, Finan MA, Fiorica JV, et al: Nonmetastatic gestational trophoblastic disease: Weekly methotrexate compared with 8-day methotrexate-folinic acid. Eur J Gynaecol Oncol 14:461–465, 1993.

Goldstein DP, Berkowitz RS, Bernstein MR: Reproductive performance after molar pregnancy and gestational trophoblastic tumor. Clin Obstet Gynecol 27:221, 1984.

Gordon AN, Gershenson DM, Copeland LJ, et al: High-risk metastatic gestational trophoblastic disease: Further stratification into two clinical entities. Gynecol Oncol 34:54, 1989.

Green DM, Zevon MA, Lowrie G, et al: Congenital anomalies in children of patients who received chemotherapy for cancer in childhood and adolescence. N Engl J Med 325:141, 1991.

Grimes DA: Epidemiology of gestational trophoblastic disease. Am J Obstet Gynecol 150:309, 1984.

Gul T, Yilmazturk A: A review of trophoblastic diseases at the medical school of Dicle University. Eur J Obstet Gynaecol Reprod Biol 74:37–40, 1997.

Ha HK, Jung JK, Jee MK, et al: Gestational trophoblastic tumors of the uterus: MR imaging pathologic correlation. Gynecol Oncol 57:340–350, 1995.

Hammond CB, Soper JT: Poor-prognostic metastatic gestational trophoblastic neoplasia. Clin Obstet Gynecol 27:228, 1984.

Hayashi K, Bracken MB, Freeman DH Jr, Hellenbrand K: Hydatidiform mole in the United States (1970–1977): A statistical and theoretical analysis. Am J Epidemiol 115:67–77, 1982.

Homesley HD: Development of single-agent chemotherapy regimens for gestational trophoblastic disease. J Reprod Med 39:185, 1994.

Homesley HD, Blessing JA, Rettenmaier M, et al: Weekly intramuscular methotrexate for nonmetastatic gestational trophoblastic disease. Obstet Gynecol 72:413, 1988.

How J, Scurry J, Grant P, et al: Placental site trophoblastic tumor: Report of three cases and review of the literature. Int J Gynecol Cancer 5:241, 1995.

Kantarjian HM, Wolf RA, Koller CA: M.D. Anderson Manual of Medical Oncology. New York, McGraw-Hill, 2006, p 594.

Kelly MP, Rustin GJS, Ivory C, et al: Respiratory failure due to choriocarcinoma: A study of 103 dyspneic patients. Gynecol Oncol 38:149, 1990.

Kim JH, Park DC, Bae SN, et al: Subsequent reproductive experience after treatment for gestational trophoblastic disease. Gynecol Oncol 71:108, 1998.

Kohorn EI: Evaluation of the criteria used to make the diagnosis of nonmetastatic gestational trophoblastic neoplasia. Gynecol Oncol 48:139, 1993.

Kohorn EI, Goldstein DP, Hancock BW, et al: Combining the staging system of the International Federation of Gynecology and Obstetrics with the scoring system of the World Health Organization for Trophoblastic Neoplasia. Report of the Working Committee of the International Society for the Study of Trophoblastic Disease and the International Gynecologic Cancer Society. Int J Gynecol Cancer 10:84, 2000.

Kohorn EI: The new FIGO 2000 staging and risk factor scoring system for gestational trophoblastic disease: Description and critical assessment. Int J Gynecol Cancer 11:73–77, 2001.

Lage JM, Berkowitz, RS, Rice LW, et al: Flow cytometric analysis of DNA content in partial hydatidiform moles with persistent gestational trophoblastic tumor. Obstet Gynecol 77:111, 1991.

Lathrop JC, Lauchlan S, Nayaf R, et al: Clinical characteristics of placental site trophoblastic tumor (PSTT). Gynecol Oncol 31:32, 1988.

Lehman E, Gershenson DM, Burke TW, et al: Salvage surgery for chemorefractory gestational trophoblastic disease. J Clin Oncol 12:2737, 1994.

Lemonnier M-C, Glezerman V, Auclair R, et al: Choriocarcinoma associated with undetectable levels of human chorionic gonadotropin. Gynecol Oncol 25:48, 1986.

Li MC, Hertz R, Spencer DB: Effect of methotrexate therapy upon choriocarcinoma and chorioadenoma. Proc Soc Exp Biol Med 93:36, 1956.

Lurain JR: High-risk metastatic gestational trophoblastic tumors: current management. J Reprod Med 39:217, 1994.

Lurain JR, Elfstrand EP: Single-agent methotrexate chemotherapy for the treatment of nonmetastatic gestational trophoblastic tumors. Am J Obstet Gynecol 172:574, 1995.

Lurain JR, Nejad B: Secondary chemotherapy for high-risk gestational trophoblastic neoplasia. Gynecol Oncol 97:618–623, 2005.

Matsuura J, Chiu D, Jacobs PA et al: Complete hydatidiform mole in Hawaii: An epidemiological study. Genet Epidemiol 1:271–284, 1984.

Montz FJ, Schlaerth JB, Morrow CP: The natural history of theca lutein cysts. Obstet Gynecol 72:247, 1988.

Morrow P, Nakamura R, Schlaerth JB, et al: The influence of oral contraceptives on the post molar hCG regression curve. Am J Obstet Gynecol 151:906, 1985.

Mortakis AE, Braga CA: "Poor prognosis" metastatic gestational trophoblastic disease: The prognostic significance of the scoring system in predicting chemotherapy failures. Obstet Gynecol 76:272, 1990.

Newlands ES, Mulholland PJ, Holden L, et al: Etoposide and cisplatin/etoposide, methotrexate, and actinomycin D (EMA) chemotherapy for patients with high-risk gestational trophoblastic tumors refractory to EMA/cyclophosphamide and vincristine chemotherapy and patients presenting with metastatic placental site trophoblastic tumors. J Clin Oncol 18:854, 2000.

Ng TY, Wong LC: Review: Diagnosis and management of gestational trophoblastic neoplasia. Best Pract Res Clin Obstet Gynaecol 6:893–903, 2003.

Ngan HY: The practicability of FIGO 2000 staging for gestational trophoblastic neoplasia. Int J Gynecol Cancer 14:202–205, 2004.

Olive DL, Lurain JR, Brewer JI: Choriocarcinoma associated with term gestation. Am J Obstet Gynecol 148:711, 1984.

Palmer JR: Advances in the epidemiology of gestational trophoblastic disease. J Reprod Med 39:155, 1994.

Palmer JR, Driscoll SG, Rosenberg L, et al: Oral contraceptive use and risk of gestational trophoblastic tumors. J Natl Cancer Inst 91:635, 1999.

Petrilli ES, Twiggs LB, Blessing JA, et al: Single-dose actinomycin D treatment for nonmetastatic gestational trophoblastic disease: A prospective phase II trial of the gynecologic oncology group. Cancer 60:2173, 1987.

Rice LW, Berkowitz RS, Lage JM, et al: Persistent gestational trophoblastic tumor after partial hydatidiform mole. Gynecol Oncol 36:358, 1990.

Rustin GJS, Booth M, Dent J, et al: Pregnancy after cytotoxic chemotherapy for gestational trophoblastic tumors. BMJ 288:103, 1984.

Rustin GJ, Newlands ES, Lutz JM, et al: Combination but not single-agent methotrexate chemotherapy for gestational trophoblastic tumors increases the incidence of second tumors. J Clin Oncol 14:2769–2773, 1996.

Rustin GJS, Newlands ES, Begent RHJ, et al: Weekly alternating etoposide, methotrexate, and actinomycin/vincristine and cyclophosphamide chemotherapy for the treatment of CNS metastases of choriocarcinoma. J Clin Oncol 7:900–903, 1989.

Schechter NR, Mychalczak B, Jones W, Sprigg D: Prognosis of patients treated with whole-brain radiation therapy for metastatic gestational trophoblastic disease. Gynecol Oncol 68:183–192, 1998.

Schink JC, Singh DK, Rademaker AW, et al: Etoposide, methotrexate, actinomycin D, cyclophosphamide, and vincristine for the treatment of metastatic, high-risk gestational trophoblastic disease. Obstet Gynecol 80:817, 1992.

Schlaerth JB, Morrow CR, Kletzky OA, et al: Prognostic characteristics of serum human chorionic gonadotropin titer regression following molar pregnancy. Obstet Gynecol 58:478, 1981.

Schlaerth JB, Morrow CP, Montz FJ, d'Ablaing G: Initial management of hydatidiform mole. Am J Obstet Gynecol 158:1299, 1988.

Schlaerth JB, Morrow CP, Nalick RH, et al: Single-dose actinomycin D in the treatment of post molar trophoblastic disease. Gynecol Oncol 19:53, 1984.

Secki MJ, Fisher RA, Salerno G, et al: Choriocarcinoma and partial hydatidiform moles. Lancet 356:36, 2000.

Smith EB, Szulman AE, Hinshaw W, et al: Human chorionic gonadotropin levels in complete and partial hydatidiform moles and in nonmolar abortuses. Am J Obstet Gynecol 149:129, 1984.

Soper JT: Surgical therapy for gestational trophoblastic disease. J Reprod Med 39:168, 1994.

Soper JT, Clarke-Pearson DL, Berchuck A, et al: 5-day methotrexate for women with metastatic gestational trophoblastic disease. Gynecol Oncol 54:76, 1994.

Soper JT, Evans AC, Conaway MR, et al: Evaluation of prognostic factors and staging in gestational trophoblastic tumor. Obstet Gynecol 84:969, 1994.

Soper JT, Evans AC, Rodriguez G, et al: Etoposide-platin combination therapy for chemorefractory gestational trophoblastic disease. Gynecol Oncol 56:421, 1995.

Szulman AE, Surti U: The syndromes of partial and complete molar gestation. Clin Obstet Gynecol 27:172, 1984.

Watson EJ, Hernandez E, Miyazawa K: Partial hydatidiform moles: A review. Obstet Gynecol Surv 42:540, 1987.

Wren BG: Hormonal therapy following female genital tract cancer. Int J Gynecol Cancer 4:217, 1994.

Young RH, Scully RE: Placental-site trophoblastic tumor: Current status. Clin Obstet Gynecol 27:248, 1984.

PART V

REPRODUCTIVE ENDOCRINOLOGY AND INFERTILITY

Primary and Secondary Dysmenorrhea, Premenstrual Syndrome, and Premenstrual Dysphoric Disorder 36

Etiology, Diagnosis, Management

Gretchen M. Lentz

KEY TERMS AND DEFINITIONS

Cervical Stenosis. Narrowing of the cervical canal, often at the level of the internal os, in such a way that menstrual flow is impeded and intrauterine pressure is increased at the time of menses.

Dysmenorrhea. Painful menstruation with a cramping sensation in the lower abdomen often accompanied by other symptoms such as sweating, tachycardia, headaches, nausea, vomiting, diarrhea, and tremulousness. These all occur just before or during the menses. Primary dysmenorrhea begins at or shortly after menarche and is usually not accompanied by pelvic pathologic conditions. Secondary dysmenorrhea arises later and usually is associated with other pelvic conditions.

Mittelschmerz. Midcycle pelvic pain usually related to ovulation. The actual mechanism is not clearly understood.

Nonsteroidal Antiinflammatory Drugs (NSAIDs). Also known as prostaglandin synthetase inhibitors. Substances that block the activity of prostaglandin synthetase, thereby preventing the effect of prostaglandins on tissue. These basically consist of two chemical groups: the arylcarboxylic acids and the arylalkanoic acids.

Pelvic Congestion Syndrome. Vascular engorgement of the uterus and the vessels of the broad ligament and lateral pelvic walls, which may lead to chronic pelvic pain.

Premenstrual Dysphoric Disorder (PMDD). A combination of marked behavioral and mood symptoms, often accompanied by physical symptoms, that occur only in the luteal phase of the menstrual cycle. Interference with social or role functioning are common when symptoms are severe.

Premenstrual Syndrome (PMS). A group of symptoms, both physical and behavioral, that occur in the second half of the menstrual cycle and often interfere with work and personal relationships. They are followed by a period entirely free of symptoms.

Dysmenorrhea, premenstrual syndrome, and premenstrual dysphoric disorder afflict a large percentage of women in the reproductive years. These conditions have a negative effect on the quality of the women's lives and on the lives of their families, and they are also responsible for a huge economic loss as a result of the cost of medications, medical care, and decreased productivity. This chapter will discuss current thinking with respect to the etiology, pathophysiology, and management of these three conditions.

DYSMENORRHEA

Dysmenorrhea is defined as a severe, painful cramping sensation in the lower abdomen often accompanied by other biologic symptoms, including sweating, tachycardia, headaches, nausea, vomiting, diarrhea, and tremulousness, all occurring just before or during the menses. The term *primary dysmenorrhea* refers to pain with no obvious pathologic pelvic disease. We currently recognize that these patients are suffering from the effects of endogenous prostaglandins. *Secondary dysmenorrhea,* on the other hand, is associated with pelvic conditions or pathology that causes pelvic pain in conjunction with the menses. Primary dysmenorrhea almost always first occurs in women younger than 20. Indeed, the patient will report pain as soon as she establishes ovulatory cycles. Secondary dysmenorrhea may, of course, occur in women younger than 20, but it is most often seen in women older than 20.

Incidence and Epidemiology

A number of studies have attempted to determine the prevalence of dysmenorrhea; a wide range (16% to 90%) has been reported. These studies have been performed on students, teenagers and their mothers, and individuals from various specific populations, such as industrial workers or college students. The best estimate of the prevalence of primary dysmenorrhea is about 75%. Andersch and Milsom surveyed all the 19-year-old women in the city of Gothenburg, Sweden. A total of 90.9% of such women responded to a randomly distributed questionnaire, and 72.4% of these stated that they suffered from dysmenorrhea. In addition, 34.3% of the total population reported mild menstrual symptoms, 22.7% cited moderate symptoms that required analgesia, and 15.4% stated that they had severe dysmenorrhea that clearly inhibited their working ability and that could not be adequately assuaged by general analgesia (Table 36-1). This study verified the work of others who found that women who had vaginally delivered a child, or who were smokers were less likely to have dysmenorrhea. Oral contraceptive (OC) use was noted by these investigators to significantly reduce the prevalence and severity of dysmenorrhea ($p = 0.01$). Pregnancy itself without actual birth did not seem to alleviate dysmenorrhea, as women who had ectopic pregnancies or spontaneous or voluntary terminations of pregnancy were not relieved of their symptoms.

Relationship to Menstruation and the Menstrual Cycle

Andersch and Milsom demonstrated a significant positive correlation between the severity of dysmenorrhea and the duration of menstrual flow, amount of menstrual flow, and early menarche. They showed no relationship with the actual duration of the menstrual cycle.

In their series, 38.3% of the patients reported that they had experienced dysmenorrhea for the first time during the first year after menarche, and only 20.8% reported that dysmenorrhea had not occurred until 4 years after menarche.

Family History

Dysmenorrhea has been reported to be increased significantly among mothers and sisters of women with dysmenorrhea.

Table 36-1 Severity of Primary Dysmenorrhea in a Population of 586 Swedish, 19-year-old Women

Severity	Number	Percent
None	162	27.6
Mild*	201	34.3
Moderate†	133	22.7
Severe‡	90	15.4

*No systemic symptoms, medication rarely required, work rarely affected.
†Few systemic symptoms, medication required, work moderately affected.
‡Multiple symptoms, poor medication response, work inhibited.
Data from Andersch B, Milsom I: An epidemiologic study of young women with dysmenorrhea. Am J Obstet Gynecol 144:655, 1982.

Pathogenesis of Primary Dysmenorrhea

The pathogenesis of dysmenorrhea is not fully understood, but there is a close association between elevated prostaglandin $F_2\alpha$ (PG $F_2\alpha$) levels in the secretory endometrium and the symptoms of dysmenorrhea, including uterine hypercontractility, complaints of severe cramping, and other prostaglandin-induced symptoms. Arachidonic acid, the precursor to prostaglandin production, has been found in increased amounts in the uterus during ovulatory cycles. Arachidonic acid is converted to PG $F_2\alpha$, PGE_2, and leukotrienes, which are involved in increasing myometrial contractions. During menses these contractions decrease uterine blood flow and cause ischemia and sensitization of pain fibers (Fig. 36-1). Both ultrasound and magnetic resonance imaging (MRI) in small studies have correlated dysmenorrhea with myometrial changes and decreased blood flow. PG $F_2\alpha$ and PGE_2 affect other organs such as the bowel and result in nausea, vomiting, and diarrhea.

Diagnosis

Primary dysmenorrhea causes midline, crampy lower abdominal pain, which begins with the onset of menstruation. The pain can be quite severe and also involve the low back and thighs. The pain gradually resolves over 12 to 72 hours. Pain does not occur at times other than menses. The diagnosis is made

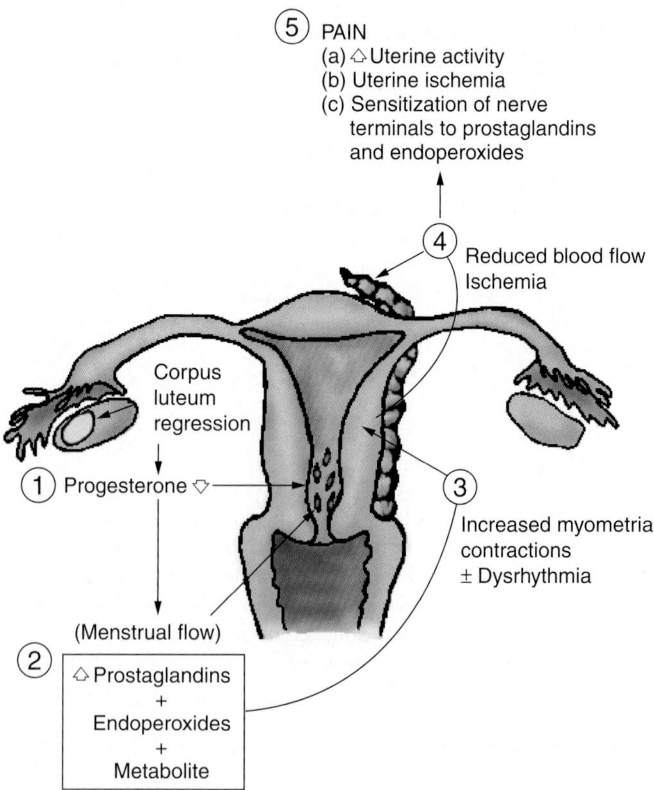

Figure 36-1. Mechanisms contributing to generation of pain in primary dysmenorrhea. (Reproduced from Dawood MY: Nonsteroidal anti-inflammatory drugs and reproduction. Am J Obstet Gynecol 169:5, 1993.)

largely by the history and physical exam. Women with primary dysmenorrhea have a normal pelvic exam.

Treatment

Nonsteroidal antiinflammatory drugs (NSAIDs) are prostaglandin synthetase inhibitors (PGSI) and have been demonstrated to alleviate these symptoms of dysmenorrhea. These substances are nonsteroidal and antiinflammatory. They are generally divided into two chemical groups: the arylcarboxylic acids, which include acetylsalicylic acid (aspirin) and fenamates (mefenamic acid), and the arylalkanoic acids, including the arylpropionic acids (ibuprofen, naproxen, and ketoprofen) and the indoleacetic acids (indomethacin). The more specific cyclooxygenase (COX-2) inhibitors such as celecoxib have similarly been shown to alleviate the primary dysmenorrheal symptoms. COX-2 expression in the uterine glandular epithelium was maximal during menstruation in one trial of ovulatory women, suggesting a possible association with the cause. The increased expression of COX-2 was eliminated with continuous use of OCs which are also an effective treatment (see the following section). The specific effect of these agents on the uterine musculature is reduction of contractility as measured by reduction of intrauterine pressure.

In 1984 Owen reviewed the effectiveness of NSAIDs in the treatment of primary dysmenorrhea. She reviewed 51 trials carried out in 1649 women. More than 72% of the women suffering from dysmenorrhea reported significant pain relief with NSAIDs, 18% reported minimal or no pain relief, and 15% showed a placebo response. Owen concluded that PGSI compounds were effective and safe for the majority of women with primary dysmenorrhea. The fenamates seemed to be more effective in relieving pain than ibuprofen, indomethacin, or naproxen. All the compounds demonstrated minimal NSAID-associated side effects, with the exception of indomethacin. In trials with indomethacin the dropout rate was higher primarily because of symptoms involving the central nervous system (CNS) and gastrointestinal tract. Efficacy with the COX-2 inhibitors is similar although several drugs in this class have been removed from the market for serious adverse cardiovascular events.

Smith has demonstrated that the effectiveness of NSAIDs is related to tissue concentration. Using meclofenamate in 18 subjects who participated in a double-blind, placebo-controlled, cross-over study, he was able to show a parallel in time response curves between the plasma levels of the drug and decrease in uterine contractility. Figure 36-2 demonstrates the average intrauterine pressure relationships between placebo-treated and drug-treated patients over time. Intrauterine pressure declined 20% to 56% in these patients during meclofenamate therapy.

NSAIDs should be given the day prior to the expected menses or at the onset of menses. If one NSAID is ineffective, switching to a different class of NSAIDs may be helpful. NSAIDs should not be given to patients who have shown previous hypersensitivity to such drugs. It is also contraindicated for women who have had nasal polyps, angioedema, and bronchospasm related to aspirin or NSAIDs. In addition, these agents are contraindicated for individuals with a history of chronic ulceration or inflammatory reaction of the upper or lower gastrointestinal tract and for those with preexisting chronic renal disease. During the use of such agents, autoimmune hemolytic anemia, rash, edema and fluid retention, and CNS symptoms, such as dizziness, headache, nervousness, and blurred vision, can occur. In up to 15% of users slight elevation of hepatic enzymes may also be found. Table 36-2 lists some of the NSAIDs in common use for the treatment of dysmenorrhea.

Other Therapy

Although NSAIDs are the standard therapy available for primary dysmenorrhea, other approaches are possible. OCs will relieve the symptoms of primary dysmenorrhea in about 90% of patients treated. This may be because OCs suppress ovulation and endometrial proliferation and the progestin component also blocks the production of the precursor to prostaglandin formation. If the patient also requires contraception, OC therapy may prove to be the treatment of choice. In small randomized controlled trials (RCTs), low-dose OCs (with 20 μg ethinyl estradiol) were effective in reducing dysmenorrhea both in adolescents and adult women. Continuous OC administration compared with traditional monthly cyclic dosing has been

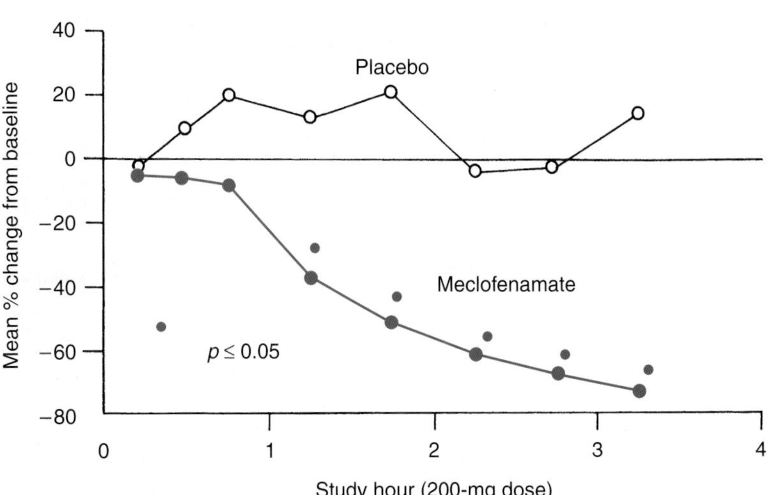

Figure 36-2. Average pressure: Meclofenamate versus placebo. (Redrawn from Smith RP: The dynamics of nonsteroidal antiinflammatory therapy for primary dysmenorrhea. Obstet Gynecol 70:785, 1987.)

Table 36-2 Commonly Used Nonsteroidal Antiinflammatory Drugs (NSAIDs)

Class	Brand Name	Generic Name	Usual Regimen (mg q6–8h)
Propronic Acids			
	Motrin	Ibuprofen	400–800
	Naprosyn	Naproxen	250–500 (bid)
	Anaprox	Naproxen sodium	275–550 (bid)
	N/A	Ketoprofen	25–50
Fenamic Acids			
	Ponstel	Mefenamic acid	250–500
Cyclooxygenase-2 Inhibitors			
	Celebrex	Celecoxib	200 (bid)

shown to reduce the menstrual pain symptoms. Breakthrough bleeding can be an undesirable side effect although a Cochrane Database Review of RCTs reported bleeding and discontinuation rates to be similar.

The levonorgestrel-releasing intrauterine system (LNG-IUS) has been shown to reduce menstrual pain in women from 60% before use to 29% when studied 3 years after insertion. A randomized comparison of microwave endometrial ablation with transcervical resection of the endometrium for menorrhagia showed both techniques reduced menstrual pain at the 5-year follow-up.

Narcotic analgesics may be necessary in treating patients with primary dysmenorrhea but should be used as backup drugs when the desired therapeutic effect is not achieved with NSAIDs or OCs.

A meta-analysis of three trials reported transcutaneous electrical nerve stimulation (TENS) was more effective than placebo in relieving dysmenorrhea although this was not as effective as analgesics. Milsom and colleagues in Sweden and Smith and Heltzel in the United States noted that TENS relieved menstrual pain without reducing intrauterine pressure, suggesting that its mode of action may be in the CNS. An abdominal patch delivering continuous topical heat was as effective as 400 mg of ibuprofen in reducing pain. Dietary and vitamin therapies may be beneficial but to date have not been studied in a rigorous fashion. A low-fat, vegetarian diet decreased menstrual pain in one study, and vitamin E was more effective than placebo in reducing dysmenorrhea in adolescents. Although the evidence is weak, exercise may be of benefit.

A 2005 Cochrane Collaborative meta-analysis of eight RCTs of surgical interruption of nerve pathways concluded that there was insufficient evidence to advise laparoscopic uterine nerve ablation (LUNA) or laparoscopic presacral neurectomy (LPSN) for primary dysmenorrhea.

Etiology and Management of Secondary Dysmenorrhea

Many other conditions cause or are associated with dysmenorrhea. Pelvic disease should be considered in cases that do not respond to NSAIDs and OCs for presumed primary dysmenorrhea. These conditions may occur at any age, and in most cases the pain experienced is either secondary to the pathologic process of the condition or a specific result of it. These constitute the so-called secondary dysmenorrhea group of problems and include cervical stenosis, ectopic endometrial tissue, pelvic inflammation, pelvic congestion, and conditioned behavior (see the following box).

Cervical Stenosis

Severe narrowing of the cervical canal, particularly at the level of the internal os, may impede menstrual flow, causing an increase in intrauterine pressure at the time of menses. In addition, retrograde menstrual flow through the fallopian tubes into the peritoneal cavity may take place. Thus severe cervical stenosis may eventually be associated with pelvic endometriosis as well. The origin of cervical stenosis may be congenital or may be secondary to cervical injury, such as with electrocautery, cryocautery, or operative trauma (i.e., conization). The condition may also result from an inflammatory process caused by infection, the application of caustic substances, or hypoestrogenism. After any of these conditions the cervical canal may narrow because of contraction of scar tissue.

The possibility of cervical stenosis should be considered if there is a history of scant menstrual flow and if severe cramping continues throughout the menstrual period. A hematometria or pyometria may occur.

The diagnosis is suspected when the external os appears scarred or when it is impossible to pass a cervical Pap smear brush or uterine sound through the internal os during the proliferative stage of the menstrual cycle. Diagnosis is generally documented by the inability to pass a thin probe of a few millimeters' diameter through the internal os or by hysterosalpingogram, which demonstrates a thin, stringy-appearing canal. If hysteroscopy and dilation and curettage (D&C) are performed, finding the passage through the internal os with a thin probe is often difficult but can frequently be accomplished with patience. The patient should be anesthetized. Ultrasound guidance may be of benefit to reduce the risk of making a false passage. Having the patient self-administer intravaginal misoprostol before the procedure has been done by the author's patients and can be helpful in relaxing the cervix, but this is not FDA-approved nor studied in large trials.

Treatment consists of dilating the cervix; this may be accomplished by D&C with progressive dilators or by the use of progressive *Laminaria japonica* tents. Unfortunately, cervical stenosis often recurs after therapy, necessitating repeat procedures. Pregnancy and vaginal delivery often afford a more lasting cure.

Causes of Secondary Dysmenorrhea

- Cervical stenosis
- Endometriosis and adenomyosis
- Pelvic infection and adhesions
- Uterine polyps
- Ovarian cyst or mass
- Pelvic congestion
- Congenital obstructed müllerian malformations
- Conditioned behavior
- Stress and tension

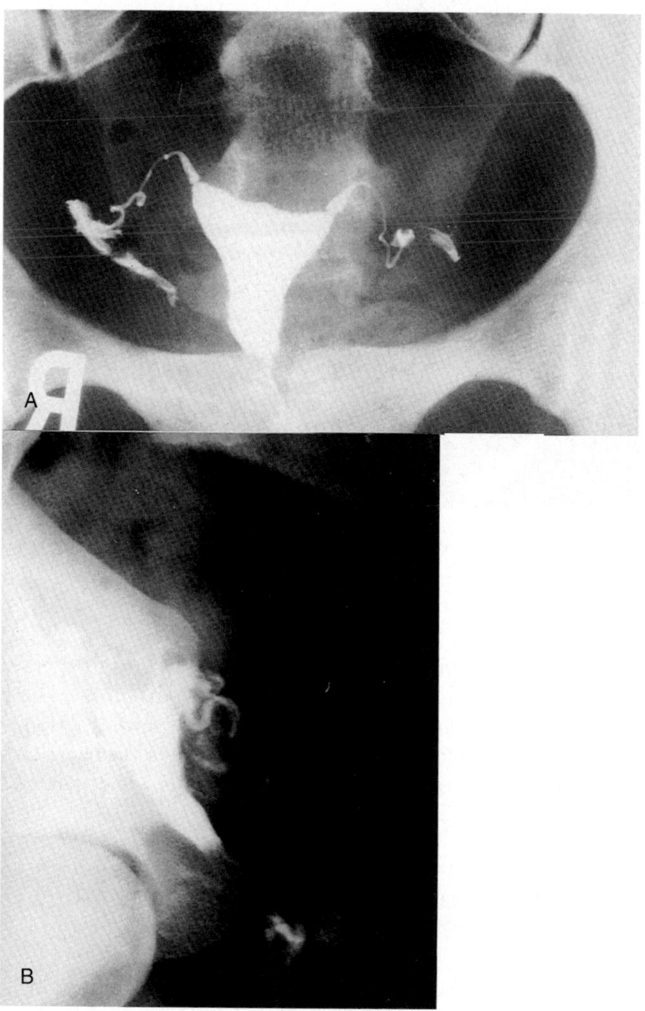

Figure 36-3. Hysterogram. Anteroposterior (**A**) view and lateral (**B**) views of an 18-year-old patient with severe disabling dysmenorrhea. At hysteroscopy she was found to have a tissue band across the internal os and an endocervical polyp at this site. Removal of the polyp and transection of the band completely relieved the dysmenorrhea.

Often other problems obstructing the cervix can have a similar presentation. Figure 36-3 shows anteroposterior and lateral views of a hysterogram in an 18-year-old nulliparous woman who had a 2-year history of severe, disabling dysmenorrhea that usually required morphine therapy with each menstrual period. At hysteroscopy she was found to have a tissue band across her internal os, at which site a large endocervical polyp had formed. Transecting the band and removing the polyp completely relieved the dysmenorrhea, and she had no further symptoms after 3 years.

Ectopic Endometrial Tissue (Endometriosis)

Ectopic endometrial tissue or endometriosis (including endometriosis and adenomyosis) should be considered when there is a history of pain becoming more severe during menses. Frequently dyspareunia and infertility are accompanying symptoms. Pertinent physical findings may include uterosacral ligament nodules, evidence for endometriosis in the vagina or cervix or lateral displacement of the cervix.

Koike and colleagues, in an in vitro experiment using tissue slices, found that prostaglandin in endometriosis implants was significantly higher than in normal endometrium, myometrium, leiomyomata, and normal ovarian tissue and that adenomyosis implants produced larger amounts of 6-keto PGF when the dysmenorrhea had been severe. They believed that prostaglandins in endometriosis increased painful menstruation.

Treatment of endometriosis is discussed in Chapter 19.

Pelvic Inflammation

Pelvic infections secondary to gonorrhea, chlamydia, or other infections may cause pelvic inflammation or pelvic abscess and with healing may be associated with pelvic adhesions and tubal damage that may cause pelvic pain. Pelvic inflammatory disease (PID) can lead to chronic pelvic pain in up to 30% of women. Often this may be aggravated at menses, causing dysmenorrhea. Infections secondary to other conditions, such as appendicitis or intrauterine device (IUD) use, may also create a similar response. The pain may be secondary to the congestion and edema that occur normally at menses, which may subsequently be aggravated by the healed inflammatory areas and adhesions.

Pelvic Congestion Syndrome and Pelvic Venous Syndromes

Pelvic congestion syndrome, which was first described by Taylor in 1949, results from engorgement of pelvic vasculature. Controversy exists regarding whether this is an actual disorder since it has been difficult to prove. However, the authors believe it exists, possibly because of past pregnancy or past inflammatory pelvic pathology. The pain is usually burning or throbbing in nature, worse at night, and worse after standing. Physical examination of the vagina and cervix usually reveals vasocongestion with evidence of some uterine enlargement and tenderness. Diagnosis is made by observation of the features noted and by laparoscopy, which not only rules out other causes of pelvic pain but also demonstrates congestion of the uterus and engorgement or varicosities of the broad ligament and pelvic side wall veins. If laparoscopy is used for diagnosis, it is important to observe the broad ligament vasculature as the pressure of the carbon dioxide or nitrous oxide is released. At full pressure during the procedure these vessels may be obliterated but will reappear as pressure is reduced.

More recently, other pelvic venous syndromes have been described that can cause pelvic pain and probably include what Taylor first described. Vulvar varices, hypogastric vein insufficiency, and gonadal venous insufficiency have been described in a review of 57 female patients ages 24 to 48. Symptoms included pelvic pain, dysuria, dysmenorrhea, and dyspareunia. These disorders are poorly understood and poorly studied so often go undiagnosed. Diagnosis in this study was made by physical exam and a variety of radiologic investigations, including Doppler scans, duplex ultrasound scans, computed tomography (CT), magnetic resonance imaging (MRI), and angiography. No standard therapeutic approach is available so therapies range from ovarian hormone suppression, local sclerotherapy (for vulvar varices), and embolization of the hypogastric vein to resection of the gonadal vein to hysterectomy.

Women with chronic pelvic pain often have psychological issues, so careful evaluation of the patient's past and present social situation and referral for counseling may be appropriate.

Behavioral Influences

In individuals with strong family histories of dysmenorrhea or when a careful history demonstrates a possibility for societal reward or control because of the symptoms of pain, a conditioned behavior should be considered. It is important to obtain a careful medical and social history and to rule out all other causes of acquired dysmenorrhea.

Treatment of patients with conditioned behavior dysmenorrhea includes reeducation so that the pain is not looked on as a rewarding experience. Teaching the patient an understanding of the pathophysiology of the problem and applying reconditioning techniques are useful. Psychologists or other similarly trained mental health workers can be consulted for this purpose.

Dysmenorrhea aggravated by stress and tension usually is accompanied by a history of gradual onset, and the pain is generally worse at times, particularly when stress is severe and when there may be a possibility for secondary gain. The pathophysiology is difficult to define; it may be a combination of prostaglandin activity and engorgement.

The treatment is centered on finding the means to relieve stress, which may include education, the teaching of relaxation techniques, counseling, and, on rare occasions, antidepressant or tranquilizing medications for short periods of time.

Relation to Functional Bowel Disease

Crowell and coworkers studied 383 women ages 20 to 40 using an NEO Personality Inventory on entry into the program, a Moos' Menstrual Distress Questionnaire, and a bowel symptom inventory every 3 months for 12 months. Dysmenorrhea was diagnosed in 19.8% of the 383 women. Functional bowel disorder, defined as abdominal pain with altered bowel function, occurred in 61% of the women with dysmenorrhea but in only 20% of the others ($p < 0.05$). Bowel symptoms were significantly correlated with dysmenorrhea even after controlling for the effects of neuroticism. Prostaglandin levels in vaginal fluid were elevated in patients with dysmenorrhea but did not consistently differentiate the diagnostic groups. These authors concluded that there was a strong covariance of menstrual and bowel symptoms, along with an overlap in their diagnosis, suggesting a common physiologic basis.

In a study of women with irritable bowel syndrome (IBS) and menstrual cycle symptoms, dysmenorrhea was twice as prevalent among women with IBS than controls (21% vs. 10%, $p = 0.09$) although this was not statistically significant. Women with IBS on OCs had significantly less dysmenorrhea than control women not on OCs (11% vs. 28%, $p = 0.02$). One case report found an association of celiac sprue and dysmenorrhea, but little is known about this finding.

Other Causes

At times dysmenorrhea may be related to unusual pathologic findings. These include small leiomyomas or polyps at the junction of the internal os and lower uterine segment (Fig. 36-4). Such a condition may produce a valvelike effect at the os at the time of menses. Frequently myomas or polyps become engorged or edematous at the time of menses, accentuating the problem. Diagnosis is generally made by history and by hysterosalpingography or hysteroscopy and D&C. Therapy consists of excising the pathologic tissue. In the case of a myoma, myomectomy or hysterectomy may be necessary.

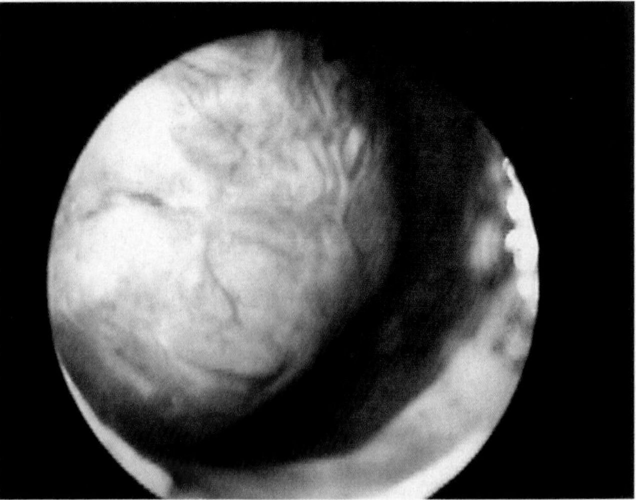

Figure 36-4. Submucus myoma blocking the internal os causing secondary dysmenorrhea.

There are nongynecologic causes for pain during menses that should be considered in the differential diagnosis. These include appendicitis, lactose intolerance, celiac sprue, abdominal mass, and multiple urinary tract conditions (urinary tract infection, interstitial cystitis, nephrolithiasis, and ureteral obstruction).

PREMENSTRUAL SYNDROME AND PREMENSTRUAL DYSPHORIC DISORDER

Premenstrual syndrome (PMS) is defined as a group of mild to moderate symptoms, both physical and behavioral, that occur in the second half of the menstrual cycle and that may interfere with work and personal relationships. These are followed by a period entirely free of symptoms. The condition was first described by Frank in 1931. That author attempted to relate symptoms of then so-called *premenstrual tension* with hormonal changes of the menstrual cycle. The term *premenstrual syndrome* was first used by Dalton in 1953. The symptoms do vary from woman to woman, and more than 150 symptoms have been linked with the disorder.

Premenstrual dysphoric disorder (PMDD) represents a more severe disorder with marked behavioral and emotional symptoms. PMS differs from PMDD in severity of symptoms, and women with PMDD must have one severe affective symptom. These include markedly depressed mood or hopelessness, anxiety or tension, affective lability, or persistent anger. Multiple physical symptoms may also be present. PMDD also differs from PMS as there is substantial impairment in personal functioning. PMS and PMDD are similar in that the symptoms manifest in the luteal phase of the menstrual cycle and resolve during menses.

Incidence and Epidemiology

Although various reports place the prevalence of PMS at 30% to 80% of menstruating women, it is generally agreed that about 40% of women are significantly affected at one time or another. Severe symptoms (PMDD) occur in only 3% to 8% of women between the ages of 18 and 48. The average age of onset is 26. Likely risk factors for PMS include family history of PMS in the mother, personal past or current psychiatric illness involving mood or anxiety disorders, history of alcohol abuse, and a history of postpartum depression. Some studies have found that nulliparity, earlier menarche, higher alcohol and caffeine intake, more stress, and higher body mass index are risk factors for certain PMS symptoms. Recent studies support earlier reports that familial and stress factors play a role in the syndrome. Little is know about racial/ethnic differences except that PMS appears to occur in all cultures studied. Data from a California HMO PMS severity study of 1194 women found Hispanics reported greater severity of symptoms than whites and blacks, and Asian women reported less.

In the Harvard Study of Moods and Cycles (Cohen and colleagues), a population-based, cross-sectional sample of 4164 premenopausal women was studied retrospectively regarding PMDD prevalence. A PMDD diagnosis was made in 6.4% of women, and PMDD was associated with lower education, a history of major depression, and current smoking. This confirms earlier studies reporting a significant lifetime comorbidity of PMDD and affective disorders.

Symptoms

In a review by O'Brien a number of common somatic and affective symptoms were enumerated. These are summarized in the following box. The most common somatic symptoms relate to abdominal bloating, breast tenderness, and various pain constellations, such as headache. Psychological symptoms vary from fatigue, irritability, and tension to anxiety, labile mood and depression. In Sternfeld and associates' severity of PMS symptoms study in an HMO population of 1194 women, consistency of symptoms was found over two consecutive cycles, especially for emotional symptoms.

Depression is a common complaint in the population in general and also in PMS/PMDD sufferers during the luteal phase. Mortola and coworkers have shown that 16 PMS patients had marked worsening of scores on the Profile of Mood States and Beck Depression Inventory during the luteal phase compared with 16 controls. However, six patients suffering from endogenous depression had scores threefold higher on both indices than PMS patients who were in the luteal phase. Also, the amplitude of cortisol secretion pulses was higher in the depressed patients than either PMS patients or control patients. The data of this study demonstrate that PMS patients do have more episodes of depression during the luteal phase compared with controls, but these episodes are distinctly different from those suffered by patients with endogenous depression.

In addition, Rapkin and colleagues have demonstrated that PMS patients show no deficit in cognitive processing and performance, as well as no loss in ability to concentrate and sustain attention and motivation. No such alterations were seen in 10 PMS patients during the luteal phase. Their performance was similar to nine controls when tested in these areas. In a later study, this group studied 30 patients with PMS and 31 controls during the follicular and luteal phases. Despite feelings of inadequacy, patients showed no statistically significant differences from controls in tests for attention, memory, cognitive flexibility, and overall mental agility.

Symptoms of Premenstrual Syndrome

Somatic Symptoms
Abdominal bloating
Feeling of weight increase
Fluid retention
Increased appetite/food cravings
Breast pain or tenderness
Skin disorders (acne)
Hot flushes
Headache
Dizziness, poor coordination, clumsiness
Change in libido
Change in bowel habits
Thirst

Affective Symptoms
Irritability
Mood lability
Angry outbursts
Poor impulse control
Tension
Anxiety
Depression
Lethargy
Insomnia
Crying, social withdrawal
Loss of concentration, confusion

Modified from O'Brien PM: The premenstrual syndrome: A review of the present status of therapy. Drugs 24:140, 1982.

A PMS diagnosis not only affects quality of life, but also economic issues. Slight increases in direct costs (medical expenses) have been noted. Indirect costs to the employer in work absences and lost productivity amount to $4333 per patient annually.

Etiology

When Frank first described the syndrome, he attributed it to estrogen excess. Others have offered theories that the disorder is related to an imbalance of estrogen and progesterone, endogenous hormone allergy, hypoglycemia, vitamin B_6 deficiency, prolactin excess, fluid retention, inappropriate prostaglandin activity, elevated monoamine oxidase (MAO) levels, endorphin malfunction, and multiple psychological disturbances. In 1981, Reid and Yen reviewed the subject and concluded that PMS was a multifactorial psychoendocrine disorder. Figure 36-5 shows a schematic of the proposed etiology. Studies indicate that cyclic gonadal hormonal alterations and serotonergic neuronal mechanisms in the CNS may interact and be major factors in the etiology of PMS in susceptible women. Evidence for this

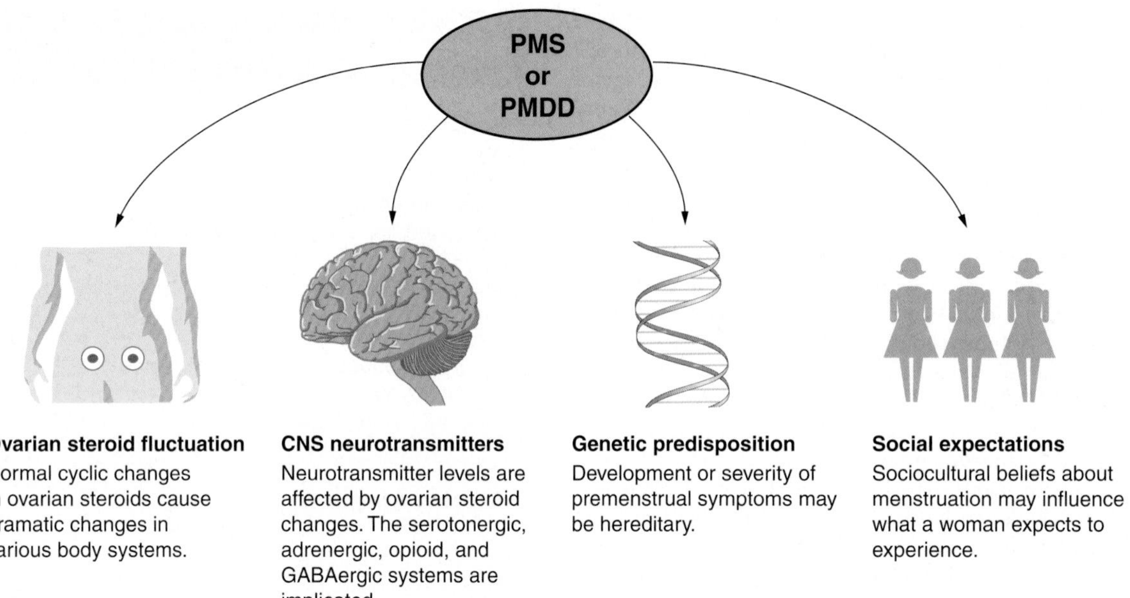

Figure 36-5. Proposed etiology of PMS and PMDD. GABA, γ-aminobutyric acid. (From Ling F, Mortola J, Pariser S, et al: Premenstrual Syndrome and Premenstrual Dysphoric Disorder: Scope, Diagnosis, and Treatment. APGO Educational Series on Women's Health Issues. Golden, CO, Medical Education Collaborative, 1998.)

is indirect but includes successful clinical trials with selective serotonin reuptake inhibitors (SSRIs) and other neurotropic agents thought to affect the serotonin pump mechanism between CNS neurons. Other indirect evidence includes the fact that platelet tritium-labeled, imipramine-binding sites are felt to be reduced in patients suffering from depression and are believed to represent receptor sites that label for a presynaptic serotonin transporter on the presynaptic nerve terminal. In some studies, binding sites have returned to normal several months after clinical remission of depression or during the response to psychotropic medications or electroconvulsive therapy. These platelet-binding sites therefore have been used as an indirect measure of the neuron receptor site. Steege and coworkers demonstrated lower platelet tritium-labeled imipramine binding in women with late luteal-phase dysphoric disorder (PMS) and felt this supported the hypothesis that such patients suffered from alterations of the central serotonergic systems.

That ovulation and therefore progesterone production is important in this syndrome has been known for some time, but studies related to the relationship of estrogen and progesterone in the circulation and the severity of the symptoms have not been fruitful. There are no consistent differences between estrogen and progesterone levels in PMS suffers and those in controls. Although symptom relief has been noted in several studies using gonadotropin-releasing hormone (GnRH) agonists to block ovulation completely, no relief was found in a study by Chan and colleagues, who blocked progesterone receptors with the progesterone antagonist RU 486. Rapkin and colleagues evaluated the anxiolytic 3-α-5-α–reduced progesterone metabolite allopregnanediol during the luteal phase of 35 women with PMS and 36 controls. Serum progesterone and allopregnanediol levels were measured on days 19 and 26 of the cycles as determined by luteinizing hormone (LH) kits. Allopregnanediol levels were significantly lower in the PMS patients than controls on day 26, but there were no significant differences with respect to progesterone itself. They concluded that since PMS patients had lower levels of this anxiolytic metabolite during the luteal phase, they could be at greater susceptibility for various mood symptoms such as anxiety, tension, and depression. Chuong and associates have recently demonstrated that β-endorphin levels throughout the periovulatory phase were lower in PMS patients than in controls, especially in postovulatory days 0 to 4. Likewise, Halbreich and coworkers demonstrated that PMS patients treated with 200 mg/day of danazol for 90 days demonstrated a complete relief of symptoms in 23 anovulatory cycles, but relief of symptoms occurred in only 6 of 32 ovulatory cycles. They concluded that the beneficial effect of danazol in the treatment of PMS was achieved only when the anovulatory state eliminated the hormonal cyclicity of the normal cycle and not because of action of drug per se. Further evidence for this was advanced by O'Brien and Abukhalil. They studied 100 women with PMS and premenstrual breast pain using a randomized, double-masked, placebo-controlled study of three menstrual cycles, using danazol 200 mg/day as the active drug. Treatment was given only during the luteal phase. Danazol did not effectively reduce the general symptoms of PMS, but did relieve mastalgia. Severe PMS has been shown to be relieved by total abdominal hysterectomy and bilateral salpingo-oophorectomy even with hormone replacement therapy using an estrogen, but some women on cyclic estrogen and progesterone therapy postmenopausally continue to complain of PMS symptoms. A recent study by Roca and colleagues suggests that women with PMS may have an abnormal response to progesterone. Women with PMS failed to show a normal increased luteal-phase hypothalamic–pituitary–adrenal axis response to exercise stress testing compared with controls. This response is distinctly different in PMS patients compared with women with major depression.

Concerning other possible causes, most dietary and vitamin deficiency theories have been difficult to prove and have not been found to be a major cause of this syndrome. However, recent data from Bertone-Johnson and colleagues' case-control study involving the Nurses' Health Study II cohort suggested a high intake of calcium and vitamin D may reduce the risk of PMS, so further research is needed in this area. Several have looked for prolactin excess since some of the patients complain of breast tenderness, but no positive findings have been found. Although some of the symptomatology seems to relate to prostaglandin activity and these symptoms are often reduced with treatment with NSAIDs, a direct cause and effect has not been established.

In summary, PMS/PMDD etiology is associated with ovulation, which seems to cause alterations in neurohormones and neurotransmitters that lead to reduction of serotonergic function during the luteal phase. The most effective evidence-based treatment for moderate to severe PMS and PMDD symptoms are SSRIs and agents that block ovulation.

Diagnosis

The diagnosis of PMS/PMDD is made by the history of two consecutive menstrual cycles demonstrating luteal-phase symptoms of PMS. The facts given by the patient may allow the physician to construct a specific treatment regimen for that patient. It is important that the physician have a clear understanding of the patient's symptoms before undertaking therapy. After a complete history and physical examination, the physician should rule out any medical problems that could be influencing the symptomatology. The physician should then ask the patient to keep a diary of her symptoms throughout two menstrual cycles. Although the patient and the physician may focus on the second half of the menstrual cycle, the patient should be encouraged to keep track of all symptoms regardless of the stage of the menstrual cycle. A number of commercial diary sheets and symptom checklists are available, but it is probably better to have the patient write the symptoms she perceives in her own words rather than clue her to specific response patterns. At the end of two cycles the physician should review the symptom diary with the patient and discuss carefully those symptoms that seem to be causing her the most difficulty.

The ACOG Practice Bulletin establishes the key elements of the PMS diagnosis as (1) symptoms characteristic of PMS, (2) luteal-phase symptoms confirmed by prospective menstrual cycle symptom charting, (3) symptoms affect the women's life, and (4) exclusion of other diagnoses.

It is important to differentiate PMS from other illnesses with similar symptomatology. Patients with depression and anxiety disorders may present believing that they have PMS. A differentiating aspect is that PMS patients suffer their symptoms *only* during the luteal phase. Diagnosis can be difficult because women with depression and anxiety disorders can have premenstrual exacerbation of their symptoms, and PMS/PMDD can coexist with psychiatric disorders.

That many women who do not actually have PMS may be self-referred to a facility that treats this condition is well appreciated. In one study, Plouffe and associates carefully analyzed 100 consecutive women prospectively entering the Uniform Diagnostic and Treatment Protocol for PMS and found that 38 women had PMS; 24 had premenstrual magnification syndrome (i.e., other conditions that were magnified during the luteal phase), and 13 had affective or other psychiatric disorders. Only 44% of the women previously given a diagnosis of PMS were found to have this syndrome. Overall, in this study, 84% of the women with PMS and premenstrual magnification syndrome responded to treatment. A variety of currently accepted therapies were used.

No laboratory tests are available to make the diagnosis. Although it has been reported that many patients with PMS suffer thyroid hypofunction, a study by Nikolai and coworkers demonstrated that there was no significant thyroid disease in 44 carefully studied PMS patients compared with 15 normal controls. In addition, treating 22 with L-thyroxine and 22 with placebo led to no differences in relief of symptoms.

Other conditions to consider based on patient symptoms include anemia, diabetes, endometriosis, autoimmune disorders, chronic fatigue syndrome, collagen vascular disorders, and many psychiatric disorders (depression, anxiety, dysthymia, bipolar disorder, etc.)

The diagnosis of PMS is therefore made by symptom diary and by the elimination of other diagnoses. The diagnosis of PMDD is made following the *Diagnostic and Statistical Manual of Mental Disorders,* 4th ed (DSM-IV) criteria, which require five symptoms of PMS including one affective symptom. Affective symptoms include (1) feeling sad or hopeless or having self-deprecating thoughts; (2) anxiety or tension; (3) mood lability and crying; or (4) persistent irritability, anger, and increased interpersonal conflicts. Prospective menstrual cycle charting is required for the diagnosis.

Management

Diet and Exercise

Although many individuals will suffer from symptomatology related to PMS, only about 3% or 8% are seriously affected. Thus the selection of medications and other regimens should be tailored to the symptomatic needs of the patient. Several dietary studies have been performed, but most were not rigorously controlled. Two trials have studied increasing complex carbohydrate intake, which reduced the severity of PMS mood symptoms. A more recent study by Barnard suggested that a low-fat vegetarian diet improved dysmenorrhea duration and intensity and duration of premenstrual symptoms. Sex hormone-binding globulin (SHBG) concentrations increased with this vegetarian diet, and SHBG binds and inactivates estrogens, which may possibly be a factor in the etiology.

A multicenter RCT of 466 women showed 1200 mg of calcium per day for three cycles reduced PMS symptoms significantly compared with placebo (48% vs. 30%, $p < .001$). This is a reasonable treatment to begin since women need adequate calcium in their diet for bone health, and it can be started while the woman completes the menstrual symptom charting. However, this trial had limitations in that other PMS treatments were allowed and one other RCT showing benefits of calcium also had study limitations. Vitamin B_6 deficiency in PMS patients has been suggested because B_6 is a coenzyme in the biosynthesis of dopamine and serotonin, and neurotransmitters have been implicated in the etiology of PMS. One double-blind study by Abraham and Hargrove demonstrated that vitamin B_6 administered at 200- to 800-mg doses daily prevented some of the symptoms of PMS in women with this affliction, significantly better than placebo. They theorized that deficiencies of vitamin B_6 and magnesium could result in lower thresholds to stress and to potential hormone imbalance. They felt that eventually the vitamin B_6 activity might lower brain serotonin levels. Although B_6 has been a conventional treatment, the effectiveness is still unknown. A review of nine RCTs of B_6 for PMS found no high-quality trials although several suggested relief of PMS symptoms over placebo. Vitamin B_6 (pyridoxine) supplement at the rate of 50 mg/day can be tried for mild PMS symptoms. Higher doses of pyridoxine should be administered with caution since neuropathy can occur in patients treated with as little as 100–200 mg/day. Such symptoms as sensory deficit, paresthesia, numbness, ataxia, and muscle weakness may occur. There is inconclusive evidence from two RCTs that magnesium (200 to 400 mg/day) reduces PMS symptoms although one trial showed a decrease in fluid retention.

Many other complementary and alternative medicines (CAM) have been studied. One of the better designed trials found chaste berry extract reduced PMS symptoms 50% from baseline in 52% of women compared with 24% of women getting placebo. However, to date calcium is the most promising dietary treatment as the research on other CAM is seriously flawed.

Patients should be encouraged to exercise at least three to four times per week for general health reasons. Small trials have suggested aerobic exercise to be beneficial for PMS sufferers, and one trial found high-intensity aerobic exercise to be superior to low-intensity aerobic exercise for PMS treatment.

Diuretics

The physician may elect to add a diuretic to the regimen if the patient complaints involve bloating, fluid retention, and perceived change in body habitus during the luteal phase of the cycle. A potassium-saving diuretic should be selected, and the lowest dose possible to achieve symptomatic relief should be used. Although many patients do report a feeling of fluid retention during the luteal phase, this has been difficult to demonstrate. Perceived swelling of the body is difficult to prove unless actual careful weight analysis is utilized. Faratian and colleagues evaluated 148 menstrual cycles in 52 women, and in each cycle various parameters were measured to determine an objective means of assessing the syndrome. These included daily mood assessment, measurement of body weight, plasma 17 β-estradiol levels, and plasma progesterone levels. The abdominal girth was measured carefully in two dimensions: at the level of the umbilicus and then 10 cm below the umbilicus. At the same time the dimensions were subjectively judged by the patient. Mood scores showed a marked shifting during the premenstrual phase of each cycle. The symptoms of bloatedness were most marked during the premenstrual phase of the cycle. Despite these elevated scores for bloatedness, there was no increase in body weight or measured body dimension changes in any plane during this period. The patient's perception of body size did increase, and a discrepancy between the perceived body size and actual body size was noted. The authors divided their patients into those with predominantly somatic symptoms and those with predominantly psychological symptoms and also studied a control group. No hormonal differences were noted in the three groups. Freeman and associates studied transcapillary fluid balance in 10 women with well-defined PMS. The capillary filtration coefficient was measured by string gauge plethysmography. They noted that from the follicular to the luteal phase, interstitial colloid osmotic pressure on the leg was significantly reduced (mean of 3.6 mm Hg), whereas the interstitial colloid osmotic pressure on the thorax remained constant. The capillary filtration coefficient increased 30% from the follicular to the luteal phase. No change was observed in body weight. The authors felt that these changes represented an instability of vascular regulation in women with PMS and that this led support to the hypothesis that redistribution of fluid rather than water retention is responsible for the subjective symptom of bloatedness in PMS. This would explain why diuretics might appear beneficial to the patient. Spironolactone (100 mg/day) has been studied in four RCTs, and three trials demonstrated moderate efficacy for breast tenderness and fluid retention and two found reduced irritability symptoms. They should be avoided in patients with chronic renal disease or in those who are suffering from diarrhea or other fluid loss.

Cognitive Behavioral Therapy

Studies in the 1950s showed that 50% of patients improved with psychotherapy alone. However, Wyatt's review of seven RCTs found significant reduction in PMS symptoms versus control treatments, but the effect was similar to the response rate of many placebo therapies. Certainly if patients have obvious psychiatric problems as detected by history, psychotherapy should be added. It is less effective as a primary therapy. Relaxation therapy may be of benefit to patients with a significant stress and anxiety components.

Psychoactive Drugs

The SSRIs have been shown to be extremely effective for treating PMS and have become first-line treatment for PMDD. Dimmock and coworkers' meta-analysis of 15 RCTs showed SSRIs to be seven times more effective than placebo in treating PMS. Relief of both physical and behavioral symptoms is noted. Intermittent treatment during just the luteal phase of the menstrual cycle was equal to continuous SSRI treatment. The doses of medications are generally lower than doses used for depression. The onset of action can be very rapid, within 1 to 2 days (for dosing, see the following box). If luteal-phase treatment is not effective after 3 months, a trial of continuous SSRIs is warranted. If one SSRI is ineffective, try other agents. Venlafaxine is a serotonin and norepinephrine reuptake inhibitor and has been studied in an RCT for PMDD. There was significant reduction in symptoms and this medication may be helpful to

FDA-approved SSRIs for PMDD

Drug	Starting Dose
Fluoxetine hydrochloride (Sarafem)	20 mg/day
Sertraline hydrochloride (Zoloft)	50 mg/day
Paroxetine hydrochloride (Paxil CR)	12.5 mg/day

patients who had side effects or had no benefit on other SSRIs. After three cycles of SSRI treatment for PMDD, symptoms recurred with the first cycle after drug discontinuation, suggesting prolonged therapy may be necessary.

Side effects include sexual dysfunction, sleep alterations, gastrointestinal distress including nausea, and CNS complaints. Some SSRIs can precipitate anxiety reactions, so caution should be used if anxiety symptoms predominate the PMS. Increased suicide rates have been observed with some SSRIs, so caution is needed if significant depressive symptoms are noted. This should be a low risk, given the low dose and intermittent luteal-phase dosing.

Continuous use of psychoactive drugs, such as tricyclics and lithium, has not yielded good PMS symptom relief. Smith and coworkers noted in a carefully performed double-blind, placebo-controlled, cross-over study of 19 patients suffering from PMS using alprazolam (Xanax) that the drug significantly relieved the severity of premenstrual nervous tension, mood swings, irritability, anxiety, depression, fatigue, forgetfulness, crying, cravings for sweets, abdominal bloating, cramps, and headaches, compared with the placebo. These investigators prescribed 0.25 mg three times a day days 20–28 of each cycle, tapering to 0.25 mg twice a day on day 1 and 0.25 mg on day 2. Several RCTs have shown doses higher than 0.75 mg/day were necessary to significantly reduce PMS symptoms. However, about 50% of women complain of drowsiness and sedation on these doses. Patients with strong tendencies to habituation should not be treated with this regimen. Buspirone has less addictive potential than alprazolam and has been found in two RCTs to reduce symptoms.

Before using psychoactive drugs, it is extremely important to be sure of the diagnosis as the drugs may not be effective and may actually be contraindicated in other psychiatric conditions that mimic PMS.

Progesterone and Estrogen

Although a common treatment previously, double-blind studies to date have not shown progestogens to be conclusively effective for PMS. Small RCTs suggest small, but significant reductions in some PMS symptoms. However, there is insufficient evidence to recommend progestogen therapy. Similarly, oral progesterone therapy showed small but significant reduction in some PMS symptoms, but the improvement was not thought to be clinically important, especially given the much greater benefit of SSRIs.

Some relief of symptoms was noted in a double-blind, placebo-controlled, cross-over study using estradiol patches (200 μg every 3 days) and norethisterone 5 mg (days 19–26 of each cycle) when compared with placebo by Watson and coworkers. The authors realized they were suppressing ovulation and that this may have been the mechanism for obtaining symptom relief. Two other small RCTs have suggested improvement from estrogen for PMS, but the magnitude of benefit is unclear.

Oral Contraceptives

Several RCTs and descriptive studies using cyclic OCs have shown mixed results for treatment of PMS, and OCs mainly help physical symptoms such as breast pain, bloating, acne and appetite. If used, monophasic OCs appear to be better. In Sulak's retrospective review of 220 patients using an extended OC regimen and a shortened hormone-free interval (3 to 4 days), 45% of patients chose this regimen for control of PMS symptoms and 40% for dysmenorrhea and pelvic pain symptoms. Continuous combined OCs should suppress ovulation and provide symptom relief. A 2005 Cochrane Database review stated few studies have reported on menstrual symptoms on continuous- or extended-use OCs, but improvement was noted in headaches, tiredness, bloating, and menstrual pain. Finally, a prospective study published in 2006 by Coffee and colleagues showed an extended regimen of 30 μg ethinyl estradiol with 3 mg of drosperinone for 168 days significantly reduced PMS symptoms compared with typical 21-day cyclic OCs.

Nonsteroidal Antiinflammatory Drugs

For patients who complain of cramping or other systemic symptoms, such as diarrhea or heat intolerance, a trial with an NSAID may be useful. RCTs with mefenamic acid and naproxen have shown improvement in pain, mood, and somatic symptoms. It should be noted, however, that a toxic complication of NSAID use is nonoliguric renal failure. Because it is more likely to occur with NSAID use associated with severe dehydration, the agent should be discontinued if severe diarrhea is present and should not be used with diuretics.

Danazol

Sarno and associates reported on the apparent effectiveness of danazol in doses of 200 mg/day, days 20 to 28 of each menstrual cycle, in relieving PMS symptoms. Studying 14 patients in a double-blind, placebo-controlled protocol, they found significant relief of symptoms in 11 of the 14 patients, compared with placebo. Because such a small dose given during only the luteal phase will not prevent pregnancy and to avoid the potential of masculinizing a female fetus, patients should be cautioned to avoid this agent if pregnancy is contemplated. As noted previously, danazol may be effective because it causes anovulation in some subjects at this dose level. One other RCT of luteal-phase danazol showed only significant reduction in premenstrual mastalgia. Because of side effects (hirsutism, deepening of the voice, acne) and treatments with more accurately known response rates are available, danazol is rarely recommended.

Bromocriptine

Bromocriptine may be used in patients with cyclic mastalgia and may be helpful for some of the other symptoms of PMS, although its use in any individual case will need to be evaluated. A dose of 2.5 to 5 mg/day during the luteal phase is appropriate.

GnRH Agonists

At least 10 RCTs have shown GnRH agonists (leuprolide 3.75 mg IM monthly) to be effective for ovulation suppression and treatment of PMS. However, they are expensive, can have marked side effects, and are limited in duration of use.

Hysterectomy and Bilateral Oophorectomy

Casper and Hearn reported complete relief of symptoms in 14 women with severe debilitating symptoms of PMS who had completed their families, had been demonstrated to have relief of symptoms with ovarian-suppressing doses of danazol, and now were treated with total hysterectomy and bilateral oophorectomy followed by continuous low-dose estrogen replacement therapy. Casson and colleagues have noted similar results. Although this approach is not offered as standard therapy for severe PMS, it may be a reasonable alternative for selective cases where all other treatments have failed. The use of a GnRH analogue for 3 to 6 months with or without estrogen add-back may be useful as therapy in severe cases or at least helpful in deciding who may benefit from surgical treatment. Hysterectomy without bilateral oophorectomy does not relieve symptoms.

The physician should be cautious in building a treatment regimen for any individual patient and should attempt to verify the patient's symptoms and to add medications only when relief has not been achieved. Medications that do not seem to be helping should be stopped. Because of the myriad of PMS symptoms, it is not surprising that individualization of treatment is essential. Many of the therapies just mentioned, however, do offer relief of most symptoms and hope for many sufferers.

KEY POINTS

- Primary dysmenorrhea almost always occurs before the age of 20. Secondary dysmenorrhea may occur at any time during the menstrual years.
- Approximately 75% of all women complain of primary dysmenorrhea. Roughly 15% have severe symptoms.
- Pregnancy without vaginal birth does not seem to alleviate primary dysmenorrhea, whereas childbirth does.
- The severity of primary dysmenorrhea correlates directly with the duration of menstrual flow, amount of menstrual flow, and age at menarche but does not correlate with the duration of the menstrual cycle.
- Among patients who had primary dysmenorrhea, 38% reported onset of symptoms within the first year after menarche.
- Nonsteroidal antiinflammatory drugs (NSAIDs) are the treatment of choice in primary dysmenorrhea, with 72% of women suffering from dysmenorrhea reporting significant pain relief.
- NSAIDs reduced intrauterine pressure 20% to 56% during treatment of patients with dysmenorrhea in one study and blocked prostaglandin production and action.
- OCs reduce the prevalence and severity of dysmenorrhea. They can be used in long cycles for better relief.
- If dysmenorrhea symptoms are not relieved with NSAIDs or OCs, consider additional evaluation for pelvic pathology.
- Approximately 40% of all women suffer considerably from premenstrual syndrome (PMS), with 3% to 8% demonstrating severe symptoms (PMDD).
- Common historical findings in PMS patients are (1) a history of maternal PMS, (2) more stress, and (3) nulliparity.
- PMS patients often suffer depression during the luteal phase but not as severe as depression noted by patients with endogenous depression when measured by standard depression scales or the amplitude of cortisol secretion pulses.
- PMS patients show no deficit in cognitive function during the luteal phase.
- Bromocriptine is effective primarily in relieving breast tenderness in PMS.
- Although fluid retention-related symptoms are prevalent in patients with PMS, it is difficult to document such retention. Redistribution of fluid may occur.
- There is no evidence that women with symptoms of PMS have impaired corpus luteal function.
- The most useful diagnostic tool in caring for PMS patients is a symptom diary.
- Calcium and aerobic exercise may be helpful in relieving PMS symptoms, but there are insufficient data to support the concept that vitamin B_6 therapy relieves PMS symptoms.
- There are limited objective data to support the concept that progesterone relieves PMS symptoms in most women.
- Therapy with psychoactive drugs, particularly the SSRIs given in relatively small doses during the luteal phase, may be helpful in relieving PMS and PMDD symptoms. Specific cautions for the use of these agents must be followed.
- In severe cases of PMS involving older women who have completed their families, hysterectomy with bilateral oophorectomy can give symptom relief.

BIBLIOGRAPHY

Key Readings

American College of Obstetricians and Gynecologists. Premenstrual syndrome. ACOG Practice Bulletin 15. American College of Obstetricians and Gynecologists, Washington, DC, 2000.

Andersch B, Milsom I: An epidemiologic study of young women with dysmenorrhea. Am J Obstet Gynecol 144:655, 1982.

Casper RF, Hearn MT: The effect of hysterectomy and bilateral oophorectomy in women with severe premenstrual syndrome. Am J Obstet Gynecol 162:105, 1990.

Casson P, Hahn PM, Van Vugt DA, Reid RL: Lasting response to ovariectomy in severe intractable premenstrual syndrome. Am J Obstet Gynecol 162:99, 1990.

Dawood MY: Nonsteroidal anti-inflammatory drugs and reproduction. Am J Obstet Gynecol 169:5, 1993.

Dimmock PW, Wyatt KM, Jones PW, et al: Efficacy of selective serotonin-reuptake inhibitors in premenstrual syndrome: A systematic review. Lancet 356:1131, 2000.

Frank RT: The hormonal causes of premenstrual tension. Arch Neurol Psychol 126:1052, 1931.

Green R, Dalton K: The premenstrual syndrome. Br Med J 1:1007, 1953.

Ling F, Mortola J, Pariser S, et al: Premenstrual Syndrome and Premenstrual Dysphoric Disorder: Scope, Diagnosis, and Treatment. 1998. APGO Educational Series on Women's Health Issues.

Plouffe L Jr, Stewart K, Craft KS, et al: Diagnostic and treatment results from a southeastern academic center-based premenstrual syndrome clinic: The first year. Am J Obstet Gynecol 169:295, 1993.

Reid RL, Yen SSC: Premenstrual syndrome. Am J Obstet Gynecol 139:85, 1981.

Taylor HC: Vascular congestion and hyperemia, their effect on the structure and function in the female reproductive system. Am J Obstet Gynecol 57:211, 1949.

Thys-Jacobs S, Starkey P, Bernstein D, Tian J: Premenstrual Syndrome Study Group. Calcium carbonate and the premenstrual syndrome: Effects on premenstrual and menstrual symptoms. Am J Obstet Gynecol 179:444, 1998.

Wyatt KM, Dimmock PW, O'Brien PMS: Vitamin B6 therapy: A systematic review of its efficacy in premenstrual syndrome. Br Med J 318:1375, 1999.

Key References

Abraham GE, Hargrove JT: Effect of vitamin B_6 on premenstrual symptomatology in women with premenstrual tension syndrome: A double blind crossover study. Infertility 3:155, 1980.

Abramson M, Torghele JR: Weight, temperature changes and psychosomatic symptomatology in relation to the menstrual cycle. Am J Obstet Gynecol 81:223, 1961.

Akin M, Price W, Rodriguez G, et al: Continuous, low-level topical heat wrap therapy as compared to acetaminophen for primary dysmenorrhea. J Reprod Med 49:739, 2004.

Andersch B: Bromocriptine and premenstrual symptoms: A survey of double blind trials. Obstet Gynecol Surv 38:643, 1983.

Babyak M, Blumenthal JA, Herman S, et al: Exercise treatment for major depression: Maintenance of therapeutic benefit at 10 months. Psychosom Med 62(5);633, 2000.

Baldaszti E, Wimmer-Puchinger B, Loschke K: Acceptability of the long-term contraceptive levonorgestrel-releasing intrauterine system (Mirena ®): A 3-year follow-up study. Contraception 67:87, 2003.

Barnard ND, Scialli AR, Hurlock D, Bertron P: Diet and sex-hormone binding globulin, dysmenorrhea, and premenstrual symptoms. Obstet Gynecol 95:245, 2000.

Bertone-Johnson ER, Hankinson SE, Bendich A, et al: Calcium and vitamin D intake and risk of incident premenstrual syndrome. Arch Intern Med 165(11):1246, 2005.

Bibi KW: The effects of aerobic exercise on premenstrual syndrome symptoms. Dissert Abstracts Int 56:6678, 1995.

Borenstein J, Chiou CF, Dean B, et al: Estimating direct and indirect costs of premenstrual syndrome. J Occup Environ Med 47:26, 2005.

Brown CS, Ling FW, Andersen RN, et al: Efficacy of depot leuprolide in premenstrual syndrome: Effect of symptom severity and type in a controlled trial. Obstet Gynecol 84:779, 1994.

Bruce J, Russell GFM: Premenstrual tension: A study of weight changes and balances of water, sodium and potassium. Lancet 2:267, 1962.

Chan AF, Mortola JF, Wood SH, Yen SSC: Persistence of premenstrual syndrome during low-dose administration of the progesterone antagonist RU 486. Obstet Gynecol 84:1001, 1994.

Chuong CJ, Hsi BP, Gibbons WE: Periovulatory beta-endorphin levels in premenstrual Syndrome. Obstet Gynecol 83:755, 1994.

Coffee AL, Kuehl TJ, Willis S, Sulak PJ: Oral contraceptives and premenstrual symptoms: Comparison of a 21/7 and extended regimen. Am J Obstet Gynecol 195:1311, 2006.

Cohen LS, Miner C, Brown E, et al: Premenstrual daily fluoxetine for premenstrual dysphoric disorder: A placebo-controlled, clinical trial using computerized diaries. Obstet Gynecol 100:435, 2002.

Cohen LS, Soares CN, Otto MW, et al: Prevalence and predictors of premenstrual dysphoric disorder (PMDD) in older premenopausal women. The Harvard Study of Moods and Cycles. J Affect Disord 70:125, 2002.

Cooper KG, Bain C, Lawrie L, Parkin DE: A randomized comparison of microwave endometrial ablation with transcervical resection of the endometrium. Br J Obstet Gynaecol 112:470, 2005.

Cronje WH, Vashist A, Studd JWW: Hysterectomy and bilateral oophorectomy for severe premenstrual syndrome. Hum Reprod 19:2152, 2004.

Crowell MD, Dubin NH, Robinson JC, et al: Functional bowel disorders in women with dysmenorrhea. Am J Gastroenterol 89:1973, 1994.

Daniels SE, Torri S, Desjardins PJ: Valdecoxib for treatment of primary dysmenorrhea. A randomized, double-blind comparison with placebo and naproxen. J Gen Intern Med 20:62, 2005.

Davis AR, Westhoff C, O'Connell K, Gallagher N: Oral contraceptives for dysmenorrhea in adolescent girls: A randomized trial. Obstet Gynecol 106:97, 2005.

Dmitrovic R, Branimir P, Cvitkovic-Kuzmic A, et al: Severity of symptoms in primary dysmenorrhea—A Doppler study. Eur J Obstet Gynecol Reprod Biol 107:191, 2003.

Doll H, Brown S, Thurston A, Vessey M: Pyridoxine (vitamin B_6) and the premenstrual syndrome: a randomized crossover trial. J R Coll Gen Pract 39:364, 1989.

Douglas S: Premenstrual syndrome. Evidence-based treatment in family practice. Can Fam Physician 48:1789, 2002.

Edelman AB, Gallo MF, Jensen JT, et al: Continuous or extended cycle vs cyclic use of combined oral contraceptives for contraception. Cochrane Database Syst Rev CD 004695, 2005.

Edwards JE, Moore RA, McQuy HF: Rofecoxib for dysmenorrhea: meta-analysis using individual patient data. BMC Womens Health 4(1):5, 2004.

Facchinetti F, Borella P, Sances G, et al: Oral magnesium successfully relieves premenstrual mood changes. Obstet Gynecol 78:177, 1991.

Facchinetti F, Fioroni L, Sances G, et al: Naproxen sodium in the treatment of premenstrual symptoms: A placebo-controlled study. Gynecol Obstet Invest 28:205, 1989.

Faratian B, Gaspar A, O'Brien PM, et al: Premenstrual syndrome, weight, abdominal swelling and perceived body image. Am J Obstet Gynecol 150:200, 1984.

Freeman E, Rickels K, Sondheimer SJ, Polansky M: Ineffectiveness of progesterone suppository treatment for premenstrual syndrome. JAMA 264:349, 1990.

Freeman EW, Kroll R, Rapkin A, et al: Evaluation of a unique oral contraceptive in the treatment of premenstrual dysphoric disorder. J Womens Health Gend Based Med 11:95, 2002.

Freeman EW, Rickels K, Sondheimer SJ, Polansky M: A double-blind trial of oral progesterone, alprazolam, and placebo in treatment of severe premenstrual syndrome. JAMA 274:51, 1995.

Freeman EW, Rickels K, Sondheimer SJ, et al: Continuous or intermittent dosing with sertraline for patients with severe premenstrual syndrome of premenstrual dysphoric disorder. Am J Psychiatry 161:343, 2004.

Freeman EW, Rickels K, Yonkers KA, et al: Venlafaxine in the treatment of premenstrual dysphoric disorder. Obstet Gynecol 98:737, 2001.

Fugh-Berman A, Kronberg F: Complementary and alternative medicine (CAM) in reproductive-age women: A review of randomized controlled trials. Reprod Toxicol 17:137, 2003.

Grady-Weliky TA: Premenstrual dysphoric disorder. N Engl J Med 348:433 2003.

Greene R, Dalton K: The premenstrual syndrome. Br Med J 1:1001–1007, 1953.

Halbreich U, Assael M, Ben-David M, et al: Serum prolactin in women with premenstrual syndrome. Lancet 2:654, 1976.

Halbreich U, Bergeron R, Yonkers KA: Efficacy of intermittent, luteal phase sertraline treatment of premenstrual dysphoric disorder. Obstet Gynecol 100:1219, 2002.

Halbreich U, Rojansky N, Palter S: Elimination of ovulation and menstrual cyclicity (with danazol) improves dysphoric premenstrual syndromes. Fertil Steril 56:1066, 1991.

Heitkemper MM, Cain KC, Jarrett ME, et al: Symptoms across the menstrual cycle in women with irritable bowel syndrome. Am J Gastroenterol 98:420, 2003.

Hendrix SL, Alexander NJ: Primary dysmenorrhea treatment with a desogestrel-containing low-dose oral contraceptive. Contraception 66:393, 2002.

Henzl MR, Ortega-Herrera E, Rodriguez C, Izu A: Anaprox in dysmenorrhea: reduction of pain in intrauterine pressure. Am J Obstet Gynecol 135:455, 1979.

Joffe H, Cohen LS, Harlow BL: Impact of oral contraceptive pill use on premenstrual mood: Predictors of improvement and deterioration. Am J Obstet Gynecol 189:1523, 2003.

Johnson NP, Farquhar CM, Crossley S, et al: A double-blind randomised controlled trial of laparoscopic uterine nerve ablation for women with chronic pelvic pain. Br J Obstet Gynaecol 111:950, 2004.

Johnson SR: Premenstrual syndrome, premenstrual dysphoric disorder, and beyond: A clinical primer for practitioners. Obstet Gynecol 104:845, 2004.

Kataoka M, Togashi K, Kido A, et al: Dysmenorrhea: Evaluation with cine-mode-display MR imaging—Initial experience. Radiology 235:124, 2005.

Koike H, Ikenoue T, Mori N: Studies on prostaglandin production relating to the mechanism of dysmenorrhea in endometriosis. Nippon Naibunpi Gakkai Zasshi. Folia Endocrinol Jpn 20:43, 1994.

Landen M, Eriksson O, Sundblad C, et al: Compounds with affinity for serotonergic receptors in the treatment of premenstrual dysphoria: A comparison of buspirone, nefazodone and placebo. Pyschopharmacologia 155:292, 2001.

Lemos D: The effects of aerobic training on women who suffer from premenstrual syndrome. Dissert Abstr Int 52:563, 1991.

Lombardi I, Luisi S, Quirici B, et al: Adrenal response to adrenocorticotropic hormone stimulation in patients with premenstrual syndrome. Gynecol Endocrinol 18:79, 2004.

Maia H Jr, Maltwz A, Studard E, et al: Effect of the menstrual cycle and oral contraceptives on cycloxygenase-2 expression in the endometrium. Gynecol Endocrinol 21(1):57, 2005.

Marjoribanks J, Proctor ML, Farquhar C: Nonsteroidal anti-inflammatory drugs for primary dysmenorrhoea. Cochrane Database Syst Rev CD001751, 2003.

Masho SW, Adera T, South-Paul J: Obesity as a risk factor for premenstrual syndrome. J Psychosom Obstet Gynaecol 26:33, 2005.

Mezrow G, Shoupe D, Spicer D, et al: Depot leuprolide acetate with estrogen and progestin add-back for long-term treatment of premenstrual syndrome. Fertil Steril 62:932, 1994.

Milsom I, Hedner N, Mannheimer C: A comparative study of the effect of high-intensity transcutaneous nerve stimulation and oral naproxen on intrauterine pressure and menstrual pain in patients with primary dysmenorrhea. Am J Obstet Gynecol 170:123, 1994.

Milsom I, Minic M, Dawood MY, et al: Comparison of the efficacy and safety of nonprescription doses of naproxen and naproxen sodium with ibuprofen, acetaminophen, and placebo in the treatment of primary dysmenorrhea: a pooled analysis of five studies. Clin Ther 24:1384, 2002.

Mira M, McNeil D, Fraser K, et al: Mefenamic acid in the treatment of premenstrual syndrome. Obstet Gynecol 68:395, 1986.

Morgan M, Rapkin AJ, D'Ella L, et al: Cognitive functioning in premenstrual syndrome. Obstet Gynecol 88:961, 1996.

Mortola JF, Girton L, Fischer U: Successful treatment of severe premenstrual syndrome by combined use of gonadotropin-releasing hormone agonist and estrogen/progestin. J Clin Endocrinol Metab 71:252A, 1991.

Mortola JF, Girton L, Yen SSC: Depressive episodes in premenstrual syndrome. Am J Obstet Gynecol 161:1682, 1989.

Nagata C, Hirokawa K, Shimizu N, Shimizu H: Soy, fat and other dietary factors in relation to premenstrual symptoms in Japanese women. BJOG 111:594, 2004.

Nikolai TF, Mulligan GM, Gribble RK, et al: Thyroid function and treatment in premenstrual syndrome. J Clin Endocrinol Metab 70:1108, 1990.

O'Brien PM: The premenstrual syndrome: a review of the present status of therapy. Drugs 24:140, 1982.

O'Brien PM, Abukhalil IEH: Randomized controlled trial of the management of premenstrual syndrome and premenstrual mastalgia using luteal phase-only danazol. Am J Obstet Gynecol 180:18, 1999.

Owen PR: Prostaglandin synthetase inhibitors in the treatment of primary dysmenorrhea: Outcome trials reviewed. Am J Obstet Gynecol 148:96, 1984.

Pearlstein T, Joliat MJ, Brown EB, Miner CM: Recurrence of symptoms of premenstrual dysphoric disorder after the cessation of luteal-phase fluoxetine treatment. Am J Obstet Gynecol 188:887, 2003.

Pearlstein TB, Stone AB, Lund SA, et al: Comparison of fluoxetine, bupropion, and placebo in the treatment of premenstrual dysphoric disorder. J Clin Psychopharmacol 17:261, 1997.

Porpora MG, Picarelli A, Porta RP, et al: Celiac disease as a cause of chronic pelvic pain, dysmenorrhea, and deep dyspareunia. Obstet Gynecol 99:937, 2002.

Proctor ML, Latthe PM, Farquhar CM, et al: Surgical interruption of pelvic nerve pathways for primary and secondary dysmenorrhoea. Cochrane Database Syst Rev CDC 001896, 2005.

Proctor ML, Roberts H, Farquhar CM: Combined oral contraceptive pill (OCP) as treatment for primary dysmenorrhoea. Cochrane Database Syst Rev CD 002120, 2001.

Rapkin AJ, Chang LI, Reading AE: Mood and cognitive style in premenstrual syndrome. Obstet Gynecol 74:644, 1989.

Rapkin AJ, Morgan M, Goldman L, et al: Progesterone metabolite allopregnanediol in women with premenstrual syndrome. Obstet Gynecol 90:709, 1997.

Roca CA, Schmidt PJ, Altemus M, et al: Differential menstrual cycle regulation of hypothalamic–pituitary–adrenal axis in women with premenstrual syndrome and controls. J Clin Endocrinol Metab 88:3057, 2003.

Rogers WC: The role of endocrine allergy in the production of premenstrual tension. West J Surg Obstet Gynecol 70:100, 1962.

Rickels K, Freeman E, Sondheimer S: Buspirone in treatment of premenstrual syndrome. Lancet 1:777, 1989.

Sampson GA: Premenstrual syndrome: a double blind control trial of progesterone and placebo. Br J Psychiatry 135:209, 1979.

Sarno AP Jr, Miller EJ, Lundblad EG: Premenstrual syndrome: beneficial effects of periodic, low-dose danazol. Obstet Gynecol 70:33, 1987.

Sayegh R, Schiff I, Wurtman J, et al: The effect of a carbohydrate-rich beverage on mood, appetite, and cognitive function in women with premenstrual syndrome. Obstet Gynecol 86:520, 1995.

Schellenberg, R. Treatment of premenstrual syndrome with agnus castus fruit extract: Prospective, randomized, placebo controlled study. BMJ 322:134, 2001.

Schmidt PJ, Grover GN, Rubinow DR: Alprazolam in the treatment of premenstrual syndrome: A double-blind, placebo-controlled trial. Arch Gen Psychiatry 50:467, 1993.

Scultetus AH, Villavicencio L, Gillespie DL, et al: The pelvic venous syndromes: Analysis of our experience with 57 patients. J Vasc Surg 36:881, 2002.

Smith RP: The dynamics of nonsteroidal anti-inflammatory therapy for primary dysmenorrhea. Obstet Gynecol 70:785, 1987.

Smith RP, Heltzel JA: Interrelation of analgesia and uterine activity in women with primary dysmenorrhea: a preliminary report. J Reprod Med 36:260, 1991.

Smith S, Rinehart JS, Ruddock VE, and Schiff I: Treatment of premenstrual syndrome with alprazolam: Results of a double-blind, placebo-controlled, randomized crossover clinical trial. Obstet Gynecol 70:37, 1987.

Steege JR, Stout AL, Knight DL, Nemeroff CB: Reduced platelet tritium-labeled imipramine binding sites in women with premenstrual syndrome. Am J Obstet Gynecol 167:168, 1992.

Steiner M, Romano SJ, Babcock S, et al: The efficacy of fluoxetine in improving physical symptoms associated with premenstrual dysphoric disorder. Br J Obstet Gynaecol 108:462, 2001.

Steiner M, Steinberg S, Stewart D, et al: Fluoxetine in the treatment of premenstrual syndrome. N Engl J Med 332:1529, 1995.

Sternfeld B, Swindle R, Chawla A, et al: Severity of premenstrual symptoms in a health maintenance organization population. Obstet Gynecol 99:1014, 2002.

Stevinson C, Ernst E: Complementary/alternative therapies for premenstrual syndrome: A systematic review of randomized controlled trials. Am J Obstet Gynecol 185:227, 2001.

Sulak PJ, Carl J, Gopalakrishnan I, et al: Outcomes of extended oral contraceptive regimens with a shortened hormone-free interval to manage breakthrough bleeding. Contraception 70:281, 2004.

Taylor JW: The timing of menstruation-related symptoms assessed by a daily symptom rating scale. Acta Psychiatr Scand 60:87, 1979.

Tollan A, Oian P, Fadness HO, Maltau JM: Evidence for altered transcapillary fluid balance in women with the premenstrual syndrome. Acta Obstet Gynecol Scand 72:238, 1993.

Walker AR, De Souza MD, Vickers MF, et al: Magnesium supplementation alleviates premenstrual symptoms of fluid retention. J Womens Health 7:1157, 1998.

Wang M, Hammarback S. Lindhe BA, et al: Treatment of premenstrual syndrome by spironolactone: A double-blind, placebo-controlled study. Acta Obstet Gynecol Scand 74:803, 1995.

Watson NR, Studd JWW, Savvas M, et al: Treatment of severe premenstrual syndrome with oestradiol patches and cyclical oral norethisterone. Lancet 2:730, 1989.

Weissman AM, Hartz AJ, Hansen MD, Johnson SR: The natural history of primary dysmenorrhoea: A longitudinal study. Br J Obstet Gynaecol 111:345, 2004.

Wyatt K: Premenstrual syndrome. Clin Evid 11:2507, 2004.

Wyatt KM, Dimmock PW, Ismail KMK, et al: The effectiveness of GnRHa with and without "add-back" therapy in treating premenstrual syndrome: a meta analysis. Br J Obstet Gynaecol 111:585, 2004.

Wyatt KM, Dimmock PW, Jones P, et al: Efficacy of progesterone and progestogens in management of premenstrual syndrome: systematic review. BMJ 323:1, 2001.

Wyatt KM, Dimmock PW, O'Brien PM: Selective serotonin reuptake inhibitors for premenstrual syndrome. Cochrane Data Base Syst Rev CD001396, 2002.

Ylikorkala O, Dawood MY: New concepts in dysmenorrhea. Am J Obstet Gynecol 130:833, 1978.

Yonkers KA, Halbreich U, Freeman E, et al: Symptomatic improvement of premenstrual dysphoric disorder with sertraline treatment. A randomized controlled trial. JAMA 278:983, 1997.

Ziaei S, Zakeri M, Kazemnejad A: A randomised controlled trial of vitamin E in the treatment of primary dysmenorrhoea. Br J Obstet Gynaecol 112:466, 2005.

Abnormal Uterine Bleeding 37

Ovulatory and Anovulatory Dysfunctional Uterine Bleeding, Management of Acute and Chronic Excessive Bleeding

Rogerio A. Lobo

KEY TERMS AND DEFINITIONS

Dysfunctional Uterine Bleeding (DUB). Excessive uterine bleeding with no demonstrable organic cause (genital or extragenital). It is most frequently due to abnormalities of endocrine origin, particularly anovulation.

Endometrial Ablation. Destruction of the endometrium by laser or electrocoagulation with instruments placed through a hysteroscope.

Intermenstrual Bleeding. Bleeding of variable amounts occurring between regular menstrual periods.

Menometrorrhagia. Prolonged uterine bleeding occurring at irregular intervals.

Menorrhagia. Prolonged (more than 7 days) or excessive (greater than 80 mL) uterine bleeding occurring at regular intervals. The term *hypermenorrhea* is synonymous.

Metrorrhagia. Uterine bleeding occurring at irregular but frequent intervals, the amount being variable.

Nonsteroidal Antiinflammatory Drugs (NSAIDs). Drugs that inhibit the synthesis of prostaglandins.

Polymenorrhea. Uterine bleeding occurring at regular intervals of less than 21 days.

Sonohysterography. Sonographic imaging of the endometrial cavity after installation of 10 to 15 mL of saline to improve contrast and facilitate diagnosis of endometrial lesions.

Abnormal uterine bleeding can take many forms: infrequent episodes, excessive flow, or prolonged duration of menses and intermenstrual bleeding. Alterations in the pattern or volume of blood flow of menses are among the most common health concerns of women. Infrequent uterine bleeding, defined as *oligomenorrhea* if the intervals between bleeding episodes vary from 35 days to 6 months, and *amenorrhea,* defined as no menses for at least 6 months, are discussed fully in Chapter 38 (Primary and Secondary Amenorrhea and Precocious Puberty). Excessive or prolonged bleeding will be discussed in this chapter. Recently several new therapeutic modalities have been successfully utilized to treat excessive uterine bleeding, and they will also be discussed in this chapter.

To define excessive abnormal uterine bleeding it is necessary to define normal menstrual flow. The mean interval between menses is 28 days (±7 days). Thus if bleeding occurs at intervals of 21 days or less, it is abnormal. The mean duration of menstrual flow is 4 days. Few women with normal menses bleed more than 7 days, thus bleeding more than 7 days is considered to be abnormally prolonged (menorrhagia). It is useful to document the duration and frequency of menstrual flow with the use of menstrual diary cards; however, it is difficult to determine the amount of menstrual blood loss (MBL) by subjective means. Several studies have shown that there is poor correlation between subjective judgment and objective measurement of MBL. Hallberg and colleagues found that 40% of women with blood loss greater than 80 mL considered their menstrual flow to be small or moderate in amount (Fig. 37-1), whereas 14% of women with blood loss less than 20 mL thought their menses was heavy. In a study by Chimbira and coworkers there was also poor correlation between a woman's perception of MBL and the actual amount lost. These investigators reported that one third of the menses described as light were more than 80 mL and that about half of those believed to be heavy were less than 80 mL. Determining the number of sanitary pads used is also an unreliable indication of MBL. There is great variability of absorption among different types of sanitary products as well as among different devices in the same package. Fraser and associates reported that the percentage contribution of blood to the total fluid volume of the menstrual discharge

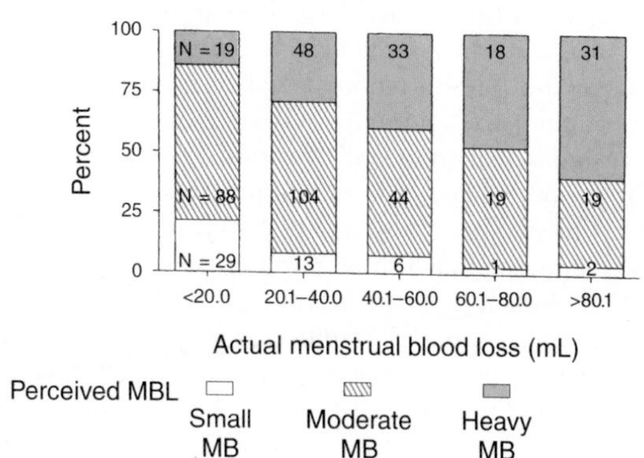

Figure 37-1. Subjective judgments of menstrual blood loss. MB, menstrual bleeding. (From Hallberg L, Högdahl AM, Nilsson L, Rybo G: Menstrual blood loss—a population study: Variation at different ages and attempts to define normality. Acta Obstet Gynecol Scand 45:320, 1966.)

varied extensively among different women, from 1.6% to 81%, with a mean of 36%. Thus the majority of fluid volume in menstrual discharge is probably derived from endometrial tissue exudate. These investigators also reported that there was a very significant correlation between the total fluid loss and blood loss. Women differ markedly in their fastidiousness in changing sanitary products. Thus queries about the passage of blood clots or the degree of inconvenience caused by the bleeding are more helpful than counting the number of pads used in order to ascertain whether menorrhagia exists.

Because of the unreliability of subjective assessment, objective methods have been developed to quantify MBL. One method involves radioisotopic labeling of the woman's red blood cells. The other, which is the most widely used technique, involves photometric measurement to quantify hematin collected onto sanitary napkins. This alkaline hematin method, originated by Hallberg and Nilsson, has been refined by Newton and colleagues and van Eijkeren and coworkers and is very accurate. Nevertheless the accuracy depends on complete collection of the sanitary napkins used by the woman. With this technique it has been found in several studies published in the 1960s and 1970s that the mean amount of MBL in normal women (women with normal hemoglobin, hematocrit, and plasma iron) is about 35 mL, with the mean in various studies ranging from 31 to 44 mL. About 95% of normal women lose less than an average of 60 mL of blood during each menses. In several recent studies in the 1990s one laboratory in Sweden reported that the mean MBL in normal women is between 55 and 60 mL. In contrast to the earlier studies in which the extraction of the blood from the sanitary napkins was performed manually, in this laboratory a machine was used to press out the hematin and the women were instructed to meticulously collect all menstrual blood. Thus it is possible that the mean amount of MBL in normal women is greater than previously reported.

In each of the studies of populations of normal women, there was a wide range of MBL with a marked positive skewness of the distribution of different volumes (Fig. 37-2). In the study by Cole and associates of 280 women using neither oral contraceptives nor an intrauterine device (IUD), about one third of women lost less than 20 mL (light) during each menstrual episode, one third lost 20 to 44 mL (medium), and one third lost more than 45 mL (heavy). These investigators also reported that there was a significant increase in MBL with increasing parity, but not with age, and that short women lost less blood than women of normal or tall height.

Hallberg and Nilsson reported that in normal women there is little variation in volume of MBL in successive menses of the same individual (standard deviation [SD] 1.9 mL) during a 1-year period, whereas the variation between women is great (SD 15.3 mL) (Fig. 37-3). In this study the average loss of iron in each menses was 13.0 mg. In normal women about 70% of the total blood loss occurs during the first 2 days of menses.

Hallberg and colleagues found that individuals with blood loss greater than 80 mL have significantly lower mean hemoglobin, hematocrit, and serum iron levels than do women with less MBL (Fig. 37-4). Therefore an MBL greater than 80 mL should be regarded as hypermenorrhea. For practical purposes, if a woman experiences a change in duration of flow (e.g., from 3 to 6 days), it must be considered abnormal, even though by definition she does not have menorrhagia.

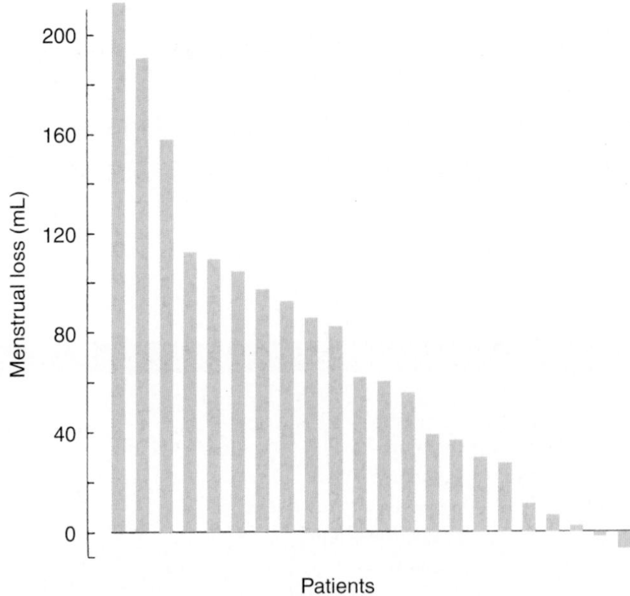

Figure 37-2. Distribution of menstrual blood loss in population sample from women living in Göteborg. (From Hallberg L, Högdahl AM, Nilsson L, Rybo G: Menstrual blood loss—a population study: Variation at different ages and attempts to define normality. Acta Obstet Gynecol Scand 45:320, 1966.)

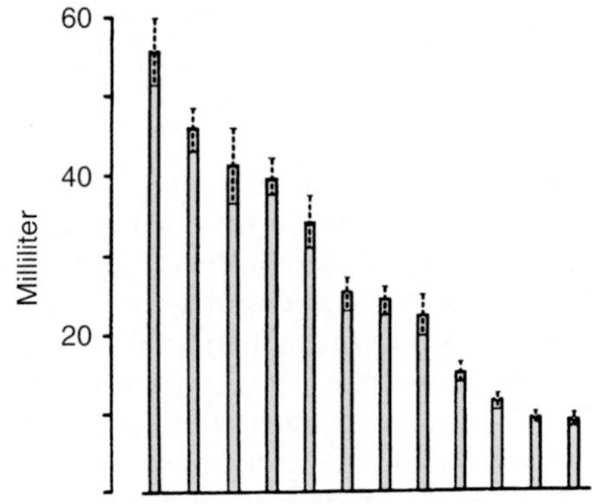

Figure 37-3. Menstrual blood loss in 12 subjects. Mean values of 12 periods and standard error of means. (From Hallberg L, Nilsson L: Constancy of individual menstrual blood loss. Acta Obstet Gynecol Scand 43:352, 1964.)

Menorrhagia has been reported to occur in 95 to 14% of healthy women who participated in the various studies of measurement of MBL. In women complaining of menorrhagia, Haynes and coworkers reported that, as with women with normal menses, 70% of the blood was lost within the first 2 days of menses and 92% by the end of the third day. Also, there was no relation between the number of days of menstrual bleeding and the total MBL. The majority of these women with menorrhagia did not have increased duration of menses but rather had a markedly increased amount of menstrual flow for the first few days of menses. Thus the mechanisms responsible for control of menses are as effective in these women as in women with normal menses. The mechanisms responsible for the increased menstrual flow are unclear but may result from alterations in prostaglandin metabolism, as discussed later.

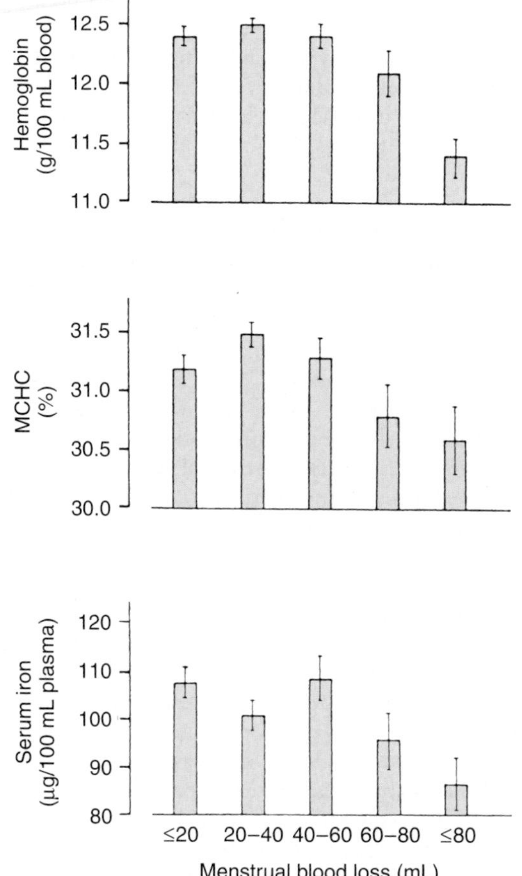

Figure 37-4. Mean values (± standard error of the mean, SEM) of hemoglobin concentration, menstrual cycle hematocrit (MCHC), and plasma iron concentration in different ranges of menstrual blood loss. (From Hallberg L, Högdahl AM, Nilsson L, Rybo G: Menstrual blood loss—a population study: Variation at different ages and attempts to define normality. Acta Obstet Gynecol Scand 45:320, 1966.)

ETIOLOGY

The causes of abnormal uterine bleeding are usually divided into two major categories: organic and dysfunctional (or endocrinologic). The organic causes of abnormal uterine bleeding are discussed in detail in other chapters of this book and will only be briefly outlined here.

Organic Causes

The organic causes can be subdivided into systemic disease and reproductive tract disease.

Systemic Disease

Systemic diseases, particularly disorders of blood coagulation such as von Willebrand's disease and prothrombin deficiency, may initially present as abnormal uterine bleeding. Other disorders that produce platelet deficiency, such as leukemia, severe sepsis, idiopathic thrombocytopenic purpura, and hypersplenism, can also cause excessive bleeding. Routine screening for coagulation defects is mainly indicated in the adolescent who has prolonged heavy menses beginning at menarche, unless otherwise indicated by clinical signs such as petechiae or ecchymosis. Claessens and Cowell reported that coagulation disorders are found in about 20% of adolescent females who require hospitalization for abnormal uterine bleeding. Coagulation defects are present in about one fourth of those whose hemoglobin levels fall below 10 g/100 mL, in one third of those who require transfusions, and in half of those whose severe menorrhagia occurred at the time of the first menstrual period. A more recent study by Falcone and associates indicated that a coagulation disorder was found in only 5% of adolescents hospitalized for heavy bleeding. Both studies indicate that the likelihood of a blood disorder in adolescents with heavy menses is sufficiently high so that they should all be evaluated to determine if a coagulopathy is present.

In the adult, abnormal bleeding may be encountered frequently in women receiving anticoagulation for a variety of medical disorders. Although the pattern of bleeding is usually menorrhagia, abnormal intracycle bleeding also occurs.

Hypothyroidism is frequently associated with menorrhagia as well as intermenstrual bleeding. Thyroid-stimulating hormone (TSH) should be measured in women with menorrhagia of undetermined origin. When standard tests of thyroid function are used to diagnose hypothyroidism, the incidence of this disorder among women with menorrhagia has been estimated to range between 0.3% and 2.5%. Wilansky and Greisman studied 67 clinically euthyroid women with normal serum thyroxine and triiodothyronine levels who had symptoms of severe menorrhagia with a thyrotropin-releasing hormone (TRH) stimulation test. They found that 15 of these women had small but significantly elevated baseline TSH levels as well as significantly elevated TSH responses (>30 mU/L) 30 minutes after TRH infusion. They characterized those women as having early or potential hypothyroidism instead of subclinical hypothyroidism. Treatment of these women with 50 to 200 mg of L-thyroxine daily resulted in normalization of their TSH levels and disappearance of the menorrhagia within 3 to 6 months in all the women treated. Although these data have not been confirmed, they suggest that a sensitive third-generation assay for TSH should be obtained in women with unexplained menorrhagia. Any elevations, even if subtle, should be evaluated further. Although hyperthyroidism is usually not associated with menstrual abnormalities, hypomenorrhea, oligomenorrhea, and amenorrhea have been reported.

Cirrhosis is associated with excessive bleeding secondary to the reduced capacity of the liver to metabolize estrogens. If hypoprothrombinemia is present, the incidence of abnormal bleeding will be increased.

Reproductive Tract Disease

The most common causes of abnormal uterine bleeding in women of reproductive age are accidents of pregnancy such as threatened, incomplete, or missed abortion and ectopic pregnancy. In addition, trophoblastic disease must be considered in the differential diagnosis of abnormal bleeding in any woman who has had a recent pregnancy. A sensitive β-human chorionic gonadotropin (β-HCG) assay should be performed as part of the diagnostic evaluation.

Any malignancy of the genital tract, particularly endometrial and cervical cancer, may present as abnormal bleeding. Less commonly, vaginal, vulvar, and fallopian tube cancer may produce abnormal bleeding. In addition, estrogen-producing ovarian tumors may become manifest by abnormal uterine bleeding. Thus granulosa-theca cell tumors may present with excessive uterine bleeding. Infection of the upper genital tract, particularly endometritis, may present as prolonged menses, although episodic intermenstrual spotting is a more common symptom. Endometriosis may also result in abnormal bleeding and frequently presents as premenstrual spotting. There are various explanations for this that relate to the location of the endometriosis implants.

Anatomic uterine abnormalities such as submucous myomas, endometrial polyps, and adenomyosis frequently produce symptoms of prolonged and excessive regular uterine bleeding. The mechanisms whereby these lesions cause menorrhagia are unclear. Makarainen and Ylikorkala reported that release of thromboxane and prostacycline from endometrial specimens of normal women and women with menorrhagia associated with leiomyomas was similar. Cervical lesions such as erosions, polyps, and cervicitis may cause irregular bleeding, particularly postcoital spotting. These lesions can usually be diagnosed by visualization of the cervix. In addition, traumatic vaginal lesions, severe vaginal infections, and foreign bodies have been associated with abnormal bleeding.

Foreign bodies in the uterus, such as the IUD, frequently produce abnormal uterine bleeding. Other iatrogenic causes include oral and injectable steroids such as those used for contraception and hormonal replacement or for the management of dysmenorrhea, hirsutism, acne, or endometriosis. Tranquilizers and other psychotropic drugs may interfere with the neurotransmitters responsible for releasing and inhibiting hypothalamic hormones, thus causing anovulation and abnormal bleeding.

Dysfunctional Causes

After organic, systemic, and iatrogenic causes for the abnormal bleeding are ruled out, the diagnosis of dysfunctional uterine bleeding (DUB) can be made. There are two types of DUB: anovulatory and ovulatory. The predominant cause of DUB in the postmenarcheal and premenopausal years is anovulation secondary to alterations in neuroendocrinologic function. In women with anovulatory DUB there is continuous estradiol production without corpus luteum formation and progesterone production. The steady state of estrogen stimulation leads to a continuously proliferating endometrium, which may outgrow its blood supply or lose nutrients with varying degrees of necrosis. In contrast to normal menstruation, uniform slough to the basalis layer does not occur, which produces excessive uterine blood flow. Ovulatory DUB occurs most commonly after the adolescent years and before the perimenopausal years. The incidence of this disorder has been reported to occur in as many as 10% of ovulatory women.

In the past, prolonged life of the corpus luteum was reported to be a cause of abnormal bleeding (Halban's syndrome). This disorder is associated with a normal-appearing secretory endometrium. A sensitive serum HCG assay should be performed to differentiate this disorder from early pregnancy loss. Irregular shedding of the endometrium has also been reported to produce menorrhagia. The diagnosis of this disorder is made if an endometrial biopsy obtained during the fourth day of the flow reveals both proliferative and secretory endometrium. No recent studies have documented the presence of these two conditions. Thus the prevalence of these disorders, if they actually exist, is uncertain.

Normal Hemostatic Mechanism

The general mechanisms of hemostasis in all blood vessels involve the following: (1) localized vasoconstriction, (2) platelet adhesion, (3) formation of a platelet plug, (4) reinforcement of the platelet plug with fibrin, and (5) removal of the coagulated material by fibrinolytic mechanisms. The process of hemostasis in the endometrial vessels differs somewhat from the response to vessel damage elsewhere in the body. Morphologic studies by Christiaens and associates have revealed that hemostatic plugs in the endometrium are smaller, have a different morphology, and persist for a shorter time than those in other tissues. The platelet plug assumes a greater importance for the initial cessation of bleeding.

These investigators found that there are two main mechanisms for hemostasis during menstruation. The first, hemostatic plug formation, is the most important mechanism in the functional endometrium. The second, vasoconstriction, is more important in the basalis layer. Since vascular occlusion by both mechanisms is never total, blood leakage continues for several days until endometrial regeneration is completed.

Sheppard and colleagues performed ultrastructural studies of samples of menstrual fluid obtained from the uterine cavity and vagina of 10 women with normal menses and 10 women with DUB. Fibrin and platelets were found in nearly all samples. No differences were found in the morphology of fibrin and platelets in the samples collected from the two groups of women. Rees and coworkers reported that there was no significant difference between the amounts of coagulation factors or fibrinolytic proteins in the menstrual fluid of women with normal blood loss and that from those with menorrhagia.

It has been reported that there is no difference in the concentrations of fibrinogen–fibrin degradation products in menstrual blood samples obtained from normal women and those with menorrhagia. Rees and coworkers reported no difference in clotting factors in menstrual fluid between the two groups of women.

Rees and coworkers performed a histologic study of the endometrium and myometrium in uteri removed by hysterectomy from women with normal and excessive amounts of uterine bleeding. No pathologic findings were found in the specimens. These investigators found no correlation between MBL and endometrial and myometrial arterial density and endometrial glandular density. Thus menorrhagia in the absence of pathologic findings does not result from an excessive number of arteries or abnormal distribution of the endometrial glands.

With the discovery that prostaglandins (PG) are involved with the regulation of vasodilation and vasoconstriction, as well as the clotting process, numerous studies were conducted in the 1980s in which various prostaglandins and their metabolites were measured in endometrial and myometrial samples obtained from normal women and women with menorrhagia. The majority of the studies were performed by two groups in the

United Kingdom, one in Oxford and the other in Edinburgh, and sometimes the results were contradictory because of differences in methodology. Since PGE_2 produces vasodilation but $PGF_2\alpha$ increases vasoconstriction, and thromboxane promotes platelet aggregation but prostacycline inhibits this process, most of the studies measured these prostaglandins or their metabolites. In women with regular ovulatory cycles with normal MBL, there was an increase in the amount of both $PGF_2\alpha$ and PGE_2 found in the endometrium in the late secretory phase and during menses, with the endometrial $PGF_2\alpha/PGE_2$ ratio steadily increasing from midcycle to menses.

Smith and associates found that the levels of $PGF_2\alpha$ in persistently proliferative endometria obtained from women with anovulatory DUB were lower than the levels in women with normal secretory endometria. They theorized that progesterone was necessary to increase levels of arachidonic acid, the precursor of $PGF_2\alpha$, whereas estradiol stimulates synthesis of prostaglandins from arachidonic acid by cyclic endoperoxides. With the absence of progesterone in anovulatory cycles, the levels of $PGF_2\alpha$ are reduced and the levels of PGE_2 are normal, resulting in a decreased $PGF_2\alpha/PGE_2$ ratio. Since $PGF_2\alpha$ binds to receptors in the spiral arteries in the late secretory phase to cause vasoconstriction and control menstrual flow, decreased levels of $PGF_2\alpha$ could cause heavier or more prolonged bleeding.

These investigators found there was an inverse correlation between the endometrial $PGF_2\alpha$/PGE ratio and the amount of MBL (Fig. 37-5). PGE_2 also stimulates contraction of the smooth muscle cells in the myometrium, and elevated levels of $PGF_2\alpha$ are found in the menstrual blood of women with dysmenorrhea. Anovulatory cycles are usually not associated with dysmenorrhea, probably because of the reduced levels of $PGF_2\alpha$. Progesterone treatment of women with anovulatory DUB rapidly reduces the amount of MBL, probably by stimulating production of arachidonic acid, the precursor of $PGF_2\alpha$.

Circulating levels of reproductive hormones are not different in women with ovulatory DUB and those with normal cycles. However several investigators have shown that the increased MBL in women with ovulatory DUB is also associated with reduced uterine synthesis of $PGF_2\alpha$ and an increase in synthesis of PGE_2 and prostacyclin. In studying uterine production of prostacyclin in women with ovulatory DUB, an increased production of the stable metabolite of prostacycline (6-keto FIX) was found.

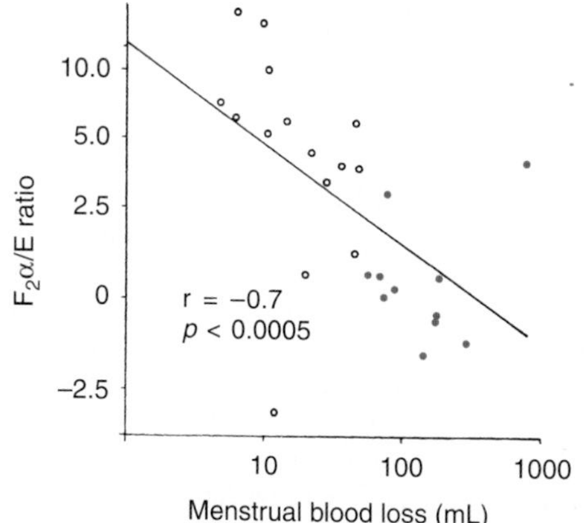

Figure 37-5. Correlation between ratio of endogenous concentrations of $PGF_2\alpha$ and PGE and menstrual blood loss (MBL). Normal secretory endometrium; persistent proliferative endometrium. (From Smith SK, Abel MH, Kelly RW, Baird DT: The synthesis of prostaglandins from persistent proliferative endometrium. J Clin Endocrinol Metab 55:284, 1982.)

Furthermore, Adelantado and colleagues reported that PGE receptor concentrations in the myometrium of hysterectomy specimens were significantly greater in women with unexplained ovulatory menorrhagia than in women with normal MBL. Also, there was a direct correlation between the concentration of myometrial PGE receptor concentration and MBL.

Makarainen and Ylikorkala reported that the ratio of release of thromboxane to prostacyclin in endometrial biopsy specimens was inversely related to the amount of MBL in a group of women with menorrhagia. They concluded that the menorrhagia could be due in part to a relative deficiency of thromboxane in the endometrium.

Bonney and coworkers reported that there was a significantly greater amount of phospholipase C, but not phospholipase A_2 types 1 and 2, in the endometrium of women with ovulatory menorrhagia. Phospholipases release arachidonic acid from cell membrane phospholipids. Several investigators have reported that there is an increased availability of arachidonic acid in the endometrium of women with ovulatory menorrhagia, in contrast to the decreased amount of this substance in the endometrium of women with anovulatory DUB.

Thus alterations in prostaglandin synthesis and release appear to occur in women with both anovulatory and ovulatory DUB. Why these changes occur and their exact causal relation with menorrhagia have not yet been determined.

DIAGNOSIS

When a woman presents with a complaint of abnormal bleeding, it is essential to take a thorough history regarding the frequency, duration, and amount of bleeding, as well as to inquire whether and when the menstrual pattern has changed. This history is extremely important for determining whether the menstrual abnormality is polymenorrhea, menorrhagia (hypermenorrhea), metrorrhagia, menometrorrhagia, or intermenstrual bleeding. Providing the woman with a calendar to record her bleeding episodes is a very helpful way to characterize definitively the bleeding episodes. Since there is a poor correlation between a woman's estimate of the amount of blood flow and the measured loss, as well as great variation in the amount of blood and fluid absorbed by different types of sanitary napkins and in the same type of napkin in different individuals, objective criteria should be used to determine if menorrhagia (blood loss more than 80 mL) is present.

Since direct measurement of MBL is not generally possible, indirect assessment by measurement of hemoglobin concentration, serum iron levels, and serum ferritin levels is useful. Serum ferritin provides a valid indirect assessment of iron stores in the bone marrow. Additional useful laboratory tests include a sensitive HCG determination and a sensitive TSH assay. For adolescent women, as well as older women with systemic disease, a coagulation profile should be performed to rule out a coagulation defect. If the woman has regular cycles, it is important to determine whether she is ovulating. However, if bleeding

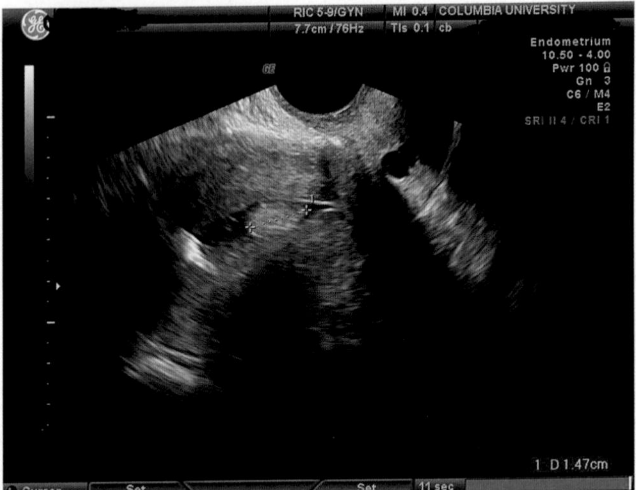

Figure 37-6. Saline sonography demonstrating a 1.4-cm diameter endometrial polyp in a woman with menorrhagia. (Courtesy of J. Lerner, MD, Columbia University Medical Center).

is very irregular, it may be difficult to determine the phase of the cycle in order to document ovulatory function, by means of serum progesterone or other methods. Classically, ovulatory DUB displays a pattern of repetition with heavy bleeding. Endometrial biopsy may be indicated and if obtained at the onset of bleeding will show secretory changes.

If a woman is ovulating and has menorrhagia, it is important to rule out the presence of a uterine lesion such as an endometrial polyp, submucous leiomyoma, or carcinoma. Endocervical curettage and pelvic sonography should be performed; then some form of cavity investigation is warranted. Evaluation of the endometrial cavity can be carried out by hysterosalpingography (HSG) or hysteroscopy. The most practical method is a sonohysterogram, by which an intracavity lesion is easily identified (Fig. 36-6). Saline, 10 to 15 mL, is usually introduced through the cervix with an insemination catheter, or with a special HSG catheter that has a balloon for inflation in the cervical canal allowing a continuous infusion to occur. If this is not available, then an HSG may be ordered. Hysteroscopy is an excellent diagnostic technique and has the potential advantage of being able to treat the abnormality at the same time, for example, removal of a polyp. However, it is not cost-effective as a diagnostic test if it cannot be carried out in an office setting.

Hysteroscopy can be performed in the office with or without local anesthesia and is clearly more accurate diagnostic procedure than a dilation and curettage (D&C). A D&C is a blind technique and does not always detect focal lesions. In a comparison of hysteroscopy with endometrial biopsy and D&C in a group of 342 women, Gimpelson and Rappold found that hysteroscopy permitted the accurate diagnosis in 60 women in whom the diagnosis was not made by D&C. Most of these individuals had the diagnosis of submucous myomas and endometrial polyps made by hysteroscopy and was missed by D&C. March reported that one fourth of women with a presumptive diagnosis of DUB were found to have uterine lesions at the time of hysteroscopy.

Bleeding Disorders

Once thought to be extremely rare as a cause for abnormal bleeding, recent data point to a fairly high prevalence of coagulation disorders in women presenting with menorrhagia. It has been estimated that the prevalence of von Willebrand's disease, the most common of these bleeding disorders, is 13% in women with menorrhagia. These data were reviewed in a consensus conference held at UCLA in August of 2005. As recommended here, history is key before a comprehensive hematologic workup is undertaken. This includes a history of menorrhagia since menarche, family history of bleeding, epistaxis, bruising, gum bleeding, postpartum hemorrhage, and surgical bleeding. In the absence of these clues, a comprehensive workup is probably unnecessary at outset but should be considered in cases refractory to treatment. Treatment involves a variety of options including oral contraceptives or the use of estrogen-free uterine contraceptive, Mirena IUS, tranexamic acid 1 g every 6 hours during menses or deamino-8-D-arginine vasopressin (DDAVP) intranasally, one puff per nostril for the first 3 days of menses.

MANAGEMENT

In the absence of an organic cause for excessive uterine bleeding, it is preferable to use medical instead of surgical treatment, especially if the woman desires to retain her uterus for future childbearing or will be undergoing natural menopause within a short time. There are several effective medical methods for treatment of DUB. These include estrogens, progestogen (delivered systemically or locally), nonsteroidal antiinflammatory drugs (NSAIDs), antifibrinolytic agents, danazol, and gonadotropin-releasing hormone (GnRH) agonists. The type of treatment utilized depends on whether it is used to stop an acute heavy bleeding episode or it is given to reduce the amount of MBL in subsequent menstrual cycles. Before instituting long-term treatment, definitive diagnosis is required and should be made on the basis of hysteroscopy or sonohysterography and directed endometrial biopsies, with definitive treatment determined by the diagnosis.

Estrogens

The rationale for the therapeutic use of estrogen for the treatment of DUB is based on the fact that estrogen in pharmacologic doses causes rapid growth of the endometrium. This strategy is for the acute management of abnormal bleeding. The bleeding that results from most causes of DUB will respond to such therapy because a rapid growth of endometrial tissue occurs over the denuded and raw epithelial surfaces. To control an acute bleeding episode, the use of oral conjugated equine estrogen (CEE) in a dose of 10 mg/day, administered in four divided doses, is a therapeutic regimen that has been found to be clinically useful. It is possible that in addition to the rapid growth mechanism of action, these large doses of CEE may alter platelet activity, thus promoting platelet adhesiveness. Livio and coworkers reported that 6 hours after infusion of an average dose of 30 mg of CEE to individuals with a prolonged bleeding time due to renal failure, the bleeding time was significantly shortened. In this study, measurements of various clotting factors were unchanged after CEE infusion. Acute bleeding from most causes is usually controlled, but if bleeding does not decrease within the first 24 hours, consideration must be given to an organic cause (e.g., an accident of pregnancy), and curettage be considered.

Intravenous administration of estrogen is also effective in the acute treatment of menorrhagia. DeVore and associates reported that, compared with women given a placebo, a significantly greater percentage of women had cessation of bleeding 2 hours after the second of two 25-mg doses of CEE were administered intravenously 3 hours apart. There was no significant difference in cessation of bleeding between women administered estrogen and those given a placebo 3 hours after the first infusion. This study indicates that at least several hours is required to induce mitotic activity and growth of the endometrium, whether the estrogen is administered orally or parenterally. Thus intravenous estrogen therapy accompanied by its rapid metabolic clearance does not appear to offer a significant advantage compared with the same dose of estrogen given orally. From a practical standpoint, if intravenous therapy is chosen it usually requires that women remain in the office or clinical area for 4 to 6 hours to receive at least a second dose.

Usually estrogen therapy reduces the amount of uterine bleeding within the first 24 hours after treatment is initiated. However, because most women with an acute heavy bleeding episode bleed because of anovulation, progestin treatment is also required. Therefore, after bleeding has ceased, oral estrogen therapy is continued at the same dosage, and a progestin, usually medroxyprogesterone acetate (MPA) 10 mg once a day, is added. Both hormones are administered for another 7 to 10 days, after which treatment is stopped to allow withdrawal bleeding, which may have an increased amount of flow but is rarely prolonged. After the withdrawal bleeding episode, one of several alternative treatment modalities should be used. Before instituting long-term treatment, a definite diagnosis should be made after reviewing the endometrial histology. Definitive treatment should be based on these findings. Oral contraceptives are usually the best long-term treatment.

A more convenient method to stop acute bleeding than the sequential high-dose estrogen–progestin regimen is the use of a combination oral contraceptive containing both estrogen and progestin. Four tablets of an oral contraceptive containing 50 μg of estrogen taken every 24 hours in divided doses will usually provide sufficient estrogen to stop acute bleeding and simultaneously provide progestin. Treatment is continued for at least 1 week after the bleeding stops. This regimen is successful and convenient and is thus the preferred method of some clinicians. However, in one study it was found not to be as effective as the use of high doses of CEE. A theoretical reason for this difference might be the fact that the combined use of estrogen and progestin does not afford as rapid endometrial growth as estrogen alone, because the progestin decreases the synthesis of estrogen receptors and increases estradiol dehydrogenase in the endometrial cell, thus inhibiting the growth-promoting action of estrogen.

It must be noted that high-dose estrogen, even for a short course, may be contraindicated for some women (e.g., those with prior thrombosis, certain rheumatologic diseases, estrogen-responsive cancer, etc.). In this instance the options are therapy with progestogen alone or given continuously or intermittently. Although invasive, curettage remains the fastest way to stop acute bleeding and should be used in women who are volume-depleted and severely anemic.

When ultrasound is available it is more logical to use estrogen therapy if there is prolonged heavy bleeding in the setting of a thin endometrium (<5 mm stripe). On the contrary if the endometrium is thick (>10 to 12 mm), or if an anatomic finding is inspected, curettage should be considered. Also unless bleeding is extremely heavy (where estrogen therapy is preferred) progestogens may be suggested and will help by organizing the endometrium as discussed later. In the setting of a thickened irregular endometrium, if curettage is not performed, an endometrial biopsy should be obtained.

Progestogens

Progestogens not only stop endometrial growth but also support and organize the endometrium in such a way that an organized slough occurs after their withdrawal. In the absence of progesterone, erratic unorganized breakdown of the endometrium occurs. With progestogen treatment, an organized slough to the basalis layer allows a rapid cessation of bleeding. In addition, progestogens stimulate arachidonic acid formation in the endometrium, increasing the $PGF_2\alpha$/PGE ratio. In general, progestogens, administered actively, do not stop bleeding but may slow it down as organization of the tissue occurs. Higher doses of norethindrone, which have been suggested to stop bleeding more acutely, may be efficacious on the basis of some conversion to ethinyl estradiol.

The mainstay of progestogen therapy is for opposing the effects of estrogen in anovulatory women. For women with the history of bothersome menometrorrhagia, it is advisable to use intermittent progestogens for several months or an oral contraceptive.

MPA in a dose of 10 mg/day for 10 days each month is a successful therapeutic regimen that produces regular withdrawal bleeding in women with adequate amounts of endogenous estrogen to cause endometrial growth. 19-Norprogestogens, such as norethindrone or norethindrone acetate (2.5 to 5 mg) may be used in the same regimen. Although more androgenic progestogens are less favorable for metabolic parameters (HDL-cholesterol, carbohydrate tolerance), short-term cyclic therapy is considered to be safe.

Adolescent anovulatory women represent an ideal model for the use of progestogens in the treatment of DUB. These women have immaturity of the hypothalamic–pituitary axis, and progestogen therapy for 10 days every month is a reasonable mode of treatment that is highly successful and produces regular cyclic withdrawal bleeding until maturity of the positive feedback system is achieved. This therapy does not interfere with the normal resumption of ovulatory cycles. Theoretically it may be better for these women not to use oral contraceptives, since this therapy inhibits hypothalamic–pituitary gonadotropin synthesis and may delay the maturation of the hypothalamic–pituitary axis. However, there are no data to support this belief. In women of reproductive age who have anovulatory DUB, long-term use of oral contraceptives is useful after the acute bleeding episode is controlled, unless the woman wishes to conceive, in which case cyclic treatment with clomiphene citrate should be used.

Ovulatory DUB

After management of the acute phase of bleeding, if there is evidence that ovulation is occurring and an endometrial lesions have been ruled out, management of menorrhagia falls into several categories which will be presented in the following sections. The pathophysiologic reasons for this abnormal bleeding is related to "idiopathic" abnormal prostaglandin metabolism, abnormalities in other cellular events, or adenomyosis that is difficult to diagnose. For all of these causes, the general strategy is to make the endometrium as thin (or atrophic) as possible to decrease the withdrawal episodes.

For women with ovulatory DUB and mean MBL more than 80 mL, administration of high doses of progestin for only 1 week each month from cycle day 19 to 26 does not reduce MBL. When norethindrone was given for 1 week at doses of either 5 mg twice or three times a day in two recent British studies, MBL was not reduced. However, Fraser reported that administration of two oral progestins (norethindrone and MPA) in high doses of 5 to 10 mg three times a day for 2 to 3 weeks each month, significantly reduced MBL by 40% to 50% in women with both ovulatory and anovulatory DUB. In women with anovulatory DUB the progestins were given from cycle days 12 to 25, whereas the ovulatory women received progestogens from days 5 to 25. Prolonged use of these high doses of progestins may cause unpleasant adverse effects, including tiredness, mood changes, and weight gain, as well as unfavorably altering the lipid profile. Several other randomized trials have shown that more prolonged progestogen treatment (21 to 25 days, each month) is beneficial and is similar in efficacy to the progestogen-IUD (described in the following section) although it is less preferred. Oral contraception will also reduce MBL by approximately 50%.

Local Progestogen Exposure: IUD

The progesterone-releasing IUD has been found to be effective in the treatment of women with ovulatory DUB. Bergqvist and Rybo inserted this device into 12 women with ovulatory DUB and found their MBL declined from an average of 138 mL to 49 mL in 1 year, a 65% reduction in MBL (Fig. 37-7). This device needs to be reinserted annually because of the rapid diffusion of progesterone through polysiloxone.

A levonorgestrol-releasing intrauterine system (LNG-IUS) has been developed that has an effective duration of action of more than 5 years. Milson and colleagues studied use of this IUS as treatment for menorrhagia and found that at the end of 3 months it caused an average 80% reduction in MBL, which increased to 100% at the end of 1 year. This reduction in MBL was significantly greater than that achieved with either an antifibrinolytic agent or a prostaglandin synthetase inhibitor in studies by the same investigators (Fig. 37-8). Several recent studies have shown that the LNG-IUS reduces MBL by 74% to 97%, is effective in increasing hemoglobin, decreasing

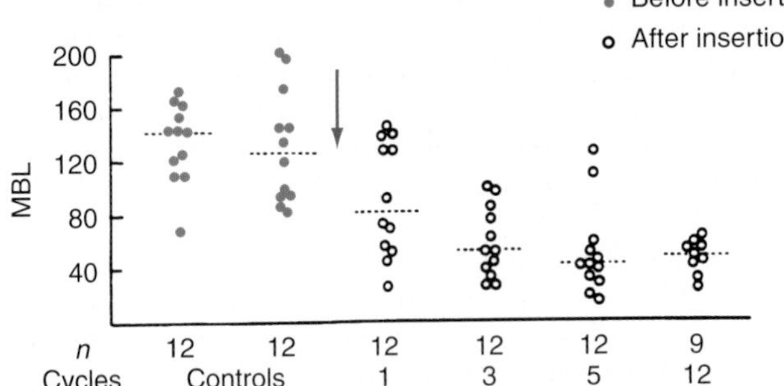

Figure 37-7. Menstrual blood loss (MBL) before and after insertion of Progestasert *(arrow)* in menorrhagic women. (Each dot marks a separate patient, and the median value is marked with a dotted line.) (From Bergqvist A, Rybo G: Treatment of menorrhagia with intrauterine release of progesterone. Br J Obstet Gynaecol 90:255, 1983.)

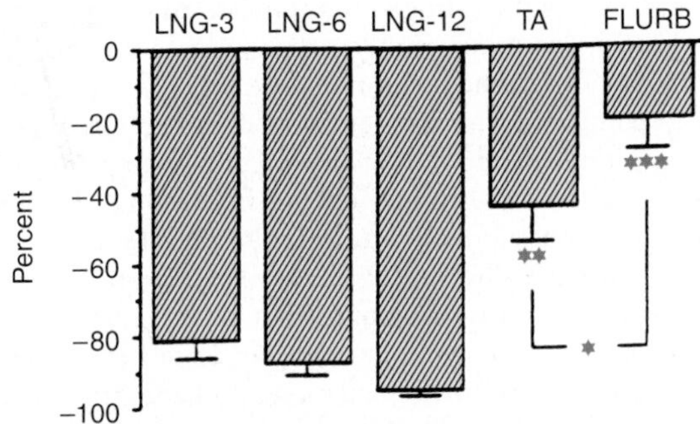

Figure 37-8. Reduction in menstrual blood loss (MBL) expressed as percentage of mean of two control cycles for each form of treatment. Significance of difference between treatment with levonorgestrel-releasing IUD (LNG) and tranexamic acid (TA) and flurbiprofen (FLURB) indicated by double asterisks ($p < 0.01$) and triple asterisks ($p < 0.001$) and between treatment with tranexamic acid and flurbiprofen indicated by a single asterisk ($p < 0.05$). (From Milson I, Andersson K, Andersch B, Rybo G: A comparison of flurbiprofen, tranexamic acid, and a levonorgestrel-releasing intrauterine contraceptive device in the treatment of idiopathic menorrhagia. Am J Obstet Gynecol 164:879, 1991.)

dysmenorrhea, and reduces blood loss due to fibroids and adenomyosis. In addition, it has also been compared with hysterectomy for menorrhagia and had been considered to be a viable alternative.

Nonsteroidal Antiinflammatory Drugs

NSAIDs are prostaglandin synthetase inhibitors that inhibit the biosynthesis of the cyclic endoperoxides, which convert arachidonic acid to prostaglandins. In addition, these agents block the action of prostaglandins by interfering directly at their receptor sites.

To decrease bleeding of the endometrium, it would be ideal to block selectively the synthesis of prostacyclin alone, without decreasing thromboxane formation, as the latter increases platelet aggregation. Presently there are no NSAIDs that possess this ability. All NSAIDs are cyclooxygenase inhibitors and thus block the formation of both thromboxane and the prostacyclin pathway. Nevertheless, NSAIDs have been shown to reduce MBL, primarily in women who ovulate. However, the

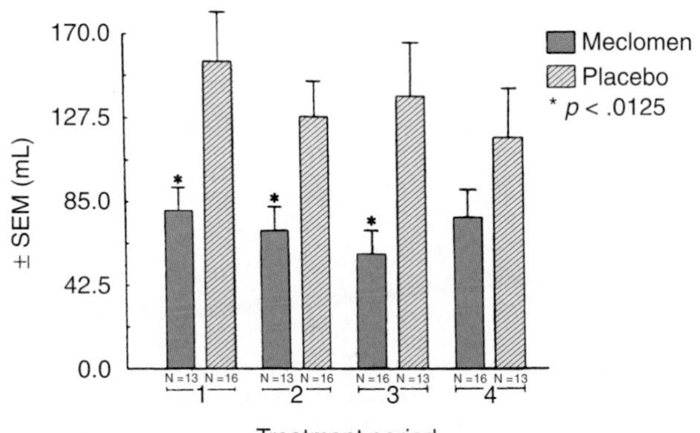

Figure 37-9. Menstrual blood loss (MBL) by treatment period and drug. (From Vargyas JM, Campeau JD, Mishell DA: Treatment of menorrhagia with meclofenamate sodium. Am J Obstet Gynecol 157:944, 1987.)

mechanisms whereby prostaglandin inhibitors reduce MBL are not yet completely understood, and their therapeutic action may take place through some as yet undiscovered mechanism. Several NSAIDs have been administered during menses to groups of women with menorrhagia and ovulatory DUB and have been found to reduce mean MBL by about 205 to 50% (Fig. 37-9). Drugs used in studies include mefenamic acid (500 mg, three times a day), ibuprofen (400 mg, three times a day), meclofenamate sodium (100 mg, three times a day), and naproxen sodium (275 mg, every 6 hours after a loading dose of 550 mg), as well as other NSAIDs. These drugs are usually given for the first 3 days of menses or throughout the bleeding episode, and they appear to have a similar level of effectiveness.

Not all women treated with these agents have reduction in blood flow, but those without a decrease usually had only a mildly increased amount of MBL. The greatest amount of MBL reduction occurs in the women with the greatest pretreatment blood loss. Fraser and coworkers reported that treatment of menorrhagia with mefenamic acid in 36 women for more than 1 year resulted in a significantly sustained reduction in amounts of MBL and a significant increase in serum ferritin. Thus this therapy can be used for long-term treatment because side effects, mainly gastrointestinal, are mild with this intermittent therapy.

Although NSAIDs have been studied by themselves to treat women with MBL who ovulate, they can also be given in combination with oral contraceptives or progestins. With this combined approach, reduction in MBL can be achieved more effectively than with use of any of these agents alone.

Antifibrinolytic Agents

ε-Aminocaproic acid (EACA), tranexamic acid (AMCA), and *para*-aminomethylbenzoic acid (PAMBA) are potent inhibitors of fibrinolysis and have, therefore, been used in the treatment of various hemorrhagic conditions. Nilsson and Rybo compared the effect on blood loss of EACA, AMCA, and oral contraceptives in 215 women with menorrhagia. EACA was given in a dose of 18 g/day for 3 days and then 12, 9, 6, and 3 g daily on successive days. The total dose was always at least 48 g. AMCA was administered in a dose of 6 g/day for 3 days followed by 4, 3, 2, and 1 g/day on successive days. The total dose of AMCA was at least 22 g. There was a significant reduction in blood loss after treatment with EACA, AMCA, and oral contraceptives, and use of each of these agents resulted in about a 50% reduction in MBL (Table 37-1). Of interest was the finding that the greatest reduction in blood loss with antifibrinolytic therapy occurred in women who exhibited the greatest MBL. Preston and colleagues compared the effects of 4 g of AMCA daily for 4 days each cycle with 10 mg of norethindrone for 7 days each cycle in a group of women with ovulatory menorrhagia with a mean MBL of 175 mL. AMCA reduced MBL by 45%, but there was a 20% increase with norethindrone. The side effects of this class of drugs in decreasing order of frequency are nausea, dizziness, diarrhea, headaches, abdominal pain, and allergic manifestations. These side effects are much more common with EACA than with AMCA. Other investigators have compared use of AMCA with placebo in double-blind studies and have found no significant differences in the occurrence of side effects. Renal failure and pregnancy are contraindications to the use of antifibrinolytic agents.

Table 37-1 Mean Menstrual Blood Loss and Reduction with Treatment with EACA, AMCA, Oral Contraceptives, and Methylergobaseimmaleate

	MEAN BLOOD LOSS (ML)		
	Before Treatment	After Treatment	% Decrease
EACA	164	87	47
AMCA	182	84	54
Oral contraceptives	158	75	52
Methylergobaseimmaleate	164	164	0

AMCA, tranexamic acid; EACA, E-ammocaproic acid.
Adapted from Nilsson L, Rybo G: Treatment of menorrhagia. Am J Obstet Gynecol 110:713, 1971.

Antifibrinolytic agents clearly produce a reduction in blood loss and may be used as therapy for women with menorrhagia who ovulate. However, their use is somewhat limited by side effects. These are mainly GI side effects and can be minimized by reducing the dose and limiting therapy to the first 3 days of bleeding. Furthermore, as with NSAIDs, they are best combined with another agent, such as oral contraceptives, for a greater effect on MBL reduction.

Ergot

Ergot derivatives are not recommended for therapy because they are rarely effective and have a high incidence of side effects (nausea, vertigo, abdominal cramps). Nilsson and Rybo demonstrated no reduction in blood loss among 82 women with menorrhagia who were treated with methylergobase immaleate (see Table 37-1).

Androgenic Steroids (Danazol)

Danazol has been used by several investigators for the treatment of menorrhagia. Doses of 200 and 400 mg daily have been given over 12 weeks after careful pretreatment observation and evaluation. MBL was markedly reduced in these studies from

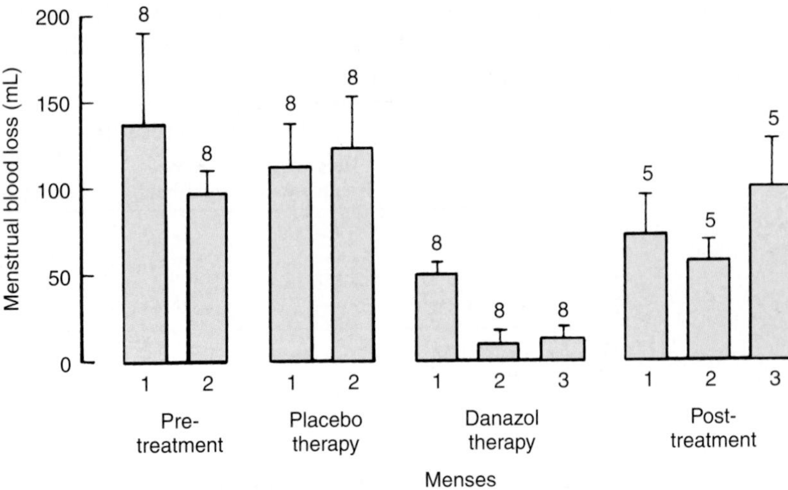

Figure 37-10. Mean (±SEM) menstrual blood loss in eight patients with menorrhagia before treatment, with placebo therapy, with 200 mg danazol daily, and after treatment. Number of patients is shown above each histogram. (From Chimbria TH, Anderson ABM, Naish C, et al: Reduction of menstrual blood loss by danazol in unexplained menorrhagia: Lack of effect of placebo. Br J Obstet Gynaecol 87:1152, 1980.)

more than 200 mL to less than 25 mL. Also, there was an increased interval between bleeding episodes (Fig. 37-10). The most common side effects of danazol treatment are weight gain and acne. Reduction of dosage from 400 to 200 mg daily decreased the side effects but did not alter the reduction in blood loss (Fig. 37-11). Some women may ovulate when receiving this dose of danazol. Further reduction to 100 mg daily did not effectively reduce MBL in most women. Although danazol is effective, it is also expensive and has moderate side effects.

Dockeray and associates treated 40 women with DUB, half with mefenamic acid (500 mg three times a day for 3 to 5 days of menses) and half with danazol (100 mg twice a day for 60 days). Danazol was more effective in reducing MBL, 60% compared with 20% for mefenamic acid (Fig. 37-12). However, adverse side effects were more severe with danazol and occurred in 75% of patients, compared with side effects in only 30% of patients treated with mefenamic acid.

A Cochrane review states that although nine RCTs were identified, studies have been generally underpowered. Nevertheless danazol appears to be more effective than placebo, progestogens, oral contraceptives and NSAIDs. However, compared with NSAIDs, the side effects of weight gain and skin problems were sevenfold greater and fourfold more when compared with progestogens.

GnRH Agonists

Although no large-scale studies have been performed, it is possible to inhibit ovarian steroid production with GnRH

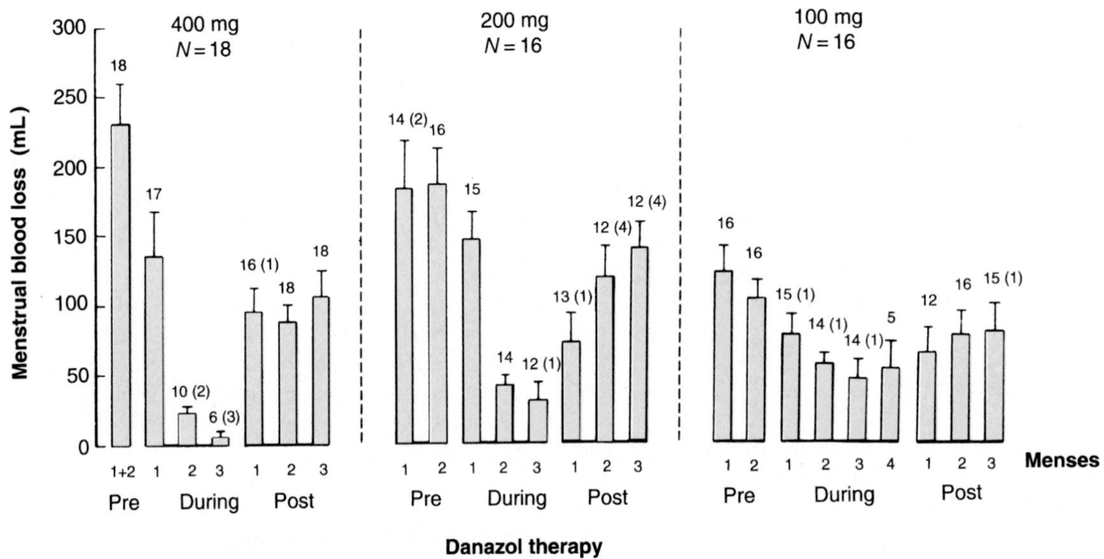

Figure 37-11. Mean (±SEM) menstrual blood loss in three groups of patients with menorrhagia treated with 400, 200, or 100 mg danazol daily for 12 weeks. Menstrual blood loss measurements are shown for each group before, during, and after danazol therapy. Number of patients menstruating is shown above each histogram, with number of missing menstrual loss collections in parentheses. (Adapted from Chimbria TH, Anderson ABM, Naish C, et al: Reduction of menstrual blood loss by danazol in unexplained menorrhagia: Lack of effect of placebo. Br J Obstet Gynaecol 87:1152, 1980.)

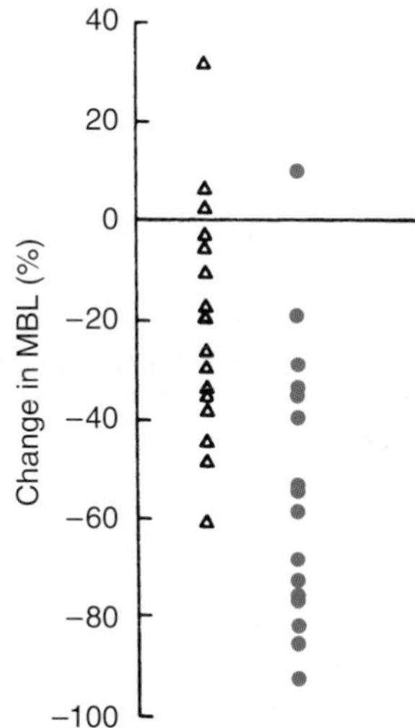

Figure 37-12. Percentage change in menstrual blood loss (MBL) between pretreatment cycles 1 and 2 and treatment cycles 3 and 4 shown for individual women treated with (triangle) mefenamic acid or (circle) danazol. Mean % change is −22.3% in the mefenamic acid group and −56.0% in the danazol-treated group. (From Dockeray CJ, Sheppard BL, Bonnard J: Comparison between mefenamic acid and danazol in the treatment of established menorrhagia. Br J Obstet Gynaecol 96:840, 1989.)

agonists. In a small study of four women, daily administration of a GnRH agonist for 3 months markedly reduced MBL from 100 to 200 mL per cycle to 0 to 30 mL per cycle. Unfortunately, after therapy was discontinued, blood loss returned to pretreatment levels (Fig. 37-13). Two other observational studies, one using sequential add-back in 20 women and another using goserelin in 60 women showed some benefit. Because of the expense and side effects of these agents, their use for menorrhagia caused by ovulatory DUB is limited to women with severe MBL who fail to respond to other methods of medical management and wish to retain their childbearing capacity. Use of an estrogen and/or progestin (add-back therapy) together with the agonist will help prevent bone loss.

Surgical Therapy

Dilation and Curettage

The performance of a D&C can be diagnostic and is therapeutic for immediate management of severe bleeding. For women with markedly excessive uterine bleeding who may be hypovolemic, the D&C is the quickest way to stop acute bleeding. Therefore it is the treatment of choice in women with DUB who suffer from hypovolemia. A D&C may be preferred as an approach to stop an acute bleeding episode in women older than 35 when the incidence of pathologic findings increases.

The use of D&C for the treatment of DUB has been reported to be curative only rarely. Temporary cure of the problem may occur in some women with chronic anovulation, since the curettage removes much of the hyperplastic endometrium; however, the underlying pathophysiologic cause is unchanged. A D&C has not proved useful for treatment of women who ovulate and have menorrhagia. Nilsson and Rybo have shown that, more than 1 month after the D&C, there was either no difference or an increase in MBL in women with menorrhagia who ovulate.

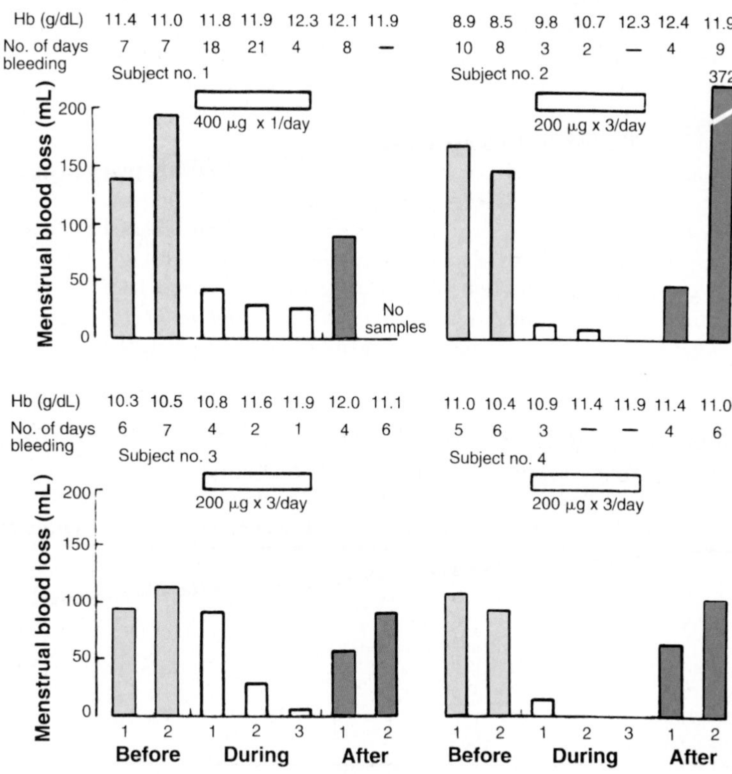

Figure 37-13. Alterations in measured monthly menstrual blood losses, number of days of menstrual bleeding, and hemoglobin (Hg) estimates before, during, and after therapy with intranasal luteinizing hormone-releasing hormone (LHRH) agonist. (From Shaw RW, Fraser HM: Use of a superactive luteinizing hormone releasing hormone (LHRH) agonist in the treatment of menorrhagia. Br J Obstet Gynaecol 9:913, 1984.)

Therefore D&C is only indicated for women with acute bleeding resulting in hypovolemia and for older women who are at higher risk of having endometrial neoplasia. All other women, after having an endometrial biopsy, sonohysteroscopy, or diagnostic hysteroscopy to rule out organic disease, are best treated with medical therapy, as outlined earlier, without a D&C.

Endometrial Ablation

Laser photovaporization of the endometrium for treatment of menorrhagia was originally reported by Goldrath and colleagues in 1981. Photovaporization of the endometrium was performed by use of a neodymium-YAG laser with hysteroscopic visualization and fluid distention of the uterine cavity. Danazol, 800 mg/day, was ingested for 2 to 3 weeks before the procedure, and an additional 2 weeks of danazol treatment was given afterward. This procedure was curative in 160 of 180 women, and follow-up biopsies showed no evidence of inflammation other than foreign body giant cells secondary to the carbon particles left after laser treatment. There was minimum endometrial regeneration. Photovaporization causes varying degrees of uterine contraction, scarring, and adhesion formation, as demonstrated by follow-up hysterosalpingograms and hysteroscopy.

Subsequently a large, prospective, 5-year, multicenter study of this technique was reported by Erian. A total of 2342 women with menorrhagia, most with ovulatory DUB, were enrolled. After producing endometrial atrophy with at least 1 month of 600 mg danazol daily, progestins, or a GnRH agonist, the endometrium was ablated with an Nd-YAG laser inserted through a hysteroscope. Complications were uncommon and minor: 0.4% fluid overload, 0.5% infection, and 0.29% uterine perforation. No major hemorrhage requiring a transfusion or laparotomy occurred. The mean duration of the procedure was 24 minutes. Of the 1866 women followed for 1 year, 56% had amenorrhea, 38% had a satisfactorily reduced amount of menses, and 7% had no reduction, requiring a second treatment (Table 37-2). Most of the latter responded to a second treatment, and only 2% required a hysterectomy.

There is good evidence from the Cochrane database that preoperative use of GnRH agonists or danazol is beneficial. Because the Nd-YAG laser is expensive, others have ablated the endometrium with electrocautery delivered by a urologic resectoscope placed through a hysteroscope. Magos and associates utilized this technique, termed *transcervical resection of the endometrium,* in 234 women with menorrhagia and produced amenorrhea in about 30%; one of the treatment groups (overall 90%) had improvement in the symptoms of heavy bleeding (Fig. 37-14).

In 1989, Vancaillie reported that thermal destruction of the endometrium could be accomplished easily and rapidly with electrocautery applied through a ball-end electrode attached to a urologic resectoscope. The ball-end electrode has several advantages compared with the loop electrode. These include a larger contact area, better fit into the cornual area, and because of the rotation, easier contact with the tissue as the ball-end electrode moves (Fig. 37-15). Paskowitz reported that in a study of 200 women treated with this technique, amenorrhea occurred in 40%, and the remainder reported decreased bleeding. The procedure was performed on an outpatient basis with general anesthesia. Preoperative endometrial suppression was accompanied with at least 1 month of danazol, GnRH analogues, or progestin. Of the 200 women, 10 (15%) had hysterectomies after the ablation.

The time to learn the roller-ball technique is shorter than for the laser, and the equipment is less expensive. However, both techniques require preoperative medications for several weeks, training and experience with operative hysteroscopy, and the use of general anesthesia. Another technique for endometrial ablation is to insert a latex balloon into the endometrial cavity, inject 5% dextrose in water into the balloon, heat the fluid to 87° C, and leave the heated filled balloon in the cavity for 8 minutes (Thermachoice, Gynecare division of Ethicon). This procedure does not require pretreatment regimens to the endometrium, does not require hysteroscopy training, and can be performed with local anesthesia. A randomized trial comparing the thermal balloon with rollerball ablating by Meyer and coworkers found that both techniques result in about an 80% return to normal bleeding. Three-year follow-up data has been reported with good results.

Several other ablation techniques may be considered. The VestaBlate system (Vesta Medical, Mountain View, CA) is a new balloon device that contains a silicone inflatable electrode carrier and a controller to monitor and distribute current. Hydrotherablator (BEI medical system, Teterborough, NJ) is another system using heated fluid in the endometrial cavity. This automated system does not allow passage of fluid into the fallopian tubes, maintaining an intrauterine pressure of 50 to 55 mm Hg. The potential advantages of this free-fluid system is that it may be used with endometrial distortions including fibroids. The reported amenorrhea rate was 35%, with 87% reporting

Table 37-2 Menstrual Bleeding at Different Ages Following Hysteroscopoic Endometrial Laser Ablation of Patients with Disabling Menorrhagia Resistant to Other Treatment

Age (years)	No. of Patients	Amenorrhea	Reduced Menses	Normal Period	No Improvement
14–19	4	0	3	1	0
20–29	35	2	11	4	18
30–34	96	18	32	20	26
35–39	242	64	55	96	27
40–44	867	502	135	194	36
45–49	510	352	112	32	14
50–56	112	105	5	1	1
Total (%)	1866	1043 (56)	353 (19)	348 (19)	122 (7)

From Erian J: Endometrial ablation in the treatment of menorrhagia. Br J Obstet Gynaecol 101(Suppl 11):19, 1994.

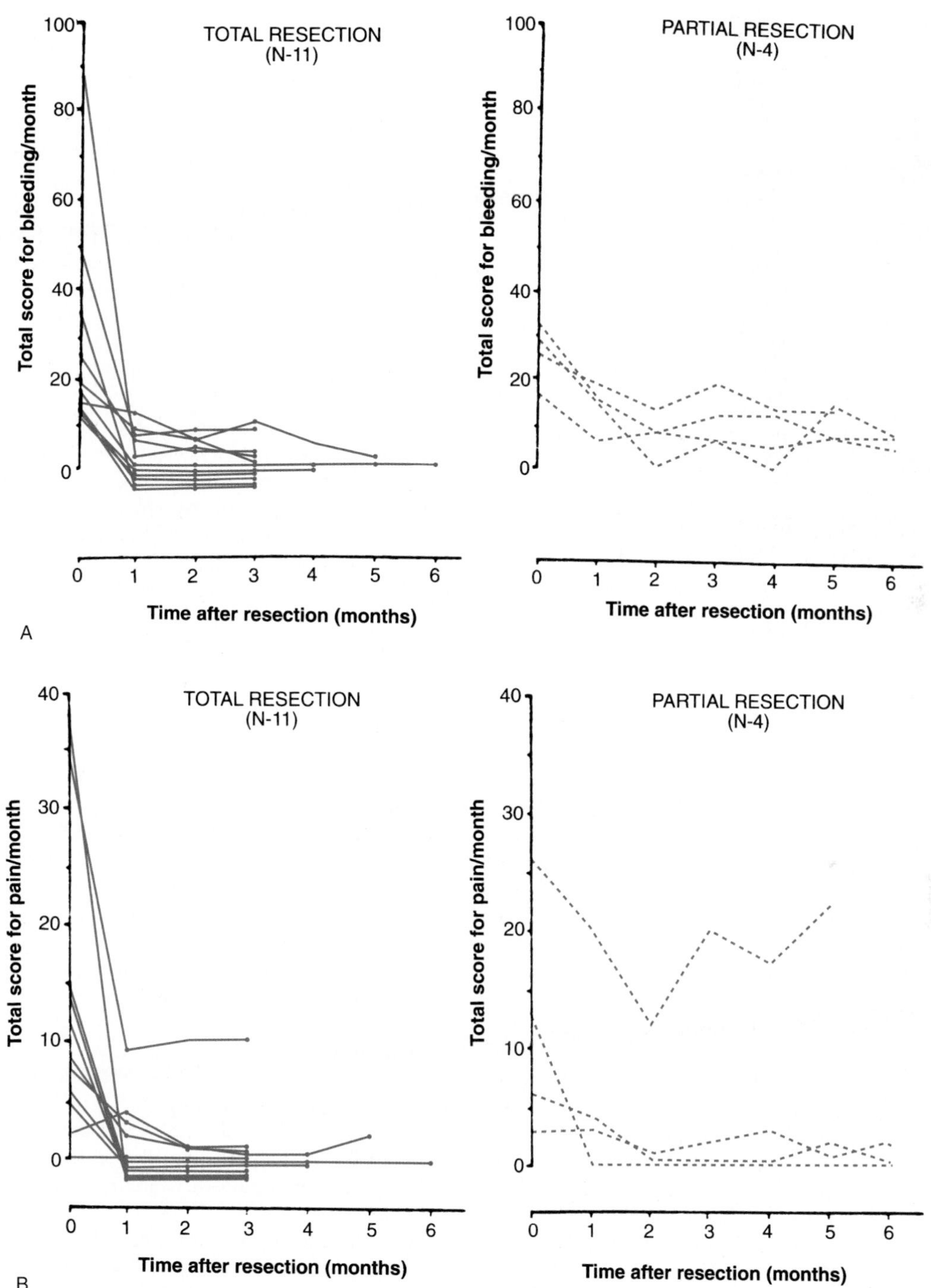

Figure 37-14. **A,** Effect of total and partial endometrial resection on total amount of menstrual bleeding each month. Blood loss was scored daily on scale of 0 to 3 (none to heavy). **B,** Effect of total and partial endometrial resection on total amount of menstrual pain each month. Pain was scored daily on score of 0 to 3 (none to severe). (From Magos AL, Baumann R, Turnbull AC: Experience with the first 250 endometrial resections for menorrhagia. Br Med J 298:1209, 1989.)

decreased blood flow. Novasure (Novacept, Palo Alto, CA) is a system containing a three-dimensional bipolar device and generator controlling the contour and depth of endometrial ablation. Suction is used to monitor the electrode surface with the endometrium. Other systems are also being used outside the United States and or under investigation. These include microwave endometrial ablation, cryoablation and photodynamic therapy. After ablation, the rates of amenorrhea in large studies vary between 25% and 60%, with most of the remainder having a decrease in the amount of menstrual bleeding. In one follow-up study in Britain 4 years after ablation, 24% of the women had a hysterectomy; older studies suggested that up to a third

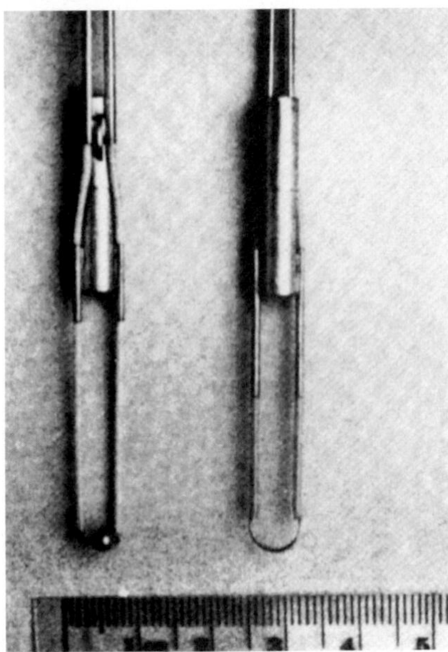

Figure 37-15. Ball-end and loop electrodes, side by side. Ball-end electrode is 2 mm in diameter and the loop, 7 mm. (From Vancaillie TG: Electrocoagulation of the endometrium with the ball-end resectoscope. Obstet Gynecol 74:425, 1989.)

of women elected to have hysterectomy within 5 years of an ablation procedure.

The various techniques of endometrial ablation are being used with increasing frequency for the treatment of women with menorrhagia without uterine lesions who are unresponsive to medical therapy, since the cost, mortality, and length of hospitalization is less than with hysterectomy. Endometrial ablation may therefore be used as an alternative to hysterectomy when other medical modalities fail or when there are contraindications to their use. Ablation is also useful in treating women with severe menorrhagia who have medical contraindications against performing a hysterectomy or for treating women with ovulatory DUB who do not wish to take medications. Obviously, ablation should not be used in women who wish to maintain their reproductive capacity. Complications of hysteroscopic endometrial ablation include fluid overload, uterine hemorrhage, uterine perforation, thermal damage to adjacent organs, and hematometria. Most of these complications occur because the ablation extends too deeply into the endometrium, opening up uterine vessels and exposing adjacent tissues to thermal injury. Guidelines for the safe and effective practice of endometrial ablation, including correct patient selection, were recently summarized by Garry after a meeting of a group of experts from several countries. They concluded that correct patient selection should be restricted to women with heavy MBL in the absence of organic distress. Ablation can be performed with either general or local anesthesia. The ablation should destroy all of the endometrium but only the superficial myometrium to reduce the rate of posttreatment problems. Similar guidelines by a British group were summarized by Lewis, who suggested that the operating surgeon perform at least 15 supervised procedures before being credentialed.

Hysterectomy

The decision to remove the uterus should be made on an individual basis and should usually be reserved for the woman with other indications for hysterectomy, such as leiomyomas or uterine prolapse. Hysterectomy should only be used to treat persistent ovulatory DUB after all medical therapy has failed and the amount of MBL has been documented to be excessive by direct measurement or by abnormally low serum ferritin levels. With increasing use of endometrial ablation to treat this problem, the incidence of hysterectomy as therapy for ovulatory DUB should decrease. It has been estimated that as many as half the women older than 40 with menorrhagia without uterine lesions are being treated by hysterectomy and that 20% of all hysterectomies in women of reproductive age are performed for excessive uterine bleeding.

As stated earlier, several reports cite the benefits (and for some women, the preference) of the LNG-IUS when hysterectomy or ablation are being considered. Uterine artery embolization is not particularly effective unless fibroids are the cause of excessive bleeding. If hysterectomy is chosen, many different options are available, including vaginal hysterectomy, laparoscopic-assisted vaginal hysterectomy (LAVH), laparoscopic supracervical hysterectomy, laparoscopic total hysterectomy, and abdominal supracervical hysterectomy.

Approach to Treatment

Having reviewed the various options as noted earlier, an important perspective is to approach the patient according to acute and chronic needs or short-term and long-term therapy.

Acute bleeding, which necessitates immediate cessation of bleeding, requires the use of pharmacologic doses of estrogen or curettage; the latter to be used more liberally in older women with risk factors or in those who are hemodynamically compromised. This approach is not dependent on whether the patient is anovulatory or ovulatory. Although estrogen will be temporarily helpful, even if there are abnormal anatomic findings, such as fibroids, it is preferable to perform curettage if pathology is suspected.

For less significant bleeding that warrants treatment, but not necessitating the immediate cessation of blood loss, high doses of progestogen alone may be used. Although this approach is used by many clinicians, there are no good data to support this approach.

After the acute episode it is imperative to know if the patient is bleeding from an anovulatory or ovulatory "dysfunctional" state. The majority of women fall into the anovulatory category.

In the adolescent, 10 mg of MPA for 10 days each month for at least 3 months should be prescribed, and the woman should be observed carefully thereafter. In this group of women additional diagnostic studies should be performed to detect possible defects in the coagulation process, particularly if bleeding is severe. For the woman of reproductive age, long-term therapy depends on whether she requires contraception, induction of ovulation, or treatment of DUB alone. In the last circumstance oral contraceptive or MPA can be administered, as stated earlier, monthly for at least 6 months, whereas oral contraceptives and clomiphene citrate are used for the other indications. For the perimenopausal woman who characteristically has lower amounts of circulating estrogen, use of cyclic progestogen alone is frequently not curative. In these women abnormal bleeding is best treated by low-dose oral contraceptives. The cyclic use of CE (0.625–1.25 mg) given for 25 days, with 10 mg of MPA or another progestogen added to the CE from days 15 to 25 can also be used after abnormal endometrial histologic findings have been ruled out.

The most difficult type of DUB to treat is chronic treatment of ovulatory women with menorrhagia. If anatomic abnormalities are not present, long-term treatment is necessary to reduce MBL. For these women NSAIDs, progestins, oral contraceptives, danazol, and GnRH analogues are all useful therapeutic modalities. A combination of two or more of these agents is often required to obviate the need for endometrial ablation or hysterectomy.

KEY POINTS

- The percentage of blood to total fluid volume of menstrual discharge averages 36%.
- The most precise method to measure menstrual blood loss (MBL) is the alkaline hematin method.
- Average loss of iron in each menses is 13 mg.
- The mean amount of MBL in one cycle in normal women was previously reported to be about 35 mL but may be as much as 60 mL.
- About 70% of total MBL occurs in the first 2 days of menses.
- Menorrhagia occurs in 9% to 14% of healthy women, and most have normal duration of menses.
- The predominant cause of dysfunctional uterine bleeding (DUB) in the postmenstrual and premenopausal years is anovulation. During the rest of the reproductive years, most DUB is associated with ovulation.
- Hemostatic plugs in the endometrium are smaller, have different morphology, and persist for a shorter time than when vessel damage occurs in other tissue.
- Following the treatment of menorrhagia in women with a normal uterus by endometrial ablation with laser or electrocoagulation, amenorrhea occurs in about half the women. About 40% have decreased bleeding, and 10% have no improvement.
- Within 4 years after endometrial ablation about 25% of women so treated will have a hysterectomy.
- There is an increase in the amount of both PGE_2 and $PGF_2\alpha$ in the endometrium in the late secretory phase and during menses, with the $PGF_2\alpha/PGE_2$ ratio steadily increasing from midcycle to menses.
- There is an inverse correlation between endometrial $PGF_2\alpha/PGE_2$ ratio and MBL.
- Anovulatory cycles are usually not associated with dysmenorrhea because of reduced levels of $PGF_2\alpha$ in the endometrium.
- Alterations in prostaglandin synthesis and release occur in women with both ovulatory and anovulatory DUB.
- Endometrial ablation by the thermal balloon technique yields similar results as electrocoagulation without the need to perform hysteroscopy.
- Diagnostic tests in women with menorrhagia include measurement of hemoglobin, serum iron, serum ferritin, HCG, TSH, endometrial biopsy, and hysteroscopy or hysterosalpingography.
- High doses of oral or intravenous estrogen will usually stop acute bleeding episodes caused by anovulatory DUB. Oral estrogen is less expensive and easier to administer than the intravenous form.
- Ergot derivatives do not reduce MBL and should not be used as therapy.
- Anovulatory DUB can be treated by cyclic use of progestins, oral contraceptives, or intermittent clomiphene citrate.
- Patients with ovulatory DUB are best treated with oral contraceptives, NSAIDs (antiprostaglandins), danazol, or progestins during the luteal phase or progesterone or progestins released locally from an IUD.
- NSAIDs administered during menses reduce MBL by 20% to 50% in women with ovulatory DUB.
- The blind technique of dilation and curettage (D&C) misses the diagnosis of uterine lesions in 10% to 25% of women.
- A D&C should be used to stop the acute bleeding episode in patients with hypovolemia or those older than 35. A D&C only treats the acute episode of excess uterine bleeding, not subsequent episodes.
- Endometrial ablation with laser or electrocautery is a useful technique to control ovulatory DUB in women who do not respond to medical management, have excessive side effects with medical therapy, or have no other indications for hysterectomy.
- Hysterectomy should be used to treat women with ovulatory DUB only after medical therapy has failed and excessive MBL has been documented by objective measurement.

BIBLIOGRAPHY

Adelantado JM, Rees CP, Bernal AL, Turnbull AC: Increased uterine prostaglandin E receptors in menorrhagic women. Br J Obstet Gynaecol 95:162, 1988.

Amso NN, for the International Collaborative Uterine Thermal Balloon Working Group: Uterine thermal balloon therapy for the treatment of menorrhagia: The first 300 patients from a multi-centre study. Br J Obstet Gynaecol 105:517, 1998.

Andersson K, Odlind V, Rybo G: Levonorgestrel-releasing and copper-releasing (Nova T) IUDs during five years of use: A randomized comparative trial. Contraception 49:56, 1994.

Beaumont H, Augood C, Duckitt K, et al: Danazol for heavy menstrual bleeding. Cochrane Database Syst Rev (2):CD001017, 2002.

Bergqvist A, Rybo G: Treatment of menorrhagia with intrauterine release of progesterone. Br J Obstet Gynaecol 90:255, 1983.
Bonney RC, Higham JM, Watson H, et al: Phospholipase activity in the endometrium of women with normal menstrual blood loss and women with proven ovulatory menorrhagia. Br J Obstet Gynaecol 98:363, 1991.
Chi IC: The TCU-380A (AG), MLCU375, and Nova-T IUDS and the IUD daily releasing 20 μg levonorgestrel-four pillars of IUD contraception for the nineties and beyond? Contraception 47:325-347, 1993.
Chimbria TH, Anderson ABM, Naish C, et al: Reduction of menstrual blood loss by danazol in unexplained menorrhagia: Lack of effect of placebo. Br J Obstet Gynaecol 87:1152, 1980.
Chimbira TH, Anderson AC, Turnbull AC: Relation between measured menstrual blood loss and patients' subjective assessment of loss, duration of bleeding, number of sanitary towels used, uterine weight and endometrial surface area. Br J Obstet Gynaecol 87:603, 1980.
Chimbria TH, Cope E, Anderson ABM, et al: The effect of danazol on menorrhagia, coagulation mechanisms, haematological indices and body weight. Br J Obstet Gynaecol 86:46, 1979.
Christiaens GC, Sixma JJ, Haspels AA: Morphology of haemostasis in menstrual endometrium. Br J Obstet Gynaecol 87:425, 1980.
Cicinelli E, Romano F, Anastasio PS, et al: Transabdominal sonohysterography, transvaginal sonography, and hysteroscopy in the evaluation of submucous myomas. Obstet Gynecol 85:42, 1995.
Claessens EA, Cowell CL: Acute adolescent menorrhagia. Am J Obstet Gynecol 139:277, 1981.
Clarke A, Black N, Rowe P, Mott S, Howle K: Indications for and outcome of total abdominal hysterectomy for benign disease: A prospective cohort study. Br J Obstet Gynecol, 102:611-20, 1995.
Cole SK, Billwicz WZ, Thomson AM: Sources of variation in menstrual blood loss. J Obstet Gynaecol Br Commonwlth 78:933, 1971.
DeVore GR, Owens O, Kase N: Use of intravenous Premarin in the treatment of dysfunctional uterine bleeding: A double-blind randomized control study. Obstet Gynecol 59:285, 1982.
Dockeray CJ, Sheppard BL, Bonnard J: Comparison between mefenamic acid and danazol in the treatment of established menorrhagia. Br J Obstet Gynaecol 96:840, 1989.
Erian J: Endometrial ablation in the treatment of menorrhagia. Br J Obstet Gynaecol 101:19, 1994.
Falcone T, Desjardins C, Bourque J, et al: Dysfunctional uterine bleeding in adolescents. J Reprod Med 39:761, 1994.
Fedele L, Bianchi S, Raffaelli R, et al: Treatment of adenomyosis-associated menorrhagia with a levonorgestrel-releasing intrauterine device. Fertil Steril 68:426, 1997.
Fong YF, Singh K: Effect of the levonorgestrel-releasing intrauterine system on uterine myomas in a renal transplant patient. Contraception, 60:51, 1999.
Fraser IS: Menorrhagia due to myometrial hypertrophy: Treatment with tamoxifen. Obstet Gynecol 70:505, 1987.
Fraser IS: Treatment of ovulatory and anovulatory dysfunctional uterine bleeding with oral progestogens. Aust N Z J Obstet Gynecol 30:353, 1990.
Fraser IS, McCarron G, Markham R: A preliminary study of factors influencing perception of menstrual blood loss volume. Am J Obstet Gynecol 149:788, 1984.
Fraser IS, McCarron G, Markham R, et al: Long-term treatment of menorrhagia with mefenamic acid. Obstet Gynecol 61:109, 1983.
Fraser IS, McCarron G, Markham R, et al: Measured menstrual blood loss in women with menorrhagia associated with pelvic disease or coagulation disorder. Obstet Gynecol 68:630, 1986.
Fraser IS, McCarron G, Markham R, Resta T: Blood and total fluid content of menstrual discharge. Obstet Gynecol 65:194, 1985.
Garry R: Good practice with endometrial ablation. Obstet Gynecol 85:144, 1995.
Garry R, Erian J, Grochmal SA: A multi-centre collaborative study into the treatment of menorrhagia by Nd-YAG laser ablation of the endometrium. Br J Obstet Gynaecol 98:357, 1991.
Garry R, Shelley-Jones D, Mooney P, Phillips G: Six hundred endometrial laser ablations. Obstet Gynecol 85:24, 1995.
Gimpelson RJ, Rappold HO: A comparative study between panoramic hysteroscopy with directed biopsies and dilatation and curettage. Am J Obstet Gynecol 158:489, 1988.
Goldrath MH, Fuller TA, Segal S: Laser photovaporization of endometrium for the treatment of menorrhagia. Am J Obstet Gynecol 140:14, 1981.
Goldstein SR: Use of ultrasonohysterography for triage of perimenopausal patients with unexplained uterine bleeding. Am J Obstet Gynecol 170:565, 1994.
Granstrom E, Swahn ML, Lundstrom V: The possible roles of prostaglandins and related compounds in endometrial bleeding. Acta Obstet Gynecol Scand (Suppl) 113:91, 1983.
Grant AM for the Aberdeen Endometrial Ablation Trials Group: A randomised trial of endometrial ablation versus hysterectomy for the treatment of dysfunctional uterine bleeding: Outcome at four years. Br J Obstet Gynaecol 106:360, 1999.
Hallberg L, Högdahl AM, Nilsson L, Rybo G: Menstrual blood loss—a population study: Variation at different ages and attempts to define normality. Acta Obstet Gynecol Scand 45:320, 1966.
Hallberg L, Nilsson L: Constancy of individual menstrual blood loss. Acta Obstet Gynecol Scand 43:352, 1964.
Hammond RH, Oppenheimer LW, Saunders PG: Diagnostic role of dilatation and curettage in the management of abnormal premenopausal bleeding. Br J Obstet Gynaecol 96:496, 1989.
Haynes PJ, Hodgson H, Anderson ABM, Turnbull AC: Measurement of menstrual blood loss in patients complaining of menorrhagia. Br J Obstet Gynaecol 84:763, 1977.
Higham JM, Shaw RW: A comparative study of danazol, a regimen of decreasing doses of danazol, and norethindrone in the treatment of objectively proven unexplained menorrhagia. Am J Obstet Gynecol 169:1134, 1993.
Hodgson DA, Feldberg IB, Sharp N, et al: Microwave endometrial ablation, development, clinical trials and outcomes at three years. Br J Obstet Gynaecol 106:684, 1999.
Hurskainen R, Teperi J, Rissanen P, et al: Quality of life and cost-effectiveness of levonorgestrel-releasing intrauterine system versus hysterectomy for treatment of menorrhagia: A randomized trial. Lancet, 357:273, 2001.
Irvine GA, Cameron IT: Medical management of dysfunctional uterine bleeding. Baillieres Best Pract Res Clin Obstet Gynaecol, 13:189, 1999.
Irvine GA, Campbell-Brolwn MB, Lumsden MA, et al: Randomised comparative trial of levonorgestrel intrauterine system and norethisterone for treatment of idiopathic menorrhagia. Br J Obstet Gynaecol 105:592, 1998.
Istre O, Trolle B: Treatment of menorrhagia with the levonorgestrel intrauterine system versus endometrial resection. Fertil Steril 76:304, 2001.
Kumar S, Suneetha PV, Dadhwal V, Mittal S: Endometrial cryoablation in the treatment of dysfunctional uterine bleeding. Int J Gynaecol Obstet, 76:189, 2002.
LaLonde A: Evaluation of surgical options in menorrhagia. Br J Obstet Gynaecol 101:8, 1994.
Lethaby AE, Cooke I, Rees M: Progesterone/progestogen releasing intrauterine systems versus either placebo or any other medication for heavy menstrual bleeding [Cochrane review]. In: The Cochrane Library. Issue 3. Chichester, UK, John Wiley, 2004.
Lethaby A, Irvine G, Cameron I: Cyclical progestogens for heavy menstrual bleeding. The Cochrane Database of Systemic Reviews. Issue 4. 1998: CD001016.
Lewis BV: Guidelines for endometrial ablation. Br J Obstet Gynaecol 101:470, 1994.
Loffer FD: Hysteroscopy with selective endometrial sampling compared with D&C for abnormal uterine bleeding: the value of a negative hysteroscopic view. Obstet Gynecol 73:16, 1989.
Loffer FD: Three-year comparison of thermal balloon and rollerball ablation in treatment of menorrhagia. J Am Assoc Gynecol Laparosc, 8:48, 2001.
Magos AL, Baumann R, Lockwood GM, Turnbull AC: Experience with the first 250 endometrial resections for menorrhagia. Lancet 337:1074, 1991.
Makarainen L, Ylikorkala O: Primary and myoma-associated menorrhagia: Role of prostaglandins and effects of ibuprofen. Br J Obstet Gynaecol 93:974, 1986.
Mercorio F, Simone RD, Sardo ADS, et al: The effect of a levonorgestrel-releasing intrauterine device in the treatment of myomarelated menorrhagia. Contraception 67:277, 2003.
Meyer WR, Walsh BW, Grainger DA, et al: Thermal balloon and rollerball ablation to treat menorrhagia: A multicenter comparison. Obstet Gynecol 92:98, 1998.
Milson I, Andersson K, Andersch B, Rybo G: A comparison of flurbiprofen, tranexamic acid, and a levonorgestrel-releasing intrauterine contraceptive device in the treatment of idiopathic menorrhagia. Am J Obstet Gynecol 164:879, 1991.

Munro MG: Dysfunctional uterine bleeding: Advances in diagnosis and treatment. Curr Opin Obstet Gynecol, 13:475, 2001.
Munro M, Lukes A, for the Abnormal Uterine Bleeding and Underlying Hemostatic Disorders Consensus Group: Abnormal uterine bleeding and underlying hemostatic disorders: Report of a consensus process. Fertil Steril 84:1335, 2005.
Newton J, Barnard G, Collins W: A rapid method for measuring menstrual blood loss using automatic extraction. Contraception 16:269, 1977.
Nilsson L, Rybo G: Treatment of menorrhagia with an antifibrinolytic agent, tranexamic acid (AMCA): A double-blind investigation. Acta Obstet Gynecol Scand 46:572, 1967.
Nilsson L, Rybo G: Treatment of menorrhagia. Am J Obstet Gynecol 110:713, 1971.
Parmer J: Long-term suppression of hypermenorrhea by progesterone intrauterine contraceptive devices. Am J Obstet Gynecol 149:578, 1984.
Paskowitz RA: "Rollerball" ablation of the endometrium. J Reprod Med 40:333, 1995.
Preston JT, Cameron IT, Adams EJ, Smith SK: Comparative study of tranexamic acid and norethisterone in the treatment of ovulatory menorrhagia. Br J Obstet Gynaecol 102:401, 1995.
Rees MCP, Cederholm-Williams SA, Turnbull AC: Coagulation factors and fibrinolytic proteins in menstrual fluid collected from normal and menorrhagic women. Br J Obstet Gynaecol 92:1164, 1985.
Rees MCP, Dunnill MS, Anderson ABM, Turnbull AC: Quantitative uterine histology during the menstrual cycle in relation to measured menstrual blood loss. Br J Obstet Gynaecol 91:662, 1984.
Romer T, Muller J, Foth D: Hyrdothermal ablation. A new simple method for coagulating endometrium in patients with therapy-resistant recurring hypermenorrhea. Contrib Gynecol Obstet, 20:154, 2000.
Ross D, Cooper AJ, Pryse-Davies J, et al: Randomized, double-blind, dose-ranging study of the endometrial effects of a vaginal progesterone gel in estrogen-treated postmenopausal women. Obstet Gynecol 1777:937, 1997.
Royal College of Obstetricians and Gynaecologists: The Initial Management of Menorrhagia-Evidence Based Clinical Guidelines, no. 1. London, RCOG Press, 1998.
Rybo G: Plasminogen activators in the endometrium. Acta Obstet Gynecol Scand 45:411, 1966.
Scottish Hysteroscopy Audit Group: A Scottish audit of hysteroscopic surgery for menorrhagia: Complications and follow up. Br J Obstet Gynaecol 102:249, 1995.
Shaw RW, Fraser HM: Use of a superactive luteinizing hormone releasing hormone (LHRH) agonist in the treatment of menorrhagia. Br J Obstet Gynaecol 9:913, 1984.
Sheppard BL, Dockeray CJ, Bonnar J: An ultrastructural study of menstrual blood in normal menstruation and dysfunctional uterine bleeding. Br J Obstet Gynaecol 90:259, 1983.
Smith SK, Abel MH, Kelly RW, Baird DT: Prostaglandin synthesis in the endometrium of women with ovular dysfunctional uterine bleeding. Br J Obstet Gynaecol 88:434, 1981.
Smith SK, Abel MH, Kelly RW, Baird DT: The synthesis of prostaglandins from persistent proliferative endometrium. J Clin Endocrinol Metab 55:284, 1982.
Smith SK, Abel MH, Kelly RW, Baird DT: A role for prostacyclin (PGI2) in excessive menstrual bleeding. Lancet 1:522, 1981.
Starczewski A, Iwanicki M: [Intrauterine therapy with levonorgestrel releasing IUD of women with hypermenorrhea secondary to uterine fibroids]. Ginekol Pol 71,1221, 2000.
Stewart A, Cummins C, Gold L, et al: The effectiveness of the levonorgestrel-releasing intrauterine system in menorrhagia: A systematic review. BJOG 108:74, 2001.
Syrop CH, Sahakian V: Transvaginal sonographic detection of endometrial polyps with fluid contrast augmentation. Obstet Gynecol 79:1041, 1992.
Unger JB, Meeks GR: Hysterectomy after endometrial ablation. Am J Obstet Gynecol 175:1432, 1996.
Vancaillie TG: Electrocoagulation of the endometrium with the ball-end resectoscope. Obstet Gynecol 74:425, 1989.
van Eijkeren MA, Christiaens GC, Sixma JJ, Haspels AA: Menorrhagia: A review. Obstet Gynecol Surv 44:421, 1989.
van Eijkeren MA, Scholten PC, Christiaens GC, et al: The alkaline hematin method for measuring menstrual blood loss—A modification and its clinical use in menorrhagia. Eur J Obstet Gynecol Reprod Biol 22:345, 1986.
Van Vugt DA, Krzemien A, Roy BN, et al: Photodynamic endometrial ablation in the nonhuman primate. J Soc Gynecol Invest, 7:125, 2000.
Vargyas JM, Campeau JD, Mishell DA: Treatment of menorrhagia with meclofenamate sodium. Am J Obstet Gynecol 157:944, 1987.
Wilansky DL, Greisman B: Early hypothyroidism in patients with menorrhagia. Am J Obstet Gynecol 160:673, 1989.

Primary and Secondary Amenorrhea and Precocious Puberty

38

Etiology, Diagnostic Evaluation, Management

Rogerio A. Lobo

KEY TERMS AND DEFINITIONS

Amenorrhea. Absence of menses during the reproductive years. It can be either physiologic (pregnancy) or pathologic.

Androgen Resistance Syndrome (Testicular Feminization). A genetically transmitted androgen receptor defect in a 46,XY individual with testes and normal male testosterone levels. These individuals have normal female phenotype, absent uterus, and scant body hair.

Anorexia Nervosa. A psychiatric disease associated with a fear of weight gain or obesity, food aversion, and a distorted body image in which the individual limits caloric intake to starvation levels. In addition to severe weight loss, there is a decreased metabolic rate and amenorrhea.

Chromophobe Adenoma. A nonhormone-secreting pituitary tumor that can disrupt normal pituitary function and thus produce low gonadotropin levels.

Congenital Absence of Uterus and Vagina. A malformation in a 46,XX individual with normal ovarian function, resulting in failure of the uterus and vagina to form. It is also called *uterovaginal agenesis* and *Rokitansky–Küster–Hauser syndrome.*

Cryptomenorrhea. Menstruation without egress of menses through the introitus.

Delayed Menarche. Onset of menses in women older than 16.5 years who have no reproductive abnormalities.

Functional Hypothalamic Amenorrhea. Amenorrhea caused by nonorganic impairment of normal hypothalamic function with slowing of normal gonadotropin-releasing hormone (GnRH) pulsatility.

Gonadal Failure. Failure of the gonads to develop. It is also called *gonadal dysgenesis* if the karyotype is abnormal and gonadal agenesis if the karyotype is normal.

Gonadal Streaks. Streaks of fibrous tissue in the normal position of the ovaries.

Gonadotropin-Resistant Ovary Syndrome. Premature ovarian failure in which the ovary contains normal-appearing primordial follicles but no follicular development. It is also called *ovarian hypofolliculogenesis.*

Hypogonadotropic Hypogonadism. Failure of the ovaries to develop as a result of low amounts of circulatory gonadotropins. When anosmia is present, the term *Kallmann's syndrome* is used.

Hypothalamic Dysfunction. Secondary amenorrhea caused by an abnormal pattern of GnRH pulsatility and normal circulatory estradiol.

Hypothalamic Failure. Secondary amenorrhea caused by an abnormal pattern of GnRH pulsatility and estradiol levels below the normal premenopausal range.

Insulin Tolerance Test. A test of adrenocorticotropic hormone function in which hypoglycemia is produced and cortisol is measured.

Intrauterine Adhesions or Synechiae. A condition in which fibrous tissue partially or completely obliterates the uterine cavity. It is also called *Asherman's syndrome.*

Isolated Gonadotropin Deficiency. The presence of hypogonadotropic hypogonadism in individuals who do not produce gonadotropins after prolonged administration of GnRH.

Leptin. A hormone secreted by fat cells that helps regulate the reproductive and GH axis. Low levels with undernutrition explains, in part, the amenorrhea.

Pituitary Destruction. Damage or necrosis of the pituitary gland caused by anoxia, thrombosis, or hemorrhage. It is called *Sheehan's syndrome* when related to pregnancy and *Simmonds' disease* when unrelated to pregnancy.

Polycystic Ovary Syndrome. An extremely common disorder in women most frequently diagnosed by anovulation, hyperandrogenism, and polycystic ovaries on ultrasound; it may also occur in women who have regular cycles and ovulation.

Precocious Puberty. Arbitrarily defined as any signs of sexual maturation at an early age (now thought to be younger than age 6 or 7). Types are divided into heterosexual or isosexual, or due to isolated conditions such as premature thelarche.

Premature Ovarian Failure. Cessation of menstruation caused by depletion of ovarian follicles or failure of primordial follicles to respond to gonadotropin before the age of 40. It is also called *hypergonadotropic hypogonadism.*

Primary Amenorrhea. Absence of any spontaneous menses in an individual older than 16.5 years of age.

Pure Gonadal Dysgenesis. Absence of the gonads in an individual with a normal 46,XX or 46,XY karyotype. It is also called *gonadal agenesis.*

Secondary Amenorrhea. Absence of menses for a variable period of time (for at least 3 to 12 months, usually 6 months or longer) in an individual who has previously had spontaneous menstrual periods.

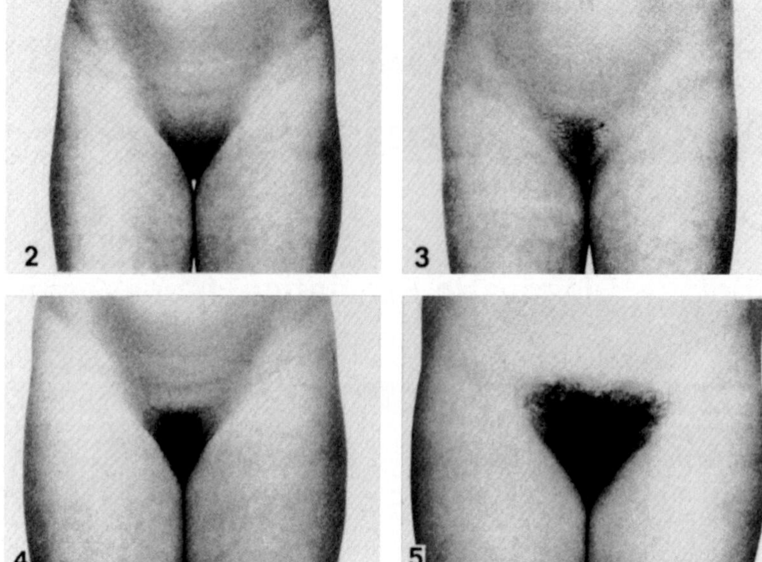

Figure 38-1. Standards for **(A)** pubic hair and **(B,** opposite page) breast ratings. The numbers correspond to parallels between pubic hair and breast development at the same age. (Modified from Tanner JM: Growth and endocrinology of the adolescent. In Gardner L [ed]: Endocrine and Genetic Diseases of Childhood, 2nd ed. Philadelphia, WB Saunders, 1975.)

Amenorrhea can be either physiologic, when it occurs during pregnancy and the postpartum period (particularly when nursing), or pathologic, when it is produced by a variety of endocrinologic and anatomic disorders. In the latter circumstance, the failure to menstruate is a symptom of these various pathologic conditions. Thus, amenorrhea itself is not a pathologic entity and should not be used as a final diagnosis.

Although the absence of menses causes no harm to the body, in a woman who is not pregnant or postpartum it is abnormal and thus is a source of concern. For this reason women usually seek medical assistance when the condition occurs. Therefore, the clinician needs to know the various etiologies of amenorrhea, how to diagnose the etiology, and how to treat the underlying pathologic condition. This chapter will present the etiology, diagnostic evaluation, and treatment of the various causes of both primary and secondary amenorrhea.

Many individuals with ambiguous external genitalia resulting from various intersex problems are raised as females and never menstruate. The cause of the intersex problem is usually determined at birth or soon thereafter. Since such disorders are discussed in Chapter 12 (Congenital Abnormalities of the Female Reproductive Tract), they will not be discussed in this chapter. Although women with cryptomenorrhea caused by anatomic disorders interfering with the outflow of menses, such as an imperforate hymen or transverse vaginal septum, have the symptom of amenorrhea, they are actually menstruating. These conditions are discussed in Chapter 12 (Congenital Abnormalities of the Female Reproductive Tract). Severe systemic diseases such as metastatic carcinoma and chronic renal failure can also cause amenorrhea; however, since amenorrhea is not the presenting symptom of these disorders, they will not be discussed in this chapter.

Primary amenorrhea is defined as the absence of menses in a woman who has never menstruated by the age of $16^1/_2$ years. The incidence of primary amenorrhea is less than 0.1%. Secondary amenorrhea is defined as the absence of menses for an arbitrary time period, usually longer than 6 to 12 months. The incidence of secondary amenorrhea of more than 6 months' duration in a survey of a general population of Swedish women of reproductive age was found to be 0.7%. The incidence was significantly higher in women younger than 25 years of age and those with a prior history of menstrual irregularity.

DELAYED MENARCHE

Before the onset of menses the normal female goes through a progressive series of morphologic changes produced by the pubertal increase in estrogen and androgen production. In 1969 Marshall and Tanner defined five stages of breast development and pubic hair development (Fig. 38-1, Table 38-1). These

Table 38-1 Classifications of Breast Growth and Pubic Hair Growth

Classification	Description
Breast Growth	
B1	Prepubertal: elevation of papilla only
B2	Breast budding
B3	Enlargement of breasts with glandular tissue, without separation of breast contours
B4	Secondary mound formed by areola
B5	Single contour of breast and areola
Pubic Hair Growth	
PH1	Prepubertal: no pubic hair
PH2	Labial hair present
PH3	Labial hair spreads over mons pubis
PH4	Slight lateral spread
PH5	Further lateral spread to form inverse triangle and reach medial thighs

Adapted from Roy S: Puberty. In Mishell DR Jr, Davajan V (eds): Infertility, Contraception and Reproductive Endocrinology, 4th ed. Copyright 1997 by Blackwell Scientific Publications, Malden, MA.

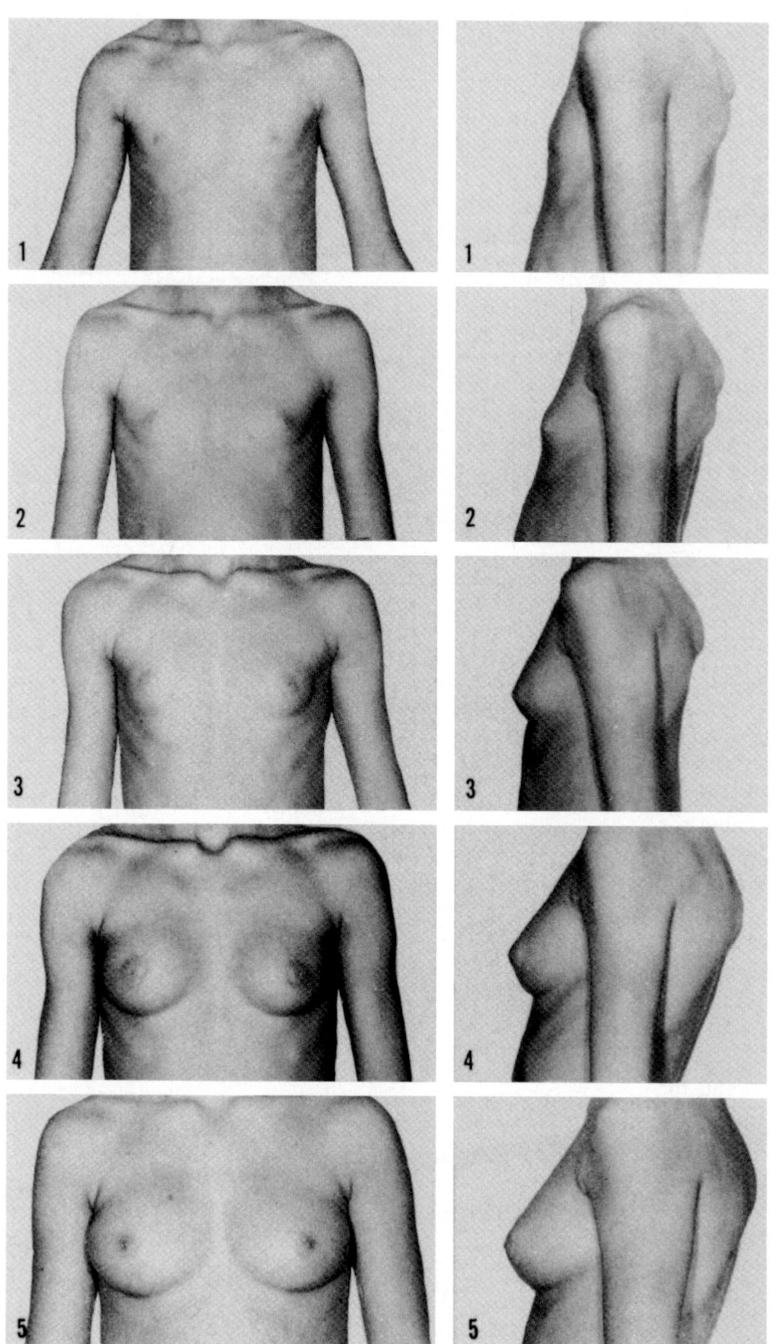

Figure 38-1. *cont'd,* B. See previous page for legend.

changes sometimes are combined and called *Tanner,* or *pubertal, stages 1 through 5.* The first sign of puberty is usually the appearance of breast budding followed within a few months by the appearance of pubic hair.

Thereafter, the breasts enlarge, the external pelvic contour becomes rounder, and the most rapid rate of growth occurs (peak height velocity). These changes precede menarche. Thus, breast budding is the earliest sign of puberty and menarche the latest. The mean ages of occurrence of these events in American women are shown in Table 38-2, and the mean intervals (with standard deviation) between initiation of breast budding and

Table 38-2 Mean Ages of Girls at the Onset of Pubertal Events (United States)

Event	Mean Age ± SD (Years)
Initiation of breast development (B2)	10.8 ± 1.10
Appearance of pubic hair (PH2)	11.0 ± 1.21
Menarche	12.9 ± 1.20

Adapted from Frisch RE, Revelle R: Height and weight in menarche and a hypothesis of menarche. Arch Dis Child 46:695, 1971.

Table 38-3 Pubertal Intervals

Interval	Mean Age ± SD (Years)
B2-peak height velocity	1.0 ± 0.77
B2-menarche	2.3 ± 1.03
B2-PH5	3.1 ± 1.04
B2-B5 (average duration of puberty)	4.5 ± 2.04

Adapted from Frisch RE, Revelle R: Height and weight in menarche and a hypothesis of menarche. Arch Dis Child 46:695, 1971.

other pubertal events are shown in Table 38-3. The mean interval between breast budding and menarche is 2.3 years, with a standard deviation of about 1 year. Some individuals can progress from breast budding to menarche in 18 months, and others may take 5 years. Thus although the arbitrary age of primary amenorrhea is 16½ years, if a woman 14 years of age or older presents to the clinician with absence of breast budding, a diagnostic evaluation should be performed at this time. The absence of breast development is indicative of a lack of estradiol (E_2) synthesis. The cause of this abnormality should be determined; then estrogen replacement can be initiated to cause breast development.

The mean time of onset of menarche was previously thought to occur when a critical body weight of about 48 kg (106 lb) was reached. However, it is now believed that body composition is more important than total body weight in determining the time of onset of puberty and menstruation. Thus, the ratio of fat to both total body weight and lean body weight is probably the most relevant factor that determines the time of onset of puberty and menstruation. Individuals who are moderately obese, between 20% and 30% above the ideal body weight, have an earlier onset of menarche than nonobese women. Malnutrition, such as occurs with anorexia nervosa or starvation, is known to delay the onset of puberty.

One of the major links between body composition and the hypothalamic–pituitary–ovarian axis, and thus menstrual cyclicity, is the adipocyte hormone leptin. Leptin is produced by adipocytes and correlates well with body weight. Leptin is also important for feedback involving gonadotropin-releasing hormone (GnRH) and luteinizing hormone (LH) pulsatility and also binds to specific receptor sites on the ovary and endometrium. Body weight and body fat content have been shown to be important for menstruation; a fatness nomogram is depicted in Figure 38-2. Well-nourished individuals with prepubertal strenuous exercise programs resulting in less total body fat have also been shown to have a delayed onset of puberty. Warren and colleagues reported that ballet dancers, swimmers, and runners had menarche delayed to about age 15 if they began exercising strenuously before menarche (Fig. 38-3). These investigators also determined that stress is not the cause of the delayed menarche in these exercising girls, as girls of the same age with stressful musical careers did not have a delayed onset of menarche. Young women with strenuous exercise programs have sufficient estrogen to produce some breast development and thus do not need extensive endocrinologic evaluation if concern arises about lack of onset of menses. Frisch and coworkers reported that for girls engaged in premenarcheal athletic training, menarche was delayed 0.4 years for each year of training. Individuals who

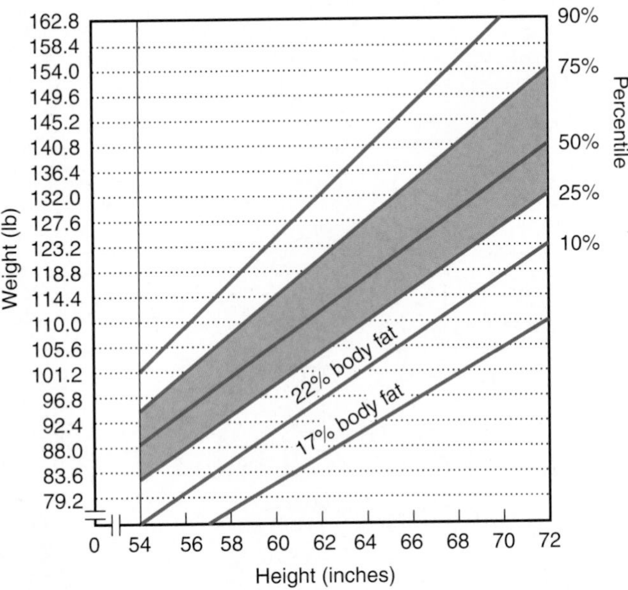

Figure 38-2. A fatness index nomogram. (Adapted from Frisch RE, Revelle R: Height and weight in menarche and a hypothesis of menarche. Arch Dis Child 46:695, 1971.)

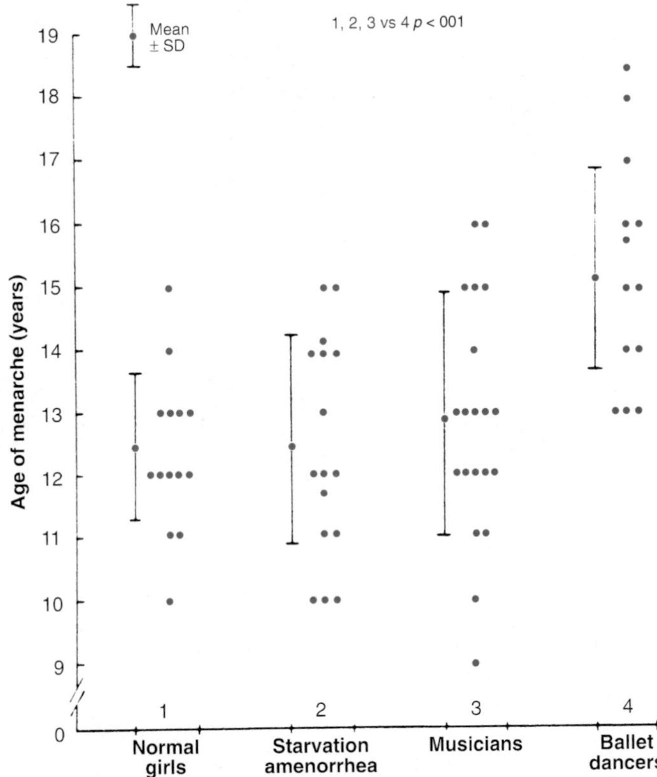

Figure 38-3. Ages of menarche in ballet dancers compared with those of three other groups. (From Warren MP: The effects of exercise on pubertal progression and reproductive function in girls. J Clin Endocrinol Metab 51:1150, 1980. Copyright 1980 by The Endocrine Society.)

exercise strenuously should be counseled that they will usually have a delayed onset of menses, but it is not a health problem. They should be told that they will most likely have regular ovulatory cycles when they either stop exercising or become older.

The metabolic features of amenorrheic athletes, who are considered to be in a state of negative energy balance, are fairly characteristic. These include elevated serum follicle-stimulating hormone (FSH), insulin-like growth factor-binding protein 1 (IGFBP-1), and lowered insulin insulin-like growth factor (IGF) levels.

Stress per se can lead to inhibition of the GnRH axis. This may be the key factor influencing amenorrhea in competitive athletes. The mechanism involves an increased secretion of corticotropin-releasing hormone (CRH) (releasing adrenocorticotropic hormone [ACTH] and cortisol). CRH itself is known to inhibit GnRH.

Before puberty, circulating levels of LH and FSH are low (FSH/LH ratio being greater than 1) because the central nervous system (CNS)–hypothalamic axis is extremely sensitive to the negative feedback effects of low levels of circulating estrogen. As the critical weight or body composition is approached, the CNS–hypothalamic axis becomes less sensitive to the negative effect of estrogen, and GnRH is secreted in greater amounts, causing an increase in both LH and to a lesser extent FSH. The initial endocrinologic change associated with the onset of puberty is the occurrence of episodic pulses of LH occurring during sleep (Fig. 38-4). These pulses are absent before the onset of puberty. After menarche the episodic secretions of LH occur both during sleep and while awake. The last endocrinologic event of puberty is activation of the positive gonadotropin response to increasing levels of E_2, which results in the midcycle gonadotropic surge and ovulation.

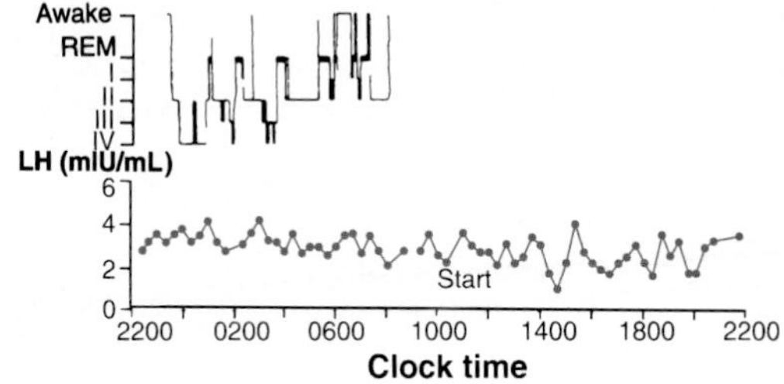

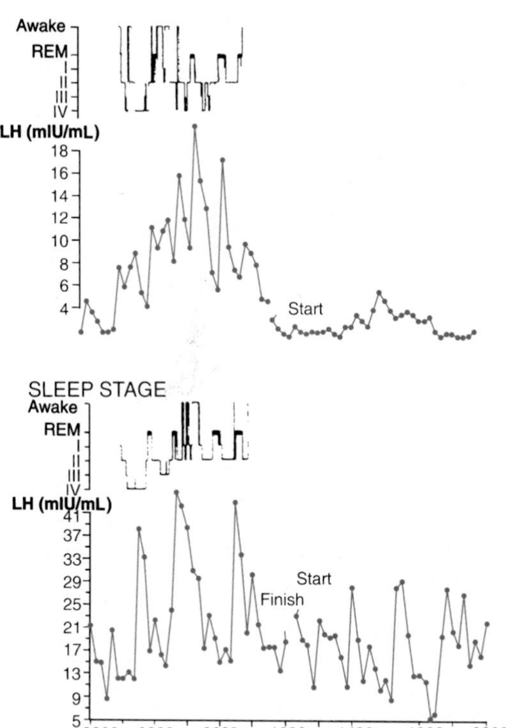

Figure 38-4. Plasma luteinizing hormone (LH) concentration measured every 20 minutes for 24 hours in normal prepubertal girl *(upper panel)*, early pubertal girl *(center panel)*, and normal late pubertal girl *(lower panel)*. In top and center panels sleep histogram is shown above period of nocturnal sleep. Sleep stages are awake, rapid eye movement (REM), and stages I–IV by depth of line graph. Plasma LH concentrations are expressed as milli international units per milliliter of Second International Reference Preparation of Human Menopausal Gonadotropin. (Modified from Boyar RM, Katz J, Finkelstein JW, et al: Anorexia nervosa: Immaturity of the 24-hour luteinizing hormone secretory pattern. N Engl J Med 291:861, 1974. Copyright 1974 Massachusetts Medical Society. All rights reserved.)

PRIMARY AMENORRHEA

It is important that the clinician understand both the sequential endocrinologic and the morphologic chronologic changes taking place during normal puberty in order to make the differential diagnosis between delayed menarche and primary amenorrhea. Although the former condition requires only reassurance, the latter requires an endocrinologic evaluation.

Etiology

Although numerous classifications have been used for the various causes of primary amenorrhea, it has been found most clinically useful to group them on the basis of whether secondary sexual characteristics (breasts) and female internal genitalia (uterus) are present or absent (see the following box). Thus, the findings of a physical examination can alert the clinician to possible causes and indicate which laboratory tests should be performed. In a series of 62 individuals reported by Maschchak and colleagues the largest subgroup with primary amenorrhea (29) were those in whom breasts were absent but who had a uterus; the second largest subgroup (22) had both breasts and uterus; lack of a uterus together with breast development accounted for the third largest category (9); and those without breasts or a uterus were the least common (2). This breakdown of the various accompanying conditions of primary amenorrhea reflects the referral pattern to the center and not necessarily the true incidence of each category.

Breasts Absent and Uterus Present

All individuals with no breast development and a uterus present have no ovarian estrogen production as a result of either a gonadal disorder or a CNS hypothalamic–pituitary abnormality. The phenotype of individuals with either of these causes of low estrogen synthesis is similar. However, because the cause of the disorder and the prognosis for fertility differs, it is important to establish the specific diagnosis.

Classification of Disorders with Primary Amenorrhea and Normal Female External Genitalia

I. Absent breast development; uterus present
  A. Gonadal failure
    1. a. 45,X (Turner's syndrome)
      b. 46,X, abnormal X (e.g., short- or long-arm deletion)
      c. Mosaicism (e.g., X/XX, X/XX,XXX)
      d. 46,XX or 46,XY pure gonadal dysgenesis
      e. 17α-hydroxylase deficiency with 46,XX
  B. Hypothalamic failure secondary to inadequate GnRH release
    1. Insufficient GnRH secretion due to neurotransmitter defect
    2. Inadequate GnRH synthesis (Kallman's syndrome)
    3. Congenital anatomic defect in central nervous system
    4. CNS neoplasm (craniopharyngioma)
  C. Pituitary failure
    1. Isolated gonadotrophin insufficiency (thalassemia major, retinitis pigmentosa)
    2. Pituitary neoplasia (chromophobe adenoma)
    3. Mumps, encephalitis
    4. Newborn kernicterus
    5. Prepubertal hypothyroidism
II. Breast development; uterus absent
  A. Androgen resistance (testicular feminization)
  B. Congenital absence of uterus (utero-vaginal agenesis)
III. Absent breast development; uterus absent
  A. 17,20-desmolase deficiency
  B. Agonadism
  C. 17α-hydroxylase deficiency with 46,XY karyotype
IV. Breast development; uterus present
  A. Hypothalamic etiology
  B. Pituitary etiology
  C. Ovarian etiology
  D. Uterine etiology

CNS, central nervous system; GnRH, gonadotropin-releasing hormone.

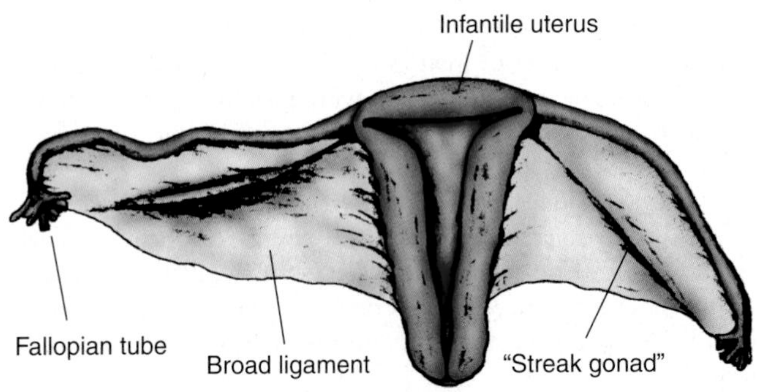

Figure 38-5. Internal genitalia of patient with gonadal dysgenesis (Turner's syndrome), featuring normal but infantile uterus, normal fallopian tubes, and pale, glistening "streak" gonads in both broad ligaments. (From Federman DD [ed]: Disorders of gonadal development: Gonadal dysgenesis [Turner syndrome]. In Abnormal Sexual Development: A Genetic and Endocrine Approach to Differential Diagnosis. Philadelphia, WB Saunders, 1967.)

Gonadal Failure (Hypergonadotropic Hypogonadism). Failure of gonadal development is the most common cause of primary amenorrhea, occurring in almost half the individuals with this symptom. Gonadal failure is most frequently due to a chromosomal disorder or deletion of all or part of an X chromosome, but it is sometimes due to a genetic defect and rarely 17α-hydroxylase deficiencies. The chromosome disorders are usually due to a random meiotic or mitotic abnormality (e.g., nondisjunction or anaphase lag) and thus are not inherited. However, if gonadal development is absent in the presence of a 46,XX or 46,XY karyotype (called pure gonadal dysgenesis), a gene disorder may be present, as it has been reported to occur in siblings. Reindollar and coworkers, in the largest single series of patients with primary amenorrhea, reported that all individuals with gonadal failure and an X chromosome abnormality were less than 63 inches in height. About one third also had major cardiovascular or renal anomalies.

Deletion of the entire X chromosome (as occurs in Turner's syndrome) or of the short arm (p) of the X chromosome results in short stature. Deletions of only the long arm (q) usually do not affect height. In place of the ovary a band of fibrous tissue called a *gonadal streak* is present (Fig. 38-5). Streaks are also present in individuals without gonads (pure gonadal dysgenesis). When ovarian follicles are absent, synthesis of ovarian steroids and inhibin does not occur. Breast development does not occur because of the very low circulating E_2 levels. Because the negative hypothalamic–pituitary action of estrogen and inhibin is not present, gonadotropin levels are markedly elevated, with FSH levels being higher than LH. Since estrogen is not necessary for müllerian duct development or wolffian duct regression, the internal and external genitalia are phenotypically normal female. Individuals with 17α-hydroxylase deficiency do have primordial follicles but cannot synthesize sex steroids.

An occasional individual with mosaicism, an abnormal X, pure gonadal dysgenesis (46,XX) or even Turner's syndrome may have a few follicles that develop under endogenous gonadotropin stimulation early in puberty and may synthesize enough estrogen to induce breast development and a few episodes of uterine bleeding, resulting early in premature ovarian failure; usually before age 25. Rarely, ovulation and pregnancy can occur.

Goldenberg and associates reported that all individuals with primary amenorrhea and plasma FSH levels greater than 40 mIU/mL had no functioning ovarian follicles in the gonadal tissue. Thus, in women with primary amenorrhea, the diagnosis of gonadal failure can be established if the FSH levels are consistently elevated without requiring ovarian tissue evaluation.

45,X Anomalies. Turner's syndrome occurs in about 1 per 2000 to 1 per 3000 live births but is much more frequent in abortuses. In addition to primary amenorrhea and absent breast development, these individuals have other somatic abnormalities, the most prevalent being short stature (less than 60 inches in height), webbing of the neck, a short fourth metacarpal, and cubitus valgus. Cardiac abnormality, renal abnormalities, and hypothyroidism are also more prevalent. The diagnosis is usually made before puberty (see Chapter 2, Reproductive Genetics).

A wide variety of chromosomal mosaics are associated with primary amenorrhea and normal female external genitalia, the most common being X/XX. In addition, individuals with X/XXX and X/XX/XXX mosaicism have primary amenorrhea. These individuals are generally taller and have fewer anatomic abnormalities than individuals with a 45,X karyotype. In addition, some of them may have a few gonadal follicles, and about 20% have sufficient estrogen production to menstruate. Occasionally, ovulation may occur as stated earlier. Isolated phenotypic features of Turner's syndrome may also occur in males, and is known as Noonan's syndrome.

Structurally Abnormal X Chromosome. Although individuals with this disorder have a 46,XX karyotype, part of one X chromosome is structurally abnormal. If there is deletion of the long arm of the X chromosome (Xq), normal height has been reported to occur, but in Reindollar's series such individuals were all relatively short. These individuals have no somatic abnormalities. However, if there is deletion of the short arm of the X chromosome (Xp), the individual phenotypically resembles those with a 45,X karyotype (Turner's syndrome). A similar phenotype occurs in persons with isochrome of the long arm of the X chromosome. Other X chromosome abnormalities include a ring X and minute fragmentation of the X chromosome.

Pure Gonadal Dysgenesis (46,XX and 46,XY with Gonad Streaks; Gonadal Agenesis). As noted earlier, this abnormality is a genetic disorder and has been reported in siblings. Abnormalities in genes involved in gonadal development are expected to be involved. These individuals have normal stature and phenotype, absence of secondary sexual characteristics, and primary amenorrhea. Some of these individuals have a few ovarian follicles, develop breasts, and may even menstruate spontaneously for a few years.

17α-Hydroxylase Deficiency with 46,XX Karyotype. A rare gonadal cause of primary amenorrhea without breast development and normal female internal genitalia is deficiency of the enzyme 17α-hydroxylase in an individual with a 46,XX karyotype (it can also occur in genetic males 46,XY). Only a few such individuals have been described in the literature, but it is important for the clinician to be aware of this entity because these individuals, in contrast to those described earlier, have hypernatremia and hypokalemia. Because of decreased cortisol, ACTH levels are elevated. The mineralocorticoid levels are also elevated, as 17α-hydroxylase is not necessary for the conversion of progesterone to deoxycortisol or corticosterone. Thus, there is excessive sodium retention and potassium excretion, leading to hypertension and hypokalemia. Serum progesterone levels are also elevated because progesterone is not converted to cortisol. In addition to sex steroid replacement, these individuals need cortisol administration. These individuals usually have cystic ovaries and viable oocytes. Pregnancies have been documented following in vitro fertilization/embryo transfer (IVF-ET) despite low levels of endogenous sex steroids.

Genetic Disorders with Hyperandrogenism. Hyperandrogenism occurs in about 10% of women with gonadal dysgenesis. Most have a Y chromosome or fragment of a Y chromosome, but some may only have a DNA fragment that contains the testes-determining gene (probably *SRY*) without a full Y chromosome. Individuals with hypergonadotropic hypogonadism and a female phenotype who have any clinical manifestation of hyperandrogenism, such as hirsutism, should have a gonadectomy even if a Y chromosome is not present because gonadal neoplasms are frequent. Although not yet considered routine, in the future all individuals with gonadal dysgenesis will be screened for the presence of *SRY* or even more specific testis-determining regions.

CNS–Hypothalamic–Pituitary Disorders. With CNS–hypothalamic–pituitary disorders the low estrogen levels are due to very low gonadotropin release. The cause of low gonadotropin production can be morphologic or endocrinologic.

Lesions. Any anatomic lesion of the hypothalamus or pituitary can be a cause of low gonadotropin production. These lesions can be congenital (stenosis of aqueduct or absence of sellar floor) or acquired (tumors). Many of these lesions, particularly pituitary adenomas, result in elevated prolactin levels (see Chapter 39, Hyperprolactinemia, Galactorrhea, and Pituitary Adenomas).

However, nonprolactin-secreting pituitary tumors (chromophobe adenomas) as well as craniopharyngiomas may not be associated with hyperprolactinemia and can rarely be the cause of primary amenorrhea with low gonadotropin levels. Thus, all individuals with primary amenorrhea and low gonadotropin levels, with or without an elevated prolactin level, should have computed tomography (CT) scanning or magnetic resonance imaging (MRI) of the hypothalamic–pituitary region to rule out the presence of a lesion.

Inadequate GnRH Release (Hypogonadotropic Hypogonadism). Individuals without a demonstrable lesion and a low gonadotropin level were previously thought to have primary pituitary failure (hypogonadotropic hypogonadism). However, when they are stimulated with GnRH, there is an increase in FSH and LH, indicating that the basic defect is either hypothalamic with insufficient GnRH synthesis or a CNS neurotransmitter defect resulting in inadequate GnRH synthesis or release or both. Although a single bolus of GnRH may not initially cause a rise in gonadotropin level in these individuals, after 4 days of GnRH administration they will have a rise in gonadotropins after a single GnRH bolus. Since GnRH secretion occurs after migration of these specific cells from the olfactory lobe to the hypothesis during embryogenesis, in some patients with gonadotropin deficiency, anosmia may also occur. This is due to specific defect of the *KAL* gene (Xp 22-3), which is responsible for neuronal migration. Other genetic defects resulting in gonadotropic deficiency may occur on the X chromosome or autosomes. Females with Kallman's syndrome and related forms of gonadotropic deficiency have normal height and an increase in growth of long bones, resulting in a greater wing span to height ratio. Men affected by gonadotropic deficiency have hypogonadism, and an increased wing span to height ratio and altered spatial orientation abilities. Anosmia in Kallman's syndrome needs to be tested for by blinded testing of certain characteristic smells, such as coffee, cocoa, or orange.

Isolated Gonadotropin Deficiency (Pituitary Disease). Rarely, individuals with primary amenorrhea and low gonadotropin levels do not respond to GnRH even after 4 days of administration. These individuals nearly always have an associated disorder such as thalassemia major (with iron deposits in the pituitary) or retinitis pigmentosa. Occasionally, this pituitary abnormality had been associated with prepubertal hypothyroidism, kernicterus, or mumps encephalitis.

Breast Development Present and Uterus Absent

Two disorders present with primary amenorrhea are associated with normal breast development and an absence of a uterus:

androgen resistance and congenital absence of the uterus. The former is a genetically inherited disorder, whereas the latter is an accident of development and is only rarely genetically inherited.

Androgen Resistance. Androgen resistance, originally termed *testicular feminization,* is a genetically transmitted disorder in which androgen receptor synthesis or action does not occur. The syndrome is due to the absence of an X-chromosomal gene responsible for the cytoplasmic or nuclear testosterone receptor function. It is either an X-linked recessive or sex-limited autosomal dominant disorder with transmission through the mother. These individuals have an XY karyotype and normally functioning male gonads that produce normal male levels of testosterone and dihydrotestosterone. However, because of a lack of receptors in target organs, there is lack of male differentiation of the external and internal genitalia. The external genitalia remain feminine, as occurs in the absence of sex steroids. Wolffian duct development, which normally occurs as a result of testosterone stimulation, fails to take place. Since müllerian duct regression is induced by antimüllerian hormone (AMH), also called müllerian-inhibiting substance (MIS, a glycoprotein synthesized by the Sertoli cells of the fetal testes), this process occurs normally in these individuals because steroid receptors are unnecessary for the action of glycoproteins. Thus, individuals with this condition have no female or male internal genitalia, normal female external genitalia, and either a short or absent vagina. Pubic and axillary hair is absent or scanty as a result of a lack of androgenic receptors, but breast development is normal or enhanced. It is known that testosterone is responsible for inhibiting breast proliferation through a receptor-mediated mechanism. Thus, in androgen resistance, absence of androgen action allows even low levels of estrogen to cause unabated breast stimulation. Estrogen levels here are in the male range but are sufficient for breast proliferative activity.

Testes that are intraabdominal or that occur in the inguinal canal have an increased risk of developing a malignancy (gonadoblastoma or dysgerminoma), with an incidence reported to be about 20%. However, these malignancies rarely occur before age 20. Therefore, it is usually recommended that the gonads be left in place until after puberty is completed, to allow full breast development and epiphyseal closure to occur. After these events occur, which is typically around age 18, the gonads should be removed. It is recommended that individuals with androgen resistance be informed that they have an abnormal sex chromosome, without specifically mentioning a Y chromosome, because it is widely known that an XY karyotype indicates maleness. In addition, because psychologically and phenotypically these individuals are female and have been raised as such, the term *gonads* should be used instead of testes. These individuals should also be informed that they can never become pregnant because they do not have a uterus and that their gonads (not testes) need to be removed after age 18 because of their high potential for malignancy.

Congenital Absence of the Uterus (Uterine Agenesis, Uterovaginal Agenesis, Rokitansky–Küster–Hauser Syndrome). This disorder is the second most frequent cause of primary amenorrhea. It occurs in 1 in 4000 to 5000 female births and accounts for about 15% of individuals with primary amenorrhea. Individuals with complete uterine agenesis have normal ovaries with regular cyclic ovulation and normal endocrine function. Women with this disorder have normal breast and pubic and axillary hair development but have a shortened or absent vagina in addition to absence of the uterus (Fig. 38-6). Congenital renal abnormalities occur in about one third of these individuals and skeletal abnormalities in about 12%. Cardiac and other congenital abnormalities also occur with increased frequency. Occasional defects in the bones of the middle ear can also occur, resulting in some degree of deafness. The overwhelming majority of these disorders are due to an isolated developmental defect, but on occasion the condition is genetically inherited. It is usually easy to differentiate these individuals from those with androgen resistance by the presence of normal pubic hair, but some individuals with incomplete androgen resistance have some pubic hair. Since women with congenital absence of the uterus are endocrinologically normal females, whereas those with androgen resistance are endocrinologically male with male testosterone levels and an XY karyotype, the differential diagnosis is easily made.

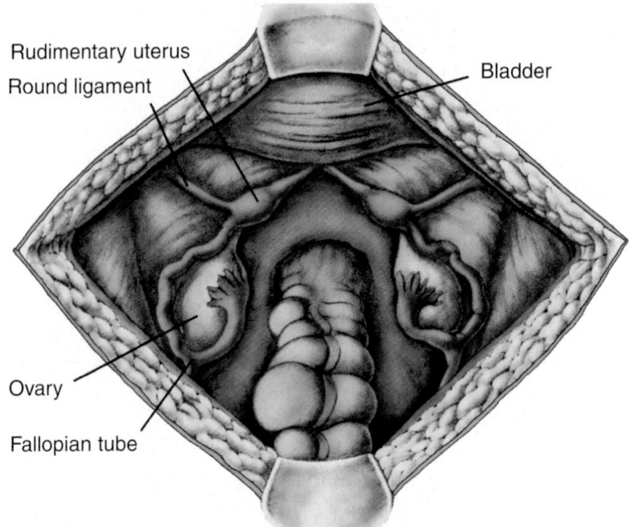

Figure 38-6. Congenital absence of vagina. Laparotomy revealed rudimentary uterus that showed evidence of failure of fusion of müllerian ducts. This is a common finding in this condition and indicates that disorder is more extensive than simple anomaly of vagina. (Redrawn from Jones HW Jr, Scott WW [eds]: Hermaphroditism, Genital Anomalies and Related Endocrine Disorders, 2nd ed. Baltimore, Williams & Wilkins, 1971.)

Absent Breast and Uterine Development

Individuals with no breast or uterine development are rare. They usually have a male karyotype, elevated gonadotropin levels, and testosterone levels in the normal or below normal female range. The differential diagnosis for this phenotype includes 17α-hydroxylase deficiency, 17,20-desmolase deficiency, and agonadism. Individuals with the first disorder have testes present but lack the enzyme necessary to synthesize sex steroids and thus have female external genitalia. Because they have testes, AMH/MIS is produced and the female internal genitalia regress; with low testosterone levels the male internal genitalia do not develop. Insufficient estrogen is synthesized to develop breasts. A similar lack of sex steroid synthesis occurs in males with a 17,20-desmolase deficiency. Individuals with agonadism, sometimes called the *vanishing testes syndrome,* have no gonads present, but since the female internal genitalia are also absent

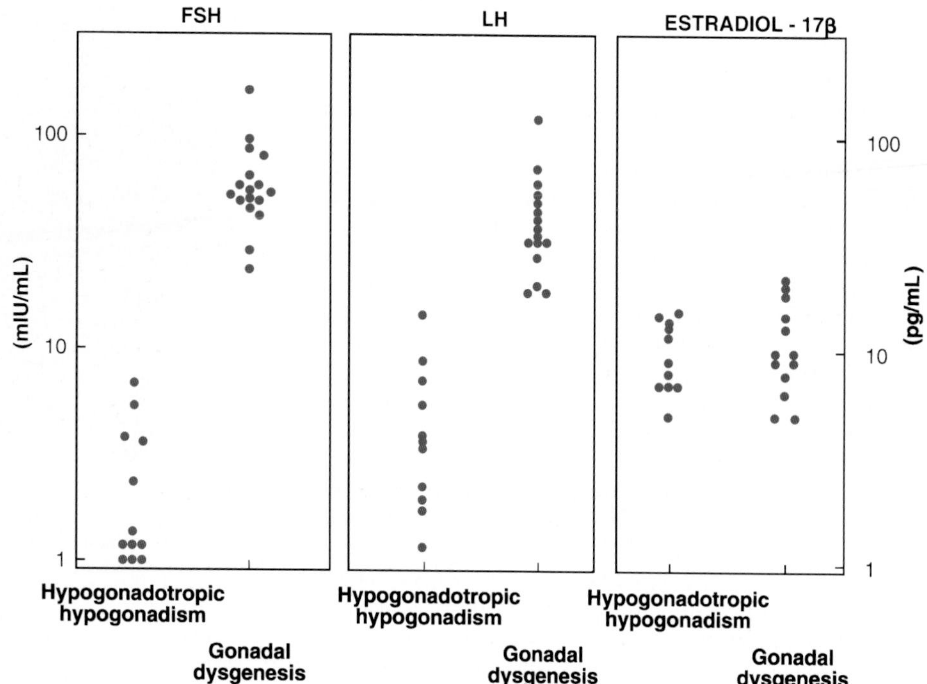

Figure 38-7. Levels of serum FSH, LH, and estradiol in patients with primary amenorrhea who have an intact uterus and no breast development. FSH, follicle-stimulating hormone; LH, luteinizing hormone. (From Mashchak CA, Kletzky OA, Davajan V, et al: Clinical and laboratory evaluation of patients with primary amenorrhea. Obstet Gynecol 57:715, 1981. Reprinted with permission from The American College of Obstetricians and Gynecologists.)

it has been postulated that testicular AMH/MIS production occurred during fetal life, but the gonadal tissue subsequently regressed.

Secondary Sex Characteristics and Female Internal Genitalia Present

This is the second largest category of individuals with primary amenorrhea, accounting for about one third of them. In the series reported by Maschchak and colleagues, about 25% of these individuals had hyperprolactinemia and prolactinomas. The remaining women had profiles similar to those with secondary amenorrhea and thus should be subcategorized and treated similarly to women with secondary amenorrhea. Secondary amenorrhea is discussed in the latter half of this chapter.

Differential Diagnosis and Management

After a history is obtained and a physical examination performed, including measurement of height, span, and weight, individuals with primary amenorrhea can be grouped into one of the four general categories listed in the previous box (on p. 938) depending on the presence or absence of breasts and a uterus.

If breasts are absent but a uterus is present, the diagnostic evaluation should differentiate between CNS–hypothalamic–pituitary disorders and failure of normal gonadal development. Although individuals with both these disorders have similar phenotypes because of low E_2 levels, a single serum FSH assay can differentiate between these two major diagnostic categories (Fig. 38-7). Women with hypergonadotropic hypogonadism (FSH > 30 mIU/ mL), not those with hypogonadotropic hypogonadism, should have a peripheral white blood cell karyotype performed to determine if a Y chromosome is present. If a Y chromosome is present, the streak gonads should be excised, as the incidence of subsequent malignancy, mainly gonadoblastomas, is relatively high. If a Y chromosome is absent, it is unnecessary to remove the gonads unless there are signs of hyperandrogenism. It is also unnecessary to perform a karyotype on the gonadal tissue to detect possible mosaicism with a Y chromosome in the gonad unless there is some evidence of hyperandrogenism.

All women with an elevated FSH level and an XX karyotype should have electrolyte and serum progesterone levels measured to rule out 17α-hydroxylase deficiency. In addition to hypernatremia and hypokalemia, individuals with 17α-hydroxylase deficiency have an elevated serum progesterone level (>3 ng/ mL), a low 17α-hydroxyprogesterone level (<0.2 ng/mL), and an elevated serum deoxycorticosterone level (>17 ng/100 mL), and usually have hypertension. Doses of conjugated equine estrogen (CEE) in the range of 0.625 mg are usually sufficient to cause breast proliferation. Those rare individuals with 17α-hydroxylase deficiency need to have adequate cortisol replacement in addition to sex steroid treatment.

Women with ovarian failure or hypergonadotropic hypogonadism who wish to become pregnant may undergo egg donation. As long as the uterus is normal, which is usually the case, high pregnancy rates close to 50% pregnancy may be expected.

If the FSH level is low, the underlying disorder is in the CNS–hypothalamic–pituitary region, and a serum prolactin measurement should be obtained. Even if the prolactin level is not elevated, all women with hypogonadotropic hypogonadism should have a cranial CT scan or MRI to rule out a lesion. It is unnecessary to perform a karyotype, as all individuals with hypogonadotropic hypogonadism are expected to be 46,XX. The use of GnRH testing is optional but is usually clinically unnecessary unless GnRH is going to be used for ovulation induction. Ovulation can be induced in women with this disorder because their ovaries are normal. Initially they should receive estrogen–progestogen treatment to induce breast development and cause epiphyseal closure. When fertility is desired, human menopausal gonadotropins or pulsatile GnRH should be administered. Clomiphene citrate will be ineffective because of low endogenous E_2 levels.

The differential diagnosis of androgen resistance from uterine agenesis can easily be made by the presence in the latter condition of normal body hair, ovulatory and premenstrual-type symptoms, a biphasic basal temperature, and a normal female testosterone level. Since women with uterine agenesis have normal female endocrine function, they do not need hormonal therapy. A renal scan should be obtained because of the high incidence of renal abnormalities. They may need surgical reconstruction of an absent vagina (McIndoe procedure), but progressive mechanical dilation with plastic dilators as described by Frank should be tried first. These women can now have their own genetic children. After ovarian stimulation and follicle aspiration, their ova can be fertilized and placed in the uterus of a surrogate recipient.

Individuals with androgen resistance have an XY karyotype and male levels of testosterone. After full breast development is obtained and epiphyseal closure occurs, the gonads should be removed because of their malignant potential. Thereafter, estrogen replacement therapy should be administered. These individuals do not need progestogen therapy in the absence of a uterus, and lower doses of estrogen are sufficient (see Chapter 42, Menopause). The rare individuals without breast development and no internal genitalia should be referred to an endocrine center for the extensive evaluation necessary to establish the diagnosis. If gonads are present, they should be removed, because a Y chromosome is present. Hormonal therapy should be administered to these individuals.

SECONDARY AMENORRHEA

Etiology

The symptom of amenorrhea associated with hyperprolactinemia or excessive androgen or cortisol production will not be considered in this chapter as these disorders are discussed in Chapters 39 (Hyperprolactinemia, Galactorrhea, and Pituitary Adenomas) and 40 (Hyperandrogenism). If amenorrhea is present without galactorrhea, hyperprolactinemia, or hirsutism, the symptom can result from disorders in the CNS–hypothalamic–pituitary axis, ovary, or uterus. In a review of 262 patients presenting with secondary amenorrhea during a 20-year period at a tertiary medical center, Reindollar and coworkers reported that 12% of cases resulted from a primary ovarian problem, 62% from a hypothalamic disorder, 16% from a pituitary problem (including prolactinomas), and 7% from a uterine disorder. The uterine cause of secondary amenorrhea is the only one in which normal endocrinologic function is present and will be discussed first.

Uterine Cause

Intrauterine adhesions (IUAs) or synechiae (Asherman's syndrome) can obliterate the endometrial cavity and produce secondary amenorrhea. Rarely, a missed abortion or endometrial tuberculosis can also cause endometrial destruction. The most frequent antecedent factor of IUAs is endometrial curettage associated with pregnancy: either evacuation of a live or dead fetus by mechanical means or postpartum or postabortal curettage. Curettage for a missed abortion results in a high (30%) incidence of IUA formation. IUAs may also occur after diagnostic dilation and curettage (D&C) in a nonpregnant individual, so this procedure should be performed only when indicated and not routinely at the time of other surgical procedures such as diagnostic laparoscopy. A less common cause of IUA is severe endometritis or fibrosis following a myomectomy, metroplasty, or cesarean delivery. This cause of amenorrhea should be considered to be most likely if a temporal relation exists between the onset of symptoms and a uterine curettage. The likelihood of the diagnosis is strengthened if a sound cannot be passed into the uterine cavity.

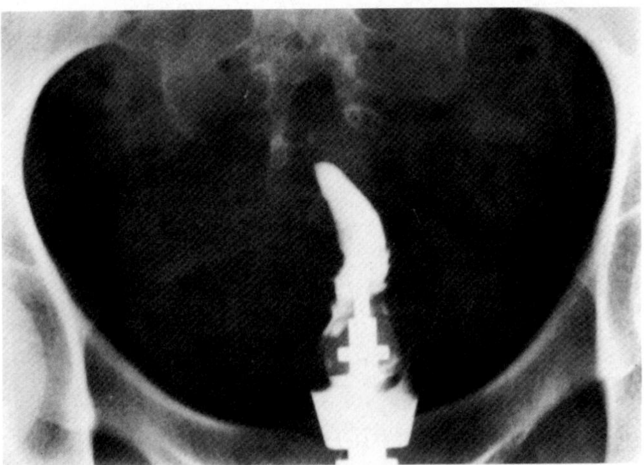

Figure 38-8. X-ray film of patient with Asherman's syndrome. Patient (33 years, gravida 3, para 0, abortus 3) had been amenorrheic for 6 months after D&C for most recent therapeutic abortion (TAB). Filling of endocervical canal and nonvisualization of endometrial cavity are consistent with complete obliteration of cavity by adhesions or with obstruction at internal os level by adhesions in lower endometrial cavity. This appearance may also be seen with advanced endometrial tuberculosis. (From Richmond JA: Hysterosalpingography. In Mishell DR Jr, Davajan V: Infertility, Contraception and Reproductive Endocrinology, 4th ed. Copyright by Blackwell Scientific Publications, Malden, MA, 1997. All rights reserved. Reproduced with permission.)

Confirmation of the diagnosis is usually made by hysterography (Fig. 38-8) or hysteroscopy. Although it has been suggested that sequential administration of estrogen–progestogen be used as the initial diagnostic procedure when IUA is suspected, withdrawal bleeding occurs following administration of the steroids in most women with IUA. Because of the lack of specificity of this test, steroid administration should not be performed prior to indirect or direct visualization of the uterine cavity.

CNS-Hypothalamic Causes

Lesions. The same anatomic lesions in the brainstem or hypothalamus that can produce primary amenorrhea by interfering with GnRH release can also cause secondary amenorrhea. Hypothalamic lesions include craniopharyngiomas, granulomatous disease (tuberculosis and sarcoidosis), and sequelae of encephalitis. When such uncommon lesions are present, circulating gonadotropin levels and E_2 levels are low, and withdrawal uterine bleeding will not occur after progestogen administration.

Drugs. Phenothiazine derivatives, certain antihypertensive agents, and other drugs listed in Chapter 39 (Hyperprolactinemia, Galactorrhea, and Pituitary Adenomas) can also produce amenorrhea without hyperprolactinemia, although usually prolactin is elevated. Therefore, every individual with secondary amenorrhea should have a detailed medication history obtained even if galactorrhea is not present. Oral contraceptive steroids inhibit ovulation by acting both on the hypothalamus to suppress GnRH and directly on the pituitary to suppress FSH and LH. Occasionally, this hypothalamic–pituitary suppression persists for several months after oral contraceptives are discontinued, producing the syndrome termed *postpill amenorrhea.* This oral contraceptive-induced suppression should not last more than 6 months. It has been reported that the incidence of amenorrhea persisting more than 6 months after discontinuation of oral contraceptives (0.8%) is about the same as the incidence of secondary amenorrhea in the general population (0.7%). Thus, the reason for amenorrhea persisting more than 6 months after discontinuation of oral contraceptives is probably unrelated to their use, except that the regular withdrawal bleeding produced by oral contraceptives masks the development of this symptom.

Stress and exercise. Stressful situations, including a sudden change in environment (e.g., going away to school), a death in the family, or divorce, can produce amenorrhea. A high percentage of women who had been placed in concentration camps or those sentenced for execution also became amenorrheic as a result of stress.

It is also now believed that the amenorrhea associated with strenuous exercise is also related to stress. Feicht and coworkers reported that the incidence of secondary amenorrhea in runners had a positive correlation with the number of miles run per week (Fig. 38-9). In a comparison of amenorrheic and eumenorrheic athletes, they reported that physical parameters such as age, weight, lean body mass, and body fat were similar. The only significant difference between the two groups was the fact that the amenorrheic athletes ran more miles per week. McArthur and associates also reported there was no significant difference in the percentage of body fat in amenorrheic runners compared with runners who were menstruating. In a longitudinal study of competitive swimmers, Russell and colleagues found that when

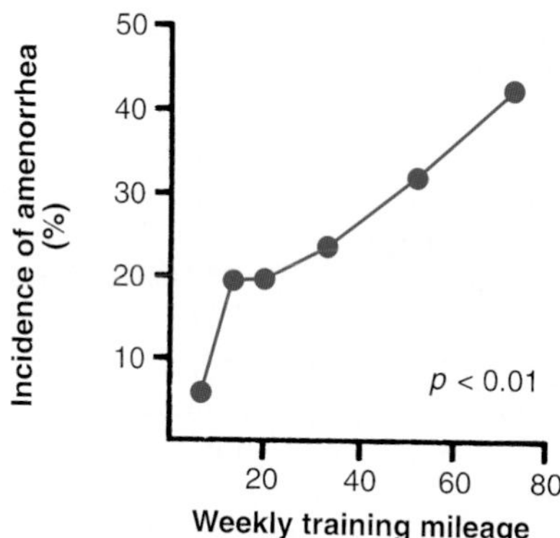

Figure 38-9. Correlation between training mileage and amenorrhea. Each point represents average of 21 respondents. Statistical significance of relationship was obtained from point-biserial correlation (1 mile [1.6 km]). (From Feicht CB, Johnson TS, Martin BJ: Secondary amenorrhoea in athletes. Lancet 2:1145, 1978.)

the training became more strenuous, their LH and FSH levels fell significantly, whereas levels of β-endorphin and catechol estrogens rose significantly as compared with levels of these hormones when the swimmers were exercising to a moderate degree (Table 38-4). Various studies in the past by Russel and coworkers, Carr and associates, Nappi and colleagues and others have pointed to a stress-induced inhibition of the GnRH axis by higher levels of catechol estrogens and opioid peptides (particularly β-endorphin [β-EP]). While Adashi and coworkers has shown that catechol estrogen infusion can suppress the release of GnRH/LH; and Reid and associates and others have demonstrated the inhibition of LH by β-EP, these measurements are difficult and unreliable in vivo in that circulating levels may not reflect brain activity. Therefore, although it is a plausible working hypothesis that exercise in general and the stress of this competitive activity in particular enhances the inhibitory effect of increased levels of catechol estrogen and β-EP on GnRH/LH, definitive proof of this link is missing.

It is probable that emotionally stressful situations such as divorce or a sudden change in environment can also cause alterations in brain chemistry. When the stressful situation (whether emotional in origin or related to strenuous exercise)

Table 38-4 Analysis* of Protein Hormones for Swimmers During Moderate and Strenuous Exercise and for Nonexercising Control Subjects

Hormone	Control Subjects	SWIMMERS: Moderate (60,000 yards)	SWIMMERS: Strenuous (100,000 yards)	GROUP COMPARISON (MEDIAN VALUES): C vs. 60	C vs. 100	100 vs. 60
Number	6	5	5			
LH (mIU/mL)	23.1 [21.4] ± 10.5 (12–13.3)	22.9 [22.2] ± 5.7 (15.9–30.7)	10.9 [11.3] ± 2.8 (7.4–13.6)	$p = 0.66$	$p = 0.02$	$p = 0.02$
FSH (mIU/mL)	10.9 [9.6] ± 3.5 (7.1–15.7)	20.2 [18.2] ± 5.1 (15.3–27.7)	6.54 [6.8] ± 2.1 (4.0–9.5)	$p = 0.05$	$p = 0.04$	$p \leq 0.001$
Prolactin (ng/mL)	20.8 [13.5] ± 15.0 (9.0–47.2)	10.6 [10.6] ± 3.6 (5.9–16.1)	1.36 [1.0] ± 0.9 (0.7–3.0)	$p = 0.18$	$p = 0.004$	$p = 0.006$

*Mean (median) value ± SD with range in parentheses.

Adapted from Fertility and Sterility, 42, Russel JB, Mitchell DE, Mussey PI, et al, The role of β-endorphins and catechol estrogens on the hypothalamic–pituitary axis in female athletes, 690. Copyright 1984, with permission from The American Society for Reproductive Medicine.

abates, normal cyclic ovarian function and regular menses usually resume in a few months.

Weight Loss. Both male and female animals who are malnourished have decreased reproductive capacity. Weight loss is also associated with amenorrhea in women and has been classified into two groups: the moderately underweight group includes individuals whose weight is 15% to 25% below ideal body weight and severely underweight women whose weight loss is greater than 25% of ideal body weight. Weight loss can occur from excessive dietary restrictions as well as malnutrition. Vigersky and colleagues have demonstrated that women with amenorrhea associated with simple weight loss have both direct and indirect evidence of hypothalamic dysfunction, but pituitary and end-organ function is normal. Mason and Sagle showed that in contrast to women with normal cycles, a group of women with weight loss amenorrhea had similar mean levels of LH as well as LH pulse amplitude but decreased frequency of LH pulses. Warren and coworkers, however, showed that when women were severely underweight, in addition to hypothalamic dysfunction, pituitary gonadotropin function was also altered because there was no increase in LH and a decreased response of FSH following GnRH administration. However, these responses could be due to a lack of prolonged GnRH secretion, because the studies were not performed after several days of GnRH priming. Thus, the amenorrhea associated with weight loss appears to be due mainly to failure of normal GnRH release, with the lack of a pituitary response under extreme conditions. Hypoleptinemia as well as GH and thyroid dysfunction contribute to these findings.

Criteria for Diagnosis of Anorexia Nervosa

Onset before 25 years of age
Anorexia with accompanying weight loss of at least 25% of original body weight
Distorted, implacable attitude toward eating, food, or weight that overrides hunger, admonitions, reassurance, and threats; for example:
- Denial of illness
- Failure to recognize nutritional needs
- Apparent enjoyment in losing weight
- Desired body image of extreme thinness
- Unusual hoarding or handling of food

No known medical illness that could account for the anorexia and weight loss
No other known psychiatric disorder
At least two of the following manifestations:
- Amenorrhea
- Lanugo
- Bradycardia (persistent resting pulse of 60 bpm or less)
- Periods of overactivity
- Episodes of bulimia
- Vomiting (may be self-induced)

From Sherman BM, Halmi KA, Zamudio R: LH and FSH response to gonadotropin–releasing hormone in anorexia nervoca: Effect of nutritional rehabilitation. J Clin Endocrinol Metab 41:135, 1975.

A severe psychiatric disorder called *anorexia nervosa* is also associated with severe weight loss and amenorrhea. Anorexia nervosa is not rare: It is estimated to occur in about 1 in 1000 white women in the United States. It is uncommon in men and rare in blacks and Asians. This disorder is most frequent in teenagers and is uncommon after the age of 25. It is one of the most important and probably the most common causes of secondary amenorrhea in adolescent women. This disorder is associated with other physical changes, including dry skin, bradycardia, hypotension, constipation, and hypothermia (see boxes). Individuals with anorexia nervosa usually have a normal thyroxine (T_4) level and an abnormally low serum triiodothyronine (T_3) level. If the clinician cannot make the differential diagnosis between amenorrhea caused by simple weight loss and that caused by anorexia nervosa on clinical findings alone, measurement of the serum T_3 level is most helpful, as individuals with simple weight loss usually have normal T_3 levels. In women with anorexia nervosa T_4 levels are normal, T_3 levels are low, and reverse T_3 (an inactive metabolite) levels are increased, indicating that peripheral conversion of T_4 to T_3 is impaired. Other endocrine changes include an elevated GH, high cortisol, but low ACTH and DHEA-S levels, suggesting altered adrenal sensitivity.

Women with anorexia nervosa have a hypothalamic disorder interfering with normal GnRH release, and their amenorrhea

DSM-IV Diagnostic Criteria for Anorexia Nervosa

A. Refusal to maintain body weight at or above a minimally normal weight for age and height (e.g., weight loss leading to maintenance of body weight less than 85% of that expected or failure to make expected weight gain during period of growth resulting in body weight than 85% of that expected).
B. Intense fear of gaining weight or becoming fat even though underweight.
C. Disturbance in the way in which one's body weight or shape is experienced, undue influence of body weight or shape on self-evaluation, or denial of the seriousness of the current low body weight.
D. In postmenarcheal females, amenorrhea (i.e., the absence of at least three consecutive menstrual cycles). A woman is considered to have amenorrhea if her periods occur following only hormone (e.g., estrogen) administration.

Specify Type:
Restricting Type: During the current episode of anorexia nervosa, the person had not regularly engaged in binge eating or purging behavior (i.e., self-induced vomiting or the misuse of laxatives, diuretics, or enemas).

Binge Eating/Purging Type: During the current episode of anorexia nervosa, the person has regularly engaged in binge eating or purging behavior (i.e., self-induced vomiting or the misuse of laxatives, diuretics, or enemas).

frequently occurs at the time of initiation of food restriction before they lose weight. However, after severe weight loss occurs in these individuals and they are less than 25% of ideal body weight, an abnormal gonadotropin response to GnRH takes place similar to that seen in individuals with severe weight loss caused by dieting. This indicates that pituitary dysfunction also occurs in persons with anorexia nervosa when the weight loss becomes severe. Boyar and associates have shown that women with anorexia nervosa have an LH secretion pattern similar to that observed in prepubertal children (absent LH pulses) (Fig. 38-10) or pubertal premenarcheal girls (nocturnal LH pulses only).

When these individuals gain weight, the normal 24-hour LH pulsatile patterns return. Weight gain results in an increase in leptin levels. However, in spite of this, feedback remains perturbed and normal GnRH and gonadotropin release only occurs after complete recovery. Weight gain in either individuals with anorexia nervosa or those with severe simple weight loss results in their gonadotropin response to GnRH infusion becoming normal or even exaggerated, with the FSH response resuming in proportion to the weight gain and the LH responsiveness returning only after the individual reaches about 85% of ideal body weight. These progressive endocrine responses are also similar to those occurring during puberty, indicating the importance of body weight in causing maturation of the CNS–hypothalamic–pituitary axis and providing additional information as to why girls who exercise strenuously before menarche and have less body fat also have a delayed onset of menstruation. Frisch and Revelle reported that undernourished girls reach menarche at an older age but at the same mean weight as well-nourished girls. Treasure and colleagues, using ultrasound scanning, showed that as women with anorexia nervosa gained weight, changes occurred in ovarian morphology. These changes progressed from small ovaries without follicles, to ovaries of normal size and multiple small follicles and finally to the appearance of a dominant follicle. These changes are similar to the changes in ovarian morphology that occur during normal pubertal development.

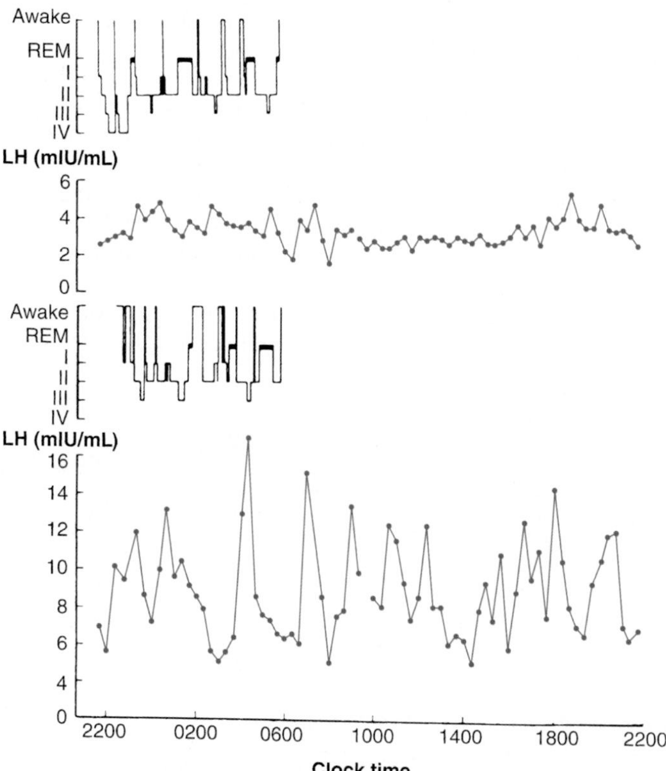

Figure 38-10. Plasma LH concentrations every 20 minutes for 24 hours during acute exacerbation of anorexia nervosa *(upper panel)* and after clinical remission with return of body weight to normal *(lower panel)*. (From Boyar RM, Katz J, Finkelstein JW, et al: Anorexia nervosa: Immaturity of the 24-hour luteinizing hormone secretory pattern. N Engl J Med 291:861, 1974. Copyright 1974 Massachusetts Medical Society. All rights reserved.)

Anorexia nervosa is a psychiatric disorder, and women with this disease should receive appropriate psychiatric treatment. These individuals, as well as those with dietary weight loss, usually resume ovulatory menstrual cycles when they gain weight and approach their ideal body weight.

Polycystic Ovary Syndrome. Polycystic ovary syndrome (PCOS) is a heterogenous disorder and may present with prolonged periods of amenorrhea although the more typical menstrual pattern is one of irregularity or oligomenorrhea. Women need not be overweight or obese, or have symptoms and signs of hyperandrogenism, which occurs classically. Although most women will have an elevated serum LH, this level may be normal and measurement of LH is not required as a diagnostic criterion. Nevertheless, confirmation of the diagnosis of PCOS may be accomplished by visualizing polycystic ovaries on ultrasound, particularly in the absence of classic findings such as hyperandrogenism. According to new European Society of Human Reproduction and Embryology/American Society for Reproductive Medicine (ESHRE/ASRM) criteria for diagnosis of PCOS, women may be diagnosed as having PCOS with only the menstrual disturbance (in this case amenorrhea) and polycystic ovaries on ultrasound. This subject is discussed in detail in Chapter 40 (Hyperandrogenism).

Functional Hypothalamic Amenorrhea. There is a group of individuals with secondary amenorrhea who do not ingest drugs, do not engage in strenuous exercise, are not undergoing environmental stress, and have not lost weight. No pituitary, ovarian, or uterine abnormalities are present in these individuals. The general term *functional hypothalamic amenorrhea* (FHA) has been used to characterize this disorder. During normal ovulatory cycles, LH is secreted in a pulsatile manner that varies in frequency and amplitude at different times of the cycle, being more rapid in the follicular phase than in the luteal phase (Fig. 38-11). Women with amenorrhea due to hypothalamic dysfunction do not exhibit these characteristic cyclic alterations in LH pulsatility. They either have no pulses (Fig. 38-12) or have a persistent pattern of pulsatility that is normally found in only one portion of the ovulatory cycle, usually the slow frequency normally found in the luteal phase, despite having a steroid milieu similar to the follicular phase (Fig. 38-13). Since each LH pulse represents a response to a pulse of GnRH, it appears that individuals with FHA have an abnormality in the normal cyclic variations of GnRH pulsatility, probably due to an abnormality in the CNS neurotransmitters and possibly produced by increased opioid activity. As reported by Ferin and colleagues, Quigley and coworkers, and Wildt and Leyendecker, administration of the opioid antagonists naloxone and naltrexone to

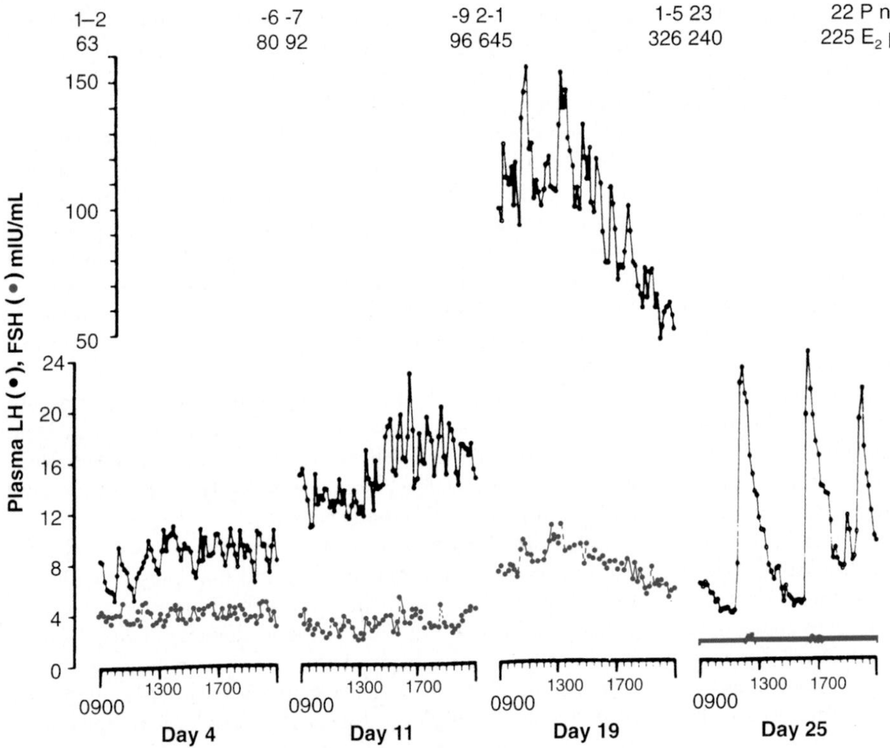

Figure 38-11. Serial measurements of plasma LH and FSH in two subjects sampled every 10 minutes at weekly intervals during cycles in which LH surge was observed on one of sampling days. E_2, estradiol; FSH, follicle-stimulating hormone; LH, luteinizing hormone; P, pregnanediol. (From Reame NE, Sauder SE, Kelch RP, et al: Pulsatile gonadotropin secretion during the human menstrual cycle: Evidence for altered frequency of gonadotropin-releasing hormone secretion. J Clin Endocrinol Metab 59:328, 1984. Copyright 1984 by The Endocrine Society.)

women with FHA is followed by an increase in frequency of LH pulses as well as induction of ovulation.

Berga and associates measured several pituitary hormones at frequent intervals in a 24-hour period in 10 women with FHA and 10 women with normal cycles. As also reported by others, they found a 53% reduction in LH pulse frequency among the women with FHA; however, the LH pulse amplitude was similar in the two groups. In addition to reduced secretion of LH, there was reduced secretion of FSH, prolactin, and thyroid-stimulating hormone (TSH), as well as altered rhythms of growth hormone (GH) and cortisol with elevated cortisol levels. However, the pituitary response to releasing hormones was unchanged. Thus, multiple hormonal alterations occur in FHA as an adaptive central neuroendocrine event. Some data from Tschugguel and Berga suggest that in stress-induced hypothalamic amenorrhea, hypnotherapy and cognitive behavior therapy may be able to restore ovarian activity. Although this is a difficult approach that is not easy to duplicate, it is a logical approach from a physiological point of view. Also, this method may be beneficial in that chronic stress reduction is generally beneficial for general health and can prevent cardiovascular problems and immune compromise.

When sufficient GnRH is produced to facilitate gonadotropin stimulation of the ovaries producing E_2 levels sufficient to prolif-

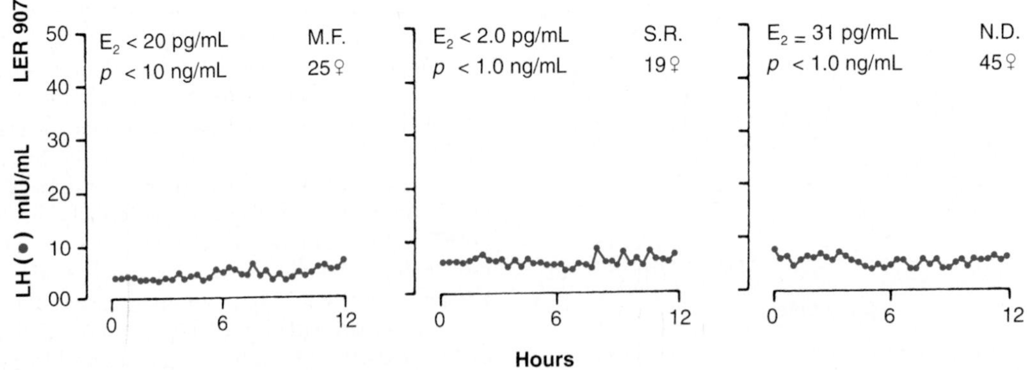

Figure 38-12. A pulsatile pattern of LH secretion in women with hypogonadotropic hypogonadism and hypothalamic amenorrhea. E_2, estradiol; LH, luteinizing hormone; M.F., S.R., and N.D. are the three patient's initials. (From Crowley WF Jr, Filicori M, Spratt DI, et al: The physiology of gonadotropin-releasing hormone (GnRH) secretion in men and women. Rec Prog Hormone Res 41:473, 1985.)

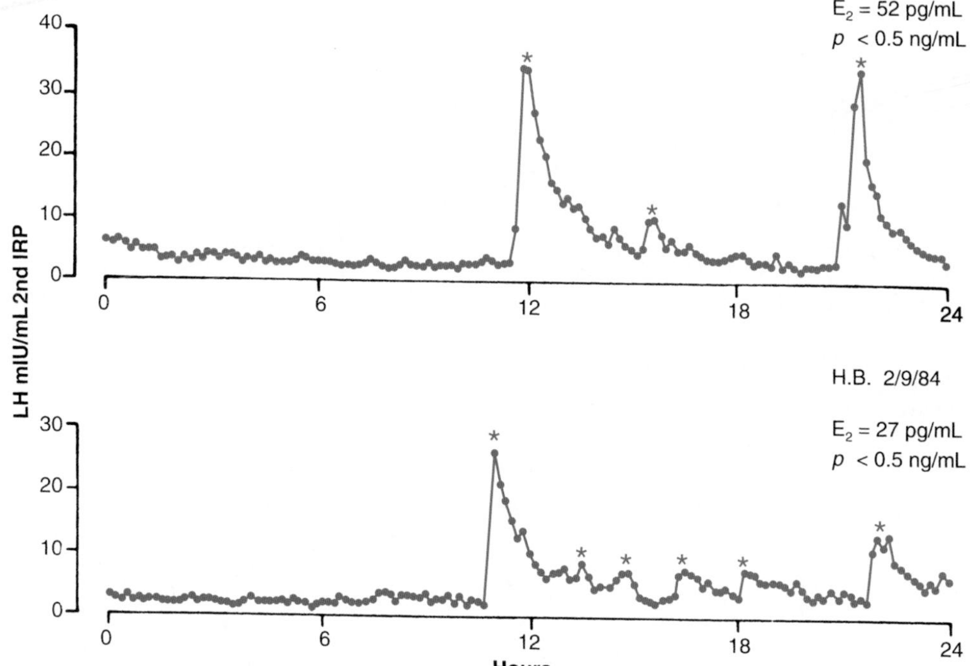

Figure 38-13. Defects in frequency of LH secretion episodes in subjects with hypothalamic amenorrhea. Asterisks indicate LH pulses. E_2, estradiol; LH, luteinizing hormone; H.B. is patient initials. (From Crowley WF Jr, Filicori M, Spratt DI, et al: The physiology of gonadotropin-releasing hormone (GnRH) secretion in men and women. Rec Prog Hormone Res 41:473, 1985.)

erate the endometrium (30–40 pg/mL), the term *hypothalamic–pituitary dysfunction* is used to characterize this disorder. However, when the E_2 levels fall below 40 pg/mL, the term *hypothalamic–pituitary failure* has been used. There is not a marked distinction between women with "dysfunction" and "failure," and this designation is merely a matter of severity of the hypothalamic suppression. Also E_2 levels may fluctuate in this narrow range, and laboratories are not often able to measure these lower levels accurately. Accordingly, it is appropriate to determine the functional or biological estrogen status of these patients by administering a progestogen. If endogenous E_2 has been sufficient to allow the endometrium to proliferate, then progestogen administration will result in withdrawal bleeding. This can also be determined by visualizing the endometrial stripe by ultrasound scans. If the thickness is less than 4 mm, hyperestrogenism is clearly present. The importance of knowing the estrogen status of these patients is that in the severe hyperandrogenism of the hypothalamic failure, bone loss occurs in these young women at a very critical time.

Pituitary Causes (Hypoestrogenic Amenorrhea)

Neoplasms. Although most pituitary tumors secrete prolactin, some do not and may be associated with the onset of secondary amenorrhea without hyperprolactinemia. Chromophobe adenomas are the most common nonprolactin-secreting pituitary tumors; however, both basophilic (ACTH-secreting) and acidophilic (GH-secreting) adenomas may be incapable of secreting prolactin. Individuals with the latter types of tumor, although having secondary amenorrhea, frequently have other symptoms produced by these lesions and present to the clinician with symptoms of acromegaly or Cushing's disease.

Nonneoplastic Lesions. Pituitary cells can also become damaged or necrotic as a result of anoxia, thrombosis, or hemorrhage. When pituitary cell destruction occurs as a result of a hypotensive episode during pregnancy, the disorder is called *Sheehan's syndrome*. When the disorder is unrelated to pregnancy, it is called *Simmonds' disease*. It is important to diagnose this cause of secondary amenorrhea, because in contrast to the hypothalamic disorders, pituitary damage can be associated with decreased secretion of other pituitary hormones, particularly ACTH and TSH, in addition to LH and FSH. Thus, these individuals may have secondary hypothyroidism or adrenal insufficiency that may seriously impair their health, in addition to their decreased estrogen levels.

Ovarian Causes (Hypergonadotropic Hypogonadism)

The ovaries may fail to secrete sufficient estrogen to produce endometrial growth if the follicles are damaged as a result of infection, interference with blood supply, or depletion of follicles caused by bilateral cystectomies. These individuals may become amenorrheic after a variable period of time has elapsed following medical treatment of bilateral tuboovarian abscess, after bilateral cystectomy for benign ovarian neoplasms, or sometimes after a hysterectomy during which the vascular supply to the ovaries is compromised (sometimes called *cystic degeneration of the ovaries*).

Occasionally, the ovaries cease to produce sufficient estrogen to stimulate endometrial growth several years before the age of the physiologic menopause. When this condition occurs before the age of 40, the term *premature ovarian failure* (POF) instead of premature menopause is best used to describe the clinical entity. Coulam and colleagues estimated that as many as 1% of women younger than age 40 have hypergonadotropic amenorrhea, with the incidence steadily increasing from ages 15 to 39. Frequently, the condition of POF is transient before permanent ovarian failure occurs; occasionally, individuals with a

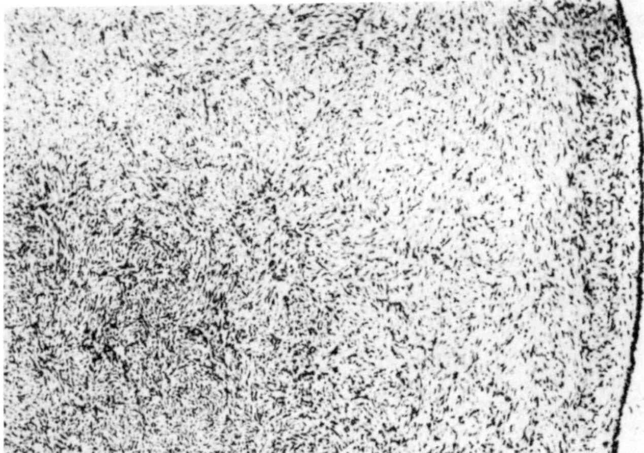

Figure 38-14. Representative section of ovary from patient with premature ovarian failure (POF). Cortex of ovary is devoid of follicles. (From Tulandi T, Kinch RAH: Premature ovarian failure. Obstet Gynecol Surv 35:521, 1981.)

diagnosis of POF may ovulate and conceive during this transition period. POF frequently occurs after gonadal irradiation or systemic chemotherapy. POF has also been reported in individuals with steroid hormonal enzyme deficiencies who menstruate temporarily and then have secondary amenorrhea.

Histologically, individuals with POF have two types of ovarian pathologic findings. In the majority there is generalized sclerosis similar to the findings of a normal postmenopausal ovary (Fig. 38-14), whereas in about 30% numerous primordial follicles with no progression past the early antrum stage are seen (Fig. 38-15). The latter condition has been called the *gonadotropin-resistant ovary syndrome* or *ovarian hypofolliculogenesis* and is histologically different from the gonadal streak, in which no follicles are seen. Women with this condition may have primary amenorrhea, but usually sufficient estrogen is produced so that they menstruate for several months or even years. Many individuals with POF, particularly those with primordial follicles that appear normal, also have an autoimmune disease such as hypoparathyroidism, Hashimoto's thyroiditis, or Addison's disease. Many individuals with POF who do not have clinical evidence of an autoimmune disease have antibodies to gonadotropins as well as to several other endocrine organs such as the thyroid and adrenal glands, suggesting an autoimmune origin.

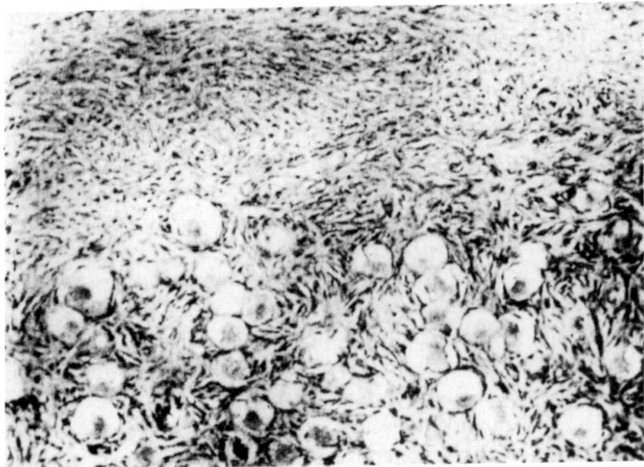

Figure 38-15. Representative section of ovary from patient with insensitive ovary syndrome. Numerous primordial follicles are seen. (From Tulandi T, Kinch RAH: Premature ovarian failure. Obstet Gynecol Surv 35:521, 1981.)

Alper and Garner estimated that about 30% to 50% of individuals with chromosomally normal POF without a history of irradiation or chemotherapy have an associated autoimmune disease, most commonly thyroid disease, which was present in 85% of the group with an autoimmune disorder. Using sophisticated immunofluorescence techniques, Mignot and coworkers demonstrated that 92% of women with POF had laboratory evidence of autosensitization. About two thirds of these were positive for nonorgan-specific antibodies, mainly antinuclear antibodies and rheumatoid factors. Fifty percent had organ-specific antibodies. Although the majority of these women had no evidence of autoimmune disease, it is recommended that immunologic screening be performed in young women with POF. In the absence of symptoms, such as weakness, lethargy, or pain, which may suggest systemic disease, it is probably sufficient to obtain a complete blood count (CBC) and sequential multiple analysis (SMA) as well as a TSH and antithyroid antibodies. If adrenal failure (weakness, etc.) are suspected, adrenal antibodies (against 21-hydroxylase) and cortisol may be obtained; rarely an ACTH stimulation test is warranted. It may be sufficient to obtain a general screen for adrenal function by obtaining levels of DHEA-S. Recent data point to the utility of DHEA-S in that finding low age-specific values in women signify decreased adrenal function.

Diagnostic Evaluation and Management

All women who consult a clinician for the symptom of secondary amenorrhea should have a diagnostic evaluation initiated at that visit, even though 6 months may not have elapsed since the last menstrual period. Amenorrhea is a source of concern to the woman, and it will relieve her concern if attempts are made to find the cause. The clinician should first take a detailed history and perform a physical examination to rule out pregnancy as a cause of the amenorrhea. In addition, he or she should determine whether there is the possibility of IUA. Any instrumentation of the endometrial cavity, particularly temporally related to pregnancy, should alert the clinician to the possibility of IUA. The initial diagnostic evaluation to determine if IUAs are present is placement of a uterine sound into the uterine cavity followed by a hysterography or hysteroscopy. The diagnosis can also be confirmed by detecting presumptive evidence of ovulation by means of either a biphasic basal temperature or an elevated serum progesterone level. If IUAs are ruled out, the history should disclose whether medications are currently being used or if oral contraceptives have been recently discontinued. In addition, questions regarding diet, weight loss, stress, and strenuous exercise are pertinent. A history of hot flushes, decreasing breast size, or vaginal dryness and physical examination of these organs are helpful in estimating the degree of estrogen deficiency. If the history and physical examination fail to reveal the cause of the amenorrhea, a CBC, urinalysis, and serum chemistries should be measured to rule out systemic disease. A sensitive

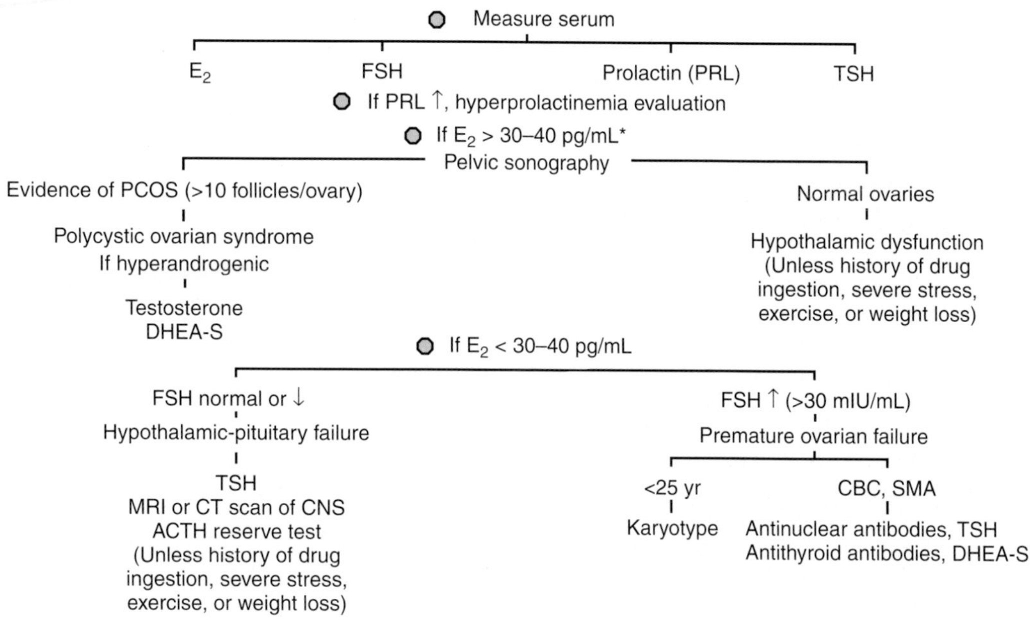

Figure 38-16. Diagnostic evaluation of secondary amenorrhea. ACTH, adrenocorticotropic hormone; CBC, complete blood count; CNS, central nervous system; CT, computed tomography; DHEA-S, dehydroeipandrosterone sulfate; E_2, estradiol; FSH, follicle-stimulating hormone; MRI, magnetic resonance imaging; PCOS, polycystic ovary syndrome; SMA, sequential multiple analysis; TSH, thyroid-stimulating hormone.

TSH assay should also be performed to rule out the uncommon asymptomatic thyroid disorders that produce secondary amenorrhea, and serum E_2, FSH, and prolactin levels should be measured (Fig. 38-16). If prolactin levels are elevated, a diagnostic evaluation for the cause of this problem should be undertaken, as discussed in Chapter 39 (Hyperprolactinemia, Galactorrhea, and Pituitary Adenomas). Administration of injectable progesterone or oral progestogen are an indirect means of determining if sufficient estrogen is present to produce endometrial growth that will slough after the progesterone levels fall (progesterone challenge test). An accurate lab assessment of E_2 level is necessary, usually with an extraction technique. Note, routine E_2 assays as used for monitoring ovulation induction and IVF cycles are not sensitive enough for this purpose. As stated earlier, imaging of the endometrial stripe is also beneficial.

Women with PCOS, moderate stress, exercise, weight loss, or hypothalamic–pituitary dysfunction will usually have E_2 levels of at least 30 to 40 pg/mL, and withdrawal bleeding after progestins usually occurs. Individuals with pituitary tumors, ovarian failure, severe dietary weight loss or anorexia nervosa, severe stress, or the rare hypothalamic lesions will usually have very low E_2 levels.

If a sensitive serum E_2 value is above 30 to 40 pg/mL, and ultrasound confirms the presence of polycystic ovaries, then the diagnosis of PCOS may be entertained, which will be discussed separately in Chapter 40 (Hyperandrogenism). If there is no sonographic evidence of polycystic ovaries and the woman has a history of drug ingestion, stress, weight loss, or strenuous exercise, she should be told that hypothalamic–pituitary dysfunction is present and the exact cause cannot be determined with current technology; as frequent LH sampling is costly and impractical. She should also be informed that hypothalamic–pituitary dysfunction is usually a self-limiting disorder and not a serious threat to health or a cause of untreatable infertility.

Women with low E_2 and low FSH levels have either a CNS lesion or hypothalamic–pituitary failure. Women with low E_2 and elevated FSH levels (>30 mIU/mL) have POF. If severe weight loss, strenuous exercise, or severe stress is not present, and FSH and E_2 levels are low, a CT or MRI scan of the hypothalamic–pituitary region should be performed to rule out a lesion, even if the prolactin level is normal. If a lesion is seen or if there is a history compatible with possible pituitary destruction (hypotension during pregnancy), a test of ACTH reserve should be performed. An insulin tolerance test in which hypoglycemia is induced should normally cause a cortisol increase of 6 μg/100 mL within 120 minutes and is a satisfactory test of ACTH function. If no lesion is identified, the term *hypothalamic–pituitary failure* may be used as a nonspecific diagnosis. Frequently, individuals with this diagnosis resume normal ovarian function without treatment.

If POF is diagnosed because of an elevated FSH level and no cause of ovarian destruction is elicited, the possibility of autoimmune disease should be considered, particularly in younger women. Therefore, antithyroid antibodies and antinuclear antibodies should be measured, and other screening should be performed as noted earlier. To rule out mosaicism or a dysgenetic gonad, including the possibility of a Y cell line, a karyotype should be obtained in women with POF who are 25 or younger. Biopsy of the gonads by laparoscopy or laparotomy is not indicated because individuals with POF are usually sterile, although occasionally a follicle may ovulate. Suppression of gonadotropin levels with estrogen, oral contraceptives, and GnRH analogues has been advocated to induce rebound ovulation following their withdrawal. Although gonadotropins are suppressed by these agents, these techniques are usually ineffective for inducing ovulation. If ovulation occurs following such treatment, it is a sporadic event and not a result of the therapy. Most cases of spontaneous pregnancy have occurred during estrogen replacement.

The appropriate treatment depends on the diagnosis and on whether conception is desired. Nonprolactin-secreting pituitary tumors should be surgically excised if possible. Individuals with weight loss should be advised to gain weight. If strenuous exercise results in low estrogen levels (<30 pg/mL), the amount of exercise should be reduced or estrogen supplementation administered to prevent possible development of osteoporosis. Several investigators have shown that amenorrheic as well as oligomenorrheic athletes with decreased E_2 levels have decreased density of trabecular bone in the lumbar spine (Fig. 38-17). Klibanski and coworkers also have shown that women with low E_2 levels caused by hypothalamic amenorrhea who have normal nutrition and activity levels have a profound reduction in spinal bone density. The reduction in bone loss is independent of whether prolactin is elevated or not. Bone loss has been found to be similar in hyperprolactinemic amenorrheic women with low estrogen levels and women with normal prolactin and low estrogen levels (Fig. 38-18). A group of women with hyperprolactinemia and regular menses did not have bone loss. If women with PCOS or hypothalamic–pituitary dysfunction desire conception, clomiphene citrate administration is very successful in inducing ovulation. If pregnancy is not desired, monthly progestin administration (medroxyprogesterone acetate 10 mg/day for the first 12 days of each month) should be given

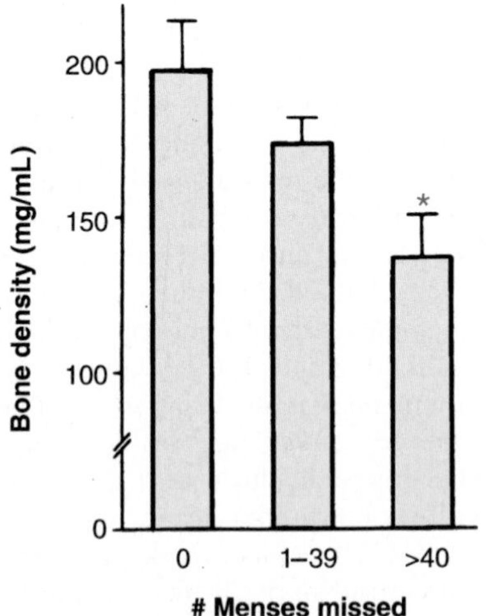

Figure 38-17. Relationship between bone density and number of missed menses in collegiate women athletes. For each subject, number of missed menses was determined from her menarche to age 19. Asterisk indicates significantly different from control group. (From Lloyd T, Myers C, Buchanan JR, et al: Collegiate women athletes with irregular menses during adolescence have decreased bone density. Obstet Gynecol 72:639, 1988.)

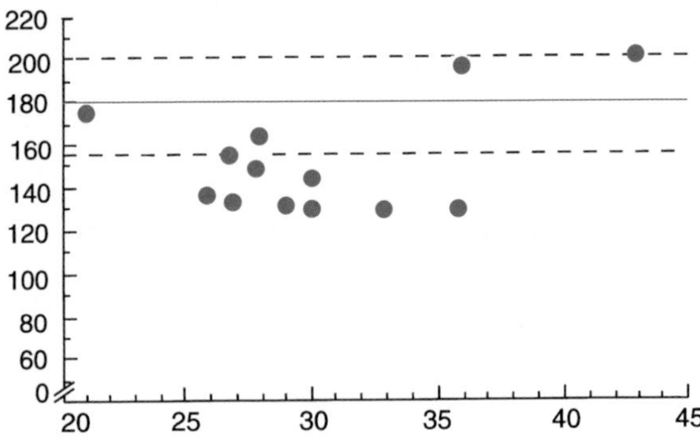

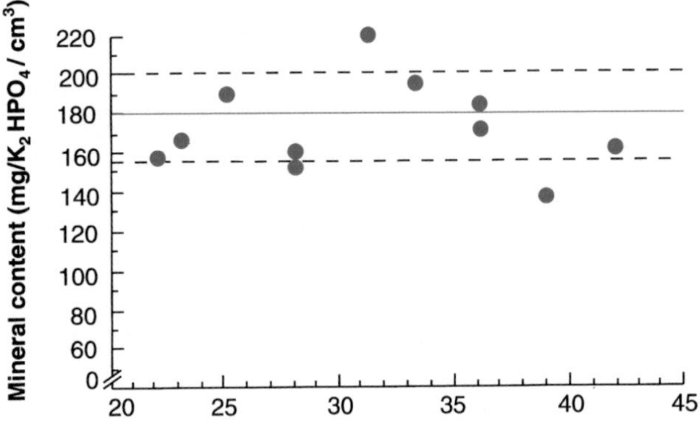

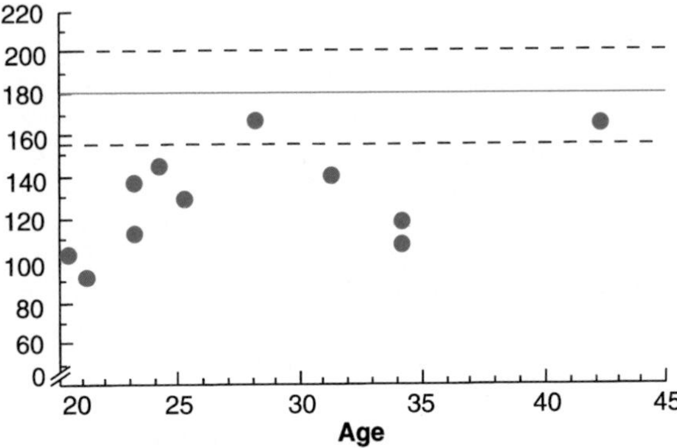

Figure 38-18. Spinal bone density in 13 women with hyperprolactinemic amenorrhea (*top panel*), 12 eumenorrheic hyperprolactinemic women (*middle panel*), and 11 women with hypothalamic amenorrhea (*bottom panel*). Mean (*solid lines*) and standard deviation (± SD, *dashed lines*) for 19 normal women are shown. (From Klibanski A, Biller BM, Rosenthal DI, et al: Effects of prolactin and estrogen deficiency in amenorrheic bone loss. J Clin Endocrinol Metab 67:124, 1988.)

to reduce the increased risk of endometrial cancer associated with unopposed estrogen. If women with hypothalamic–pituitary failure desire fertility, ovulation can be induced with exogenous gonadotropins or intermittent GnRH. Clomiphene is not successful if the estrogen levels are low. If pregnancy is not desired, then estrogen–progestogen replacement is indicated for all amenorrheic women with low E_2 levels, including those with POF, to reduce the risk of osteoporosis. Women with POF are also vulnerable to accelerated atherosclerosis. There's no increased cardiovascular risk in prescribing estrogen to these women. Women with POF may become pregnant with the use of donor oocytes and the priming of their endometrium with estrogen and progesterone for embryo transfer.

PRECOCIOUS PUBERTY

Puberty in the female is the process of biologic change and physical development after which sexual reproduction becomes possible. This is a time of accelerated linear skeletal growth and development of secondary sexual characteristics, such as breast development and the appearance of axillary and pubic hair. The usual sequence of the physiologic events of puberty begins with breast development, the subsequent appearance of pubic and axillary hair, followed by the period of maximal growth velocity, and lastly, menarche. Menarche may occur before the appearance of axillary or pubic hair in 10% of normal females. Normal puberty occurs over a wide range of ages.

Precocious puberty is arbitrarily defined as the appearance of any signs of secondary sexual maturation at an early age. Puberty in girls is now recognized to be occurring earlier than in previous studies (Table 38-5). In an article by Kaplowitz and associates, it was suggested that girls with either breast development or pubic hair should be evaluated when these signs occur before age 7 in whites and age 6 in black girls. Thus, evaluation of precocious puberty need not be performed for whites older than 7 years of age and for blacks older than 6 years of age. Precocious puberty is associated with a wide range of disorders. It should be emphasized that regardless of the cause, precocious puberty is a very rare disorder. The incidence of this condition in the United States is estimated to be approximately 1 in 10,000 young girls. When it is diagnosed, the physician should undertake a detailed investigation of the etiology of the condition in order not to overlook a potentially correctable pathologic lesion. The two primary concerns of parents of children with precocious puberty are the social stigma associated with the child being physically different from her peers and the diminished ultimate height caused by the premature closure of epiphyseal growth centers.

Puberty is a time of accelerated growth, skeletal maturation, and resulting epiphyseal closure. Although precocious puberty occurs early in a child's life, it usually develops in the normal sequence. This produces the paradox of precocious puberty. Early in the course of the disease the girls are taller and heavier than their chronologic peers who have not experienced the growth spurt (Fig. 38-19). However, although the patient is tall as a child, her eventual adult height will be shorter than normal. Without therapy, approximately 50% of females with precocious puberty will not reach a height of 5 feet. The pathophysiology of this short stature is related to the limited duration of the rapid growth spurt. There is accelerated bone maturation and premature closure of the distal epiphyseal growth centers.

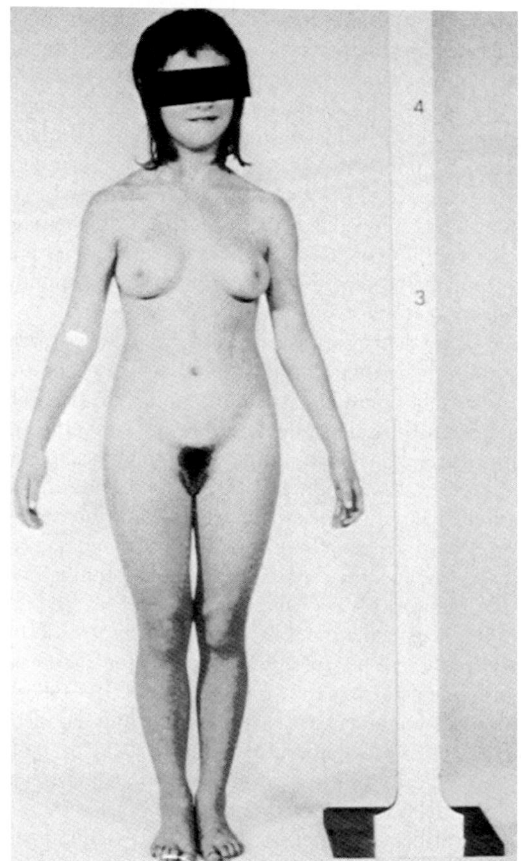

Figure 38-19. Child age 7 years with constitutional precocious puberty. Note increased height for age. (From Dewhurst CJ: Practical Pediatric and Adolescent Gynecology. New York, Marcel Dekker, 1980. Reprinted courtesy of Marcel Dekker, Inc.)

The syndrome of precocious puberty is subdivided into GnRH-dependent (complete, true) or GnRH-independent (incomplete, pseudo) and isosexual and heterosexual disorders. These categories are of clinical value only after the eventual

Table 38-5 Prevalence of Breast and Pubic Hair Development in White and Black Girls Between 5 and 10 Years of Age

Age Range in Years	5.00–5.99	6.00–6.99	7.00–7.99	8.00–8.99	9.00–9.99
Prevalence of breast development at Tanner stage 2 or greater (%)					
White	1.6	2.9	5.0	10.5	32.1
African American	2.4	6.4	15.4	37.8	62.6
Prevalence of pubic hair development at Tanner stage 2 or greater (%)					
White	0.4	1.4	2.8	7.7	20.0
African American	3.4	9.5	17.7	34.3	62.6

From Kaplowitz PB, Oberfield SE, and the Drug and Therapeutics and Executive Committees of the Lawson Wilkins Pediatric Endocrine Society: Reexamination of the age limit for determining when puberty is precocious in girls in the United States: Implications for evaluation and treatment. Pediatrics 104:937, 1999.

diagnosis has been established. The pathophysiology and corresponding categories of precocious puberty may change during the course of the disease; for example, congenital adrenal hyperplasia initially is GnRH-independent but subsequently, over many months, eventually becomes a GnRH-dependent form of precocious puberty. The pathophysiology of precocious puberty is divided into two distinct categories: a normal physiologic process involving GnRH secretion with an integrated hypothalamic–pituitary axis, which occurs at an abnormal time, or an abnormal physiologic process independent of an integrated hypothalamic–pituitary–ovarian axis.

GnRH-dependent precocious puberty involves premature maturation of the hypothalamic–pituitary–ovarian axis and includes normal menses, ovulation, and the possibility of pregnancy. GnRH-independent precocious puberty involves premature female sexual maturation, which may lead to estrogen-induced uterine stimulation and bleeding without any normal ovarian follicular activity. Both categories have increased circulating levels of estrogen. In the latter syndrome, secretion of estrogens is independent of hypothalamic–pituitary control. Obviously, depending on when the patient is first seen in relationship to the natural history of her disease, it may be necessary to observe her at regular intervals for 2 to 3 years to distinguish one syndrome from another (Table 38-6). Prolonged follow-up is sometimes necessary to rule out subtle, slow-growing lesions of the brain, ovary, or adrenal gland.

The vast majority of females with precocious puberty (70%) develop a GnRH-dependent process. The exact cause of most cases of GnRH-dependent precocious puberty is unknown (constitutional); however, approximately 30% are secondary to CNS disease. A definitive diagnosis is established more often for pseudoprecocious puberty, which is usually related to an ovarian or adrenal disorder. If the secondary sex characteristics are discordant with the genetic and phenotypic sex, the condition is termed *heterosexual precocious puberty.* This is premature virilization in a female child and includes development of masculine secondary sexual characteristics. The androgens that cause heterosexual precocious puberty usually come from the adrenal gland.

Premature Thelarche

Premature thelarche is defined as isolated unilateral or bilateral breast development as the only sign of secondary sexual maturation. It is not accompanied by other associated evidence of pubertal development, such as axillary or pubic hair or changes in vaginal epithelium. Breast hyperplasia is a normal physiologic phenomenon in the neonatal period, and it may persist up to 6 months of age. Premature thelarche usually occurs between 1 and 4 years of age. The breast buds enlarge to 2 to 4 cm, and sometimes this process is asymmetrical. Nipple development is absent. This is a benign, self-limiting condition that does not require treatment. Often the breast enlargement spontaneously regresses. It is important to observe these children closely for other signs of precocious puberty. The cause of premature thelarche is not understood. Although it is postulated to be related to a slight increase in circulating estrogen levels, these levels are normally low to undetectable. This disorder may be associated with female infants who had extremely low birth weights. The child should be seen at regular intervals in follow-up to rule out progression of the symptoms to precocious puberty. This is frequently an isolated event, but accumulating evidence suggests that ovarian follicular activity may occur and that this may be part of the continuum with cases of GnRH-dependant precocious puberty.

Table 38-6 Physical Findings Among Patients with Various Syndromes of Precocious Puberty

			GNRH-DEPENDENT AND GNRH-INDEPENDENT			
Findings	**Premature Thelarche**	**Premature Adrenarche**	**Idiopathic**	**Central Nervous System Tumor**	**McCune–Albright Syndrome**	**Hypothyroid**
Breast enlargement	Yes	No	Yes	Yes	Yes	Yes
Pubic hair	No	Yes	Yes	Yes	Yes	Unusual
Vaginal bleeding	No	No	Yes	Yes	Yes	Yes
Virilizing signs	No	No	No	No	No	No
Bone age	Normal	Normal to minimally advanced	Advanced	Advanced	Advanced	Normal or retarded
Neurologic deficit	No	No	No	Yes	Yes	No
Abdominopelvic mass	No	No	Occ'l	No	No	Occ'l

	ISOSEXUAL		HETEROSEXUAL			
Findings	**Ovarian Tumors**	**Adrenal Tumors**	**Factitious**	**Ovarian Tumors**	**Adrenal Tumors**	**Adrenal Hyperplasia**
Breast enlargement	Yes	Yes	Yes	Yes	Yes	Yes
Pubic hair	Yes	Yes	Yes	Yes	Yes	Yes
Vaginal bleeding	Yes	Yes	Yes	Yes	Yes	Yes
Virilizing signs	No	Yes	No	Yes	Yes	Yes
Bone age	Advanced	Advanced	Advanced	Advanced	Advanced	Advanced
Neurologic deficit	No	No	No	No	No	No
Abdominopelvic mass	Usually	No	No	Occ'l	No	No

GnRH, gonadotropin-releasing hormone.
From Ross GT: Disorders of the ovary and female reproductive tract. In Wilson JD, Foster DW (eds): Williams Textbook of Endocrinology, 7th ed. Philadelphia, WB Saunders, 1985.

Premature Pubarche or Adrenarche

Premature pubarche is early isolated development of pubic hair without other signs of secondary sexual maturation. Premature adrenarche is isolated early development of axillary hair. Neither of these conditions is progressive, and the girls do not have clitoral hypertrophy. However, it is important to differentiate premature pubarche from the virilization produced by congenital adrenal hyperplasia. Some children with premature pubarche have abnormal electroencephalograms (EEGs) without significant neurologic disease. The bone age should not be advanced in this disorder. The cause is poorly understood but believed to be related to increased androgen production by the adrenal glands (DHEA and DHEA-S). Similar to premature the larche, the child should have periodic follow-up visits to confirm that the condition is not progressive. Many cases of premature adrenarche evolve into PCOS.

GnRH-Dependent Precocious Puberty

Idiopathic development is responsible for approximately 70% of the cases of GnRH-dependent precocious puberty. Some of these children are simply at the earliest limits of the normal distribution of the biologic curve (see Table 38-5). Most idiopathic cases are sporadic in distribution; however, some are familial.

A high incidence of abnormal EEGs in children with idiopathic precocious puberty has raised the question of potential CNS disease. With increasing use of high-resolution imaging techniques, such as cranial CT scan and MRI, the number of truly idiopathic cases is declining.

These girls have no genital abnormality except for early development. Occasionally, follicular cysts of the ovary may form secondary to increased levels of pituitary gonadotropins (Fig. 38-20). In these cases the cysts are the result of, not the cause, of precocious puberty. Gonadotropin levels, sex steroid levels, and response of LH after administration of GnRH are similar to those in normal puberty. The cause of premature maturation of the hypothalamic–pituitary–ovarian axis is unknown. The syndrome may appear as early as age 3 to 4 years. When observed for several decades, these women have normal menopausal ages. Emotional problems are a cause for concern because the young girls suffer from extreme social pressures. The intellectual, behavioral, and psychosocial development of girls with precocious puberty is appropriate for their chronologic age. Most are shy and withdrawn from their peers.

A wide range of inflammatory, degenerative, neoplastic, or congenital defects that involve the CNS may produce GnRH-dependent precocious puberty. This occurs in at least 30% of cases and warrants a careful evaluation. Usually, symptoms of a neurologic disease, especially headaches and visual disturbances, precede the manifestations of precocious puberty. A most unusual neurologic symptom that may be associated with precocious puberty is seizures with inappropriate laughter (gelastic seizures). Anatomically, most CNS lesions are located near the hypothalamus in the region of the third ventricle, tuber cinereum, or mammillary bodies. Major CNS diseases associated with true precocious puberty include tuberculosis, encephalitis, trauma, secondary hydrocephalus, neurofibromatosis, granulomas, hamartomas of the hypothalamus, teratomas, craniopharyngiomas, cranial irradiation, and congenital brain defects, such as hydrocephalus and cysts in the area of the third ventricle. These children have markedly fluctuating estrogen levels and low gonadotropin concentrations that are independent of GnRH stimulation. These CNS space-occupying masses are most difficult to successfully treat surgically. The pathophysiology by which CNS disease produces precocious puberty is poorly understood. It is known that hamartomas may secrete GnRH; this secretion is not subject to the normal physiologic inhibition that occurs during childhood.

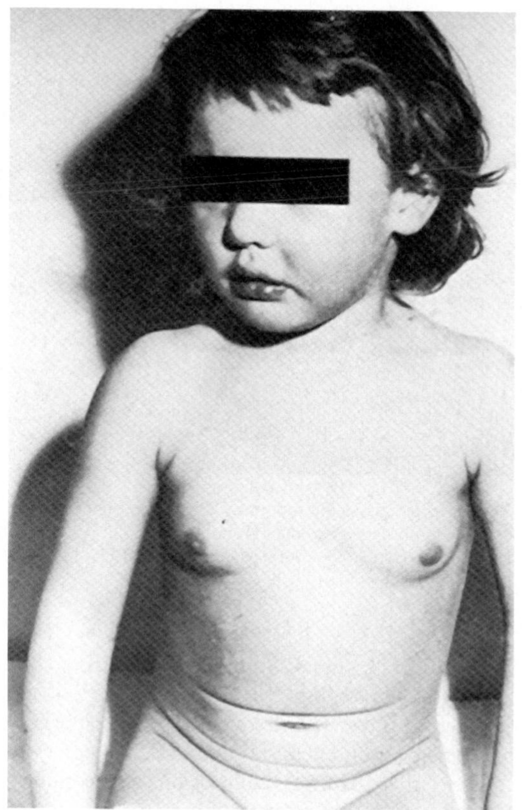

Figure 38-20. Precocious puberty in young girl. The child had large lower abdominal swelling, which at operation was shown to be bilateral follicular cysts (result of premature ovarian stimulation and not cause of condition). (From Dewhurst CJ: Practical Pediatric and Adolescent Gynecology. New York, Marcel Dekker, 1980. Reprinted courtesy of Marcel Dekker, Inc.)

GnRH-Independent Precocious Puberty

The most common cause of pseudoprecocious puberty is an estrogen-secreting ovarian tumor. Among ovarian tumors, granulosa cell tumors are the most common type, accounting for approximately 60%. These tumors are usually greater than 8 cm in diameter when associated with precocious puberty; 80% can be palpated abdominally. Other ovarian tumors that may be associated with precocious puberty include thecomas, luteomas, teratomas, Sertoli–Leydig tumors, choriocarcinomas, and benign follicular cysts. Thecomas and luteomas are usually much smaller than granulosa cell tumors and usually cannot

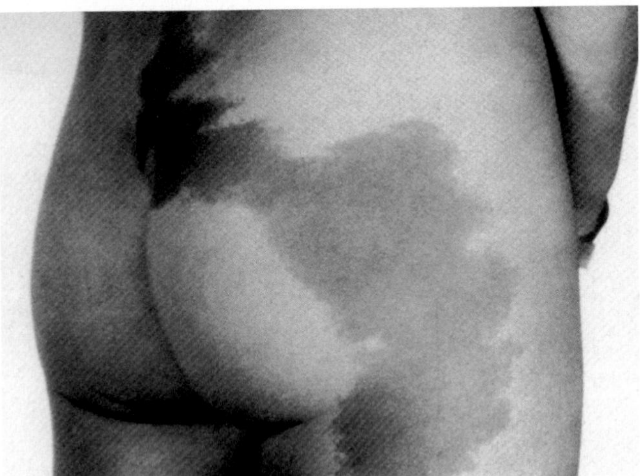

Figure 38-21. Large café-au-lait spot in child with precocious puberty as result of McCune–Albright syndrome. (From Dewhurst CJ: Practical Pediatric and Adolescent Gynecology. New York, Marcel Dekker, 1980. Reprinted courtesy of Marcel Dekker, Inc.)

be palpated. Overall, these tumors are rare during childhood, with only 5% of granulosa cell tumors and 1% of thecomas occurring before puberty. Infrequently, follicular cysts of the ovary may emerge spontaneously and secrete enough estrogen to be the cause, rather than the result, of precocious puberty. It is speculated that these benign cysts function in an autonomous fashion. The ability of many tumors, including teratomas, choriocarcinomas, and dysgerminomas, to secrete estrogen, human chorionic gonadotropin (HCG), α-fetoprotein, and other markers has been established.

McCune–Albright syndrome (MAS, polyostotic fibrous dysplasia) is a rare triad of café-au-lait spots, fibrous dysplasia, and cysts of the skull and long bones (Fig. 38-21). These patients also have facial asymmetry. Approximately 40% of girls with MAS have associated isosexual precocious puberty.

Adrenocortical neoplasms may produce either isosexual or heterosexual precocious puberty. The relationship between congenital adrenal hyperplasia and puberty depends on the time of initial diagnosis and therapy. If the disease is diagnosed in the neonatal period and treated, normal puberty ensues. If the disease is untreated, the girl over time usually develops heterosexual precocious puberty (signs of androgen excess) from the adrenal androgens. However, if congenital adrenal hyperplasia is diagnosed late in childhood, isosexual precocious puberty may follow initial treatment of the adrenal disease.

Hypothyroidism most commonly is associated with delayed pubertal development. However, in rare instances untreated hypothyroidism results in isosexual, GnRH-dependent, or GnRH-independent precocious puberty. The hypothyroidism associated with precocious puberty is due to primary thyroid insufficiency, usually Hashimoto's thyroiditis, and not a deficiency in pituitary TSH. The pathophysiology of this syndrome is caused by the diminished negative feedback of thyroxine, resulting in an increased production of TSH, which may be accompanied by an increase in production of gonadotropins. Interestingly, hypothyroidism is the only cause of precocious puberty in which the bone age is retarded. This syndrome is observed usually in girls between the ages of 6 and 8 years.

Iatrogenic or factitious precocious puberty results when a young female has used hormonal cream or ingested adult medication such as oral estrogen or birth control pills. The secondary sexual characteristics regress after discontinuation of the medication.

Diagnosis

The diagnostic workup of a young child with precocious puberty begins with a meticulous history and physical examination. The primary emphasis should be to rule out life-threatening neoplasms of the ovary, adrenal gland, or CNS. The secondary emphasis is to delineate the speed of the maturation process, for this is crucial in making decisions concerning therapy. The height of the girl and exact stage of pubertal development, including Tanner stage, should be recorded. Similar to other syndromes with a long list of causes, a battery of tests, including imaging studies of the brain, serum estradiol levels, FSH levels, and thyroid function tests, may be needed to establish the diagnosis (Table 38-7). With this acceleration of development, the sex steroids and adrenal androgen (DHEA-S) are elevated regardless of the cause. Acceleration of growth is one of the earliest clinical features of precocious puberty. Thus, bone age should be determined by hand–wrist films and compared with standards for a patient's age (Fig. 38-22). Usually these films are repeated at 6-month intervals to evaluate the rate of skeletal maturation and correspondingly the need for active treatment of the disease. Advancement of bone age more than 95% of the norm for the child's chronologic age is indicative of an estrogen effect.

Diseases of the CNS are suggested during the history by symptoms such as headaches, seizures, trauma to the head, and encephalitis. These conditions are confirmed or excluded by a series of tests, including neurologic and ophthalmologic examinations, EEGs, and brain imaging.

Hypothalamic hamartomas can be classified based on the tumor topology on MRI. This classification has been shown to correlate with the clinical manifestations of precocious puberty. Ultrasound, CT, or MRI of the abdomen and pelvis should

Table 38-7 Laboratory Findings in Disorders Producing Precocious Puberty

	Gonadal Size	Basal FSH/LH	Estradiol or Testosterone	DHAS	GnRH Response
Idiopathic	Increased	Increased	Increased	Increased	Pubertal
Cerebral	Increased	Increased	Increased	Increased	Pubertal
Gonadal	Unilat. incr.	Decreased	Increased	Increased	Flat
Albright	Increased	Decreased	Increased	Increased	Flat
Adrenal	Small	Decreased	Increased	Increased	Flat

Adapted from Speroff L, Glass RH, Kase NG: Clinical Gynecology Endocrinology and Infertility, 6th ed. Baltimore, Lippincott Williams & Wilkins, 1999, p 396.

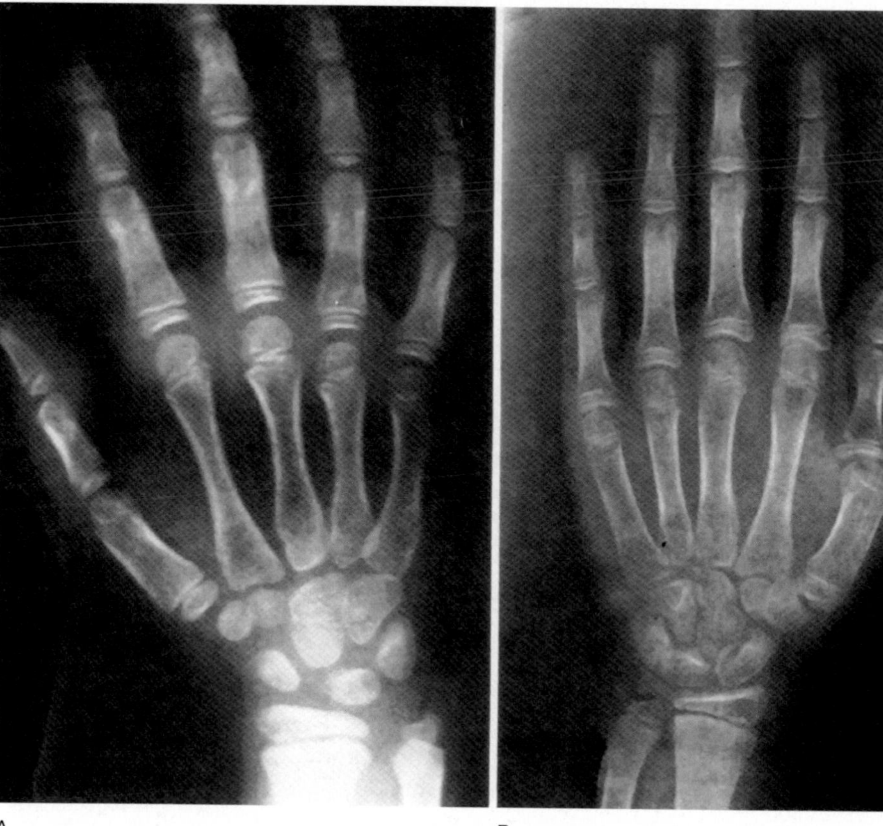

Figure 38-22. X-ray films demonstrating bone age. **A,** Normal for 7 years of age. **B,** Advanced bone age in a girl 7 years of age who also shows other signs of isosexual precocity. (From Huffman JW: The Gynecology of Childhood and Adolescence, 2nd ed. Philadelphia, WB Saunders, 1981.)

be performed to evaluate enlargement of the ovaries (ovarian volume), uterus, or adrenal glands.

Serum levels of FSH, LH, prolactin, TSH, E_2, testosterone, DHEA or DHEA-S, HCG, androstenedione, 17-hydroxyprogesterone, T_3, and T_4 may be of value in establishing the differential diagnosis. Sometimes a GnRH stimulation test is diagnostic in differentiating incomplete from true precocious puberty, but this test does not specifically identify children with CNS lesions. The LH responses to gonadotropin stimulation after reaching a basal level are similar in cases of true precocious puberty to the responses of a mature adult. In contrast, a child with precocious puberty secondary to a feminizing ovarian neoplasm does not have a significant elevation in LH response to exogenous gonadotropins. In summary, a stimulation test with exogenous GnRH is fundamental in helping to delineate the underlying pathophysiology.

Management

The treatment of precocious puberty depends on the cause, the extent and progression of precocious signs, and whether the cause may be removed operatively. For example, extirpation of a granulosa cell tumor and subtotal removal of a hypothalamic hamartoma are successful treatments because they remove hormone-secreting tumors. Because most cases involve premature maturation of the hypothalamic–pituitary–ovarian axis without a lesion, this discussion focuses on the medical management of this condition. Girls with menarche before age 8 years, progressive thelarche and pubarche, and bone age more than 2 years greater than their chronologic ages definitely should be treated. The goals of therapy are to reduce gonadotropin secretions and reduce or counteract the peripheral actions of the sex steroids, decrease growth rate to normal, and slow skeletal maturation to allow development of maximal adult height.

The present drug of choice for GnRH-dependent precocious puberty is one of the potent GnRH agonists. These drugs are typically given by monthly injections or, rarely, intranasally. A 3-month depo form is also available. GnRH agonists are safe and effective treatments for children with the disease secondary to disturbances in the hypothalamic–pituitary–ovarian axis. Therapy should be initiated as soon as possible after the diagnosis is established in order to achieve maximal adult height. The effect on adult height depends on the chronologic age at which therapy is initiated. The therapy is most effective in 4- to 6-year-olds. Continuous chronic administration of the drug is maintained until the median age of puberty. The optimal dosage of medication may be confirmed by determining that peripheral E_2 levels are in a normal prepubertal range. Medical therapy produces involution of secondary sexual characteristics, with amenorrhea and regression of both breast development and amount of pubic hair. LH and FSH pulsations are abolished. Most importantly the drug not only reverses the ovarian cycle but definitely changes the growth pattern. Growth velocity is usually decreased by approximately 50% (Fig. 38-23). In one series the predicted adult height increased a mean of 6.5 cm in girls who were age 6 years or less when therapy was initiated.

Multiple studies have documented that agonist therapy decreases gonadotropins within 1 week and decreases sex steroids to the prepubertal range within the first 2 weeks of therapy

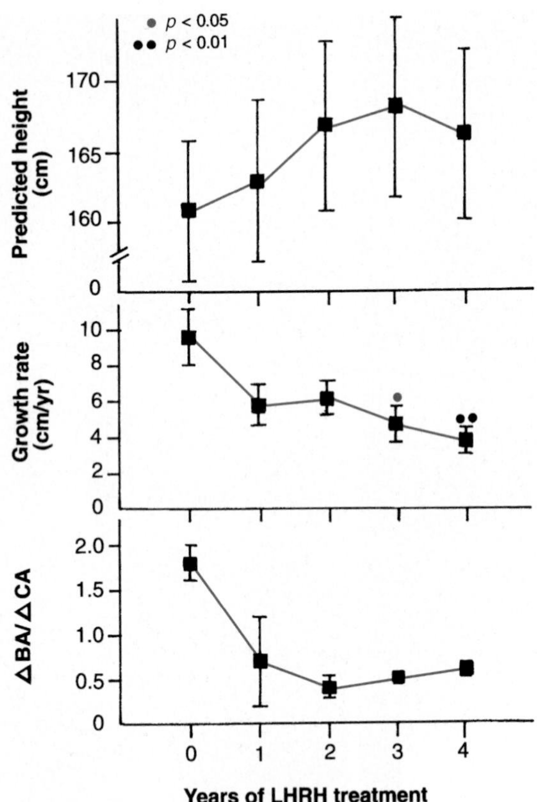

Figure 38-23. Predicted height, growth rate, and rate of bone age advancement in six children with central precocious puberty who have received 4 years of therapy with the long-acting analogue of luteinizing hormone releasing hormone (LHRH). Asterisks indicate significant differences compared with pretreatment value. ΔBA/ΔCA, change in bone age/change in chronological age. (Redrawn from Comite F, Cassorla F, Barnes KM, et al: Luteinizing hormone releasing hormone analogue therapy for central precocious puberty. Long-term effect on somatic growth, bone maturation, and predicted height. JAMA 255:2615, 1986.)

(Fig. 38-24). Serial ultrasound examinations have documented that the size of the ovaries and uterus regresses to normal prepubertal shape and size. The most common observed side effect to agonists was cutaneous reaction at the site of injection. However, approximately one in four girls experienced recurrent and sometimes prolonged vaginal bleeding while receiving GnRH agonists. The effects of these drugs are quite reversible when the agonists are discontinued after normal height is achieved. The effect on final adult height has not been clearly established.

There has been a suggestion that rare forms of GnRH-independent precocious puberty that do not respond to agonist therapy may be successfully treated using a GnRH antagonist. Here there may be a direct antagonist effect on the ovary mediated through gonadotropin receptors. Recently, small studies have suggested a minimal benefit from adding growth hormone to GnRH agonist therapy in girls with suboptimal growth. The initial observations of combination therapy are encouraging, but the clinical data is from small series and of a preliminary nature.

Patients with McCune–Albright syndrome may be treated with aromatase inhibitors, which prevent the conversion to biologically active estrogens. This treatment leads to diminished circulating estrogen levels, diminished frequency of menses, and a decreased rate of growth and skeletal maturation.

Both the child with precocious puberty and her family need intensive counseling. The child will have the psychosocial and behavioral maturation of children of her chronologic age, not the age reflected by her physical appearance. She may be exposed to ridicule by her peers and to sexual exploitation. Thus, the child needs extensive sex education and help in anticipating and confronting various social experiences. Often it is possible to dress the child in clothes that diminish the recognition of her advanced sexual maturation until the effects of her disease are inhibited by drug therapy.

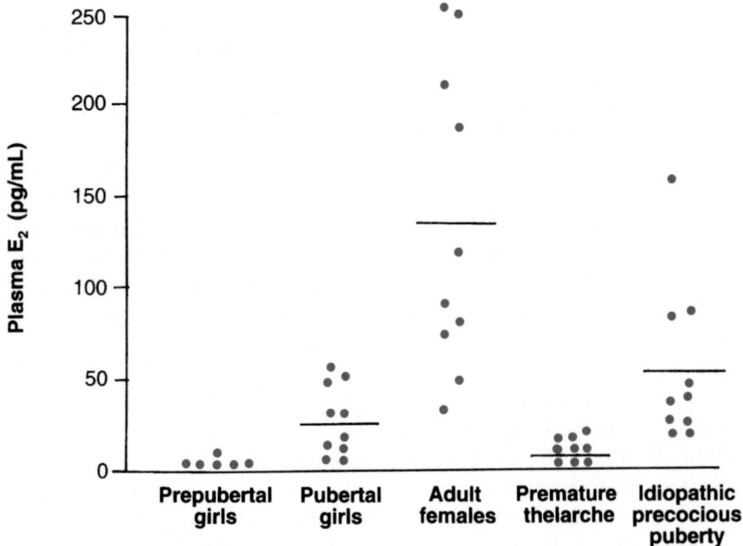

Figure 38-24. Estradiol values in normal females and in patients with premature thelarche and idiopathic precocious puberty. Horizontal lines depict mean levels. (Redrawn from Escobar ME, Rivarola MA, Bergada C: Plasma concentration of oestradiol-17beta in premature thelarche and in different types of sexual precocity. Acta Endocrinol 81:351, 1976.)

KEY POINTS

- The incidence of secondary amenorrhea of more than 6 months' duration in the general population is 0.7%.
- The incidence of amenorrhea lasting more than 6 months after discontinuation of oral contraceptives is 0.8%.
- The most important and probably most common cause of amenorrhea in adolescent girls is anorexia nervosa.
- A woman 13 years of age or older without any breast development has estrogen deficiency due to a severe abnormality and needs a diagnostic evaluation.
- Menarche is delayed about 0.4 year for each year of premenarcheal athletic training.
- Gonadal failure is the most common cause of primary amenorrhea, accounting for nearly half the patients with this syndrome.
- Individuals with gonadal failure and an X chromosome abnormality are shorter than 63 inches in height.
- The testes of individuals with androgen resistance have about a 20% chance of becoming malignant after age 20 years.
- Uterovaginal agenesis is the second most common cause of primary amenorrhea, with an incidence of about 15% of individuals with this symptom.
- About one third of individuals with gonadal failure have major cardiovascular or renal abnormalities.
- Congenital renal abnormalities occur in about one third of women with uterovaginal agenesis.
- The differential diagnosis between estrogen deficiency caused by gonadal failure and hypogonadotropic hypogonadism is best established with measurement of serum follicle-stimulating hormone (FSH).
- The diagnosis of gonadal failure, or hypergonadotropic hypogonadism, can be established if the FSH levels exceed 30 mIU/mL.
- Individuals with gonadal failure should have a peripheral karyotype performed to determine if a Y chromosome is present. If it is present, or signs of hyperandrogenism are present, the gonads should be excised to prevent development of malignancy, mainly a gonadoblastoma.
- Individuals with primary amenorrhea and hypogonadotropic hypogonadism do not need karyotyping but need a cranial CT scan to rule out a CNS tumor.
- The most frequent cause of intrauterine adhesions (IUAs) is curettage performed during pregnancy or shortly thereafter.
- The amenorrhea associated with strenuous exercise is related to stress, not weight loss, and is most probably caused by an increase in CNS opioids (β-endorphin) and catechol estrogens, both of which interfere with gonadotropin-releasing hormone (GnRH) release.
- When women lose 15% below ideal body weight, amenorrhea can occur due to CNS-hypothalamic dysfunction. When weight loss decreases below 25% of ideal body weight, pituitary gonadotropin function can also become abnormal.
- Anorexia nervosa occurs in about 1 in 1000 white women. It is uncommon in men and women older than 25 and rare in blacks and Asians.
- Individuals with anorexia nervosa have impaired peripheral conversion of thyroxine (T_4) to triiodothyronine (T_3), resulting in normal T_4 levels, decreased T_3 levels, and increased reverse T_3 levels.
- The normal cyclic pattern of LH pulsatility is not present in individuals with functional hypothalamic amenorrhea. Either no pulse or pulses of slow frequency, similar to those in the normal luteal phase, are usually observed.
- The GnRH alterations as reflected in LH pulsatility in persons with severe weight loss and anorexia nervosa are similar to those seen in normal prepubertal girls. When such individuals gain weight, GnRH changes similar to those occurring during puberty take place.
- When uterine bleeding fails to occur after progestin is administered, E_2 levels are usually lower than 40 pg/mL.
- In contrast to hypothalamic disorders, pituitary causes of amenorrhea can be associated with ACTH and TSH deficiency.
- Individuals with premature ovarian failure have two different histologic findings: generalized sclerosis or primordial follicles scattered through the stroma.
- Individuals with premature ovarian failure frequently have antibodies to gonadotropins and other endocrine organs, indicating an autoimmune origin.
- A karyotype should be obtained in women with premature ovarian failure younger than 25 but not in those who are older.
- Amenorrhea with low estrogen levels is associated with decreased density of trabecular bone.
- The most frequent cause of secondary amenorrhea is hypothalamic dysfunction.
- Physiologic development in females with precocious puberty usually follows the normal sequence of changes of secondary sexual characteristics.
- The two primary concerns of parents of children with precocious puberty are the social stigma associated with the child being physically different from her peers and the diminished ultimate height caused by the premature closure of epiphyseal growth centers.
- The exact cause of the majority of cases of GnRH-dependent (true or complete) precocious puberty is unknown; however, approximately 30% of cases are secondary to CNS disease.
- A definitive diagnosis is established more often for GnRH-independent (pseudoprecocious or incomplete) puberty, and it is usually related to an ovarian or adrenal disorder.
- Breast hyperplasia is a normal phenomenon in neonates and may persist up to 6 months of age.
- The most common cause of GnRH-independent precocious puberty is a functioning ovarian tumor. Granulosa cell tumors are the most common type, accounting for approximately 60%.
- The primary emphasis of the diagnostic workup on a child with precocious puberty should be to rule out life-threatening neoplasms of the ovary, adrenal glands, or CNS. The

Continued

KEY POINTS *Continued*

secondary emphasis is to delineate the speed of the maturation process, for this fact is crucial in decisions concerning therapy.

- The goals of therapy of precocious puberty are to reduce gonadotropin secretions and reduce or counteract the peripheral actions of sex steroids, decreasing growth rate to normal and slowing skeletal maturation. This is best accomplished by GnRH agonists.
- The effect on adult height depends on the chronologic age at which the GnRH therapy is initiated. The therapy is most effective in 4- to 6-year-olds.
- Both the child with precocious puberty and her family need intensive counseling.

BIBLIOGRAPHY

Adashi EY, Casper RF, Fishman J, et al: Stimulatory effect of 2-hydroxyestradiol on prolactin release in hypogonadal women. J Clin Endocrinol Metab 51:413, 1980.

Adashi EY, Rakoff J, Divers W, et al: The effect of acutely administered 2-hydroxyestrone on the release of gonadotropins and prolactin before and after estrogen priming in hypogonadal women. Obstet Gynecol Surv 35:363, 1980.

Albright AL, Lee PA: Hypothalamic hamartomas and sexual precocity. Pediatr Neurosurg 18:315, 1992.

Alper MM, Garner PR: Premature ovarian failure: Its relationship to autoimmune disease. Obstet Gynecol 66:27, 1985.

Ambrosino MM, Hernanz-Schulman M, Genieser NB, et al: Monitoring of girls undergoing medical therapy for isosexual precocious puberty. J Ultrasound Med 13:501, 1994.

American College of Obstetricians and Gynecologists: Pediatric gynecologic disorders. ACOG Tech Bull 201:1, 1995.

Arita K, Ikawa F, Jurisu K, et al: The relationship between magnetic resonance imaging findings and clinical manifestations of hypothalamic hamartoma. J Neurosurg 91:212, 1999.

Bell TA, Stamm WE, Wang S, et al: Chronic *Chlamydia trachomatis* infections in infants. JAMA 267:400, 1992.

Berga SL, Loucks TL: The Diagnosis and treatment of stress-induced anovulation. Minerva Ginecol 57:45, 2005.

Berga SL, Marcus MD, Loucks TL, et al: Recovery of ovarian activity in women with functional hypothalamic amenorrhea who were treated with cognitive behavior therapy. Fertil Steril 80:976, 2003.

Berga SL, Mortola JF, Girton BS, et al: Neuroendocrine aberrations in women with functional hypothalamic amenorrhea. J Clin Endocrinol Metab 68:301, 1989.

Beumont PJ, George GC, Pimstone BL, Vinick AI: Body weight and the pituitary response to hypothalamic releasing hormones in patients with anorexia nervosa. J Clin Endocrinol Metab 43:487, 1976.

Blake J: Gynecologic examination of the teenager and young child. Obstet Gynecol Clin North Am 19:27, 1992.

Boepple PA, Frisch LS, Wierman ME, et al: The natural history of autonomous gonadal function, adrenarche, and central puberty in gonadotropin-independent precocious puberty. J Clin Endocrinol Metab 75:1550, 1992.

Bonazzi C, Peccatori F, Colombo N, et al: Pure ovarian immature teratoma, a unique and curable disease: 10 years' experience of 32 prospectively treated patients. Obstet Gynecol 84:598, 1994.

Bond GR, Dowd MD, Landsman I, Rimsza M: Unintentional perineal injury in prepubescent girls: A multicenter, prospective report of 56 girls. Pediatrics 95:628, 1995.

Boyar RM, Katz J, Finkelstein JW, et al: Anorexia nervosa: Immaturity of the 24-hour luteinizing hormone secretory pattern. N Engl J Med 291:861, 1974.

Brenner PF: Precocious puberty in the female. In Lobo R, Mishell DR Jr, Paulson RJ, Shoupe D (eds): Mishell's Textbook of Infertility, Contraception and Reproductive Endocrinology, 4th ed. Malden, MA, Blackwell Science, 1997.

Bridges NA, Cooke A, Healy MJR, et al: Standards for ovarian volume in childhood and puberty. Fertil Steril 60:456, 1993.

Brown MF, Hebra A, McGeehin K, Ross AJ III: Ovarian masses in children: A review of 91 cases of malignant and benign masses. J Pediatr Surg 28:930, 1993.

Buchta RM: Use of chaperons during pelvic examinations of female adolescents. Am J Dis Child 141:666, 1987.

Capraro VJ: Pediatric gynecology. In Danforth DN (ed): Obstetrics and Gynecology, 4th ed. Philadelphia, Harper & Row, 1982.

Carpenter SE, Rock JA (eds): Pediatric and Adolescent Gynecology. New York, Raven Press, 1992.

Carr DB, Bullen BA, Skrinar GS, et al: Physical conditioning facilitates the exercise-induced secretion of beta-endorphin and beta-lipotropin in women. N Engl J Med 305:560, 1981.

Chan JL, Mantzoros CS: Role of leptin in energy-deprivation states: Normal human physiology and clinical implications for hypothalamic amenorrhea and anorexia. Lancet 366(9479):74, 2005.

Cohen HL, Eisenberg P, Mandel F, Haller JO: Ovarian cysts are common in premenarchal girls: A sonographic study of 101 children 2-12 years old. AJR 159:89, 1992.

Comite F, Cassorla F, Barnes KM, et al: Luteinizing hormone releasing hormone analogue therapy for central precocious puberty: Long-term effect on somatic growth, bone maturation, and predicted height. JAMA 255:2613, 1986.

Coulam CB, Adamson SC, Annegers JF: Incidence of premature ovarian failure. Obstet Gynecol 67:604, 1986.

Crofton PM, Evans NEM, Wardhaugh B, et al: Evidence for increased ovarian follicular activity in girls with premature thelarche. J Clin Endocrinol 62:205, 2005.

Cronjé HS, Niemand I, Bam RH, Woodruff JD: Granulosa and theca cell tumors in children: A report of 17 cases and literature review. Obstet Gynecol Surv 53:240, 1998.

Crowley WF Jr, Filicori M, Spratt DI, et al: The physiology of gonadotropin-releasing hormone (GnRH) secretion in men and women. Rec Prog Hormone Res 41:473, 1985.

Cushing B, Giller R, Ablin A, et al: Surgical resection alone is effective treatment for ovarian immature teratoma in children and adolescents: A report of the Pediatric Oncology Group and the Children's Cancer Group. Am J Obstet Gynecol 181:353, 1999.

DiMartino-Nardi J, Wu R, Varner R, et al: The effect of luteinizing hormone-releasing hormone analog for central precocious puberty on growth hormone (GH) and GH-binding protein. J Clin Endocrinol Metab 78:664, 1994.

DiMartino-Nardi J: Premature adrenarche: Findings in prepubertal African-American and Caribbean-Hispanic girls. Acta Paediatr (Suppl) 433:67, 1999.

Djurovic M, Pekic S, Petakov M, et al: Gonadotropin response to clomiphene and plasma leptin levels in weight recovered but amenorrhoeic patients with anorexia nervosa. J Endocrinol Invest 6:523, 2004.

Drinkwater BL, Nilson K, Chestnut CH III, et al: Bone mineral content of amenorrheic and eumenorrheic athletes. N Engl J Med 322:277, 1984.

Ehren IM, Mahour GH, Isaacs H: Benign and malignant ovarian tumors in children and adolescents. Am J Surg 147:339, 1984.

Ehrhardt AA, Meyer-Bahlburg HFL: Psychosocial aspects of precocious puberty. Horm Res 41(S2):30, 1994.

Emans SJ, Goldstein DP: The gynecologic examination of the prepubertal child with vulvovaginitis: Use of the knee-chest position. Pediatrics 65:758, 1980.

Emans SJ, Woods ER, Allred EN, Grace E: Hymenal findings in adolescent women: Impact of tampon use and consensual sexual activity. J Pediatr 125:153, 1994.
Emans SJH, Goldstein DP: Pediatric and Adolescent Gynecology, 4th ed. Philadelphia, Lippincott-Raven, 1998.
Eugster EA: Aromatase inhibitors in precocious puberty: Rationale and experience to date. Treat Endocrinol 3(3):141, 2004.
Farrington PF: Pediatric vulvo-vaginitis. Clin Obstet Gynecol 40:135, 1997.
Feicht CB, Johnson TS, Matrin BJ: Secondary amenorrhea in athletes. Lancet 1:1145, 1978.
Ferin M, Van Vugt D, Wardlaw S: The hypothalamic control of the menstrual cycle and the role of endogenous opioid peptides. Recent Prog Horm Res 40:441, 1984.
Feuillan PP, Foster CM, Pescovitz OH, et al: Treatment of precocious puberty in the McCune-Albright syndrome with the aromatase inhibitor testolactone. N Engl J Med 315:1115, 1986.
Freud E, Golinsky D, Steinberg RM, et al: Ovarian masses in children. Clin Pediatr 38:573, 1999.
Friedman CI, Barrows H, Kim MH: Hypergonadotropic hypogonadism. Am J Obstet Gynecol 145:360, 1983.
Fries H, Nillius SJ, Pettersson F: Epidemiology of secondary amenorrhea. Am J Obstet Gynecol 118:473, 1974.
Frisch RE, Gotz-Welbergen AV, McArthur JW, et al: Delayed menarche and amenorrhea of college athletes in relation to onset of training. JAMA 246:1559, 1981.
Frisch RE, Revelle R: Height and weight at menarche and a hypothesis of critical body weights and adolescent events. Science 169:397, 1970.
Frisch RE, Revelle R: Height and weight at menarche and a hypothesis of menarche. Arch Dis Child 46:695, 1971.
Frisch RE, Rose E, Wyshak G, et al: Delayed menarche and amenorrhea in ballet dancers. N Engl J Med 303:17, 1980.
Galatzer A, Laron Z: Behavior in girls with true precocious puberty. J Pediatr 108:790, 1986.
Goff CW, Burke KR, Rickenback C, Buebendorf DP: Vaginal opening measurement in prepubertal girls. Am J Dis Child 143:1366, 1989.
Goldenberg RL, Grodin JM, Aodbard D, Ross GT: Gonadotropins in women with amenorrhea. Am J Obstet Gynecol 116:1003, 1973.
Goodpasture JC, Ghai K, Cara JF, Rosenfield RL: Potential of gonadotropin-releasing hormone agonists in the diagnosis of pubertal disorders in girls. Clin Obstet Gynecol 36:773, 1993.
Griffin JE, Edwards C, Madden JD, et al: Congenital absence of the vagina. Ann Intern Med 85:224, 1976.
Hairston L: Physical examination of the prepupertal girl. Clin Obstet Gynecol 40:127, 1997.
Hammerschlag MR: Sexually transmitted diseases in sexually abused children: Medical and legal implications. Sex Trans Inf 74:167, 1998.
Handley J, Dinsmore W, Maw R, et al: Anogenital warts in prepubertal children: Sexual abuse or not? Int J STD AIDS 4:271, 1993.
Heger S, Sippell WG, Partsch CJ: Gonadotropin-releasing hormone analogue treatment for precocious puberty. Twenty years of experience. Endocr Dev 8:94, 2005.
Hill NCW, Oppenheimer LW, Morton KE: The aetiology of vaginal bleeding in children: A 20-year review. Br J Obstet Gynaecol 96:467, 1989.
Hintz RL, Attie KM, Baptista J, Roche A for the Genentech Collaborative Group: Effect of growth hormone treatment on adult height of children with idiopathic short stature. N Engl J Med 340:502, 1999.
Huffman JW: The Gynecology of Childhood and Adolescence, 2nd ed. Philadelphia, WB Saunders, 1981.
Ibánez L, Potau N, de Zegher F: Endocrinology and metabolism after premature pubarche in girls. Acta Paediatr Suppl 433:73, 1999.
Ibánez L, Potau N, Francois I, de Zegher F: Precocious pubarche, hyperinsulinism, and ovarian hyperandrogenism in girls: Relation to reduced fetal growth. J Clin Endocrinol Metab 83:3558, 1998.
Ingram JM: The bicycle stool in the treatment of vaginal agenesis and stenosis: A preliminary report. Am J Obstet Gynecol 140:867, 1981.
Jabra AA, Fishman EK, Taylor GA: Primary ovarian tumors in the pediatric patient: CT evaluation. Clin Imaging 17:199, 1993.
Jay N, Mansfield MJ, Blizzard RM, et al: Ovulation and menstrual function of adolescent girls with central precocious puberty after therapy with gonadotropin-releasing hormone agonists. J Clin Endocrinol Metab 75:890, 1992.
Jenkinson SD, Mackinnon AE: Spontaneous separation of fused labia minora in prepubertal girls. BMJ 289:160, 1984.
Kao SCS, Cook JS, Hansen JR, Simonson TM: MR imaging of the pituitary gland in central precocious puberty. Pediatr Radiol 22:481, 1992.
Kaplowitz PB, Oberfield SE, and the Drug and Therapeutics and Executive Committees of the Lawson Wilkins Pediatric Endocrine Society: Reexamination of the age limit for defining when puberty is precocious in girls in the United States: Implications for evaluation and treatment. Pediatrics 104:936, 1999.
King LR, Siegel MJ, Solomon AL: Usefulness of ovarian volume and cysts in female isosexual precocious puberty. J Ultrasound Med 12:577, 1993.
Klein VR, Willman SP, Carr BR: Familial posterior labial fusion. Obstet Gynecol 73:500, 1989.
Kletter GB, Kelch RP: Effects of gonadotropin-releasing hormone analog therapy on adult stature in precocious puberty. J Clin Endocrinol Metab 79:331, 1994.
Kletzky OA, Davajan V, Nakamura RM, et al: Clinical categorization of patients with secondary amenorrhea using progesterone-induced uterine bleeding and measurement of serum gonadotropin levels. Am J Obstet Gynecol 121:695, 1975.
Klibanski A, Biller BMK, Rosenthal DI, et al: Effects of prolactin and estrogen deficiency in amenorrheic bone loss. J Clin Endocrinol Metab 67:124, 1988.
Kreiter M, Burstein S, Rosenfield RL, et al: Preserving adult height potential in girls with idiopathic true precocious puberty. J Pediatr 117:364, 1990.
LaBarbera AR, Miller MM, Ober C, et al: Autoimmune etiology in premature ovarian failure. Am J Reprod Immunol Microbiol 16:115, 1988.
Layman LC: Mutations in human gonadotropin genes and their physiologic significance in puberty and reproduction. Fertil Steril 71:201, 1999.
Ledger WL, Thomas EJ, Browning D, et al: Suppression of gonadotrophin secretion does not reverse premature ovarian failure. Br J Obstet Gynaecol 96:196, 1989.
Lee PA: Laboratory monitoring of children with precocious puberty. Arch Pediatr Adolesc Med 148:369, 1994.
Lee PA, Page JG, and the Leuprolide Study Group: Effects of leuprolide in the treatment of central precocious puberty. J Pediatr 114:321, 1989.
Leung AKC, Robson WLM: Labial fusion and asymptomatic bacteriuria. Eur J Pediatr 152:250, 1993.
Leung AKC, Robson WLM, Tay-Uyboco J: The incidence of labial fusion in children. J Paediatr Child Health 29:235, 1993.
Liapi C, Evain-Brion D: Diagnosis of ovarian follicular cysts from birth to puberty: A report of twenty cases. Acta Paediatr Scand 76:91, 1987.
Lieblich JM, Rogol AD, White BJ, et al: Syndrome of anosmia with hypogonadotropic hypogonadism (Kallmann syndrome): Clinical laboratory studies in 23 cases. Am J Med 73:506, 1982.
Lloyd T, Myers C, Buchanan JR, et al: Collegiate women athletes with irregular menses during adolescence have decreased bone density. Obstet Gynecol 72:639, 1988.
Mansfield MJ, Beardsworth DE, Loughlin JS, et al: Long-term treatment of central precocious puberty with a long-acting analogue of luteinizing hormone-releasing hormone. N Engl J Med 309:1286, 1983.
Marshall WA, Tanner JM: Variations in pattern of pubertal changes in girls. Arch Dis Child 44:291, 1969.
Maschchak CA, Kletzky OA, Davajan V, et al: Clinical and laboratory evaluation of patients with primary amenorrhea. Obstet Gynecol 57:715, 1981.
Mason HD, Sagle M: Reduced frequency of luteinizing hormone pulses in women with weight loss-related amenorrhea and multifollicular ovaries. Clin Endocrinol 280:611, 1988.
McArthur JW, Bullen BA, Beitins IZ, et al: Hypothalamic amenorrhea in runners of normal body composition. Endocr Res Commun 7:13, 1980.
McCann J, Voris J, Simon M: Labial adhesions and posterior fourchette injuries in childhood sexual abuse. Am J Dis Child 142:659, 1988.
McCann J, Voris J, Simon M, Wells R: Comparison of genital examination techniques in prepubertal girls. Pediatr 85:182, 1990.
McCrea RS: Uterine adnexal torsion with subsequent contralateral recurrence. J Reprod Med 25:123, 1980.
Meffert JJ, Davis BM, Grimwood RE: Lichen sclerosus. J Am Acad Derm 32:393, 1995.
Mignot MH, Schoemaker J, Kleingeld M, et al: Premature ovarian failure. I. The association with autoimmunity. Eur J Obstet Gynecol Reprod Biol 30:59, 1989.
Millar DM, Blake JM, Stringer DA, et al: Prepubertal ovarian cyst formation: 5 years' experience. Obstet Gynecol 81:434, 1993.

Miller WL: The molecular basis of premature adrenarche: An hypothesis. Acta Paediatr Suppl 433:60, 1999.

Misra M, Miller KK, Kuo K, et al: Secretory dynamics of leptin in adolescent girls with anorexia nervosa and healthy adolescents. Am J Physiol Endocrinol Metab 289:E373, 2005.

Moraes-Ruehsen M de, Blizzard RM, Garcia-Bunuel R, et al: Autoimmunity and ovarian failure. Am J Obstet Gynecol 112:693, 1972.

Muram D, Elias S: Child sexual abuse-genital tract findings in prepubertal girls. II. Comparison of colposcopic and unaided examinations. Am J Obstet Gynecol 160:333, 1989.

Muram D, Laufer MR: Limitations of the medical evaluation for child sexual abuse. J Reprod Med 44:993, 1999.

Muram D: Child sexual abuse-genital tract findings in prepubertal girls. I. The unaided medical examination. Am J Obstet Gynecol 160:328, 1989.

Nappi RE, DÁmbrogio G, Petraggia F, et al: Hypothalamic amenorrhea: Evidence for a central derangement of hypothalamic-pituitary-adrenal cortex axis activity. Fertil Steril 59:571, 1993.

Pacheco BP, Di Paola G, Ribas JMM, et al: Vulvar infection caused by human papilloma virus in children and adolescents without sexual contact. Adolesc Pediatr Gynecol 4:136, 1991.

Pasquino AM, Tebaldi L, Cives C, et al: Precocious puberty in the McCune-Albright syndrome. Acta Paediatr Scand 76:841, 1987.

Penny R, Goldstein IP, Frasier SD: Gonadotropin excretion and body composition. Pediatrics 61:294, 1978.

Pescovitz OH, Comite F, Hench K, et al: The NIH experience with precocious puberty: Diagnostic subgroups and response to short-term luteinizing hormone releasing hormone analogue therapy. J Pediatr 108:47, 1986.

Pescovitz OH, Hench KD, Barnes KM, et al: Premature thelarche and central precocious puberty: The relationship between clinical presentation and the gonadotropin response to luteinizing hormone-releasing hormone. J Clin Endocrinol Metab 67:474, 1988.

Pettersson F, Fries H, Nillius SJ: Epidemiology of secondary amenorrhea. Am J Obstet Gynecol 117:80, 1973.

Pokorny SF: Prepubertal vulvovaginopathies. Obstet Gynecol Clin North Am 19:39, 1992.

Pokorny SF: Long-term intravaginal presence of foreign bodies in children: A preliminary study. J Reprod Med 39:931, 1994.

Pokorny SF: Genital trauma. Clin Obstet Gynecol 40:219, 1997.

Pokorny SF, Pokorny WJ, Kramer W: Acute genital injury in the prepubertal girl. Am J Obstet Gynecol 166:1461, 1992.

Pucarelli I, Segni M, Ortore M, et al: Effects of combined gonadotrophin-releasing hormone agonist and growth hormone therapy on adult height in precocious puberty: A further contribution. J Pediatr Endocrinol Metab 16:1005, 2003.

Quigley ME, Sheehan KL, Casper RF, Yen SSC: Evidence for increased dopaminergic and opioid activity in patients with hypothalamic hypogonadotropic hypogonadism. J Clin Endocrinol Metab 50:949, 1980.

Reame NE, Sauder SE, Case GD, et al: Pulsatile gonadotropin secretion in women with hypothalamic amenorrhea: Evidence that reduced frequency of gonadotropin-releasing hormone secretion is the mechanism of persistent anovulation. J Clin Endocrinol Metab 61:851, 1985.

Reame NE, Sauder SE, Kelch RP, et al: Pulsatile gonadotropin secretion during the human menstrual cycle: Evidence for altered frequency of gonadotropin-releasing hormone secretion. J Clin Endocrinol Metab 59:328, 1984.

Rebar RW, Connolly HV: Clinical features of young women with hypergonadotropic amenorrhea. Fertil Steril 53:804, 1990.

Rebar RW, Erickson GF, Yen SSC: Idiopathic premature ovarian failure: clinical and endocrine characteristics. Fertil Steril 137:35, 1982.

Reid RL, Hoff JD, Yen SSC, et al: Effects of exogenous β-endorphin on pituitary hormone secretion and its disappearance rate in normal human subjects. J Clin Endocrinol Metab 52:1179, 1981.

Reindollar RH, Byrd JR, McDonough PG: Delayed sexual development: A study of 252 patients. Am J Obstet Gynecol 140:371, 1981.

Reindollar RH, Novak M, Tho SPT, McDonough PG: Adult-onset amenorrhea: A study of 262 patients. Am J Obstet Gynecol 155:531, 1986.

Robinson AJ: Sexually transmitted organism in children and child sexual abuse. Int J STD AIDS 9:501, 1998.

Rosen GF, Vermesh M, dÁblaing G, et al: The endocrinologic evaluation of a 45,X true hermaphrodite. Am J Obstet Gynecol 157:1272, 1987.

Rosenfield RL: Normal and almost normal precocious variations in pubertal development, premature pubarche and premature thelarche revisited. Horm Res 41(S2):7, 1994.

Rosenfield RL: Selection of children with precocious puberty for treatment with gonadotropin releasing hormone analogs. J Pediatr 124:989, 1994.

Russell JB, DeCherney AH, Collins DC: The effect of naloxone and metoclopramide on the hypothalamic pituitary axis in oligomenorrheic and eumenorrheic swimmers. Fertil Steril 52:583, 1989.

Russell JB, Mitchell D, Musey PI, et al: The relationship of exercise to anovulatory cycles in female athletes: Hormonal and physical characteristics. Obstet Gynecol 63:452, 1984.

Russell JB, Mitchell DE, Musey PI, et al: The role of β-endorphins and catechol estrogens on the hypothalamic-pituitary axis in female athletes. Fertil Steril 42:690, 1984.

Sanfilippo JS (ed): Pediatric and Adolescent Gynecology. Philadelphia, WB Saunders, 1994.

Sankila R, Olsen JH, Anderson H, et al: Risk of cancer among offspring of childhood-cancer survivors. N Engl J Med 338:1339, 1998.

Schenker JG, Margalioth EJ: Intrauterine adhesions: An updated appraisal. Fertil Steril 37:593, 1982.

Schlechte JA, Sherman B, Martin R: Bone density in amenorrheic women with and without hyperprolactinemia. J Clin Endocrinol Metab 56:1120, 1983.

Shawis RN, El Gohary AE, Cook RCM: Ovarian cysts and tumors in infancy and childhood. Ann R Coll Surg Engl 67:17, 1985.

Sherman BM, Halmi KA, Zamudio R: LH and FSH response to gonadotropin-releasing hormone in anorexia nervosa: Effect of nutritional rehabilitation. J Clin Endocrinol Metab 41:135, 1975.

Siegel MJ: Pediatric gynecologic sonography. Radiology 179:593, 1991.

Siegel MJ, Carel C, Surratt S: Ultrasonography of acute abdominal pain in children. JAMA 266:1987, 1991.

Siegel MJ, Surratt JT: Pediatric gynecologic imaging. Obstet Gynecol Clin North Am 19:103, 1992.

Siegel SF, Finegold DN, Urban MD, et al: Premature pubarche: etiological heterogeneity. J Clin Endocrinol Metab 74:239, 1992.

Sonis WA, Comite F, Pescovitz OH, et al: Biobehavioral aspects of precocious puberty. J Am Acad Child Psychiatry 25:674, 1989.

Speroff L, Glass RH, Kase NG: Clinical Gynecologic Endocrinology and Infertility, 6th ed. Philadelphia, Lippincott Williams & Wilkins, 1999.

Thorp JM, Wells SR, Droegemueller W: Ovarian suspension in massive ovarian edema. Obstet Gynecol 76:912, 1990.

Traggiai C, Perucchin PP, Zerbini K, et al: Outcome after depot gonadotropin-releasing hormone agonist treatment for central precocious puberty: Effects on body mass index and final height. Eur J Endocrinol 153:463, 2005.

Treasure JL, King EA, Gordon PAL, et al: Cystic ovaries: A phase of anorexia nervosa. Lancet 28:1379, 1985.

Tschugguel W, Berga SL: Treatment of functional hypothalamic amenorrhea with hypnotherapy. Fertil Steril 80:982, 2003.

Tulandi T, Finch RA: Premature ovarian failure. Obstet Gynecol Surv 36:521, 1981.

Valerie E, Gilchrist BF, Frischer J, et al: Diagnosis and treatment of ureteral prolapse in children. Urology 54:1082, 1999.

Van Winter JT, Simmons PS, Podratz KC: Surgically treated adnexal masses in infancy, childhood, and adolescence. Am J Obstet Gynecol 170:1780, 1994.

Vance ML, Mauras N: Growth hormone therapy in adults and children. N Engl J Med 341:1206, 1999.

Vigersky RA, Andersen AE, Thompson RG, et al: Hypothalamic dysfunction in secondary amenorrhea associated with simple weight loss. N Engl J Med 297:1141, 1977.

Vigersky RA, Loriaux DL, Andersen AE, et al: Delayed pituitary hormone response to LRF and TRF in patients with secondary amenorrhea associated with simple weight loss. J Clin Endocrinol Metab 43:893, 1976.

Walvoord EC, Pescovitz OH: Combined use of growth hormone and gonadotropin-releasing hormone analogues in precocious puberty: Theoretic and practical considerations. Pediatrics 104:1010, 1999.

Warren MP: The effects of exercise on pubertal progression and reproductive function in girls. J Clin Endocrinol Metab 51:1150, 1980.

Warren MP, Jewelwicz R, Dyrenfurth I, et al: The significance of weight loss in the evaluation of pituitary response to LH-RH in women with secondary amenorrhea. J Clin Endocrinol Metab 40:601, 1975.

Wildt L, Leyendecker G: Indication of ovulation by the chronic administration of naltrexone in hypothalamic amenorrhea. J Clin Endocrinol Metab 64:1334, 1987.

Witchel SF, Plant TM: Puberty: Gonadarche and adrenarche. In Yen and Jaffe's Reproductive Endocrinology-Physiology, Pathophysiology and Clinical Management, 5th ed. Philadelphia, Elsevier Saunders, 2004.

Wu M-H, Lin S-J, Wu L-H, et al: Clinical suppression of precocious puberty with cetrorelix after failed treatment with GnRH agonist in a girl with gonadotropin-independent precocious puberty. Rep BioMed Online 11:18, 2005.

Yeshaya A, Kauschansky A, Orvieto R, et al: Prolonged vaginal bleeding during central precocious puberty therapy with a long-acting gonadotropin-releasing hormone agonist. Acta Obstet Gynaecol Scand 77:327, 1998.

Zalel Y, Piura B, Elchalal U, et al: Diagnosis and management of malignant germ cell ovarian tumors in young females. Int J Gynaecol Obstet 55:1, 1996.

Zitsman JL, Cirincione E, Margossian H: Vaginal bleeding in an infant secondary to sliding inguinal hernia. Obstet Gynecol 89:840, 1997.

Hyperprolactinemia, Galactorrhea, and Pituitary Adenomas

39

Etiology, Differential Diagnosis, Natural History, Management

Rogerio A. Lobo

KEY TERMS AND DEFINITIONS

Bromocriptine (2-Bromo-α-Ergocryptine Mesylate). Semisynthetic ergot alkaloid that is a dopamine receptor agonist used to treat hyperprolactinemia.

Cabergoline. A long-acting dopamine receptor agonist that directly inhibits secretion of prolactin from the pituitary and is an effective treatment for hyperprolactinemia.

Computed Tomography (CT). An imaging technique for detecting soft tissue abnormalities that uses a computer to integrate differences in X-ray beam attenuation resulting from varying densities in adjacent tissue.

Craniopharyngioma. A rare hypothalamic tumor that can produce hyperprolactinemia.

Empty Sella Syndrome. An intrasellar extension of the subarachnoid space resulting in compression of the pituitary gland and an enlarged sella turcica that may be associated with galactorrhea and hyperprolactinemia.

Galactorrhea. Nonpuerperal secretion from the breast of watery or milky fluid that contains neither pus nor blood.

Hyperprolactinemia. Levels of circulating prolactin above normal (>20 to 25 ng/mL) that can cause galactorrhea or amenorrhea or both.

Hypocycloidal Tomography. Multiple radiographs of the sella turcica at intervals of 2 to 3 mm with a hypocycloidal movement.

Macroadenoma. An uncommon type of prolactin-secreting pituitary adenoma (prolactinoma) greater than 1 cm in diameter, usually with extrasellar extension.

Magnetic Resonance Imaging (MRI). Technique for soft tissue imaging that uses resonance of hydrogen nuclei in a static magnetic field exposed to low-frequency radiowaves.

Microadenoma. The common type of prolactinoma less than 1 cm in diameter.

Prolactin. Polypeptide hormone secreted by anterior pituitary lactotrophs that has mammotrophic and lactogenic functions.

Prolactin-Inhibiting Factor. The neurotransmitter (believed to be dopamine) that inhibits prolactin synthesis and release.

Prolactinoma. The most common pituitary tumor arising from chromophobic cells that secrete prolactin.

Prolactin (PRL) is a polypeptide hormone containing 198 amino acids and having a molecular weight of 22,000 daltons. It circulates in different molecular sizes: a monomeric (small) form (mol wt 22,000 daltons), a polymeric (big) form (mol wt 50,000 daltons), and an even larger polymeric (big-big) form (mol wt > 100,000 daltons). Big PRL is presumed to be a dimer, and big-big PRL may represent an aggregation of monomeric molecules. The larger forms also contain added sugar moieties (glycosylation) which decreases biologic activity. The small form is biologically active, and about 80% of the hormone is secreted in this form. Most immunoassays measure both the small and large forms of PRL. As stated earlier, the polymeric forms have reduced biologic activity and reduced binding to mammary tissue membranes. Women have been identified with high levels of PRL on routine immunoassay who are completely normal and have been found to have circulating polymeric forms on gel electrophoresis.

PRL is synthesized and stored in the pituitary gland in chromophobe cells called *lactotrophs,* which are located mainly in the lateral areas of the gland. PRL is encoded by its gene (10 kb) on chromosome 6. At the molecular level, it is stimulated and suppressed by multiple factors. The principal stimulating factor is thyroid-releasing hormone (TRH), and the major inhibiting factor is dopamine. Estrogen also enhances PRL secretion by enhancing the effects of TRH and inhibiting the effects of dopamine. A potential direct effect may also be mediated via galanin. The principal receptor dopamine interacts with is D2, which is the target for various dopamine agonists used in the treatment of hyperprolactinemia.

In addition, PRL is synthesized in decidualized stroma of endometrial tissue. From these tissues PRL is secreted into the circulation and, in the event of pregnancy, into the amniotic fluid. The control of decidual PRL is different from that of the pituitary and does not respond to dopamine. PRL is normally present in measurable amounts in serum, with mean levels of about 8 ng/mL in adult women. It circulates in an unbound form, has a 20-minute half-life, and is cleared by the liver and kidney. The main function of PRL is to stimulate the growth of mammary tissue as well as to produce and secrete milk into the alveoli; thus, it has both mammogenic and lactogenic functions. Specific receptors for PRL are present in the plasma membrane of mammary cells as well as many other tissues.

PHYSIOLOGY

PRL synthesis and release from the lactotrophs are controlled by central nervous system neurotransmitters, which act on the pituitary via the hypothalamus. The major control mechanism is inhibition, as pituitary stalk section results in increased PRL secretion. It appears that the major physiologic inhibitor of PRL release is the neurotransmitter dopamine, which acts directly on the pituitary gland. There are specific dopamine receptors on the lactotrophs, and dopamine inhibits PRL synthesis and release in pituitary cell cultures. Thus dopamine appears to be the prolactin-inhibiting factor (PIF). Although a hypothalamic prolactin-releasing factor (PRF) has not been isolated, it is known that both the neurotransmitter serotonin and thyrotropin-releasing factor stimulate PRL release. Since the latter stimulates PRL release only minimally unless infused, it appears that serotonin is PRF or is responsible for its secretion. The rise in PRL levels during sleep appears to be controlled by serotonin.

PRL is secreted episodically, and serum levels fluctuate throughout the day and throughout the menstrual cycle, with peak levels occurring at midcycle. Although changes in PRL levels are not as marked as the pulsatile episodes of luteinizing hormone (LH), Bäckström and colleagues reported a decline in both basal concentration and pulse frequency of PRL in the luteal phase of the cycle. Estrogen stimulates PRL production and release. Under the influence of estrogen, PRL levels increase in females at the time of puberty.

During pregnancy, as estrogen levels increase, there is a concomitant hypertrophy and hyperplasia of the lactotrophs. The maternal increase in PRL occurs soon after implantation, concomitant with the increase in circulating estrogen. Circulating levels of PRL steadily increase throughout pregnancy, reaching about 200 ng/mL in the third trimester, and the rise is directly related to the increase in circulating levels of estrogen. Despite the elevated PRL levels during pregnancy, lactation does not occur because estrogen inhibits the action of PRL on the breast, most likely blocking PRL's interaction with its receptor. A day or two following delivery of the placenta, both estrogen levels and PRL levels decline rapidly and lactation is initiated. PRL levels reach basal levels in nonnursing women in 2 to 3 weeks. Although basal levels of circulating PRL decline to the nonpregnant range about 6 months after parturition in nursing women, following each act of suckling, PRL levels increase markedly and stimulate milk production for the next feeding.

Nipple and breast stimulation also increase PRL levels in the nonpregnant female. Other physiologic stimuli that increase PRL release are exercise, sleep, and stress. In addition, PRL levels normally rise following ingestion of the noonday meal. For these reasons PRL levels normally fluctuate throughout the day, with maximal levels observed during nighttime while asleep and a smaller increase occurring in the early afternoon (Fig. 39-1). When the amount measured in the circulation in the nonpregnant woman exceeds a certain level, usually 20 to 25 ng/mL, the condition is called *hyperprolactinemia.* The optimal time to obtain a blood sample for assay to diagnose hyperprolactinemia is during the midmorning hours. Increases in PRL levels above the normal range can occur without a pathologic condition if the serum sample is drawn from a patient who has recently awakened, has exercised, or has had recent breast stimulation, such as breast palpation, during a physical examination.

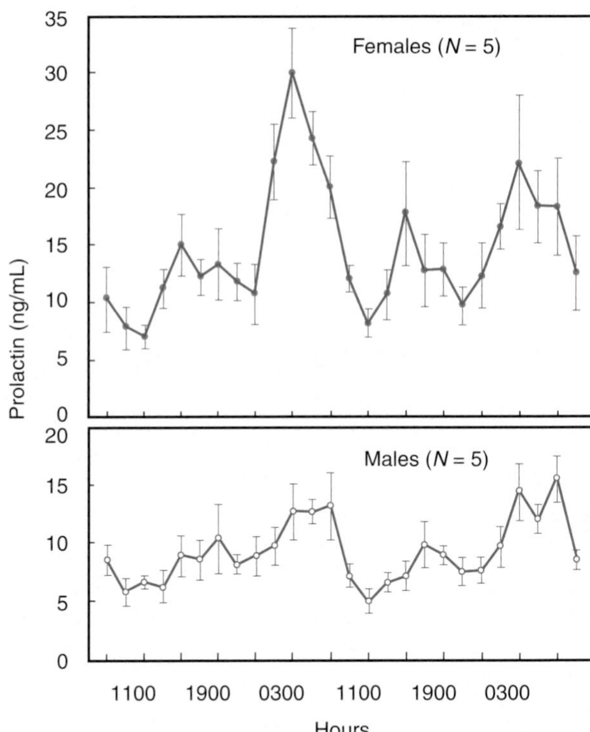

Figure 39-1. Hour-to-hour variation of serum prolactin concentration in normal women and men studied throughout 48 consecutive hours. (From Kletzky OA, Davajan V: Hyperprolactinemia: Diagnosis and treatment. In Mishell DR Jr, Davajan V: Infertility, Contraception and Reproductive Endocrinology, 4th ed. © Copyright 1997 by Blackwell Scientific Publications, Malden, MA. All rights reserved. Reproduced with permission.)

The most frequent cause of slightly elevated PRL levels is stress, particularly the stress caused by visiting the physician's office. An excellent study demonstrating that most mildly elevated PRL levels are not caused by pathologic hyperprolactinemia was performed by Muneyyirci-Delale and coworkers. These investigators studied 50 women without radiologic evidence of a prolactinoma who had elevated PRL levels (23 to 156 ng/mL) measured in two consecutive blood samples obtained 1 to 2 weeks apart. When these women had serial blood sampling subsequently performed in a quiet room, 20 had normal PRL levels in the 1-hour blood sample (Fig. 39-2). The initial PRL levels in these 20 women ranged from 26 to 69 ng/mL. The results of this study indicate that stress-related hyperprolactinemia is a common cause of a mild increase in PRL. All women with initial PRL levels less than 70 ng/mL should have subsequent samples drawn 60 minutes after resting in a quiet room to determine whether true pathologic hyperprolactinemia is present.

Hyperprolactinemia can produce disorders of gonadotropin sex steroid function, resulting in menstrual cycle derangement (oligomenorrhea and amenorrhea) and anovulation, as well as inappropriate lactation or galactorrhea. The mechanism whereby elevated PRL levels interfere with gonadotropin release appears to be related to abnormal gonadotropin-releasing hormone (GnRH) release. Women with hyperprolactinemia have abnormalities in the frequency and amplitude of LH pulsations, with

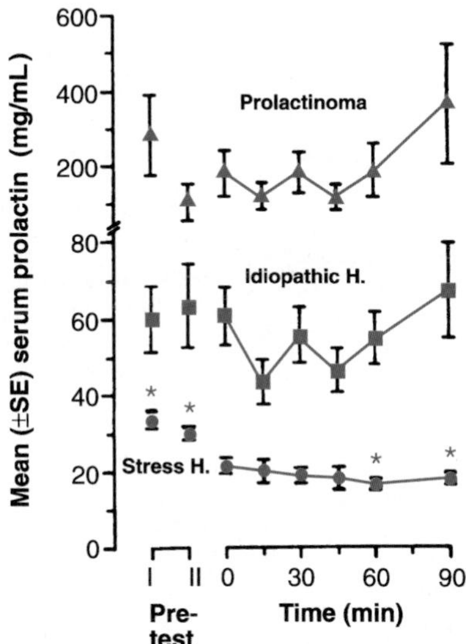

Figure 39-2. Mean plus or minus standard error (± SE) serum prolactin levels in women with prolactinoma (N = 20) and idiopathic (N = 30) and stress-related (N = 20) hyperprolactinemia before (pretest I and II) and during hyperprolactinemia test. Differences (*$p < 0.01$) are in relation to time zero values. (Mean prolactin values among groups were also significantly different [$p < 0.01$] at all times.) (From Muneyyirci-Delale O, Goldstein D, Reyes FI, et al: Diagnosis of stress-related hyperprolactinemia: evaluation of the hyperprolactinemia rest test. NY State J Med 89:205, 1989.)

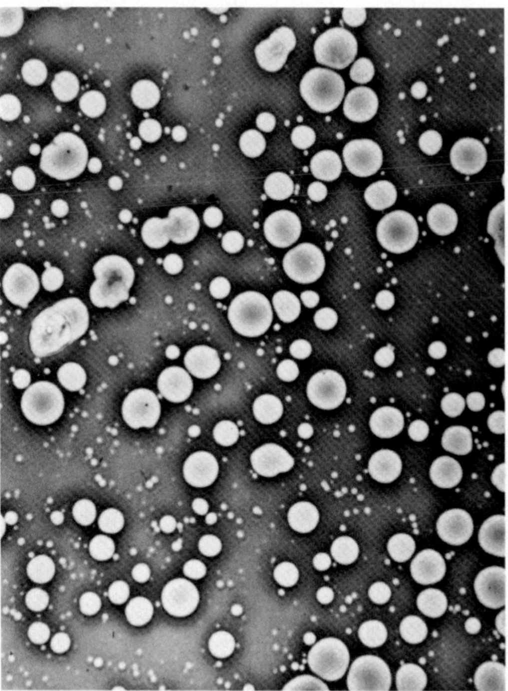

Figure 39-3. Fat droplets seen under microscope from a patient with galactorrhea. (From Kletzky OA, Davajan V: Hyperprolactinemia: Diagnosis and treatment. In Mishell DR, Davajan V, Lobo RA [eds]: Infertility, Contraception and Reproductive Endocrinology, 3rd ed. Cambridge, MA, Blackwell Scientific Publications, 1991.)

a normal or increased gonadotropin response following GnRH infusion.

This abnormality of GnRH cyclicity thus inhibits gonadotropin release but not its synthesis. The reason for this abnormal secretion of GnRH is an inhibitory effect of dopamine opioid peptides at the level of the hypothalamus. In addition, elevated PRL levels have been shown to interfere with the positive estrogen effect on midcycle LH release. It has also been shown that elevated levels of PRL directly inhibit basal as well as gonadotropin-stimulated ovarian secretion of both estradiol and progesterone. However, this mechanism is probably not the primary cause of anovulation, because women with hyperprolactinemia can have ovulation induced with various agents, including pulsatile GnRH. Some women with moderate hyperprolactinemia as determined by radioimmunoassay have a greater than normal proportion of the big-big forms. Because of the reduced bioactivity of this form of PRL, these individuals can have normal pituitary and ovarian function.

The clinician should measure serum PRL levels in all women with galactorrhea, as well as those with oligomenorrhea and amenorrhea without the presence of an elevated level of follicle-stimulating hormone (FSH). Hyperprolactinemia has been reported to be present in 15% of all anovulatory women and 20% of women with amenorrhea of undetermined cause. Galactorrhea is defined as the nonpuerperal secretion from the breast of watery or milky fluid that contains neither pus nor blood. The fluid may appear spontaneously or after palpation. To determine if galactorrhea is present, the clinician should palpate the breast, moving from the periphery toward the nipple in an attempt to express any secretion. The diagnosis of galactorrhea can be confirmed by observing multiple fat droplets in the fluid when it is examined under low-power magnification (Fig. 39-3). The incidence of galactorrhea in women with hyperprolactinemia has been reported to range from 30% to 80%, and these differences probably reflect variations in the techniques used to detect mammary excretion. Unless there has been continued breast stimulation after a pregnancy, the presence of galactorrhea serves as a biologic indicator that the PRL level is abnormally elevated. Davajan and associates reported that 62% of women with galactorrhea have hyperprolactinemia. Some individuals with galactorrhea and normal immunoassayable PRL levels may have elevated biologically active PRL. The incidence of hyperprolactinemia is higher (88%) in those women with galactorrhea who have amenorrhea and low estrogen levels than in those women with galactorrhea and normal estrogen levels (49%), regardless of menstrual status.

ETIOLOGY

Pathologic causes of hyperprolactinemia, in addition to a PRL-secreting pituitary adenoma (prolactinoma) and other pituitary tumors that produce acromegaly and Cushing's disease, include hypothalamic disease, various pharmacologic agents, hypothyroidism, chronic renal disease, or any chronic type of breast nerve stimulation, such as may occur with thoracic operation, herpes zoster, or chest trauma. The following box provides a list of the various causes of hyperprolactinemia.

One of the most frequent causes of galactorrhea and hyperprolactinemia is the ingestion of pharmacologic agents, particularly tranquilizers, narcotics, and antihypertensive agents (see the following box). Of the tranquilizers, the phenothiazines and

Causes of Hyperprolactinemia

Pituitary Disease
Prolactinomas
Acromegaly
"Empty sella syndrome"
Lymphocytic hypophysitis
Cushing's disease

Hypothalamic Disease
Craniopharyngiomas
Meningiomas
Dysgerminomas
Nonsecreting pituitary adenomas
Other tumors
Sarcoidosis
Eosinophilic granuloma
Neuraxis irradiation
Vascular
Pituitary stalk section

Medications
See next box

Neurogenic
Chest wall lesions
Spinal cord lesions
Breast stimulation

Other
Pregnancy
Hypothyroidism
Chronic renal failure
Cirrhosis
Pseudocyesis
Adrenal insufficiency
Ectopic
Polycystic ovary syndrome
Idiopathic

From Molitch ME: Prolactinoma. In Melmed S (ed): The Pituitary, 2nd ed. Malden, MA, Blackwell Publishing, 2002, pp 455–495.

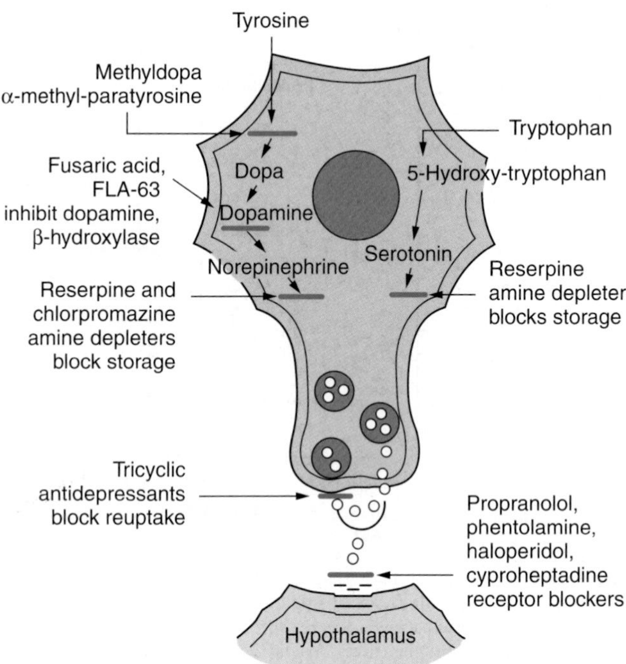

Figure 39-4. Schematic representation of inhibitory effects of drugs on synthesis and release of neurotransmitters. (From Kletzky OA, Davajan V: Hyperprolactinemia: Diagnosis and treatment. In Mishell DR, Davajan V, Lobo RA [eds]: Infertility, Contraception and Reproductive Endocrinology, 3rd ed. Cambridge, MA, Blackwell Scientific Publications, 1991.)

diazepam can produce hyperprolactinemia either by depleting the hypothalamic circulation of dopamine or by blocking its binding sites and thus decreasing dopamine action (Fig. 39-4). The tricyclic antidepressants block dopamine uptake, and propranolol, haloperidol, phentolamine, and cyproheptadine block hypothalamic dopamine receptors. The antihypertensive agent reserpine depletes catecholamines, and methyldopa blocks the conversion of tyrosine to dihydroxyphenylalanine (dopa). Ingestion of oral contraceptive steroids can also increase PRL levels, with a greater incidence of hyperprolactinemia occurring with higher estrogen formulations. Nevertheless, galactorrhea does not usually occur during oral contraceptive ingestion because the exogenous estrogen blocks the binding of PRL to its receptors.

Women who develop galactorrhea while ingesting oral contraceptives or any of the other drugs just listed should ideally discontinue the medication, and PRL should be measured 1 month thereafter to determine if the level has returned to normal. If the medication cannot be discontinued, the PRL level should be measured, and if it is elevated above 100 ng/mL, imaging of the sella turcica should be performed to determine whether a macroadenoma is present.

Primary hypothyroidism can also produce hyperprolactinemia and galactorrhea because of decreased negative feedback of thyroxine (T_4) on the hypothalamic–pituitary axis. The resulting increase in TRH stimulates PRL secretion as well as thyroid-stimulating hormone (TSH) secretion from the pituitary. About 3% to 5% of individuals with hyperprolactinemia have hypothyroidism, and thus TSH, the most sensitive indicator of hypothyroidism, should be measured in all individuals with hyperprolactinemia. If the TSH level is elevated, triiodothyronine (T_3) and T_4 should be measured to confirm the diagnosis of primary hypothyroidism, as occasionally a TSH-secreting pituitary adenoma will be present. Treatment with appropriate thyroid replacement usually returns the TSH and PRL levels to normal within a short time.

Hyperprolactinemia can occur in those individuals with abnormal renal disease resulting from decreased metabolic clearance as well as increased production rate. The cause of the latter is not known.

Mild hyperprolactinemia (30 to 50 ng/mL) may occur in women with PCOS. This occurs in up to 30% of women and may be related to the chromic state of unopposed estrogen stimulation.

Central Nervous System Disorders

Hypothalamic Causes

Diseases of the hypothalamus that produce alterations in the normal portal circulation of dopamine can result in hyperprolactinemia. Such diseases include craniopharyngioma and infiltration of the hypothalamus by sarcoidosis, histiocytosis, leukemia, or carcinoma. All these conditions are rare, with craniopharyngioma being the most common. These tumors arise from remnants of Rathke's pouch along the pituitary stalk. Grossly they can be cystic, solid, or mixed, and calcification is usually visible on radiograph. They are most frequently diagnosed during the second and third decades of life and usually result in impairment of secretion of several pituitary hormones.

Pituitary Causes

Various types of pituitary tumors, lactotroph hyperplasia, and the empty sella syndrome can be associated with hyperprolactinemia. It has been estimated that as many as 80% of all pituitary adenomas secrete PRL. The most common pituitary tumor associated with hyperprolactinemia is the prolactinoma, arbitrarily defined as a microadenoma if its diameter is less than 1 cm and as a macroadenoma if it is larger. Hyperprolactinemia has been reported to occur in about 25% of individuals with acromegaly and 10% of those with Cushing's disease, indicating that these pituitary adenomas, which mainly secrete growth hormone (GH) and adrenocorticotropic hormone (ACTH), frequently also secrete PRL. Hyperplasia of lactotrophs has been reported to occur in about 8% of pituitary glands examined at autopsy. Individuals with hyperplasia of the lactotrophs cannot be distinguished from those having a microadenoma by any clinical, laboratory, or radiologic method. It is a diagnosis that can be made only at the time of surgical exploration of the pituitary gland. Pituitary enlargement with suprasellar extension caused by lactotroph hyperplasia has been reported. *Functional hyperprolactinemia* is the term used for the clinical diagnosis of cases of elevated PRL levels without evidence of an adenoma. This condition may occur because of decreased dopamine inhibition or the presence of an adenoma that is too small to be visualized.

Another cause of hyperprolactinemia is the primary empty sella syndrome. The term *primary empty sella syndrome* describes a clinical situation in which an intrasellar extension of the subarachnoid space results in compression of the pituitary gland and an enlarged sella turcica. The cause is believed to result from a congenital or acquired (by radiation or surgery) defect in the sella diaphragm that allows the subarachnoid membrane to herniate into the sella turcica (Fig. 39-5). The syndrome is usually associated with normal pituitary function except for hyperprolactinemia. Although some individuals with primary empty sella syndrome have a coexistent prolactinoma, Gharib and colleagues reported a series of 11 persons with an empty sella and hyperprolactinemia who had no histologic evidence of a prolactinoma or hyperplasia of the lactotrophs. They stated that about 5% of individuals with the empty sella have hyperprolactinemia or amenorrhea–galactorrhea or both. It is theorized that with this syndrome distortion of the infundibular stalk results in decreased levels of dopamine reaching the pituitary to inhibit PRL. Serum PRL levels are usually less than 100 ng/mL with the empty sella syndrome, and some women with this syndrome have galactorrhea with normal PRL levels. Kleinberg and coworkers reported that about 10% of all individuals with an enlarged sella turcica have the empty sella syndrome. The best modality for diagnosing this condition is magnetic resonance imaging (MRI). Computed tomographic (CT) scanning with intrathecal injection of metrizamide can also be used. It is important to establish the diagnosis because the syndrome has a benign course.

Pharmacologic Agents Affecting Prolactin Concentrations

Stimulators

- Anesthetics including cocaine
- Psychoactive
  - Phenothiazines
  - Tricyclic antidepressants
  - Opiates
  - Chlordiazepoxide
  - Amphetamines
  - Diazepams
  - Haloperidol
  - Fluphenazine
  - Chlorpromazine
  - SSRIs
- Hormones
  - Estrogen
  - Oral-steroid contraceptives
  - Thyrotropin-releasing hormone
- Antihypertensives
  - α-Methyldopa
  - Reserpine
  - Verapamil
- Dopamine receptor antagonists
  - Metoclopramide
- Antiemetics
  - Sulpride
  - Promazine
  - Perphenazine
- Others
  - Cimetidine
  - Cyproheptiadine
  - Protease inhibitors

Inhibitors

- L-Dopa
- Dopamine
- Bromocriptine
- Pergolide
- Cabergoline
- Depot bromocriptine

SSRIs, selective serotonin reuptake inhibitors.
From Shoupe D, Mishell DR Jr: Hyperprolactinemia: Diagnosis and treatment. In Lobo RA, Mishell DR Jr, Paulson RJ, Shoupe D (eds): Mishell's Textbook of Infertility, Contraception and Reproductive Endocrinology, 4th ed. Cambridge, MA, Blackwell Scientific Publications, 1997.

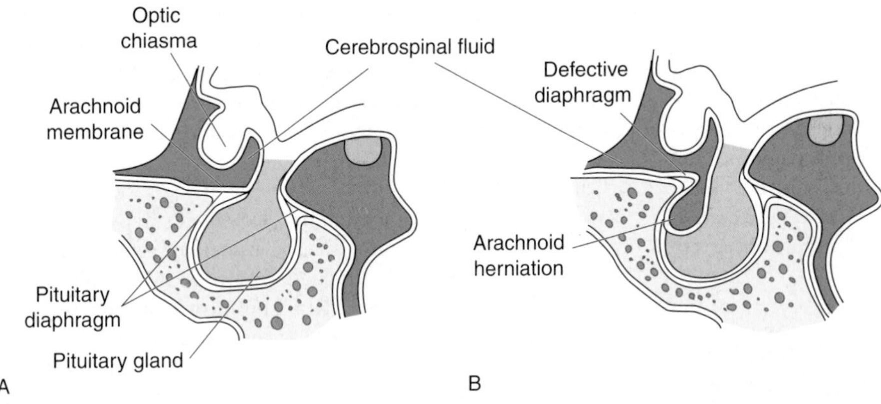

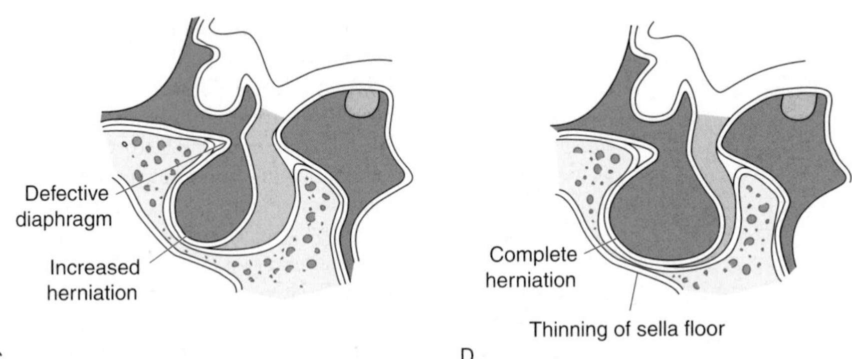

Figure 39-5. Diagrammatic representation of empty sella syndrome. **A,** Normal anatomic relationship. **B, C,** and **D,** Progression in development of empty sella syndrome. Note thinning of floor and symmetrical enlargement of sella turcica. (From Kletzky OA, Davajan V: Hyperprolactinemia: Diagnosis and treatment. In Mishell DR, Davajan V, Lobo RA [eds]: Infertility, Contraception and Reproductive Endocrinology, 3rd ed. Cambridge, MA, Blackwell Scientific Publications, 1991.)

Prolactinomas

In an unselected series of 120 autopsies of persons who had had no clinical evidence of pituitary disease, Burrow and associates found pituitary microadenomas to be present in 32 (27%). More recently Molitch described that PRL incidentalomas occur in 11% of subjects at autopsy. Abd El-Hamid and colleagues also reported that adenomas were found in 78 of 486 (16%) pituitary glands examined after unselected autopsies. In all series PRL was found in about half the glands, indicating that more than 1 in 10 individuals in the general population have a prolactinoma.

Overall about 50% of women with hyperprolactinemia have a prolactinoma. The incidence is higher when the PRL levels exceed 100 ng/mL, and nearly all individuals with PRL levels greater than 200 ng/mL have a prolactinoma. The vast majority of prolactinomas in women are microadenomas. Kleinberg and coworkers reported that overall 20% of individuals with galactorrhea and 35% of women with amenorrhea–galactorrhea had radiologic evidence of pituitary tumors. Tumors are also present in about 20% of women with hyperprolactinemia and menstrual irregularities without galactorrhea. The incidence of prolactinoma is greater in those individuals with a more profound disturbance of normal hypothalamic–pituitary–ovarian function. Davajan and associates reported that 70% of women with hyperprolactinemia, galactorrhea, and secondary amenorrhea with low estrogen levels had radiologic evidence of a pituitary adenoma. Evidence of a tumor occurred in only 20% to 30% of those with hyperprolactinemia and normal menses, oligomenorrhea, or secondary amenorrhea who had sufficient estrogen to undergo withdrawal bleeding after progesterone administration. In both these studies no evidence of tumor was found in individuals with normal menses, galactorrhea, and normal PRL levels. Therefore radiologic studies do not need to be performed if galactorrhea is present and PRL levels are normal.

Figure 39-6 depicts various possible causes of prolactinoma formation. In the past it was firmly believed that adenomas or hyperplasia were the result of hypothalamic dopamine dysregulation, which was either a functional defect or the result of altered blood supply. Current thinking is that adenomas arise from single cell mutations, with clonal proliferation occurring subsequently. However, a search for mutations in oncogenes, the dopamine D2 or TRH receptor, signal transduction mechanisms or transcription factors have not been very rewarding to date. Prolactinomas that occur in 20% of patients with multiple endocrine neoplasia type 1 (MEN-1) may be due to an inactivating mutation of the *MENIN* gene, although this special case is clearly different from the usual type of prolactinomas.

It is also important to note that prolactinomas may also secrete other hormones; GH is the most frequent combination. Also, up to 40% of GH-secreting adenomas also secrete PRL. Combinations of PRL and ACTH, PRL and TSH, and PRL and FSH have been described.

Long-term studies of individuals with microadenomas demonstrate that enlargement is uncommon and that many of these tumors regress spontaneously. In a longitudinal retrospective study of 43 women with hyperprolactinemia and a radiologic

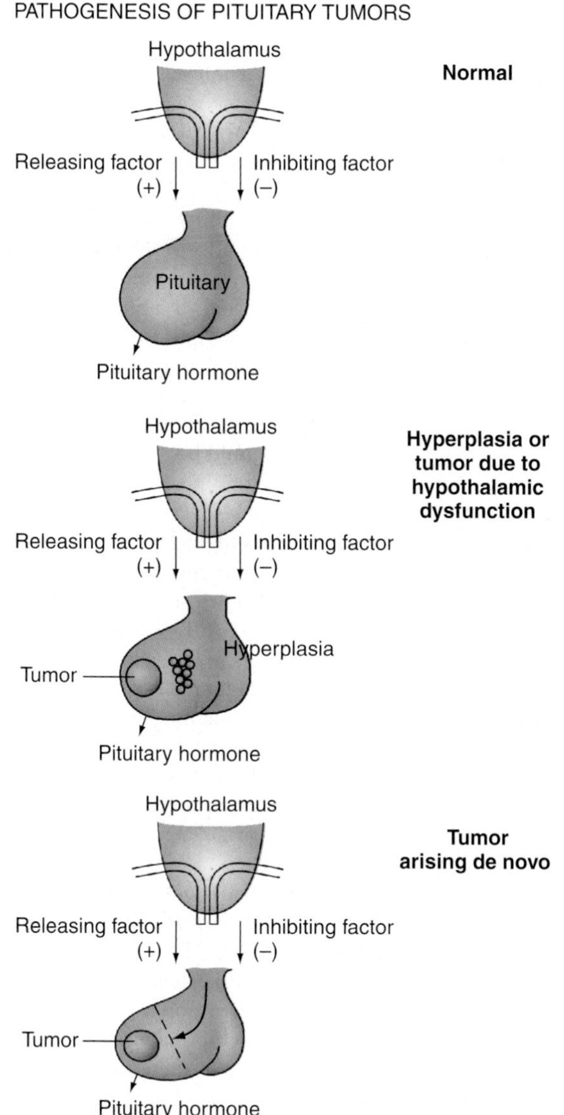

Figure 39-6. Possible mechanisms leading to the formation of a prolactinoma. Top: normal regulation. Middle: tumors could arise because of an increase in PRL-releasing factor (PRF) or a decrease in PRL-inhibiting factor (dopamine). Bottom: tumors could arise de novo without hypothalamic influence. (From Molitch ME: Clinical features and epidemiology of prolactinomas in women. In Olefsky JM, Robbins RJ [eds]: Prolactinomas: Practical Diagnosis and Management. New York, Churchill Livingstone, 1986, pp 67–95.)

diagnosis of microadenoma, March and colleagues found that only 2 women had evidence of enlargement of the adenoma, with a mean duration of follow-up of 5 years. Of these 43 women, 3 had spontaneous regression of their hyperprolactinemia and resumption of normal menses. Koppelman and coworkers reported similar results. Of 25 women with prolactinomas (18 with microadenomas and 7 with minimally enlarged sella) followed up for a mean duration of 11 years without treatment, only 1 woman had slight progression of a sella abnormality. None had visual field or other pituitary function changes, seven resumed normal menses spontaneously, and galactorrhea spontaneously resolved in six.

The results of these retrospective studies have been confirmed by two prospective studies of untreated microprolactinomas. In a 3- to 7-year prospective longitudinal study of 30 hyperprolactinemic women, Schlechte and associates found that of 13 women with initially abnormal radiographic findings, 4 became normal, 7 did not change, and 2 had evidence of tumor growth. Of 17 women with initially normal radiographic findings, 4 became minimally abnormal. None of the 30 developed a macroadenoma or pituitary hypofunction. In this study, as in the two retrospective studies just reported, more sensitive radiographic techniques (tomograms, followed by CT) were used as the study progressed and could account for the minimal evidence of tumor growth. Sisam and colleagues overcame this problem by prospectively following a group of 38 women with hyperprolactinemia and microprolactinomas by serial CT scans for a mean duration of 50 months. None of these women had evidence of tumor progression, even the 2 who had a marked increase in PRL levels. In this group, nine (25%) had spontaneous improvement of their symptoms. Martin and coworkers followed the natural history of 41 women with idiopathic hyperprolactinemia and amenorrhea–galactorrhea for up to 11 years. During this time, 9 women conceived spontaneously, and 16 have resumed spontaneous menses with cessation of galactorrhea. Only one woman developed a microadenoma. Thus, hyperprolactinemia with or without a microadenoma follows a benign clinical course in most women, and therapy is unnecessary unless pregnancy is desired or estrogen levels are low.

The combination of six studies in 139 women observed for at least 8 years without treatment showed that the progression rate is only 6.5%. Several studies have reported that pregnancy is beneficial for women with functional hyperprolactinemia or PRL-secreting microadenomas. Following pregnancy, PRL levels decrease in about half the women. Crosignani and associates reported that PRL levels became normal in about 30% of 176 hyperprolactinemic women after pregnancy. PRL levels decreased to normal in 36% of women with functional hyperprolactinemia and 17% of those with adenomas. Therefore if women with hyperprolactinemia desire to become pregnant they should be encouraged to do so, as pregnancy is likely to result in normal or lowered PRL levels.

DIAGNOSTIC TECHNIQUES

Because most prolactinomas are microadenomas that do not cause enlargement of the sella turcica, the diagnosis usually cannot be made by ordinary anteroposterior and lateral coned X-ray examination of the sella turcica. With the development of more precise radiologic methods of detecting soft tissue pituitary abnormalities, it is now possible to detect even small adenomas.

Initially detection of microadenomas was accomplished by obtaining tomographic radiographic examination of the sella turcica at intervals of 2 to 3 mm in the anteroposterior and lateral projections with a hypocycloidal movement. These are called *hypocycloidal tomograms.* Comparing the results of tomograms with the findings of microadenoma at autopsy, Burrow and coworkers found that the incidence of both false-positive and false-negative tomographic findings was about 20% each, with an overall accuracy rate of 61%. Furthermore, radiation exposure with polytomography may be in excess of 20 rads.

Current recommended techniques are to obtain a CT scan with IV contrast, or an MRI with gadolinium enhancement. The latter provides better soft tissue definition, and the CT scan principally shows bony structural abnormalities.

The MRI provides 1-mm resolution and thus should be able to detect all microadenomas. Stein and associates compared results of CT and MRI in 22 individuals with suspected pituitary adenomas. MRI was found to be the superior diagnostic modality because of its greater soft tissue contrast (Fig. 39-7). In addition the MRI does not have the radiation exposure of the CT scan (23 rads, 0.03 Gy).

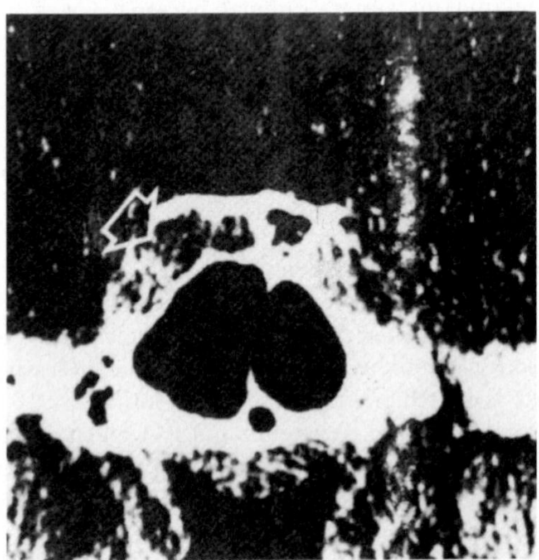
A

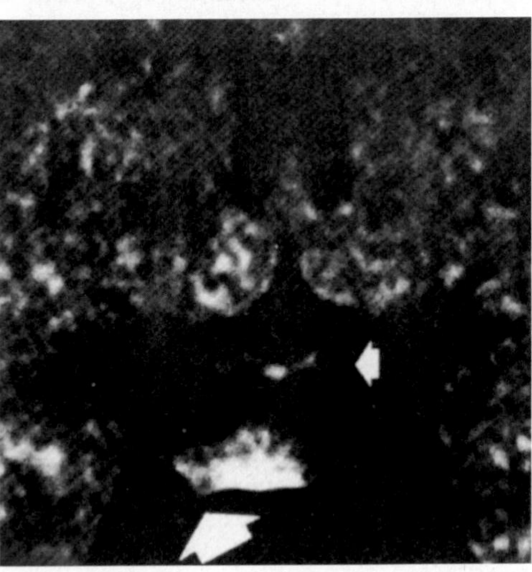
B

Figure 39-7. Images were selected to best demonstrate pathology and do not exactly correspond in level of section through sella turcica. **A,** CT scan (coronal section) showing bony erosion of right sella turcica (*arrowhead*) with possible soft tissue extension into right cavernous sinus. Height of pituitary gland (not shown) is 9 mm. **B,** MRI (coronal section) showing soft tissue mass extending into right cavernous sinus near carotid artery *(large arrowhead).* Height of pituitary gland is 9 mm. Normal optic chiasm is seen *(small arrowhead).* (From Stein AL, Levenick MN, Kletzky OA: Computer tomography versus magnetic resonance imaging for the evaluation of suspected pituitary adenomas. Obstet Gynecol 73:996, 1989.)

Recommended Diagnostic Evaluation

It is currently recommended that PRL levels be measured in all women with galactorrhea, oligomenorrhea, or amenorrhea who do not have an elevated FSH level. If PRL is elevated, a TSH assay should be performed to rule out the presence of primary hypothyroidism. If TSH is elevated, T_3 and T_4 should be measured to rule out the rare possibility of a TSH-secreting pituitary adenoma. If TSH is elevated and hypothyroidism is present, appropriate thyroid replacement should begin, and the PRL level will usually return to normal. If TSH is normal and the woman has a normal PRL level with galactorrhea, no further tests are necessary if she has regular menses. Because some women with galactorrhea, abnormal menstrual function, and normal PRL levels have been found to have the empty sella syndrome, an MRI or a CT scan should be obtained to establish the diagnosis in women with these findings.

If PRL levels are elevated and the TSH is normal, an MRI if available or CT scan should be obtained to detect a microadenoma or macroadenoma. Macroadenomas are uncommon and rarely are present with a PRL level less than 100 ng/mL. If the PRL level is more than 100 ng/mL or the woman complains of headaches or visual changes, the likelihood of a tumor extending beyond the sella turcica is increased. Microadenomas are a common cause of hyperprolactinemia, but rarely enlarge. Neither pregnancy, oral contraceptives, nor hormone replacement therapy stimulates the growth of these small tumors, and therapy is unnecessary unless ovulation induction is desired or hypoestrogenism is present.

Visual field determination and tests of ACTH and thyroid function are not necessary if a microadenoma is present, as these small tumors do not interfere with overall pituitary function and do not extend beyond the sella. However, these evaluations should be performed in individuals with macroadenomas because suprasellar extension of the tumor may exert pressure on the optic chiasm, resulting in bitemporal visual field defects and interference with vision. The size of these tumors may also affect other aspects of pituitary function. Thus a test of ACTH reserve, such as insulin-induced hypoglycemia (insulin tolerance test), as well as tests of thyroid function, should be performed on all individuals with a macroadenoma.

MANAGEMENT

Expectant Treatment

Women with radiologic evidence of a microadenoma or functional hyperprolactinemia who do not wish to conceive may be followed without treatment by measuring PRL levels once yearly. Many of these women have deficient estrogen, and low estrogen levels in combination with hyperprolactinemia have been shown to be associated with the early onset of osteoporosis. If the woman has low estrogen levels, exogenous estrogen should be administered. Either replacement estrogen–progestin therapy, as is used for postmenopausal women, or oral contraceptives can be utilized. Corenblum and Donovan reported that a group of women with both functional hyperprolactinemia and PRL-secreting pituitary microadenomas who were treated with either cyclic estrogen and progestin or oral contraceptives for several years did not have an increase in the size of the adenomas or a marked increase in PRL levels. Mean PRL levels actually declined with both treatment regimens. Testa reported that 2 years of oral contraceptive use in a group of women with hyperprolactinemia with microadenoma did not alter the size of the adenoma. Since side effects and cost are less and compliance is better with exogenous estrogen than with bromocriptine, it is not necessary to use the latter agent unless ovulation and pregnancy are desired. Individuals with hyperprolactinemia with or without microadenomas who have adequate estrogen levels as shown by the presence of oligomenorrhea or amenorrhea with follicular phase estradiol levels who do not wish to conceive should be treated with periodic progestin withdrawal (e.g., medroxyprogesterone acetate 5–10 mg/day for 10 days each month) or combination oral contraceptives to prevent endometrial hyperplasia.

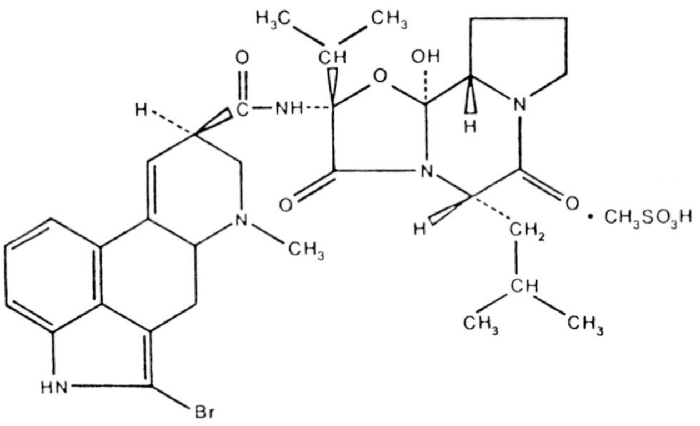

Figure 39-8. Formula of bromocriptine.

Medical Therapy

The initial treatment for macroadenomas, as well as for women with hyperprolactinemia who are anovulatory and wish to conceive, should be administration of a dopamine receptor agonist. Bromocriptine, pergolide, and cabergoline have been used with success for treating hyperprolactinemia; bromocriptine and cabergoline are approved for use in the United States). The greatest amount of clinical experience has been with use of bromocriptine (Fig. 39-8). This semisynthetic ergot alkaloid was developed in 1967 to inhibit PRL secretion. It directly stimulates dopamide 2 receptors, and as a dopamine receptor agonist it inhibits PRL secretion both in vitro and in vivo. After ingestion, bromocriptine is rapidly absorbed, with blood levels reaching a peak 1 to 3 hours later. Serum PRL levels remain depressed for about 14 hours after ingestion of a single dose, after which time the drug is not detectable in the circulation. For this reason the drug is usually given at least twice daily, with initial therapy being started at one half of the 2.5-mg tablet to minimize side effects. The most frequent side effects are orthostatic hypotension (with an incidence of 15%), which can produce fainting and dizziness as well as nausea and vomiting. To minimize these symptoms the initial dose should be taken in bed and with food at nighttime. Less frequent adverse symptoms include headache, nasal congestion, fatigue, constipation, and diarrhea. Most of these reactions are mild, occur early in the course of treatment, and are transient. To reduce the adverse symptoms, the dose should be gradually increased every 1 to 2 weeks until PRL levels fall to normal. The usual therapeutic dose is 2.5 mg twice or three times a day, but larger doses are sometimes used when a macroadenoma is present.

Adverse effects, such as nausea, vomiting, and nasal congestion, occur in about half the women taking oral bromocriptine and may cause them to discontinue treatment. Vermesh and colleagues reported that the drug was very well absorbed vaginally without the presence of side effects. Furthermore, when a single tablet was placed deep in the posterior vaginal fornix, therapeutic blood levels persisted for more than 24 hours, during which time PRL levels remained suppressed (Fig. 39-9). Ginsburg and coworkers subsequently reported that this method of bromocriptine administration was well accepted, effective, and well tolerated in a group of 31 hyperprolactinemic women, 17 of whom could not tolerate oral bromocriptine. Minor side effects occurred in only three women. The tablet is placed digitally deep in the vagina nightly at bedtime. A single 2.5-mg dose reduced PRL concentrations in 90% of patients treated and brought the levels to normal in one third of women. Higher doses do not appear to be more effective. Ginsburg and coworkers recommended that the drug be administered vaginally instead of orally for all women as a smaller dose of drug can be

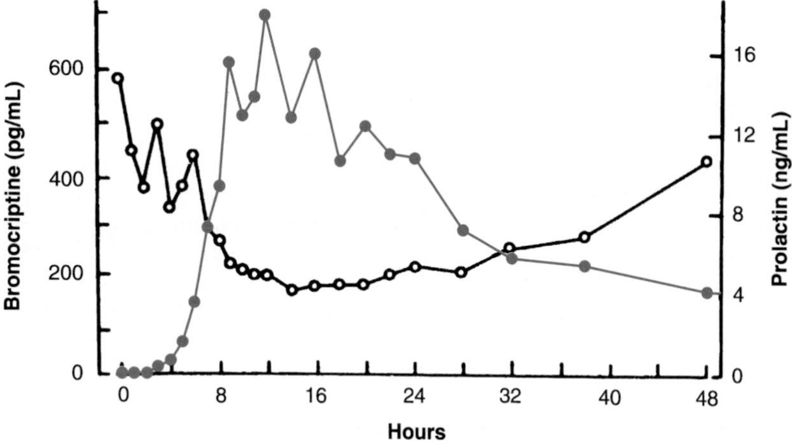

Figure 39-9. Mean (± SEM) plasma levels of bromocriptine *(blue circles)* and prolactin *(open circles)* in a single study, extended to 48 hours, after vaginal bromocriptine (2.5 mg). (From Vermesh M, Fossum GT, Kletzky OA: Vaginal bromocriptine: Pharmacology and effect on serum prolactin in normal women. Obstet Gynecol 72:693, 1988.)

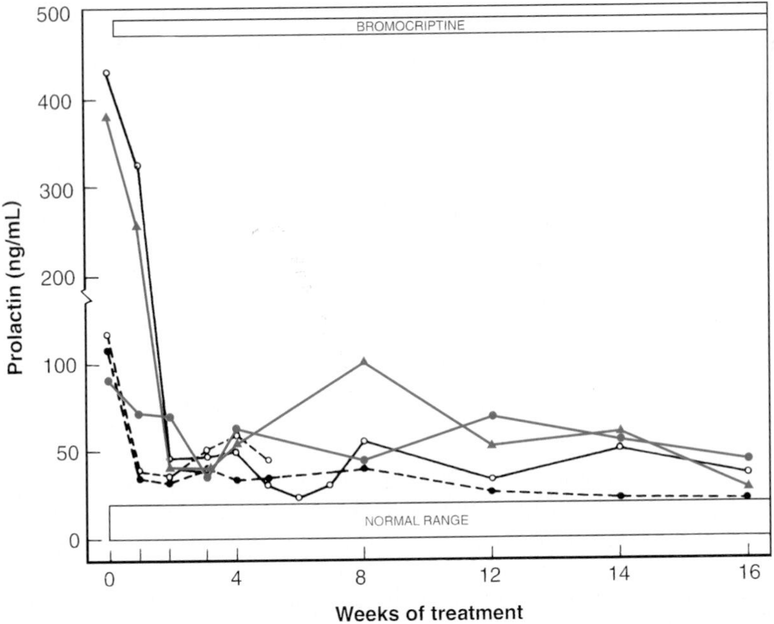

Figure 39-10. Mean serum prolactin response to bromocriptine therapy in five patients with radiographic evidence of pituitary adenoma and residual hyperprolactinemia. All five ovulated, and four conceived. (From Kletzky OA, Marrs RP, Davajan V: Management of patients with hyperprolactinemia and normal or abnormal tomograms. Am J Obstet Gynecol 147:528, 1983.)

used, once-daily administration is more convenient, and side effects are fewer.

Bromocriptine is approved for treatment of adverse symptoms associated with hyperprolactinemia, such as galactorrhea, as well as anovulatory infertility with and without the presence of a PRL-secreting adenoma. In hyperprolactinemic women without adenomas, PRL levels return to normal in more than 90%, fertility is restored in 80%, and galactorrhea is eradicated in 60% with bromocriptine therapy. In women with hyperprolactinemia and a microadenoma, similar rates of success have been reported. Therefore, a dopamine agonist such as bromocriptine or cabergoline is the treatment of choice for women with PRL-secreting microadenomas who wish to ovulate or are bothered by galactorrhea.

Despite administration of up to 20 mg of bromocriptine per day orally, about 10% of individuals with microadenomas fail to have PRL levels return to normal, probably because of individual differences in the sensitivity of lactotrophs to bromocriptine. Nevertheless, despite the persistently elevated PRL levels, many of these women ovulate and conceive (Fig. 39-10).

If pregnancy occurs after ovulation is induced with bromocriptine, therapy is usually discontinued, although there is no evidence that the drug is teratogenic or adversely affects pregnancy outcome. If pregnancy is not desired but bromocriptine is used to treat galactorrhea, therapy is usually continued for at least 12 months, after which it should be discontinued for a few weeks. Most women with microadenomas have recurrence of hyperprolactinemia, amenorrhea, and galactorrhea, although about 10% to 20% have permanent remission after discontinuing bromocriptine treatment. Moriondo and associates reported that after 1 year of bromocriptine treatment, 11% of women with microadenomas had persistent normalization of PRL, with return of regular menses after the drug was discontinued (Fig. 39-11). This incidence of permanent remission reached 22% after 2 years of treatment. A higher rate of permanent remission occurred in women treated with 10 mg/day than with lower dosages, but higher doses of drug increase the incidence of adverse reactions and cause discontinuation of treatment. These investigators found that after bromocriptine was discontinued, there was a 40% reduction in mean PRL levels in all women treated, and about 60% had a greater than 30% reduction from pretreatment PRL levels after the drug was discontinued. Rasmussen and colleagues reported the results of discontinuation of long-term (median of 2 years) bromocriptine therapy in 75 hyperprolactinemic women. In about half the women it was necessary to reinstate treatment because PRL levels rose. However, in the other half further treatment was unnecessary because mean PRL levels decreased more than 60% and either returned to normal or were only slightly elevated (Fig. 39-12). More than half of these 33 women resumed regular menses without further treatment. These data indicate that the remissions were drug-related and not spontaneous. Using CT scans before and during bromocriptine therapy, Bonneville and coworkers found that about 75% of individuals with microadenomas had reduction in tumor size during bromocriptine treatment, and in 40% the tumor had disappeared (Fig. 39-13). To determine if permanent remission has occurred, the PRL level should be measured about 6 weeks after discontinuation of treatment because the levels plateau at this time.

Bromocriptine treatment has also been shown to reduce tumor mass in 80% to 90% of individuals with macroadenomas. In addition, visual disturbances, if present, are usually promptly relieved. Following subsequent surgical removal of these bromocriptine-treated tumors, histologic examination revealed a reduction of tumor cell size, with shrinkage of the cytoplasm being greater than the nucleus. In addition, there are modifications of cell structure and morphology as compared with tumors removed without prior medical treatment. The organelles responsible for PRL synthesis shrink, indicating that bromocriptine impairs PRL synthesis as well as release. The reduction in size of macroadenomas usually occurs rapidly, within a few weeks after starting treatment, but following withdrawal of drug the

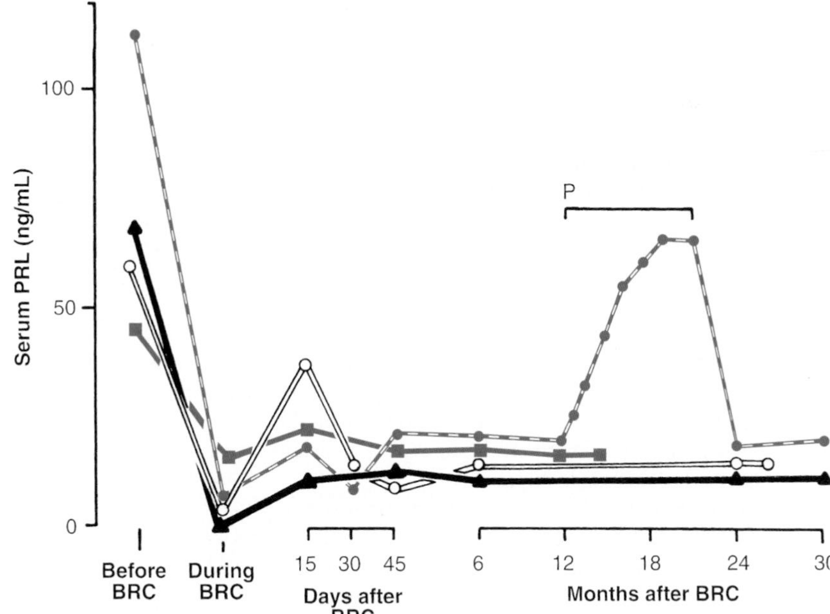

Figure 39-11. Serum prolactin levels in four patients who had persistently normal prolactin levels after bromocriptine *(BRC)* treatment for 12 months. *P,* Pregnancy. (From Moriondo P, Travaglini P, Nissim M, et al: Bromocriptine treatment of microprolactinomas: Evidence of stable prolactin decrease after drug withdrawal. J Clin Endocrinol Metab 60:764, 1985. © Copyright 1985 by The Endocrine Society.)

tumor size may increase just as rapidly; thus the drug should be withdrawn cautiously. In contrast to the frequent occurrence of pituitary insufficiency, including diabetes insipidus, after surgical or radiologic treatment of large tumors, bromocriptine treatment is not accompanied by any type of pituitary insufficiency.

Because permanent remission rarely occurs following withdrawal of bromocriptine treatment from individuals with large tumors, long-term treatment is usually necessary. The drug has been administered in some individuals for up to 12 years without problems, and once biochemical, radiologic, and clinical responses to treatment are established, they are generally maintained over a long-term period. Bromocriptine has also been successfully used to treat individuals with failure of, or recurrence after, operation or irradiation therapy.

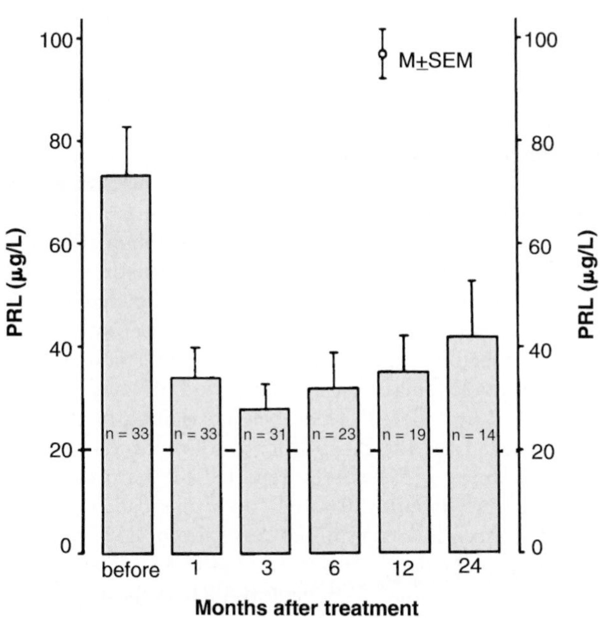

Figure 39-12. Geometric mean serum prolactin levels before and after discontinuation of bromocriptine treatment in 33 women with hyperprolactinemic amenorrhea. (Reprinted from Fertility and Sterility, 48, Rasmussen C, Bergh T, Wide L, Prolactin secretion and menstrual function after long-term bromocriptine treatment, 550. Copyright 1987, with permission from The American Society for Reproductive Medicine.)

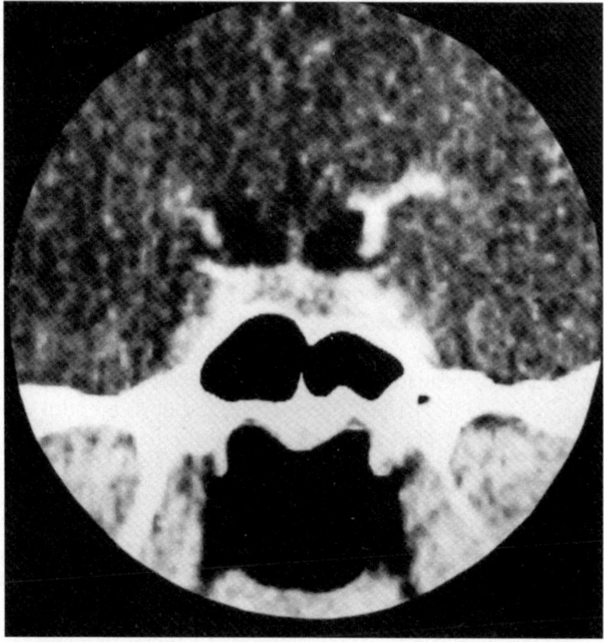

Figure 39-13. Coronal CT scan of a woman with microadenoma 4 months after bromocriptine therapy (5 mg per day). Clinical and biologic results were excellent; pituitary gland is nearly normal, with reconstruction of sellar floor. (From Bonneville JF, Poulignot D, Cattin F, et al: Computed tomographic demonstration of the effects of bromocriptine on pituitary microadenoma size. Radiology 143:451, 1982.)

Molitch and associates reported the results of a 1-year prospective multicenter study of the use of bromocriptine as primary therapy for PRL-secreting macroadenomas in 27 individuals. Bromocriptine dosage ranged from 5 to 12.5 mg daily, with 7.5 mg being the most frequent dose. PRL levels fell in all individuals, and to 11% or less of pretreatment values in all but one. Of this group, two thirds had PRL levels decrease to normal during treatment. Tumor shrinkage was observed in all individuals, being reduced by more than 50% in half the patients and by about 50% in an additional 20% of the study group. Visual field impairment disappeared in 9 of the 10 individuals with abnormalities. In two thirds of the individuals reduction in tumor size occurred by 6 weeks, but in one third it was not evident until 6 months, indicating there were both rapid and slow responses of tumor to drug treatment. Therefore at least a 6-month trial of medical therapy is warranted for individuals with a macroadenoma.

Because of these excellent results, the poor initial results of operation, and the high recurrence rates, these investigators concluded that bromocriptine should be used as the initial management of individuals with PRL-secreting macroadenomas. After maximal shrinkage of tumor, medical therapy can be continued or operative treatment used. The cost of continuing bromocriptine treatment is considerable; it is inconvenient to take medication several times a day, and some individuals have unpleasant side effects with the higher dosages that may be necessary. Therefore some individuals prefer operative treatment. If they elect to have an operation, the drug should be continued until the time of operation to prevent tumor expansion. The rates of success after operation are no different among individuals who received or did not receive bromocriptine before the operation.

Cabergoline is a long-acting dopamine receptor agonist. This agent directly inhibits pituitary lactotrophs, thereby decreasing PRL secretion. It is given orally in doses of 0.25–1.0 mg twice a week. The initial dose is half a 0.5-mg tablet twice a week. Peak plasma levels occur in 2 to 3 hours, and this drug has a half-life of 65 hours. Its slow elimination and long half-life produces a prolonged PRL-lowering effect. The initial dose is 0.25 mg twice weekly and the dosage may be increased at intervals of 4 weeks to achieve a satisfactory response. In a randomized trial with bromocryptine, cabergoline lowered PRL levels to normal in 83% of women, induced ovulation in 72%, and eliminated galactorrhea in 90%. The effectiveness of cabergoline was greater than that of bromocryptine. Adverse effects, particularly nausea, headaches, and dizziness, occurred with both agents but were less frequent, less severe, and of shorter duration with cabergoline. Therefore cabergoline is better tolerated than bromocryptine and has higher continuation rates. Recent evidence suggests that cabergoline is more effective in lowering PRL than bromocryptine. Even in patients who had been treated previously with bromocryptine, cabergoline has been found to be effective (Table 39-1).

Cabergoline has been compared with other agents in effectiveness for reducing tumor size (see Table 39-1). It may be concluded that in women who have never been treated, cabergoline is currently the agent of choice for reducing PRL levels and effecting tumor shrinkage. It is recommended that after serum PRL levels have remained normal for 6 months cabergoline be discontinued to determine if the PRL levels stay low without therapy.

Table 39-1 Comparison of Efficacy of Dopamine Agonists in Affecting Tumor Size Reduction*

Dopamine Agonist	Number of Cases	TUMOR SIZE REDUCTION >50%	25%–50%	<25%	No Change
Bromocriptine	112	40.2%	28.6%	12.5%	18.7%
Pergolide	61	75.4%	9.8%	8.2%	6.5%
Quinagolide	105	48.1%	20.2%	17.3%	14.4%
Cabergoline	130	25.4%	46.9%	6.9%	21.5%

*It should be noted that in many of the studies of pergolide, quinagolide, and cabergoline, many of the patients had previously been found to be resistant to or intolerant of bromocriptine.

Adapted from Molitch ME: Prolactin in human reproduction. In Strauss JF III, Barbieri R (eds): Yen and Jaffe's Reproductive Endocrinology. Philadelphia, Elsevier, 2004, p 109.

Operative Approaches

Transsphenoidal microsurgical resection of prolactinoma has been widely used for therapy, and numerous reports of large series of individuals treated by this technique have been published. In general, transsphenoidal operations have minimal risk, with a mortality of less than 0.5%; however, the majority of deaths have been reported to occur after treatment of macroadenomas. The risk of temporary postoperative diabetes insipidus is 10% to 40%, but the risk of permanent diabetes insipidus and iatrogenic hypopituitarism is less than 2%. The initial cure rate, with normalization of PRL levels and return of ovulation, is relatively high for microadenomas (65% to 85%) and less so with macroadenomas (20% to 40%). Vision can return to normal in 85% of patients with loss of acuity and visual field defects.

The initial cure rate is related to the pretreatment PRL levels. Those tumors with levels less than 100 ng/mL have an excellent prognosis (85%), and those with levels greater than 200 ng/mL have a poor prognosis (35%). Operative treatment of tumors in individuals older than 26 with amenorrhea for more than 6 months carries a poorer prognosis than tumors in younger women with a shorter duration of amenorrhea. Nevertheless, long-term follow-up of patients after operation indicates that late recurrence of hyperprolactinemia is common. Serri and colleagues followed 28 women with microadenomas and 16 with macroadenomas for 6 years after operation. Although PRL levels normalized and menses resumed in 24 (85%) of those with microadenomas and 5 (31%) of those with macroadenomas who had a good initial postoperative response, hyperprolactinemia recurred in half of those with microadenoma and 4 of the 5 with macroadenomas after a mean period of 4 and 2.5 years, respectively (Fig. 39-14). There was no significant difference in recurrence rates for those who conceived and those who did not. Rodman and coworkers reported a lower postoperative recurrence rate (about 20% for both microadenomas and macroadenomas) following initial cure rates of 85% and 37%, respectively. The risk of recurrence in both series appeared to be related to the immediate postoperative PRL levels, being greater in persons with a PRL level greater than 10 ng/mL.

Overall it can be concluded that after surgery, recurrence rates for micro- or macroadenoma are similar (21% and 19.8%, respectively). Long-term surgical cure rates are 58% of microadenomas and only 26% macroadenomas using a normal PRL level as a criterion.

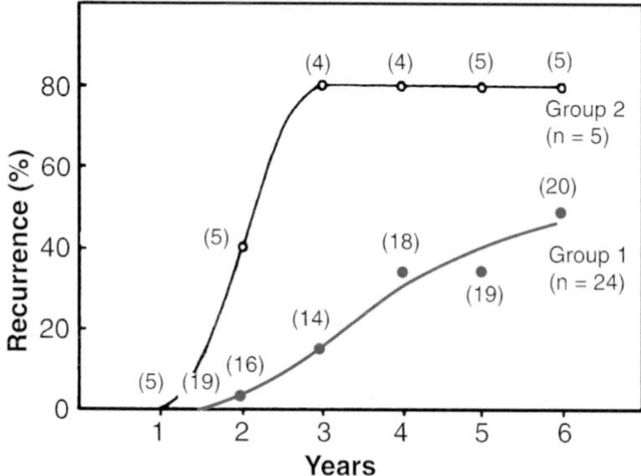

Figure 39-14. Cumulative recurrence rate in patients with microprolactinoma (group 1) or macroprolactinoma (group 2) after initially successful operation. Figures in parentheses indicate numbers of patients who were seen at each yearly interval. (From Serri O, Rasio E, Beauregard H, et al: Recurrence of hyperprolactinemia after selective transsphenoidal adenomectomy in women with prolactinoma. N Engl J Med 309:280, 1983. Copyright 1983 Massachusetts Medical Society. All rights reserved.)

Because of the good results with medical therapy, surgery is recommended only for women with macroadenoma who fail to respond to medical therapy or have poor compliance with this regimen. It is best to reduce the size of macroadenomas maximally with bromocriptine before surgical removal of these extrasellar tumors.

Radiation Therapy

External radiation with cobalt, proton beam, or heavy-particle therapy and brachytherapy with yttrium-90 rods implanted in the pituitary have all been used to treat macroadenomas but are not the primary mode of treatment. Results of such therapy have been inconsistent, and there is a delay of several months between treatment and resumption of ovulation. Furthermore, damage to normal pituitary tissue occurs, frequently leading to abnormal anterior pituitary function as well as diabetes insipidus. Damage to the optic nerves may also occur. Thus radiation therapy should be used only as adjunctive management following incomplete operative removal of large tumors.

Pregnancy

Many women with hyperprolactinemia with or without adenomas wish to become pregnant. A small percentage of these women conceive spontaneously, but most require treatment to induce ovulation. Barbieri and Ryan compiled a literature review of the pregnancy courses of 275 women with adenomas, the majority of whose conceptions had been induced by bromocriptine. They reported that of 215 women with microprolactinomas, less than 1% had changes in visual fields, radiologic evidence of tumor enlargement, or neurologic signs. About 5% developed headaches during pregnancy. Of 60 women with macroprolactinomas, 20% developed adverse changes in visual fields and polytomographic or neurologic signs during pregnancy, and some of them required bromocriptine or operative treatment during pregnancy or shortly postpartum. Overall, although only 1.4% of women with microadenomas have symptoms during pregnancy, 24.4% of women with macroadenomas have symptoms. However, only about 3% of women with macroadenomas have symptoms if they are treated prior to pregnancy. For this reason excision of macroprolactinomas before pregnancy has been recommended in some cases. Nevertheless, because pituitary function is usually diminished after operation, induction of ovulation must be performed with complicated and expensive gonadotropin treatment. Bromocriptine treatment does not interfere with pituitary function and is thus the therapy of choice for women with macroadenomas who wish to conceive. Continuous bromocriptine treatment throughout pregnancy for women with macroadenomas has been recommended by some, because with this therapy visual disturbances are rare. Despite a lowering of PRL levels, there is no effect on placental hormone production, and pregnancy outcome does not appear to be affected.

Nevertheless, since bromocriptine crosses the placenta and suppresses fetal PRL levels, its long-term effects on the newborn are unknown. Therefore it is now advised that women with macroadenomas discontinue the drug after conception (as is the case for those with microadenomas) and have therapy reinitiated if and when symptoms of visual disturbance or severe headaches occur. Most women who conceive after bromocriptine treatment have ingested the drug for a few weeks after conception. In a review of 1410 such pregnancies compiled by Turkalj and associates there was a spontaneous abortion rate of 11%, ectopic pregnancy rate of 0.7%, and twin pregnancy rate of 1.8%. The incidence of minor (2.5%) and major (1%) congenital defects was similar to pregnancy outcomes in untreated populations of women. The mean amount of drug ingested and duration of postconception treatment were similar in mothers who had normal children and those with defects. Thus ingestion of bromocriptine during pregnancy does not appear to increase the risk of congenital abnormalities, spontaneous abortion, or multiple gestation. Postnatal surveillance of more than 200 children born in this series has revealed no adverse effects to date.

Ruiz-Velasco and Tolis compiled the obstetric histories of nearly 2000 pregnancies occurring in hyperprolactinemic women that have been reported in the literature. Most of these pregnancies were induced with bromocriptine. There was a full-term delivery rate of 85%, an abortion rate of 11%, a prematurity rate of 2%, and a multiple pregnancy rate of 1.2%. Although PRL levels increased during pregnancy, after delivery the levels returned to pretreatment values in about 85%. A postpartum increase over pretreatment levels was uncommon (3%), and PRL levels returned to normal in 13%. Likewise, among women who had postpartum radiologic sellar examination, 84% showed no change, 9% improved, and 7% worsened. Thus stopping treatment during pregnancy only occasionally results in tumor growth. It is advised that women with macroadenomas have monthly visual field examination and neurologic testing during pregnancy, but this is probably unnecessary for women with microadenomas unless they develop symptoms of headache or visual disturbances.

Following delivery, breast-feeding may be initiated without adverse effects on the tumors. Godo and associates reported that use of bromocriptine before conception and during pregnancy did not affect the incidence of persistent lactation following discontinuation of nursing. The incidence of menstrual abnormalities and degree of galactorrhea were usually similar to the state that existed before starting bromocriptine therapy. Therefore, following completion of nursing, as well as for women who do not breast-feed at all, bromocriptine should be ingested for 2 to 3 weeks and then discontinued. At that time serum PRL measurement should be performed and treatment reinstituted according to the findings.

Women with Hyperprolactinemia Who Do Not Wish to Conceive

For women who do not wish to conceive and for whom galactorrhea is not a problem, no therapy is necessary unless estrogen levels are low. Thus, to prevent osteoporosis in this clinical situation, estrogen–progestin hormone replacement or oral contraceptives should be given regardless of whether an adenoma is present. Long-term evaluation of all women with hyperprolactinemia should be performed. Unless a macroadenoma is present, measurement of PRL levels once a year is advisable. Repeat imaging studies are unnecessary unless symptoms of headaches or visual disturbances occur or PRL levels increase substantially. If bromocriptine therapy is used, temporary discontinuation of medication every year is advisable, with PRL measurement 6 weeks later. If the level is normal, repeat PRL measurements should be made semiannually. If the level is increased, therapy may be reinitiated. During medical treatment of macroadenomas, MRI or CT and visual field examination should be performed every 6 months to determine the effect of medication on the tumor. At these intervals a decision can be made about whether to continue long-term bromocriptine treatment or to remove the tumor surgically.

KEY POINTS

- Estrogen stimulates PRL release but blocks its action at the receptor in the breast.
- Physiologic stimuli for PRL release include breast and nipple palpation, exercise, stress, sleep, and the noonday meal.
- The main symptoms of hyperprolactinemia are galactorrhea and amenorrhea, the latter caused by alterations in normal gonadotropin-releasing hormone (GnRH) release.
- Hyperprolactinemia is present in 15% of all anovulatory women and 20% of women with amenorrhea of undetermined cause.
- About 60% of all women with galactorrhea have hyperprolactinemia, but almost 90% of women with galactorrhea, amenorrhea, and low estrogen levels have hyperprolactinemia.
- Pathologic causes of hyperprolactinemia include pharmacologic agents (tranquilizers, narcotics, and antihypertensive drugs), hypothyroidism, chronic renal disease, chronic neurostimulation of the breast, hypothalamic disease, and pituitary tumors (prolactinoma, acromegaly, Cushing's disease).
- About 3% to 5% of individuals with hyperprolactinemia have hypothyroidism.
- About 80% of all pituitary tumors secrete PRL.
- About 25% of individuals with acromegaly and 10% of those with Cushing's disease have hyperprolactinemia.
- About 10% of individuals with an enlarged sella have the empty sella syndrome.
- Autopsy studies reveal that prolactinomas are present in about 10% of the population.
- About 50% of women with hyperprolactinemia will have a prolactinoma, as will nearly all of those with PRL levels greater than 200 ng/mL.
- About 20% of women with galactorrhea and 35% of those with amenorrhea and galactorrhea have prolactinomas.
- About 70% of women with hyperprolactinemia, galactorrhea, and amenorrhea with low estrogen levels will have a prolactinoma.
- Women with regular menses, galactorrhea, and normal PRL levels do not have prolactinomas.
- About 13% of women with prolactinomas do not have galactorrhea.
- Most macroadenomas enlarge with time; nearly all microdenomas do not.
- The initial operative cure rate for microadenomas is about 80% and for macroadenomas 30%, but the long-term recurrence rate is at least 20% for each.
- Most frequent side effects of bromocriptine are orthostatic hypotension, nausea, and vomiting.
- In women with hyperprolactinemia and no macroadenoma, bromocriptine treatment returns PRL levels to normal in 90%, induces ovulatory cycles in 80%, and eradicates galactorrhea in 60%.
- After 1 year of bromocriptine treatment, PRL levels remain normal in 11% of women with microadenomas; after 2 years permanent remission reaches 22%. After longer use, remissions of 50% have been reported.
- Bromocriptine shrinks 80% to 90% of macroadenomas.
- When pregnancy occurs in women with microadenomas, less than 1% have visual field changes, tumor enlargement, or neurologic signs; about 20% of women with macroadenomas have such adverse changes.
- Pregnancy increases the likelihood that PRL levels will decrease or become normal over time.
- Estrogen replacement therapy or oral contraceptives will not stimulate growth of PRL-secreting microadenomas and can be used for therapy of hyperprolactinemia and hypoestrogenism.
- Bromocriptine induction of pregnancy is not associated with an increased risk of congenital abnormalities, spontaneous abortion, or multiple gestation.
- About 85% of patients with prolactinomas have no change in PRL levels or tumor size after delivery, 10% improve, and 5% worsen.
- The most frequent cause of mildly elevated PRL levels is stress.

KEY POINTS *Continued*

- The best modality to diagnose pituitary adenomas or empty sella syndrome is MRI.
- The natural history of nearly all microprolactinomas is to stay the same size, with adverse menstrual problems resolving spontaneously in about one fourth of patients.
- Surgical treatment of prolactinomas is recommended only for patients who fail to respond or do not comply with medical management.
- For women who develop side effects with oral bromocriptine, vaginal administration usually alleviates the problem.
- Cabergoline appears to be more effective and better tolerated than bromocriptine.

BIBLIOGRAPHY

Abd El-Hamid MW, Joplin EF, Lewis PD: Incidentally found small pituitary adenomas may have no effect on fertility. Acta Endocrinol (Copenh) 117:361, 1988.

Ampudia X, Pulig-Domingo M, Schwarzstein D, et al: Outcome and long-term effects of pregnancy in women with hyperprolactinaemia. Eur J Obstet Gynecol Reprod Biol 46:101, 1992.

Asa S: Pathology of pituitary adenomas. Endocrinol Metab Clin North Am 28:13, 1999.

Bäckstrüm CT, McNeilly AS, Leash RM, et al: Pulsatile secretion of LH, FSH, prolactin oestradiol and progesterone during the human menstrual cycle. Clin Endocrinol 17:29, 1982.

Barbieri RL, Ryan KJ: Bromocriptine: endocrine pharmacology and therapeutic applications. Fertil Steril 39:727, 1983.

Biller BMK, Molitch ME, Vance ML, Cannistraro KB, et al: Treatment of prolactin-secreting macroadenomas with the once-weekly dopamine agonist cabergoline. J Clin Endocrinol Metab 81:2338, 1996.

Bonneville JF, Poulignot D, Cattin F, et al: Computed tomographic demonstration of the effects of bromocriptine on pituitary microadenoma size. Radiology 143:451, 1982.

Burrow GN, Wortzman G, Rewcastle NB, et al: Microadenomas of the pituitary and abnormal sellar tomograms in an unselected autopsy series. N Engl J Med 304:156, 1981.

Ciccarelli E, Giusti M, Miola C, et al: Effectiveness and tolerability of long-term treatment with cabergoline, a new long-lasting ergoline derivative, in hyperprolactinemic patients. J Clin Endocrinol Metab 69:725, 1989.

Ciccarelli E, Miola C, Avateneo T, et al: Long-term treatment with a new repeatable injectable form of bromocriptine, Parlodel LAR, in patients with tumorous hyperprolactinemia. Fertil Steril 52:930, 1989.

Corenblum B, Donovan L: The safety of physiological estrogen plus progestin replacement therapy and with oral contraceptive therapy in women with pathological hyperprolactinemia. Fertil Steril 59:671, 1993.

Corenblum B, Taylor PJ: Long-term follow-up of hyperprolactinemic women treated with bromocriptine. Fertil Steril 40:596, 1983.

Crosignani PG, Mattei AM, Scarduelli C, et al: Is pregnancy the best treatment for hyperprolactinemia? Hum Reprod 4:910, 1989.

Crosignani PG, Mattei AM, Severini V, et al: Long-term effects of time, medical treatment and pregnancy in 176 hyperprolactinemic women. Eur J Obstet Gynecol Reprod Biol 44:175, 1992.

Davajan V, Kletzky O, March CM, et al: The significance of galactorrhea in patients with normal menses, oligomenorrhea, and secondary amenorrhea. Am J Obstet Gynecol 130:894, 1978.

Fahy UM, Foster PA, Torode HW, et al: The effect of combined estrogen/progestogen treatment in women with hyperprolactinemic amenorrhea. Gynecol Endocrinol 6:183, 1992.

Gharib H, Frey HM, Laws ER Jr, et al: Coexistent primary empty sella syndrome and hyperprolactinemia: report of 11 cases. Arch Intern Med 143:1383, 1983.

Ginsburg J, Hardiman P, Thomas M: Vaginal bromocriptine: clinical and biochemical effects. Gynecol Endocrinol 6:119, 1992.

Godo G, Kolosziar S, Szilagyi I, et al: Experience related to pregnancy, lactation, and the after-weaning condition of hyperprolactinemic patients treated with bromocriptine. Fertil Steril 51:529, 1989.

Kleinberg DL, Noel GL, Frantz AG: Galactorrhea: a study of 235 cases, including 48 with pituitary tumors. N Engl J Med 296:589, 1977.

Kletsky OA, Vermesh M: Effectiveness of vaginal bromocriptine in treating women with hyperprolactinemia. Fertil Steril 51:269, 1989.

Klibanski A. Further evidence for a somatic mutation theory in the pathogenesis of hyman pituitary tumors. J Clin Endocrinol Metab 71;1415, 1990.

Koppelman MCS, Jaffe MJ, Rieth KG, et al: Hyperprolactinemia, amenorrhea, and galactorrhea: A retrospective assessment of 25 cases. Ann Intern Med 100:115, 1984.

March CM, Kletzky OA, Davajan V, et al: Longitudinal evaluation of patients with untreated prolactin-secreting pituitary adenomas. Am J Obstet Gynecol 139:835, 1981.

Martin TL, Kim M, Malarkey WB: The natural history of idiopathic hyperprolactinemia. J Clin Endocrinol Metab 60:855, 1985.

Melmed S: Pathogenesis of pituitary tumors. Endocrinol Metab Clin North Am 28:1, 1999.

Molitch ME, Elton RL, Blackwell RE, et al: Bromocriptine as primary therapy for prolactin-secreting macroadenomas: Results of a prospective multicenter study. J Clin Endocrinol Metab 60:698, 1985.

Molitch ME: Pituitary incidentalomas. Endocrinol Metab Clin North Am 26:727, 1997.

Moriondo P, Travaglini P, Nissim M, et al: Bromocriptine treatment of microprolactinomas: Evidence of stable prolactin decrease after drug withdrawal. J Clin Endocrinol Metab 60:764, 1985.

Mornex R, Hugues B: Remission of hyperprolactinemia after pregnancy. N Engl J Med 324:60, 1991.

Muneyyirci-Delale O, Goldstein D, Reyes FI, et al: Diagnosis of stress-related hyperprolactinemia: evaluation of the hyperprolactinemia rest test. NY State J Med 89:205, 1989.

Rasmussen C, Bergh T, Wide L: Prolactin secretion and menstrual function after long-term bromocriptine treatment. Fertil Steril 48:550, 1987.

Rasmussen C, Bergh T, Nillius SJ, and Wide L: Return of menstruation and normalization of prolactin in hyperprolactinemic women with bromocriptine-induced pregnancy. Fertil Steril 44:31, 1985.

Rodman EF, Molitch ME, Post KD, et al: Long-term follow-up of transsphenoidal selective adenomectomy for prolactinoma. JAMA 252:921, 1984.

Ruiz-Velasco V, Tolis G: Pregnancy in hyperprolactinemic women. Fertil Steril 41:793, 1984.

Schlechte J, Dolan K, Sherman B, et al: The natural history of untreated hyperprolactinemia: A prospective analysis. J Clin Endocrinol Metab 68:412, 1989.

Serri O, Rasio E, Beauregard H, et al: Recurrence of hyperprolactinemia after selective transsphenoidal adenomectomy in women with prolactinoma. N Engl J Med 309:280, 1983.

Shoupe D, Mishell DR Jr: Hyperprolactinemia: Diagnosis and treatment. In Lobo RA, Mishell DR Jr, Paulson RJ, Shoupe D (eds): Mishell's Textbook of Infertility, Contraception and Reproductive Endocrinology, 4th ed. Blackwell Scientific Publications, Cambridge, MA, 1997.

Sisam DA, Sheehan JP, Sheeler LR: The natural history of untreated microprolactinomas. Fertil Steril 48:67, 1987.

Slujmer AV, Lappohn RE: Clinical history and outcome of 59 patients with idiopathic hyperprolactinemia. Fertil Steril 50:72, 1992.

Stein AL, Levenick MN, Kletzky OA: Computer tomography versus magnetic resonance imaging for the evaluation of suspected pituitary adenomas. Obstet Gynecol 73:996, 1989.

Testa G, Vegetti W, Motta T, et al: Two-year treatment with oral contraceptives in hyperprolactinemic patients. Contraception 58:69, 1998.

Turkalj I, Brain P, Krupp P: Surveillance of bromocriptine in pregnancy. JAMA 247:1589, 1982.

Vermesh M, Fossum GT, Kletzky OA: Vaginal bromocriptine: Pharmacology and effect on serum prolactin in normal women. Obstet Gynecol 72:693, 1988.

Webster J, Piscitelli G, Polli A, Ferrari CI, et al: A comparison of cabergoline and bromocriptine in the treatment of hyperprolactinemic amenorrhea. N Engl J Med 331:904, 1994.

Hyperandrogenism 40

Physiology, Etiology, Differential Diagnosis, Management

Rogerio A. Lobo

KEY TERMS AND DEFINITIONS

Acanthosis Nigricans. Dark, raised hyperpigmentation of the skin, found particularly on the nape of the neck and axilla.

5α-Androstane-3α,17β-diol Glucuronide (3α-diol-G). A metabolite of 5α-reductase conversion of testosterone (T) to dihydrotestosterone (DHT) that can be measured in serum and is the most accurate indicator of peripheral androgen metabolism.

Cryptic Hyperandrogenism. Elevated levels of circulatory androgens without clinical manifestations of hirsutism or acne. It is usually accompanied by anovulation.

Dehydroepiandrosterone Sulfate (DHEA-S). An androgen secreted nearly exclusively by the adrenal gland. Serum levels are used as a marker of adrenal androgen activity.

Free Androgen Index (ng/nmol). Measurement of biologically active testosterone, calculated as follows: total testosterone (ng/mL) times 1000 divided by sex hormone-binding globulin (SHBG) (nmol/L).

Free Testosterone. Small portion of circulating testosterone that is not bound to sex hormone-binding globulin or albumin.

Hilus Cell Tumor. Small testosterone-secreting ovarian tumors that most frequently develop after menopause.

Hirsutism. Presence of hair in locations where it is not normally found in a woman, specifically in the midline of the body (upper lip, chin, back, and intermammary region).

Hypertrichosis. A generalized increase in the amount of body hair in its normal location.

Idiopathic Hirsutism (Constitutional or Familial Hirsutism). This is an extremely common cause of hirsutism which is characterized by the findings of normal circulating androgens in otherwise normal ovulatory women. Hirsutism in these women is explained by an enhancement of the end organ (hair follicle) response to androgen; mostly because of enhanced 5α-reductase activity.

17-Ketosteroids. Urinary metabolites of DHEA, DHEA-S, androstenedione, and testosterone. They consist of DHEA, androsterone, and etiocholanolone.

Late-Onset Congenital Adrenal Hyperplasia/Late-Onset 21-Hydroxylase Deficiency (LOHD). Also called *late-onset hyperplasia,* nonclassic congenital adrenal hyperplasia attenuated, or acquired adrenal hyperplasia. Mild degree of enzymatic 21-hydroxylase deficiency of cortisol biosynthesis that produces signs of androgen excess after puberty without external sexual ambiguity being present at birth. This genetically acquired entity can be present in multiple forms depending on genetic factors.

Metformin. An oral antihyperglycemic agent that improves glucose tolerance by decreasing hepatic glucose production and other less clear effects which decreases serum insulin. This agent induces ovulation whether or not a woman is glucose-intolerant, probably through a direct ovarian effect

Nonsex Hormone-Binding Globulin Bound Testosterone. Biologically active component of circulatory testosterone, consisting of free testosterone and albumin-bound testosterone.

Pilosebaceous Unit. Structure in skin from which sebaceous glands and hair are derived. Found in the skin in every area of the body except the palms and soles.

Polycystic Ovarian Syndrome (PCOS). Probably the most common endocrine disorder in women. PCOS is classically characterized by the findings of irregular (anovulatory) cycles, symptoms or signs of androgen excess and polycystic ovaries on ultrasound. Newer criteria from a meeting in Rotterdam only require two of the three findings to establish the diagnosis. Although this is not universally accepted, the definition of PCOS can include women with normal ovulatory function

5α-Reductase. The enzyme that converts testosterone to its more active metabolite, dihydrotestosterone.

Sertoli–Leydig Cell Tumor. Testosterone-secreting ovarian tumor that usually is unilateral and palpably enlarged and occurs most frequently in the second to fourth decades of life. It was previously termed arrhenoblastoma.

Spironolactone. An aldosterone antagonist that acts as an antiandrogen by binding to the peripheral androgen receptor without inducing androgenic activity. It also inhibits steroidogenesis by interfering with ovarian enzymatic activity as well as inhibiting 5α-reductase activity in the pilosebaceous unit.

Stromal Hyperthecosis. An ovarian disorder characterized by nests of luteinized theca cells within the stroma of bilaterally enlarged ovaries. Clinically this condition is associated with slowly but progressively increasing signs of virilization.

Virilization. Presence of signs of masculinization in a woman. These signs include temporal balding, voice deepening, clitoral enlargement, and increased muscle mass.

The clinical signs associated with excessive androgen production in women include acne, hirsutism, alopecia, and rarely virilization.

These skin disorders may be understood by understanding the pilosebaceous unit. The pilosebaceous unit is composed of a sebaceous component and a pilary component from which the hair shaft arises. Abnormalities of the sebaceous component lead to acne and abnormalities of the pilary unit lead to excessive growth (hirsutism) or shedding (alopecia). There are two types of hair: Vellus hair is soft, fine, and unpigmented, whereas the terminal hair is coarse, thick, pigmented, and undergoes cyclic changes. *Anagen* is the growth phase of hair. It is followed by the transitional *catagen* phase and finally by a resting, or *telogen,* phase, after which the hair sheds. Androgen is necessary to produce development of terminal hair, and the duration of the anagen phase is directly related to the levels of circulating androgen.

The level of activity of the enzyme 5α-reductase in the hair follicle directly influences the level of androgenic effect on hair growth. With elevated levels of circulating androgen or increased activity of 5α-reductase, terminal hair appears where normally only vellus hair is present. With these alterations the length of the anagen phase is prolonged and the hair becomes thicker. Excessive 5α-reductase activity also may lead to acne as well as scalp hair loss (alopecia).

The presence of hirsutism without other signs of virilization is associated with relatively mild disorders of androgen production or increased 5α-reductase activity, and circulating testosterone levels are either normal or mildly to moderately elevated (less than 1.5 ng/mL). Hirsutism usually has a gradual onset and if unaccompanied by signs of virilization is not caused by a severe enzymatic defect or a neoplasm. The amount and location of the central hair growth found in women with hirsutism vary. In the milder forms hair is found only on the upper lip and chin, whereas with increasing severity it appears on the cheeks, chest (intermammary), abdomen (superior to the umbilicus), inner aspects of thighs, lower back, and intergluteal areas. The severity of the hirsutism can be roughly quantified by means of the scoring system of Ferriman and Gallwey (Fig. 40-1 and Table 40-1). Increased hair growth only on the extremities (hypertrichosis) should not be considered hirsutism, as terminal hair is normally found in this location in women. Women with hirsutism can have normal ovulatory menstrual cycles, oligomenorrhea, or amenorrhea.

Virilization is a relatively uncommon clinical finding, and its presence is usually associated with markedly elevated levels of circulating testosterone (≥2 ng/mL). In contrast to the gradual development of hirsutism, signs of virilization usually occur over a relatively short time. These signs are due to both the masculinizing and the defeminizing (antiestrogenic) action of testosterone and include temporal balding, clitoral hypertrophy, decreased breast size, dryness of the vagina, and increased muscle mass. Women with virilization are nearly always amenorrheic. The presence of androgen-secreting neoplasms should always be suspected in any woman who develops signs of virilization, particularly if the onset is rapid.

Table 40-1 Definition of Hair Gradings at 11 Sites*

Site	Grade	Definition
Upper lip	1	Few hairs at outer margin
	2	Small moustache at outer margin
	3	Moustache extending halfway from outer margin
	4	Moustache extending to midline
Chin	1	Few scattered hairs
	2	Scattered hairs with small concentrations
	3 & 4	Complete cover, light and heavy
Chest	1	Circumareolar hairs
	2	With midline hair in addition
	3	Fusion of these areas, with three-quarters cover
	4	Complete cover
Upper back	1	Few scattered hairs
	2	Rather more, still scattered
	3 & 4	Complete cover, light and heavy
Lower back	1	Sacral tuft of hair
	2	With some lateral extension
	3	Three-quarters cover
	4	Complete cover
Upper abdomen	1	Few midline hairs
	2	Rather more, still midline
	3 & 4	Half and full cover
Lower abdomen	1	Few midline hairs
	2	Midline streak of hair
	3	Midline band of hair
	4	Inverted V-shaped growth
Arm	1	Sparse growth affecting not more than one quarter of limb surface
	2	More than this; cover still incomplete
	3 & 4	Complete cover, light and heavy
Forearm	1, 2, 3, 4	Complete cover of dorsal surface; 2 grades of light and 2 of heavy growth
Thigh	1, 2, 3, 4	As for arm
Leg	1, 2, 3, 4	As for arm

*Grade 0 at all sites indicates absence of terminal hair.
From Ferriman D, Gallwey JD: Clinical assessment of body hair growth in women. J Clin Endocrinol Metab 21:1440, 1961. Copyright 1961 by The Endocrine Society.

PHYSIOLOGY

Androgen production in women can be discussed in terms of three separate sources of production: the ovaries and the adrenal glands, which are glandular sources, and the peripheral compartment, which comprises all extrasplanchnic and nonglandular areas of androgen production. The peripheral compartment includes many tissues, the largest of which is the skin. The peripheral compartment modulates androgens produced by the ovaries and the adrenals.

The sources of androgen glandular production are the ovaries and the adrenal glands. The major androgen produced by the ovaries is testosterone and that of the adrenal glands is dehydroepiandrosterone sulfate (DHEA-S). Measurement of the amount of these two steroids in the circulation provides clinically relevant information regarding the presence and source of increased androgen production. In addition to glandular production of androgens, conversion of androstenedione and DHEA to testosterone occurs in peripheral tissues.

The ovaries secrete only about 0.1 mg of testosterone each day, mainly from the theca–stroma cells. Other androgens secreted by the ovary are androstenedione (1 to 2 mg/day) and DHEA (<1 mg/day). The adrenal glands, in addition to secreting large quantities of DHEA-S (6 to 24 mg/day), secrete about the same daily amount of androstenedione (1 mg/day) as the ovaries and less than 1 mg of DHEA per day. The normal adrenal gland secretes little testosterone, although some uncommon adrenal tumors may secrete testosterone directly.

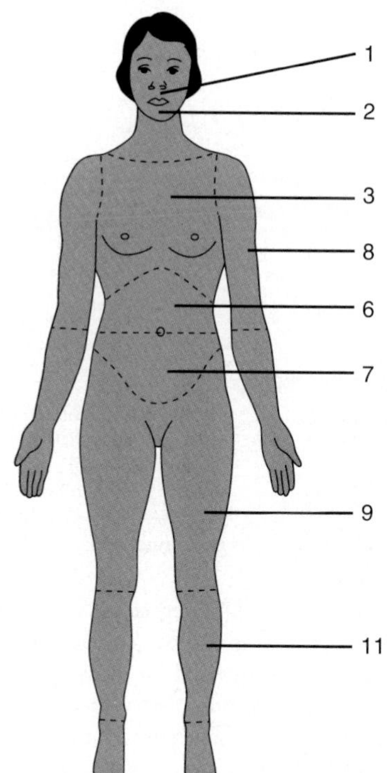

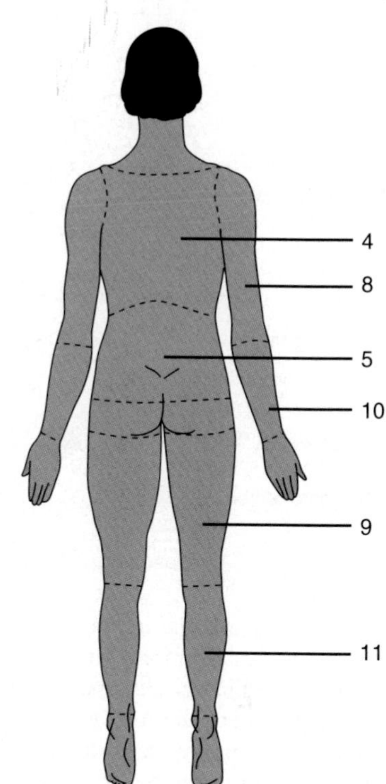

Figure 40-1. Demarcation of 11 sites used for numerically grading amount of hair growth-anterior and posterior views. (From Ferriman D, Gallwey JD: Clinical assessment of body hair growth in women. J Clin Endocrinol Metab 21:1440, 1961. Copyright 1961 by The Endocrine Society.)

Androstenedione and DHEA do not have androgenic activity but are peripherally converted at a slow rate to the biologically active androgen, testosterone. Only about 5% of androstenedione and a smaller percentage of DHEA are converted to testosterone. The total daily production of testosterone in women is normally about 0.35 mg. Of this, 0.1 mg comes from direct ovarian secretion, 0.2 mg from peripheral conversion of androstenedione, and 0.05 mg from peripheral conversion of DHEA (Table 40-2). Since the ovary and adrenal gland secrete about equal amounts of androstenedione and DHEA, about two thirds (0.22 mg) of the daily testosterone produced in a woman originates from the ovaries. Thus increased circulating levels of testosterone usually indicate abnormal ovarian androgen production. Normal circulating levels of these androgens in women of reproductive age are shown in Table 40-3. Only a small amount of testosterone is metabolized to testosterone glucuronide and then excreted in the urine. Testosterone, which is not a 17-ketosteroid (17-KS), is mainly metabolized to androstenedione and then excreted as androsterone and etiocholanolone, both of which are 17-KS. DHEA, DHEA-S, and androstenedione are excreted as DHEA, androsterone, and etiocholanolone, respectively, all of which are 17-KS. The origin of the major amount of urinary 17-KS is the precursor androgen produced in the greatest amounts, DHEA-S. Because DHEA-S has a long half-life in serum, serum levels of DHEA-S correlate well with amounts of 17-KS excreted in the urine. Urinary 17-KS levels were previously measured to assess adrenal androgenic activity. Now DHEA-S levels are measured directly in the serum.

For practical purposes circulatory levels of DHEA-S reflect an adrenal source of production in that in normal women more than 95% is adrenal-derived. Occasionally in women who have increased production of ovarian DHEA, such as in some women with polycystic ovary syndrome (PCOS), the elevated levels of DHEA-S might have an ovarian component as DHEA may be converted to DHEA-S in the circulation. Another very specific marker of adrenal androgen production, used for research purposes, is 11β-hydroxyandrostenedione.

Table 40-2 Origin of Testosterone in Women

Origin	Amount (mg/day)
Ovarian secretion	0–1
Peripheral conversion	
Androstenedione → testosterone	0.2
Dehydroepiandrosterone → testosterone	0.05
Total testosterone production	0.35

From Lobo RA: Androgen excess. In Mishell DR Jr, Davajan V, Lobo RA (eds): Infertility, Contraception and Reproductive Endocrinology, 3rd ed. Cambridge, MA, Blackwell Scientific, 1991.

Table 40-3 Plasma Concentrations of Androgens During Menstrual Cycle

Steroid Hormone	Phase of Cycle	PLASMA CONCENTRATION Mean	Range
Androstenedione (ng/mL)	*	1.4	0.7–3.1
Testosterone (ng/mL)	*	0.35	0.15–0.55
Dehydroepiandrosterone (ng/mL)	*	4.2	2.7–7.8
Dehydroepiandrosterone sulfate (μg/mL)	*	1.6	0.8–3.4

*Unspecified; no major changes during menstrual cycle.
From Goebelsmann U: Steroid hormones. In Mishell DR Jr, Davajan V (eds): Infertility, Contraception and Reproductive Endocrinology, 2nd ed. Oradell, NJ, Medical Economics Books, 1986.

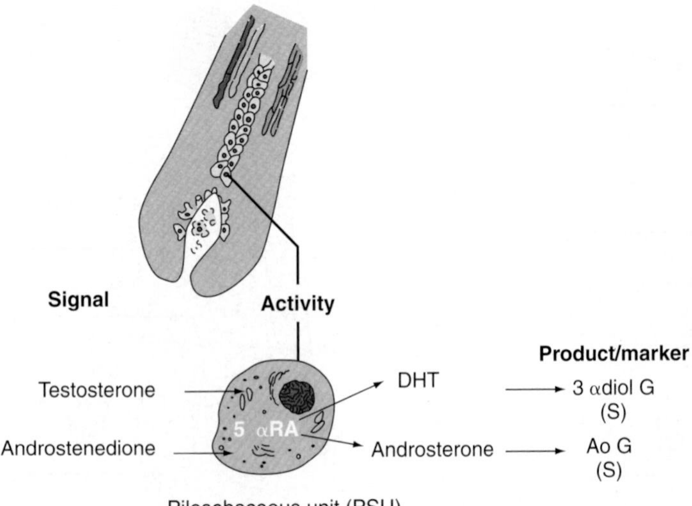

Figure 40-2. Peripheral androgen metabolism and markers of this activity. 5α RA, 5α-Reductase; DHT, dihydrotestosterone; 3α-diol-G, 3α-androstanediol glucuronide; Ao G, androsterone glucuronide; (S), serum. (From Lobo RA: Androgen excess. In Mishell DR Jr, Davajan V, Lobo RA [eds]: Infertility, Contraception and Reproductive Endocrinology, 3rd ed. Cambridge, MA, Blackwell Scientific, 1991.)

Most testosterone in the circulation (about 85%) is tightly bound to sex hormone-binding globulin (SHBG) and is believed to be biologically inactive. An additional 10% to 15% is loosely bound to albumin, with only about 1% to 2% not bound to any protein (free testosterone). Both the free and albumin-bound fractions are biologically active. Serum testosterone can be measured either as the total amount, the amount that is believed to be biologically active (non-SHBG bound), and as the free form.

To exert a biologic effect, testosterone is metabolized peripherally in target tissues to the more potent androgen 5α-dihydrotestosterone (DHT) by the enzyme 5α-reductase. After further 3-keto reduction, DHT is converted to its distal metabolite, 5α-androstane-3α,17β-diol (3α-diol). 3α-diol is conjugated to 5α-androstane-3α,17β-diol glucuronide (3α-diol-G), which is a stable, irreversible product of intracellular 5α-reductase activity (Fig. 40-2).

Even with normal circulatory levels of androgen, increased 5α-reductase activity in the pilosebaceous unit will result in increased androgenic activity, producing hirsutism (Fig. 40-3). We measured 5α-reductase activity in skin biopsies and found the level of activity correlated very well with the degree of hirsutism present.

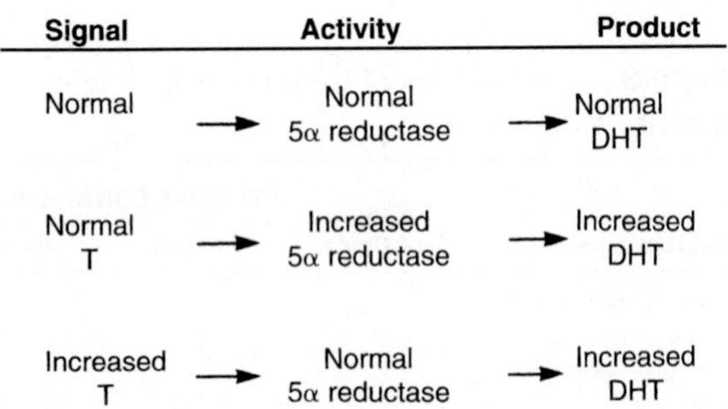

Figure 40-3. Influence of androgen substrate (signal, e.g., testosterone or androstenedione) and 5α-reductase activity (in pilosebaceous units) on local production of biologically active androgens. T, Testosterone; DHT, dihydrotestosterone. (From Lobo RA: Androgen excess. In Mishell DR Jr, Davajan V, Lobo RA [eds]: Infertility, Contraception and Reproductive Endocrinology, 3rd ed. Cambridge, MA, Blackwell Scientific, 1991.)

The degree of 5α-reductase activity can be measured in skin biopsies by a variety of methods. Currently this technique is only used for investigational purposes; if necessary for diagnostic reasons, 3-α-diol-G levels can be directly measured in serum. We have shown measurement of this metabolite to be the most accurate indicator of the degree of peripheral androgen metabolism in women. Although serum levels of total testosterone are similar in normal and hirsute women, there are significant differences in the amounts of non-SHBG-bound testosterone as well as 3α-diol-G (Fig. 40-4). Non-SHBG-bound testosterone

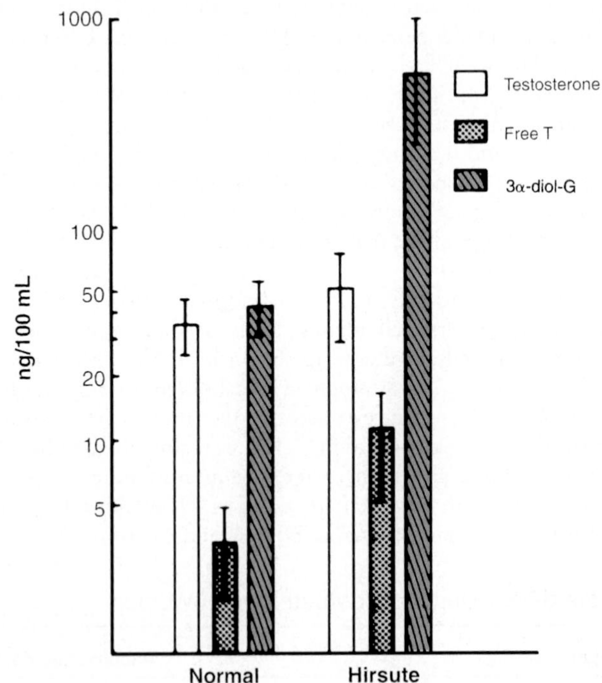

Figure 40-4. Plasma total testosterone, unbound testosterone (free T) and 5α-androstane-3α, 17β-diol glucuronide (3α-diol-G) in normal and hirsute women. Note insignificant elevation with overlap for testosterone and free T testosterone and highly significant increase in 3α-diol-G without overlap between two groups of women. (Reproduced from Horton R, Hawks D, Lobo RA: 3α,17β-androstanediol glucuronide in plasma: A marker of androgen action in idiopathic hirsutism. J Clin Invest 69:1203, 1982. By copyright permission of The American Society for Clinical Investigation.)

Table 40-4 Markers of Androgen Production

Source	Marker
Ovary	Testosterone
Adrenal gland	DHEA-S
Periphery	3α-diol-G

DHEA-S, dehydroepiandrosterone sulfate; 3α-diol-G, 5α-androstane-3α, 17β-diol glucuronide.
From Lobo RA: Androgen excess. In Mishell DR Jr, Davajan V, Lobo RA (eds): Infertility, Contraception and Reproductive Endocrinology, 3rd ed. Cambridge, MA, Blackwell Scientific, 1991.

is elevated in about 60% to 70% of hirsute women, but 3α-diol-G is elevated in more than 80% of such individuals. Thus increased levels of non-SHBG-bound testosterone indicate increased ovarian production. If levels of non-SHBG-bound testosterone are normal and levels of 3α-diol-G are elevated, testosterone production is not increased, but peripheral conversion of testosterone to its active metabolite (DHT) is increased above normal. Either of these processes can cause symptoms and signs of androgen excess. Thus there are three markers of androgen production in serum, one for each compartment where androgens are produced (Table 40-4). Interpretation of levels of 3α-diol-G is controversial because these levels are highly dependant on circulating levels of precursor androgens such as testosterone. A reasonable argument may be that if testosterone and DHEA-S are "normal" yet there is significant hirsutism, then measuring 3α-diol-G may not be necessary and one may merely assume a peripheral source of androgen excess.

ETIOLOGY

There are 10 currently recognized causes of androgen excess in women. One frequent cause is administration of androgenic medication. In addition to testosterone itself, various anabolic steroids, 19-norprogestins, and danazol have androgenic effects. Thus a careful history of medication intake is important for all women with hirsutism.

Hirsutism or virilization can also be associated with some forms of abnormal gonad development. With this cause, individuals have signs of either external sexual ambiguity or primary amenorrhea, in addition to findings of androgen excess and a Y chromosome present in the gonad. These conditions are discussed in Chapter 38 (Primary and Secondary Amenorrhea and Precocious Puberty) and will not be further described in the discussion of the differential diagnosis of androgen excess in this chapter.

Signs of androgen excess during pregnancy can be caused by increased ovarian testosterone production. This is usually caused by either a luteoma of pregnancy or hyperreactio luteinalis. The former is a unilateral or bilateral solid ovarian enlargement, whereas the latter is bilateral cystic ovarian enlargement. After pregnancy is completed, the excessive ovarian androgenic production resolves spontaneously and the androgenic signs regress.

A diagnosis of these three causes of androgen excess can usually be easily made by means of a careful history and physical examination. The remaining causes of androgen excess, together with the origin of hyperandrogenism, are listed in Table 40-5. Details of each of these causes will be described in decreasing order of their frequency.

Table 40-5 Differential Diagnosis of Hirsutism and Virilization*

Source	Diagnosis
Nonspecific	Exogenous/iatrogenic
	Abnormal gonadal or sexual development
Pregnancy	Androgen excess in pregnancy: luteoma or hyperreactio luteinalis
Periphery	Idiopathic hirsutism
Ovary	Polycystic ovary syndrome
	Stromal hyperthecosis
	Ovarian tumors
Adrenal gland	Adrenal tumors
	Cushing syndrome
	Adult-onset congenital adrenal hyperplasia

*Idiopathic hirsutism and polycystic ovary syndrome do not present with virilizations.

Idiopathic Hirsutism (Peripheral Disorder of Androgen Metabolism)

"Idiopathic" hirsutism is manifested by signs of hirsutism and regular menstrual cycles in conjunction with normal circulatory levels of androgens (both testosterone and DHEA-S). Because this type of disorder is frequently present in several individuals in the same family, particularly those of Mediterranean descent, it has also been called *familial,* or *constitutional, hirsutism.* Since neither ovarian nor adrenal androgen production is increased in these individuals, the cause of the androgen excess was not determined until recently, hence the term *idiopathic hirsutism.* This is a very common cause of hirsutism and is second in frequency only to polycystic ovary syndrome (PCOS). We have shown that about 80% of these individuals have increased levels of 3α-diol-G, indirectly indicating that the cause of hirsutism is increased 5α-reductase activity (5α-RA) (Fig. 40-5). Also we have directly measured the percent conversion of testosterone to DHT in genital skin as an assessment of 5α-RA in the skin of women with idiopathic hirsutism. The amount of 5α-RA was increased in hirsute women as compared with normal women and correlated well with both the degree of hirsutism and serum levels of 3α-diol-G. Thus idiopathic hirsutism is actually a disorder of peripheral androgen metabolism in the pilosebaceous apparatus of the skin and is possibly genetically determined although it is also possible that early exposure to androgens can "program" increased 5α-RA. Antiandrogens that block peripheral testosterone action or interfere with 5α-RA are effective therapeutic agents for this disorder. We have shown that hirsutism is largely a disorder of the peripheral compartment, and the most effective treatments involve peripheral blockade (described below).

Polycystic Ovary Syndrome

Polycystic ovary syndrome was originally described in 1935 by Stein and Leventhal as a syndrome consisting of amenorrhea, hirsutism, and obesity in association with enlarged polycystic ovaries. The classic definition of PCOS includes women who are anovulatory and have irregular periods as well as hyperandrogenism (as determined by signs such as hirsutism or elevated blood levels of androgens: testosterone or DHEA-S. This should

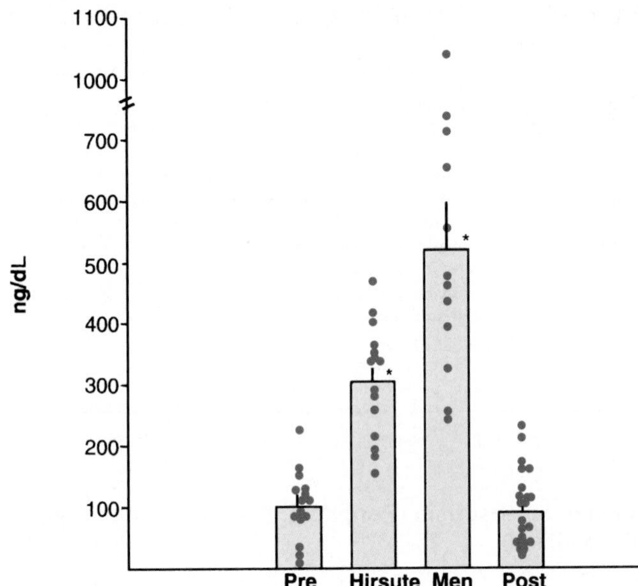

Figure 40-5. Serum 3α-diol-G in premenopausal nonhirsute women (Pre), hirsute women, normal men, and postmenopausal nonhirsute women (Post). The asterisks denote $p < 0.05$, as compared with Pre. (Reprinted from Fertility and Sterility, 42, Paulson RJ, Serafini PC, Catalino JA, Lobo RA, Measurements of 3α,17β-androstanediol glucuronide in serum and urine and the correlation with skin 5α-reductase activity, 422. Copyright 1986, with permission from The American Society for Reproductive Medicine.)

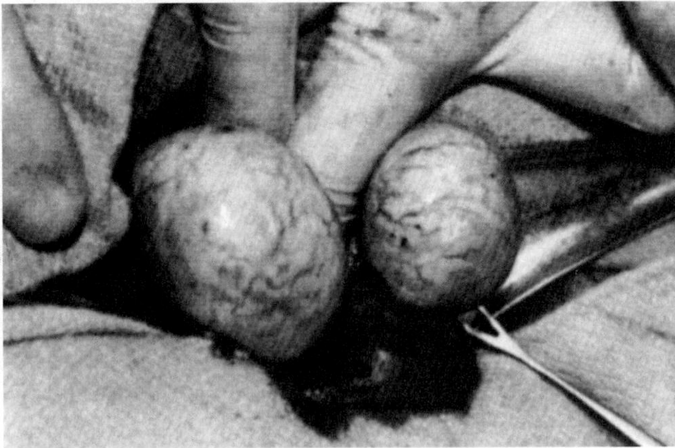

Figure 40-6. Gross characteristics of polycystic ovaries. Bilateral enlarged ovaries with smooth and thickened capsule. (From Yen SSC: Chronic anovulation caused by peripheral endocrine disorders. In Yen SSC, Jaffe RB [eds]: Reproductive Endocrinology, 2nd ed. Philadelphia, WB Saunders, 1986.)

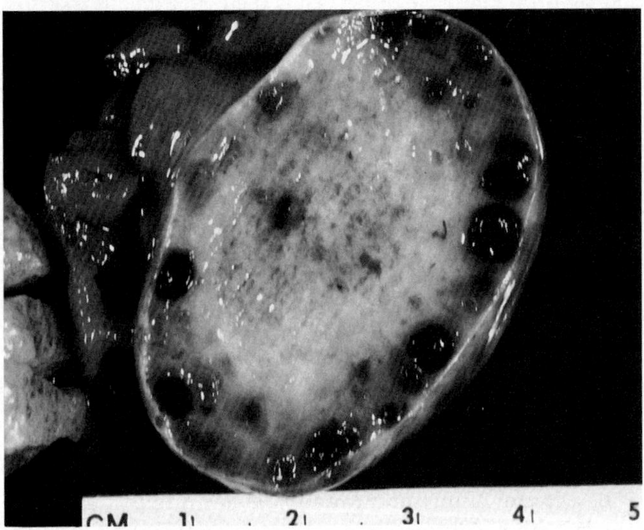

Figure 40-7. Sagittal section of a polycystic ovary illustrating large number of follicular cysts and thickened stroma.

be in the absence of enzymatic disorders (such as 21-hydroxylase deficiency) or tumors.

This diagnosis does not require findings on ultrasound (US) of characteristic polycystic ovaries. For the past 15 years, this non-US-based definition has been referred to as the "NIH consensus" definition because it followed an NIH conference in 1989. However this was not a consensus conference and there was no true consensus among attendees.

Over time there was been increasing evidence that some women with all the features of PCOS may be ovulatory and have regular menstrual cycles. Also there has been renewed emphasis placed on finding polycystic ovaries on US. Accordingly, a conference in Rotterdam has come up with a new definition, which was published simultaneously in the journals *Human Reproduction* and *Fertility and Sterility* in 2004. This definition places an emphasis on finding polycystic ovaries on US as an important criterion. Other significant findings are the classic features of anovulation/menstrual irregularity and hyperandrogenism. Women with PCOS may have all three findings, but it requires any two out of the three to make a diagnosis of PCOS. Thus, hyperandrogenic women with normal ovulatory cycles and polycystic ovaries on US may be diagnosed as having PCOS. We have found that approximately 95% of women who have classic symptoms (NIH criteria) of anovulation and hyperandrogenism have polycystic ovaries on US. Therefore it may be unnecessary to "confirm" the diagnosis by US in this setting. Figures 40-6 and 40-7 show the classic appearing polycystic ovary at surgery in a sagittal section, which is nearly identical to what is seen by US in a sagittal plane. The US diagnosis of polycystic ovaries has been made on the basis of finding enlarged ovaries (>10 cm^3) and the presence of 10 or more peripherally oriented cystic structures (2 to 8 mm) surrounding a dense stroma. Since the Rotterdam conference, however, ovarian size alone has been suggested to be sufficient, with ovaries larger than 10 cm^3 being diagnostic, and recent evidence suggesting that this lower limit may be 7 cm^3.

It is also important to note that anywhere from 10% to 25% of the normal reproductive-age population (no symptoms or signs of PCOS) may have polycystic ovaries found on US. These ovaries have been called "polycystic-appearing ovaries" (PAO) or "polycystic ovarian morphology" (PCOM) in the literature. This isolated finding should not be confused with the diagnosis of PCOS, but may be a risk factor for other traits of PCOS (insulin resistance, cardiovascular risk factors) discussed later.

Using the classic definition of PCOS, which can also be quite heterogeneous in terms of the severity of the findings of menstrual irregularity and hyperandrogenism, approximately 3% to 7% of the reproductive-age population will have PCOS. Thus

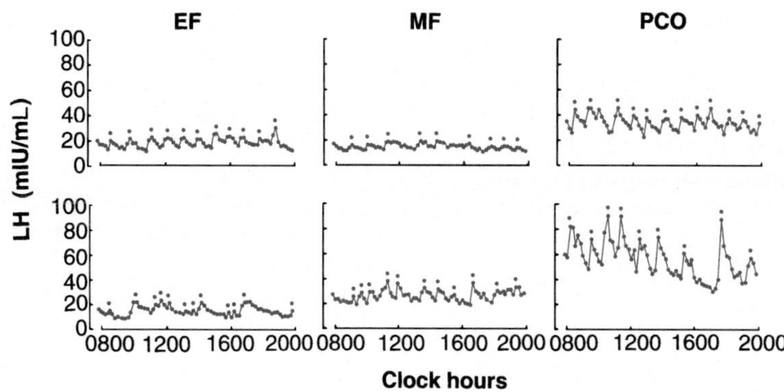

Figure 40-8. Patterns of pulsatile luteinizing hormone (LH) secretion in patients with polycystic ovarian syndrome (PCO) and in control subjects with normal early follicular (EF) and midfollicular (MF) phases. The asterisks indicate significant pulses. (From Kazer AR, Kessel B, Yen SSC: Circulating luteinizing hormone pulse frequency in women with polycystic ovary syndrome. J Clin Endocrinol Metab 65:233, 1987.)

PCOS is an extremely common disorder, and its diagnosis is important because of its consequences (see section on consequences of PCOS).

Depending on the women' country of origin, 30% to 70% of women with PCOS are overweight, although it's clear that thin women may also have PCOS. All symptoms of PCOS will be worse in women who are overweight or obese. This relates most strongly to insulin resistance, which is a key factor of PCOS and will be described later. The degree of menstrual irregularity may also relate to the finding of insulin resistance.

Characteristic endocrinologic features include abnormal gonadotropin secretion caused by either increased gonadotropin-releasing hormone (GnRH) pulse amplitude or increased pituitary sensitivity to GnRH. These abnormalities result in tonically elevated levels of luteinizing hormone (LH) in about two thirds of the women with this syndrome (Fig. 40-8). After a bolus of GnRH, there is usually an exaggerated response of LH, but not of follicle-stimulating hormone (FSH) (Fig. 40-9). In addition, there are increased circulating levels of androgens produced by both the ovaries and the adrenal glands (Fig. 40-10). Serum testosterone levels usually range between 0.7 to 1.2 ng/mL, and androstenedione levels are usually between 3 and 5 ng/mL. In addition, about half the women with this syndrome have elevated levels of DHEA-S, suggesting adrenal androgen involvement. Evidence also exists for adrenal hyperactivity in at least a third of women with PCOS. Although nearly all women with PCOS have elevated levels of circulating androgens, we have found that the presence or absence of hirsutism depends on whether those androgens are converted peripherally by 5α-reductase to the more potent androgen DHT, as reflected by increased circulating levels of 3α-diol-G. Nonhirsute women with PCOS have elevated circulatory levels of testosterone or DHEA-S or both but not 3α-diol-G. The tonically elevated levels of LH are usually above 15 mIU/mL.

Because FSH levels in women with PCOS are normal or low, an elevated LH–FSH ratio has been used to diagnose PCOS.

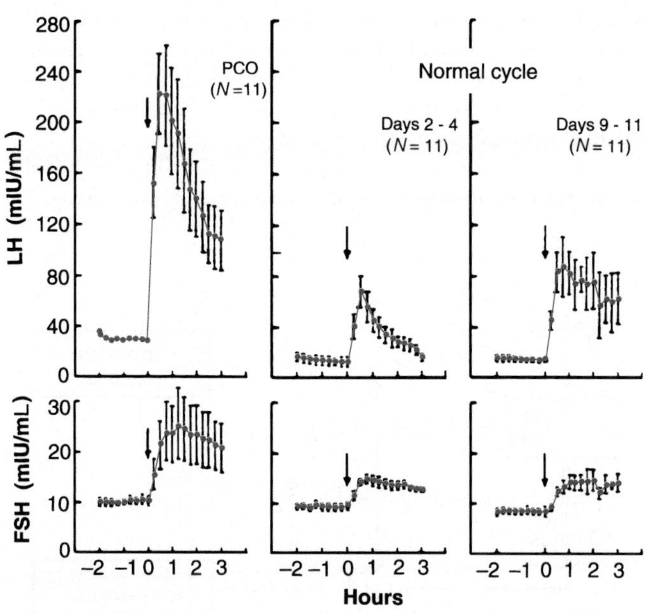

Figure 40-9. Comparison of quantitative luteinizing hormone (LH) and follicle-stimulating hormone (FSH) release in response to a single bolus of 150 μg of GnRH in patients with polycystic ovarian syndrome (PCO) and in normal women during low-estrogen (early follicular) and high-estrogen (late follicular) phases of their cycles. (From Rebar R, Judd HL, Yen SSC, et al: Characterization of the inappropriate gonadotropin secretion in polycystic ovary syndrome. J Clin Invest 57:1320, 1976.)

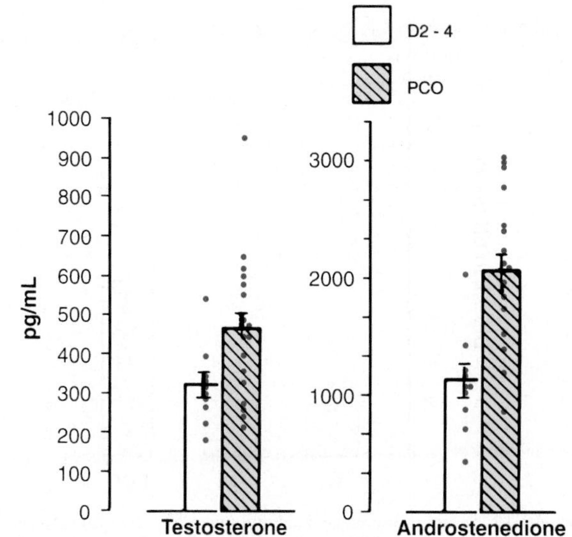

Figure 40-10. Mean (±SD) concentrations of testosterone and Δ^4-androstenedione in 19 patients with polycystic ovarian syndrome (PCO) and 10 normal subjects between days 2 and 4 (D2–4) of their menstrual cycles. (From DeVane GW, Czekala NM, Judd HL, et al: Circulating gonadotropins, estrogens, and androgens in polycystic ovarian disease. Am J Obstet Gynecol 121:496, 1975.)

However, we reported that among women with a clinical diagnosis of PCOS, only 70% had an elevated level of immunoreactive LH or an immunologic LH–FSH ratio greater than 3. Although almost all women with PCOS had elevated serum levels of biologically active LH (Fig. 40-11), use of LH or the LH–FSH ratio should not be part of the diagnostic evaluation of PCOS.

In addition to increased levels of circulatory androgens, we have found that women with PCOS have increased levels of biologically active (non-SHBG-bound) estradiol, although total circulating levels of estradiol were not increased (Fig. 40-12). The increased amount of non-SHBG-bound estradiol is caused by a decrease in SHBG levels, which is brought about by the increased levels of androgens and obesity with high insulin levels present in many of these women. Estrone is also increased because of increased peripheral (adipose) conversion of androgen. The tonically increased levels of biologically active estradiol may stimulate increased GnRH pulsatility and produce tonically elevated LH levels and anovulation. In addition, the lowered SHBG level increases the biologically active fractions of the elevated androgens in the circulation. The importance of the decreased levels of SHBG is shown schematically in Figure 40-13. This relative hyperestrogenism (elevated estrone and non-SHBG-bound estradiol), which is unopposed by progesterone because of anovulation, increases the risk of endometrial hypoplasia.

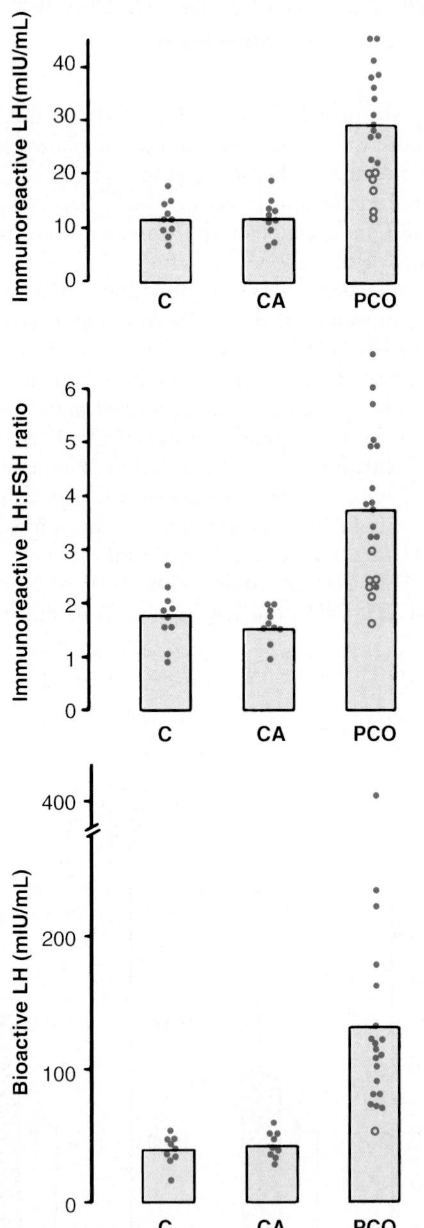

Figure 40-11. Serum measurements of immunoreactive luteinizing hormone (LH), immunoreactive LH: follicle-stimulating hormone (FSH) ratios, and bioactive LH in control subjects (C), women with chronic anovulation (CA), and women with PCOS (PCO). Boxes represent the mean ±3 standard deviation (SD) of control levels. (Reprinted from Fertility and Sterility, 39, Lobo RA, Kletzky OA, Campeau JD, et al, Elevated bioactive luteinizing hormone in women with the polycystic ovary syndrome, 674. Copyright 1983, with permission from The American Society for Reproductive Medicine.)

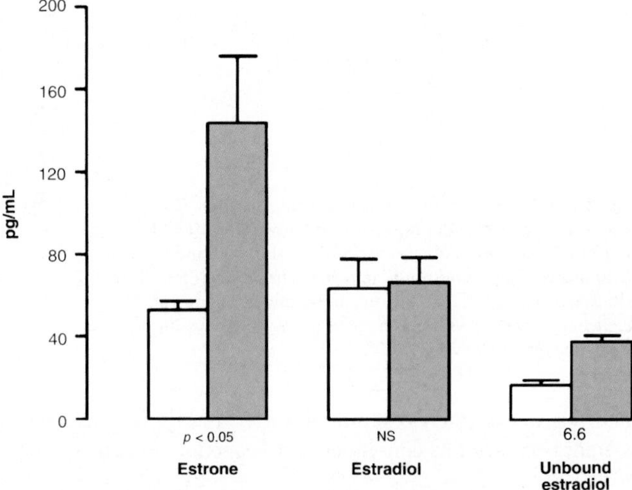

Figure 40-12. Serum estrogen concentrations in 13 normal women and 22 PCOS patients (shaded areas). (From Lobo RA, Granger L, Goebelsmann U, et al: Elevation in unbound serum estradiol as a possible mechanism for inappropriate gonadotropin secretion in women with PCO. J Clin Endocrinol Metab 52:156, 1981. Copyright 1981 by The Endocrine Society.)

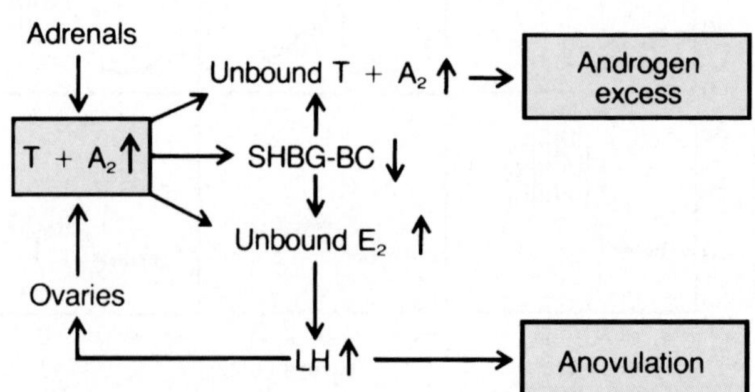

Figure 40-13. Scheme depicting the possible role of adrenal-derived androgen (A_2, androstanediol; E_2, estradiol; LH, luteinizing hormone; SHBG-BC, sex hormone-binding globulin binding capacity; T, testosterone.) In initiating androgen excess and anovulation. (From Lobo RA, Goebelsmann U: Effect of androgen excess on inappropriate gonadotropin secretion as found in polycystic ovary syndrome. Am J Obstet Gynecol 142:394, 1982.)

About 20% of women with PCOS also have mildly elevated levels of prolactin (20 to 30 ng/mL), possibly related to increased pulsatility of GnRH, to a relative dopamine deficiency, or tonic stimulation from unopposed estrogen.

It is well established that some degree of insulin resistance occurs in most women with PCOS even those of normal weight. Insulin and insulin-like growth factor-I (IGF-I) enhance ovarian androgen production by potentiating the stimulatory action of LH on ovarian androstenedione and testosterone secretion. High levels of insulin bind with the receptor for IGF-I as a result of the significant homology of the IGF-I receptor with the insulin receptor. The granulosa cells also produce IGF-I and IGF-binding proteins (IGFBP). This local production of IGF-I and IGFBP may result in paracrine control and enhancement of LH stimulation and production of androgens by the theca cells in women with PCOS. Since IGFBP levels are lower in women with PCOS, this leads to increased bioavailable IGF-I, which increases stimulation of the theca cells in combination with LH to produce higher levels of androgen production. Insulin resistance and the resultant hyperinsulinemia stimulate ovarian androgen production. It is not clear why women with PCOS have insulin resistance; the insulin resistance in PCOS is greater than in age-matched and weight-matched controls.

Dunaif and colleagues studied a group of hyperandrogenic women with and without PCOS and obesity using glucose tolerance tests and insulin levels. They found that hyperinsulinemia occurred only in the women with PCOS, whether or not they were obese, but only the obese women with PCOS had impaired glucose tolerance. In a subsequent study they found that nonobese women with PCOS also had glucose intolerance, but the incidence was less than in the obese women. In a prospective evaluation of 254 women with PCOS who had an oral glucose tolerance test, they found that 31% had impaired glucose tolerance and 7.5% had undiagnosed diabetes. In nonobese women with PCOS, 10% had impaired glucose tolerance and 1.5% had diabetes. Norman and coworkers showed that over a mean follow-up time period of 6.2 years 9% of women with PCOS in Australia progressed to having impaired glucose tolerance and 8% became diabetic. Thus, the negative effect of obesity and PCOS on insulin resistance is additive. Fasting glucose levels are a poor predictor of diabetes in PCOS. It would appear advisable to perform an oral glucose tolerance test at the time of diagnosis in overweight women with PCOS and periodically thereafter. If abnormalities in glucose metabolism are found, appropriate interventions should be recommended.

Acanthosis nigricans (AN) has been found in about 30% of hyperandrogenic women. About half of the hyperandrogenic women who had PCOS and were obese had AN. Although it has been suggested that the presence of *hy*per*a*ndrogenism *i*nsulin *r*esistance, and *AN* constitute a special syndrome (the HAIR-AN syndrome), most investigators believe that women with PCOS who have AN are a subgroup of those with PCOS and do not have a distinct endocrine disorder. No causal relation among PCOS, obesity, insulin resistance, and hyperandrogenism has been elucidated to date. It is clear, however, that the combination of insulin and IGF-I (which enhance AN) leads to the hyperandrogenism.

Although the ovaries of women with PCOS produce excessive amounts of androgen, particularly androstenedione, there is no inherent endocrinologic abnormality in the ovaries. The tonically elevated levels of LH cause the stromal tissue to produce more androstenedione and other androgens, which in turn produces premature follicular atresia. Furthermore, the ovaries are deficient in aromatase, a deficiency that results in less conversion of androstenedione to estrogen in the ovary. The polycystic ovary does not secrete increased amounts of estrone or estradiol, but the increased levels of androstenedione are peripherally converted to estrone, thereby increasing circulating estrone levels.

Whatever the cause, the endocrinologic effects of PCOS produce a cycle of events, as shown by Yen and associates (Fig. 40-14). The increased pulsatility of GnRH produces

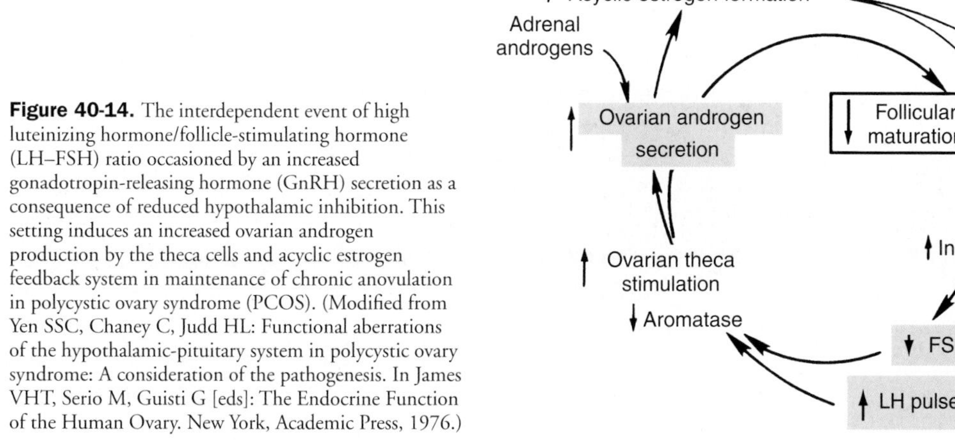

Figure 40-14. The interdependent event of high luteinizing hormone/follicle-stimulating hormone (LH–FSH) ratio occasioned by an increased gonadotropin-releasing hormone (GnRH) secretion as a consequence of reduced hypothalamic inhibition. This setting induces an increased ovarian androgen production by the theca cells and acyclic estrogen feedback system in maintenance of chronic anovulation in polycystic ovary syndrome (PCOS). (Modified from Yen SSC, Chaney C, Judd HL: Functional aberrations of the hypothalamic-pituitary system in polycystic ovary syndrome: A consideration of the pathogenesis. In James VHT, Serio M, Guisti G [eds]: The Endocrine Function of the Human Ovary. New York, Academic Press, 1976.)

tonically elevated LH levels and increased ovarian androgen production. Peripheral conversion of androstenedione to estrone in conjunction with the decreased SHBG levels causes tonic hyperestrogenism, which increases the pituitary sensitivity to GnRH and leads to increased LH release.

Some Insights into Pathophysiology

It is clear that there is a genetic predisposition to PCOS. However, it is likely that several genes are involved. A susceptibility gene for PCOS has been suggested to lie in the region of 19p 3.2 although this needs confirmation. Environmental factors are clearly involved as well, based on twin studies, where PCOS is not always concordant on a genetic basis. Maternal exposure to androgen has been shown in a monkey model to contribute to the development of PCOS.

It is clear from the cycle model of Yen (see Fig. 40-14) that the syndrome may evolve from any point. Thus it was attractive to postulate that dopamine deficiency in the hypothalamus might give rise to the exaggerated LH responses in PCOS, and there are several similar hypotheses. However, it has been observed that morphologically identifiable polycystic ovaries are seen in children. This occurrence predicts puberty and other normal endocrinologic events, suggesting a central role for altered PCOM in the disorder. Furthermore not all women with isolated polycystic ovaries have PCOS as stated earlier. Thus a pathophysiologic model can be put together as follows:

An ovary is polycystic in up to a fifth of girls according to data from Bridges and colleagues. Thus the ovary transitions early in life from normal to polycystic-appearing (PAO). This influence occurs in a specific way by genetic factors, by environmental factors, or is induced by other endocrine disturbances (Fig. 40-15). The woman who develops PAO may have normal menses, normal androgen levels, and normal ovulatory function and parity. However, if subjected to various susceptibility factors or "insults" with various degrees of severity, women with PAO may develop a full-blown syndrome (PCOS). The syndrome, if full-blown, will exhibit the full extent of hyperandrogenism and anovulation, with the most extreme form of this menstrual disturbance being amenorrhea. However, in this spectrum of disorders, the androgen disturbances may also be near normal. Similarly, the menstrual disturbance may be very mild (Fig. 40-16).

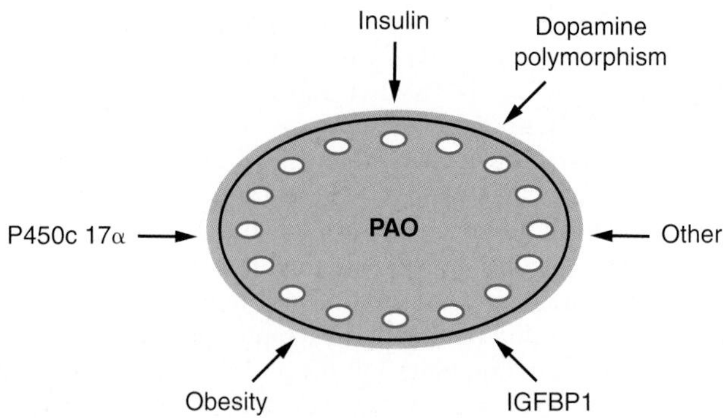

Figure 40-15. Pathophysiology of polycystic ovary syndrome (PCOS): The syndrome develops when one or more "insults" persist. IGFBG1, insulin-like growth factor-binding protein 1; P450c 17α, cytochrome 450.

This model requires that normal homeostatic factors may be able to ward off stressors or insults in some women who can go through life without PCOS but have a PAO which does not change morphologically. Alternatively, with varying degrees of success a woman's homeostatic mechanism may at any time, early or later in reproductive life, allow symptoms or PCOS to emerge with varying degrees of severity. Two of the major insults are thought to be weight gain and psychological stress. Thus, the typical teenager born with PAO may develop PCOS fairly quickly; yet a PCOS picture may develop only later in life in some women even after having children. Because of hyperandrogenism and obesity, women with PCOS have abnormal lipoprotein profiles. The increase in triglycerides and the decrease in low-density lipoprotein (LDL) cholesterol and high-density lipoprotein (HDL) may be related to the increased body weight or hyperandrogenism (Fig. 40-17). If PCOS is not treated, the endocrinologic abnormalities persist and gradually worsen until the ovary stops functioning at the menopause. Long-term sequelae of PCOS were examined in 33 women ages 40 to 59 who had undergone ovarian wedge resection 22 to 31 years previously. Compared with age-matched controls, they had a significantly greater incidence of hypertension and diabetes mellitus (Fig. 40-18). Using multiple logistic regression analysis it was predicted that women with PCOS have an increased risk

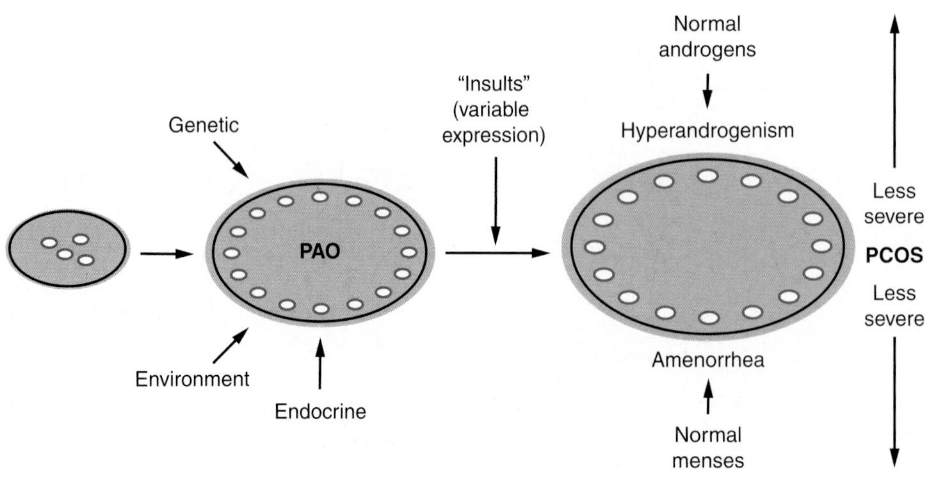

Figure 40-16. Pathophysiology of polycystic ovary syndrome (PCOS): Differences in presentation. PAO, polycystic-appearing ovaries.

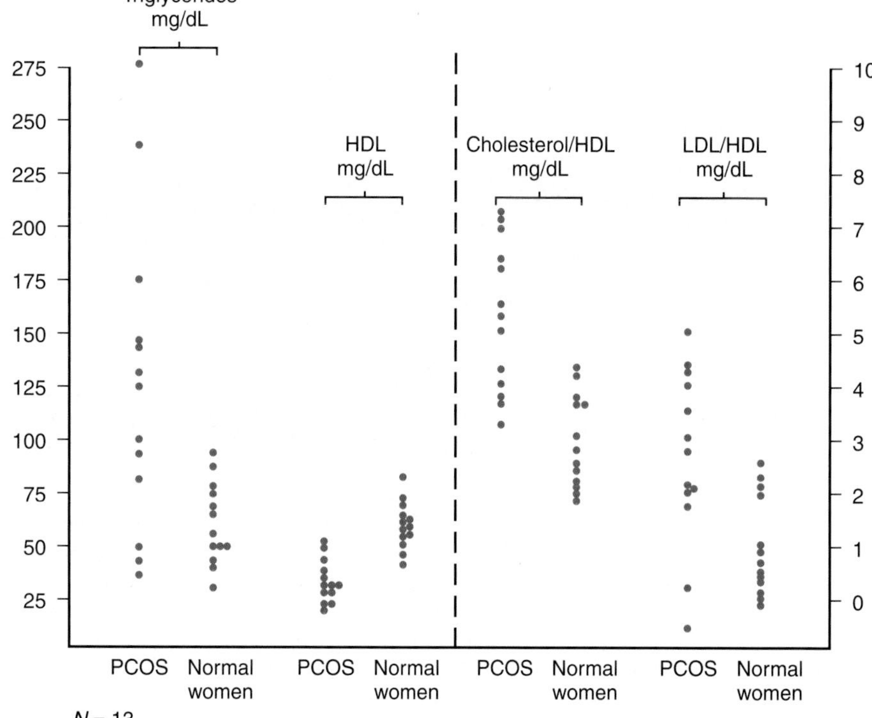

Figure 40-17. Lipid and lipoprotein profiles in 13 women with polycystic ovary syndrome (PCOS) versus control group when matched for percent ideal body weight. Differences are evident in all measures ($p < 0.01$). HDL, high-density lipoprotein; LDL, low-density lipoprotein. (From Wild RA, Bartholomew MJ: The influence of body weight on lipoprotein lipids in patients with polycystic ovary syndrome. Am J Obstet Gynecol 159:423, 1988.)

of developing cardiovascular disease compared with controls. Many studies show increased cardiovascular risk factors in PCOS, including elevations in homocysteine, C-reactive protein (CRP), endothelin-1, reductions in plasminogen activator inhibitor-1 (PA-1), increased coronary Ca^{2+}, increased carotid intima media thickness, and endothelial dysfunction. However, retrospective studies by Pierpont and Wild and colleagues reported that women with PCOS do not have an increased risk of death due to cardiovascular disease, unless they were diabetic. This issue is not clear at present.

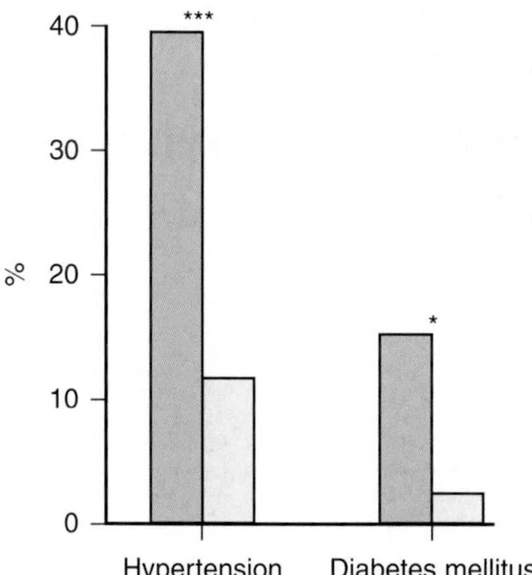

Figure 40-18. Prevalence of hypertension (medically treated) and manifest diabetes mellitus in 33 PCOS subjects and 132 referents. The dark-shaded bars illustrate the polycystic ovary syndrome (PCOS) subjects. The light-shaded bars illustrate the referents. Statistical comparisons were made between the women with PCOS and referents. Differences were considered significant at $^{*}p = 0.05$ and $^{***}p = 0.001$. (Reprinted from Fertility and Sterility, 57, Dahlgren E, Janson PO, Johansson S, et al, Women with polycystic ovary syndrome wedge resected in 1956 to 1965: A long-term follow-up focusing on natural history and circulating hormones, 505. Copyright 1992, with permission from The American Society for Reproductive Medicine.)

Isolated Polycystic Ovaries

We have shown that normal ovulatory women with PAO or PCOM have a subtle form of ovarian hyperandrogenism (when stimulated with GnRH-A or human chorionic gonadotropin [HCG]). We have also found subtle changes in insulin sensitivity and altered lipoproteins in these women. There may also be some reduction in fertility in these ovulatory women. Therefore although many women with isolated PAO/PCOM may not have any problems, we view this finding as a risk for developing the consequences of PCOS.

Consequences of PCOS

The importance of diagnosing PCOS is that there are known long-term consequences of the diagnosis warranting lifelong surveillance. Figure 40-19 shows the ages at which various consequences may emerge. Although in the early reproductive years abnormal bleeding and infertility are common, later in life, concerns relate to cardiovascular disease, diabetes mellitus, and ovarian cancer. The risk of ovarian cancer has been suggested to be increased twofold, a finding seen in women with general infertility. This risk is normalized with the use of oral contraceptives (OCs).

Stromal Hyperthecosis

Stromal hyperthecosis is an uncommon benign ovarian disorder in which the ovaries are bilaterally enlarged to about 5 to 7 cm

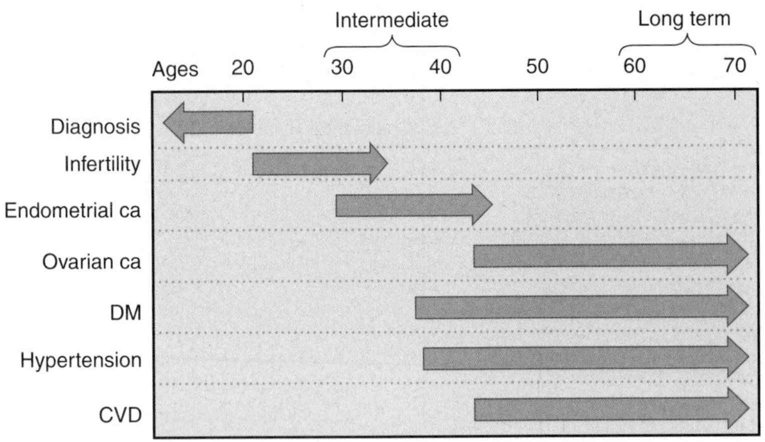

Figure 40-19. Consequences of polycystic ovary syndrome (PCOS). ca, cancer; CVD, cardiovascular disease; DM, diabetes mellitus.

in diameter. Histologically there are nests of luteinized theca cells within the stroma (Fig. 40-20). The capsules of these ovaries are thick, similar to those found in PCOS, but unlike PCOS, subcapsular cysts are uncommon. The theca cells produce large amounts of testosterone as determined by retrograde ovarian vein catheterization. Like PCOS, this disorder has a gradual onset and is initially associated with anovulation or amenorrhea and hirsutism. However, unlike PCOS, with increasing age the ovaries secrete steadily increasing amounts of testosterone. Thus when women with this disorder reach the fourth decade of life, the severity of the hirsutism increases, and signs of virilization, such as temporal balding, clitoral enlargement, deepening of the voice, and decreased breast size, appear and gradually increase in severity. By this time serum testosterone levels are usually greater than 2 ng/mL, similar to levels found in ovarian and adrenal testosterone-producing tumors. However, with the latter conditions the symptoms of virilization appear and progress much more rapidly than with ovarian hyperthecosis, in which symptoms progress gradually over many years.

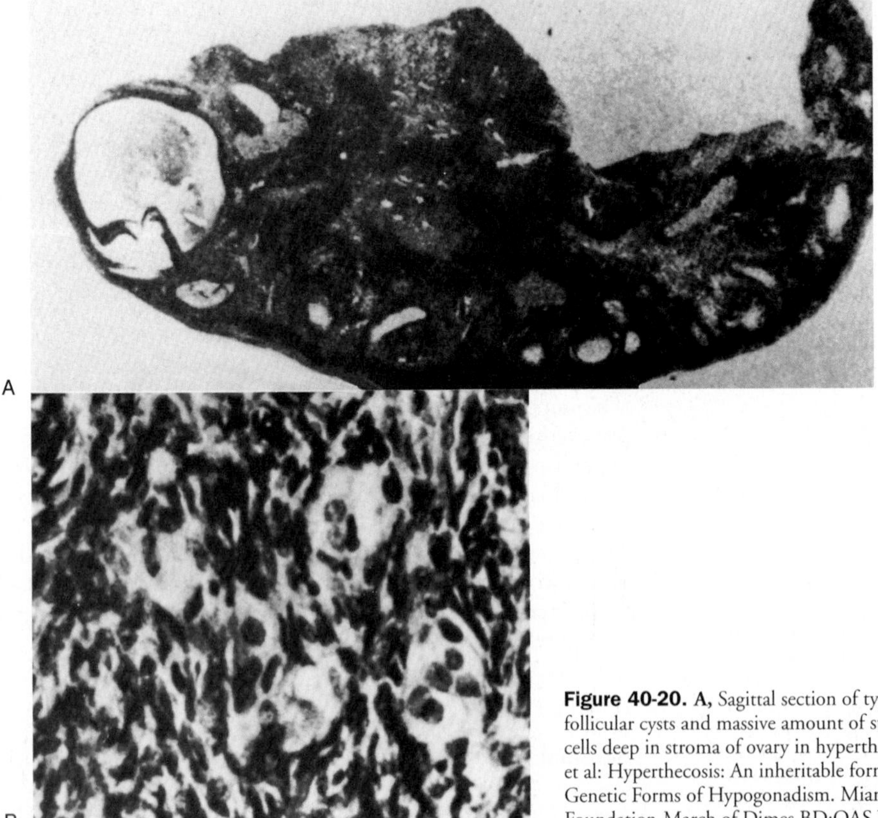

Figure 40-20. **A,** Sagittal section of typical hyperthecotic ovary illustrating small number of follicular cysts and massive amount of stromal hyperplasia. **B,** Islands of luteinized theca-like cells deep in stroma of ovary in hyperthecosis. (From Wilroy RS Jr, Givens JR, Wiser WL, et al: Hyperthecosis: An inheritable form of polycystic ovarian disease. In Bergsma D [ed]: Genetic Forms of Hypogonadism. Miami, FL, Symposia Specialists for the National Foundation-March of Dimes BD:OAS XI(4):81, 1975, with permission.)

Androgen-Producing Tumors

Ovarian Neoplasms

It is possible for nearly every type of ovarian neoplasm to have stromal cells that secrete excessive amounts of testosterone and cause signs of androgen excess. Thus on rare occasions excess testosterone produced by both benign and malignant cystadenomas, Brenner's tumors, and Krukenberg's tumors has caused hirsutism or virilization or both. Certain germ cell tumors contain many testosterone-producing cells. The testosterone produced by two of these neoplasms, Sertoli–Leydig cell tumors and hilus cell tumors, nearly always causes virilization. In addition, lipoid cell (adrenal rest) tumors can produce increased amounts of testosterone or DHEA-S or both. Rarely granulosa/theca cell tumors can also produce testosterone in addition to increased levels of estradiol.

Androgen-producing ovarian tumors usually produce rapidly progressive signs of virilization. Sertoli–Leydig cell tumors usually develop during the reproductive years (second to fourth decades), and by the time they produce detectable signs of androgen excess, the tumor is nearly always (more than 85% of the time) palpable during bimanual examination. These tumors are uncommon. Less than 1% of solid ovarian neoplasms are Sertoli–Leydig cell tumors. Hilus cell tumors most often occur after menopause. They are usually small and not palpable during bimanual examination; however, the history of rapid development of signs of virilization and the presence of markedly elevated levels of testosterone (more than two and a half times the upper limits of the normal range) with normal levels of DHEA-S usually facilitate the diagnosis.

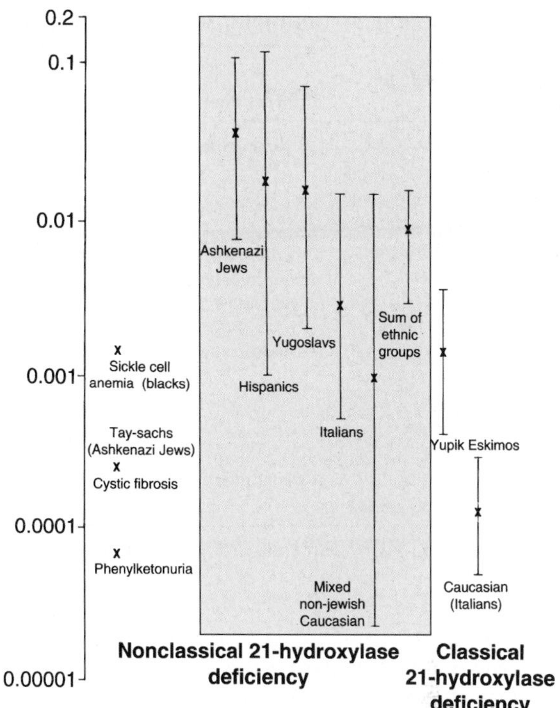

Figure 40-21. Relative frequencies of nonclassic 21-hydroxylase deficiency, classic 21-hydroxylase deficiency, and other autosomal recessive disorders. (From Speiser PW, Dupont B, Rubenstein P, et al: High frequency of nonclassical steroid 21-hydroxylase deficiency. Am J Hum Genet 37:650, 1985.)

Adrenal Tumors

Nearly all the androgen-producing adrenal tumors are adenomas or carcinomas that generate large amounts of the C_{19} steroids normally produced by the adrenal gland: DHEA-S, DHEA, and androstenedione. Although these tumors do not usually directly secrete testosterone, testosterone is produced by extraglandular conversion of DHEA and androstenedione. Women with these tumors usually have markedly elevated serum levels of DHEA-S (>8 μg/mL). Women with these laboratory findings and a history of rapid onset of signs of androgen excess should undergo a computerized tomography (CT) scan or magnetic resonance imaging (MRI) of the adrenal glands to confirm the diagnosis. In addition to these uncommon tumors, a few testosterone-producing adrenal adenomas have been reported. The cellular patterns of these tumors resemble those of ovarian hilus cells, and the tumors secrete large amounts of testosterone. Because adrenal adenomas also secrete DHEA-S, an adrenal adenoma is highly likely when DHEA-S levels are greater than 8 μg/mL and testosterone levels are more than 1.5 ng/mL.

Late-Onset 21-Hydroxylase Deficiency

Congenital adrenal hyperplasia (CAH) is an inherited disorder caused by an enzymatic defect (usually 21-hydroxylase [21-OHase] or less often 11β-hydroxylase), resulting in decreased cortisol biosynthesis. As a consequence, adrenocorticotropic hormone (ACTH) secretion increases and adrenal cortisol precursors produced proximal to the enzymatic block accumulate and are converted mainly to DHEA and androstenedione. These C_{19} steroids are in turn peripherally converted to testosterone, which produces signs of androgen excess.

Because the enzymatic defects are congenital, the classic severe form (complete block) usually becomes clinically apparent in fetal life by producing masculinization of the female external genitalia. The severe form of CAH is the most common cause of sexual ambiguity in the newborn. The more attenuated (mild) block of 21-OHase activity usually does not produce physical signs associated with increased androgen production until after puberty. Thus this condition, termed late-onset 21-hydroxylase deficiency (LOHD) or late-onset congenital adrenal hyperplasia, is associated with the development of signs of hyperandrogenism in a woman in the second or early third decade of life.

Although the incidence of classic CAH is only 1 per 14,500 live births worldwide, Speiser and coworkers, using histocompatibility locus antigen (HLA)-B genotyping of families with LOHD-affected individuals, concluded that the incidence of LOHD varied among different ethnic groups but overall was probably the most frequent autosomal genetic disorder in humans. The incidence of LOHD was estimated to be 0.1% among a diverse white population; among Yugoslavians, Hispanics, and Ashkenazi Jews, however, the incidence was 1.6%, 1.9%, and 3.7%, respectively (Fig. 40-21). Both classic CAH and LOHD are transmitted in an autosomal recessive manner at the *CYP21B* locus and are linked to the HLA-B locus.

The molecular basis of the disease is complex. The gene for CYP21 is located on 6p near the HLA complex. In proximity

Table 40-6 Genotypic Characterization of the Forms of 21-Hydroxylase Deficiency

Form of 21-Hydroxylase Deficiency	Clinical Phenotype	Hormonal Phenotype (in Response to ACTH)	Genotype
Classic (CAH)	Prenatal virilization, fully symptomatic	Marked elevation of precursors (serum 17-hydroxyprogesterone and Δ-androstenedione)	21-OH-def^{severe} / 21-OH-def^{severe}
Nonclassic (LOHD)	Symptomatic: later development of virilization; milder symptoms Asymptomatic: no virilization or other symptoms	Moderate elevation of precursors	21-OH-def^{severe} / 21-OH-def^{mild} 21-OH-def^{mild} / 21-OH-def^{mild}
Carrier	Asymptomatic	Precursor level greater than normal	21-OH-def^{severe} / 21-OHase (normal) 21-OH-def^{mild} / 21-OHase (normal)
Normal	Asymptomatic	Lowest levels—some overlap seen with carriers	21-OHase (normal) / 21-OHase (normal)

From New MI, White PC, Pang S, et al: The adrenal hyperplasias. In Scriver CR, Beaudet AL, Sly S, Valle D (eds): Metabolic Basis of Inherited Diseases, 6th ed. New York, McGraw-Hill, 1989.

to this gene is a nonfunctional or pseudogene (CYP21P). Depending on the population, one fourth to one fifth of individuals with classic CAH have a deletion of the *CYP21* locus or a rearrangement between *CYP21* and *CYP21P*. Current molecular techniques of genotyping can pick up well over 95% of these abnormalities, with the majority of cases being one of 10 common mutations. A spectrum of mutations results in the enzymatic defects and clinical presentations shown in Table 40-6.

LOHD is a phenotype that is symptomatic after adolescence and does not define the genotype. Affected individuals may be homozygous for alleles, yielding mildly abnormal enzymatic activity, or compound heterozygotes with a combination of defective alleles. The so-called cryptic 21-OHase deficiency, on the other hand, represents mild or asymptomatic individuals with biochemically identified defects that, with the advent of molecular diagnostic techniques, have been redefined as belonging to several different clinical presentations.

New and associates have proposed a schema for identifying and classifying the clinical spectrum of disease shown in Table 40-6. Since there are three possible manifestations of *CYP21Y* alleles (normal, mildly defective, or severely defective), there are six possible genotypes representing three clinical phenotypes (asymptomatic, LOHD, and classic CAH). Individuals with LOHD may be compound heterozygotes, with one mildly and one severely defective allele, or homozygous, with two mildly defective alleles. Although biochemical differences in the hormonal response to ACTH have been shown between these two genotypes, their phenotypes are similar. Carriers can be identified among family members who are heterozygous with one normal allele. These individuals have normal basal 17-hydroxyprogesterone (17-OHP) levels, a mild degree of hirsutism, if present, and smaller increases of 17-OHP after ACTH stimulation, usually between 3.5 and 10 ng/mL.

LOHD is also usually associated with menstrual irregularity. It has been hypothesized that the mechanism for anovulation is similar to that which occurs with PCOS. The increased levels of androgen lower SHBG levels, thus increasing the amount of biologically active circulating estradiol. The increased estradiol stimulates tonic LH release, which increases ovarian androgen production and locally inhibits follicular growth and ovulation. Thus women with this disorder present with postpubertal onset of hirsutism and oligomenorrhea or amenorrhea, similar to women with PCOS. However, women with LOHD, unlike those with PCOS, commonly have a history of prepubertal accelerated growth (ages 6 to 8 years) with later decreased growth and a short ultimate height. A history of this growth pattern, a family history of postpubertal onset of hirsutism, and findings of mild virilization are indicators of the presence of CAH.

To differentiate LOHD from PCOS, measurement of basal (early-morning) serum 17-OHP levels should be performed. If basal levels of 17-OHP are greater than 8 ng/mL, the diagnosis of LOHD is established. If 17-OHP is above normal (2.5 to 3.3 ng/mL) but less than 8 ng/mL, an ACTH stimulation test should be performed. A baseline 17-OHP should be measured and 0.25 mg of synthetic ACTH infused as a single bolus. One hour later another serum sample of 17-OHP should be measured. If the level of 17-OHP increases more than 10 ng/mL, the diagnosis of LOHD is established (Fig. 40-22). Individuals with LOHD should be treated with continuous corticosteroids to arrest the signs of androgenicity and restore ovulatory menstrual cycles.

Cushing's Syndrome

Excessive adrenal production of glucocorticoids due to increased ACTH secretion (Cushing's disease) or adrenal tumors produces the signs and symptoms of Cushing's syndrome. These findings include hirsutism and menstrual irregularity in addition to the classic findings of central obesity, dorsal neck fat pads, abdominal striae, and muscle wasting and weakness. The latter catabolic effect of glucocorticoid excess differs from the anabolic effects of testosterone excess, but some women with PCOS may have other clinical findings that are similar to those found with Cushing's syndrome. In such instances Cushing's syndrome can be easily excluded by performing an overnight dexamethasone suppression test. To perform this test, 1 mg of dexamethasone

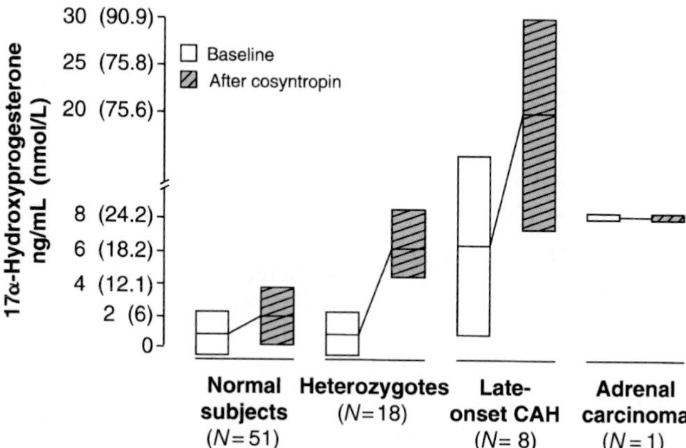

Figure 40-22. Means and ranges of 17α-hydroxyprogesterone levels before and after cosyntropin administered intramuscularly in normal subjects, suspected heterozygotes, patients with late-onset congenital adrenal hyperplasia (CAH), and one patient with adrenal carcinoma. (From Baskin HJ: Screening for late-onset congenital adrenal hyperplasia in hirsutism or amenorrhea. Arch Intern Med 147:847, 1987.)

is ingested at 11 PM, and plasma cortisol is measured the following morning at 8 AM (Fig. 40-23). If the cortisol level is less than 5 μg/100 mL, Cushing's syndrome is ruled out. If the cortisol level fails to suppress to this degree, the diagnosis of Cushing's syndrome is not established. It is necessary to perform a complete dexamethasone suppression test (Liddle's test) or measurement of urinary free cortisol and plasma ACTH to determine whether Cushing's syndrome exists.

Depression and other conditions can cause failure to suppress with the dexamethasone screening test just described. Accordingly many endocrinologists prefer to depend on measurements of 24-hour urinary free cortisol. A creatinine is also measured to gauge completeness of collection. Values above 100 μg/ 24 hr are abnormal, and values greater than 240 μg are virtually diagnostic of Cushing's syndrome. Cushing's syndrome may result from a pituitary tumor producing ACTH (Cushing's disease), from an ectopic tumor in the body, from adrenal neoplasms or hyperplasia. Various algorithms have been developed for this differential diagnosis.

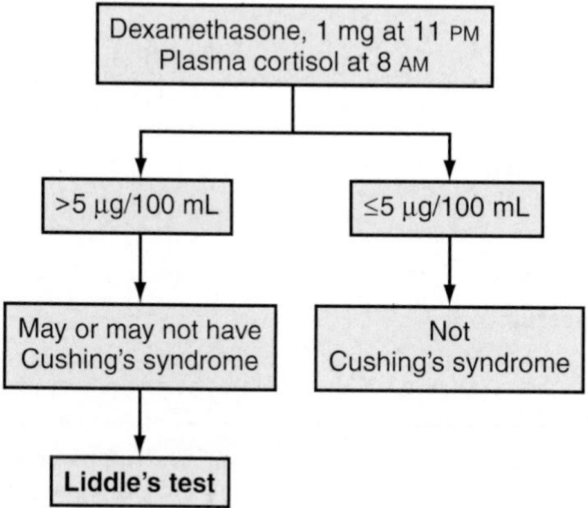

Figure 40-23. Outline of overnight dexamethasone suppression test. (From Goebelsmann U, Lobo RA: Androgen excess. In Mishell DR Jr, Davajan V, Lobo RA [eds]: Infertility, Contraception and Reproductive Endocrinology, 2nd ed. Cambridge, MA, Blackwell Scientific, 1986.)

DIFFERENTIAL DIAGNOSIS

The differential diagnosis of the various causes of androgen excess can usually be made without difficulty by means of a complete history, a careful physical examination, and measurement of serum levels of testosterone and DHEA-S to determine if there is an ovarian or adrenal source of excess androgen production.

Measurement of total testosterone, free testosterone, the free androgen index, and non-SHBG-bound testosterone (unbound testosterone) have all been advocated to assist in the diagnosis of hyperandrogenism. Loric and colleagues measured all these serum parameters in a group of hirsute women and age-matched control subjects. Slopes of the first two of these parameters overlapped between the two groups, whereas no overlap of values occurred with the last two assays. It has been suggested by these and other investigators that measurement of the free androgen index or non-SHBG-bound testosterone is a more specific discriminator of hyperandrogenism than total or free testosterone. Clinically, however, measurement of total testosterone is all that is necessary. It is not clinically important whether a hirsute woman has a total testosterone level in the highest portion of the normal range or a mildly elevated level of non-SHBG-bound testosterone. Schwartz and coworkers reported that when total testosterone levels are elevated, there is an excellent correlation with free testosterone levels. Thus, to determine the magnitude of elevated androgens, as well as their source, measurement of total testosterone is more cost-effective than the other assays and provides the clinician with the information necessary to establish the diagnosis.

As mentioned earlier, androgen excess due to iatrogenic causes, sexual ambiguity, or pregnancy-associated ovarian tumors can usually be easily determined by the history and physical examination. Masculinizing ovarian or adrenal tumors are associated with rapidly progressive signs of hirsutism and virilization. Serum testosterone levels greater than 2 ng/mL with normal DHEA-S levels indicate the probable presence of an ovarian tumor. The diagnosis can be confirmed by bimanual pelvic examination and ultrasonography, CT scan, or MRI. Women with a rapid progression of virilization and DHEA-S levels greater than 8 μg/mL most likely have an androgen-producing adrenal adenoma, and the diagnosis can be confirmed by CT scan or MRI. A long history of gradually increasing hirsutism, even if accompanied by virilization, is not consistent with the diagnosis of adrenal or ovarian tumors. The diagnosis of ovarian stromal hyperthecosis should be suspected for individuals with these signs and testosterone levels greater than 1.5 ng/mL. Women with physical findings consistent with Cushing's syndrome should have the diagnosis ruled out. PCOS, LOHD, and idiopathic hirsutism may be associated with a similar history and findings at physical examination. Menstrual irregularity, however, is uncommon among women with idiopathic hirsutism, and testosterone and DHEA-S levels are normal. Women with LOHD commonly have a family history of androgen excess, and often belong to an ethnic group with a higher gene frequency for an abnormality. The diagnosis of LOHD is established by measurement of 17-OHP either by an early-morning serum sample or following ACTH stimulation. Treatment of hirsutism depends on whether the androgen excess is ovarian, adrenal, or peripheral.

MANAGEMENT

Ovarian and Adrenal Tumors

Nearly all Sertoli–Leydig cell tumors are unilateral. If the woman has not completed her family and these tumors are well differentiated and confined to one ovary, the tumors may be treated by unilateral salpingo-oophorectomy. Since most hilus cell tumors occur after menopause, they are best treated by bilateral salpingo-oophorectomy and total abdominal hysterectomy. Adrenal adenomas and carcinomas also should be treated by operative removal. Adrenal carcinomas frequently have metastasized to the liver by the time the androgenic signs have developed. Despite chemotherapy the prognosis is poor after metastases have occurred. Stromal hyperthecosis is also best treated by bilateral salpingo-oophorectomy together with total abdominal hysterectomy. After removal of the ovaries of women with stromal hyperthecosis or any of the androgen-producing tumors, the acne and oiliness of the skin disappear, breast size increases, and clitoral size decreases. The excess central hair becomes finer and grows less rapidly but does not disappear. Electrolysis can remove the facial hair, and depilatories, bleaches, or shaving can be used to treat the body hair.

Late-Onset 21-Hydrolase Deficiency

The treatment of individuals with LOHD depends on their primary complaint. The androgen excess and menstrual irregularity can be treated as they are in PCOS. However, if these women wish to conceive, it is preferable to use glucocorticoids such as hydrocortisone (15 to 20 mg), prednisone (5 to 7.5 mg), or dexamethasone (0.5 to 0.75 mg) in divided doses. Doses as low as 2.5 mg of prednisone or 0.25 mg dexamethasone may be used initially. The aim of treatment is to suppress androstenedione and bring 17-OHP and progesterone levels into the normal range. Ovulation usually resumes rapidly.

Polycystic Ovarian Syndrome

Before ovulation induction, it is necessary to normalize overt abnormalities in glucose tolerance and to encourage weight loss if BMI is excessive (>28). Ovulation induction may be accomplished by a variety of agents including metformin, clomiphene, letrozole (and other aromatase inhibitors), gonadotropins, and pulsatile GnRH as well as ovarian diathermy or drilling. Adjunctive measures include the use of dexamethasone, dopamine agonists, thiadolazimediones, and various combinations of these. In vitro fertilization (stimulated or unstimulated) may be indicated in difficult to manage cases or if other fertility factors are present.

Metformin has emerged as a first-line treatment for infertility although not all women with PCOS will respond. A recent Cochrane review reported an odds ratio of 3.88 (CI 2.25–6.69) for restoration of ovulatory function. In a recent randomized trial of metformin (1700 mg/day vs. clomiphene 150 mg for 5 days), the cumulative pregnancy rate for metformin (68.9%) was significantly better than for clomiphene (34%, $p < 0.01$); and the abortion rate was lower with metformin (9.7% vs. 37.5%, $p = 0.045$). Even when metformin is not able to induce ovulation, its continued use may be beneficial when combined with clomiphene or gonadotropins. An improvement in oocyte quality with metformin has been suggested, but the effect has not been proven.

Clomiphene has been the mainstay for ovulation induction, but its use as a first-line therapy has been challenged recently. Most pregnancies occur within the first few cycles. Accordingly it is reasonable to continue to use clomiphene, with or without metformin, as an initial approach, but not for more than three or four ovulatory cycles.

Letrozole (2.5 to 5 mg/day for 5 days) has proven to be efficacious as a first-line agent and is particularly suited for women who have side effects with clomiphene. However, there are no long-term data to date, and although unlikely, an increased fetal anomaly rate has been suggested.

Low-dose gonadotropin therapy is highly effective as a second-line treatment, and there is no evidence that any one gonadotropin preparation is better than another. Pulsatile GnRH therapy is rarely used currently primarily because its use is cumbersome. Ovarian drilling (diathermy) is a reasonable second-line therapy, particularly in clomiphene failures and when gonadotropin therapy has proven difficult (Table 40-7). In randomized trials against standard gonadotropin therapy ovarian drilling resulted in similar pregnancy rates but with a lower rate of multiple pregnancies.

As adjunctive treatment, thiadolazimediones have been found to be similar in effectiveness to metformin for ovulation

Table 40-7 Ovulation and Pregnancy After Electrocautery and Laser Treatment of Polycystic Ovaries

N	Ovulation (%)	Pregnancy (%)	Authors and year of Publication*
Electrocautery			
35	92	69†	Gjønnaess (1984)
6	83	67	Greenblatt and Casper (1987)
14	64	36	v.d. Weiden et al (1989)
21	81	52	Armar et al (1990)
29	71	52	Abdel Gadir (1990)
7	71	57	Gürgan et al (1991)
10	70		Kovacs et al (1991)
22		86	Armar and Lachelin (1993)
104	76	70	Naether et al (1993)
10	70		Tiitinen et al (1993)
Laser vaporization			
85	53	56	Daniell and Miller (1989)
19	80	37	Keckstein et al (1990)
10	70		Gürgan et al (1991)
Wedge resection			
8	65	0	Huber et al (1988)
12	83	58	Kojima et al (1989)

*References are from the original source. Before laparascopy, some *patients* had been resistant to hormonal stimulation therapy. After inclusion of patients made responsive to clomiphene citrate (CC) by electrocautery, the pregnancy rate increased to 80%.

From Gjønnaess H: Ovarian electrocautery in the treatment of women with polycystic ovary syndrome (PCOS): Factors affecting the results. Acta Obstet Gynecol Scand 73:407, 1994.

induction. However, there is a concern with its use because of the risk of teratogenicity.

Treatment of Skin Disorders

Hirsutism, acne, and alopecia are related to hyperandrogenism in women with PCOS. Although ovarian or adrenal androgen excess increases the likelihood of these complaints, enhancement of these effects due to increased 5α-reductase activity largely explains the abnormalities. Accordingly, successful strategy usually requires an antiandrogen added to ovarian suppressive therapy, usually with an OC. Clearly women with PCOS who are interested in pregnancy are not candidates for suppressive therapy or the use of antiandrogens.

Peripheral androgen blockade with antiandrogens is dose-related, and spironolactone and flutamide are the most frequently used agents although finasteride, a specific 5α-2 inhibitor also has efficacy. Cyproterone acetate (2 mg) is most frequently used in combination with ethinyl estradiol as an OC, although larger doses have been used as well. A recent review on hirsutism suggested that spironolactone (100 mg daily) is superior to finasteride (5 mg) and cyproterone acetate (12.5 mg).

Flutamide, a "pure" androgen, should only be used in lower doses because of hepatic toxicity. This antiandrogen may have particular efficacy for androgenic alopecia, although there is only limited success with any therapy for this disorder.

Use of a nonandrogenic progestogen (desogestrel, norgestimate, or drospirenone) in an OC in combination with spironolactone (100 to 200 mg) is suggested to be the first-line treatment. Adjuncts or other antiandrogens can be used if necessary. In very severe cases, use of a GnRH agonist with estrogen or an OC "add-back" has been shown to be successful. However, this therapy is difficult to maintain long term. Androgenic acne responds more quickly to treatment and is more successful than the treatment of hirsutism: Alopecia is least responsive to therapy, with responses rates only in the range of 30%.

Treatment of Metabolic and Weight Concerns

The key management strategy should be directed at altering lifestyle variables. Exercise regimens, particularly when coordinated with a group of similar women, have been shown to be beneficial. Details of these approaches may be found elsewhere. However, this philosophy should be part and parcel of all therapies for PCOS, acknowledging that some thin and normal weight women with PCOS probably already have a healthy lifestyle.

Metabolic syndrome (MBS), driven largely by weight in the United States, is usually treated by a combination of diet and metformin. Six- to 12-month therapies have been shown to reduce weight by 5% to 7%, as well as to reduce insulin resistance and improve metabolic parameters. Most recently, positive results also have been reported with the use of bariatric surgery as well in obese women with PCOS. Clearly this approach carries risks and should not be considered as first line.

Some data suggest that the use of antiandrogens (specifically flutamide) may also be efficacious for reducing body weight and visceral fat in women with PCOS. A combination of drospirenone/EE_2 with flutamide and metformin has been used successfully in adolescents. This multidrug regimen has not been tested in an adult population. Although therapy for women with PCOS should be directed at a woman's specific complaint, improvement of lifestyle variables including weight reduction and fitness should be the mainstay of all treatments. Metformin is emerging as a first-line management strategy for fertility and as an adjunct for metabolic concerns, particularly when MBS is present. For skin manifestations of androgen excess, first-line treatment should encompass the combination of an OC with an antiandrogen.

A summary of various treatments for specific complaints is provided in (Table 40-8).

Table 40-8 Treatment for Women with PCOS

Complaint	Treatment Options
Infertility	Metformin; clomiphene; letrozole; gonadotropins; ovarian cautery
Skin manifestations	Oral contraceptive + antiandrogen (spironolactone, flutamide, finestride); GnRH agonists
Dysfunctional bleeding	Cyclic progestogen; oral contraceptives
Weight/metabolic concerns	Diet/lifestyle management; metformin

Idiopathic Hirsutism

Although hirsutism is a benign condition, it is frequently of great concern to the woman. Women with idiopathic hirsutism have normal circulating levels of testosterone and DHEA-S. Nearly all individuals with symptomatic hirsutism who have normal testosterone and DHEA-S levels have elevated skin 5α-RA, which may by reflected in elevated levels of 3α-diol-G. It is not necessary to measure 3α-diol-G in women with hirsutism without elevated circulating androgen levels, because the presence of hirsutism is itself evidence of increased peripheral androgen activity. An agent that inhibits peripheral androgen activity should be administered to women with these findings.

Because of the length of the hair growth cycle, responses to treatment should not be expected to occur within the first 3 months of therapy. Objective methods of assessing changes of hair growth, such as photographs, are useful. With use of various therapies, a successful response should occur in about 70% of women with 1 year of therapy. Remaining excess hair can be removed by electrolysis. Treatment should be continued for 4 years and then stopped to determine if hirsutism recurs. If so, therapy can be reinitiated.

Many agents are available to inhibit the various sources of androgen production that may lead to hirsutism. OCs suppress LH and ovarian testosterone production by the inhibitory action of the progestational component. The estrogenic component in OCs increases SHBG levels in the circulation, which decreases free testosterone levels. The progestins in the OCs also inhibit 5α-reductase activity in the skin. Women in whom OCs are contraindicated or produce side effects may be treated with medroxyprogesterone acetate. This agent also inhibits LH, which causes decreased testosterone production, although to a lesser extent than occurs with combined OCs. Treatment with GnRH agonists is expensive and reserved for severe clinical manifestations of ovarian hyperandrogenism, not hirsutism alone.

Ketoconazole, which blocks adrenal and gonadal steroidogenesis by inhibiting cytochrome P-450-dependent enzyme pathways, has been used in dosages of 200 mg twice a day to treat hyperandrogenism associated with PCOS and idiopathic hirsutism. This potent drug effectively decreases hair growth and acne, but major side effects and complications (including hepatitis) occur in the majority of women treated. These problems limit the use of ketoconazole to very select women, who require careful monitoring. In these severe cases it is probably preferable to use a GnRH agonist.

Spironolactone has been used and studied extensively and should be considered the treatment of choice in the United States for women with idiopathic hirsutism as well as many with PCOS. This agent, in addition to being an androgen receptor blocker, also decreases ovarian testosterone production and inhibits 5α-RA. Various dosages from 50 to 200 mg daily have been used. We reported that a dose of 200 mg/day of spironolactone is more effective than 100 mg/day. Barth and associates found a clinically evident response of decreased hair after 3 months of 200 mg/day of spironolactone. After 1 year of treatment a 15% to 25% reduction occurred in both hair shaft diameter and linear growth rate at all body sites. With the higher dose of spironolactone, liver function tests and plasma electrolytes are usually unchanged, and side effects occur infrequently except for irregular uterine bleeding. The latter can be controlled with concomitant use of OCs. Electrolytes and blood pressure should be monitored for the first few weeks of therapy to be certain hypotension and hyperkalemia do not occur. Finasteride, a 5α-reductase inhibitor (5 mg/day), and flutamide, a nonsteroidal antiandrogen (250 to 500 mg/day) have also been used to treat hirsutism and have a similar level of effectiveness as spironolactone (100 mg/day). If flutamide is used, doses should be kept as low as possible and liver function tests should be obtained regularly. None of these agents, however, is approved for treatment in the United States. Antiandrogen therapy has been shown to be the most important modality for hirsutism treatment.

KEY POINTS

- The three cyclic changes of hair development include a growth phase called anagen, followed by a transitional phase called catagen and a resting phase called telogen.
- Testosterone levels in women with hirsutism without virilization are lower than 1.5 ng/mL.
- Circulating testosterone levels in the presence of virilization are usually greater than 2 ng/mL.
- The major androgen provided by the ovaries is testosterone, and that of the adrenal glands is DHEA-S.
- Total daily testosterone production is 0.35 mg: 0.1 mg from ovarian secretion, 0.2 mg from peripheral conversion of androstenedione, and 0.05 mg from peripheral conversion of DHEA.
- About two thirds of the daily testosterone production in a woman originates in the ovaries.
- There are three markers of androgen production, one for each compartment where androgens are produced. In the ovary it is testosterone; in the adrenal gland, DHEA-S; and in the periphery, 3α-diol-G.
- About 85% of testosterone is bound to SHBG and is biologically inactive, 10% to 15% is bound to albumin, and 1% to 2% is not bound. Both of the latter fractions are biologically active.
- Non-SHBG-bound testosterone is elevated in about 60% to 70% of women with hirsutism, and 3α-diol-G is elevated in about 98%.
- About 80% of individuals with idiopathic hirsutism have elevated levels of 3α-diol-G.
- Individuals with idiopathic hirsutism have increased 5α-RA.
- Women with PCOS usually have testosterone levels between 0.7 and 1.2 ng/mL and androstenedione levels of 3 to 5 ng/mL; about half have elevated levels of DHEA-S.
- About 30% of women with PCOS do not have hirsutism.
- About 70% of women with PCOS have elevated levels of immunologic LH or an immunologic LH–FSH ratio greater than 3, and nearly all have elevated levels of biologically active LH and biologically active estradiol and increased amplitude of LH pulse.
- About 40% of women with PCOS have hyperinsulinemia and impaired glucose tolerance.
- Acanthosis nigricans is a common finding in obese women who have PCOS. It is generally unnecessary to measure free testosterone, free androgen, free androgen index, or non-SHBG-bound testosterone. Only total testosterone needs to be measured.
- If untreated, women with PCOS have an increased risk of developing diabetes mellitus and hypertension after menopause.
- Women with ovarian neoplasms have testosterone levels more than two and a half times the upper limits of the normal range.
- The diagnosis of LOHD is established if the basal (early morning) serum 17-hydroxyprogesterone (17-OHP) levels are greater than 5 ng/mL or if the level at 1 hour after infusion of 0.25 μg ACTH is more than 10 ng/mL.
- About 40% of women with PCOS have impaired glucose tolerance (30%) or undiagnosed noninsulin-dependent diabetes mellitus (10%).
- Metformin given to women with PCOS decreases glucose and may increase insulin sensitivity. It frequently causes ovulation to occur and increases the frequency of ovulation when clomiphene citrate is given to women with PCOS.
- Women with LOHD have a block in cortisol biosynthesis of 11β-hydroxylase or 21-hydroxylase, resulting in increased circulating levels of 17-OHP.

KEY POINTS *Continued*

- Because of the length of the hair growth cycle, response should not be expected until after 3 months of therapy. Successful responses should occur in about 70% of those patients treated.
- If after an overnight dexamethasone suppression test serum cortisol levels are lower than 5 μg/100 mL, Cushing's syndrome may be ruled out.
- The best treatment for hirsutism due to increased peripheral androgen metabolism is the antiandrogen spironolactone.
- Women with PCOS who desire fertility should be treated with agents that stimulate ovulation, starting with metformin, clomiphene citrate and, if the condition is unresponsive, proceeding to gonadotropins. An alternative treatment for unresponsive patients is ovarian drilling.
- Spironolactone, an aldosterone antagonist, is the most effective treatment for idiopathic hirsutism, but is dose-related. The major side effect is abnormal bleeding, which can be controlled with use of OCs. Spironolactone should be administered in a dose of 100 to 200 mg/day.

BIBLIOGRAPHY

Andreyko JL, Monroe SE, Jaffe RB, et al: Treatment of hirsutism with a gonadotropin-releasing hormone agonist (nafarelin). J Clin Endocrinol Metab 63:854, 1986.

Ardaens Y, Robert Y, Leemaitre L, et al: Polycystic ovarian disease: contribution of vaginal endosonography and reassessment of ultrasonic diagnosis. Fertil Steril 55:1062, 1991.

Azziz R, Zacur HA: 21-Hydroxylase deficiency in female hyperandrogenism: Screening and diagnosis. J Clin Endocrinol Metab 69:577, 1989.

Balen AH, Conway GS, Kaltsas G, et al: Polycystic ovary syndrome: The spectrum of the disorder in 1741 patients. Hum Reprod 10:2107, 1995.

Barth JH, Cherry CA, Wojnarowska F, Dawber RPR: Spironolactone is an effective and well tolerated systematic antiandrogen therapy for hirsute women. J Clin Endocrinol Metab 68:966, 1989.

Baskin HJ: Screening for late-onset congenital adrenal hyperplasia in hirsutism or amenorrhea. Arch Intern Med 147:847, 1987.

Boyers P, Buster JE, Marshall JR: Hypothalamic-pituitary-adrenocortical function during long-term low-dose dexamethasone therapy in hyperandrogenized women. Am J Obstet Gynecol 142:330, 1982.

Bridges NA, Cooke A, Healy MJ, Hindmarsh PC, Brook CG.: Standards for ovarian volume in childhood and puberty. Fertil Steril 60(3):456, 1993.

Burger CW, Korsen T, van Kessel H, et al: Pulsatile luteinizing hormone patterns in the follicular phase of the menstrual cycle, polycystic ovarian disease (PCOD) and non-PCOD secondary amenorrhea. J Clin Endocrinol Metab 61:1126, 1985.

Carlstrom K, Gershagen S, Marcolin G, et al: Free testosterone and testosterone/SHBG index in hirsute women: A comparison of diagnostic accuracy. Gynecol Obstet Invest 24:256, 1987.

Chang RJ, Mandel FP, Wolfsen AR, et al: Circulating levels of plasma adrenocorticotropin in polycystic ovary disease. J Clin Endocrinol Metab 54:1265, 1982.

Chapman AJ, Wilson M, Obhrai M, et al: Effect of bromocriptine on pulsatility in the polycystic ovary syndrome. Clin Endocrinol 27:571, 1987.

Chapman G, Dowsett M, Dewhurst CJ, Jeffcoate SL: Spironolactone in combination with an oral contraceptive: An alternative treatment for hirsutism. Br J Obstet Gynaecol 92:983, 1985.

Chez RA: Clinical aspects of three new progestogens: Desogestrel, gestodene, and norgestimate. Am J Obstet Gynecol 160:1296, 1989.

Conway GS, Jacobs HS: Clinical implications of hyperinsulinemia in women. Clin Endocrinol 39:623, 1993.

Cumming DC, Wall SR: Non-sex hormone-binding globulin-bound testosterone is a marker for hyperandrogenism. J Clin Endocrinol Metab 61:873, 1985.

Cumming D, Yang JC, Rebar RW, et al: Treatment of hirsutism with spironolactone. JAMA 247:1295, 1982.

Dahlgren E, Janson PO, Johansson S, et al: Women with polycystic ovary syndrome wedge resected in 1956 to 1965: A long-term follow-up focusing on natural history and circulating hormones. Fertil Steril 57:505, 1992.

DeVane GW, Czekala NM, Judd HL, et al: Circulating gonadotropins, estrogens, and androgens in polycystic ovarian disease. Am J Obstet Gynecol 121:496, 1975.

Dewailly D, Vantyghem-Haudiquet MC, Sainsard C, et al: Clinical and biological phenotypes in late-onset 21-hydroxylase deficiency. J Clin Endocrinol Metab 63:418, 1986.

Dibbelt L, Knuppen R, Jutting G, et al: Group comparison of serum ethinyl estradiol, SHGB and CBG levels in 83 women using 2 low-dose combination oral contraceptives for 3 months. Contraception 43:1, 1991.

Dolzan V, Solyom J, Fekete G, et al: Mutational spectrum of steroid 21-hydroxylase and the genotype-phenotype association in Middle European patients with congenital adrenal hyperplasia. Eur J Endocrinol 153:99, 2005.

Dunaif A, Graf M, Mandeli J, et al: Characterization of groups of hyperandrogenic women with acanthosis nigricans, impaired glucose tolerance, and/or hyperinsulinemia. J Clin Endocrinol Metab 65:499, 1987.

Ehrmann DA, Cavaghan MK, Barnes RB: Prevalence of impaired glucose tolerance and diabetes in women with polycystic ovary syndrome. Diabetes Care 22:141, 1999.

Felemban A, Tan SL, Tulandi T: Laparoscopic treatment of polycystic ovaries with insulated needle cautery: A reappraisal. Fertil Steril 73:266, 2000.

Ferriman D, Gallwey JD: Clinical assessment of body hair growth in women. J Clin Endocrinol Metab 21:1440, 1961.

Filicori M, Flamigni C, Campaniello E, et al: The abnormal response of polycystic ovarian disease patients to exogenous pulsatile gonadotropin-releasing hormone: characterization and management. J Clin Endocrinol Metab 69:825, 1989.

Fox R, Corrigan E, Thomas PA, Hull MGR: The diagnosis of polycystic ovaries in women with oligo-amenorrhoea: predictive power of endocrine tests. Clin Endocrinol (Oxf) 34:127, 1991.

Givens JR, Andersen RN, Wiser WL, et al: A gonadotropin responsive adrenocortical adenoma. J Clin Endocrinol Metab 38:126, 1974.

Gjønnaess H: Late endocrine effects of ovarian electrocautery in women with polycystic ovary syndrome. Fertil Steril 69:697, 1998.

Gjønnaess H: Ovarian electrocautery in the treatment of women with polycystic ovary syndrome (PCOS): Factors affecting the results. Acta Obstet Gynecol Scand 73:407, 1994.

Goldzieher JW: Polycystic ovarian syndrome. Fertil Steril 35:371, 1981.

Goldzieher JW, Axelrod LR: Clinical and biochemical features of polycystic ovarian disease. Fertil Steril 14:631, 1963.

Hann LE, Hall DA, McArdle CR, Seibel M: Polycystic ovarian disease: Sonographic spectrum. Radiology 150:531, 1984.

Helfer EL, Miller JL, Rose LI: Side effects of spironolactone therapy in the hirsute woman. J Clin Endocrinol Metab 66:208, 1988.

Hensleigh PA, Woodruff JD: Differential maternal-fetal response to androgenizing luteoma or hyperreactio luteinalis. Obstet Gynecol Surv 33:262, 1978.

Hoffman D, Klove K, Lobo RA: The prevalence and significance of elevated dehydroepiandrosterone sulfate levels in anovulatory women. Fertil Steril 42:76, 1984.

Horton R, Hawks D, Lobo RA: 3α,17β-androstanediol glucuronide in plasma: A marker of androgen action in idiopathic hirsutism. J Clin Invest 69:1203, 1982.

Horton R, Lobo RA: Peripheral androgens and the role of androstanediol glucuronide. Clin Endocrinol Metab 15:293, 1986.

Hull MGR: Epidemiology of infertility and polycystic ovarian disease: Endocrinological and demographic studies. Gynecol Endocrinol 1:235, 1987.

Ireland K, Woodruff JD: Masculinizing ovarian tumors. Obstet Gynecol Surv 31:83, 1976.

Judd HL, Rigg LA, Anderson DC, et al: The effects of ovarian wedge resection on circulating gonadotropin and ovarian steroid levels in patients with polycystic ovary syndrome. J Clin Endocrinol Metab 43:347, 1976.

Judd HL, Scully RE, Herbst AL, et al: Familial hyperthecosis: Comparison of endocrinologic and histologic findings with polycystic ovarian disease. Am J Obstet Gynecol 117:976, 1973.

Kazer AR, Kessel B, Yen SSC: Circulating luteinizing hormone pulse frequency in women with polycystic ovary syndrome. J Clin Endocrinol Metab 65:233, 1987.

Kirschner MA, Samojlik E, Szmal E: Clinical usefulness of plasma androstanediol glucuronide measurements in women with idiopathic hirsutism. J Clin Endocrinol Metab 65:597, 1987.

Klove KL, Roy S, Lobo RA: The effect of different contraceptive treatments on the serum concentration of dehydroepiandrosterone sulfate. Contraception 29:319, 1984.

Knochenhauer ES, Key TJ, Kahsar-Miller, et al: Prevalence of the polycystic ovary syndrome in unselected black and white women of the southeastern United States: a prospective study. J Clin Endocrinol Metab 83:3078, 1998.

Kohn B, Levine MS, Pollack MS, et al: Late-onset steroid 21-hydroxylase deficiency: A variant of classical congenital adrenal hyperplasia. J Clin Endocrinol Metab 55:817, 1982.

Koivunen R, Laatikainen T, Tomas C, et al: The prevalence of polycystic ovaries in healthy women. Acta Obstet Gynecol Scand 78:137, 1999.

Kokaly W, McKenna TJ: Relapse of hirsutism following a long-term successful treatment with oestrogen. Clin Endocrinol 52:379, 2000.

Koskinen P, Erkkota R, Penttila T-A, et al: Optimal use of hormone determinations in the biochemical diagnosis of the polycystic ovary syndrome. Fertil Steril 65:517, 1996.

Kuttenn F, Couillin P, Girard F, et al: Late-onset adrenal hyperplasia in hirsutism. N Engl J Med 313:224, 1985.

Legro RS, Kunselman AR, Dodson WC, Dunaif A: Prevalence and predictors of risk for type 2 diabetes mellitus and impaired glucose tolerance in polycystic ovary syndrome: A prospective controlled study in 254 affected women. J Clin Endocrinol Metab 84:165, 1999.

Li TC, Saravelos H, Chow MS, et al: Factors affecting the outcome of laparoscopic ovarian drilling for polycystic ovarian syndrome in women with anovulatory infertility. Br J Obstet Gynaecol 105:338, 1998.

Lobo RA, Goebelsmann U: Adult manifestation of congenital adrenal hyperplasia due to incomplete 21-hydroxylase deficiency mimicking polycystic ovarian disease. Am J Obstet Gynecol 138:720, 1980.

Lobo RA, Goebelsmann U: Evidence for reduced 3β-ol-hydroxysteroid dehydrogenase activity in some hirsute women thought to have polycystic ovary syndrome. J Clin Endocrinol Metab 53:394, 1981.

Lobo RA, Goebelsmann U: Effect of androgen excess on inappropriate gonadotropin secretion as found in polycystic ovary syndrome. Am J Obstet Gynecol 142:394, 1982.

Lobo RA, Goebelsmann U, Horton R: Evidence for the importance of peripheral tissue events in the development of hirsutism in polycystic ovary syndrome. J Clin Endocrinol Metab 57:393, 1983.

Lobo RA, Granger L, Goebelsmann U, et al: Elevation in unbound serum estradiol as a possible mechanism for inappropriate gonadotropin secretion in women with PCO. J Clin Endocrinol Metab 52:156, 1981.

Lobo RA, Granger LR, Paul WL, et al: Psychological stress and increases in urinary norepinephrine metabolites, platelet serotonin and adrenal androgens in women with polycystic ovary syndrome. Am J Obstet Gynecol 145:496, 1983.

Lobo RA, Kletzky OA, Campeau JD, et al: Elevated bioactive luteinizing hormone in women with the polycystic ovary syndrome. Fertil Steril 39:674, 1983.

Lobo RA, Paul WL, Goebelsmann U: Dehydroepiandrosterone sulfate as an indicator of adrenal androgen function. Obstet Gynecol 57:69, 1981.

Lobo RA, Paul WL, Goebelsmann U: Serum levels of DHEA-S in gynecologic endocrinopathy and infertility. Obstet Gynecol 57:607, 1981.

Lobo RA, Shoupe D, Serafini P, et al: The effects of two doses of spironolactone on serum androgens and anagen hair in hirsute women. Fertil Steril 43:200, 1985.

Loric S, Guechot J, Duron F, et al: Determination of testosterone in serum not bound by sex-hormone-binding globulin: Diagnostic value in hirsute women. Clin Chem 34:1826, 1988.

Mandel FP, Chang RJ, Dupont B, et al: HLA genotyping in family members and patients with familial polycystic ovarian disease. J Clin Endocrinol Metab 56:862, 1983.

Michelmore KF, Balen AH, Dunger DB, Vessey MP: Polycystic ovaries and associated clinical and biochemical features in young women. Clin Endocrinol 51:779, 1999.

Milewicz A, Silber D, Kirschner MA: Therapeutic effects of spironolactone in polycystic ovary syndrome. Obstet Gynecol 61:429, 1983.

Moghetti P, Castello R, Negri C, et al: Metformin effects on clinical features, endocrine and metabolic profiles, and insulin sensitivity in polycystic ovary syndrome: A randomized, double-blind, placebo-controlled 6-month trial, followed by open, long-term clinical evaluation. J Clin Endocrinol Metab 85:139, 2000.

Mornet E, Crete P, Kuttenn F, et al: Distribution of deletions and seven point mutations on CYP21-genes in three clinical forms of steroid 21-hydroxylase deficiency. Am J Hum Genet 48:79, 1991.

Murdoch AP, McClean KG, Watson MJ, et al: Treatment of hirsutism in polycystic ovary syndrome with bromocriptine. Br J Obstet Gynaecol 94:358, 1987.

Nestler JE, Jakubowicz DJ, Evans WS, et al: Effects of metformin on spontaneous and clomiphene-induced ovulation in the polycystic ovary syndrome. N Engl J Med 338:1876, 1998.

New MI, Lorenzen F, Lerner AJ, et al: Genotyping steroid 21-hydroxylase deficiency: hormonal reference data. J Clin Endocrinol Metab 57:320, 1983.

New MI, White PC, Pang S, et al: The adrenal hyperplasias. In Scriver CR, Beaudet AL, Sly S, and Valle D (eds): Metabolic Basis of Inherited Diseases, 6th ed. New York, McGraw-Hill, 1989.

Nicolini U, Ferrazzi E, Bellotti M, et al: The contribution of sonographic evaluation of ovarian size in patients with polycystic ovarian disease. J Ultrasound Med 4:342, 1985.

Norman RJ, Hague WM, Masters SC, Wang XJ: Subjects with polycystic ovaries without hyperandrogenaemia exhibit similar disturbances in insulin and lipid profiles as those with polycystic ovary syndrome. Hum Reprod10:2258, 1995.

Norman RJ, Davies MJ, Lord J, Moran LJ: The role of lifestyle modification in polycystic ovary syndrome. Trends Endocrinol Metab 13:251, 2002.

Pache TD, Wladimiroff JW, Hop WC, Fauser BC: How to discriminate between normal and polycystic ovaries: Transvaginal US study. Radiology 183:421, 1992.

Pang S, Wallace MA, Hofman L, et al: Worldwide experience in newborn screening for classical congenital adrenal hyperplasia due to 21-hydroxylase deficiency. Pediatrics 81:866, 1988.

Parisi L, Tramonti M, Casciano S, et al: The role of ultrasound in the study of polycystic ovarian disease. J Clin Ultrasound 10:167, 1982.

Paulson RJ, Serafini PC, Catalino JA, Lobo RA: Measurements of 3α,17β-androstanediol glucuronide in serum and urine and the correlation with skin 5α-reductase activity. Fertil Steril 46:222, 1986.

Phocas I, Chryssikopoulos A, Sarandakou A, et al: A contribution to the classification of cases of non-classic 21-hydroxylase-deficient congenital adrenal hyperplasia. Gynecol Endocrinol 9:229, 1995.

Plymate SR, Fariss BL, Bassett ML, et al: Obesity and its role in polycystic ovary syndrome. J Clin Endocrinol Metab 52:1246, 1981.

Polson DW, Adams J, Wadsworth J, Franks S: Polycystic ovaries: A common finding in normal women. Lancet 1:870, 1988.

Raj SG, Thompson IE, Berger MJ, et al: Clinical aspects of the polycystic ovary syndrome. Obstet Gynecol 49:552, 1977.

Rebar R, Judd HL, Yen SSC, et al: Characterization of the inappropriate gonadotropin secretion in polycystic ovary syndrome. J Clin Invest 57:1320, 1976.

Rittmaster RS: Differential suppression of testosterone and estradiol in hirsute women with the superactive gonadotropin-releasing hormone agonist leuprolide. J Clin Endocrinol Metab 67:651, 1988.

Rittmaster RS, Loriaux DL, Cutler GB: Sensitivity of cortisol and adrenal androgens to dexamethasone suppression in hirsute women. J Clin Endocrinol Metab 61:462, 1985.

Rittmaster RS, Thompson DL: Effect of leuprolide and dexamethasone on hair growth and hormone levels in hirsute women: The relative importance of the ovary and the adrenal in the pathogenesis of hirsutism. J Clin Endocrinol Metab 70:1096, 1990.

Schwartz U, Moltz L, Brotherton J, Hammerstein J: The diagnostic value of plasma free testosterone in non-tumorous and tumorous hyperandrogenism. Fertil Steril 40:66, 1983.

Serafini P, Ablan R, Lobo RA: 5α-Reductase activity in the genital skin of hirsute women. J Clin Endocrinol Metab 60:349, 1985.

Speiser PW, Dupont B, Rubenstein P, et al: High frequency of nonclassical steroid 21-hydroxylase deficiency. Am J Hum Genet 37:650, 1985.

Speiser PW, New MI, White PC: Molecular genetic analysis of nonclassic steroid 21-hydroxylase deficiency associated with HLA-B14, DR1. N Engl J Med 319:19, 1988.

Speiser PW: Molecular diagnosis of CYP21 mutations in congenital adrenal hyperplasia: Implications for genetic counseling. Review. Am J Pharmacogenomics 1:101, 2001.

Stein IF, Leventhal ML: Amenorrhea associated with bilateral polycystic ovaries. Am J Obstet Gynecol 29:181, 1935.

Swanson M, Sauerbrei EE, Cooperberg PL: Medical implications of ultrasonically detected polycystic ovaries. J Clin Ultrasound 9:219, 1981.

Urbanek M, Woodroffe A, Ewens KG, et al: Candidate gene region for polycystic ovary syndrome on chromosome 19p13.2. J Clin Endocrinol Metab 90(12):6623, 2005.

Velazquez E, Acosta A, Mendoza SG: Menstrual cyclicity after metformin therapy in polycystic ovary syndrome. Obstet Gynecol 90:392, 1997.

Venturoli S, Fabbri R, Dal Prato L, et al: Ketoconazole therapy for women with acne and/or hirsutism. J Clin Endocrinol Metab 71:335, 1990.

Wild RA, Bartholomew MJ: The influence of body weight on lipoprotein lipids in patients with polycystic ovary syndrome. Am J Obstet Gynecol 159:423, 1988.

Wild RA, Demers LM, Applebaum-Bowden D, Lenker R: Hirsutism: Metabolic effects of two commonly used oral contraceptives and spironolactone. Contraception 44:113, 1991.

Wild RA, Umstot ES, Andersen RN, et al: Adrenal function in hirsutism. II. Effect of an oral contraceptive. J Clin Endocrinol Metab 54:676, 1981.

Williams IA, Shaw RW, Burford G: An attempt to alter the pathophysiology of polycystic ovary syndrome using a gonadotropin hormone releasing hormone agonist-nafarelin. Clin Endocrinol 31:345, 1989.

Wilroy RS Jr, Givens JR, Wiser WL, et al: Genetic forms of hypogonadism. Birth Defects 11:81, 1975.

Yeh HC, Futterweit W, Thornton JC: Polycystic ovarian disease: US features in 104 patients. Radiology 163:111, 1987.

Yen SSC: Chronic anovulation caused by peripheral endocrine disorders. In Yen SSC, Jaffe RB (eds): Reproductive Endocrinology, 2nd ed. Philadelphia, WB Saunders, 1986.

Yen SSC, Chaney C, Judd HL: Functional aberrations of the hypothalamic–pituitary system in polycystic ovary syndrome: A consideration of the pathogenesis. In James VHT, Serio M, Guisti G (eds): The Endocrine Function of the Human Ovary. New York, Academic Press, 1976.

Infertility

41

Etiology, Diagnostic Evaluation, Management, Prognosis

Rogerio A. Lobo

KEY TERMS AND DEFINITIONS

Artificial Insemination. Method to place sperm in the female reproductive tract by means other than sexual intercourse. If the sperm are from the husband, the technique is called artificial insemination husband (AIH). If the sperm are from another man, the method has been called artificial insemination donor (AID). Other terms are *donor insemination* and *therapeutic donor insemination* (TDI).

Assisted Reproductive Technology. Various techniques utilized to increase fecundability by nonphysiologic methods of enhancing probability of fertilization. Categories include in vitro fertilization, gamete intrafallopian tube transfer, zygote intrafallopian tube transfer, and tubal embryo transfer.

Asthenospermia. Loss or reduction of the motility of the spermatozoa.

Azoospermia. Absence of sperm in the semen.

Clomiphene Citrate. A weak synthetic estrogenic compound with three benzene rings given orally to induce ovulation in anovulatory women with circulating estradiol levels more than 40 pg/mL.

Controlled Ovarian Hyperstimulation (COH). Inducing development of more than one dominant follicle with pharmacologic agents, usually clomiphene citrate or gonadotropins, also called *superovulation or multiple follicular recruitment* (MFR). COH is usually combined with intrauterine insemination to treat unexplained infertility.

Fecundability. Probability of conception occurring in a population of couples in a given period of time, usually 1 month.

Fimbrioplasty. Surgical technique of removing adhesions between fimbrial fronds of the partially occluded distal end of the oviduct.

Gamete Intrafallopian Transfer (GIFT). Placement of human ova and sperm into the distal end of the oviduct.

Hamster Egg Penetration Assay (Sperm Penetration Assay). Test of the fertilizing ability of human sperm based on their ability to penetrate zona-free hamster ova.

Human Menopausal Gonadotropin (HMG). Formulation made up of equal amounts of follicle-stimulating hormone (FSH) and luteinizing hormone (LH) derived from urine obtained from postmenopausal women. The injectable agent is used to stimulate follicular development in both anovulatory and ovulatory women.

Several urinary extracts are available including one with proportionality greater FSH activity. Recombinant (pure) FSH is often used and recombinant (pure) LH is also available as a supplement.

Hysterosalpingogram (HSG). Fluoroscopic and radiographic visualization of the interior of the female upper genital tract after instillation of radiopaque dye.

Intracytoplasmic Sperm Injection (ICSI). Technique by which a single spermatozoon is injected into the cytoplasm of an ovum.

Infertility. Inability of couples of reproductive age to establish a pregnancy by having sexual intercourse within a certain period of time, usually 1 year. Infertility is considered primary if the woman has never been pregnant and secondary if it occurs after one or more pregnancies.

Intrauterine Insemination. Placement of spermatozoa that have been separated from the seminal fluid into the endometrial cavity through a small catheter.

In Vitro Fertilization. Fertilization of human ova by sperm in a laboratory environment.

Luteal Phase Deficiency (Inadequate Luteal Phase). Deficient progesterone secretion or action resulting in a delay of normal endometrial development.

Microsurgery. Operative technique using magnification and fine, nonreactive suture material.

Oligozoospermia (Oligospermia). Presence of fewer than 20 million sperm per milliliter of semen.

Ovarian Hyperstimulation Syndrome (OHSS). Ovarian enlargement to a diameter of more than 6 cm as a result of stimulation of multiple follicles. In the mild form there is abdominal pain, distention, and weight gain. In the moderate form ovarian enlargement is more than 10 cm in diameter with ascites, nausea, and vomiting. Severe OHSS is associated with hemoconcentration, oliguria, and elevated serum creatine. Pleural effusions and ascites can be present; OHSS becomes critical when hypercoagulability and hypotension occur. This condition may be fatal.

Postcoital Test. Examination of the cervical mucus to evaluate the presence of sperm several hours after sexual intercourse.

Pronuclear Stage Tubal Transfer (PROST) or Zygote Intrafallopian Transfer (ZIFT). In vitro fertilization with transfer of the zygote to the oviducts by transabdominal cannulation.

Salpingitis Isthmica Nodosa. Diverticula of the endosalpinx in the muscularis of the isthmic portion of the oviduct.

Continued

KEY TERMS AND DEFINITIONS *Continued*

Salpingolysis. Removal of adhesions attached to an oviduct that appears normal on gross inspection.

Salpingostomy. Surgical creation of a new opening of a completely occluded distal end of the oviduct.

Semen Analysis. Quantitation of various parameters of a recently ejaculated semen specimen analyzed after liquefaction has occurred.

Spinnbarkeit. Property of elasticity (distensibility) of cervical mucus.

Teratozoospermia. Greater-than-normal (50%) incidence of abnormal forms of sperm in semen analysis.

Treatment-Independent Pregnancy. Infertile women conceiving without use of infertility therapy.

Tubal Embryo Transfer (TET) or Tubal Embryo Stage Transfer (TEST). Same as ZIFT, except additional incubation to embryo stage occurs before transfer to the oviducts.

Unexplained Infertility. The diagnosis of an infertile couple when ovulation and tubal patency, as well as a normal semen analysis, are all present.

Testicular Sperm Extraction. Retrieval of sperm from the testis by biopsy or aspiration from men with azoospermia due to obstruction of the vas deferens or epididymis (obstructive azoospermia) or without such obstruction (nonobstructive azoospermia). The sperm are injected into ova retrieved by follicle aspiration by the ICSI procedure.

The term *infertility* is generally used to indicate that a couple has a reduced capacity to conceive as compared with the mean capacity of the general population. In a group of normal fertile couples, the monthly conception rate, or fecundability, is about 20%. This figure is important for all couples seeking fertility to know, because it will alleviate unrealistic expectations of immediate success with various therapies, which can only approach 20% per cycle (with the exception of in vitro fertilization/embryo transfer [IVF-ET]). For most couples the correct term should be *subfertility*, suggesting a decreased capacity for pregnancy but not an impossible feat.

INCIDENCE OF INFERTILITY

Results from the three U.S. National Surveys of Family Growth performed under the direction of U.S. government agencies provide information about infertility in this country. Analysis of the data obtained from the surveys performed in 1982, 1988, and 1995 indicate that the proportion of U.S. women ages 15 to 44 with impaired fecundity increased from 8% in 1982 and 1988 to 10% in 1995, a 20% rise. It was estimated that the number of women with impaired fecundity in the United States increased from 4.6 million to 6.2 million between 1982 and 1995, a 35% rise. Most of this increase occurred among nulliparous women in the oldest age group (35 to 44) due to women of the Baby-Boom generation reaching this age. Many in this group had delayed their childbearing. The percentage of women with impaired fecundity seeking medical assistance for this problem remained stable, about 44% between 1988 and 1995. However because more women had impaired fecundity there was a 30% increase in women who utilized medical help for this problem in the United States, an increase from 2.1 to 2.7 million women.

INFERTILITY AND AGE

Data from both older and more recent studies indicate that the percentage of infertile couples increases with increasing age of the female partner. Analysis of data from three national surveys in the United States revealed that the percentage of presumably fertile married women not using contraception who failed to conceive in 1 year steadily increased from ages 25 to 44 (Table 41-1). Data from a study of presumably fertile nulliparous women married to husbands with azoospermia who underwent donor artificial insemination revealed that the percentage who conceived after 12 cycles of insemination declined substantially after age 30 (Table 41-2). With IVF, recent data show the percentage of deliveries per oocyte retrieval procedure to be 36.9% in women younger than 35, 20.5% by ages 38 to 40 and only 10.7% by ages 41 to 42. In general terms, about one in seven couples are infertile if the wife is 30–34 years of age, one in five is infertile if she is 35 to 40, and one in four is infertile if she is 40 to 44. Another way to interpret these data is to state that as compared with women ages 20 to 24, fertility is reduced

Table 41-1 Percentage of Married Women Who Are Infertile, by Age, from Three National U.S. Surveys

Age	Infertile (%)
20–24	7.0
25–29	8.9
30–34	14.6
35–39	21.9
40–44	28.7

From Menken J, Trussell IJ, Larsen U: Age and infertility. Science 23:1389, 1986.

Table 41-2 Percentage of Pregnancy Rates by Age at 1 Year in Normal Women with Azoospermatic Husbands After Donor Insemination

Age	Pregnancy Rate (%)
<25	73.0
26–30	74.1
31–35	61.5
36–40	55.8

From Schwartz D, Mayaux MJ: Female fecundity as a function of age: Results of artificial insemination in 2193 nulliparous women with azoospermic husbands. N Engl J Med 306:404, 1982.

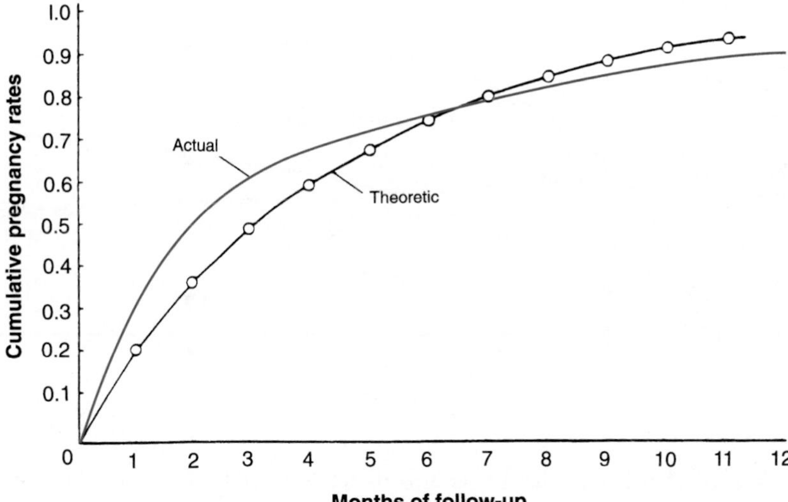

Figure 41-1. Curve of theoretic time to pregnancy in women with a monthly fecundability of 0.2 (*open circles*) and curve of actual time to pregnancy in fertile women discontinuing contraception (*solid line*). (Open-circle data from Hull MGR, Glazener CMA, Kelly NJ, et al: Population study of causes, treatment, and outcome of infertility. Br Med J 291:1693, 1985; solid-line data from Murray DL, Reich L, Adashi EY: Oral clomiphene citrate and vaginal progesterone suppositories in the treatment of luteal phase dysfunction: A comparative study. Fertil Steril 51:35, 1989.)

by 6% in the next 5 years, by 14% between ages 30 and 34, by 31% between ages 35 and 39, and to a much greater extent after age 40.

Because human reproduction is an inefficient process, it takes time to become pregnant. Therefore, because a woman's reproductive life span is limited to a certain number of years, if couples intend to have children, they should be counseled to maximize the length of time during which they attempt to conceive. Because the percentage of couples with decreased rates of fecundity increases with age of the female partner, couples should be informed that the probability of conception is substantially reduced by delaying childbearing until later in life. This reduction is caused by two factors: (1) the incidence of infertility increases with increasing age of the woman and (2) the total length of time during which conception is possible is less in older women. Because the occurrence of monthly ovulation decreases greatly after age 45, as a woman becomes older, a corresponding decrease occurs in the total duration of time during which she may conceive.

FECUNDABILITY

Analysis of data from presumably fertile couples who stop using contraception in order to conceive reveals that about only half the couples will conceive in 3 months, three fourths will conceive in 6 months, and by 1 year about 90% will have conceived (Fig. 41-1). Statistical analysis of these data indicates that normal monthly fecundability is about 0.2.

This information is extremely important when analyzing data concerning the results of various treatment methods applied to a group of infertile couples. This group includes those with hypofertility due to presumed causes (e.g., mild endometriosis) as well as those with idiopathic (unexplained) infertility. For example, Leridon and Spira estimated that if the mean fecundability of the population is 0.2, 14% of the couples will not have conceived after 12 months; during the following year, however, 69% of the nonsterile couples in this population will conceive without treatment (Table 41-3). Analysis of these statistical tables reveals that after 2 years of trying to conceive, about 4% of these couples will not have done so. Their mean monthly fecundability is about 0.08, and 57% will conceive in the next year. Of the 2% still not pregnant at this time, 3 years after trying to conceive, the monthly fecundability drops to about 0.06, 0.05, and 0.04 in the next 3 years, respectively. Thus in the fourth, fifth, and sixth years of attempting to conceive, 48%, 42%, and 37% of the nonpregnant women should conceive without treatment. Infertility is usually defined as inability to conceive in 1 year. When so defined, the group of infertile couples includes those who have difficulty in conceiving quickly (hypofertile) or subfertile as well as those who will "never" be able to conceive (sterile). In another analysis,

Table 41-3 Incidence of Conception over Time Among Nonsterile Couples with Mean Fecundability of 0.2

Months without Conception	Proportion (%) of Couples Not Yet Having Conceived	Mean Fecundability of Couples Not Yet Having Conceived	Proportion (%) of Couples Who Will Conceive within 12 Months among Couples Not Yet Having Conceived
0	100.0	0.20	86.0
6	31.9	0.14	77.0
12	14.0	0.11	69.2
24	4.3	0.08	57.0
36	1.9	0.06	48.2
48	1.0	0.05	41.7
60	0.6	0.04	36.7

Adapted from Fertility and Sterility, 41, Leridon H, Spira A, Problems in measuring the effectiveness of infertility therapy, 580. Copyright 1984, with permission from The American Society for Reproductive Medicine.

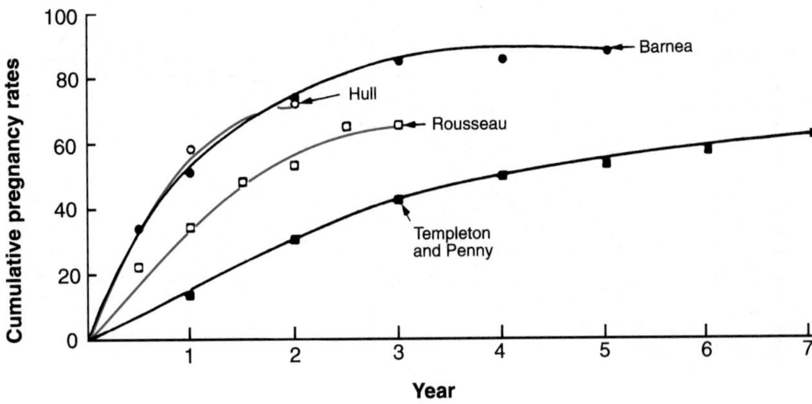

Figure 41-2. Pregnancy rates over time in untreated couples with normal basic (five-step) infertility investigation-results of four studies. (Adapted from Barnea ER, Holford TR, McInnes DRA: Long-term prognosis of infertile couples with normal basic investigations: A life-table analysis. Obstet Gynecol 66:24, 1985; Hull MGR, Glazener CMA, Kelly NJ, et al: Population study of causes, treatment, and outcome of infertility. Br Med J 291:1963, 1985; Rousseau S, Lora J, Lepage Y, Van Campenhout J: The expectancy of pregnancy for "normal" infertile couples. Fertil Steril 40:768, 1983; and Templeton AA, Penney GC: The incidence, characteristics, and prognosis of patients whose infertility is unexplained. Fertil Steril 37:175, 1982.)

it was calculated that after 12 months the cycle fecundability without treatment is in the range of 0 to 0.04.

Several studies have reported the incidence of spontaneous conception among infertile couples without a specifically diagnosed cause of infertility (unexplained infertility). Four long-term studies have reported fecundity rates in couples with unexplained infertility of at least 1 year's duration without treatment. In all four studies there was indirect documentation of ovulation, evidence of fallopian tubal patency, and the presence of a normal semen analysis. In three of the four studies a normal postcoital test and normal laparoscopic evaluation of the pelvis were also present. Thus the most meaningful diagnostic tests of the infertility evaluation were normal in the couples studied. The cumulative pregnancy rates at the end of 2 to 7 years without any treatment ranged from 43% to 87% (Fig. 41-2). Collins and colleagues reported that the live-birth rate of 873 infertile couples in several Canadian centers observed without treatment for 18,364 months steadily rose to more than 35% at 3 years and 45% after 7 years (Fig. 41-3). Of the 562 couples in this group with unexplained infertility who received no treatment, one third had a live birth during the first 3 years of observation without treatment.

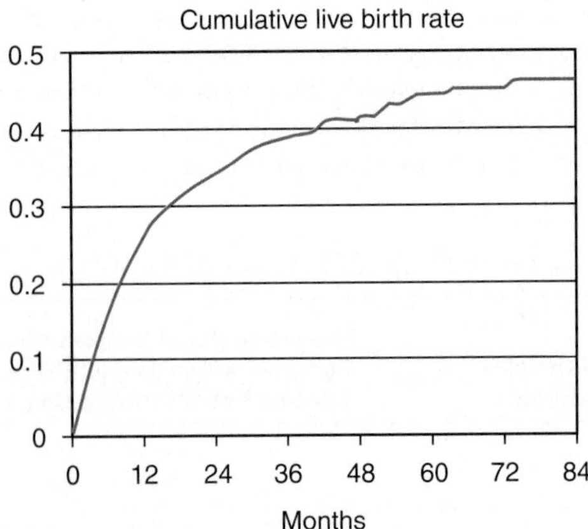

Figure 41-3. Cumulative rate of conceptions leading to live birth. Couples (873) who remained untreated throughout follow-up; cumulative rate of live birth conception at 36 months was 38.2% (95% CI 34.2, 42.3). (Modified from Fertility and Sterility, 64, Collins JA, Burrows EA, Willan AR, The prognosis for live birth among untreated infertile couples, 22. Copyright 1995, with permission from The American Society for Reproductive Medicine.)

Thus, to determine that any method of treatment of infertility is superior to no treatment, the treatment results on the incidence of pregnancy over time need to be statistically analyzed. Ideally, these results should be compared with a nontreated control group. At the least, these pregnancy rates should be compared with the rates of the nontreated women with a normal diagnostic evaluation reported in the four studies mentioned. Various statistical formulas for performing such analyses based on life table analysis have been described. This statistical approach is necessary to determine if treatment methods are indeed beneficial, since data from uncontrolled studies can give a false impression of treatment effectiveness. These formulas provide mathematical techniques to determine the monthly probability of conception and the cumulative conception rate.

After using these techniques of analysis, therapy should be offered to the couple only if it is found that such therapy hastens the time in which conception will take place as compared with untreated controls or couples with a similar duration of infertility and a normal diagnostic infertility evaluation. Furthermore, couples should be counseled that with sufficient time the likelihood of eventually conceiving without empiric treatment (and its associated expense) may be similar to that occurring in a shorter time period with use of certain therapies. For couples with unexplained infertility, treatment with controlled ovarian hyperstimulation and intrauterine insemination has been shown to increase fecundability compared with no treatment, as has in vitro fertilization.

CAUSES OF INFERTILITY

The exact incidence of the various factors causing infertility varies among different populations and cannot be precisely determined. Collins reported that among 14,141 couples in 21 publications, ovulatory disorders occurred 27% of the time; male factors, 25%; tubal disorders, 22%; endometriosis, 5%; other, 4%; and unexplained factors, 17%. It has not been shown that other abnormalities, such as antisperm antibodies, luteal-phase deficiency, subclinical genital infection, or subclinical endocrine abnormalities such as hypothyroidism or hyperprolactinemia in ovulatory women are actual causes of infertility. No prospective randomized studies demonstrate that treatment of these latter entities results in greater fecundability than occurs without treatment. If any of these entities do cause infertility, they do so infrequently. With current techniques of investigation, it is impossible to diagnose the cause of infertility in up to 20% of couples, and they are considered to have unexplained infertility. Other reports have suggested this figure to be as low as 10% after a rigorous investigation. However, it is unclear if subtle abnormalities as previously noted have much to do with infertility. Also as explained previously, most of the couples with unexplained infertility are hypofertile and some are able to conceive without treatment although it may take several years and with a diminishing probability of this occurrence as time goes on.

DIAGNOSTIC EVALUATION

The diagnostic evaluation of infertility should be thorough and completed as rapidly as possible. During the initial interview the couple should be informed about normal human fecundability and how these probabilities decrease with increasing age of the female partner over age 30 and duration of infertility for more than 3 years. The various tests in the diagnostic evaluation and the reasons why they are performed should be thoroughly explained. In addition, the sequence of performing these tests, their degree of discomfort, cost, and time in the cycle at which they should be performed should also be discussed. The available therapies and the prognosis for treatment of the various causes of infertility should also be included in the dialogue. The couple should be informed that after a complete diagnostic infertility evaluation, the cause for infertility cannot be determined in up to 20% of couples. Methods to increase the fecundity of couples with a normal diagnostic evaluation such as controlled ovarian hyperstimulation and intrauterine insemination, as well as assisted reproductive techniques (ARTs), should also be covered.

Each couple should be instructed about the optimal time in the cycle for conception to occur and should be encouraged to have intercourse on the day before ovulation.

Unless the husband has oligospermia, daily intercourse for 3 consecutive days at midcycle should be encouraged. When ovulation is more precisely determined as with luteinizing hormone (LH) monitoring (see the following discussion), intercourse should occur for 2 consecutive days around the LH surge. Because the egg disintegrates less than a day after it reaches the ampulla of the oviduct, it is best that sperm be present in this area when the egg arrives so that fertilization can occur. Since normal sperm retains its fertilizing ability for up to 72 hours, it is preferable to have sperm in the oviduct prior to the arrival of the oocyte.

A study was performed by Wilcox and coworkers among fertile couples who stopped contraception in order to conceive and recorded the cycle day when they had sexual intercourse. Hormone analysis was performed to determine the day of ovulation. None of the women became pregnant in the group of couples who had intercourse after ovulation occurred. The pregnancy rate was about 30% if intercourse occurred on the day of ovulation as well as 1 and 2 days prior to ovulation. The pregnancy rate was about 10% if coitus occurred 3, 4, or 5 days before ovulation. No pregnancies occurred when intercourse took place 6 days or more before ovulation (Fig. 41-4). It is therefore considered optimal to perform insemination or have sexual intercourse on the day before ovulation.

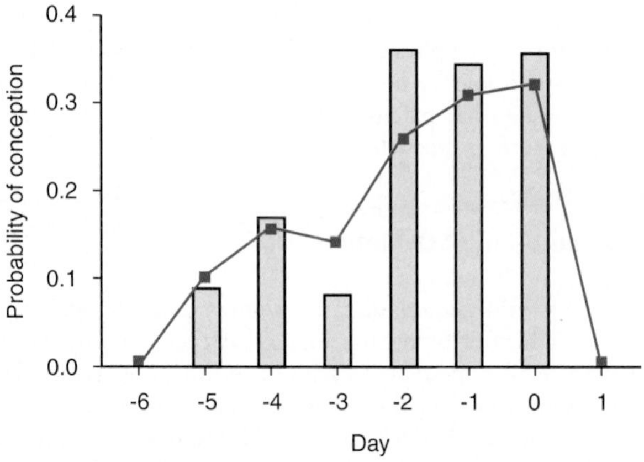

Figure 41-4. Probability of conception on specific days near the day of ovulation. The bars represent probabilities calculated from data on 129 menstrual cycles in which sexual intercourse was recorded to have occurred on only a single day during the 6-day interval ending on the day of ovulation (day 0). The solid line shows daily probabilities based on all 625 cycles, as estimated by the statistical model. (From Wilcox AJ, Weinberg CR, Baird DD: Timing of sexual intercourse in relation to ovulation. N Engl J Med 333:1517, 1995. Copyright 1995 Massachusetts Medical Society. All rights reserved.)

Because peak levels of LH occur 1 day before ovulation, measurement of LH by urinary LH immunoassays is the best way to determine the optimal time to have intercourse or insemination. Tests that measure LH in a random daily urine specimen are usually more convenient for planning natural or artificial insemination than the tests that detect LH in the first morning urine specimen. Ovulation most commonly occurs on the day following the detection of LH in a random specimen (12 to 24 hours later), and it occurs on the day when LH is detected in the first morning specimen, which contains urine formed during the prior night. Several types of commercial kit are available for determining peak LH, so women who find it difficult to determine a hormone change using one type can try another system or kit. Use of basal body temperature (BBT) charts are not as precise in determining ovulation, with ovulation occurring over a span of several days of the thermogenic shift.

In some instances, women produce less-than-adequate amounts of vaginal lubricant. Various vaginal lubricants and chemicals, as well as saliva, used to improve coital satisfaction may interfere with sperm transport. Some men experience midcycle impotence because of the pressure of performing intercourse on demand. In such cases the intercourse schedule should be less rigorous. The couple should also be told that among fertile couples there is only about a 20% chance of conceiving in each ovulatory cycle even with optimally timed coitus, and that it takes time to become pregnant. Thus the two terms *time* and *timing* should be emphasized during the initial counseling session. Couples should also be advised to cease smoking cigarettes and drinking caffeinated beverages, if they do so, since both cigarette smoking and caffeine consumption have been shown independently in several studies to decrease the chances of conception. Baird and associates reported that the common practice of vaginal douching also reduces the chance of conception by about 30%. Therefore infertile women should be advised to discontinue all vaginal douching.

All couples should have a complete history taken, including a sexual history, and a physical examination. After this initial evaluation, tests should be undertaken to determine if the woman is ovulating and has patent oviducts and if a semen sample of the male partner is normal.

Documentation of Ovulation

Preliminary information that the woman is ovulatory is provided by a history of regular menstrual cycles. If the woman is having regular menstrual cycles, a serum progesterone level should be measured in the midluteal phase to provide indirect evidence of ovulation as well as normal luteal function. Although in the normal luteal phase serum progesterone levels vary in a pulsatile manner, a serum progesterone level above 10 ng/mL is indicative of adequate luteal function. Progesterone levels of 10 ng/mL or higher are found during at least 1 day of the luteal phase of normal ovulatory cycles in which conception occurred. Measurement of daily BBT also provides indirect evidence that ovulation has taken place. The BBT graph also provides information concerning the approximate day of ovulation and duration of the luteal phase. The BBT should be taken shortly after awakening only after at least 6 hours of sleep and prior to ambulating, with sublingual placement of a special thermometer with gradients between 96° and 100° F.

Women with oligomenorrhea (menses at intervals of 35 days or longer) or amenorrhea who wish to conceive should be treated with agents that induce ovulation regardless of whether they have occasional ovulatory cycles. Therefore, for such women direct or indirect measurement of progesterone is unnecessary until after therapy is initiated.

Semen Analysis

While information about ovulation is being obtained, the male partner's reproductive system should be evaluated by means of semen analysis. The male partner should be advised to abstain from ejaculation for 2 to 3 days before collection of the semen sample, because frequent ejaculation lowers seminal volume and occasionally the sperm count in some individuals. It is best to collect the specimen in a clean (not necessarily sterile), wide-mouthed jar after masturbation. It is important that the entire specimen be collected, because the initial fraction contains the greatest density of sperm. Ideally, collection should take place in the location where the analysis will be performed. The degree of sperm motility should be determined as soon as possible after liquefaction, which usually occurs 15 to 20 minutes after ejaculation. Sperm motility begins to decline 2 hours after ejaculation, and it is best to examine the specimen within this time period. Semen should not be exposed to marked changes in temperature, and if collected at home during cold weather, the specimen should be kept warm during transport to the laboratory.

Parameters used to evaluate the semen include volume, viscosity, sperm density, sperm morphology, and sperm motility. The last parameter should be evaluated in terms of percentage of total motile sperm as well as quality of motility (rapidity of movement and amount of progressive motility). Sperm morphology is an extremely important parameter, which is correlated to fertilizing ability. Using strict criteria (Kruger) only approximately 15% or more of the sperm in an ejaculate may be considered normal. It should be remembered that the sperm analysis is a subjective test and that there is a fair degree of variability from test to test in the same man. Also the semen profile reflects sperm production, which occurred 3 months earlier, which is important to note if there were illness at that time. Table 41-4 lists the parameters that are generally considered "normal" for a semen analysis. It is beyond the scope of this text to fully discuss the etiology and diagnostic evaluation of semen abnormalities. The various causes of semen abnormalities are cited in Table 41-5.

Table 41-4 Semen Analysis: Normal Reference Values

Volume	1.5–5.0 mL
pH	>7.2
Viscosity	<3 (Scale 0–4)
Sperm concentration	>20 million mL
Total sperm number	>40 million ejaculate
Percent motility	>50%
Forward progression	>2 (scale 0–4)
Normal morphology	>50% normal >30% normal >14% normal
Round cells	<5 million mL
Sperm agglutination	< (Scale 0–3)

As reported by Barratt and colleagues, when semen analyses were performed on a group of men whose wives had conceived within the past 4 months, about 75% had at least one abnormal characteristic and 25% had two abnormalities. These results confirm that there is normally a wide variability in the parameters used to characterize semen. Because the characteristics of semen may vary over time and undergo normal biological variability, if an abnormality is found, it is best to repeat the test on two or three occasions.

Evaluation and Laboratory Tests

Aspects of the woman's medical history that should be highlighted include the following: any pregnancy complications if previously pregnant; previous pelvic surgery of any type; significant dysmenorrhea; dyspareunia or sexual dysfunction; abnormal cervical cytology or procedures to treat cervical abnormalities; and use of medication, drugs, and tobacco. Family history should be explored for genetically related illnesses, birth defects, and most importantly the history of age of menopause in female family members. Finally any symptoms suggestive of endocrine disorders should be solicited (weight changes, skin changes, etc.).

The physical exam should focus on extremes of body mass, skin changes, thyroid size, breast secretion, abnormal pain on abdominal or pelvic exam, and assessment of the vagina and cervix. In addition, if available, vaginal ultrasound obtained at the same time may be extremely valuable in picking up abnormalities of the uterus (e.g., fibroids) endometrial thickness, pelvic masses, and ovarian morphology (polycystic appearance or unusually small). These may provide a guide for further testing.

Table 41-5 Causes of Semen Abnormalities

Finding	Cause
Abnormal count	
Azoospermia	Klinefelter's syndrome or other genetic disorders
	Sertoli-cell-only syndrome
	Seminiferous tubule or Leydig cell failure
	Hypogonadotrophic hypogonadism
	Ductal obstruction, including Young's syndrome
	Varicocele
	Exogenous factors
Oligozoospermia	Genetic disorder
	Endocrinopathies, including androgen receptor defects
	Varicocele and other anatomic disorders
	Maturation arrest
	Hypospermatogenesis
	Exogenous factors
Abnormal volume	
No ejaculate	Ductal obstruction
	Retrograde ejaculation
	Ejaculatory failure
	Hypogonadism
Low volume	Obstruction of ejaculatory ducts
	Absence of seminal vesicles and vas deferens
	Partial retrograde ejaculation
	Infection
High volume	Unknown factors
Abnormal motility	Immunologic factors
	Infection
	Varicocele
	Defects in sperm structure
	Metabolic or anatomic abnormalities of sperm
	Poor liquefaction of semen
Abnormal viscosity	Etiology unknown
Abnormal morphology	Varicocele
	Stress
	Infection
	Exogenous factors
	Unknown factors
Extraneous cells	Infection or inflammation
	Shedding of immature sperm

From Bernstein GS, Siegel MS: Male factor in infertility. In Mishell DR Jr, Davajan V, Lobo RA (eds): Infertility, Contraception and Reproductive Endocrinology, 3rd ed. Cambridge, MA, Blackwell Scientific, 1991, p 629.

In a healthy asymptomatic woman, only a complete blood count (CBC), blood type, RH, and rubella status are needed together with a Pap smear obtained within 12 months of the previous test. Cystic fibrosis screening is currently recommended in all women. Infections disease screening (for chlamydia and gonorrhea) is carried out routinely in most practices at the time of the Pap smear. Further infectious disease screening (syphilis, HIV, hepatitis, etc.) is warranted only on a selective basis and is required for all couples undergoing insemination or IVF.

In women older than 35, serum follicle-stimulating hormone (FSH) and estradiol (E_2) should be obtained on cycle day 2 or 3. Values over 15 mU/mL are abnormal, suggesting decreased ovarian reserve, which is the pool of viable oocytes remaining in the ovary; values over 20 miU/mL are particularly bad prognostically. However, although FSH levels tend to fluctuate from cycle to cycle, once FSH has been elevated in a given cycle, the overall prognosis is reduced. E_2 levels if elevated on days 2 and 3 (>70 pg/mL) do not allow for a valid interpretation of FSH values and may independently suggest a decreased prognosis regarding ovarian reserve.

Some specialists have suggested obtaining antibody titers for *Chlamydia trachomatis,* which if elevated this may signify the possibility of tubal disease. Thomas and coworkers have suggested that if the immunoglobulin G (IgG) antibody titer is greater than 1:32, 35% of patients had evidence of tubal damage. Whether this type of evaluation is routinely warranted as a focus for the infertility investigation continues to be debated. Routine measurement of thyroid-stimulating hormone (TSH) and prolactin in women with regular ovulatory cycles at the time of the initial visit may not be cost-effective. These tests are usually normal, and even if abnormalities are present in women with regular ovulatory cycles, these hormones may not be associated with infertility. Treatment with thyroid replacement and bromocriptine has not been shown to increase the chance of conception in women with ovulatory cycles compared with no therapy.

If an abnormality is found in one of the first two noninvasive diagnostic procedures (documentation of ovulation and semen analysis), it should be treated before proceeding with the more costly and invasive procedures, unless there is a history or findings suggestive of tubal disease. For example, if the woman has oligomenorrhea and does not ovulate each month, after a normal semen analysis is observed, ovulation should be induced with clomiphene citrate before performing the other diagnostic measures. Provided no other infertility factors are present, most anovulatory women (80%) conceive after induction of ovulation with therapeutic agents and half the couples will conceive during the first three ovulatory cycles.

If these initial diagnostic tests are normal, the more uncomfortable and costly hysterosalpingography (HSG) should be performed in the follicular phase of the next cycle.

Hysterosalpingogram

It is best to schedule the HSG during the week following the end of menses to avoid irradiating a possible pregnancy. The HSG should be avoided if there has been a history of salpingitis in the recent past or if there is tenderness on pelvic exam. As noted earlier, most practices routinely screen for chlamydia and gonorrhea during the initial examination. However, we still routinely advise using prophylactic antibiotics at the time of HSG. We prescribe doxycycline (100 mg twice a day for 4 days starting 1 day before the procedure), but this recommendation is not universally followed. If a hydrosalpinx is seen at HSG, doxycycline should be continued for 1 week. The examination should be performed with use of a water-soluble contrast medium and image-intensified fluoroscopy. A water-soluble contrast medium enables better visualization of the tubal mucosal folds and vaginal markings than does an oil-based medium. It is important to be able to evaluate the appearance of the intratubal architecture to determine the extent of damage to the oviduct. A meta-analysis by Watson and associates of clinical studies, including four randomized trials, indicated that a therapeutic benefit is more likely to occur when oil-soluble contrast media are used in an HSG performed for the diagnostic evaluation of infertility. The odds of pregnancy occurring after the procedure were twofold higher when oil-soluble media were used compared with water-soluble media. These results differ from those of a recently published large randomized trial by

Spring and colleagues that found no difference in pregnancy rates when the HSG was performed with oil-soluble or water-soluble contrast media. Thus the therapeutic benefit of oil-soluble contrast media remains inconclusive. Because oil-soluble contrast media have a greater number of complications, including pain resulting from peritoneal irritation and formation of granulomas than do water-soluble media, it is probably best to perform routine HSGs with water-based media. The diagnostic HSG will not only determine whether the tubes are patent but also, if disease is present, will help to determine the magnitude of the disease process as well as provide information about the lining of the oviduct and uterine cavity that cannot be obtained by laparoscopic visualization. The procedure can also determine whether salpingitis isthmica nodosa is present in the interstitial portion of the oviduct. Mol and coworkers reported that if one oviduct is patent, fecundability is only minimally reduced compared with that in women with two patent oviducts. When an HSG shows lack of patency in one tube, this has been shown to be falsely positive 50% to 60% of the time at laparoscopy. Therefore it is not necessary to perform tubal reconstructive surgery on a woman with one patent oviduct. However, a diagnostic laparoscopy may be considered to detect the presence of peritubal adhesions. The finding of a normal endometrial cavity at the time of HSG obviates the need for hysteroscopy. Fayes and associates reported that women with infertility and a normal HSG had no abnormalities of the uterine cavity when subsequently examined by hysteroscopy.

If severe tubal disease, such as a large hydrosalpinx, is found at the time of HSG, based on success rates it is preferable for the couple to undergo IVF-ET than for the woman to have tubal surgery. If the hydrosalpinx is large and clearly visible on ultrasound, it is preferable to perform laparoscopic salpingectomy prior to IVF-ET, as the pregnancy rate with IVF-ET may be decreased by as much as 40%. When the extent of tubal disease is unclear or the couple prefers not to undergo IVF/ET, diagnostic laparoscopy should be carried out in the follicular phase of the cycle. In general, the goal should be to have all tubal reconstruction carried out laparoscopically.

Previously a postcoital test and a laparoscopy were routinely performed as part of the initial infertility evaluation. After an abnormal postcoital test, controlled ovarian hyperstimulation and intrauterine insemination are recommended. Since this is the same therapy for infertile couples with a normal postcoital test and tubal patency, it does not appear to be cost-effective or necessary to continue to perform a postcoital test. A diagnostic laparoscopy was also previously performed routinely as part of the diagnostic evaluation of all women with infertility. Since this invasive procedure usually requires general anesthesia and is costly, it should only be performed if there is a likelihood of visualizing peritubal adhesions or pelvic endometriosis. Ovarian endometriomas can usually be visualized by pelvic sonography. If the sonographic appearance of the ovaries is normal and the HSG is normal, it is unlikely that peritubal adhesions that restrict ovarian pickup are present, particularly if the *Chlamydia* antibody titer is normal. Meikle and colleagues reported that only 4 of 74 infertile women with a normal HSG and a negative *Chlamydia* antibody titer had evidence of tubal disease at the time of diagnostic laparoscopy. The probability that peritubal adhesions of sufficient severity to cause infertility will be found at the time of laparoscopy is therefore much less than 5% in a woman with no history of salpingitis or symptoms of dysmenorrhea, a normal bimanual pelvic examination, and normal antibody titers. Provided the woman is younger than 40 and having ovulatory cycles and there are more than 5 million motile sperm in the ejaculate of the male partner, several cycles of controlled ovarian hyperstimulation and intrauterine insemination should be undertaken before performing diagnostic laparoscopy or going directly to IVF-ET. This therapy has been shown to increase fecundability (see Prognosis) and is thus a useful initial therapy for hypofertile couples.

At the time of laparoscopy following a normal HSG, neither a dilation and curettage nor hysteroscopy should be routinely performed. However, hysteroscopic tubal cannulation and other adjunctive procedures may be indicated on an individual basis. At the time of laparoscopy, indigo carmine should be introduced through the cervix into the peritoneal cavity to confirm tubal patency. Performing the laparoscopy in the follicular phase of the cycle before maximal endometrial growth enables the dye to pass into the oviducts with less chance of obstruction.

Additional Testing

The following additional laboratory procedures have been advocated by some to assist in determining the cause of the infertility: (1) measurement of serum TSH and prolactin in ovulatory women, (2) luteal-phase endometrial biopsy, (3) measurement of antisperm antibodies in both the male and female partner, (4) bacteriologic cultures of the cervical mucus and semen, and (5) hamster egg penetration test.

If abnormalities are discovered in any of the initial three steps of the infertility evaluation, treatment has been found to increase the incidence of pregnancy significantly as compared with no treatment, particularly treatment of anovulation or total tubal obstruction. Treatment of abnormalities found in the five diagnostic procedures just mentioned has not been documented to be more effective than withholding therapy. Therefore the necessity and cost-effectiveness of performing these additional tests and correcting the abnormalities found by them have not been demonstrated. Until it is demonstrated conclusively that treatment of abnormalities diagnosed by these additional tests results in a significantly improved pregnancy rate compared with placebo or no treatment, the advisability of continuing the diagnostic evaluation beyond the initial three diagnostic steps remains unproven as elaborated later.

Measurement of TSH and Prolactin in Ovulatory Women

If women with anovulation have hypothyroidism or hyperprolactinemia, treatment with thyroid replacement or dopamine agonists, respectively, have been shown to cause resumption of ovulation and enhanced fecundity. However, if women with regular ovulatory cycles have mild hyperprolactinemia, Glazener and coworkers reported that pregnancy rates 1 year after the diagnostic evaluation without treatment were similar to those in ovulatory women without hyperprolactinemia. Several investigators have performed randomized clinical trials with bromocriptine and placebo that have shown that treatment with bromocriptine does not increase fecundity rates in ovulatory infertile women. Lincoln and colleagues reported that less than 1% of women with infertility and normal ovulatory cycles had elevated TSH levels. None of these women became pregnant when treated with thyroxine.

Luteal Deficiency

Although suggested for many years, it has never been established that luteal-phase defects cause infertility. The diagnosis of luteal deficiency can be determined by finding serum progesterone levels consistently below 10 ng/mL a week before menses or finding consistent histologic evidence of a delay in development of the normal secretory endometrial pattern, indicating an inadequate effect of progesterone production on the endometrium. Using classic criteria to establish the diagnosis histologically, secretory endometrial development (usually obtained in the late luteal phase) must lag *3 days* or more behind the expected pattern for the time of the cycle as originally described by Noyes and associates. Furthermore, this finding must be consistent and found in *at least two cycles.* Dating needs to be calculated using indicators that will detect the day of ovulation, rather than by subtracting 14 days from the onset of the next menses.

Because the onset of the next menses is the least accurate parameter for determining if luteal deficiency exists, the diagnosis of this entity occurs more frequently when this technique is used to establish the diagnosis than when pelvic sonography is used (Fig. 41-5). Peters and coworkers reported that the percentage of out-of-phase endometrial biopsies among both fertile and infertile women was similar, being nearly 50% when dating from the day of onset of last menses was used, about 30% when subtracting 14 days from the onset of the next menses was used, and about 25% when the urinary LH peak was used to estimate the day of ovulation (Figs. 41-6 and 41-7). When the most precise method of detecting ovulation (pelvic sonography) was used, out-of-phase endometrial biopsies occurred in 3.5% of infertile women and 10% of fertile women.

Erroneous diagnosis of this entity also occurs because of the subjective interpretation of histologic dating criteria. Li and colleagues reported that a 10% disagreement of more than 2 days occurred when the same observer dated the specimens on two separate occasions. Scott and coworkers reported that there was great interobserver variation in dating endometrial biopsy specimens, even when performed by five experienced pathologists.

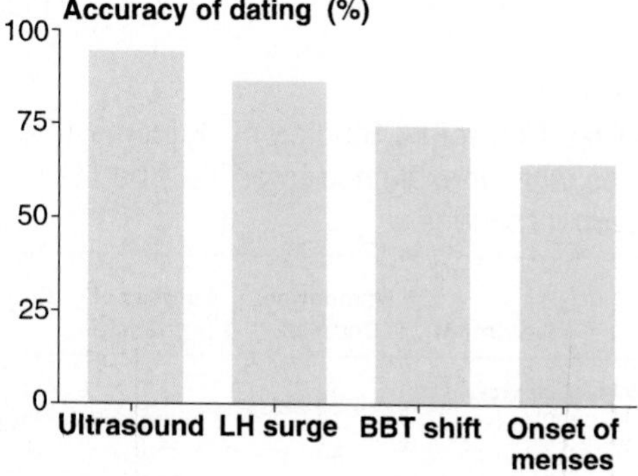

Figure 41-5. Percentage of endometrial biopsy interpretations that correlated within 2 days using four different methods of ovulation prediction. Onset of menses: $p < 0.05$ compared with ultrasonography. (From Shoupe D, Mishell DR Jr, LaCarra M, et al: Correlation of endometrial maturation with four methods of estimating day of ovulation. Obstet Gynecol 73:88, 1988.)

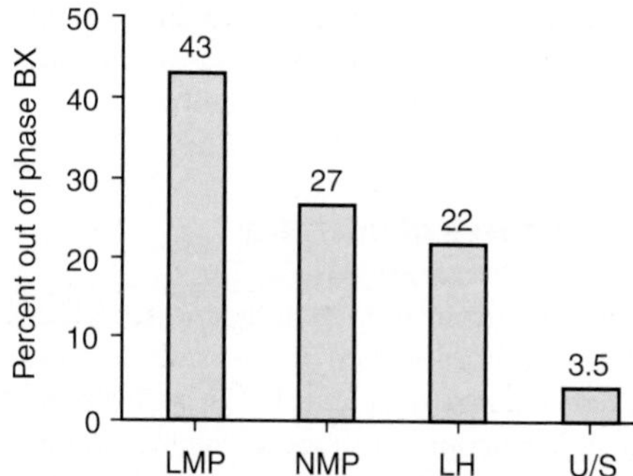

Figure 41-6. Prevalence of out-of-phase endometrial biopsy specimens among 340 infertile women: biopsies are on basis of onset of last menstrual period (LMP), next menstrual period (NMP), urinary LH testing, and documentation of follicle rupture by ultrasonographic examination (ultrasound, US). BBT, basal body temperature; LH, luteinizing hormone. (From Peters AJ, Lloyd RP, Coulam CB: Prevalence of out-of-phase endometrial biopsy specimens. Am J Obstet Gynecol 166:1738, 1992.)

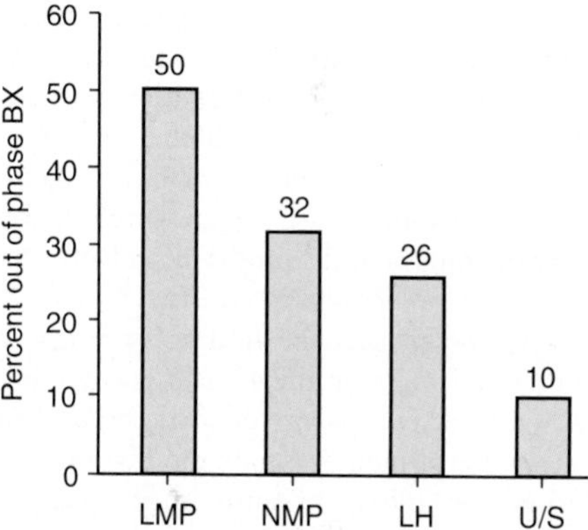

Figure 41-7. Prevalence of out-of-phase endometrial biopsy (BX) specimens among 30 fertile women on basis of onset of LMP, next menstrual period (NMP), urinary testing, and documentation of follicle rupture by ultrasonography examination (ultrasound, US). (From Peters AJ, Lloyd RP, Coulam CB: Prevalence of out-of-phase endometrial biopsy specimens. Am J Obstet Gynecol 166:1738, 1992.)

Davis and associates reported that the incidence of luteal-phase defect in normal fertile women, as determined by serial endometrial biopsies, was 31.4% if a single biopsy was 3 or more days out of phase and 6.6% if sequential biopsies were analyzed.

The data from these and other studies indicate that the diagnosis of luteal-phase inadequacy by the use of subjective histologic observations of endometrial biopsy specimens is imprecise, and when used, the incidence of this entity is similar in fertile and infertile populations. These results indicate that luteal-phase deficiency, when diagnosed by the currently used imprecise criterion of histologic maturation of the endometrium, is more a normal biologic variant than a true cause of infertility. Accordingly, this entity is diagnosed and treated much more often than it actually exists.

Conception rates as high as 75% with the use of progestins, clomiphene citrate, and human chorionic gonadotropin (HCG) have been reported by certain investigators, but as summarized by Karamardian and Grimes no randomized, placebo-controlled trials have been conducted that demonstrate a significantly greater conception rate of women with luteal deficiency as a result of treatment. Similar conception rates have been observed among infertile couples without treatment.

Immunologic Causes of Infertility

Substantial evidence from animal studies indicates that antibodies can be induced in females from antigens obtained from organs in the male reproductive tract and that these antibodies interfere with normal reproduction. Both sperm-agglutinating and sperm-immobilizing antibodies have been found in the serum of some infertile women, but also in the serum of fertile control subjects. Agglutinating antibodies are found more frequently than immobilizing antibodies in most series, and in some series the incidence of sperm-agglutinating antibodies in infertile women is similar to that in the control group. Even with the finding of sperm agglutination or immobilization in serum, it has not been demonstrated that a similar degree of sperm inactivation occurs in the lower genital tract. Thus there is no definitive evidence that sperm agglutination or immobilization in the serum of infertile women is the cause of their infertility. One of the reasons for this discrepancy is the fact that both serum assays measure mainly IgM and IgG antibodies, whereas the antibodies locally produced in the genital tract are mainly IgA. For this reason some investigators have measured antisperm antibodies in cervical mucus and found a correlation between the presence of such antibodies and infertility.

No data have shown that the finding of antibodies against sperm in either the male or the female partner is a cause of infertility. A retrospective analysis of corticosteroid therapy and no treatment was performed by Smarr and Hammond in women with high titers of antisperm antibodies. Even though the analysis was retrospective and therapy was administered in a nonrandomized manner, the results are in agreement with those of a randomized study in males, indicating that corticosteroid treatment of either the male or female partner does not significantly increase the pregnancy rate compared with no therapy.

Autoimmunity to sperm in both semen and serum has been found in some infertile men, particularly those who have had testicular infection, injury, or a surgical procedure such as vasectomy reversal. Men with these antibodies have been treated with corticosteroid therapy and sperm-washing techniques. The effectiveness of such treatment remains to be established, since a study by Haas and Beer failed to show that corticosteroid therapy given to men with antisperm antibodies resulted in significantly greater pregnancy rates than occurred when the men were not given such treatment.

In 1993, four prospective studies reported the incidence of fertility occurring after a diagnostic infertility evaluation was performed in which the presence of antisperm antibodies was documented. These studies were performed in four different laboratories in three different countries. Several different techniques for immunoassay were used. All four studies showed no correlation between the presence of antisperm antibodies in either member of the couples and the chance of conception. Pregnancy rates over time were similar in couples who had or did not have antisperm antibodies. Therefore tests to detect these antibodies as part of the diagnostic infertility evaluation are not justified since their presence does not affect fecundity.

Infection

Some researchers have suggested that asymptomatic, or occult, infection of the upper female genital tract and the male genital tract is a cause of infertility. Friberg and Gnarpe suggested in 1973 that infection with what was then called T. mycoplasma in the male could interfere with normal sperm function, and infection of the female reproductive tract could interfere with normal sperm transport. The current name now used for those organisms is *Ureaplasma urealyticum.* Two other microorganisms of the genus *Mycoplasma* that are found in the female genital tract are *M. hominis* and *M. fermentans.* Although Friberg and Gnarpe and others have reported that treatment of infertile couples with antibiotics, such as tetracycline or doxycycline, that eradicate these organisms resulted in high pregnancy rates, controlled studies have reported no difference in pregnancy rates between couples treated with antibiotics and those not treated. Harrison and colleagues studied 88 infertile couples with no demonstrable cause of infertility. One third were treated with doxycycline, one third received placebo, and one third received no treatment. *T. mycoplasma* was isolated from about two thirds of the couples in each group and was eradicated only in the group treated with doxycycline. Nevertheless, conception rates were similar in each group (Table 41-6). Matthews and coworkers performed a similar study and obtained similar results. Other investigators have suggested that asymptomatic *C. trachomatis* infection may also cause infertility, but the dosage of doxycycline used in these randomized studies would also have eradicated these organisms. Thus there is no evidence that asymptomatic infection of the genital tract of the human male or female can cause infertility.

Fertilization Abnormality: Zona-Free Hamster Egg Penetration Test

The zona-free hamster egg penetration test originally described by Yanagimachi and associates was a test developed to predict the fertilizing ability of sperm and provides an additional, perhaps more sensitive parameter for assessing sperm function than the routine semen analysis. However, many variables factors affect the test results.

Vazquez-Levin and colleagues reported that this test did not correlate well with in vitro fertilization (IVF) of human eggs.

Table 41-6 Controlled Studies of Outcome of Therapy of Couples with Unexplained Infertility and *U. urealyticum* infections

Author	Treatment	Number of Couples	Number of Pregnancies	Conceptions (%)
Harrison et al	Doxycycline	30	5	17
	Placebo	28	4	14
	None	30	5	17
Matthews et al	Treated	51	10	20
	None	18	4	22

From Bernstein GS: Occult genital infection and infertility. In Mishell DR Jr, Davajan V, Lobo RA (eds): Infertility, Contraception and Reproductive Endocrinology, 3rd ed. Cambridge, MA, Blackwell Scientific, 1991.

Mao and Grimes surveyed the literature written about this test and concluded the sensitivity and specificity of the sperm penetration assay was too low to justify its routine use as part of the infertility investigation.

O'Shea and coworkers reported that 6-month fecundity rates were not statistically different among couples whose male partner had a normal amount of motile sperm but different percentages of hamster egg penetration. Even couples with penetration scores of 0 did not conceive significantly less often than those with higher percentages of penetration. Therefore the value of performing the zona-free test as part of the evaluation of the infertile couple has not been satisfactorily demonstrated, and this expensive assay should no longer be part of the infertility diagnostic evaluation.

PROGNOSIS

All infertile couples should be informed of the prognosis for pregnancy associated with treatment of their particular cause of infertility. The highest probability of conception with treatment other than ARTs occurs among couples in whom anovulation is the only abnormality, with a substantially lower probability of pregnancy with tubal disease or sperm abnormalities (Fig. 41-8). Although these data are older, this information from Hull still provides the best available. Among a group of infertile couples with unexplained infertility who were followed for 2 years without treatment after the evaluation was completed, it was found that the chances of becoming pregnant were greater in women younger than 35 (about 75%) than in women older than 35 (50%) (Fig. 41-9). The cumulative conception rate at the end of 2 years without therapy for those couples was much greater for those who had tried to conceive for less than 3 years before evaluation (about 75%) than in those who had tried to conceive for more than 3 years (about 30%) (Fig. 41-10). In three of the four studies of infertile couples who received no therapy mentioned earlier, more than half the couples that eventually conceived did so in the first year after completing the infertility evaluation, and the vast majority of those who conceived, which was greater than 50% of the entire group,

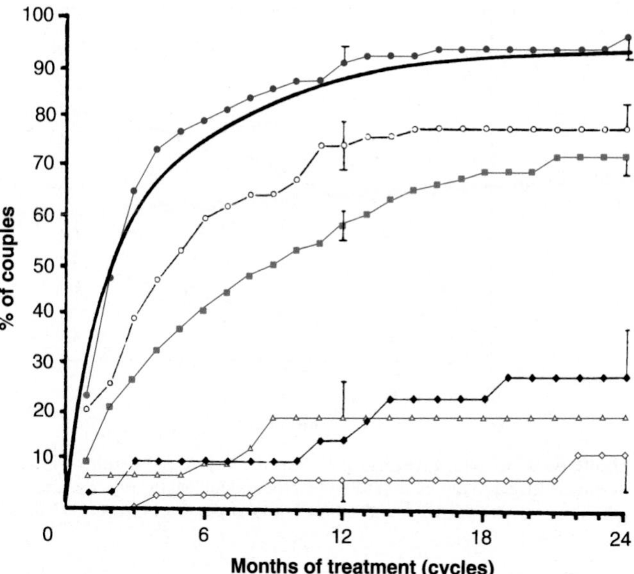

Figure 41-8. Cumulative rates of conception in couples with a single cause of infertility treated appropriately, excluding use of donor insemination or in vitro fertilization, as compared with normal rates (highest rates reported in couples with proved fertility). Rates for couples with each cause shown as solid line, normal; blue circles, amenorrhea; open circles, oligomenorrhea; blue squares, unexplained infertility; open triangles, tubal damage (moderate or severe); black diamonds, failure of sperm penetration of mucus (normal semen); open diamonds, oligospermia and failure to penetrate mucus. Standard errors of proportions are given at 12 and 24 months. (From Hull MGR, Glazener CMA, Kelly NJ, et al: Population study of causes, treatment, and outcome of infertility. Br Med J 291:1693, 1985.)

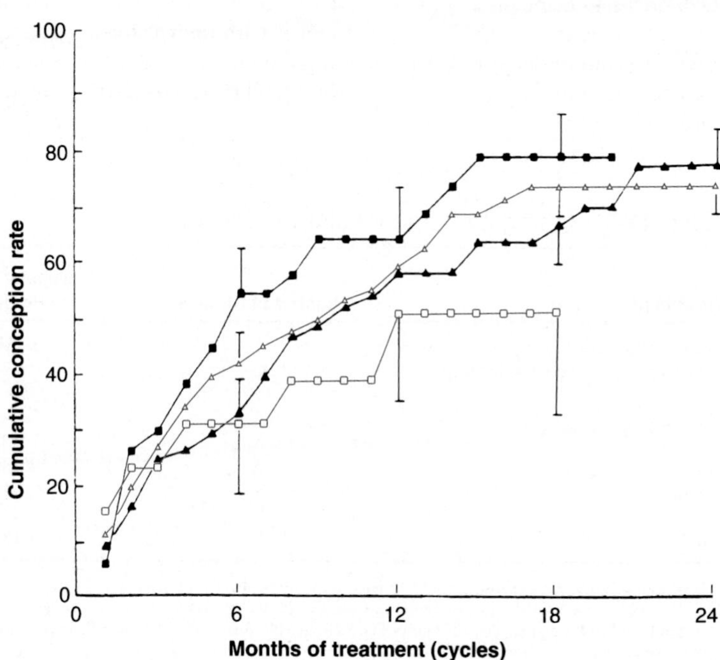

Figure 41-9. Cumulative rates of conception from first attendance at clinic in couples with unexplained infertility related to age of woman. Rates for each age group are shown as solid squares, <25 years; blue triangles, 25 to 29 years; solid triangles, 30 to 34 years; blue squares, >35 years. Standard errors of proportions are given at 6, 12, 18, and 24 months. (From Hull MGR, Glazener CMA, Kelly NJ, et al: Population study of causes, treatment, and outcome of infertility. Br Med J 291:1693, 1985.)

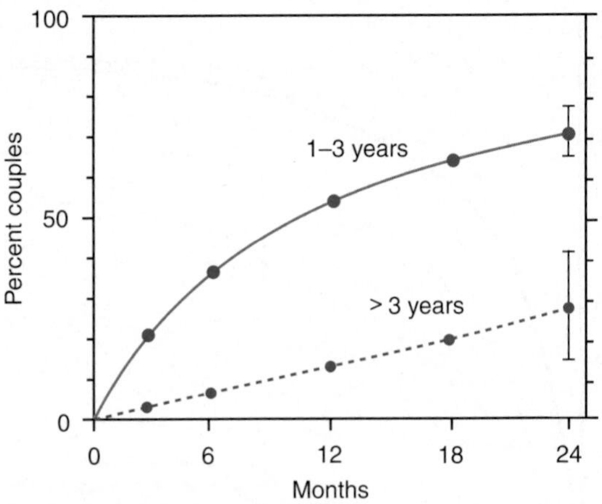

Figure 41-10. Cumulative pregnancy rates in unexplained infertility without treatment related to duration of infertility. (From Hull MGR: Effectiveness of infertility treatments: Choice and comparative analysis. Int J Gynaecol Obstet 47:99, 1994.)

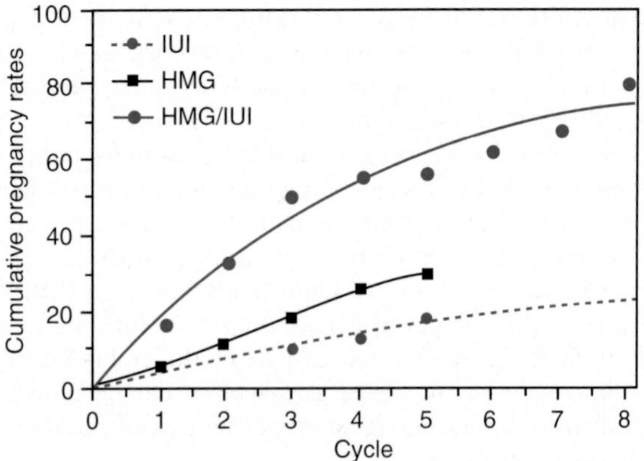

Figure 41-11. Overall cumulative proportion of pregnant patients comparing HMG, IUI, and combined HMG/IUI therapies. Life-table analysis was calculated by the method of Cramer et al., and the curves were fitted by computer analysis of the individual data points. (Reprinted from Fertility and Sterility, 55, Chaffkin LM, Nulsen JC, Luciano AA, Metzger DA, A comparative analysis of the cycle fecundity rates associated with combined human menopausal gonadotropin (HMG) and intrauterine insemination (IUI) versus either HMG or IUI alone, 252. Copyright 1991, with permission from The American Society for Reproductive Medicine.)

who did conceive without treatment, did so within 2 years (see Fig. 41-2). Thus infertile couples with no demonstrable cause of infertility have their best prognosis for conception without treatment for about 2 years after the initial infertility evaluation is completed, and a poor prognosis thereafter. To increase their chances of conception or to shorten the time interval until conception takes place, various treatment methods have been advocated.

For examples with unexplained infertility, IVF and gamete intrafallopian transfer (GIFT) afford the highest pregnancy rates. Although GIFT was considered to be more effective than IVF taking into account patient selection, these therapies are equivalent. Noting that the normal cycle fecundability is in the range of 20% to 25%, IVF provides a cycle rate of approximately 28% on a national basis according to Society for Assisted Reproductive Technology (SART) data. In couples, with unexplained infertility who undergo IVF, fertilization failure has been documented, explaining, at least in part, the inability to conceive naturally.

Controlled ovarian hyperstimulation (COH) with either clomiphene citrate or human menopausal gonadotropin (HMG) followed by intrauterine insemination (IUI) also increase pregnancy rates compared with no treatment during short time intervals. Chaffkin and coworkers reported that treatment with HMG plus IUI enhanced fecundability to a greater degree than treatment with HMG or IUI alone (Fig. 41-11).

Data compiled by Guzick from several studies show considerably lower cycle fecundability (Table 41-7). This should be considered the conservative estimate in counseling patients regarding therapy.

After four to six cycles of COH and IUI in couples with unexplained fertility, the cumulative pregnancy rate is about 50%. Because cycle fecundability and cumulative pregnancy rates are enhanced with COH and IUI, this combined therapy should be tried for several cycles prior to initiating ARTs. However, in woman older than 40 or in couples with marked abnormalities in the semen analysis, IVF with or without intracytoplasmic sperm injection (ICSI) should be recommended.

Table 41-7 Aggregate Data for Each Treatment

Treatment	Number of Studies	Number (%) Pregnancies Per Initiated Cycle	Percentage of Quality-Adjusted Pregnancies Per Initiated Cycle
Control groups	11	64/3539 (1.8)	1.3
Control groups, randomized studies	6	23/597 (3.8)	4.1
IUI	9	15/378 (4)	3.8
CC	3	37/617 (6)	5.6
CC + IUI	5	21/315 (6.7)	8.3
HMG	13	139/1806 (7.7)	7.7
HMG + IUI	14	207/1133 (18)	17.1
IVF	9	378/683 (22.5)	20.7
GIFT	9	158/607 (26.0)	27.0

*Many studies appear in more than 1 row if they reported on more than 1 treatment.

CC, clomiphene citrate; GIFT, gamete intrafallopian transfer; HMG, gonadotropins; IUI, intrauterine insemination; IVF, in vitro fertilization.

Modified from Fertility and Sterility, 70, Guzick DS, Sullivan MW, Adamson GD, et al, Efficacy of treatment for unexplained infertility, 207. Copyright 1998, with permission from The American Society for Reproductive Medicine.

OUTCOME OF PREGNANCY

Several studies have reported the pregnancy outcome of women with long-standing infertility who conceive after treatment. Ovulation-inducing drugs and reconstructive tubal surgery have independently been shown to be associated with an increased incidence of ectopic pregnancy compared with the normal population. Use of ovulation-inducing drugs alone, as well as when combined with IVF and GIFT, has been shown to increase the incidence of multiple gestations. Therefore, if conception occurs after treatment with either ovulation induction or tubal reconstructive surgery, monitoring of the early gestation with serial HCG measurements and ultrasonography assists in determining whether or not the pregnancy is intrauterine and how many gestational sacs are present. Varma and associates reported that infertile couples who conceive do not have a higher rate of spontaneous abortion or perinatal mortality than occurs in normal couples. However, because cycles are monitored closely, the detection early of biochemical pregnancies leads to the perception of a higher loss rate. This is particularly prevalent in older women in whom aneuploidy does result in a higher loss rate normally.

MANAGEMENT OF THE CAUSES OF INFERTILITY

The management of the various causes of infertility will be presented in the order generally followed in an infertility investigation.

Anovulation

Therapeutic agents currently available to induce ovulation are clomiphene citrate, urinary gonadotropins (HMG and other more FSH-enriched preparations), recombinant FSH recombinant LH and colleagues *Ureaplasma urealyticum* and coworkers and associates gonadotropin-releasing hormone (GnRH). In addition, there is growing experience with the use of letrozole and metformin. In addition, as discussed in Chapter 39 (Hyperprolactinemia, Galactorrhea, and Pituitary Adenomas), if anovulation is due to hyperprolactinemia, dopamine agonists are an effective means of inducing ovulation. As noted in Chapter 40 (Hyperandrogenism), in women with congenital adrenal hyperplasia or anovulation accompanied by excessive production of androgens, ovulation may be induced by corticosteroid therapy.

Clomiphene Citrate

Clomiphene citrate is the usual first-line pharmacologic agent for treating women with oligomenorrhea as well as those with amenorrhea who have sufficient ovarian E_2 production. This synthetic, weak estrogen acts by competing with endogenous circulating estrogens for estrogen-binding sites on the hypothalamus, thereby blocking the negative feedback of endogenous estrogen. GnRH is then released in a normal manner, stimulating FSH and LH, which in turn cause oocyte maturation with increased E_2 production. The drug is usually given daily for 5 days beginning 3 to 5 days after the onset of spontaneous menses or withdrawal bleeding induced with progesterone in oil or an oral progestin.

During the days the drug is ingested, serum levels of LH and FSH rise, accompanied by a steady increase in serum E_2 (Fig. 41-12). After ingestion of clomiphene citrate is discontinued, E_2 levels continue to increase, and the negative feedback on the hypothalamic-pituitary axis causes a decrease in FSH and LH, similar to the change seen in the late follicular phase of a normal ovulatory cycle. About 5 to 9 days (mean 7 days) after the last clomiphene citrate tablet has been ingested, the exponentially rising level of E_2 from the dominant follicle has a positive feedback effect on the pituitary or hypothalamus, producing a surge in LH and FSH, which usually results in ovulation and luteinization of the follicle.

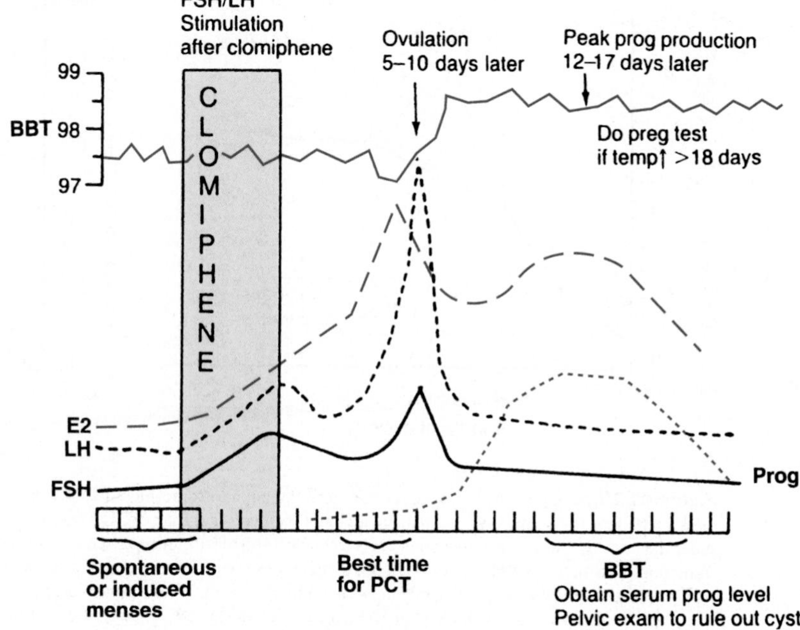

Figure 41-12. Luteinizing hormone (LH), follicle-stimulating hormone (FSH), estradiol (E_2), and progesterone (prog) levels before, during, and after successful treatment with clomiphene citrate. BBT, basal body temperature; PCT, postcoital test. (From March CM, Mishell DR Jr: Induction of ovulation. In Mishell DR Jr, Davajan V, Lobo RA [eds]: Infertility, Contraception and Reproductive Endocrinology, 3rd ed. Cambridge, MA, Blackwell Scientific, 1991.)

Presumptive evidence of ovulation can be obtained by observation of a sustained rise in BBT or measurement of an elevation of serum progesterone. It is best to obtain the serum sample for progesterone measurement about 2 weeks after the last clomiphene tablet has been ingested, because this will usually be in the middle of the luteal phase, about 1 week after ovulation. A rise in serum progesterone level above 3 ng/mL correlates well with the finding of secretory endometrium on an endometrial biopsy sample, but Hull and colleagues Hammond and coworkers have reported that maximal midluteal progesterone levels in clomiphene citrate-induced ovulatory conception cycles are consistently above 15 ng/mL. These levels are higher than the 10 ng/mL level, which is the minimum concentration of progesterone found in spontaneous ovulatory conception cycles because following pharmacologic ovulation induction, more than one follicle usually matures and undergoes luteinization.

Various treatment regimens have been advocated for the use of clomiphene citrate. Most start with an initial dosage of 50 mg per day for 5 days beginning on the fifth day of spontaneous or induced menses. If presumptive evidence of ovulation occurs with this dosage, the same dosage of clomiphene citrate is ingested in subsequent cycles until conception occurs. If ovulation fails to occur with the initial dosage, a sequential, graduated, increasing dosage regimen has proven to be effective with a minimum of side effects. With this regimen if ovulation does not occur with the 50-mg dose, the dosage of drug is increased in the next treatment cycle to 100 mg/day for 5 days. If ovulation does not occur with 100 mg/day in subsequent cycles, the dosage is sequentially increased to 150 mg, 200 mg, and finally 250 mg for 5 days. If ovulation is induced with any of these dosages, the woman is maintained on her individualized ovulatory dosage until conception occurs. If ovulation does not occur with 250 mg, in the next cycle 250 mg is given daily for 5 days, and 1 week after the last tablet has been ingested, 5000 IU of HCG is given to increase the chances of inducing ovulation by simulating the LH surge. In the 10 years' experience with this treatment regimen reported by Gysler and associates about half the women who ovulated and half those who conceived did so following treatment with the 50 mg/day regimen, and an additional one fifth did so with the 100 mg/day dosage. However, about one fourth of all women who ovulated or conceived did so following treatment with a higher dosage regimen, indicating the value of the individualized sequential treatment regimen. However, from a practical standpoint it is unusual to use doses higher than 150 mg, particularly when adjuncts are available such as metformin or switching to letrozole.

With this dosage regimen of clomiphene citrate more than 90% of women with oligomenorrhea and 66% with secondary amenorrhea and normal estrogen status will have presumptive evidence of ovulation. Although only about half the patients who ovulate with this treatment will conceive, Gysler and associates reported that 85% of those with no other causes of infertility conceived after such treatment. Hammond and coworkers, by calculating the fecundability during several months of treatment, reported that if ovulation is induced with clomiphene citrate and no other causes of infertility are present, conception rates over time are similar to those of a normal fertile population who stop using barrier methods of contraception in order to conceive (Fig. 41-13). Using life-table analysis these investigators reported that the monthly pregnancy rate (fecundability) of women treated with clomiphene citrate who had no other infertility factor was 22%, compared with a rate of 25% calculated for women discontinuing diaphragm use. The monthly fecundability remained constant throughout nearly 1 year of treatment. Nearly all of the anovulatory women without other infertility factors in this series, as well as other women with correctable infertility factors, had conceived after 10 cycles of treatment. These data indicate that discontinuation of therapy is the major reason for the reported difference in ovulation and conception rates in anovulatory women treated with clomiphene

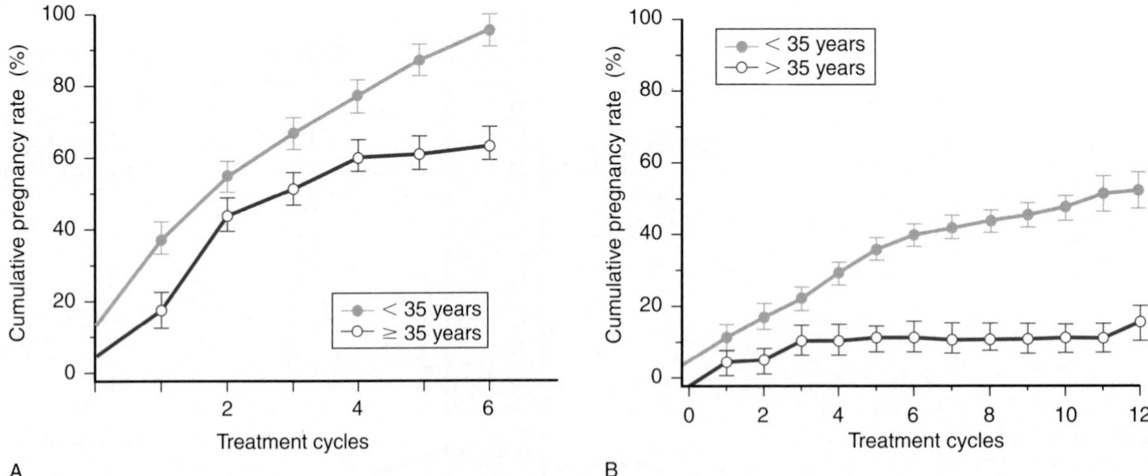

Figure 41-13. **A,** Cumulative pregnancy rates for hypogonadotropic anovulatory women (WHO Group I) treated with gonadotropins. Solid circles represent the cumulative pregnancy rate in women younger than 35. Open circles represent the cumulative pregnancy rate in women older than 35. **B,** Cumulative pregnancy rates following gonadotropin treatment for anovulatory women who did not respond to clomiphene induction of ovulation (WHO Group II). Solid circles represent the cumulative pregnancy rate in women younger than 35. Open circles represent the cumulative pregnancy rate in women older than 35. (From Lunenfeld B, Insler V. Human gonadotropins. In Wallach EE, Zacur HA [eds]: Reproductive Medicine and Surgery. St. Louis, Mosby, 1995, p 617, figs. 20-6, 20-7.)

citrate. However, despite these data, many investigators feel that pregnancy rates are lower with clomiphene than might be expected based on ovulation rates, and other factors (in some women) such as cervical mucus and endometrial problems explains this discrepancy. Clomiphene citrate does not itself cause infertility, as has been stated in some reports. If other causes of infertility are found, they should be treated and induction of ovulation with clomiphene citrate continued.

When conception occurs after ovulation has been induced with this drug, the incidence of multiple gestation is increased to about 5%, with nearly all being twin gestations. However, when the drug is used in normally ovulating women with unexplained infertility, the rate increases to almost 20%. The incidence of clinical spontaneous abortion ranges between 15% and 20%, similar to the rate in the general population. The rates of ectopic gestation, intrauterine fetal death, and congenital malformation are also not significantly increased. Animal data indicate that if the drug is given in high dosages during the time of embryogenesis, there is an increased incidence of fetal anomalies. However, limited human data indicate that if the drug is ingested during the first 6 weeks after conception has occurred, the incidence of fetal malformation, although higher (5.1%) than normal, is not significantly increased. Although no definitive data show that the drug is teratogenic in humans, it is best that the woman be reexamined before each course of treatment to be certain that she is not pregnant. It is also important to determine that the ovaries have not become enlarged, because formation of ovarian cysts is the major side effect of clomiphene treatment.

If cysts are present, they will regress spontaneously without therapy, but if additional clomiphene citrate is given and further gonadotropin release is induced, stimulation and further enlargement of the cyst may occur. Clinically palpable ovarian cysts occur in about 5% of women treated with clomiphene citrate but in less than 1% of treatment cycles. The cysts usually range in size from 5 to 10 cm and do not require surgical excision as they nearly always regress spontaneously. Cysts can occur in any treatment cycle with any dosage, and the incidence is not increased with the higher dosages of drug. Recurrence of cyst formation with the same dosage is uncommon. Other side effects, which occur in less than 10% of women treated with this drug, include vasomotor flushes, blurring of vision, abdominal pain or bloating, urticaria, and a slight degree of hair loss.

About 5% to 10% of women treated with the individually graduated, sequential regimen of clomiphene citrate fail to ovulate with the highest dosage. Because treatment with gonadotropins or GnRH is expensive and time-consuming, other treatment regimens have been used with success.

Some data suggest that in women with elevated levels of dehydroeipandrosterone sulfate (DHEA-S), use of low doses of dexamethasone may enhance the ovulation-inducing effect of clomiphene. This approach is less frequently used today.

Metformin and Other Insulin Sensitizers

Metformin can be considered an adjunctive treatment for ovulation induction and for most women with polycystic ovary disease (PCOS) is being considered now as first-line therapy. Metformin is a biguanine, which is used for diabetes. Its principal role is in reducing hepatic glucose production and thus commensurately decreasing hyperinsulinemia. However, it also has a direct effect on the ovary. Accordingly metformin has been shown to induce ovulation in women with PCOS as well as in other anovulatory women who do not meet the criteria for the diagnosis. Its mechanism of action in inducing ovulation is both through reducing insulin resistance (and thereby affecting gonadotropins and androgens (see Chapter 4, Reproductive Endocrinology) as well as directly stimulating the ovary.

The typical dose of metformin is 1500 mg/day. It is preferable to use long-acting tablets (XR or ES) in 500- and 750-mg tablets and to ingest them all at the same time at dinner. It should be begun, however, only at 500 mg and titrated up over several weeks. This is because of gastrointestinal effects (nausea, vomiting), which is the primary concern with metformin and which precludes its use in up to 20% of women.

Lactic acidosis is a very rare complication that occurs primarily in older individuals. However, checking chemistry blood levels after 3 months of metformin is good practice, and women also should be reminded not to drink alcohol heavily, although the occasional drink is acceptable.

When metformin alone is prescribed for anovulatory women who wish to conceive, the ovulation rate is approximately 60% among adherent women. In clomiphene-resistant patients, (those who fail to ovulate with 150 mg/day), although the data are mixed about 25% of women will respond to clomiphene with metformin. Metformin is a category B substance for pregnancy and has been continued through the first trimester and beyond in selected patients (See Chapter 7, History, Physical Examination, and Preventive Health Care).

Rosiglitazone and Pioglitazone

In insulin-resistant patients with PCOS, the diabetic drugs (thiadolazimediones) may induce ovulation by improving the insulin-hormone axis as well as through direct effort on the ovary. These drugs have also been added to clomiphene therapy. However, this therapy should be reserved for short-term use under special circumstances. There is only a small risk of hepatic enzyme changes (unlike troglitazone, which is no longer available), but there is also a tendency for weight gain with long-term treatment.

Letrozole

Aromatase inhibitors are efficacious as primary agents for ovulation induction. There is the most experience with letrozole. The mechanism of action is that of inhibition of E_2 production during the 5 days of administration, with a negative feedback causing an increase in the LH:FSH ratio, much like the response to clomiphene. Intraovarian androgens are also increased, which may enhance FSH sensitivity. Letrazole (2.5 mg or 5 mg; there is no good evidence for a dose difference) is administered for 5 days like clomiphene, beginning on cycle days 3 to 5.

Because letrozole is short-acting, the problems of thick cervical mucus or a thin endometrium associated with clomiphene have not been reported with letrozole; however E_2 levels are usually lower at ovulation. Pregnancy rates are comparable or better than those with clomiphene alone and there is a reduced incidence of multiple pregnancies. There is sparse information about the effects of letrozole in clomiphene-resistant patients, but anecdotally it has been found to be effective in this regard in many women. Letrozole with gonadotropin have also been used for COH.

Weight and Lifestyle Management

Particularly in women who are clomiphene-resistant, weight loss will often ameliorate the situation. In overweight women it is important to ensure that abnormalities in glucose and lipid metabolism are normalized, as much as possible, before induction of ovulation. To this point there is evidence from Norman that lifestyle changes in diet and exercise may improve overall fitness and metabolic parameters, as well as ovulatory responses, even in the absence of true weight loss although there could be a redistribution of body fat with lifestyle changes.

Gonadotropin Therapy

Gonadotropin therapy is indicated for ovulation induction when estrogen levels are low. Low serum E_2 levels (usually < 30 pg/mL) or lack of withdrawal bleeding after progestogen administration signifies a state that will be unresponsive to oral therapies (clomiphene, letrozole) that are dependent on a negative feedback system. Apart from this indication in usually amenorrheic women, it is appropriate to use gonadotropins in clomiphene/letrozole failures, rather than on the basis of persistent anovulation or the inability to conceive after severe cycles (four to six) ovulatory cycles.

The original preparations of gonadotropin (HMG) were urinary extracts of postmenopausal urine. Although purified, it contained large amounts of protein contaminants. These preparations are less used today but are still available (Pergonal, Humegon). More modern preparations with additional purification have allowed them to be administered subcutaneously as well as intramuscularly (the only option for the older preparations). These preparations are titrated to provide on equal quantity of LH (75 IU) and FSH (75 IU) in one ampule.

Further modifications of these urinary products have eliminated most of the LH activity and provided a relatively "pure" FSH urinary preparation (Bravelle, Metrodin: containing 75 IU FSH per ampule). All nonrecombinant preparations, since they are extracted from human sources, have batch-to-batch variability in terms of biological activity. Recombinant pure FSH preparations (from Chinese hamster ovarian cells) are currently available for subcutaneous administration (Gonal-F, Follistim, 75 IU FSH). Recently, recombinant pure LH has also become available as a supplement (Luveris 75 IU LH), although it is unclear if the addition of LH is really necessary in most individuals.

Because each woman responds individually to the dosage of gonadotropins—even the same woman in different treatment cycles—it is essential to monitor treatment carefully with frequent measurement of estrogen levels and ovarian ultrasonography. Monitoring needs to take place frequently, because there is little difference between the minimal degree of ovarian follicular development necessary to induce ovulation and the amount of follicular development that results in hyperstimulation. Close monitoring requires ultrasound to determine the number of follicles and the maturity status (ultrasound and E_2).

A regimen is described in the following box showing the traditional dosing with HMG. This should consistently induce ovulation, with an overall pregnancy rate of about 60%. The pregnancy rate per cycle is similar to that following clomiphene therapy (22%). Therefore, with sufficient duration of treatment and no other infertility factors, cumulative pregnancy rates should be greater than 90%. It has been reported that the cumulative pregnancy rate after nine cycles of HMG therapy is approximately 77%. However, the incidence of spontaneous abortion after HMG therapy is high (25% to 35%), cumulative pregnancy rates with gonadotropins are influenced by age and the cause of anovulation. The pregnancy rates are highest for young women who are hypoestrogenic with low to normal gonadotropin levels and worse in older women and those with anovulation with normal estrogen status, such as women who are clomiphene-resistant who have PCOS (see Fig. 41-13*A* and *B*). The overall multiple pregnancy rate (usually twins) is in the range of 15%.

Ovarian Hyperstimulation Syndrome

Although enlarged ovaries are frequently encountered after gonadotropin administration, the incidence of significant ovarian hyperstimulation syndrome (OHSS) occurs in approximately 0.5% of women receiving gonadotropin. OHSS can be life-threatening, causing massive fluid shifts, ascites, pleural effusion, electrolyte disturbances, and thromboembolism. The cause has not been completely elucidated but is related to the large cystic ovaries, high E_2 levels and the ovarian elaboration of substances such as VEGF, which increase vascularity and vascular permeability. OHSS has been classified by several investigators into mild, moderate, and severe forms. A representative categorization by Schenken may be found in Table 41-8. HCG triggers the syndrome and blood levels of HCG continue to stimulate the ovaries in OHSS and therefore the syndrome is worse if pregnancy occurs and abates within a week in the absence of pregnancy. For this reason, if severe OHSS is anticipated, HCG injection is withheld, and in IVF cycles the embryo may be frozen rather then replaced to avoid pregnancy.

Treatment of OHSS is largely supportive with judicious use of fluids and the prevention of thrombosis. Correction of electrolyte disturbances and maintenance of urine output are of

Table 41-8 Comparison of Pregnancy Outcome After Terminal Neosalpingostomy Using Careful Conventional Techniques (1978) Versus Microsurgical Techniques (1989)

	1978	1989
Mild	15	10
Pregnant*	13 (86)	7 (70)
Ectopic†	1 (7/8)	1 (10/14)
Moderate	30	29
Pregnant*	9 (30)	9 (31)
Ectopic†	4 (13/44)	4 (14/44)
Severe	42	56
Pregnant*	2 (5)	9 (16)
Ectopic†	0 (0/0)	2 (4/22)
Total	87	95
Pregnant*	24 (28)	26 (27)
Ectopic†	5 (6/21)	7 (7/27)

*Values in parentheses are percentages.
†Values in parentheses are percentages of total patients in the category/percentages of only those patients in the category who became pregnant.
Reprinted from Fertility and Sterility, 54, Schlaff WD, Hassiakos DK, Damewood MD, Rock JA, Neosalpingostomy for distal tubal obstruction: Prognostic factors and impact of surgical technique, 984. Copyright 1990, with permission from The American Society for Reproductive Medicine.

"Step-Up" Treatment Protocol with Human Menopausal Gonadotropin (HMG)

1. Perform baseline ultrasonography of ovaries.
2. Administer HMG, 150 IU/day for 3–5 days.
3. Repeat estradiol measurement. If level has doubled, continue same HMG dosage; if not, increase HMG by 50% for 3 days.
4. Repeat step 3 until estradiol doubles.
5. Perform ovarian scan every 2–3 days until the dominant follicle is = 14 mm.
6. Perform daily ultrasonography until the follicle is = 18 mm.
7. Stop HMG and perform postcoital test.
8. Twenty-four hours later give 10,000 IU of HCG. If the postcoital test result is poor, perform intrauterine insemination.

HCG, human chorionic gonadotropin; HMG, human menopausal gonadotropin.
From March CM: Induction of ovulation. In Lobo RA, Mishell DR Jr, Paulson RJ, Shoupe D (eds): Mishell's Textbook of Infertility, Contraception, and Reproductive Endocrinology, 4th ed. Malden, MA, Blackwell Scientific, 1997, p 520.

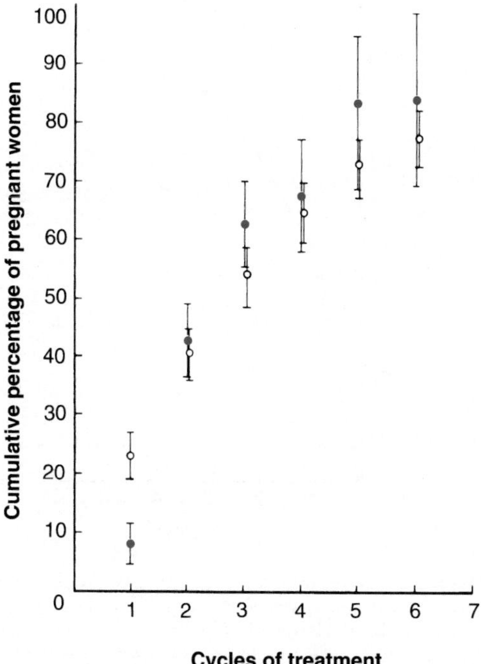

Figure 41-14. Comparison of therapy with gonadotropin-releasing hormone (solid circles) to that with human pituitary gonadotropin (open circles) (mean ± SE). (From Kovacs GT, Phillips S, Healy DL, Burger HG: Induction of ovulation with gonadotrophin-releasing hormone-life-table analysis of 50 courses of treatment. Med J Aust 151:21, 1989.)

greatest importance. Occasionally admission for ICU monitoring is necessary.

Although two epidemiologic studies have suggested that there may be an association between the use of ovulation-inducing agents and an increased risk of developing ovarian cancer later in life, other studies have reported no change in the risk. Because of methodologic problems in two observational studies that showed an association, there is no firm evidence that the association was causally related to the use of ovulation-inducing agents. It should be noted that being infertile (without treatment) increases the risk of ovarian cancer about twofold.

Gonadotropin-Releasing Hormone

An alternative to administration of HMG is GnRH treatment. Because continuous administration of GnRH will saturate the receptors and thus inhibit gonadotropin release to induce ovulation, GnRH needs to be administered in a pulsatile manner at intervals of 1 to 2 hours. Because GnRH is a peptide, it cannot be administered orally, and the two routes of administration in current use are intravenous and subcutaneous. A greater amount of drug must be administered by the subcutaneous route than by the intravenous route; however, the subcutaneous route avoids use of an intravenous catheter with its accompanying problems. The medication is administered by means of a small portable pump, which is usually worn attached to an article of clothing. Ovulation rates of about 75% to 85% per treatment cycle have been reported. Kovacs and coworkers and Braat and associates administered pulsatile GnRH by the subcutaneous route and intravenous route to 41 and 49 anovulatory women, respectively. Each reported that the conception rate per cycle of treatment was 22%. The cumulative pregnancy rate at the end of six cycles of treatment was 85% in the first study and 78% in the second. These pregnancy rates are similar to that reported with use of HMG (Fig. 41-14). One advantage of GnRH therapy is that hyperstimulation occurs less often with it than with HMG and therefore less monitoring is required. However, many women find wearing the pump, which is needed for intermittent pulsing, to be inconvenient. Therefore the woman can choose whether she wishes to receive HMG or GnRH. However, pretreatment with GnRH analogues followed by either HMG or GnRH has resulted in higher pregnancy rates than when GnRH analogues are not administered.

Fleming and colleagues reported that use of this combination treatment in women with polycystic ovaries who had not ovulated after treatment with clomiphene citrate or HMG resulted in a cumulative pregnancy rate of 77% after six cycles of treatment (Fig. 41-15). Dodson and coworkers reported that in a small group of anovulatory women with polycystic ovaries use of HMG alone resulted in a cycle fecundity of 0.16, but with a GnRH agonist together with HMG the cycle fecundity was 0.27. Thus use of a GnRH agonist together with HMG may result in conception in those women with PCOS who fail to respond to HMG alone. However, from a practical standpoint this more difficult protocol is not used routinely unless IVF-ET is anticipated. There is an increased risk of hyperstimulation with this regimen.

Because these medications are expensive, endoscopic partial ovarian destruction with electrocautery or laser has also been used by several groups to treat women with polycystic ovaries who do not ovulate with clomiphene citrate. Ovarian wedge resection was previously used to induce ovulation in women with PCOS before ovulation-inducing drugs became available. However, severe postoperative adhesion formation often occurred, and this technique should no longer be used. To avoid this

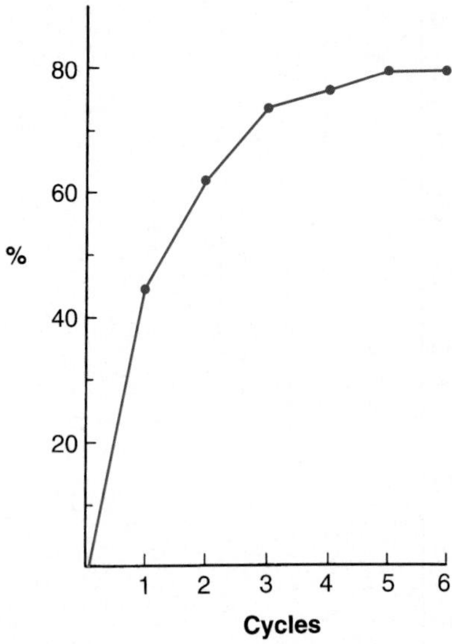

Figure 41-15. Cumulative pregnancy rates in patients with polycystic ovary syndrome receiving combined gonadotropin agonist and HMG therapy. (Modified from Fleming R, Haxton MJ, Hamilton MPR, et al: Combined gonadotropin-releasing hormone analog and exogenous gonadotropins for ovulation induction in infertile women: Efficacy related to ovarian function assessment. Am J Obstet Gynecol 159:376, 1988.)

problem, partial ovarian destruction with electrocauterization or laser ablation of multiple sites has been performed. This laparoscopic technique has resulted in a high rate of spontaneous ovulation and pregnancy. Even the women who do not ovulate spontaneously after this therapy usually ovulate when treated with clomiphene citrate, which was ineffective before partial ovarian destruction. Gjønnaess, who initially described this technique in 1984, reported that after treating 252 women with PCOS with ovarian electrocautery during a 12-year period, 92% ovulated and 89% conceived. The ovulation rate after treatment was influenced by body weight, being 97% in slim women and only 70% in obese women. If the treatment results in ovulatory cycles only about 4% of the women cease having ovulatory cycles in each of the first 3 years after treatment, and 10 or more years after ovarian electrocautery 80% of the women who initially ovulated were still having regular ovulatory cycles. Gjønnaess summarized the results of several investigators who have reported ovulation and pregnancy rates after electrocautery and laser treatment of PCOS (Table 41-9). More recently he has shown that the endocrine changes may persist for at least 10 years. A recent Cochrane review reported an overall term pregnancy rate of 50% after surgery and a low multiple pregnancy rate.

Nevertheless ovulation induction in women with PCOS should still be a medical treatment, particularly with the use of adjuncts, if necessary. Ovarian electrocautery should be reserved for those patients who have difficulties with gonadotropin stimulation (failure of dominant follicle selection or hyperstimulation risk).

Table 41-9 Ovulation and Pregnancy After Electrocautery and Laser Treatment of Polycystic Ovaries

N	Ovulation (%)	Pregnancy (%)	Authors and Year of Publication*
Electrocautery			
35	92	69	Gjønnaess (1984)†
6	83	67	Greenblatt and Casper (1987)
14	64	36	v.d. Weiden et al (1989)
21	81	52	Armar et al (1990)
29	71	52	Abdel Gadir (1990)
7	71	57	Gürgan et al (1991)
10	70		Kovacs et al (1991)
22	86		Armar and Lachelin (1993)
104	76	70	Naether et al (1993)
10	70		Tirtinen et al (1993)
Laser Vaporization			
85	53	56	Daniell and Miller (1989)
19	80	37	Keckstein et al (1990)
10	70		Gürgan et al (1991)
Wedge Resection			
8	65	0	Huber et al (1988)
12	83	58	Kojima et at (1989)

*References appear in the original source.

†Before the laparoscopy, some of the patients had been resistant to hormonal stimulation therapy. After inclusion of patients made responsive to clomiphene citrate by the electrocautery, the pregnancy rate increased to 80% (1).

From Gjønnaess H: Ovarian electrocautery in the treatment at women with polycystic ovary syndrome (PCOS). Acta Obstet Gynecol Scand 73:407, 1994.

Male Cause of Infertility

All gynecologists who care for infertile couples should understand how to interpret a semen analysis as well as how to offer a prognosis for a disorder of abnormal semen. Although gynecologists usually do not perform a diagnostic evaluation or treat the male with a reproductive disorder, they should be able to provide counsel regarding the use of intrauterine insemination with either the husband's or a donor's semen, as well as with treatment by ICSI, testicular sperm extraction (TESE), or microsurgical epididymal serum aspiration (MESA).

Intrauterine insemination has been used to treat oligospermia, as well as abnormalities of semen volume or viscosity. Cruz and associates reported that in a group of infertile couples whose male partner had oligoasthenospermia, the pregnancy rate was significantly greater with intrauterine inseminations, 14.3%, than with intracervical inseminations, 2.0%, of their husband's semen.

McGovern and colleagues reported that the prognosis for pregnancy after intrauterine insemination was significantly greater if the original semen analysis had greater than 30% motility and after swim-up there was a motility rate greater than 70% than for samples with lower percentages of motility. Berg and coworkers reported that if more than 800,000 motile sperm are present after swim-up separation, the pregnancy rate following intrauterine insemination in couples with unexplained infertility treated with controlled ovarian hyperstimulation was about 10% per cycle, but if fewer than this number of sperm was present, the pregnancy rate was only 1% per cycle.

The technique of intrauterine insemination of sperm following their separation from the semen by centrifugation should be used to treat mild to moderate abnormalities in the semen analysis and unexplained infertility. This procedure is associated with higher pregnancy rates if it is combined with COH than when used in natural ovulatory cycles. Intrauterine insemination is also of benefit to women with cervical stenosis, such as that sometimes found following cervical conization. Ideally, insemination should take place on the day of or 1 day before ovulation. It is advisable to utilize urinary LH enzyme-linked immunosorbent assay (ELISA) kits to determine the optimal date to perform insemination since the urinary LH peak occurs on the day prior to ovulation. Insemination should be scheduled for the morning after LH is initially detected in an afternoon urine specimen.

Separation of sperm from the seminal fluid by double centrifugation, the swim-up technique, or use of a density gradient should be performed before intrauterine insemination. Intrauterine insemination of seminal fluid can produce severe uterine cramps as a result of prostaglandin release.

Until a few years ago, if there were severe abnormalities in the semen analysis, the prognosis for fertility was less than that for any other cause of infertility, even with the use of IVF techniques. Attempts to enhance fertilization rates of aspirated oocytes with the technique of subzonal insemination of sperm were unsuccessful because fertilization rates remained low, about 15%. After Van Steirteghem and associates developed the technique of ICSI, fertilization rates of oocytes injected with a single spermatozoon that was obtained from men with severe abnormalities in the semen analysis were increased to about 50%. Pregnancy rates per embryo transfer were about 35%, significantly greater than the 16% rate of pregnancy with embryos fertilized by subzonal insemination techniques.

In a study by Palermo and colleagues similar fertilization rates of about 60% of the oocytes injected were achieved with sperm from semen samples containing no motile sperm, few motile sperm, and high numbers of motile sperm. In addition, a fertilization rate of about 60% was obtained whether the sperm were freshly obtained by masturbation, by electroejaculation, or were previously frozen. Nearly a 50% fertilization rate of oocytes was also achieved when the sperm were aspirated directly from the epididymal fluid.

In this study, fewer than 1% of the couples studied failed to achieve fertilization of at least one oocyte with this technique. High ongoing pregnancy rates of 30% or more were also achieved, regardless of the number of motile sperm identified in the original semen analysis.

The excellent results obtained with ICSI by the group that originally described the technique have now been replicated in other centers. By using this technique, the pregnancy rate of couples whose male partner has an extremely low concentration of motile sperm in the semen samples (<100,000/mL) can reach 35% per treatment cycle. With a loss rate of 25%, the live-birth rate of 27% is similar to that for couples with other causes of infertility that are treated by IVF. Studies of pregnancies resulting from ICSI and standard IVF reveal a similar rate of pregnancy loss and multiple gestation. Therefore, ICSI is now the ART of choice for all causes of male infertility, as well as for those couples with no known cause of infertility in whom fertilization does not occur with standard IVF procedures. It has been suggested that a sperm concentration of less than 2 million per milliliter of semen is an indicator for initial use of ICSI.

Similarly, significant reductions in motility (10%) and morphology (5%) are indications for ICSI, although these criteria are relatively arbitrary. With the technique of ICSI the probability of achieving a viable pregnancy is inversely correlated with the age of the woman. Oehninger and coworkers reported that the fertilizability of human ova with ICSI remained constant, at about 60%, in women in different age groups, but ongoing pregnancy rates decreased from about 50% when the woman was younger than 35 to 23% among women ages 35 to 40 to less than 6% for women older than 40. Use of donor eggs should be considered in women older than 40 or those with elevated circulating levels of FSH who are candidates for ICSI. A few years ago, the finding of azoospermia in seminal fluid was considered an untreatable cause of infertility. After development of the techniques of ICSI as an adjunct to IVF, it was found that spermatozoa retrieved from the testes of azoospermic men could fertilize ova retrieved from their partner's ovaries. Palermo and colleagues reported that the clinical pregnancy rate is higher when testicular or epididymal sperm is retrieved from men with obstruction in their vas deferens (obstructive azoospermia) than when testicular sperm is retrieved from men with azoospermia without reproductive tract obstruction (nonobstructive azoospermia). The rates were 57% and 49%, respectively. Shulman and associates reported that even if the sperm retrieved from the testes remains immotile, the pregnancy rate after ICSI is about 16% per cycle of oocyte retrieval. Jezek and coworkers reported that the likelihood of retrieval of spermatozoa from testicular tissue of men with azoospermia and normal FSH levels is nearly 100%. Even if the FSH levels are markedly elevated, there is at least a 50% likelihood that spermatozoa can be retrieved from the testes and used to perform an ICSI procedure. Thus the presence of a combination of azoospermia and an elevated FSH level is not a contraindication for performing a TESE procedure. Although controversial, there is probably a slight but significant increase in chromosomal structural defects in children born after ICSI. In 8319 live births, Van Steirteghem showed a rate of sex chromosomal aneuploidy of 0.6% versus 0.2%, and structural autosomal abnormalities in 0.4% versus 0.07% as well as an increase in structural aberrations related to the infertile fathers. A Danish study by Mau suggested that although 2 papers have suggested abnormalities, 9 of 11 publications on this topic do not, suggesting that if there truly is an increased risk of chromosomal abnormalities after ICSI, the rate is low. Follow-up of the children; however, does suggest an increased rate of urogenital abnormalities, which may be related to the male subfertility. Counseling of patients before ICSI about these findings is important.

Some couples, particularly those whose male partner has azoospermia, may choose to utilize donor sperm insemination. If they do so, the attitudes of both partners regarding the use of donor semen and the stability of the marriage need to be thoroughly discussed before the procedure is performed. Donors from sperm banks are carefully screened for infectious diseases, and all semen samples are quarantined for at least 6 months because of the long time it takes for positive antibodies to HIV to appear after infection. A set of guidelines for semen donor insemination has been published by the Association for Reproductive Medicine. These guidelines provide information regarding indications for donor insemination, as well as suggested procedures for selection and screening of possible semen donors.

Most centers using frozen semen for insemination have reported that the pregnancy rate per cycle is less than with fresh semen. Hammond and associates reported that a 50% cumulative pregnancy rate after insemination with previously frozen

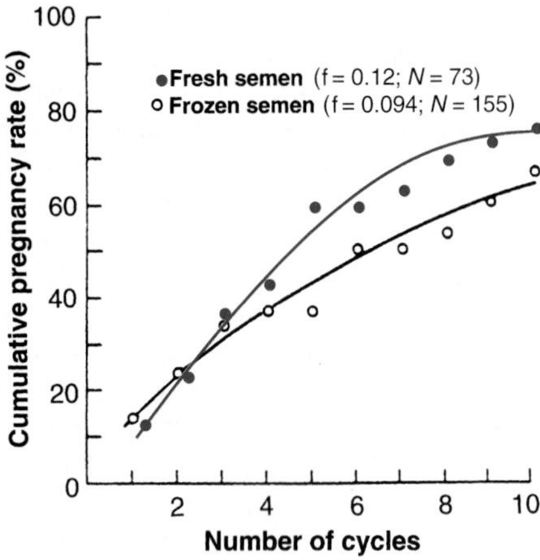

Figure 41-16. Cumulative fecundability curves for fresh or frozen semen (fresh: $f = 0.12$, $n = 73$; frozen: $f = 0.094$, $n = 155$). (From Hammond MG, Jordan S, Sloan CS: Factors affecting pregnancy rates in a donor insemination program using frozen semen. Am J Obstet Gynecol 155:480, 1986.)

sperm was only reached after 6 months of treatment, and the monthly fecundity rate was only 9% (Fig. 41-16). However, in the study by Gillett and colleagues with use of frozen semen from donors the monthly fecundity rate was 18%, with a 45% cumulative pregnancy rate at 3 months. Although it is clear that pregnancy rates are much lower with frozen rather than fresh sperm, variation of semen quality (after thaw) are more important than insemination timing issues, although these are also important variables.

Uterine Causes of Infertility

Intrauterine Adhesions

In addition to menstrual abnormalities and recurrent abortion, some women may not be able to conceive because of the presence of intrauterine adhesions (IUA). As mentioned in Chapter 16 (Spontaneous and Recurrent Abortion), most women with IUA have had a previous curettage of the uterine cavity, most often during or shortly following a pregnancy. If the only abnormal finding in the infertility investigation is the presence of IUA, the prognosis for conception after hysteroscopic lysis of the adhesions is good. March reported that of 69 infertile women with IUA and no other infertility factors, 52 (75%) conceived after hysteroscopic treatment.

Leiomyoma

Congenital uterine defects rarely cause infertility, and the uterine anomalies associated with maternal ingestion of diethylstilbestrol (DES) have not been shown in randomized studies to be a cause of infertility. It is also difficult to assess the effect of leiomyomas on conception, since so many women with leiomyomas have no difficulty conceiving. Nevertheless, it is plausible that cervical myomas could cause distortion of the endocervix, interfering with normal sperm transport, and that some submucous leiomyomas may interfere with sperm transport or normal implantation of the blastocyst. There is evidence that certain myomas (depending on location) can increase the risk of abortion. Large intrauterine leiomyomas can also occlude the interstitial portion of the oviduct and prevent normal sperm transport. If no other cause of infertility is found and myomas of moderate size and position that may interfere with sperm transport are present, then a myomectomy is justified. More recent data from the IVF literature point to a decreased pregnancy rate with submucous fibroids, intramural fibroids which are large (74 cm) and which distort the cavity. Vercellini and colleagues reviewed all studies published about the effect of myomectomy on infertility published between 1982 and 1996. The overall conception rate after myomectomy among seven prospective studies of women with no other causes of infertility was 61%. However, no study included a comparison group of infertile women with leiomyomas treated expectantly.

Tuberculosis

If the HSG reveals findings consistent with pelvic tuberculosis, then endometrial biopsy and culture should be performed to confirm the diagnosis. The radiographic features of pelvic tuberculosis that are virtually diagnostic of the disease include (1) calcified lymph nodes or granulomas in the pelvis, (2) tubal obstruction in the distal isthmus or proximal ampulla, sometimes resulting in a "pipe-stem" configuration of the tube proximal to the obstruction, (3) multiple strictures along the course of the tube, (4) irregularity to the contour of the ampulla, and (5) deformity or obliteration of the endometrial cavity without a previous curettage (Fig. 41-17). Appropriate antituberculosis medication should be initiated, but women with pelvic tuberculosis should be considered sterile, as pregnancies after therapy are rare. Tubal reconstructive surgical procedures are therefore pointless. If tuberculosis is present in the oviduct but not the uterus, pregnancies have been reported following IVF.

Tubal Causes of Infertility

During the past two decades the incidence of infertility caused by damage to the oviduct has increased because of an increased incidence of salpingitis. Obstructions occur at either the distal or proximal portion of the oviduct and sometimes in both regions. Distal obstruction is much more common than proximal obstruction. In a Swedish study, only 15% of the women with tubal disease had proximal tubal obstruction. The prognosis for fertility after surgical tubal reconstruction depends on the amount of damage to the oviduct as well as the location of the obstruction. If there is extensive damage, the chances for conception after tubal reconstruction are very unlikely. Women with extensive tubal disease have a greater chance of conceiving with an IVF procedure, and thus the extent and location of the intrinsic and extrinsic tubal disease should be ascertained by HSG and possibly laparoscopy in an effort to determine whether tubal reconstruction or IVF offers the better prognosis. As stated earlier, if large hydrosalpinges are seen at the time of the HSG, it is best to suggest that the woman have IVF rather than undergo tubal reconstructive surgery. It is recommended that hydrosalpinges be excised before IVF if it is large and visible by ultrasound. If both proximal and distal obstructions of the oviduct exist, the damage to the oviduct is usually so extensive that the oviduct cannot function normally. Therefore, although it is possible to achieve tubal patency after surgical repair of a tube with both proximal and distal blockage, subsequent

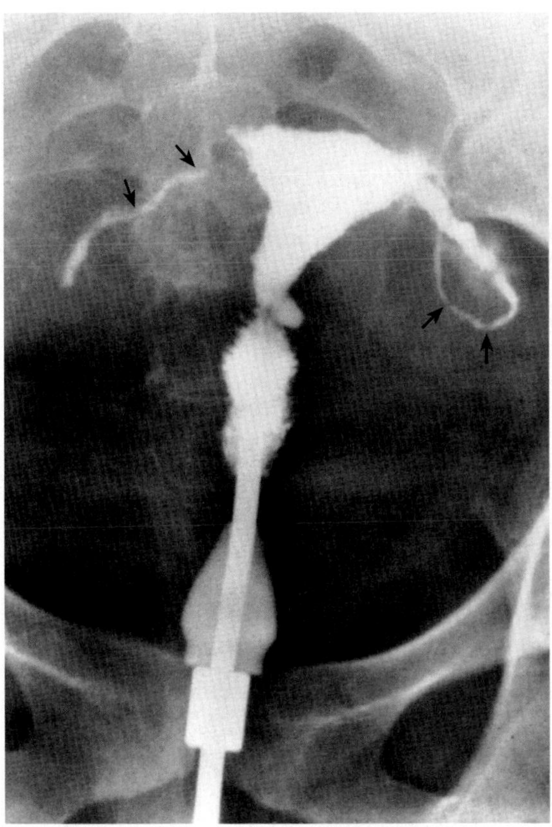

Figure 41-17. Tuberculous salpingitis in 37-year-old nulligravida with primary infertility for 15 years. Right tube is obstructed in the zone of transition between the isthmus and the ampulla. Arrows indicate multiple strictures in both tubes. Nodular contour of endometrial cavity may also be related to tuberculosis and is analogous to the pattern found in the ampulla in other cases. Small diverticulum near internal os probably represents adenomyosis. Diagnosis of tuberculosis was confirmed by endometrial culture. (From Richmond JA: Hysterosalpingography. In Mishell DR Jr, Davajan V, Lobo RA [eds]: Infertility, Contraception and Reproductive Endocrinology, 3rd ed. Cambridge, MA, Blackwell Scientific, 1991.)

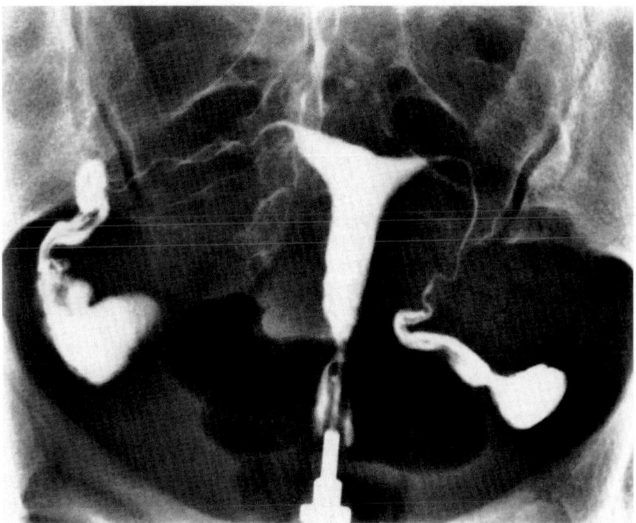

Figure 41-18. HSG showing bilateral hydrosalpinges with dilation, clubbing, and obstruction at fimbriated ends. Patient was 32-year-old woman with 10-year history of primary infertility. (From Richmond JA: Hysterosalpingography. In Mishell DR Jr, Davajan V, Lobo RA [eds]: Infertility, Contraception and Reproductive Endocrinology, 3rd ed. Cambridge, MA, Blackwell Scientific, 1991.)

intrauterine pregnancy is uncommon. Therefore, surgical reconstruction should not be performed in such instances.

Distal Tubal Disease

HSG will determine whether the tubal obstruction is complete or partial, the size of the distal sacculation, and the appearance of the mucosal folds and rugal pattern of the endosalpinx (Fig. 41-18). Laparoscopy will assist in determining the size of the hydrosalpinx, the amount of muscularis, and the thickness of the wall of the oviduct after distention with dye. Laparoscopic examination will determine whether pelvic adhesions are present and the extent of such adhesions. Women with fimbrial obstruction are not a homogeneous group, and the prognosis for intrauterine pregnancy following distal tubal reconstruction is related to the extent of the disease process. Therefore, it is important to perform both HSG and laparoscopy before surgical reconstruction to provide an individualized prognosis.

If the fimbriae of the distal end of the oviduct are relatively normal with only partial occlusion by adhesions or fimbrial bridges, removal of these adhesions by means of a fimbrioplasty procedure will result in higher conception rates (≅60%) than if the distal end is completely occluded and a cuff salpingostomy procedure is required. Overall conception rates following salpingostomy are in the 30% range, with a high percentage (about one fourth) being tubal pregnancies. As reported by Schlaff and associates, with the use of microsurgical techniques for the treatment of distal tubal disease the intrauterine pregnancy rate has not increased when compared with the results following conventional macrosurgery, but the rate of ectopic pregnancy appears to be somewhat greater following microsurgery (see Table 41-8). The incidence of ectopic pregnancy after surgical reconstruction for distal tubal disease is directly related to the amount of tubal damage existing before the operative procedure.

Boer-Meisel and colleagues correlated the results of tubal reconstruction with the degree of tubal damage according to the severity of five factors: (1) extent of adhesions, (2) nature of adhesions, (3) diameter of the hydrosalpinx, (4) appearance of the endosalpinx, and (5) thickness of the tubal wall. Utilizing these criteria they developed three prognostic categories: good—with a cumulative pregnancy rate of about 75%; intermediate—about 20%; and poor—less than 5%. In the good category, only 1 of 22 pregnancies was ectopic, but in the intermediate group half of the pregnancies were tubal, and in the poor prognostic group 6 of 7 pregnancies were ectopic. They concluded that if there were fixed adhesions with absent rugal folds and a thick, fixed tubal wall, distal tubal reconstructive surgery should not be performed.

Donnez and Casanas-Roux classified the degree of distal tubal occlusion into four categories on the basis of HSG (Fig. 41-19). Following microscopic tubal reconstruction the cumulative pregnancy rate was directly related to the degree of occlusion. If the distal tubal ostium was completely normal but peritubal adhesions were present, lysis of these adhesions by a procedure called salpingolysis resulted in a 64% intrauterine pregnancy rate, similar to that obtained with a fimbrioplasty for partial obstruction.

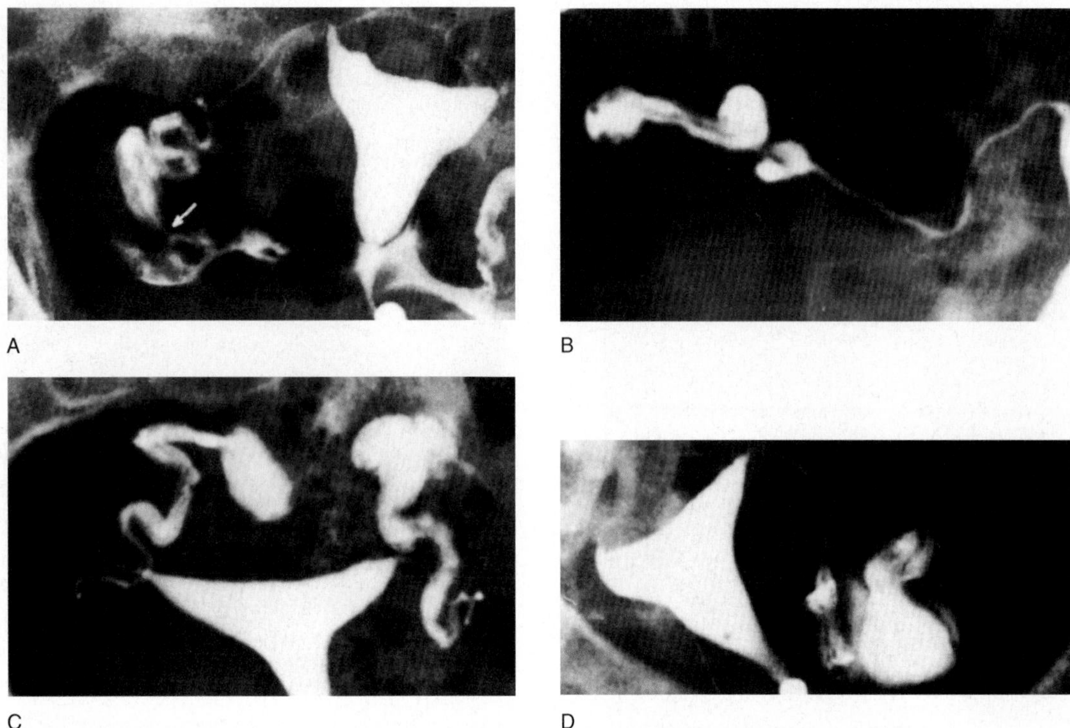

Figure 41-19. Classification of distal tubal occlusion based on degree of dilation seen on HSG. **A,** Degree I: Conglutination of the fimbrial folds *(arrow)* with tubal patency. **B,** Degree II: Complete distal occlusion with normal ampullary diameter. **C,** Degree III: Complete distal occlusion with ampullary dilation of 15 to 25 mm in diameter. **D,** Degree IV: Occlusion with ampullary distention greater than 25 mm. (Reprinted from Fertility and Sterility, 46, Donnez J, Casanas-Roux F, Prognostic factors influencing the pregnancy rate after microsurgical cornual anastomosis, 200. Copyright 1986, with permission from The American Society for Reproductive Medicine.)

About half the women who underwent salpingostomy for degree II occlusion conceived, with no ectopic pregnancies, but only about one fourth of those with degree III or IV occlusions had subsequent intrauterine pregnancies, and the ectopic pregnancy rate was about 10% (Fig. 41-20 and Table 41-10). Thus following operation for more extensive distal tubal disease, nearly one third of the pregnancies that occurred were ectopic.

In both these studies the best prognostic factor was thickness of the tubal wall. If there was a hydrosalpinx greater than 2 cm in diameter with a thick tubal wall, the prognosis for a term pregnancy following distal tubal reconstruction was extremely poor. Hulka reported that when more than one half of the ovary was involved with adhesions, no woman had a term pregnancy following salpingostomy.

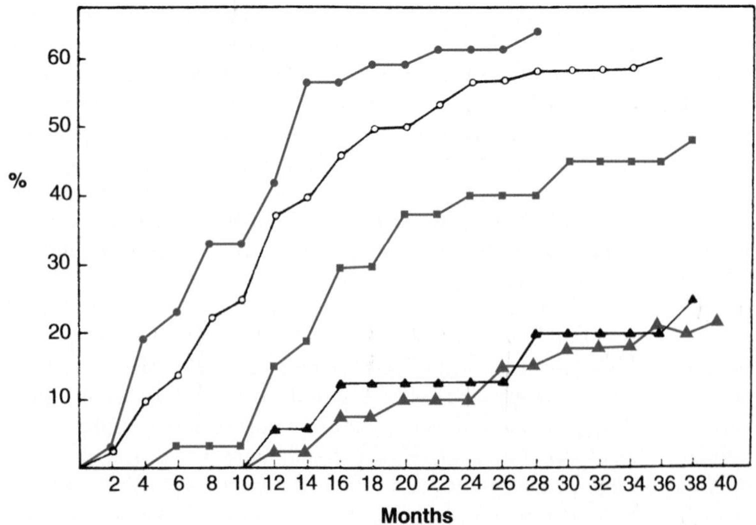

Figure 41-20. Cumulative pregnancy rates following microsurgical repair of these lesions are depicted. Solid circles, salpingolysis; open circles, fimbrioplasty; squares, salpingostomy (degree II); black triangles, salpingostomy (degree III); blue triangles, salpingostomy (degree IV). (Reprinted from Fertility and Sterility, 46, Donnez J, Casanas-Roux F, Prognostic factors influencing the pregnancy rate after microsurgical cornual anastomosis, 200. Copyright 1986, with permission from The American Society for Reproductive Medicine.)

Table 41-10 Pregnancy Rate After Microsurgery and Ciliated Cell Percentage in Cases of Distal Tubal Occlusion

Type of Operation	Number of Patients	Number of Intrauterine Pregnancies	Ectopic Pregnancies
Fimbrioplasty			
Occlusion of degree I	132	79 (60%)	2 (2%)
Salpingostomy			
Occlusion of degree II	27	13 (48%)	0
Occlusion of degree III	16	4 (25%)	1 (6%)
Occlusion of degree IV	40	9 (22%)	5 (12%)
Total	83	26 (31%)	6 (7%)
Salpingolysis	42	27 (64%)	1 (2%)

Modified from Fertility and Sterility, 46, Donnez J, Casanas-Roux F, Prognostic factors of fimbrial microsurgery, 200. Copyright 1986, with permission from The American Society for Reproductive Medicine.

Rock and coworkers classified women with distal fimbrial occlusion into three categories based on the extent of tubal disease (see the following box). Schlaff and associates then performed a life table analysis of couples in these three categories with no other causes of infertility after the female partner underwent neosalpingostomy. They found that 80% of those women with mild tubal disease conceived, whereas only 31% of those with moderate disease and 16% of those with severe disease conceived (Fig. 41-21). The ectopic pregnancy rate was higher in the latter two categories. Thus this information should be presented to the woman when she is counseled, and if the prognosis for term pregnancy is poor, she should be advised to undergo IVF instead of surgical tubal reconstruction.

Distal tubal reconstructive surgery should be carried out by operative laparoscopy. Dubuisson and colleagues reported the results of a series of 65 consecutive distal tuboplasties, both fimbrioplasties and neosalpingostomies performed endoscopically. The intrauterine pregnancy rate was 26% after fimbrioplasty and 29% after neosalpingostomy, similar to the success rate after microsurgery. Canis and coworkers reported similar results. Of 87 women who had a distal tuboplasty performed by laparoscopy, one third had intrauterine pregnancies, nearly all of whom had mild or moderate disease (Fig. 41-22). A comparison of the pregnancy rates obtained after laparoscopic surgery with those obtained in an earlier series by the same investigators after laser microsurgical distal tuboplasty performed through a laparotomy incision revealed no statistical difference in the pregnancy rates between the two treatment modalities. It appears

Classification of the Extent of Tubal Disease with Distal Fimbrial Obstruction

Mild

Absent or small hydrosalpinx less than 15 mm diameter
Inverted fimbriae easily recognized when patency is achieved
No significant peritubal or periovarian adhesions
Preoperative hysterogram reveals a rugal pattern

Moderate

Hydrosalpinx 15–30 mm in diameter
Fragments of fimbriae not readily identified
Periovarian or peritubular adhesions without fixation, minimal cul-de-sac adhesions
Absence of a rugal pattern on preoperative hysterogram

Severe

Large hydrosalpinx greater than 30 mm diameter
No fimbriae
Dense pelvic or adnexal adhesions with fixation of the ovary and tube to the broad ligament, pelvic sidewall, omentum, or bowel
Obliteration of the cul-de-sac
Frozen pelvis (adhesion formation so dense that limits of organs are difficult to define)

From Rock JA, Katayama P, Martin EJ, et al: Factors influencing the success of salpingostomy techniques for distal fimbrial obstruction. Obstet Gynecol 52:591, 1978.

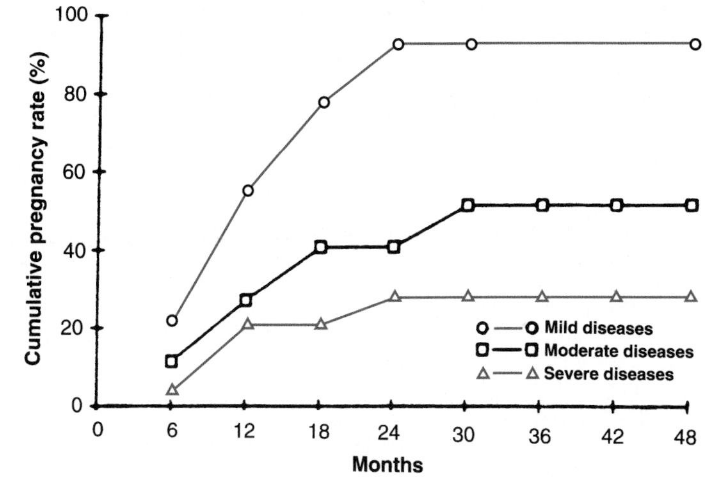

Figure 41-21. Life-table analysis of pregnancy outcome after neosalpingostomy by extent of disease. (Reprinted from Fertility and Sterility, 54, Schlaff WD, Hassiakos DK, Damewood MD, Rock JA, Neosalpingostomy for distal tubal obstruction: Prognostic factors and impact of surgical technique, 984. Copyright 1990, with permission from The American Society for Reproductive Medicine.)

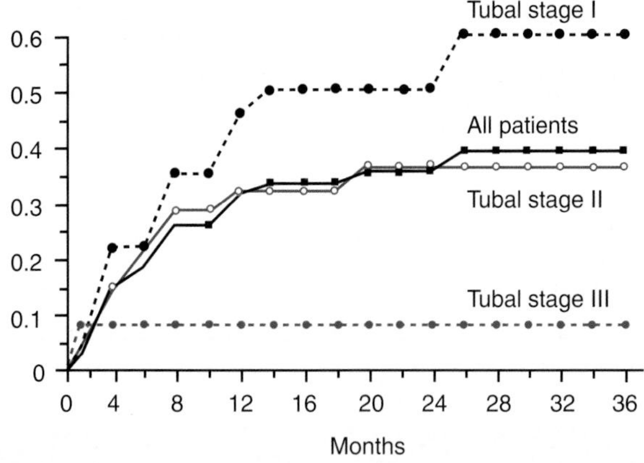

Figure 41-22. Cumulative pregnancy rates with laparoscopic distal tuboplasty after 4 years. (Reprinted from Fertility and Sterility, 56, Canis M, Manhes H, Mage G, et al, Laparoscopic distal tuboplasty: Report of 87 cases and a 4-year experience, 616. Copyright 1991, with permission from The American Society for Reproductive Medicine.)

that the prognoses for fertility after salpingostomy by any operative technique is correlated more with the extent of disease than with the type of surgical procedure. Because laparoscopic salpingostomy results in less morbidity, length of hospitalization, and cost than performing the procedure by laparotomy, the former technique is the procedure of choice to treat distal tubal disease.

Proximal Tubal Blockage

If no dye reaches the oviduct during an HSG, the diagnosis of proximal tubal blockage is likely. However, since spasm of the intrauterine portion of the oviduct can occur, the diagnosis cannot be confirmed unless laparoscopy is performed with general anesthesia. Here at least half of the time the tube is found to be patent. Laparoscopy also allows examination of the distal portion of the oviduct, which cannot be visualized radiographically if there is proximal blockage. Proximal tubal blockage is most commonly due to residual damage after infection, but it can be due to plugs of material or endometriosis. Frequently, tubal diverticula, also called *salpingitis isthmica nodosa (SIN),* are present.

Unlike the results of distal tubal reconstruction, the use of microsurgery has improved intrauterine rates for proximal tubal disease. Before the use of microsurgery, tubal intrauterine blockage was treated by reimplantation of the patent portion of the oviduct into the endometrial cavity. Term pregnancy rates following tubocornual implantation were in the 30% range. This procedure has now been replaced by a microsurgical tubocornual reanastomosis procedure in which the diseased portion of oviduct is excised and the patent distal oviduct is reanastomosed to the portion of the interstitial segment of the oviduct that is patent. With this technique various authors have reported term pregnancy rates of about 50%, with ectopic pregnancy rates of less than 10%.

Donnez and Casanas-Roux reported that the pregnancy rate following tubocornual reanastomosis was related to the extent of preexisting disease as determined at the time of HSG (Fig. 41-23). The best pregnancy rate (55%) was obtained when the interstitial portion of the oviduct was not damaged and less than 1.5 cm of occluded tube needed to be removed. The pregnancy rate declined to 33% when the interstitial portion of the tube was occluded and still further with the presence of some (25%) or numerous (16%) diverticular lesions. The ectopic pregnancy rate of all women treated was 7%, but of those who conceived, 15% had an ectopic pregnancy.

The surgical treatment of a proximal tubal blockage has now been replaced in most centers by the use of transcervically placed probes, catheters, or balloons, which are placed under fluoroscopic or hysteroscopic guidance in an outpatient setting with or without local anesthesia and sedation (Fig. 41-24). This is frequently carried out independently by an experienced radiologist. After a cannula is placed at the tubal ostium, radiographic dye is injected through the oviduct. This technique is called *selective salpingography.* If this technique does not produce tubal patency then a catheter is inserted into the interstitial portion of the oviduct to achieve patency. Results from several centers indicate that this outpatient procedure of selective salpingography and tubal cannulation, provided it is performed by well-trained, capable individuals, yields patency and pregnancy rates similar to those achieved by microsurgical reanastomosis (Table 41-11). Patency rates after these procedures range from 60% to 85%, with subsequent pregnancy rates

Table 41-11 Review of Pregnancy Rates and Outcomes After Hysteroscopic Cannulation

		NUMBER OF PREGNANCIES (%)			
Author and Year of Publication*	**Number of Patients**	**Total**	**Ongoing†**	**SAB**	**Ectopic**
Ransom et al, 1997	17‡	10 (59)	8 (47)	1 (5.9)	1 (5.9)
Das et al, 1995	21	15 (71.4)	12 (57)	2 (9.5)	1 (3.6)
Sakumoto et al, 1993	88	38 (43)	NA	NA	NA
Deaton et al, 1990	7	2 (29)	2 (29)	0	0
Subtotal	133	65 (48.9)	22 (48.9)	3 (6.7)	2 (4.4)
Excluded (small series)					
Sulak et al, 1987	2	1 (50)	1 (50)	0	0
Daniell et al, 1987	1	1 (100)	1 (100)	0	0

NA, not available; SAB, spontaneous abortion.
*References are from original source.
†Ongoing pregnancies are all those of > 20 weeks' gestation. Some investigators reported term pregnancies.
‡Seventeen patients in this study had bilateral occlusion; five others had unilateral blockage.
Modified from Fertility and Sterility, 71, Honoré GM, Holden AEC, Schenken RS, Pathophysiology and management of proximal tubal blockage, 785. Copyright 1999, with permission from The American Society for Reproductive Medicine.

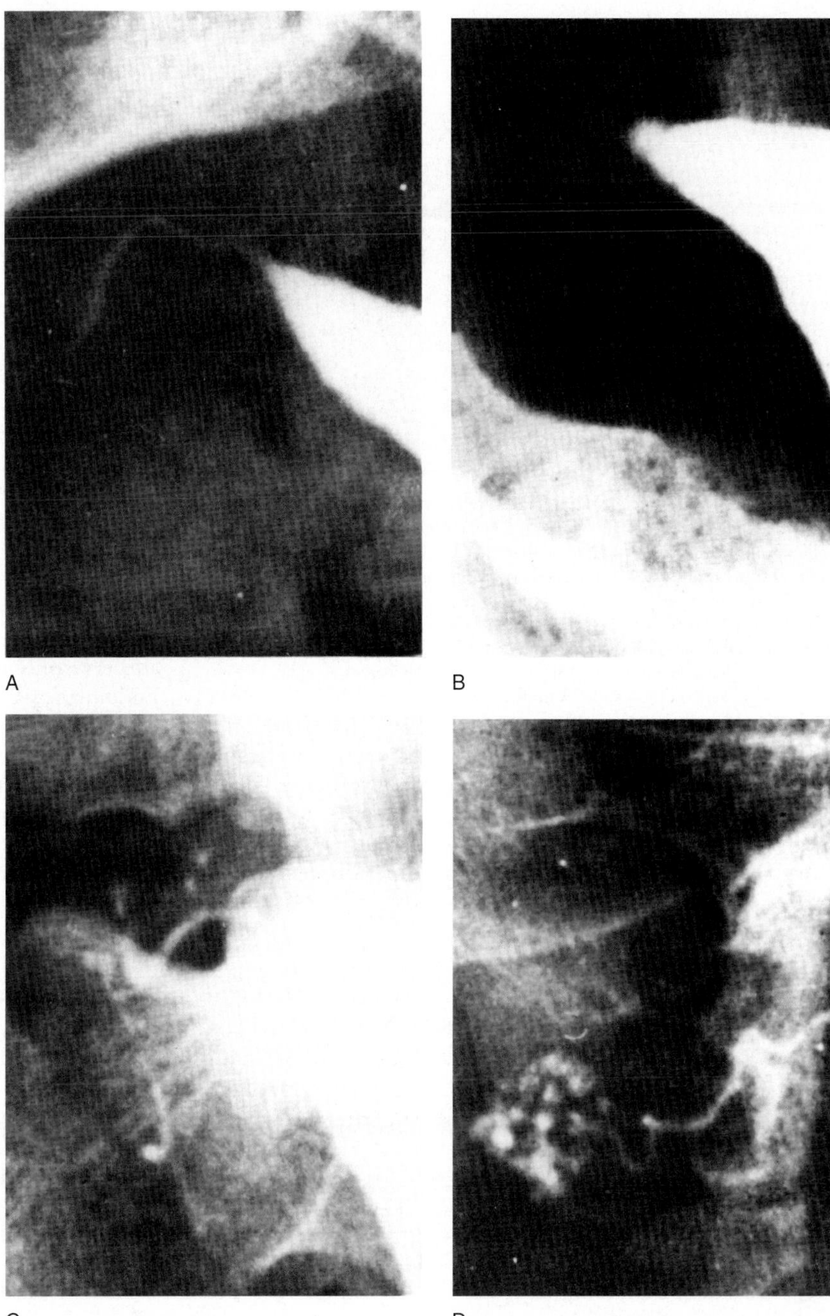

Figure 41-23. Types of occlusion following HSG. **A,** Undamaged intramural portion. **B,** Occluded intramural portion. **C,** Cornual occlusion with contrast extravasation in tubal wall. **D,** Occlusion with numerous diverticular lesions. (Reprinted from Fertility and Sterility, 46, Donnez J, Casanas-Roux F, Prognostic factors influencing the pregnancy rate after microsurgical cornual anastomosis, 1089. Copyright 1986, with permission from The American Society for Reproductive Medicine.)

in the 20% to 50% range in different series of small numbers of women. These relatively easy outpatient procedures, whether performed under fluoroscopic or hysteroscopic visualization, should now be considered the initial treatment of choice for proximal tubal obstruction. Indeed if tubal obstruction persists, IVF-ET is usually the procedure of choice.

Adjunctive Therapy

Adjunctive procedures for surgical tubal reconstruction previously included prophylactic antibiotics, intraperitoneal corticosteroids, postoperative hydrotubation, and placement of tubal stents. Prospective studies have not demonstrated postoperative hydrotubation to have any benefit, and tubal stents should not be used because they may cause mucosal damage. Recent data from the Nordic Adhesion Prevention Study Group reported that intraperitoneal corticosteroids failed to reduce adhesion scores in infertility patients.

It is important to stress surgical technique, attention to hemostasis and irrigation of blood and debris away from the surgical site with Ringers' lactate solution. The only barriers currently used with some efficacy are Interceed (to be used only in areas which are "dry" and not bleeding) and barriers impregnated with hyaluronic acid (Seprafilm). Gore-Tex requires suturing and removal and is therefore rarely used and not applicable for tubal disease. A recent Cochrane review supported the use of Interceed but not Seprafilm.

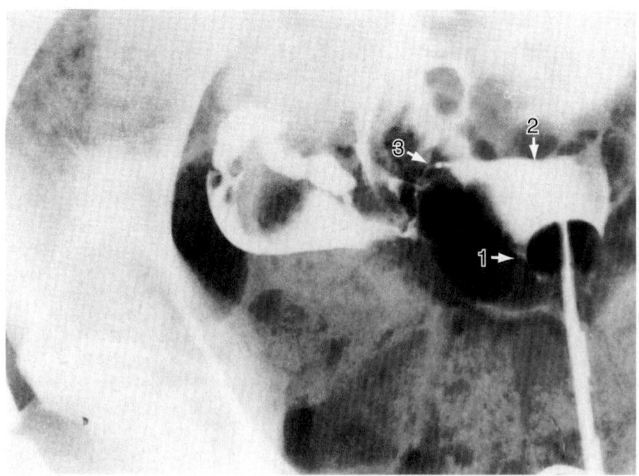

Figure 41-24. HSG demonstrating transcervical balloon tuboplasty system in place following successful balloon dilation of a cornual occlusion. Two tandem balloons of the introductory catheter are inflated in lower uterine segment and in the endocervical canal *(1)*. The selective salpingography catheter is wedged into the cornual angle *(2)*. Balloon marker of the transcervical balloon tuboplasty catheter is shown *(3)*. Injection of contrast medium through transcervical balloon tuboplasty catheter demonstrates tubal patency and peritoneal spillage. (From Confino E, Tur-Kaspa I, DeCherney A, et al: Transcervical balloon tuboplasty: A multicenter study. JAMA 264:2079, 1990.)

Tulandi and colleagues, in a randomized prospective study, demonstrated that second-look laparoscopy 1 year after failure of terminal salpingostomy or salpingo-ovariolysis to achieve pregnancy was not beneficial in achieving higher pregnancy rates. The benefit of second-look laparoscopy performed within a few weeks or months after tubal reconstructive surgery has also not been demonstrated in a prospective randomized trial. Thus a second-look laparoscopy performed at some time interval after tubal reconstructive surgery is not cost-effective.

If pregnancy does not occur within 6 to 12 months after tubal reconstruction, another HSG should be performed. If tubal obstruction has recurred, a repeat surgical procedure is not advised because pregnancy rates are less than 10%.

Endometriosis

Some investigators have estimated that as many as 40% of infertile women have endometriosis. If endometriosis is found at the time of laparoscopy, the extent of the disease should be classified according to the stages recommended by the American Society of Reproductive Medicine (Fig. 41-25). The etiology, diagnosis, and treatment of endometriosis are presented in detail in Chapter 19.

Mild Endometriosis

An inflammatory/immune reaction occurs in endometriosis that affects fertility status even if the process is "mild" (Chapter 19, Endometriosis). Although Schenken and Malinak, as well as Garcia and David, reported that pregnancy rates following conservative surgical treatment of mild endometriosis were nearly identical to the rates of groups of women in the same institution who had no surgical corrective treatment, these rates are lower than in normal fertile women. Inoue and coworkers reported that if electrocoagulation of mild or moderate endometriosis

Patient's Name ______________________ Date ______________________

Stage I (Minimal) = 1–5 Laparoscopy __________ Laparotomy __________ Photography __________

Stage II (Mild) = 6–15 Recommended Treatment ______________________

Stage III (Moderate) = 16–40

Stage IV (Severe) = >40 ______________________

Total __________ Prognosis ______________________

PERITONEUM	ENDOMETRIOSIS		<1 cm	1–3 cm	>3 cm
		Superficial	1	2	4
		Deep	2	4	6
OVARY	R	Superficial	1	2	4
		Deep	4	16	20
	L	Superficial	1	2	4
		Deep	4	16	20
	POSTERIOR CULDESAC OBLITERATION		Partial		Complete
			4		40
	ADHESIONS		<1/3 Enclosure	1/3–2/3 Enclosure	>2/3 Enclosure
OVARY	R	Filmy	1	2	4
		Dense	4	8	16
	L	Filmy	1	2	4
		Dense	4	8	16
TUBE	R	Filmy	1	2	4
		Dense	4*	8*	16
	L	Filmy	1	2	4
		Dense	4*	8*	16

***If the fimbriated end of the fallopian tube is completely enclosed, change the point assignment to 16.**

Figure 41-25. American Fertility Society classification of endometriosis. (Reprinted from Fertility and Sterility, 43, Andrews WC, Buttram VC, Behrman SJ, et al, Revised American Fertility Society classification of endometriosis, 1985, 351. Copyright 1985, with permission from The American Society for Reproductive Medicine.)

was performed at the time of diagnostic laparoscopy, then conception rates were slightly lower in women in whom the endometriotic lesions were not coagulated. In the Canadian study by Marcoux and associates twice as many women conceived when the endometrial implants were resected or ablated compared with those who received no therapy of implants, but in the treated group the fecundity rate was only 6% per cycle. A subsequent and smaller clinical trial from Italy reported no difference in pregnancy rate whether minimal to mild endometriosis was ablated or not. If only mild endometriosis is found at the time of laparoscopy and no other cause of infertility is present, then it is advisable to treat these individuals with controlled ovarian hyperstimulation and intrauterine insemination similar to the treatment of unexplained infertility. Simpson and colleagues reported results of a nonrandomized, prospective, multicenter cohort analysis in Canada that analyzed results of different therapies of 297 women with endometriosis and regular cycles and patent oviducts whose partners had more than 5 million motile sperm in their ejaculate. They found that the relative likelihood of pregnancy with the use of clomiphene citrate supraovulation was 2.9 times that of women who received no treatment. Use of danazol was associated with the same likelihood of pregnancy as occurred with no treatment.

Moderate Endometriosis

If pelvic adhesions that cannot be lysed at the time of laparoscopy or ovarian endometriomas larger than 1 cm in diameter are present, medical therapy will not cause sufficient regression to improve fertility rates, and surgical treatment should be undertaken. For women with moderate disease without ovarian endometriomas and minimal adhesions that can be cut at the time of laparoscopy, no evidence indicates that medical treatment improves fertility rates compared with no treatment.

The use of danazol, GnRH agonists, progestins, or oral contraceptives has not been shown to increase fertility rates compared with observation without treatment.

Hughes and coworkers performed a meta-analysis of four randomized clinical trials and five cohort studies of women who had mild or moderate endometriosis treated with either danazol or progestins compared with a control group who received a placebo or no therapy. No individual study showed a significantly greater pregnancy rate with treatment, and the common odds ratio for pregnancy occurring with treatment compared with no treatment was 0.85 (Fig. 41-26). They also performed a meta-analysis of six randomized clinical trials in which ovulation suppression with GnRH agonists or progestins was compared with danazol. The common odds ratio was 1.07, an insignificant difference.

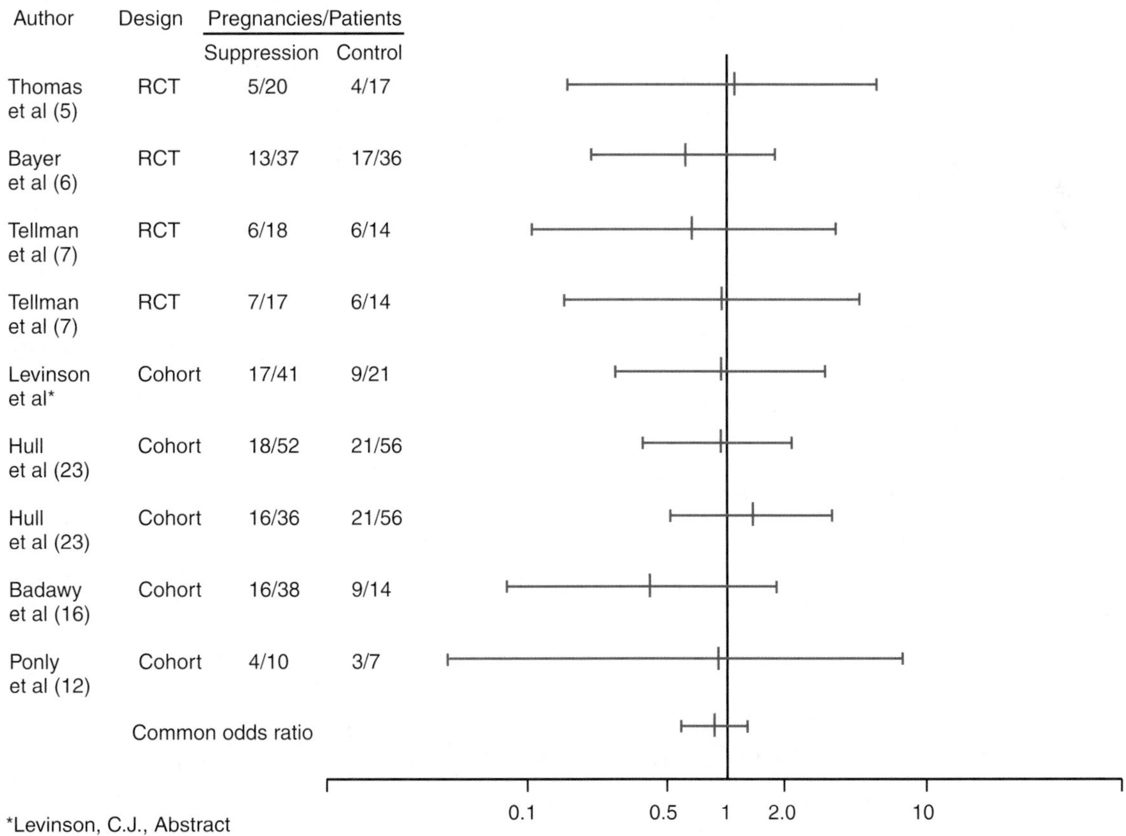

Figure 41-26. Controlled studies comparing ovulation suppression versus no treatment in women with endometriosis-associated infertility: Odds Ratio for pregnancy. References are from the original source. (Reprinted from Fertility and Sterility, 59, Hughes EG, Fedorkow DM, Collins JA, A quantitative overview of controlled trials in endometriosis-associated infertility, 963. Copyright 1993, with permission from The American Society for Reproductive Medicine.)

Severe Endometriosis

Conservative operative resection of endometriosis should be performed for women with infertility and moderate or severe disease with adhesions that cannot be cauterized or lysed at the time of laparoscopy or those with endometriomas more than 1 cm in diameter. Preoperative treatment with danazol or GnRH agonists for 6 weeks to 3 months is advised by some authorities to facilitate the surgical resection, but there appears to be no benefit from postoperative danazol or GnRH agonist treatment. Conception rates for women treated operatively have been reported to be in the 50% to 60% range for those with moderate disease and 30% to 40% for those with severe disease. These rates are better than those reported for expectant management. Three of five cohort studies reported that pregnancy rates following laparoscopic surgical treatment of endometriosis was significantly greater than use of danazol or no treatment. The common odds ratio for pregnancy was 2.67 times greater with use of laparoscopic surgery.

Of the women who do conceive after surgical resection, about half will do so in the first 6 months, and nearly all in the first 15 months after the operative procedure, similar to what occurs after discontinuation of medical therapy.

Olive and Martin reported that women with severe endometriosis had a 50% pregnancy rate after being treated with carbon dioxide laser laparoscopy, similar to the rates of those treated with laparotomy (Fig. 41-27). In the absence of significant pain, if women have such severe disease that it cannot be treated adequately by endoscopic surgery, IVF should be utilized instead of performing a laparotomy. Pregnancy rates after IVF for endometriosis are about 20% per treatment cycle. Therefore both treatment options should be offered to individual women with severe endometriosis.

Operative treatment of endometriosis has for many years included the use of electrocautery as well as microsurgical techniques. In the past 15 years argon and carbon dioxide lasers have been used to vaporize adhesions and endometrial implants. Studies in animals and humans have shown no difference in the results of treatment of periadnexal adhesions with carbon dioxide laser or electrocautery. In a prospective randomized study Tulandi reported that pregnancy rates were similar following the use of each of these two techniques for lysis of periadnexal adhesions. The duration of operating time may be reduced with the laser, but the technique has the disadvantages of higher cost and necessity for additional training, because it is more difficult to use the laser than electrocautery.

Unexplained Infertility

For couples in whom the female member ovulates and has patent oviducts and the male member has at least 20 million motile sperm in the ejaculate, the diagnosis of unexplained infertility should be made and treatment initiated with COH and appropriately timed preovulatory IUI with a sample of freshly prepared, recently ejaculated sperm or IVF. COH should be performed with either clomiphene citrate or HMG. Insemination is best performed on the day prior to spontaneous ovulation, on the morning following the day that LH is initially detected in a random urine specimen, or 36 hours after intramuscular HCG is given to induce ovulation. A meta-analysis of several randomized trials by Zeyneloglu and associates comparing IUI with timed intercourse after COH in couples with unexplained infertility revealed that the pregnancy rate per cycle with IUI is about 20%, whereas with timed intercourse it is

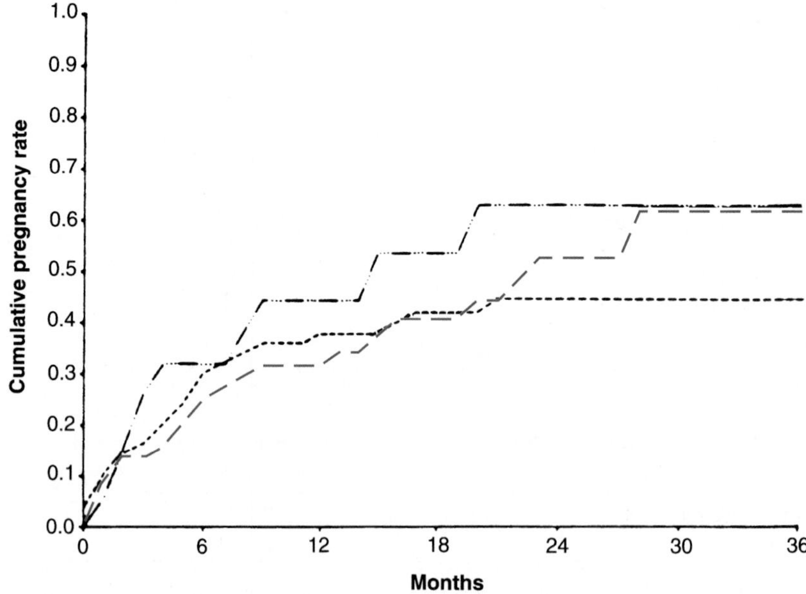

Figure 41-27. Cumulative pregnancy rates for women with endometriosis using life-table analysis. The long dashed line indicates patients with stage I endometriosis, the short dashed line indicates patients with stage II endometriosis, and dash and triple dot line indicates those with stage III disease. (Reprinted from Fertility and Sterility, 48, Olive DL, Martin DC, Treatment of endometriosis-associated infertility with CO2 laser laparoscopy: The use of one- and two-parameter exponential models, 18. Copyright 1987, with permission from The American Society for Reproductive Medicine.)

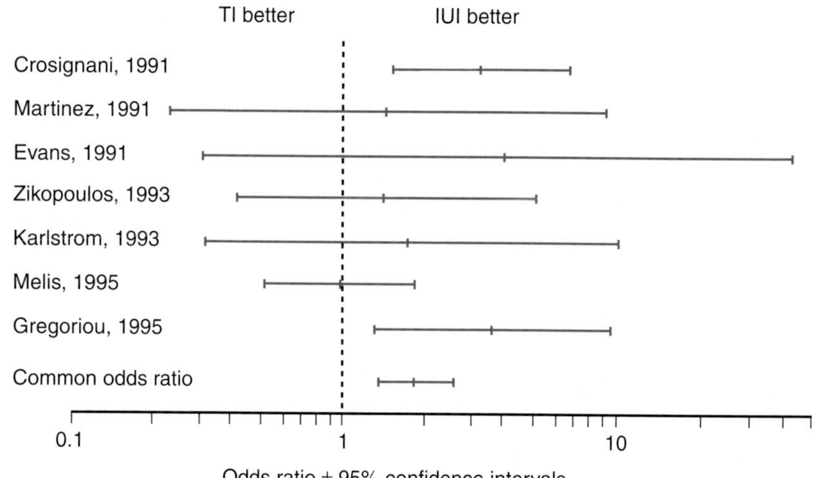

Figure 41-28. The odds ratio of the studies included in the meta-analysis. References are from the original source. (Reprinted from Fertility and Sterility, 69, Zeyneloglu HB, Arici A, Olive DL, et al, Comparison of intrauterine insemination with timed intercourse in superovulated cycles with gonadotropins: A meta-analysis, 486. Copyright 1998, with permission from The American Society for Reproductive Medicine.)

about 11% (Fig. 41-28). Dodson and colleagues reported results of a randomized trial of COH and IUI using various methods of sperm separation. There were no significant differences in per cycle pregnancy rates with any of the methods.

It is much easier for the clinician and woman to undergo ovarian stimulation with clomiphene citrate than with HMG because use of the former drug is less expensive and requires less monitoring. Monitoring is necessary with HMG to reduce the possibility of developing the ovarian hyperstimulation syndrome as well as multiple gestations. When clomiphene citrate is used to cause ovarian hyperstimulation in ovulatory women, treatment should be initiated on cycle day 2 or 3 before the dominant follicle is recruited. A dose of 100 mg/day for 5 days usually results in the development of two or three dominant follicles, which release eggs shortly after the endogenous LH surge or after giving exogenous HCG.

Deaton and coworkers performed a prospective, randomized, clinical trial comparing the use of clomiphene citrate and timed intrauterine insemination with timed periovulatory sexual intercourse in an unstimulated cycle in 67 couples with unexplained infertility or mild endometriosis. The monthly fecundability in the treatment cycles was 0.095 compared with 0.033 in the control cycles, a significant difference.

In 1998 Guzick and associates published a review of data from 45 published studies of various therapies of unexplained infertility including mild endometriosis. After adjustment for study quality, pregnancy rates per initiated treatment cycle were 1.3% to 4.1% for no treatment, 8.3% for clomiphene citrate plus IUI, 17.1% for HMG plus IUI, and 20.7% for IVF (see Table 41-7). Although the pregnancy rate in this analysis of nonrandomized studies was higher with HMG plus IUI than with clomiphene citrate plus IUI, use of HMG is more costly, requires frequent sonographic and hormone monitoring, and has a higher complication rate than clomiphene citrate. In a prospective randomized trial comparing HMG plus IUI with HMG and intracervical insemination, and intracervical or intrauterine insertion without HMG Guzick and associates found the pregnancy rate per treatment cycle with HMG plus IUI was 9%, about twice as high as for the other three treatment regimens. One third of the couples treated with HMG plus IUI conceived after four treatment cycles (Table 41-12). Unfortunately, even with monitoring, 20% of the pregnancies that

Table 41-12 Pregnancy Rates Per Couple

Treatment Group	Number of Couples	Number of Insemination Cycles	Number of Pregnancies	Pregnancy Rate per Couple* (%)	Pregnancies During Insemination Cycle† Number of Pregnancies/ Number of Insemination Cycles (%)
Intracervical insemination	233	706	23	10	14/706 (2)
Intrauterine insemination	234	717	42	18	35/717 (5)
Superovulation and intracervical insemination	234	637	44	19	26/637 (4)
Superovulation and intrauterine insemination	231	618	77	33	54/618 (9)

*The results of tests of a χ^2 priori comparison, adjusted for center, are as follows: intracervical insemination as compared with superovulation and intracervical insemination, $p = 0.006$; intracervical insemination as compared with intrauterine insemination, $p = 0.01$; intracervical insemination as compared with superovulation and intrauterine insemination: $p < 0.001$; intrauterine insemination as compared with superovulation and intrauterine insemination, $p < 0.001$; superovulation and intracervical insemination as compared with superovulation and intrauterine insemination, $p < 0.001$. The p value that indicates statistical significance after the Bonferroni correction is 0.01.

†The results of χ^2 tests of a priori comparison, adjusted for center, are as follows: intracervical insemination as compared with superovulation and intracervical insemination, $p = 0.024$; intracervical insemination as compared with intrauterine insemination, $p = 0.003$; intracervical insemination as compared with superovulation and intrauterine insemination, $p < 0.001$; intrauterine insemination as compared with superovulation and intrauterine insemination, $p < 0.001$; superovulation and intracervical insemination as compared with superovulation and intrauterine insemination, $p = 0.005$. The p value that indicates statistical significance after the Bonferroni correction is 0.01.

Modified from Guzick DS, for the National Cooperative Reproductive Medicine Network: Efficacy of superovulation and intrauterine insemination in the treatment of infertility. N Engl J Med 340:177, 1999. Modified with permission.

occurred with use of HMG were multiple gestations. It therefore appears best to initially treat unexplained infertility in a younger woman with clomiphene citrate and IUI for four to six cycles. If pregnancy fails to occur then referral to an infertility specialist for treatment with HMG plus IUI or IVF is advisable.

Several authors have reported that with the use of COH and IUI fecundability declines dramatically after age 40. Pregnancy rates with IVF also decrease substantially after age 40. In several reports, the pregnancy rate per cycle with COH and IUI in women older than 40 was only 5% compared with 10% to 15% in younger women. Some studies report no pregnancies in women older than 42 treated with COH plus IUI. Even if pregnancy occurs the pregnancy loss rate doubles in conceptions occurring in women older than 40, compared with those for younger women. The more expensive IVF procedure in women older than 40 is also not as effective as it is in younger women. Live-birth rates of about 10% per cycle with IVF have been reported in women of this age with use of their own oocytes. With the use of donor oocytes live-birth rates increase to approximately 50% per IVF embryo transfer cycle.

In Vitro Fertilization

The technique of IVF-ET is now being widely used to treat infertility. Although the method was originally restricted to women who had no functioning oviducts as a result of severe tubal disease, it is now being used for women with severe endometriosis and couples with male factor or unexplained infertility. Because the rate of pregnancy after IVF is directly related to the number of embryos placed in the uterine cavity, nearly all IVF clinics currently utilize some form of ovarian hyperstimulation to increase the number of oocytes obtained at the time of follicle aspiration. Stimulation protocols utilizing clomiphene citrate, HMG or FSH, or a combination of agents are being used. These agents are usually given after a period of suppression with a GnRH agonist. GnRH antagonists are increasing being used only at midcycle, particularly in older women with poor responses. Monitoring of follicle growth is usually performed by both daily ultrasonography and estrogen measurement.

Some centers perform IVF with a single ovum retrieved from an unstimulated follicle. There are two main advantages for performing IVF with eggs collected from the dominant follicle in a normal, unstimulated ovulatory cycle. First, the substantial cost of administering gonadotropin and additional days of monitoring that are necessary in stimulated cycles are avoided. Second, more aspiration cycles can be performed in the same time period. Thus aspirating eggs from unstimulated cycles is both cost-effective and time-efficient. In addition, the problems associated with multiple gestation and cryopreservation of excess embryos are avoided. Foulet and colleagues reported a similar pregnancy rate, 22.5% per cycle, with this technique as others have with hyperstimulation. However, the pregnancy rate per cycle reported by most others is in the 15% range.

Originally, oocyte retrieval was done by laparoscopic visualization. Follicle aspiration is now being performed routinely through the vagina into the cul-de-sac with sonographic guidance of needle placement.

Following aspiration of the oocytes they are cultured in a rigidly controlled, sterile laboratory environment. Various culture media are used in different clinics. The media are freshly prepared at frequent intervals, and sterility is ensured. The eggs are incubated in an atmosphere of 5% carbon dioxide and high humidity.

A few hours after egg retrieval, sperm that has been separated from semen are added to the culture medium. About 18 hours later the oocytes are observed to determine if fertilization has occurred. The oocytes that are fertilized are then cultured for an additional 48 to 96 hours, and from one to four normally cleaving embryos are then placed into the uterus of the patient in a sterile environment without the use of general anesthesia. Embryo placement is performed through a small catheter placed through the cervical canal. With the development of sequential culture media it has become possible to allow embryos to develop in vitro to the blastocyst stage, 5 days after fertilization, prior to transfer into the endometrial cavity. Several centers report per cycle pregnancy rates of 40% to 60% with blastocyst culture and transfer. Most centers are freezing the embryos not utilized and transferring them in subsequent spontaneous ovulatory cycles, if pregnancy does not occur in the initial treatment cycle. Since women older than 40 have decreased implantation rates compared with younger women, most centers transfer four or more embryos to those women unless donor oocytes are used.

Pregnancy rates with IVF vary among different centers, and one of the reasons for the variability is the lack of precision in the definition of the term *pregnancy rate.* If women who exhibit a transitory increase in HCG following embryo transfer but who have no clinical or ultrasound-demonstrated evidence of pregnancy are defined as pregnant, then the size of the numerator will be increased. The denominator will be highest if all women starting the process are included, but most centers report pregnancy rates per number of women with follicle aspiration or number of women with embryo transfer. Use of the latter two categories will decrease the size of the denominator and thus increase the pregnancy rates reported.

A modification of IVF, called *gamete intrafallopian transfer (GIFT),* can be used if the infertile woman has functioning oviducts. With this technique both oocytes and sperm are placed into the oviduct through a catheter at the time of laparoscopy or minilaparotomy. Although IVF, embryo culturing, and embryo transfer into the uterus are avoided by this technique, ovarian hyperstimulation and laparoscopy are still required. Modifications of GIFT include *zygote intrafallopian transfer (ZIFT)* and *tubal embryo stage transfer (TEST).* With ZIFT the oocytes are fertilized in vitro and transferred 24 hours later. Tubal embryo transfer (TET) is similar to ZIFT except the embryos are transferred 8 to 72 hours after fertilization. SART performs annual surveys of the various techniques of assisted reproduction. These annual surveys provide useful information for infertile couples who wish to consider use of assisted reproductive technology to conceive. The data from the most recent survey can be used to counsel couples about the expected outcomes of pregnancy. The 2002 SART survey reported that the live-delivery rate per cycle in which ova were retrieved was 40.7% in women younger than 35 years and 35.1% in women between age 35 and 37 years (Table 41-13). The rate of deliveries per IVF embryo transfer cycle has been steadily increasing each year.

In 2002, about one third of the IVF cycles in the United States were accompanied by an ICSI procedure. With all techniques of

Table 41-13 Comparison of Reported Outcomes for All Assisted Reproductive Technology Procedures

2002 ART CYCLE PROFILE

TYPE OF ART				PATIENT DIAGNOSIS			
IVF	>99%	**Procedural Factors:**		Tubal factor	13%	Other factor	7%
GIFT	<1%	With ICSI	53%	Ovulatory dysfunction	6%	Unknown factor	10%
ZIFT	<1%	Unstimulated	<1%	Diminished ovarian reserve	9%	Multiple factors	
Combination	<1%	Used gestational carrier	<1%	Endometriosis	6%	Female factors only	13%
				Uterine factor	1%	Female and male factors	18%
				Male factor	17%		

2002 PREGNANCY SUCCESS RATES

TYPE OF CYCLE	AGE OF WOMAN			
Fresh Embryos from Nondonor Eggs	**<35**	**35–37**	**38–40**	**41–42[‡]**
Number of cycles	37,591	19,110	17,454	7,733
Percentage of cycles resulting in pregnancies	42.5	36.4	27.5	17.3
Percentage of cycles resulting in live births[†]	36.9	30.6	20.5	10.7
Percentage of retrievals resulting in live births[†]	40.7	35.1	24.7	13.4
Percentage of transfers resulting in live births[†]	43.0	37.1	26.4	14.7
Percentage of transfers resulting in singleton live births	26.3	24.0	19.3	11.9
Percentage of cancellations	9.2	12.6	16.8	19.9
Average number of embryos transferred	2.7	3.0	3.3	3.5
Percentage of pregnancies with twins	33.2	28.9	22.6	15.5
Percentage of pregnancies with triplets or more	7.2	8.2	5.1	3.0
Percentage of live births having multiple infants[†]	38.9	35.4	26.9	18.6
Frozen Embryos from Nondonor Eggs				
Number of transfers	7680	3463	2327	699
Percentage of transfers resulting in live births[†]	27.9	24.1	20.0	16.6
Average number of embryos transferred	2.8	2.8	2.9	3.1

	ALL AGES COMBINED[§]	
Donor Eggs	**Fresh Embryos**	**Frozen Embryos**
Number of transfers	8394	3476
Percentage of transfers resulting in live births[†]	50.0	28.8
Average number of embryos transferred	2.7	2.9

*Donor includes known or anonymous but not surrogate.
[†]Cryopreserved embryo transfer cycles not done in combination with fresh embryo transfers and not with donor egg-embryo.
[‡]Includes all cycles regardless of age and diagnosis.
[§]Birth defect reporting did not account for all neonatal outcomes.
GIFT, gamete intrafallopian transfer; ICSI, intracytoplasmic sperm injection; IVF, in vitro fertilization; ZIFT, zygote intrafallopian transfer.
Modified from American Society for Reproductive Medicine: Assisted reproductive technology in the United States: 2002 results generated from the American Society for Reproductive Medicine/Society for Assisted Reproductive Technology Registry. CDC National Summary 2002.

assisted reproduction about 60% of the pregnancies are singleton gestations, 32% twins, 6% triplets, and the rest higher order births. Schieve and colleagues analyzed data from 300 U.S. clinics that reported data about IVF to the Centers for Disease Control and Prevention in 1991. The risk of multiple birth varied directly with the number of embryos transferred and inversely with maternal age. The analysis indicated that it is not beneficial in terms of greater pregnancy rates to transfer more than two embryos after IVF if the woman is younger than 35 years of age. In this age group the multiple-birth rate increased to 40% or more when three or more embryos were transferred. When two embryos were transferred in this age group, the twin rate was still 20%. Transfer of three embryos in women age 35 to 39 increased the multiple birth rate from 11.6% to 29.4%. It would appear best to limit the number of embryos transferred to two for women younger than age 35 and three for women 35–39. No limit of numbers of embryos transferred should be undertaken for women over age 40 because the multiple birth rate was less than 25% even if five embryos were transferred.

Data from several large centers in three different countries indicate that the pregnancy rate per IVF treatment cycle remains relatively constant for about six cycles. After six cycles the cumulative pregnancy rate is about 60% (Fig. 41-29). After six cycles of IVF the procedure is associated with a significant decrease in pregnancy rates. Women should be counseled that chances of pregnancy occurring with IVF after six failed cycles of IVF are very low.

An important factor when counseling couples about any ART concerns the pregnancy outcome. With any form of ART resulting in a singleton gestation advancing to the second trimester, perinatal outcome, gestational age, mean birth weight, congenital malformations, and complications of pregnancy or labor are no different from those in the normal fertile population. Therefore viable singleton pregnancies occurring after ART should not be considered high-risk pregnancies. However, there is an increased risk of spontaneous abortion and preterm delivery among women with multiple gestations conceived by ART. All types of ART with ovarian stimulation are followed

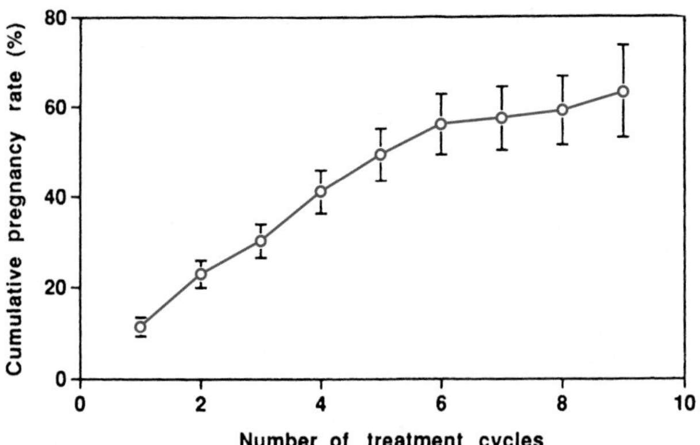

Figure 41-29. Overall cumulative pregnancy rate in IVF treatment (with 95% confidence interval). (From Dor J, Seidman DS, Ben-Shlomo I, et al: Cumulative pregnancy rate following in-vitro fertilization: The significance of age and infertility aetiology. Hum Reprod 11:425, 1996.)

by about 40% incidence of multiple gestations. The majority of these pregnancies are twins (25%), and 5% are higher order gestations. These multiple gestations can be as high as 40% and are usually 25% to 30%. Furthermore about 4% of all pregnancies with IVF are tubal pregnancies, with 1% being combined ectopic and intrauterine pregnancies. Therefore these pregnancies need to be closely monitored, as described in Chapter 17 (Ectopic Pregnancy).

Cryopreservation of embryos that have undergone IVF is being used in most assisted reproductive centers. Cryopreservation allows embryos that cannot be immediately transferred to the woman to be stored for future use. If more than four eggs are fertilized in a given cycle, the excess embryos can be frozen if they are of good quality. In addition, if there are indications that the woman is at risk of developing ovarian hyperstimulation syndrome, which would be enhanced by endogenous HCG production from pregnancy, the fertilized embryos can be frozen and transferred to the endometrial cavity at a later date. Frozen embryo pregnancy rates are in the range of 25%.

Wada and coworkers studied the outcome of 283 infants conceived from cryopreserved embryos. If a pregnancy takes place after a transfer of a frozen embryo, there is no evidence of a deleterious effect on the fetus. As a matter of fact, the incidence of fetal malformations appears to be significantly reduced compared with the normal IVF process. Furthermore, there is no increased risk of perinatal mortality or preterm delivery. Even in twin gestations after cryopreservation, the incidence of preterm birth was significantly lower than in twin gestations resulting from the normal IVF process. This reassuring information should be conveyed to those infertile couples undergoing IVF with cryopreservation of the fertilized embryo.

In some instances biopsy of the four- to eight-cell blastomere can be done for (preimplantation genetic diagnosis) PGD. Although PGD is most useful for specific genetic diseases, it can also be used in couples with Robertsonian translocations which are responsible for recurrent pregnancy loss. PGD has not proven useful for women older than 40, in whom the rate of aneuploidy is increased. In this setting, it is advisable to transfer multiple embryos.

FINAL COUNSELING

If intensive treatment of the infertile couple with various techniques fails to result in conception after 2 years, the couple should be informed that the chances for conception are much reduced. It is best to inform the couple of the prognosis for fertility and the duration beyond which conception should not be expected at the time of the initial consultation, and this information should be restated at subsequent visits. When the period during which conception should be expected has been exceeded, the couple should be informed that further testing and treatment are not warranted and other alternatives such as adoption should be considered.

Finally, it is important for the couple to consider psychological counseling, because the prospect of permanent infertility can cause severe mental trauma.

KEY POINTS

- In 1995 about 10% of all U.S. couples with women in the reproductive age group were infertile—6.2 million women.
- The incidence of infertility steadily increases in women after age 30.
- Among fertile couples who have coitus in the week before ovulation, there is only about a 20% (monthly fecundability of 0.2) chance of developing a clinical pregnancy in each ovulatory cycle.
- In about half of fertile couples attempting to conceive the woman will become pregnant in 3 months, 75% in 6 months, and 90% at the end of 1 year.
- Infertile couples who conceive do not have higher rates of spontaneous abortion or perinatal mortality than age-matched control subjects.
- In the United States approximately 10% to 15% of cases of infertility are caused by anovulation, 30% to 40% by an abnormality of semen production, 30% to 40% by pelvic disease, and 10% to 15% by abnormalities of sperm transport through the cervical canal. About 10% to 20% of cases are unexplained.
- The primary diagnostic tests for infertility are documentation of ovulation, semen analysis, and hysterosalpingogram (HSG).
- The basal body temperature (BBT) increases when circulating levels of progesterone increase, and a sustained increase of BBT occurs following ovulation.
- A sustained rise in BBT or a serum progesterone level greater than 5 ng/mL is presumptive evidence of ovulation.

KEY POINTS *Continued*

- A midluteal-phase serum progesterone level above 10 ng/mL is an indication of adequate luteal function.
- A high percentage of fertile men will have at least one abnormal parameter in their semen analysis.
- In women with a normal HSG, a hysteroscopy is unnecessary because it will not detect additional abnormality.
- Other diagnostic tests for infertility, including (1) measurement of serum prolactin and TSH in ovulatory women, (2) a late luteal-phase endometrial biopsy, (3) immunologic tests to detect sperm antibodies, and (4) bacterial culture of cervical mucus and semen.
- There is no evidence that treatment of an abnormality in the tests just listed significantly improves pregnancy rates compared with withholding therapy.
- Of all the causes of infertility, treatment of anovulation results in the greatest success.
- When ovulation is induced with clomiphene citrate and no other causes of infertility are present, conception rates over time are similar to those of a normal fertile population.
- Discontinuation of therapy is the major reason for the reported difference in ovulation and conception rates in anovulatory women treated with clomiphene.
- More than 90% of women with oligomenorrhea and 66% with secondary amenorrhea and E_2 levels of 40 pg/mL or higher will have presumptive evidence of ovulation following clomiphene therapy.
- When conception occurs after clomiphene treatment in anovulatory women, the incidence of multiple gestation is increased to about 8%, nearly all of them being twin gestations. The incidences of clinical spontaneous abortion, ectopic gestation, intrauterine fetal death, and congenital malformation are not significantly increased.
- Formation of ovarian cysts is the major side effect of clomiphene treatment.
- About 5% to 10% of women treated with the individualized, graduated, sequential regimen of clomiphene citrate fail to ovulate with the highest dosage.
- Treatment of anovulation with gonadotropin effects an ovulatory rate of about 100%.
- The pregnancy rate per cycle with gonadotropins is similar to that following clomiphene therapy (22%).
- The incidence of spontaneous abortion after HMG therapy is high (25% to 35%), and clinically detectable ovarian enlargement occurs in about 5% to 10% of treatment cycles.
- If GnRH is used for ovulation induction it needs to be administered in a pulsatile manner at intervals of 1 to 2 hours.
- For women with polycystic ovaries who do not ovulate following administration of clomiphene citrate, partial ovarian destruction by electrocautery or laser through the laparoscope is effective in inducing ovulation.
- Pregnancy rates for oligospermia following intrauterine insemination are in the 25% to 35% range.
- Semen donors need to be carefully screened to be certain that they are in good health, do not have a potentially inherited disorder, and will not transmit an infectious agent in the semen.
- Because antibodies to HIV may not develop for several months after infection, it is recommended that all donor insemination be performed with frozen sperm that has been stored for at least 6 months at which time negative antibodies to HIV should be observed in the donor before the sperm is used for insemination.
- The prognosis for fertility after tubal reconstruction depends on the amount of damage to the oviduct as well as the location of the obstruction.
- If both proximal and distal obstructions of the oviduct exist, intrauterine pregnancy is uncommon, and operative reconstruction should not be performed, IVF is the best therapy.
- Women with pelvic tuberculosis should be considered sterile, and no tubal reconstructive procedures should be attempted. IVF may be attempted if the endometrial cavity is not infected.
- Overall conception rates following salpingostomy are in the 30% range, with a high percentage (about one fourth) being tubal pregnancies.
- The pregnancy rate after salpingolysis and fimbrioplasty for partial distal obstruction is about 65%.
- Unlike the results of distal tubal reconstruction, the use of microsurgery has improved intrauterine pregnancy rates for proximal tubal disease.
- Proximal tubal obstruction is now usually treated by cannulation of the oviducts with catheters or balloons placed under hysteroscopic visualization.
- The benefit of second-look laparoscopy after tubal surgery has not been established.
- No medical therapy for endometriosis has proved to increase pregnancy rates compared with no treatment.
- Pregnancy rates for women with mild endometriosis can be increased with the use of controlled ovarian hyperstimulation and intrauterine insemination but not with danazol.
- About 65% of women with mild endometriosis and no other cause of infertility conceive without treatment. With moderate or severe disease, pregnancy rates with expectant management are 25% and 0%, respectively.
- Conception rates for women treated surgically have been reported to be in the 50% to 60% range for those with moderate endometriosis and 30% to 40% for those with severe endometriosis.
- About half of infertile women with myomas conceive after myomectomy.
- Luteal-phase deficiency, as currently diagnosed histologically, is probably a normal biologic variant and not a true cause of infertility.
- No data conclusively demonstrate that the finding of antisperm antibodies in either member of the couple is a cause of infertility.
- In women with unexplained infertility the use of controlled ovarian hyperstimulation (COH) and intrauterine insemination (IUI) yields monthly fecundity rates of 10% to 15%. Therefore COH and IUI should be the initial treatment

Continued

KEY POINTS *Continued*

for women who ovulate, have patent oviducts, and whose male partner has at least 5 million motile sperm in the ejaculate.

- For IVF with and without ICSI the delivery rate per cycle in which ova are retrieved is as high as 40% depending on the age of the woman.
- The rate of pregnancy following IVF is directly related to the number of embryos placed in the uterine cavity.
- The pregnancy rate per cycle of IVF remains relatively constant for about six cycles after which it declines. After six cycles the cumulative pregnancy rate is about 60%.
- There is a high spontaneous abortion rate (about 30%) for pregnancies after IVF.
- If an infertile couple fails to conceive after 2 years of therapy, they should be informed the chances for conception are remote.
- The optimal treatment for all causes of sperm abnormalities is ICSI. With this technique, pregnancy rates per cycle are similar to that of IVF performed for other causes of infertility.

BIBLIOGRAPHY

Ahmed Ebbiary NA, Llenton EA, Salt C, et al: The significance of elevated basal follicle stimulating hormone in regularly menstruating infertile women. Hum Reprod 9:245, 1994.

Aitken RJ, Comhaire FH, Eliasson R, et al: WHO laboratory manual for the examination of human semen and semen-cervical mucus interaction. Cambridge, Cambridge University Press, 1987.

Alper MM, Garner PR, Spence JEH, et al: Pregnancy rates after hysterosalpingography with oil- and water-soluble contrast media. Obstet Gynecol 68:6, 1986.

American Society for Reproductive Medicine: Assisted reproductive technology in the United States: 1996 results generated from the American Society for Reproductive Medicine/ Society for Assisted Reproductive Technology Registry. Fertil Steril 71:798, 1999.

Andrews WC, Buttram VC, Behrman SJ, et al: Revised American Fertility Society classification of endometriosis 1985. Fertil Steril 43:351, 1985.

Argawal SK, Buyalos RP: Clomiphene citrate with intrauterine insemination: Is it effective therapy in women above the age of 35 years? Fertil Steril 65:759, 1996.

Armar NA, McGarrible HHG, Honour J, et al: Laparoscopic ovarian diathermy in the management of anovulatory infertility in women with polycystic ovaries: Endocrine changes and clinical outcome. Fertil Steril 53:45, 1990.

Artini PG, Fasciani A, Cela V, et al: Fertility drugs and ovarian cancer. Gynecol Endocrinol 11:59, 1997.

Baird DD, Weinberg CR, Voigt LF, et al: Vaginal douching and reduced fertility. Am J Public Health 86:844, 1996.

Balash J, Fabregues F, Creus M, Vanrell JA: The usefulness of endometrial biopsy for luteal phase evaluation in infertility. Hum Reprod 7:973, 1992.

Barnea ER, Holford TR, McInnes DRA: Long-term prognosis of infertile couples with normal basic investigations: A life-table analysis. Obstet Gynecol 66:24, 1985.

Bayer SR, Seibel MM, Saffan DS, et al: Efficacy of danazol treatment for minimal endometriosis infertile women: A prospective randomized study. J Reprod Med 33:179, 1988.

Berg U, Brucker C, Berg FD: Effect of motile sperm count after swim-up on outcome of intrauterine insemination. Fertil Steril 67:747, 1997.

Boer-Meisel ME, te Velde ER, Habbema JDF, et al: Predicting the pregnancy outcome in patients treated for hydrosalpinx: A prospective study. Fertil Steril 45:23, 1986.

Bolumar F, and the European Study Group on Infertility and Subfecundity: Caffeine intake and delayed conception: A European multicenter study on infertility and subfecundity. Am J Epidemiol 145:324, 1997.

Bonduelle M, Legein J, Buysse A, et al: Prospective follow-up study of 423 children born after intracytoplasmic sperm injection. Hum Reprod 11:1558, 1996.

Bongain A, Castillon JM, Isnard V, et al: In vitro fertilization in women over 40 years of age: A study on retrospective data for eight years. Eur J Obstet Gynecol Reprod Biol 76:225, 1998.

Canis M, Manhes H, Mage G, et al: Laparoscopic distal tuboplasty: Report of 87 cases and a 4-year experience. Fertil Steril 56:616, 1991.

Chaffkin LM, Nulsen JC, Luciano AA, Metzger DA: A comparative analysis of the cycle fecundity rates associated with combined human menopausal gonadotropin (HMG) and intrauterine insemination (IUI) versus either HMG or IUI alone. Fertil Steril 55:252, 1991.

Chandra A, Stephen EH: Impaired fecundity in the United States: 1982–1995. Fam Plann Perspect 30:34, 1998.

Chung CC, Fleming R, Jamieson ME, et al: Randomized comparison of ovulation induction with and without intrauterine insemination in the treatment of unexplained infertility. Hum Reprod 10:3139, 1995.

Collins JA. Unexplained infertility: In Keye WR, Chang RJ, Rebar RW, Soules MR (eds): Infertility: Evaluation and Treatment. Philadelphia, WB Saunders, 1995, pp 249–262.

Collins JA, Burrows EA, Willan AR: The prognosis for live birth among untreated infertile couples. Fertil Steril 64:22, 1995.

Collins JA, Burrows EA, Yeo J, Young LAI EV: Frequency and predictive value of antisperm antibodies among infertile couples. Hum Reprod 8:592, 1993.

Collins JA, Wrixon W, Janes LB, et al: Treatment-independent pregnancy among infertile couples. N Engl J Med 309:1201, 1983.

Confino E, Tur-Kaspa I, DeCherney A, et al: Transcervical balloon tuboplasty: A multicenter study. JAMA 264:2079, 1990.

Corson G, Trias A, Trout S, et al: Ovulation induction combined with intrauterine insemination in women 40 years of age and older: Is it worthwhile? Hum Reprod 11:1109, 1996.

Cramer DW, Walker AM, Schiff I: Statistical methods in evaluating the outcome of infertility therapy. Fertil Steril 32:80, 1979.

Cruz JR, Dubey AK, Patel J, et al: Is blastocyst transfer useful as an alternative treatment for patients with multiple in vitro fertilization failures? Fertil Steril 72:218, 1999.

Cruz RI, Kemmann E, Brandeis VT, et al: A prospective study of intrauterine insemination of processed sperm from men with oligoasthenospermia in superovulated women. Fertil Steril 46:673, 1986.

Daly DC, Walters CA, Soto-Albors CE, et al: A randomized study of dexamethasone in ovulation induction with clomiphene citrate. Fertil Steril 41:844, 1984.

Daniell JF, Miller W; Hysteroscopic correction of cornual occlusion with resultant term pregnancy. Fertil Steril 48:490, 1987.

Daniell JF, Miller W: Polycystic ovaries treated by laparoscopic laser vaporization. Fertil Steril 51:232, 1989.

Das K, Nagel TC, Malo JW: Hysteroscopic cannulation for proximal tubal obstruction: A change for the better? Fertil Steril 63:1009, 1995.

Davis OK, Berkeley AS, Naus GJ, et al: The incidence of luteal phase defect in normal, fertile women, determined by serial endometrial biopsies. Fertil Steril 51:582, 1989.

Deaton JL, Gibson M, Riddick DH, Brumsted JR. Diagnosis and treatment of cornual obstruction using a flexible tip guidewire. Fertil Steril 53:232, 1990.

Deaton JL, Nakajima ST, Gibson M, et al: A randomized, controlled trial of clomiphene citrate and intrauterine insemination in couples with unexplained infertility of surgically corrected endometriosis. Fertil Steril 54:1083, 1990.

Dodson WC, Hughes CL, Yancy SE, Haney AF: Clinical characteristics of ovulation induction with human menopausal gonadotropins with and without leuprolide acetate in polycystic ovary syndrome. Fertil Steril 42:915, 1989.

Dodson WC, Moessner J, Miller J, et al: A randomized comparison of the methods of sperm preparation for intrauterine insemination. Fertil Steril 70:574, 1998.

Donderwinkel PF, van der Vaart Hester H, Wolters VM, et al: Treatment of patients with long-standing unexplained subfertility with in vitro fertilization. Fertil Steril 73:334, 2000.

Donnez J, Casanas-Roux F: Prognostic factors influencing the pregnancy rate after microsurgical cornual anastomosis. Fertil Steril 46:1089, 1986.

Donnez J, Casanas-Roux F: Prognostic factors of fimbrial microsurgery. Fertil Steril 46:200, 1986.

Dor J, Seidman DS, Ben-Shlomo I, et al: Cumulative pregnancy rate following in vitro fertilization: The significance of age and infertility aetiology. Hum Reprod 11:425, 1996.

Dubuisson JB, Bouquet de Joliniere J, Zubriot FX, et al: Terminal tuboplasties by laparoscopy: 65 consecutive cases. Fertil Steril 54:401, 1990.

Dubuisson JB, Chapron C, Morice P, et al: Laparoscopic salpingostomy: Fertility results according to the tubal mucosal appearance. Hum Reprod 9:334, 1994.

Eggert-Kruse W, Huber K, Rohr G, Runnebaum B: Determination of antisperm antibodies in serum samples by means of enzyme-linked immunosorbent assay: A procedure to be recommended during infertility investigation? Hum Reprod 8:1405, 1993.

Farquhar C, Lilford RJ, Marjoribanks J, Vandekerckhove P: Laproscopic "drilling" by diathermy or laser for ovulation induction in anovulatory polycystic ovary syndrome; Review Abstract and plain language summary. The Cochrane Database of Systematic Reviews, Issue 4, 2005.

Fayes JA, Mutie G, Schneider PJ: The diagnostic value of hysterosalpingography and hysteroscopy in infertility investigation. Am J Obstet Gynecol 156:558, 1987.

Fedele L, Bianchi S, Arcaini L, et al: Buserelin versus danazol in the treatment of endometriosis-associated infertility. Am J Obstet Gynecol 161:871, 1989.

Filmar S, Gomel V, McComb P: The effectiveness of CO_2 laser and electromicrosurgery in adhesiolysis: A comparative study. Fertil Steril 45:407, 1986.

Fisch P, Collins JA, Casper RF, et al: Unexplained infertility: Evaluation of treatment with clomiphene citrate and human chorionic gonadotropin. Fertil Steril 51:441, 1987.

Fleischer AC, Pennell RG, McKee MS, et al: Ectopic pregnancy: Features at transvaginal sonography. Radiology 174:375, 1990.

Fluker MR, Wang IY, Rowe TC: An extended 10-day course of clomiphene citrate (CC) in women with CC-resistant ovulatory disorders. Fertil Steril 66:761, 1996.

Frederick JL, Denker MS, Rojas A, et al: Is there a role for ovarian stimulation and intra-uterine insemination after age 40? Hum Reprod 9:2284, 1994.

Friberg J, Gnarpe H: *Mycoplasma* and human reproductive failure. III. Pregnancies in "infertile" couples treated with doxycycline for T-mycoplasmas, Am J Obstet Gynecol 116:23, 1973.

Friedler S, Strassburger D, Raziel A, et al: Intracytoplasmic injection of fresh and cryopreserved testicular spermatozoa in patients with nonobstructive azoospermia. A comparative study, Fertil Steril 68:892, 1997.

Gadir AA, Mowafi RS, Alnaser HMI, et al: Ovarian electrocautery versus human menopausal gonadotrophins and pure follicle stimulating hormone therapy in treatment of patients with polycystic ovarian disease. Clin Endocrinol 33:585, 1990.

Geber S, Paraschos T, Atkinson G, et al: Results of IVF in patients with endometriosis: The severity of the disease does not affect outcome, or the incidence of miscarriage. Hum Reprod 10: 1507, 1995.

Gil-Salom M, Minguez Y, Rubio C, et al: Intracytoplasmic sperm injection: A treatment for extreme oligospermia. J Urol 156: 1001, 1996.

Gjønnaess H: Ovarian electrocautery in the treatment of women with polycystic ovary syndrome (PCOS). Acta Obstet Gynecol Scand 73:407, 1994.

Gjønnaess H: Late endocrine effects of ovarian electrocautery in women with polycystic ovary syndrome. Fertil Steril 69 (4):697, 1998.

Glazener CMA, Coulson C, Lambert PA, et al: Clomiphene treatment for women with unexplained infertility: Placebo-controlled study of hormonal responses and conception rates. Gynecol Endocrinol 4:75, 1990.

Glazener CMA, Kelly NJ, Hull MGR: Prolactin measurement in the investigation of infertility in women with a normal menstrual cycle. Br J Obstet Gynaecol 94:535, 1987.

Gurgan T, Urman B, Yarali H, et al: The results of in vitro fertilization-embryo transfer in couples with unexplained infertility failing to conceive with superovulation and intrauterine insemination. Fertil Steril 64:93, 1995.

Guzick DS, Sullivan MW, Adamson GD, et al: Efficacy of treatment for unexplained infertility. Fertil Steril 70:207, 1998.

Guzick DS, for the National Cooperative Reproductive Medicine Network: Efficacy of superovulation and intrauterine insemination in the treatment of infertility. N Engl J Med 340:177, 1999.

Gysler M, March CM, Mishell DR Jr, et al: A decade's experience with an individualized clomiphene treatment regimen including its effect on the postcoital test. Fertil Steril 37:161, 1982.

Hammond MG, Halme JK, Talbert LM: Factors affecting the pregnancy rate in clomiphene citrate induction of ovulation. Obstet Gynecol 62:196, 1983.

Hammond MG, Jordan S, Sloan CS: Factors affecting pregnancy rates in a donor insemination program using frozen semen. Am J Obstet Gynecol 155:480, 1986.

Harrison RF, DeLouvois J, Blades M, et al: Doxycycline treatment and human infertility. Lancet 1:605, 1975.

Hatch EE and Bracken MB: Association of delayed conception with caffeine consumption. Am J Epidemiol 138:1082, 1993.

Hendershot GE, Mosher WD, Pratt WF: Infertility and age: an unresolved issue. Fam Plann Perspect 14:287, 1982.

Holtz G, Kling OR: Effect of surgical technique on peritoneal adhesion reformation after lysis. Fertil Steril 37:494, 1982.

Homburg R: Clomiphene citrate-end of an era? a mini-review. Hum Reprod 20:2043, 2005.

Homburg R, Eshel A, Kilborn J, et al: Combined luteinizing hormone releasing hormone analogue and exogenous gonadotrophins for the treatment of infertility associated with polycystic ovaries. Hum Reprod 5:32, 1990.

Honoré GM, Holden AEC, Schenken RS: Pathophysiology and management of proximal tubal blockage. Fertil Steril 71:785, 1999.

Howe G, Westhoff C, Vessey M, et al: Effects of age, cigarette smoking, and other factors on fertility: Findings in a large prospective study. Br Med J 290:1697, 1985.

Howe RS, Sayegh RA, Durinzi KL, Tureck RW: Perinatal outcome of singleton pregnancies conceived by in vitro fertilization: a controlled study. J Perinatol 10:261, 1990.

Hughes EG, Fedorkow DM, Collins JA: A quantitative overview of controlled trials in endometriosis-associated infertility. Fertil Steril 59:963, 1993.

Hull MGR: Effectiveness of infertility treatments: Choice and comparative analysis. Int J Gynaecol Obstet 47:99, 1994.

Hull MGR, Eddowes HA, Fahy U, et al: Expectations of assisted conception for infertility. Br Med J 304:1465, 1992.

Hull MGR, Glazener CMA, Kelly NJ, et al: Population study of causes, treatment, and outcome of infertility. Br Med J 291:1984, 1985.

Hull MGR, Savage PE, Bromham DR, et al: The value of a single serum progesterone measurement in the midluteal phase as a criterion of a potentially fertile cycle ("ovulation") derived from treated and untreated conception cycles. Fertil Steril 37:355, 1982.

Inoue M, Kobayashi Y, Honda I, et al: The impact of endometriosis on the reproductive outcome of infertile patients. Am J Obstet Gynecol 157:278, 1992.

Jansen RPS: Failure of intraperitoneal adjuncts to improve the outcome of pelvic operations in young women. Am J Obstet Gynecol 153:363, 1985.

Jezek D, Knuth UA, Schulze W: Successful testicular sperm extraction (TESE) in spite of high serum follicle stimulating hormone and azoospermia: correlation between testicular morphology, TESE results, semen analysis and serum hormone values in 103 infertile men. Hum Reprod 13:1230, 1998.

Jones WR: Immunologic infertility: fact or fiction? Fertil Steril 33:577, 1980.

Karamardian LM, Grimes DA: Luteal phase deficiency: effect of treatment on pregnancy rates. Am J Obstet Gynecol 167:1391, 1992.

Kohl B, Kohl H, Krause W, Deichert U: The clinical significance of antisperm antibodies in infertile couples. Hum Reprod 7:1384, 1992.

Kovacs GT, Phillips S, Healy DL, Burger HG: Induction of ovulation with gonadotrophin-releasing hormone-life-table analysis of 50 courses of treatment. Med J Aust 151:21, 1989.

Kurachi K, Aono T, Minagawa J, et al: Congenital malformations of newborn infants after clomiphene-induced ovulation. Fertil Steril 40:187, 1983.

Lalich RA, Marut EL, Prins GS, Scommegna A: Life table analysis of intrauterine insemination pregnancy rates. Am J Obstet Gynecol 158:980, 1988.

Land JA, Evers JLH, Goossens VJ: How to use chlamydia antibody testing in subfertility patients. Hum Reprod 13:1094, 1998.

Lang EK, Dunaway HE, Roniger WE: Selective osteal salpingography and transvaginal catheter dilatation in the diagnosis and treatment of fallopian tube obstruction. AJR 154:735, 1990.

Larsen T, Larsen JF, Schioler V, et al: Comparison of urinary human follicle-stimulating hormone and human menopausal gonadotropin for ovarian stimulation in polycystic ovarian syndrome. Fertil Steril 53:426, 1990.

Leeton J, Healy D, Rogers P, et al: A controlled study between the use of gamete intrafallopian transfer (GIFT) and in vitro fertilization and embryo transfer in the management of idiopathic and male infertility. Fertil Steril 48:605, 1987.

Lenton EA, Sobowale OS, Cooke ID: Prolactin concentrations in ovulatory but infertile women: treatment with bromocriptine. Br Med J 2:1179, 1977.

Leridon H, Spira A: Problems in measuring the effectiveness of infertility therapy. Fertil Steril 41:580, 1984.

Lewin A, Reubinoff B, Poratl-Katz A, et al: Testicular fine needle aspiration: The alternative method for sperm retrieval in non-obstructive azoospermia. Hum Reprod 14:1785, 1999.

Li TC, Dockery P, Rogers AW, Cooke ID: How precise is histologic dating of endometrium using the standard dating criteria? Fertil Steril 51:759, 1989.

Lincoln SR, Ke RW, Kutteh WH. Screening for hypothyroidism in infertile women. J Reprod Med 44:455, 1999.

Lobo RA, Granger LR, Davajan V, et al: An extended regimen of clomiphene citrate in women unresponsive to standard therapy. Fertil Steril 37:762, 1982.

Lobo RA, Paul W, March CM, et al: Clomiphene and dexamethasone in women unresponsive to clomiphene alone. Obstet Gynecol 60:497, 1982.

Loft A, Peterson K, Erb K, et al: A Danish national cohort of 730 infants born after intracytoplasmic sperm injection (ICSI) 1994–1997. Hum Reprod 14:2143, 1999.

Luciano AA, Hauser KS, Benda J: Evaluation of commonly used adjuvants in the prevention of postoperative adhesions. Am J Obstet Gynecol 146:88, 1983.

Luciano AA, Turksoy RN, Carleo J: Evaluation of oral medroxyprogesterone acetate in the treatment of endometriosis. Obstet Gynecol 72:323, 1988.

Mau C, Juul A, Main KM, Loft A: Children conceived after intracytoplasmic sperm injection (ICSI): Is there a role for the paedriatrician? Acta Paediatr 93 (9):123, 2004.

Mao C, Grimes DA: The sperm penetration assay: Can it discriminate between fertile and infertile men? Am J Obstet Gynecol 159:279, 1988.

March CM, Israel R: Gestational outcome following hysteroscopic lysis of adhesions. Fertil Steril 36:455, 1981.

Marcoux S, and the Canadian Collaborative Group on Endometriosis: Laparoscopic surgery in infertile women with minimal or mild endometriosis. N Engl J Med 337:217, 1997.

Martin JS, Nisker JA, Parker JI, et al: The pregnancy rates of cohorts of idiopathic infertility couples gives insights into the underlying mechanism of infertility. Fertil Steril 64:98,1995.

Martinez AR, Bernardus RE, Vermeiden JPW, Schoemaker J: Basic questions on intrauterine insemination: An update. Obstet Gynecol 48:811, 1992.

Martinez AR, Bernardus RE, Voorhorst FJ, et al: Intrauterine insemination does and clomiphene citrate does not improve fecundity in couples with infertility due to male or idiopathic factors: A prospective, randomized, controlled study. Fertil Steril 53:847, 1990.

Matthews CD, Clapp KH, Tansing JA, et al: T-mycoplasma genital infection: The effect of doxycycline therapy on human unexplained infertility. Fertil Steril 30:98, 1978.

McFaul PB, Traub AI, Thompson W: Treatment of clomiphene citrate-resistant polycystic ovarian syndrome with pure follicle-stimulating hormone or human menopausal gonadotropin. Fertil Steril 53:792, 1990.

McGovern P, Quagliarello J, Arny M: Relationship of within-patient semen variability to outcome of intrauterine insemination. Fertil Steril 51:1019, 1989.

Meikle SF, Zhang X, Marine WM, et al: Chlamydia trachomatis antibody titers and hysterosalpingography in predicting tubal disease in infertility patients. Fertil Steril 62:305, 1994.

Menken J, Trussell IJ, Larsen U: Age and infertility. Science 23:1389, 1986.

Merek D, Langley M, Gardner DK, et al: Introduction of blastocyst culture and transfer for all patients in an in vitro fertilization program. Fertil Steril 72:1035, 1999.

Milki AA, Fisch JD, Behr B: Two-blastocyst transfer has similar pregnancy rates and a decreased multiple gestation rate compared with three-blastocyst transfer. Fertil Steril 72:225, 1999.

Milki AA, Hinckley MD, Fisch JD, et al: Comparison of blastocyst transfer with day 3 embryo transfer in similar patient populations. Fertil Steril 73:126, 2000.

Mills MS, Eddowes HA, Cahill DJ, et al: A prospective controlled study of in-vitro fertilization, gamete intrafallopian transfer and intrauterine insemination combined with superovulation. Hum Reprod 7:490, 1992.

Mitwally MF MD, Biljan MM MD, Casper RF MD: Pregnancy outcome after the use of an aromatase inhibitor for ovarian stimulation. Am J Obstet Gynecol 192:381, 2005.

Mol BW, Hajenius PJ, Engelsbel S, et al: Serum human chorionic gonadotropin measurement in the diagnosis of ectopic pregnancy when transvaginal sonography is inconclusive. Fertil Steril 70:972, 1998.

Mol BWJ, Swart P, Bossuyt PMM, et al: Is hysterosalpingography an important tool in predicting fertility outcome? Fertil Steril 67:663, 1997.

Mosgaard BJ, Schou G, Lidegaard O, et al: Infertility, fertility drugs, and invasive ovarian cancer: A case-control study. Fertil Steril 67:1005, 1997.

Motta ELA, Nelson J, Batzofin J, Serafini P: Selective salpingography with an insemination catheter in the treatment of women with cornual fallopian tube obstruction. Hum Reprod 10:1156, 1995.

MRC Working Party on Children Conceived by In Vitro Fertilisation: Births in Great Britain resulting from assisted conception, 1978–1987. Br Med J 300:1299, 1990.

Murray DL, Reich L, Adashi EY: Oral clomiphene citrate and vaginal progesterone suppositories in the treatment of luteal phase dysfunction: A comparative study. Fertil Steril 51:35, 1989.

Norman RJ, Noakes M, Wu R, et al: Improving reproductive performance in overweight/obese women with effective weight management. Hum Reprod Update May-Jun; 10 (3):267, 2004.

Noyes RW, Hertig AT, Rock J: Dating the endometrial biopsy. Fertil Steril 39:277, 1983.

Oehninger S, Malaoney M, Veeck L, et al: Intracytoplasmic sperm injection: Achievement of high pregnancy rates in couples with severe male factor infertility is dependent primarily upon female and not male factors. Fertil Steril 64:977, 1995.

O'Herlihy C, Pepperell JR, Brown JB, et al: Incremental clomiphene therapy: A new method for treating persistent anovulation. Obstet Gynecol 58:535, 1981.

Ombelet W, Vandeput H, Van de Putte G, et al: Intrauterine insemination after ovarian stimulation with clomiphene citrate: Predictive potential of inseminating motile count and sperm morphology. Hum Reprod 12:1458, 1997.

Osada H, Fijii I, Tsunoda I, et al: Outpatient evaluation and treatment of tubal obstruction with selective salpingography and balloon tuboplasty. Fertil Steril 73:1032, 2000.

O'Shea DL, Odem RR, Cholewa C, Gast MJ: Long-term follow-up of couples after hamster egg penetration testing. Fertil Steril 60:1040, 1993.

Osmanagaoglu K, Tournaye H, Camus M, et al: Cumulative delivery rates after intracytoplasmic sperm injection: 5 year follow-up of 498 patients. Hum Reprod 14(10):2651, 1999.

Palermo GD, Adler A, Cohen J, et al: Intracytoplasmic sperm injection: A novel treatment of all forms of male factor infertility. Fertil Steril 63:1231, 1995.

Palermo GD, Schliegel PN, Hariprashad JJ, et al: Fertilization and pregnancy outcome with intracytoplasmic sperm injection for azoospermic men. Hum Reprod 14:741, 1999.

Parazzini F, Negri E, La Vecchia C, et al: Treatment of infertility and risk of invasive epithelial ovarian cancer. Hum Reprod 12:2159, 1997.

Parazzini F, for the Gruppo Italiano per lo Studio dell'Endometriosi: Ablation of lesions or no treatment in minimal-mild endometriosis in infertile women: a randomized trial. Hum Reprod 14:1332, 1999.

Patton GW Jr: Pregnancy outcome following microsurgical fimbrioplasty. Fertil Steril 37:150, 1982.

Patton PE, Williams TJ, Coulam CB: Microsurgical reconstruction of the proximal oviduct. Fertil Steril 47:35, 1986.

Peters AJ, Lloyd RP, Coulam CB: Prevalence of out-of-phase endometrial biopsy specimens. Am J Obstet Gynecol 166: 1738, 1992.

Peterson CM, Poulson AM Jr, Hatasaka HH, et al: Ovulation induction with gonadotropins and intrauterine insemination compared with in vitro fertilization and no therapy: A prospective, nonrandomized cohort study and meta-analysis. Fertil Steril 62:535, 1994.

Plosker SM, Jacobson W, Amato P: Predicting and optimizing success in an intrauterine insemination programme. Hum Reprod 9:2014, 1994.
Rammar E, Freidrich F: The effectiveness of intrauterine insemination in couples with sterility caused by male infertility with and without a female hormone factor. Fertil Steril 69:31, 1998.
Ranieri M, Beckett VA, Marchant S, et al: Gamete intra-fallopian transfer or in-vitro fertilization after failed ovarian stimulation and intrauterine insemination in unexplained infertility? Hum Reprod 10:2023, 1995.
Ransom M, Garcia A: Surgical management of cornual- isthmic tubal obstruction. Fertil Steril 68:887, 1997.
Rock JA, Katayama P, Martin EJ, et al: Factors influencing the success of salpingostomy techniques for distal fimbrial obstruction. Obstet Gynecol 52:591, 1978.
Rossing MA, Daling JR, Weiss NS, et al: Ovarian tumors in a cohort of infertile women. N Engl J Med 331:771, 1994.
Rousseau S, Lord J, Lepage Y, Van Campenhout J: The expectancy of pregnancy for "normal" infertile couples. Fertil Steril 40:768, 1983.
Ruiz A, Remohi J, Minguez Y, et al: The role of in vitro fertilization and intracytoplasmic sperm injection in couples with unexplained infertility after failed intrauterine insemination. Fertil Steril 68:171, 1997.
Sadek AL, Schiotz HA: Transvaginal sonography in the management of ectopic pregnancy. Acta Obstet Gynecol Scand 74:293, 1995.
Sahakyan M, Harlow BL, Hornstein MD: Influence of age, diagnosis, and cycle number on pregnancy rates with gonadotropin-induced controlled ovarian hyperstimulation and intrauterine insemination. Fertil Steril 72:500, 1999.
Sakumoto T, Shinkawa T, Izena H, et al: Treatment of infertility associated with endometriosis by selective tubal catheterization under hysteroscopy and laparoscopy. Am J Obstet Gynecol 169:744, 1993.
Schenken RS, Malinak LR: Conservative surgery versus expectant management for the infertile patient with mild endometriosis. Fertil Steril 37:183, 1982.
Schieve LA, Peterson HB, Meikle SF, et al: Live-birth rates and multiple-birth risk using in vitro fertilization. JAMA 282: 1832, 1999.
Schlaff WD, Hassiakos DK, Damewood MD, Rock JA: Neosalpingostomy for distal tubal obstruction: prognostic factors and impact of surgical technique. Fertil Steril 54:984, 1990.
Schoolcraft WB, Gardner DK, Lane M, et al: Blastocyst culture and transfer: Analysis of results and parameters affecting outcome in two in vitro fertilization programs. Fertil Steril 72:604, 1999.
Schwarz D, Mayaux MJ: Female fecundity as a function of age: Results of artificial insemination in 2193 nulliparous women with azoospermic husbands, Fédération des Centres d'Etude et de Conservation du Sperme Humain. N Engl J Med 306:404, 1982.
Scott RT, Snuder RR, Strickland DM, et al: The effect of interobserver variation in dating and endometrial histology on the diagnosis of luteal phase defects. Fertil Steril 50:888, 1988.
Seiler JC, Gidwani G, Ballard L: Laparoscopic cauterization of endometriosis for fertility: A controlled study. Fertil Steril 46:1098, 1986.
Sherins RJ, Thorsell LP, Dorfmann A, et al: Intracytoplasmic sperm injection facilitates fertilization even in the most severe forms of male infertility: Pregnancy outcome correlates with maternal age and number of eggs available. Fertil Steril 64:369, 1995.
Shoupe D, Mishell DR Jr, LaCarra M, et al: Correlation of endometrial maturation with four methods of estimating day of ovulation. Obstet Gynecol 73:88, 1988.
Shulman A, Feldman B, Madgar I, et al: In-vitro fertilization treatment for severe male factor: The fertilization potential of immotile spermatozoa obtained by testicular extraction. Hum Reprod 14:749, 1999.
Silber SJ, Nagy Z, Devroey P, et al: The effect of female age and ovarian reserve on pregnancy rate in male infertility: Treatment of azoospermia with sperm retrieval and intracytoplasmic sperm injection. Hum Reprod 12:2693, 1997.
Simon A, Avidan B, Mordel N, et al: The value of menotrophin treatment for unexplained infertility prior to an in-vitro fertilization attempt. Hum Reprod 6:222, 1991.
Simpson CW, Taylor PJ, Collins JA: A comparison of ovulation suppression and ovulation stimulation in the treatment of endometriosis-associated infertility. Int J Obstet Gynecol 38:207, 1992.
Smarr SC, Hammond MG: Effect of therapy on infertile couples with antisperm antibodies. Am J Obstet Gynecol 158:969, 1988.
Spring DB, Barka HE, Pruyn SC: Potential therapeutic effects of contrast materials in hysterosalpingography: A prospective randomized clinical trial. Radiology 214:53, 2000.
Steirteghem A, Bonduelle M, Devroey P, Liebaera I: Follow-up of children born after ICSI. Hum Reprod 8:111, 2002.
Stumpf PG, March CM: Febrile morbidity following hysterosalpingography: Identification of risk factors and recommendations for prophylaxis. Fertil Steril 33:487, 1980.
Sulak PJ, Letterie GS, Hayslip CC, et al: Hysteroscopic cannulation and lavage in the treatment of proximal tubal occlusion. Fertil Steril 48:493, 1987.
Telimaa S: Danazol and medroxyprogesterone acetate inefficacious in the treatment of infertility in endometriosis. Fertil Steril 50:872, 1988.
Templeton AA, Penney GC: The incidence, characteristics, and prognosis of patients whose infertility is unexplained. Fertil Steril 37:175, 1982.
Te Velde ER, Van Kooy RJ, Waterreus JJH: Intrauterine insemination of washed husband's spermatozoa: A controlled study. Fertil Steril 51:182, 1989.
Thomas K, Coughlin L, Mannion PT, Haddad NG: The value of chlamydia trachomatis antibody testing as part of routine infertility investigations. Hum Reprod 15:1079, 2000.
Thurmond AS, Rosch J: Nonsurgical fallopian tube recanalization for treatment of infertility. Radiology 174:371, 1990.
Tomlinson MJ, Barratt CLR, Cooke ID: Prospective study of leukocytes and leukocyte subpopulations in semen suggests they are not a cause of male infertility. Fertil Steril 60:1069, 1993.
Tsirgotis M, Nicholson N, Yang D, et al: Assisted fertilization with intracytoplasmic sperm injection. Fertil Steril 62:781, 1994.
Tulandi T: Salpingo-ovariolysis: A comparison between laser surgery and electrosurgery. Fertil Steril 45:489, 1986.
Tulandi T, Guralnick M: Treatment of tubal ectopic pregnancy by salpingotomy with or without tubal suturing and salpingectomy. Fertil Steril 55:53, 1991.
Tummon IS, Asher LJ, Martin JSB, et al: Randomized controlled trial of superovulation and insemination for infertility associated with minimal or mild endometriosis. Fertil Steril 68:8, 1997.
Van Steirteghem AC, Liu J, Joris H, et al: Higher success rate by intracytoplasmic sperm injection than by subzonal insemination: Report of a second series of 300 consecutive treatment cycles. Hum Reprod 8:1055, 1993.
Varma TR, Patel RH, Bhathenia RK: Outcome of pregnancy after infertility. Acta Obstet Gynecol Scand 67:115, 1988.
Vazquez-Levin M, Kaplan P, Sandler B, et al: The predictive value of zona-free hamster egg sperm penetration assay for failure of human in vitro fertilization and subsequent successful zona drilling. Fertil Steril 53:1055, 1990.
Vercellini P, Maddalena S, De Giorgi O, et al: Abdominal myomectomy for infertility: A comprehensive review. Hum Reprod 13(4):873, 1998.
Vermesh M, Kletzky OA, Davajan V, Israel R: Monitoring techniques to predict and detect ovulation. Fertil Steril 147:259, 1987.
Wada I, Macnamee MCX, Wick K, et al: Birth characteristics and perinatal outcome of babies conceived from cryopreserved embryos. Hum Reprod 9:543, 1994.
Watson A, Vail A, Vandekerckhove P, et al: A meta-analysis of the therapeutic role of oil soluble contrast media at hystersalpingography: A surprising result? Fertil Steril 61:470, 1994.
Weiner S, DeCherney AH, Polan ML: Human menopausal gonadotropins: A justifiable therapy in ovulatory women with long-standing idiopathic infertility. Am J Obstet Gynecol 158:111, 1988.
Wilcox AJ, Weinberg CR, Baird DD: Timing of sexual intercourse in relation to ovulation. New Engl J Med 333:1517, 1995.
Wilcox A, Westhoff C, Vessey M, et al: Effects of age, cigarette smoking, and other factors on fertility: Findings in a large prospective study. Br Med J 290:1697, 1985.
Winston RM: Microsurgical tubocornual anastomosis for reversal of sterilization. Lancet 1:284, 1977.
Winston RM: Microsurgery of the fallopian tube: From fantasy to reality. Fertil Steril 34:521, 1980.
Yanagimachi R, Yanagimachi H, Rogers BT: The use of zona-free animal ova as a test system for the assessment of the fertilizing capacity of human spermatozoa. Biol Reprod 15:471, 1976.
Zeyneloglu HB, Arici A, Olive DL, et al: Comparison of intrauterine insemination with timed intercourse in superovulated cycles with gonadotropins: A meta-analysis. Fertil Steril 69:486, 1998.

Menopause

42

Endocrinology, Consequences of Estrogen Deficiency, Effects of Hormone Replacement Therapy, Treatment Regimens

Rogerio A. Lobo

KEY TERMS AND DEFINITIONS

Atrophic Vaginitis. Inflammation of the vaginal epithelium due to atrophy secondary to decreased levels of circulating estrogen.

Bisphosphonates. A new class of compounds characterized by two carbon–phosphorous bonds that inhibit the rate of bone resorption and osteoporotic fractures Bisphosphonates approved for prevention and treatment of osteoporosis include alendronate and risedronate.

Climacteric. The physiologic period in a woman's life during which there is regression of ovarian function.

Continuous Combined Hormone Replacement. Administration of a small dose of progestin every day together with daily estrogen orally or transdermally to postmenopausal women.

Cortical Bone. Bone in the limbs (axial skeleton). With estrogen deficiency bone density decreases more slowly in cortical than in trabecular bone.

Estrogen Replacement Therapy (ERT). Administration of physiologic doses of estrogen orally or transdermally to postmenopausal women without addition of a progestin (also called unopposed estrogen therapy).

Hormone Replacement Therapy (HRT). Administration of an estrogen and a progestin to postmenopausal women.

Hot Flush. Pathognomonic symptom of the menopause; an abrupt physiologic phenomenon brought about by changes in hypothalamic thermoregulation to induce loss of body heat. Each episode lasts about 3 to 4 minutes and occurs at unpredictable, irregular intervals. During the symptomatic flush there is increased digital perfusion and increased vascular peripheral skin temperature and sweating.

Menopause Permanent cessation of menstruation caused by failure of ovarian follicular development and estradiol production in the presence of elevated gonadotropin levels.

Osteopenia. Decreased quantity of bone mass of a lesser amount than osteoporosis. An early state of osteoporosis with a bone mineral density T score between −1 and −2.5.

Osteoporosis. A systematic skeletal disease characterized by low bone mass and microarchitectural deterioration of bone tissue with a consequent increase in bone fragility and susceptibility to fractures The bone mineral density T score is less than −2.5.

Perimenopausal Transition. The time between the onset of irregular menses and permanent cessation of menstruation. The average duration is about 4 years.

Premature Ovarian Failure. Cessation of menstruation due to depletion of ovarian follicles before the age of 40. It is also called premature menopause

Raloxifene. A benzothiophene SERM that has an estrogen agonist effect on bone by suppressing bone resorption and an estrogen antagonist effect on the endometrium and breast tissue.

Selective Estrogen Receptor Modulator (SERM). Agents that bind to estrogen receptors and have estrogen agonist effects on certain tissues and estrogen antagonist effects on other tissues. SERM compounds include raloxifene, clomiphene citrate, and tamoxifen.

Sequential Hormone Replacement (also referred to as cyclic hormone replacement). Administration of relatively high daily doses of a progestin for 2 weeks or less per month together with daily estrogen for part or all of the remainder of the month.

Tibolone. A synthetic steroid with estrogenic, progestogenic, and androgenic activity. When given orally this agent reduces hot flushes, increases bone density, and does not stimulate endometrial proliferation.

Trabecular Bone. Bone in the spinal column and distal radius. With estrogen deficiency osteoporosis develops more rapidly in trabecular than in cortical bone.

T score. The difference between bone mineral density of the individual at a specific site and the mean bone density of young adults of the same gender divided by the standard deviation of this mean. The T score is expressed as the difference in standard deviations of the measured bone density from the mean value of young adults.

Unopposed Estrogen Therapy. Postmenopausal estrogen therapy given without the addition of a progestin.

Z Score. The difference between bone mineral density of the individual at a specific site and the mean normal value of adults of the same age and gender divided by the standard deviation of this mean. The Z score is expressed as the difference in standard deviations of the measured bone density from the mean normal value of age- and gender-matched controls.

Menopause is defined by the last menstrual period. Because cessation of menses is variable and many of the symptoms thought to be related to menopause may occur prior to cessation of menses, there is seldom a precise timing of this event. Other terms used are *perimenopause,* which refers to a variable time beginning a few years before and continuing after the event of menopause, and *climacteric,* which merely refers to the time after the cessation of reproductive function. Although the terms *menopausal* and *postmenopausal* are used interchangeably, the former term is less correct because *menopausal* should only relate to the time around the cessation of menses. As life expectancy increases beyond the eighth decade worldwide, particularly in developed countries, an increasing proportion of the female population is postmenopausal. With the average age of menopause being at 51 years, more than a third of a woman's life is now spent after menopause. Here, symptoms and signs of estrogen deficiency merge with issues encountered with natural aging. As the world population increases and a larger proportion of this population is made up of individuals older than 50, medical care specifically directed at postmenopausal women becomes an important aspect of modem medicine. Between the years 2000 and 2005, the world population older than 60 years is expected to double, from 590 million to 1 billion. In the United States, the number of women entering menopause will almost double in the 30 years between 1990 and 2020 (Table 42-1). Age of menopause, which is a genetically programmed event, is subject to some variability. The age of menopause in western countries (between 51 and 52 years) is thought to correlate with general health status: Socioeconomic status is associated with an earlier age of menopause. Higher parity, on the other hand, has been found to be associated with a later menopause. Smoking has consistently been found to be associated with menopause onset taking place 1 to 2 years earlier. Although body mass has been thought to be related to age of menopause (greater body mass index [BMI] with later menopause); the data have not been consistent. However, physical or athletic activity has not been found consistently to influence the age of menopause. There also appear to be ethnic differences in the onset of menopause. In the United States, black and Hispanic women have been found to have menopause approximately 2 years earlier than white women. Although parity is generally greater around the world than in the United States, the age of menopause appears to be somewhat earlier outside the United States. Malay women have menopause at approximately age 45, Thai women at age 49.5, and Filipina women between ages 47 and 48. Countries at higher altitude (Himalayas or Andes) have been shown to have menopause 1 to 1.5 years earlier. Because the average age of menopause in the United States is 51 to 53 years, with an age distribution weighted toward white women, menopause prior to age 40 is considered premature. Conversely, by age 58, 97% of women will have gone through menopause. The primary determinate of age of menopause is genetic. Based on family studies, de Bruin and colleagues showed that heritability for age of menopause averaged 0.87—suggesting that genetics explains up to 87% of the variance in menopausal age. Other than gene mutations that cause premature ovarian failure (explained later in this chapter), no specific genes have been discovered to date that account for this genetic influence. However, several genes are likely involved in aging, including genes coding telomerase.

Table 42-1 U.S. Population Entering the Postmenopausal Years, Ages 55 Through 64

Year	Population
1990	10.8 million
2000	12.1 million
2010	17.1 million
2020	19.3 million

Adapted from U.S. Bureau of the Census: Current Population Reports: Projections of the Population of the United States 1977 to 2050. Washington, DC, U.S. Government Printing Office, 1993.

PREMATURE OVARIAN FAILURE

Premature ovarian failure (POF) is defined as hypergonadotropic ovarian failure occurring prior to age 40. POF has occurred in 5% to 10% of women who are evaluated for amenorrhea, thus the incidence varies according to the prevalence of amenorrhea in various populations. Estimates of the overall prevalence of POF in the general population range between 0.3% and 0.9% of women. Throughout life, there is an ongoing rate of atresia of oocytes. Because this process is accelerated with various forms of gonadal dysgenesis due to defective X chromosomes, one possible cause of POF is an increased rate of atresia that has yet to be explained. A decreased germ cell endowment or an increased rate of germ cell destruction can also explain POF. Nevertheless, about 1000 (of the original 2 million) primarily follicles may remain. While most of these oocytes are likely to be functionally deficient, occasionally spontaneous pregnancies occur in young women in the first few years after the diagnosis of POF. There are several possible etiologies of POF (Table 42-2). Defects in the X chromosome may result in various types of gonadal dysgenesis with varied times of expression of ovarian failure. Even patients with classical gonadal dysgenesis (e.g., 45,XO) may undergo a normal puberty, and occasionally a pregnancy may ensue as a result of genetic mosaicism. Very small defects in the X chromosome may be sufficient to cause POF. Familial forms of POF may be related to either autosomal dominant or sex-linked modes of inheritance. Mutations in the gene encoding the follicle-stimulating hormone (FSH) receptor (e.g., mutation in exon 7 in the gene on chromosome 2p) have been described, but these are extremely rare outside of the Finnish population in which these mutations were originally described. An expansion of a trinucleotide repeat sequence in the first exon on the FMR1 gene (Xq 27.3) leads to fragile X syndrome, a major cause of developmental disabilities in males.

Table 42-2 Possible Causes of Premature Ovarian Failure

Genetic
Enzymatic
Immune
Gonadotropin defects
Ovarian insults
Idiopathic

The permutation in fragile X syndrome has been shown to be associated with POF. Type 1 blepharophimosis/ptosis/epicanthus inversus (BPES) syndrome, an autosomal dominant disorder due to mutations in the forkhead transcription factor FOXL2, includes POF. Triple X syndrome has also been associated with POF. Dystrophic myotonia has also been linked to POF, although the mechanism underlying this relationship is unclear. Under the category of enzymatic defects, galactosemia is a major cause of POF that is related to the toxic buildup of galactose in women who are unable to metabolize the sugar. Even in women with fairly well controlled galactose-free diets, POF tends to occur. Another enzymatic defect linked to POF is 17α-hydroxylase deficiency. This rare condition manifests differently from the other causes discussed here because the defect in the production of sex steroids leads to sexual infantilism and hypertension. Because of the prevalence of autoimmune disorders in women, the degree to which autoimmunity may be responsible for POF is unclear. La Barbera has suggested an association in 17.5% of cases. Virtually all autoimmune disorders have been found to be associated with POF, including autoimmune polyendocrinopathies like autoimmune polyendocrinopathy/candidiasis/ectodermal dystrophy (APECED), which is caused by mutations in the autoimmune (AIRE) gene on band 21 q22. The presence of the thymus gland appears to be required for normal ovarian function as PDF has been associated with hypoplasia of the thymus. In patients who have undergone ovarian biopsy as part of their evaluation, lymphocytic infiltration surrounding follicles has been described, as well as resumption of menses after immunosuppression. Immunoassays utilizing antibodies directed at ovarian antigens have been developed and have demonstrated positive findings in some patients with POF, although the relevance of these findings remains unsettled. Ovarian autoantibodies could also conceivably be a secondary phenomenon to a primary cell-mediated form of immunity. Specific enzymes such as 3β-hydroxysteroid dehydrogenase (3βHSD) may also be the target of ovarian autoimmunity. From a practical standpoint, screening for the common autoimmune disorders is appropriate in women found to have POF. More from a theoretical standpoint, abnormalities in the structure of gonadotropins, in their receptors, or in receptor binding could be associated with POF. Although abnormal urinary forms of gonadotropins have been reported in women with POF, these data have not been replicated. Abnormalities of FSH receptor binding, as mediated by a serum inhibitor, have been described. A genetic defect that may lead to alterations in FSH receptor structure was mentioned previously. Under the category of ovarian insults, POF may be induced by ionizing radiation, chemotherapy, or overly aggressive ovarian surgery. Although not well documented, viral infections have been suggested to play a role, particularly mumps. A dose of 400 to 500 rads is known to cause ovarian failure 50% of the time, and older women are more vulnerable to experiencing permanent failure. A dose of approximately 800 rads is associated with failure in all women. Ovarian failure (transient or permanent) may be induced by chemotherapeutic agents, although younger women receiving this insult have a better prognosis. Alkalizing agents, particularly cyclophosphamide, appear to be most toxic. By exclusion, the majority of women are considered to have idiopathic POF because no demonstrable cause can be pinpointed. Among these women, small mutations in genes lying on the X chromosome or yet to be identified autosomal genes may be the cause.

Management of Premature Ovarian Failure

Evaluation of POF in women younger than 30 should include screening for autoimmune disorders and a karyotype; detailed recommendations for screening of such women are available. In addition, vaginal ultrasound may be useful for assessing the size of the ovaries and the degree of follicular development, which, if present, may signify an immunologic defect. Treatment usually consists of estrogen replacement. If fertility is a concern, the most efficacious treatment is oocyte donation. Various attempts at ovarian stimulation are usually unsuccessful, and the sporadic pregnancies that may occur are just as likely to occur spontaneously as with any intervention. A spontaneous pregnancy rate as high as 5% has been suggested.

THE MENOPAUSAL TRANSITION (PERIMENOPAUSE)

A workshop was convened in 2001 to build consensus on describing various stages of the menopausal transition. As depicted in Figure 42-1, the menopausal transition (perimenopause) is divided into early and late phases according to menstrual acyclicity. These changes signify a varying period of time (years) during which rapid oocyte depletion occurs, followed by hypoestrogenism. The ovary changes markedly from birth to the onset of menopause (Fig. 42-2). The greatest number of primordial follicles is present in utero at 20 weeks' gestation and undergoes a regular rate of atresia until around the age of 37. After this time, the decline in primordial follicles appears to become more rapid between age 37 and menopause (Fig. 42-3) when no more than a thousand follicles remain. These remaining follicles are primarily atretic in nature.

Types of Ovarian Changes

Although perimenopausal changes are generally thought to be endocrine in nature and result in menstrual changes, a marked diminution of reproductive capacity precedes this period by several years. This decline may be referred to as gametogenic ovarian failure. The concept of dissociation in ovarian function is appropriate. Gametogenic failure is signified by reduced early follicular phase inhibin secretion, rising serum FSH levels, and a marked reduction in fecundity. These changes may occur with normal menstrual function and no obvious endocrine deficiency; however, they may occur in some women as early as age 35 (10 or more years before endocrine deficiency ensues). Although subtle changes in endocrine and menstrual function can occur for up to 3 years before menopause, it has been shown that the major reduction in ovarian estrogen production does not occur until approximately 6 months before menopause (Fig. 42-4). There is also a very slow decline in androgen status (i.e., androstenedione and testosterone), which cannot be adequately detected at the time of the perimenopause. The decline in androgen is largely a phenomenon of aging. Products of the granulosa cell are most important for the feedback control of FSH. As the

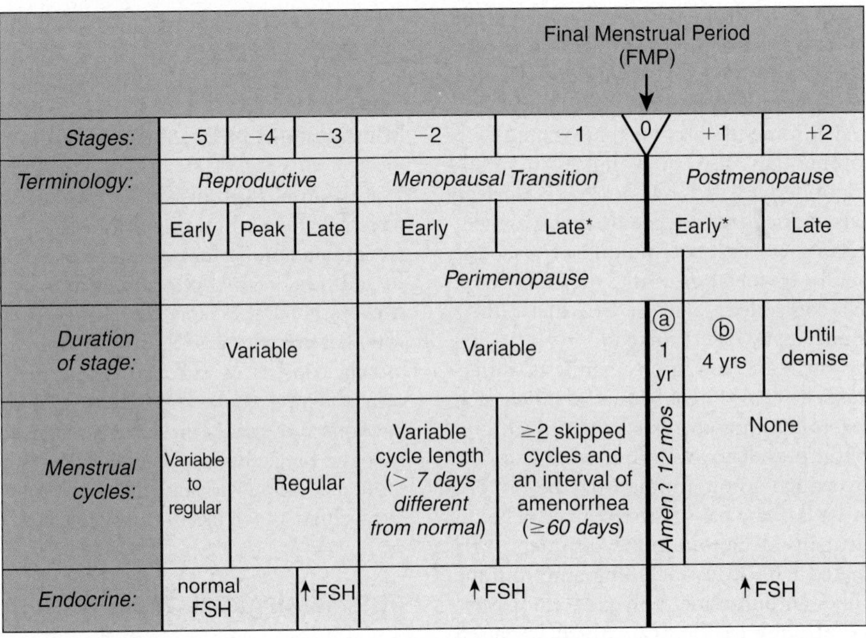

Final Menstrual Period
(FMP)
Stages: −5 −4 −3 −2 −1 0 +1 +2
Terminology: Reproductive
Menopausal Transition
Postmenopause
Early Peak Late Early Late* Early* Late
Perimenopause
Duration of stage: Variable
Variable
ⓐ 1 yr
ⓑ 4 yrs
Until demise
Menstrual cycles: Variable to regular
Regular
Variable cycle length (> 7 days different from normal)
≥2 skipped cycles and an interval of amenorrhea (≥60 days)
Amen ? 12 mos
None
Endocrine: normal FSH
↑FSH
↑FSH
↑FSH
*Stages most likely to be characterized by vasomotor symptoms ↑ = elevated

Figure 42-1. The Stages of Reproductive Aging Workshop (STRAW) staging system. (Reprinted from Fertility and Sterility, 76, Soules MR, Sherman S, Parrott E, et al, Executive summary: Stages of Reproductive Aging Workshop [STRAW], 874. Copyright 2001, with permission from The American Society for Reproductive Medicine.)

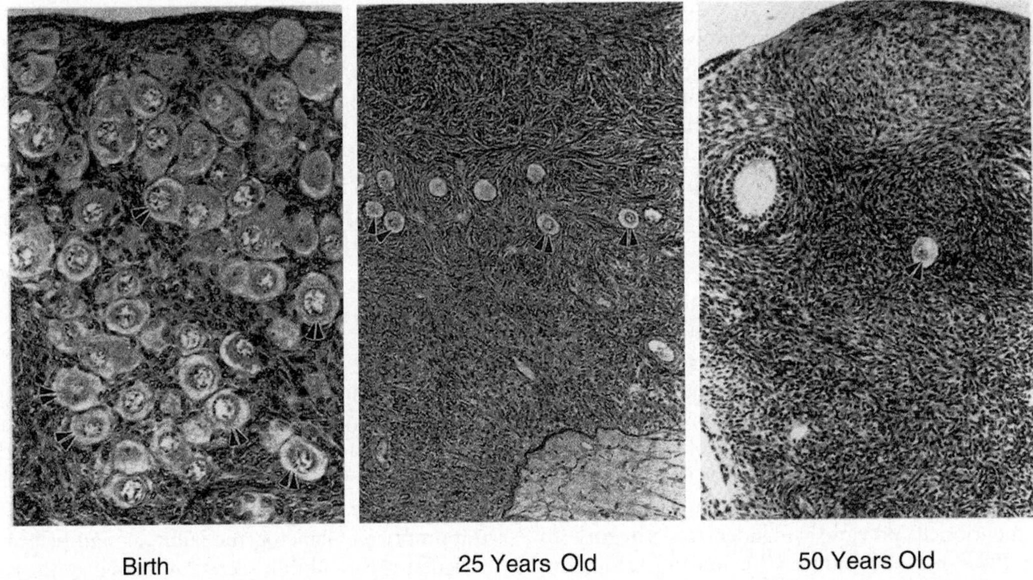

Figure 42-2. Photomicrographs of the cortex of human ovaries from birth to 50 years of age. Small nongrowing primordial follicles *(arrowheads)* have a single layer of squamous granulosa cells. (Adapted from Erickson GF: An analysis of follicle development and ovum maturation. Semin Reprod Endocrinol 4:233, 1986.)

functional capacity of the follicular units decreases, secretion of substances that suppress FSH also decrease. Most notably, inhibin B levels are lower in the early follicular phase in women in their late 30s (Fig. 42-5). Indeed, FSH levels are higher throughout the cycle in older ovulatory women than in younger women (Fig. 42-6). The functional capacity of the ovary is also diminished as women enter into the perimenopause. With gonadotropin stimulation, although estradiol (E_2) levels are not very different between younger and older women, total inhibin production by granulosa cells is decreased in women older than 35. From a clinical perspective, subtle increases in FSH on day 3 of the cycle, or increases in the clomiphene challenge test, correlate with decreased ovarian responses to stimulation and decreased fecundability. An excellent new marker of ovarian reserve is müllerian inhibiting hormone (MIH) or antimüllerian hormone (AMH). Levels decrease throughout life, being undetectable at menopause day 3 values less than 0.2 ng/mL generally indicate poor ovarian reserve. Although there is a

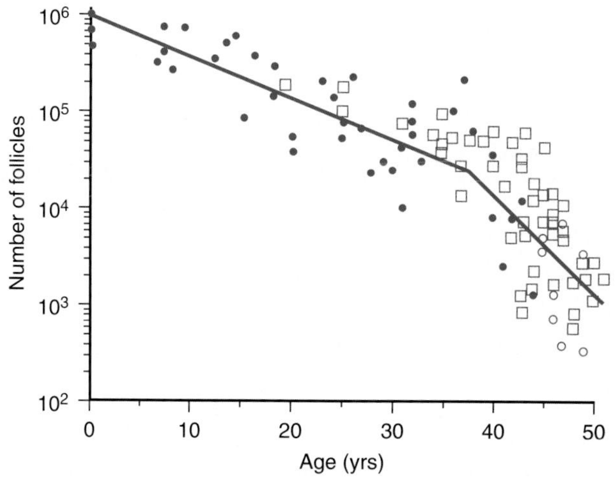

Figure 42-3. The age-related decrease in the total number of primordial follicles (PF) within both human ovaries from birth to menopause. As a result of recruitment (initiation of PF growth), the number of PF decreases progressively from about 1 million at birth to 25,000 at 37 years. At 37 years, the rate of recruitment increases sharply, and the number of PF declines to 1000 at menopause (about 51 years of age). (Adapted from Faddy MJ, Gosden RJ, Gougeon A, et al: Accelerated disappearance of ovarian follicles in mid-life: Implications for forecasting menopause. Hum Reprod 7:1342, 1992.)

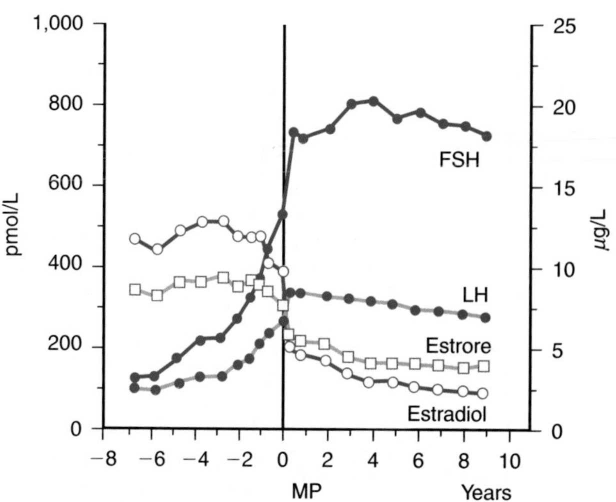

Figure 42-4. Mean serum levels of follicle-stimulating hormone, luteinizing hormone, estradiol, and estrone, showing the perimenopausal transition. MP, menopause. (Adapted from Rannevik G, Jeppsson S, Johnell O, et al: A longitudinal study of the perimenopausal transition: Altered profiles of steroid and pituitary hormones-SHBG and bone mineral density. Maturitas 21:103, 1995.)

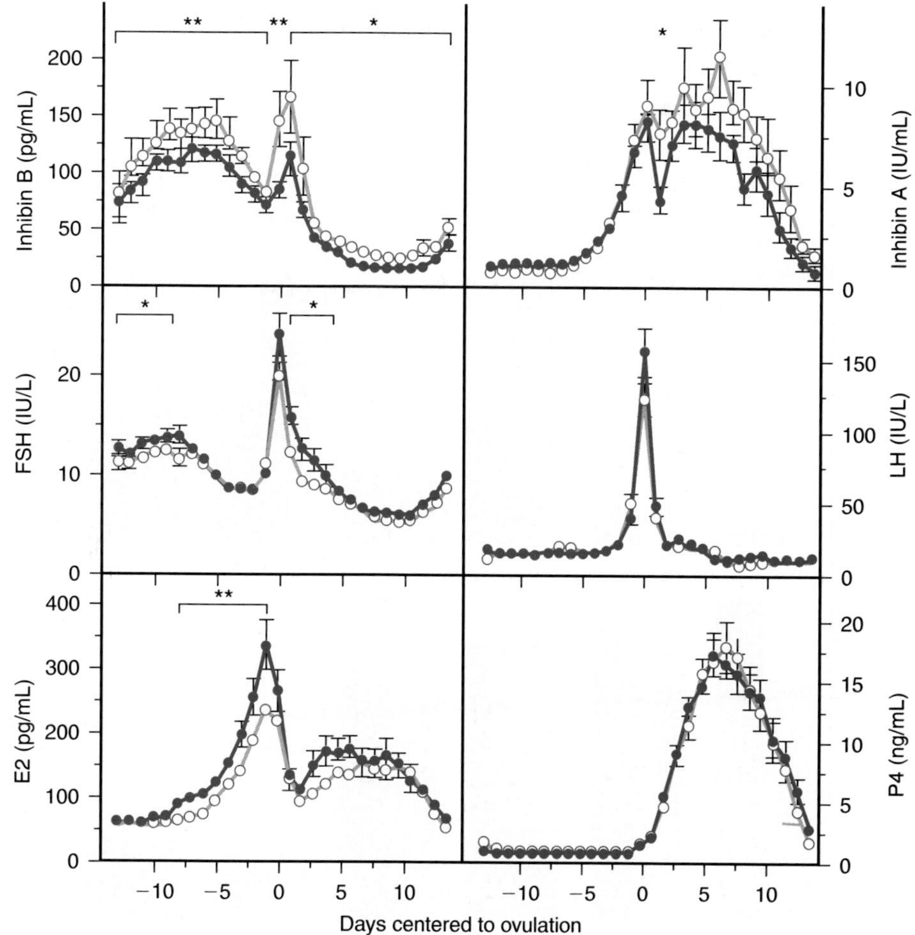

Figure 42-5. An inhibin B, follicle-stimulating hormone (FSH), estradiol (E_2), inhibin A, and progesterone (P_4) levels in cycling women 20 to 34 years old (○) and 35 to 46 years old (●). Hormone levels are depicted as centered to the day of ovulation (*, $p < 0.04$; **, $p < 0.02$) when comparing the two age groups. (Adapted from Welt CK, McNicholl DJ, Taylor AE, Hall JE: Female reproductive aging is marked by decreased secretion of dimeric inhibin. J Clin Endocrinol Metab 84:105, 1999.)

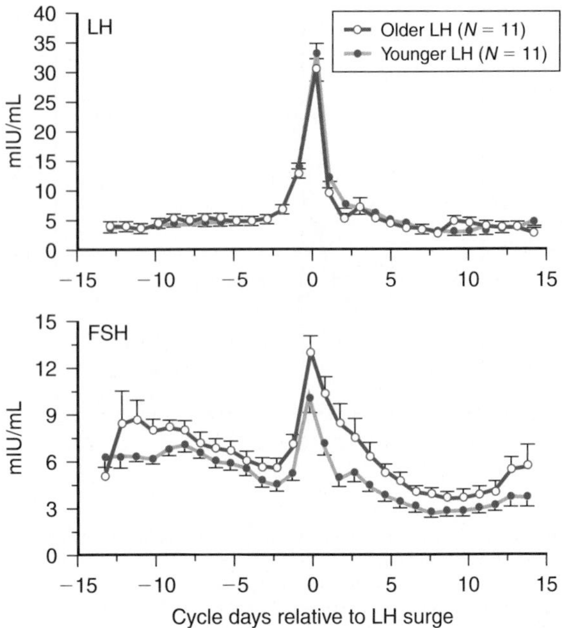

Figure 42-6. The daily serum follicle-stimulating hormone (FSH) and luteinizing hormone (LH) levels throughout the menstrual cycle of 11 women in each group (mean ± SE). The gonadotropin secretion pattern in normal women of advanced reproductive age in relation to the monotropic FSH rise. (Adapted from Klein NA, Battaglia DE, Clifton DK, et al: The gonadotropin secretion pattern in normal women of advanced reproductive age in relation to the monotropic FSH rise. J Soc Gynecol Investig 3:27, 1996.)

general decline in oocyte number with age, an accelerated atresia occurs around age 37 or 38 (see Fig. 42-3). Although the reason for this acceleration is not clear, one possible theory relates to activin secretion. Because granulosa cell-derived activin is important for stimulating FSH receptor expression, the rise in FSH levels could result in more activin production, which in turn enhances FSH action. A profile of elevated activin with lower inhibin B has been found in older women (Fig. 42-7). This autocrine action of activin, involving enhanced FSH action, might be expected to lead to accelerated growth and differentiation of granulosa cells. Furthermore, activin has been shown to increase the size of the pool of preantral follicles in the rat. At the same time, these follicles become more atretic. Clinical treatment of women in the perimenopause should address three general areas of concern: (1) irregular bleeding, (2) symptoms of early menopause, such as hot flushes, and (3) the inability to conceive. Treatment of irregular bleeding is complicated by the fluctuating hormonal status. Estrogen levels may be higher than normal in the early follicular phase and progesterone secretion may be normal, although not all cycles are ovulatory. For these reasons, short-term use of an oral contraceptive (usually 20 μg ethyinl estradiol) may be an option for otherwise healthy women who do not smoke to help them cope with irregular bleeding. Early symptoms of menopause, particularly vasomotor changes, may occur as the result of fluctuating hormonal levels. In this setting, an oral contraceptive again may be an option if symptoms warrant therapy. Alternatively, lower doses of estrogen used alone may be another option. Reproductive concerns often require more aggressive treatment because of decreased cycle

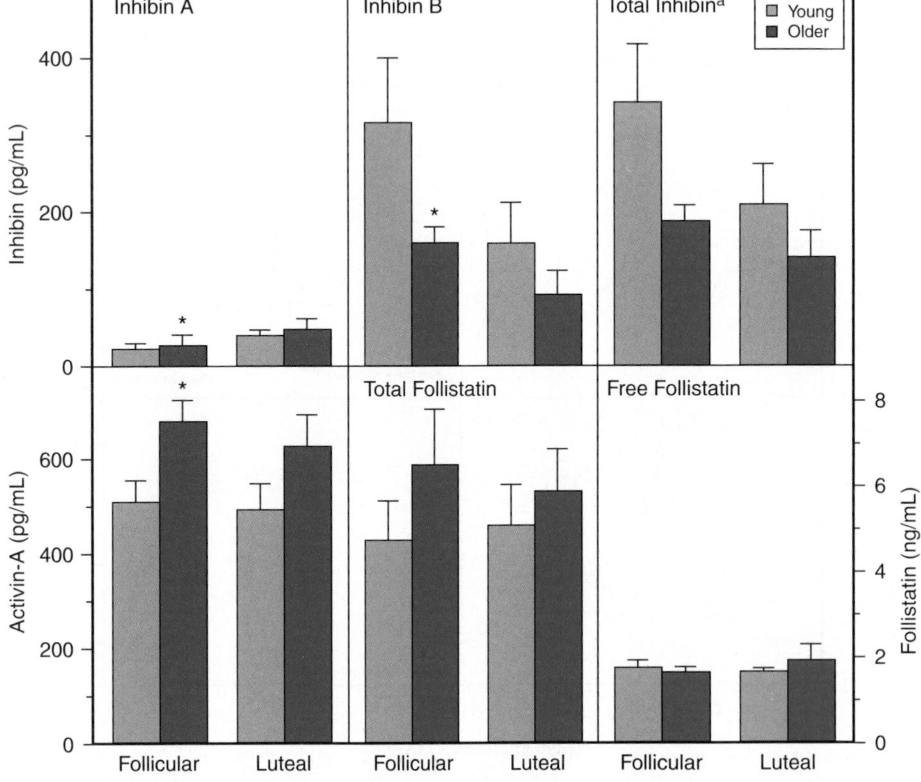

Figure 42-7. Mean concentrations of gonadal proteins from the same subjects. Total inhibin is a derived number from the sum of inhibin A and inhibin B. *Group differences; $p < 0.05$. Net increase in stimulatory input resulting from a decrease in inhibin B and an increase in activin A may contribute in part to the rise in follicular phase follicle-stimulating hormone of aging cyclic women. (Adapted from Reame NE, Wyman TL, Phillips DJ, et al: Net increase in stimulatory input resulting from a decrease in inhibin B and an increase in activin A may contribute in part to the rise in follicular phase follicle-stimulating hormone of aging cyclic women. J Clin Endocrinol Metab 83:3302, 1998.)

fecundity. Once day 3 FSH levels increase, the prognosis for pregnancy is markedly reduced.

Hormonal Changes with Established Menopause

Depicted in Figure 42-8 are the typical hormonal levels of postmenopausal women compared with those of ovulatory women in the early follicular phase. The most significant findings are the marked reductions in E_2 and estrone (E_1). Serum E_2 is reduced to a greater extent than E_1. Serum E_1, on the other hand, is produced primarily by peripheral aromatization from androgens, which decline principally as a function of age. Levels of E_2 average 15 pg/mL and range from 10 to 25 pg/mL, but are closer to 10 pg/mL in women who have undergone oophorectomy. Serum E_1 values average 30 pg/mL but may be higher in obese women because aromatization increases as a function of the mass of adipose tissue. Estrone sulfate (E_1 S) is an estrogen conjugate that serves as a stable circulating reservoir of estrogen, and levels of E_1 S are the highest among estrogens in postmenopausal women. In premenopausal women, values are usually above 1000 pg/mL; in postmenopausal women, levels average 350 pg/mL. Apart from elevations in FSH and luteinizing hormone (LH), other pituitary hormones are not affected. The rise in FSH, beginning in stage −3 as early as age 38 (see Fig. 42-1), fluctuates considerably until approximately 4 years after menopause (stage +1) when values are consistently greater than 20 mIU/mL. Specifically, growth hormone (GH), thyroid-stimulating hormone (TSH), and adrenocorticotropic hormone (ACTH) levels are normal. Serum prolactin levels may be very slightly decreased because prolactin levels are influenced by estrogen status. Both the postmenopausal ovary and the adrenal gland continue to produce androgen. The ovary continues to produce androstenedione and testosterone but not E_2, and this production has been shown to be at least partially dependent on LH. Androstenedione and testosterone levels are lower in women who have experienced bilateral oophorectomy, with values averaging 0.8 ng/mL and 0.1 ng/mL, respectively. The adrenal gland also continues to produce androstenedione, dehydroepiandrosterone (DHEA), and dehydroepiandrosterone sulfate (DHEA-S); primarily as a function of aging, these values decrease somewhat (adrenopause), although cortisol secretion remains unaffected. Recent data by Couzinet suggest that much "ovarian" testosterone production may actually arise from the adrenal. Most likely, this production is by indirect mechanisms due to the adrenal supplying precursor substrate (DHEA and androstenedione). Although DHEA-S levels decrease with age (approximately 2% per year), recent data have suggested that

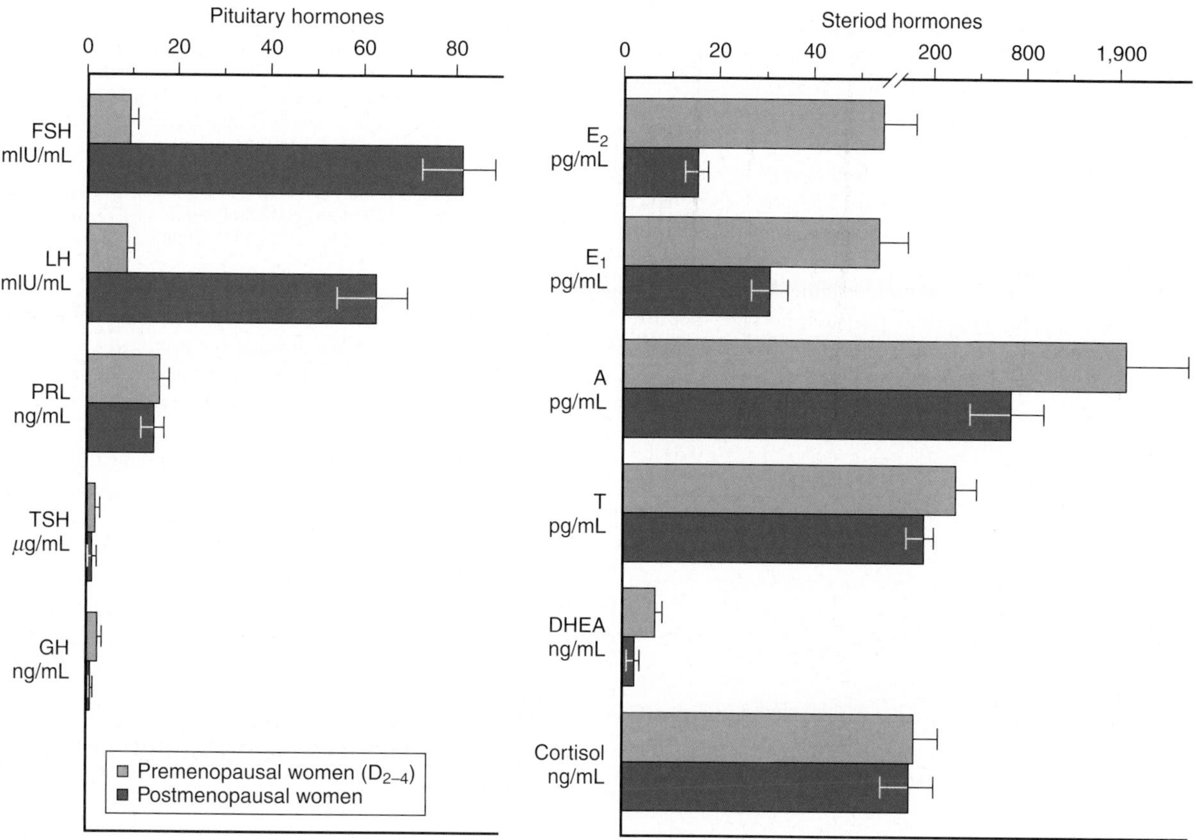

Figure 42-8. Circulating levels of pituitary and steroid hormones in postmenopausal women compared with levels in premenopausal women studied during the first week (days 2 to 4 [D_{2-4}] of the menstrual cycle. A, androstenedione; DHEA, dehydroepiandrosterone; E_1, estrogen; E_2, estradiol; FSH, follicle-stimulating hormone; GH, growth hormone; LH, luteinizing hormone; PRL, prolactin; T, testosterone; TSH, thyroid-stimulating hormone. (Adapted from Yen SSC: The biology of menopause. J Reprod Med 18:287, 1977.)

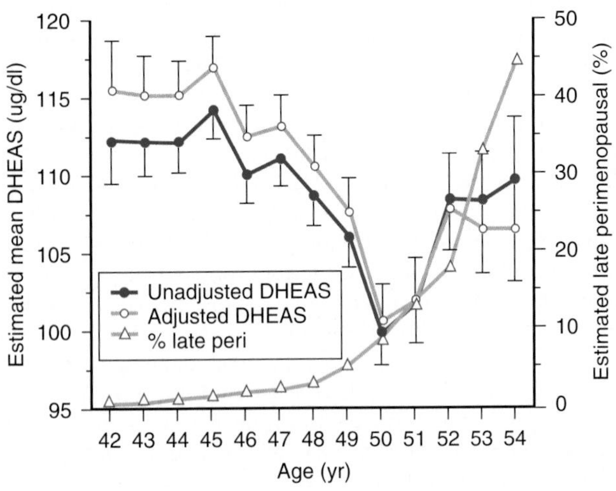

Figure 42-9. Mean (± SE) circulating DHEAS at each year of age of the entire study population before (solid circles) and after (open circles) adjustment for age, current smoking, menopausal status, log body mass index (BMI), ethnicity, site, and the interaction between ethnicity and log BMI. Also shown is the percentage of women at each year of age who have transitioned to late perimenopausal status (triangles). (Adapted from Lasley BL, Santoro N, Randolf JF, et al: The relationship of circulating dehydroepiandrosterone, testosterone, and estradiol to stages of the menopausal transition and ethnicity. J Clin Endocrinol Metab 87:3760, 2002.)

levels transiently rise in the perimenopause before the continuous decline thereafter (Fig. 42-9). This interesting finding from the Study of Women Across the Nation (SWAN) also suggested that DHEA-S levels are highest in Chinese women and lowest in black women.

Testosterone levels also decline as a function of age, which is best demonstrated by the reduction in 24-hour means levels (Fig. 42-10). Because of the role of the adrenal in determining levels of testosterone after menopause, adrenalectomy or dexamethasone treatment results in undetectable levels of serum testosterone. Compared with total testosterone, the measurement of bioavailable, or "free," testosterone is more useful in

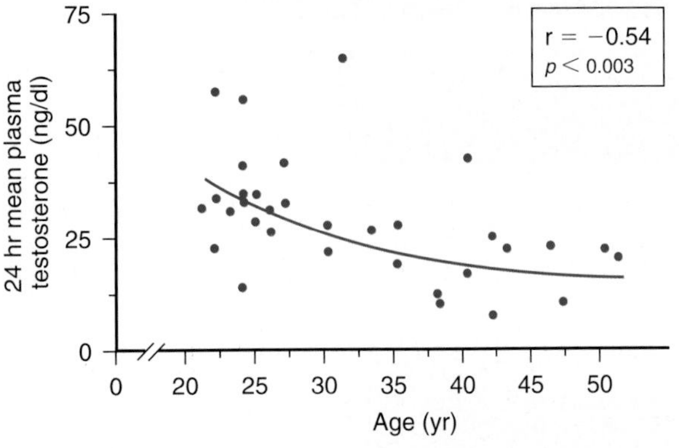

Figure 42-10. The 24-hour mean plasma total testosterone (T) level compared with age in normal women. The regression equation was T (nmol/L) = 37.8 × age (years) – 1.12 ($r = -0.54$; $p < 0.003$). (Adapted from Zumoff B, Strain GW, Miller LK, et al: Twenty-four hour mean plasma testosterone concentration declines with age in normal premenopausal women. J Clin Endocrinol Metab 80:1429, 1995.)

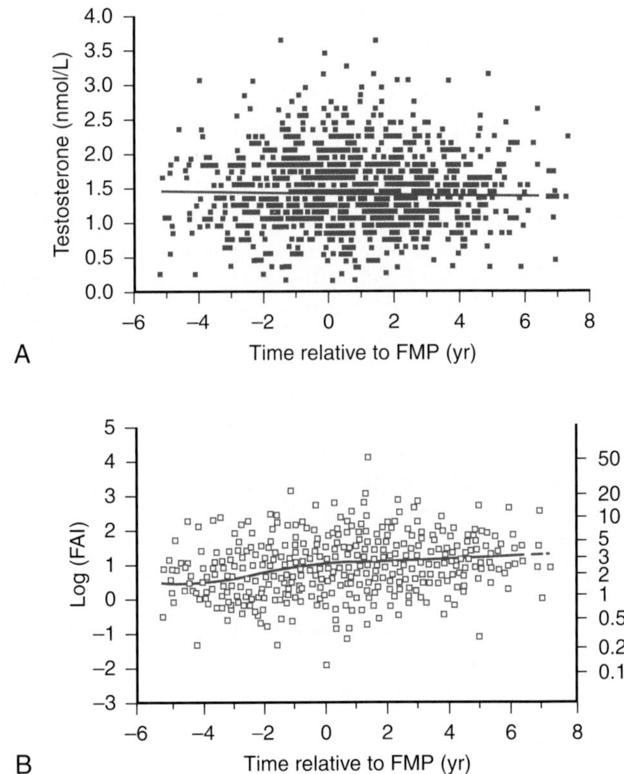

Figure 42-11. **A,** Linear regression model: Observed testosterone (T) and fitted levels of mean T across the menopausal transition. **B,** Double logistic model: Observed free androgen index (FAI) and fitted levels of mean FAI across the menopausal transition. The left and right axes show FAI levels on the log and antilog scales, respectively. The horizontal axis represents time (years) with respect to first menstrual period (FMP); negative (positive) numbers indicate time before (after) FMP. (From Burger HG, Dudley EC, Cui J, et al: A prospective longitudinal study of serum testosterone, dehydroepiandrosterone sulfate, and sex hormone-binding globulin levels through the menopause transition. J Clin Endocrinol Metab 85:2832, 2000.)

postmenopausal women. After menopause, sex hormone-binding globulin (SHBG) levels decrease, resulting in relatively higher levels of bioavailable testosterone or a higher free androgen index (Fig. 42-11). In women receiving oral estrogen, bioavailable testosterone levels are extremely low because SHBG levels are increased. How this relates to the decision to consider androgen therapy in postmenopausal women will be discussed later in this chapter.

Elevated gonadotropin (FSH/LH) levels arise from reduced secretion of E_2 and inhibin as described earlier. Although some aging effects of the brain are likely to exist, there is abundant human evidence for menopause in women to be an ovarian-induced event.

EFFECTS OF MENOPAUSE ON VARIOUS ORGAN SYSTEMS

Central Nervous System

The brain is an active site for estrogen action as well as estrogen formation. Estrogen activity in the brain is mediated via estrogen receptor (ER) α and ER β. Whether or not a novel membrane

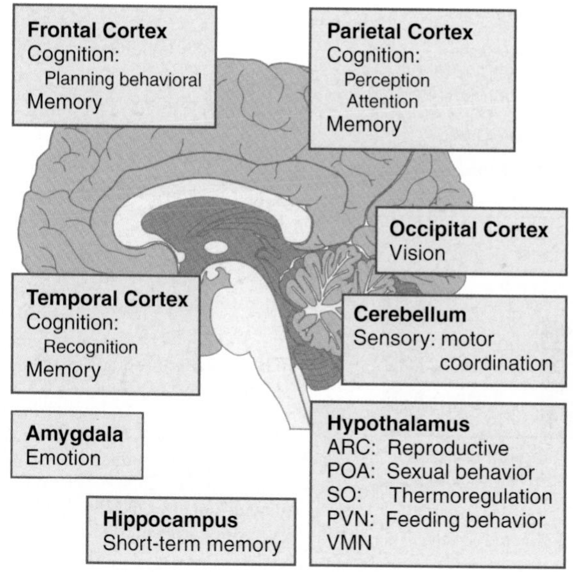

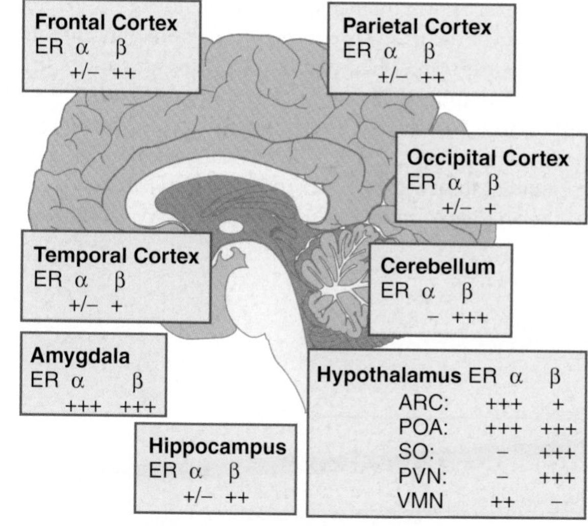

Figure 42-12. **A,** Each region of the brain has an important role in specific brain functions. Optimal brain activity is maintained by means of the integration of different areas by neural tracts. ARC, arcuate nucleus; POA, preoptic area; PVN, paraventricular nucleus; SO, supraoptic nucleus; VMN, ventromedial nucleus. **B,** Distribution of estrogen receptors ER α and ER β mRNA in the rat brain. (**B,** adapted from Cela V, Naftolin F: Clinical effects of sex steroids on the brain. In Lobo RA [ed]: The Treatment of the Postmenopausal Woman: Basic and Clinical Aspects, 2nd ed. Philadelphia, Lippincott Williams & Wilkins, 1999, pp 247–262.)

receptor (non-ER α/ER β) exists is still being debated. However, both genomic and nongenomic mechanisms of estrogen action clearly exist in the brain. Figure 42-12 illustrates the predominance of ER β in the cortex (frontal and parietal) and the cerebellum, based on work in the rat. While 17β E_2 is a specific ligand for both receptors, certain synthetic estrogens (e.g., diethylstilbestrol) have greater affinity for ER α, whereas phytoestrogens have a greater affinity for ER β.

There are multiple actions of estrogen on the brain as reviewed by Henderson (Table 42-3), thus some important functions linked to estrogen contribute to well-being in general and, more specifically, to cognition and mood. The hallmark feature of declining estrogen status in the brain is the hot flush, which is more generically referred to as a vasomotor episode. The hot flash usually refers to the acute sensation of heat, and the flush or vasomotor episode includes changes in the early perception of this event and other skin changes (including diaphoresis). Hot flushes usually occur for 2 years after the onset of estrogen deficiency, but can persist for 10 or more years. In 10% to 15% of women these symptoms are severe and disabling. In the United States the incidence of these episodes varies in different ethnic groups. Symptoms are greatest in Hispanic and black women, intermediate in white women, and lowest among Asian women (Fig. 42-13). The severity of hot flushes decreases with time, but it is known that in some women they may be bothersome for 10 or more years as shown by Oldenhave. As modulated by severity, hot flushes may cause a series of "irregular" symptoms, such as irritability, which may affect quality of life. The fall in estrogen levels precipitate the vasomotor symptoms. It has been found that some women who experience hot flushes have a thermoregulatory disruption with a much narrower temperature range between sweating and shivering. Although the proximate cause of the flush remains elusive, the episodes result from a hypothalamic response (probably mediated by catecholamines) to the change in estrogen status.

Table 42-3 Effects of Estrogen on Brain Function

Organizational Actions
Effects on neuronal number, morphology, and connections occurring during critical stages of development
Neurotrophic Actions
Neuronal differentiation
Neurite extension
Synapse formation
Interactions with neurotrophins
Neuroprotective Actions
Protection against apoptosis
Antioxidant properties
Antiinflammatory properties
Augmentation of cerebral blood flow
Enhancement of glucose transport into the brain
Blunting of corticosteroid response to behavioral stress
Interactions with neurotrophins
Effects on Neurotransmitters
Acetylcholine
Noradrenaline
Serotonin
Dopamine
Glutamate
Gamma aminobutyric acid
Neuropeptides
Effects on Glial Cells
Effects on Proteins Involved in Alzheimer's Disease
Amyloid precursor protein
Tau protein
Apolipoprotein E

Adapted from Henderson VW: Estrogen, cognition, and a woman's risk of Alzheimer's disease. Am J Med 103(Suppl 3A):11, 1997.

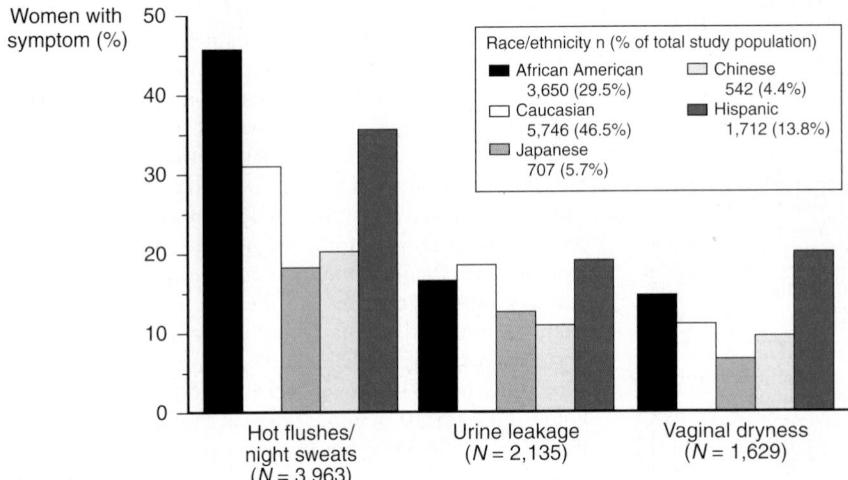

Figure 42-13. A Study of Women's Health Across the Nation (SWAN): Symptom severity. (Adapted from Gold EB, Sternfeld B, Kelsey JL, et al: Relation of demographic and lifestyle factors to symptoms in a multi-racial/ethnic population of women 40 to 55 years of age. Am J Epidemiol 152:463, 2000.)

The flush has been well characterized physiologically. It results in heat dissipation as witnessed by an increase in peripheral temperature (fingers, toes); a decrease in skin resistance, associated with diaphoresis; and a reduction in core body temperature (Fig. 42-14). There are hormonal correlates of flush activity, such as an increase in serum LH and in plasma levels of pro-opiomelanocortin peptides (ACTH, β-endorphin) at the time of the flush, but these occurrences are thought to be epiphenomena that result as a consequence of the flush and are not related to its cause. One of the primary complaints of women with hot flushes is sleep disruption. They may awaken several times during the night and require a change of bedding and clothes because of diaphoresis. Nocturnal sleep disruption in postmenopausal women with hot flushes has been well documented by electroencephalographic (EEG) recordings. Sleep efficiency is lower, and the latency to rapid eye movement (REM) sleep is longer in

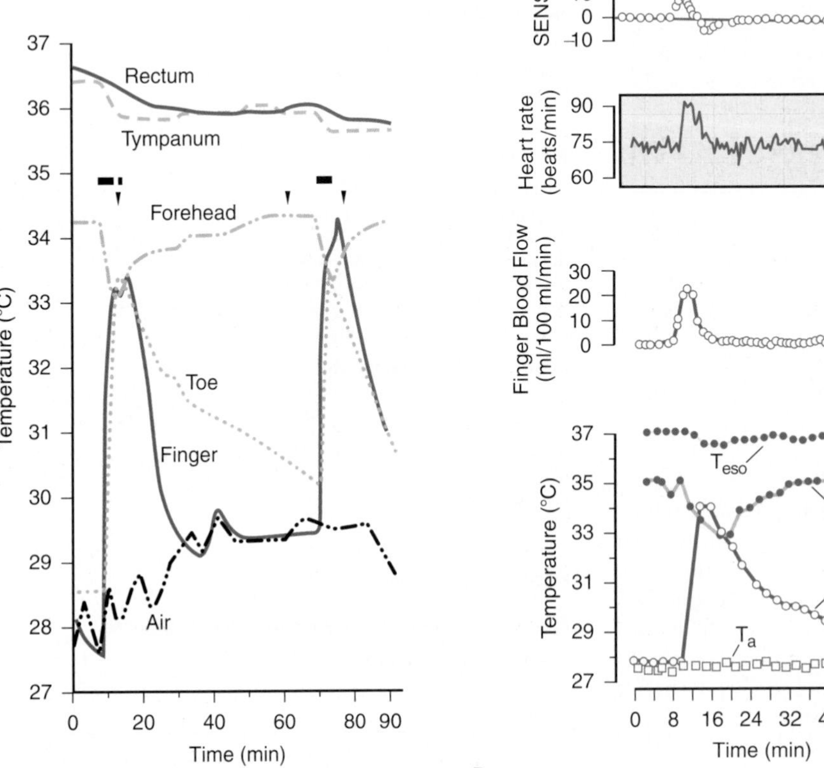

Figure 42-14. Temperature responses to two spontaneous flashes **(A)** and evoked flash **(B)**. Down arrowhead indicates finger stab for blood sample. (Data adapted from Molnar GW: Body temperature during menopausal hot flashes. J Appl Physiol 38:499, 1975.)

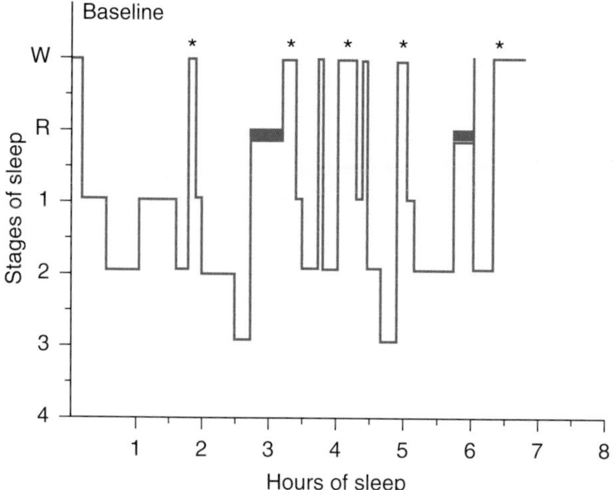

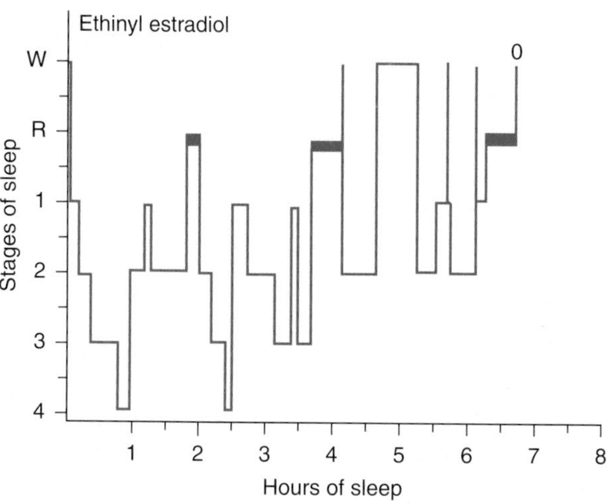

Figure 42-15. Sleepgrams measured in symptomatic patient before and after 30 days' administration of ethinyl estradiol, 50 µg four times daily. (Adapted from Erlik Y, Tataryn IV, Meldrum DR, et al: Association of waking episodes with menopausal hot flushes. JAMA 245:1741, 1981.)

women with hot flushes compared with asymptomatic women. This disturbed sleep often leads to fatigue and irritability during the day. The frequency of awakenings and of hot flushes are reduced appreciably with estrogen treatment (Fig. 42-15). Sleep may be disrupted even if the woman is not conscious of being awakened from sleep. In this setting, EEG monitoring has indicated sleep disruption in concert with physiologic measures of vasomotor episodes.

In postmenopausal women, estrogen has been found to improve depressed mood regardless of whether or not this is a specific complaint (critics of some of this work point out that mood is affected by the symptomatology and by sleep deprivation). Blinded studies carried out in asymptomatic women have also shown benefit. In an estrogen-deficient state such as occurs after the menopause, a higher incidence of depression (clinical or subclinical) is often manifest. However, menopause per se does not cause depression, and although estrogen does generally improve depressive mood, it should not be used for psychiatric disorders. Nevertheless, very high pharmacologic doses of estrogen have been used to treat certain types of psychiatric depression in the past. Progestogens as a class generally attenuate the beneficial effects of estrogen on mood, although this effect is highly variable.

Cognitive decline in postmenopausal women is related to aging as well as to estrogen deficiency. The literature is somewhat mixed about whether there are benefits of estrogen in terms of cognition. In more recent studies, verbal memory appears to be enhanced with estrogen and has been found to correlate with acute changes in brain imaging signifying brain activation. Dementia increases as women age, and the most common form of dementia is Alzheimer's disease (AD). Table 42-3 lists several neurotropic and neuroprotective factors related to how estrogen deficiency may be expected to result in the loss of protection against the development of AD. In addition, estrogen has a positive role in enhancing neurotransmitter function, which is deficient in women with AD. This function of estrogen has particular importance and relevance for the cholinergic system that is affected in AD. Estrogen use after menopause appears to decrease the likelihood of developing or delaying the onset of AD (Fig. 42-16) However, once a woman is affected by AD, estrogen is unlikely to provide any benefit. In that data from the Women's Health Initiative (WHI) suggested a lack of benefit of estrogen or estrogen/progestogen, or even a worsening of cognition, suggests that timing of initiation of hormone therapy is critical. Recent data by Espeland from WHI showed that prior users of estrogen before entering the WHI trial had less dementia at follow up. Early treatment in younger women at the onset of menopause may be beneficial, (although not proven yet), but later treatment (e.g., after age 65) has no benefit.

Collagen

Estrogen has a positive effect on collagen, which is an important component of bone and skin and serves as a major support tissue for the structures of the pelvis and urinary system. Both estrogen and androgen receptors have been identified in skin fibroblasts. Nearly 30% of skin collagen is lost within the first 5 years after menopause, and collagen decreases approximately 2% per year for the first 10 years after menopause. This statistic, which is similar to that of bone loss after menopause, strongly suggests a link between skin thickness, bone loss, and the risk of osteoporosis. Although the literature is not entirely consistent, estrogen therapy generally improves collagen content after menopause and improves skin thickness substantially after about 2 years of treatment. There is a possible biomodal effect with high doses of estrogen causing a reduction in skin thickness. The supportive effect of estrogen on collagen has important implications for bone homeostasis and for the pelvis after menopause. Here, reductions in collagen support and atrophy of the vaginal and urethral mucosa have been implicated in a variety of symptoms, including prolapse and urinary symptoms.

Symptoms of urinary incontinence and irritative bladder symptoms occur in 20% to 40% of perimenopausal and postmenopausal women. Uterine prolapse and other gynecologic symptoms related to poor collagen support, as well as urinary complaints, may improve with estrogen therapy. Although estrogen generally improves symptoms, urodynamic changes have not been shown to be altered. Estrogen has also been shown to

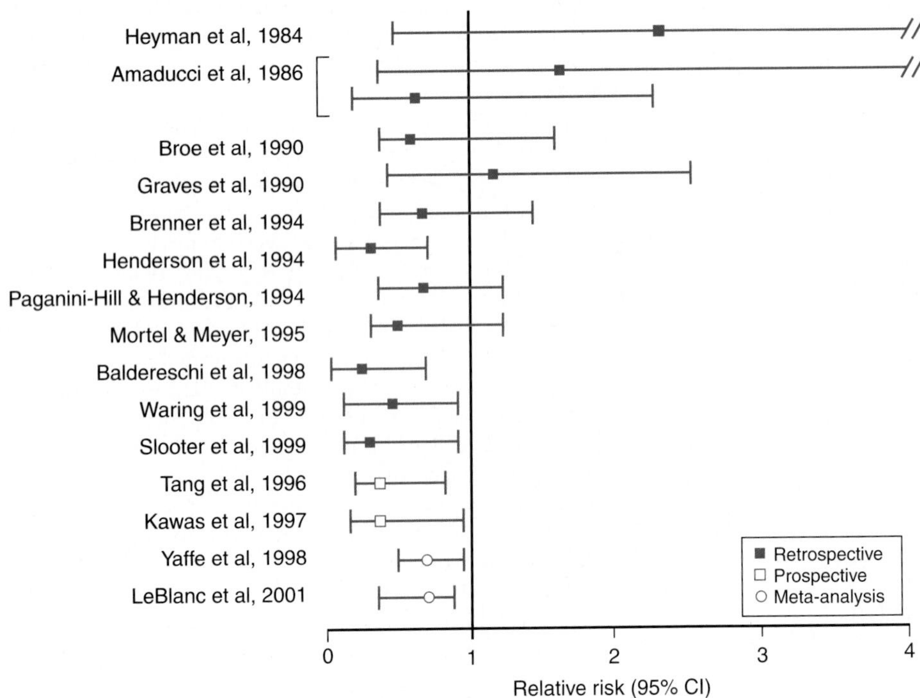

Figure 42-16. Estrogen replacement therapy/hormone replacement therapy use and risk of Alzheimer's disease. References are from the original source. (Adapted from LeBlanc ES, Janowsky J, Chan BK, Nelson HD: Hormone replacement therapy and cognition: Systematic review and meta-analysis. JAMA 285:1489, 2001.)

decrease the incidence of recurrence of urinary tract infections. Restoration of bladder control in older women with estrogen has been shown to decrease the need for admission to nursing homes in Sweden. Estrogen may also have an important role in normal wound healing. In this setting, estrogen enhances the effects of growth factors such as transforming growth factor-β (TGF-β). Although still not completely settled, it appears that oral estrogen does not improve stress urinary incontinence in postmenopausal women and may even cause such symptoms in previously asymptomatic older women. Estrogen may, however, improve urge and other irritative urinary symptoms.

Genital Atrophy

Vulvovaginal complaints are often associated with estrogen deficiency. In the perimenopause, symptoms of dryness and atrophic changes occur in 21% and 15% of women, respectively. However, these findings increase with time, and by 4 years these incidences are 47% and 55%, respectively. With this change, an increase in sexual complaints also occurs, with an incidence of dyspareunia of 41% in sexually active 60-year-old women. Estrogen deficiency results in a thin, paler vaginal mucosa. The moisture content is low, the pH increases (usually greater than 5), and the mucosa may exhibit inflammation and small petechiae. With estrogen treatment, vaginal cytology changes have been documented, transforming from a cellular pattern of predominantly parabasal cells to one with an increased number of superficial cells. Along with this change, the vaginal pH decreases, vaginal blood flow increases, and the electropotential difference across the vaginal mucosa increases to that found in premenopausal women.

Bone Loss

Estrogen deficiency has been well established as a cause of bone loss. This loss can be noted for the first time when menstrual cycles become irregular in the perimenopause from 1.5 years before the menopause to 1.5 years after menopause, spine bone mineral density has been shown to decrease by 2.5% per year, compared with a premenopausal loss rate of 0.13% per year. Loss of trabecular bone (spine) is greater with estrogen deficiency than is loss of cortical bone.

Postmenopausal bone loss leading to osteoporosis is a substantial health care problem. In white women, 35% of all postmenopausal women have been estimated to have osteoporosis based on bone mineral density. Furthermore, the lifetime fracture risk for these women is 40%. The morbidity and economic burden of osteoporosis is well documented. Interestingly, some data suggest that up to 19% of white men also have osteoporosis. Bone mass is substantially affected by sex steroids through classic mechanisms to be described later in this chapter. Attainment of peak bone mass in the late second decade (Fig. 42-17) is key to ensuring that the subsequent loss of bone mass with aging and estrogen deficiency does not lead to early osteoporosis. E_2, together with GH and insulin-like growth factor-1 act to double bone mass at the time of puberty, beginning the process of attaining peak bone mass. Postpubertal estrogen deficiency (amenorrhea from various causes) substantially jeopardizes peak bone mass. Adequate nutrition and calcium intake are also key determinants. Although estrogen is of predominant importance for bone mass in both women and men, testosterone is important in stimulating periosteal apposition; as a result, cortical bone in men is larger and thicker. Estrogen receptors are present in osteoblasts, osteoclasts, and

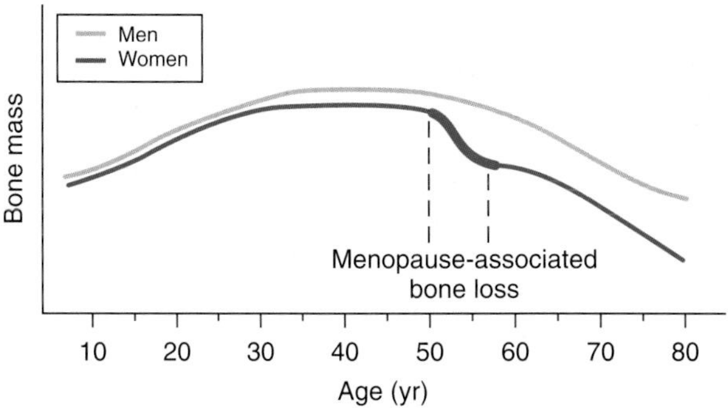

Figure 42-17. Bone mass by age and sex. (Adapted from Finkelstein JS: Osteoporosis. In Goldman L, Bennet JC [eds]: Cecil Textbook of Medicine, 21st ed. Philadelphia, Saunders, 1999, pp 1366–1373; Riggs BL, Melton LJ III: Involutional osteoporosis. N Engl J Med 314:1676, 1986, adapted with permission.)

osteocystes. Both ER α and ER β are present in cortical bone, whereas ER β predominates in cancellous or trabecular bone. However, the more important actions of estradiol are believed to be mediated via ER α. Estrogens suppress bone turnover and maintain a certain rate of bone formation. Bone is remodeled in functional units, called bone multicenter units (BMUs), where resorption and formation should be in balance. Multiple sites of bone go through this turnover process over time. Estrogen decreases osteoclasts by increasing apoptosis and thus reduces their lifespan. The effect on the osteoblast is less consistent, but E_2 antagonizes glucocorticoid-induced osteoblast apoptosis. Estrogen deficiency increases the activities of remodeling units, prolongs resorption, and shortens the phase of bone formation. It also increases osteoclast recruitment in BMUs, thus resorption outstrips formation. The molecular mechanisms of estrogen action on bone involve the inhibition of production of pro-inflammatory cytokines, including interleukin-1, interleukin-6, tumor necrosis factor-α, colony-stimulating factor-1, macrophage colony-stimulating factor, and prostaglandin E2, which lead to increased resorption. Estradiol also up-regulates TGF-β in bone, which inhibits bone resorption. Receptor activation of nuclear factor kappa (NFκB) ligand (RANKL) is responsible for osteoclast differentiation and action: A scheme for how all these factors interact has been proposed by Riggs (Fig. 42-18). In women, Riggs has suggested that bone loss occurs in two phases. With estrogen levels declining at the onset of menopause (leading to an accelerated phase of bone loss) predominantly cancellous bone loss occurs. Here 20% to 30% of cancellous bone and 5% to 10% of cortical bone can be lost in a span of 4 to 8 years. Thereafter a slower phase of loss (1% to 2%/year) ensues during which more cortical bone is lost. This phase is thought to be induced primarily by secondary hyperparathyroidism. The first phase is also accentuated by the decreased influence of stretching or mechanical factors, which generally promote bone homeostasis, as a result of estrogen deficiency: Genetic influences on bone mass are more important for attainment of peak bone mass (heritable component, 50% to 70%) than for bone loss. Polymorphisms of the vitamin D receptor gene, TGF-β gene, and the Spl-binding site in the collagen type 1 Al gene have all been implicated as being important for bone mass. Although testosterone is important for bone formation and stimulation of bone mass, even in men estrogen action is of paramount importance. Bone mass, which was in the osteoporosis range in an aromatase-deficient man was shown to increase on estrogen administration.

Bone mass can be detected by a variety of radiographic methods (Table 42-4). Dual-energy X-ray absorptiometry (DEXA) scans have become the standard of care for detection of osteopenia and osteoporosis. By convention, the T score is used to reflect the number of standard deviations of bone loss

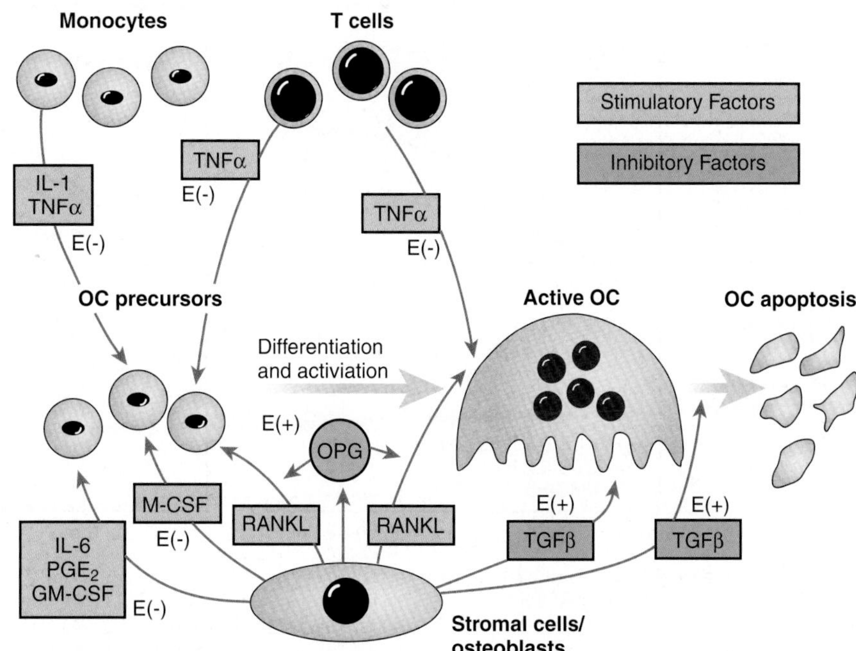

Figure 42-18. Model for mediation of effects of estrogen (E) on osteoclast formation and function by cytokines in bone marrow microenvironment. Stimulatory factors are shown in orange and inhibitory factors are shown in blue. Positive (+) or negative (−) effects of E on these regulatory factors are shown in red. The model assumes that regulation is accomplished by multiple cytokines working together in concert. IL, interleukin; PGE_2, prostaglandin E_2; GM-CSF, granulocyte macrophage/colony-stimulating factor; M-CSF, macrophage/colony-stimulating factor; RANKL, Receptor activation of B ligand; OC, osteoclast; OPG, osteoprotegerin; TGF-β, transforming growth factor β. (Adapted from Riggs BL: The mechanisms of estrogen regulation of bone resorption. J Clin Invest 106:1203, 2000.)

Table 42-4 Techniques for the Detection of Bone Mass

Technique	Anatomic Site of Interest	Precision in vivo (%)	Examination and Analysis Time (min)	Estimated Effective Dose Equivalent (uSv)
Conventional radiographs	Spine, hip	NA	< 5	2000
Radiogrammetry	Hand	1–3	5–10	< 1
Radiographic absorptiometry	Hand	1–2	5–10	< 1
Single X-ray absorptiometry	Forearm, heel	1–2	5–10	< 1
Dual X-ray absorptiometry	Spine, hip, forearm, total body	1–3	5–20	1–10
Quantitative computed tomography	Spine, forearm, hip	2–4	10–15	50–100
Quantitative ultrasound	Heel, hand, lower leg	1–3	5–10	none

NA, not applicable.
Adapted from van Kuijk C, Genant HK: Detection of osteopenia. In Lobo RA (ed): Treatment of the Postmenopausal Woman: Basic and Clinical Aspects, 2nd ed. Philadelphia, Lippincott Williams & Wilkins, 1999, pp 287–292.

from the peak bone mass of a young adult. Osteopenia is defined by a T score of –1 to –2.5 standard deviations; osteoporosis is defined as greater than 2.5 standard deviations. Various biochemical assays are also available to assess bone resorption and formation in both blood and urine (Table 42-5). At present, serum markers appear to be most useful for assessing changes with antiresorptive therapy. Many agents are now available for preventing osteoporosis. The use of estrogen will depend on whether there are other indications for estrogen treatment and any possible contraindications. Estrogen has been shown to reduce the risk of osteoporosis as well as to reduce osteoporotic fractures. A dose equivalent of 0.625 mg of conjugated equine estrogens (CEE) was once thought to prevent osteoporosis, but we now know that lower doses (0.3 mg of CEE or its equivalent) in combination with progestogens can prevent bone loss although there are no fracture data (Fig. 42-19). Whether the addition of progestogens by stimulating bone formation

Table 42-5 Biochemical Markers of Bone Formation and Bone Resorption

Markers of Bone Formation	Markers of Bone Resorption
Serum	Serum
Total and bone-specific	Tartrate-resistant acid phosphatase
Alkaline phosphatase	Free pyridinium crosslinks
Osteocalcin	Telopeptides of type 1 collagen
Propeptides of type 1 procollagen	
	Urine
	Hydroxyproline
	Calcium
	Pydridinoline and deoxypuridinoline
	Telopeptides of type 1 collagen
	Galactosyl hydroxylysine

Adapted from Eastell R, Hannon RA: Biochemical markers of bone turnover. In Lobo RA (ed): Treatment of the Postmenopausal Woman: Basic and Clinical Aspects, 2nd ed. Philadelphia, Lippincott Williams & Wilkins, 1999, pp 293–303.

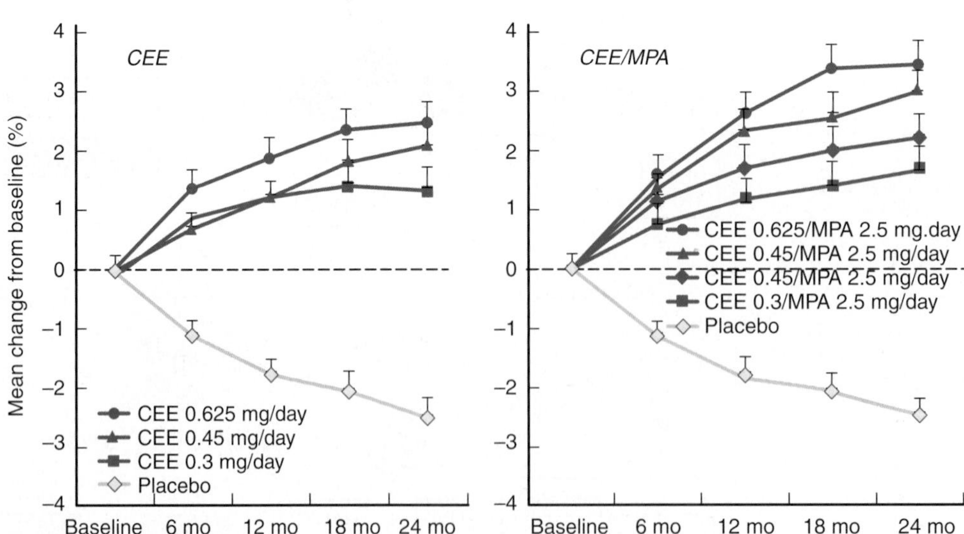

Figure 42-19. Changes in spine bone mineral density (BMD) with hormone therapy (HT). Intent-to-treat population only. The Women's HOPE Study. CEE, conjugated equine estrogens; HOPE, Heart, Osteoporosis, Progestin, Estrogen; MPA, medroxyprogesterone. (From Lindsay R, Gallagher JC, Kleerekoper M, Pickar JH: Effect of lower doses of conjugated equine estrogens with and without medroxyprogesterone acetate on bone in early postmenopausal women. JAMA 287:2668, 2002.)

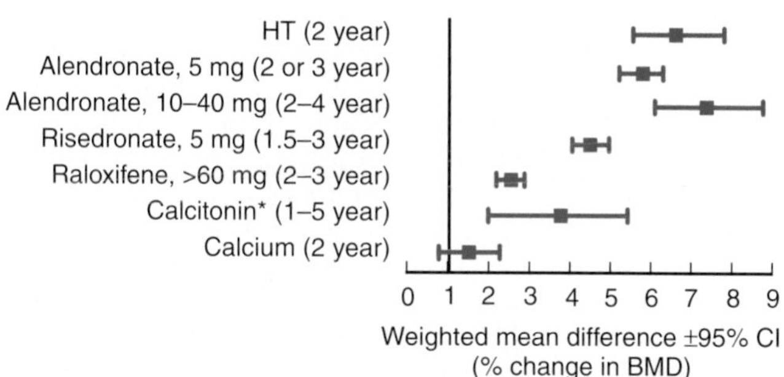

Figure 42-20. Meta-analysis of osteoporosis therapies: Spine bone mineral density (BMD). CI, confidence interval; HT, hormone therapy. (From Cranney A, Guyatt G, Griffith L, et al: Meta-analyses of therapies for postmenopausal osteoporosis. IX: Summary of meta-analyses of therapies for postmenopausal osteoporosis. Endocr Rev 23:570, 2002; Cranney A, Tugwell P, Wells G, et al: Meta-analyses of therapies for postmenopausal osteoporosis. I. Systematic reviews of randomized trials in osteoporosis: introduction and methodology. Endocrine Rev 23:496, 2002.)

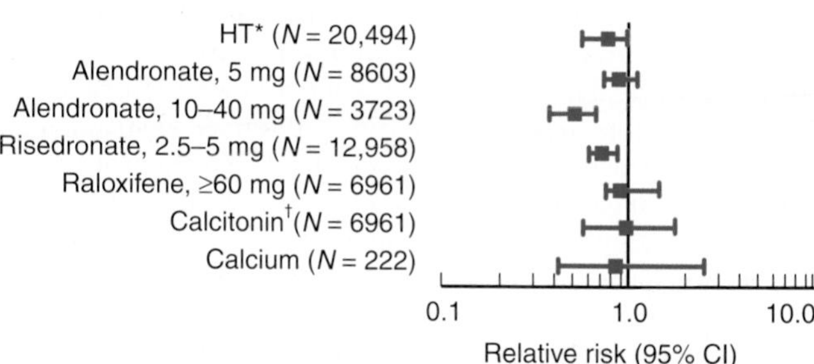

Figure 42-22. Meta-analysis of osteoporosis therapies: Nonvertebral fractures. CI, confidence interval; HT, hormone therapy. (From Cranney A, Guyatt G, Griffith L, et al: Meta-analyses of therapies for postmenopausal osteoporosis. IX: Summary of meta-analyses of therapies for postmenopausal osteoporosis. Endocr Rev 23:570, 2002; Cranney A, Tugwell P, Wells G, et al: Meta-analyses of therapies for postmenopausal osteoporosis. I. Systematic reviews of randomized trials in osteoporosis: introduction and methodology. Endocrine Rev 23:496, 2002; Rosen C: Presentation for ASBMR at NIH Scientific Workshop: Menopausal Hormone Therapy, October 23–24, 2002. Available at http//www4.od.nih.gov/orwh/htslides/rosen2.ppt.)

increases bone mass beyond that produced by estrogen alone is unclear. The androgenic activity of certain progestogens such as norethindrone acetate (NET) also has been suggested to play a role. Figures 42-20 and 42-21 provide data on changes in bone mineral density (BMD) at the spine and hip using various agents. Selective estrogen receptor modulators (SERMs) such as raloxifene, droloxifene, and tamoxifen have all been shown to decrease bone resorption. Raloxifene has been shown to decrease vertebral fractures in a large prospective trial.

However, SERMs that acts as low-dose estrogen on the skeleton have not been shown to prevent hip fractures (Fig. 42-22). Tibolone has also been shown to be an effective treatment for osteoporosis. Tibolone (not marketed in the United States) has SERM-like properties, but it is not specifically a SERM because it has mixed estrogenic, antiestrogenic, androgenic, and progestogenic properties. The drug does not seem to cause uterine or breast cell proliferation but is beneficial for vasomotor symptoms. It prevents osteoporosis and has been shown to be beneficial in treatment of osteoporosis as well. Bisphosphonates have been shown to have a significant effect on the prevention and treatment of osteoporosis. With this class of agents (etidronate, alendronate, risedronate, ibandronate), incorporation of the bisphosphonate with hydroxyapatite in bone increases bone mass. The skeletal half-life of bisphosphonates in bone can be as long as 10 years. These agents reduce both spine and hip fractures (see Fig. 42-22). Most data have been derived with alendronate, which, at a dosage of 5 mg daily (35 mg weekly) prevents bone loss; at 10 mg daily (70 mg weekly), alendronate is an effective treatment for osteoporosis, with evidence available that this treatment reduces vertebral and hip fractures Similar data are available for risedronate (35 mg weekly). Ibandronate has been approved as a once-a-month treatment (150 mg), and some data to date support the reduction in vertebral fractures. Calcitonin (50 IU subcutaneous injections daily, or 200 IU intranasally) has been shown to inhibit bone resorption. Vertebral fractures have been shown to decrease with calcitonin therapy. Long-term effects, however, have not been established.

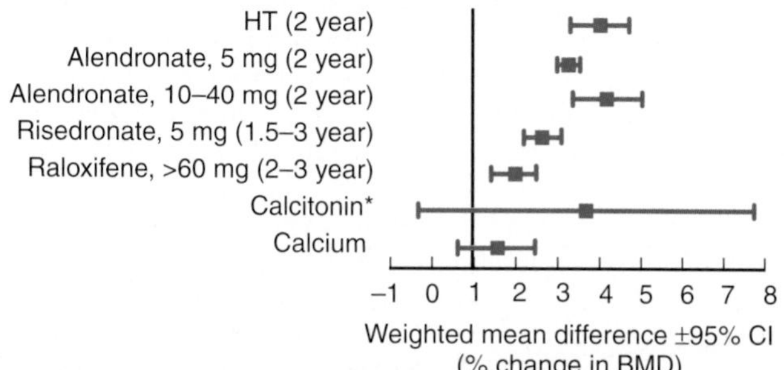

Figure 42-21. Meta-analysis of osteoporosis therapies: Total hip bone mineral density (BMD). CI, confidence interval. (From Cranney A, Guyatt G, Griffith L, et al: Meta-analyses of therapies for postmenopausal osteoporosis. IX: Summary of meta-analyses of therapies for postmenopausal osteoporosis. Endocr Rev 23:570, 2002; Cranney A, Tugwell P, Wells G, et al: Meta-analyses of therapies for postmenopausal osteoporosis. I. Systematic reviews of randomized trials in osteoporosis: introduction and methodology. Endocrine Rev 23:496, 2002.)

Fluoride has been used for women with osteoporosis because it increases bone density. Currently, a lower dose (50 μg daily) of slow-release sodium fluoride does not seem to cause adverse effects (gastritis) and has efficacy in preventing vertebral fractures.

Intermittent parathyroid hormone (PTH) offers promise as an agent to increase bone mass in women with osteoporosis. In a randomized trial lasting 3 years, average bone density increased in the hip and spine with fewer fractures observed. This therapy is now available in the United States. Teriparatide 20 μg needs to be injected subcutaneously on a daily basis for no longer than 18 months. It should be reserved for severe osteoporosis.

Adjunctive measures for prevention of osteoporosis are calcium, vitamin D, and exercise. Calcium with vitamin D treatment has been shown to increase bone only in older individuals. It will not prevent bone loss in younger women at the onset of menopause. These modalities alone are not thought to be effective for the treatment of osteoporosis. A woman's total intake of elemental calcium should be 1500 mg daily if no agents are being used to inhibit resorption, and 400 to 800 IU of vitamin D should also be ingested. Exercise has been shown to be beneficial for building muscle and bone mass and for reducing falls.

Although it is clear that women with established osteoporosis (fractures or a T score of −2.5 or greater) should receive an antiresorptive agent (usually a bisphosphonate), there is more controversy with initiating preventative strategies with T scores in the osteopenia range (−1.0 to −2.5). Many women, however, may sustain fractures in this range of T scores. Age and risk factors (thinness, immobilization, nutritional deficiencies, family history, etc.) largely help determine the need to treat those with osteopenia. In this setting, depending on the age of the woman and whether she has vasomotor symptoms, she may be offered hormone therapy, a SERM, or a bisphosphonate.

CARDIOVASCULAR EFFECTS

Clearly after menopause, the risk of cardiovascular disease in women is increased. Data from the Framingham study have shown that the incidence is three times lower in women before menopause than in men (3.1 per 1000 per year in women ages 45 to 49) The incidence is approximately equal in men and women ages 75 to 79 (53 and 50.4 per 1000 per year, respectively). This trend also pertains to gender differences in mortality due to cardiovascular disease. Coronary artery disease is the leading cause of death in women, and the lifetime risk of death is 31% in postmenopausal women versus a 3% risk of dying of breast cancer.

Although cardiovascular disease becomes more prevalent only in the later years following a natural menopause, premature cessation of ovarian function (before the average age of menopause) constitutes a significant risk. Premature menopause, occurring before age 35, has been shown to increase the risk of myocardial infarction two- to three-fold, and oophorectomy before age 35 increases the risk sevenfold.

When the possible reasons for the increase in cardiovascular disease are examined, the most prevalent finding is an accelerated rise in total cholesterol in postmenopausal women. The changes of weight, blood pressure, and blood glucose with aging, although important, are not thought to be as important as the rate of rise in total cholesterol, which is substantially different in women versus men. This increase in total cholesterol is explained by increases in levels of low-density lipoprotein cholesterol (LDL-C). The oxidation of LDL-C is also enhanced, as are levels of very low density lipoproteins and lipoprotein (a) lipoprotein. HDL-C levels trend downward with time, but these changes are small and inconsistent relative to the increases in LDL-C.

Coagulation balance is not substantially altered as a counterbalance of changes occurs. Some procoagulation factors increase (factor VII, fibrinogen), but so do counterbalancing factors like antithrombin III, plasminogen, protein C, and protein S. Blood flow in all vascular beds decreases after menopause; prostacyclin production decreases, endothelin levels increase, and vasomotor responses to acetylcholine are constrictive, reflecting reduced nitric oxide synthetase activity. With estrogen, all these parameters (generally) improve, and coronary arterial responses to acetylcholine are dilatory with a commensurate increase in blood flow.

Circulating plasma nitrites and nitrates have also been shown to increase with estrogen, and angiotensin-converting enzyme levels tend to decrease. Estrogen and progesterone receptors have been found in vascular tissues, including coronary arteries (predominantly ER β). In addition, some membrane effects are mediated by estrogen, which may or may not relate to either ER α or ER β.

Overall, the direct vascular effects of estrogen are viewed to be as important, or more important, than the changes in lipid and lipoproteins after menopause. Although replacing estrogen has been thought to be beneficial for the mechanisms previously cited, these beneficial arterial effects may only be seen in younger (stage +1) postmenopausal women. Women with significant atherosclerosis or risk factors such as those studied in a secondary prevention trial do not respond well to this treatment. Some of this lack of effect may be accounted for by increased methylation of the promoter region of ER α, which occurs with atherosclerosis and aging.

In normal, nonobese postmenopausal women, carbohydrate tolerance also decreases as a result of an increase in insulin resistance. This, too, may be partially reversed by estrogen, although the data are mixed and high doses of estrogen with or without progestogen cause a deterioration in insulin sensitivity. Biophysical and neurohormonal responses to stress (stress reactivity) are exaggerated in postmenopausal women compared with premenopausal women, and this heightened reactivity is blunted by estrogen. Whether these changes influence cardiovascular risk with estrogen deficiency is not known, but clearly estrogen treatment returns many parameters into the range of premenopausal women in early postmenopausal women.

These consistently strong basic science and clinical data for the protective effects of estrogen on the cardiovascular system, together with strong epidemiological evidence for a protective effect of estrogen (Fig. 42-23) led to the belief that estrogen should be prescribed to prevent cardiovascular disease in women. Recent clinical trial data, however, have refuted this notion in women with established disease as noted previously. Results from several randomized trials in women have failed to show a protective effect, including the 3-year extension of the Heart and Estrogen/Progestin Replacement Study (HERS), called HERS-II.

Furthermore, a trend toward increased cardiovascular events (early harm) has been observed in this setting in some women within the first 1 to 2 years. The Women's Health Initiative (WHI) trial, which compared CEE/medroxyprogesterone acetate (MPA) with placebo, came to similar conclusions. This trial was considered to be a primary prevention trial, but it studied a large range of ages, with risk factors occurring in an older cohort of women (mean age 63). These women did not have vasomotor symptoms and had more risk factors than the healthy women studied in observational cohorts.

The protective effect of estrogen demonstrated in the observational trials such as the Nurse's Health Study (NHS) (see

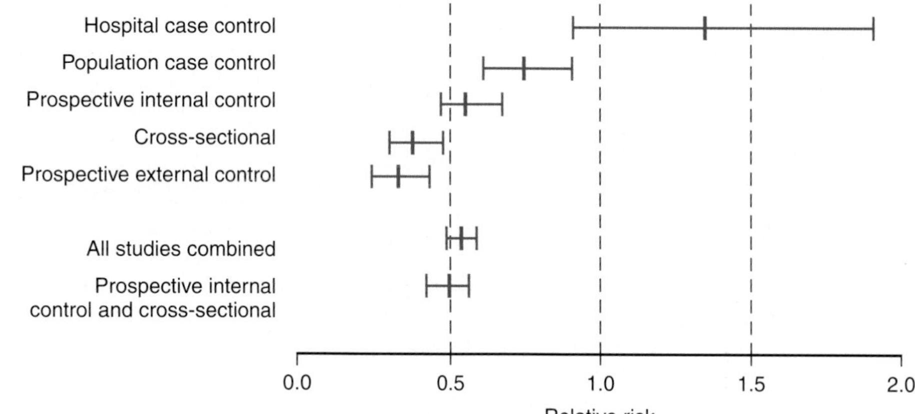

Figure 42-23. Estrogen replacement therapy and coronary heart disease. Relationship between relative risk and study type. (Adapted from Stampfer MJ, Colditz GA: Estrogen replacement therapy and coronary heart disease: A quantitative assessment of the epidemiologic evidence. Prev Med 20:47, 1991.)

Fig. 42-23) occurred predominantly in young, healthy, symptomatic women. Table 42-6 compares the demographics of the participants of WHI and the NHS. Trials carried out in the monkey model have shown a 50% to 70% protective effect against coronary atherosclerosis when estrogen is begun at the time of oophorectomy, with or without an atherogenic diet; delaying the initiation of hormonal therapy for even 2 years (in the monkey) prevents this protective effect (Fig. 42-24).

Table 42-6 Baseline Characteristics: Nurse's Health Study (NHS) Versus Women's Health Initiative (WHI)

	WHI	NHS
Mean age or age range at enrollment (years)	63	30–55
Smokers (past and current)	49.9%	55%
Body mass index (BMI:mean)	28.5 kg/m^2	25.1 kg/m^2
Aspirin users	19.1%	43.9%
Menopausal symptoms	Rare	Common

Observations in HERS (a secondary prevention trial in older women with established disease) demonstrated that hormone therapy (HT) was ineffective in preventing the progression of coronary heart disease (CHD), particularly if statins and other cardiac medications were already in use. Lack of an effect of estrogen therapy (ET) or HT was also demonstrated in an angiographic endpoint trial and another secondary prevention trial in the United Kingdom.

The differences in types and regimens of HT in these trials suggest that this lack of benefit in secondary prevention is not dependent on the hormonal preparation. Why aging and progressive atherosclerosis impede the ability of estrogen to be protective is unclear, but it is likely to be due to a variety of mechanisms:

- The inability to alter the endothelium after it is covered substantially by atherosclerotic plaque
- The inability to improve further on the beneficial effect that occurs with powerful cardiovascular medications

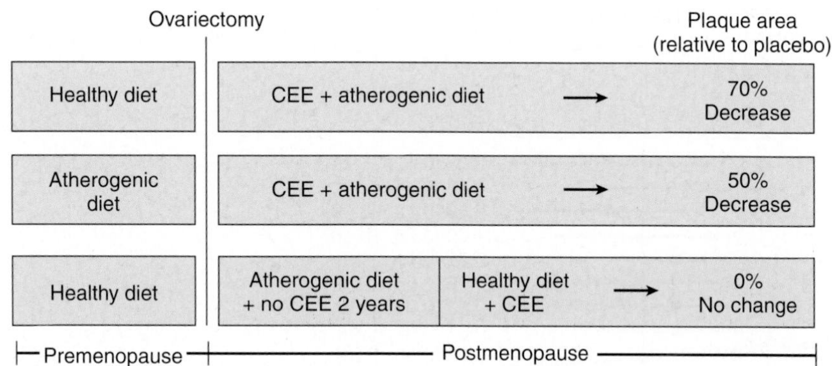

Figure 42-24. Importance of timing of intervention on the effect of estrogens on atherogenesis in nonhuman primates. CEE, conjugated equine estrogen. (Adapted from Clarkson TB, Anthony MS, Jerome CP: Lack of effect of raloxifene on coronary artery atherosclerosis of postmenopausal monkeys. J Clin Endocrinol Metab 83:721, 1998; Adams MR, Register TC, Golden DL, et al: Medroxyprogesterone acetate antagonizes inhibitory effects of conjugated equine estrogens on coronary artery atherosclerosis. Arterioscler Thromb Vasc Biol 17:217, 1997; Clarkson TB, Anthony MS, Morgan TM: Inhibition of postmenopausal atherosclerosis progression: A comparison of the effects of conjugated equine estrogens and soy phytoestrogens. J Clin Endocrinol Metab 86:41, 2001; Williams JK, Anthony MS, Honore EK, et al: Regression of atherosclerosis in female monkeys. Arterioscler Thromb Vasc Biol 15:827, 1995.)

- Inability of estrogen to work as effectively, due to methylation of the promoter region of ER α
- The inability to demonstrate any overall benefit when an early detrimental effect is experienced by some women (described below)

In the WHI, two thirds of the women were older than 60 (at least 10 years postmenopausal). We do not know the age at menopause for participants, but it is likely that women between age 50 and 59 in WHI, who were largely without menopausal symptoms, were several years postmenopausal. With aging, even in the absence of a documented cardiac event such as myocardial infarction, we know that women have substantial atherosclerosis. Extrapolating from the monkey model, we can estimate that the diminished ability of estrogen to inhibit coronary atherosclerosis can occur as early as 6 years after menopause if no hormones have been administered. This effect, of course, is aggravated if there are cardiovascular risk factors.

In the first year of the HT (CEE + MPA) trial of WHI, more cardiac events occurred. This finding is consistent with the other secondary prevention trials mentioned earlier, including the NHS, in which a subgroup analysis was carried out to examine only those women with documented coronary disease. Here there was an increase in cardiovascular events in the first year in that group (not statistically significant), followed by a reduction in events and mortality with time. No clear explanation exists for what the observed "early harm" may be due to, but these effects were not observed in those women receiving statins concurrently. This finding suggests that HT (in the doses used) may lead to plaque destabilization and thrombosis in some women with established (although possibly silent) coronary disease. The molecular mechanisms for this may be due to estrogen up-regulating matrix metalloproteinase-9 and inhibiting its natural inhibitor within the mural area of the plaque; the resultant disruption of the gelatinous covering then leads to thrombosis. This process is inhibited by statins. In women who had been receiving estrogen for a prolonged time, mortality rates decreased in those who sustained a myocardial infarction. No increase in cardiovascular events has been found in young, healthy, symptomatic women during the first 2 years of various ET/HT regimens in clinical trials. In the WHI, the estrogen alone trial did not find any evidence of "early harm," and there was no overall effect over the 6 years of observation in the trial. However, there was a significant trend for a decrease in events with time, and this was also seen in the HT trial. Moreover, with estrogen alone the 50- to 59-year-old group had a reduction in events, which was almost statistically significant, and when global coronary scores for this group were computed, this did achieve a statistical beneficial effect. Thus, in younger women, and particularly with estrogen alone, the randomized controlled trial data parallel the findings from the observational studies, all suggesting a beneficial effect. A recent pooled analysis by Salpeter and colleagues, looking at 25 prospective trials, showed that in women within 10 years of menopause who received HT, there was a significant reduction in CHD (Fig. 42-25). Newer prospective randomized trials (some of which are underway) will be necessary to prove that young, healthy women receiving hormones at the onset of menopause experience a cardioprotective effect.

Two more areas of CVD need to be discussed regarding their interactions with HT, stroke, and venous thrombosis. Stroke (ischemic, not hemorrhagic) was found to be increased in the WHI (both HT and ET) trials. This increase was approximately a 30% increase over the 5 to 6 years of the trial but was confined to older women in the trial. This was not an early harm phenomenon but tended to occur as the trial progressed. These data are similar to data from the NHS trial when dose is taken into account (women using CEE at 0.625 mg or more). Lower doses (e.g., CEE 0.3 mg) were not associated with an increased risk of stroke.

It is now accepted that there is a two- to threefold increase in venous thrombosis risk with oral hormonal therapy. However, the prevalence of this risk is low, particularly in young, healthy women. This two- to threefold risk is similar to that

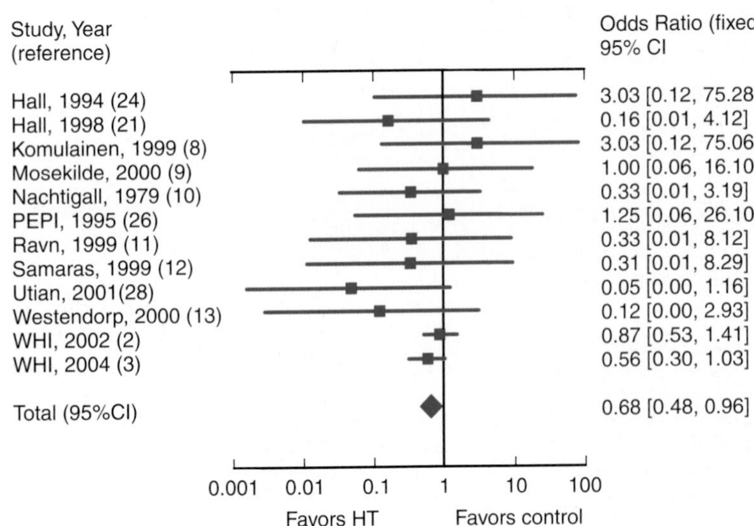

Figures 42-25. Pooled analysis from 23 randomized trials: Younger women (younger than 10 years or younger than 60 years). CI, confidence interval; HT, hormone therapy. References are from the original source. (From Salpeter SR, Walsh JM, Greyber E, Salpeter EE: Brief report: Coronary heart disease events associated with hormone therapy in younger and older women. A meta-analysis. J Gen Intern Med 21:363, 2006.)

with the use of oral contraceptives. For pulmonary embolism risk, in women at age 50 to 60 years, the background risk is approximately 10 to 20 events /100,000 women-years. Thus, with HT, the twofold increase may result in 40 events/100,000 women-years, which is less than the rate in normal pregnancy (approximately 60/100,000 women).

In summary, there should be no concern regarding increased cardiovascular risk for young, healthy women at the onset of menopause who are contemplating HT/ET for treatment of symptoms. In this setting there is no evidence of increased risk, and, indeed, these women may be found to benefit from a cardiovascular standpoint.

CANCER RISKS IN POSTMENOPAUSAL WOMEN

Although breast cancer is generally believed to be the leading cause of death in postmenopausal women, in fact it is lung cancer. Indeed, mortality from breast cancer tends to decrease after menopause, on an age-specific basis, but cardiovascular mortality increases, and these lines transect around the time of menopause (Fig. 42-26). The gynecologist should be well versed in the epidemiology and preventative strategies for breast, lung, cervical, endometrial, ovarian, and colorectal cancer. Further discussions of these cancers may be found in Part IV (Gynecologic Oncology) of this text. What follows is the potential effects of ET and HT on endometrial, breast, ovarian, and colorectal cancer.

Endometrial disease occurs with unopposed ET in women who have a uterus. Although a woman's risk for endometrial cancer with unopposed estrogen use is twofold to eightfold higher than that for the general population, precursor lesions (primarily endometrial hyperplasia) signal the presence of an abnormality in most patients. Thus, the risk is far less for endometrial cancer than it is for varying degrees of hyperplasia.

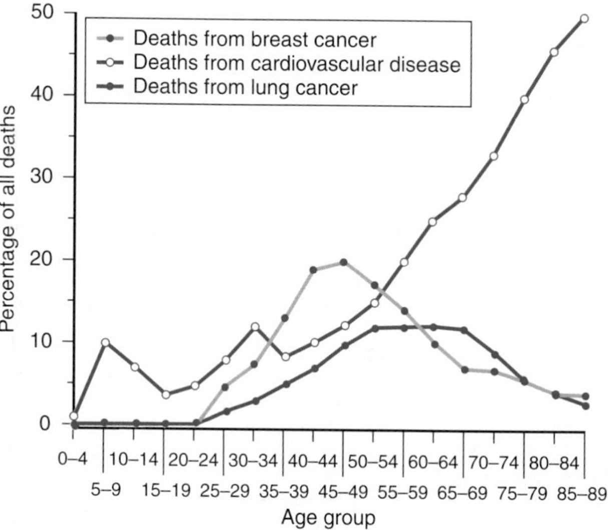

Figure 42-26. Risks of breast cancer and lung cancer versus cardiovascular disease in various age categories. (Adapted from Phillips KA, Glendon G, Knight JA: Putting the risk of breast cancer in perspective. N Engl J Med 340:141, 1999. Copyright 1999 Massachusetts Medical Society. All rights reserved. Adapted with permission.)

One study showed that the risk of endometrial hyperplasia was 20% after 1 year of use of 0.625 mg of oral CEE. In another study, the 3-year postmenopausal Estrogen/Progestin Interventions Trial, this risk was approximately 40% at the end of 3 years. No cancers were reported in either of these two studies, and the addition of a progestin essentially eliminated the hyperplasia risk. Use of CEE alone at 0.3 mg/day for 2 to 3 years results in a hyperplasia risk of 5% to 10%. With the same dose of esterified estrogens (which is less potent), no hyperplasia was found after 2 years.

The risk for endometrial cancer in women taking estrogen and progestogen is similar to that of women in the general population because combination therapy merely eliminates the excess risk attributed to estrogen; a few studies, however, have suggested a lower risk of endometrial cancer with continuous combined HT. It is important to remember that some endometrial cancers occurring in postmenopausal women are not hormonally related; thus some women may develop a serious type of cancer while on HT, making continuous surveillance important.

Although the risk for endometrial cancer is increased substantially in estrogen users, the risk of death from this type of endometrial cancer does not increase proportionately. Endometrial cancers associated with estrogen use are thought to be less aggressive than spontaneously occurring cancers, in part because tumors in women taking estrogen are more likely to be discovered and treated at an earlier stage, thus improving survival rates.

More controversial is the risk of breast cancer with estrogen use. Several studies and meta-analyses have shown a borderline or small statistical increase in the risk of breast cancer (relative risk [RR] 1.2–1.4) after approximately 5 years of use. This risk is related to the dose of estrogen, as well as duration of use. Recent data have pointed to the addition of progestogen as a major contribution to this increased risk of breast cancer. There is some biologic plausibility to this notion in that progesterone in the normal luteal phase increases breast mitotic activity and HT increases mammographic tissue density relative to ET alone. Several recent small case-control studies found no increase with ET alone, but the same studies showed a statistically significant increase with progestogen use (in the range of 1.3 or 1.4 RR). In the WHI trial, the increase in breast cancer risk was of borderline significance (hazard ratio [HR] 1.24, 1.01–1.54). A recent analysis by Anderson and coworkers found that when correcting for variables known to affect breast cancer risk, the average risk was no longer statistically significant: 1.20 (0.94–1.53). A large collaborative case-control study also has shown that continuous combined estrogen–progesterone therapy is associated with increased breast cancer risk over time.

In the estrogen only area of WHI, after $6^1/_2$ years there was a *decrease* in breast cancer risk of borderline significance HR = 0.77 (0.59 - 1.01). In a more complete analysis of these findings Stephanick and associates found the risk to be significantly decreased for ductal cancer (0.71 [0.52–0.99]), and in a sensitivity analysis among adherent women the decrease was statistically significant (0.67 [0.47–0.9]) (Fig. 42-27). Thus, although it is unclear why there should be a decrease in breast cancer risk, we may conclude that standard dose ET (0.625 mg CEE) is not associated with a risk of breast cancer except for very long term users. In a recent analysis from the NHS, Chen and colleagues found that this risk only increases significantly after 20 years (Table 42-7).

CUMULATIVE HAZARD FOR INVASIVE BREAST CANCER: SENSITIVITY ANALYSIS

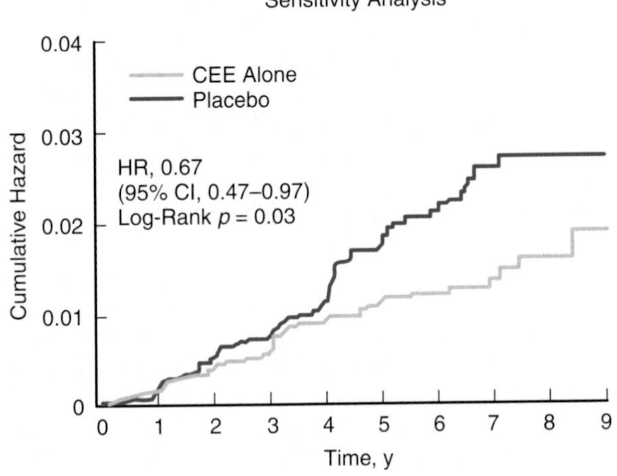

No. at Risk						
CEE	5310	3399	2448	1718	469	161
Placebo	5429	3638	2540	1760	422	168

Figure 42-27. Cumulative hazard for invasive breast cancer: Sensitivity analysis. CEE, conjugated equine estrogen; CI, confidence interval; HR, (From Stefanick ML, Anderson GL, Margolis KL, et al: Effects of conjugated equine estrogens on breast cancer and mammography screening in postmenopausal women with hysterectomy. JAMA 295:1647, 2006.)

Putting these risks into perspective is important for patient treatment. The background risk for breast cancer in a woman between the ages of 50 and 60 is 2.8/100 women. According to data from the WHI, the overall risk for women taking CEE/MPA for 5 years was approximately a relative risk of 1.24. This 24% increase translates into an overall risk of 3.47/100; less than 1% above the background risk. This risk would be less for never users who did not have an increased risk of the 5 years of the trial; and possibly may be lower still with low-dose therapy. A relative risk of 1.24 for breast cancer is less than that for obesity alone (3.3) or being a flight attendant (1.87). Furthermore, for estrogen alone, there is probably no increased risk at moderate to low doses for up to 20 years of exposure, as noted by Chen and colleagues.

It is generally thought that HT is linked to breast cancer through a promotional effect; that is, by causing the growth of undetectable preexisting small tumors. There is no evidence that estrogen actually causes new cancers. Thus, dose and duration of therapy is important, and particularly the use of a progestogen, which may potentiate growth. The normal time needed for the average breast cancer to be clinically detectable from a microscopic stage is approximately 10 years. Thus, the promotional effect of HT on breast cancer in susceptible women takes several years for clinical detection. With some exceptions in the literature, most reports have shown that the mortality rate in users of ET/HT is improved compared with those women not receiving hormones who are diagnosed with breast cancer. Furthermore, since women on HT/ET are likely (and should) have closer surveillance (exams and mammography) most tumors detected are at an early stage.

Family history and genetic mutations (*BRCA* 1 and 2, etc.) substantially increases the risk of a woman developing breast cancer. However, the literature suggests that the use of ET/HT does not increase this risk further. Nevertheless, for many women it is unacceptable to consider a potentially promotional effect of using HT and they may opt for risk reduction strategies such as use of tamoxifen or other SERMs.

If there is a concern regarding hormones and breast cancer, it is with larger doses, a longer duration, and specifically the use of a progestogen. Accordingly, for longer term therapy, if warranted (>5 years) lower doses of estrogen should be used, and progestogen exposure should be minimized.

Table 42-7 Risk of Invasive Breast Cancer by Duration of ET Use Among All Postmenopausal Women Who Had Undergone Hysterectomy and Those With ER+/PR+ Cancer Only*

	ALL POSTMENOPAUSAL WOMEN WHO HAD UNDERGONE HYSTERECTOMY				ER+/PR+ CANCERS ONLY			
	ALL		SCREENED COHORT†		ALL		SCREENED COHORT†	
ET Use and Duration (years)	**Cases**	**Risk**	**Cases**	**Risk**	**Cases**	**Risks**	**Cases**	**Risks**
Never	226	1.00	104	1.00	87	1.00	48	1.00
Current								
< 5	99	0.96 (0.75–1.22)	59	1.06 (0.76–1.47)	38	1.00 (0.67–1.49)	26	1.04 (0.64–1.70)
5–9.9	145	0.90 (0.73–1.12)	95	0.91 (0.68–1.21)	70	1.19 (0.86–1.66)	50	1.08 (0.72–1.62)
10–14.9	190	1.06 (0.87–1.30)	141	1.11 (0.85–1.44)	85	1.27 (0.93–1.73)	77	1.29 (0.89–1.86)
15–19.9	129	1.18 (0.95–1.48)	95	1.19 (0.89–1.58)	61	1.48 (1.05–2.07)	58	1.50 (1.02–2.21)
≥ 20	145	1.42 (1.13–1.77)	127	1.58 (1.20–2.07)	69	1.73 (1.24–2.43)	74	1.83 (1.25–2.68)
p for trend for current use		<.001		<.001		<.001		<.001

BMI, body mass index; CI, confidence interval; ER+/PR+, positive for both estrogen and progesterone receptors; ET, unopposed estrogen therapy.
*All cases are reported as number of cases; risks are reported as multivariate relative risk (95% CI), controlled for age (continuous), age at menopause (continuous), age at menarche (continuous), BMI (quintiles), history of benign breast disease (yes or no), family history of breast cancer in first-degree relative (yes or no), average daily alcohol consumption (0, 0.5–5, 5–10, 10–20, or ≥ 20 g/day), parity/age at first birth (nulliparous; 1–2 children and age at first birth ≤ 22 years; 1–2 children and age at first birth 23–25 years; 1–2 children and age at first birth > 25 years; ≥ 3 children and age at first birth ≤ 22 years; ≥ 3 children and age at first birth 23–25 years; ≥ 3 children and age at 1st birth > 25 years).
†Screened cohort defined as those women starting in 1988 who reported either a screening mammogram or clinical breast examination in the previous 2 years. All cases before 1988 are excluded.
From Chen WY, Manson JE, Hankinson SE, et al: Unopposed estrogen therapy and the risk of invasive breast cancer. Arch Intern Med 166:1027, 2006.

Ovarian Cancer

Several studies have also suggested an increased risk of ovarian cancer with long-duration use of ET/HT. However, the data are inconsistent, and the purported risk is in the range of less than a twofold relative risk. A recent analysis also found no association. In the WHI, there was no statistical increase in risk.

Colorectal Cancer

This is the third most frequent cancer in women and is often preventable by the detection and treatment of polyps. Women older than 50 should have a colorectal evaluation by some means (detection of occult blood, sigmoidoscopy, or a colonoscopy). Data have been fairly consistent for a reduction in risk with the use of HT/ET. Nanda showed a 33% decrease in risk in a meta-analysis as did data from the NHS and the HT arm of WHI. It is unclear why in the ET arm of WHI, a decrease was not seen. No definitive mechanism for this protective effect has been found, although several theories have been advanced (changes in the composition of bile acids, antiinflammatory effects, etc.).

THE DECISION TO USE ESTROGEN

Whether hormonal therapy should be considered is a very individual decision. The woman must take into account symptoms, risk factors, and individual preferences and needs. The predominant indication for estrogen is for symptoms (vasomotor, vulvovaginal, or urinary). Alternatives should also be considered. If hormonal therapy is chosen, there should be flexibility in prescribing because there is no ideal regimen for every woman, and each woman has individual risks and needs.

Risk–Benefit Assessment

The WHI was conceived in an attempt to determine the overall risks and benefits of ET/HT in a prospective randomized trial. The premise to be tested in an asymptomatic population of postmenopausal women was that ET/HT reduces cardiovascular disease and may increase the risk of breast cancer (primary endpoints). Several other secondary endpoints were also assessed: venous thromboembolism, stroke, osteoporotic fracture, colon cancer, and mortality). The HT arm of the trial (CEE 0.625 mg with MPA 2.5 mg) was terminated at 5.2 years because the event rates for breast cancer exceeded a preset monitoring boundary and because there was increased cardiovascular risk encountered (as previously discussed).

A tally of the various endpoints pointed to overall risks rather than benefit, although there was protection of osteoporotic fracture and colon cancer (Table 42-8). The ET randomized trial (hysterectomized women) did not have the same risk profile, and data are available for 6$^1/_2$ years (Table 42-9). Although there have been several analyses and critiques of the WHI data, the size of the trial sheds important light on the decision to use this

Table 42-8 WHI Results: Overall Relative and Attributable Risk in Women 50 to 79 Years of Age at Baseline

	Overall HR	CONFIDENCE INTERVALS 95% Nominal	CONFIDENCE INTERVALS 95% Adjusted	Attributable Risk per 10,000 Women/Year	Benefit per 10,000 Women/Year
CHD	1.24	1.00–1.54	0.85–1.97	7	
Breast cancer	1.26	1.01–1.59	0.83–1.92	8	
Stroke	1.41	1.07–1.85	0.86–2.31	8	
VTE	2.11	1.58–2.82	1.26–3.55	18	
PE	2.13	1.39–3.25	0.99–4.56	8	
Colorectal cancer	0.63	0.43–0.92	0.32–1.24		6
Hip fractures	0.66	0.45–0.98	0.33–1.33		5
Total fractures	0.76	0.69–0.85	0.63–0.92		44

CHD, coronary heart disease; PE, pulmonary embolism; VTE, venous thromboembolism.
From Writing Group for the Women's Health Initiative Investigators: Risks and benefits of estrogen plus progestin in healthy postmenopausal women: Principal results from the Women's Health Initiative randomized controlled trial. JAMA 288:321, 2002.

Table 42-9 WHI CEE Alone Results: Overall Relative and Attributable Risk

Event	Overall HR	CONFIDENCE INTERVALS 95% Nominal	CONFIDENCE INTERVALS 95% Adjusted	Attributable Risk per 10,000 Women/Year	Benefit per 10,000 Women/Year
CHD	0.91	0.75–1.12	0.72–1.15		5
Breast cancer	0.77	0.59–1.01	0.57–1.06		7
Stroke	1.39	1.10–1.77	0.97–1.99	12	
VTE	1.33	0.99–1.79	0.86–2.08	7	
PE	1.34	0.87–2.06	0.70–2.55	3	
Colorectal cancer	1.08	0.75–1.55	0.63–1.86	1	
Hip fractures	0.61	0.41–0.91	0.33–1.11		6
Total fractures	0.70	0.63–0.79	0.59–0.83		56

CHD, coronary heart disease; PE, pulmonary embolism; VTE, venous thromboembolism.
Women's Health Initiative Steering Committee: Effects of conjugated equine estrogen in postmenopausal women with hysterectomy: The Women's Health Initiative randomized controlled trial. JAMA 291:1701, 2004.

form of HT in asymptomatic women. The results of the trial were consistent with observational studies in all areas except for cardiovascular disease, which have been discussed previously.

The WHI trials computed an arbitrary "global index" adding up various changes in the eight major areas. Although this approach has not been validated, it provides a rough assessment that for older asymptomatic women of these specific regimens, there was more risk than benefit. However, the risk assessment clearly shifts toward benefit in younger symptomatic women as discussed earlier. Also for some women, protection from osteoporotic fractures becomes a significant benefit overriding some other concerns.

It is important that patients understand the "attributable" risk as described in Tables 42-8 and 42-9. This is the risk per year for 10,000 women exposed. Thus, an attributable risk of 8/10,000 women/year from cancer with HT is a very small risk and according to WHO terminology has been described as "rare." This concept has been lost by the media and others who have misinterpreted both relative risk and attributable risk.

Recently there has been a trend to reduce potential risks and adverse effects by using lower doses of ET/HT, which have been shown to be beneficial. The NHS demonstrated a protective effect with a lower dose of CEE (0.3 mg) and no increased risk of stroke. These lower doses have also been found to be sufficient to treat vasomotor symptoms.

Changes in Mortality Rates with Estrogen Use

In several cohort studies, an overall 40% reduction in all-cause mortality has been observed with long-term estrogen use. Two studies have shown that the benefit in mortality is related to the duration of use; one study has suggested that the effect is decreased beyond 10 years of use because of an increase in breast cancer mortality (only reported in this cohort and not in the others). Most studies have shown either no change in breast cancer mortality rates with estrogen use or a decrease.

In these observational cohorts looking at all-cause mortality, the overall reduction was found to be attributable to a reduction in cardiovascular mortality, although there was a small effect in cancer mortality as well. It is important to note that the women in these observational (epidemiologic) trials received therapy at the onset of menopause, and the women observed were healthier. In older women (10 or more years after menopause) who may have silent or established cardiovascular disease, there may not be a protective effect on mortality. In the WHI trial, total mortality was similar in HT/ET and placebo groups.

Other Risks Associated with Estrogen Therapy

A discussion of the relationship with cancer was described earlier. One of the concerns of women receiving estrogen is the return of menstrual bleeding. Somatic complaints such as breast tenderness and bloating may also occur with ET/HT, but these can be alleviated by alterations in dose and the type of preparation. Such concerns should be discussed with the patient, and the choice of the regimen should remain flexible.

Idiosyncratic reactions like hypertension and allergic manifestations have been observed in users of estrogen, particularly oral estrogen. Hypertension with estrogen use, the cause of which is not entirely clear, occurs in about 5% of women using the oral route. Otherwise, estrogen usually causes no change in blood pressure; it may actually reduce blood pressure, a finding that has relevance for normotensive as well as hypertensive individuals and is rapidly reversible with discontinuation of the regimen. A different form of estrogen may eliminate the problem, and alterations in the route of estrogen administration have also resulted in normal blood pressure responses in such individuals.

In unsusceptible individuals, ET does not increase procoagulant factors outside the normal range; for many years, ET was not considered to increase the risk of venous thrombosis—unlike oral contraceptive use. However, several recent observational studies and the results of HERS and WHI have suggested a twofold increase in venous thromboembolic phenomena with oral estrogen. This risk has not been definitively related to an unknown thrombophilia, but some women, based on an individual sensitivity, are clearly at increased risk for thrombosis. The observed events all tend to occur in the first two years of estrogen exposure. This increased risk does not increase mortality, however, and the rate is low.

A recent meta-analysis estimated that the absolute increased risk for venous thromboembolic events is 15 per 100,000 women per year. Nevertheless, all patients must be informed of these findings. Data from France by Scarabin and colleagues found no increased risk with transdermal estrogen therapy confirmed the increased risk with oral hormones. Women who have a family history of thrombosis or have had thrombotic events linked to oral contraceptives or any prior estrogen use should be counseled very carefully and monitored closely. A low-dose, nonoral form of estrogen would be a consideration for these patients; again, the need for choosing estrogen as a treatment should be clearly documented.

As noted previously, the risk of unstable angina and potential myocardial infarction is increased within the first 2 years of initiating hormones in older women with silent or established coronary disease. There is evidence that concurrent statin use may decrease or eliminate this early risk. However, it is unlikely that these other women would ever need any HT or ET.

APPROACH TO THERAPY

In developed countries, much of what women know about health care is gleaned from the mass media. In general, the more sensational an item is, the more noteworthy. For example, breast cancer risk is a real and serious concern for all women, but the fear of breast cancer seems to drive all decision-making, particularly regarding hormonal options.

American women believe that the leading cause of death in women is breast cancer and attribute only a small percentage of deaths to cardiovascular disease. In reality, the opposite is true. Statistics indicate that one in three women older than 65 has some evidence of cardiovascular disease. Despite public perception, the overall incidence of breast cancer has remained constant in recent years. Nevertheless, what is not commonly appreciated by those health care professionals counseling patients is the age-associated relationship in the incidence of breast cancer.

Table 42-10 Women Who Will Develop Breast Cancer: Risk According to Age

Decade of Life	Incidence
Third	1 of 250
Fourth	1 of 77
Fifth	1 of 42
Sixth	1 of 36
Seventh	1 of 34
Eighth	1 of 45

From Cancer Care Ontario; adapted from Lobo RA: Treatment of the postmenopausal woman: Where we are today. In Lobo RA (ed): Treatment of the Postmenopausal Woman: Basic and Clinical Aspects, 2nd ed. Philadelphia, Lippincott Williams & Wilkins, 1999, pp 655–659.

Although it has been widely asserted that the incidence of breast cancer in women is approximately one in eight, this is the lifetime risk. The age-specific data are quite different: 1 of 77 in the fourth decade and 1 of 32 in the fifth decade, rising to 1 of 45 when a woman is in her eighth decade (Table 42-10). Misperceptions about the magnitude of cancer risk may lead some women not to consider ET/HT for the prevention of other conditions that actually have greater morbidity and mortality, as well as for the alleviation of menopausal symptoms.

Because the case fatality rate of cardiovascular disease is several times greater than that of breast cancer, many more women would die of cardiovascular disease even if the incidence of these two diseases were similar as mentioned earlier. Figure 42-26 shows the death rate according to different ages. Soon after menopause, at age 50 to 54, the death rate for breast cancer decreases, but the death rate for cardiovascular disease rises steadily. The leading cause of caner death in women is lung cancer. By age 55, 20% of all deaths are caused by cardiovascular disease; overall, 30% to 40% of women eventually will die of cardiovascular disease. The rationale for choosing estrogen at the onset of menopause for symptom control is expected to have a minimal effect on breast cancer incidence, particularly if the dose of estrogen is lowered. Whether there is also some cardiovascular benefit in this setting cannot be determined at this time.

Hormone Regimens

The various hormonal preparations available for treatment are listed in (Table 42-11). Also included are the SERM raloxifene and other compounds like bisphosphonates, tibolone, and human parathyroid hormone. For the clinician and patient, the decision to start estrogen therapy need not involve a long-term commitment. For short-term treatment of symptoms, estrogen should be used at the lowest dose that can control hot flushes or can be administered via the vaginal route for symptoms of dryness or dyspareunia.

Oral ET results in higher levels of estrone (E_1) than estradiol (E_2); this is true for oral micronized E_2 as well as E_1 products. CEE is a mixture of at least 10 conjugated estrogens derived from equine pregnant urine. Estrone sulfate is the major component, but the biologic activities of equilin, 17α-dihydroequilin, and several other B-ring unsaturated estrogens, including Δ5 dehydroestrone, have been documented. Table 14-12 compares the standard doses of the most frequently prescribed oral estrogens and the levels of E_1 and E_2 achieved. Much of the following clinical information may be found in systematic reviews.

Synthetic estrogens, given orally, are more potent than natural E_2. Ethinyl estradiol is used in oral contraceptives, with a dose of 5 μg being equivalent to the standard ET doses used

Table 42-11 Hormonal Treatment Available for Postmenopausal Women

Estrogens

Oral
Oral CEE, 0.3, 0.45, 0.625, 0.9, 1.25, and 2.5 mg
Piperazine estrone sulfate, equivalent of 0.625, 1.25, and 2.5 mg
Esterified, 0.3, 0.625, 0.9, 1.25, and 2.5 mg
Micronized estradiol, 0.5, 1, and 2 mg

Transdermal
Estradiol patches, 0.014, 0.025, 0.0375, 0.05, 0.75, and 0.10 mg/d
Estradiol gel, 1.5 and 3 mg

Vaginal
Cream, CEE (0.0625%), estradiol (0.01%)
Estradiol ring, 2 mg; vaginal tablets, 25 μg

Parenteral
Intramuscular injections should be avoided

Progestins

Oral
Medroxyprogesterone acetate, 2.5, 5, and 10 mg
Norethindrone acetate, 5 mg
Micronized progesterone, 100 and 200 mg

Vaginal
Micronized progesterone, 100 mg
Progesterone gel, 4% and 8%

Combinations

Oral
CEE + MPA (0.625 mg) + MPA (2.5 or 5 mg)
CEE + MPA (0.3 mg + MPA, 1.5 mg)
Micronized estradiol (1 mg) + norethindrone, acetate (0.5 mg)
Micronized estradiol (1 mg) + 0.5 mg drosperinone
Ethinyl estradiol 5 μg, norethindrone, 1 mg

Transdermal
Patch, 0.05 mg estradiol with 140 μg or 250 μg norethindrone acetate
Patch, 0.045 mg estradiol with levonorgestrel 0.05 mg

Androgens

Oral
Esterified estrogen and methyl testosterone (0.625/1/25 mg and 1.25/2.5 mg)

Transdermal
Patch, 150 μg/300 μg in development

Bisphosphonates

Alendronate, 5 and 10 mg daily; 35 and 70 mg weekly
Risedronate, 5 mg; 35 mg weekly
Ibandronate, 150 mg monthly
Etidronate, 200 mg (intermittent)

Selective estrogen receptor modulators

Raloxifene, 60 mg
Others for osteoporosis
Tibolone, 2.5 mg (not approved in the United States)
Human parathyroid hormone 1–34; 20 μg subcutaneously daily

CEE, conjugated equine estrogens; MPA, medroxyprogesterone acetate.

Table 42-12 Mean Serum Estradiol (E_2) and Estrone (E_1)

Estrogen Dose (mg)	Level (pg/mL) E_2	E_1
CEE (0.3)*	18	76
CEE (0.625)	39	153
CEE (1.25)	60	220
Micronized E_2 (1)	35	190
Micronized E_2 (2)	63	300
E_1 sulfate (0.625)	34	125
E_1 sulfate (1.25)	42	220

*Conjugated equine estrogen (CEE) contains biologically active estrogens other than E_2 and E_1.

(0.625 mg CEE or 1 mg micronized E_2). Standard ET doses are five or six times less than the amount of estrogen used in oral contraceptives.

Oral estrogens have a potent hepatic "first-pass" effect that results in the loss of approximately 30% of their activity with a single passage after oral administration. However, this results in stimulation of hepatic proteins and enzymes. Some of these changes are not particularly beneficial, for example, an increase in procoagulation factors and an increase in C-reactive protein, whereas other changes are beneficial (an increase in HDL-C and a decrease in fibrinogen and plasminogen activator inhibitor-1).

E_2 can be administered in patches, gels, and subcutaneously. These routes of administration are not subject to major hepatic effects as with oral therapy. Accordingly, there is no increase in C-reaction protein and minimal if any change in coagulation factors, but also only a minimal increase in HDL-C. Doses of patches are available from 0.014 mg to 0.1 mg, available for administration once or twice weekly. The new ultralow-dose patch of 0.014 mg/day has been marketed for osteoporosis prevention in older women and not for treating hot flushes. Matrix patches are preferable to the older alcohol-based preparations because there is less skin reaction and estrogen delivery is more reliable. Whereas levels of E_2 with oral therapy may vary widely between women and within the day (peaks and valleys) levels with transdermal therapy are more constant within each woman, yet values achieved may vary from woman to woman based on absorption and metabolic characteristics. With the 0.05-mg patch, E_2 levels should be in the 40 to 50-pg/mL range, but an occasional woman can have values as high as 200 pg/mL. Note also that many commercial essays for E_2 are not very reliable.

In women with vulvovaginal or urinary complaints, vaginal therapy is most appropriate. Creams of E_2 or CEE are available, as well as tablets and an estrogen ring. With creams, systemic absorption occurs but with levels that are one fourth of that achieved after similar doses administered orally. Absorption decreases as the mucosa becomes more estrogenized. For CEE, only 0.5 g (0.3 mg) or less is necessary; for micronized E_2, doses as low as 0.25 mg are sufficient. Other products (tablets and rings) are available that have been designed to limit systemic absorption. A Silastic ring is available that delivers E_2 to the vagina for 3 months with only minimal systemic absorption.

Estrogen may be administered continuously (daily) or for 21 to 26 days each month. If the woman has a uterus, a progestogen should be added to the regimen (see Table 42-2). For women who are totally intolerant of progestogens (regardless of the dose and route of administration) and take unopposed estrogen, even at lower doses, periodic endometrial sampling is necessary. In this setting endometrial thickness by ultrasound may be a guide.

Use of a Progestogen

There are many ways to administer progestogens. The most commonly used oral progestins are MPA in doses of 2.5 and 5 to 10 mg, NET in doses of 0.3 to 1 mg, and micronized progesterone in doses of 100 to 300 mg. Equivalent doses to prevent hyperplasia when administered for at least 10 days in a woman receiving ET (equivalent to 0.625 mg CEE) are as follows: MPA, 5 mg; NET, 0.35 mg; and micronized progesterone, 200 mg. Larger doses of estrogen may require larger doses and more prolonged regimes of progestins. In the sequential administration of progestogens, the number of days (length of exposure) is more important than the dose. Thus, if a woman is receiving oral ET continuously, a regimen of at least 10 to 12 days exposure is preferable to a 7-day regimen.

When progestogens are administered sequentially (10 to 14 days each month), withdrawal bleeding occurs in about 80% of women. Continuous administration of both estrogen and progestogen (continuous combined therapy) was developed to achieve amenorrhea. In the first 3 to 6 months, breakthrough bleeding and spotting is common. In some women on this regimen, amenorrhea is never completely achieved. The most common combinations in the United States are single tablets containing 0.45 or 0.625 mg CEE with 1.5 and 2.5 mg of MPA, respectively; 5 μg of E_2 with 1 mg NET and 1 mg micronized E_2 with 0.5 mg NET. A patch with E_2 and NET or E_2 and levonorgestrel is also available.

Progesterone administered vaginally (in low doses) avoids systemic effects and results in high concentrations of progesterone in the uterus. This can be accomplished with capsules, suppositories, or a 4% gel. Intrauterine delivery of progestogens is ideal for targeting the uterus and minimizing systemic effects. However, the only marketed product, the 20-μg Mirena IUS delivers too high a dose of levonorgestrel for lower dose estrogen therapy, and the 10-μg system is not available.

Progestogens, particularly when taken orally, may lead to problems of continuance or compliance because of adverse effects, including mood alterations and bleeding. This requires flexibility in prescribing habits. Most short-term clinical trials have demonstrated an attenuating effect of progestogens on cardiovascular endpoints that are improved with estrogen; these effects include lipoprotein changes (an attenuation of the rise in HDL-C) and arterial and metabolic effects. A reduction in blood flow and some brain effects may also be found. As noted earlier, it is most likely progestogen exposure that increases the risk of breast cancer with HT. Progestogens should not be used in women who have had a hysterectomy.

Androgen Therapy

In a very subtle way, some women are relatively androgen-deficient. Clinicians have proposed adding androgen to ET or HT for complaints or problems relating to libido and energy, which are not relieved by adequate estrogen. Although well-controlled trials using parenteral testosterone have shown benefit in younger oophorectomized women, there have been few data showing benefit using more physiologic therapy, until recently. Recent data using a testosterone patch or pellet (with near physiologic levels) have shown improvement in several scales of well-being and sexual function. An oral preparation (esterified estrogens 0.625 mg with 1.25 mg of methyl testosterone) was shown to improve sexual motivation and enjoyment in women with hypoactive sexual desire who were unresponsive to estrogen alone. The latter findings correlated with an increase in circulating unbound testosterone levels. As newer forms and doses of androgen become available, perhaps more women may benefit from this approach. At present, androgen therapy should be individualized and considered for those women who have symptoms that are not adequately relieved with traditional hormonal therapies. It is important to note that there are no approved products for androgen therapy in the United States.

At lower doses, androgenizing side effects are very infrequent. At present, small doses of methyltestosterone (1.25 and 2.5 mg) added to esterified estrogens are available in tablets, which only have the indication of relief of vasomotor symptoms. As testosterone patches are only available for men, as are gels and creams, considerable dose titration needs to be considered in administering testosterone to women. Administration of dehydroepiandrosterone at 25 to 50 mg/day may also be an option for raising endogenous testosterone.

Another SERM-like compound that is used worldwide but is not yet approved in the United States if tibolone. This progestogen-like compound exhibits estrogenic, antiestrogenic, and androgenic effects by virtue of its structure and metabolites. At 2.5 mg, tibolone suppresses hot flushes, prevents osteoporosis, and has a positive effect on mood and sexual function. There is also very limited (or no) uterine stimulation. However, there is suppression of HDL-C, but at the same time a decrease in triglycerides. In the monkey, there is no deleterious effect of tibolone on coronary arteries.

ALTERNATIVE THERAPIES FOR MENOPAUSE

Phytoestrogens

Phytoestrogens are a class of plant-derived estrogen-like compounds conjugated to glycoside moieties. Phytoestrogens are not biologically active in their native forms unless taken orally. After oral ingestion, colonic bacteria cleave the glycosides, producing active compounds that are subject to the enterohepatic circulation These compounds can produce estrogen-agonistic effects in some tissues, whereas in other tissues they produce antagonistic effects.

Few randomized trials have examined the efficacy of phytoestrogens. For large daily doses (60 mg isoflavone) there appears to be some limited efficacy in relieving hot flushes although the literature on this issue is mixed in placebo-controlled trials. With doses of 30 to 40 mg. cholesterol levels may be reduced, but this is not a consistent finding. It should be noted that there is an important reduction in hot flushes with any placebo treatment. Phytoestrogens do not appear to have much of an effect on bone loss or on vaginal atrophy.

Estimates are that between 30% and 60% of women use so-called alternative interventions for the symptoms of menopause, including "natural" estrogens, plant estrogens, herbal medicines, and acupuncture. Botanicals, herbals, and many steroid products are sold over the counter, and some do in fact exert significant hormonal activity. The use of botanicals to alleviate the symptoms of menopause is extremely popular. This popularity is fostered by the notion that plant sterols might provide all the benefits of estrogen replacement therapy without the risks. However, most plant products recommended for menopause have performed poorly in clinical trials. The Dietary Supplement Health and Education Act of 1994 classifies most botanical medicines as food supplements and removes them from regulatory oversight and scrutiny by the U.S. Food and Drug Administration (FDA). Adulteration, contamination, and poor quality control in their harvesting, manufacture, and formulation yield products of questionable efficacy and safety.

The FDA has determined that more than 25% of Chinese patent medicines are adulterated with hidden pharmaceutical drugs. These kinds of deficiencies make it difficult for consumers and practitioners to employ botanicals with confidence and security. Furthermore, clinical trial data obtained using one brand of herbal product cannot necessarily be extrapolated to other brands using the same plant. DHEA is marketed as a dietary supplement for a variety of purported benefits. There are no data in women to support its role in well-being or immune function. As an androgen, DHEA is converted to androstenedione and testosterone. Doses of 25 to 50 mg raised testosterone and has been mentioned as an option for androgen therapy. However, these doses can reduce HDL-C levels.

KEY POINTS

- The median age of the onset of perimenopause is 47.5 years, and its median length is about 4 years.
- The initial endocrinologic change signaling the onset of menopause is decreased ovarian inhibin production accompanied by an increase in pituitary FSH release.
- Ovarian estradiol secretion does not begin to significantly diminish until 6 months to 1 year before the menopause.
- There is only a slight decrease in circulating testosterone and androstenedione levels immediately postmenopausally, and between 3 and 8 years postmenopausally levels of these two hormones remain relatively constant.
- Measurement of FSH cannot be used to determine the physiologic amount of estrogen replacement needed.
- Postmenopausally there is an increase in body weight and total body fat that is unaffected by estrogen administration.
- Postmenopausally there is a distribution of fat from peripheral sites to the abdomen. This change of fat distribution is prevented by exogenous estrogen.

Continued

KEY POINTS *Continued*

- About 50% of postmenopausal women experience hot flushes, and the incidence decreases to 20% 4 years after menopause
- Estrogen is the best therapy for the hot flush; other effective therapies are progestogens, SSRIs, gabapentin, and clonidine.
- Physiologic replacement doses of estrogen include 0.625 mg of conjugated equine estrogen and estrone sulfate, 1 mg of micronized estradiol, and transdermal administration of 0.05 mg of estradiol daily. Current practice suggests using lower than these doses for initial therapy.
- According to observational data, exogenous estrogen reduces the overall death rate in postmenopausal women, mainly because of the reduction in risk of death from cardiovascular disease, the major cause of death among women.
- Estrogen and estrogen/progestogen therapy has been shown to increase the risk of venous thrombosis.
- Estrogen plus progestogen may increase the risk of breast cancer.
- Survival rates of breast cancer have been shown in most studies to be greater among women who have this disease diagnosed while taking estrogen therapy than among age-matched controls who are not taking estrogen therapy.
- Estrogen therapy does not further increase the risk of diagnosis of breast cancer in women with a family history of breast cancer compared with that of nonusers.
- Estrogen and estrogen/progestogen therapy appears to reduce the risk of colon cancer and has no effect on the risk of ovarian cancer.
- If sonographic measurement of the endometrial echo complex (thickness) is 4 mm or less, the chance of endometrial cancer being present is about 0.25%.
- Contraindications to estrogen include the presence of breast or endometrial cancer, active thrombophlebitis, and undiagnosed abnormal bleeding.
- The mean age of menopause is about 51 years.
- Age at menopause is genetically predetermined and is not related to the number of ovulations, race, socioeconomic conditions, education, height, weight, age at menarche, or age at last pregnancy.
- The basic feature of menopause is depletion of ovarian follicles with degeneration of the granulosa and theca cells while stromal cells continue to produce the androgens androstenedione and testosterone.
- Androstenedione is converted to estrone in the peripheral body fat, and its rate of conversion increases as women age. Obese postmenopausal women have higher levels of estrone than thin women and are less likely to have hot flushes or osteoporosis and more likely to develop endometrial cancer.
- About 1% to 1.5% of bone mass is lost each year after menopause in nonobese white and Asian women. Fractures begin to occur about age 60 to 65 in trabecular bone, such as the vertebral spine, and by age 60, 25% of these women develop spinal compression fractures. Hip fractures begin to increase after age 70.
- By age 80, 20% of all white women will develop hip fractures, and 15% of these fractures are fatal within 6 months. In the United States each year osteoporosis causes about 300,000 hip fractures, 100,000 radius fractures, and 400,000 other fractures.
- Women with postmenopausal osteoporosis have a higher bone resorption rate than normal, whereas the rate of bone formation with osteoporosis is normal.
- In terms of equivalent weight, when an increase in liver globulins is used as the parameter of estrogenic activity, ethinyl estradiol is about 90 times as potent as conjugated equine estrogen.
- Levels of LDL cholesterol have a positive correlation with coronary heart disease, and levels of HDL cholesterol have an inverse relation to coronary heart disease. Postmenopausal estrogen users have decreased levels of LDL cholesterol as well as increased levels of HDL cholesterol compared with postmenopausal nonestrogen users.
- The risk of developing endometrial cancer is 2 to 10 times greater in postmenopausal women who are ingesting estrogen without progestogens compared with nonestrogen users. The risk is increased with higher dosages and prolonged use of estrogen and can be reduced below the incidence in nonusers by the addition of continuous progestogens.
- Estrogen increases the synthesis of both estrogen and progesterone receptors in the endometrium; progesterone and synthetic progestins decrease the synthesis of both these receptors and thus have an antimitotic, antiproliferative action.
- Indications for estrogen therapy in menopause include the presence of vasomotor symptoms as well as prevention of atrophic vaginitis, atrophic urethritis, and osteoporosis.
- Before estrogen therapy is instituted, a pretreatment mammogram should be performed and repeated annually thereafter.
- At least 25% of bone needs to be lost before osteoporosis can be diagnosed by routine radiographic examination.
- Dual-energy X-ray absorptiometry (DEXA) is the most accurate method to measure bone density. The bone mineral density is usually expressed as T scores and Z scores.
- Bone mass measurements are indicated only when clinical decisions will be influenced by the information gained.
- In addition to estrogen, alendronate, risendronate, ibandronate, raloxifene, and calcitonin will reduce postmenopausal bone loss.
- Postmenopausal oral estrogen use increases the risk of gallbladder disease.
- Addition of a progestogen to estrogen does not inhibit the beneficial effect of estrogen on reducing the rate of bone reabsorption.
- Estrogen increases calcium absorption and reduces the rate of bone reabsorption postmenopausally. It does not stimulate bone formation.
- In young women several small studies have shown that estrogen retards the development of coronary atherosclerosis.

KEY POINTS *Continued*

- The endometrial cancer that develops among estrogen users is usually well differentiated and nearly always cured by hysterectomy.
- Estrogen without a progestogen is recommended for postmenopausal women who have had a hysterectomy.
- Progestogens can be given cyclically or continuously with estrogen to reduce the risk of endometrial cancer. When given cyclically about 80% of women have regular withdrawal bleeding. When given continuously most women bleed during the first 6 months but become amenorrheic after 1 year.
- Most herbal products have not been shown to decrease menopausal symptoms.
- Soy extracts help prevent hot flushes to a variable degree but have no effect on the vaginal epithelium or bone.

BIBLIOGRAPHY

Abel TW, Voytko ML, Rance NE: The effects of hormone replacement therapy on hypothalamic neuropeptide gene expression in a primate model of menopause J Clin Endocrinol Metab 84:2111, 1999.

Adami S, Zamberlan N, Mian M, et al: Duration of the effects of intravenous alendronate in postmenopausal women and in patients with primary hyperparathyroidism and Paget's disease of bone. Bone Miner 25:75, 1994.

Adams MR, Register TC, Golden DL, et al: Medroxyprogesterone acetate antagonizes inhibitory effects of conjugated equine estrogens on coronary artery atherosclerosis. Arterioscler Thromb Vasc Biol 17:217, 1997.

Aiman J, Smentek C: Premature ovarian failure. Obstet Gynecol 66:9, 1985.

Aittomaki K, Lucena JLD, Pakarinen P, et al: Mutation in the follicle-stimulating hormone receptor gene causes hereditary hypergonadotropic ovarian failure. Cell 82:959, 1995.

Alexander KP, Newby LK, Hellkamp AS, et al: Initiation of hormone replacement therapy after acute myocardial infarction is associated with more cardiac events during follow up. J Am Coll Cardiol 38:1, 2001.

Alper MM, Garner PR, Cher B, et al: Premature ovarian failure. J Reprod Med 31:699, 1986.

Alper MM, Jolly EE, Garner PB: Pregnancies after premature ovarian failure. Obstet Gynecol 67:595, 1986.

Alvarado G, Rivera R, Ruix R, et al: Characteristicas del; patron de sangrado menstrual; en un grupo de mujeres normales de Durango. Ginecol Obstet Mex 56:127, 1998.

Amaducci LA, Henderson AS, Creasey H, et al: Risk factors for clinically diagnosed Alzheimer's disease: A case-control study of an Italian population. Neurology 36:922, 1986.

Anderson GL, Chlebowdki RT, Rossouw JE, Rodabough RJ, et al: Prior hormone therapy and breast cancer risk in the Women's Health Initiative randomized trial of estrogen plus progestin. Maturitas 55(2):103, 2006.

Andreyko JL, Monroe SE, Marshall LA, et al: Concordant suppression of serum immunoreactive luteinizing hormone (LH), follicle-stimulating hormone, alpha subunit, bioactive LH, and testosterone in postmenopausal women by a potent gonadotropin releasing hormone antagonist (detirelix). J Clin Endocrinol Metab 74:399, 1992.

Arif S, Vallian S, Farazneh F, et al: Identification of 3 beta-hydroxysteroid dehydrogenase as novel target of steroid-producing cell autoantibodies: Association of autoantibodies with endocrine autoimmune disease. J Clin Endocrinol Metab 81:4439, 1996.

Arisawa M, De Palatis L, Ho R, et al: Stimulatory role of substance P on gonadotropin release in ovariectomized rats. Neuroendocrinology 51:523, 1990.

Ash P: The influence of radiation on fertility in man. Br J Radiol 1980; 53:271-278.

Ashcroft GS, Dodsworth J, van Boxtel E, et al: Estrogen accelerates cutaneous wound healing associated with an increase in TGF-beta 1 levels. Nat Med 3:1209, 1997.

Ashcroft GS, Greenwell-Wild T, Horan MA, et al: Topical estrogen accelerates cutaneous wound healing in aged humans associated with an altered inflammatory response. Am J Pathol 155:1137, 1997.

Bachmann G, Bancroft J, Braunstein G, et al: Female androgen insufficiency: The Princeton consensus statement on definition, classification, and assessment. Fertil Steril 77:660, 2002.

Baird DD, Tylavsky FA, Anderson JJB: Do vegetarians have earlier menopause? Proc Soc Epidemiol Res 128:907, 1988.

Baldereschi M, Di Carlo A, Lepore V, et al: Estrogen-replacement therapy and Alzheimer's disease in the Italian Longitudinal Study on Aging. Neurology 50:996, 1998.

Barlow DH, Samsioe G, van Geelen JM: A study of European women's experience of the problems of urogenital ageing and its management. Maturitas 27:239, 1997.

Bateman BG, Nunley WC, Kitchin JD III: Reversal of apparent premature ovarian failure in a patient with myasthenia gravis. Fertil Steril 39:108, 1983.

Beall CM: Ages at menopause and menarche in a high altitude Himalayan population. Ann Hum Biol 10:365, 1983.

Best NR, Rees MP, Barlow DH, Cowen PJ: Effect of estradiol implant on noradrenergic function and mood in menopausal subjects. Psychoneuroendocrinology 17:87, 1992.

Beyene Y: Cultural significance and physiological manifestations of menopause, a bicultural analysis. Cult Med Psychol 10:47, 1986.

Bigleri EG, Herron MA, Brust N: 17-Hydroxylation deficiency in man. J Clin Invest 45:1946, 1996.

Bilezikian JP, Morishima A, Bell J, Grumbach MM: Increased bone mass as a result of estrogen therapy in a man with aromatase deficiency. N Engl J Med 339:599, 1998.

Bjarnason NH, Bjarnason K, Haarbo J, et al: Tibolone: Prevention of bone loss in late postmenopausal women. J Clin Endocrinol Metab 81:2419, 1996.

Bjorses P, Aaltonen J, Horelli-Kuitunen N, et al: Gene defect behind APECED: A new clue to autoimmunity. Hum Mol Genet 7:1547, 1998.

Bord S, Horner A, Beavan S, Compston J: Estrogen receptors alpha and beta are differentially expressed in developing human bone. Endocrinology 86:2309, 2001.

Braidman I, Baris C, Wood L, et al: Preliminary evidence for impaired estrogen receptor-a protein expression in osteoblasts and osteocytes from men with idiopathic osteoporosis. Bone 26:423, 2000.

Brenner DE, Kukull WA, Stergachis A, et al: Postmenopausal estrogen replacement therapy and the risk of Alzheimer's disease: A population-based case-control study. Am J Epidemiol 140:262, 1994.

Brincat M, Kabalan S, Studd JWW, et al: A study of the relationship of skin collagen content, skin thickness and bone mass in the postmenopausal woman. Obstet Gynecol 70:840, 1987.

Brincat M, Moniz CJ, Studd JWW, et al: Sex hormones and skin collagen content in postmenopausal women. Br Med J 287:1337, 1983.

Brincat M, Moniz CJ, Studd JWW, et al: Long term effects of the menopause and sex hormones on skin thickness. Br J Obstet Gynaecol 92:256, 1985.

Broe GA, Henerson AS, Creasy H, et al: A case-control study of Alzheimer's disease in Australia. Neurology 40:1698, 1990.

Bromberger JT, Matthews KA, Kuller LH, et al: Prospective study of the determinants of age at menopause Am J Epidemiol 145:124, 1997.

Burger HG, Dudley EC, Cui J, et al: A prospective longitudinal study of serum testosterone, dehydroepiandrosterone sulfate, and sex hormone-binding globulin levels through the menopause transition. J Clin Endocrinol Metab 85:2832, 2000.

Burger HG, Hailes J, Menelaus M: The management of persistent menopausal symptoms with oestradiol-testosterone implants: Clinical, lipid and hormonal results. Maturitas 6:351, 1984.

Campisi R, Nathan L, Pampaloni MH, et al: Noninvasive assessment of coronary microcirculatory function in postmenopausal women and effects of short-term and long-term estrogen administration. Circulation 105:425, 2002.

Carani C, Quin K, Simoni M, et al: Effect of testosterone and estradiol in a man with aromatase deficiency. N Engl J Med 337:91, 1997.

Cassidenti DL, Vijod AG, Vijod MA, et al: Short-term effects of smoking on the pharmacokinetic profiles of micronized estradiol in postmenopausal women. Am J Obstet Gynecol 163:1953, 1990.

Castelo-Branco C, Duran M, Gonzalez-Merlo J: Skin collagen changes related to age and hormone replacement therapy. Maturitas 15:113, 1992.

Chen C-L, Weiss NS, Newcomb P, et al: Hormone replacement therapy in relation to breast cancer. JAMA 287:734, 2002.

Chen WY, Manson JE, Hankinson SE, et al: The menstrual age and climacteric complaints in Thai women in Bangkok. Maturitas 17:63, 1993.

Civitelli R, Pilgram TK, Dotson M: Alveolar and postcranial bone density in postmenopausal women receiving hormone/estrogen replacement therapy. Arch Intern Med 162:1409, 2002.

Clarke SC, Kelleher J, Lloyd-Jones H, et al: A study of hormone replacement therapy in postmenopausal women with ischaemic heart disease: The Papworth HRT atherosclerosis study. Br J Obstet Gynaecol 109:1056, 2002.

Clarkson TB: The new conundrum: Do estrogens have any cardiovascular benefits? Int J Fertil 47:61, 2002.

Clarkson TB, Anthony MS, Jerome CP: Lack of effect of raloxifene on coronary artery atherosclerosis of postmenopausal monkeys. J Clin Endocrinol Metab 83:721, 1988.

Clarkson TB, Anthony MS, Morgan TM: Inhibition of postmenopausal atherosclerosis progression: A comparison of the effects of conjugated equine estrogens and soy phytoestrogens. J Clin Endocrinol Metab 86:41, 2001.

Clarkson TB, Anthony MS, Wagner JD: A comparison of tibolone and conjugated equine estrogens effects on coronary artery atherosclerosis and bone density of postmenopausal monkeys. J Clin Endocrinol Metab 86:5396, 2001.

Collaborative Group on Hormonal Factors in Breast Cancer Breast cancer and hormone replacement therapy: Collaborative analyses of data from 51 epidemiological studies of 52,705 women with breast cancer and 108,411 women without breast cancer. Lancet 350:1047, 1997.

Collins JA, Allen I, Donner A, Adams O: Oestrogen use and survival in endometrial cancer. Lancet 2:961, 1980.

Collins P, Rosano GMC, Sarrel PM, et al: Estradiol-17β attenuates acetylcholine-induced coronary arterial constriction in women but not men with coronary heart disease. Circulation 92:24, 1995.

Conway GS, Hettiarachchi S, Murray A, Jacobs PA: Fragile X permutations in familial premature ovarian failure. Lancet 346:309, 1995.

Cooper C, Campion G, Melton LJ: Hip fractures in the elderly: A world-wide projection. Osteoporosis Int 2:285, 1992.

Cooper GS, Sandler DP: Age at natural menopause and mortality. Ann Epidemiol 1998;8:229-235.

Coulam CB, Adamson SC, Annegers JF. Incidence of premature ovarian failure. Obstet Gynecol 67:604, 1986.

Coulam CB, Kempers RD, Randall RV: Premature ovarian failure: evidence for the autoimmune mechanism. Fertil Steril 36:238, 1981.

Coulam CB, Stringfellow SS, Hoefnagel D: Evidence for a genetic factor in the etiology of premature ovarian failure. Fertil Steril 40:693, 1983.

Couzinet B, Meduri G, Lecce MG, et al: The postmenopausal ovary is not a major androgen-producing gland. J Clin Endocrinol Metab 86:5060, 2001.

Coyle JT, Price DL, DeLong MR: Alzheimer's disease: A disorder of cortical cholinergic innervation. Science 219:1184, 1983.

Cummings SR, Black DM, Rubin SM: Lifetime risks of hip, Colles', or vertebral fracture and coronary heart disease among white postmenopausal women. Arch Intern Med 14:2445, 1989.

Cummings SR, Black DM, Thompson DE, et al: Effect of alendronate on risk of fracture in women with low bone density but without vertebral fractures: Results from the fracture intervention trial. JAMA 280:2077, 1998.

Damewood MD, Grochow LB: Prospects for fertility after chemotherapy or radiation for neoplastic disease. Fertil Steril 45:443, 1986.

Dawson-Hughes B, Harris SS, Krall EA, Dalla GE: Effect of calcium and vitamin D Supplementation on bone density in men and women 65 years of age or older. N Engl J Med 337:670, 1997.

De Baere E, Dixon MJ, Small KW, et al: Spectrum of FOXL2 gene mutations in blepharophimosis-ptosis-epicanthus inversus (BPES) families demonstrates a genotype–phenotype correlation. Hum Mol Genet 15:1591, 2001.

de Bruin JP, Bovenhuis H, van Noord PA, et al: The role of genetic factors in age at natural menopause Hum Reprod 16:2014, 2001.

de Moraes M, Jones GS: Premature ovarian failure. Fertil Steril 18:440, 1967.

Dennerstein L, Dudley EC, Hopper JL, et al: A prospective population-based study of menopausal symptoms. Obstet Gynecol 96:351, 2000.

Deutsch S, Ossowski R, Benjamin I: Comparison between degree of systemic absorption of vaginally and orally administered estrogens at different dose levels in postmenopausal women. Am J Obstet Gynecol 139:967, 1981.

Diokno AC, Brock BM, Brown MB, Herzog AR: Prevalence of urinary incontinence and other urological symptoms in the noninstitutionalized elderly. J Urol 136:1022, 1986.

Ditkoff EC, Crary WG, Cristo M, Lobo RA: Estrogen improves psychological function in asymptomatic postmenopausal women. Obstet Gynecol 78:991, 1991.

Dowsett M, Cantwel B, Lal A, et al: Suppression of postmenopausal ovarian steroidogenesis with the luteinizing hormone-releasing hormone agonist goserelin. J Clin Endocrinol Metab 66:672, 1988.

Dunn LB, Damesyn M, Moore AA, et al: Does estrogen prevent skin aging? Results from the First National Health and Nutrition Examination Survey (NHANESI). Arch Dermatol 133:339, 1997.

Eastell R, Hannon RA: Biochemical markers of bone turnover. In Lobo RA (ed): Treatment of the Postmenopausal Woman: Basic and Clinical Aspects, 2nd ed. Philadelphia, Lippincott Williams & Wilkins, 1999, pp 293–303.

Elia G, Bergman A: Estrogen effects on the urethra: Beneficial effects in women with genuine stress incontinence. Obstet Gynecol Surv 48:509, 1993.

Erdman JW Jr: Soy protein and cardiovascular disease: A statement for healthcare professionals from the Nutrition Committee of the AHA. Circulation 102:2555, 2000.

Ericksen EF, Colvard DS, Berg NJ, et al: Evidence of estrogen receptors in normal human osteoblast-like cells. Science 241:84, 1988.

Erickson GF: An analysis of follicle development and ovum maturation. Semin Reprod Endocrinol 4:233, 1986.

Erickson GF, Kokka S, Rivier C: Activin causes premature superovulation. Endocrinology 136:4804, 1995.

Erlik Y, Tataryn IV, Meldrum DR, et al: Association of waking episodes with menopausal hot flushes. JAMA 245:1741, 1981.

Ettinger B, Black DM, Mitlak BH, et al: Reduction of vertebral fracture risk in postmenopausal women with osteoporosis treated with raloxifene: Results from a 3-year randomized clinical trial. Multiple Outcomes of Raloxifene Evaluation (MORE) investigators. JAMA 282:637, 1999.

Ettinger B, Friedman GD, Bush T, Quesenberry CP Jr: Reduced mortality associated with long-term postmenopausal estrogen therapy. Obstet Gynecol 87:6, 1996.

Eye-Disease Case-Control Study Group: Risk factors for neovascular age-related macular degeneration. Arch Ophthalmol 110:1701, 1992.

Faddy MJ, Gosden RG, Gougeon A, et al: Accelerated disappearance of ovarian follicles in mid-life: Implications for forecasting menopause Hum Reprod 7:1342, 1992.

Falconer C, Ekman Orderberg G, Ulmasten U, et al: Changes in paraurethral connective tissue at menopause are counteracted by estrogen. Maturitas 24:197, 1996.

Fantl JA, Bump RC, Robinson D, et al: Efficacy of estrogen Supplementation in the treatment of urinary incontinence: The Continence Program for Women Research Group. Obstet Gynecol 88:745, 1996.

Fedor-Freybergh P: The influence of oestrogens on the well being and mental performance in climacteric and postmenopausal women. Acta Obstet Gynecol Scand 64(Suppl):1, 1977.

Feldman BM, Voda AM, Gronseth E: The prevalence of hot flash and associated variables among perimenopausal women. Res Nurs Health 8:261, 1985.

Ferguson DJP, Anderson TJ: Morphological evaluation of cell turnover in relation to menstrual cycle in the "resting" human breast. Br J Cancer 44:177, 1981.

Ficicioglu C, Kutlu T, Baglam E, Bakacak Z: Early follicular antimullerian hormone as an indicator of ovarian reserve. Fertil Steril 85(3):592, 2006.

Frost HM: The role of changes in mechanical usage set points in the pathogenesis of osteoporosis. J Bone Miner Res 7:253, 1992.

Frost HM: On rho, a marrow mediator, and estrogen: Their roles in bone strength and "mass" in human females, osteopenias, and osteoporosis—insights from a new paradigm. J Bone Miner Metab 16:113, 1998.

Frost HM: Perspective on the estrogen-bone relationship and postmenopausal bone loss. J Bone Miner Res 14:1473, 1999.

Ganger KF, Vyas S, Whitehead M, et al: Pulsatility index in internal carotid artery in relation to transdermal oestradiol and time since menopause Lancet 338:839, 1991.

Genazzani AR, Petraglia F, Facchinetti F, et al: Increase of proopiomelanocortin-related peptides during subjective menopausal flushes. Am J Obstet Gynecol 149:775, 1984.

Geusens P, Dequeker J, Gielen J, Schot LPC: Non-linear increase in vertebral density induced by a synthetic steroid (Org OD14) in women with established osteoporosis. Maturitas 13:155, 1991.

Gilligan DM, Quyyumi AA, Cannon RO III: Effects of physiological levels of estrogen on coronary vasomotor function in postmenopausal women. Circulation 89:2545, 1994.

Giustina A, Veldhuis JD: Pathophysiology of the neuroregulation of growth hormone secretion in experimental animals and the human. Endocr Rev 19:717, 1998.

Gold EB, Sternfeld B, Kelsey JL, et al: Relation of demographic and lifestyle factors to symptoms in a multi-racial/ethnic population of women 40-55 years of age. Am J Epidemiol 152:463, 2000.

Golditz GA, Hankinson SE, Hunter DJ, et al: The use of estrogen and progestins and the risk of breast cancer in postmenopausal women. N Engl J Med 332:1589, 1995.

Goldsmith O, Solomon DH, Horton R: Hypogonadism and mineralcorticoid excess. The 17-hydroxylayse deficiency syndrome. N Engl J Med 277:673, 1967.

Gonzalez GF, Villena A: Age at menopause in central Andean Peruvian women. Menopause 4:32, 1997.

Gougeon A, Ecochard R, Thalabard JC: Age-related changes of the population of human ovarian follicles: Increase in the disappearance rate of non growing and early growing follicles in aging women. Biol Reprod 50:653, 1994.

Grady D, Herrington D, Bittner V, et al: Cardiovascular disease outcomes during 6.8 years of hormone therapy: Heart and estrogen/progestin replacement study follow-up (HERS II). JAMA 288:49, 2002.

Graves AB, White E, Koepsell TD, et al: A case-control study of Alzheimer's disease. Ann Neurol 28:766, 1990.

Greendale G, Hogan P, Kritz-Silverstain D, et al: Age at menopause in women participating in the Postmenopausal Estrogen/Progestin Interventions (PEPI) trial: An example of bias introduced by selection criteria. Menopause 2:27, 1995.

Greendale GA, Reboussin BA, Sie A, et al: Effects of estrogen and estrogen-progestin on mammographic parencymal density: Postmenopausal Estrogen/Progestin Interventions (PEPI) investigators. Ann Intern Med 130:262, 1999.

Grimes DA, Lobo RA: Perspectives on the Women's Health Initiative trial of hormone replacement therapy. Obstet Gynecol 100:1344, 2002.

Grodstein F, Manson JE, Colditz GA: A possible observational study of postmenopausal hormone therapy and primary prevention of cardiovascular disease. Ann Intern Med 133:933, 2000.

Grodstein F, Manson JE, Stampfer MJ: Postmenopausal hormone use and secondary prevention of coronary events in the Nurses' Health Study. Ann Intern Med 135:1, 2001.

Grodstein F, Manson JE, Stampfer MJ: Hormone therapy and coronary heat disease: The role of time since menopause and age at hormone initiation. J Womens Health (Larchmont) 15(1):35, 2006.

Grodstein F, Stampfer MJ, Colditz GA, et al: Postmenopausal hormone therapy and mortality. N Engl J Med 336:1769, 1997.

Harper PS, Dyken PR: Early onset dystrophic myotonia. Lancet 2:53, 1972.

Harwood DG, Barker WW, Loewenstein DA, et al: A cross-ethnic analysis of risk factors for AD in white Hispanics and white non-Hispanics. Neurology 52:551, 1999.

Healy DL, Bacher J, Hodgen GD: Thymic regulation of primate fetal ovarian-adrenal differentiation. Biol Reprod 32:1127, 1985.

Heaney RP: Fluoride and osteoporosis. Ann Intern Med 120:689, 1994.

Heimer G, Samsioe G: Effects of vaginally delivered estrogens. Acta Obset Gynecol Scand 163(Suppl):1, 1996.

Henderson BE, Paganini-Hill A, Ross RK: Decreased mortality in users of estrogen replacement therapy. Arch Intern Med 151:75, 1991.

Henderson VW: Estrogen, cognition and a woman's risk of Alzheimer's disease. Am J Med 103:11, 1997.

Henderson VW, Paganini-Hill A, Emanuel CK, et al: Estrogen replacement therapy in older women: Comparisons between Alzheimer's disease cases and nondemented control subjects. Arch Neurol 51:896, 1994.

Herrington DM, Reboussin DM, Brosnihan KB, et al: Effects of estrogen replacement on the progression of coronary-artery atherosclerosis. N Engl J Med 343:522, 2000.

Herrington DM, Vittinghoff E, Lin F: Statin therapy, cardiovascular events and total mortality in the Heart and Estrogen/Progestin Replacement Study (HERS). Circulation 105:2962, 2002.

Heyman A, Wilkinson WE, Stafford JA, et al: Alzheimer's disease: A study of epidemiological aspects. Ann Neurol 15:335, 1984.

Hilton P, Stanton SL: The use of intravaginal estrogen cream in genuine stress incontinence: A double blind clinical trial. Urol Int 33:136, 1978.

Hilton P, Tweddel AL, Mayne C: Oral and intravaginal oestrogens alone and in combination with alpha adrenergic stimulation in genuine stress incontinence. Int Urogynecol J 12:80, 1990.

Hoefnagel D, Wurster–Hili D, Child EL: Ovarian failure in galactosemia. Lancet 2:1197, 1979.

Hoek A, Shoemaker J, Drexhage HA: Premature ovarian failure and ovarian autoimmunity. Endocr Rev 18:107, 1997.

Hofbauer LC, Khosla S, Dunstan CR, et al: The roles of osteoprotegerin and osteoprotegerin ligand in the paracrine regulation of bone resorption. J Bone Miner Res 15:2, 2000.

Holst J, Backstrom T, Hammarback S, von Schoultz B: Progestogen addition during oestrogen replacement therapy: Effects on vasomotor symptoms and mood. Maturitas 11:13, 1989.

Hsia J, Langer RD, Manson JE, et al: Conjugated equine estrogens and coronary heart disease: The Women's Health Initiative. Arch Intern Med 166(3):357, 2006.

Hughes EG, Robertson DM, Handelsman DJ, et al: Inhibin and estradiol responses to ovarian hyperstimulation: Effects of age and predictive value for in vitro fertilization outcome. J Clin Endocrinol Metab 70:358, 1990.

Hulley S, Grady D, Bush T, et al: Randomized trial of estrogen plus progestin for secondary prevention of coronary heart disease in postmenopausal women. JAMA 280:605, 1998.

Jacobs DM, Tang MX, Stern Y, et al: Cognitive function in nondemented older women who took estrogen after menopause. Neurology 50:368, 1998.

Jacobs PA: Fragile X syndrome. J Med Genet 28:809, 1991.

Kannel WB, Hjortland MC, McNamara PM, Gordon T: Menopause and the risk of cardiovascular disease. The Framingham study. Ann Intern Med 85:447, 1976.

Kasperk CH, Wergedak JE, Farley JR, et al: Androgens directly stimulate proliferation of bone cells in vitro. Endocrinology 124:1576, 1989.

Kaufman FR, Kogut MD, Donnell GN, et al: Hypergonadotropic hypogonadism in female patients with galactosemia. N Engl J Med 304:994, 1981.

Kawas C, Resnick S, Morrison A, et al: A prospective study of estrogen replacement therapy and the risk of developing Alzheimer's disease: The Baltimore Longitudinal Study of Aging. Neurology 48:1517, 1997.

Kinch RAH, Plunkett ER, Smout MS, Carr DH: Primary ovarian failure: A clinicopathological and cytogenetic study. Am J Obstet Gynecol 91:630, 1965.

King RJ, Whitehead JH: Assessment of the potency of orally administered progestins in women. Fertil Steril 46(6):1062, 1986.

Klaiber EL, Broverman DM, Vogel W, Kobayashi Y: Estrogen therapy for severe persistent depressions in women. Arch Gen Psychiatry 36:550, 1979.

Klaiber EL, Broverman DM, Vogel W, et al: Individual differences in changes in mood and platelet monoamine oxidase (MAO) activity during hormonal replacement therapy in menopausal women. Psychoneuro Endocrinol 21:575, 1996.

Klein NA, Battaglia DE, Clifton DK, et al: The gonadotropin secretion pattern in normal women of advanced reproductive age in relation to the monotropic FSH rise. J Soc Gynecol Invest 3:27, 1996.

Klein NA, Illingworth PJ, Groome NP, et al: Decreased inhibin B secretion is associated with the menotropic FSH rise in older, ovulatory women: a study of serum and follicular fluid levels of dimeric inhibin A and B in spontaneous menstrual cycles. J Clin Endocrinol Metab 81:2742, 1996.

Komm BS, Terpening CM, Benz DJ, et al: Estrogen binding receptor mRNA, and biologic response in osteoblast-like osteosarcoma cells. Science 241:81, 1988.

Krall EA, Dawson-Hughes B, Hannan MT, et al: Postmenopausal estrogen replacement and tooth retention. Am J Med 102:536, 1997.

Krauss CM, Turksoy RN, Atkins L, et al: Familial premature ovarian failure due to an interstitial deletion of the long arm of the X chromosome. N Engl J Med 317:125, 1987.

Kronenberg F. Hot flashes: Epidemiology and physiology. Ann N Y Acad Sci 592:52, 1990.

LaBarbera AR, Miller MM, Ober C, Rebar RW: Autoimmune etiology in premature ovarian failure. Am J Reprod Immunol Microbiol 16:115, 1988.

Lacey JV, Mink PJ, Lubin JH, et al: Menopausal hormone replacement therapy and risk of ovarian cancer. JAMA 288:368, 2002.

Laflamme N, Nappi R, Drolet G, et al: Expression and neuropeptidergic characterization of estrogen receptor (ER alpha and beta) throughout the rat brain: Anatomical evidence of district role of each subtype. J Neurobiol 36:357, 1998.

Lasley BL, Santoro N, Randolf JF, et al: The relationship of circulating dehydroepiandrosterone, testosterone, and estradiol to stages of the menopausal transition and ethnicity. J Clin Endocrinol Metab 87:3760, 2002.

LeBlanc ES, Janowsky J, Chan BK, Nelson HD: Hormone replacement therapy and cognition. Systematic review and meta-analysis. JAMA 285:1489, 2001.

Ledger WL, Thomas EJ, Browning D, et al: Suppression of gonadotropin secretion does not reverse premature ovarian failure. J Obstet Gynecol 96:196, 1989.

Li CL: Hormone replacement therapy in relation to risk of lobular and ductal breast carcinoma in middle-aged women. Cancer 88:2570, 2000.

Licciardi FL, Liu HC, Rosenwaks Z: Day 3 estradiol serum concentrations as prognosticators of ovarian stimulation response and pregnancy outcome in patients undergoing in vitro fertilization. Fertil Steril 64:991, 1995.

Lindheim SR, Legro RS, Bernstein L, et al: Behavioral stress responses in premenopausal and postmenopausal women and the effects of estrogen. Am J Obstet Gynecol 67:1831, 1992.

Lindheim SR, Presser SC, Ditkoff EC, et al: A possible bimodal effect of estrogen on insulin sensitivity in postmenopausal women and the attenuating effect of added progestin. Fertil Steril 60:664, 1993.

Lindsay R, Gallagher JC, Kooper M, Pickar JH: Effect of lower doses of conjugated equine estrogen with and without medroxyprogesterone acetate on bone in early postmenopausal women. JAMA 287:2668, 2002.

Lindsay R, Nieves J, Formica C, et al: Randomized controlled study of effect of parathyroid hormone on vertebral-bone mass and fracture incidence among postmenopausal women on oestrogen with osteoporosis. Lancet 350:550, 1997.

Lobo RA: Clinical aspects of hormonal replacement—Routes of administration. In Lobo RA (ed): Treatment of Postmenopausal Women: Basic and Clinical Aspects, 2nd ed. Philadelphia, Lippincott Williams & Wilkins, 1999, pp 125–139.

Lobo RA: Treatment of the postmenopausal woman: where we are today. In Lobo RA (ed): Treatment of Postmenopausal Women: Basic and Clinical Aspects, 2nd ed. Philadelphia, Lippincott Williams & Wilkins, 1999, pp 655–659.

Lobo RA: Progestogens. In Lobo RA, Kelsey J, Marcus R (eds): Menopause: Biology and Pathobiology. New York, Academic Press, 2000, pp 429–458.

Lobo RA: Androgens in postmenopausal women: Production, possible role and replacement options (CME review article). Obstet Gynecol Surv 56:361, 2001.

Lobo RA: Evaluation of cardiovascular event rates with hormone therapy in healthy postmenopausal women: Results from four large clinical trials. Arch Intern Med 164:482, 2004.

Lobo RA, Whitehead M: Is low-dose hormone replacement for postmenopausal women efficacious and desirable? Climacteric 4:110, 2001.

Lobo RA, Brenner P, Mishell DR Jr: Metabolic parameters and steroid levels in postmenopausal women receiving lower doses of natural estrogen replacement. Obstet Gynecol 62:94, 1983.

Lobo RA, Rosen RC, Yang H-M, et al: Comparative effects of oral esterified estrogens with and without methyltestosterone on endocrine profiles and dimensions of sexual function in postmenopausal women with hypoactive sexual desire. Fertil Steril 79:1341, 2002.

Lu LJ, Tice JA, Bellino FL: Phytoestrogens and healthy aging: Gaps in knowledge (a workshop report). Menopause 8:157, 2001.

Lucky AW, Rebar RW, Blizzard RM, Goren EM: Pubertal progression in the presence of elevated serum gonadotropins in girls with multiple endocrine deficiencies. J Clin Endocrinol Metab 45:673, 1977.

Luoto R, Laprio J, Uutela A: Age at natural menopause and sociodemographic status in Finland. Am J Epidemiol 139:64, 1994.

MacLusky N, Naftolin F: Sexual differentiation of central nervous system. Science 211:1294, 1981.

Magnusson C, Baron JA, Correira N, et al: Breast cancer risk following long term oestrogen and oestrogen-progestin replacement therapy. Int J Cancer 31:339, 1999.

Maki PM, Resnick SM: Longitudinal effects of estrogen replacement therapy on PET cerebral blood flow and cognition. Neurobiol Aging 21:373, 2000.

Maki PM, Zonderman AB, Resnick SM: Enhanced verbal memory in nondemented elderly estrogen users. Am J Psychiatry 158:227, 2001.

Mallin SR: Congenital adrenal hyperplasia secondary to 17-hydroxylase deficiency: Two sisters with amenorrhea, hypokalemia, hypertension and cystic ovaries. Ann Intern Med 70:69, 1969.

Mandel FP, Geola FL, Meldrum DR, et al: Biological effects of various doses of vaginally administered conjugated equine estrogens in postmenopausal women. J Clin Endocrinol Metab 57:133, 1983.

Manolagas SC: Birth and death of bone cells: basic regulatory mechanisms and implications for the pathogenesis and treatment of osteoporosis. Endocr Rev 21:115, 2000.

Mashchak CA, Lobo RA, Dozono-Takano R, et al: Comparison of pharmacodynamic properties of various estrogen formulations. Am J Obstet Gynecol 144:511, 1982.

Matthews KA, Meilahn E, Kuller LH, et al: Menopause and risk factors for coronary heart disease. N Engl J Med 321:641, 1989.

Mattison DR, Evans MI, Schwimmer WB, et al: Familial premature ovarian failure. Am J Hum Genet 36:1341, 1984.

McCrohon JA, Walters WA, Robinson JT, et al: Arterial reactivity is enhanced in genetic males taking high dose estrogens. J Am Coll Cardiol 29:1437, 1997.

Meldrum DR, Tataryn IV, Frumar AM, et al: Gonadotropins, estrogens, and adrenal steroids during the menopausal hot flash. J Clin Endocrinol Metab 50:685, 1980.

Melton LJ, Chrischilles EA, Cooper C, et al: Perspective: How many women have osteoporosis? J Bone Miner Res 7:1005, 1992.

Mendelsohn ME: Nongenomic, estrogen receptor-mediated activation of endothelial nitric oxide synthase. How does it work? What does it mean? Circ Res 87:956, 2000.

Mendelsohn ME, Karas RH: The protective effects of estrogen on the cardiovascular system. N Engl J Med 340:1801, 1999.

Miller J, Chan BK, Nelson HD: Postmenopausal estrogen replacement and risk for venous thromboembolism: A systematic review and meta-analysis for the U.S. Preventive Services Task Force. Ann Intern Med 136:680, 2002.

Million Women Study Collaboration: Breast cancer and hormone-replacement therapy in the Million Women Study. Lancet 362:419, 2003.

Montgomery JC, Appleby L, Brincat M, et al: Effect of oestrogen and testosterone implants on psychological disorders in the climacteric. Lancet 1:297, 1987.

Morales AJ, Nolan JJ, Nelson JC: Effects of replacement dose of dehydroepiandrosterone in men and women of advancing age. J Clin Endocrinol Metab 78:1360, 1994.

Morishima A, Grumbach MM, Simpson ER, et al: Aromatase deficiency in male and female siblings caused by a novel mutation and the physiological role of estrogens. J Clin Endocrinol Metab 80:3689, 1995.

Morrison JC, Givens JR, Wiser WL, Fisk SA: Mumps oophoritis: A cause of premature menopause Fertil Steril 26:655, 1975.

Mortel KF, Meyer JS: Lack of postmenopausal estrogen replacement therapy and the risk of dementia. J Neuropsychiatry Clin Neurosci. 1995;7:334–337.

Mosca L, Collins P, Herrington DM, et al: Hormone replacement therapy and cardiovascular disease: A statement for healthcare professionals from American Heart Association. Circulation 104:499, 2001.

Mulnard RA, Cotman CW, Kawas C, et al: Estrogen replacement therapy for treatment of mild to moderate Alzheimer disease: A randomized controlled trial. Alzheimer's Disease Cooperative Study. JAMA 283:1007, 2000.

Nelson HD: Assessing benefit and harms of hormone replacement therapy: Clinical applications. JAMA 288:882, 2002.

Nguyen TV, Blangero J, Eisman JA: Genetic epidemiological approaches to the search for osteoporosis genes. J Bone Miner Res 15:392, 2000.

Notelovitz M, Ware M: Coagulation risks with postmenopausal oestrogen therapy. In Studd J (ed): Progress in Obstetrics and Gynecology. Edinburgh, Churchill Livingston, 1982.

Oldenhave A, Jaszmann LJ, Haspels AA, Everaerd WT: Impact of climacteric on well-being. A study based on 5213 women 39 to 60 years old. Am J Obstet Gynecol 168:772, 1993.

Oursler MJ, Cortese C, Keeting PE, et al: Modulation of transforming growth factor beta production in normal human osteoblast-like cells by 17 beta estradiol and parathyroid hormone. Endocrinology 129:3313, 1991.

Oursler MJ, Osdoby P, Pyfferoen J, et al: Avian osteoclasts as estrogen target cells. Proc Natl Acad Sci USA 88:6613, 1991.

Oursler MJ, Pederson L, Fitzpatrick L, Riggs BL: Human giant cell tumors of the bone (osteoclastomas) are estrogen target cells. Proc Natl Acad Sci USA 91:5227, 1994.

Overgaard K, Hansen MA, Jensen SB: Effects of salcatonin given intranasally on bone mass and fracture rates in established osteoporosis: a dose-response study. Br Med J 305:556, 1992.

Pacifici R: Estrogen, cytokines, and pathogenesis of postmenopausal osteoporosis. J Bone Miner Res 11:1043, 1996.

Paganini-Hill A, Henderson VW: Estrogen deficiency and risk of Alzheimer's disease in women. Am J Epidemiol 140:256, 1994.

Paganini-Hill A, Henderson VW: Estrogen replacement therapy and risk of Alzheimer's disease. Arch Intern Med 156:2213, 1996.

Paganini-Hill A, Chao A, Ross RK, Henderson BE: Exercise and other factors in the prevention of hip fracture: the Leisure World study. Epidemiology 2:16, 1991.

Pak CYC, Sakhaee K, Adams-Huet B, et al: Treatment of postmenopausal osteoporosis with slow-release sodium fluoride: Final report of a randomized controlled trial. Ann Intern Med 23:401, 1995.

PEPI Trial Writing Group: Effects of hormone replacement therapy on endometrial histology in postmenopausal women. JAMA 275:370, 1996.

Phillips KA, Glendon G, Knight JA: Putting the risk of breast cancer in perspective. N Engl J Med 340:141, 1999.

Pines A, Fisman EZ, Drory Y, et al: Menopause-induced changes in Doppler-derived parameters of aortic flow in healthy women. Am J Cardiol 69:1104, 1992.

Post WS, Goldschmidt-Clermont PJ: Methylation of the estrogen receptor gene is associated with aging and atherosclerosis in the cardiovascular system. Cardiovasc Res 43:985, 1999.

Proudler AJ, Hasib Ahmed AJ, Crook D, et al: Hormone replacement therapy and serum angiotensin-converting-enzyme activity in postmenopausal women. Lancet 346:89, 1995.

Punnonen R: Effect of castration and peroral therapy on skin. Acta Obstet Gynaecol Scand 21(Suppl):1, 1973.

Rabinowe SL, Berger MJ, Welch WR, et al: Lymphocyte dysfunction in autoimmune oophoritis: Resumption of menses with corticosteroids. Am J Obstet Gynecol 81:348, 1986.

Ramoso-Jalbuena J: Climacteric Filipino women: A preliminary survey in the Philippines. Maturitas 19:183, 1994.

Rance NE, Uswandi SV: Gonadotropin-releasing hormone gene expression is increased in the medial basal hypothalamus of postmenopausal women. J Clin Endocrinol Metab 81:3540, 1996.

Rance NE, Young WS: Hypertrophy and increased gene expression of neurons containing neurokinin-B and substance-P messenger ribonucleic acids in the hypothalami of postmenopausal women. Endocrinology 128:2239, 1991.

Rance NE, Young WS, McMullen NT: Topography of neurons expressing luteinizing hormone-releasing hormone gene transcripts in the human hypothalamus and basal forebrain. J Comp Neurol 339:573, 1994.

Rannevik G, Jeppsson S, Johnell O, et al: A longitudinal study of the perimenopausal transition: Altered profiles of steroid and pituitary hormones-SHBG and bone mineral density. Maturitas 21:103, 1995.

Ray GR, Trueblood HW, Enright LP, et al: Oophoropexy: A means of preserving ovarian function following pelvic megavoltage radiotherapy for Hodgkin's disease. Radiology 96:175, 1970.

Ray NF, Chan JK, Thamer M, Melton LJ: Medical expenditures for the treatment of osteoporotic fractures in the United States in 1995: Report from the National Osteoporosis Foundation. J Bone Miner Res 12:24, 1997.

Raz R, Stamm WE: A controlled trial of intravaginal estriol in postmenopausal women with recurrent urinary tract infections. N Engl J Med 329:753, 1993.

Reame N, Luckas J, Ansbacher R, et al: The hypothalamic GnRH pulse generator is altered in ovulatory, premenopausal women: Evidence from 24 hr pulsatile LH studies. Fertil Steril 255:S97, 2002.

Reame NE, Wyman TL, Phillips DJ, et al: Net increase in stimulatory input resulting from a decrease in inhibin B and an increase in activin A may contribute in part to the rise in follicular phase follicle-stimulating of hormone of aging cyclic women. J Clin Endocrinol Metab 83:3302, 1998.

Rebar RW: Premature ovarian failure. In Lobo RA, Kelsey J, Marcus R (eds): Menopause—Biology and Pathobiology. New York, Academic Press, 2000, pp 135–146.

Rebar RW, Erickson GF, Coulam CB: Premature ovarian failure. In Gondos B, Riddick D (eds): Pathology of Infertility. New York, Thieme, 1987, pp 123–141.

Reis SE, Gloth ST, Blumenthal RS, et al: Ethinyl estradiol acutely attenuates abnormal coronary vasomotor responses to acetylcholine in postmenopausal women. Circulation 89:52, 1994.

Resnick SM, Makii PM, Golski S, et al: Effects of estrogen replacement therapy on PET cerebral blood flow and neuropsychological performance. Hormone Behav 34:171, 1998.

Rico H, Hernandez ER, Revilla M, Gomez-Castresana F: Salmon calcitonin reduces vertebral fracture rates in postmenopausal crush fracture syndrome. Bone Miner 16:131, 1992.

Riggs BL: The mechanisms of estrogen regulation of bone resorption. J Clin Invest 106:1203, 2000.

Riggs BL, Hodgson SF, O'Fallon WM, et al: Effect of fluoride treatment on the fracture rate in postmenopausal women with osteoporosis. N Engl J Med 322:802, 1990.

Riggs BL, Khosla S, Melton JL III: A unitary model for involutional osteoporosis: Estrogen deficiency causes both type I and type II osteoporosis in postmenopausal women and contributes to bone loss in aging men. J Bone Miner Res 13:763, 1998.

Riggs BL, Khosla S, Melton JL III: Sex steroids and the construction and conservation of the adult skeleton. Endocr Rev 23:279, 2002.

Riggs BL, Melton LJ: Involutional osteoporosis. N Engl J Med 314:1676, 1986.

Riggs BL, Wahmer HW, Melton L, et al: Rates of bone loss in the appendicular and axial skeletons of women: Evidence of substantial vertebral bone loss before menopause J Clin Invest 77:1487, 1986.

Riis BJ, Lehmann HJ, Christiansen C: Norethindrone acetate in combination with estrogen: Effects on the skeleton and other organs. Am J Obstet Gynecol 187:1101, 2002.

Riman T, Dickman RT, Nilsson S, et al: Hormone replacement therapy and the risk of invasive epithelial ovarian cancer in Swedish women. J Natl Cancer Inst 4:497, 2002.

Rosano GMC, Caixeta AM, Chierchia SL, et al: Acute anti-ischemic effect of estradiol-17β in postmenopausal women with coronary artery disease. Circulation 96:2837, 1997.

Rosen GE, Kaplan B, Lobo RA: Menstrual function and hirsutism in patients with gonadal dysgenesis. Obstet Gynecol 71:677, 1988.

Rosenberg L, Hennekens CH, Rosner B: Early menopause and the risk of myocardial infarction. Am J Obstet Gynecol 139:47, 1981.

Ross LA, Alder EM: Tibolone and climacteric symptoms. Maturitas 21:127, 1995.

Ross RK, Paganini-Hill A, Wan PC, et al: Effect of hormone replacement therapy on breast cancer risk: Estrogen versus estrogen plus progestin. J Natl Cancer Inst 92:328, 2000.

Salpeter SR, Walsh JM, Greyber E, Salpeter EE: Brief report: Coronary heart disease events associated with hormone therapy in younger and older women. A meta-analysis. J Gen Intern Med 21(4):363, 2006.

Samuelsson EC, Victor FT, Svardsudd KF: Five-year incidence and remission rates of female urinary incontinence in a Swedish population less than 65 years old. Am J Obstet Gynecol 183:568, 2000.

Scarabin PY, Oger E, Plu-Bureau G, and the EStrogen and THromboEmbolism risk Study Group: Differential association of oral and transdermal oestrogen-replacement therapy with venous thromboembolism risk. Lancet 62(9382):428, 2003.

Schaiirer C, Lubin J, Troisi R, et al: Menopausal estrogen and estrogen-progestin replacement therapy and breast cancer risk. JAMA 283:485, 2000.

Schiff I, Regestein Q, Tulchinsky D, Ryan KJ: Effects of estrogens on sleep and psychological state of hypogonadal women. JAMA 242:2405, 1979.

Schmidt G, Anderson SB, Nordle O, et al: Release of 17-beta-oestradiol from a vaginal ring in postmenopausal women: Pharmacokinetic evaluation. Gynecol Obstet Invest 38:253, 1994.

Schneider HP: The view of the International Menopause Society on the Women's Health Initiative. Climacteric 5:211, 2002.

Schneider MA, Brotherton PL, Hailes J: The effect of exogenous oestrogens on depression in menopausal women. Med J Aust 2:162, 1977.

Schwartzbaum JA, Hulka BS, Fowler WC, et al: The influence of exogenous estrogen use on survival after diagnosis of endometrial cancer. Am J Epidemiol 126:851, 1987.

Scott RT, Leonardi MR, Hofmann GE, et al: A prospective evaluation of clomiphene citrate challenge test screening of the general infertility population. Obstet Gynecol 82:539, 1993.

Scragg RFR: Menopause and reproductive span in rural Nulgini. Proc Ann Symp (Papua, New Guinea Medical Society) 1973, pp 126–144.

Semmens JP, Tsai CC, Semmens EF, Loadholt CB: Effects of estrogen therapy on vaginal physiology during menopause. Obstet Gynecol 66:15, 1985.

Shahrad P, Marks RA: Pharmacological effect of oestrone on human epidermis. Br J Dermatol 97:383, 1977.

Shaver J, Giblin E, Lentz M, Lee K: Sleep patterns and stability in perimenopausal women. Sleep 11:556, 1988.

Shaywitz SE, Shaywitz BA, Pugh KR, et al: Effect of estrogen on brain activation patterns in postmenopausal women during working memory task. JAMA 281:1197, 1999.

Sherwin BB: Affective changes with estrogen and androgen replacement therapy in surgically menopausal women. J Affective Disord 14:177, 1988.

Sherwin BB: The impact of different doses of estrogen and progestin on mood and sexual behavior in postmenopausal women. J Clin Endocrinol Metab 72:336, 1991.

Sherwin RB, Gelfand MM: Sex steroids and affect in the surgical menopause: A double-blind cross-over study. PsychoneurolEndocrinol 10:325, 1985.

Shifren JL, Braunstein GD, Simon JA: Transdermal testosterone treatment in women with impaired sexual function after oophorectomy. N Engl J Med 343:682, 20002.

Shlipak M, Angeja BG, Go AS, et al: Hormone therapy and in-hospital survival after myocardial infarction in postmenopausal women. Circulation 104:2300, 2002.

Shughrue P, Lane M, Merchenthaler I: Comparative distribution of estrogen receptor-alpha and-beta mRNA in the rat central nervous system. J Comp Neurol 388:507, 1997.

Silva de Sa MF, Matthews MJ, Rebar RW: Altered forms of immunoreactive urinary FSH and LH in premature ovarian failure. Infertility 11:1, 1988.

Siris ES, Leventhal BG, Vaitukaitis JL: Effects of childhood leukemia and chemotherapy on puberty and reproductive function in girls. N Engl J Med 294:1143, 1976.

Sit AS, Modugno F, Weissfeld JL, et al: Hormone replacement therapy formulations and risk of epithelial ovarian carcinoma. Gynecol Oncol 86:118, 2002.

Slemenda C, Huise, Longcope C, Johnston CC: Sex steroids and bone mass: A study of changes about the time of menopause. J Clin Invest 80:1261, 1987.

Slooter AJ, Bronzova J, Witteman JC, et al: Estrogen use and early onset Alzheimer's disease: A population-based study. J Neurol Neurosurg Psychiatry 67:779, 1999.

Sluss PM, Schneyer AL: Low molecular weight follicle-stimulating hormone receptor binding inhibitor in sera from premature ovarian failure patients. J Clin Endocrinol Metab 74:1242, 1992.

Smith EP, Boyd J, Frank GR, et al: Estrogen resistance caused by a mutation in the estrogen-receptor gene in a man. N Engl J Med 331:1056, 1994.

Snowdon DA, Kane RL, Besson WL, et al: Is early natural menopause a biologic marker of health and aging? Am J Public Health 79:709, 1989.

Soules MR, Sherman S, Parrott E, et al: Executive summary: Stages of Reproductive Aging Workshop (STRAW). Fertil Steril 76:874, 2001.

Stampfer MJ, Colditz GA: Estrogen replacement therapy and coronary heart disease: A quantitative assessment of the epidemiologic evidence. Prev Med 20:47, 1991.

Stanczyk FZ, Shoupe D, Nunez V, et al: A randomized comparison of nonoral estradiol delivery in postmenopausal women. Am J Obstet Gynecol 159:1540, 1988.

Stanford L, Hartge P, Brinton LA, et al: Factors influencing the age at natural menopause. J Chron Dis 40:995, 1987.

Starup J, Philip J, Sele V: Oestrogen treatment and subsequent pregnancy in two patients with severe hypergonadotropic ovarian failure. Acta Endocrinol (Copenhagen) 89:149, 1978.

Stefanick ML, Anderson GL, Margolis KL, Hendrix SL, et al: Effects of conjugated equine estrogens on breast cancer and mammography screening in postmenopausal women with hysterectomy. JAMA 295(14):1647, 2006.

Stenburg A, Heimer G, Ulmsten U, Cnattingius S: Prevalence of genitourinary and other climacteric symptoms in 61-year-old women. Maturitas 24:31, 1996.

Stillman RJ, Schiff I, Schinfeld J: Reproductive and gonadal function in the female after therapy for childhood malignancy. Obstet Gynecol Surv 37:385, 1982.

Suda T, Takahashi N, Udagawa N, et al: Modulation of osteoclast differentiation and function by the new members of the tumor necrosis factor receptor and ligand families. Endocr Rev 20:345, 1999.

Tang M-X, Jacobs D, Stern Y, et al: Effect of oestrogen during menopause on risk and age at onset of Alzheimer's disease. Lancet 348:429, 1996.

Thomson J, Oswald I: Effect of oestrogen on the sleep, mood, and anxiety of menopausal women. Br Med J 2:1317, 1977.

Tinetti ME, Baker DI, McAvay G, et al: A multifactorial intervention to reduce the risk of falling among elderly people living in the community. N Engl J Med 331:821, 1994.

Tomkinson A, Gevevers EF, Wit JM, et al: The role of estrogen in the control of rat osteocyte apoptosis. J Bone Miner Res 13:1243, 1998.

Toran-Allerand CD, Guan X, MacLusky NJ, et al: ER-X: A novel, plasma membrane-associated, putative estrogen receptor that is regulated during development and after ischemic brain injury. J Neurosci 22:8391, 2002.

Toran-Allerand CD, Miranda RC, Bentham WDL, et al: Estrogen receptors colocalize with low-affinity nerve growth factor receptors in cholinergic neurons of the basal forebrain. Proc Natl Acad Sci 89:4668, 1992.

Turner G, Robinson H, Wake S, Martin S: Dizygous twinning and premature menopause in fragile X syndrome. Lancet 344:1500, 1994.

US Bureau of the Census: Current Population Reports: Projections of the Population of the United States 1977 to 2050. Washington, DC: US Government Printing Office, 1993.

van Kuijk C, Genant HK: Detection of osteopenia. In Lobo RA (ed): Treatment of the Postmenopausal Woman: Basic and Clinical Aspects, 2nd ed. Philadelphia, Lippincott Williams & Wilkins, 1999, pp. 212.

van Noord PA, Dubas JS, Dorland M, et al: Age at natural menopause in a population-based screening cohort: The role of menarche, fecundity, and lifestyle factors. Fertil Steril 68:95, 1997.

Varila E, Rantala I, Ikarinem A, et al: The effect of topical oestriol on skin collagen of postmenopausal women. Br J Obstet Gynaecol 102:985, 1995.

Veldhuis JD, Iranmanesh A, Johnson ML, Lizarralde G: Twenty-four hour rhythms in plasma concentrations of adrenohypophyseal hormones are generated by distinct amplitude and/or frequency modulation of underlying pituitary secretory bursts. J Clin Endocrinol Metab 71:1616, 1990.

Vermuelen A: Dehydroepiandrosterone and aging. Ann N Y Acad Sci 774:121, 1995.

Versi E, Caradozo LD, Brincat M, et al: Correlation of urethral physiology and skin collagen in postmenopausal women. Br J Obstet Gynaecol 95:147, 1988.

Versi E, Harvey MA, Cardozo L, et al: Urogenital prolapse and atrophy at menopause: A prevalence study. Int Urogynecol J Pelvic Floor Dysfunct 12:107, 2001.

Wakley GK, Schutter HD Jr, Hannon KS, Turner RT: Androgen treatment prevents loss of cancellous bone in the orchidectomized rat. J Bone Miner Res 6:325, 1991.

Wang SC, Rocca WA, Petersen RC, et al: Postmenopausal estrogen replacement therapy and risk of AD: A population-based study. Neurology 52:965, 1995.

Weiss LK, Burkman RT, Cushing-Haugen KL, et al: Hormone replacement therapy regimens and breast cancer. Obstet Gynecol 100:1148, 2002.

Welt CK, McNicholl DJ, Taylor AE, Hall JE: Female reproductive aging is marked by decreased secretion of dimeric inhibin. J Clin Endocrinol Metab 84:105, 1999.

Whitehead E, Shalet SM, Blackledge G, et al: The effect of combination chemotherapy on ovarian function in women treated for Hodgkin's disease. Cancer 52:988, 1983.

Willett W, Stampfer MJ, Bain C, et al: Cigarette smoking, relative weight and menopause. Am J Epidemiol 117:651, 1983.

Williams JK, Anthony MS, Honore EK, et al: Regression of atherosclerosis in female monkeys. Arterioscler Thromb Vasc Biol 15:827, 1995.

Wilson PD, Paragher B, Butler B, et al: Treatment with oral piperalzine oestrone sulphate for genuine stress incontinence in postmenopausal women. Br J Obstet Gynaecol 94:568, 1987.

Wise PM: Menopause and the brain. Sci Am 9(special issue):79, 1998.

Wise PM, Krajnak KM, Kashon ML: Menopause: the aging of multiple pacemakers. Science 273:67, 1996.

Wise PM, Scarbrough K, Lloyd J, et al: Neuroendocrine concomitants of reproductive aging. Exp Gerontol 29:275, 1994.

Wollter-Sevensson L-O, Stadberg E, Anderson K, et al: Intrauterine administration of levonorgestrel 5 and 10 mg/24 h in perimenopausal hormone replacement therapy: A randomized clinical trial during one year. Acta Obstet Gynecol Scand 76:449, 1997.

Woodruff JD, Pickar JH: Incidence of endometrial hyperplasia in postmenopausal women taking conjugated estrogens (Premarin) with medroxyprogesterone acetate or conjugated estrogens alone. Am J Obstet Gynecol 170:1213, 1994.

Writing Group for the Women's Health Initiative Investigators: Risks and benefits of estrogen plus progestin in healthy postmenopausal women: Principal results from the Women's Health Initiative randomized controlled trial. JAMA 288:321, 2002.

Xiao S, Robertson DM, Findlay JK: Effects of activin and follicle-stimulating hormone (FSH) suppression protein/follistatin on FSH receptors and differentiation of cultured rat granulosa cells. Endocrinology 131:1009, 1992.

Yaffe K, Sawaya G, Lieberburg I, Grady D: Estrogen therapy in postmenopausal women: Effects on cognitive function and dementia. JAMA 279:688, 1998.

Yen SSC: Neuroendocrine rhythms of gonadotropin secretion in women. In Ferin M, Halber F, Richart RM, et al (eds): Biorhythms and Human Reproduction. New York, John Wiley & Sons, 1977, pp 219–238.

Yen SSC. The biology of menopause. J Reprod Med 18:287, 1977.

Zumoff B, Strain GW, Miller LK, et al: Twenty-four hour mean plasma testosterone concentration declines with age in normal premenopausal women. J Clin Endocrinol Metab 80:1429, 1995.

Zweifel JE, O'Brien WH: A meta-analysis of the effect of hormone replacement therapy upon depressed mood. Psychoneurol Endocrinol 22:189, 1997.

Index

Note: Page numbers followed by f indicate figures; those followed by t indicate tables; those followed by b indicate boxed material.

D

G

H

N

Q

R

T

W

X

Y

Z